HAINES & TAYLOR

OBSTETRICAL AND GYNAECOLOGICAL PATHOLOGY

FIFTH EDITION

VOLUME 2

Commissioning Editor: Michael J Houston
Project Development Manager: Sheila Black
Project Manager: Camilla Rockwood
Designer: Sarah Russell
Illustration Manager: Mick Ruddy
Illustrator: Jenni Miller

HAINES & TAYLOR

OBSTETRICAL AND GYNAECOLOGICAL PATHOLOGY

FIFTH EDITION

VOLUME 2

Edited by

Harold Fox

Emeritus Professor of Reproductive Pathology
Department of Pathological Sciences
University of Manchester Medical School
Manchester, UK

Michael Wells

Professor of Gynaecological Pathology
Academic Unit of Pathology, Section of Oncology and Pathology
Division of Genomic Medicine
University of Sheffield Medical School
Honorary Consultant Histopathologist, Sheffield Teaching Hospitals
Sheffield, UK

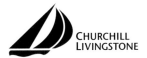

CHURCHILL
LIVINGSTONE

CHURCHILL LIVINGSTONE

An imprint of Elsevier Science Limited

First edition 1962
Second edition 1975
Third edition 1987
Fourth edition 1995
Fifth edition 2003

ISBN 0 443 06385 0

British Library Cataloguing in Publication Data
A catalogue record for this book is available from the British Library

Library of Congress Cataloging in Publication Data
A catalog record for this book is available from the Library of Congress

Note
Medical knowledge is constantly changing. As new information
becomes available, changes in treatment, procedures, equipment and
the use of drugs become necessary. The editors and the publishers
have taken care to ensure that the information given in this text is
accurate and up to date. However, readers are strongly advised to
confirm that the information, especially with regard to drug usage,
complies with the latest legislation and standards of practice.

ELSEVIER
SCIENCE
your source for books,
journals and multimedia
in the health sciences

www.elsevierhealth.com

The
publisher's
policy is to use
**paper manufactured
from sustainable forests**

Printed in Spain

Contents

Preface   vii

Preface to the fourth edition   ix

Preface to the third edition   xi

List of contributors   xiii

Volume 1

1. **Embryology and anatomy of the female genital tract**   1
   J M McLean

2. **Congenital malformation of the female genital tract**   41
   H Fox

3. **Non-neoplastic pathology of the vulva and related structures**   53
   S Neill, M Ridley

4. **Neoplastic disease of the vulva and associated structures**   95
   H Fox, C H Buckley

5. **Pathology of the vagina**   147
   W A Schmidt

6. **Anatomy of the cervix and physiological changes in cervical epithelium**   247
   A Singer, C Chow

7. **Non-neoplastic conditions of the cervix**   273
   P Craig, D Lowe

8. **Premalignant and malignant squamous lesions of the cervix**   297
   C S Herrington, M Wells

9. **Malignant and premalignant glandular lesions of the cervix**   339
   L J R Brown, M Wells

10. **Miscellaneous primary tumours and metastatic tumours of the uterine cervix**   369
    P B Clement

11. **Normal endometrium and non-proliferative conditions of the endometrium**   391
    C H Buckley

12. **Endometrial hyperplasia and carcinoma**   443
    R J Zaino

13. **Non-neoplastic conditions of the myometrium and pure mesenchymal tumours of the uterus**   497
    T P Rollason, N Wilkinson

14. **Mixed tumours of the uterus**   549
    A G Östör, T P Rollason

15. **Pathology of the Fallopian tube and broad ligament**   585
    L H Honoré

16. **Embryology and anatomy of the ovaries**   635
    J M McLean

17. **Non-neoplastic disorders of the ovary**   663
    R H Young, R E Scully

18. **Ovarian tumours: classification, histogenesis and aetiology**   693
    H Fox, M Wells

19. **Surface epithelial-stromal tumours of the ovary**   713
    H Fox, M Wells

20. **Sex cord-stromal tumours of the ovary**   745
    L M Roth

21. **Germ cell tumours of the ovary**   771
    F F Nogales

Volume 2

22. Mixed germ cell sex cord-stromal tumours of the ovary   821
A Talerman

23. Steroid cell tumours of the ovary   845
R H Young, R E Scully

24. Mesenchymal tumours of the ovary   857
J Prat, H Fox

25. Metastatic tumours of the ovary   879
H Fox

26. Ovarian tumours of uncertain origin   897
A J Tiltman

27. Pathology of the peritoneum and secondary Müllerian system   913
D A Bell

28. Lymphoproliferative disease of the female genital tract   935
E Benjamin, P Isaacson

29. Endometriosis   963
B Czernobilsky, H Fox

30. Pathology of infertility   989
L H Honoré

31. Ectopic pregnancy   1045
H Fox

32. Pathology of contraception and hormonal therapy   1071
C H Buckley, S M Ismail

33. Tropical pathology of the female genital tract and ovaries   1133
S B Lucas

34. Pathology of the female genital tract and ovaries in childhood and adolescence   1157
A M Kelsey, M J Newbould

35. Interrelationships of non-gynaecological and gynaecological disease   1181
C H Buckley

36. Pathology of abnormal sexual development   1209
S J Robboy, R C Bentley, P Russell, M C Anderson

37. Development and anatomy of the placenta   1233
B Huppertz, M Castellucci, P Kaufmann

38. General pathology of the placenta, umbilical cord and fetal membranes   1273
H Fox

39. Pathology of the pregnant uterus   1327
J Hustin, M Wells

40. Gestational trophoblastic diseases   1359
F J Paradinas, C W Elston

41. Pathology of miscarriage   1431
H Fox, L Regan

42. Non-trophoblastic tumours of the placenta   1449
H Fox

43. Pathology of the liver and gallbladder in pregnancy   1465
S G Hübscher

44. Pathology of the kidney in pregnancy   1495
D R Turner

45. Pathology of the nervous system in pregnancy   1523
H Reid

46. Pathology of the cardiovascular system in pregnancy   1541
E G J Olsen, H Fox

47. Pathology of maternal death   1559
H Fox

48. The pathology of multiple pregnancy   1575
H Fox

49. The application of new techniques to gynaecological pathology   1595
A Cheung, H Fox, M Wells

Index   1627

Preface

The years that have ensued since the last edition of this book have seen exciting, even dramatic, changes in the discipline of pathology. In particular, molecular and genetic studies have given us an increasing understanding of, and insight into, the pathogenesis of many disease processes. It is admitted, however, that molecular and genetic techniques have, as yet, yielded relatively little that is of practical value in the daily diagnostic work of most pathologists, though it is almost certain that we are on the brink of a massive change in this respect. At the same time there has been no slackening of interest in the classical discipline of histopathology; new entities continue to be defined, older concepts re-evaluated and diagnostic criteria refined and sharpened. Gynaecological and obstetrical pathology have shared fully in this almost explosive advance in our knowledge and it has been our concern that this should be reflected in this new edition in terms of both basic and diagnostic pathology.

The overall pattern of the volume is similar to that of its predecessors and, as before, because we feel that each chapter should stand in its own right we have not discouraged overlap between chapters. Some relatively minor changes have been made in the format of some of the chapters and, using the "rotation system" now employed by leading football clubs, there are a number of changes in authorship, changes which in no way reflect upon the previous authors but which represent a "freshening" process.

Harold Fox
Michael Wells

Manchester
Sheffield
August 2002

Preface to the fourth edition

During the years which have elapsed since the last edition of this text new information has continued to accrue, in an ever increasing flow, about all aspects of gynaecological and obstetrical pathology and this fresh material has been fully covered in the thorough updating to which every chapter of this book has been subjected.

This present edition represents, however, more than a simple updating. The aims and intent of the previous edition have been retained but there are several structural alterations, some of which have stemmed from the constructive criticism afforded that edition and some of which reflect changing pathological practice. I have, with some reluctance, excluded the contributions on perinatal pathology for with the advantage of hindsight I can appreciate that they distract from the main theme of this book and these topics are, furthermore, fully covered in the now quite numerous admirable texts devoted to perinatal pathology. I have also reversed my stance concerning gynaecological cytopathology because I became convinced that an authorative overview of this topic could be achieved in a single chapter and would be of value. I have included chapters on immunocyto-chemistry, quantitative analysis and molecular biology, not simply as an obeisance to the onward march of medical technology but because such techniques have now passed from the province of the research laboratory to become routine diagnostic tools and I thought it useful to collate, into single chapters, the information about the application of these techniques to gynaecological pathology.

As before, and for reasons detailed in the Preface to the third edition, I have allowed considerable freedom to my contributors and accepted, even welcomed, some degree of overlap between chapters.

One sad event has been the death of Elizabeth Ramsey who contributed two chapters to the last edition. She was not only an embryologist of the highest international renown but also a joy and an inspiration to all those who had the privilege of knowing her.

A further, and on a personal level even sadder event, has been the death of Frederick Langley, who was my mentor and guide in the study of gynaecological pathology. He was a man of great scientific insight, allied to considerable personal kindness, and is much missed.

Manchester, 1995   H.F.

Preface to the third edition

This is the third edition of Haines and Taylor's text on Gynaecological Pathology. It is readily admitted, however, that this edition departs so radically from the format of its two predecessors that it represents new entity rather than a simple revision and updating. Despite this lack of any evolutionary continuity, I wished to retain the names of Claude Taylor and Magnus Haines in the title as a tribute to two men who did much to establish the scientific respectability and intellectual credibility of gynaecological pathology in Great Britain.

The primary aim of this book is to give a full account of the pathology of both gynaecological and obstetrical disorders. There are, of course, many other texts devoted to this topic, but it has appeared to me that few have given sufficient attention to obstetrical pathology. The clinical chimerism of obstetrics and gynaecology should be, but is often not, reflected in pathological texts, and it is hoped that the detailed attention given in this volume will help to correct the imbalance which has tended to lead to a relative neglect of this topic.

The chapters in this multi-author book vary in length and style, and there is some repetition between the various contributions. All these features are usually considered to be defects in the format of a multi-author volume resulting from a lack of editorial control. These apparent faults are, however, the direct result of editorial decisions based upon my own concept of the strengths and weaknesses of a large and complex multi-author volume.

Thus I did not impose any minimum or maximum limits on the number of words allowed for each contribution. This decision was based on two factors, of which the first was my confidence in the ability of the invited contributors to decide for themselves the number of words required for a comprehensive consideration of their subject. A second factor was my belief that decisions as to chapter length in multi-author volumes often reflect editorial interests and thus result in an arbitrary and biased view of the relative importance of various topics: this has often resulted in certain aspects of gynaecological pathology, such as the consideration of vulvar, vaginal and tubal disease, receiving relatively inadequate attention, a fault which I hope is rectified in this volume. I have also not insisted upon any unity of style, approach or presentation from the various contributors. The major merit of literary style in a scientific text is that it allows for a lucid and easily comprehensive exposition: I therefore limited my stylistic interventions to the clarification of any obscure passages, and have not attempted to submerge the individualism or flair of my contributors by the editorial imposition of the dead hand of stylistic conformity. I have allowed, and even encouraged, some degree of repetition between chapters. This is because I felt that a book of this length is unlikely to be read in its entirely at a single sitting and that, each chapter should therefore be able to stand as a discrete entity which could be read as a review of a particular topic without the frequent necessity of following cross references to other chapters. My aim was, therefore, to ensure that each chapter was comprehensive, complete in itself and retained the authentic voice of the author.

Certain omissions and commissions in this book require comment. No chapter on gynaecological cytopathology has been included, largely because I felt this to be a subject worthy of a volume in its own right and one which could be considered only in a superficial and sketchy manner when restricted by the confines of a single chapter. By contrast I specifically asked for a rather lengthy description of the embryology and anatomy of the female genital tract; this is perhaps unusual in a textbook of pathology, but reflects my view that many gynaecological lesions can only be fully understood when placed in the context of a sound knowledge of female genital tract development and structure. Some aspects of perinatal pathology have also been included in this book, but these represent, to my mind, only those aspects of this topic which are logical extensions of obstetrical pathology. I have also included discussions of such subjects as the pathology of infertility, the pathology of contraception, the histogenesis of ovarian tumours, the immunopathology of the female genital tract and reproductive immunology: to some, these topics may appear to be out of place in a text devoted primarily to histopathology but their inclusion reflects my feeling that the pathologist must be concerned with all aspects of disorders of the female genital tract and should not be restricted by the limits of the microscope. There has also been a deliberate inclusion of two chapters on abnormalities of sexual differentiation. This was because I wished to have a general overview of this topic which could be set in apposition to chapters on normal development and on malformations of the female genital tract, together with a separate chapter devoted principally to gonadal pathology in patients with abnormal sexual development.

In most general hospitals, biopsies and surgical specimens from gynaecological and obstetrical patients constitute approximately one third of the total workload of departments of surgical pathology. It is hoped that this book will, despite its imperfections, be of assistance to the pathologist in dealing with this massive inflow of material. I hope also that this volume will indicate some of the scientific and intellectual satisfaction that can be gained from a study of this branch of pathology.

Manchester, 1987   H.F.

Contributors

Malcolm C Anderson FRCPath FRCOG
Emeritus Consultant Histopathologist
Department of Histopathology
University Hospital
Queen's Medical Centre
Nottingham, UK

Debra A Bell MD
Associate Professor of Pathology
Harvard Medical School
Associate Pathologist, Department of Pathology
Massachusetts General Hospital
Boston, MA
USA

Elizabeth Benjamin MBBS FRCPath
Senior Clinical Lecturer and Consultant Pathologist
Department of Histopathology
Royal Free and University College of London
Medical School
London, UK

Rex C Bentley MD
Associate Professor of Pathology
Duke University Medical Center
Durham, NC
USA

Laurence J R Brown BSc MBBS FRCPath
Consultant Gynaecological Pathologist
Department of Histopathology
Leicester Royal Infirmary
Leicester, UK

C Hilary Buckley MD FRCPath
Honorary Consultant Gynaecological Pathologist
St Mary's Hospital
Manchester, UK

Mario Castellucci MD PhD
Instituto di Morfologia
Ancona
Italy

Annie Cheung MBBS MD FRCPath (UK) FHKAM(Path) FIAC
Associate Professor of Pathology
Department of Pathology
University of Hong Kong
Hong Kong

Carl Chow MB BS BSc MRCOG
Clinical Research Fellow
Department of Obstetrics & Gynaecology
The Whittington Hospital
London, UK

Phillip B Clement MD
Professor of Pathology
Department of Pathology
Vancouver General Hospital
Vancouver, Canada

Paul Craig BSc MB BS
Specialist Registrar in Histopathology
Department of Histopathology
St Bartholomew's Hospital
London, UK

Bernard Czernobilsky MD
Professor of Pathology
Patho-Lab Laboratories
Ness-Ziona
Israel

Christopher W Elston MD FRCPath
Professor of Tumour Pathology and Consultant
Histopathologist
Department of Histopathology
Nottingham City Hospital NHS Trust
Nottingham, UK

Harold Fox MD FRCPath FRCOG
Emeritus Professor of Reproductive Pathology
Department of Pathological Sciences
University of Manchester Medical School
Manchester, UK

C S Herrington MA MBBS DPhil MRCP MRCPath
Professor of Pathology
Department of Pathology, Duncan Building
Royal Liverpool University Hospital
Liverpool, UK

Louis H Honoré BSc(Hons) MB ChB FRCP(C)
Emeritus Professor of Laboratory Medicine
  and Pathology
University of Alberta
Department of Laboratory Medicine
Cross Cancer Institute
Edmonton, Alberta
Canada

Stefan G Hübscher MB ChB FRCPath
Consultant Histopathologist and Reader
in Hepatic Pathology
Department of Pathology
University of Birmingham Medical School
Birmingham, UK

Berthold Huppertz PD
Associate Professor of Anatomy
Department of Anatomy
University Hospital RWTH Aachen
Aachen, Germany

Jean Hustin MD
Faculty Professor of Pathology
Department of Pathology
Institut de Morphologie Pathologique
Belgium

Peter G Isaacson DM FRCPath
Professor of Pathology
Department of Histopathology
Royal Free and University College of London
  Medical School
London, UK

Sezgin M Ismail MBChB MRCP FRCPath
Senior Lecturer/Honorary Consultant in Pathology
Department of Pathology
University of Wales College of Medicine
Cardiff, UK

Peter Kaufmann
Professor of Anatomy
Department of Anatomy II
Aachen, Germany

Anna M Kelsey MRCS LRCP FRCPath
Consultant Paediatric Histopathologist
Department of Pathology
Royal Manchester Children's Hospital
Manchester, UK

David Lowe MD FRCS FRCPath FIBiol
Professor of Surgical Pathology
Formerly of St Bartholomew's Hospital
London, UK

Sebastian Lucas FRCP FRCPath
Professor of Clinical Histopathology
Department of Histopathology
St Thomas's Hospital
London, UK

John M McLean BSc MD
Formerly Senior Lecturer in Anatomy and Embryology
The University of Manchester
Manchester, UK

Sarah Neill MB ChB FRCP
Consultant Dermatologist
St John's Institute of Dermatology
St Thomas' Hospital
London, UK

Melanie J Newbould MBBS FRCPath
Consultant Paediatric Histopathologist
Department of Pathology
Royal Manchester Children's Hospital
Manchester, UK

Francisco F Nogales MD
Professor of Pathology
University of Granada
Granada, Spain

Eckhardt G J Olsen AKC MD FRCPath FACC (deceased)
Late Consultant and Director
Cardiovascular Division
Department of Histopathology
Royal Brompton National Heart Hospital
London, UK

Andrew G Östör MBBS MD FRCPA MIAC
Associate Professor of Pathology, and Obstetrics
and Gynecology
Department of Pathology
The Royal Women's Hospital
Melbourne, Australia

Fernando J Paradinas LMS LRCP LRCS FRCPath MRCR
Emeritus Professor of Trophoblastic Pathology
Department of Histopathology
Charing Cross Hospital
London, UK

Jaime Prat MD FRCPath
Professor and Chairman
Department of Pathology
Hospital de la Santa Creu i Sant Pau
Barcelona
Spain

Lesley Regan MD MBBS FRCOG
Professor of Obstetrics and Gynaecology
Department of Reproductive Science and Medicine
Imperial College School of Medicine
London, UK

Helen Reid MBBS FRCPath
Consultant Neuropathologist
Department of Cellular Pathology
Hope Hospital
Salford, UK

Marjorie Ridley MA BM FRCP (deceased)
Late Honorary Consultant Dermatologist
St John's Dermatology Centre
St Thomas' Hospital
London, UK

Stanley J Robboy MD FCAP
Professor of Pathology and Vice Chairman for Diagnostic
Services
Professor of Obstetrics and Gynecology
Duke University Medical Center
Durham, NC
USA

Terence Rollason BSc MB ChB FRCPath
Consultant Pathologist
Department of Pathology
Birmingham Women's Hospital
Birmingham, UK

Lawrence M Roth MD
Emeritus Professor of Pathology
Indiana University School of Medicine
Indiana University Hospital
Indianapolis, IN
USA

Peter Russell MD BS BSc(Med), FRCPA
Professor of Pathology
Department of Anatomical Pathology
Royal Prince Alfred Hospital
Camperdown, NSW
Australia

Waldemar A Schmidt MD PhD
Professor of Pathology
Department of Pathology
School of Medicine
Oregon Health and Science University
Portand, OR
USA

Robert E Scully MD
Professor Emeritus, Harvard Medical School
Pathologist, Massachusetts General Hospital
Boston, MA
USA

Albert Singer PhD DPhil FRCOG
Professor of Gynaecological Research
The Whittington Hospital
London, UK

Aleksander Talerman MD FRCPath MB ChB
Peter A Herbut Professor of Pathology and Cell Biology
Department of Pathology
Thomas Jefferson University
Philadelphia, PA
USA

Andrew J Tiltman MD MMed(Path) FCPath
Emeritus Professor, University of Cape Town
Cape Town
South Africa

David R Turner MB BS PhD FRCPath
Emeritus Professor of Pathology
Department of Cellular Pathology
Musgrove Park Hospital
Taunton
Somerset, UK

Michael Wells BSc(Hons) MD FRCPath
Professor of Gynaecological Pathology, Consultant
Histopathologist Sheffield Teaching Hospitals
Academic Unit of Pathology, Section of Oncology
and Pathology
Division of Genomic Medicine
University of Sheffield Medical School
Sheffield, UK

Nafisa Wilkinson MA MB BChir MRCPath
Honorary Senior Lecturer University of Leeds
Consultant Gynaecological Pathologist
Department of Histopathology
St James NHS Trust
Leeds, UK

Robert H Young MD FRCPath
Professor of Pathology, Harvard Medical School
Pathologist, Massachusetts General Hospital
Boston, MA
USA

Richard J Zaino MD
Professor of Pathology
Pennsylvania State University/Milton S. Hershey
Medical Center
Hershey, PA
USA

Mixed germ cell sex-cord–stromal tumours of the ovary

A. Talerman

Gonadoblastoma   821
Incidence   822
Clinical findings   823
Familial aspects   823
Genetic findings   824
Hormonal findings   824
Pathology   825
Differential diagnosis   831
Therapy   831
Behaviour and prognosis   832

Mixed germ cell sex-cord–stromal tumour   832
Terminology   832
Incidence   832
Clinical findings   833
Genetic findings   833
Hormonal findings   833
Pathology   834
Differential diagnosis   840
Behaviour and prognosis   840
Treatment   841

Germ cell tumours and sex-cord–stromal tumours form two separate and well-established groups of ovarian neoplasms, both showing a remarkable homology with testicular neoplasms. Neoplasms composed of germ cells intimately admixed with sex-cord–stromal elements have become recognised as specific entities during the last 50 years, although occasional examples corresponding to these lesions had been noted earlier (Masson 1922; Schapiro 1927; Schiller 1934; Reifferscheid 1935; Lindvall & Wahlgren 1940). The presence of neoplasms composed of two distinct cell types intimately admixed with each other is a remarkable phenomenon in gonadal pathology. Neoplasms of this type occur both in the ovary and in the testis and thus exhibit the same remarkable homology which is a feature of the two well-established groups of gonadal neoplasms mentioned above.

Although originally it was considered that neoplasms composed of germ cells intimately admixed with sex-cord–stromal elements represented a single histopathological entity, it has become evident that this group of neoplasms consists of two specific types, the gonadoblastoma and the mixed germ cell sex-cord–stromal tumour, which exhibit different histopathological appearances, and are associated with different anatomical, genetic and endocrine findings, and with different clinical and biological behaviour. These neoplasms have been the subject of considerable interest and controversy due to their unique histological appearances and their frequent association with unusual somatic, genetic and endocrine findings. Of these two entities gonadoblastoma is much the more common and will be discussed first.

GONADOBLASTOMA

Synonyms: Dysgenetic gonadoma (Melicow & Uson 1959); gonocytoma 3 (Teter 1960); tumour of dysgenetic gonad (Collins & Symington 1964)

Although neoplasms exhibiting features consistent with a gonadoblastoma had been noted earlier (Schapiro 1927; Schiller 1934; Reifferscheid 1935; Lindvall & Wahlgren

1940), it was not until 1953, when it was described in detail by Scully, that this tumour became recognised as a specific histopathological entity. Scully (1953) described the gonadoblastoma as a gonadal tumour composed of germ cells and sex-cord derivatives resembling immature granulosa and Sertoli cells and, in one of the two reported cases, also containing Leydig or lutein-like cells in the surrounding stroma. In both cases the tumours were bilateral and were overgrown by a dysgerminoma. The tumours were located at the site of normal ovaries, but normal ovarian tissue was not discernible and the exact nature of the gonads in which the tumours had arisen could not be determined. The affected patients were young phenotypic females, who exhibited abnormal sexual development, and it was considered that the tumour was capable of steroid hormone production. It was subsequently demonstrated that both patients were chromatin negative and the older of the two showed virilisation. Scully (1953) named the tumour gonadoblastoma because it appeared to recapitulate gonadal development and occurred in gonads the nature of which was indeterminate and in individuals showing abnormal sexual development. A few years later Melicow & Uson (1959) reported the presence of gonadoblastoma in two phenotypic male pseudohermaphrodites under the term of 'dysgenetic gonadoma' and emphasised the relationship between this lesion, the development of malignancy (seminoma) and abnormal sexual development.

In 1960 Teter formulated a classification of neoplasms containing germ cells, according to their endocrine relationships, based on the term 'gonocytoma', which had been introduced earlier by Teilum (1946). Teter (1960) divided these neoplasms into four groups depending on the number of cell types present and on their endocrine properties:

Gonocytoma 1: A tumour composed entirely of germ cells and corresponding to dysgerminoma or seminoma. This tumour was not associated with hormonal activity.

Gonocytoma 2: A tumour composed of germ cells and sex-cord derivatives resembling immature granulosa or Sertoli cells. This tumour when hormonally active was feminising; otherwise it was inert.

Gonocytoma 3: A tumour composed of germ cells, sex-cord derivatives resembling immature granulosa or Sertoli cells and lutein or Leydig-like cells. When hormonally active the tumour was virilising. This tumour was considered to correspond to classical gonadoblastoma.

Gonocytoma 4: A pure germ cell tumour (dysgerminoma) with clinical findings of virilisation produced by overgrowth of androgenic Leydig (interstitial) cells adjacent to the germ cell tumour, or present in the contralateral gonad.

This classification attempted to correlate the hormonal, clinical and genetic findings with the histological appearances of the tumour. Unfortunately, in practice the differences between the various groups were not very well defined as the histological findings often did not correlate well with the endocrine and clinical aspects of the cases. In an extensive review of the subject, Scully (1970b) presented convincing arguments against Teter's classification, indicating that it was unjustifiable on both pathological and clinical grounds. Scully's views (1970b) are strongly supported by the present-day concept that the classification of gonadal neoplasms should be based as far as possible on histogenesis and morphological features and not on endocrinological, clinical, and genetic factors. Over the years the term gonadoblastoma has become fully established as the only one to describe this entity and it has been used in this context in the classifications of ovarian and testicular neoplasms produced by the World Health Organization tumour panels (Serov et al 1973; Mostofi & Sobin 1978; Mostofi & Sesterhenn 1998, Scully 1999).

The neoplastic nature of the gonadoblastoma has been questioned because some of the lesions are very small, composed of two or three cell types and may undergo complete regression by the process of hyalinisation and calcification. The facts that when overt malignancy supervenes it manifests itself as germ cell neoplasia, and that gonadoblastoma as such never metastasises, have also been used as arguments in this context. In spite of these arguments it has been shown that gonadoblastoma exhibits exactly the same histological picture in the very small lesions, 'the bisexual formations' (Teter & Boczkowski 1967), as in the larger ones or in those associated with dysgerminoma or other neoplastic germ cell elements, including the presence of mitotic activity in the germ cell element. The frequent association of a gonadoblastoma with a dysgerminoma, which is seen in at least 50% of cases, or with other neoplastic germ cell elements, observed in 10% of cases (Scully 1970b; Talerman 1974; Talerman 1980), supports the concept that the gonadoblastoma represents an in situ germ cell neoplasm and that the lesion has a considerable malignant potential.

INCIDENCE

Although the majority of reports describing patients with gonadoblastomas originate from Europe and North America, cases of gonadoblastoma have been reported from all parts of the world and in all races. The exact incidence of gonadoblastoma is not known, but it is considered to be uncommon.

More than 200 cases have been reported, the majority during the last 30 years, and although some individual cases are still being recorded, the number of unreported cases is considerable.

Gonadoblastomas are seen in young patients, being encountered most frequently during the second decade and somewhat less frequently during the third and first decade, in that order. Although the age of patients ranges from 6 months (Damjanov & Klauber 1980) to 52 years (Scully 1982 personal communication), a gonadoblastoma is very rare in patients beyond the third decade. Two patients, who were noted to have ambiguous genitalia at four days and six weeks of age, but were treated conservatively, were found to have gonadoblastomas when explored surgically at 22 months and four years, respectively (Park et al 1972; Mandell et al 1977), this suggesting that the lesion was congenital.

CLINICAL FINDINGS

Gonadoblastomas are most frequently found in patients who are being investigated because of primary amenorrhoea, virilisation or developmental anomalies of the external genitalia. Another common mode of presentation is the presence of abdominal enlargement caused by a gonadal tumour. In the great majority of these latter cases the gonadoblastoma is overgrown by a malignant germ cell neoplasm, most frequently a dysgerminoma. The gonadoblastoma, which in these cases forms only a small part of the tumour, is usually found only on histological examination.

The majority (80%) of patients with a gonadoblastoma are phenotypic females and the remaining 20% are phenotypic male pseudohermaphrodites with cryptorchidism, hypospadias, ambiguous external genitalia and female internal secondary sex organs. Of the phenotypic females with a gonadoblastoma, the majority (60%) are virilised and, although the remaining 40% appear normal, most patients exhibit poor genital development. Breast development is also frequently poor even among the non-virilised phenotypic females (Scully 1970b).

While the majority of patients with a gonadoblastoma present with primary amenorrhoea, some have sporadic episodes of spontaneous cyclical menstrual bleeding, although usually these episodes are infrequent and the bleeding is scanty (Scully 1970b). Occasional patients menstruate normally (Scully 1970b; Pratt-Thomas & Cooper 1976; Talerman et al 1981) and some, having menstruated normally, present later with secondary amenorrhoea (Muhlenstedt et al 1979; Dewhurst & Ferreira 1982).

Although most patients with a gonadoblastoma have various forms of gonadal dysgenesis, a gonadoblastoma has been encountered in a patient who, subsequent to the excision of the tumour, which was overgrown by dysgerminoma, had two normal pregnancies (Bergher de Bacalao & Dominquez 1969), as well as in a patient with a ruptured ectopic tubal pregnancy (Pratt-Thomas & Cooper 1976). Gonadoblastomas have been encountered in at least eight true hermaphrodites (Park et al 1972; McDonough et al 1976a; Szokol et al 1977; Radhakrishnan et al 1978; Quigley et al 1981; Talerman et al 1981; Talerman et al 1990; Tanaka et al 2000). One of these patients, who had an ovotestis containing gonadoblastoma and dysgerminoma excised during childhood, subsequently, at the age of 30, had a normal pregnancy. One year later she developed abdominal enlargement. The remaining gonad was excised and was found to be an ovotestis largely overgrown by dysgerminoma and containing a gonadoblastoma. Although originally the karyotype was found to be 46,XX, a more detailed study showed a 97% 46,XX/3% 46,XY composition. The patient is well and disease free 10 years following surgery and radiation therapy (Talerman et al 1990). Another case of a true hermaphrodite, who developed a dysgerminoma in a right-sided ovotestis, which also showed evidence of a 'burnt out' gonadoblastoma was reported recently (Tanaka et al 2000). Nine months after the excision of the right gonad and wedge biopsy of the left gonad, which showed normal ovarian tissue, the patient became pregnant and delivered a normal male infant at term. The patient had a 20%, 46XX/80% 46,XY chromosomal composition indicating that true hermaphrodites with a predominance of 46,XY karyotype may be fertile (Tanaka et al 2000). Gonadoblastomas have also been observed in patients with normally descended testes (Hughesdon & Kumarasamy 1970; Talerman unpublished observations; Talerman & Delemarre 1975; Chapman et al 1990), two of whom fathered children following excision of the affected testis. A gonadoblastoma has been observed within normal ovaries (Goldsmith & Hart 1975; Mikulowski & Talerman unpublished observations; Pratt-Thomas & Cooper 1976; Richmond, personal communication; Nakashima et al 1989; Magyar & Talerman unpublished observations), as well as in patients with Turner's syndrome (Muhlenstedt et al 1979; Shah et al 1988). Gonadoblastoma has been encountered in at least two patients with ataxia-telangiectasia (Goldsmith & Hart 1975; Buyse et al 1976). It has also been observed in patients with a syndrome of aniridia, cataract, growth and mental retardation, and chromosome anomalies (Andersen et al 1978; Dufier et al 1981; Martinez-Mora et al 1989), as well as in patients with Drash syndrome (Manivel et al 1987).

FAMILIAL ASPECTS

A family history of gonadal dysgenesis has been described in more than a dozen reports of patients with a gonadoblastoma (Frazier et al 1964; Cohen & Shaw, 1965; Bartlett et al 1968; Sternberg et al 1968; Talerman 1971; Allard et al 1972; Boczkowski et al 1972; Anderson

& Carlson 1975; Govan et al 1977; Ionescu & Maximilian 1977; Phansey et al 1980; Moltz et al 1981; Szamborski et al 1981). In two instances gonadal dysgenesis was observed in three generations in the family of a patient with a gonadoblastoma (Bartlett et al 1968; Allard et al 1972). At least seven pairs of siblings with gonadoblastoma have been reported (Talerman 1971; Allard et al 1972; Boczkowski et al 1972; Anderson & Carlson 1975; Govan et al 1977; Ionescu & Maximilian 1977; Kingsbury et al 1987), as well as one pair of twins (Frazier et al 1964). All these patients had a 46,XY karyotype. These findings indicate that there is a high incidence of gonadoblastoma in families with gonadal dysgenesis. They also call for a careful study of the family history in patients with gonadoblastoma and investigation of the patient's relatives because of the increased familial incidence of the lesion. It has been suggested that the mode of inheritance of gonadoblastoma is either an X-linked recessive gene or an autosomal sex-linked mutant gene (Bartlett et al 1968; Sternberg et al 1968; Schellhas 1974a; Wachtel 1979).

GENETIC FINDINGS

Nearly all the reported cases of gonadoblastoma have occurred in phenotypic female patients with pure or mixed gonadal dysgeneis or in male pseudohermaphrodites. Occasional patients are of short stature and exhibit complete or incomplete forms of Turner's syndrome (Dominquez & Greenblatt 1962; Schellhas 1974a; Muhlenstedt et al 1979; Bonakdar & Peisner 1980; Shah et al 1988). The majority of patients are chromatin negative, and 96% of patients with a gonadoblastoma whose karyotype has been determined were found to have a Y chromosome. The most common karyotype observed was 46,XY (50%), followed by 45,X/46,XY mosaicism (25%), while the remainder consisted of various other forms of mosaicism (Schellhas 1974a). Recent studies using banding techniques indicate the presence of many complicated cases of mosaicism with deletions of portions of the sex chromosomes, as well as autosomes, presence of chromosomal fragments, ring chromosomes or chromosomal translocations (Malkova et al 1975; Ishida et al 1976; Piazza et al 1977; Ying et al 1977; Anderson et al 1978; Blair 1978; Khodr et al 1979; Rary et al 1979; Herva et al 1980; Seki et al 1981; Shah et al 1988; Martinez-Mora et al 1989). More than 15 patients with gonadoblastoma have had a normal female 46,XX karyotype (Bergher de Bacalao & Dominquez 1969; Salet et al 1970; Drobnjak et al 1971; Stolecke et al 1974; Goldsmith & Hart 1975; McDonough et al 1976a; Mikulowski & Talerman unpublished observations; Talerman et al 1981; Hoffman et al 1987; Nakashima et al 1989; Richmond personal communication; Talerman et al 1990; Erhan et al 1992; Obata et al 1995). Three of the patients were true hermaphrodites (McDonough et al 1976a; Talerman et al 1981, 1990). Three patients had 45,X/46,XX mosaicism (Patel & Prentice 1972; Pratt-Thomas & Cooper 1976; Dewhurst & Ferreira 1982).

A number of unreported cases of gonadoblastoma occurring in histologically normal ovaries are known to the author. All occurred in anatomically normal non-virilised females with normal 46,XX karyotype, when studied by conventional techniques. Although the presence of fragments of Y chromosomal material cannot be entirely excluded without more detailed studies, it is likely that most of these patients had at least a marked predominance of 46,XX karyotype. A report by Letterie & Page (1995) is of interest in this context. They described a case of a 17-year-old patient with a left-sided streak gonad and dysgerminoma replacing the right gonad. The patient was found to have a normal 46,XX karyotype in peripheral blood lymphocytes, cultivated skin fibroblasts and cells from the left streak gonad. No Y-chromosomal material was detected when blood DNA was examined for Y-specific sequences.

The presence of H-Y antigen has been noted in a number of patients with gonadoblastoma, gonadal dysgenesis and a 46,XY karyotype (Dorus et al 1977; Wolf 1979; Moltz et al 1981). These findings indicate that aberrant testicular differentiation may occur in the presence of H-Y antigen (Dorus et al 1977; Wachtel 1979; Moltz et al 1981).

The practice of genotyping and karyotyping of patients with gonadal dysgenesis, genital anomalies, primary amenorrhoea, as well as those with gonadoblastoma, is considered to be an essential part of the investigation of these patients and needs no further emphasis. Although the majority of patients with a gonadoblastoma have karyotypes containing a Y chromosome, the absence of a Y chromosome does not exclude the presence of the lesion and its malignant potential.

HORMONAL FINDINGS

The presence of hormonal abnormalities in patients with a gonadoblastoma was noted when the tumour was first described. Scully (1953) reported the presence of virilisation in one of his cases and considered that the tumour was capable of steroid hormone production. Since then the presence of virilisation has been observed in numerous cases of gonadoblastoma, indicating a close association. The partial or complete regression of virilisation following the excision of the tumour, observed in some cases, indicates that the virilisation and thus steroid hormone secretion are related to the presence of the tumour.

The frequent presence of virilisation in patients with a gonadoblastoma should not be confused with the finding of gonadal dysgenesis and defective gonadal development, which are observed in the great majority of patients with gonadoblastoma. The virilisation, which is a hormonal manifestation, is related to the presence of the tumour and is not the result of the abnormal gonadal development, the latter being unaffected by excision of the tumour. There is no further gonadal development and the gonadal abnormalities persist.

Originally the evidence for the presence of steroid hormone production in patients with a gonadoblastoma was mainly clinical, as many patients did not have hormonal studies performed prior to excision of the tumour. Histologically the lutein or Leydig-like cells were considered to be the most likely source of the steroids producing virilisation in the patient (Scully, 1953). Further studies revealed that the presence of lutein or Leydig-like cells was not always associated with virilisation, and, although these cells were found more frequently in tumours from virilised phenotypic females and male pseudohermaphrodites, this relationship was far from absolute. It has been shown that the presence of these cells is age related, and they are observed much more frequently in tumours from postpubertal patients than from those who have not reached puberty (Scully 1970b). The virilisation found in postpubertal patients with gonadoblastoma manifests itself mainly as masculine body contour, hirsutism and clitoromegaly. Further studies have also revealed the possibility that the tumour may be associated with oestrogen synthesis, as some patients with gonadoblastoma experienced hot flushes and other postmenopausal symptoms following excision of the tumour (Scully 1970b; Schellhas 1974b).

Biochemical tests providing more concrete evidence of steroid hormone production by the tumour were not performed initially in many cases. When they were performed preoperatively the urinary 17-ketosteroid and 17-ketogenic steroids were usually normal although slight elevation of 17-ketosteroid excretion was observed in some cases (McDonough et al 1967; Cooperman et al 1968). The most important finding was the frequent, although not invariable, elevation of the gonadotrophins, and this was considered an important diagnostic criterion (Teter 1960).

More recently, due to improved methodology and greater availability of hormonal tests, gonadoblastomas have been shown to be capable of producing various steroid hormones both in vivo and in vitro. Gonadoblastoma tissue is capable of producing testosterone (Griffiths et al 1966; Bardin et al 1968; Bartlett et al 1968; Mackay et al 1974; Rose et al 1974; Anderson & Carlson 1975; Quigley et al 1981) and oestrogens (Griffiths et al 1966; Mackay et al 1974; Quigley et al 1981). Increased synthesis of testosterone (Judd et al 1970; McDonough et al 1976b), oestrogens and progesterone (McDonough et al 1976b) in vivo has also been demonstrated. Determinations of steroid hormones in ovarian and peripheral venous blood have shown that in a patient with bilateral gonadoblastomas, one tumour, which was obliterated by calcification and hyalinisation,

was not associated with increased steroid synthesis, while the contralateral tumour, which was viable, was associated with increased testosterone and oestradiol levels (McDonough et al 1976b). The actual source of the steroid hormone production is still a matter of debate and contoversy: the Leydig-like or lutein cells have long been considered to be responsible for the steroid synthesis, but a stromal reaction has also been implicated. It appears reasonable to consider that both types of cells are capable of steroid hormone production and may be involved in the steroid synthesis associated with gonadoblastomas.

PATHOLOGY

Macroscopical findings

The pure gonadoblastoma is a small lesion varying in size from microscopic up to 8 cm in the longest diameter, most of the macroscopically apparent lesions measuring between 1 and 2 cm. When a gonadoblastoma becomes overgrown by a dysgerminoma or other neoplastic germ cell elements the tumour may reach a very large size, and neoplasms in excess of 20 cm in diameter and weighing more than 1000 g have been reported (Scully 1970b). It is possible that even the tumour measuring 8 cm in diameter (Scully 1970b) may have been overgrown by dysgerminoma, as most pure gonadoblastomas do not exceed 3 cm in the longest diameter.

The macroscopical appearances of gonadoblastomas vary depending on the amount of hyalinisation and calcification present, and whether the tumour is overgrown by a dysgerminoma or other neoplastic germ cell elements. A pure gonadoblastoma is solid, round or oval and has a smooth or slightly lobulated surface. It may vary from soft

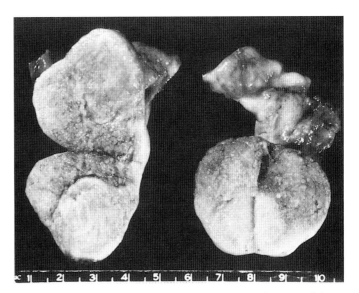

Fig. 22.1 Bilateral gonadoblastoma. Note the solid nature of the tumour, the slightly lobulated surface and the shiny specks of calcification. Both tumours were associated with dysgerminoma. (Courtesy of Dr. R. E. Scully.)

and fleshy to firm, or hard. On cross-section it is solid and varies from grey–white to yellow, or light brown. It is speckled with calcific granules (Fig. 22.1) and may be completely calcified. The calcification has been recognised on gross examination in 45% of cases and in 20% on radiological examination.

Gonadoblastomas have been found more frequently in the right gonad than the left (Scully 1970b), although some dispute this finding (Hart & Burkons 1979). The frequent bilaterality of gonadoblastomas is beyond dispute; although found to be present in 38% of cases in the largest reported series (Scully 1970b), subsequent experience indicates the presence of bilateral involvement in at least 50% of cases and emphasises that a careful search for the presence of a lesion in the contralateral gonad must always be made. In a considerable number of cases overgrowth of the lesion by a neoplastic germ cell element may occur. In some of these cases the gonadoblastoma may be found only on histological examination, while in others it may remain undetected even in spite of careful histological examination.

The nature of the gonad in which a gonadoblastoma originates is frequently indeterminate because it is often overgrown by the gonadoblastoma or a neoplastic germ cell element, most frequently a dysgerminoma. When the nature of the gonad is discernible it is usually a fibrous streak (gonadal streak) or a testis, and the contralateral gonad may be a streak, a testis, or it may be indeterminate and may also contain a gonadoblastoma (Scully 1970b). In a number of cases the affected gonad as well as the contralateral gonad has been a normal ovary (Bergher de Bacalao & Dominquez 1969; Goldsmith & Hart 1975; Mikulowski & Talerman unpublished observations; Pratt-Thomas & Cooper 1976; Hoffman et al 1987; Nakashima et al 1989; Talerman unpublished observations) (Fig. 22.2). Gonadoblastomas have also been

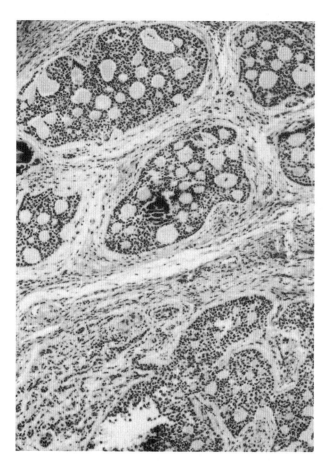

Fig. 22.3 Gonadoblastoma. The tumour is composed of cellular nests surrounded by dense connective tissue stroma. Note the hyaline bodies (white) and calcification (black) within the nests.

encountered in ovotestes of true hermaphrodites (Park et al 1972; McDonough et al 1976a; Szokol et al 1977; Talerman et al 1981; Talerman et al 1990; Tanaka et al 2000).

The external sex organs in patients with a gonadoblastoma exhibit a wide range of appearances and vary from normal to completely ambiguous. A certain degree of clitoromegaly is common. The secondary sex organs usually consist of a hypoplastic uterus and two normal or slightly hypoplastic Fallopian tubes. Male internal sex organs, such as the epididymis, vas deferens, and prostate, are sometimes found in virilised phenotypic females and are nearly always present in phenotypic male pseudohermaphrodites.

Histological findings

A gonadoblastoma is composed of multiple cellular nests surrounded by a connective tissue stroma (Fig. 22.3). The latter is usually dense and fibrous, but may be cellular, resembling ovarian cortex, or loose and oedematous. The cellular nests are solid, round, or oval and though usually small, may occasionally be large and elongated. They are composed of germ cells intimately admixed with sex-cord

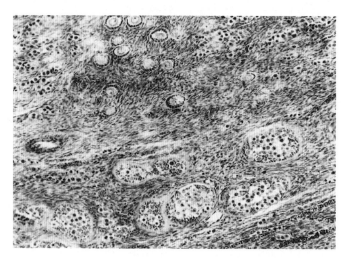

Fig. 22.2 Gonadoblastoma overgrown by dysgerminoma present in an otherwise normal ovary. Note the numerous primordial follicles (top).

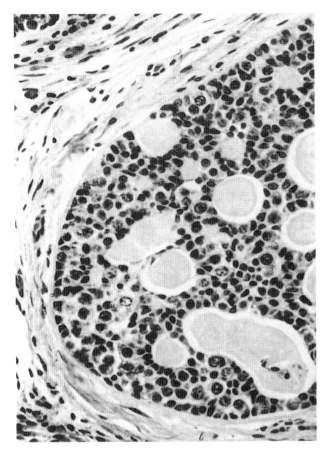

Fig. 22.4 Gonadoblastoma nests showing the hyaline Call–Exner-like bodies and the cellular composition. The surrounding dense connective tissue stroma contains a few somewhat distorted Leydig-like or lutein cells.

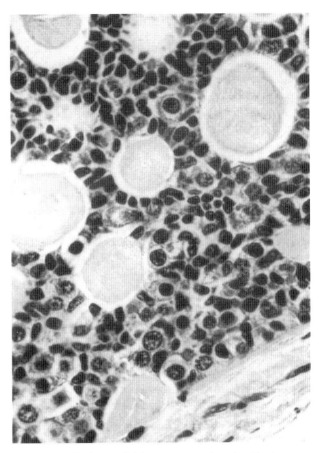

Fig. 22.5 Detail of gonadoblastoma nest showing the large germ cells with clear cytoplasm and round vesicular nuclei, and the smaller sex-cord derivatives with ovoid or elongated nuclei.

derivatives resembling immature Sertoli and granulosa cells (Fig. 22.4). The germ cells are large, round with clear or pale, slightly granular cytoplasm, and contain round vesicular nuclei, often with prominent nucleoli (Fig. 22.5).

These cells show histological appearances similar to those of germ cells in dysgerminomas or seminomas. They also show similar ultrastructural appearances and histochemical reactions to those observed in dysgerminoma cells, as well as in primordial germ cells. The germ cells of gonadoblastomas show mitotic activity, which may be marked in some cases. The extent of the mitotic activity tends to reflect the proliferative activity of the germ cell component and it is greater in tumours showing overgrowth of the tumour nests by the germ cell element. The germ cells are intimately admixed with the sex-cord derivatives resembling immature Sertoli and granulosa cells. These cells are round or oval and have hyperchromatic oval, round, slightly elongated or carrot-shaped nuclei. They are smaller than the germ cells, epithelial-like in appearance (Figs 22.4 and 22.5) and devoid of mitotic activity. The sex-cord derivatives resembling Sertoli and granulosa cells form three typical patterns within the cellular nests (Fig. 22.4 and 22.5).

1. They line the periphery of the nest in a coronal pattern.
2. They surround individual, or collections of, germ cells in the same way as the follicular epithelium surrounds the ovum of the primary follicle.
3. They surround small round amorphous hyaline eosinophilic, PAS-positive, diastase-resistant Call–Exner-like bodies which are present within the cellular nests.

Collections of cells indistinguishable from Leydig cells or luteinized ovarian stromal cells are frequently present within the connective tissue surrounding the cellular nests (Figs 22.4, 22.6). These cells may contain lipochrome granules and exhibit vacuolation associated with the presence of a lipid substance, but have never been found to contain Reinke crystals, which are considered to be specifically diagnostic of Leydig cells. The collections of these cells vary from very small, sometimes represented by individual cells (Fig. 22.4), to large (Fig. 22.6). The Leydig or lutein-like cells have been identified in 66% of gonadoblastomas and have been detected nearly twice as frequently in patients older than 15 years than in those 15 years or younger (Scully 1970b). The presence of these

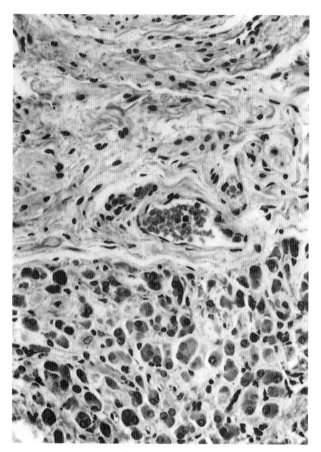

Fig. 22.6 Collection of Leydig-like, or lutein, cells in the vicinity of a gonadoblastoma nest.

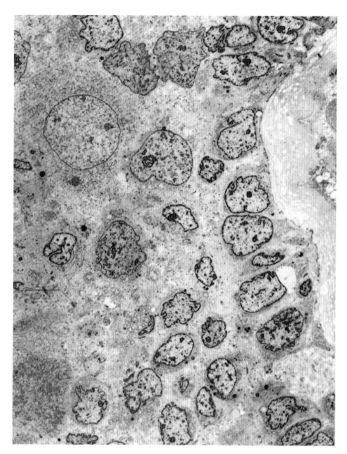

Fig. 22.7 Ultrastructural appearances of gonadoblastoma showing the two cell types: the germ cells with large round nuclei and smaller sex-cord derivatives with irregularly shaped light or dark nuclei. Hyaline material is seen at the periphery of the nest. Uranyl acetate and lead citrate. (Courtesy of Dr T Okagaki.)

cells is not necessary for the diagnosis of a gonadoblastoma and, conversely, they may be identified in gonadal streaks which do not contain gonadoblastoma nests.

Ultrastructural studies in a number of cases have confirmed the basic composition of the gonadoblastoma, consisting of the two cell types within the cellular nests (Fig. 22.7) and the Leydig or lutein-like cells within the surrounding connective tissue (Hou-Jensen & Kempson 1974; Mackay et al 1974; Damjanov et al 1975; Garvin et al 1976; Ishida et al 1976; Bjersing & Cajander 1977; Damjanov & Klauber 1980; Bolen 1981). These studies show complete agreement as to the nature of the germ cells, but the nature of the sex-cord cells continues to be a matter of dispute and controversy. Some consider them as Sertoli cells or their precursors (Mackay et al 1974; Ishida et al 1976), others as granulosa cells or their precursors (Damjanov & Klauber 1980), while the majority regard them as primitive sex-cord derivatives which cannot be further differentiated (Scully 1970b; Hou-Jensen & Kempson 1974; Garvin et al 1976; Bjersing & Cajander 1977; Talerman 1980; Bolen 1981). Ishida et al (1976), on the basis of an ultrastructural study, considered that the Leydig or lutein-like cells may in fact represent precursors of Leydig cells but there has been no further confirmation of these findings. The hyaline mate-

rial present within the cellular nests (Fig. 22.7) and forming the Call–Exner-like bodies is considered to be of basement membrane origin (Mackay et al 1974; Damjanov et al 1975; Garvin et al 1976; Ishida et al 1976; Damjanov & Klauber 1980; Bolen 1981).

The basic histological pattern of a gonadoblastoma may be altered by two different processes:

1. Hyalinisation, usually associated with calcification (Fig. 22.8), the latter often supervening and becoming the predominant feature
2. Overgrowth by a neoplastic germ cell element, usually a dysgerminoma (Fig. 22.9).

These two processes have completely opposite effects: the former is a regressive process leading to the complete obliteration of the lesion, whilst the latter is a proliferative process representing the activation of the malignant potential of the lesion and the formation of a malignant germ cell tumour. In a number of cases both processes may, however, coexist. Hyalinisation takes place by extension and coalescence of the hyaline Call–Exner-like bodies present within the cellular nests and of the basement membrane-like band present in the periphery and

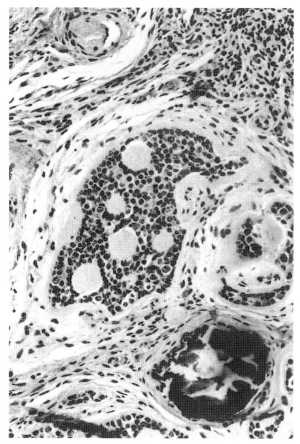

Fig. 22.8 Gonadoblastoma nests showing hyalinisation and calcification. This process often leads to obliteration of the lesion.

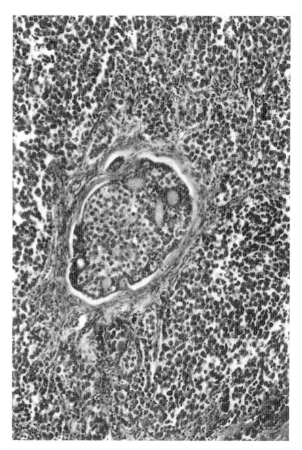

Fig. 22.9 Gonadoblastoma overgrown by a dysgerminoma.

surrounding the nest. The hyaline material extends and replaces the cells present within the nest, resulting in the obliteration of the whole nest. Calcification takes place in the hyalinised areas (Fig. 22.8): it first appears in the Call–Exner-like bodies with the formation of small calcific spherules which are frequently laminated and resemble psammoma bodies. The process of calcification extends by fusion and replacement of the hyalinised material, resulting in the formation of a calcified mass replacing the whole nest. The calcification and hyalinisation may extend to the connective tissue surrounding the cellular nests. In such cases the only evidence that a gonadoblastoma has been present is the finding of a large rounded smooth calcified mass or masses (Fig. 22.10). Such a finding has been designated 'burnt out' gonadoblastoma (Scully 1970b) and although not diagnostic of the lesion (Hughesdon & Kumarasamy 1970; Scully 1970b; Talerman 1971; Talerman 1980) is very suggestive that a gonadoblastoma may be present and demands a study of all the material available and a careful search for more viable areas. When regressive changes are observed within the cellular nests of a gonadoblastoma, the germ cell component is affected first, showing lack of cellular proliferation, and cell loss. Ultimately it may disappear entirely, while the sex-cord element may still be present

(Fig. 22.11). Persistence of the Leydig, or lutein-like, cells within the surrounding connective tissue may be occasionally observed even when the gonadoblastoma nests have undergone complete obliteration (Garvin et al 1976) and these cells may be hormonally active. Sometimes complete hyalinisation and calcification of the entire lesion may occur.

A gonadoblastoma is frequently overgrown by a neoplastic germ cell element, this being observed in more than 60% of cases (Scully 1970b; Garvin et al 1976; Govan et al 1977; Talerman 1980). In at least 50% of cases a gonadoblastoma is overgrown by a dysgerminoma (Scully 1970b), and in a further 10% by other more malignant neoplastic germ cell elements (Scully 1970b; Talerman 1974; Talerman 1980). The earliest stage of the process of overgrowth by the germ cell element manifests itself as an increased proliferation of germ cells within the cellular nest, resulting in a decrease of the sex-cord elements and a preponderance of germ cells (Fig. 22.12). This process results in the virtual disappearance of the sex-cord elements and their complete overgrowth by the germ cells. Following this the malignant germ cells penetrate the basement membrane of the nest and extend into the surrounding connective tissue, forming a microscopic dysgerminoma. Further extension of this process results

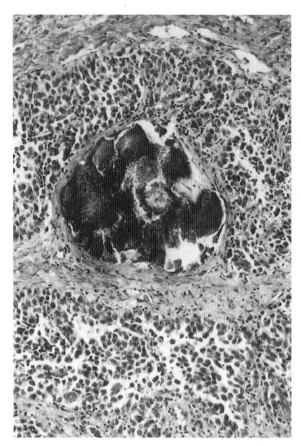

Fig. 22.10 Large rounded calcific concretion surrounded by dysgerminoma cells. Such a finding is highly suggestive of the presence of gonadoblastoma, and has been called 'burnt out' gonadoblastoma.

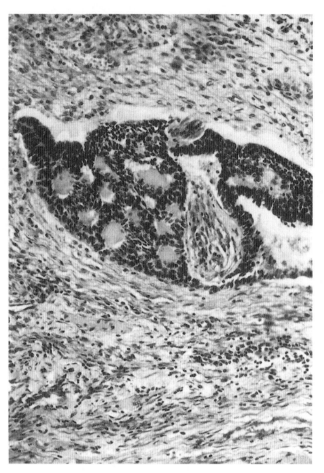

Fig. 22.11 Gonadoblastoma nest showing regressive changes with disappearance of the germ cell component and persistence of the sex-cord derivatives.

in more obvious invasion of the surrounding connective tissue, followed by its replacement, enlargement of the tumour and formation of a tumour mass composed either of dysgerminoma in which occasional nests of gonadoblastoma are discernible (Fig. 22.9) or of pure dysgerminoma. The dysgerminoma in these cases shows appearances which are indistinguishable histologically, histochemically and ultrastructurally from dysgerminomas, or seminomas, unassociated with gonadoblastoma and occurring in otherwise normal individuals (Scully 1970b; Hou-Jensen & Kempson 1974; Damjanov et al 1975; Garvin et al 1976; Bjersing & Cajander 1977; Damjanov & Klauber 1980; Talerman 1980; Bolen 1981).

A gonadoblastoma may be associated with, or overgrown by, other malignant neoplastic germ cell elements, either individually or in combination. Gonadoblastomas have been associated with immature teratoma (Frazier et al 1964; Scully 1970b; Stolecke et al 1974; Govan et al 1977), embryonal carcinoma (Talerman 1974; Talerman & Delemarre 1975; Ben-Romdhane et al 1988), yolk sac tumour (Santesson & Marrubini 1957; Scully 1970b; Hart & Burkons 1979; Muzsnai & Feinberg 1980) and choriocarcinoma (Drobnjak et al 1971; Gallager & Lewis 1973; Zuntova et al 1992b).

A case of a 19-year-old phenotypic female with 46,XY karyotype and a gonadal tumour composed of gonadoblastoma overgrown by dysgerminoma and containing a proliferation suggestive of a Sertoli cell tumour was reported by Nomura et al (1999). The contralateral gonad was described as hypoplastic. The authors stated that the gonadoblastoma in parts showed extensive regressive changes including loss of germ cells and that the Sertoli cell tumour-like lesion formed an intimate part of the gonadoblastoma and dysgerminoma. In view of this, the possibility that the Sertoli cell tumour-like lesion represents a regressing gonadoblastoma and not a true Sertoli cell tumour arising from the gonadoblastoma as suggested by the authors (Nomura et al 1999) must be seriously considered.

Gonadoblastoma has never been detected within metastatic lesions, and has never been encountered outside the gonads. Although Bhathena et al (1985) described a case of gonadoblastoma coexisting with mixed germ cell sex-cord–stromal tumour, review of the case revealed that the tumour was in fact a pure gonadoblastoma. A similar conclusion can be reached as regards the case reported by Colafranceschi & Massi (1995)

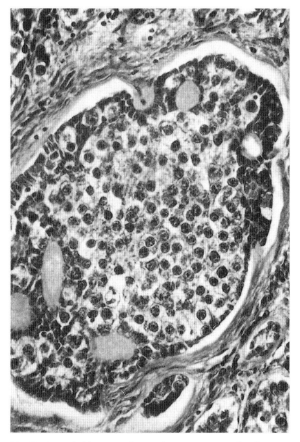

Fig. 22.12 Gonadoblastoma becoming overgrown by the germ cell component. Note the increase in germ cells within the nest and paucity of the sex-cord derivatives.

occurring in a 14-year-old phenotypic female with 46,XY karyotype and bilateral gonadal tumours. One of the tumours was described as a pure dysgerminoma, while the other, which was illustrated, shows appearances more in keeping with gonadoblastoma becoming overgrown by dysgerminoma than with a mixed germ cell-sex-cord stromal tumour.

DIFFERENTIAL DIAGNOSIS

Because the gonadoblastoma has a distinctive histological appearance and a unique cellular constitution, being composed of germ cells intimately admixed with sex-cord elements, it should not be easily confused with any of the well-established gonadal neoplasms. Failure to recognise the presence of one of the elements and the histological pattern may of course lead to an erroneous diagnosis of a germ cell tumour or a sex-cord–stromal neoplasm. The importance of careful examination of the lesion, especially when it is undergoing regressive changes or is being overgrown by a neoplastic germ cell element, cannot be overemphasised.

A gonadoblastoma is most likely to be confused with other entities which exhibit a similar cellular composition or similar histological pattern. It may be confused with the mixed germ cell sex-cord–stromal tumour (Talerman 1972a,b) which, like the gonadoblastoma, is composed of germ cells intimately admixed with sex-cord derivatives, but shows a different histological pattern, a less uniform appearance and much more marked proliferative activity, involving also the sex-cord element, resulting in large tumours. The tumours are unilateral and occur in normal ovaries and testes. The patients with this tumour also show genetic, anatomical and hormonal differences from patients with gonadoblastoma. Another lesion which may be confused with gonadoblastoma is the ovarian sex-cord tumour with annular tubules (Scully 1970a; Young et al 1982), which is often found in patients with the Peutz–Jeghers syndrome. This tumour has a similar histological pattern to a gonadoblastoma and consists of round tubular structures lined by Sertoli and granulosa-like cells and contains similar round, hyaline eosinophilic, PAS-positive Call–Exner-like bodies and laminated calcific concretions. It may undergo extensive hyalinisation and calcification. The main difference between these two entities is the complete absence of germ cells in the ovarian sex-cord tumour with annular tubules.

THERAPY

There is general agreement that a gonadoblastoma may act as a source of origin of malignant germ cell neoplasms and that it nearly always occurs in dysgenetic gonads (Hughesdon & Kumarasamy 1970; Scully 1970b; Teter 1970; Schellhas 1974a,b; Talerman 1974; Garvin et al 1976; Govan et al 1977; Hart & Burkons 1979; Talerman 1980). Even when a gonadoblastoma occurs in a normal gonad it may be a source of origin of a malignant germ cell neoplasm (Hughesdon & Kumarasamy 1970; Goldsmith & Hart 1975; Talerman & Delemarre 1975; Pratt-Thomas & Cooper 1976; Magyar & Talerman unpublished observations). These findings indicate that gonads harbouring a gonadoblastoma are not only a danger to the patient but, because of a lack of normal function, are expendable, and there is nowadays full agreement that the treatment of choice is the excision of the gonads (Scully 1970b; Teter 1970; Schellhas 1974a,b; Talerman 1974; Garvin et al 1976; Govan et al 1977; Hart & Burkons 1979; Talerman 1980). Both gonads must be excised, not only the gonad which appears to be abnormal, because the contralateral gonad, however small or normal appearing it might be, may harbour a microscopic gonadoblastoma from which a malignant neoplasm may originate (Scully 1970b; Talerman 1971; Gallager & Lewis 1973; Schellhas 1974a). There is at present no complete agreement on whether the uterus should be excised together with the gonads or left in situ for psychological reasons with the option of inducing cyclical bleeding by oestrogen, or oestrogen-progestagen, replacement therapy. Because long-term oestrogen administration has been associated with a risk of development of endometrial adenocarcinoma (Cutler et al 1972; Schellhas 1974b), leaving the uterus in situ at the time of gonadectomy may pose a certain risk to the patient. Because of this the view that hysterectomy should also be undertaken during gonadectomy appears to be more favoured nowadays.

BEHAVIOUR AND PROGNOSIS

Patients with a pure gonadoblastoma have an excellent prognosis provided both gonads are excised. The prognosis of patients with gonadoblastoma associated with, or overgrown by, dysgerminoma is also very good. In these cases metastases tend to occur less frequently and somewhat later than in patients who have a dysgerminoma unassociated with a gonadoblastoma (Scully 1970b; Teter 1970; Talerman 1971; Schellhas 1974a; Garvin et al 1976; Hart & Burkons 1979; Talerman 1980). Except for three patients who died with disseminated dysgerminoma (Teter 1970; Govan et al 1977; Hart & Burkons 1979), all patients with a gonadoblastoma associated with dysgerminoma with a known follow-up, including occasional cases with metastases (Teter 1970; Schellhas et al 1971; Govan et al 1977; Hart & Burkons 1979), are alive and well following adequate therapy. When a gonadoblastoma is associated with malignant neoplastic germ cell elements other than dysgerminoma, such as immature teratoma, yolk sac tumour, embryonal carcinoma or choriocarcinoma, the prognosis in the past was poor, none of the patients surviving longer than 18 months (Santesson & Marrubini 1957; Frazier et al 1964; Scully 1970b; Gallager & Lewis 1973; Talerman 1974; Hart & Burkons 1979; Muzsnai & Feinberg 1980; Talerman 1980). The administration of new chemotherapeutic regimens, such as the cisdiaminoplatinum, etopoxide (VP 16) and bleomycin combination, which has been successful in the treatment of patients with malignant germ cell tumours of the testis and ovary, has altered this dismal outcome, even if metastases are present (LaPolla et al 1990).

MIXED GERM CELL SEX-CORD–STROMAL TUMOUR

Synonyms: epithelioma pflugerien (Masson 1922); Pflugerome (Cabanne 1971); mixed germ cell tumour (Hughesdon & Kumarasamy 1970); gonocytoma 2 (Teter 1960); atypical gonadoblastoma (Serment et al 1970; Mostofi & Sobin 1977).

TERMINOLOGY

The designation mixed germ cell sex-cord–stromal tumour (Talerman 1972a,b) could be used to describe all neoplams composed of germ cells intimately admixed with sex-cord–stromal derivatives, including the gonadoblastoma; however, since the latter is now so well established it is considered appropriate that this term should be reserved to denote neoplasms composed of these cell types other than gonadoblastoma. The term mixed germ cell sex-cord–stromal tumour is preferable to the terms 'epithelioma pflugerien' (Masson 1922), or 'Pflugerome' (Cabanne 1971), which have been used to describe this entity, because they imply that the tumour originates from Pflüger's tubes, described as germ cell clusters in a granulosal envelope, which are formed in the embryo during gonadal development. In view of the fact that there is even some doubt as to the presence of Pflüger's tubes in the human during fetal life, and as there is no good evidence that this tumour could originate in this way, these terms are considered to be unsatisfactory. The term 'mixed germ cell tumour' (Hughesdon & Kumarasamy 1970) is unsuitable because it is used to describe tumours of germ cell origin composed of several neoplastic germ cell elements and it was used in this context in the 1973 histological classification of ovarian tumours formulated by the World Health Organization (Serov et al, 1973). The term 'gonocytoma 2' (Teter 1960) is unsatisfactory because the tumour is not only composed of gonocytes, or germ cells, but contains sex-cord–stromal derivatives which form an integral and important part of the tumour. Although the mixed germ cell sex-cord–stromal tumour shares with the gonadoblastoma a similar cellular composition it shows considerable histopathological as well as other differences which are important enough to merit a designation as a specific histopathological entity distinctive from gonadoblastoma. In view of this the term 'atypical gonadoblastoma' (Serment et al 1970; Mostofi & Sobin 1978) is incorrect. The term mixed germ cell sex-cord–stromal tumour has now become the accepted term and the entity has been included as such in the revised World Health Organization classifications of ovarian and testicular neoplasms (Mostofi and Sesterhenn 1998; Scully 1999).

INCIDENCE

A mixed germ cell sex-cord–stromal tumour is encountered less frequently than is a gonadoblastoma, and is considered to be uncommon. Its true incidence is not, however, known, for it is likely that some cases have not been recognised and have been classified with other types of ovarian neoplasms. During the three decades since this neoplasm was first described as a specific histopathological entity (Talerman 1972a,b) additional cases have been recorded (Talerman & van der Harten 1977; Talerman 1980; Bolen 1981; Tavassoli 1983; Tokuoka et al 1985; Lacson et al 1988; Matoska & Talerman 1989; Minh et al 1990; Jacobsen et al 1991; Zuntova et al 1992a) and a number of well-documented cases have been seen (Talerman unpublished observations). Most cases have occurred in phenotypically and genetically normal female infants and children in the first decade of life (Diligent 1971; Talerman 1972a,b; Talerman & van der Harten 1977; Talerman 1980; Talerman unpublished observations; Tavassoli 1983; Tokuoka et al 1985; Lacson et al 1988; Zuntova et al 1992a). Twenty patients presented during the first year of life, their ages ranging from a few days to nine months (Diligent 1971; Talerman 1972a; Talerman 1980; Talerman unpublished observations; Tavassoli 1983; Tokuoka et al 1985), whilst a further 12 patients presented between three and 10 years of age (Cabanne 1971; Talerman 1972b; Talerman & van der Harten 1977; Talerman unpublished observations; Lacson et al 1988; Zuntova et al 1992a). Six cases occurred in phenotypic and genotypic females aged between 16 and 31 years (Hughesdon & Kumarasamy 1970; Szymanska et al 1981; Jacobsen et al 1991; Talerman unpublished observations). Two of these patients had normal pregnancies prior to the excision of the tumour (Talerman 1980; Talerman unpublished observations). A 46-year-old normal phenotypic female with a 46,XX karyotype had two normal pregnancies prior to the diagnosis of ovarian mixed germ cell sex-cord–stromal tumour (Minh et al 1990). It is likely that some cases described as gonocytoma 2 by Teter (1960) may have been examples of this entity. Mixed germ cell sex-cord–stromal tumours have been encountered in at least 20 normal males, many of whom have fathered children. Although most patients were adult males (Talerman 1980; Bolen 1981; Matoska & Talerman 1989; Talerman unpublished observations), an 8-year-old boy affected by this tumour is also known to the author (Talerman & Harms unpublished observations).

CLINICAL FINDINGS

The majority of patients with mixed germ cell sex-cord–stromal tumours, in contrast to those with gonadoblastoma, are normal phenotypic females, mainly infants and children, or normal adult males. The most common presenting symptom in female patients is the presence of a tumour mass in the lower abdomen, which may be affected by torsion and therefore associated with pain, and the patient may present with signs of an acute abdominal emergency. Signs of isosexual precocious pseudopuberty have been observed in five infants under one year, and a girl aged eight years showed signs of isosexual precocious pseudopuberty for three years prior to the excision of a large ovarian tumour (Talerman & van der Harten 1977). Other female patients did not have any hormonal abnormalities. Male patients with this tumour presented with testicular enlargement. None of the patients with a mixed germ cell sex-cord–stromal tumour showed any evidence of developmental abnormalities affecting the gonads, the external genitalia, or body build.

GENETIC FINDINGS

The majority of patients with a mixed germ cell sex-cord–stromal tumour had genotype and karyotype determinations. This applies to nearly all the female patients, who were chromatin positive, had a normal female chromosome complement with a 46,XX karyotype and showed normal somatosexual development. Three of the older patients had normal full-term pregnancies and delivered normal children (Talerman 1980; Talerman unpublished observations; Minh et al 1990).

Many of the male patients with this tumour are known to have fathered children. All the male patients who had chromosomal studies performed were found to have a normal male 46,XY karyotype. These findings indicate that patients with mixed germ cell sex-cord–stromal tumours have no evidence of chromosomal abnormalities or of gonadal dysgenesis.

HORMONAL FINDINGS

Although a few patients with a mixed germ cell sex-cord–stromal tumour have shown evidence of abnormal hormonal function, manifesting itself as isosexual precocious pseudopuberty, most patients with this neoplasm do not exhibit clinical evidence of abnormal hormonal activity. Determinations of endocrine function have not been performed preoperatively in the majority of patients with this tumour, and when they were performed after the operation the findings were normal. Abnormal hormonal manifestations have, however, been noted in five patients. One otherwise normal 8-year-old girl exhibited signs of precocious isosexual pseudopuberty manifesting itself as breast development and vaginal bleeding for three years prior to the excision of a large ovarian tumour. The urinary oestrogens were elevated and vaginal smears showed an oestrogen effect. Following the excision of the ovarian tumour the urinary oestrogens returned to normal, the vaginal bleeding ceased and there was no further increase in the size of the breasts during the following three years (Talerman & van der Harten 1977). Four infants aged under one year also exhibited isosexual precocious pseudopuberty which manifested itself as breast development and vaginal bleeding. The urinary oestrogens were elevated and vaginal smears showed an oestrogenic effect. Excision of the tumour resulted in the disappearance of the symptoms and a complete return to normal.

None of the patients exhibited any evidence of virilisation or defeminisation. The males with this tumour did not show any hormonal abnormalities.

These findings indicate that the majority of patients with a mixed germ cell sex-cord–stromal tumour do not have any associated hormonal abnormalities, but that when these occur they manifest themselves as feminisation. Because of the young age of the majority of patients with this tumour precocious isosexual pseudopuberty is induced.

A patient who was found to have a mixed germ cell sex-cord–stromal tumour at the age of 10 years (Talerman 1972b), when followed postoperatively, was found to develop normally and commenced menstruating at the age of 15 years.

PATHOLOGY

Macroscopical findings

Mixed germ cell sex-cord–stromal tumours, unlike gonadoblastomas, are large neoplasms (Figs 22.13, 22.14) and vary in size from 7.5–18 cm in the longest diameter, their weight ranging from 100–1050 g (Talerman 1980).

In the great majority of patients, the tumours have been unilateral and the contralateral gonad appeared normal. In patients where biopsy was performed, these findings were confirmed histologically. The gonad in which the tumour originated was normal in all cases, showing normal ovarian structure in all female patients and normal testicular morphology in males. In two cases the tumour was bilateral (Jacobsen et al 1991; Talerman unpublished observations). In one case the contralateral

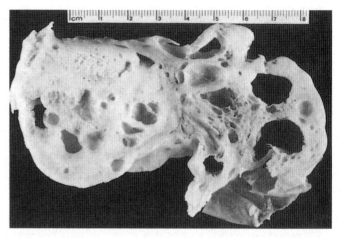

Fig. 22.14 Mixed germ cell sex-cord–stromal tumour. The tumours are mainly solid, but may contain cystic areas, which in this case are large (right).

ovary contained a sex-cord tumour with annular tubules (Szymanska et al 1981). A case of a normal female infant whose ovary contained a mixed germ cell sex-cord–stromal tumour and a sex-cord tumour with annular tubules is known to the author. The two tumours were in close proximity but were completely separated by a fibrous band. The contralateral gonad was a normal ovary (Talerman unpublished observations).

The tumour is usually oval or round, firm in consistency, smooth, may be somewhat lobulated and has a smooth slightly glistening surface (Fig. 22.13). In the majority of cases the tumour is solid, but in some cases it may contain cystic areas, some of which may be large (Talerman & van der Harten 1977). The cut surface of the tumour is solid, except for tumours with cystic areas (Fig. 22.14), and varies in colour from uniformly grey–white to grey–pink, or pale yellow to light tan. In the larger tumours slightly softer oedematous areas are present which may show early necrotic changes. Large foci of necrosis have not been observed and calcification has not been encountered. When cysts are present they vary in size, and occasionally may be large (Fig. 22.14). They have smooth walls and contain pale, translucent, watery fluid, which in some of the larger cysts may be slightly opalescent.

All patients with this tumour have had normal external genitalia. The Fallopian tubes and the uterus did not show any abnormalities and there was no evidence of gonadal dysgenesis.

Histological findings

The mixed germ cell sex-cord–stromal tumour is composed of germ cells intimately admixed with sex-cord derivatives resembling Sertoli and granulosa cells and shows much greater variability in its histological appearance than does a gonadoblastoma. Collections of Leydig or lutein-like cells have been observed only in occasional

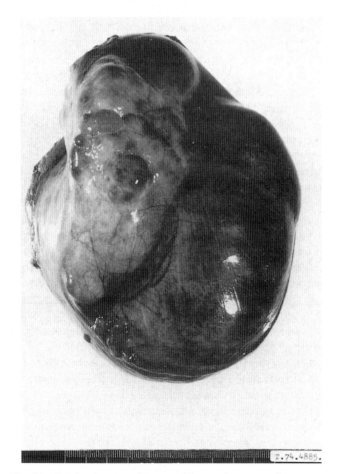

Fig. 22.13 Mixed germ cell sex-cord–stromal tumour. The tumour is large, and has a glistening slightly lobulated surface.

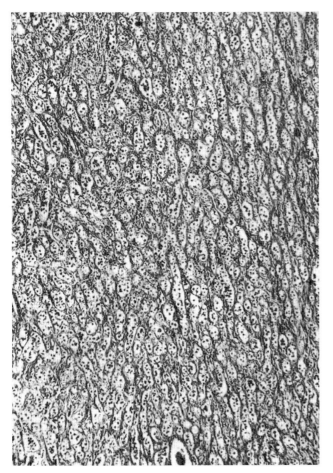

Fig. 22.15 Mixed germ cell sex-cord–stromal tumour showing tubular pattern. The tumour is composed of tubules without a lumen containing germ cells and sex-cord derivatives.

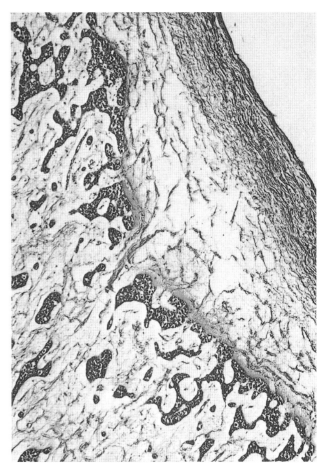

Fig. 22.16 Mixed germ cell sex-cord–stromal tumour showing trabecular or cord-like pattern. The tumour is composed of cords or trabeculae which are surrounded by loose connective tissue. A narrow rim of unaffected ovarian tissue is seen at the right of the picture.

cases (Talerman 1972b; Szymanska et al 1981) and are not considered to be an integral component of the tumour. Although originally the tumour was considered to exhibit two distinct histological patterns — the tubular (Fig. 22.15) (Talerman 1972a) and the cord-like or trabecular (Fig. 22.16) (Talerman 1972b) — it has been established subsequently that both patterns may be seen in the same tumour, as well as a third pattern which consists of a haphazard arrangement of germ cells surrounded by sex-cord elements, the latter sometimes predominating (Fig. 22.17).

The three histological patterns observed in mixed germ cell sex-cord–stromal tumours are:

1. Composed of long, narrow ramifying cords or trabeculae (Fig. 22.18) which in places expand and form wider columns and larger round or oval cellular aggregates or clusters surrounded by a connective tissue stroma (Fig. 22.19). Some of the clusters may resemble the nests seen in a gonadoblastoma and may occasionally contain small, round, eosinophilic hyaline Call–Exner-like bodies, but do not contain calcific concretions (Fig. 22.20). These clusters are usually very

much more abundant and less well circumscribed than the nests observed in gonadoblastomas and exhibit no evidence of regressive changes.

2. Composed of tubular structures devoid of a lumen and surrounded by a fine connective tissue network (Figs 22.15, 22.21). In some places the tubular pattern is less obvious, and the tumour is composed of small clusters of larger round, or oval, solid cellular aggregates surrounded by connective tissue similar to those described above.

3. Composed of scattered, haphazardly arranged, individual or collections of germ cells surrounded by sex-cord derivatives, which may be very abundant (Fig. 22.22). The proportions of the two components, the germ cells and the sex-cord elements, may vary widely when this pattern is observed, although usually the sex-cord derivatives tend to predominate.

There is a frequent admixture between these patterns, but tumours may be observed where only one of these patterns can be demonstrated, or shows marked predominance. The two cellular elements comprising this

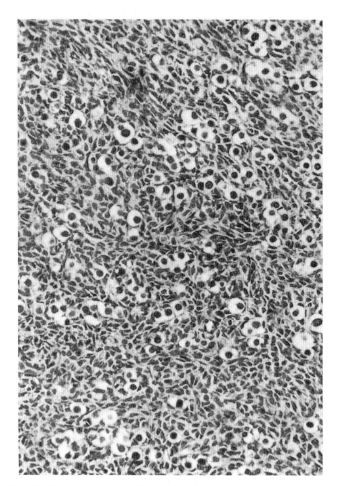

Fig. 22.17 Mixed germ cell sex-cord–stromal tumour showing germ cells intermingled with sex-cord elements forming a haphazard arrangement.

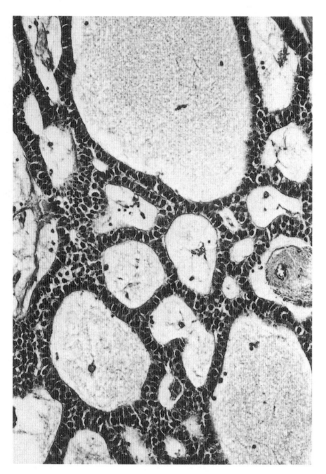

Fig. 22.18 Mixed germ cell sex-cord–stromal tumour showing cord-like pattern. The cords of tumour cells are surrounded by loose connective tissue.

tumour, the germ cells and the sex-cord derivatives, are always intimately admixed.

There may be considerable variation in the cellular content in some parts of the tumour, and in some areas there is a preponderance of sex-cord derivatives, while in other parts of the tumour germ cells may predominate. The sex-cord derivatives, which resemble Sertoli and granulosa cells, are arranged peripherally in a single file forming long rows on the outer side of the cords (Fig. 22.23), or lining peripherally the tubular structures (Figs 22.21, 22.24), as well as surrounding individual, or collections of, germ cells within the small clusters or larger cellular aggregates comprising the tumour (Fig. 22.22). The germ cell component of the mixed germ cell sex-cord–stromal tumour shows a similar appearance to the germ cells seen in dysgerminomas or gonado-blastomas, including brisk mitotic activity and abnormal mitoses (Fig. 22.24). The ultrastructural appearances as well as the histochemical reactions are similar and also resemble those observed in primordial germ cells. In a number of tumours some germ cells appear to be more mature than those observed in gonadoblastomas and dys-germinomas, tending to resemble primordial germ cells

even on lightmicroscopy. In view of this it is possible that they may represent a more advanced stage in the matura-tion process of the germ cell as compared with those observed in a dysgerminoma or gonadoblastoma. Although these findings have received support from the ultrastructural study of a single case (Bolen 1981), studies of several other cases have not confirmed these observations (Lacson et al 1988; Matoska & Talerman 1989; Talerman & Okagaki unpublished observations; Zuntova et al 1992a). The sex-cord derivatives tend to resemble Sertoli cells rather than granulosa cells, both lightmicroscopically and ultrastructurally, but in many tumours they resemble immature sex-cord derivatives (Fig. 22.25) which can be considered as precursors of both Sertoli and granulosa cells. The sex-cord derivatives, unlike those seen in a gonadoblastoma, show proliferative changes and exhibit a variable degree of mitotic activity.

There is no evidence of hyalinisation, calcification or other regressive changes. The connective tissue sur-rounding the tumour cells varies from a very fine reti-culin network surrounding the tubules, seen in tu-mours exhibiting mainly or entirely the tubular pattern (Figs 22.14, 22.21), to dense fibrous tissue which may be

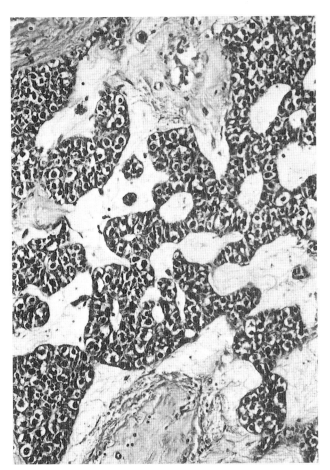

Fig. 22.19 Mixed germ cell sex-cord–stromal tumour showing trabeculae and larger cellular aggregates surrounded by dense connective tissue.

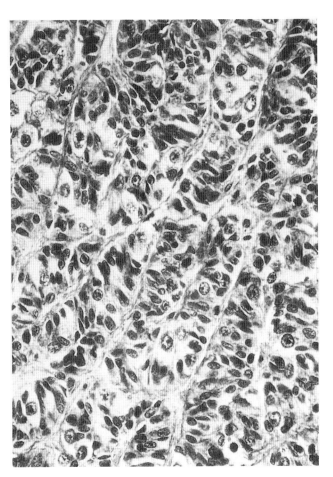

Fig. 22.21 Mixed germ cell sex-cord–stromal tumour showing a tubular pattern. Note the cellular composition and the fine connective tissue network. The large germ cells with round nuclei are surrounded by sex-cord derivatives.

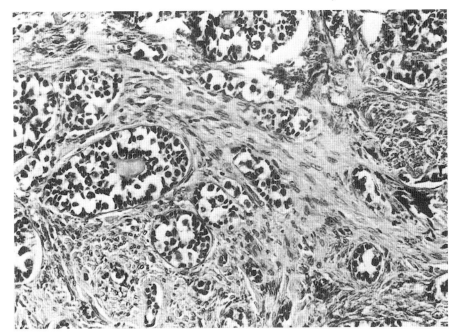

Fig. 22.20 Mixed germ cell sex-cord–stromal tumour showing nest-like pattern. A hyaline body, an uncommon finding, is seen within the largest nest. This pattern is usually admixed with the tubular pattern. Note the dense connective tissue surrounding the tumour nests.

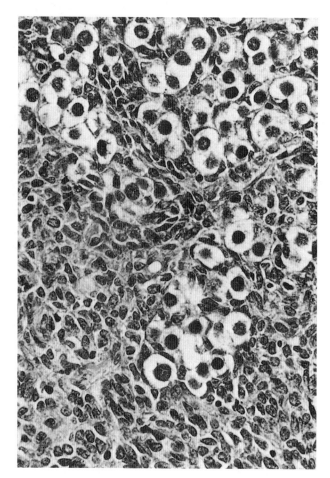

Fig. 22.22 Mixed germ cell sex-cord–stromal tumour composed of haphazardly arranged germ cells surrounded by sex-cord elements.

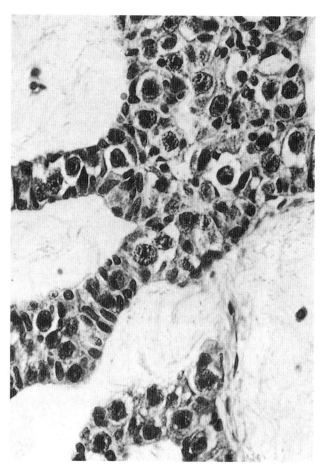

Fig. 22.23 Mixed germ cell sex-cord–stromal tumour showing cord-like pattern. Note the peripherally arranged sex-cord derivatives surrounding the larger germ cells.

somewhat hyalinised (Figs 22.19 and 22.20) and is mainly seen in tumours composed of small clusters or larger aggregates of tumour cells. The connective tissue may also be loose and oedematous and this is usually seen in tumours showing the cord-like or trabecular pattern (Figs 22.16, 22.18).

Most tumours show a solid pattern although occasionally small clefts or spaces may be present. In occasional tumours more numerous and larger cystic spaces may be seen which vary in size and can sometimes be observed on gross examination. These spaces are either devoid of an epithelial lining or lined by small flattened epithelial-like cells. They may also be lined by sex-cord derivatives and resemble the cystic spaces seen in typical cystic and retiform sex-cord–stromal tumours. In some cases the spaces may be lined by cells resembling those lining the cystic spaces of a serous cystadenoma. Occasionally there may be extensive proliferation of these cells and the tumour shows the same resemblance to borderline and malignant serous tumours as do some retiform Sertoli–Leydig cell tumours (Young & Scully 1983; Talerman 1987). The pale eosinophilic fluid present within the cystic spaces is similar to the material present within

cystic spaces in sex-cord–stromal tumours. Although originally it was believed that some of these changes were reactive, it is considered that they represent cystic and retiform differentiation within the sex-cord component of the tumour. Thus the epithelial component of the gonadal germ cell stromal epithelial tumour of the ovary reported by Tavassoli (1983) represents precisely this type of differentiation and the tumour was a typical mixed germ cell sex-cord–stromal tumour.

All the tumours occurring in female patients originated in normal ovaries, as shown by the presence of normal ovarian tissue containing primordial and Graafian follicles. The ovaries of the postpubertal patients contained corpora albicantia, indicating ovulatory activity, and the contralateral ovaries, when biopsied, showed normal histological appearances. In male patients the testicular tissue surrounding the tumour was histologically normal.

In four patients the mixed germ cell sex-cord–stromal tumour was associated with a dysgerminoma, which showed typical histological appearances (Fig. 22.26). There were no metastases in two of these cases.

All the patients, including the two with metastatic disease, are well and disease-free for periods ranging from

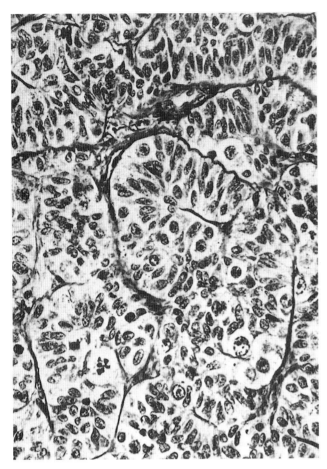

Fig. 22.24 Mixed germ cell sex-cord–stromal tumour showing tubular pattern. The sex-cord derivatives line the tubular structures and surround the germ cells. A germ cell showing a quadripolar mitosis is seen (bottom).

three to five years following excision of the tumour and radiation therapy. In four additional cases the tumour was admixed with other malignant germ cell elements. In one case in a 5-year-old girl the tumour was admixed with choriocarcinoma, while in another case in an 8-year-old girl it was admixed with choriocarcinoma, yolk sac tumour, immature teratoma and dysgerminoma. Both these patients died with disseminated metastatic disease (Talerman unpublished observations). A similar course was seen in a 16-year-old girl whose tumour, in addition to a dysgerminoma, also contained what, from the description and illustrations, appears to be a yolk sac tumour (Hughesdon & Kumarasamy 1970 — Case 2). In a more recent case occurring in a 16-year-old girl, mixed germ cell sex-cord–stromal tumour was admixed with yolk sac tumour. The patient was treated successfully with surgery and cisdiaminoplatinum, vinblastine, and bleomycin combination chemotherapy and is well and disease free five years following diagnosis.

A unique, well-documented case of a mixed germ cell sex-cord–stromal tumour occurring in a 5-year-old girl with isosexual precocious pseudopuberty, where the tumour metastasised to the retroperitoneal lymph nodes and the peritoneal cavity, has been reported by Lacson et al (1988). Unlike the other cases of mixed germ cell sex-cord–stromal tumour, where the metastatic lesions were composed of malignant germ cell elements, in this case the metastases were composed of pure mixed germ cell sex-cord–stromal tumour. The patient was treated successfully with surgery and combination chemotherapy and was well and disease free more than two years following the excision of the tumour (Lacson personal

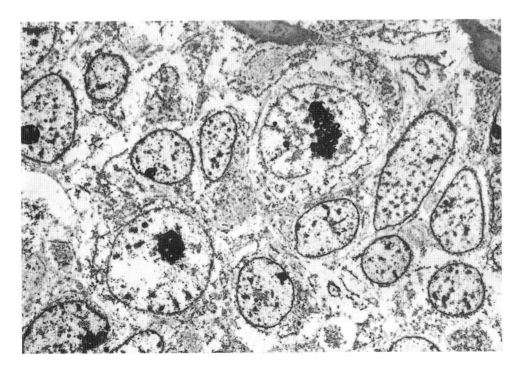

Fig. 22.25 The ultrastructural appearance of mixed germ cell sex-cord–stromal tumour. Note the germ cells with large round nuclei and prominent nucleolonema (centre) and the smaller more numerous sex-cord derivatives with ovoid or elongated nuclei. Uranyl acetate and lead citrate.

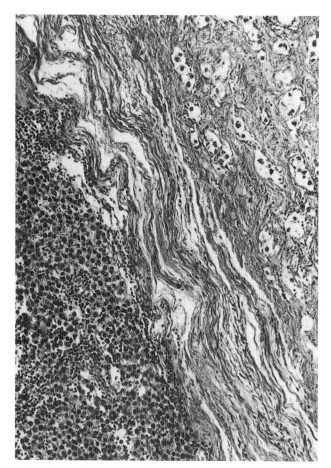

Fig. 22.26 Mixed germ cell sex-cord–stromal tumour associated with dysgerminoma.

communication). The diagnosis of mixed germ cell sex-cord–stromal tumour could not be substantiated in the second case reported by these authors (Lacson et al 1988). Another case of a mixed germ cell sex-cord–stromal tumour associated with metastases has been reported by Arroyo et al (1998). The patient was a 30-year-old woman with a right-sided ovarian tumour showing a mixed germ cell sex-cord–stromal tumour with an unusual histological pattern resembling the sex-cord tumour with annular tubules containing germ cells. Three years after the excision of the tumour, a large mass was noted in the region of the uterine fundus. The mass and a number of peritoneal inplants were excised together with the uterus and the left ovary. The metastatic tumours showed identical appearances to the original ovarian tumour. The left ovary and the uterus were normal. Chemotherapy was administered and the patient was well and disease free one year following the operation (Arroyo et al 1998).

Although it has been suggested by Bhathena et al (1985) and Colafranceschi & Massi (1995) that gonadoblastoma may coexist with mixed germ cell sex-cord–stromal tumour, the documentation in the two cases describing such an association is considered to be unsatis-

factory. The tumour described and depicted is in reality a conventional gonadoblastoma.

DIFFERENTIAL DIAGNOSIS

Due to their similar cellular composition, mixed germ cell sex-cord–stromal tumours are most likely to be confused with gonadoblastoma. They can be differentiated from this by the presence of a totally different histological pattern, more marked proliferative activity, including mitotic activity and proliferation of the sex-cord component, and absence of regressive changes such as calcification and hyalinisation. Macroscopically, the mixed germ cell sex-cord–stromal tumours are larger than gonadoblastomas. The gonad of origin in female patients with this tumour, unlike in patients with gonadoblastoma, is a normal ovary and there are no stigmata of gonadal dysgenesis or any abnormalities affecting the internal or external sex organs. There is no evidence of virilisation and when there are abnormal hormonal manifestations they are feminising and present as isosexual precocious pseudopuberty.

The female patients with a mixed germ cell sex-cord–stromal tumour are normal phenotypic and genotypic females with a 46,XX karyotype, unlike patients with a gonadoblastoma who are usually chromatin negative and have either a 46,XY karyotype or various forms of mosaicism.

When the germ cell element of a mixed germ cell sex-cord–stromal tumour appears to predominate, and especially in the occasional cases when the tumour is associated with a dysgerminoma, confusion with the latter may arise. The finding of sex-cord derivatives, in addition to the germ cells, which are intimately admixed with and surround the germ cells, should alert the observer to the fact that the tumour is not a pure dysgerminoma. If the germ cells are relatively scanty and their presence is not identified, the tumour may be confused with sex-cord–stromal tumours of the ovary such as androblastoma, sex-cord tumour with annular tubules or granulosa cell tumour. In such cases the identification of germ cells within the tumour should help to achieve the correct diagnosis.

Occasionally mixed germ cell sex-cord–stromal tumour may exhibit pronounced cystic and retiform patterns affecting the sex-cord component. In such cases the tumour may be confused with retiform Sertoli–Leydig cell tumours (androblastomas) or with serous tumours of the ovary. The recognition of the retiform pattern and the detection of germ cells provide the correct diagnosis.

BEHAVIOUR AND PROGNOSIS

At the time when this neoplasm was first described in detail (Talerman 1972a,b) it was thought not to be associated with other neoplastic germ cell elements. The identification of some cases where the tumour was associated with dysgerminoma and other neoplastic germ cell elements (Talerman 1980; Talerman unpublished observation; Szymanska et al 1981; Minh et al 1990; Zuntova et al 1992a) has disproved this assumption. The recognition of new cases has helped to identify the type of patient more likely to have a mixed germ cell sex-cord–stromal tumour associated with a malignant germ cell neoplasm. The presence of malignant germ cell elements was noted in nine of ten postpubertal patients whose age ranged from 16 to 46 years. In four of these patients the tumour was associated with a dysgerminoma, while in the remaining four it was associated with other malignant germ cell elements. These included yolk sac tumour, choriocarcinoma, and immature teratoma or a combination of these elements and dysgerminoma (Talerman 1980; Talerman unpublished observations; Szymanska et al 1981; Minh et al 1990). Of the four patients with mixed germ cell sex-cord–stromal tumour associated with dysgerminoma only one had metastases in the contralateral ovary, abdominal cavity, and para-aortic lymph nodes. All the other tumours were not associated with metastases. All these patients are alive and disease free for periods of one to 12 years following surgery and radiation therapy (Talerman 1980; Talerman unpublished observations; Szymanska et al 1981; Minh et al 1990). Three patients with mixed germ cell sex-cord–stromal tumour associated with yolk sac tumour, choriocarcinoma, and immature teratoma died of disseminated metastatic disease prior to the introduction of effective combination chemotherapy (Hughesdon & Kumarasamy 1970; Talerman unpublished observations). In a more recent case of a 16-year-old girl with mixed germ cell sex-cord–stromal tumour admixed with yolk sac tumour the patient was treated with surgery and combination chemotherapy (cisdiaminoplatinum, vinblastine, and bleomycin) and is well and disease free five years following diagnosis (Talerman unpublished observations). In one case the tumour was admixed with mature teratoma and the patient is well and disease free three and a half years following excision of the tumour (Zuntova et al 1992a). Two patients with metastasising mixed germ cell sex-cord–stromal tumour are well and disease free two years following excision of the tumour and combination chemotherapy (Lacson et al 1988; Arroyo et al 1998). Two patients with bilateral pure mixed germ cell sex-cord–stromal tumours are well and disease free following excision of the tumours and, in one case, radiation therapy (Jacobsen et al 1991; Talerman unpublished observations).

In the majority of the prepubertal patients with mixed germ cell sex-cord–stromal tumour, the tumour occurred in pure form, and there was no evidence of dysgerminoma or any other malignant neoplastic elements. This includes a case of an 8-year-old girl, who had a large ovarian tumour for at least three years prior to its excision (Talerman & van der Harten 1977). There was no evidence of metastases and the contralateral ovary was normal. The patient was well and free from disease 12 years following excision of the tumour.

All the patients with mixed germ cell sex-cord–stromal tumour occurring in the testes had unilateral tumours unassociated with other neoplasms or metastatic disease, and the patients are well and disease free following orchidectomy (Talerman unpublished observations).

TREATMENT

As the majority of patients with mixed germ cell sex-cord–stromal tumours are normally developed phenotypic female infants or children in the first decade, and as in this group the prognosis is favourable in spite of the fact that the tumour may be large, the therapy of choice should be conservative, consisting of excision of the tumour or unilateral salpingo-oophorectomy. The tumours in all the known cases in the prepubertal group, although of considerable size, were freely mobile and not attached to the surrounding structures. Careful examination of the abdominal cavity and biopsy of the contralateral ovary, especially if it shows any abnormality, are recommended. The patient should be fully investigated and this should include chromosomal studies. If the karyotype is normal 46,XX and the tumour is a pure mixed germ cell sex-cord–stromal tumour, further therapy is not indicated, though long-term follow-up is advisable. In postpubertal patients the tumour should be carefully examined and evaluated in view of the possibility of admixture with other neoplastic germ cell elements. If the tumour is not associated with other neoplastic components the treatment of choice is conservative. When the tumour is associated with a dysgerminoma or other malignant neoplastic germ cell elements the patient should be treated by the best therapeutic modalities currently used to treat the most malignant elements present within the tumour. Thus dysgerminoma may be treated by chemotherapy or radiation therapy in addition to surgery, while if other more malignant neoplastic germ cell elements are present, such as yolk sac tumour, they must be treated by a combination of surgery and the best chemotherapeutic regimen currently available.

REFERENCES

Allard S, Cadotte M, Boivin Y 1972 Dysgenesie gonadique pure familiare et gonadoblastome. L'Union Medicale du Canada 101: 448–452

Andersen S R, Geertinger P, Larsen H W et al 1978 Aniridia, cataract, and gonadoblastoma in a mentally retarded girl with deletion of chromosome 11: clinicopathological case report. Ophthalmologica 176: 171–177

Anderson C T, Carlson I H 1975 Elevated plasma testosterone and gonadal tumors in two 46,XY 'sisters'. Archives of Pathology 99: 360–363

Arroyo J G, Harris W, Laden S A 1998 Recurrent mixed germ cell-sex-cord stromal tumor of the ovary in an adult. International Journal of Gynecological Pathology 17: 281–283

Bardin C W, Rosen S, Le Maire W J et al 1968 In vivo and in vitro studies of androgen metabolism in a patient with pure gonadal dysgenesis and Leydig cell hyperplasia. Journal of Clinical Endocrinology and Metabolism 29: 1429–1437

Bartlett D J, Grant J K, Pugh M A, Aherne W 1968 A familial feminising syndrome: a family showing intersex characteristics with XY chromosomes in three female members. Journal of Obstetrics and Gynaecology of the British Commonwealth 75: 199–210

Ben-Romdhane K, Bessrrour A, Amor M S B, Ben-Ayed M 1988 46 XY pure gonadal dysgenesis (Swyer's syndrome) with gonadoblastoma, dysgerminoma and embryonal carcinoma. Bulletin de Cancer 75: 263–269

Bergher de Bacalao E, Dominquez I 1969 Unilateral gonadoblastoma in a pregnant woman. American Journal of Obstetrics and Gynecology 105: 1279–1281

Bhathena D, Haning R V, Shapiro S, Hafez G R 1985 Coexistence of a gonadoblastoma and mixed germ cell-sex-cord stromal tumour. Pathology Research and Practice 180: 203–206

Bjersing L, Cajander S 1977 Ultrastructure of gonadoblastoma and dysgerminoma (Seminoma) in a patient with XY gonadal dysgenesis. Cancer 40: 1127–1137

Blair J D 1978 Gonadoblastoma: cytogenetic and histopathologic study of seven cases. Laboratory Investigation 38: 334–335

Boczkowski K, Teter J, Sternadel Z 1972 Sibship occurrence of XY gonadal dysgenesis with dysgerminoma. American Journal of Obstetrics and Gynecology 113: 952–955

Bolen J W 1981 Mixed germ cell sex-cord-stromal tumour: a gonadal tumor distinct from gonadoblastoma. American Journal of Clinical Pathology 75: 563–573

Bonakdar M I, Peisner D B 1980 Gonadoblastoma with a 45, XO karyotype. Obstetrics and Gynecology 56: 748–750

Buyse M, Hartman C T, Wilson M G 1976 Gonadoblastoma and dysgerminoma with ataxia-telangiectasia. Birth Defects 12: 165–169

Cabanne F 1971 Gonadoblastoma et tumeures de l'ebauche gonadique. Annales d'Anatomie Pathologique 16: 387–404

Chapman W H, Plymyer M R, Dresner M L 1990 Gonadoblastoma in an anatomically normal man: a case report and literature review. Journal of Urology 144: 1472–1474

Cohen M, Shaw M W 1965 Two XY siblings with gonadal dysgenesis and female phenotype. New England Journal of Medicine 272: 1083–1088

Colafranceschi M, Massi D 1995 Gonadoblastoma with coexistent features of mixed germ cell-sex-cord stromal tumor: a case report. Tumori 81: 215–218

Collins D H, Symington T 1964 Sertoli cell tumour. British Journal of Urology (suppl) 36: 52–64

Cooperman L R, Hamlin J, Elmer N 1968 Gonadoblastoma: a rare ovarian tumor with characteristic roentgen appearance. Radiology 90: 322–324

Cutler B S, Forbes A P, Ingersoll F, Scully R E 1972 Endometrial carcinoma after stilbestrol therapy in gonadal dygenesis. New England Journal of Medicine 287: 628–631

Damjanov I, Klauber G 1980 Microscopic gonadoblastoma in a dysgenetic gonad of an infant: an ultrastructural study. Urology 15: 605–609

Damjanov I, Drobnjak P, Grizelj V 1975 Ultrastructure of gonadoblastoma. Archives of Pathology 99: 25–31

Dewhurst J, Ferreira H P 1982 Gonadoblastoma in a patient with gonadal dysgenesis with a Y chromosome. Obstetrics and Gynecology 59: 247–249

Diligent E 1971 Gonadoblastomes et dysgenesies pseudo-gonadoblastiques. Thesis. University of Nancy.

Dominquez C J, Greenblatt R G 1962 Dysgerminoma of the ovary in a patient with Turner's syndrome. American Journal of Obstetrics and Gynecology 83: 674–677

Dorus E, Amarose A P, Koo G C, Wachtel S S 1977 Clinical, pathologic, and genetic findings in a case of 46, XY pure gonadal dysgenesis (Swyer's syndrome) II. Presence of H-Y antigen. American Journal of Obstetrics and Gynecology 127: 829–831

Drobnjak P, Damjanov I, Grizelj V, Kalafatic Z N 1971 Precocious puberty with masculinization due to terato-chorio-gonadoblastoma. Journal of Obstetrics and Gynaecology of the British Commonwealth 78: 845–852

Dufier J L, Le-Hoang-Phug, Schmelck P et al 1981 Intercalary deletion of the short arm of chromosome 11. Aniridia, glaucoma, growth and mental retardation, sexual ambiguity, gonadoblastoma and catalase deficiency. Bulletin des Societes d'Ophthalmologie de France 81: 747–749

Erhan Y, Toprak A S, Ozdemir N, Tiras B 1992 Gonadoblastoma and fertility. Journal of Clinical Pathology 45: 828–829

Frazier S D, Bashore R A, Mosier H D 1964 Gonadoblastoma associated with pure gonadal dysgenesis in monozygous twins. Journal of Pediatrics 64: 740–745

Gallager H S, Lewis R P 1973 Sequential gonadoblastoma and choriocarcinoma. Obstetrics and Gynecology 41: 123–128

Garvin A J, Pratt-Thomas H R, Spector M, Spicer S, Williamson H O 1976 Gonadoblastoma: histologic, ultrastructural, and histochemical observations in five cases. American Journal of Obstetrics and Gynecology 125: 459–471

Goldsmith C I, Hart W R 1975 Ataxia-telangiectasia with ovarian gonadoblastoma and contralateral dysgerminoma. Cancer 36: 1838–1842

Govan A D T, Woodcock A S, Gowing N F C, Langley F A, Neville A M, Anderson M C 1977 A clinicopathological study of gonadoblastoma. British Journal of Obstetrics and Gynaecology 84: 222–228

Griffiths K, Grant J K, Browning M C K, Whyte W G, Sharp J L 1966 Steroid synthesis in vitro by tumor tissue from a dysgenetic gonad. Journal of Endocrinology 34: 155–162

Hart W R, Burkons D M 1979 Germ cell neoplasms arising in gonadoblastomas. Cancer 43: 669–678

Herva R, Saarinen I, Savikurki H, de la Chapelle A 1980 Dicentric Y chromosome arising via tandem translocation. American Journal of Medical Genetics 7: 115–122

Hoffman W H, Gala R R, Kovacs K, Subramanian M G 1987 Ectopic prolactin secretion from a gonadoblastoma. Cancer 60: 2690–2695

Hou-Jensen K, Kempson R L 1974 The ultrastructure of gonadoblastoma and dysgerminoma. Human Pathology 5: 155–162

Hughesdon P E, Kumarasamy T 1970 Mixed germ cell tumours (gonadoblastomas) in normal and dygenetic gonads: case reports and review. Virchows Archiv Abt. A. Pathologische Anatomie 349: 258–280

Ionescu B, Maximilian C 1977 Three sisters with gonadoblastoma. Journal of Medical Genetics 14: 194–199

Ishida T, Tagatz G E, Okagaki T 1976 Gonadoblastoma: ultrastructural evidence for testicular origin. Cancer 37: 1770–1781

Jacobsen G K, Braendstrup O, Talerman A 1991 Bilateral mixed germ cell sex-cord-stromal tumour in a young adult woman: case report. Acta Pathologica Microbiologica Immunologica Scandinavica (suppl) 23: 132–137

Judd H L, Scully R E, Atkins L, Neer R M, Kliman B 1970 Pure gonadal dysgenesis with progressive hirsutism. New England Journal of Medicine 282: 881–885

Khodr G S, Cadena G D, Ong T C, Siler-Khodr T M 1979 Y-autosome translocation, gonadal dysgenesis and gonadoblastoma. American Journal of Diseases of Childhood 133: 277–282

Kingsbury A C, Frost F, Cookson W O 1987 Dysgerminoma, gonadoblastoma and testicular germ cell neoplasia in phenotypically female and male siblings with 46 XY genotype. Cancer 59: 288–291

Lacson A G, Gillis D A, Shawwa A 1988 Malignant mixed germ cell-sex-cord stromal tumors of the ovary associated with isosexual precocious puberty. Cancer 61: 2122–2133

LaPolla J P, Fiorica J V, Turnquist D, Nicosia S, Wilson J, Cavanagh D 1990 Successful therapy of metastatic embryonal carcinoma coexisting with gonadoblastoma in a patient with 46, XY pure gonadal dysgenesis (Swyer's syndrome). Gynecologic Oncology 37: 417–421

Letterie G S, Page D C 1995 Dysgerminoma and gonadal dysgenesis in 46,XX female with no evidence of Y chromosomal DNA. Gynecologic Oncology 57: 423–425

Lindvall S, Wahlgren F 1940 Beitrag zur Discussion uber die Genese der sexuellen Zwischenstufen beim Menschen. Acta Pathologica et Microbiologica Scandinavica 17: 60–99

McDonough P G, Greenblatt R B, Byrd J R, Hastings E V 1967 Gonadoblastoma (gonocytoma III): report of a case. Obstetrics and Gynecology 29: 54–58

McDonough P G, Byrd J R, Tho P T, Otken L 1976a Gonadoblastoma in a true hermaphrodite with a 46, XX karyotype. Obstetrics and Gynecology 47: 355–358

McDonough P G, Ellegood J O, Byrd J R, Mahesh V B 1976b Ovarian and peripheral venous steroids in XY gonadal dysgenesis and gonadoblastoma. Obstetrics and Gynecology 47: 351–355

Mackay A M, Pettigrew W, Symington T, Neville A M 1974 Tumors of dysgenetic gonad (gonadoblastoma): ultrastructural and steroidogenic aspects. Cancer 34: 1108–1125

Magyar E, Talerman A Unpublished observations Magyar E, Talerman A, unpublished observations

Malkova J, Michalova K, Chrz R, Kobilkova J, Motlik K, Starka L 1975 Dicentric Y P chromosome in a patient with gonadal dysgenesis and gonadoblastoma. Humangenetik 27: 251–253

Mandell J, Stevens P S, Fried F A 1977 Childhood gonadoblastoma and seminoma in a dysgenetic cryptorchid gonad. Journal of Urology 117: 674–675

Manivel J C, Sibley R K, Dehner L P 1987 Complete and incomplete Drash syndrome: a clinicopathologic study of five cases of a dysontogenetic-neoplastic complex. Human Pathology 18: 80–89

Martinez-Mora J, Audi L, Toran N et al 1989 Ambiguous genitalia, gonadoblastoma, aniridia, and mental retardation with deletion of chromosome 11. Journal of Urology 142: 1298–1300

Masson P 1922 Epitheliomas Pflugeriens. In: Diagnostics de laboratoire. Les tumeurs, 1st edn. Maloine Editions, Paris, pp 477–478

Matoska J, Talerman A 1989 Mixed germ cell sex-cord-stromal tumor of the testis: a report with ultrastructural findings. Cancer 64: 2146–2153

Melicow M M, Uson A C 1959 Dysgenetic gonadomas and other gonadal neoplasms in intersexes: report of 5 cases and review of the literature. Cancer 12: 552–572

Mikulowski P, Talerman A Unpublished observations

Minh H N, Smadja A, Delteil C, Sevestre C 1990 A case of pflugeroma or mixed germ cell sex-cord-stromal tumor. Archives d'Anatomie et de Cytologie Pathologiques 38: 11–17

Moltz L, Schwartz U, Pickartz H, Hammerstein J, Wolf U 1981 XY gonadal dysgenesis: aberrant testicular differentiation in the presence of H-Y antigen. Obstetrics and Gynecology 58: 17–25

Mostofi F K, Sesterhenn I A 1998 World Health Organization International Histological Classification of Tumours. Histological Typing of Testis Tumours, 2nd edn. Springer-Verlag, Berlin

Mostofi F K, Sobin L H 1977 International histological classification of tumours, no 16. Histological typing of testicular tumours. World Health Organization, Geneva

Muhlenstedt D, Bohnet H G, Pawlowitzki I H, Schneider H P 1979 Gonadoblastoma with overgrowing dysgerminoma in Turner mosaicism (45, XO/46, XI (XQ). Archiv fur Gynakologie 227: 47–54

Muzsnai D, Feinberg M 1980 Mixed endodermal sinus tumor of the ovary in a Swyer's syndrome patient. Gynecologic Oncology 10: 230–234

Nakashima N, Nagasaka T, Fukata S et al 1989 Ovarian gonadoblastoma with dysgerminoma in a woman with two normal children. Human Pathology 20: 814–816

Nomura K, Matsui T, Aizawa S 1999 Gonadoblastoma with proliferation resembling Sertoli cell tumor. International Journal of Gynecological Pathology 18: 91–93

Obata N H, Nakashima N, Kawai M, Kikkawa F, Mamba S, Tomoda Y 1995 Gonadoblastoma with dysgerminoma in one ovary and gonadoblastoma with dysgerminoma and yolk sac tumor in the contralateral ovary in a girl with 46,XX karyotype. Gynecologic Oncology 58: 124–128

Park I J, Pyeatte J C, Jones H W Jr, Woodruff J D 1972 Gonadoblastoma in a true hermaphrodite with 46, XY genotype. Obstetrics and Gynecology 40: 466–472

Patel S K, Prentice R S A 1972 Gonadoblastoma: distinctive ovarian tumor. Archives of Pathology 94: 165–170

Phansey S A, Salterfield R, Jorgenson R J et al 1980 XY gonadal dygenesis in three siblings. American Journal of Obstetrics and Gynecology 138: 133–138

Piazza M J, Teixeira A C, Amaral M F, Netto A S, Marcallo F A 1977 Bilateral gonadoblastoma with chromosomal aberration. Obstetrics and Gynecology (suppl) 50: 355–385

Pratt-Thomas H R, Cooper J M 1976 Gonadoblastoma with tubal pregnancy. American Journal of Clinical Pathology 65: 121–125

Quigley M M, Vaughan T C, Hammond C B, Haney A F 1981 Production of testosterone and estrogen in vitro by gonadal tissue from a 46, XY true hermaphrodite with gonadal failure and gonadoblastoma. Obstetrics and Gynecology 58: 253–259

Radhakrishnan S, Sivaraman L, Natarajan P S 1978 True hermaphrodite with multiple gonadal neoplasms: report of a case with cytogenetic study. Cancer 42: 2726–2732

Rary J M, Middleton A, Mulivor R A, Green A E, Corriel L L 1979 A (Y; 17) translocation in a fibroblast culture from a female with 46 chromosomes. Cytogenetics and Cell Genetics 24: 198

Reifferscheid W 1935 Uber Sieben neue Falle von 'Disgerminoma Ovarii' (R. Meyer) davon einen mit kleine Einschlussen von folliculoiden Bildungen. Zeitschrift fur Geburtshilfe und Gynakologie 110: 273–290

Richmond H 1978 Personal communication

Rose L I, Underwood R H, Williams G H, Pincus G S 1974 Pure gonadal dysgenesis: studies of in vitro androgen metabolism. American Journal of Medicine 57: 957–961

Salet J, De Gennes J L, De Grouchy J et al 1970 A propos d'un cas de gonadoblastome 46 XX. Annales d'Endocrinologie 31: 927–938

Santesson L, Marrubini G 1957 Clinical and pathological survey of ovarian embryonal carcinomas, including so called 'Mesonephromas' (Schiller) or 'mesoblastomas' (Teilum) treated at the Radiumhemmet. Acta Obstetricia et Gynecologica Scandinavica 36: 399–410

Schapiro G 1927 Zur Frage des Hermaphroditismus. Virchows Archiv Pathologische Anatomie 266: 392–406

Schellhas H F 1974a Malignant potential of the dysgenetic gonad. Part I. Obstetrics and Gynecology 44: 298–309

Schellhas H F 1974b Malignant potential of the dysgenetic gonad. Part II. Obstetrics and Gynecology 44: 455–462

Schellhas H F, Trujillo J M, Rutledge F N, Cork A 1971 Germ cell tumor associated with XY gonadal dysgenesis. American Journal of Obstetrics and Gynecology 109: 1197–1204

Schiller W 1934 Disgerminom und Tuberculose. Archiv für Gynakologie 156: 513–533

Scully R E 1953 Gonadoblastoma: a gonadal tumor related to the dysgerminoma (seminoma) and capable of sex hormone production. Cancer 6: 455–463

Scully R E 1970a Sex-cord tumor with annular tubules: a distinctive tumor of the Peutz–Jeghers syndrome. Cancer 25: 1107–1121

Scully R E 1970b Gonadoblastoma: a review of 74 cases. Cancer 25: 1340–1356

Scully R E 1982 Personal communication

Scully R E 1999 World Health Organization International Histological Classification of Tumours. Histological Typing of Ovarian Tumours, 2nd edn. Springer-Verlag, Berlin

Seki T, Fujimoto S, Abe S et al 1981 Long arm deletion of the X chromosome, 46, X, DEL (X) (Q21) associated with gonadoblastoma. Jinrui Idengaku Zasshi 26: 307–312

Serment H, Laffargue P, Piana L, Blanc B 1970 Ovarian hormone tumors of female children. International Journal of Gynaecology and Obstetrics 8: 409–456

Serov S F, Scully R E, Sobin L H 1973 International histological classification of tumours, no 9. Histological typing of ovarian tumours. World Health Organization, Geneva

Shah K D, Kaffe S, Gilbert F, Dolgin S, Gertner M 1988 Unilateral microscopic gonadoblastoma in a prepubertal Turner mosaic with Y chromosome material identified by restriction fragment analysis. American Journal of Clinical Pathology 90: 622–627

Sternberg W H, Barclay D L, Kloepfer H W 1968 Familial XY gonadal dysgenesis. New England Journal of Medicine 278: 695–700

Stolecke H, Muller W, Hienz H A 1974 The endocrine and histological pattern of a gonadoblastoma with teratoid elements and normal female karyotype. Zeitschrift für Kinderheilkunde 117: 213–222

Szamborski J, Obrebski T, Starzynska J 1981 Germ cell tumors in monozygous twins with gonadal dysgenesis and 46, XY karyotype. Obstetrics and Gynecology 58: 120–122

Szokol M, Kondrai G, Papp Z 1977 Gonadal malignancy and 46, XY karyotype in a true hermaphrodite. Obstetrics and Gynecology 49: 358–360

Szymanska K, Starzynski S, Miechowiecka N, Piotrowski J 1981 Ovarian tumor composed of gonocytes and sex-cord cells. Ginekologia Polska 52: 651–659

Talerman A 1971 Gonadoblastoma and dysgerminoma in two siblings with dysgenetic gonads. Obstetrics and Gynecology 38: 416–426

Talerman A 1972a A mixed germ cell sex-cord-stromal tumor of the ovary in a normal female infant. Obstetrics and Gynecology 40: 473–478

Talerman A 1972b A distinctive gonadal neoplasm related to gonadoblastoma. Cancer 30: 1219–1224

Talerman A 1974 Gonadoblastoma associated with embryonal carcinoma. Obstetrics and Gynecology 43: 138–142

Talerman A 1980 The pathology of gonadal neoplasms composed of germ cells and sex-cord-stromal derivatives. Pathology Research and Practice 170: 24–38

Talerman A 1987 Ovarian Sertoli–Leydig cell tumor (androblastoma) with retiform pattern: a clinicopathologic study. Cancer 60: 3056–3064

Talerman A Unpublished observations

Talerman A, Delemarre J F M 1975 Gonadoblastoma associated with embryonal carcinoma in an anatomically normal male. Journal of Urology 113: 355–359

Talerman A, van der Harten J J A 1977 A mixed germ cell sex-cord-stromal tumor of the ovary associated with isosexual precocious puberty in a normal girl. Cancer 40: 889–894

Talerman A, Harms D Unpublished observations

Talerman A, Okagaki T Unpublished observations

Talerman A, Jarabak J, Amarose P A 1981 Gonadoblastoma and dysgerminoma in a true hermaphrodite with a 46, XX karyotype. American Journal of Obstetrics and Gynecology 140: 475–477

Talerman A, Verp M, Senekjian E, Gilewski T, Vogelzang N 1990 True hermaphrodite with normal female 46, XX karyotype, bilateral gonadoblastomas and dysgerminomas and normal pregnancy. Cancer 66: 2668–2672

Tanaka Y, Fujiwara K, Yamauchi H, Mikami Y, Kohno I 2000 Pregnancy in a woman with a Y chromosome after removal of an ovarian dysgerminoma. Gynecologic Oncology 79: 519–521

Tavassoli F A 1983 A combined germ cell gonadal stromal epithelial tumor of the ovary. American Journal of Surgical Pathology 7: 73–84

Teilum G 1946 Gonocytoma; homologous ovarian and testicular tumours; 1; With discussion of 'mesonephroma ovarii' (Schiller: American Journal of Cancer 1939). Acta Pathologica et Microbiologica Scandinavica 23: 242–251

Teter J 1960 A new concept in classification of gonadal tumours arising from germ cells (gonocytoma) and their histogenesis. Gynaecologia 150: 84–102

Teter J 1970 Prognosis, malignancy and curability of germ cell tumor occurring in dysgenetic gonads. American Journal of Obstetrics and Gynecology 115: 894–900

Teter J, Boczkowski K 1967 Occurrence of tumors in dysgenetic gonads. Cancer 20: 1301–1310

Tokuoka S, Aoki Y, Hayashi J, Yokoyama T, Ishii T 1985 A mixed germ cell-sex-cord-stromal tumor of the ovary with retiform tubular structure: a case report. International Journal of Gynecological Pathology 4: 161–170

Wachtel S S 1979 The genetics of intersexuality: clinical and theoretic perspectives. Obstetrics and Gynecology 54: 671–685

Wolf U 1979 XY gonadal dysgenesis and the H-Y antigen: report on 12 cases. Human Genetics 47: 269–277

Ying K L, Ives E J, Stephenson O D 1977 Gonadal dysgenesis with 45X/46X DIC (YP) mosaicism. Clinical Genetics 11: 402–408

Young R H, Scully R E 1983 Ovarian Sertoli–Leydig cell tumors with a retiform pattern: a problem in histopathologic diagnosis: a report of 25 cases. American Journal of Surgical Pathology 7: 755–771

Young R H, Welch W R, Dickersin G R, Scully R E 1982 Ovarian sex-cord tumor with annular tubules: review of 74 cases, including 27 with Peutz–Jeghers syndrome and four with adenoma malignum of the cervix. Cancer 50: 1384–1402

Zuntova A, Motlik K, Horejsi J, Eckschlager T 1992a Mixed germ cell sex-cord-stromal tumor with heterologous structures. International Journal of Gynecological Pathology 11: 227–233

Zuntova A, Motlik K, Horejsi J, Weinreb M 1992b Ovarialni nador se strukturami gonadoblastomu, dysgerminomu a choriokarcinomu. Ceskoslovenska patologie 28: 175–181

23

Steroid cell tumours of the ovary

R. H. Young   R. E. Scully

Introduction   845

Stromal luteoma   846

Leydig cell tumours   848

Steroid cell tumours not otherwise specified   850

Differential diagnosis of steroid cell tumours from tumours of other types   853

Extraovarian steroid cell tumours in the female genital tract   855

INTRODUCTION

These tumors, until recently most often referred to as 'lipoid' or 'lipid' cell tumours, are composed entirely, or almost entirely, of cells resembling typical steroid-hormone secreting cells, i.e. lutein cells, Leydig cells, and adrenocortical cells. The term 'steroid cell tumour' was proposed as most appropriate for them some years ago by one of us (RES) and has been accepted by the World Health Organization (Scully 1999). This designation reflects both the morphological features of the neoplastic cells and their propensity to secrete steroid hormones. Although they typically contain intracytoplasmic lipid, its absence in up to 25% of cases makes the older terms suboptimal.

Steroid cell tumours account for 0.1% of all ovarian neoplasms, and are derived in almost all the cases from ovarian stromal cells or their luteinized derivatives, or from Leydig cells of hilar or stromal origin. An origin from the cells of adrenocortical rests is unlikely, as the latter have been reported within the fetal ovary only rarely (Symmonds & Driscoll 1973) and have not been identified within the postnatal ovary. Even in cases in which elevated cortisol levels or Cushing's syndrome, or both, have been associated with a steroid cell tumour, the intraovarian location of the tumours in such cases and their similarity to other tumours in this category without such associations favour the interpretation that the adrenal-type hormones were secreted ectopically by steroid cells of gonadal rather than of adrenocortical rest origin. Adrenocortical rests have been found in the broad ligament, however, in up to 27% of hysterectomy specimens and occasionally within the ovarian hilus (Falls 1955). Therefore, it is possible that some steroid cell tumours in these locations arise in such rests.

Steroid cell tumours have been subclassified as stromal luteoma, Leydig cell tumours (hilus cell tumour and Leydig cell tumour, non-hilar type), and steroid cell tumour not otherwise specified (NOS) on the basis of knowledge, or lack of knowledge, of their cell of origin.

Table 23.1 Clinical and pathological features of steroid cell tumours. (From Paraskevas & Scully 1989.)

	Stromal luteoma	C+Hilus cell tumour	C–Hilus cell tumour	Steroid cell tumour NOS
No. of cases	25	12	9	63
Age range (mean)	28–74 (58)	32–75 (57)	34–82 (61)	2–80 (43)
Virilisation/hirsutism	12%	83%	33%	52%
Oestrogenic manifestations	60%	0	44%	8%
Duration of androgenic manifestations	1.5–5 yr	2–20 yr	1–24 yr	0.5–30 yr
No endocrine abnormality	20%	17%	23%	27%
Cushing's syndrome	0	0	0	6%
Diameter cm (mean)	1.3	2.4	1.8	8.4
Stromal hyperthecosis	92%	42%	67%	23%
Endometrial hyperplasia or carcinoma	88%	8%	33%	24%

C = Reinke crystal

The major clinical and pathological features of these neoplasms are compared in Table 23.1. Tumours composed of steroid cells arising on the background of a thecomatous or fibromatous tumour, luteinized thecomas and stromal Leydig cell tumours (Zhang et al 1982), which are closely related to steroid cell tumours, are discussed in conjunction with other sex cord–stromal tumours in Chapter 20.

STROMAL LUTEOMA

Stromal luteomas (Scully 1964; Hayes & Scully 1987a) account for approximately 25% of steroid cell tumours. They are characterised by a location within the ovarian stroma and an absence of crystals of Reinke, the distinctive inclusions of Leydig cells. These neoplasms are by definition small because large tumours in the steroid cell category are no longer identifiable as arising within the ovarian stroma and must be designated steroid cell tumour not otherwise specified in the absence of crystals of Reinke. In view of its topography the stromal luteoma must arise from luteinized stromal cells or their precursors, the spindle cells of the ovarian stroma. The presence of luteinized stromal cells (stromal hyperthecosis) elsewhere in the same or contralateral ovary in 90% of the cases supports a stromal origin (Hayes & Scully 1987a), as does the rare occurrence of a lesion intermediate between stromal hyperthecosis and the stromal luteoma: nodular hyperthecosis. The latter is characterised by multiple nests of stromal lutein cells that are large enough to be visible on very careful gross examination, but do not form a single tumour mass.

Eighty per cent of stromal luteomas occur in postmenopausal women (Table 23.1) (Hayes & Scully 1987a). The initial symptom in 60% of cases is abnormal vaginal bleeding which is probably related to associated hyperoestrinism, although whether the tumour secretes

oestrogen directly or secretes an androgen that is converted peripherally to an oestrogen is unknown. Androgenic manifestations are present in only 12% of cases. This profile of hormonal function is the opposite of that associated with other categories of steroid cell tumour, which are usually androgenic and only occasionally oestrogenic. Underlying stromal hyperthecosis may contribute to the clinical picture in some cases, particularly those in which there is a very long history of hormonal disturbance. At least one case of stromal luteoma was associated with the insulin resistance-acanthosis nigricans-hyperandrogenism syndrome (Givens et al 1974), in which the ovaries are polycystic with stromal hyperthecosis (Dunaif et al 1985). All of the reported

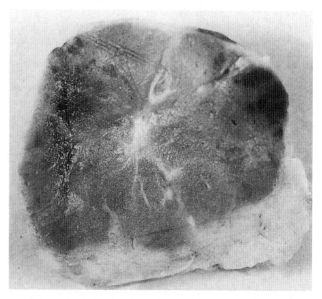

Fig. 23.1 Stromal luteoma. The tumour measured 2.0 cm in greatest dimension and was brown in the fresh state. (Courtesy of Philip B. Clement, MD)

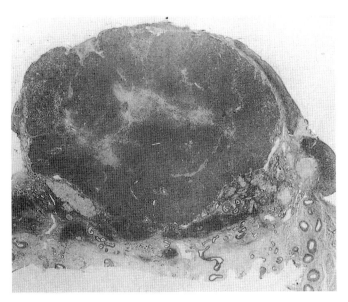

Fig. 23.2 Stromal luteoma. The tumour is confined within the ovarian stroma.

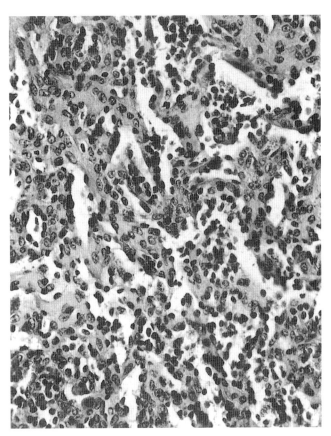

Fig. 23.4 Stromal luteoma. Degenerative changes have produced irregular spaces containing red blood cells and simulating vascular spaces. (Reproduced with permission from Young & Scully, 1987c.)

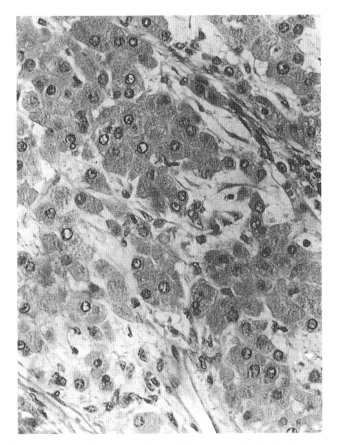

Fig. 23.3 Stromal luteoma. The cells have abundant cytoplasm that was granular and eosinophilic. The nuclei are round and regular; some of them have a prominent nucleolus.

stromal luteomas have been benign, as would be expected because of their small size and bland cytological features.

Stromal luteomas are almost always under 3 cm in diameter and, with rare exceptions, are unilateral. They are well circumscribed, solid, and usually grey–white or yellow, but one-third have red or brown areas (Fig. 23.1). Microscopic examination reveals an unencapsulated, rounded nodule (Fig. 23.2) composed of polyhedral cells arranged diffusely, in small nests (Fig. 23.3), and least commonly in cords, more or less completely surrounded by ovarian stroma. Degenerative changes occur in 20% of cases resulting in the presence of spaces that vary from elongated and slit-like (Fig. 23.4) to rounded and cystically dilated. The spaces may contain, or be separated by, lipid-laden cells and chronic inflammatory cells and may be associated with fibrosis. In some cases these spaces contain red blood cells (Fig. 23.4). The stroma is typically sparse and consists of delicate connective tissue but in about 20% of cases it is more prominent and fibrous or hyalinised. The cytoplasm of the neoplastic cells is abundant and usually eosinophilic and slightly granular but occasionally it is pale or foamy; it often contains lipochrome granules. The nuclei are typically small and round with single prominent nucleoli; mitotic figures are generally rare. As noted above, stromal hyperthecosis is also present in the stroma of one or both ovaries in almost all cases, and hilus cell hyperplasia is additionally seen in 25% of cases (Hayes & Scully 1987a).

LEYDIG CELL TUMOURS

Leydig cells cannot be distinguished from lutein or adrenocortical cells unless they contain intracytoplasmic Reinke crystals, and a steroid cell tumour cannot be demonstrated conclusively to be of Leydig cell nature unless these inclusions are found on either lightmicroscopic or electronmicroscopic examination. Since only 35–40% of Leydig cell tumours of the testis contain crystals on lightmicroscopic examination (Kim et al 1985), it is probable that a number of steroid cell tumours not otherwise specified are crystal-negative Leydig cell tumours that cannot be specifically identified as such. Some ovarian Leydig cell tumours arise in the hilus from hilar Leydig cells (hilus cells), which can be identified in over 80% of normal adult ovaries that are sampled extensively for microscopic examination (Sternberg 1949). Other Leydig cell tumours that are located within the ovarian stroma are referred to as Leydig cell tumours, non-hilar type. When a Leydig cell tumour lies deep in the medullary stroma of the ovary, abutting the hilus, it may be impossible to be certain whether it originated within the stroma or arose from hilus cells close to the medulla and expanded into the medullary stroma. In such cases, as well as in cases of large tumours that no longer have discernible topographical relations, the term Leydig cell tumour, not otherwise specified is appropriate.

Hilus cell tumours and tumours designated as probable (crystal-negative) hilus cell tumours account for approximately 20% of steroid cell tumours (Paraskevas & Scully 1989) and, like stromal luteomas, usually occur in postmenopausal patients (Table 23.1). They are only rarely palpable (Dunnihoo et al 1966; Salm 1974; Motlik et al 1988; Ichinohasama et al 1989; Paraskevas & Scully 1989). Androgenic manifestations are present in approximately 80% of cases (Paraskevas & Scully 1989), and in some patients have been present for many years prior to diagnosis; the androgenic changes are typically less abrupt in onset and milder than those associated with Sertoli–Leydig cell tumours (Young & Scully 1987a). The patients usually have a high serum level of testosterone. Virilising changes regress but may not disappear after removal of the tumour. Oestrogenic changes may also be present and can be attributed to secretion of oestrogens by the tumour, peripheral conversion of androgens produced by the tumour, associated stromal hyperthecosis or a combination of these factors. Almost all the hilus cell tumours that have been reported have been benign; only one purported malignant case in the literature merits serious consideration, but Reinke crystals were not convincingly documented in the illustrations of that tumour (Echt & Hadd 1968).

Hilus cell tumours are typically reddish-brown to yellow but may be dark brown or almost black (Fig. 23.5). They are characteristically small (mean diameter, 2.4 cm), circumscribed nodules centred in the ovarian hilus (Fig. 23.5) but may extend for varying distances into the ovarian stroma (Paraskevas & Scully 1989). Rare tumours are bilateral (Baramki et al 1983). Microscopic examination reveals an unencapsulated nodule composed of steroid cells typically growing diffusely but occasionally growing as nests (Fig. 23.6) or nodules separated by fibrous stroma. Perivascular nuclear clustering with pooling of cytoplasm or hyalinised stroma is present in half the cases (Fig. 23.6). An unusual feature in one-third of cases is fibrinoid replacement of the walls

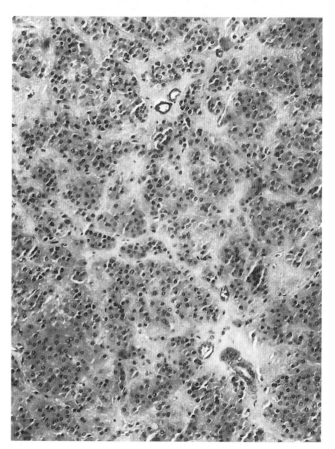

Fig. 23.6 Hilus cell tumour. The Leydig cells are aggregated and separated by acellular tissue.

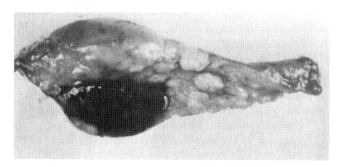

Fig. 23.5 Leydig cell tumour (hilar cell type). The small tumour is located in the hilus and was black.

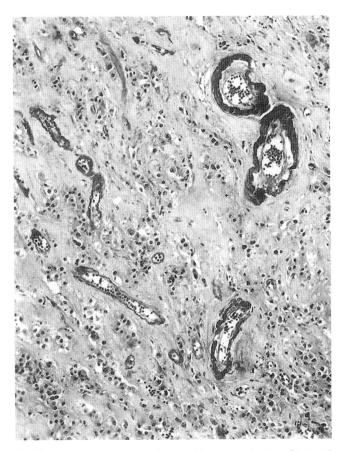

Fig. 23.7 Leydig cell tumour. Several blood vessels show fibrinoid change of their walls.

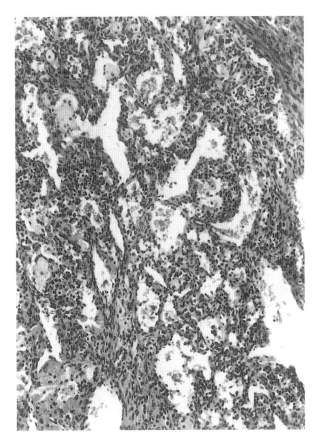

Fig. 23.8 Leydig cell tumour. Degenerative spaces, which are irregular in size and shape, are conspicuous.

of moderate-sized vessels unaccompanied by inflammatory cell infiltration (Fig. 23.7). Degenerative spaces similar to those seen in stromal luteomas may be present (Fig. 23.8). The tumour cells typically contain abundant granular eosinophilic cytoplasm (Fig. 23.9); occasional cells have spongy cytoplasm indicating the presence of lipid. Cytoplasmic lipochrome pigment, which is usually sparse, is present in most cases. The typically round nuclei are often hyperchromatic and contain single small nucleoli. There may be slight to moderate variation in nuclear size and shape; occasional bizarre nuclei (Fig. 23.10) and multinucleated cells may be present. Pseudoinclusions of cytoplasm into the nucleus may be present. Mitotic figures are usually infrequent. Elongated eosinophilic Reinke crystals of varying sizes are present in varying numbers in the cytoplasm (Fig. 23.9), or sometimes in the nucleus, but are often found only after prolonged search. They have tinctorial properties that differ slightly from those of red blood cells, which can be confused with crystals when compressed and elongated within capillaries. Special stains such as iron haematoxylin and trichrome stains may make the crystals more conspicuous. On electronmicroscopic examination crystals of Reinke typically appear as needle-shaped structures when cut longitudinally, or as hexagonal structures

when cut in cross-section (Schnoy 1982). The interior of the crystal has a cross-hatched appearance. Intracytoplasmic eosinophilic spheres, which may be crystal precursors, are also typically present, but are not specific for hilus cell tumours. Stromal hyperthecosis, hilus cell hyperplasia, or both, are associated findings in occasional cases.

A diagnosis of crystal-negative or probable hilus cell tumour is occasionally made if a crystal-free steroid cell tumour has a predominant location in the hilus and one or more of the following features: a juxtaposition to non-medullated nerve fibres similar to that of normal hilus cells, a background of hilus cell hyperplasia, nuclear clustering with intervening anuclear zones, and fibrinoid change in vessel walls (Paraskevas & Scully 1989). These tumours have clinical and laboratory features similar to those of definite hilus cell tumours.

Only four non-hilar Leydig cell tumours have been reported, and their features are similar to those of hilus cell tumours except for their location (Roth & Sternberg 1973). An ovarian stromal derivation of these tumours is supported by the finding of rare stromal Leydig cells in otherwise typical cases of stromal hyperthecosis (Sternberg & Roth 1973).

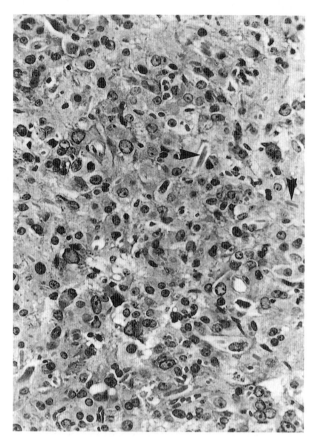

Fig. 23.9 Leydig cell tumour. The tumour cells have abundant cytoplasm that was eosinophilic and crystals of Reinke are seen in the cytoplasm of occasional cells (arrows). Many of the nuclei have a prominent nucleolus.

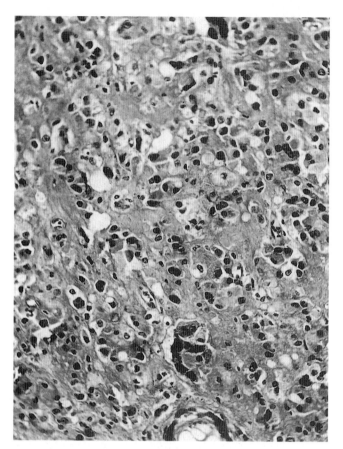

Fig. 23.10 Leydig cell tumour. The stroma between the cells is hyalinised and some of the nuclei are enlarged and bizarre.

STEROID CELL TUMOURS NOT OTHERWISE SPECIFIED

These tumours account for approximately 60% of steroid cell tumours (Taylor & Norris 1967; Hayes & Scully 1987b). They occur at any age but the patients are typically younger (mean age 43 years) than those with other types of steroid cell tumours. In contrast to stromal luteomas and Leydig cell tumours these tumours occasionally occur in children, in whom they may cause heterosexual pseudoprecocity (Case Records of the Massachusetts General Hospital 1982) and, less commonly, isosexual pseudoprecocity (Campbell & Danks 1963; Hayes & Scully 1987b). Steroid cell tumours not otherwise specified are associated with androgenic changes, which may be of many years' duration, in approximately half the cases, oestrogenic changes in approximately 10% of cases, and occasionally progestogenic changes. Four tumours have secreted cortisol and caused Cushing's syndrome (Marieb et al 1983, Young & Scully 1987a; Hayes & Scully 1987b), and occasional other tumours have been accompanied by elevated cortisol levels in the absence of clinical manifestations of the syndrome. Rare tumours have been associated with hypercalcaemia,

erythrocytosis or ascites (Hayes & Scully 1987b). One has been responsible for aldosterone production (Kulkarni et al 1990). The remaining cases have been unassociated with endocrine or paraendocrine manifestations. Hormone studies performed in patients with androgenic changes, Cushing's syndrome, or both, typically show elevated urinary levels of 17-ketosteroids and 17-hydroxycorticosteroids as well as increased serum levels of testosterone and androstenedione. The tumours that resulted in Cushing's syndrome have been associated with elevated levels of free cortisol in the blood or urine. In 20% of cases, extraovarian spread of tumour is apparent at the time of operation; three of the four patients with Cushing's syndrome had extensive intra-abdominal spread of tumour (Young & Scully 1987a). In the two largest series in the literature, the proportion of tumours that were clinically malignant was 25% (Taylor & Norris 1967) and 43% (Hayes & Scully 1987b); rare tumours recur late, in one case 19 years postoperatively. Patients with clinically malignant tumours were on average 16 years older than patients with benign tumours in one series (Hayes & Scully 1987b); no malignant steroid cell tumours have been reported in patients in the first two decades.

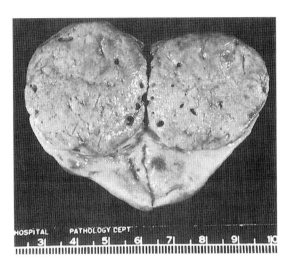

Fig. 23.11 Steroid cell tumour, not otherwise specified. The tumour, which was virilising, is predominantly solid with rare cysts and was yellow in the fresh state.

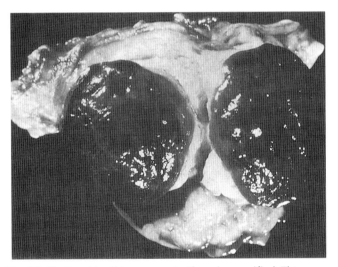

Fig. 23.12 Steroid cell tumour, not otherwise specified. The tumour, which was virilising, is well circumscribed and was dark brown in the fresh state.

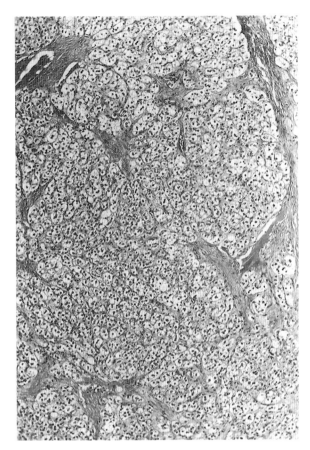

Fig. 23.13 Steroid cell tumour, not otherwise specified. Large aggregates of cells with abundant pale cytoplasm are intersected by fibrous bands.

The tumours are typically solid and well circumscribed (Figs 23.11, 23.12), are occasionally lobulated, and have ranged in diameter from 1.2 to 45 cm (mean 8.4 cm); only about 5% are bilateral. The sectioned surfaces are typically yellow (Fig. 23.11) or orange if large amounts of intracytoplasmic lipid are present, red to brown if the cells are lipid-poor, or dark brown to black (Fig. 23.12) if large quantities of intracytoplasmic lipochrome pigment are present. Necrosis, haemorrhage, and cystic degeneration are occasionally observed. On microscopic examination, the cells are typically arranged diffusely but occasionally they grow in large aggregates (Fig. 23.13), small nests, irregular clusters (Fig. 23.14), thin cords (Fig. 23.14) or columns. The stroma is inconspicuous in most cases but in approximately 15% it is more prominent. A minor fibromatous component may be seen indicating, as suggested by Hughesdon, that some steroid cell

tumours may be completely luteinized thecomas (Hughesdon 1983). Rarely the stroma is oedematous or myxoid, with tumour cells loosely dispersed within it. Exceptionally, the stroma exhibits calcification and even psammoma body formation. Necrosis and haemorrhage may be prominent, particularly in tumours that have significant cytological atypia.

The polygonal to rounded tumour cells have distinct cell borders, central nuclei, and moderate to abundant amounts of cytoplasm that varies from eosinophilic and granular (lipid-free or lipid-poor) to vacuolated and spongy (lipid-rich) (Fig. 23.15); lipid was present in 75% of the tumours stained for this material in one series (Hayes & Scully 1987b). Steroid cell tumours not otherwise specified have lipid-rich cytoplasm more often than do other subtypes of steroid cell tumour. Rarely, cells with large fat droplets have a signet-ring appearance. Intracytoplasmic lipochrome pigment has been found in 40% of the tumours. In 60% of the cases in the largest published series (Hayes & Scully 1987b), nuclear atypia was absent or slight, and mitotic activity was low (less than 2 mitotic figures/10 high-power fields). In the remaining cases, grade 1–3 nuclear atypia (Fig. 23.16), usually associated with a parallel increase in mitotic activity (up to 15 mitotic figures/10 high-power fields), was

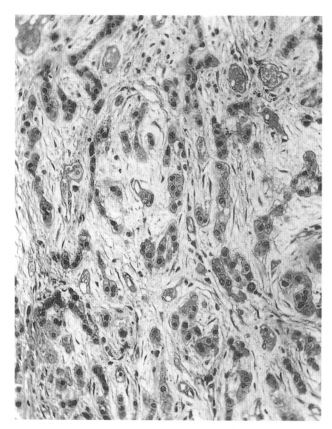

Fig. 23.14 Steroid cell tumour, not otherwise specified. The tumour cells are growing in small clusters and cords are separated by an oedematous stroma.

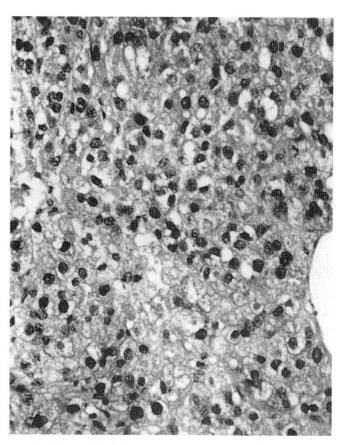

Fig. 23.16 Steroid cell tumour, not otherwise specified. The tumour cells exhibit moderate nuclear atypicality. This tumour was clinically malignant and associated with Cushing's syndrome.

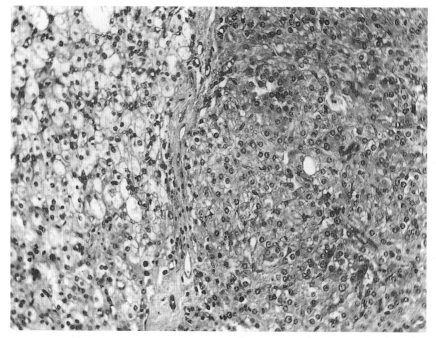

Fig. 23.15 Steroid cell tumour, not otherwise specified. This illustration shows two characteristic cell types — cells with abundant lipid-rich vacuolated cytoplasm on the left and smaller cells with abundant lipid-poor dense cytoplasm on the right.

present. Ultrastructural examination in rare cases has demonstrated abundant smooth endoplasmic reticulum in the cytoplasm of the tumour cells (Koss et al 1969).

Immunohistochemical staining is positive for α-inhibin, vimentin (75%); CAM 5.2 (46%) (globoid, paranuclear); AE1/AE3, CK1 (37%); epithelial membrane antigen (8%); and S-100 protein (7%). There is no staining for carcinoembryonic antigen, chromogranin A, alpha-fetoprotein, or HMB-45. These findings occasionally help in the differential diagnosis which is discussed below (Seidman et al 1995; Rishi et al 1997; Zheng et al 1997).

The best pathological correlates with a malignant behaviour in one series (Hayes & Scully 1987b) were: 2 or more mitotic figures per 10 high-power fields (92% malignant); necrosis (86% malignant); a diameter of 7 cm or greater (78% malignant); haemorrhage (77% malignant); and grade 2 or 3 nuclear atypia (64% malignant); occasional tumours that appear cytologically benign, however, may be clinically malignant. The metastatic tumour appears similar to the primary tumour in some cases (Fig. 23.17) but more poorly differentiated in others.

Because of the high frequency of malignancy of steroid cell tumours not otherwise specified careful staging should be performed. In a young patient with a stage Ia tumour, unilateral oophorectomy is adequate, but careful

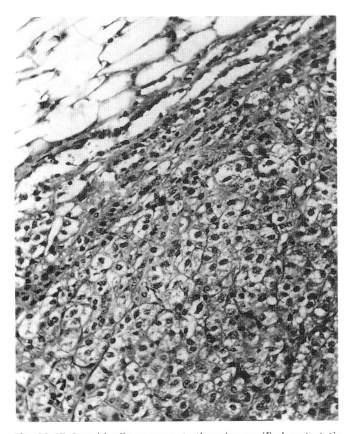

Fig. 23.17 Steroid cell tumour, not otherwise specified, metastatic in the omentum. Same case as Fig. 23.16.

follow-up is essential and should include measurement of hormone levels, particularly those demonstrated to have been elevated before removal of the primary tumour. In perimenopausal or postmenopausal patients hysterectomy with bilateral salpingo-oophorectomy is the procedure of choice. In patients with high-stage disease tumour debulking is advisable. Radiation therapy and chemotherapy have been generally disappointing, but effective in occasional cases (Hayes & Scully 1987b).

DIFFERENTIAL DIAGNOSIS OF STEROID CELL TUMOURS FROM TUMOURS OF OTHER TYPES

Stromal luteomas and Leydig cell tumours usually do not pose much diagnostic difficulty for the pathologist because of their characteristic locations, uniform appearances and composition of steroid-type cells, with those of Leydig cell tumours containing crystals of Reinke. The extensive formation of degenerative spaces in occasional tumours in these categories (Figs 23.4, 23.8), however, may cause confusion with an adenocarcinoma or, more often, a vascular tumour. Awareness of this degenerative phenomenon and its association with inflammatory cell infiltration and fibrosis, as well as the finding of typical steroid cell neoplasia elsewhere in the specimen, should facilitate the diagnosis.

Steroid cell tumours in the not otherwise specified category vary more widely in appearance than the stromal luteoma and Leydig cell tumour from both architectural and cytological viewpoints and are accordingly the cause of greater diagnostic difficulty. The tumours that may enter the differential diagnosis of these neoplasms include extensively luteinized granulosa cell tumours and thecomas, lipid-rich Sertoli cell tumours, clear cell carcinomas, including those of the oxyphil type, rare oxyphilic endometrioid carcinomas, hepatoid yolk sac tumours and hepatoid carcinomas, endocrine tumours such as oxyphilic Sertoli cell tumour, struma ovarii with a Hürthle cell content, pituitary-type tumours and paragangliomas (phaeochromocytoma), metastatic renal cell, adrenocortical, and hepatocellular carcinomas, other metastatic tumours with an oxyphilic appearance, and primary and metastatic melanomas. The presence of characteristic non-luteinized cells in both luteinized granulosa cell tumours and thecomas, as well as the typical cytological features and patterns of these neoplasms, and the finding of abundant reticulin in thecomas, are of help in the identification of these tumours. The recognition of areas with a solid tubular pattern helps distinguish a usually oestrogenic lipid-rich Sertoli cell tumour with a predominant diffuse pattern (Young & Scully 1984) from a typically androgenic steroid cell tumour. In contrast to steroid cell tumours, the clear cells of clear cell carcinomas and metastatic renal cell carcinomas (Young & Hart

1992) have glycogen-rich cytoplasm and eccentric nuclei. Also, the presence of other patterns such as tubular, glandular, and papillary, inconsistent with a steroid cell tumour, generally facilitates the differential diagnosis. Radiological studies to rule out a renal cell carcinoma may be additionally helpful. Oxyphilic clear cell carcinomas (Young & Scully 1987b) and endometrioid carcinomas, and hepatoid yolk sac tumours (Prat et al 1982), hepatoid carcinomas (Ishikura & Scully 1987) and metastatic hepatocellular carcinoma (Young et al 1992) are all characterised by neoplastic cells with abundant eosinophilic cytoplasm. The first two tumours generally exhibit epithelial patterns, may contain glandular lumens and are almost always accompanied by more easily recognised patterns. The oxyphilic clear cell carcinoma is almost always accompanied by a variable component of other distinctive cell types not seen in steroid cell tumours. The hepatoid tumours also have epithelial patterns and may contain glandular lumens and bile; they are characterised by immunohistochemical staining for alphafetoprotein. We are not aware of any case of adrenocortical carcinoma that has presented in the form of a metastatic mass involving the ovary but the possibility exists. Primary and metastatic melanomas can simulate steroid cell tumours if amelanotic, and if they are pigmented the pigment granules may be confused with the lipochrome granules of a steroid cell tumour (Young & Scully 1991). Melanomas generally have more malignant nuclear features than steroid cell tumours. Special staining, including staining for melanin and lipochrome granules and immunohistochemical staining for S-100 protein and HMB-45, may be helpful in difficult cases. Although we have seen oxyphilic

change occurring extensively in struma ovarii it has always been accompanied by areas of more typical struma. An association with other teratomatous elements, the presence of colloid and immunostaining for thyroglobulin are features that should enable one to distinguish these two tumours. A rare pituitary-type tumour containing cells with abundant eosinophilic cytoplasm that arose in the wall of a dermoid cyst secreted ACTH and caused Cushing's syndrome (Axiotis et al 1987). Such a tumour might be confused with a steroid cell tumour. In that case immunostaining for several pituitary hormones was positive. Finally, we have seen a case of apparently primary phaeochromocytoma of the ovary in which the diagnosis of a steroid cell tumour was a consideration. Phaeochromocytoma of the ovary, although rare, has been reported elsewhere as well (Fawcett & Kimbell 1971). In our case immunohistochemical staining of the tumour cells for chromogranin was helpful in establishing the diagnosis. Electronmicroscopic examination of most of the neoplasms that simulate steroid cell tumours should disclose strikingly different features. Finally, the presence or absence of endocrine manifestations and their nature may be important clinical clues to the diagnosis.

The pregnancy luteoma, a non-neoplastic lesion (Norris & Taylor 1966; Sternberg & Barclay 1966), can also closely resemble a steroid cell tumour. Pregnancy luteomas are hyperplastic nodules of lutein cells that are dependent on the hCG stimulation of pregnancy, are discovered almost exclusively during the third trimester, and involute spontaneously after the termination of pregnancy. They may measure up to 30 cm. They may also be associated with

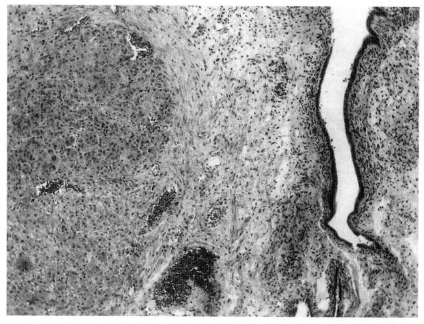

Fig. 23.18 Paratubal steroid cell nodule in a patient with Nelson's syndrome. A portion of Fallopian tube is seen at the right and a hyperplastic aggregate of steroid cells at the left.

virilisation of the mother, female infant, or both. Unlike steroid cell tumours, however, pregnancy luteomas are bilateral in about one-third of the cases and multiple in almost half of them. On microscopical examination, the cells have abundant eosinophilic cytoplasm with little or no cytoplasmic lipid, and the nuclei, although not significantly atypical, often show mitotic activity, with up to 7 mitotic figures/10 high-power fields (mean 2–3). In contrast, a steroid cell tumour with minimal cytological atypicality that resembles a pregnancy luteoma usually contains only rare mitotic figures. It may be impossible to distinguish a lipid-poor or lipid-free steroid cell tumour not otherwise specified in a pregnant patient from a solitary pregnancy luteoma, but if the lesion is encountered during the third trimester it is usually presumed to be the latter unless clearly proven otherwise.

EXTRAOVARIAN STEROID CELL TUMOURS IN THE FEMALE GENITAL TRACT

Exceptionally, steroid cell tumours originate in the broad ligament (Roth et al 1996; Sasano et al 1997). Adrenocortical rests in the broad ligament (Falls 1955) could be the source of these rare tumours. Adrenocortical rests may also undergo hyperplasia in the congenital adrenogenital syndrome simulating a small steroid cell tumour. Multiple hyperplastic nodules in the vicinity of the ovaries, presumably of adrenal rest origin, can develop in Nelson's syndrome (development of a pituitary tumour after bilateral adrenalectomy for ACTH-dependent adrenal hyperplasia), sometimes associated with virilisation (Baranetsky et al 1979; Wild et al 1988), and resemble small steroid cell tumours on microscopic examination (Fig. 23.18). The clinical background and location of these lesions enable one to differentiate them from ovarian steroid cell tumours.

The possibility that steroid cell tumours of the broad ligament may arise from an accessory ovary is supported by a recently documented case (Roth et al 1996). In that case, a 29-year-old woman who presented with evidence of virilisation was found to have a 21 cm broad ligament tumour and a separate normal ovary on the same side. Microscopic examination disclosed a Graafian follicle and a primordial follicle at the periphery of the steroid cell tumour providing evidence for the presence of an accessory ovary. The tumour mass was connected to the surface of the eutopic ovary on that side by thin membranous tissue.

REFERENCES

Axiotis C A, Lippes H A, Merino M J, deLanerolle N C, Stewart A F, Kinder B 1987 Corticotroph cell pituitary adenoma within an ovarian teratoma: a new cause of Cushing's syndrome. American Journal of Surgical Pathology 11: 218–224

Baramki T A, Leddy A L, Woodruff J D 1983 Bilateral hilus cell tumors of the ovary. Obstetrics and Gynecology 62: 128–131

Baranetsky N G, Zipser R D, Goebelsmann U et al 1979 Adrenocorticotropin-dependent virilizing paraovarian tumors in Nelson's syndrome. Journal of Clinical Endocrinology and Metabolism 49: 381–386

Campbell P E, Danks D M 1963 Pseudoprecocity in an infant due to a luteoma of the ovary. Archives of Diseases in Childhood 38: 519–523

Case Records of the Massachusetts General Hospital Case 22, 1982 New England Journal of Medicine 306: 1348–1352

Dunaif A, Hoffman A R, Scully R E et al 1985 Clinical, biochemical, and ovarian morphologic features in women with acanthosis nigricans and masculinization. Obstetrics and Gynecology 66: 545–552

Dunnihoo D R, Grieme D L, Woolf R B 1966 Hilar cell tumors of the ovary: report of 2 new cases and a review of the world literature. Obstetrics and Gynecology 27: 703–713

Echt C R, Hadd H E 1968 Androgen excretion patterns in a patient with a metastatic hilus cell tumor of the ovary. American Journal of Obstetrics and Gynecology 100: 1055–1061

Falls J L 1955 Accessory adrenal cortex in the broad ligament: incidence and functional significance. Cancer 8: 143–150

Fawcett F J, Kimbell N K B 1971 Phaeochromocytoma of the ovary. Journal of Obstetrics and Gynaecology of the British Commonwealth 78: 458–459

Givens J R, Kerber I J, Wiser W L, Andersen R N, Coleman S A, Fish S A 1974 Remission of acanthosis nigricans associated with polycystic ovarian disease and a stromal luteoma. Journal of Clinical Endocrinology and Metabolism 38: 347–355

Hayes M C, Scully R E 1987a Stromal luteoma of the ovary: a clinicopathological analysis of 25 cases. International Journal of Gynecological Pathology 6: 313–321

Hayes M C, Scully R E 1987b Ovarian steroid cell tumour (not otherwise specified): a clinicopathological analysis of 63 cases. American Journal of Surgical Pathology 11: 835–845

Hughesdon P E 1983 Lipid cell thecomas of the ovary. Histopathology 7: 681–692

Ichinohasama R, Teshima S, Kishi K et al 1989 Leydig cell tumor of the ovary associated with endometrial carcinoma and containing 17 beta-hydroxysteroid dehydrogenase. International Journal of Gynecological Pathology 8: 64–71

Ishikura H, Scully R E 1987 Hepatoid carcinoma of the ovary: a newly described tumor. Cancer 60: 2775–2784

Kim I, Young R H, Scully R E 1985 Leydig cell tumors of the testis: a clinicopathological analysis of 40 cases and review of the literature. American Journal of Surgical Pathology 9: 177–192

Koss L G, Rothschild E O, Fleisher M, Francis J E Jr 1969 Masculinizing tumor of the ovary, apparently with adrenocortical activity. Cancer 23: 1245–1258

Kulkarni J N, Mistry R C, Kamat M R, Chinoy R, Lotlikar R G 1990 Case report of autonomous aldosterone-secreting ovarian tumor. Gynecologic Oncology 37: 284–289

Marieb H J, Spangler S, Kashgarian M, Heiman A, Schwartz M L, Schwartz P E 1983 Cushing's syndrome secondary to ectopic cortisol production by an ovarian carcinoma. Journal of Clinical Endocrinology and Metabolism 57: 737–740

Motlik K, Stejskalova A, Stejskal J, Kobilkova J, Starka L 1988 Hilus cell tumours of the ovary. Ceskoslovenska Patologie 24: 144–160

Norris H J, Taylor H B 1966 Nodular theca-lutein hyperplasia of pregnancy (so-called 'pregnancy luteoma'): a clinical and pathological study of 15 cases. American Journal of Clinical Pathology 47: 557–566

Paraskevas M, Scully R E 1989 Hilus cell tumor of the ovary: a clinicopathological analysis of 12 Reinke-crystal-positive and 9 crystal-negative cases. International Journal of Gynecological Pathology 8: 299–310

Prat J, Bhan A K, Dickersin G R, Robboy S J, Scully R E 1982 Hepatoid yolk sac tumor of the ovary (endodermal sinus tumor with hepatoid differentiation): a light microscopic, ultrastructural and immunohistochemical study of seven cases. Cancer 50: 2355–2368

Rishi M, Howard L N, Bratthauer G L, Tavassoli F A 1997 Use of monoclonal antibody against human inhibin as a marker for sex cord-stromal tumors of the ovary. American Journal of Surgical Pathology 21: 583–589

Roth L M, Sternberg W H 1973 Ovarian stromal tumors containing Leydig cells. II. Pure Leydig cell tumour, non-hilar type. Cancer 32: 952–960

Roth L M, Davis M M, Sutton G P 1996 Steroid cell tumor of the broad ligament arising in an accessory ovary. Archives of Pathology and Laboratory Medicine 120: 405–409

Salm R 1974 Ovarian hilus-cell tumours: their varying presentations. Journal of Pathology 13: 117–127

Sasano H, Sato S, Yajima A, Akama J, Nagura H 1997 Adrenal rest tumor of the broad ligament: Case report with immunohistochemical study of steroidogenic enzymes. Pathology International 47: 493–496

Scully R E 1964 Stromal luteoma of the ovary: a distinctive type of lipoid cell tumor. Cancer 17: 769–778

Scully R E 1999 Histological typing of ovarian tumors. World Health Organization International Histological Classification of Tumours. Springer-Verlag, Berlin

Schnoy N 1982 Ultrastructure of a virilizing ovarian Leydig-cell tumor. Hilar cell tumor. Virchows Archiv A Pathological Anatomy and Histology 397: 17–27

Seidman J D, Abbondanzo S L, Bratthauer G L 1995 Lipid cell (steroid cell) tumor of the ovary. Immunophenotype with analysis of potential pitfalls due to endogenous biotin-like activity. International Journal of Gynecological Pathology 14: 331–338

Sternberg W H 1949 The morphology, androgenic function, hyperplasia and tumors of the human ovarian hilus cells. American Journal of Pathology 25: 493–521

Sternberg W H, Barclay D L 1966 Luteoma of pregnancy. American Journal of Obstetrics and Gynecology 95: 165–184

Sternberg W H, Roth L M 1973 Ovarian stromal tumors containing Leydig cells. I. Stromal-Leydig cell tumor and non-neoplastic transformation of ovarian stroma to Leydig cells. Cancer 12: 940–951

Symmonds D A, Driscoll S G 1973 An adrenal cortical rest within the fetal ovary: report of a case. American Journal of Clinical Pathology 60: 562–564

Taylor H B, Norris H J 1967 Lipid cell tumors of the ovary. Cancer 20: 1953–1962

Wild R A, Albert R D, Zaino R J, Abrams C S 1988 Virilizing paraovarian tumors: a consequence of Nelson's syndrome? Obstetrics and Gynecology 71: 1053–1056

Young R H, Hart W R 1992 Renal cell carcinoma metastatic to the ovary: a report of three cases emphasizing possible confusion with ovarian clear cell adenocarcinoma. International Journal of Gynecological Pathology 11: 96–104

Young R H, Scully R E 1984 Ovarian Sertoli cell tumors: a report of ten cases. International Journal of Gynecological Pathology 2: 349–363

Young R H, Scully R E 1987a Ovarian steroid cell tumors associated with Cushing's syndrome: a report of three cases. International Journal of Gynecological Pathology 6: 40–48

Young R H, Scully R E 1987b Oxyphilic clear cell carcinoma of the ovary: a report of nine cases. American Journal of Surgical Pathology 11: 661–667

Young R H, Scully R E 1987c Sex cord-stromal tumors, steroid cell tumors and other ovarian tumors with endocrine, paraendocrine and paraneoplastic manifestations. In: Kurman R J (ed) Blaustein's Pathology of the female genital tract. Springer-Verlag, New York, pp 607–658

Young R H, Scully R E 1991 Malignant melanoma metastatic to the ovary: a clinicopathologic analysis of 20 cases. American Journal of Surgical Pathology 15: 849–860

Young R H, Gersell D J, Clement P B, Scully R E 1992 Hepatocellular carcinoma metastatic to the ovary: a report of three cases discovered during life with discussion of the differential diagnosis of hepatoid tumors of the ovary. Human Pathology 23: 574–580

Zhang J, Young R H, Arseneau J, Scully R E 1982 Ovarian stromal tumors containing lutein or Leydig cells (luteinized thecomas and stromal Leydig cell tumors): a clinicopathological analysis of fifty cases. International Journal of Gynecological Pathology 1: 275–285

Zheng W, Sung C J, Hanna I et al 1997 α and β subunits of inhibin/activin as sex cord-stromal differential markers. International Journal of Gynecological Pathology 16: 263–271

24

Mesenchymal tumours of the ovary

J. Prat   H. Fox

Introduction   857

Tumours of fibrous tissue   858
Fibroma   858
Cellular fibroma   860
Fibrosarcoma   861

Tumours of smooth muscle   862
Leiomyoma   862
Leiomyosarcoma   862

Tumours of striated muscle   864
Rhabdomyoma   854
Rhabdomyosarcoma   864

Tumours of cartilage   866
Chondroma   866
Chondrosarcoma   866

Tumours of bone   866
Osteoma   866
Giant cell tumour (osteoclastoma)   866
Osteogenic sarcoma   866

Tumours of neural origin   867
Neurofibroma   867
Schwannoma   867
Ganglioneuroma   867
Malignant schwannoma   867
Phaeochromocytoma   867

Myxoma   867

Tumours of fat   868

Tumours of vascular origin   868
Haemangioma   868
Haemangiopericytoma   869
Angiosarcoma   869

Tumours of lymphatic vessels   870
Lymphangioma   870
Lymphangiosarcoma   870

Endometrioid stromal sarcoma   870

Undifferentiated 'stromal' sarcoma   872

Combined sarcoma and epithelial tumour   873

Adenomatoid tumours   873

INTRODUCTION

Many of the neoplasms considered in this chapter arise from those tissue elements in the ovary, such as blood vessels, nerves or lymphatics, which are not committed to the specific gonadal function of the organ. The situation is, however, complicated by the fact that such tumours, particularly those which are malignant, may have other quite different origins.

1. The tumour may arise in, and from, pre-existing foci of ovarian endometriosis: as the neoplasm grows it may destroy all evidence of the endometriotic focus from which it evolved.
2. A tissue which was originally a component of a mixed Müllerian tumour may subsequently become totally dominant and thus appear as a monomorphic tumour.
3. Mesenchymal neoplasms may arise in ovarian teratomas, either because of malignant change in a mature teratoma or as a component of an immature teratoma: in either case the mesenchymal tumour may overgrow and obliterate all other teratomatous elements.
4. A mesenchymal neoplasm may develop from heterologous elements in a Sertoli–Leydig cell tumour: again, such a neoplasm may totally obscure the sex-cord components and thus masquerade as a pure mesenchymal neoplasm.
5. Mesenchymal tumours may arise in the wall of a cystic epithelial neoplasm: the theoretical possibility exists once again of progressive mesenchymal dominance.

It is thus apparent that in many examples of pure mesenchymal tumours of the ovary it is virtually impossible to reach any decision as to their original histogenesis. Consider, for example, an oncological curiosity such as a pure ovarian rhabdomyosarcoma: this could have arisen in any of the above described fashions, for whilst the most obvious tumour to develop from endometriosis is the endometrioid stromal sarcoma there is no theoretical reason why a rhabdomyosarcoma should not have a similar origin as a form of pure heterologous sarcoma. Conversely, if endometrioid adenocarcinoma can arise either from endometriotic foci or from the surface epithelium of the ovary then it is at least possible that endometrioid sarcomas, including by extrapolation pure heterologous sarcomas such as a rhabdomyosarcoma, could also originate from this site. Clearly a rhabdomyosarcoma could have developed from a mixed Müllerian neoplasm whilst a teratomatous origin for a rhabdomyosarcoma is undoubtedly possible as is an evolution from a Sertoli–Leydig cell tumour. Whether a neoplasm such as a rhabdomyosarcoma can originate directly from ovarian stroma is a debatable point but such a possibility can certainly not be excluded.

Faced with this histogenetic maze the most that a pathologist can do is to sample all apparently pure mesenchymal tumours very extensively so as to be able to exclude with some degree of confidence other tissue components. The application of common sense will, of course, suggest that mesenchymal tumours occurring in elderly women are unlikely to have originated either from ovarian endometriosis or from immature teratomas and that a similar neoplasm in a prepubertal girl may well be of teratomatous origin. Beyond that, however, the pathologist usually cannot go.

In this chapter the pure mesenchymal tumours of the ovary will be discussed, as will sarcomas associated with epithelial neoplasms; sarcomas arising in teratomas (see Chapter 21) and mixed Müllerian tumours (see Chapter 14) will not be considered. Endometrioid stromal sarcomas are briefly discussed in Chapter 14 and could be considered further under the heading of Müllerian tumours or that of endometrioid neoplasms; they will be reviewed here in greater detail, partly because of their importance in the differential diagnosis of malignant mesenchymal tumours of the ovary and partly because, in some cases at least, they may arise from ovarian stromal cells.

TUMOURS OF FIBROUS TISSUE

FIBROMA

The origin of fibromas is far from clear. It is possible that they arise from non-specialised ovarian tissues, such as the connective tissue of the capsule or blood vessels, in which case they merit their place in this chapter. On the other hand, there is a continuous histological spectrum between thecomas and fibromas (Scully et al 1998) and it is quite legitimate to consider that many, or even most, fibromas are 'burnt out' thecomas; electronoptical studies have also supported the concept of the fibroma developing from specialised ovarian stroma (Amin et al 1971) and hence it would be more logical to consider these neoplasms as sex cord–stromal tumours. The consideration of fibromas in this chapter is undertaken largely because

they fit more tidily into a discussion of mesenchymal neoplasms and should not be taken as implying that they should be excluded from the sex cord–stromal category.

In most series of ovarian neoplasms fibromas account for about 4% of the total: an incidence as high as 10% has been quoted (Duchini & Menegaldo 1967) and this indicates that the reported frequency with which fibromas occur is in part dependent upon the criteria used for differentiating them from thecomas and on how 'fibrothecomas' are categorized. Between 4 and 8% of fibromas are bilateral (Dockerty & Masson 1944; Driscoll 1964) and most appear as moderately well defined, but not encapsulated, intraovarian nodules of variable size with an average diameter of 6 cm; a proportion totally replace the ovary and a few occur as nodules or plaques on the ovarian surface. They tend to have a smooth, lobulated or nodular outer surface and on section are usually formed of uniformly white or greyish-white solid tissue (Fig. 24.1);

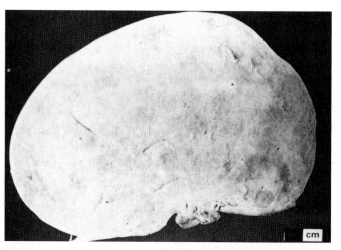

Fig. 24.1 A typical fibroma.

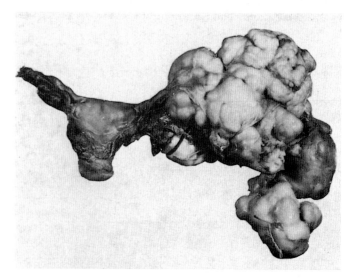

Fig. 24.2 Multiple ovarian fibromas of the type characteristically seen in women with the basal cell naevus syndrome.

sometimes, however, the cut surface has a whorled or lob-ulated appearance. Some degree of cystic change is seen in about 20% of these neoplasms whilst calcification is not uncommon and is sometimes massive (Sengupta et al 1979); rarely a fibroma may show ossification.

Ovarian fibromas occur in a high proportion of young women with the basal cell naevus syndrome (Glenden-ning et al 1963; Gorlin & Sedano 1971; Burkett & Rauh 1976; Raggio et al 1983) and in these patients the fibromas are characteristically bilateral, multiple and calcified (Fig. 24.2).

Histologically (Fig. 24.3), fibromas are formed of interlacing bundles of cells which often show a 'feather-tail' pattern: they are small, thin and spindle-shaped with narrow ovoid nuclei running parallel to their long axis. Nuclear palisading is sometimes seen whilst occasionally a storiform pattern, similar to that encountered in fibrous histiocytomas, is present. The cells are regular and mitotic figures are absent. The cytoplasm of the tumour cells often contains a small amount of lipid and occasionally there are eosinophilic cytoplasmic hyaline droplets. Sharply delineated hyaline plaques are sometimes present whilst a more diffuse hyalinisation is not uncommon: many fibromas show a variable degree of intercellular oedema or myxoid change. Occasional fibromas contain a few scattered foci of sex-cord cells (Fig. 24.4) which may be represented by nests of undifferentiated cells, by small aggregates of granulosa cells or by tubules lined by Sertoli cells (Young & Scully 1983). The sex-cord component usually exhibits a stronger immunoreaction for alpha-inhibin than does that of the surrounding fibromatous element.

Fibromas occur in women of all ages though they are most commonly found in those aged between 50 and 60 years; examples have been recorded of their occurrence in premenarchal girls (Charache 1959; Martins & Klinger

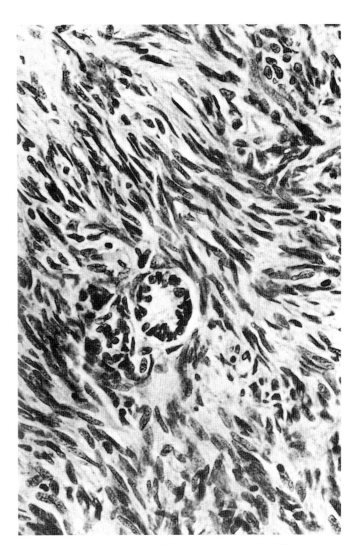

Fig. 24.4 A sex-cord epithelial element in an ovarian fibroma. Tubules lined by sertoliform cells were seen in only one of 14 blocks from this tumour.

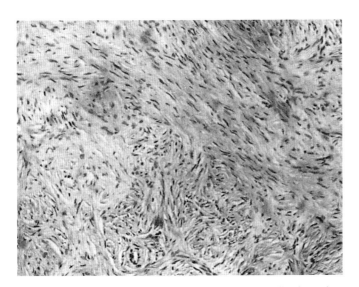

Fig. 24.3 Ovarian fibroma formed of elongated spindle-shaped cells.

1964; Bower & Erikson 1967), but it should be noted that all these cases were described before the association of these tumours with the basal cell naevus syndrome became well known. Small tumours, i.e. those measuring less than 4 cm in diameter, appear to be invariably asymptomatic, whilst many larger fibromas have also been incidental findings: in various series the incidence of asymptomatic tumours has ranged from 30–54% (Dockerty & Masson 1944; Biggart & Macafee 1955; Driscoll 1964).

When symptoms do occur the most common are abdominal pain, abdominal enlargement or urinary dis-turbances; in about 5% of cases there is an acute onset of abdominal pain because of torsion of the neoplasm. It has been claimed by some that these tumours are associated with a high incidence of menstrual abnormalities, postmenopausal bleeding and infertility (Duchini & Menegaldo 1967; Grosieux 1970); others have suggested that although such symptoms are atypical they do occur in association with, and are apparently caused by, isolated examples of fibroma (Destro 1958; Mazella 1963). In most series of fibromas, however, such symptoms have either been completely absent or have been clearly due to some other factor.

Ascites is a relatively common accompaniment of fibromas, being found in between 15 and 30% of cases: it appears only to complicate those with a diameter greater than 6 cm. A typical Meigs' syndrome, though classically associated with this neoplasm, is far from common and is found in only between 1 and 2% of cases (Dockerty & Masson 1944; Kleitsman 1949b; Biggart & Macafee 1955; Driscoll 1964); nevertheless, when a fibroma is associated with Meigs' syndrome and elevated CA-125 levels the clinical picture is very similar to that of an ovarian carcinoma and it may be only after laparotomy and surgical staging that the final diagnosis is achieved (Siddiqui & Toub 1995; Spinelli et al 1999). Very exceptionally, fluid accumulates elsewhere to produce oedema of the legs, anterior abdominal wall or vulva.

Fibromas are benign and oophorectomy will result in rapid resolution of any ascites or hydrothorax that may be present. One patient has been described in whom recurrent attacks of hypoglycaemia were permanently cured by removal of an ovarian fibroma (Michael 1966). Although fully benign, these tumours may, in exceptional cases, seed implants on to the peritoneum (Lyday 1952): if both these and the ovarian neoplasm appear histologically benign the prognosis is excellent and the peritoneal nodules should not be taken as evidence of malignancy.

CELLULAR FIBROMA

Prat & Scully (1981) categorised as cellular fibromas those fibromatous tumours of the ovary which are unduly cellular but contain fewer than 4 mitotic figures per 10 high-power fields. These authors described 11 such neoplasms which ranged in size from 4.5–21.5 cm in diame-

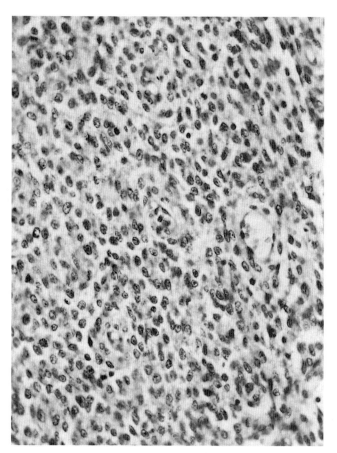

Fig. 24.6 A cellular fibroma. The neoplasm is hypercellular and there is a moderate degree of pleomorphism. There were fewer than 4 mitotic figures per 10 high-power fields.

ter, with an average diameter of 12 cm. The outer surface of the tumour is generally smooth or bosselated and on section most of the neoplasms are solid throughout (Fig. 24.5), a minority being partly cystic and very occasional examples being predominantly cystic. On section, these tumours have a greyish-white whorled appearance with multiple foci of haemorrhage and necrosis; the cystic areas in a minority of these tumours contain clear watery fluid.

Histologically (Fig. 24.6), cellular fibromas are composed largely of densely cellular tissue interspersed with a few areas of hypocellular fibrous tissue. The cells are spindle-shaped and arranged in intersecting bundles or in a storiform pattern. The cells are small and thin with ill-defined cytoplasmic borders and round to oval hyperchromatic nuclei; in some tumours rounded cells with abundant cytoplasm are present. The nuclei are slightly or moderately atypical, and between 1 and 3 mitotic figures per 10 high-power fields are present. A gain of trisomy 12 cells has been demonstrated by fluorescence in situ hybridisation in eight cases of cellular fibroma (Tsuji et al 1998).

Patients with cellular fibromas have ranged in age from 14–82 years with an average of 49 years. The symptoms are generally those of a pelvic mass, and follow-up of Prat

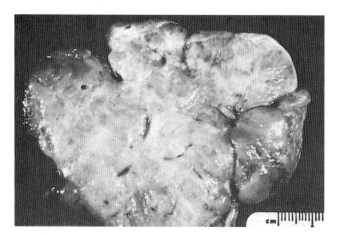

Fig. 24.5 A cellular fibroma of the ovary. This is predominantly solid but a few small cystic areas are present.

& Scully's (1981) 11 cases showed no evidence of recurrence in nine patients: one patient died seven years postoperatively of pneumonia and at autopsy recurrent tumour was found adherent to the small bowel and sigmoid colon with several smaller nodules in the small bowel mesentery; a further patient died of massive pelvic recurrence 33 months after incomplete removal of the tumour which was adherent to the pelvic wall and omentum. Because of the typically benign course and infrequent bilaterality of cellular fibromas they can justifiably be treated by unilateral salpingo-oophorectomy in a young woman desirous of retaining her fertility. If the tumour is adherent it should be removed as completely as is technically feasible. Patients with ruptured tumours should be followed carefully because of the possibility of intra-abdominal recurrence.

FIBROSARCOMA

There had been sporadic reports in the literature of ovarian fibrosarcomas (Variati & Donatelli 1966; Nieminen et al 1969; Azoury & Woodruff 1971; Toth et al 1971) but it was Prat & Scully (1981) who rendered a definitive account of these neoplasms. They described six ovarian fibrosarcomas which ranged in size from 9–35 cm in diameter with a mean diameter of 17.5 cm. The tumours were soft and lobulated and completely replaced the ovary: on section they varied from greyish-white to tan and showed numerous areas of haemorrhage and necrosis.

Histologically, the neoplasms were densely cellular, the spindle-shaped cells being arranged in a herring-bone or storiform pattern: the tumour cells had indistinct borders, eosinophilic cytoplasm, and hyperchromatic nuclei with prominent nucleoli. There was a moderate to marked degree of pleomorphism and the number of mitotic figures ranged from 4–25 per 10 high-power fields (Fig. 24.7).

The MIB-1 labelling index and the proliferative index (percentage of cells in S + G2 + M phases) have been found to be higher in fibrosarcomas than in cellular fibromas of the ovary (Tsuji et al 1997). It has been claimed that the presence of trisomy 8 cells is an effective marker of fibrosarcomas (Tsuji et al 1997) but the specificity of this finding has been questioned (Dal Cin et al 1998). The formal mitotic count is therefore still the best indicator of malignant behaviour in this group of tumours though it should be noted that it is not an absolute indicator because a tumour with a low mitotic count can occasionally metastasise (McCluggage et al 1998).

The patients with ovarian fibrosarcoma in the series reported by Prat & Scully (1981) ranged in age from 42–73 years with an average of 58 years; the principal presenting complaints were of pelvic pain, abdominal enlargement or awareness of an abdominal mass. Of the six patients, five died within four years of the initial diag-

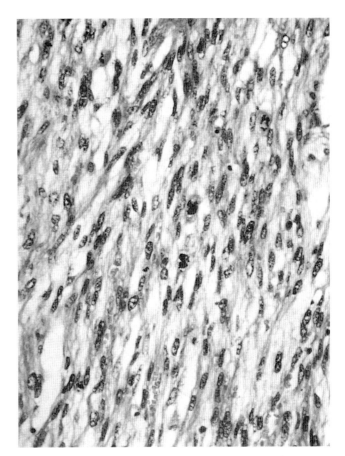

Fig. 24.7 An ovarian fibrosarcoma. There is considerable pleomorphism and many mitotic figures are present.

nosis: in four of these cases death was due to the tumour whilst the fifth patient died of cardiac disease but had a massive pelvic recurrence. The sixth patient was lost to follow-up at 15 months but had extensive metastases at that time. The ovarian fibrosarcoma is thus seen to be a lethal neoplasm.

In a recent case of ovarian fibrosarcoma with thecomatous features that presented with metastatic disease in the small intestine and peritoneum, positive immunostaining with anti-inhibin was of value in confirming the sex cord–stromal nature of the tumour and in excluding other lesions (McCluggage et al 1998).

There is a general impression that ovarian fibrosarcomas develop as a result of malignant change within a fibroma rather than occurring as a malignant tumour de novo and strength is lent to this view by a report of a fibrosarcoma which developed in an 8-year-old girl with multiple ovarian fibromas as a component of the naevoid basal cell carcinoma syndrome (Kraemer et al 1984); this neoplasm had a high mitotic count and a metastasis developed two years later, after removal of which, however, the patient was alive and well four years later. An ovarian fibrosarcoma has also been reported in a patient with Maffucci's syndrome (Christman & Ballon 1990).

TUMOURS OF SMOOTH MUSCLE

LEIOMYOMA

Ovarian leiomyomas appear to be rare, for fewer than 60 examples have been reported (Kleitsman 1949a; Wellman 1961; Fallahzadeh et al 1972; Thay et al 1973; Kalra et al 1981; Tsalacopoulos & Tiltman 1981; Matamala et al 1988; Vierhout et al 1990; Prayson & Hart 1992; Randrianjafisamindrakotroka et al 1994; Morgante et al 1995; Sari et al 1995; Kobayashi et al 1998; Sato & Tanaka 1998; Kohno et al 1999; Doss et al 1999b): it is highly probable, however, that most cases go unrecorded. The tumours are usually unilateral, only very occasional bilateral cases having been reported (Kandalaft & Esteban 1992; Danihel et al 1995), and usually range in size from 1–24 cm in diameter; one exceptional ovarian leiomyoma which weighed over 11 kilogrammes has been described (Khaffaf et al 1996). It has been noted that small leiomyomas appear to originate in the hilum and that the attenuated cortex is stretched over their surface but in the larger neoplasms this topographical relationship is not discernible. Leiomyomas, though lacking a true capsule, tend to be sharply delineated: they are solid and firm and on section have a white, grey or brown cut surface which often shows central bulging.

They have a whorled or multinodular structure and although commonly solid throughout may show areas of myxoid or pseudocystic change, the latter sometimes being sufficiently marked for the tumour to resemble a cystadenoma. Foci of haemorrhage, necrosis or calcification are common.

Histologically, these neoplasms show the usual features of a leiomyoma with interlacing bundles of smooth muscle fibres which are often admixed with collagenous septa. The muscle cells have elongated blunt-ended or cigar-shaped nuclei and although occasional multinucleated giant cells may be present there is otherwise no pleomorphism, and as a rule mitotic figures are either absent or extremely sparse. Two examples of 'mitotically active', but otherwise unremarkable, ovarian leiomyomas have, however, been noted (Prayson & Hart 1992). As in uterine leiomyomas, the appearances may be altered by degenerative changes such as cystic change, hyalinisation or oedema. A lipoleiomyomatous pattern has been occasionally observed (Dodd et al 1989; Mira 1991).

The histogenesis of ovarian leiomyomas is uncertain but they could arise from the smooth muscle fibres of the ovarian ligaments which run into the gonad, from the musculature of the ovarian blood vessels or from the smooth muscle fibres which have been demonstrated, by electronmicroscopy (Okamura et al 1972) and immunohistochemistry (Doss et al 1999a) in the corpus luteum and in the cortical stroma.

Ovarian leiomyomas have been encountered in women aged between 20 and 65 years, with only about one-sixth of cases occurring in those who have passed their menopause. Most leiomyomas have been asymptomatic incidental findings at autopsy or surgery but about a third have produced non-specific pelvic mass symptoms such as abdominal pain or swelling. Rarely, torsion of the tumour leads to presentation with acute abdominal pain. Ascites has developed in a few patients but hydrothorax has not been noted. These tumours do not appear to cause menstrual disturbances or abnormal vaginal bleeding, for although such symptoms have often been a feature of the clinical picture of women with ovarian leiomyomas these have invariably been explicable by the presence of coexistent uterine leiomyomas, a common finding in these patients. Ovarian leiomyomas have been noted in pregnant women (Moore 1945) but no information is available about the effects of the gravid state on the growth and vascularity of these neoplasms.

Ovarian leiomyomas are benign, including those which are 'mitotically active', and can be treated by the least radical surgery necessary for their complete removal. It has to be accepted, however, that no definite criteria have been established for distinguishing between benign and malignant smooth muscle tumours of the ovary and the criteria used for uterine smooth muscle tumours have usually been applied (Nielsen & Young 2001). In a not yet fully reported study of 53 ovarian smooth muscle tumours it was found that moderate to severe cytological atypia, a mitotic count of more than 5 per 10 high-power fields, tumour cell necrosis and infiltrative margins correlated with malignant behaviour (Fan et al 2001a,b). The only other diagnostic problem posed by ovarian leiomyomas, not one of any great practical importance, is their differentiation from a pedunculated subserosal uterine leiomyoma which has separated off and become secondarily attached to the ovary, from which it receives its blood supply.

LEIOMYOSARCOMA

Ovarian leiomyosarcomas of non-teratoid origin are extremely uncommon, less than 25 examples having been reported (Balazs & Lazlo 1965; Nieminen et al 1969; Bettendorf & Zimmermann 1975; Mani et al 1975; Raj-Kumar 1982; Balaton et al 1987; Cortes et al 1987; Karogozov et al 1990; Friedman & Mazur 1991; Monk et al 1993; O'Sullivan et al 1998; Piura et al 1998; Nasu et al 2000) though Prat & Scully (unpublished observations) have recently reviewed a series of 14 cases. The tumours usually occur in elderly women: in Prat & Scully's series the ages of the patients ranged from 30–71 years with a mean of 53 years. The presenting symptoms are usually of abdominal pain or an awareness of an abdominal mass, and a history of menstrual abnormalities is most uncommon. The tumours are nearly always unilateral (bilaterality being noted in only one of Prat & Scully's cases) and are generally large, varying in Prat & Scully's series from 7.5–20 cm in

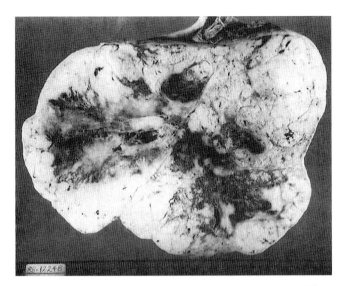

Fig. 24.8 Ovarian leiomyosarcoma. This is predominantly solid and focally haemorrhagic.

diameter with a mean of 12.4 cm. Grossly, ovarian leiomyosarcomas have a nodular outer surface and on section most are predominantly solid but with foci of cystic change; there may be extensive areas of haemorrhage and necrosis (Fig. 24.8). Their cut surface tends to be greyish-white and generally has a rather more fleshy texture than does a leiomyoma. The histological appearances (Fig. 24.9) are variable and range from very well-differentiated tumours, differing from a leiomyoma only by containing an excessive number of mitotic figures (such neoplasms now probably being regarded as mitotically active leiomyomas), to highly pleomorphic sarcomas with only a few small areas that are recognisably smooth muscle in nature. The mitotic counts in Prat & Scully's cases ranged from four to twenty-five mitotic figures per 10 high-power fields. One of Prat & Scully's tumours had extensive myxoid change and resembled a myxoid leiomyosarcoma whilst a further neoplasm showed leiomyoblastomatous (or epithelioid) differentiation (Fig. 24.10). The former case was included in a series of three myxoid leiomyosarcomas of the ovary reported by Nogales et al (1991). They were large gelatinous tumours

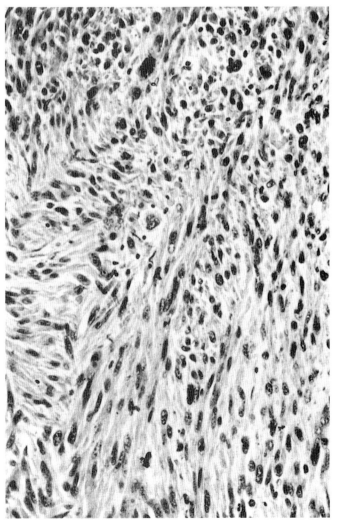

Fig. 24.9 An ovarian leiomyosarcoma.

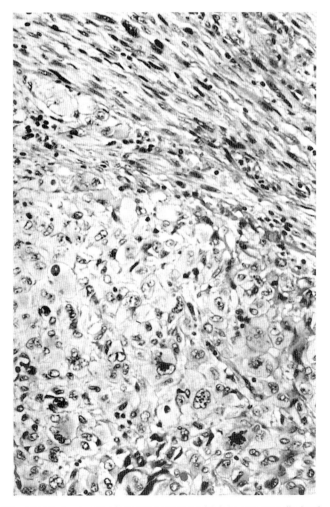

Fig. 24.10 An ovarian leiomyosarcoma which in one area (below) showed an epithelioid (or 'leiomyoblastomatous') pattern.

with cystic change, necrosis and haemorrhage. Microscopically, they exhibited a reticular meshwork of elongated cells surrounded by abundant basophilic myxoid material. The use of immunohistochemical stains against smooth muscle actin demonstrated a smooth muscle type of differentiation. The differential diagnosis of this rare ovarian neoplasm includes ovarian oedema, myxoma, yolk sac tumour and the myxoid sarcomatous component of malignant mixed Müllerian tumour and carcinosarcoma. Due to decreased cellular density, mitotic counts are usually low; clinical stage seems to be a more reliable prognostic indicator. Like its uterine counterpart, myxoid leiomyosarcoma of the ovary is a highly aggressive tumour. Two of the three patients reported by Nogales et al (1991) died of tumour at 13 and 24 months after diagnosis.

Ovarian leiomyosarcomas are aggressive neoplasms and have commonly spread beyond the ovary at the time of initial diagnosis. Thus, in Prat & Scully's 14 cases, the tumour was confined to the ovary in only two patients whilst in the remainder there was involvement of the omentum, peritoneum, diaphragm and, in one woman, the heart and adrenal glands. The treatment of choice is probably radical surgery though radiotherapy or chemotherapy may prolong survival in some instances. Most of the reported cases of ovarian leiomyosarcoma have led to death within two years, the longest survival being three and a half years after initial diagnosis (Nasu et al 2000). Of the eight patients in Prat & Scully's series for whom follow-up information was available, five died from widespread metastases, two were alive but with metastases one and two years postoperatively, whilst one was alive and well one year after surgery.

TUMOURS OF STRIATED MUSCLE

RHABDOMYOMA

A single example of an ovarian rhabdomyoma has been reported (Iizuka et al 1992).

RHABDOMYOSARCOMA

Fewer than 40 acceptable cases of pure primary ovarian rhabdomyosarcoma have been recorded (Vignard 1889; Himwich 1920; Barris & Shaw 1928; La Manna 1936; Rio 1956; Payan 1965; Dubey & Agrawal 1967; Srinivasa Roa & Subuadra Devi 1967; Spies & Lorenz 1973; Guerard et al 1983; Kanajet & Pirkic 1988; Chan et al 1989; Nielsen et al 1998): one example has also been reported which was associated with, but apparently independent of, an ovarian clear cell carcinoma (Sant 'Ambrogio et al 2000). Obeisance is usually paid to Virchow (cited by Sandison 1955) as having first described an ovarian rhabdomyosarcoma in 1850, but his report was notably lacking in both clinical and pathologi-

cal documentation, whilst a reappraisal of the frequently quoted case of Sandison (1955) shows clearly that it was a mixed Müllerian tumour.

Ovarian rhabdomyosarcomas are usually unilateral and range in size from relatively small lesions of 5 cm diameter to huge masses that extend up to the umbilicus: most are, however, more than 10 cm in diameter. They are smooth and lobulated and small villiform processes may project from their surfaces. The tumours are generally solid with a firm or rubbery texture but fleshy, soft or gelatinous areas may be focally present and are sometimes dominant; the cut surface is usually greyish-white or tan. Focal cystic change is common as are areas of haemorrhage and necrosis.

Histologically, ovarian rhabdomyosarcomas in children and young adults tend to show a mixed embryonal and alveolar pattern whilst those occurring in older individuals more commonly exhibit pleomorphic features; all three morphological patterns can, however, be present in a single tumour. Embryonal rhabdomyosarcomas are

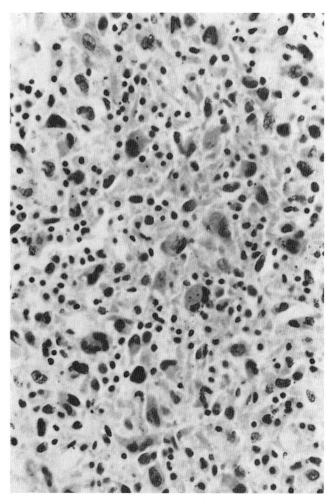

Fig. 24.11 An embryonal rhabdomyosarcoma of the ovary. Small, rounded cells are admixed with poorly differentiated rhabdomyoblasts.

formed largely of small, rounded or ovoid cells with hyperchromatic nuclei and scanty cytoplasm. Intermingled with these undifferentiated cells are larger cells with ample, strongly eosinophilic, granular cytoplasm and eccentric nuclei (Fig. 24.11). Better-differentiated rhabdomyoblasts with cross-striations may also be present but the finding of such striations is not a strict diagnostic prerequisite. Areas of typical embryonal rhabdomyosarcoma usually blend with alveolar areas in which the cellular elements are separated by fibrovascular septa to form alveolar lobules. The pleomorphic rhabdomyosarcoma is formed of spindle cells, rhabdomyoblasts in all stages of differentiation, multinucleated giant cells and racquet-shaped cells (Fig. 24.12). The diagnosis of a rhabdomyosarcoma is aided by electronmicroscopic detection of myofilaments and associated Z-band material, whilst immunohistological demonstration of myosin is also of great diagnostic value.

Ovarian rhabdomyosarcomas occur at any age, the youngest reported patient being 13 months and the oldest 86 years: in the 13 cases of ovarian rhabdomyosarcomas reported by Nielsen et al (1998) the mean age of the patients was 37 years. Patients usually complain of symptoms directly referable to a rapidly expanding pelvic mass but occasionally they present as an acute abdominal catastrophe following rupture of the neoplasm: one patient, aged 16 years, presented with a leukaemia-like syndrome (Nunez et al 1981) whilst another, aged 14 years, complained of bone pain and was found to have diffuse marrow involvement by the tumour (Nielsen et al 1998). The neoplasm is highly aggressive and has commonly extended beyond the ovary at the time of diagnosis: thus, in Nielsen et al's series of 13 cases, only four were confined to the ovary whilst the other 8 in which the stage was known were either infiltrating the pelvic organs or had given rise to peritoneal implants. The prognosis is poor and all the reported patients have died within two and a half years of initial diagnosis: all six patients for whom over a year's follow-up details were available in Nielsen et al's series died of tumour metastases between 10 days and 26 months.

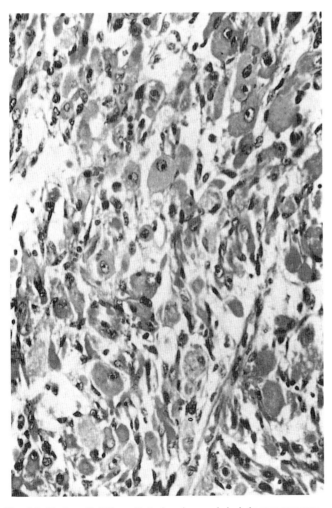

Fig. 24.12 A well-differentiated embryonal rhabdomyosarcoma of the ovary. Numerous rhabdomyoblasts with abundant eosinophilic cytoplasm are present.

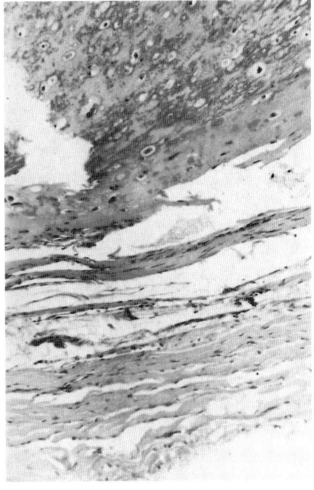

Fig. 24.13 An ovarian chondroma formed solely of mature cartilaginous tissue.

TUMOURS OF CARTILAGE

CHONDROMA

Most, probably all, ovarian chondromas which have been reported appear to have been either fibromas showing cartilaginous metaplasia or mature cystic teratomas with a prominent cartilaginous component. The lesion illustrated in Fig. 24.13 did, however, appear to be a true chondroma. The patient, an elderly woman, presented with non-specific pelvic tumour symptoms, and an ovarian mass measuring 12 cm was removed. Histologically, this consisted solely of mature cartilaginous tissue with a thin compressed surrounding rim of ovarian cortex.

CHONDROSARCOMA (Fig. 24.14)

Nearly all reported ovarian chondrosarcomas have either arisen in a mature cystic teratoma or have been unusually conspicuous components of a malignant mixed Müllerian tumour. Talerman et al (1981) have, however, described

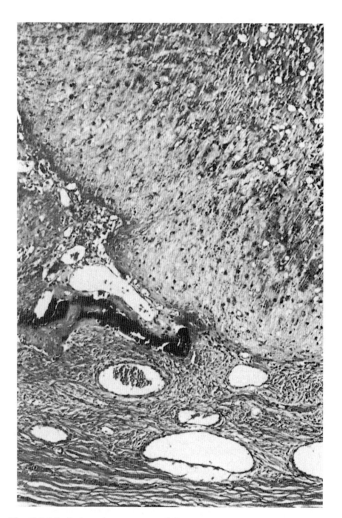

Fig. 24.14 A chondrosarcoma of the ovary.

an apparently pure, primary chondrosarcoma of the ovary which occurred in a 61-year-old woman who presented with a pelvic mass. The ovarian tumour was large, solid and firm; it consisted histologically of islands of cartilage containing chondrocytes in many stages of differentiation: cellular atypia and mitotic activity were manifest.

Following surgical removal the patient was alive and well four years later.

TUMOURS OF BONE

OSTEOMA

Occasional osteomas of the ovary have been described but all would more correctly be considered either as fibromas showing extensive osseous metaplasia or as examples of heterotopic bone formation in the ovarian stroma (Shipton & Meares 1965).

GIANT CELL TUMOUR (OSTEOCLASTOMA)

Virtually all of the ovarian giant cell tumours reported in the literature have been associated with mucinous cyst-adenomas and would now be regarded as pseudosarcomatous mural nodules. An exception to this, however, is the neoplasm described by Lorentzen (1980). This was an asymptomatic mass in a 31-year-old woman which was discovered incidentally during investigation of infertility. The tumour was small, solid and yellow–brown: histologically, it had the characteristics of a giant cell tumour with mononuclear ovoid or spindle-shaped stromal cells interspersed with multinucleated giant cells, the latter containing up to 100 nuclei. Trabeculae of osteoid and bone were present and there was a sprinkling of mitotic figures. There was no evidence of any other tumour component and following surgery the patient was alive and well four and a half years later.

OSTEOGENIC SARCOMA

Four apparently pure primary osteogenic sarcomas of the ovary (Azoury & Woodruff 1971; Hirakawa et al 1988; Hines et al 1990; Sakata et al 1991) have been recorded. The first occurred in a 41-year-old woman, had the typical histological appearances of an osteogenic sarcoma as seen in the skeleton, contained no other tissue elements and led to the patient's death within five months. One, in a perimenopausal woman, was noted as a calcified adnexal mass on abdominal radiography: the patient was alive and well after eight courses of chemotherapy. Two other osteosarcomas, one of which had a telangiectatic pattern (Hirakawa et al 1988), led to the death of the patients within a few months.

TUMOURS OF NEURAL ORIGIN

NEUROFIBROMA

Only two ovarian tumours of this type have been fully documented (Smith 1931; Hegg & Flint 1990). The first was an incidental finding in a woman with von Recklinghausen's disease and its histological appearances were similar to neurofibromas occurring elsewhere in more conventional sites. The second, also in a patient with von Recklinghausen's syndrome, was symptomatic and simulated a malignant neoplasm.

SCHWANNOMA

Three ovarian schwannomas have been described (Meyer 1943; Mishura 1963; De Franchis & Galliani 1964). In each case the patient presented with non-specific symptoms suggestive of a pelvic mass. Histologically, the tumours showed the typical appearance of a schwannoma as seen elsewhere in the body and all the patients were alive and symptom-free after extirpation of the neoplasm.

GANGLIONEUROMA

A number of very small ovarian ganglioneuromas have been noted (Meyer 1943), but these hilar clusters of ganglion cells are almost certainly hamartomatous in nature rather than neoplastic. One undoubtedly neoplastic ganglioneuroma was, however, found in a 4-year-old girl who presented with abdominal swelling (Schmeisser & Anderson 1938); the tumour, which had almost totally replaced the ovary, was solid, weighed 200 g and was formed of well-differentiated ganglion cells.

MALIGNANT SCHWANNOMA

Only one apparently non-teratomatous ovarian malignant schwannoma has been reported (Dover 1950): this was in a 38-year-old woman with von Recklinghausen's disease who, whilst being treated for postabortal bleeding, was found to have a pelvic mass. The neoplasm was solid, had replaced the ovary and had the typical appearances of a malignant schwannoma with some degree of pleomorphism and mitotic activity; the patient was alive and well one year after treatment with surgery and radiotherapy.

PHAEOCHROMOCYTOMA

Small groups of paraganglion cells have been occasionally noted in the ovarian hilum but only one phaeochromocytoma of the ovary has been described (Fawcett & Kimbell 1971). This was in a 15-year-old girl who presented with severe hypertension, fits and an abdominal mass. An ovarian tumour, which weighted 970 g and had undergone torsion, was removed from the left ovary: this had the typical histological appearances of a phaeochromocytoma and contained considerable quantities of adrenaline and noradrenaline. The patient was well and normotensive 15 months later.

MYXOMA

Twelve ovarian myxomas have been reported (Dutz & Stout 1961; Masubuchi et al 1970; Majmudar et al 1978; Brady et al 1987; Eichhorn & Scully 1991; Tetu & Bonenfant 1991; Costa et al 1992). The patients ranged in age from 16–45 years and all presented with adnexal masses; the tumours were moderately large and partly solid and partly cystic with a gelatinous or mucinous texture. None had ruptured. Histologically, they were composed of scattered stellate or spindle-shaped cells set in a loose, abundant myxoid stroma (Fig. 24.15) which stained intensely positively with Alcian Blue due to the presence of hyaluronic acid. The tumours were richly vascularised by vessels of capillary size and contained a network of delicate reticulum fibres. The tumour cells

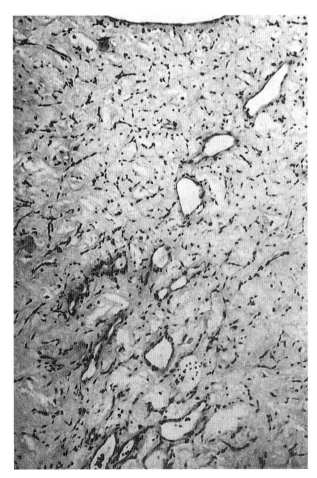

Fig. 24.15 Ovarian myxoma. Parvicellular tumour with abundant pale intercellular matrix that mimics the appearance of massive oedema of the ovary. (Courtesy of Dr Eichhorn, Boston, Ma.)

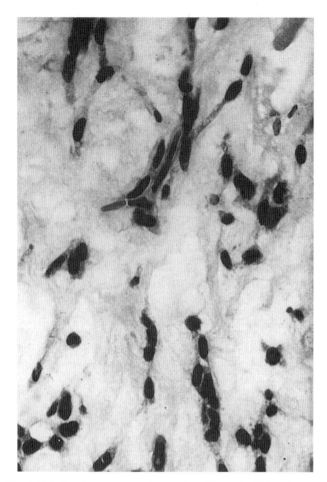

Fig. 24.16 Ovarian myxoma. Focus of capillary-sized blood vessels in a plexiform arrangement simulating myxoid liposarcoma. (Courtesy of Dr Eichhorn, Boston, Ma.)

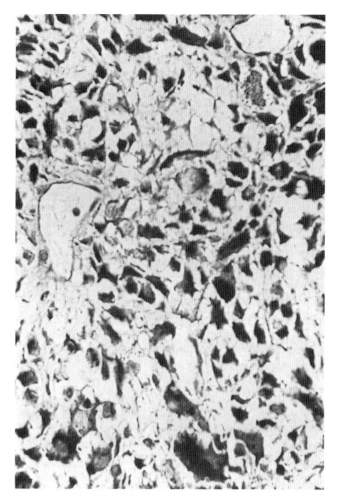

Fig. 24.17 A pleomorphic liposarcoma of the ovary.

were immunoreactive for vimentin and usually for actin, but not for desmin (Eichhorn & Scully 1991; Costa et al 1992). All the patients were treated by unilateral adnexectomy and none of seven tumours, with a follow-up period of 1–13 years (mean 5 years), recurred.

The histogenesis of ovarian myxoma is obscure but these neoplasms require extensive sampling to exclude other tissue components such as lipoblasts or muscle; the differential diagnosis includes massive oedema, myxoid change in a fibroma, myxoid liposarcoma (Fig. 24.16), myxoid leiomyosarcoma and sarcoma botryoides.

TUMOURS OF FAT

Although a few ovarian lipomas have been described (Fahr 1941) these seem to have been teratomas with a conspicuous adipose element, self-amputated epiploic appendages which have become adherent to the ovary or examples of the non-neoplastic accumulations of fat cells sometimes seen in the ovary and known variously as 'adipose prosoplasia' (Hart & Abell 1970) or 'adipocytic infiltration' (Honoré & O'Hara 1980). The very occasional liposarcomas which have been reported all appear

to have been ovarian metastases from extragonadal liposarcomas, though the neoplasm illustrated in Fig. 24.17 was a primary ovarian neoplasm which was considered to be a pleomorphic liposarcoma.

TUMOURS OF VASCULAR ORIGIN

HAEMANGIOMA

Whether haemangiomas are hamartomas or true neoplasms is a moot point but the ovary has a complex and abundant vasculature and it is surprising that these lesions are so rare at this site, only about 40 examples having been reported (Baryluk et al 1966; Gaal 1967; Talerman 1967; Gay & Janovski 1969; Ebrahimi et al 1971; Griffin 1971; Caresano 1977; Kela & Aurdra 1980; Betta et al 1988; Gunes et al 1990; Pethe et al 1991; Prus et al 1997). Even this small number may, however, exaggerate the true incidence of ovarian haemangiomas, for the difficulties that may be encountered in distinguishing a small lesion of this type from dilated, congested hilar vessels do not always appear to have been taken into account and reports of small hilar haemangiomas must be regarded with some scepticism. It is difficult to define absolute criteria for the recognition of an ovarian haemangioma but it does seem reasonable to suggest that hilar lesions should only be so regarded if there is a visible and well-demarcated nodule; less strict requirements apply only to those lesions situated in the cortex.

Haemangiomas are usually unilateral, though occasional bilateral examples have been recorded (Payne 1869; Shearer 1935; Fundaro 1969; Miyauchi et al 1987). They usually have a smooth, glistening outer surface, are well demarcated from the surrounding ovarian tissue and although generally small can attain a diameter of 12 cm. On section, haemangiomas tend to be of spongy texture and often have a honeycomb appearance; characteristically, they are red or purplish and, not uncommonly, focal calcification is noted. Nearly all ovarian haemangiomas show, histologically, a cavernous or a mixed cavernous-capillary pattern with large vascular spaces, lined by a single layer of regular endothelial cells, being separated from each other by a variable amount of fibrous tissue which is often hyalinised.

Ovarian haemangiomas have been noted in patients ranging from 4 months to 81 years in age (Rodriguez 1979) and in approximately two-thirds of cases the tumour has been an asymptomatic incidental finding at surgery or autopsy. In the relatively few women with symptoms the principal complaints have been of abdominal pain, abdominal swelling or awareness of a mass. In these patients abdominal pain was due to torsion of a large haemangioma, this occurring chronically in one (Mann & Metrick 1961) and acutely in two (Schaeffer & Cancelmo 1939; Scheinman et al 1982). Ascites has developed, and been the principal cause of symptoms, in three patients (Keller 1927; Presno-Bastiony & Puente-Duany 1929; McBurney & Trumbull 1955) whilst only in a few women have symptoms been due solely to the presence of an expanding ovarian mass unaccompanied by torsion or ascites. In one patient, bilateral ovarian haemangiomas were one component of diffuse haemangioendotheliomatosis (Miyauchi et al 1987). Simple oophorectomy is curative and it is followed by rapid regression of any ascites that may be present.

HAEMANGIOPERICYTOMA

The literature, particularly that before 1920, is replete with accounts of ovarian 'perithelioma'. These have usually been too inadequately described for their true nature to be apparent and it is probable that some were endometrioid stromal sarcomas of low-grade malignancy.

ANGIOSARCOMA

Less than 25 cases of ovarian angiosarcoma have been reported (Rice et al 1943; Meylan 1958; Cunningham et al 1994; Nara et al 1996; Nielsen et al 1997; Furihata et al 1998; Lifschitz-Mercer et al 1998; Nucci et al 1998; Platt et al 1999; Twu et al 1999). The angiosarcoma described by Ongkasuwan et al (1982) was associated with a mucinous cystadenoma and is discussed under the separate heading of 'Sarcomas associated with epithelial tumours'. Two of the seven cases reported by Nielsen et al (1997) arose in mature cystic teratomas.

The tumours are usually unilateral and tend to be large, soft, friable and spongy; cystic change is common and can be extensive whilst foci of haemorrhage and necrosis are common. Histologically, these tumours are formed of proliferating vascular spaces of all degrees of development lined by endothelial cells showing atypia, pleomorphism and mitotic activity (Fig. 24.18). In some areas tumour cells may grow in solid cords whilst undifferentiated spindle or epithelioid cells may sometimes be present. In occasional cases the sarcomatous pattern predominates and any proliferating neoplastic vascular structures may be misinterpreted as being part of an inflammatory response to bleeding from the tumour.

The diagnosis of an angiosarcoma of the ovary may be difficult if the vascular nature of the tumour is not

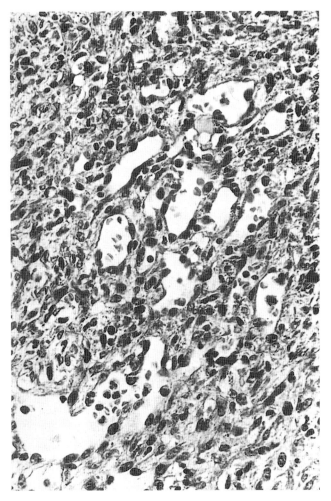

Fig. 24.18 An angiosarcoma of the ovary.

obvious at first microscopic examination. The differential diagnosis includes other primary and metastatic ovarian tumours such as sarcomatoid carcinoma, leiomyosarcoma, yolk sac tumour, clear cell carcinoma, retiform Sertoli–Leydig cell tumour, choriocarcinoma and metastatic melanoma. Immunostaining for CD31, CD34 and von Willebrand factor is helpful in establishing the correct diagnosis. Angiosarcomas with epithelioid cells may stain focally for keratin.

Patients with ovarian angiosarcomas have ranged in age from 19–69 years and have usually presented solely with non-specific symptoms indicative of a pelvic mass; one striking feature of the clinical picture is a tendency for the tumour to rupture and cause severe intraperitoneal bleeding, this sometimes being a consequence of torsion of the tumour.

The prognosis for ovarian angiosarcomas with extraovarian spread is poor, but if the tumour is confined to the ovary at the time of operation the outlook appears to be reasonably good (Nielsen et al 1997).

TUMOURS OF LYMPHATIC VESSELS

LYMPHANGIOMA

Lesions of this type, the neoplastic nature of which is debatable, occur with extreme rarity in the ovary, only a handful of cases having been described (Siddall & Clinton 1937; Ferrari & de Angelis 1953; Bieniasz & Sierant 1961; Loubiere et al 1968; Paliez et al 1970; Khanna et al 1979; Evans et al 1999). They are usually unilateral with a smooth, grey outer surface and rarely attain a diameter of more than 6 cm; on section numerous tiny cystic spaces are seen from which clear straw-coloured fluid oozes out. They are formed of closely packed lymphatic vessels lined by a flattened layer of endothelial cells.

Lymphangiomas closely resemble an adenomatoid tumour from which, however, they can usually be distinguished by the absence of solid cords of cells between the vessels, by their lack of PAS- or Alcian Blue-positive material and by their positive immunostaining for Factor VIII, CD34 and CD31. Care also has to be taken not to confuse the sieve-like areas often found in mature cystic teratomas with a lymphangioma.

These tumours are usually asymptomatic incidental findings and are fully benign.

LYMPHANGIOSARCOMA

There has been only one report of an ovarian lymphangiosarcoma (Rice et al 1943). This was a mass measuring 15 cm in diameter which was found in the ovary of a 31-year-old woman who gave a short history of abdominal enlargement. Histologically, the appearances were similar to those seen in a benign lymphangioma, but in a few

areas the endothelial cells lining the lymphatic vessels showed focal proliferation with some degree of pleomorphism and nuclear hyperchromatism. The patient died within a year of widespread metastases.

ENDOMETRIOID STROMAL SARCOMA

Forty-five cases of endometrioid stromal sarcoma of the ovary have been reported in detail (Benjamin & Campbell 1960; Keller & Rygh 1964; Palladino & Trousdell 1969; Gruskin et al 1970; Azoury & Woodruff 1971; Silverberg & Nogales 1981; Young et al 1984; Shakfeh & Woodruff 1987; Baiocchi et al 1990; Young & Scully 1990; Shiraki et al 1991; Chang et al 1993; Fukunaga et al 1998). The neoplasms may derive from foci of ovarian endometriosis (concomitant endometriosis being present in 40% of the reported cases), from foci of gland-free endometrial stroma in the ovary (ovarian stromatosis — Hughesdon 1972, 1976) or, possibly, may arise directly from the ovarian stromal cells following metaplasia into endometrial stromal-type cells.

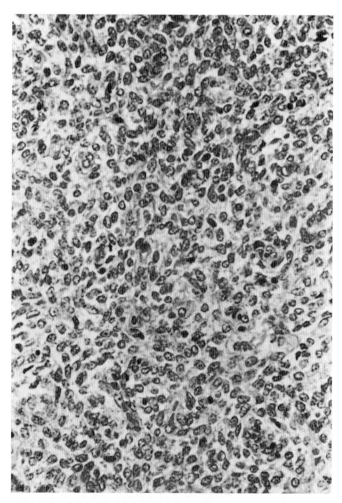

Fig. 24.19 An endometrioid stromal sarcoma of the ovary. This is composed of sheets of cells which resemble the stromal cells of normal proliferative endometrium.

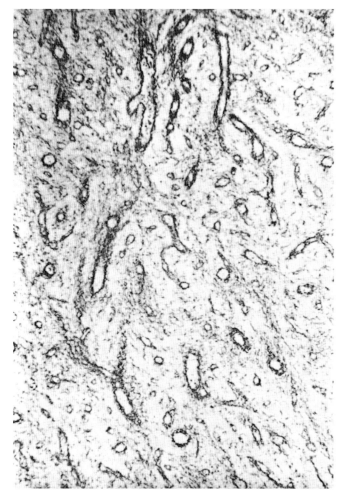

Fig. 24.20 Endometrioid stromal sarcoma of the ovary. A reticulin stain demonstrates the rich vascular network.

The tumours commonly measure less than 15 cm in diameter and were unilateral in 75% of the described cases. They are predominantly solid, though foci of cystic change are present in over half; on section they usually have a homogeneous appearance, with foci of necrosis or haemorrhage being relatively uncommon. Histologically, the ovarian tumours, like their more common uterine counterparts, are composed of sheets of uniform cells resembling the stromal cells of normal proliferative endometrium (Fig. 24.19). Fibromatous areas are, however, also frequently present, this not being a feature of uterine neoplasms of this type. An important diagnostic feature is the presence of a prominent network of small arterioles, these closely resembling the spiral vessels seen in normal late secretory endometrium: this network is most clearly seen in reticulin-stained sections (Fig. 24.20). The focal intravascular growth characteristic of uterine endometrial sarcomas of low-grade malignancy is not seen within the ovarian tumours but is typically present when the neoplasm extends beyond the confines of the ovary (Fig. 24.21). The tumour cells may contain abundant intracellular lipid and, although usually growing in uniform sheets, can, like similar uterine tumours, show an epithelial or sex-cord tumour-like pattern in some areas.

The nature of the cells in an endometrioid stromal sarcoma and the presence of a rich vascular network allow for the differentiation of these neoplasms from other types of ovarian sarcoma. A Müllerian adenosarcoma may, however, be mimicked if endometriotic glands are trapped within the tumour: in such circumstances the focal presence of the glands, as opposed to their uniform

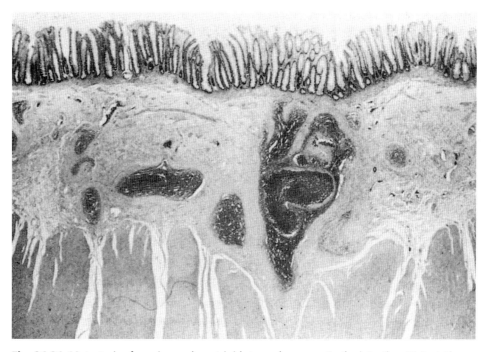

Fig. 24.21 Metastasis of ovarian endometrioid stromal sarcoma to the intestine. Metastatic deposits of this neoplasm typically show intravascular growth.

distribution throughout an adenosarcoma, together with the absence of any stromal condensation around the glands (cambium layer), usually indicates the correct diagnosis. If a sex-cord-like pattern is a prominent feature of an endometrioid stromal sarcoma this may lead to confusion with a granulosa cell tumour: the epithelial-like cells do not, however, have the nuclear features of granulosa cells and a lack of staining for alpha-inhibin is helpful in identifying the tumour as a stromal sarcoma (Zheng et al 1997).

The patients with endometrioid stromal sarcomas ranged in age from 11–76 years with slightly over half of the tumours being diagnosed in women in their fifth or sixth decades. The presenting symptoms are of a non-specific nature and are entirely related to the presence of a pelvic mass. In the series of Young et al (1984) the tumour was, at the time of operation, confined to the ovary in only four patients: in nine cases the tumour involved other pelvic structures, whilst eight tumours had spread into the abdomen and had metastasised to the lungs.

The behaviour of ovarian endometrioid stromal sarcomas is analogous to that of their uterine counterparts with the degree of mitotic activity being of major prognostic significance. Tumours with fewer than 10 mitotic figures per 10 high-power fields are associated with a good prognosis, even if there is extrauterine spread: thus in Young et al's (1984) series only two of 19 patients whose neoplasms contained less than 10 mitotic figures per 10 high-power fields died of their disease and nine patients with spread beyond the ovary at the time of presentation were alive one or more years postoperatively. The prognosis for those tumours containing more than 10 mitotic figures per 10 high-power fields is comparable to that of other ovarian sarcomas, and three of the four women in Young et al's (1984) series with tumours showing this degree of mitotic activity were dead within four years.

It should be noted that ovarian endometrioid stromal sarcomas are associated with a prior, synchronous or subsequent uterine endometrial stromal sarcoma in approximately 30% of patients. This was the case in nine of the 23 patients reported by Young et al (1984): in at least two of these cases, in which the uterine lesions preceded the ovarian neoplasm by many years, there was strong circumstantial evidence to suggest independent primary tumours of each organ. In synchronous cases it is, of course, usually impossible to exclude metastasis from one organ to the other, especially if other pelvic structures are involved. Chang et al (1993) believe that an endometrial stromal sarcoma can only be considered as primarily ovarian in origin if the tumour is confined to the ovary and the uterus has been shown to be free of tumour on pathological examination. Scully et al (1998) accept, however, continuity with ovarian endometriosis as evidence for an ovarian origin of an endometrial stromal sarcoma even if there is also a histologically similar uterine neoplasm. From a practical point of view, it is of value to review any prior hysterectomy specimen in a patient with an ovarian endometrioid stromal sarcoma; it is also important to recognise that if the uterus is not removed at the time of operation for an ovarian endometrioid stromal sarcoma it is possible that a uterine stromal sarcoma may have been left behind or will subsequently develop.

The primary therapeutic approach to ovarian endometrioid stromal sarcoma is surgical. If the patient is menopausal or postmenopausal, hysterectomy with bilateral salpingo-oophorectomy is the treatment of choice and, because of the high frequency of bilateral ovarian involvement and the possibility of synchronous or subsequent uterine endometrial stromal sarcoma, a similar approach may be optimal even for younger women. Both progestagens and radiotherapy have been used for residual or recurrent disease, but in assessing the value of such therapy it has to be remembered that those tumours of low-grade malignancy (less than 10 mitotic figures per 10 high-power fields) typically run a very indolent course and that patients with untreated residual disease may remain free of signs or symptoms for many years: indeed, in some cases the extraovarian lesions appear to regress spontaneously.

UNDIFFERENTIATED 'STROMAL' SARCOMA

This term has been applied to those ovarian sarcomas which appear to arise from the ovarian stromal mesenchyme but which do not show any specific differentiation (Azoury & Woodruff 1971). How common such tumours are is a moot point: the literature is replete with reports of 'spindle cell' or 'round cell' sarcomas, most of which have clearly been examples of leiomyosarcoma, malignant lymphoma, granulosa cell tumour or endometrioid stromal sarcoma. Some quite convincing reports have appeared, however, of sarcomas which seemed to have originated in the stroma and have shown no obvious differentiation along either leiomyosarcomatous or fibrosarcomatous lines (Foda et al 1958; Variati & Donatelli 1966; Azoury & Woodruff 1971) and Prat & Scully have reviewed a series of six such tumours (unpublished observations).

Azoury & Woodruff (1971) thought that these neoplasms had a predilection for relatively young females, for five of their seven tumours occurred in patients aged less than 20 years. This was not the case, however, in Prat & Scully's series, in which the age range was from 35–65 years. The tumours are generally large, measuring up to 20 cm in diameter, and may be firm, fleshy, soft or friable; histologically, they are formed of ovoid or elongated cells which have relatively large vesicular nuclei and show varying degrees of pleomorphism and mitotic activity (Fig. 24.22): there is often an admixture of multinucleated giant cells.

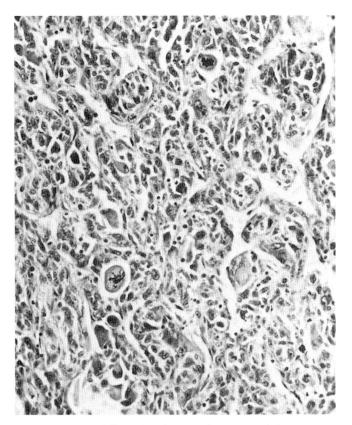

Fig. 24.22 An undifferentiated 'stromal' sarcoma of the ovary.

In Azoury & Woodruff's (1971) series four patients whose tumours were thought to be of only low-grade malignancy were alive and well at periods ranging from six to 14 years after removal of the tumour, whilst two patients with neoplasms showing considerable pleomorphism and abundant mitotic activity were dead within two years. A rather more gloomy outlook prevailed in Prat & Scully's series, for all of the five patients for whom follow-up information was available were dead from metastatic disease within two and a half years of initial diagnosis.

COMBINED SARCOMA AND EPITHELIAL TUMOUR

There have been occasional reports of ovarian sarcomas occurring in combination with an epithelial neoplasm. Thus Prat & Scully (1979) described two sarcomas, each of which presented as a distinct solitary nodule in the wall of an ovarian mucinous cystic tumour: one was a fibrosarcoma in the wall of a mucinous cystadenoma and the other was an undifferentiated sarcoma in conjunction with a mucinous cystadenocarcinoma. A second example of fibrosarcoma arising as a well-circumscribed 9 cm nodule in the wall of a mucinous cystadenoma has been described by de Nictolis et al (1990). The tumour, though well-differentiated, was adherent to the omentum and contained four mitoses per 10 high-power fields. The patient received radiotherapy, but she died with clinical evidence of peritoneal and hepatic metastases 18 months postoperatively. The findings in this case support the validity of the two diagnostic criteria proposed to separate cellular fibromas from fibrosarcomas, namely, the finding of four or more mitoses per 10 high-power fields and the extension of the tumour beyond the ovary (Prat & Scully 1979). Ongkasuwan et al (1982) reported an angiosarcoma associated with a mucinous cystadenoma whilst there have been two recorded examples of leiomyosarcomas coexisting with serous tumours, one a serous cystadenoma (von Numers & Mikkonen 1960) and the other a serous adenocarcinoma (Walts & Lichtenstein 1977). A single case of rhabdomyosarcoma associated with a mucinous cystic tumour of the ovary has been reported (Tsujimura & Kawano 1992). The sarcoma, a solid mass 15 cm in greatest diameter, contained pleomorphic rhabdomyoblasts with occasional cross-striations. The exact nature of these apparently combined tumours is debatable: they are probably collision tumours but the possibility of malignant change in the stroma of an epithelial neoplasm cannot be totally discounted.

ADENOMATOID TUMOURS

Adenomatoid tumours are virtually confined to the genital tract but the ovary is one of the least common sites for such a neoplasm to occur (Masson et al 1942; Lee et al 1950; Teel 1958; Serrapiao & Serrapiao 1964; Jones & Donova 1965; Ferenczy et al 1972; Boczkowski et al 1977). Ovarian tumours of this type are nearly always small and asymptomatic incidental findings. They are usually seen as unilateral, well-delineated but non-encapsulated, firm grey–white nodules which on section are honeycombed by numerous small cystic spaces. Histologically, the tumour is formed of cystic or gland-like spaces lined by flattened or cuboidal cells having abundant vacuolated eosinophilic cytoplasm and ovoid nuclei. Cords of similar cells are also usually present and these may contain slit-like clefts. The epithelial structures are set in a variable amount of connective tissue stroma which is often hyalinised and may contain smooth muscle fibres. Alcian Blue-positive material is usually present but PAS-positive material is often absent.

REFERENCES

Amin H K, Okagaki T, Richart R M 1971 Classification of fibroma and thecoma of the ovary: an ultrastructural study. Cancer 27: 438–446

Azoury R S, Woodruff J D 1971 Primary ovarian sarcomas: report of 43 cases from the Emil Novak ovarian tumour registry. Obstetrics and Gynecology 37: 920–941

Baaiocchi G, Kavanagh J J, Wharton J T 1990 Endometrioid stromal sarcomas arising from ovarian and extraovarian endometriosis: report of two cases and review of the literature. Gynecologic Oncology 36: 147–151

Balaton A, Vaury P, Imbert M C, Mussy M A 1987 Primary leiomyosarcoma of the ovary: a histological and immunocytochemical study. Gynecologic Oncology 28: 116–120

Balazs M, Lazlo J 1965 Das Leiomyosarkome des Ovar. Zentralblatt fur Gynakologie 87: 633–638

Barris J, Shaw W 1928 Rhabdomyosarcoma of the ovary. Proceedings of the Royal Society of Medicine 22: 320–322

Baryluk V L, Lui H, Horn R C 1966 Hemangioma of the ovary. Henry Ford Hospital Medical Bulletin 14: 167–172

Benjamin F, Campbell J A H 1960 Stromal 'endometriosis' with possible ovarian origin. American Journal of Obstetrics and Gynecology 80: 449–453

Betta P G, Robutti F, Spinoglio G 1988 Hemangioma of the ovary. European Journal of Gynaecological Oncology 9: 184–185

Bettendorf U, Zimmermann H 1975 Leiomyosarkoma de Ovarium. Medizinische Welt 26: 429–430

Bieniasz A, Sierant A 1961 A case of lymphangioma cavernosum of the ovary. Ginekologica Polska 32: 667–669

Biggart J H, Macafee C H G 1955 Tumours of the ovarian mesenchyme: a clinicopathological study. Journal of Obstetrics and Gynaecology of the British Empire 62: 829–837

Boczkowski Z, Czuczwar S, Pakula H, Sikorska-Haliniare W 1977 Benign adenomatoid tumour of the ovary. Ginekologica Polska 48: 913–915

Bower J F, Erikson E R 1967 Bilateral ovarian fibroma in a 5 year old. American Journal of Obstetrics and Gynecology 99: 880–882

Brady K, Page D V, Benn L E, de las Morenas A, O'Brien M 1987 Ovarian myxoma. American Journal of Obstetrics and Gynecology 156: 1240–1242

Burkett R L, Rauh J L 1976 Gorlin's syndrome: ovarian fibromas at adolescence. Obstetrics and Gynecology 47: 43s–46s

Caresano G 1977 L'emangioma cavernosa dell'ovaio: presentazione di un caso e rassegna della bibiliografia. Minerva Ginecologica 29: 103–106

Chan Y F, Leung C S, Ma L 1989 Primary embryonal rhabdomyosarcoma of the ovary in a 4-year-old girl. Histopathology 15: 309–311

Chang K L, Crabtree G S, Lim-Tan S K, Kempson R L, Hendrickson M R 1993 Primary extrauterine endometrial stromal neoplasms: a clinico-pathologic study of 20 cases and review of the literature. International Journal of Gynecological Pathology 12: 282–296

Charache H 1959 Ovarian tumours in childhood: report of six new cases and review of the literature. Archives of Surgery 79: 573–580

Christman J E, Ballon S C 1990 Ovarian fibrosarcoma associated with Mafucci's syndrome. Gynecologic Oncology 37: 290–291

Cortes J, Cuartero M L, Rossello J J et al 1987 Ovarian pure leiomyosarcoma: case report. European Journal of Gynaecological Oncology 8: 19–22

Costa M J, Thomas W, Majmudar B, Hewan-Lowe K 1992 Ovarian myxoma: ultrastructural and immunohistochemical findings. Ultrastructural Pathology 16: 429–438

Cunningham M J, Brooks J S, Noumoff J S 1994 Treatment of primary ovarian angiosarcoma with ifosfamide and doxorubicin. Gynecologic Oncology 53: 265–268

Dal Cin P, Pauwels P, van der Berghe H 1998 Fibrosarcoma versus cellular fibroma of the ovary (Letter to Editor). American Journal of Surgical Pathology 22: 508–510

Danihel L, Losch A, Kainz C, Feldmar T, Breiteneckerg G 1995 Bilaterales primares Leiomyom des Ovars. Wien Klinische Wochenschrift 107: 436–438

De Franchis M, Galliani A 1964 Neurinoma dell ovaio. Rivista di Pathologia e Clinica 19: 567–574

de Nictolis M, di Loreto C, Clinti S, Prat J 1990 Fibrosarcomatous mural nodule in an ovarian mucinous cystadenoma. Surgical Pathology 3: 309–315

Destro F 1958 Contributo allo studio de fibroma ovarico in metropatia emorragica. Archivio Italiano di Pathologia 2: 329–344

Dockerty M B, Masson J V 1944 Ovarian fibromas: a clinical and pathologic study of two hundred and eighty three cases. American Journal of Obstetrics and Gynecology 47: 741–752

Dodd G D, Lancaster K T, Moulton J S 1989 Ovarian lipoleiomyoma: a fat-containing mass in the female pelvis. American Journal of Roentgenology 153: 1007–1008

Doss B J, Wanek S M, Jacques S M, Qureshi F, Ramirez N C, Lawrence W D 1999a Ovarian smooth muscle metaplasia: an uncommon and possibly underrecognised entity. International Journal of Gynecological Pathology 18: 58–62

Doss B J, Wanek S M, Jacques S M, Qureshi F, Ramirez N C, Lawrence W D 1999b Ovarian leiomyomas: clinicopathologic features in fifteen cases. International Journal of Gynecological Pathology 18: 63–68

Dover H 1950 Malignant schwannoma of the ovary, associated with neurofibromatosis. Canadian Medical Association Journal 63: 488–490

Driscoll J A 1964 Ovarian fibroma. Journal of the Irish Medical Association 53: 184–187

Dubey M M, Agrawal S 1967 Rhabdomyosarcoma of ovary: a case report. Journal of Obstetrics and Gynaecology of India 17: 724–725

Duchini L, Menegaldo R 1967 I fibroma dell'ovaio. Archivio de Vechhi per l'anatomia Patologica e la Medicina Clinica 48: 973–997

Dutz W, Stout A P 1961 The myxoma in childhood. Cancer 14: 629–635

Ebrahimi T, Goldsmith J W, Okagaki J 1971 Hemangioma of the ovary: a case report. Obstetrics and Gynecology 38: 477–479

Eichhorn J H, Scully R E 1991 Ovarian myxoma: clinicopathologic and immunocytologic analysis of five cases and a review of the literature. International Journal of Gynecological Pathology 10: 156–169

Evans A, Lytwyn A, Urbach G, Chapman W 1999 Bilateral lymphangiomas of the ovary: an immunohistochemical characterization and review of the literature. International Journal of Gynecological Pathology 18: 87–90

Fahr E 1941 Eigenartige Fetgeschwulst des Ovariums. Zentralblatt fur allgemeine Pathologie und fur pathologischen Anatomie 77: 264–266

Fallahzadeh H, Dockerty M B, Lee R A 1972 Leiomyoma of the ovary: report of five cases and review of the literature. American Journal of Obstetrics and Gynecology 113: 394–398

Fan M J, Sung R, Oliva E, Young R H, Scully R E 2001a Morphological spectrum and differential diagnosis of 63 ovarian smooth muscle tumors (Abstract). Modern Pathology 14: 136A

Fan J M, Sung R, Oliva E, Young R H, Scully R E 2001b Spindle cell smooth muscle tumors: a study of 53 cases evaluating prognostic criteria (Abstract). Modern Pathology 14: 136A

Fawcett F J, Kimbell N K B 1971 Phaeochromocytoma of the ovary. Journal of Obstetrics and Gynaecology of the British Commonwealth 78: 456–459

Ferenczy A, Fenoglio J, Richart R M 1972 Observations of benign mesothelioma of the genital tract (adenomatoid tumour): a comparative ultrastructural study. Cancer 30: 244–260

Ferrari W, de Angelis V 1953 Linfangioma do ovario. Revista Brasileira of Cirugia 25: 329–334

Foda M S, Shafeek M A, Hashem M 1958 Sarcoma of the ovary. Gazette of the Egyptian Society of Obstetrics and Gynaecology 7: 15–37

Friedman H D, Mazur M T 1991 Primary ovarian leiomyosarcoma: an immunohistochemical and ultrastructural study. Archives of Pathology and Laboratory Medicine 115: 941–945

Fukunaga M, Ishihara A, Ushigome S 1998 Extrauterine low-grade endometrial stromal sarcoma: report of three cases. Pathology International 48: 297–302

Fundaro P 1969 Emangiomi cavernoso bilaterale del'ovai: presentazione di un caso e rassegna della letteratura. Folia Hereditaria et Patologica 18: 45–49

Furihata M, Takeuchi T, Iwata J et al 1998 Primary ovarian angiosarcoma: a case report and literature review. Pathology International 48: 967–973

Gaal M 1967 Die Hamangiome der weiblichen Geschlechtsorgane. Gynaecologia 164: 307–315

Gay R M, Janovski N A 1969 Cavernous hemangioma of the ovary. Gynaecologia 168: 248–257

Glendenning W E, Herdt J E, Black T B 1963 Ovarian fibromas and mesenteric cysts: their association with hereditary basal cell cancer of the skin. American Journal of Obstetrics and Gynecology 87: 1008–1012

Gorlin R D, Sedano H O 1971 The multiple nevoid basal cell carcinoma syndrome. Birth Defects 7: 140–148

Griffin N B 1971 Hemangiomas of the female genital tract. Southern Medical Journal 64: 104–117

Grosieux P 1970 Les fibromes de l'ovaire. Revue Francaise de Gynecologie 65: 95–100

Gruskin P, Osborne N G, Morley G W, Abell M R 1970 Primary endometrial stromatosis of ovary: report of a case. Obstetrics and Gynecology 36: 702–707

Guerard M J, Arguelles M A, Ferenczy A 1983 Rhabdomyosarcoma of the ovary: ultrastructural study of a case and review of the literature. Gynecologic Oncology 15: 325–339

Gunes H A, Egilmez R, Dulger M 1990 Ovarian haemangioma. British Journal of Clinical Practice 44: 734–735

Hart W R, Abell M R 1970 Adipose prosoplasia of ovary. American Journal of Obstetrics and Gynecology 106: 929–931

Hegg C A, Flint A 1990 Neurofibroma of the ovary. Gynecologic Oncology 37: 437–438

Himwich H E 1920 Rhabdomyoma of the ovary. Journal of Cancer Research 5: 227–241

Hines J F, Compton D M, Stacy C G, Potter M E 1990 Pure primary osteosarcoma of the ovary presenting as an extensively calcified adnexal mass: a case report and review of the literature. Gynecologic Oncology 39: 258–263

Hirakawa T, Tsuneyoshi M, Enjoji M, Shigyo R 1988 Ovarian sarcoma with features of telangiectatic osteosarcoma of the bone. American Journal of Surgical Pathology 12: 567–572

Honoré L H, O'Hara K E 1980 Subcapsular adipocytic infiltration of the human ovary: a clinicopathological study of eight cases. European Journal of Obstetrics, Gynecology and Reproductive Biology 10: 13–20

Hughesdon P E 1972 The origin and development of benign stromatosis of the ovary. Journal of Obstetrics and Gynaecology of the British Commonwealth 79: 348–359

Hughesdon P E 1976 The endometrial identity of benign stromatosis of the ovary and its relation to other forms of endometriosis. Journal of Pathology 119: 201–209

Iizuka S, Nagata J, Fukuo S, Kosaka J 1992 A case of rhabdomyoma arising from the ovary. Nippon Sanka Fujinka Gakkai Zasshi 44: 1197–2000

Jones E G, Donova A J 1965 Adenomatoid tumor of the ovary versus mesothelial reaction. American Journal of Obstetrics and Gynecology 92: 694–698

Kalra V B, Kalra R, Sareen P M, Lodra S K, Utreja R K 1981 Leiomyoma of ovary: case report with brief review. Journal of Obstetrics and Gynaecology of India 31: 1037–1038

Kanajet O, Pirkic A 1988 Rhabdomiosarkom ovarija s kasnijim ispadima centrainog nervnog sistema. Jugoslavenska Ginekologija Perinatologisa (Zagreb) 28: 44–47

Kandalaft P L, Esteban J L 1992 Bilateral massive ovarian leiomyomata in a young woman: a case report with review of the literature. Modern Pathology 5: 586–589

Karogozov A, Chakalova G, Ganchev G 1990 Riaduk sluchai na gigantski ovarialen leiomiosarkom. Akush Erstvo Ginekologiia (Sofia) 29: 70–72

Kela K, Aurdra A L 1980 Haemangioma of the ovary. Journal of the Indian Medical Association 75: 201–202

Keller O, Rygh O 1964 A case of stromal endometriosis originating from ovarian endometriosis. Acta Obstetricia et Gynecologica Scandinavica 39: 178–183

Keller R 1927 L'hemangiome de l'ovaire. Gynecologie et Obstetrique 16: 405–407

Khaffaf N, Khaffaf H, Wuketich S 1996 Giant ovarian leiomyoma as a rare cause of acute abdomen and hydronephrosis. Obstetrics and Gynecology 87: 872–873

Khanna S, Mehrota M L, Basumallik M 1979 Lymphangioma cavernosum of the ovary. International Surgery 63: 104–105

Kleitsman R J 1949a Ein Beitrag zur Kenntnis der Leiomyomes des Ovariums. Acta Obstetricia et Gynecologica Scandinavica 29: 161–174

Kleitsman R J 1949b Zur Kasuistik der Eierstocksfibroma. Acta Obstetricia et Gynecologica Scandinavica 29: 234–245

Kobayashi Y, Murakami R, Sugizaki K et al 1998 Primary leiomyoma of the ovary: a case report. European Radiology 8: 1444–1446

Kohno A, Yoshikawa W, Yunoki M, Yanagida T, Fukunaga S 1999 MR findings in degenerated ovarian leiomyoma. British Journal of Radiology 72: 1213–1215

Kraemer B B, Silva E G, Sneige N 1984 Fibrosarcoma of ovary: a new component in the nevoid basal-cell carcinoma syndrome. American Journal of Surgical Pathology 8: 231–236

La Manna D 1936 Ueber Myoblastome. Virchows Archiv A Pathological Anatomy and Histology 294: 663–691

Lee M J, Dockerty M B, Thompson G J, Waugh J M 1950 Benign mesotheliomas (adenomatoid tumors) of the genital tract. Surgery, Gynecology and Obstetrics 91: 221–231

Lifschitz-Mercer B, Leider-Trejo L, Messer G, Peyser M R, Czernobilsky B 1998 Primary angiosarcoma of the ovary: a clinicopathologic, immuno-histochemical and electronmicroscopic study. Pathology Research and Practice 194: 183–187

Lorentzen M 1980 Giant cell tumour of the ovary. Virchows Archiv A Pathological Anatomy and Histology 388: 113–122

Loubiere R, Ette M, Boury-Heyler G, Sangaret M, Chesney Y, Reynaud R 1968 Sur deux cas de tumeurs lymphangiomateuses de l'ovaire. Annales d'Anatomie Pathologique 16: 133–177

Lyday R O 1952 Fibroma of the ovary with abdominal implants. American Journal of Surgery 84: 737–738

McBurney R C, Trumbull M 1955 Hemangioma of the ovary with ascites. Mississippi Doctor 32: 271–274

McCluggage W G, Sloan J M, Boyle D D, Toner P G 1998 Malignant fibrothecomatous tumour of the ovary: diagnostic value of anti-inhibin immunostaining. Journal of Clinical Pathology 51: 868–871

Majmudar B, Kapernick P S, Phillips R S 1978 Ovarian myxoma. Human Pathology 9: 723–725

Mani M, Okamury H, Takenaka A et al 1975 A light and electron microscopic study of ovarian leiomyosarcoma. Acta Obstetrica et Gynecologica Japonica 30: 671–677

Mann L S, Metrick S 1961 Hemangioma of the ovary: report of a case. Journal of International College of Surgeons 36: 500–502

Martins S M, Klinger O J 1964 Bilateral ovarian fibromas before the menopause. American Journal of Obstetrics and Gynecology 87: 381–390

Masson P, Riopelle J L, Simard L C 1942 Le mesotheliome benin de la sphere genital. Revue Canadienne de Biologie 1: 720–751

Masubuchi K, Kumura M, Suzumura H 1970 Case of ovarian myxoma. Japanese Journal of Cancer Clinics 16: 156–159

Matamala M F, Nogales F F, Aneiros J, Herraiz M A, Caracuel M D 1988 Leiomyomas of the ovary. International Journal of Gynecological Pathology 7: 190–196

Mazella G 1963 Sul fibroma del ovaio. Rassegna Internazionale di Clinica e Terapia 43: 28–38

Meyer R 1943 Nerve tumors of the female genitals and pelvis. Archives of Pathology 36: 437–464

Meylan J 1958 Hemangio-endotheliome de l'ovaire (a propos des tumeurs ovariennes d'origine vasculaire). Annales d'Anatomie Pathologique 3: 558–594

Michael C A 1966 Pelvic fibroma causing recurrent attacks of hypoglycemia in a post-menopausal patient. Proceedings of the Royal Society of Medicine 59: 835

Mira J L 1991 Lipoleiomyoma of the ovary: report of a case and review of the English literature. International Journal of Gynecological Pathology 10: 198–202

Mishura V I 1963 Report of large benign tumour: three cases. Voprosy Onkologii 9: 102–106

Miyauchi J, Mukai M, Yamazaki K et al 1987 Bilateral ovarian hemangiomas associated with diffuse hemangioendotheliomatosis: a case report. Acta Pathologica Japonica 37: 1347–1355

Monk B J, Nieberg R, Berek J S 1993 Primary leiomyosarcoma of the ovary in a perimenarchal female. Gynecologic Oncology 48: 389–393

Moore J H 1945 Leiomyoma of the ovary complicating pregnancy. American Journal of Obstetrics and Gynecology 50: 244

Morgante G, Bernabei A, Facchini C, Mazzini M Fava A 1995 Leiomyoma of the ovary: case report. Clinical and Experimental Obstetrics and Gynecology 22: 312–314

Nara M, Sasaki T, Shimura S et al 1996 Diffuse alveolar hemorrhage caused by lung metastasis of ovarian angiosarcoma. Internal Medicine 35: 653–656

Nasu M, Inoue J, Matsui M, Minoura S, Matsubara O 2000 Ovarian leiomyosarcoma: an autopsy case report. Pathology International 50: 162–165

Nielsen G P, Young R E 2001 Mesenchymal tumors and tumor-like lesions of the female genital tract: a selective review with emphasis on recently described entities. International Journal of Gynecological Pathology 20: 105–127

Nielsen G P, Young R H, Prat J, Scully R E 1997 Primary angiosarcoma of the ovary: a report of 7 cases and review of the literature. International Journal of Gynecological Pathology 16: 378–382

Nielsen G P, Oliva A, Young R H, Rosenberg A E, Prat J, Scully R E 1998 Primary ovarian rhabdomyosarcoma: a report of 13 cases. International Journal of Gynecological Pathology 17: 113–119

Nieminen U von, Numers C, Parola E 1969 Primary sarcoma of the ovary. Acta Obstetricia et Gynecologica Scandinavica 48: 423–432

Nogales F F, Ayala A, Ruiz-Avila I, Sirvent J J 1991 Myxoid leiomyosarcoma of the ovary: analysis of three cases. Human Pathology 22: 1268–1273

Nucci M R, Krausz T, Lifschitz-Mercer B, Chan J K C, Fletcher C D M 1998 Angiosarcoma of the ovary: clinicopathologic and immunohistochemical analysis of four cases with a broad morphologic spectrum. American Journal of Surgical Pathology 22: 620–630

Nunez C, Abboud S L, Lemon N C, Kemp J A 1981 Ovarian rhabdomyosarcoma presenting as leukemia: case report. Cancer 52: 297–300

Okamura H, Virutamasen P, Wright K H, Wallach E E 1972 Ovarian smooth muscle in the human being, rabbit and cat: histochemical and electron microscopic study. American Journal of Obstetrics and Gynecology 112: 183–191

Ongkasuwan C, Taylor J E, Tang C K, Prempree T 1982 Angiosarcomas of the uterus and ovary: clinicopathologic report. Cancer 49: 1469–1475

O'Sullivan S G, Das-Narla L, Ferraro E 1998 Primary ovarian leiomyosarcoma in an adolescent following radiation for medulloblastoma. Pediatric Radiology 28: 468–470

Paliez R, Delecour M, Duponi A, Monnier J C, Begueri F, Houcke M 1970 Lymphangiome ovarien: a propos d'une observation. Bulletin de la Federation des Societies de Gynecologie et d'Obstetrique de Langue Francaise 22: 51–53

Palladino V S, Trousdell M 1969 Extra-uterine Mullerian tumors: a review of the literature and the report of a case. Cancer 23: 1413–1422

Patel T, Ohri S K, Sundaresan M et al 1991 Metastatic angiosarcoma of the ovary. European Journal of Gynaecological Oncology 17: 295–299

Payan H 1965 Rhabdomyosarcoma of the ovary. Obstetrics and Gynecology 26: 393–395

Payne J F 1869 Vascular tumours of the liver, suprarenal capsule and other organs. Transactions of the Pathological Society of London 20: 203–205

Pethe V V, Chitale S V, Godbole R N, Bidaye S V 1991 Haemangioma of the ovary: case report and review of literature. Indian Journal of Pathology and Microbiology 34: 290–292

Pezullo G 1960 Endothelioma ovarico. Rassegna Internazionale di Clinica e Terapia 40: 481–488

Piura B, Rabinovich A, Yanal-Invar I, Cohen Y, Glezernan M 1998 Primary sarcoma of the ovary: report of five cases and review of the literature. European Journal of Gynaecological Oncology 19: 257–261

Platt J S, Rogers S J, Flynn E A, Taylor R R 1999 Primary angiosarcoma of the ovary: a case report and review of the literature. Gynecologic Oncology 73: 443–446

Prat J, Scully R E 1979 Sarcomas in ovarian mucinous tumors: a report of two cases. Cancer 44: 1327–1331

Prat J, Scully R E 1981 Cellular fibromas and fibrosarcoma of the ovary: a comparative clinicopathologic analysis of seventeen cases. Cancer 47: 2663–2670

Prayson R A, Hart W R 1992 Primary smooth-muscle tumors of the ovary: a clinicopathologic study of four leiomyomas and two mitotically active leiomyomas. Archives of Pathology and Laboratory Medicine 116: 1068–1071

Presno-Bastiony J A, Puente-Duany S 1929 Consideraciones sobre un caso de hemangioma del ovario. Revista de Medicina v Cirugia Habana 34: 165–173

Prus D, Rosenberg A E, Blumenfeld A et al 1997 Infantile hemangioendothelioma of the ovary: a monodermal teratoma or a neoplasm of ovarian somatic cells? American Journal of Surgical Pathology 21: 1231–1235

Raggio M, Kaplan A L, Harberg J F 1983 Recurrent ovarian fibromas with basal cell nevus syndrome (Gorlin syndrome). Obstetrics and Gynecology 60: 955–965

Raj-Kumar G 1982 Leiomyosarcoma of probable ovarian or broad ligament origin. British Journal of Obstetrics and Gynaecology 89: 327–329

Randrianjafisamindrakotroka N S, Chadli-Debbiche A, Philipe E 1994 Les leiomyomes de l'ovaire: a propos de douze cas. Archive de Annatomie, Cytologie et Pathologie 42: 26–28

Rice M, Pearson B, Treadwell W B 1943 Malignant lymphangioma of the ovary. American Journal of Obstetrics and Gynecology 45: 884–889

Rio F 1956 Contributo allo studio di rare neoplasie ovariche (rhab-domyosarcoma). Rivista Italiana di Ginecologia 39: 218–228

Rodriguez M A 1979 Hemangioma of the ovary in an 81-year-old woman. Southern Medical Journal 72: 503–504

Sakata H, Hirahara T, Ryu A et al 1991 Primary osteosarcoma of the ovary: a case report. Acta Pathologica Japonica 41: 311–317

Sandison A T 1955 Rhabdomyosarcoma of the ovary. Journal of Pathology and Bacteriology 70: 433–438

Sant'Ambrogio S, Malpica A, Schroeder B, Silva E G 2000 Primary ovarian rhabdomyosarcoma associated with clear cell carcinoma of the ovary: a case report and review of the literature. International Journal of Gynecological Pathology 19: 169–173

Sari I, Kurt A, Kadanali S, Gundogdu C, Bitiren M 1995 Leiomyoma of the ovary: report of two cases and review of the literature. Acta Obstetricia et Gynecologica Scandinavica 74: 480–482

Sato Y, Tanaka T 1998 An ovarian leiomyoma: a case report. Journal of Obstetric and Gynecologic Research 24: 349–354

Schaeffer M H, Cancelmo J J 1939 Cavernous hemangioma of ovary in a girl twelve years of age. American Journal of Obstetrics and Gynecology 38: 723–772

Scheinman H Z, McKenna A J, Rutner N 1982 Ovarian hemangioma with acute abdominal pain. Mount Sinai Journal of Medicine 49: 133–135

Schmeisser H C, Anderson W A D 1938 Ganglioneuroma of the ovary. Journal of the American Medical Association 111: 2005–2007

Scully R E, Young R H, Clement P B 1998 Tumors of the ovary, maldeveloped gonads, Fallopian tube, and broad ligament. Atlas of tumour pathology, third series, fascicle 23. Armed Forces Institute of Pathology, Washington DC

Sengupta S, Daita P, Pal A 1979 Ovarian fibroma with massive calcification. Journal of the Indian Medical Association 72: 64–65

Serrapiao C J, Serrapiao M J 1964 'Tumour adenomatoid' de ovario. Hospital (Rio) 66: 177–182

Shakfeh S M, Woodruff J D 1987 Primary ovarian sarcomas: report of 46 cases and review of the literature. Obstetrical and Gynecological Survey 42: 331–349

Shearer J P 1935 Hemangioma of the ovary: reported in a child 3 years of age. Medical Annals of the District of Columbia 4: 223–224

Shipton E A, Meares S D 1965 Heterotopic bone formation in the ovary. Australian and New Zealand Journal of Obstetrics and Gynaecology 5: 100–102

Shiraki M, Otis C N, Powell J L 1991 Endometrial stromal sarcoma arising from ovarian and extraovarian endometriosis-report of two cases and review of the literature. Surgical Pathology 4: 333–343

Siddall R S, Clinton W R 1937 Lymphangioma of the ovary. American Journal of Obstetrics and Gynecology 34: 306–310

Siddiqui M, Toub D B 1995 Cellular fibroma of the ovary with Meigs' syndrome and elevated CA-125: a case report. Journal of Reproductive Medicine 40: 817–819

Silverberg S G, Nogales F 1981 Endolymphatic stromal myosis of the ovary: a report of three cases and literature review. Gynecologic Oncology 12: 129–138

Smith F R 1931 Neurofibroma of the ovary associated with Recklinghausen's disease. American Journal of Cancer 15: 859–862

Sovak F W, Carabba V 1931 Hemangioendothelioma intravasculare of the ovary. American Journal of Obstetrics and Gynecology 21: 544–550

Spies H, Lorenz G 1973 Rhabdomyosarkom bei Ovars in Kindesalter. Zentralblatt für Gynekologie 95: 1322–1325

Spinelli C, Gadducci A, Bonadio A G, Berti P, Miccoli P 1999 Benign ovarian fibroma associated with free peritoneal fluid and elevated serum CA 125 levels. Minerva Ginecologica 51: 403–407

Srinivasa Rao K, Subuadra Devi N 1967 Rhabdomyosarcoma of ovary. Journal of Obstetrics and Gynaecology of India 17: 93–95

Talerman A 1967 Hemangiomas of the ovary and the uterine cervix. Obstetrics and Gynecology 30: 108–113

Talerman A, Ayerbach W M, van Meurs A J 1981 Primary chondrosarcoma of the ovary. Histopathology 5: 319–324

Teel P 1958 Adenomatoid tumor of the genital tract with special reference to the female. American Journal of Obstetrics and Gynecology 75: 1347–1355

Tetu B, Bonenfant J L 1991 Ovarian myxoma: a study of two cases with long-term follow-up. American Journal of Clinical Pathology 95: 340–346

Thay T Y, Orizaga M, Campbell J S, de Saint Victor H 1973 Leiomyoma of ovary. European Journal of Obstetrics, Gynecology and Reproductive Biology 3: 51–55

Toth F, Csomor S, Zambo A 1971 Primares Ovarialfibrosarkome bei einer 71 jahrigen Patientin. Strahlentherapie 141: 44–46

Tsalacopoulos G, Tiltman A T 1981 Leiomyoma of the ovary: a report of 3 cases. South African Medical Journal 59: 574–575

Tsuji T, Kawauchi S, Utsunomiya T, Nagata Y, Tsuneyoshi M 1997 Fibrosarcoma versus cellular fibroma of the ovary: a comparative study of their proliferative activity and chromosome aberrations using MIB-1 immunostaining, DNA flow cytometry, and fluorescence in situ hybridization. American Journal of Surgical Pathology 21: 52–59

Tsujimura T, Kawano K 1992 Rhabdomyosarcoma coexistent with ovarian mucinous cystadenocarcinoma: a case report. International Journal of Gynecological Pathology 11: 58–62

Twu N F, Juang C M, Yeng M S, Lu C J, Lai C Z, Chao K C 1999 Treatment of primary pure angiosarcoma of ovary with multiple lung metastases: a case report. European Journal of Gynaecological Oncology 20: 383–385

Variati G, Donatelli G F 1966 Il sarcoma dell ovaio (contributo casistico anatomo-clinico) Annali di Obstetricia e Ginecologia 88: 440–453

Vierhout H E, Pijpers L, Tham M N, Chadha-Ajwani S 1990 Leiomyoma of the ovary. Acta Obstetricia et Gynecologica Scandinavica 69: 445–447

Vignard E 1889 Tumeur solide de l'ovaire a fibres striees chez une jeune fille de 17 ans. Bulletin de Societe d'Anatomie 64: 33–36

von Numers C, Mikkonen R 1960 Leiomyosarcoma arising in serous cystadenoma of ovary. Annales Chirurgiae et Gynaecologiae Fenniae 49: 240–244

Walts A E, Lichtenstein I 1977 Primary leiomyosarcoma associated with serous cystadenocarcinoma of the ovary. Gynecologic Oncology 5: 81–86

Wellman K F 1961 Leiomyoma of the ovary: report of an unusual case and review of the literature. Canadian Medical Association Journal 85: 429–432

Young R H, Scully R E 1983 Ovarian stromal tumors with minor sex cord elements: a report of seven cases. International Journal of Gynecological Pathology 2: 277–284

Young R H, Scully R E 1990 Sarcomas metastatic to the ovary: a report of 21 cases. International Journal of Gynecological Pathology 9: 231–252

Young R H, Prat J, Scully R E 1984 Endometrioid stromal sarcomas of the ovary: a clinicopathologic analysis of 23 cases. Cancer 53: 1143–1155

Zheng W, Sung C J, Hanna I et al 1997 Alpha and beta subunits of inhibin/activin as sex cord-stromal differentiation markers. International Journal of Gynecological Pathology 16: 263–271

25

Metastatic tumours of the ovary

H. Fox

Mechanisms of tumour spread to the ovary   879

Incidence of metastatic ovarian tumours   880

Pathology and clinical aspects of metastatic ovarian
   neoplasms   881
Specific forms of metastatic ovarian neoplasia   881
Krukenberg tumours   890

The ovary shares with the liver and the lung the dubious distinction of being a common, indeed often a preferential, site of tumour metastasis. Just why this should be so is unknown for there are no obvious features of the ovary which make it such a suitable 'soil' for secondary tumour growth.

MECHANISMS OF TUMOUR SPREAD TO THE OVARY

There are four possible pathways by which extragonadal tumours may spread to the ovary:

1. Direct spread
Direct extension of tumour from a primary site to the ovary occurs most commonly in cases of carcinoma of the Fallopian tube, endometrium and colon. This form of spread is sometimes along bridges provided by adhesions.
2. Surface implantation
Transcoelomic spread with surface implantation accounts for most cases of ovarian involvement in generalised peritoneal metastases but is sometimes an isolated phenomenon, this latter being particularly true for metastatic breast carcinoma. Surface implantation also occurs when an endometrial adenocarcinoma metastasises to the ovary via the tubal lumen.
3. Lymphatic spread
This is a common pathway of ovarian metastasis, partly because of the rich network of lymphatic channels in the pelvis. Blaustein (1982) has pointed out that metastatic breast carcinoma in the ovary may be limited to clumps of tumour cells in the lymphatic vessels of the ovarian medulla, a finding which suggests that spread of mammary carcinoma to the ovary may well be, at least partly, via the lymphatic system. It is possible that gastric carcinoma also spreads to the ovary via the lumbar lymphatics, which connect with both the lymphatic vessels of the upper gastrointestinal tract and those of the ovary.
4. Haematogenous spread
This is probably a very common mode of ovarian metastasis, for metastatic tumour is often seen within ovarian

blood vessels. The high incidence of ovarian metastases in young women with cancer may well be a reflection of the rich vascularisation of the gonads during the reproductive years.

INCIDENCE OF METASTATIC OVARIAN TUMOURS

The true frequency with which metastases occur in the ovary is extremely difficult to establish, for some surveys have been restricted to autopsy cases, others to tumours encountered at operation and yet others to the incidence of clinically silent metastases from breast carcinomas in ovaries removed for therapeutic purposes (Scully 1979). In theory, autopsy studies should produce the most accurate figures but, unfortunately, data derived from many autopsy series are of little value — either because the cases studied have included both males and females without giving any indication as to the proportions of each or because they have included women dying from both malignant and non-malignant disease without stating the numbers in each group. Even some of the surveys limited solely to women with malignant disease have blurred the issue by including cases of lymphoma. In Manchester, Fox & Langley (1976) found that amongst 272 women dying of malignant disease, ovarian metastases were present in 4.4%: if only women with metastatic malignant disease were included the incidence of ovarian involvement rose to just over 6%. This is a figure which is roughly comparable to that found in other autopsy studies of women dying of malignant disease (Warren & Macomber 1935; Walther 1948; Willis 1952) though in none of these series were the ovaries studied histologically in all, or even most, cases. The significance of this deficiency was shown by Virieux (1962) who found ovarian metastases in 37% of women succumbing to malignant disease: in 60% of the patients with ovarian involvement the ovaries were, however, not obviously abnormal on naked-eye examination and metastatic tumour was only detectable on histological examination. Luisi (1968), in a similar study, found ovarian metastases in 29% of women dying of carcinoma whilst Fujiwara et al (1995) found metastases in the ovaries of 19.2% of women dying from malignant non-lymphomatous disease and in nearly a quarter of these cases the metastases were occult, being of microscopic size and being present in macroscopically normal ovaries. Taken together these three series suggest that the true incidence of ovarian involvement in women with malignant disease is between 20 and 30%. The incidence varies, of course, with the site of the primary tumour: thus ovarian metastases have been noted in 50% of women with gastric carcinoma (Virieux 1962) or renal carcinoma (Fujiwara et al 1995), in 44% of fatal cases of breast carcinoma (Turksoy 1960; Virieux 1962; Luisi 1968), in 30% with colonic carcinomas (Virieux 1962)

and in 16% of women with malignant melanomas (DasGupta & Brasfield 1964). Figures quoted for the incidence of metastasis of genital tract cancer to the ovaries are very variable, those for cervical carcinoma ranging from less than 1% to over 40% and those for endometrial carcinoma from nil to 60% (Finn 1951; Luisi 1968; Fox & Langley 1976).

Of more importance both to the pathologist and the gynaecologist is the proportion of apparently primary malignant ovarian tumours which eventually turn out to be metastases. Studies from England, Scandinavia and the United States suggest that between 13 and 18% of malignant ovarian carcinomas are metastatic rather than primary (Parnanen & Vataja 1954; von Numers 1960; Israel et al 1965; Fox & Langley 1976) though a much lower incidence of 6–7% has also been quoted (Santesson & Kottmeier 1968; Ulbright et al 1984; Perucchini et al 1996). By contrast, in a series from Turkey metastatic tumours accounted for 21.5% of all malignant ovarian neoplasms (Ayhan et al 1995), though this series contained a suspiciously high proportion of metastases from endometrial carcinomas. Metastatic tumours

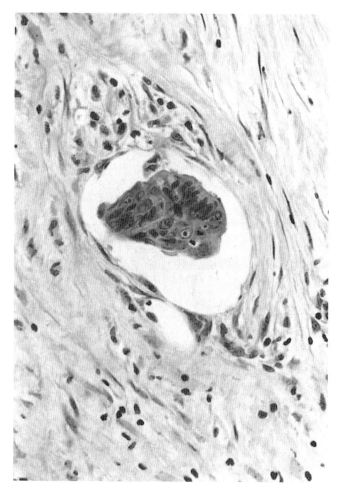

Fig. 25.1 Vascular invasion in a metastatic carcinoma of the ovary.

masquerading as primary ovarian neoplasms stem most commonly from the stomach, large intestine and breast (Johansson 1960; Mazur et al 1984; Ulbright et al 1984; Perucchini et al 1996).

PATHOLOGY AND CLINICAL ASPECTS OF METASTATIC OVARIAN NEOPLASMS

Only those neoplasms which do not show the typical and specific features of a Krukenberg tumour are discussed in this section: Krukenberg tumours are a distinctive and specific form of metastatic neoplasm which merit, and will receive, separate consideration.

Metastatic tumours are commonly bilateral (about 60% of cases) and may appear as a diffusely solid tumour, as multiple solid nodules of tumour, as a partly cystic mass or, rather uncommonly, as entirely cystic lesions; extensive areas of haemorrhage and/or necrosis are common. Histologically, the tumours show a variety of patterns which depend, to some extent, on the site of the primary tumour: most are adenocarcinomas and the ovarian deposits may have a similar appearance to the primary tumour, may be less well differentiated or can be better differentiated. Features indicative of a metastatic tumour include extensive areas of necrosis, surface implants, a multifocal pattern and vascular invasion (Fig. 25.1), this latter feature being highly suggestive, though not pathognomonic, of secondary neoplasia. Stromal luteinization occurs much more commonly with metastatic tumours than it does with primary ovarian neoplasms.

SPECIFIC FORMS OF METASTATIC OVARIAN NEOPLASIA

Metastasis from mammary carcinoma

In both autopsy series and in studies of ovaries removed for therapeutic purposes in women with disseminated breast carcinoma the incidence of ovarian metastases is in the region of 24–40% (Saphir 1951; Johansson 1960; Brickman & Ferreira 1967; Harris et al 1984): in women in whom the ovaries have been removed prophylactically in the absence of overt metastatic disease the incidence of ovarian involvement has ranged from 2–11% (Scully 1979). Ovarian metastases are rarely the initial clinical manifestation of a mammary carcinoma, the ovarian tumours usually becoming manifest at intervals ranging from six months to 19 years after the initial diagnosis of carcinoma of the breast. Young et al (1981) have described a small series of cases of mammary cancer in which the initial manifestation was an ovarian tumour, but the very fact that such cases merit recording attests to their rarity.

Metastatic breast carcinoma in the ovary is bilateral in about 60% of cases and the involved ovary either contains multiple nodules of firm or gritty white tissue or is completely replaced by a smooth or bosselated mass; very rarely the metastatic neoplasm is predominantly cystic. Histologically, the metastatic tumour often replicates the pattern seen in the primary breast neoplasm. Lobular carcinoma of the breast has a particular tendency to metastasise to the ovary where it tends to retain its characteristic 'Indian-file' pattern (Fig. 25.2), the tumour cells often being found, in early cases, in the walls of follicles or corpora lutea (Scully 1979). Metastatic tumour of ductal origin may closely resemble an undifferentiated primary ovarian carcinoma but tends to have a more multifocal pattern. Metastatic ductal carcinoma commonly grows in nests, cords, solid tubules or diffuse sheets but glandular and microacinar patterns may also be encountered (Gagnon & Tetu 1989; Young & Scully 1991b). Ovarian metastases of breast carcinoma usually stain positively for gross cystic disease fluid protein-15 and are often positive for oestrogen receptors (Monteagudo et al 1991; Lagendijk et al 1999).

Death usually ensues in less than 12 months after detection of clinically apparent ovarian metastases of

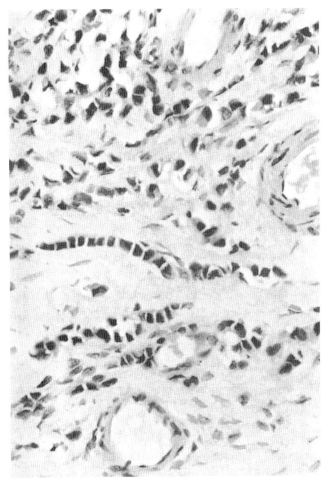

Fig. 25.2 An ovarian metastasis from a lobular carcinoma of the breast. The metastasis replicates the 'Indian-file' pattern seen in primary breast neoplasms of this type.

mammary carcinoma (Johansson 1960) though Osborne & Pitts (1961) noted a mean survival time of over 20 months in patients in whom metastases were diagnosed only by histological examination of therapeutic oophorectomy specimens.

Metastases from large intestinal carcinoma

The overall incidence of metastasis of colorectal cancer to the ovary is probably in the region of 30% (Virieux 1962) and in a small proportion of cases (probably about 3%) an ovarian mass is the presenting symptom or sign of an intestinal neoplasm (Harcourt & Dennis 1968; Herrera-Ornelas et al 1983). The incidence of overt ovarian metastases at the time of initial surgery for an intestinal neoplasm is 3.7% but if prophylactically removed, microscopically normal, ovaries are examined histologically, metastatic deposits will be found in a further 4.5% (Graffner et al 1983): this has prompted the suggestion that prophylactic oophorectomy should be undertaken at the time of initial surgery in all women with intestinal carcinoma (Harcourt & Dennis 1968; O'Brien et al 1981; Cutait et al 1983; Graffner et al 1983; Morrow & Enker 1984), a course of action that has not achieved any success, in terms of survival, in recent series (Sielezneff et al 1997; Young-Fadok et al 1998).

The metastatic tumours (Fig. 25.3) may be solid but are usually either partly or wholly cystic (Scully & Richardson 1961; Scully 1979; Ulbright et al 1984; Lash & Hart 1987; Daya et al 1992); on section they are formed of soft yellowish, red or grey tissue with cystic areas that may contain necrotic material, old or fresh blood, clear fluid or mucinous fluid (Scully 1979). The tumours are unilateral in a high proportion of cases. Histologically, the metastatic tumour tends to show either

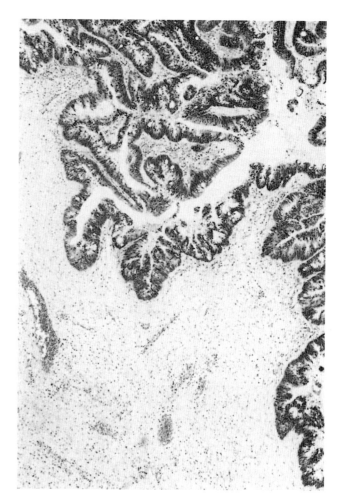

Fig. 25.4 Histological appearances of a typical ovarian metastasis from an intestinal adenocarcinoma. The pattern is virtually identical to that of a primary mucinous adenocarcinoma of the ovary.

a mucinous or, more commonly, an endometrioid pattern whilst the stroma, which is usually of ovarian type, may be oedematous or show a desmoplastic reaction. A small proportion of metastatic colonic carcinomas have a pattern which mimics that of a primary ovarian clear cell carcinoma (Young & Hart 1998).

The histological distinction between a metastasis from an intestinal neoplasm showing a mucinous pattern (Fig. 25.4) and a primary ovarian mucinous adenocarcinoma can be extremely difficult and is sometimes impossible. Ulbright et al (1984) noted that a mucus cell predominant pattern occurred at least locally in 82% of primary ovarian mucinous adenocarcinomas whereas this pattern was found in only 11% of metastatic intestinal neoplasms: a transition from benign-appearing epithelium to atypical or frankly malignant epithelium was found in 90% of primary mucinous neoplasms but this feature does not unequivocally rule out a metastatic tumour, for a similar appearance was found in 11% of metastases from intestinal carcinomas. Other features noted by Ulbright et al (1984) as indicating a metastatic rather than a

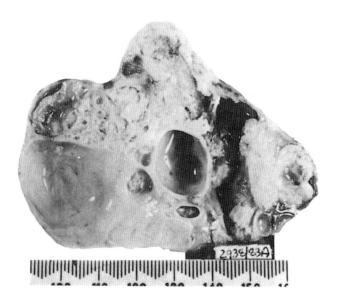

Fig. 25.3 Macroscopic appearances of an ovarian metastasis from an intestinal carcinoma.

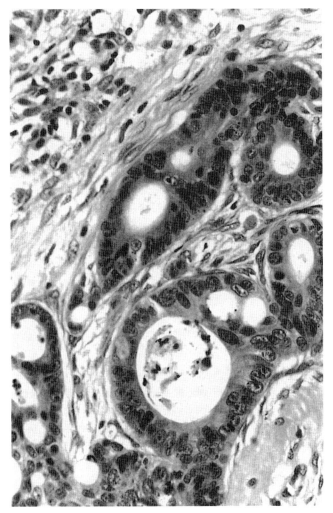

Fig. 25.5 An ovarian metastasis from an intestinal adenocarcinoma which has an 'endometrioid' pattern and resembles closely a primary endometrioid adenocarcinoma of the ovary.

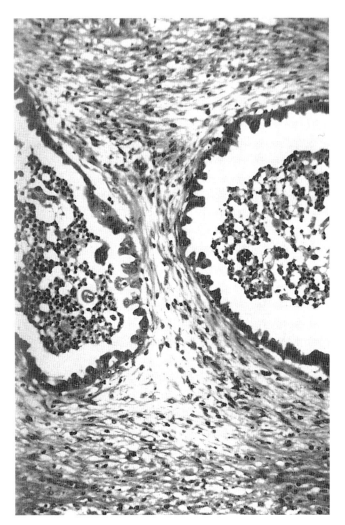

Fig. 25.6 An ovarian metastasis from an intestinal adenocarcinoma. The lumens of the neoplastic glands contain 'dirty' necrotic and inflammatory debris.

primary mucinous neoplasm were bilaterality, extensive areas of necrosis, denser more eosinophilic cytoplasm and a more frequent and prominent striated border.

The distinction between a metastatic intestinal tumour with an endometrioid pattern (Fig. 25.5) and a primary endometrioid carcinoma of the ovary can also be extremely difficult. It has been suggested that histological features indicative of a metastatic neoplasm include extensive confluent necrosis, the presence (Fig. 25.6) within gland lumena and cysts of eosinophilic debris containing nuclear fragments ('dirty necrosis'), focal segmental necrosis of glandular epithelium (Fig. 25.7) and a so-called 'garland' pattern in which there is a clustering of glands around an area of necrosis (Lash & Hart 1987; Daya et al 1992). DeCostanzo et al (1997) found, however, that over two-thirds of primary ovarian carcinomas showed a variable degree of 'dirty' necrosis and concluded that this feature was of no value in distinguishing primary ovarian carcinoma from metastatic colonic carci-

noma. In contrast, the presence of endometriosis or of squamous metaplasia will favour the diagnosis of a primary endometrioid carcinoma (Young & Scully 1991b).

The problems encountered in attempting to differentiate between primary ovarian carcinomas and ovarian metastases of colonic carcinoma on histological grounds alone have prompted an intensive search for immunohistochemical markers that could aid in this differential diagnosis. The antibody HAM 56, first used to identify macrophages and endothelial cells, stains many primary ovarian carcinomas and it was proposed that this allowed for a distinction from colonic metastases which stained negatively with this antibody (Loy & Abshier 1993: Fowler et al 1994; Younes et al 1994). Cheung et al (1997) found, however, that although HAM 56 stained ovarian carcinomas most commonly it also stained adenocarcinomas arising from several other sites and, more particularly, gave a positive reaction in 21% of colonic carcinomas, these findings diminishing considerably the

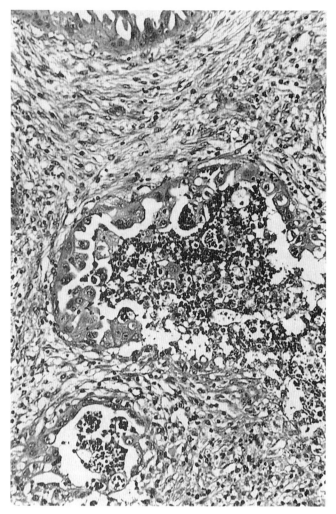

Fig. 25.7 An ovarian metastasis from an intestinal adenocarcinoma. The centrally placed gland shows segmental necrosis of its lining epithelium.

diagnostic value of this antibody. Immunohistochemical staining for carcino-embryonic antigen (CEA) is of help in distinguishing metastatic intestinal cancer with an endometrioid pattern from a primary ovarian endometrioid adenocarcinoma, the former showing strong immunoreactivity and the latter either no, or only weak, focal reactivity; unfortunately, however, CEA immunostaining is of no value in the differentiation between metastatic tumours showing a mucinous pattern and primary mucinous adenocarcinomas, both showing equally strong staining (Lash & Hart 1987). Staining for CEA is also of value in distinguishing those metastatic colonic carcinomas having a clear cell pattern, which stain positively for this antigen, from primary clear cell carcinomas of the ovary which are usually CEA negative. Staining for cytokeratins (CK) has proved to be of considerable diagnostic value for primary ovarian carcinomas are usually CK 7 positive and CK 20 negative whilst metastatic colonic carcinomas are usually CK 7 negative and CK 20 positive (Wauters et al 1995; Berezowski et al

1996; Loy et al 1996; DeCostanzo et al 1997; Lagendijk et al 1998). The value of these anticytokeratin antibodies is greatest when dealing with tumours showing an endometrioid or a clear cell pattern for a small proportion of primary ovarian mucinous adenocarcinomas are CK 7 negative and/or CK 20 positive (McCluggage 2000). A further aid in distinguishing primary ovarian adenocarcinomas from metastatic colonic adenocarcinomas may be the differential expression of mucin genes. The expression of these genes is relatively organ specific and in a recent study 9 out of 10 metastatic colonic adenocarcinomas stained positively for MUC2 apomucin and none expressed MUC5AC apomucin: by contrast all primary mucinous adenocarcinomas expressed MUC5AC (Albarracin et al 2000).

Nearly all women with untreated ovarian metastases from an intestinal carcinoma are dead within three years of diagnosis and over 50% succumb within one year (Johansson 1960; Richardson 1967). These gloomy figures do not necessarily imply, however, that surgical resection of an ovarian metastasis is of no value: Morrow & Enker (1984) found that whilst the mean survival for women with non-resectable ovarian metastases from large bowel cancer was 9.8 months, that for patients with resectable tumours was 48 months. Taylor et al (1995), by contrast, found a very poor survival rate for women with surgically treated metastatic colorectal cancer and noted a very poor response to chemotherapy. A few women (probably about 5%) do, however, survive for five or more years following simple surgical resection (Webb et al 1975) whilst a 23% five-year survival rate has been achieved with aggressive surgery (Petru et al 1992): others have also found that prolonged survival could be achieved in occasional patients by aggressive surgery (Miller et al 1997; Huang et al 1998).

Metastases from appendiceal carcinomas

Ovarian metastases from carcinoma of the appendix are not commonly encountered, largely because primary neoplasms at this site are relatively rare; nevertheless ovarian metastases are present in 10% of women with appendiceal carcinomas and amongst such patients the ovarian lesion is the presenting feature in 25–30% (Merino et al 1985; Thorsen et al 1991; Ronnett et al 1997a). The ovarian tumours are usually bilateral and histologically they may have a signet ring cell pattern, with or without glandular or goblet cell differentiation, which mimics metastases from a gastric carcinoma, may mimic a primary mucinous carcinoma of the ovary, may simulate metastatic colorectal cancer or may resemble an endometrioid adenocarcinoma (Ronnett et al 1997a). All ovarian metastases from appendiceal carcinomas appear to be positive for CK 20 but about 50% are also positive for CK 7. Because small appendiceal tumours, which may not be macroscopically obvious, can give rise to large

METASTATIC TUMOURS OF THE OVARY

ovarian metastases it has been suggested that appendicectomy should always be performed in women with apparently primary ovarian neoplasms (Merino et al 1985).

A particular problem is posed by patients in whom a mucinous tumour is present in both the appendix and the ovary in association with pseudomyxoma peritonei. In these cases both the appendiceal and ovarian neoplasms have a histological appearance which resembles either that of a mucinous cystadenoma or, much more commonly in the case of the ovary, a mucinous tumour of borderline malignancy: the ovarian tumours are usually cystic whilst the appendiceal neoplasms appear as mucoceles. Young et al (1991) reviewed 22 such cases and concluded that the ovarian tumours were, despite their bland appearance, metastases from a low-grade mucinous adenocarcinoma of the appendix, basing this view upon the common bilaterality of the ovarian tumours, the predominance of right-sided ovarian involvement and the presence of mucin and atypical cells on the ovarian surfaces. Others disagreed with this concept, maintaining that the ovarian and appendiceal neoplasm are usually independent of each other (Seidman et al 1993). Further histological, immunohistochemical and genetic studies have, however, largely confirmed the original view of Young et al (1991) and it is now widely agreed that in most, though admittedly not all, cases of pseudomyxoma peritonei with concomitant appendiceal and ovarian neoplasms the ovarian tumour is a metastasis from the appendix (Prayson et al 1994; Ronnett et al 1995; Chuaqui et al 1996; Cuatrecasai et al 1996; Guerrieri et al 1997; Ronnett et al 1997b; Seidman et al 2000).

Metastases from pancreatic adenocarcinoma

Ovarian metastases are rarely encountered in patients with pancreatic adenocarcinoma but Young & Hart (1989) described seven women in whom pancreatic adenocarcinomas spread to the ovary and there mimicked primary ovarian mucinous neoplasms: six of the pancreatic tumours were ductal adenocarcinomas whilst one was a mucinous adenocarcinoma. The pancreatic and ovarian neoplasms occurred synchronously in five patients whilst in two the ovarian lesion developed after diagnosis of the pancreatic adenocarcinoma: the clinical features were suggestive of a primary ovarian adenocarcinoma in four cases. The ovarian metastatic tumours were characteristically bilateral, large, cystic and multilocular and histologically usually contained areas resembling mucinous cystadenoma, mucinous tumour of borderline malignancy and mucinous adenocarcinoma. When such an ovarian neoplasm is encountered in the absence of any knowledge that the patient has a pancreatic adenocarcinoma it may be only the bilaterality that serves to raise a suspicion of metastatic tumour, a suspicion hardened if desmoplastic surface implants are present.

Young & Scully (1991b) have also described an ovarian metastasis from a pancreatic microadenocarcinoma: this closely resembled metastatic carcinoid tumour but did not contain argyrophil cells.

Metastases from carcinoma of the gallbladder and extrahepatic bile ducts

The very scanty literature on this topic suggests that between 6 and 12% of biliary neoplasms metastasise to the ovary (Brandt-Rauf et al 1982; Albores-Saavedra & Henson 1986; Lashgari et al 1992). Six examples of ovarian metastases from biliary tract neoplasms were reported by Young & Scully (1990a): in one case the ovarian neoplasm was detected before the biliary tumour became clinically overt but in the other five the ovarian lesion occurred either synchronously with, or developed after, diagnosis of the primary neoplasm. Five of the metastatic ovarian tumours were bilateral and whilst most were solid one was cystic. Two of the metastatic ovarian tumours resembled mucinous neoplasms, one simulated an endometrioid adenocarcinoma and yet another bore a close resemblance to a Sertoli–Leydig cell neoplasm. The three remaining tumours showed appearances resembling closely those of a biliary adenocarcinoma.

Metastases from bronchial carcinoma

Only 5% of bronchial carcinomas metastasise to the ovaries (Galluzzi & Payne 1955; Budinger 1958; Warren & Gates 1964). In most cases the ovarian metastases are an incidental unsuspected finding at autopsy and it is distinctly uncommon for a bronchial neoplasm to present initially as an ovarian tumour. Malviya et al (1982) described, however, a patient in whom an ovarian mass was the initial presentation of a small cell carcinoma of the bronchus whilst Young & Scully (1985) have reported six examples of bronchial neoplasms presenting as ovarian tumours: two of Young & Scully's patients were suffering from undifferentiated small cell carcinomas, one from an undifferentiated carcinoma, one from an adenocarcinoma and one from an atypical carcinoid tumour. Three of these patients had radiological evidence of a pulmonary neoplasm at the time of diagnosis of the ovarian lesion but in the other women evidence of a bronchial tumour did not appear until two, four and 26 months, respectively, after surgical removal of the ovarian metastasis. Notable features of these cases were the relatively young age of the patients (mean age 42 years) and the high incidence, unusual for ovarian metastatic disease, of unilaterality of the ovarian tumours. These two features make diagnosis difficult and in most cases only the application of the general criteria for metastatic disease, e.g. multinodularity, vascular invasion, will assist in the differential diagnosis from primary ovarian adenocarcinoma or, in the case of the metastatic undifferentiated bronchial small cell carcinoma, from the primary ovarian small cell carcinoma with hypercalcaemia: distinction from this latter entity is, however, aided by the fact that most bronchial small cell carcinomas are aneuploid whilst ovarian small cell carcinomas with hypercalcaemia are diploid (Scully 1993). The only histological difference between an ovarian metastasis from a pulmonary small cell carcinoma and the primary ovarian small cell carcinoma of pulmonary type (Eichhorn et al 1992) is the not infrequent presence in the latter of an epithelial component, such as endometrioid carcinoma. In the absence of this feature only a rigorous exclusion of a pulmonary neoplasm will allow for the differentiation of these two entities.

Metastases from carcinoid tumours

Carcinoid tumours of the gastrointestinal tract, pancreas or bronchus may metastasise to the ovary (Robboy et al 1974; Brown et al 1980; Heisterberg et al 1982) where they commonly present as bilateral solid tumours with smooth or bosselated surfaces; the cut surface usually shows multiple, often confluent, masses of firm white or yellow tissue though small cysts containing clear watery fluid may also be present (Robboy et al 1974).

Histologically (Fig. 25.8), metastatic carcinoid tumours usually have either a trabecular or insular pattern but acinar and solid tubular patterns may also be seen: features suggestive of a metastatic, rather than a primary lesion in such cases include bilaterality, multinodularity, the absence of other teratomatous elements and vascular invasion.

Metastatic goblet cell or mucinous carcinoids (Fig. 25.9) form rounded nests containing goblet cells and argentaffin or argyrophil cells (Zirkin et al 1980; Heisterberg et al 1982): this pattern may be admixed with that of a typical mucinous adenocarcinoma (Ikeda et al 1991).

In the 25 non-autopsied cases of metastatic ovarian carcinoid tumour studied by Robboy et al (1974), one-third of the patients died within a year of diagnosis and three-quarters within five years. Six women were, however, well and free of symptoms for periods varying from six months to 29 years (mean of 5.6 years) and this

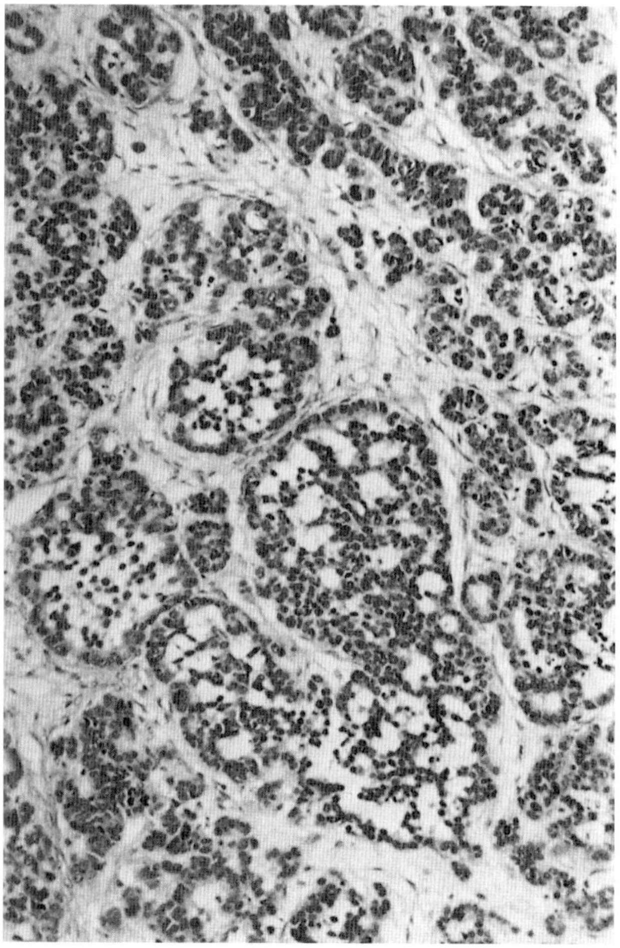

Fig. 25.8 Histological appearances of an ovarian metastasis from an intestinal carcinoid tumour.

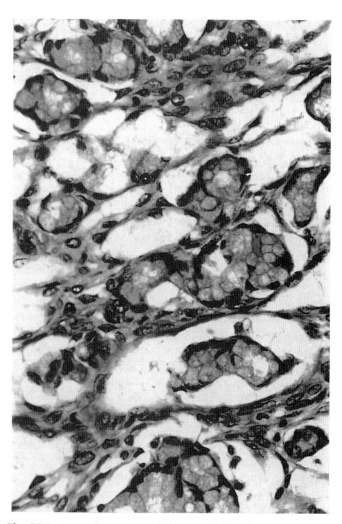

Fig. 25.9 An ovarian metastasis from a goblet cell carcinoid tumour of the terminal ileum.

has led Scully (1979) to suggest that both the metastases and the primary tumour should, if feasible, be removed: Scully further argued that menopausal or postmenopausal women with intestinal carcinoid tumours should have a prophylactic bilateral salpingo-oophorectomy and that all women with bilateral ovarian carcinoid tumours should be subjected to an intensive search for an extraovarian primary lesion.

Metastases from hepatocellular carcinoma

Ovarian metastases from hepatocellular carcinoma are extremely rare but Young et al (1992) have reported three such cases. The ovarian tumours were bilateral in two patients and locally cystic in one case: they ranged from 4–11 cm in maximum diameter and were yellow–green or yellow on section. Histologically, they were composed of cells with moderate to abundant eosinophilic cytoplasm growing diffusely or in nodules, nests or trabeculae (Fig. 25.10); cysts or glandular structures were prominent in two cases and bile was present in one tumour.

In the presence of a known hepatocellular carcinoma, which is usually the case, the diagnosis of an ovarian metastasis is straightforward. If, however, the presentation is with an ovarian tumour, a metastatic hepatocellular carcinoma has to be differentiated from, depending upon the patient's age, a yolk sac tumour showing a hepatoid pattern and from a hepatoid carcinoma. Bilaterality and the presence of bile help in the distinction from a hepatoid carcinoma whilst bilateral ovarian involvement also argues against a diagnosis of a yolk sac neoplasm.

Metastases from renal adenocarcinoma

Renal adenocarcinomas rarely metastasise to the ovary and, indeed, in one autopsy study of 324 women with renal adenocarcinoma no ovarian metastases were encountered (Saitoh 1981). Nevertheless, there have been a number of reports of clinically apparent ovarian metastases from renal adenocarcinoma (Martzloff & Manlove 1949; Vorder-Bruegge et al 1957; Buller et al 1983; Young

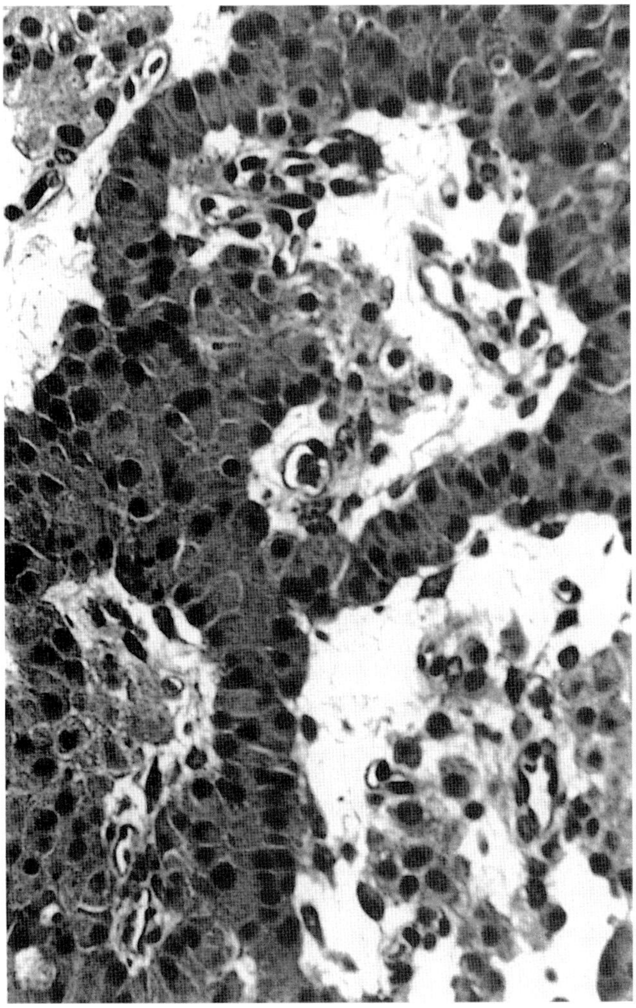

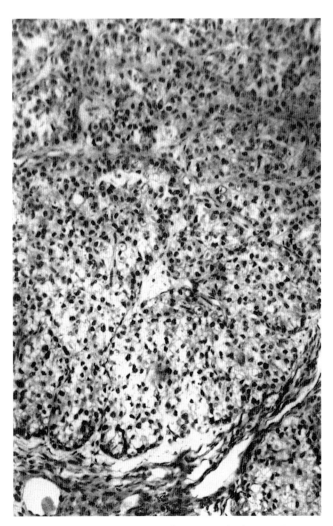

Fig. 25.10 An ovarian metastasis from a well-differentiated hepatocellular carcinoma.

Fig. 25.11 An ovarian metastasis from a renal adenocarcinoma.

& Hart 1992). Most of these neoplasms have been unilateral and in over half of the patients the ovarian tumour occurred before the renal neoplasm was detected. Because of the histological similarity between metastatic renal adenocarcinoma and primary ovarian clear cell adenocarcinoma (Fig. 25.11), a diagnostic difficulty is clearly posed by such cases. Young & Hart (1992) considered that the principal features of metastatic renal adenocarcinoma that allow for its distinction from an ovarian clear cell adenocarcinoma are the presence of a striking sinusoidal vascular pattern, the absence of hobnail cells, a lack of hyaline basement membrane-like material, a negative stain for intraluminal mucin and a homogeneous clear cell pattern rather than the melange of cystic, glandular, papillary, solid, tubular and glandular patterns that characterises ovarian clear cell adenocarcinomas.

Metastases from bladder, ureteric and urethral carcinomas

The ovary is a rare locus of tumour spread from these sites (Fetter et al 1959; Babaian et al 1980) but metastases have been recorded from signet-ring cell carcinomas of the bladder (Ulbright et al 1984; Bowlby & Smith 1986), and from transitional cell carcinomas of the bladder (Fossa et al 1977; Svenes & Eide 1984; Ulbright et al 1984; Andriole et al 1985; Young & Scully 1988b), ureter (Batata et al 1975), renal pelvis (Hsiu et al 1991) and urethra (Graves & Guiss 1941).

Signet-ring cell carcinomas of the bladder metastasise to the ovary as Krukenberg tumours and do not provoke any diagnostic dilemmas. The presence, however, of simultaneous transitional cell neoplasms in the urinary tract and in the ovary raises the question as to whether there are two synchronous and independent primary neoplasms (Van der Weiden & Gratama 1987; Young & Scully 1988a). In the absence of the general features of a metastatic ovarian tumour this distinction may be impossible.

Metastases from malignant melanoma

Metastases of malignant melanoma in the ovary are usually from a primary cutaneous lesion and may become apparent many years (up to 13) after removal of the skin melanoma (Fitzgibbons et al 1987; Young & Scully 1991a)

The tumours are usually large (10–20 cm in diameter) and are bilateral in about 45% of cases: only about one-third are obviously pigmented. Extraovarian tumour is commonly present, usually in the pelvis and upper abdomen. Histologically, a multinodular pattern is usually apparent. About 50% of the tumours are amelanotic and in most the predominant appearance is either of large cells with amphophilic or eosinophilic cytoplasm or of small cells with scanty cytoplasm; a sarcoma-like pattern is uncommon. Rounded or ovoid nests of cells having a

somewhat 'naevoid' appearance are seen in some cases. Follicle-like spaces are present in about 40% of metastatic melanomas and may lead to an erroneous diagnosis of either small cell carcinoma with hypercalcaemia or juvenile granulosa cell tumour. Specific cytological features seen in metastatic melanomas include prominent nucleoli, cytoplasmic pseudoinclusions within the nuclei and, rather uncommonly, nuclear grooving; cytoplasmic melanin granules, are, of course, a diagnostic feature when present. Metastatic malignant melanoma usually stains positively for S-100 and HMB-45, the latter being the more specific (Remadi et al 1997).

Very often the clinical history will point strongly to a diagnosis of melanoma but in the absence of such a history the most important element in diagnosing this neoplasm is an awareness of its possibility by the pathologist. If the tumour is unilateral and there is no history of a preceding cutaneous lesion a careful search should be made for teratomatous elements.

Most patients with ovarian metastatic malignant melanoma die within a few years of diagnosis but occasional women have remained well and apparently tumour-free for as long as eight years after surgical extirpation of the ovarian metastases.

Metastases from endometrial adenocarcinoma

There is no doubt that endometrial adenocarcinomas can, and do, metastasise to the ovary and ovarian secondary deposits have been reported as occurring in between 5 and 60% of women with an endometrial neoplasm (Finn 1951; Luisi 1968; Takeshema et al 1998). An endometrial adenocarcinoma with ovarian metastases would be classed as stage III and thus expected to have a gloomy prognosis; over the years it has, however, become clear that the outlook for such cases is unusually favourable (Dockerty 1954; Woodruff et al 1970; Bruckman et al 1980; Jambhekar & Sampat 1988) and this has increasingly led to the belief that many instances of endometrial adenocarcinoma with apparent ovarian metastases are in reality examples of synchronous dual primary neoplasms of the ovary and endometrium (Scully 1979; Choo & Naylor 1982; Zaino et al 1984; Ulbright & Roth 1985; Piura & Glezerman 1989; Prat et al 1991). This raises the question of whether the pathologist can distinguish between dual synchronous primary ovarian and endometrial neoplasms of the same histological type and endometrial adenocarcinomas with ovarian metastases. In some cases this is, as Silverberg (1984) has pointed out, relatively easy: thus if the endometrial tumour arises superficially in a polyp or is clearly seen to be emerging from a background of 'atypical hyperplasia' and the ovarian carcinoma is in direct continuity with a focus of endometriosis, it will be reasonably obvious that the ovarian lesion is not a metastasis from the endometrial neoplasm. Conversely, direct extension of a large endometrial tumour to the ovary, bilateral ovarian tumours, a multinodular ovarian tumour, extensive vascular permeation by tumour within the ovary, the presence of tumour cells in ovarian hilar lymphatics, tubal involvement with ovarian surface implantation and deep invasion of the myometrium together with involvement of vascular spaces by the endometrial tumour are all features which point to a true ovarian metastasis (Ulbright & Roth 1985).

In some cases, however, the decision as to whether one is dealing with an ovarian metastasis or a second primary neoplasm has to be taken on grounds other than those outlined above, grounds which are of a largely circumstantial nature. Eifel et al (1982) suggested that if the tumour in both ovary and endometrium is of the endometrioid type and if the uterine neoplasm is of grade 1 differentiation and shows no, or minimal, myometrial invasion, then it is almost certain that both neoplasms are primary tumours. A similar conclusion can, according to these workers, also be drawn if the endometrial tumour is grade 2 or 3 but is not invading the myometrium: if there is deep myometrial invasion, and especially if the tumour is of grade 2 or 3 differentiation, then it would be prudent to regard the ovarian tumour as metastatic in nature, this being a view in accord with that of Zaino et al (1984). Eifel et al (1982) also thought that if both the uterine and ovarian neoplasms are of the serous papillary or clear cell types it would be reasonable to consider, for practical purposes, the ovarian lesion to be secondary to these aggressive forms of endometrial neoplasia. By contrast, Ulbright & Roth (1985) maintained that whilst all ovarian lesions found in association with a grade 3 endometrioid adenocarcinoma or an adenosquamous carcinoma of the endometrium should be regarded as metastases, independent dual primary neoplasms of papillary serous or clear cell type could be recognised and treated as such. Currently, both immunohistochemistry and flow cytometry appear to be of very limited value in resolving the problems posed by concurrent endometrial and ovarian carcinoma (Prat et al 1991). Molecular genetic techniques may, however, be of some value if they show different loss of heterozygosity patterns between the endometrial and the ovarian neoplasm (Shenson et al 1995; Emmert-Buck et al 1997).

Metastases from tubal carcinoma

Adenocarcinoma of the Fallopian tube commonly involves the ovary, either by direct extension or via inflammatory adhesions (Scully 1979). In many such cases, however, it may be impossible to distinguish between a tubal neoplasm invading the ovary and an ovarian serous adenocarcinoma which has spread to the tube: in the face of this dilemma the non-committal, but useful, diagnosis of 'tubo-ovarian' carcinoma is often resorted to. Perhaps the only hint in such cases of a primary tubal origin is if the contralateral tube also contains carcinoma which has not spread to the ovary, tubal carcinomas being not infrequently bilateral.

Metastases from cervical carcinoma

Ovarian metastases occur in only about 0.5% of squamous cell carcinomas of the uterine cervix (Tabata et al 1986; Toki et al 1991; Sutton et al 1992), with the metastases not uncommonly being of only microscopic size and localised to the ovarian hilus (Toki et al 1991). Somewhat rarely, however, the ovarian lesion may be not only large but also responsible for the presenting symptoms (Young et al 1993b). Cervical carcinomas giving rise to ovarian metastases are usually quite advanced with most patients also having nodal metastases or involvement of the corpus but an ovarian metastasis has occurred in a woman with early Stage IBI disease (Nguyen et al, 1998).

The incidence of ovarian spread is highest in patients with a cervical adenocarcinoma and has been variously estimated at between 1.3 and 7.7% (Kjorstadt & Bond 1984; Tabata et al 1986; Mann et al 1987; Brown et al 1990; Sutton et al 1992). There appears to be a particular tendency for mucinous adenocarcinomas of the cervix to metastasise to the ovary (Kaminski & Norris 1984) and the coexistence of mucinous tumours in both the cervix and the ovary may give rise to difficulties in deciding whether the ovarian lesion is a metastasis or a synchronous second primary neoplasm (LiVolsi et al 1983; Young & Scully 1988a). The finding within the ovarian tumour of areas of apparently benign or borderline epithelium is not a conclusive indication of its primary nature whilst bilaterality, the presence of desmoplastic surface implants and vascular space invasion are all suggestive of a metastatic lesion (Young & Scully 1988a).

Metastases from sarcomas

Young & Scully (1990b) described 21 sarcomas metastasising to the ovaries and reviewed the few previous reports of sporadic examples of this phenomenon. Included in Young & Scully's series were three uterine leiomyosarcomas, eight endometrial stromal sarcomas, four extragenital leiomyosarcomas and single instances of fibrosarcoma, neural sarcoma, haemangiosarcoma, osteosarcoma, chondrosarcoma and Ewing's sarcoma. In only three cases did the ovarian tumour precede diagnosis of the primary neoplasm. A further example of osteogenic sarcoma metastatic in the ovary 7 years after removal of the primary tumour was later reported by Eltabbakh et al (1997).

In 11 of the 21 cases described by Young & Scully the ovarian metastases were bilateral, and histologically the metastatic tumours usually recapitulated the microscopic appearances of the primary sarcoma: diagnostic difficulties were encountered only in cases of metastatic endometrial stromal sarcoma, which proved difficult to distinguish both from primary ovarian neoplasms of this type and, in a few instances, from a sex cord–stromal tumour.

Young & Scully (1989) also described two examples of alveolar rhabdomyosarcoma which had metastasised to the ovary and reviewed the previously reported six cases of ovarian metastatic rhabdomyosarcoma. Metastases from an alveolar rhabdomyosarcoma occur predominantly as small cell tumours and a distinction from the small cell carcinoma with hypercalcaemia depends upon recognition of the retained alveolar pattern in the metastasis. Young et al (1993a) have subsequently described a further three examples of rhabdomyosarcoma metastasising to the ovaries in children.

Metastases from miscellaneous unusual sites

Tumours of any site in the body can, on occasion, metastasise to the ovary though often the ovarian involvement is only apparent at autopsy. Amongst such oncological exotica may be mentioned ovarian metastases from thyroid carcinoma (Luisi 1968; Woodruff et al 1970; Young et al 1994), thymoma (Yoshida et al 1981), cerebellar medulloblastoma (Paterson 1961), Merkel cell tumour (George et al 1985), hepatoblastoma (Green & Silva 1989), Wilms' tumour (Jereb et al 1977), adrenal neuroblastoma (Sty et al 1980; Young et al 1993a), renal rhabdoid tumour (Young et al 1993a), retinoblastoma (Moore et al 1967), adenoid cystic carcinoma of the salivary gland (Young & Scully 1991b), chordoma (Zukerberg & Young 1990) and extragenital non-pulmonary small cell carcinomas (Eichhorn et al 1993).

Probably, with the passage of time, every known tumour will eventually have been recorded as having metastasised to the ovaries and it is a moot point whether such cases should continue to be documented.

KRUKENBERG TUMOURS

The eponymous fame of Krukenberg rests upon his description, in 1896, of five tumours which he thought were primary neoplasms of the ovary and to which he gave the name 'fibrosarcoma ovarii mucocellulares (carcinomatoides)'. Schlagenhauffer (1902) recognised these tumours as metastases from epithelial neoplasms, but since then the term 'Krukenberg tumour' has been variously interpreted as:

1. A pathological entity in which solid, usually bilateral, ovarian tumours are formed of mucus-containing signet-ring cells set in a hyperplastic cellular stroma
2. A purely histological diagnosis which is applicable to any tumour showing the above histological characteristics irrespective of its macroscopic appearances

3. Any metastatic ovarian tumour
4. Any ovarian metastasis from a primary gastric carcinoma
5. Any ovarian metastasis from a primary tumour in any part of the gastrointestinal tract.

The diagnosis of a Krukenberg tumour should rest solely on histological grounds and although neoplasms with the characteristic histological features of a Krukenberg tumour usually also show a typical macroscopic appearance, the absence of characteristic gross features should not be allowed to detract from the diagnosis.

Krukenberg tumours (Fig. 25.12), which account for 3–4% of all ovarian neoplasms (Soloway et al 1956), are bilateral in over 80% of cases and range in size from 5–20 cm in diameter: they are solid with a smooth nodular or bosselated outer surface and on section are formed of firm, white, yellow or pinkish tissue which is often coarsely lobulated. The tumour is sometimes locally myxoid or mucinous in texture and whilst foci of necrosis are common, cystic change is unusual. Occasional Krukenberg tumours are, however, predominantly cystic, the large thin-walled cysts being filled with mucinous or watery fluid.

Histologically, the Krukenberg tumour is formed of a varying number of plump, rounded epithelial cells set in dense cellular stroma. The epithelial cells occur singly or in clumps, and a proportion, sometimes small but usually considerable, contain mucus and have their nuclei displaced laterally to give a signet-ring appearance

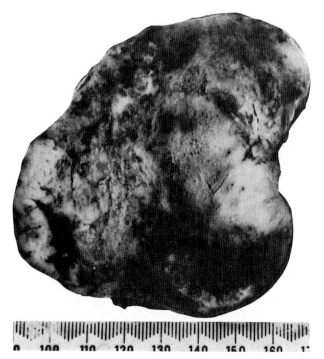

Fig. 25.12 Macroscopic appearances of an ovarian Krukenberg tumour.

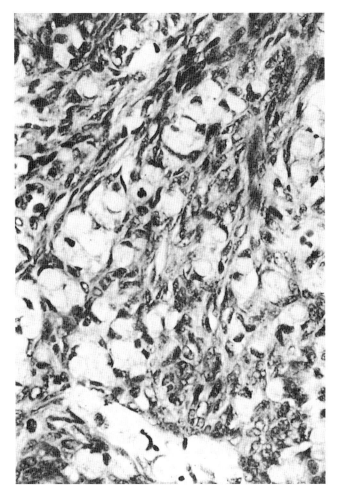

Fig. 25.13 Histological appearances of a typical ovarian Krukenberg tumour. Signet-ring, mucus-containing cells are set in a proliferating stroma.

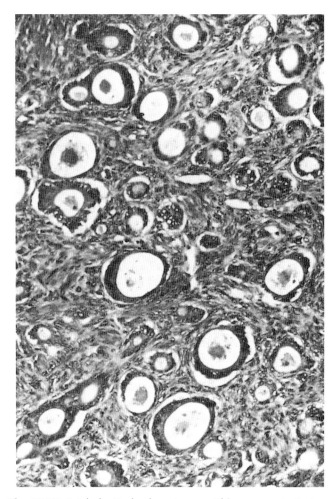

Fig. 25.14 A tubular Krukenberg tumour. This was a metastasis from a gastric adenocarcinoma and elsewhere showed a transition to a more conventional signet-ring cell appearance.

(Fig. 25.13). Poorly formed acinar structures are present in many cases and occasionally (Fig. 25.14) there is a predominantly tubular pattern (Bullon et al 1981). In some cases mucin-poor cells are arranged in trabeculae or large clumps whilst, very infrequently, cysts lined by apparently innocuous mucinous epithelium are a conspicuous component of the tumour (Scully 1979). Carcinomatous cells may be suspended in pools of extracellular mucus.

The tumour stroma is of ovarian type and its constituent cells are plump and spindle-shaped; there may be a moderate number of mitotic figures in the stromal cells and these, together with a not uncommon degree of pleomorphism, may impart a 'pseudosarcomatous' pattern to the stromal component. The proliferating stromal cells may assume a storiform pattern in some areas and this may be associated with dense collagenisation; if tumour cells are sparsely dispersed in such areas the appearances may resemble those of a fibrous histiocytoma (Holtz & Hart 1982). Foci of stromal oedema are not uncommon and stromal luteinization is often a conspicuous feature. Tumour emboli can be found in lymphatic and vascular

spaces of the hilum, mesovarium, and mesosalpinx in about 50% of cases (Holtz & Hart 1982).

The vast majority of Krukenberg tumours are metastases from a gastric carcinoma; other much less commonly encountered primary carcinomas giving rise to metastatic Krukenberg tumours occur in the large intestine, breast, gallbladder, endocervix, appendix and urinary bladder (McDuff 1950; Karsh 1951; Soloway et al 1956; Woodruff & Novak 1960; Hale 1968; Paone et al 1978; Scully 1979; Kashani & Levy 1983; Mazur et al 1984; Savey et al 1996). It should not be assumed, however, that any histological type of carcinoma can give rise to a Krukenberg tumour and that the typical signet-ring appearance of the cells in such a neoplasm represents a structural modification imposed by their ovarian environment. Krukenberg tumours are metastases of signet-ring carcinomas and such neoplasms have a particular tendency to spread to the ovary (Saphir 1951; Amorn & Knight 1978; Duarte & Llanos 1981); the reasons for this propensity are totally obscure but the predominance of the stomach as the site of origin of Krukenberg tumours simply reflects the fact that signet-ring carcinomas occur most commonly at this site and does not indicate a general tendency for all adenocarcinomas of the stomach to metastasise to the ovary.

The question arises as to whether Krukenberg tumours of the ovary are always metastatic in nature. It has been maintained that a typical Krukenberg tumour can arise as a primary neoplasm of the ovary; indeed, not only have approximately 40 such tumours been reported (Joshi 1968), but in one series of 48 Krukenberg tumours no less than 10 were thought to have arisen de novo in the ovary (Woodruff & Novak 1960). There is certainly no inherent reason why a primary signet-ring carcinoma should not occur in the ovary but extreme caution should be exercised before making such a diagnosis. The diagnosis of a primary Krukenberg tumour rests not on any special characteristics of the ovarian neoplasm but on the absence of any primary lesion elsewhere; the lack of a primary extraovarian tumour may, however, be very difficult to prove and in many of the reported cases the evidence for this has been solely that the patient survived in apparently good health for two or three years after removal of an ovarian Krukenberg tumour. This is too short a follow-up period, as is shown by the salutary case reported by McGoogan & Hatch (1972) in which a gastric carcinoma did not become apparent until four and a half years after removal of an ovarian Krukenberg tumour. Any suggested period of follow-up is, of course, arbitrary but it is widely accepted that a Krukenberg tumour should not be regarded as primary unless either the patient has lived in good health for at least five years after removal of the ovarian neoplasm or has died and been subjected to a thorough autopsy examination which has excluded a primary extraovarian lesion. Application of these criteria to the reported cases of primary Krukenberg tumours reduces their number to less than 20 (Fox & Langley 1976) though even these are regarded with considerable scepticism by Holtz & Hart (1982), who note that some primary neoplasms may remain occult for many years and that small carcinomas of the stomach can be difficult to detect at autopsy; nevertheless, of the 27 cases of Krukenberg tumours in their series a detailed autopsy failed to identify a primary extraovarian carcinoma in two patients.

The age of women with an ovarian Krukenberg tumour tends to be unusually low for patients with metastatic carcinoma; most are between 30 and 50 years of age at the time of initial diagnosis (Diddle 1955) and the mean age is about 45 years (Berens 1951; Karsh 1951; Bernier & Bonnenfant 1955; Soloway et al 1956; Woodruff & Novak 1960; Hale 1968; Holtz & Hart 1982; Savey et al 1996): these mean figures conceal, however, the fact that in some series nearly half the patients have been under the age of 40 years at initial diagnosis and that a significant proportion have been in their twenties (Linard 1946; Holtz & Hart 1982). The youngest patient

in whom a Krukenberg tumour has been described was aged 13 years (Berens 1951).

The symptoms of a Krukenberg tumour are generally non-specific and related solely to the presence of a pelvic mass, abdominal discomfort or pain being the most commonly encountered complaints. Accompanying ascites may cause abdominal enlargement whilst occasional Krukenberg tumours are associated with a hydrothorax which resolves after removal of the ovarian tumour (Dick et al 1950; Bernier & Bonnenfant 1955; Woodruff & Novak 1960). Because of the relative youth of many of the women with this tumour it is not surprising that occasional Krukenberg tumours have occurred during pregnancy (Fox & Stamm 1965; Spadoni et al 1965; Ward 1966; Connor et al 1968; Forest et al 1978). Menstrual disturbances and postmenopausal bleeding are common, though rarely dominant, complaints in women with a Krukenberg tumour, whilst a much smaller proportion of women with such neoplasms show evidence of virilisation: the endocrine effects are regarded as being due to an associated stromal luteinization (Scully & Richardson 1961; Ober et al 1962; Forest et al 1978; Schoenfeld et al 1982). It is worth noting, however, that pregnant women with a Krukenberg tumour show a particular tendency to become virilised (Fox & Langley 1976; Bullon et al 1981): this is thought to be due to stimulation of the luteinized cells by hCG, and the maternal virilisation may be associated with partial masculinisation of female children resulting from such pregnancies (Bell 1977; Vicens et al 1980).

Only between 20 and 30% of patients with an ovarian Krukenberg tumour have a history of a previously removed extraovarian neoplasm (Johansson 1960; Scully 1979): in such cases the time interval between diagnosis of the extraovarian tumour and presentation of an ovarian metastasis is usually less than six months (Johansson 1960), with very few cases having an apparently tumour-free interval of more than two years (Hale 1968). Nevertheless, in occasional cases there may be a long time interval, up to 12 years, between diagnosis of an extraovarian neoplasm and the appearance of an ovarian metastasis (Hale 1968). In most cases the extraovarian neoplasm is diagnosed at the time of presentation of the ovarian tumour, even though it may have been, until then, clinically silent. In a proportion of cases a Krukenberg tumour is the initial presentation of an extraovarian primary neoplasm and in such circumstances the extragonadal tumour may not become apparent for anything up to six years (Johansson 1960).

The prognosis for a woman with a Krukenberg tumour is extremely poor, with most patients surviving only between three and ten months (Leffel et al 1942; Soloway et al 1956; Hale 1968); only 10% of patients survive for more than two years after diagnosis of the ovarian tumour.

REFERENCES

Albarracin C T, Jafri J, Montag A G, Hart J, Kuan S F 2000 Differential expression of MUC2 and MUC5AC mucin genes in primary ovarian and metastatic colonic carcinoma. Human Pathology 31: 672–677

Albores-Saavedra A, Henson D E 1986 Tumors of the gallbladder and extrahepatic bile ducts. In: Atlas of tumour pathology, second series, fascicle 22. Armed Forces Institute of Pathology, Washington, DC

Amorn Y, Knight W A 1978 Primary linitis plastica of the colon: report of two cases and review of the literature. Cancer 41: 2420–2425

Andriole G L, Garnick M B, Richie J P 1985 Unusual behaviour of low grade, low stage transitional cell carcinoma of bladder. Urology 25: 524–526

Ayhan A, Tuncer Z S, Bukulmez O 1995 Malignant tumors metastatic to the ovaries. Journal of Surgical Oncology 60: 268–276

Babaian R J, Johnson D E, Llamas L, Ayala A G 1980 Metastases from transitional cell carcinoma of urinary bladder. Urology 16: 142–144

Batata M A, Whitmore W F, Hilaris B S, Tokita N, Grabstald H 1975 Primary carcinoma of the ureter: a prognostic study. Cancer 35: 1616–1632

Bell R J M 1977 Fetal virilization due to maternal Krukenberg tumour. Lancet 1: 1162–1163

Berens J J 1951 Krukenberg tumors of the ovary. American Journal of Surgery 81: 484–491

Berezowski K, Stasny J F, Kornstein M J 1996 Cytokeratins 7 and 20 and carcinoembryonic antigen in ovarian and colonic carcinoma. Modern Pathology 9: 426–429

Bernier L, Bonnenfant J L 1955 La tumeur de Krukenberg. Gynecologie et Obstetrique 54: 615–621

Blaustein A 1982 Metastatic carcinoma in the ovary. In: Blaustein A (ed) Pathology of the female genital tract, 2nd edn. Springer-Verlag, New York, pp 705–715

Bowlby L S, Smith M L 1986 Signet-ring cell carcinoma of the urinary bladder: presentation as a Krukenberg tumor. Gynecologic Oncology 25: 376–381

Brandt-Rauf P W, Pincus M, Adelson S 1982 Cancer of the gallbladder: a review of forty-three cases. Human Pathology 13: 48–53

Brickman M, Ferreira B 1967 Metastasis of breast carcinoma to the ovaries — incidence, significance and relationship to survival: a preliminary study. Grace Hospital Bulletin 45: 44–49

Brown B L, Sharifker D A, Gordon R, Deppe G, Cohen C J 1980 Bronchial carcinoid tumor with ovarian metastasis: a light microscopic and ultrastructural study. Cancer 46: 543–546

Brown J W, Fu Y S, Berek J S 1990 Ovarian metastases are rare in Stage 1 adenocarcinoma of the cervix. Obstetrics and Gynecology 76: 623–626

Bruckman J E, Bloomer W D, Marck A, Ehrmann R L, Knapp R C 1980 Stage III adenocarcinoma of the endometrium: two prognostic groups. Gynecologic Oncology 9: 12–17

Budinger J M 1958 Untreated bronchogenic carcinoma: a clinicopathological study of 250 autopsied cases. Cancer 11: 106–116

Buller R E, Braga C A, Tanagho E A, Miller T 1983 Renal cell carcinoma metastatic to the ovary: a case report. Journal of Reproductive Medicine 28: 217–220

Bullon A, Arseneau J, Prat J, Young R H, Scully R E 1981 Tubular Krukenberg tumor: a problem in histopathologic diagnosis. American Journal of Surgical Pathology 5: 225–232

Cheung A N, Chiu P M, Khoo U S 1997 Is immunostaining with HAM56 antibody useful in identifying ovarian origin of metastatic adenocarcinoma? Human Pathology 28: 91–94

Choo Y C, Naylor B 1982 Multiple primary neoplasms of the ovary and uterus. International Journal of Gynaecology and Obstetrics 20: 327–334

Chuaqui R F, Zhuang Z, Emmert-Buck M R et al 1996 Genetic analysis of synchronous mucinous tumors of the ovary and appendix. Human Pathology 27: 165–171

Connor T B, Ganis F M, Levin H S, Migeon C J, Martin L G 1968 Gonadotrophic-dependent Krukenberg tumor causing virilization during pregnancy. Journal of Clinical Endocrinology and Metabolism 28: 198–214

Cuatrecasai M, Marias-guiu X, Prat J 1996 Synchronous mucinous tumors of the appendix and the ovary associated with pseudomyxoma peritonei: a clinicopathologic study of six cases with comparative analysis of c-Ki-ras mutations. American Journal of Surgical Pathology 20: 739–746

Cutait R, Lesser M, Enker W E 1983 Prophylactic oophorectomy in surgery for large bowel cancer. Diseases of the Colon and Rectum 26: 6–11

DasGupta T, Brasfield R 1964 Metastatic melanoma: a clinicopathological study. Cancer 17: 1323–1339

Daya D, Nazerali L, Frank G L 1992 Metastatic ovarian carcinoma of large intestinal origin simulating primary ovarian carcinoma: a clinicopathologic study of 25 cases. American Journal of Clinical Pathology 27: 751–758

DeCostanzo D C, Elias J M, Chumas J C 1997 Necrosis in 84 ovarian carcinomas: a morphologic study of primary versus metastatic colonic carcinoma with a selective immunohistochemical analysis of cytokeratin subtypes and carcinoembryonic antigen. International Journal of Gynecological Pathology 16: 245–249

Dick H J, Spire L J, Worboys C S 1950 Association of Meig's syndrome with Krukenberg tumors. New York State Journal of Medicine 50: 1842–1846

Diddle A W 1955 Krukenberg tumors: diagnostic problem. Cancer 8: 1026–1034

Dockerty M B 1954 Primary and secondary ovarian adenoacanthoma. Surgery, Gynecology and Obstetrics 99: 392–400

Duarte I, Llanos O 1981 Patterns of metastases in intestinal and diffuse types of carcinoma of the stomach. Human Pathology 12: 237–242

Eichhorn J H, Young R H, Scully R E 1992 Primary ovarian small cell carcinoma of pulmonary type: a clinicopathologic, immunohistologic and flow cytometric analysis of 11 cases. American Journal of Surgical Pathology 16: 926–938

Eichhorn J H, Young R H, Scully R E 1993 Non-pulmonary small cell carcinomas of extragenital origin metastatic to the ovary: a report of seven cases. Cancer 71: 177–186

Eifel P, Hendrickson M, Ross J, Ballon S, Martinez A, Kempson R 1982 Simultaneous presentation of carcinoma involving the ovary and the uterine corpus. Cancer 50: 163–170

Eltabbakh G H, Belinson J L, Biscotti C V 1997 Osteosarcoma metastatic to the ovary: a case report and review of the literature. International Journal of Gynecological Pathology 16: 76–78

Emmert-Buck M R, Chuaqui R, Zhuang Z, Nogales F, Liotta L A, Merino M J 1997 Molecular analysis of synchronous uterine and ovarian endometrioid tumors. International Journal of Gynecological Pathology 16: 143–148

Fetter T R, Bogaev J H, McCuskey B, Seres J L 1959 Carcinoma of the bladder: sites of metastases. Journal of Urology 81: 746–748

Finn W F 1951 Diagnostic confusion of ovarian metastases from endometrial carcinoma with primary ovarian cancer. American Journal of Obstetrics and Gynecology 62: 403–408

Fitzgibbons P L, Martin S E, Simmons T J 1987 Malignant melanoma metastatic to the ovary. American Journal of Surgical Pathology 11: 959–964

Forest M G, Orgiazzi J, Tranchant D, Mornex R, Bertrand J 1978 Approach to the mechanism of androgen overproduction in a case of Krukenberg tumour responsible for virilization during pregnancy. Journal of Clinical Endocrinology and Metabolism 47: 428–434

Fossa S D, Schjolseth J A, Miller A 1977 Multiple urothelial tumours with metastases to uterus and left ovary: a case report. Scandinavian Journal of Urology and Nephrology 11: 81–84

Fowler L J, Maygarden S J, Novotny D B 1994 Human alveolar macrophage-56 and carcinoembryonic antigen monoclonal antibodies in the differential diagnosis between primary ovarian and metastatic gastrointestinal carcinomas. Human Pathology 25: 666–670

Fox H, Langley F A 1976 Tumours of the ovary. Heinemann, London

Fox L P, Stamm W J 1965 Krukenberg tumor complicating pregnancy: report of a case with androgenic activity. American Journal of Obstetrics and Gynecology 92: 702–709

Fujiwara K, Ohishi Y, Koike H, Sawada S, Moriya T, Kohno I 1995 Clinical implications of metastases to the ovary. Gynecologic Oncology 59: 124–128

Gagnon Y, Tetu B 1989 Ovarian metastases of breast carcinoma: a clinicopathologic study of 59 cases. Cancer 64: 892–898

Galluzzi S, Payne P M 1955 Bronchial carcinoma: a statistical study of 741 necropsies with special reference to the distribution of bloodborne metastases. British Journal of Cancer 9: 511–527

George T K, di Sant'Agnese P A, Bennett J M 1985 Chemotherapy for metastatic Merkel cell carcinoma. Cancer 56: 1034–1038

Graffner H D L, Alm P O R, Oscarson J E A 1983 Prophylactic oophorectomy in colorectal cancer. American Journal of Surgery 146: 233–235

Graves R C, Guiss L W 1941 Tumors of the urethra. Journal of Urology 46: 925–947

Green L K, Silva E G 1989 Hepatoblastoma in an adult with metastasis to the ovaries. American Journal of Clinical Pathology 92: 110–115

Guerrieri C, Franlund B, Fristedt S et al 1997 Mucinous tumors of the vermiform appendix and ovary, and pseudomyxoma peritonei: histogenetic implications of cytokeratin 7 expression. Human Pathology 28: 1039–1045

Hale R W 1968 Krukenberg tumor of the ovary: a review of 81 records. Obstetrics and Gynecology 32: 221–225

Harcourt K F, Dennis D L 1968 Laparotomy for 'ovarian tumors' in unsuspected carcinoma of the colon. Cancer 21: 1244–1246

Harris M, Howell A, Chrissohou M et al 1984 A comparison of the metastatic pattern of infiltrating lobular carcinoma and infiltrating duct carcinoma of the breast. British Journal of Cancer 50: 23–30

Heisterberg L, Wahlin A, Nieldsen K S 1982 Two cases of goblet cell carcinoid tumour of the appendix with bilateral ovarian metastases. Acta Obstetricia et Gynecologica Scandinavica 61(2): 153–156

Herrera-Ornelas L, Natarajan N, Tsukada I et al 1983 Adenocarcinoma of the colon masquerading as primary ovarian neoplasia: an analysis of ten cases. Diseases of the Colon and Rectum 26: 377–380

Holtz F, Hart W R 1982 Krukenberg tumours of the ovary: a clinicopathologic analysis of 27 cases. Cancer 50: 2438–2447

Hsiu J-G, Kemp G A, Singer G A, Rawis W H, Siddiky M A 1991 Transitional cell carcinoma of the renal pelvis with ovarian metastasis. Gynecologic Oncology 41: 178–181

Huang P P, Weber T K, Mendoza C, Rodriguez-Bigaz M A, Petrelli N J 1998 Long-term survival in patients with ovarian metastases from colorectal carcinoma. Annals of Surgical Oncology 5: 695–698

Ikeda E, Tsutsumi Y, Yoshida H, Yanagi K 1991 Goblet cell carcinoid of the vermiform appendix with ovarian metastasis. Acta Pathologica Japonica 41: 455–460

Israel S L, Helsel E W, Hausman D H 1965 The challenge of metastatic ovarian carcinoma. American Journal of Obstetrics and Gynecology 93: 1094–1101

Jambhekar N, Sampat M B 1988 Simultaneous endometrioid carcinoma of the uterine corpus and ovary: a clinicopathologic study of 15 cases. Journal of Surgical Oncology 37: 20–23

Jereb B, Golough R, Havlicek S 1977 Ovarian cancer in children and adolescents: a review of 15 cases. Medical Pediatric Oncology 3: 339–343

Johansson M 1960 Clinical aspects of metastatic ovarian cancer of extragenital origin. Acta Obstetricia et Gynecologica Scandinavica 39: 681–697

Joshi V V 1968 Primary Krukenberg tumor of the ovary: review of literature and case report. Cancer 22: 1199–1207

Kaminski P F, Norris H J 1984 Coexistence of ovarian neoplasms and endocervical adenocarcinoma. Obstetrics and Gynecology 64: 553–556

Karsh J 1951 Secondary malignant disease of the ovaries: a study of 72 autopsies. American Journal of Obstetrics and Gynecology 61: 154–160

Kashani M, Levy M 1983 Primary adenocarcinoma of the appendix with bilateral Krukenberg ovarian tumors. Journal of Surgical Oncology 22: 101–105

Kjorstad K E, Bond B 1984 Stage 1b adenocarcinoma of the cervix: metastatic potential and patterns of dissemination. American Journal of Obstetrics and Gynecology 54: 553–556

Krukenberg F E 1896 Ueber das Fibrosarcoma ovarii mucocellulare (carcinomatides). Archiv fur Gynakologie 50: 287–321

Lagendijk J H, Mullink H, van Diest P J, Meijer G A, Meijer C J 1998 Tracing the origin of adenocarcinomas with unknown primary using immunohistochemistry: differential diagnosis between colonic and ovarian carcinoma as primary sites. Human Pathology 29: 491–497

Lagendijk J H, Mullink H, van Diest P J, Meijer G A, Meijer C J 1999 Immunohistochemical differentiation between primary adenocarcinomas of the ovary and ovarian metastases of colonic and breast origin: a statistical and intuitive approach. Journal of Clinical Pathology 52: 283–290

Lash R H, Hart W R 1987 Intestinal adenocarcinomas metastatic to the ovaries: a clinicopathologic evaluation of 22 cases. American Journal of Surgical Pathology 11: 114–121

Lashgari M, Bemmaram B, Hoffman J S et al 1992 Primary biliary carcinoma with metastasis to the ovary. Gynecologic Oncology 47: 272–274

Leffel J M, Masson J C, Dockerty M B 1942 Krukenberg's tumors: a survey of forty-four cases. Annals of Surgery 115: 102–113

Linard P 1964 Carcinomes metastatiques bilateraux des ovaries du tumeurs du Krukenberg. Journal de Chirurgie 62: 15–29

LiVolsi V A, Merino M J, Schwarz P E 1983 Coexistent endocervical adenocarcinoma and mucinous adenocarcinoma of ovary: a clinicopathological study of four cases. International Journal of Gynecological Pathology 1: 391–402

Loy T S, Abshier J 1993 Immunostaining with HAM56 in the diagnosis of adenocarcinomas. Modern Pathology 6: 473–475

Loy T S, Calaluce R D, Keeney G L 1996 Cytokeratin immunostaining in differentiating primary ovarian carcinoma from metastatic colonic adenocarcinoma. Modern Pathology 9: 1040–1044

Luisi A 1968 Metastatic ovarian tumours. In: Junqueira A C, Gentil F (eds) Ovarian cancer. UICC monograph series, vol 11. Springer-Verlag, Berlin, pp 87–104

McDuff H C 1950 Metastatic Krukenberg tumor of the ovary: primary in the breast with six-year survival. Rhode Island Medical Journal 33: 589–593

McCluggage W G 2000 Recent advances in immunohistochemistry in the diagnosis of ovarian neoplasms. Journal of Clinical Pathology 53: 327–334

McGoogan L S, Hatch K D 1972 Krukenberg tumor: report of two cases. Nebraska Medical Journal 57: 409–415

Malviya V K, Baysal M, Chayiuiau P, Deppe G, Lauersen H, Gordon R E 1982 Small cell anaplastic lung cancer presenting as an ovarian metastasis. International Journal of Gynaecology and Obstetrics 20: 487–493

Mann W J, Chumas J, Amalfitano T, Westermann C, Patsner C 1987 Ovarian metastases from Stage 1B adenocarcinoma of the cervix. Cancer 60: 1123–1126

Martzloff K H, Manlove C H 1949 Vaginal and ovarian metastases from hypernephroma: report of a case and review of the literature. Surgery, Gynecology and Obstetrics 88: 145–154

Mazur M T, Hsueh S, Gersell D J 1984 Patterns of metastasis to the female genital tract: analysis of 325 cases. Cancer 53: 1978–1984

Merino M J, Edmonds P, LiVolsi V 1985 Appendiceal carcinoma metastatic to the ovaries and mimicking primary ovarian tumors. International Journal of Gynecological Pathology 4: 110–120

Miller B E, Pittman B, Wan J Y, Fleming M 1997 Colon cancer with metastasis to the ovary at time of initial diagnosis. Gynecologic Oncology 66: 368–371

Monteagudo C, Merino M J, LaPorte N, Neumann R D 1991 Value of gross cystic disease fluid protein-15 in distinguishing metastatic breast carcinomas amongst poorly differentiated neoplasms involving the ovary. Human Pathology 22: 368–372

Moore J G, Schifrin B S, Erez S 1967 Ovarian tumors in infancy, childhood and adolescence. American Journal of Obstetrics and Gynecology 99: 913–922

Morrow M, Enker W E 1984 Late ovarian metastases in carcinoma of the colon and rectum. Archives of Surgery 119: 1385–1388

Nguyen L, Brewer C A, DiSaia P J 1998 Ovarian metastasis of stage IB1 squamous cell cancer of the cervix after radical parametrectomy and oophoropexy. Gynecologic Oncology 68: 198–200

Ober W B, Pollak A, Gerstmann K E, Kupperman H S 1962 Krukenberg tumor with androgenic and progestational activity. American Journal of Obstetrics and Gynecology 84: 739–744

O'Brien P H, Newton B B, Metcalfe J S, Rittenburg M S 1981 Oophorectomy in women with carcinoma of the colon and rectum. Surgery, Gynecology and Obstetrics 153: 827–830

Osborne M P, Pitts R M 1961 Therapeutic oophorectomy for advanced breast cancer: the significance of metastases to the ovary and of ovarian cortical stromal hyperplasias. Cancer 14: 128–130

Paone J F, Bixler T J, Imbembo A L 1978 Primary mucinous adenocarcinoma of appendix with bilateral ovarian Krukenberg tumors. Johns Hopkins Medical Journal 143: 43–47

Parnanen P O, Vataja U 1954 Metastatic carcinoma of the ovary. Annales Chirurgie Fennae 43 (suppl 5): 322–331

Paterson E 1961 Distant metastases from medulloblastoma of the cerebellum. Brain 84: 301–309

Perucchini D, Caduff R, Schar G, Fink D, Kochli O R 1996 Ovarielle Metastasierung extragenitaler Tumoren an der Universitatsfrauenklinik Zurich 1978–1990. Geburtshilfe und Frauenheilkunde 56: 351–356

Petru E, Pickel H, Haydarfadai M et al 1992 Nongenital cancer metastatic to the ovary. Gynecologic Oncology 44: 83–86

Piura B, Glezerman M 1989 Synchronous carcinomas of endometrium and ovary. Gynecologic Oncology 33: 261–264

Prat J, Matias-Guiu X, Barreto J 1991 Simultaneous carcinoma involving the endometrium and the ovary: a clinicopathologic, immunohistochemical and DNA flow cytometric study of 18 cases. Cancer 68: 2455–2459

Prayson R A, Hart W R, Petras R E 1994 Pseudomyxoma peritonei: a clinicopathologic study of 19 cases with emphasis on site of origin and nature of associated ovarian tumors. American Journal of Surgical Pathology 18: 591–603

Remadi S, McGee W, Egger J F, Ismail A 1997 Ovarian metastatic melanoma: a diagnostic pitfall in histopathologic examination. Archives d'Anatomie Cytologie et Pathologie 45: 43–46

Richardson G S 1967 Ovariectomy in cancer of the colon. New England Journal of Medicine 276: 526

Robboy S J, Scully R E, Norris H J 1974 Carcinoid metastatic to the ovary: a clinicopathologic analysis of 35 cases. Cancer 33: 798–811

Ronnett B M, Kurmam R J, Zahn C M et al 1995 Pseudomyxoma peritonei in women; a clinicopathologic analysis of 30 cases with emphasis on site of origin, prognosis and relationship to ovarian mucinous tumors of low malignant potential. Human Pathology 26: 509–524

Ronnett B M, Kurman R J, Shmookler B M, Sugarbaker P N, Young R H 1997a The morphological spectrum of ovarian metastases of appendiceal adenocarcinomas: a clinicopathological and immunohistological analysis of tumors often misinterpreted as primary ovarian tumors or metastatic tumors from other gastrointestinal sites. American Journal of Surgical Pathology 21: 805–815

Ronnett B M, Shmookler B M, Diener-West M et al 1997b Immunohistochemical evidence supporting the appendiceal origin of pseudomyxoma peritonei. International Journal of Gynelogical Pathology 16: 1–9

Saitoh H 1981 Distant metastasis of renal adenocarcinoma. Cancer 48: 1487–1491

Santesson L, Kottmeier H L 1968 General classification of ovarian tumours. In: Junqueira A C, Gentil F (eds) Ovarian cancer. UICC monograph series, vol 11. Springer-Verlag, Berlin, pp 1–8

Saphir O 1951 Signet-ring cell carcinoma. Military Surgeon 105: 360–369

Savey L, Lasser P, Castaigne D, Michel G, Bognel C, Colau J C 1996 Tumeurs de Krukenberg: analyse d'une serie de 28 observations. Journal de Chirurgie Paris 133: 427–431

Schlagenhauffer F 1902 Ueber das metastatiche Ovarialcarcinoma nach Krebs des Magens, Darmes und anderer Bauchorgane. Monatschrift fur Geburtshilfe und Gynakologie 15: 485–528

Schoenfeld A, Pistiner M, Pitlik S, Rosenfeld J B, Ovadia J 1982 Long-interval maculinizing Krukenberg tumor of the ovary. European Journal of Obstetrics, Gynaecology and Reproductive Biology 14: 49–53

Scully R E 1979 Tumors of the ovary and maldeveloped gonads. Atlas of tumor pathology, second series, fascicle 16. Armed Forces Institute of Pathology, Washington, DC

Scully R E 1993 Small cell carcinoma of hypercalcemic type. International Journal of Gynecological Pathology 12: 148–152

Scully R E, Richardson G S 1961 Luteinization of the stroma of metastatic cancer involving the ovary and its endocrine significance. Cancer 14: 827–840

Seidman J D, Elsayed A M, Sobin L H et al 1993 Association of mucinous tumours of the ovary and appendix: clinicopathologic study of 25 cases. American Journal of Surgical Pathology 17: 85–90

Seidman J D, Ronnett B M, Kurman R K 2000 Evolution of the concept and terminology of borderline ovarian tumours. Current Diagnostic Pathology 6: 31–37

Shenson D, Gallion H H, Powell D E, Pietetti M 1995 Loss of heterozygosity and genomic instability in synchronous endometrioid tumors of the ovary and endometrium. Cancer 76: 650–657

Sielezneff I, Salle E, Antoine K, Thirion X, Brunet C, Sastre B 1997 Simultaneous bilateral oophorectomy does not improve prognosis of postmenopausal women undergoing colorectal resection for cancer. Diseases of the Colon and Rectum 40: 1299–1302

Silverberg S G 1984 New aspects of endometrial carcinoma. Clinics in Obstetrics and Gynaecology 11: 189–208

Soloway I, Latour J P A, Young M H V 1956 Krukenberg tumors of the ovary. Obstetrics and Gynecology 8: 636–638

Spadoni L R, Linoberg M C, Mottet N K, Herman W L 1965 Virilization co-existing with Krukenberg tumor during pregnancy. American Journal of Obstetrics and Gynecology 92: 198–201

Sty J R, Kum L F, Casper J T 1980 Bone scintigraphy in neuroblastoma with ovarian metastasis. Wisconsin Medical Journal 79: 28–29

Sutton G P, Bundy B N, Delgado G et al 1992 Ovarian metastases in Stage 1b carcinoma of the cervix: a Gynecologic Oncology Group study. American Journal of Obstetrics and Gynecology 166: 50–53

Svenes K B, Eide J 1984 Proliferative Brenner tumor or ovarian metastases? A case report. Cancer 53: 2692–2697

Tabata M, Ichinoe K, Skuragi N et al 1986 Incidence of ovarian metastasis in patients with cancer of the uterine cervix. Gynecologic Oncology 28: 255–261

Takeshima N, Hirai Y, Kano K, Tanaka N, Yamauchi K, Hasumi K 1998 Ovarian metastasis in endometrial carcinoma. Gynecologic Oncology 70: 183–187

Taylor A E, Nicolson V M, Cunningham D 1995 Ovarian metastases from primary gastrointestinal malignancies: the Royal Marsden Hospital experience and implications for adjuvant treatment. British Journal of Cancer 71: 92–96

Thorsen P, Dybdahl H, Sogaard H, Moller B R 1991 Ovarian tumors caused by metastatic tumors of the appendix: two case reports. European Journal of Obstetrics, Gynecology and Reproductive Biology 40: 67–71

Toki N, Tsukamoto N, Kaku T et al 1991 Microscopic ovarian metastasis of uterine cervical cancer. Gynecologic Oncology 41: 46–51

Turksoy N 1960 Ovarian metastasis of breast carcinoma: a surgical surprise. Obstetrics and Gynecology 15: 573–578

Ulbright T M, Roth L M 1985 Metastatic and independent cancers of the endometrium and ovary: a clinicopathologic study of 34 cases. Human Pathology 16: 28–34

Ulbright T M, Roth L M, Stehman F B 1984 Secondary ovarian neoplasms: a clinicopathologic study of 35 cases. Cancer 53: 1164–1174

Van der Weiden R M F, Gratama S 1987 Proliferative and malignant Brenner tumors (BT) and their differentiation from metastatic transitional cell carcinoma of the bladder: a case report and review of the literature. European Journal of Obstetrics, Gynecology and Reproductive Biology 26: 251–260

Vicens E, Martinez-Mora J, Potau N, Sans M, Boix-Ochoa J 1980 Masculinization of a female fetus by Krukenberg tumor during pregnancy. Journal of Pediatric Surgery 15: 188–190

Virieux C 1962 Untersuchungen uber Haufgkeit und Enstehungweise von Krebsmetastasen in den Eirstocken. Gynaecologia (Basel) 153: 209–224

von Numers C 1960 Sind die Krukenberg Tumoren wirklich metastatiche. Eierstockgeschwulste. Geburtshilfe und Frauenheilkunde 20: 726–731

Vorder-Bruegge C G, Hobbl J E, Weener C R, Wintemute R W 1957 Bilateral ovarian metastases from renal adenocarcinoma. Obstetrics and Gynecology 9: 198–205

Walther H 1948 Krebsmetastasen. Schwabe Verlag, Basel

Ward R T H 1966 Krukenberg tumours in pregnancy. Australian and New Zealand Journal of Obstetrics and Gynaecology 6: 312–315

Warren S, Gates O 1964 Lung cancer and metastases. Archives of Pathology 78: 467–473

Warren S, Macomber W B 1935 Tumor metastasis. VI. Ovarian metastasis of carcinoma. Archives of Pathology 19: 75–82

Wauters C C, Smedts F, Gerrrits L G, Bosman F T, Ramaekers F C 1995 Keratins 7 and 20 as diagnostic markers of carcinomas metastatic to the ovary. Human Pathology 26: 852–855

Webb M G, Decker D G, Mussey E 1975 Cancer metastatic to the ovary: factors influencing survival. Obstetrics and Gynecology 45: 391–396

Willis R A 1952 The spread of tumours in the human body, 2nd edn. Butterworths, London

Woodruff J D, Novak E R 1960 The Krukenberg tumor: study of 48 cases from the ovarian tumor registry. Obstetrics and Gynecology 15: 356–360

Woodruff J D, Murphy Y S, Bhaskar T N, Borobar F, Tseng S S 1970 Metastatic ovarian tumors. American Journal of Obstetrics and Gynecology 107: 202–209

Yoshida A, Shigematsu T, Mori H, Yoshida H, Fukunishi R 1981 Non-invasive thymoma with widespread blood-borne metastasis. Virchows Archives A Pathological Anatomy 390: 121–126

Younes M, Katikaneni P R, Lechago L V, Lechago J 1994 HAM56 antibody: a tool in the differential diagnosis between colorectal and gynecological malignancy. Modern Pathology 7: 396–400

Young R H, Hart W R 1989 Metastases from carcinoma of the pancreas simulating primary mucinous tumours of the ovary: a report of seven cases. American Journal of Surgical Pathology 13: 748–756

Young R H, Hart W R 1992 Renal cell carcinoma metastatic to the ovary: a report of three cases emphasizing possible confusion with ovarian clear cell adenocarcinoma. International Journal of Gynecological Pathology 11: 96–104

Young R H, Hart W R 1998 Metastatic intestinal carcinomas simulating primary ovarian clear cell carcinoma and secretory endometrioid carcinoma: a clinicopathologic and immunohistochemical study of five cases. American Journal of Surgical Pathology 22: 805–815

Young R H, Scully R E 1985 Ovarian metastases from cancer of the lung: problems in interpretation: a report of seven cases. Gynecologic Oncology 21: 337–350

Young R H, Scully R E 1988a Mucinous ovarian tumors associated with mucinous adenocarcinoma of the cervix: a clinicopathologal anaalysis of 16 cases. International Journal of Gynecological Pathology 7: 99–111

Young R H, Scully R E 1988b Urothelial and ovarian carcinomas of identical cell types: problems in interpretation: a report of three cases and review of the literature. International Journal of Gynecological Pathology 7: 197–211

Young R H, Scully R E 1989 Alveolar rhabdomyosarcoma metastatic to the ovary: a report of two cases and discussion of the differential diagnosis of small cell malignant tumors of the ovary. Cancer 64: 899–904

Young R H, Scully R E 1990a Ovarian metastases from carcinoma of the gallbladder and extrahepatic bile ducts simulating primary tumors of the ovary: a report of six cases. International Journal of Gynecological Pathology 9: 60–72

Young R H, Scully R E 1990b Sarcomas metastatic to the ovary; a report of 21 cases. International Journal of Gynecological Pathology 9: 231–252

Young R H, Scully R E 1991a Malignant melanoma metastatic to the ovary: a clinicopathologic analysis of 20 cases. American Journal of Surgical Pathology 15: 849–860

Young R H, Scully R E 1991b Metastatic tumors of the ovary: a problem-orientated approach and review of the recent literature. Seminars in Diagnostic Pathology 8: 250–276

Young R H, Carey R W, Robboy S J 1981 Breast carcinoma masquerading as primary ovarian neoplasm. Cancer 48: 210–212

Young R H, Gilks C B, Scully R E 1991 Mucinous tumors of the appendix associated with mucinous tumors of the ovary and pseudomyxoma peritonei: a clinicopathological analysis of 22 cases supporting an origin in the appendix. American Journal of Surgical Pathology 15: 415–429

Young R H, Gersell D J, Clement P B, Scully R E 1992 Hepatocellular carcinoma metastatic to the ovary: a report of three cases discovered during life with discussion of the differential diagnosis of hepatoid tumors of the ovary. Human Pathology 23: 574–580

Young R H, Kozakewich H P W, Scully R E 1993a Metastatic ovarian tumors in children: a report of 14 cases and review of the literature. International Journal of Gynecological Pathology 12: 8–19

Young R H, Gersell D J, Roth L M, Scully R E 1993b Ovarian metastases from cervical carcinomas other than pure adenocarcinomas: a report of 12 cases. Cancer 71: 407–418

Young R H, Jackson A, Wells M 1994 Ovarian metastasis from thyroid carcinoma twelve years after thyroidectomy mimicking struma ovarii. International Journal of Gynecological Pathology 13: 181–185

Young-Fadok T M, Wolff B G, Nivatvongs S, Metzger P P, Ilstrup D M 1998 Prophylactic oophorectomy in colorectal carcinoma: preliminary results of a randomized, prospective trial. Diseases of the Colon and Rectum 41: 277–283

Zaino R J, Unger E R, Whitney C 1984 Synchronous carcinomas of the uterine corpus and ovary. Gynecological Oncology 19: 329–335

Zirkin R, Brown S, Hertz M 1980 Adenocarcinoid of appendix presenting as bilateral ovarian tumors. Diagnostic Gynecology and Obstetrics 2: 269–274

Zukerberg L R, Young R H 1990 Chordoma metastatic to the ovary. Archives of Pathology and Laboratory Medicine 114: 208–210

26

Ovarian tumours of uncertain origin

A. J. Tiltman

Introduction 897

Tumours of possible mesonephric origin 897
Ovarian tumours of probable Wolffian origin 898
Tumours of the rete ovarii 902
Wilms' tumour 903

Small cell tumours 903
Small cell undifferentiated carcinoma — hypercalcaemic
  type 903
Small cell carcinoma — pulmonary type 905
Desmoplastic small round cell tumour 906

Miscellaneous tumours 907
Adenomatoid tumours 907
Hepatoid carcinoma 908
Oncocytic tumour 909
Adenoid cystic carcinoma 909

INTRODUCTION

This chapter gathers together a number of miscellaneous, uncommon, primary tumours of the ovary which cannot be readily classified among the major categories of ovarian neoplasms. In some the histogenesis is presumed but in others it remains unknown. They can be divided broadly into three groups.

1. Those possibly of mesonephric or displaced renal blastemic origin
   a. Tumour of probable Wolffian origin
   b. Tumours of the rete ovarii
   c. Wilms' tumour
2. Small cell tumours
   a. Small cell undifferentiated carcinoma of hypercalcaemic type
   b. Small cell carcinoma of pulmonary type
   c. Desmoplastic small round cell tumour
3. A miscellaneous group, possibly of mesothelial or epithelial origin
   a. Adenomatoid tumour
   b. Hepatoid carcinoma
   c. Oncocytoma
   d. Adenoid cystic carcinoma.

TUMOURS OF POSSIBLE MESONEPHRIC ORIGIN

The mesonephros and the mesonephric ducts arise within the intermediate mesoderm early in embryogenesis. The mesonephric ducts are destined to form the trigone of the urinary bladder, the posterior wall of the urethra and, in the male, the epididymis and vas deferens. In the female, the mesonephric ducts degenerate at about 75 days gestation but remnants may be found in the uterine corpus, cervix and vagina as Gartner's duct, in the broad ligament as the paroophoron and adjacent to the ovary as the epoophoron (Duthie 1925) and the rete ovarii (Wenzel & Odend'hal 1985). The indifferent gonad develops medial to the mesonephros and the mesonephric blastema is thought to play a rôle in the development of both the testis and ovary (Wartenberg 1982).

A. OVARIAN TUMOURS OF PROBABLE WOLFFIAN ORIGIN

In 1973 Kariminejad & Scully described nine distinctive paraovarian tumours which they called female adnexal tumours of probable Wolffian origin. Later, Hughesdon (1982) and Young & Scully (1983) described morphologically similar tumours arising in the ovary itself. Because of this similarity, the ovarian and paraovarian tumours are regarded as of the same histogenesis.

Morphology

Both ovarian and paraovarian tumours have been described as being solid or solid with cystic areas (Fig. 26.1) and have varied in size from 2–25 cm in great-

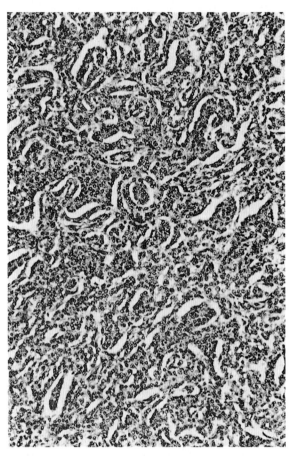

Fig. 26.3 Ovarian tumour of probable Wolffian origin. Cords and tubules with papillary formations giving a retiform appearance.

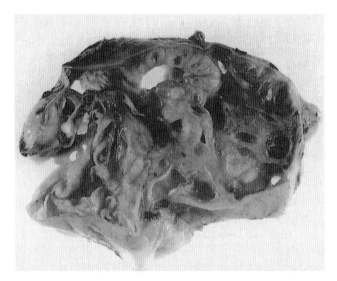

Fig. 26.1 Ovarian tumour of probable Wolffian origin which is mainly cystic with solid areas.

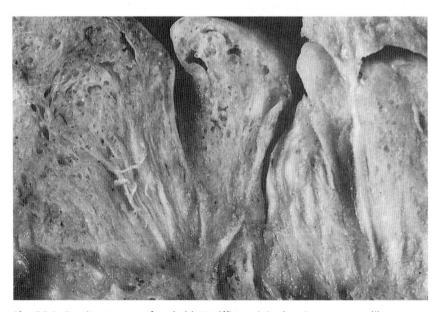

Fig. 26.2 Ovarian tumour of probable Wolffian origin showing a sponge-like appearance produced by numerous small cysts.

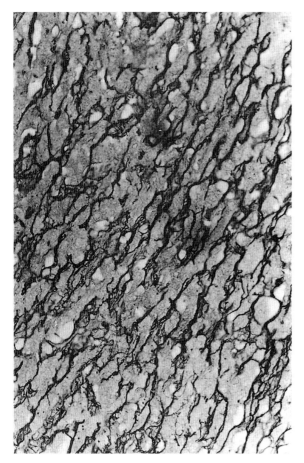

Fig. 26.4 Ovarian tumour of probable Wolffian origin. Reticulin stain showing cord-like structures.

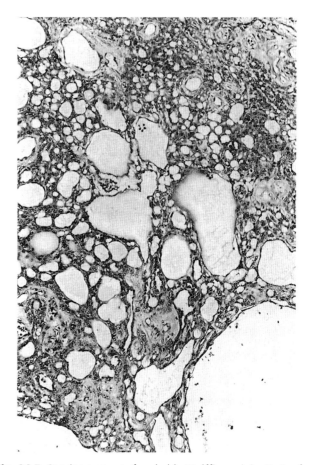

Fig. 26.5 Ovarian tumour of probable Wolffian origin. Cysts of varying sizes producing a sieve-like appearance.

est diameter. The cysts contain clear yellow or haemorrhagic fluid. The solid areas may be lobulated and consist of white or cream-coloured tissue. Haemorrhage may be present. In some instances close inspection may show a spongy appearance produced by smaller cysts (Fig. 26.2).

Microscopy shows a variety of appearances with epithelial cells arranged in tubules, as multiple dilated cysts or as diffuse sheets. All these may be present in the same tumour but one pattern often dominates.

The tubular pattern is formed by tubules or solid cords of cuboidal cells with central nuclei. The nuclei show diffuse chromatin and small nucleoli. Columnar cells and vacuolated cells have also been described. The tubules may be interwoven and branching, sometimes exhibiting a papillary or retiform appearance (Fig. 26.3), or may be so tightly packed as to resemble solid sheets on H&E-stained sections. A well-delineated PAS-positive basement membrane may be seen and reticulin stains reveal the true tubular or nested architecture (Fig. 26.4).

The cysts vary in size from very small to large and are separated by fibrous stroma or solid tumour. In places they have been described as imparting a sieve-like appearance (Fig. 26.5). In other areas, closely packed small spaces may resemble the appearance of an adenomatoid tumour (Fig. 26.6). The cells lining these spaces are flat, sometimes cuboidal and sometimes show a hobnail appearance with loss of cytoplasm. Occasionally the cells may contain coarse eosinophilic cytoplasmic granules (Fig. 26.7). The material within the cysts may stain weakly with PAS after digestion with diastase.

The solid sheets of tumour cells may be composed of polygonal cells (Fig. 26.8) or spindle cells resembling stroma. Reticulin stains usually delineate groups of cells. Small amounts of intracytoplasmic glycogen have been demonstrated. A small number of mitoses may be present but pleomorphism is usually absent.

A moderate vasculature is present throughout the tumour. The intervening stroma is fibrous and may become hyalinised, entrapping tumour cells within it (Fig. 26.9).

The recent immunohistochemical studies on probable Wolffian tumours are tabulated in Table 26.1. In general the tumours are positive for cytokeratin and vimentin and negative for EMA (Rahilly et al 1995; Devouassoux-Shisheboran et al 1999; Tiltman & Allard, 2000). Inhibin-α is positive in about two thirds of cases (Kommoss et al 1998;

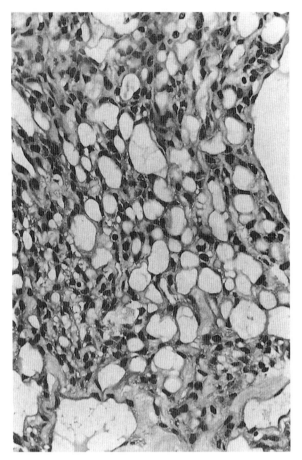

Fig. 26.6 Ovarian tumour of probable Wolffian origin. Small dilated tubules resembling an adenomatoid tumour.

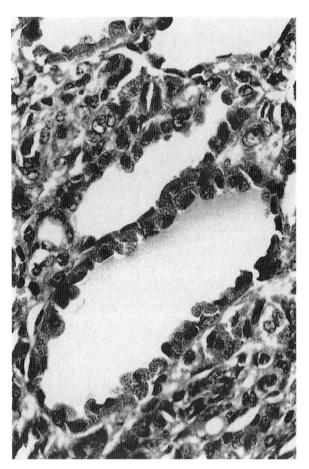

Fig. 26.7 Ovarian tumour of probable Wolffian origin. Small cystic spaces lined by cells with coarse granular cytoplasm.

Table 26.1 Immunohistochemical profile of adnexal tumours of probable Wolffian origin

| Antibody | No. positive/no. tested | | | |
	Rahilly et al 1995	**Devouassoux-Shisheboran et al 1999**	**Tiltman & Allard 2000**	**Total**
AE-1/AE-3		25/25		25/25
CAM 5.2	3/3	25/25	4/6	32/34
CK 7		22/25	2/6	24/31
CK 19			5/6	5/6
CK 20		2/25	0/6	2/31
Calretenin		20/25	0/6	33/34[a]
EMA	0/3	3/25	1/6	4/34
Vimentin	3/3	25/25	5/6	33/34
α-inhibin		17/25		26/35[b]
S-100	3/3		3/6	6/16[c]

AE-1/AE-3 = all basic and acidic cytokeratins; CAM 5.2 = CK 8 & 18; EMA = epithelial membrane antigen.
a — different antibodies used in two studies; *b* — includes 9/10 cases from Kommoss et al 1998;
c — includes 0/7 cases from Tavassoli et al 1990.

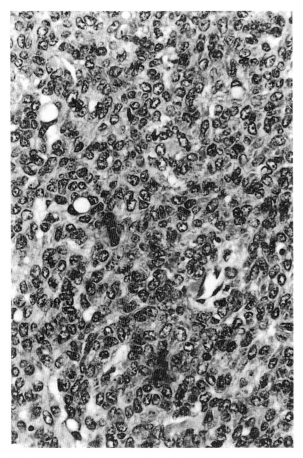

Fig. 26.8 Ovarian tumour of probable Wolffian origin. Solid sheets of polygonal cells.

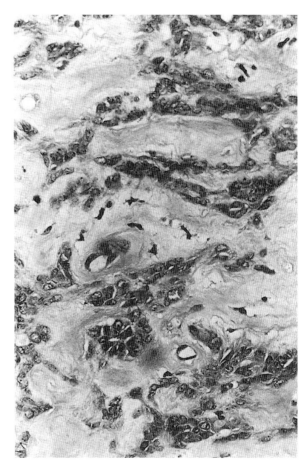

Fig. 26.9 Ovarian tumour of probable Wolffian origin. Hyalinised collagenous stroma with entrapped epithelial elements.

Devouassoux-Shisheboran et al 1999). Staining for cal-retenin appears to depend on the antibody used.

Clinical presentation and behaviour

The patients with tumours arising in the ovary have been between 28 and 79 years of age, with most patients in the sixth decade (mean 52 years). Those patients with para-ovarian tumours have been younger (13–62 years; mean 40 years) with several being less than 30 years. Presenting symptoms include lower abdominal pain, an enlarging abdomen or frequency of micturition. Most tumours are, however, discovered during pelvic examination for unrelated symptoms or are incidental findings at laparotomy. They are generally regarded as hormonally inert but there have been 4 reported cases associated with endometrial hyperplasia (Kariminejad & Scully 1973; Sivathondan et al 1979; Hughesdon 1982) and an additional postmenopausal patient had endometrial hyperplasia and a significantly raised serum estradiol level which returned to normal after surgery (Inoue et al 1995).

Ovarian and paraovarian Wolffian tumours are generally regarded as benign but a number of malignant ovarian (Hughesdon 1982; Young & Scully 1983) and paraovarian tumours have been reported (Taxy & Battifora 1976; Abbot et al 1981; Brescia et al 1985; Prasad et al 1992; Daya 1994; Sheyn et al 2000; Tiltman & Allard 2000). These malignant tumours have shown increased mitotic activity (> 10/10 high-power fields) or nuclear pleomorphism. One case showed areas described as undifferentiated carcinoma. The age range of malignant tumours varies from 13–81 years. Recurrences generally present years after removal of the primary tumour suggesting that malignancy, when present, is usually of low grade.

Histogenesis

The belief that these tumours are of Wolffian (mesonephric) remnant origin is based on:

a. the observation that although epithelial in nature they do not resemble any of the ovarian tumours of

Müllerian origin and have not been described in association with the common epithelial tumours;

b. the fact that they are morphologically distinguishable from sex cord–stromal tumours such as Sertoli–Leydig or granulosa cell tumours;

c. the finding that the extraovarian tumours occur at sites where Wolffian remnants are often found and that some of the ovarian tumours arise in the ovarian hilus where the rete ovarii could be the source;

d. the presence of a prominent basement membrane around the epithelial tubules which is structurally consistent with the Wolffian but not Müllerian ducts (Gardner et al 1948; Lamb et al 1960);

e. Ultrastructural examinations show features compatible with a Wolffian, and do not support a Müllerian, origin (Taxy & Battifora 1976; Demopoulos et al 1980);

f. Immunohistochemistry has done little more than support the compatibility between the tumour and Wolffian remnants (Tavassoli et al 1990; Rahilly et al 1995; Devouassoux-Shisheboran et al 1999; Tiltman & Allard 2000). Antibody to glutathione S-transferase-μ, a putative marker for mesonephric remnants, was positive in only 50% of probable Wolffian tumours in one study (Tiltman & Allard 2000).

Differential diagnosis

Tumours of probable Wolffian origin need to be differentiated from Sertoli–Leydig cell tumours, granulosa cell tumours, clear cell carcinomas and adenomatoid tumours. Focal areas within the Wolffian tumours may closely mimic each of the above but if sufficient tissue is examined the variations in morphology become apparent.

Sertoli–Leydig cell tumours may show tubules, cords and solid areas composed of oval cells but the mixed composition is not as variable as that seen in the Wolffian tumour. The retiform type of Sertoli–Leydig tumour may, however, show larger spaces superficially resembling the cystic areas in the Wolffian tumour. Sertoli–Leydig tumours usually contain luteinized stromal or Leydig cells and the patients may show virilisation.

On low-power examination, the solid areas of a Wolffian tumour may resemble the diffuse form of granulosa cell tumour and, when admixed with cystic spaces, may superficially resemble the juvenile granulosa cell tumour. Granulosa cell tumours either show the typical cytological morphology of the adult type or the vacuolated cytoplasm of the juvenile form, both of which differ from the Wolffian tumour.

The cystic spaces lined by hobnail-like cells resemble those seen in the Müllerian clear cell carcinoma but the remainder of the Wolffian morphology is quite unlike that seen in the clear cell carcinoma.

The sponge-like areas and small cystic spaces may resemble the canalicular pattern of an adenomatoid tumour

but the solid tubules and cords of the Wolffian tumour differ from the solid cords of the adenomatoid tumour, and solid spindle cell areas are not present in the latter. Adenomatoid tumours are generally much smaller and hyaluronic acid may be demonstrable in cytoplasmic vacuoles.

B. TUMOURS OF THE RETE OVARII

The rete ovarii is a small irregular tubular structure, of mesonephric origin, located in the hilus of the ovary (Wenzel & Odend'hal 1985). There is, therefore, a close, if not inseparable, histogenetic relationship between tumours arising from the rete and the tumours of probable Wolffian origin. In an early report, a tumour arising in the ovarian hilus and later accepted as a Wolffian tumour was initially called an adenoma of the rete body (Greene & Dilts 1965) and the review by Tavassoli et al (1990) referred to the Wolffian tumours as 'retiform' because of the close immunohistochemical and ultrastructural similarities. There are, however, a small group of morphologically distinct tumours of the rete ovarii.

Adenomas of the rete are rare, small tumours measuring up to 5 mm in diameter (Janovski & Paramanandhan 1973). Microscopically they consist of tubules lined by a single layer of cuboidal or columnar cells morphologically

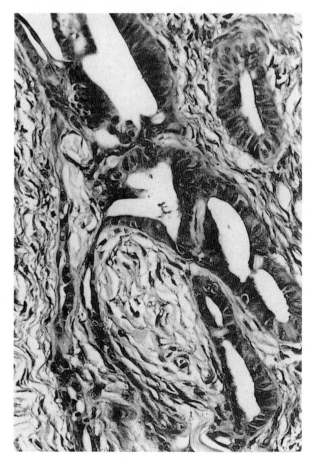

Fig. 26.10 Hyperplasia of rete ovarii. Tubules and cords lined by columnar cells within a fibrous stroma.

resembling those of the rete (Rutgers & Scully 1988). These tubules are separated and usually distorted by the supporting fibrous stroma and may contain intraluminal fibropapillary projections. Luteinization of the stromal cells to resemble hilus cells may be present giving a morphology that needs to be distinguished from retiform Sertoli–Leydig cell tumours (Nogales et al 1997). Adenomatous hyperplasia of the rete is morphologically similar on high-power examination (Fig. 26.10) but is not as well circumscribed as the adenoma. The dividing line between the two is not well defined. Cysts of the rete ovarii may measure up to 27 cm in diameter. Most of these are probably non-neoplastic but some cysts show stratification of the lining cells and have been regarded as cystadenomas (Rutgers & Scully 1988). Adenocarcinoma of the rete is extremely rare. The case described by Rutgers & Scully (1988) showed a papillary and tubular pattern and also contained areas of urothelial-like cells.

C. WILMS' TUMOUR

Very rare examples of extrarenal adult Wilms' tumours have been described in the ovary (Sahin & Benda 1988; Gursoy et al 1995) where they consist of blastematous tissue with tubules or glomeruloid structures surrounded

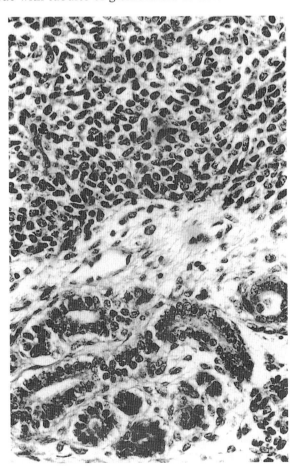

Fig. 26.11 Wilms' tumour showing blastema and tubular structures.

by small spindle cells morphologically typical of Wilms' tumour in the kidney (Fig. 26.11). A single case described as cystic partially differentiated Wilms' tumour of the ovary has been reported in a 21-year-old patient (Isaac et al 2000). Nephroblastematous elements may be present in teratomas of the ovary (Nogales et al 1980) and have also been described in association with a juvenile granulosa cell tumour where it was not certain whether it represented an independent tumour or was part of a mixed sex cord–stromal/germ cell neoplasm (O'Dowd & Ismail 1990).

The histogenetic theories of extrarenal Wilms' tumour include derivation from misplaced renal blastema, primitive extrarenal mesoderm or as part of a teratoma. A diagnosis of primary Wilms' tumour of the ovary requires that no teratomatous elements be present. The differential diagnosis includes other small cell tumours, Sertoli–Leydig cell tumours and malignant mixed Müllerian tumour.

SMALL CELL TUMOURS

A number of ovarian neoplasms consist of small cells with little cytoplasm. Some of these are metastatic to the ovary. Others are primary ovarian neoplasms of known histogenesis such as primitive neuroectodermal tumour and granulosa cell tumours. A third group of uncertain histogenesis includes:

a. Small cell undifferentiated carcinoma — hypercalcaemic type
b. Small cell carcinoma — pulmonary type
c. Desmoplastic small round cell tumour.

A. SMALL CELL UNDIFFERENTIATED CARCINOMA — HYPERCALCAEMIC TYPE

Small cell undifferentiated carcinoma of the ovary in young women, in association with hypercalcaemia, was first described by Dickersin et al in 1982. Since then there have been several reports of morphologically similar tumours, not always accompanied by raised serum calcium levels. While the tumour is most frequently found in younger patients it is also described in older women.

Morphology

The tumours are generally large and unilateral. The cut surface shows solid tissue which is grey–white, grey–yellow or tan coloured. Haemorrhage and necrosis are frequently present and cystic degeneration or small cysts may be seen.

Microscopically the tumours are composed of small epithelial cells with little cytoplasm (Fig. 26.12). The cells may be arranged in diffuse sheets, as smaller islands or as anastomosing cords. Small cystic, follicle-like, spaces

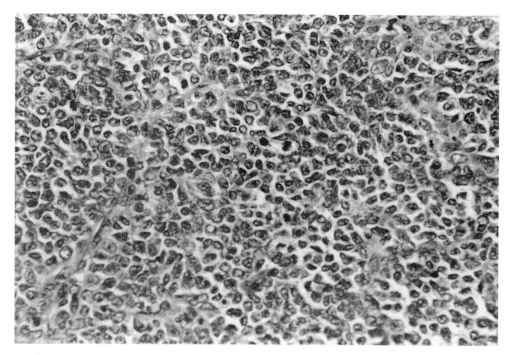

Fig. 26.12 Ovarian small cell carcinoma with hypercalcaemia. Small cells with little cytoplasm are lying in sheets. Elsewhere in the neoplasm there was extensive haemorrhage and necrosis.

Table 26.2 Immunohistochemistry of small cell carcinomas — hypercalcaemic type (SCC. HT) (Ulbright et al 1987; Abeler et al 1988; Aguirre et al 1989; Young et al 1994); small cell carcinoma — pulmonary type (SCC. PT)) Eichhorn et al 1992a) and desmoplastic small round cell tumour (DSRCT) (Young et al 1992)

	No. positive/no. tested		
Antibody	SCC.HT	SCC.PT	DSRCT
Cytokeratin	5/6	6/9	
AE-1/AE-3	6/14		2/3
CAM 5.2	15/15		2/3
EMA	8/25	5/9	3/3
Vimentin	16/28	0/8	3/3*
NSE	15/21	6/9	1/3
Chromogranin	5/11	2/9*	0/3

AE-1/AE-3 = high molecular weight cytokeratin; CAM 5.2 = CK 8 & 18; EMA = epithelial membrane antigen; NSE = neurone-specific enolase.
* = focal only.

surrounded by tumour cells are usually present. Necrosis is common. The tumour cell nuclei are generally round or polygonal with some clumping of chromatin and a small nucleolus. Mitoses are easily found but nuclear pleomorphism is not a feature and flow cytometric analysis has shown a diploid DNA content in all tumours examined (Eichhorn et al 1992a). Cells with abundant eosinophilic cytoplasm may be present in up to half the tumours and dominant in about 10% of cases — the so-called large cell variant (Young et al 1994). Cells containing intracytoplasmic mucin either admixed with tumour cells or lining

glandular spaces may be found in up to 10% of cases (Young et al 1994).

Immunohistochemistry has shown varying results (Ulbright et al 1987; Abeler et al 1988; Aguirre et al 1989; Young et al 1994) which are summarised in Table 26.2. Tumour cells stain for both cytokeratins and vimentin. Neurone-specific enolase (NSE) is generally positive. Chromogranin may be present in some instances. Parathormone has been demonstrated in 4 of 26 patients, 11 of whom were hypercalcaemic (Abeler et al 1988; McMahon & Hart 1988; Aguirre et al 1989). Parathyroid hormone related protein has been demonstrated in 5 of 7 cases (Matias-Guiu et al 1994).

Electronmicroscopy confirms the epithelial nature of the cell with desmosome-like junctions and a basal lamina surrounding groups of cells (Dickersin et al 1982; McMahon & Hart 1988). Cells may be arranged around a central space and microvilli and cilia have been demonstrated. The cytoplasm typically contains prominent dilated rough endoplasmic reticulum. Dense core granules are usually not found (Dickersin & Scully 1998) but have been described in occasional examples (Abeler et al 1988; Nesland & Abeler 1989).

Clinical presentation and behaviour

The age at presentation ranges from 9–55 years with a mean age of about 23 years. Few patients are over the age of 40 years. The presenting symptoms are typically abdominal swelling and/or pain. Hypercalcaemia, up to

4.5 mmol/l, which returns to normal after resection of the tumour and is not associated with bone involvement by tumour, occurs in about two-thirds of the patients (Young et al 1994).

Although tumours are frequently stage I at presentation, small cell carcinoma of the ovary has generally behaved in a very aggressive manner. In the only large series reported, only 33% of patients with stage IA remained disease free and almost all of those with higher stage died of disease, usually within a year (Young et al 1994). As with other ovarian carcinomas, spread is predominantly into the peritoneal cavity and retroperitoneal lymph nodes.

Histogenesis

Despite detailed morphological and immunohistochemical investigations the histogenesis of ovarian small cell carcinomas remains an enigma. While they are regarded as epithelial they do not resemble the common epithelial tumours of the ovary, are not seen in combination with them and generally occur at a younger age. This last factor has suggested a germ cell origin but other germ cell elements have not been seen in these tumours and the arguments presented by Ulbright et al (1987) in favour of a germ cell origin are not convincing. Dense core granules have only been demonstrated by electronmicroscopy on rare occasions but chromogranin and NSE have been positive by immunohistochemistry. These have suggested a neuroendocrine cell origin but the overall morphology is not in keeping with such a conclusion.

Differential diagnosis

Small cell undifferentiated carcinoma needs to be distinguished from other small cell tumours.

- Primary ovarian small cell carcinoma of pulmonary type and desmoplastic small round cell tumour as discussed below.
- The diffuse forms of adult granulosa cell tumour can resemble small cell carcinomas but the nuclei may show nuclear grooving and mitoses are infrequent. Juvenile granulosa cell tumour, which occurs in the same age group as small cell carcinoma, is usually distinctive. The follicles of the juvenile granulosa cell tumour are less regular in outline, sometimes appear to be surrounded by a collar of cells and contain weakly staining mucicarminophilic material. The cells show some pleomorphism and may contain lipid.
- Primary malignant neuroectodermal tumour of the ovary is considered to be of germ cell origin and may show focal glial or ependymal differentiation (Aguirre & Scully 1982; Kleinman et al 1993).
- Primary ovarian rhabdomyosarcoma usually has some diagnostic morphological feature such as striated

muscle cells or an alveolar pattern to indicate its myosarcomatous nature which can be confirmed by immunohistochemistry (Nielsen et al 1998). Rhabdomyosarcoma may also be an uncommon metastasis to the ovary and may show bilateral involvement (Young & Scully 1989).
- Metastatic oat cell carcinoma from the lung may be recognised by the clinical history, pulmonary involvement and the widespread distribution of metastases. The cells are smaller and may show nuclear smearing. The nuclei show more diffuse chromatin and the nucleoli are generally inconspicuous. Small cell carcinomas of the oat cell type may also arise in the endometrium and cervix and metastasise to the ovary. Nonpulmonary extragenital small cell carcinomas may also metastasise to the ovary (Eichhorn et al 1993).
- Metastatic lobular carcinoma of the breast which may maintain its 'single file' growth pattern or show nests of small cells with central nuclei. Mucin may be demonstrable. Ovarian involvement is usually late and the presence of the breast primary obvious.
- Metastatic melanomas may present as small cell tumours but may show areas of pleomorphism. Melanin is usually demonstrable and the tumour cells are S-100 positive.
- Lymphomas and leukaemia may present as ovarian neoplasms (Osborne & Robboy 1983; Fox et al 1988; Monterroso et al 1993). Their recognition may be confirmed by immunohistochemistry.

B. SMALL CELL CARCINOMA — PULMONARY TYPE

Eichhorn et al (1992b) have described primary small cell carcinomas of the ovary that microscopically resembled small cell carcinomas of the lung and differed from the small cell undifferentiated carcinoma of hypercalcaemic type described above.

Morphology

As described by these authors, the tumours are bilateral in about half the cases and vary from 4.5–26 cm in greatest diameter. The cut surface shows solid tumour with cystic spaces. Microscopically the tumours are composed of small cells with little cytoplasm arranged in sheets, closely packed nests or islands. The nuclei are small, oval and generally monomorphic with evenly dispersed chromatin and small nucleoli. Flow cytometry has shown aneuploidy in five of the eight tumours investigated. The immunohistochemical findings are shown in Table 26.1. Occasional cells may demonstrate argyrophilia. Dense core granules have been demonstrated by electron microscopy (Dickersin & Scully 1998).

Clinical presentation and behaviour

The 11 cases reported by Eichhorn et al (1992b) presented at ages between 28 and 85 years (mean 59 years) with symptoms referable to the mass. Endocrine abnormalities were not present and no patient had hypercalcaemia. Six of the neoplasms were stage III on presentation but even the stage I tumours behaved in an aggressive fashion, with most patients either dead of disease or alive with recurrence within a year of presentation.

Histogenesis

Ovarian small cell carcinomas of pulmonary type are considered to be neuroendocrinal but are frequently associated with ovarian epithelial tumours. Of the 11 cases of small cell carcinoma of pulmonary type reported by Eichhorn et al, four had an associated endometrioid carcinoma and two a benign Brenner tumour. As argyrophilic cells have been demonstrated in a range of ovarian epithelial tumours small cell carcinomas of pulmonary type might represent a divergent neuroendocrine differentiation in other, more common neoplasms.

Differential diagnosis

The differential diagnosis includes all those listed under small cell undifferentiated carcinoma — hypercalcaemic type. The small cell carcinoma of pulmonary type, which occurs at a mean age of 59 years, differs from the small cell undifferentiated carcinoma of hypercalcaemic type with a mean age of 23 years. In addition the pulmonary type is bilateral in about half the cases, may be associated with another epithelial component and is not associated with hypercalcaemia. In contrast to the hypercalcaemic type, the pulmonary type tumours may be aneuploid and are vimentin negative. Ovarian small cell carcinoma of pulmonary type must be distinguished from metastatic carcinoma from the lung. If both lung and ovary are involved it is better regarded as a lung primary.

C. DESMOPLASTIC SMALL ROUND CELL TUMOUR

The tumour designated intra-abdominal desmoplastic small round cell tumour with divergent differentiation occurs, as its name implies, within the abdominal cavity in young patients — mainly in the first and second decades but up to the age of 30 years with occasional cases in the fourth decade (Gerald et al 1991). It is more common in males but occasional cases involving the ovary have been reported (Young et al 1992a; Zaloudek et al 1995).

Morphology

Multiple tumour nodules are present within the abdominal cavity. The ovaries contain solid tan–white tumour (Fig. 26.13). Microscopically there are nests of small tumour cells separated by a fibrous stroma (Fig. 26.14). Necrosis may be present in the centre of these islands and at the periphery there may be palisading of tumour cells. The tumour cells are small, with little cytoplasm and round to polygonal hyperchromatic nuclei with some chromatin clumping (Fig. 26.15). Mitoses are frequent. The fibrous stroma varies in cellularity with collagenous and occasional myxoid areas.

Immunohistochemistry shows positive staining with a wide spectrum of antibodies. Table 26.1 compares the findings to other small cell tumours of the ovary. In addition to those shown in the table, desmin characteristically stains as a paranuclear globule.

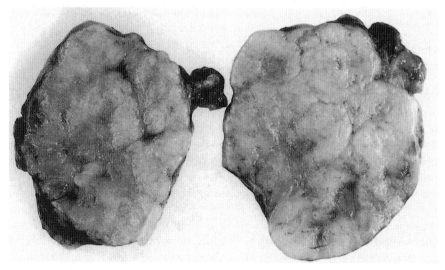

Fig. 26.13 Desmoplastic small round cell tumour. Two slices through a solid tumour showing a lobulated structure and small areas of haemorrhage.

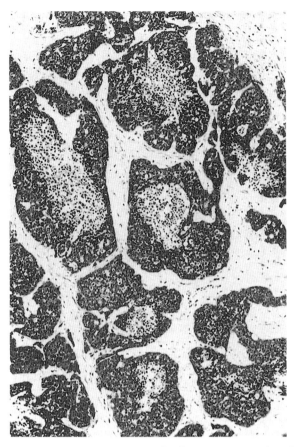

Fig. 26.14 Desmoplastic small round cell tumour. Nests of small tumour cells surrounded by fibrous stroma and showing central necrosis.

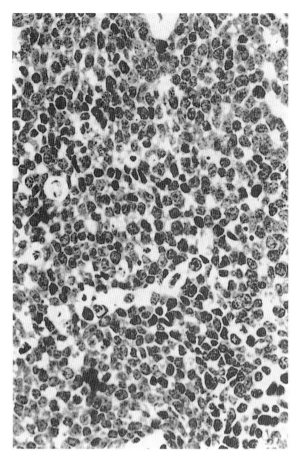

Fig. 26.15 Desmoplastic small round cell tumour. Nests consist of small cells with little cytoplasm.

Electronmicroscopy shows cells with tight junctions, arranged in groups, sometimes with poorly formed lumina at the centre and surrounded at the periphery by a basal lamina. The cytoplasm contains numerous ribosomes, a few mitochondria and some glycogen.

Clinical presentation and behaviour

Desmoplastic small round cell tumour generally occurs in young patients. The 4 documented ovarian cases were 14, 15, 15 and 22 years old (Young et al 1992a; Zaloudek 1995). Other intra-abdominal cases, without ovarian involvement, have ranged in age from 3–38 years of age with a mean of about 18 years (Gonzalez-Crussi et al 1990; Gerald et al 1991; Variend et al 1991). The tumours behave in a malignant fashion with death occurring within four years.

Histogenesis

The origin of desmoplastic small round cell tumour is not known. Some have considered a neuroectodermal (Variend et al 1991) and others a mesothelial origin (Gerald et al 1991).

Differential diagnosis

Desmoplastic small round cell tumour needs to be differentiated from other small cell tumours, as discussed under both hypercalcaemic and pulmonary types of small cell undifferentiated carcinoma. A striking feature of the desmoplastic tumour is the low-magnification appearance of nests of cells separated by fibrous stroma.

MISCELLANEOUS TUMOURS

A. ADENOMATOID TUMOURS

Adenomatoid tumours are not infrequently found in the uterine corpus or adjacent to the Fallopian tube but are an uncommon finding in the ovary. Ovarian adenomatoid tumours have been reported in patients between 23 and 79 years of age and are usually incidental findings at surgery for some unrelated reason.

Morphology

Adenomatoid tumours of the ovary are generally small grey lesions measuring less than 1 cm in diameter and are usually present in the ovarian hilus extending into the

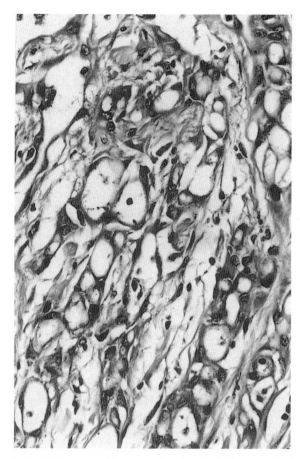

Fig. 26.16 Adenomatoid tumour showing both short cords of vacuolated cuboidal cells and dilated spaces lined by flattened cells.

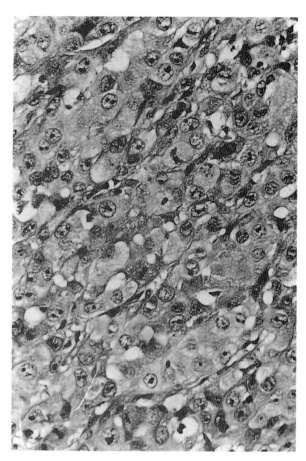

Fig. 26.17 Hepatoid carcinoma. Cells with abundant eosinophilic cytoplasm arranged in trabeculae.

medulla. Williamson & Moore (1964) describe a tumour measuring 3 cm in diameter occurring within the ovary, and a 5 cm juxtaovarian tumour is reported by Young et al (1991). The diffuse involvement of the ovary described by Morehead (1946) is not a convincing example of adenomatoid tumour.

Microscopically the typical features of adenomatoid tumours seen elsewhere may be present, either alone or in combination (Fig. 26.16). A plexiform pattern is produced by nests or cords of eosinophilic cuboidal cells, some of which may be vacuolated. A tubular pattern contains spaces lined by cuboidal cells. Vacuolation within the cytoplasm is usual. A canalicular pattern is produced by spaces of varying size lined by flattened cells. Scattered lymphocytes are frequently seen. Small amounts of smooth muscle may be present. Focal, intracytoplasmic positivity for Alcian Blue can be eliminated by prior digestion with hyaluronidase. Mucicarmine stain is negative.

Adenomatoid tumours are benign. It is generally held that they are of mesothelial origin but the almost exclusive occurrence within the genital tract has not been adequately explained.

B. HEPATOID CARCINOMA

There are a small number of primary ovarian carcinomas which morphologically resemble hepatocellular carcinoma and have hence been labelled hepatoid carcinomas (Ishikura & Scully 1987). These tumours have occurred in women between 35 and 78 years of age with no specific clinical presentation. One case presented during pregnancy (Maymon et al 1998).

The tumours are solid or solid and cystic and have measured up to 20 cm in greatest diameter. Microscopically they are composed of cells with abundant eosinophilic cytoplasm and central nuclei. The cells are arranged in sheets or trabeculae (Fig. 26.17). Intra- and extracytoplasmic PAS-positive hyaline globules are present but sometimes only in small numbers (Fig. 26.18a). Variable numbers of giant cells are scattered throughout the tumour (Fig. 26.18b). Small amounts of glycogen may be demonstrated. Alpha-fetoprotein is present in the tumour cells and serum and is considered essential for the diagnosis.

The histogenesis of hepatoid carcinoma is unknown but it has been described in association with a 'tubular' adeno-carcinoma (Matsuta et al 1991) and serous carcinoma

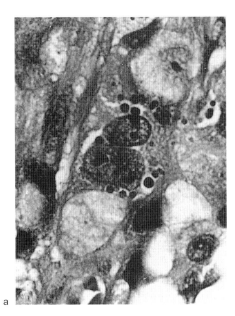 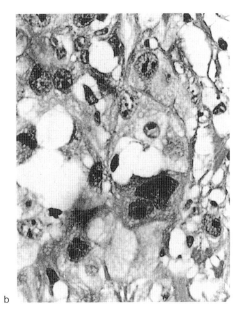

Fig. 26.18 Hepatoid carcinoma.
a Hyaline globules. **b** Giant cell.

(Scurry et al 1996). This suggests a similar histogenesis to the common epithelial tumours of the ovary

Ovarian hepatoid carcinoma needs to be distinguished from:

- Hepatocellular carcinoma metastatic to the ovary (Young et al 1992b).
- Hepatoid yolk sac tumour, which is of germ cell origin, occurs at an earlier age and also contains areas showing more typical yolk sac features.
- Sertoli–Leydig cell tumours with hepatocytic differentiation (Mooney et al 1999).

C. ONCOCYTIC TUMOUR

There have been two reports of oncocytic tumours of the ovary. One was a solid and cystic tumour measuring 15 cm in greatest diameter occurring in a 39-year-old woman (Takeda et al 1983) and the other a solid tumour, 11 cm in diameter, in a 22-year-old woman (Yoshida et al 1984). Microscopically, both showed cells with a granular eosinophilic cytoplasm and electronmicroscopy showed numerous mitochondria. In the first case, the cells were arranged in a tubular or papillary arrangement and in the second they were in solid sheets. The first tumour showed stromal invasion and was diagnosed as a carcinoma. The second was regarded as benign.

Ovarian oncocytoma may represent an oncocytic metaplasia within a common epithelial ovarian tumour such as endometrioid carcinoma (Pitman et al 1994) and not a specific tumour type.

D. ADENOID CYSTIC CARCINOMA

Eichhorn and Scully (1995) described 6 cases of adenoid cystic carcinoma of the ovary and Feczo et al (1996) described a seventh. They have occurred in patients from 45–78 years of age. Microscopically they resemble adenoid cystic carcinoma of the salivary glands or those found elsewhere in the female genital tract. Their histogenesis is uncertain but 5 of the 7 described cases have been associated, either syn- or metachronously, with malignant common epithelial ovarian tumours. Metastatic adenoid cystic carcinoma, from the submandibular gland to the ovary has been reported (Longacre et al 1996).

REFERENCES

Abbot R L, Barlogie B, Schmidt W A 1981 Metastasizing malignant juxtaovarian tumor with terminal hypercalcemia. Cancer 48: 860–865

Abeler V, Kjorstad K E, Nesland J M 1988 Small cell carcinoma of the ovary. International Journal of Gynecological Pathology 7: 315–329

Aguirre P, Scully R E 1982 Malignant neuroectodermal tumor of the ovary, a distinctive form of monodermal teratoma. American Journal of Surgical Pathology 6: 283–292

Aguirre P, Thor A D, Scully R E 1989 Ovarian small cell carcinoma: histogenetic considerations based on immunohistochemical and other findings. American Journal of Clinical Pathology 92: 140–149

Brescia R J, Cardoso de Almeida P C, Fuller A F, Dickersin G R, Robboy S J 1985. Female adnexal tumor of probable Wolffian origin with multiple recurrences over 16 years. Cancer 56: 1456–1461

Daya, D 1994 Malignant female adnexal tumor of probable Wolffian origin with review of the literature. Archives of Pathology and Laboratory Medicine 118: 310–312

Demopoulos R I, Sitelman A, Flotte T, Bigelow B 1980 Ultrastructural study of a female adnexal tumor of probable Wolffian origin. Cancer 46: 2273–2280

Devouassoux-Shisheboran M, Silver S A, Tavassoli F A 1999 Wolffian adnexal tumor, so called female adnexal tumor of probable Wolffian origin (FATWO): Immunohistochemical evidence in support of a Wolffian origin. Human Pathology 30: 856–863

Dickersin G R, Scully R E 1998 Ovarian small cell tumors: an electron microscopic review. Ultrastructural Pathology 22: 199–226

Dickersin G R, Kline I W, Scully R E 1982 Small cell carcinoma of the ovary with hypercalcemia. Cancer 49: 188–197

Duthie G M 1925 An investigation of the occurrence, distribution and histological structure of the embryonic remains in the human broad ligament. Journal of Anatomy 59: 410–431

Eichhorn J H, Scully R E 1995 Adenoid cystic and basaloid carcinomas of the ovary: evidence for a surface epithelial lineage. A report of 12 cases. Modern Pathology 8: 731–740

Eichhorn J H, Bell D A, Young R H et al 1992a DNA content and proliferative activity in ovarian small cell carcinomas of the hypercalcemic type: implications for diagnosis, prognosis and histogenesis. American Journal of Clinical Pathology 98: 579–586

Eichhorn J H, Young R H, Scully R E 1992b Primary ovarian small cell carcinoma of pulmonary type: a clinicopathologic, immunohistologic and flow cytometric analysis of 11 cases. American Journal of Surgical Pathology 18: 926–938

Eichhorn J H, Young R H, Scully R E 1993 Nonpulmonary small cell carcinoma of extragenital origin metastatic to the ovary. Cancer 71: 177–186

Feczko J D, Jentz D L, Roth L M 1996 Adenoid cystic ovarian carcinoma compared with other adenoid cystic carcinomas of the female genital tract. Modern Pathology 9: 413–417

Fox H, Langley F A, Govan A D T, Hill A S, Bennett M H 1988 Malignant lymphoma presenting as an ovarian tumour: a clinicopathological analysis of 34 cases. British Journal of Obstetrics and Gynaecology 95: 386–390

Gardner G H, Greene R R, Peckham B M 1948 Normal and cystic structures of the broad ligament. American Journal of Obstetrics and Gynecology 55: 917–939

Gerald W L, Miller H K, Battifora H, Miettinen M, Silva E G, Rosai J 1991 Intra-abdominal desmoplastic small round-cell tumor. American Journal of Surgical Pathology 15: 499–513

Gonzalez-Crussi F, Crawford S E, Sun C-C J 1990 Intra-abdominal desmoplastic small-cell tumors with divergent differentiation. American Journal of Surgical Pathology 14: 633–642

Greene R R, Dilts P V 1965 Adenoma of the rete body. American Journal of Obstetrics and Gynecology 93: 886–888

Gursoy R, Akyol G, Tiras B et al 1995 Adult extrarenal Wilms' tumor. A case report. Gynecological and Obstetric Investigation 40: 141–144

Hughesdon P E 1982 Ovarian tumours of Wolffian or allied nature: their place in ovarian oncology. Journal of Clinical Pathology 35: 526–535

Inoue H, Kikuchi Y, Hori T, Nabuchi K, Kobayashi M, Nagata I 1995. An ovarian tumor of probable Wolffian origin with hormonal function. Gynecologic Oncology 59: 304–308

Isaac M A, Vijayalakshni S, Madhu C S, Bosincu L, Nogales F F 2000 Pure cystic nephroblastoma of the ovary with a review of extrarenal Wilms' tumors. Human Pathology 31: 761–764

Ishikura H, Scully R E 1987 Hepatoid carcinoma of the ovary. Cancer 60: 2775–2784

Janovski N A, Paramanandhan T L 1973 Ovarian tumors. In: Friedman E A (ed) Major problems in obstetrics and gynecology, vol 4. Saunders, Philadelphia, pp 104–105

Kariminejad M H, Scully R E 1973 Female adnexal tumor of probable Wolffian origin: a distinctive pathologic entity. Cancer 31: 671–677

Kleinman G M, Young R H, Scully R E 1993 Primary neuroectodermal tumors of the ovary. A report of 25 cases. American Journal of Surgical Pathology 17: 764–778

Kommoss F, Oliva E, Bhan A K, Young R H, Scully R E 1998 Inhibin expression in ovarian tumors and tumor like lesions: an immunohistochemical study. Modern Pathology 11: 656–664

Lamb E J, Fucilla I, Greene R R 1960 Basement membranes in the female genital tract. American Journal of Obstetrics and Gynecology 79: 79–85

Longacre T A, O'Hanlan K, Hendrickson M R 1996 Adenoid cystic carcinoma of the submandibular gland with symptomatic ovarian metastases. International Journal of Gynecological Pathology 15: 349–355

McMahon J T, Hart W R 1988 Ultrastructural analysis of small cell carcinomas of the ovary. American Journal of Clinical Pathology 90: 523–529

Matias-Guiu X, Prat J, Young R H et al 1994 Human parathyroid hormone related protein in ovarian small cell carcinoma. An immunohistochemical study. Cancer 73: 1878–1881

Matsuta M, Ishikura H, Murakami K, Kagabu T, Nishiya I 1991 Hepatoid carcinoma of the ovary. International Journal of Gynecological Pathology 10: 302–310

Maymon E, Piura B, Mazor M, Bashiri A, Silberstein T, Yanai-Inbar I 1998 Primary hepatoid carcinoma of ovary in pregnancy. American Journal of Obstetrics and Gynecology 179: 820–822

Monterroso V, Jaffe E S, Merino M J, Medeiros L J 1993 Malignant lymphoma involving the ovary: a clinicopathological analysis of 39 cases. American Journal of Surgical Pathology 17: 154–170

Mooney E E, Nogales F F, Tavassoli F A 1999 Hepatocytic differentiation in retiform Sertoli–Leydig cell tumors: distinguishing a heterologous element from Leydig cells. Human Pathology 30: 611–617

Morehead R P 1946 Angiomatoid formations in the genital organs with and without tumor formation. Archives of Pathology and Laboratory Medicine 42: 56–63

Nesland J M, Abeler V 1989 Response to letter by Scully R E and Dickersen G R. International Journal of Gynecological Pathology 8: 296–297

Nielsen G P, Oliva E, Young R H, Rosenberg A E, Prat J, Scully R E 1998 Primary ovarian rhabdomyosarcoma: a report of 13 cases. International Journal of Gynecological Pathology 17: 113–119

Nogales F F, Ortega I, Rivera F, Armas J R 1980 Metanephrogenic tissue in immature ovarian teratoma. American Journal of Surgical Pathology 4: 297–299

Nogales F F, Carvia R E, Donne C, Campello T R, Vidal M, Martin A 1997 Adenomas of the rete ovarii. Human Pathology 28: 1428–1433

O'Dowd J, Ismail S M 1990 Juvenile granulosa cell tumour of the ovary containing a nodule of Wilm's tumour. Histopathology 17: 468–470

Osborne B M, Robboy S J 1983 Lymphomas or leukemia presenting as ovarian tumors: an analysis of 42 cases. Cancer 52: 1933–1943

Pitman M B, Young R H, Clement P B, Dickersin G R, Scully R E 1994 Endometrioid carcinoma of the ovary and endometrium, oxyphil cell type: a report of nine cases. International Journal of Gynecological Pathology 13: 290–301

Prasad C J, Ray J A, Kessler S 1992 Female adnexal tumor of Wolffian origin. Archives of Pathology and Laboratory Medicine 116: 189–191

Rahilly M A, Williams A R, Krausz T, Nafussi A A 1995 Female adnexal tumour of probable Wolffian origin: a clinicopathological and immunohistochemical study of three cases. Histopathology 26: 69–74

Rutgers J L, Scully R E 1988 Cysts (cystadenomas) and tumors of the rete ovarii. International Journal of Gynecological Pathology 7: 330–342

Sahin A, Benda J A 1988 Primary ovarian Wilm's tumor. Cancer 61: 1460–1463

Scurry J P, Brown R W, Jobling T 1996. Combined ovarian serous papillary and hepatoid carcinoma. Gynecologic Oncology 63: 138–142

Sheyn I, Mira J L, Bejarano P A, Husseinzadeh N 2000 Metastatic female adnexal tumor of probable Wolffian origin: a case report and review of the literature. Archives of Pathology and Laboratory Medicine 124: 431–434

Sivathondan Y, Salm R, Hughesdon P E, Faccini J M 1979. Female adnexal tumour of probable Wolffian origin. Journal of Clinical Pathology 32: 616–624

Takeda A, Matsuyama M, Sugimoto Y et al 1983 Oncocytic adenocarcinoma of the ovary. Virchows Archiv A Pathological Anatomy and Histology 399: 345–353

Tavassoli F A, Andrade R, Merino M 1990 Retiform Wolffian adenoma. In: Fenoglio-Preizer C (ed) Progress in surgical pathology 11: 121–136

Taxy J B, Battifora H 1976 Female adnexal tumor of probable Wolffian origin: evidence for a low grade malignancy. Cancer 37: 2349–2354

Tiltman A J, Allard U 2001 Female adnexal tumours of probable Wolffian origin: An immunohistochemical profile of tumours, mesonephric remnants and paramesonephric derivatives. Histopathology 38: 237–242

Ulbright T M, Roth L M, Stehman F B, Talerman A, Senekjian E K 1987 Poorly differentiated (small cell) carcinoma of the ovary in young women: evidence supporting a germ cell origin. Human Pathology 18: 175–184

Variend S, Gerrard M, Norris P D, Goepel J R 1991 Intra-abdominal neuroectodermal tumour of childhood with divergent differentiation. Histopathology 18: 45–51

Wartenberg H 1982 Development of the early human ovary and role of the mesonephros in the differentiation of the cortex. Anatomy and Embryology 165: 253–280

Wenzel J G, Odend'hal S 1985 The mammalian rete ovarii: a literature review. Cornell Veterinarian 75: 411–425

Williamson H O, Moore M P 1964 Ovarian and paraovarian adenomatoid tumors. American Journal of Obstetrics and Gynecology 90: 388–394

Yoshida Y, Tenzaki T, Ishiguro T, Kawanami D, Ohshima M 1984 Oncocytoma of the ovary: light and electron microscopic study. Gynecologic Oncology 18: 109–114

Young R H, Scully R E 1983 Ovarian tumors of probable Wolffian origin: a report of 11 cases. American Journal of Surgical Pathology 7: 125–135

Young R H, Scully R E 1989 Alveolar rhabdomyosarcoma metastatic to the ovary. A report of two cases and discussion of the differential diagnosis of small cell malignant tumors of the ovary. Cancer 64: 899–904

Young R H, Silva E G, Scully R E 1991 Ovarian and juxtaovarian adenomatoid tumors: a report of 6 cases. International Journal of Gynecological Pathology 10: 364–371

Young R, Eichhorn J H, Dickersin G R, Scully R E 1992a Ovarian involvement by the intra-abdominal desmoplastic small round cell tumour with divergent differentiation: a report of three cases. Human Pathology 23: 454–464

Young R H, Gersell D J, Clement P B, Scully R E 1992b Hepatocellular carcinoma metastatic to the ovary: a report of three cases discovered during life with discussion of the differential diagnosis of hepatoid tumors of the ovary. Human Pathology 23: 574–580

Young R H, Oliva E, Scully R E, 1994 Small cell carcinoma of the ovary, hypercalcemic type. A clinicopathological analysis of 150 cases. American Journal of Surgical Pathology 18: 1102–1116

Zaloudek C, Miller T R, Stern J L, 1995. Desmoplastic small cell tumor of the ovary: a unique polyphenotypic tumor with an unfavourable prognosis. International Journal of Gynecological Pathology 14: 260–265

27

Pathology of the peritoneum and secondary Müllerian system

D. A. Bell

Introduction   913

Mesothelial lesions   913
Mesothelial hyperplasia   913
Multioculated peritoneal inclusion cysts (multicystic
    mesothelioma)   914
Well-differentiated papillary mesothelioma   915
Diffuse malignant mesothelioma   916
Deciduoid mesothelioma   918
Intra-abdominal desmoplastic small round cell tumour   919

Lesions of the secondary Müllerian system   920
Serous lesions   921
Mucinous lesions   925
Transitional-like lesions   926
Squamous lesions   927
Clear cell lesions   927
Ectopic decidua   927
Diffuse peritoneal leiomyomatosis   928

INTRODUCTION

The female peritoneum is the site of a diverse group of benign and malignant lesions, many of which are seen only rarely in men. A number of these lesions maintain a peritoneal or mesothelial appearance and cellular phenotype; others show definitive Müllerian differentiation. This chapter will focus on gynaecologically related pathology. Other intra-abdominal lesions have been recently and excellently reviewed elsewhere (Al-Nafussi & Wong 2001).

MESOTHELIAL LESIONS

MESOTHELIAL HYPERPLASIA

Perhaps the most common lesion of the peritoneum seen in surgical pathology specimens is mesothelial hyperplasia. In general, these benign mesothelial proliferations which occur as a reaction to serosal injury cause few diagnostic problems. Occasional florid cases, however, may be difficult to distinguish from diffuse malignant mesothelioma or primary or secondary carcinoma or borderline tumours involving the peritoneum.

Mesothelial hyperplasia of the peritoneal surfaces most often is noted as an incidental finding, but in rare cases may be visible grossly as small nodules measuring up to several millimetres in diameter (Rosai & Dehner 1975; McCaughey & Al-Jabi 1986; Daya & McCaughey 1991; Clement & Young 1993). Microscopically, the mesothelial proliferation usually is located on the surfaces of the peritoneum but may extend for variable distances into underlying tissue. When the mesothelial surface is affected, the mesothelial cells form a single layer of enlarged polygonal cells, solid sheets of cells or papillae with delicate or prominent fibrovascular cores (Fig. 27.1). When the proliferation contains fibrous tissue or extends superficially into underlying tissue, the mesothelial cells are arranged in papillae, tubulopapillary structures, tubules, cords, or trabeculae, often in linear arrays parallel to the overlying mesothelial

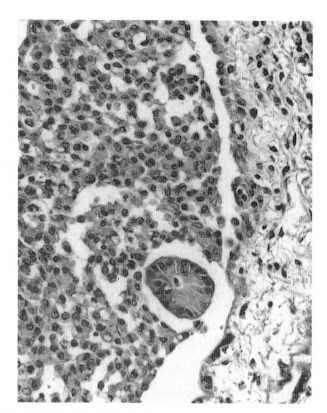

Fig. 27.1 Mesothelial hyperplasia. Bland polygonal mesothelial cells are present in sheets and a papillary cluster on the peritoneal surface.

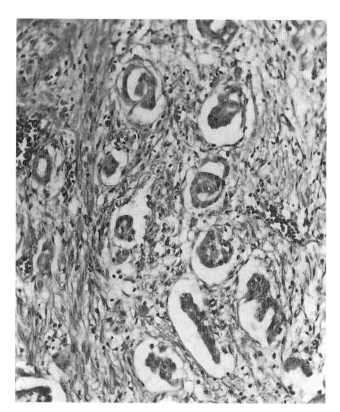

Fig. 27.2 Mesothelial hyperplasia. Tubules and papillary structures composed of polygonal mesothelial cells are present in a linear array in fibrous tissue.

surface (Fig. 27.2). The cells show minimal to moderate nuclear atypia and are polygonal or cuboidal with abundant amphophilic cytoplasm. Focally, large cytoplasmic vacuoles may be present.

Mesothelial hyperplasia must be distinguished from diffuse malignant mesothelioma and primary or secondary carcinomas or borderline tumours involving the peritoneum. Features that aid in distinguishing mesothelial hyperplasia from diffuse malignant mesothelioma are the presence of an extensive proliferation with marked cytological atypia, necrosis, prominent cytoplasmic vacuolisation, and deep extension or invasion into underlying tissues in the latter. It should be noted, however, that marked cytological atypia may be present only focally in diffuse malignant mesothelioma and for this reason the absence of cytological atypia in a biopsy specimen does not exclude diffuse malignant mesothelioma absolutely (McCaughey et al 1985; McCaughey & Al-Jabi 1986; Daya & McCaughey 1990). Mesothelial hyperplasia may be mistaken for primary or secondary adenocarcinoma or ovarian borderline tumours involving the peritoneum, especially when papillae or extension into underlying tissue is present (Bell & Scully 1989; Clement & Young 1993). The major features that favour a diagnosis of mesothelial hyperplasia over adenocarcinoma are the absence of marked cytological atypia or deep infiltration of underlying tissue. Mesothelial hyperplasia may be especially difficult to distinguish from serous borderline tumours because both may show minimal

cytological atypia. The cells of serous borderline tumours, however, usually show a greater degree of nuclear variation, and tend to be columnar with delicate cytoplasm; the cells of mesothelial hyperplasia usually have more uniform nuclei and are polygonal, with well-defined cytoplasm. Serous borderline tumours often show a greater degree of papillarity and a more haphazard arrangement of cell nests than usually is seen in mesothelial hyperplasia. Psammoma bodies may be seen in either lesion, although they are more numerous in serous borderline tumours (Bell & Scully 1989; Clement & Young 1993).

MULTILOCULATED PERITONEAL INCLUSION CYSTS (MULTICYSTIC MESOTHELIOMA)

These grossly cystic mesothelial proliferations of the peritoneum have been described by a variety of terms including, among others, peritoneal inclusion cysts (McFadden & Clement 1986; Ross et al 1989), cystic or multicystic mesothelioma (Mennemeyer & Smith 1979; Moore et al 1980; Katsube et al 1982; Weiss & Tavassoli 1988) and postoperative peritoneal cysts (Gussman et al 1986), these reflecting the numerous theories regarding their pathogenesis.

Multiloculated peritoneal inclusion cysts occur predominantly in reproductive aged women although up to 17% of reported cases have been in men (Weiss &

Tavassoli 1988; Ross et al 1989). The patients usually present with abdominal pain and the sensation of a mass; a small number have presented with symptoms of an acute abdomen. Up to 84% of patients have a history of prior abdominal surgery, endometriosis or pelvic inflammatory disease (Ross et al 1989). On physical examination, a palpable mass is often present (Katsube et al 1982; McFadden & Clement 1986; Weiss & Tavassoli 1988; Ross et al 1989).

Grossly, localised aggregates or diffuse studding of the peritoneal surfaces by translucent fluid-filled cysts is usually seen. In a small number of cases, the translucent cysts are found floating free in the abdominal cavity. The cysts primarily involve the pelvic peritoneum but may involve the serosa of the intra-abdominal viscera, omentum or retroperitoneum (Weiss & Tavassoli 1988; Ross et al 1989). In one study, all cases with upper abdominal, peritoneal or retroperitoneal involvement also had involvement of the pelvic peritoneum (Ross et al 1989).

Microscopically, the cysts are lined by one to two layers of flattened, cuboidal, or hobnail-shaped mesothelial cells that show minimal cytological atypia. Small detached groups or papillary clusters of similar cells are often present in the cyst lumens focally. The cysts are separated by scantly to moderately cellular connective tissue that is often infiltrated by lymphocytes (Fig. 27.3). Extension of mesothelial cells into the stroma of multi-loculated peritoneal inclusion cysts is common; this phenomenon has been termed 'mural mesothelial proliferation' (McFadden & Clement 1986) or 'adenomatoid change' (Weiss & Tavassoli 1988). In cases with this feature, tubules, microcysts, plexiform nests, small nests, and cords of focally vacuolated mesothelial cells are present in the stroma. These structures are often arranged in a zonal pattern or in linear arrays parallel to the mesothelial cells lining the adjacent cysts. Squamous or tubal metaplasia of the lining epithelium is seen in a small number of cases (Ross et al 1989).

The therapy of multiloculated peritoneal inclusion cysts is excision. Although there have been no well-documented examples of fatal multiloculated peritoneal inclusion cysts, postoperative recurrences have been reported in up to 50% of patients (Ross et al 1989). Thus far, neither the size of the lesion nor the presence of mural mesothelial proliferations have been predictive of recurrence (Ross et al 1989). It has been suggested that antioestrogens or long-acting GnRH agonists may play a rôle in the conservative management of these lesions (Letterle & Yon 1995; Letterle & Yon 1998).

The pathogenesis of multiloculated peritoneal inclusion cysts has yet to be determined; features favouring a reactive or neoplastic pathogenesis have been summarised in several publications (Weiss & Tavassoli 1988; Ross et al 1989). The microscopic presence of inflammation and fibrosis, the historical association with serosal injury and a benign clinical course are cited as evidence that these lesions are reactive (Ross et al 1989), whereas the absence of a history of peritoneal injury in a substantial number of patients in many series and the microscopic association of multiloculated peritoneal inclusion cysts with diffuse malignant mesothelioma in one case are felt to support a neoplastic origin (Weiss & Tavassoli 1988).

Multiloculated peritoneal inclusion cysts are most often confused with lymphangiomas microscopically. In contrast to multiloculated peritoneal inclusion cysts, lymphangiomas occur in children with a male predominance and are located in the mesentery or retroperitoneum. Microscopically, they are lined by flattened endothelial cells and the stroma contains lymphoid aggregates or smooth muscle, features not generally present in multiloculated peritoneal inclusion cysts. Also, the lining cells do not form papillae or detached papillary clusters as is commonly seen in multiloculated peritoneal inclusion cysts (Weiss & Tavassoli 1988; Ross et al 1989). Immunohistochemical stains or ultrastructural studies are useful in establishing a definitive mesothelial or endothelial origin in questionable cases (Mennemeyer & Smith 1979; Moore et al 1980).

WELL-DIFFERENTIATED PAPILLARY MESOTHELIOMA

This mesothelial neoplasm occurs predominantly in reproductive aged women with a smaller number occurring

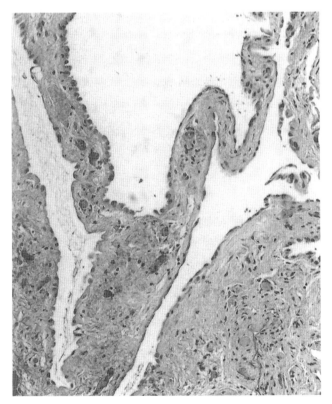

Fig. 27.3 Multiloculated peritoneal inclusion cysts. The cysts are lined by a single layer of flattened and polygonal mesothelial cells.

in men (Goepel 1981; Addis & Fox 1983; Daya & McCaughey 1990; Daya & McCaughey 1991) and young girls (Lovell & Cranston 1990). The tumours are usually incidental findings; patients occasionally present with chronic pelvic pain, an acute abdomen or ascites. Possible exposure to asbestos has been documented in rare cases (Daya & McCaughey 1990).

On gross examination, solitary or multiple peritoneal nodules, some with a papillary appearance, measuring up to several centimetres in diameter, are usually noted. The nodules may involve the omentum, pelvic and upper abdominal peritoneum (Goepel 1981; Daya & McCaughey 1990) or more rarely the tunica vaginalis (Chetty 1992). Ovarian surface involvement is often present (Daya & McCaughey 1990).

Histologically, the lesions show well-developed, often coarse, papillae lined by a single layer of uniform flattened to cuboidal mesothelial cells (Fig. 27.4). The papillary areas may be adjacent to tubules, branching cords or focal solid nests of similar cells. Extensive fibrosis may entrap and compress tubules resulting in an irregular gland-like appearance. Solid sheets of cells are focal or absent. Psammoma bodies have been described in up to 25% of cases in some series (Goepel 1981; Daya & McCaughey 1990).

Although follow-up information is scant and in some cases is indeterminant, many tumours with this appear-

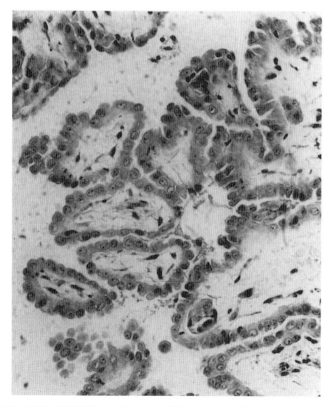

Fig. 27.4 Well-differentiated papillary mesothelioma. The papillae are lined by a single layer of cuboidal mesothelial cells.

ance have behaved in a benign fashion. Several deaths, possibly secondary to tumour, have been reported (Daya & McCaughey 1990; Burrig et al 1990). The most convincing of these was in a 51-year-old man who died of extensive intra-abdominal tumour five years after the diagnosis of well-differentiated papillary mesothelioma. The recurrent tumour had the appearance of a diffuse malignant mesothelioma; however, the degree of sampling of the initial lesions was not discussed in the report (Burrig et al 1990). Several other patients have died, but it is unclear whether their deaths resulted from intercurrent disease, complications of therapy or tumour (Daya & McCaughey 1990). It is presently recommended that these neoplasms should be resected as completely as possible with careful clinical follow-up and that additional therapy should be withheld unless tumour progression is documented (Daya & McCaughey 1990).

A recent study of genital and peritoneal mesotheliomas found that predictably benign mesotheliomas were characteristically small, solitary polypoid or nodular lesions and were localised to one site. They were purely or predominantly tubulopapillary; solid sheets of cells were focal or absent. Nuclear atypia was absent or slight (Goldblum & Hart 1995). These authors (Goldblum & Hart 1997) and others (Swan et al 1997) have described individual cases of diffuse peritoneal mesotheliomas with uniformly benign cytological features and uneventful short-term follow-up. Thus, the long-term clinical behaviour of these diffuse lesions remains uncertain. Since diffuse malignant mesotheliomas may contain focal areas with bland cytological features, a diagnosis of benign mesothelioma should be made only after extensive sampling.

DIFFUSE MALIGNANT MESOTHELIOMA

Diffuse malignant mesothelioma of the peritoneum is less common than its pleural counterpart, accounting for 6–20% of cases in both sexes (Chahinian et al 1982; Lerner et al 1983; Daya & McCaughey 1991; Sridhar et al 1992). The percentage of female patients with such tumours varies in the literature from 7 to 57% (Kannerstein et al 1977; Casey Jones & Silver 1979; Piccigallo et al 1988; Plaus 1988; Asensio et al 1990; Dawson et al 1993; Goldblum & Hart 1995; Roggli et al 1997). The great variation in incidence may reflect the erroneous classification of peritoneal serous carcinomas or well-differentiated papillary mesotheliomas as diffuse malignant mesothelioma. The frequency of asbestos exposure in patients with peritoneal diffuse malignant mesothelioma ranges from zero to 79% (Casey Jones & Silver 1979; Chahinian et al 1982; Plaus 1988; Piccigallo et al 1988; Dawson et al 1993; Roggli et al 1997). Eighty-three per cent of patients had asbestos exposure in one large series: however, most of the patients in that study were identified through records of occupational exposure to asbestos thus creating substantial selection bias (Kannerstein et al 1977). Many women do not have direct occupational exposure but are exposed indirectly through household contact with asbestos workers (Roggli et al 1997). Peritoneal diffuse malignant mesothelioma has also been reported after radiation therapy (Babcock & Powell 1976; Antman et al 1983; Gilks et al 1990; Roggli et al 1997) or recurrent peritonitis (Riddell et al 1981). Peritoneal diffuse malignant mesothelioma is most commonly diagnosed in the fifth to seventh decades of life (Kannerstein et al 1977; Casey Jones & Silver 1979; Piccigallo et al 1988; Plaus 1988; Asensio et al 1990; Dawson et al 1993; Goldblum & Hart 1995; Roggli et al 1997), although they may occur in younger women, especially those with childhood asbestos exposure (Kane et al 1990). The presenting symptoms are relatively nonspecific including abdominal pain, distention and weight loss (Kannerstein et al 1977; Casey Jones & Silver 1979; Piccigallo et al 1988; Plaus 1988; Asensio et al 1990; Kane et al 1990; Goldblum & Hart 1995). Ascites is usually present and an abdominal or pelvic mass is often palpable (Kannerstein et al 1977; Casey Jones & Silver 1979; Piccigallo et al 1988; Plaus 1988; Asensio 1990; Kane et al 1990; Goldblum & Hart 1995).

Grossly, both the parietal and visceral peritoneal surfaces are studded with nodules or plaques of tumour measuring from several mm in diameter up to 25 cm in greatest dimension. Diffuse thickening of the peritoneum or omentum may also be seen (Kannerstein et al 1977; Goldblum & Hart 1995). As the tumour spreads, it may encase the viscera, frequently infiltrating the bowel wall. Occasionally, the retroperitoneum, including the pancreas, may be extensively involved by tumour. Rarely the only site of involvement is the ovary, or a dominant mass is present in the ovary with lesser involvement of the peritoneum (Goldblum & Hart 1995; Clement et al 1996). Sites of metastatic tumour include lymph nodes, liver and lung; the pleura as well as the peritoneum is involved in a minority of cases (Kannerstein et al 1977; McCaughey et al 1985).

Microscopically, diffuse malignant mesotheliomas have a varied histologic appearance and are classified as epithelial, biphasic or mixed, and sarcomatous (Kannerstein et al 1977; McCaughey et al 1985; Daya & McCaughey 1991). The majority of peritoneal diffuse malignant mesotheliomas are of epithelial type which accounted for 56–84% of cases, the biphasic type for 15–53% and the sarcomatous type for 0–11% of cases in several large studies (Dawson et al 1993; Roggli et al 1997; Goldblum & Hart 1995).

Epithelial tumours or the epithelial component of biphasic neoplasms are characterised by tubules, branching tubules or clefts, broad fibrous papillae with anastomosing interconnections, or tubulopapillary structures lined by cuboidal, columnar, hobnailed or polygonal cells. Solid sheets of round or polygonal non-overlapping cells are also seen in the majority of cases. The nuclei are

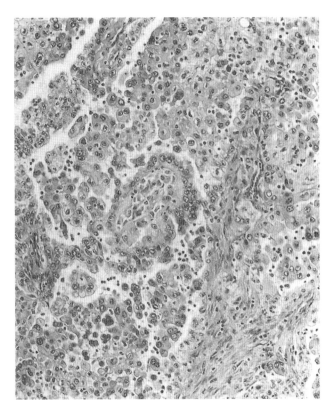

Fig. 27.5 Diffuse malignant mesothelioma. Nests, sheets and papillae are present. The cells are round or polygonal with hyperchromatic pleomorphic nuclei.

round or oval and nuclear atypia ranges from mild to marked (Fig. 27.5). Marked atypia is seen in the majority of cases at least focally (Goldblum et al 1995). The cytoplasm is generally amphophilic; large cytoplasmic vacuoles that do not stain with PAS with diastase or mucicarmine are often present, at least focally. In rare cases the epithelial component may form nests and cords of small hyperchromatic cells similar to those of a small cell carcinoma. In pure epithelial diffuse malignant mesotheliomas, the tubules and papillae are separated by a mildly cellular, oedematous or myxoid stroma.

Pure sarcomatous diffuse malignant mesothelioma generally has the appearance of nonspecific sarcomas of spindle cell type although it may have the appearance of malignant fibrous histiocytoma, fibrosarcoma, rhabdomyosarcoma or malignant schwannoma. Focally, diffuse malignant mesotheliomas may be extensively fibrotic or desmoplastic and the tumour cells in these areas may be small, irregular, and hyperchromatic.

Diffuse malignant mesotheliomas are classified as biphasic when both the epithelial and stromal components are clearly malignant. The two components may be intimately intermixed or, more commonly, form separate areas of the neoplasm (Kannerstein et al 1977; McCaughey et al 1985; Daya & McCaughey 1991).

The histological differential diagnosis of epithelial peritoneal diffuse malignant mesothelioma generally includes mesothelial hyperplasia, multiloculated peritoneal inclusion cysts, well-differentiated papillary mesothelioma, metastatic carcinoma and primary Müllerian tumours of the peritoneum. The features that distinguish between diffuse malignant mesotheliomas and other mesothelial lesions have been discussed in the previous sections. Features that favour a diagnosis of serous carcinoma over diffuse malignant mesotheliomas either primarily or secondarily involving the peritoneum include the presence of markedly pleomorphic cells, overlapping pleomorphic nuclei, the presence of slit-like spaces and complex glands, numerous psammoma bodies and intracytoplasmic epithelial mucin (Kannerstein et al 1977; Foyle et al 1981; White et al 1985; Truong et al 1990; Goldblum & Hart 1995).

Numerous studies have demonstrated that special stains, electronmicroscopy and immunohistochemical stains are valuable adjuncts in differentiating between epithelial diffuse malignant mesotheliomas and adenocarcinomas involving the serosal surfaces (Dabbs & Geisinger 1988; Bollinger et al 1989; Tickman et al 1990; Wick et al 1990; Sheibani et al 1991; Gaffey et al 1992; Leong et al 1992; Flynn et al 1993; Weiss & Battifora 1993). Adenocarcinomas often contain neutral epithelial mucin, as demonstrated by mucicarmine and PAS-diastase stains, and diffuse malignant mesotheliomas frequently contain hyaluronic acid demonstrated as hyaluronase digestible Alcian Blue or colloidal-iron positive material (McCaughey et al 1985; Bollinger et al 1989; Leong et al 1992). The practical usefulness of such stains is limited, however, by the substantial proportion of tumours in both categories that do not stain for these (Bollinger et al 1989; Leong et al 1992).

Ultrastructural analysis may also distinguish between diffuse malignant mesotheliomas and adenocarcinoma. The epithelial elements of diffuse malignant mesotheliomas have abundant, long, branching, 'bushy' circumferential microvilli and tonofilaments whereas adenocarcinomas contain gland lumens, short microvilli and mucin droplets (McCaughey et al 1985; Bedrossian et al 1992).

Immunohistochemical stains are the most widely used aid in distinguishing diffuse malignant mesothelioma from adenocarcinoma. Most of the immunoperoxidase studies in the literature have focused on defining the best diagnostic panel for differentiating pulmonary adenocarcinoma from pleural diffuse malignant mesothelioma. These studies have suggested various panels of antibodies as optimal for this differential diagnosis. Most of these panels have included antibodies to CEA, CD 15 (Leu M1), BER-EP4 and B72.3 as epithelial markers and cytokeratins 5/6, calretinin, and thrombomodulin as mesothelial markers (Brown et al 1993; Weiss & Battifora 1993; Moran et al 2000; Carella et al 2001; Comin et al 2001).

A smaller number of studies have attempted to determine the most sensitive and specific combination of anti-

bodies to distinguish peritoneal diffuse malignant mesotheliomas from the neoplasms that commonly involve the peritoneum of women. Antibodies against CEA are not as useful in this differential because only 6 to 52% of serous carcinomas of ovarian or peritoneal origin stain positively with this antibody (Dabbs & Geisinger 1988; Bollinger et al 1989; Tickman et al 1990). Antibodies against B72.3, PLAP, S-100, Leu M1 and BER-EP4 are more useful in indicating the presence of serous carcinoma and calretinin, thrombomodulin and keratin 5/6 as indicators of mesothelioma (Bollinger et al 1989; Delahaye et al 1997; Riera et al 1997; Ordonez 1998a).

The prognosis of peritoneal diffuse malignant mesothelioma is very poor, with a median survival of 7–8 months (Chahinian et al 1982; Piccigallo et al 1988; Sridhar et al 1992). Most patients die of tumour within 18 months (Casey Jones & Silver 1979; Chahinian et al 1982; Plaus 1988; Spirtas et al 1988; Sridhar et al 1992; Asensio et al 1990; Kane et al 1990; Goldblum & Hart 1995; Roggli et al 1997).

DECIDUOID MESOTHELIOMA

Rarely, diffuse malignant mesotheliomas may have a morphological appearance that mimics ectopic decidua. Such tumours have been termed 'deciduoid' mesotheliomas. Approximately six cases have been reported in the peritoneum in girls and women ranging from 13 to 53 years of age. In most of the cases, grossly apparent plaques or nodules of tumour are present on the peritoneum. The tumours are characterised histologically by sheets of cells with abundant eosinophilic glassy cytoplasm with well defined cell borders and round to oval nuclei showing mild to moderate pleomorphism (Fig. 27.6). Focal necrosis is usually present. Some tumours have had a purely deciduoid morphology and others have had areas of coexisting typical diffuse malignant mesotheliomas. The tumour has a very poor prognosis; all of the patients with follow-up information have died within one year of

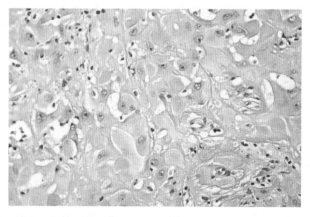

Fig. 27.6 Deciduoid malignant mesothelioma. Sheets of cells with abundant cytoplasm and atypical nuclei resembling ectopic decidua are present.

presentation (Talerman et al 1985; Nascimento et al 1994; Orosz et al 1999; Shanks et al 2000).

These tumours may be differentiated from decidua by the presence of a grossly visible mass, greater nuclear pleomorphism and focal necrosis in deciduoid mesotheliomas.

INTRA-ABDOMINAL DESMOPLASTIC SMALL ROUND CELL TUMOUR

This distinctive small cell neoplasm that has a characteristic chromosomal abnormality most commonly arises in or near serosal surfaces and occurs in children and young adults (Gonzales-Crussi et al 1990; Gerald et al 1991; Layfield & Lenarsky 1991; Young et al 1992; Ordonez et al 1993; Gerald et al 1998; Ordonez 1998b). Although these tumours were originally reported to have a strong predilection for adolescent males, approximately 18% of reported cases in the literature have been in female patients (Ordonez et al 1993; Gerald et al 1998; Ordonez 1998b) and ovarian involvement was prominent in several of them (Young et al 1992). The histological and clinical features of male and female patients are similar.

Several large series have found that intra-abdominal desmoplastic small round cell tumours occur in patients ranging in age from 3 to 49 years with a mean age of 18 to 25 years (Gerald et al 1998; Ordonez 1998b). Most of the patients present with abdominal pain, distention and a palpable mass (Gerald et al 1998; Ordonez 1998b); occasional patients present with an acute abdomen (Gonzales-Crussi et al 1990; Gerald et al 1998) Extra-abdominal disease has been reported in a minority of cases in the paratesticular region (Cummings et al 1997; Ordonez 1998) ovary (Young et al 1992; Furman et al 1997), prostate (Furman et al 1997), thoracic cavity, lung, hand, lymph node, and cranial fossa (Gerald et al 1998) and liver (Ordonez 1998b).

Macroscopic examination reveals numerous tumour nodules involving the abdominal and pelvic peritoneal surfaces. In most cases a large or dominant peritoneal mass is associated with smaller peritoneal nodules or implants. The nodules are firm with smooth or bosselated outer surfaces and are tan–white or grey with areas of necrosis or haemorrhage on cut surface. Direct invasion of the intestinal wall or intra-abdominal viscera occasionally occurs; involvement of the retroperitoneum as well as the peritoneum has been reported in 22 to 25% of cases. Large ovarian masses have been reported in a small number of female patients (Gerald et al 1991; Young et al 1992; Ordonez et al 1993; Gerald et al 1998; Ordonez 1998b).

Microscopically, intra-abdominal desmoplastic small round cell tumour is characterised by nests or trabeculae of small cells separated by a fibrous or desmoplastic stroma, that are present in equal proportions, at least focally (Fig. 27.7). The cells are small with round to oval

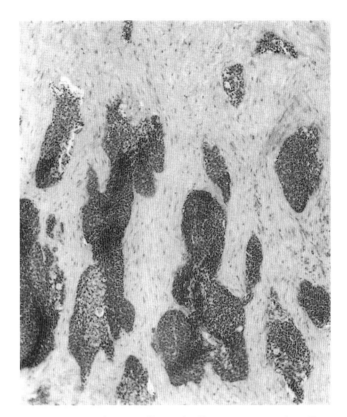

Fig. 27.7 Desmoplastic small round cell tumour. Nests of small cells are separated by a desmoplastic stroma.

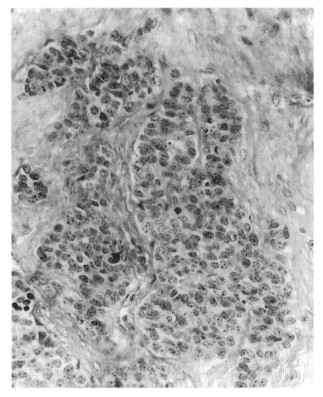

Fig. 27.8 Desmoplastic small round cell tumour. The cells are small with scant cytoplasm. Focal peripheral palisading of tumour cells is present at the periphery of the nests.

hyperchromatic nuclei and scant cytoplasm. Peripheral palisading of tumour cells is apparent focally and necrosis in the centre of tumour nests is common (Fig. 27.8). Unusual histological features may be identified in a substantial minority of cases and include spindling of the neoplastic cells, formation of gland lumens, rosettes or tubules, pleomorphic cells with cytological atypia, signet-ring like cells and 'rhabdoid' cells with eosinophilic cytoplasm and eccentric nuclei (Gerald et al 1991; Ordonez et al 1993; Gerald et al 1998; Ordonez 1998b).

Although the histological appearance is distinctive, the diagnosis is confirmed by identification of the unusual immunohistochemical profile expressed by these tumours or by their specific translocation or chimeric protein. Immunohistochemically, the tumours most frequently stain with antibodies to the following: keratin (86–92%), desmin (90–100%), EMA (93–98%), vimentin (81–97%), and NSE (72–81%). The tumours also have been positively stained with antibodies to the following less frequently: Leu 7 (67%), synaptophysin (16%), chromogranin (2–5%), S-100 (20%), muscle specific actin (16%), and Leu M1 (69%). The tumours have been negative for myogenin, cytokeratin 5/6 and thrombomodulin (Gerald et al 1998; Ordonez 1998c).

The specific translocation t(11;22)(p13;12) associated with these tumours results in the formation of a functional fusion gene (EWS/WT1) that encodes for a chimeric transcript. This transcript can be detected by reverse transcriptase–polymerase chain reaction (RT–PCR) in virtually all cases and the fusion protein can be detected immunohistochemically utilising an antibody to the carboxy terminus of WT1 in 93–100% of cases (Charles et al 1997; Gerald et al 1998; Ordonez 1998c; Barnoud et al 2000; Hill et al 2000).

Ultrastructurally, the tumour cell nests are surrounded by basal lamina which may be discontinuous and the cells have intermediate junctions, desmosomes and, less commonly, tight junctions. Many cells contain cytoplasmic aggregates of intermediate-sized filaments and cell processes have been reported infrequently (Gerald et al 1991; Young et al 1992; Ordonez et al 1993; Ordonez 1998c). Dense core granules (Gerald et al 1991; Young et al 1992; Ordonez et al 1993; Ordonez 1998c) and a suggestion of lumens or well-developed small lumens containing microvilli have been reported in a small number of cases (Gerald et al 1991; Ordonez et al 1993).

Although the clinical features suggest a primary peritoneal origin for this neoplasm, the histogenesis of the tumour remains uncertain. The tumour shares many features with the 'small round cell tumours' of childhood (Gerald et al 1991; Gerald et al 1998; Ordonez 1998c). One group has suggested that the tumour arises from embryonal mesenchyme of the coelomic cavities because of the involvement of WT1 (Gerald et al 1998).

The differential diagnosis includes small cell neoplasms that may involve the peritoneum either primarily or secondarily. Diffuse malignant mesothelioma occurs predominantly in older individuals but has been reported, rarely, in children and young adults (Grundy & Miller 1972; Fraire et al 1988; Kane et al 1990). Uncommonly, the epithelial element of a diffuse malignant mesothelioma may be composed of small cells that mimic small cell carcinoma (McCaughey et al 1985): however, further sampling of such a diffuse malignant mesothelioma usually reveals more typical areas of mesothelioma. Additionally, the immunohistochemical profiles of diffuse malignant mesothelioma and intra-abdominal desmoplastic small round cell tumour are distinctive. Although intra-abdominal desmoplastic small round cell tumour resembles other small cell tumours of childhood, such as Wilms' tumour, primitive neuroectodermal tumour, malignant rhabdoid tumour, and Ewing's sarcoma, these neoplasms rarely develop diffuse peritoneal disease and have different genetic, ultrastructural and immunohistochemical characteristics. Desmoplastic small round cell tumour must also be differentiated from ovarian small cell carcinoma of the type often associated with hypercalcaemia which occurs in young females and may spread widely throughout the abdomen. Small cell carcinoma of the type associated with hypercalcaemia, in contrast to intra-abdominal desmoplastic small round cell tumour, usually has a more diffuse growth pattern with inconspicuous stroma as well as the formation of 'follicle-like' spaces lined by tumour cells (Young et al 1992).

The prognosis of intra-abdominal desmoplastic small round cell tumour is very poor with a median survival of only 17 months and only very rare long-term survivors in the initial literature (Gonzales-Crussi et al 1990; Gerald et al 1991). Recent trials with aggressive tumour debulking surgery, radiation and chemotherapy have resulted in a somewhat better, but still poor, survival rate of 18–28% at 3 to 5 years (Schwarz et al 1998; Kurre et al 2000; Quaglia & Brennan 2000).

LESIONS OF THE SECONDARY MÜLLERIAN SYSTEM

It has been amply demonstrated that the female peritoneum is frequently the site of Müllerian epithelial lesions that exhibit the full spectrum of differentiation from benign to malignant (Lauchlan 1984). The presence of Müllerian lesions beyond the direct derivatives of the Müllerian ducts (the cervix, endometrium and Fallopian tubes), primarily in the ovary and lower abdominal and pelvic peritoneum, has been ascribed to the existence of a 'secondary Müllerian system' of peritoneum with an increased propensity toward Müllerian differentiation. It has been speculated that the peritoneum and subperitoneal mesenchyme at these sites retains a potential for Müllerian differentiation due to its proximity to the coelomic epithelium from which the Müllerian ducts are derived. Alternatively, there may be 'nothing intrinsically specialised about peritoneum in this location' (Lauchlan 1994). The development of Müllerian lesions may be secondary to the proximity of the pelvic peritoneum to the fimbriated end of the Fallopian tube which allows exposure of the peritoneal and ovarian surfaces to the outside environment. It has been postulated that entry of a variety of external agents via the tube may initiate Müllerian differentiation or 'Müllerianosis' of the proximate peritoneum (Lauchlan, 1972, 1984, 1994; Russell & Bannatyne 1989).

SEROUS LESIONS

Endosalpingiosis

Endosalpingiosis is defined as the presence of glandular inclusions lined by tubal-appearing epithelium located in ectopic sites. It has been identified histologically in 84% of aymptomatic women undergoing laparoscopy for elective sterilisation (Hesseling & De Wilde 2000). It most commonly involves the superficial layers of the peritoneum of the uterus, Fallopian tubes, ovaries or cul-de-sac (Sinykin 1960; Schuldenfrei & Janovsky 1962; Burmeister et al 1969; Tutschka & Lauchlan 1980; Holmes et al 1981; Bryce et al 1982; Zinsser & Wheeler 1982; McCaughey et al 1984; Dallenbach 1987). Less frequent sites of involvement are the omentum (Tutschka & Lauchlan 1980; Zinsser & Wheeler 1982; McCaughey et al 1984), bladder (Chen 1981; Young 1997), bowel serosa (Chen 1981; Dallenbach 1987; Cajigas & Axiotis 1990), skin (Dore et al 1980), gastric lymph nodes (Tsuchiya et al 1999), pelvic or para-aortic lymph nodes (Shen et al 1983; Ryuko et al 1992) and uterine wall (Young 1997; Clement & Young 1999; Heatley & Russell 2001).

Endosalpingiosis occurs in women ranging in age from 12 to 66 years, with a peak frequency in the third and fourth decades of life (Sinykin 1960; Schuldenfrei & Janovsky 1962; Burmeister et al 1969; Dore et al 1980; Tutschka & Lauchlan 1980; Holmes et al 1981; Bryce et al 1982; Zinsser & Wheeler 1982; Shen et al 1983; McCaughey et al 1984; Dallenbach 1987; Cajigas & Axiotis 1990; Ryuko et al 1992). The patients present with pelvic pain although in many cases the lesions are asymptomatic (Laufer et al 1998). The majority of these women have clinical or pathological evidence of tubal disease such as chronic salpingitis with or without hydrosalpinx, prior tubal pregnancies, or salpingitis isthmica nodosum (Sinykin 1960; Schuldenfrei & Janovsky 1962; Holmes et al 1981; Zinsser & Wheeler 1982; Shen et al 1983; McCaughey et al 1984; McCaughey et al 1985; Bell & Scully 1988). Endosalpingiosis has been identified in up to 56% of women with stage II or III ovarian serous borderline tumours (Sinykin 1960; Burmeister et al 1969; Zinsser & Wheeler 1982; McCaughey et al 1984; Ryuko et al 1992); it has also been noted in

association with benign (Sinykin 1960; Tutschka & Lauchlan 1980; Zinsser & Wheeler 1982) and malignant serous tumours of the ovary (Zinsser & Wheeler 1982).

On gross examination, endosalpingiosis is usually inapparent but can occasionally be appreciated as fine granularity or small cysts on the peritoneal surfaces (Sinykin 1960; Schuldenfrei & Janovsky 1962; Burmeister et al 1969; Tutschka & Lauchlan 1980; Holmes et al 1981; Bryce et al 1982; Shen et al 1983; Dallenbach 1987). Rarely, cystic endosalpingiosis may present as cystic masses involving the peritoneum or cervix and lower uterine segment and simulate a neoplasm (Laufer et al 1998; Clement & Young 1999; McCluggage & Weir 2000; Heatley & Russell 2001). In some cases it is associated with pelvic fibrous adhesions, which may be related to tubal inflammatory disease.

Histological examination reveals the presence of single smoothly contoured, round or oval glands, or clusters of them beneath the serosa of the uterus or Fallopian tubes, the pelvic or extrapelvic parietal peritoneum, or the peritoneal surfaces of the omentum. The glands are lined by one to two layers of columnar cells that are commonly ciliated (Fig. 27.9). Less often, the lining epithelium is identical to that of the Fallopian tube, containing ciliated cells, secretory nonciliated cells, and peg-shaped cells. The nuclei are generally round, oval or pencil-shaped, uniform, basally oriented, and show no cytological

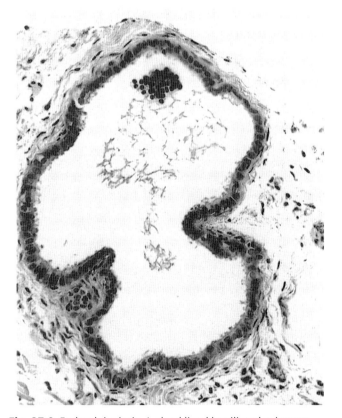

Fig. 27.9 Endosalpingiosis. A gland lined by ciliated columnar cells is present beneath the peritoneal surface.

atypicality. Rarely, blunt papillae with prominent fibrovascular cores lined by similar epithelial cells are present within the glands. Mitotic figures are usually absent. Psammoma bodies are often present in the glands, in the stroma beneath the epithelium of the glands, or unassociated with epithelial cells. The glands are usually surrounded by several layers of delicate connective tissue infiltrated with scattered lymphocytes. In occasional cases, a dense lymphocytic infiltrate or prominent rim of fibroblasts may be present (Sinykin 1960; Schuldenfrei & Janovsky 1962; Burmeister et al 1969; Dore et al 1980; Tutschka & Lauchlan 1980; Holmes et al 1981; Bryce et al 1982; Zinsser & Wheeler 1982; Shen et al 1983; McCaughey et al 1984; Dallenbach 1987; Cajigas & Axiotis 1990; Ryuko et al 1992).

The histological differential diagnosis of endosalpingiosis includes endometriosis, mesothelial hyperplasia, peritoneal inclusion cysts, implants of ovarian serous borderline tumours, primary peritoneal serous borderline tumour, and metastatic adenocarcinoma. Although the cellular features of the glandular epithelium in endosalpingiosis and endometriosis may be similar, the obvious periglandular endometrial stroma that is usually identified in endometriosis in premenopausal women is not apparent in endosalpingiosis. It may be difficult, however, to distinguish these entities in postmenopausal women, when endometrial stroma is not discernible due to atrophy and fibrosis. The presence of stroma around some of the glands should not preclude a diagnosis of endosalpingiosis if typical endosalpingiotic glands without stroma are present as well, since endosalpingiosis and endometriosis are commonly found in continuity or in adjacent tissue (Zinsser & Wheeler 1982). In mesothelial hyperplasia, cords, gland-like spaces and papillae may be present, although they are often arranged in rows parallel to the mesothelial surface (Rosai & Dehner 1975; Bryce et al 1982). The cells lining these mesothelial structures are typically not columnar or ciliated. Peritoneal inclusion cysts, in contrast to endosalpingiosis, are lined by one to several layers of flat-to-cuboidal mesothelial cells. Focally the cysts may be lined by columnar cells characteristic of endosalpingiosis; however, this is considered evidence of tubal metaplasia of the lining mesothelium (Ross et al 1989). Endosalpingiosis may be differentiated from implants of ovarian serous borderline tumour and primary peritoneal serous borderline tumour by both architectural and cytological features. The papillarity, tufting, and especially detached buds of epithelial cells that are characteristic of serous borderline tumours are not seen in endosalpingiosis; also, the cells of endosalpingiosis show little or no cytological atypia. Endosalpingiosis can be distinguished from metastatic adenocarcinoma by the regular arrangement of simple glands in a noninfiltrative pattern and by the absence of cytological atypia or a significant stromal response in the former. Cilia may be prominent in endosalpingiosis but

are very rare in metastatic adenocarcinoma (Zinsser & Wheeler 1982).

The histogenesis of endosalpingiosis remains in dispute. Theories of its origin are similar to those suggested for the origin of endometriosis (Holmes et al 1981; Zinsser & Wheeler 1982; Shen et al 1983). It has been suggested that endosalpingiosis results from direct extension of proliferating tubal epithelium into surrounding tissue, from implantation of sloughed tubal epithelium into the peritoneal cavity, from 'Müllerian' metaplasia of the coelomic epithelium, or from lymphatic or haematogenous spread to lymph nodes. The two most widely accepted theories currently are that of Müllerian metaplasia of the peritoneum, which would also explain the common coexistence of endosalpingiosis and endometriosis, and that of peritoneal implantation by sloughed tubal epithelium, which would explain in part the strong association between endosalpingiosis and diseases of the Fallopian tubes (Zinsser & Wheeler 1982). One group (Moore et al 2000) has suggested that endosalpingiosis, especially involving lymph nodes, may represent differentiated metastases from ovarian tumours.

Although endosalpingiosis is presumed to be benign, few reports with long-term follow-up are available. Zinsser & Wheeler (1982) reported that subsequent tumour did not develop in any of their 16 patients with endosalpingiosis who were followed from 1 to 16 years. Dubeau (1999) has suggested that endosalpingiosis may be the precursor lesion of many ovarian carcinomas.

Rare cases of endosalpingiosis with architectural and cytological atypia ranging in severity from mild nuclear pleomorphism and cellular stratification to moderate nuclear atypia with prominent stratification, tufting and detachment of solid clusters of atypical epithelial cells have been reported (Zinsser & Wheeler 1982; Fievez et al 1983; Dallenbach 1987). Lesions spanning this spectrum of histological appearance have been termed 'atypical endosalpingiosis' by some authors (Zinsser & Wheeler 1982; Fievez et al 1983; Dallenbach 1987); we classify the former lesions as endosalpingiosis with atypia and the latter as peritoneal serous borderline tumours.

Peritoneal serous borderline tumours

In a small number of patients peritoneal lesions histologically identical to the noninvasive peritoneal implants associated with ovarian serous borderline tumours are seen in the absence of ovarian involvement, in the presence of only a minimal degree of ovarian involvement or in association with a serous cystadenoma. Three series of 25, 17, and 19 patients each with these lesions which have been designated as 'serous borderline tumour of the peritoneum' or 'peritoneal serous micropapillomatosis of low malignant potential (serous borderline tumours of the peritoneum)' have been reported (Bell & Scully 1990; Biscotti & Hart 1992; Weir et al 1998).

Peritoneal serous borderline tumours occur in women ranging from 16 to 77 (mean, 31–33) years of age. Infertility and abdominal pain are the most common presenting complaints, although many lesions are discovered as incidental findings (Bell & Scully 1990; Biscotti & Hart 1992; Weir et al 1998).

Grossly, adhesions or granularity of the peritoneal surfaces is present. A mass is only rarely seen. In two-thirds of the cases only the pelvic peritoneum is involved with the upper abdominal peritoneum also being affected in the remainder. Histologically, the tumours have the typical appearance of noninvasive implants of ovarian serous borderline tumours. Papillae, glands or nests of moderately atypical columnar, cuboidal or polygonal cells are present on the peritoneal surfaces, in subperitoneal invaginations, or in crevices between omental fat lobules, either without an accompanying stromal response or compressed within a dense or reactive fibrous stroma. The glands contain detached clusters of atypical epithelial cells (Fig. 27.10). Invasion of underlying tissue is not seen (Bell & Scully 1990; Biscotti & Hart 1992; Weir et al 1998).

The histological differential diagnosis of peritoneal serous borderline tumour includes endosalpingiosis and florid papillary mesothelial hyperplasia. The features that differentiate between these entities have been discussed earlier in this chapter.

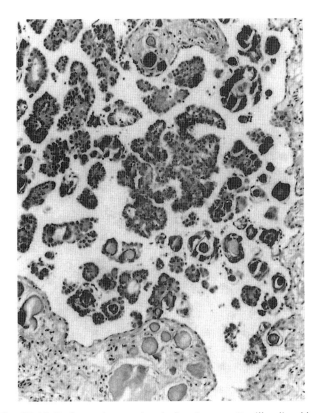

Fig. 27.10 Peritoneal serous borderline tumour. Papillae lined by cuboidal to columnar cells are present in a subperitoneal invagination.

Most women with peritoneal serous borderline tumour have been treated by hysterectomy with bilateral salpingo-oophorectomy and omentectomy and some also received chemotherapy. Twenty-three of the patients had a limited operation to conserve fertility. Follow-up information from 47 patients revealed no clinical evidence of persistent disease in 41 of them (Bell & Scully 1990; Biscotti & Hart 1992; Weir et al 1998). Borderline tumour recurred in two patients, who remained well for 1.7 and 2 years after re-excision of the recurrent tumour, and two additional patients developed small bowel obstruction and were living without progressive disease 11 and 16 years after diagnosis. Invasive low-grade serous carcinoma of the peritoneum developed in three women, two of whom were living with extensive intra-abdominal tumour at the last follow-up examination; the third woman was without evidence of disease after therapy and short-term follow-up (1.6 years). An additional woman died of disseminated serous tumour which was diagnosed cytologically, but not confirmed by biopsy. This very good prognosis, even with limited operative therapy, indicates that conservation of the reproductive organs may be considered in a young women after careful clinical evaluation to exclude a primary ovarian serous borderline tumour.

Although most extraovarian serous borderline tumours are of the diffuse type and do not form grossly visible cysts, occasional cases in which the tumour has the typical gross features of a serous papillary cystadenoma of borderline malignancy have been reported, most frequently in the broad ligament (Aslani et al 1988). These tumours have all been stage Ia, have been unassociated with ovarian involvement, and have been cured by cystectomy.

Serous psammocarcinoma

Although it is classified separately, a tumour that shows many features similar to serous borderline tumour is the rare serous psammocarcinoma of the peritoneum (McCaughey et al 1986; Gilks et al 1990; Weir et al 1998). This diagnosis has been proposed for serous tumours with the following microscopic features: 1. invasion of omentum, intraperitoneal viscera or their vascular spaces; 2. no more than moderate nuclear atypia; 3. solid epithelial nests no greater than 15 cells in diameter; 4. at least 75% of the papillae or nests contain psammoma bodies (Fig. 27.11). Except for invasion and striking calcification, these tumours are very similar in appearance to serous borderline tumours.

Only a small number of cases that fulfill these stringent criteria have been reported in the literature; approximately 9 of peritoneal and 10 of ovarian origin. The ages of the patients with both ovarian and peritoneal tumours ranged from 18 to 76 years with a mean age of 48 to 57 years. The patients usually present with an abdominal mass or increasing abdominal girth, but many cases have

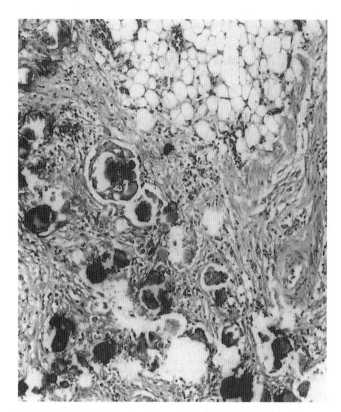

Fig. 27.11 Peritoneal serous psammocarcinoma. Papillary groups of moderately atypical epithelial cells, most associated with psammoma bodies, infiltrate the omentum.

Rothacker & Mobius 1995; Zhou et al 1995; Ben-Baruch et al 1996; Liapis et al 1996). The frequency of primary peritoneal serous carcinoma is highly variable, due to the lack of widely accepted criteria for separating these tumours from ovarian serous carcinomas with extensive peritoneal involvement. Recently, many authors have utilised the criteria proposed by the Gynecologic Oncology Group. These criteria are as follows: 1. Both ovaries are normal in size or enlarged by a benign process; 2. The involvement of extraovarian sites is greater than the involvement of the ovarian surfaces; 3. Microscopically, tumour involving the ovary is absent, is confined to the surface without cortical involvement or with cortical involvement less than 5×5 mm^2, or tumour measuring less than 5×5 mm^2 involves the ovarian stroma without surface involvement; 4. Histologically, the tumour is predominantly of serous type. The age and clinical presentation of women with serous carcinoma arising from the peritoneum are similar to those of women with advanced-stage serous carcinoma of ovarian origin (Ben-Baruch et al 1996; Piura et al 1998).

On gross examination, the appearance of the peritoneal tumour is similar to that of metastatic serous ovarian carcinoma; the peritoneum is usually diffusely involved by small nodules or warty excrescences as well as by larger masses that often involve the omentum. In most cases the ovaries are grossly normal in size and shape but

been incidental findings. Occasionally the calcifications are so massive that they are visible radiologically. Operative findings include a dominant mass, adhesions or small nodules, excrescences or granularity of the peritoneum. The tumour typically has a solid or solid and cystic gritty or granular cut surface.

All of the patients with peritoneal tumours were without evidence of postoperative tumour: however one patient developed a recurrence at 4 years but was without evidence of tumour four years later. Thus, despite the small number of cases reported, it is felt that these tumours probably have a similar prognosis to ovarian serous borderline tumours (McCaughey et al 1986; Gilks et al 1990; Weir et al 1998).

Primary peritoneal serous carcinoma

Many studies have examined the clinicopathological features of this variant of serous carcinoma that extensively involves peritoneal surfaces with minimal or no ovarian parenchymal involvement (Kannerstein et al 1977; Foyle et al 1981; Gooneratne et al 1982; Tobacman et al 1982; Hochster et al 1984; August et al 1985; White et al 1985; Chen & Flam 1986; Lele et al 1988; Mills et al 1988; Dalrymple et al 1989; Raju et al 1989; Rutledge et al 1989; Fromm et al 1990; Ransom et al 1990; Truong et al 1990; Bloss et al 1993; Killackey & Davis 1993;

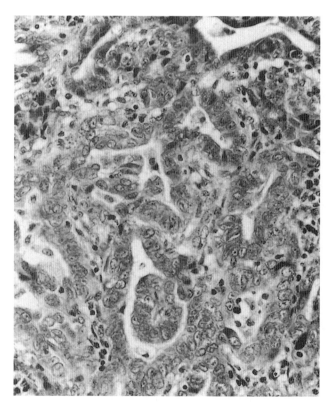

Fig. 27.12 Peritoneal serous carcinoma. Glands, papillae and slit-like spaces are lined by cuboidal to columnar cells with pleomorphic, overlapping nuclei.

closer examination in many cases reveals fine granularity, small nodules or warty excrescences on their surfaces. On microscopic examination, the peritoneal tumour has the typical histological appearance of serous carcinoma which, in the majority of reported cases, has been moderately or poorly differentiated (Fig. 27.12) (Gooneratne et al 1982; White et al 1985; Dalrymple et al 1989; Rutledge et al 1989; Ransom et al 1990). Psammoma bodies are present in most cases. A small number of low-grade peritoneal serous carcinomas have been described (Gooneratne et al 1982; Dalrymple et al 1989; Weir et al 1998).

Much of the controversy surrounding these neoplasms has focused on their biological behaviour and their histogenesis. Although it has been suggested that serous surface carcinomas are highly aggressive and have a less favourable prognosis than their ovarian counterparts of similar grade and stage (Gooneratne et al 1982; White et al 1985; Mills et al 1988; Killackey & Davis 1993; Rothacker & Mobius 1995), a number of studies have reported no differences in survival between these two tumours when patients were matched for extent of disease and treated with standard ovarian carcinoma chemotherapeutic protocols (Lele et al 1988; Dalrymple et al 1989; Fromm et al 1990; Ransom et al 1990; Truong et al 1990; Bloss et al 1993; Ben-Baruch et al 1996; Liapis et al 1996; Piura et al 1998; Schorge et al 1998; Schorge, Muto, Welch 2000). Small numbers of long-term survivors have been reported after such therapy (Hochster et al 1984; Chen & Flam 1986). One study found a significantly longer survival in patients treated with cisplatin-containing treatment protocols compared with non-cisplatin-containing regimens, possibly accounting for the differing conclusions among various investigators (Fromm et al 1990). Currently, chemotherapy with platinum-paclitaxel is recommended (Kennedy et al 1998). The little data available regarding the prognosis of well-differentiated primary peritoneal serous carcinomas indicate that these tumours appear to have a much better prognosis than typical higher-grade peritoneal serous carcinomas, at least after relatively short follow-up intervals (Gooneratne et al 1982; Dalrymple et al 1989; Weir et al 1998).

Although it has been suggested that these tumours represent massive peritoneal spread from small ovarian primary carcinomas (Gooneratne et al 1982), the extent of peritoneal involvement, the absence of ovarian involvement in some women, and the development of these neoplasms in patients whose ovaries were normal at the time of prior bilateral oophorectomies for benign disease or a family history of ovarian carcinoma indicate that they arise from extraovarian peritoneum (Tobacman et al 1982; Lele et al 1988; Dalrymple et al 1989; Fromm et al 1990). Electronmicroscopic and immunohistochemical studies have failed to allow definitive conclusions regarding the histogenesis of these tumours. Several groups report features common to both serous carcinomas and mesotheliomas (Gooneratne et al 1982; August et al 1985; White et al 1985) and other groups report features identical to those of serous carcinoma (Raju et al 1989; Truong et al 1990). A single study using flow cytometry has shown that 29% of serous surface carcinomas exhibit heterogeneity of DNA content at various sites (Rutledge et al 1989), a finding that supports a multifocal peritoneal origin of these neoplasms given the high rate of agreement of DNA content, ranging from 87 to 100% between primary ovarian carcinomas and their peritoneal metastases (Erba et al 1985; Volm et al 1985; Blumenfeld et al 1987; Iversen & Skaarland 1987; Rodenburg et al 1987). A variety of genetic techniques have been applied to these tumours, including examination of mutation patterns of *p53* and *k-ras*, patterns of allelic loss at various loci and X-inactivation of the androgen receptor locus, to determine if they are clonal or multifocal. These studies have demonstrated that many peritoneal serous carcinomas are multifocal, whereas most metastatic ovarian serous carcinomas are clonal (Muto et al 1995; Schorge et al 1998; Huang et al 2000; Nishimura et al 2000). One study has noted that peritoneal serous carcinomas in patients with BRCA1 mutations are more often polyclonal or multifocal (63 versus 7%) and have a greater frequency of p53 mutations (89 versus 47%) than tumours in women without such mutations (Schorge et al 2000b). These findings suggest a unique molecular pathogenesis for peritoneal serous carcinoma in these women that may create a peritoneal field defect (Schorge et al 2000b). One familial ovarian cancer early detection surveillance study found that 7 of 10 carcinomas detected were peritoneal serous carcinomas (Karlan et al 1999), lending support to this view.

Peritoneal serous carcinomas can be distinguished from peritoneal serous borderline tumours by the presence of invasion of omentum or underlying intra-abdominal viscera and the greater degree of nuclear atypicality in the former; the degree of nuclear atypicality also distinguishes serous carcinomas from the much rarer serous psammocarcinomas of peritoneal origin. Peritoneal serous carcinomas may be differentiated from malignant mesotheliomas by the presence of columnar cells with overlapping nuclei, slit-like spaces, numerous psammoma bodies, and intracytoplasmic neutral mucin as demonstrated by mucicarmine or period acid–Schiff stains after diastase digestion in the former (Kannerstein et al 1977; Foyle et al 1981; White et al 1985; Truong et al 1990; Goldblum & Hart 1995).

MUCINOUS LESIONS

Endocervicosis

Subperitoneal glandular inclusions lined by benign mucinous epithelium have been reported only rarely involving the posterior uterine serosa, cul-de-sac (Lauchlan 1972),

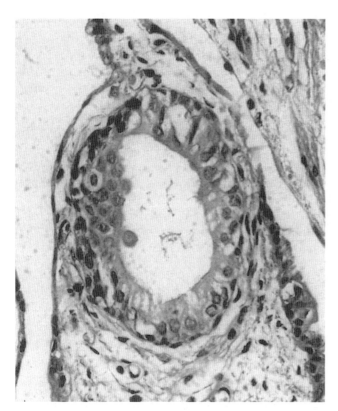

Fig. 27.13 Endocervicosis. A gland lined by mucin-containing columnar cells is present beneath the peritoneum.

subserosa of the vermiform appendix, and urinary bladder (Fig. 27.13) (Clement & Young 1992). Similar lesions have also been reported in cutaneous scars (Lauchlan 1965), and pelvic lymph nodes (Ferguson et al 1969; Baird & Reddick 1991). These lesions may be distinguished from metastatic adenocarcinoma by the absence of cytological atypia.

A small number of cases in which endocervicosis extended into underlying bladder or cervical wall have been reported (Clement & Young 1992; Nada et al 2000; Young & Clement 2000; Kim et al 2001). The patients were reproductive age women who presented with pelvic pain or a mass. Each of them had a mass measuring up to 4 cm in diameter predominantly involving the outer wall of the bladder or cervix. Microscopically the lesions were composed of glands of variable sizes and shapes lined by bland endocervical-type epithelium. The major differential diagnosis is with primary adenocarcinoma. The main features that may aid in this distinction are the deep involvement of the wall of the involved organ with a spared zone of normal stroma or muscle between the normal epithelium and the endocervicosis and the bland cytological appearance of the cells lining the glands.

Mucinous neoplasms

The clinicopathologic features of pseudomyoma peritonei are discussed elsewhere. Thus far, a well documented primary mucinous tumour of the peritoneum has not been reported.

Localised cystic mucinous tumours have been described rarely in the retroperitoneum, primarily as isolated case reports (Douglas et al 1965; Williams et al 1971; Lauchlan 1972; Banerjee & Gough 1988; Pennell & Gusdon 1989; Park et al 1990; Gotoh et al 1992; Tenti et al 1994; Papadogiannakis et al 1997; Kehagias et al 1999; Uematsu et al 2000; Subramony et al 2001). These neoplasms occur in women ranging in age from 18 to 58 years. The spectrum of histological abnormalities in these tumours mimics that seen in primary cystic mucinous neoplasms of the ovary, ranging from benign to borderline to frankly malignant. All of the mucinous cystadenomas behaved in a benign fashion, several of the mucinous cystadenocarcinomas metastasised widely resulting in the death of the patient (Douglas et al 1965; Roth & Ehrlich 1977), and one tumour with a borderline histology metastasised to mediastinal lymph nodes (Banerjee & Gough 1988). Although it has been postulated that retroperitoneal cystic tumours may arise from teratomas or ectopic ovarian tissue (Williams et al 1971), the absence of residual teratomatous elements or ovarian tissue in these neoplasms would support their origin from coelomic epithelium (Banerjee & Gough 1988; Pennell & Gusdon 1989; Park et al 1990). The presence of flattened calretinin-positive cells interspersed between the mucin-containing columnar cells raises the possibility that the tumours arise from mucinous metaplasia of mesothelial cysts (Subramony et al 2001). It has also been suggested that the neoplasms may arise from endometriosis (Carabias et al 1995).

TRANSITIONAL-LIKE LESIONS

Walthard nests

Solid nests, cysts and surface plaques composed of transitional-like cells termed Walthard nests are common on the pelvic peritoneum. These lesions measure up to several millimetres in greatest dimension and are most frequently identified on the postero-lateral serosa of the Fallopian tubes, on the posterior surface of the mesosalpinx and less often in the meso-ovarium or ovary (Teoh 1953; Bransilver et al 1974). They have also been described involving the serosa of the appendix testis and epididymis in men (Hartz 1947; Sundarasivarao 1953). Histologically, the nests are composed of polygonal cells with oval nuclei and scant to moderate amounts of cytoplasm that resemble urothelial cells. The nuclei focally contain longitudinal nuclear grooves; the cysts often contain eosinophilic or amorphous material (Fig. 27.14) (Teoh 1953; Bransilver et al 1974; Roth 1974).

Because of the light and electron microscopic similarities of Walthard nests to urothelium, and because of their frequently documented continuity with the surface

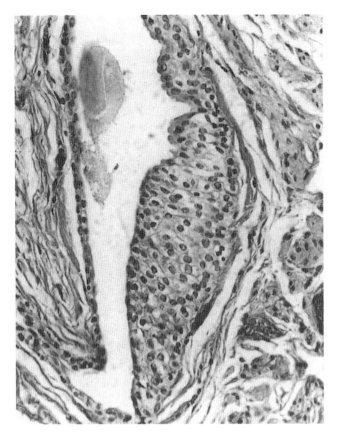

Fig. 27.14 Walthard nest. The cyst is lined by polygonal cells with bland nuclei that resemble urothelial cells. Amorphous material is present in the lumen.

mesothelium, these lesions have long been felt to arise from transitional or urothelial metaplasia of the mesothelium (Bransilver et al 1974; Roth 1974). However, several recent studies have failed to demonstrate convincing immunohistochemical staining of Walthard nests with urothelial markers such as uroplakin or cytokeratins 13 or 20 (Soslow et al 1996; Ogawa et al 1999; Riedel et al 2001).

Transitional cell neoplasms

Although Walthard nests of the peritoneum are common, extraovarian Brenner tumours have been reported as individual case reports only rarely. These tumours have been identified as solid masses in older women; most have been located in the broad ligament. Borderline or malignant Brenner tumours or peritoneal transitional cell carcinomas have not been described thus far (Pschera & Wikstrom 1991; Hampton et al 1992).

SQUAMOUS LESIONS

Very few examples of squamous metaplasia of otherwise normal peritoneum have been reported (Crome 1950; Schatz & Colgan 1991), although squamous metaplasia of peritoneal inclusion cysts is not uncommon (Ross et al

1989). True squamous metaplasia may be distinguished from the much more common transitional metaplasia by the orderly maturation of the epithelial cells to superficial cells, prominent intercellular bridges and presence of cytoplasmic keratinisation or keratohyaline granules in the former.

CLEAR CELL LESIONS

Although focal clear cell differentiation is observed in a substantial number of peritoneal serous carcinomas (Mills et al 1988; Truong et al 1990), pure clear cell carcinoma of the peritoneum without coexisting evidence of endometriosis has been reported only once in a 67-year-old woman (Lee et al 1991) and we have observed an additional case in a patient from our institution. A small number of localised clear cell carcinomas of the retroperitoneum has been reported (Brooks & Wheeler 1977; Goldberg et al 1978; Mostoufizadeh & Scully 1980; Evans et al 1990); most of them were felt to arise from endometriosis.

ECTOPIC DECIDUA

Extrauterine decidua formation is common in pregnant women and occurs rarely in nonpregnant patients in association with progestational therapy, trophoblastic neoplasia, hormonally active lesions of the ovary and adrenal, in proximity to a corpus luteum or after radiation therapy. Occasionally ectopic decidua is observed without an apparent underlying cause in either premenopausal or postmenopausal women (Ober et al 1957; Boss et al 1965; Buttner et al 1993; Clement & Young 1993). Ectopic decidua has been reported in the ovary, cervix (Zaytsev & Taxy 1987), uterine, bowel and appendiceal serosa (Suster & Moran 1990), omentum, renal pelvis (Bettinger 1947) and para-aortic and pelvic lymph nodes (Zaytsev & Taxy 1987; Cobb 1988). The patients are usually asymptomatic, although a small number of women has presented with intra-abdominal haemorrhage (Sabatelle & Winger 1973; Richter et al 1983; Bashir et al 1995) or pain (Hulme-Moir & Ross 1969; Suster & Moran 1990).

Ectopic decidua involving peritoneal surfaces usually is not evident grossly although in a few cases the peritoneal surfaces are studded with greyish-white granules or plaques measuring up to several millimetres in diameter (O'Sullivan & Heffernan 1960). Microscopically, single cells, nodules or ill-defined aggregates of cells are present beneath the mesothelium. The decidual cells have abundant amphophilic cytoplasm and round to oval, uniform nuclei with delicate chromatin and prominent nucleoli (Fig. 27.15). Smooth muscle cells or fibroblasts are occasionally interspersed among the decidual cells.

Ectopic decidua can be distinguished from deciduoid malignant mesothelioma, metastatic carcinoma or

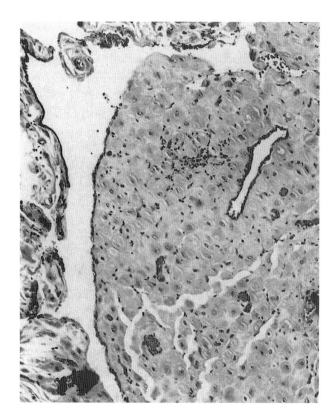

Fig. 27.15 Ectopic decidua. A nodule of decidual cells with abundant cytoplasm and uniform nuclei is present beneath the mesothelium.

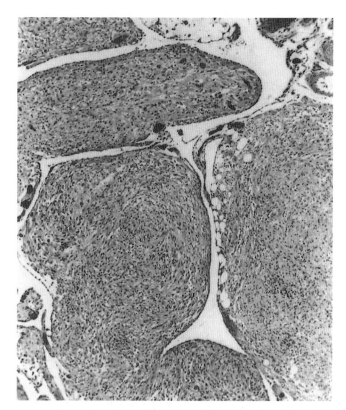

Fig. 27.16 Diffuse peritoneal leiomyomatosis. Nodules of interlacing bundles of smooth muscle cells are located beneath the mesothelium.

sarcoma by the uniformity and bland appearance of the nuclei in the former.

DIFFUSE PERITONEAL LEIOMYOMATOSIS

Diffuse peritoneal leiomyomatosis is characterised by multiple subperitoneal nodules of smooth muscle that occur in reproductive-aged women (Parmley et al 1975; Winn et al 1976; Nogales et al 1978; Herr et al 1979; Pieslor et al 1979; Kaplan et al 1980; Kuo et al 1980; Fujii et al 1981; Hsu et al 1981; Ceccacci et al 1982; Tavassoli & Norris 1982; Akkersdijk et al 1990; Hales et al 1992) and rarely in postmenopausal women (Nigojevic et al 1997; Bekkers et al 1999; Danikas et al 2000; Strinic et al 2000). The patients are usually pregnant, postpartum, on oral contraceptives, have an oestrogen producing tumour, or have uterine leiomyomas, although cases have been reported in women with none of these conditions (Fujii et al 1981; Tavassoli & Norris 1982; Bekkers et al 1999). Clinically, diffuse peritoneal leiomyomatosis is usually an asymptomatic incidental finding. Approximately half of the patients have abdominal pain or vaginal bleeding, which is usually attributable to coexisting uterine leiomyomas (Tavassoli & Norris 1982; Bekkers et al 1999).

Grossly, diffuse peritoneal leiomyomatosis is seen as numerous white or tan, firm peritoneal nodules ranging in size from less than 1 mm to 10 cm (Nogales et al 1978; Pieslor et al 1979; Kuo et al 1980; Tavassoli & Norris 1982; Akkersdijk et al 1990; Hales et al 1992), although the majority of lesions measure less than several centimetres in diameter. Microscopically, the nodules are located beneath the mesothelium and are composed of interlacing bundles of spindle cells with elongated, uniform nuclei (Fig. 27.16). Cytological atypia and mitotic figures are not generally identified, although Tavassoli and Norris (1982) reported up to 3 mitotic figures per 10 high-power fields in two of their 20 cases. Decidual cells are often intermixed with smooth muscle cells in pregnant patients (Tavassoli & Norris 1982), and coexisting endometriosis has been reported in a small number of patients (Herrero et al 1998; Zotalis et al 1998). Ultrastructurally, the cells in the nodules have been shown to have features of smooth muscle cells; myofibroblasts, fibroblasts and decidual cells have also been identified (Winn et al 1976; Nogales et al 1978; Pieslor et al 1979; Kuo et al 1980; Ceccacci et al 1982; Tavassoli & Norris 1982).

Despite the aggressive clinical appearance of diffuse peritoneal leiomyomatosis only a small number of cases have been reported in which patients originally diagnosed with diffuse peritoneal leiomyomatosis subsequently developed leiomyosarcomas, most within 2 years of the diagnosis of diffuse peritoneal leiomyomatosis (Akkersdijk et al 1990; Raspagliesi et al 1996; Fulcher & Szucs 1998;

Bekkers et al 1999; Morizaki et al 1999). Most of the patients who developed sarcoma had no history of hormonal stimulation and their diffuse peritoneal leiomyomatosis was often negative for oestrogen and progesterone receptors. One group has suggested that diffuse peritoneal leiomyomatosis with these characteristics may have a low malignant potential (Bekkers et al 1999). Persistence or recurrence of benign-appearing diffuse peritoneal leiomyomatosis in later pregnancies has been reported in a small number of women (Tavassoli & Norris 1982; Hales et al 1992). The majority of patients have a benign clinical course (Tavassoli & Norris 1982; Bekkers et al 1999). Follow-up laparotomy or laparoscopy has documented complete or partial regression of the lesions in some patients after cessation of hormone stimulation (Tavassoli & Norris 1982; Bekkers et al 1999).

The majority of authors have suggested that diffuse peritoneal leiomyomatosis results from hormonally related smooth muscle metaplasia of subperitoneal mesenchyme. The development of diffuse peritoneal leiomyomatosis in pregnant women or women taking oral contraceptives, the regression of the lesions postpartum or after discontinuation of exogenous hormones (Tavassoli & Norris 1982) or after treatment with a gonadotropin-releasing agonist (Hales et al 1992), and the production of lesions resembling diffuse peritoneal leiomyomatosis in guinea pigs (Fujii et al 1981) all support this hypothesis. Conversely, one study has demonstrated that the nodules of diffuse peritoneal leiomyomatosis are monoclonal with non-random inactivation of the same parental X-chromosome in the cells both within an individual nodule and among multiple nodules in the same patient, raising the possibility that the lesions are neoplastic and possibly a diffusely metastatic unicentric neoplasm (Quade et al 1997).

Diffuse peritoneal leiomyomatosis may be distinguished from metastatic leiomyosarcoma by both microscopic and gross features. Grossly, the nodules of diffuse peritoneal leiomyomatosis tend to be numerous and small whereas leiomyosarcomas usually present as one or several large masses. Histologically, diffuse peritoneal leiomyomatosis is cytologically bland with few mitotic figures; marked atypia, mitotic activity and necrosis characterise metastatic leiomyosarcoma.

REFERENCES

Addis B J, Fox H 1983 Papillary mesothelioma of ovary. Histopathology 7: 287–298

Akkersdijk G J M, Flu P K, Giard R W M, van Lent M, Wallenburg H C S 1990 Malignant leiomyomatosis peritonealis disseminata. American Journal of Obstetrics and Gynecology 163: 591–593

Al-Nafussi A, Wong N A C S 2001 Intra-abdominal spindle cell lesions: a review and practical aids to diagnosis. Histopathology 38: 387–402

Antman K H, Corson J M, Li F P 1983 Malignant mesothelioma following radiation exposure. Journal of Clinical Oncology 1: 695–700

Asensio J A, Goldblatt P, Thomford N R 1990 Primary malignant peritoneal mesothelioma. A report of seven cases and a review of the literature. Archives of Surgery 125: 1477–1481

Aslani M, Ahn G H, Scully R E 1988 Serous papillary cystadenoma of borderline malignancy of broad ligament. A report of 25 cases. International Journal of Gynecological Pathology 7: 131–138

August C Z, Murad T M, Newton M 1985 Multiple focal extraovarian serous carcinoma. International Journal of Gynecological Pathology 1985; 4: 11–23

Babcock T L, Powell D H 1976 Radiation induced peritoneal mesothelioma. Journal of Surgical Oncology 8: 369–372

Baird D B, Reddick R L 1991 Extraovarian mucinous metaplasia in a patient with bilateral mucinous borderline tumours: A case report. International Journal of Gynecological Pathology 10: 96–103

Banerjee R, Gough J 1988 Cystic mucinous tumours of the mesentery and retroperitoneum: report of three cases. Histopathology 12: 527–532

Barnoud R, Sabourin S J, Pasquier D et al 2000 Immunohistochemical expression of WT1 by desmoplastic small round cell tumor: a comparative study with other small round cell tumors. American Journal of Surgical Pathology 24: 830–836

Bashir R M, Montgomery E A, Gupta P K et al 1995 Massive gastrointestinal hemorrhage during pregnancy caused by ectopic decidua of the terminal ileum and colon. American Journal of Gastroenterology 90: 1325–1327

Bedrossian C W, Bonsib S, Moran C 1992 Differential diagnosis between mesothelioma and adenocarcinoma: a multimodal approach based on ultrastructure and immunocytochemistry. Seminars in Diagnostic Pathology 9: 124–140

Bekkers R L, Willemsen W N, Schijf C P, Massuger L F, Bulten J, Merkus J M 1999 Leiomyomatosis peritonealis disseminata: does malignant transformation occur? A literature review. Gynecologic Oncology 75: 158–163

Bell D A, Scully R E 1989 Benign and borderline serous lesions of the peritoneum in women. Pathology Annual 2: 1–21

Bell D A, Scully R E 1990 Serous borderline tumors of the peritoneum. American Journal of Surgical Pathology 14: 230–239

Bell D A, Weinstock M A, Scully R E 1988 Peritoneal implants of ovarian serous borderline tumors. Histologic features and prognosis. Cancer 62: 2212–2222

Ben-Baruch G, Sivan E, Moran O, Rizel S, Menczer J, Seidman D S 1996 Primary peritoneal serous papillary carcinoma: a study of 25 cases and comparison with stage III–IV ovarian papillary serous carcinoma. Gynecologic Oncology 60: 393–396

Bettinger H F 1947 Ectopic decidua in the renal pelvis. Journal of Pathology and Bacteriology 59: 686–687

Biscotti C V, Hart W R 1992 Peritoneal serous micropapillomatosis of low malignant potential (serous borderline tumors of the peritoneum). A clinicopathologic study of 17 cases. American Journal of Surgical Pathology 16: 467–475

Bloss J D, Liao S-Y, Buller R E et al 1993 Extraovarian peritoneal serous papillary carcinoma: a case-control retrospective comparison to papillary adenocarcinoma of the ovary. Gynecologic Oncology 50: 347–351

Blumenfeld D, Braly P S, Ben E J, Klevecz R R 1987 Tumor DNA content as a prognostic feature in advanced epithelial ovarian carcinoma. Gynecologic Oncology 27: 389–402

Bollinger D J, Wick M R, Dehner L P, Mills S E, Swanson P E, Clarke R E 1989 Peritoneal malignant mesothelioma versus serous papillary adenocarcinoma. A histochemical and immunohistochemical comparison. American Journal of Surgical Pathology 13: 659–670

Boss J H, Scully R E, Wegner K H, Cohen R B 1965 Structural variations in the adult ovary — clinical significance. Obstetrics and Gynecology 1965; 25: 747–763

Bransilver B R, Ferenczy A, Richart R M 1974 Brenner tumors and Walthard cell nests. Archives of Pathology 98: 76–86

Brooks J J, Wheeler J E 1977 Malignancy arising in extragonadal endometriosis. Cancer 40: 3065–3073

Brown J V, Karlan B Y, Greenspoon J S, Rosove M H, Lagasse L D 1993 Perioperative coagulopathy in patients undergoing primary cytoreduction. Cancer 71: 2557–2561

Bryce R L, Barbatis C, Charnock M 1982 Endosalpingiosis in pregnancy. Case report. British Journal of Obstetrics and Gynaecology 89: 166–168

Burmeister R E, Fechner R E, Franklin R R 1969 Endosalpingiosis of the peritoneum. Obstetrics and Gynecology 34: 310–318

Burrig K F, Pfitzer P, Hort W 1990 Well-differentiated papillary mesothelioma of the peritoneum: a borderline mesothelioma. Report of two cases and review of literature. Virchows Archives A Pathological Anatomy and Histopathology 417: 443–447

Buttner A, Bassler R, Theele C 1993 Pregnancy-associated ectopic decidua (deciduosis) of the greater omentum. An analysis of 60 biopsies with cases of fibrosing deciduosis and leiomyomatosis peritonealis disseminata. Pathology Research and Practice 189: 352–359

Cajigas A, Axiotis C A 1990 Endosalpingiosis of the vermiform appendix. International Journal of Gynecological Pathology 9: 291–295

Carabias E, Garcia Munoz H, Dihmes F P, Pino L, Ballestin C 1995 Primary mucinous cystadenocarcinoma of the retroperitoneum. Report of a case and literature review. Virchows Archives A Pathological Anatomy and Histopathology 426: 641–645

Carella R, Deleonardi G, D'Errico A et al 2001 Immunohistochemical panels for differentiating epithelial malignant mesothelioma from lung adenocarcinoma: a study with logistic regression analysis. American Journal of Surgical Pathology 25: 43–50

Casey Jones D E, Silver D 1979 Peritoneal mesotheliomas. Surgery 86: 556–560

Ceccacci L, Jacobs J, Powell A 1982 Leiomyomatosis peritonealis disseminata: Report of a case in a nonpregnant woman. American Journal of Obstetrics and Gynecology 144: 105–109

Chahinian A P, Pajak T F, Holland J F, Norton L, Ambinder R M, Mandel E M 1982 Diffuse malignant mesothelioma. Prospective evaluation of 69 patients. Annals of Internal Medicine 96: 746–755

Charles A K, Moore I E, Berry P J 1997 Immunohistochemical detection of the Wilm's tumour gene WT1 in desmoplastic small round cell tumour. Histopathology 30: 312–314

Chen K T 1981 Benign glandular inclusions of the peritoneum and periaortic lymph nodes. Diagnostic Gynecology and Obstetrics 3: 265–268

Chen K T, Flam M S 1986 Peritoneal papillary serous carcinoma with long-term survival. Cancer 58: 1371–1373

Chetty R 1992 Well differentiated (benign) papillary mesothelioma of the tunica vaginalis. Journal of Clinical Pathology 45: 1029–1030

Clement P B 1993 Tumor-like lesions of the ovary associated with pregnancy. International Journal of Gynecological Pathology 12: 108–115

Clement P B, Young R H 1993 Florid mesothelial hyperplasia associated with ovarian tumors: A potential source of error in tumour diagnosis and staging. International Journal of Gynecological Pathology 12: 51–58

Clement P B, Young R H 1992 Endocervicosis of the urinary bladder. A report of six cases of a benign mullerian lesion that may mimic adenocarcinoma. American Journal of Surgical Pathology 16: 533–542

Clement P B, Young R H 1999 Florid cystic endosalpingiosis with tumor-like manifestations: a report of four cases including the first reported cases of transmural endosalpingiosis of the uterus. American Journal of Surgical Pathology 23: 166–175

Clement P B, Young R H, Scully R E 1996 Malignant mesotheliomas presenting as ovarian masses. A report of nine cases, including two primary ovarian mesotheliomas. American Journal of Surgical Pathology 20: 1067–1080

Cobb C J 1988 Ectopic decidua and metastatic squamous carcinoma: presentation in a single pelvic lymph node. Journal of Surgical Oncology 38: 126–129

Comin C E, Novelli L, Boddi V, Paglierani M, Dini S 2001 Calretinin, thrombomodulin, CEA, and CD15: a useful combination of immunohistochemical markers for differentiating pleural epithelial mesothelioma from peripheral pulmonary adenocarcinoma. Human Pathology 32: 529–536

Crome L 1950 Squamous metaplasia of the peritoneum. Journal of Pathology and Bacteriology 62: 61–68

Cummings O W, Ulbright T M, Young R H, Dei Tos A P, Fletcher C D M, Hull M T 1997 Desmoplastic small round cell tumors of the

paratesticular region: a report of six cases. American Journal of Surgical Pathology 21: 219–225

Dabbs D J, Geisinger K R 1988 Common epithelial ovarian tumours. Immunohistochemical intermediate filament profiles. Cancer 62: 368–374

Dallenbach H G 1987 Atypical endosalpingiosis: a case report with consideration of the differential diagnosis of glandular subperitoneal inclusions. Pathology Research and Practice 182: 180–182

Dalrymple J C, Bannatyne P, Russell P et al 1989 Extraovarian peritoneal serous papillary carcinoma. A clinicopathologic study of 31 cases. Cancer 64: 110–115

Danikas D, Goudas V T, Rao C V, Brief D K 2000 Luteininzing hormone receptor expression in leiomyomatosis peritonealis disseminata. Obstetrics and Gynecology 95: 1009–1011

Dawson A, Gibbs A R, Pooley F D, McGriffiths D M, Hoy J 1993 Malignant mesothelioma in women. Thorax 48: 269–274

Daya D, McCaughey W T E 1990 Well-differentiated papillary mesothelioma of the peritoneum. A clinicopathologic study of 22 cases. Cancer 65: 292–296

Daya D, McCaughey W T E 1991 Pathology of the peritoneum: a review of selected topics. Seminars in Diagnostic Pathology 8: 277–289

Delahaye M, Van der Ham F, Van der Kwast T H 1997 Complementary value of five carcinoma markers for the diagnosis of malignant mesothelioma, adenocarcinoma metastasis, and reactive mesothelium in serous effusions. Diagnostic Cytopathology 17: 115–120

Dore N, Landry M, Cadotte M, Schurch W 1980 Cutaneous endosalpingiosis. Archives of Dermatology 116: 909–912

Douglas G W, Kastin A J, Huntington R W 1965 Carcinoma arising in a retroperitoneal mullerian cyst, with widespread metastasis during pregnancy. American Journal of Obstetrics and Gynecology 91: 210–216

Dubeau L 1999 The cell of origin of ovarian epithelial tumors and the ovarian surface epithelium dogma: does the emperor have no clothes? Gynecologic Oncology 72: 437–442

Erba E, Vaghi M, Pepe S et al 1985 DNA index of ovarian carcinomas from 56 patients: in vivo in vitro studies. British Journal of Cancer 52: 565–573

Evans H, Yates W A, Palmer W E, Cartwright R L, Antemann R W 1990 Clear cell carcinoma of the sigmoid mesocolon: a tumor of the secondary Müllerian system. American Journal of Obstetrics and Gynecology 162: 161–163

Ferguson B R, Bennington J L, Haber S L 1969 Histochemistry of mucosubstances and histology of mixed mullerian pelvic lymph node glandular inclusions. Evidence for histogenesis by mullerian metaplasia of coelomic epithelium. Obstetrics and Gynecology 33: 617–625

Fievez M, Lambot P, Dewin B 1983 Endosalpingosis of the peritoneum and chronic salpingitis. Archives of Anatomy and Cytological Pathology 31: 355–558

Flynn M K, Johnston W, Bigner S 1993 Carcinoma of ovarian and other origins in effusions. Immunocytochemical study with a panel of monoclonal antibodies. Acta Cytologica 37: 441–447

Foyle A, Al-Jabi M, McCaughey W T E 1981 Papillary peritoneal tumors in women. American Journal of Surgical Pathology 5: 241–249

Fraire A E, Cooper S, Greenberg S D, Buffler P, Langston C 1988 Mesothelioma of childhood. Cancer 62: 838–847

Fromm G L, Gershenson D M, Silva E G 1990 Papillary serous carcinoma of the peritoneum. Obstetrics and Gynecology 75: 89–95

Fujii S, Nakashima N, Okamura H et al 1981 Progesterone-induced smooth muscle-like cells in the subperitoneal nodules produced by estrogen. Experimental approach to leiomyomatosis peritonealis disseminata. American Journal of Obstetrics and Gynecology 139: 164–172

Fulcher A S, Szucs R A 1998 Leiomyomatosis peritonealis disseminata complicated by sarcomatous transformation and ovarian torsion: presentation of two cases and review of the literature. Abdominal Imaging 23: 640–644

Furman J, Murphy W M, Wajsman Z, Berry A D 1997 Urogenital involvement by desmoplastic small round-cell tumor. Journal of Urology 158: 1506–1509

Gaffey M J, Mills S E, Swanson P E, Zarbo R J, Shah A R, Wick M R 1992 Immunoreactivity for BER-EP4 in adenocarcinomas, adenomatoid tumors, and malignant mesotheliomas. American Journal of Surgical Pathology 16: 593–599

Gerald W L, Miller H K, Battifora H, Miettinen M, Silva E G, Rosai J 1991 Intra-abdominal desmoplastic small round-cell tumor. Report of 19 cases of a distinctive type of high-grade polyphenotypic malignancy affecting young individuals. American Journal of Surgical Pathology 15: 499–513

Gerald W L, Ladanyi M, de Alava E et al 1998 Clinical, pathologic, and molecular spectrum of tumors associated with t(11;22)(p13;q12): desmoplastic small round-cell tumor and its variants. Journal of Clinical Oncology 16: 3028–3036

Gilks C B, Bell D A, Scully R E 1990 Serous psammocarcinoma of the ovary and peritoneum. International Journal of Gynecological Pathology 9: 110–121

Goepel J R 1981 Benign papillary mesothelioma of peritoneum: a histological, histochemical and ultrastructural study of six cases. Histopathology 5: 21–30

Goldberg M I, Ng A B P, Belinson J L, Hutson E D, Nordquist S R B 1978 Clear cell adenocarcinoma arising in endometriosis of the rectosigmoid septum. Obstetrics and Gynecology 51: 385–405

Goldblum J, Hart W R 1995 Localized and diffuse mesotheliomas of the genital tract and peritoneum in women: a clinicopathologic study of nineteen true mesothelial neoplasms, other than adenomatoid tumors, multicystic mesotheliomas, and localized fibrous tumors. American Journal of Surgical Pathology 19: 1124–1137

Goldblum J R, Hart W R 1997 Author's reply. American Journal of Surgical Pathology 21: 123–124

Gonzales-Crussi F, Crawford S E, Sun C-C J 1990 Intraabdominal desmoplastic small-cell tumors with divergent differentiation. Observations on three cases of childhood. American Journal of Surgical Pathology 14: 633–642

Gooneratne S, Sassone M, Blaustein A, Talerman A 1982 Serous surface papillary carcinoma of the ovary: a clinicopathologic study of 16 cases. International Journal of Gynecological Pathology 1: 258–269

Gotoh K, Konaga E, Arata A, Takeuchi H, Mano S 1992 A case of primary retroperitoneal mucinous cystadenocarcinoma. Acta Medica Okayama 46: 49–52

Grundy G W, Miller R W 1972 Malignant mesothelioma in childhood. Report of 13 cases. Cancer 30: 1216–1218

Gussman D, Thickman D, Wheeler J E 1986 Postoperative peritoneal cysts. Obstetrics and Gynecology 68: 53S–55S

Hales H A, Peterson C M, Jones K P, Quinn J D 1992 Leiomyomatosis peritonealis disseminata treated with a gonadotropin-releasing hormone agonist. American Journal of Obstetrics and Gynecology 167: 515–516

Hampton H L, Huffman H T, Meeks G R 1992 Extraovarian Brenner tumor. Obstetrics and Gynecology 79: 844–846

Hartz P H 1947 Occurrence of Walthard cell rests in Brenner-like epithelium in the serosa of the epididymis. American Journal of Clinical Pathology 17: 654–656

Heatley M K, Russell P 2001 Florid cystic endosalpingiosis of the uterus. Journal of Clinical Pathology 2001; 54: 399–400

Herr J C, Platz C E, Heidger P M, Curet L B 1979 Smooth muscle within ovarian decidual nodules: a link to leiomyomatosis peritonealis disseminata? Obstetrics and Gynecology 53: 451–456

Herrero J, Kamali P, Kirschbaum M 1998 Leiomyomatosis peritonealis disseminata associated with endometriosis: a case report and literature review. European Journal of Obstetrics, Gynecology and Reproductive Biology 76: 189–191

Hesseling M H, De Wilde R L 2000 Endosalpingiosis in laparoscopy. Journal of the American Association of Gynecologic Laparoscopists 7: 215–219

Hill D A, Pfeifer J D, Marley E F et al 2000 WT1 staining reliably differentiates desmoplastic small round cell tumor from Ewing sarcoma/primitive neuroectodermal tumor. An immunohistochemical and molecular diagnostic study. American Journal of Clinical Pathology 114: 345–353

Hochster H, Wernz J C, Muggia F M 1984 Intra-abdominal carcinomatosis with histologically normal ovaries [letter]. Cancer Treatment Reports 68: 931–932

Holmes M D, Levin H S, Ballard L A J 1981 Endosalpingiosis. Cleveland Clinic Quarterly 48: 345–352

Hsu Y K, Rosenshein N B, Parmley T H, Woodruff J D, Elberfeld H T 1981 Leiomyomatosis in pelvic lymph nodes. Obstetrics and Gynecology 57: 91S–93S

Huang L W, Garrett A P, Muto M G et al 2000 Identification of a novel 9 cM deletion unit on chromosome 6q23–24 in papillary serous carcinoma of the peritoneum. Human Pathology 2000; 31: 367–373

Hulme-Moir I, Ross M S 1969 A case of early postpartum abdominal pain due to haemorrhagic deciduosis peritonei. Journal of Obstetrics and Gynaecology of the British Commonwealth 76: 746–749

Iversen O E, Skaarland E 1987 Ploidy assessment of benign and malignant ovarian tumors by flow cytometry. A clinicopathologic study. Cancer 60: 82–87

Kane M J, Chahinian A P, Holland J F 1990 Malignant mesothelioma in young adults. Cancer 65: 1449–1455

Kannerstein M, McCaughey W T, Churg J, Selikoff I J 1977 A critique of the criteria for the diagnosis of diffuse malignant mesothelioma. Mt Sinai Journal of Medicine 44: 485–494

Kannerstein M, Churg J, McCaughey W T, Hill D P 1997 Papillary tumors of the peritoneum in women: mesothelioma or papillary carcinoma. American Journal of Obstetrics and Gynecology 127: 306–314

Kaplan C, Benirschke K, Johnson K C 1980 Leiomyomatosis peritonealis disseminata with endometrium. Obstetrics and Gynecology 55: 119–122

Karlan B Y, Baldwin R L, Lopez-Luevanos E et al 1999 Peritoneal serous papillary carcinoma, a phenotypic variant of familial ovarian cancer: implications for ovarian cancer screening. American Journal of Obstetrics and Gynecology 180: 917–928

Katsube Y, Mukai K, Silverberg S G 1982 Cystic mesothelioma of the peritoneum. A report of five cases and review of the literature. Cancer 50: 1615–1622

Kehagias D T, Karvounis E E, Fotopoulos A, Gouliamos A D 1999 Retroperitoneal mucinous cystadenoma. European Journal of Obstetrics, Gynecology and Reproductive Biology 82: 213–215

Kennedy A W, Markman M, Webster K D et al 1998 Experience with platinum-paclitaxel chemotherapy in the initial management of papillary serous carcinoma of the peritoneum. Gynecologic Oncology 71: 288–290

Killackey M A, Davis A R 1993 Papillary serous carcinoma of the peritoneal surface: matched-case comparison with papillary serous ovarian carcinoma. Gynecologic Oncology 51: 171–174

Kim H J, Lee T J, Kim M K et al 2001 Mullerianosis of the urinary bladder, endocervicosis type: a case report. Journal of Korean Medical Science 16: 123–126

Kuo T, London S N, Dinh T V 1980 Endometriosis occurring in leiomyomatosis peritonealis disseminata. Ultrastructural study and histogenetic consideration. American Journal of Surgical Pathology 1980: 197–204

Kurre P, Felgenhauer J L, Miser J S, Patterson K, Hawkins D S 2000 Successful dose-intensive treatment of desmoplastic small round cell tumor in three children. Journal of Pediatric Hematology and Oncology 22: 446–450

Lauchlan S C 1965 Two types of mullerian epithelium in an abdominal scar. American Journal of Obstetrics and Gynecology 93: 89

Lauchlan S C 1972 The secondary mullerian system. Obstetrical and Gynecological Survey 27: 133–146

Lauchlan S C 1984 Metaplasias and neoplasias of mullerian epithelium. Histopathology 1984; 8: 543–557

Lauchlan S C 1994 The secondary mullerian system revisited. International Journal of Gynecological Pathology 13: 73–79

Laufer M R, Heerema A E, Parsons K E, Barbieri R L 1998 Endosalpingiosis: clinical presentation and follow-up. Gynecologic & Obstetric Investigation 46: 195–198

Layfield L J, Lenarsky C 1991 Desmoplastic small cell tumors of the peritoneum coexpressing mesenchymal and epithelial markers. American Journal of Clinical Pathology 96: 536–543

Lee K R, Verma U, Belinson J 1991 Primary clear cell carcinoma of the peritoneum. Gynecologic Oncology 41: 259–262

Lele S B, Piver M S, Matharu J, Tsukada Y 1988 Peritoneal papillary carcinoma. Gynecologic Oncology 31: 315–320

Leong A S, Stevens M W, Mukherjee T M 1992 Malignant mesothelioma: Cytologic diagnosis with histologic immunohistochemical and ultrastructural correlation. Seminars in Diagnostic Pathology 9: 141–150

Lerner H J, Schoenffeld D A, Martin A, Falkson G, Borden E 1983 Malignant mesothelioma: the eastern clinical oncology group (ECOG) experience. Cancer 52: 1981–1985

Letterle G S, Yon J L 1995 Use of a long acting GnRH agonist for benign cystic mesothelioma. Obstetrics and Gynecology 85: 901–903

Letterle G S, Yon J L 1998 The antiestrogen tamoxifen in the treatment of recurrent benign cystic mesothelioma. Gynecologic Oncology 70: 131–133

Liapis A, Condi-Paphiti A, Pyrgiotis E, Zourlas P A 1996 Ovarian surface serous papillary carcinomas: a clinicopathologic study. European Journal of Gynaecological Oncology 17: 79–82

Lovell F A, Cranston P E 1990 Well-differentiated papillary mesothelioma of the peritoneum. American Journal of Roentgenology 155: 1245–1246

McCaughey W T E, Al-Jabi M 1986 Differentiation of serosal hyperplasia and neoplasia in biopsies. Pathology Annual 21: 271–292

McCaughey W T, Kirk M E, Lester W, Dardick I 1984 Peritoneal epithelial lesions associated with proliferative serous tumours of ovary. Histopathology 8: 195–208

McCaughey W T E, Kannerstein M, Churg J 1985 Tumors and pseudotumors of the serous membranes. Atlas of tumor pathology. Fascicle 20. Armed Forces Institute of Pathology, Washington, DC

McCaughey W T, Schryer M J, Lin X S, Al Jabi M 1986 Extraovarian pelvic serous tumor with marked calcification. Archives of Pathology and Laboratory Medicine 110: 78–80

McCluggage W G, Weir P E 2000 Paraovarian cystic endosalpingiosis in association with tamoxifen therapy. Journal of Clinical Pathology 53: 161–162

McFadden D E, Clement P B 1986 Peritoneal inclusion cysts with mural mesothelial proliferation. A clinicopathological analysis of six cases. American Journal of Surgical Pathology 10: 844–854

Mennemeyer R, Smith M 1979 Multicystic peritoneal mesothelioma. A report with electron microscopy of a case mimicking intra-abdominal cystic hygroma (lymphangioma). Cancer 44: 692–698

Mills S E, Andersen W A, Fechner R E, Austin M B 1988 Serous surface papillary carcinoma. A clinicopathologic study of 10 cases and comparison with stage III–IV ovarian serous carcinoma. American Journal of Surgical Pathology 12: 827–834

Moore J H, Crum C P, Chandler J G, Feldman P S 1980 Benign cystic mesothelioma. Cancer 45: 2395–2399

Moore W F, Bentley R C, Berchuck A, Robboy S J 2000 Some mullerian inclusion cysts in lymph nodes may sometimes be metastases from serous borderline tumors of the ovary. American Journal of Surgical Pathology 24: 710–718

Moran C A, Wick M R, Suster S 2000 The role of immunohistochemistry in the diagnosis of malignant mesothelioma. Seminars in Diagnostic Pathology 17: 178–183

Morizaki A, Hayashi H, Ishikawa M 1999 Leiomyomatosis peritonealis disseminata with malignant transformation. International Journal of Gynaecology and Obstetrics 66: 43–45

Mostoufizadeh G H M, Scully R E 1980 Malignant tumors arising in endometriosis. Clinical Obstetrics and Gynecology 23: 951–963

Muto M G, Welch W R, Mok S C et al 1995 Evidence for a multifocal origin of papillary serous carcinoma of the peritoneum. Cancer Research 55: 490–492

Nada W, Parker J, Wong F, Cooper M, Reid G 2000 Laparoscopic excision of endocervicosis of the urinary bladder. Journal of the American Association of Gynecological Laparoscopists 7: 135–137

Nascimento A G, Keeney G L, Fletcher D M 1994 Deciduoid peritoneal mesothelioma: an unusual phenotype affecting young females. American Journal of Surgical Pathology 18: 439–445

Nigojevic S, Kapural L, Scukanec-Spoljar M et al 1997 Leiomyomatosis peritonealis disseminata in a postmenopausal woman. Acta Obstetricia et Gynecologica Scandinavaca 76: 893–894

Nishimura M, Wakabayashi M, Hashimoto T et al 2000 Papillary serous carcinoma of the peritoneum: analysis of clonality of peritoneal tumors. Journal of Gastroenterology 35: 540–547

Nogales F F, Matilla A, Carrascal E 1978 Leiomyomatosis peritonealis disseminata. An ultrastructural study. American Journal of Clinical Pathology 69: 452–457

Ober W B, Grady H G, Schoenbucher A K 1957 Ectopic ovarian decidua without pregnancy. American Journal of Pathology 33: 199–217

Ogawa K, Johansson S L, Cohen S M 1999 Immunohistochemical analysis of uroplakins, urothelial specific proteins, in ovarian Brenner tumors, normal tissues, and benign and metaplastic lesions of the female genital tract. American Journal of Pathology 155: 1047–1050

Ordonez N G 1998a Role of immunohistochemistry in distinguishing epithelial peritoneal mesotheliomas from peritoneal and ovarian serous carcinomas. American Journal of Surgical Pathology 22: 1203–1214

Ordonez N G 1998b Desmoplastic small round cell tumor. I: A histopathologic study of 39 cases with emphasis on unusual histological patterns. American Journal of Surgical Pathology 22: 1303–1313

Ordonez N G 1998c Desmoplastic small round cell tumor: II: an ultrastructural and immunohistochemical study with emphasis on new immunohistochemical markers. American Journal of Surgical Pathology 22: 1314–1327

Ordonez N G, El-Naggar A K, Ro J Y, Silva E G, Mackay B 1993 Intra-abdominal desmoplastic small cell tumor: A light microscopic, immunocytochemical, ultrastructural, and flow cytometric study. Human Pathology 24: 850–865

Orosz Z, Nagy P, Szentirmay Z, Zalatnai A, Hauser P 1999 Epithelial mesothelioma with deciduoid features. Virchows Archiv 434: 263–266

O'Sullivan D, Heffernan C K 1960 Deciduosis peritonei in pregnancy. Report of two cases respectively simulating carcinoma and tuberculosis. Journal of Obstetrics and Gynaecology of the British Empire 67: 1013–1016

Papadogiannakis N, Gad A, Ehliar B 1997 Primary retroperitoneal mucinous tumor of low malignant potential: histogenetic aspects and review of the literature. APMIS 105: 483–486

Park U, Han K C, Chang H K, Huh M H 1990 A primary mucinous cystadenocarcinoma of the retroperitoneum. Gynecologic Oncology 42: 64–67

Parmley T H, Woodruff J D, Winn K, Johnson J W C, Douglas P H 1975 Histogenesis of leiomyomatosis peritonealis disseminata (disseminated fibrosing deciduosis). Obstetrics and Gynecology 46: 511–516

Pennell T C, Gusdon J P J 1989 Retroperitoneal mucinous cystadenoma. American Journal of Obstetrics and Gynecology 160: 1229–1231

Piccigallo E, Jeffers L J, Reddy K R, Caldironi M W, Parenti A, Schiff E R 1988 Malignant peritoneal mesothelioma. A clinical and laparoscopic study of ten cases. Digestive Diseases and Sciences 33: 633–639

Pieslor P C, Orenstein J M, Hogan D L, Breslow A 1979 Ultrastructure of myofibroblasts and decidualized cells in leiomyomatosis peritonealis disseminata. American Journal of Clinical Pathology 72: 875–882

Piura B, Meirovitz M, Bartfeld M, Yanai-Inbar I, Cohen Y 1998 Peritoneal papillary serous carcinoma: study of 15 cases and comparison with stage III–IV ovarian papillary serous carcinoma. Journal of Surgical Oncology 68: 173–178

Plaus W J 1988 Peritoneal mesothelioma. Archives of Surgery 123: 763–766

Pschera H, Wikstrom B 1991 Extraovarian Brenner tumor coexisting with serous cystadenoma. Case report. Gynecological and Obstetrical Investigation 31: 185–187

Quade B J, McLachlin C M, Soto-Wright V, Zuckerman J, Mutter G L, Morton C C 1997 Disseminated peritoneal leiomyomatosis. Clonality analysis by X chromosome inactivation and cytogenetics of a clinically benign smooth muscle proliferation. American Journal of Pathology 150: 2153–2166

Quaglia M P, Brennan M F 2000 The clinical approach to desmoplastic small round cell tumor. Surgical Oncology 9: 77–81

Raju U, Fine G, Greenawald K A, Ohorodnik J M 1989 Primary papillary serous neoplasia of the peritoneum: a clinicopathologic and ultrastructural study of eight cases Human Pathology 20: 426–436

Ransom D T, Patel S R, Keeney G L, Malkasian G D, Edmonson J H 1990 Papillary serous carcinoma of the peritoneum. A review of 33 cases treated with platin-based chemotherapy. Cancer 66: 1091–1094

Raspagliesi F, Quattrone P, Grosso G, Cobellis L, Di Re E 1996 Malignant degeneration in leiomyomatosis peritonealis disseminata. Gynecologic Oncology 61: 272–274

Richter M A, Choudhry A, Barton J J, Merrick R E 1983 Bleeding ectopic decidua as a cause of intraabdominal hemorrhage. A case report. Journal of Reproductive Medicine 28: 430–432

Riddell R H, Goodman M J, Moose A R 1981 Peritoneal malignant mesothelioma in a patient with recurrent peritonitis. Cancer 48: 134–139

Riedel I, Czernobilsky B, Lifschitz-Mercer B et al 2001 Brenner tumors but not transitional cell carcinomas of the ovary show urothelial differentiation: immunohistochemical staining of urothelial markers, including cytokeratins and uroplakins. Virchows Archiv 438: 181–191

Riera J R, Astengo-Osuma C, Longmate J A, Battifora H 1997 The immuno-histochemical diagnostic panel for epithelial mesothelioma: A reevaluation after heat-induced epitope retrieval. American Journal of Surgical Pathology 21: 1409–1419

Rodenburg C J, Cornelisse C J, Heintz P A, Hermans J, Fleuren G J 1987 Tumor ploidy as a major prognostic factor in advanced ovarian cancer. Cancer 59: 317–323

Roggli V L, Oury T D, Moffatt E J 1997 Malignant mesothelioma in women. Anatomy and Pathology 2: 147–163

Rosai J, Dehner L P 1975 Nodular mesothelial hyperplasia in hernia sacs. A benign reactive condition simulating a neoplastic process. Cancer 35: 165–175

Ross M J, Welch W R, Scully R E 1989 Multilocular peritoneal inclusion cysts (so-called cystic mesotheliomas). Cancer 64: 1336–1346

Roth L M 1974 The Brenner tumor and the Walthard cell nest. An electron microscopic study. Laboratory Investigation 31: 15–23

Roth L M, Ehrlich C E 1977 Mucinous cystadenocarcinoma of the retroperitoneum. Obstetrics and Gynecology 1977; 49: 486–488

Rothacker D, Mobius G 1995 Varieties of serous surface papillary carcinoma of the peritoneum in Northern Germany: a thirty-year autopsy study. International Journal of Gynecological Pathology 14: 310–318

Russell P, Bannatyne P 1989 Surgical pathology of the ovaries. Churchill Livingstone, London

Rutledge M L, Silva E G, McLemore D, El N A 1989 Serous surface carcinoma of the ovary and peritoneum. A flow cytometric study. Pathology Annual 2: 227–235

Ryuko K, Miura H, Abu M A, Iwanari O, Kitao M 1992 Endosalpingiosis in association with ovarian surface papillary tumor of borderline malignancy. Gynecologic Oncology 46: 107–110

Sabatelle R, Winger E 1973 Postpartum intraabdominal hemorrhage caused by ectopic deciduosis. Obstetrics and Gynecology 41: 873–875

Schatz J E, Colgan T J 1991 Squamous metaplasia of the peritoneum. Archives of Pathology and Laboratory Medicine 115: 397–398

Schorge J O, Muto M G, Welch W R et al 1998 Molecular evidence for multifocal papillary serous carcinoma of the peritoneum in patients with germline BRCA1 mutations. Journal of the National Cancer Institute 90: 841–845

Schorge J O, Miller Y B, Qi L J et al 2000a Genetic alterations of the WT1 gene in papillary serous carcinoma of the peritoneum. Gynecologic Oncology 76: 369–372

Schorge J O, Muto M G, Lee S J et al 2000b BRCA1-related papillary serous carcinoma of the peritoneum has a unique molecular pathogenesis. Cancer Research 60: 1361–1364

Schuldenfrei R, Janovsky N A 1962 Disseminated endosalpingiosis associated with bilateral papillary serous cystadenocarcinoma of the ovaries. A case report. American Journal of Obstetrics and Gynecology 84: 382–389

Schwarz R E, Gerald W L, Kushner B H, Coit D G, Brennan M F, La Quaglia M P 1998 Desmoplastic small round cell tumors: prognostic indicators and results of surgical management. Annals of Surgical Oncology 5: 416–422

Shanks J H, Banerjee S S, Joglekar V M, Hasleton P S, Nicholson A G 2000 Mesotheliomas with deciduoid morphology: a morphologic spectrum and a variant not confined to young females. American Journal of Surgical Pathology 24: 285–294

Sheibani K, Shin S S, Kezirian J, Weiss L M 1991 Ber-EP4 antibody as a discriminant in the differential diagnosis of malignant mesothelioma versus adenocarcinoma. American Journal of Surgical Pathology 15: 779–784

Shen S C, Bansal M, Purrazzella R, Malviya V, Strauss L 1983 Benign glandular inclusions in lymph nodes, endosalpingiosis, and salpingitis isthmica nodosa in a young girl with clear cell adenocarcinoma of the cervix. American Journal of Surgical Pathology 7: 293–300

Sinykin M B 1960 Endosalpingiosis. Minnesota Medicine 43: 759–761

Soslow R A, Rouse R V, Hendrickson M R, Silva E G, Longacre T A 1996 Transitional cell neoplasms of the ovary and urinary bladder: a comparative immunohistochemical analysis. International Journal of Gynecological Pathology 15: 257–265

Spirtas R, Connelly R R, Tucker M A 1988 Survival patterns for malignant mesothelioma: the SEER experience. International Journal of Cancer 41: 525–530

Sridhar K S, Doria R, Raub W A, Thurer R J, Saldana M 1992 New strategies are needed in diffuse malignant mesothelioma. Cancer 70: 2969–2970

Strinic T, Kuzmic–Prusac I, Eterovic D, Jakic J, Scukanec M 2000 Leiomyomatosis peritonealis disseminata in a postmenopausal woman. Archives of Gynecology and Obstetrics 264: 97–98

Subramony C, Habibpour S, Hashimoto L A 2001 Retroperitoneal mucinous cystadenoma. Archives of Pathology and Laboratory Medicine 125: 691–694

Sundarasivarao D 1953 The mullerian vestiges and benign epithelial tumors of the epididymis. Journal of Pathology 66: 417–432

Suster S, Moran C A 1990 Deciduosis of the appendix. American Journal of Gastroenterology 85: 841–845

Swan N, Cottell D C, Sheahan K 1997 Peritoneal mesotheliomas. American Journal of Surgical Pathology 21: 122–123

Talerman A, Chilcote R R, Montero J R, Okagaki T 1985 Diffuse malignant peritoneal mesothelioma in a 13-year-old girl: report of a case and review of the literature. American Journal of Surgical Pathology 9: 73–80

Tavassoli F A, Norris H J 1982 Peritoneal leiomyomatosis (leiomyomatosis peritonealis disseminata): a clinicopathologic study of 20 cases with ultrastructural observations. International Journal of Gynecological Pathology 1: 59–74

Tenti P, Carnevali L, Tateo S, Durola R 1994 Primary mucinous cystadenocarcinoma of the retroperitoneum: two cases. Gynecologic Oncology 55: 308–312

Teoh T B 1953 The structure and development of Walthard nests. Journal of Pathology and Bacteriology 66: 433–439

Tickman R J, Cohen C, Varma V A, Fekete P S, DeRose P B 1990 Distinction between carcinoma cells and mesothelial cells in serous effusions. Usefulness of immunohistochemistry. Acta Cytologica 34: 491–496

Tobacman J K, Greene M H, Tucker M A, Costa J, Kase R, Fraumeni J F J 1982 Intra-abdominal carcinomatosis after prophylactic oophorectomy in ovarian-cancer-prone families. Lancet 2: 795–797

Truong L D, Maccato M L, Awalt H, Cagle P T, Schwartz M R, Kaplan A L 1990 Serous surface carcinoma of the peritoneum: a clinicopathologic study of 22 cases. Human Pathology 21: 99–110

Tsuchiya A, Kikuchi Y, Matsuoka T, Yashima R, Abe R, Suzuki T 1999 Endosalpingiosis of nonmetastatic lymph nodes along the stomach in a patient with early gastric cancer: report of a case. Surgery Today 29: 264–265

Tutschka B G, Lauchlan S C 1980 Endosalpingiosis. Obstetrics and Gynecology 55: 575–605

Uematsu T, Kitamura H, Iwase M et al 2000 Ruptured retroperitoneal mucinous cystadenocarcinoma with synchronous gastric carcinoma and a long postoperative survival: a case report. Journal of Surgical Oncology 73: 26–30

Volm M, Bruggemann A, Gunther M, Kleine W, Pfleiderer A, Vogt S M 1985 Prognostic relevance of ploidy, proliferation, and resistance-predictive tests in ovarian carcinoma. Cancer Research 45: 5180–5185

Weir M M, Bell D A, Young R H 1998 Grade 1 peritoneal serous carcinomas: a report of 14 cases and comparison with 7 peritoneal serous psammocarcinomas and 19 peritoneal serous borderline tumors. American Journal of Surgical Pathology 22: 849–862

Weiss L M, Battifora H 1993 The search for the optimal immunohistochemical panel for the diagnosis of malignant mesothelioma. Human Pathology 24: 345–346

Weiss S W, Tavassoli F A 1988 Multicystic mesothelioma. An analysis of pathologic findings and biologic behavior in 37 cases. American Journal of Surgical Pathology 12: 737–746

White P F, Merino M J, Barwick K W 1985 Serous surface papillary carcinoma of the ovary: a clinical, pathologic, ultrastructural, and immunohistochemical study of 11 cases. Pathology Annual 1: 403–418

Wick M R, Mills S E, Swanson P E 1990 Expression of 'myelomonocytic' antigen in mesotheliomas and adenocarcinomas involving the serosal surfaces. American Journal of Clinical Pathology 94: 18–26

Williams P P, Gall S A, Prem K A 1971 Ectopic mucinous cystadenoma. A case report. Obstetrics and Gynecology 38: 831–837

Winn K J, Woodruff J D, Parmley T H 1976 Electronmicroscopic studies of leiomyomatosis peritonealis disseminata. Obstetrics and Gynecology 48: 225–227

Young R H 1997 Pseudoneoplastic lesions of the urinary bladder and urethra: a selective review with emphasis on recent information. Seminars in Diagnostic Pathology 14: 133–146

Young R H, Clement P B 1996 Müllerianosis of the urinary bladder. Modern Pathology 9: 731–737

Young R H, Clement P B 2000 Endocervicosis involving the uterine cervix: a report of four cases of a benign process that may be confused with deeply invasive endocervical adenocarcinoma. International Journal of Gynecological Pathology 19: 322–328

Young R H, Eichhorn J H, Dickersin G R, Scully R E 1992 Ovarian involvement by the intra-abdominal desmoplastic small round cell tumor with divergent differentiation: a report of three cases. Human Pathology 23: 454–464

Zaytsev P, Taxy J B 1987 Pregnancy-associated ectopic decidua. American Journal of Surgical Pathology 11: 526–530

Zhou J, Iwasa Y, Konishi I et al 1995 Papillary serous carcinoma of the peritoneum in women: a clinicopathologic and immunohistochemical study. Cancer 76: 429–436

Zinsser K R, Wheeler J E 1982 Endosalpingiosis in the omentum: a study of autopsy and surgical material. American Journal of Surgical Pathology 6: 109–117

Zotalis G, Nayar R, Hicks D G 1998 Leiomyomatosis peritonealis disseminata, endometriosis, and multicystic mesothelioma: an unusual association. International Journal of Gynecological Pathology 17: 178–182

28

Lymphoproliferative disease of the female genital tract

E. Benjamin   P. Isaacson

Introduction   935

Classification of non-Hodgkin's lymphomas   936

Subtypes of malignant lymphoma   936
Low-grade B-cell lymphomas   937
High-grade B-cell lymphomas   937
T-cell lymphomas   937
Rare forms of malignant lymphoma   937
Lymphomas of mucosa-associated lymphoid tissue
  (MALT)   938

Staging   938

Ovary   939
Non-Hodgkin's lymphoma   939
Hodgkin's disease   945
Leukaemia   946
Granulocytic sarcoma   946

Fallopian tube   948

Uterus and cervix   948
Non-Hodgkin's lymphoma   948
Stage and survival   951
Hodgkin's disease   951
Granulocytic sarcoma (myelosarcoma)   951

Vagina   953
Non-Hodgkin's lymphoma   953

Vulva   954
Non-Hodgkin's lymphoma   954

Langerhans' cell histiocytosis   957

Lymphoma and pregnancy   957

Conclusions   958

INTRODUCTION

The term lymphoproliferative disease refers to a wide variety of conditions including Hodgkin's disease, non-Hodgkin's lymphoma and conditions which may mimic lymphoma including certain non-lymphoid haematological proliferations and various florid chronic inflammatory conditions. This group of disorders uncommonly presents in the female genital tract but, when it does so, it is important that it is correctly discriminated from the more common gynaecological neoplasms and that a precise diagnosis is made since treatment, which is often curative, is closely related to the histopathological diagnosis. Because malignant lymphoma presenting as primary tumours of the female genital tract is rare, these tumours are frequently undiagnosed or misdiagnosed (Harris & Scully 1984). From a clinical perspective extirpative surgery is the primary mode of treatment for most gynaecological malignancies whereas malignant lymphomas are usually managed with chemotherapy or radiotherapy or a combination of the two, and radical surgery is inappropriate. This assumes increased significance in young patients in whom preservation of sexual function and reproductive capacity may be a prime consideration (Sandvei et al 1990).

It is arguable whether Hodgkin's disease ever arises primarily in the female genital tract and indeed it seldom arises or presents outside the lymph nodes. Non-Hodgkin's lymphoma, on the other hand, frequently arises or presents extranodally and may do so in the female genital tract where it may manifest as any one of its various subtypes. Presentation of lymphoma in the female genital tract is often a manifestation of disseminated disease and is, therefore, an indication of an advanced stage requiring systemic treatment. Careful staging is necessary before making a diagnosis of those rare cases of early stage, true primary extranodal lymphomas which may be treated more conservatively.

Advances in immunohistochemistry in recent years, such as the introduction of antibodies reactive in routinely processed paraffin-embedded tissues, and of techniques for antigen retrieval (Cattoretti et al 1993; Cuevas et al 1994), facilitate the identification and categorisation of malignant lymphomas and their separation from other neoplasms and reactive processes. Molecular biological techniques can now also be applied to routinely processed and paraffin-embedded tissues and may be of value in supporting or confirming a diagnosis of non-Hodgkin's lymphoma.

CLASSIFICATION OF NON-HODGKIN'S LYMPHOMAS

In the 1960s it became evident that the clinical behaviour and response to treatment of non-Hodgkin's lymphoma varied according to the histological features. After many years of confusion and differing classifications being used on either side of the Atlantic an international lymphoma study group composed of haematopathologists mainly from Europe and North America put forward a proposal for an international consensus on the classification of lymphoid neoplasms (Table 28.1) (Harris et al 1994). This group defined entities that can be recognised with currently available morphological, immunological and genetic techniques. Many of these entities are associated with distinctive clinical presentations and natural histories. Cases that do not fit into these defined categories have been left unclassified or provisionally classified. The terminology used is mainly that of the Kiel classification (Stansfeld et al 1988).

An important feature of this proposed consensus classification is that it identifies defined clinicopathological entities based on their morphological, immunological, genetic molecular biological and clinical features. The recognition of clinicopathological entities is important in understanding the nature and probable behaviour of malignant lymphomas at any particular site. Thus, most low-grade B-cell lymphomas are usually widespread diseases and therefore involvement of the female genital tract by, for example, follicular lymphoma, is more likely to be part of a disseminated disease process than a primary tumour. Amongst the high-grade lymphomas, lymphoblastic tumours are, similarly, part of a widespread, often leukaemic, neoplastic process and should never be interpreted as a stage 1 or primary tumour. Most of the entities and concepts incorporated in the consensus classification (REAL Classification) have been included in the proposed WHO Classification of Lymphoid Malignancies (Harris et al 2000).

SUBTYPES OF MALIGNANT LYMPHOMA

Non-Hodgkin's lymphomas are categorised into systemic lymphomas and those derived from mucosa-associated lymphoid tissue (MALT lymphomas). This influences their presentation and pattern of dissemination. For a

Table 28.1 List of lymphoid neoplasms recognised by the International Lymphoma Study Group (Harris et al 1994)

B-CELL NEOPLASMS

I. Precursor B-cell neoplasm: Precursor B-lymphoblastic leukaemia/lymphoma

II. Peripheral B-cell neoplasm
1. B-cell chronic lymphocytic leukaemia/prolymphocytic leukaemia/small lymphocytic lymphoma
2. Lymphoplasmacytoid lymphoma/immunocytoma
3. Mantle cell lymphoma
4. Follicle centre lymphoma, follicular
   Provisional cytologic grades: I (small cell), II(mixed small and large cell), III(large cell)
   Provisional subtype: diffuse, predominantly small cell type
5. Marginal zone B-cell lymphoma
   Extranodal (MALT type +/– monocytoid B cells)
   Provisional subtype: Nodal (+/– monocytoid B cells)
6. Provisional entity: Splenic marginal zone lymphoma (+/– villous lymphocytes)
7. Hairy cell leukaemia
8. Plasmacytoma/plasma cell myeloma
9. Diffuse large B-cell lymphoma
   Subtype: Primary mediastinal (thymic) B-cell lymphoma
10. Burkitt's lymphoma
11. Provisional entity: High-grade B-cell lymphoma, Burkitt-like

T-CELL AND PUTATIVE NK-CELL NEOPLASMS

I. Precursor T-cell neoplasm: Precursor T-lymphoblastic lymphoma/leukaemia

II. Peripheral T-cell and NK-cell neoplasms
1. T-cell chronic lymphocytic leukaemia/prolymphocytic leukaemia
2. Large granular lymphocyte leukaemia (LGL)
   T-cell type
   NK-cell type
3. Mycosis fungoides/Sezary syndrome
4. Peripheral T-cell lymphomas, unspecified
   Provisional cytologic categories: Medium-sized cell, mixed
   Medium and large cell, large cell, lymphoepithelial cell
   Provisional subtype: Hepatosplenic γδ T-cell lymphoma
   Provisional subtype: Subcutaneous panniculitic T-cell lymphoma
5. Angioimmunoblastic T-cell lymphoma (AILD)
6. Angiocentric lymphoma
7. Intestinal T-cell lymphoma (+./–enteropathy associated)
8. Adult T-cell lymphoma/leukaemia (ATL/L)
9. Anaplastic large cell lymphoma (ALCL), CD30+, T-and null-cell types
10. Provisional entity: Anaplastic large-cell lymphoma, Hodgkin's-like

HODGKIN'S DISEASE (HD)

I. Lymphocyte predominance

II. Nodular sclerosis

III. Mixed cellularity

IV. Lymphocyte depletion

V. Provisional entity: Lymphocyte-rich classical HD
   These categories are thought likely to include more than one disease entity

fuller account the reader is referred to Isaacson (1992) and Stansfeld & D'Ardenne (1992). Both types may involve the female genital tract, although systemic lymphomas are far more common.

LOW-GRADE B-CELL LYMPHOMAS

The main types of low-grade B-cell lymphomas of systemic lymphoid tissue include: lymphocytic lymphoma (which in most cases is associated with chronic lymphocystic leukaemia), lymphoplasmacytic lymphoma (in which evidence of plasma cell differentiation is present); plasmacytic lymphoma; follicular or follicular/diffuse centroblastic/centrocytic lymphoma (follicular, mixed small cleaved and large cell); and centrocytic or mantle cell lymphoma (diffuse small cleaved cell). These lymphomas tend to be widely disseminated at presentation (stages 3 and 4) but may follow an indolent course despite their widespread dissemination. They are, in the ma-jority of cases, associated with long survival, sometimes even without treatment. They are, however, generally not as sensitive to chemotherapy as are high-grade lymphomas. Some may transform into high-grade lymphomas.

HIGH-GRADE B-CELL LYMPHOMAS

These may arise by transformation of low-grade lymphomas but more commonly arise de novo. Lymphomas in this category now designated as diffuse large B-cell lymphoma are heterogeneous in terms of their histogenesis, immunophenotype and cytogenetic characteristics. These lymphomas are frequently localised tumours at presentation (stages 1 and 2). They may show aggressive behaviour and rapid dissemination. Many tumours, however, respond well to chemotherapy. The term 'Burkitt-like' is used for a type of lymphoma which resembles Burkitt's lymphoma but which does not meet the stringent histological criteria for that diagnosis.

T-CELL LYMPHOMAS

T-cell lymphomas are far less common than B-cell tumours in the Western world, comprising 10–15% of non-Hodgkin's lymphoma. They include lymphoblastic lymphomas which arise from early T-cell precursors and are well characterised. The cutaneous forms include mycosis fungoides and Sezary's syndrome and are also well defined. Those arising from mature T cells, the peripheral T-cell lymphomas, however, are a less well-understood group. Their classification and definition is still a matter of debate and controversy. Tumours which are considered low grade in the Kiel classification include chronic lymphocytic leukaemia (T-CLL); mycosis fungoides and Sezary's syndrome; lymphoepithelioid lymphoma (Lennert's lymphoma); angioimmunoblastic lymphoma; T-zone lymphoma and pleomorphic, small cell lymphoma (HTLV-1 positive or negative); immunoblastic (HTLV-1 positive or negative) and large cell anaplastic (Ki-1 positive). The proposed classification of T-cell lymphomas in the consensus classifica-

Table 28.2 The World Health Organisation Classification of Lymphoid Neoplasms (Harris et al 2000)

B-cell Neoplasms
Precursor B-cell neoplasm
Precursor B-lymphoblastic leukaemia/lymphoma (Precursor B-cell acute lymphoblastic leukaemia)
Mature (peripheral) B-cell neoplasms
B-cell chronic lymphocytic leukaemia/small lymphocytic lymphoma
B-cell prolymphocytic leukaemia
Lymphoplasmacytic lymphoma
Splenic marginal zone B-cell lymphoma (+/− villous lymphocytes)
Hairy cell leukaemia
Plasma cell myeloma/plasmacytoma
Extranodal marginal zone B-cell lymphoma of MALT type
Mantle cell lymphoma
Follicular lymphoma
Nodal marginal B-cell lymphoma (+/− monocytoid B-cells)
Diffuse large B-cell lymphoma
Burkitt lymphoma/Burkitt cell leukaemia

T and NK-cell Neoplasms
Precursor T-cell neoplasm
Precursor T-lymphoblastic lymphoma/leukaemia (precursor T-cell acute lymphoblastic leukaemia)
Mature (peripheral) T-cell neoplasms
T-cell prolymphocytic leukaemia
T-cell granular lymphocytic leukaemia
Aggressive NK-cell leukaemia
Adult T-cell lymphoma/leukaemia (HTLVI+)
Extranodal NK/T-cell lymphoma nasal type
Enteropathy type T-cell lymphoma
Hepatosplenic gamma/delta T-cell lymphoma
Subcutaneous panniculitis-like T-cell lymphoma
Mycosis fungoides/Sezary syndrome
Anaplastic large cell lymphoma, primary cutaneous type
Peripheral T-cell lymphoma, not otherwise specified (NOS)
Angioimmunoblastic T-cell lymphoma
Anaplastic large cell lymphoma, primary systemic type

Hodgkin's Disease (Hodgkin's lymphoma)
Nodular lymphocyte predominance Hodgkin's Disease
Classical Hodgkin's Disease
Nodular sclerosis Hodgkin's disease
Lymphocyte-rich classical Hodgkin's disease
Mixed cellularity Hodgkin's disease
Lymphocyte depletion Hodgkin's disease

tion is shown in Table 28.1) and in the proposed WHO Classification in Table 28.2.

RARE FORMS OF MALIGNANT LYMPHOMA

These include malignant lymphoma, histiocytic (ML, miscellaneous, histiocytic). These lesions have been over-diagnosed in the past. The term 'histiocytic' has also been applied to large cell lymphomas, in the older literature. True histiocytic neoplasms do occur and present either as a disseminated malignancy or as a localised lymph node tumour. Stringent immunohistochemical requirements must be fulfilled before a diagnosis of a histiocytic malignancy is made. These include immunoreactivity with one or more macrophage-specific monoclonal antibodies and the synthesis of lysozyme by tumour cells. Reactive macrophages present in both B- and T-cell lymphomas should not be mistaken for the tumour cell population.

LYMPHOMAS OF MUCOSA-ASSOCIATED LYMPHOID TISSUE (MALT)

It was noted that certain primary extranodal lymphomas did not fit into any of the established categories of systemic lymphomas. The concept of lymphomas of mucosa-associated lymphoid tissue is now widely accepted (Isaacson & Wright 1983, 1984; Isaacson & Spencer 1987). Such lymphomas recapitulate the properties of mucosa-associated lymphoid tissue (MALT). Unlike nodal low-grade B-cell lymphomas, MALT lymphomas tend to remain localised for long periods and have a good prognosis. The concept of lymphomas of mucosa-associated lymphoid tissue is probably of particular relevance to the understanding of primary lymphomas of the female genital tract. In rodents, migration of mucosal B-lymphocytes to the lower female genital tract has been shown to occur in pregnancy (McDermott et al 1980) and it is likely that the female genital tract is part of the mucosal immune system. MALT lymphomas are thought to be derived from marginal zone B cells and are composed of marginal zone cells that have variable morphology but often resemble centrocytes. These centrocyte-like cells invade epithelia to form characteristic lymphoepithelial lesions. They frequently colonise pre-existing reactive germinal centres and they may show plasmacytic differentiation. The latter two features may lead to the miscategorisation of MALT lymphoma as either follicular lymphoma or as lymphoplasmacytic or plasmacytic lymphoma. The natural history of MALT lymphomas is to progress from a low-grade to a high-grade B-cell lymphoma. In the stomach, coexistent low-grade lymphomas with the same immunoglobulin phenotype may be found (Chan et al 1990). When transformation to a high-grade lymphoma occurs the tumours cannot be distinguished from other high-grade B-cell lymphomas, in the absence of coexisting low-grade tumour. In the stomach, stage rather than grade appears to be important in determining the good prognosis of MALT lymphomas (Cogliatti et al 1991).

MALT lymphomas usually arise in a setting of pre-existing inflammation. Thus, thyroid MALT lymphomas arise in glands affected by Hashimoto's or lymphocytic thyroiditis, salivary MALT lymphomas arise in glands affected by autoimmune sialadenitis and gastric MALT lymphomas arise on a background of *Helicobacter pylori* gastritis. This may be of significance in determining the frequency of lymphomas arising in the cervix in comparison with other part of the female genital tract.

STAGING

Staging is performed for most neoplastic diseases for the purpose of determining treatment regimens and of predicting survival. In gynaecological oncology, the staging system introduced by the Federation Internationale de Gynaecologists and Obstetricians, FIGO, in 1979 and in

Table 28.3 Ann Arbor staging system for Hodgkin's disease (Adapted from Carbone et al 1971)

Stage 1
Involvement of a single lymph node region (1) or a single extralymphatic organ or site (1E).

Stage 2
Involvement of two or more lymph node regions on the same side of the diaphragm (2) or localised involvement of an extralymphatic organ or site and one or more lymph node regions on the same side of the diaphragm (2E).

Stage 3
Involvement of lymph node regions on both sides of the diaphragm (3) which may also be accompanied by localised involvement of an extra-lymphatic organ or site (3E) or by involvement of the spleen (3S) or both (3SE).

Stage 4
Diffuse or disseminated involvement of one or more extra-lymphatic organs or tissues with or without associated lymph node enlargement.

Note: Each stage is further divided into A and B categories. B is for those patients with any of (a) unexplained weight loss or more than 10% of body weight over the previous 6 months, (b) unexplained fever with temperatures 38°C and (c) night sweats.

1986 is widely used (Ulfelder 1981). This system was, however, designed for the staging of primary epithelial neoplasms of the ovary and is therefore inappropriate for primary lymphomas at this site. The Ann Arbor system (Carbone et al 1971) is a staging classification for Hodgkin's disease that is also used for the staging of non-Hodgkin's lymphomas (Table 28.3). Staging data must of course be interpreted in the context of the histopathology. As stated above, most low-grade B-cell lymphomas form widespread (stage 3 and 4) disease processes. This is a characteristic of these lymphoma and with few exceptions does not affect the management of the disease nor the relatively good prognosis of these neoplasms.

Ziegler (1981) found that the Ann Arbor staging system was not well suited to the management of patients with Burkitt's lymphoma. He introduced a staging scheme that reflected the poor prognosis associated with bulky abdominal tumours compared with involvement of single or multiple non-abdominal sites and the serious prognosis accompanying a combination of intra-abdominal and multiple extra-abdominal sites (Ziegler & Magrath 1974).

In a study of 42 lymphomas and leukaemias presenting as ovarian tumours, Osborne & Robboy (1983) staged their cases using the FIGO system, stating that the Ann Arbor staging method for non-Hodgkin's lymphomas was less sensitive and that no differentiation is made between ulilateral and bilateral ovarian involvement. However, Fox et al (1988), in their study of 34 patients with lymphoma presenting as ovarian tumour, found the Ann Arbor system to be a more sensitive prognostic indicator than the FIGO system. Monterroso et al (1993) investigated the problems associated with the staging of non-Hodgkin's lymphoma of the ovary. They noted that the

Ann Arbor staging system was designed for Hodgkin's disease and has inherent deficiencies in the staging of non-Hodgkin's lymphomas, particularly those neoplasms arising at extranodal sites. They noted the failure of the Ann Arbor staging system to take into account tumour bulk, which appears to be of paramount importance in the management and prognosis of Burkitt's lymphoma (Ziegler & Magrath 1974). Finally, the Ann Arbor system does not address the issue whether patients with bilateral ovarian involvement are best considered as having stage 4 disease. To resolve these issue Monterroso et al (1993) staged 39 patients with malignant lymphomas of the ovary using the FIGO system, the Ann Arbor system and the modification proposed by Ziegler & Magrath (1974). The conclusion of this study was that the FIGO and Ziegler systems did not offer any significant advantage over the Ann Arbor system in the staging of ovarian lymphoma and that bilateral ovarian involvement indicated stage 4 disease.

OVARY

NON-HODGKIN'S LYMPHOMA

Incidence and pathogenesis

Primary ovarian lymphomas are rare. In a study of 1467 extranodal lymphomas, 47% of which were in female patients, Freeman et al (1972) found only two cases. Chorlton et al (1974a) identified only 19 cases with disease localised to the ovary in a review of 9500 cases of lymphoma in female patients accessioned at the Armed Forces Institute of Pathology. It is possible that the number of cases in this series was boosted by the inclusion of cases of Burkitt's lymphoma, reflecting the referral bias of the Armed Forces Institute of Pathology. Norris & Jensen (1972), in a study of 353 ovarian tumours in females under the age of 20, found only two cases of ovarian lymphoma. Chorlton (1987) recorded 165 cases of lymphoma presenting initially in the ovary and either published or known personally to the author. The current number of documented primary ovarian lymphomas is in the region of 200 cases. This does not fully represent the prevalence of this type of lymphoma presentation since the tumour is not so rare that individual cases or small series are likely to be published.

In contrast to the rare presentation of lymphomas in the ovary, the ovaries are the most common site of involvement of the female genital tract by lymphoma found at autopsy (Lathrop 1967). Autopsy studies of women dying of lymphomas have found an incidence of lymphoma in one or both ovaries of between 7 and 18% (Lucia et al 1952; Woodruff et al 1963).

There has been considerable debate in the literature as to whether ovarian lymphomas can ever be considered as primary tumours or whether they are always part of a more widespread disease process. One argument advanced against the possibility that ovarian lymphomas could be primary tumours is that lymphoid tissue is not a normal constituent of the ovary (Nelson et al 1958). Others have argued that ovarian lymphomas could arise from hilar lymphoid tissue (Woodruff et al 1963), from lymphocytes in an inflammatory infiltrate (Walther 1934) or from lymphoid tissue in a teratoma (Durfee et al 1937). With respect to the last suggestion, it is of interest that a lymphoma arising in the thyroid tissue in a mature cystic teratoma of the ovary has been reported (Seifer et al 1986). A case of histiocytic lymphoma, transforming later to a monoblastic leukaemia, has been reported as arising in a malignant teratoma in the ovary of a patient with 46,XY gonadal dysgenesis (Koo et al 1992). This mode of origin is, however, unlikely to account for many ovarian lymphomas.

As part of their study of ovarian lymphomas, Monterroso et al (1993) reviewed the histology of 35 ovaries removed at autopsy from 24 women aged from 18–58 years. Lymphoid cells were found in the hilus or medulla of 13 individuals (54%), and in two of these formed distinct aggregates. It would appear therefore that lymphoid aggregates are not uncommon in the ovary and could provide a possible origin for primary ovarian lymphomas.

Fox & Langley (1976) proposed the following criteria for the diagnosis of primary ovarian lymphomas:

1. At the time of diagnosis the lymphomas is clinically confined to the ovary and full investigation fails to reveal evidence of lymphoma elsewhere.
   A lymphoma can still, however, be considered as primary if spread has occurred to immediately adjacent lymph nodes or if there has been direct spread to infiltrate immediately adjacent structures.
2. The peripheral blood and bone marrow should not contain any abnormal cells.
3. If further lymphomatous lesions occur at a site remote from the ovary, then at least several months should have elapsed between the appearance of the ovarian and extraovarian lesions.

Application of these criteria to reported cases of ovarian lymphoma (Chorlton 1987) indicates that approximately 54 examples of primary lymphoma of the ovary had been reported up to that time. Paladugu et al (1980), however, suggested that the above criteria for the designation of primary ovarian lymphomas were insufficiently stringent and they proposed that there should be a disease-free interval of at least 60 months following treatment of the ovarian lesion by surgery alone. If this more restrictive definition had been adopted, there would have been only five acceptable reported cases of primary ovarian lymphomas up to 1987 (Chorlton 1987). It is likely that many more cases with survival exceeding 60 months now exist.

The above arguments are, however, to some extent unrealistic since they do not take into account the nature of the lymphoma under consideration. Most low-grade B-cell lymphomas, with the exception of lymphomas of MALT, are widespread at the time of diagnosis. The findings of a stage 1, low-grade, B-cell lymphoma of the ovary should therefore raise suspicions of a MALT lymphoma. High-grade B-cell lymphomas might present with stage 1 disease but it is unlikely that they would be treated with surgery alone and it is very probable that they would receive chemotherapy. If the criteria of Paladugu et al are applied, such cases would never be diagnosed as primary ovarian lymphomas. Fox et al (1988) state, 'it would be reasonable to conclude therefore that an ovarian lymphoma should always be considered for therapeutic purposes as a local manifestation of systemic disease and that to rely upon the possibility of such a lesion being primary to the ovary is unduly optimistic'. In practical terms all ovarian lymphomas should be graded histologically and staged using the Ann Arbor system, and both histology and stage should be taken into account in determining further management.

Age

Five large series of ovarian lymphomas (Paladugu et al 1980; Rotmensch & Woodruff 1982; Osborne & Robboy 1983; Fox et al 1988; Monterroso et al 1993), totalling 181 cases, show an age range of 3 months to 77 years with a mean of approximately 35 years. Two-thirds of the patient are under the age of 40 years (Fox et al 1988). This contrasts with testicular lymphomas which occur predominantly in older age groups with a mean age of 64 years (Paladugu et al 1980).

Clinical features

The common presenting features of ovarian lymphomas are as abdominal and pelvic masses causing abdominal distension. Fox et al (1988) noted three main patterns of clinical presentation: (1) acute presentation with abdominal pain and distension, sometimes accompanied by vomiting; (2) chronic onset of symptoms with abdominal pain and distension of 1–6 months duration; (3) with non-specific gynaecological symptoms such as menorrhagia and oligomenorrhoea. Those patients presenting with rapid onset of abdominal distension and pain more frequently had symptoms of fever and weight loss and had a worse prognosis than those in whom onset of symptoms was more gradual. A smaller number of patients present with symptoms of menorrhagia or oligomenorrhoea. Presentation with amenorrhoea and resumption of periods after removal of tumour occurred in a patient whose B-cell lymphoma was associated with ovarian stromal luteinization (Mittal et al 1992). In the series of cases reported by Monterroso et al (1993), all of the tumours

that were thought to be primary in the ovary were discovered incidentally on clinical examination or at surgery performed for other reasons. A number of cases have been discovered during pregnancy with presentations ranging from first-trimester miscarriages to full-term deliveries (Finkle & Goldman 1974; Armon 1976; Rotmensch & Woodruff 1982; Monterroso et al 1993).

Gross pathology

In most reported series of ovarian lymphomas over half the tumours have been bilateral. When unilateral they show no consistent predilection for either side. The tumours are frequently described as smooth-surfaced and bosselated. They may be associated with ascites, which is sometimes blood-stained. Tumour size varies widely, from a maximum of 5280 g reported by Rotmensch & Woodruff (1982), to a tumour of only 15 g discovered as an incidental finding (Monterroso et al 1993); tumour diameters have ranged from microscopic to 25 cm (Osborne & Robboy 1983).

Grossly, on section the tumours have a mainly solid, creamy, white 'fish-flesh' appearance with areas of necrosis and haemorrhage in the larger tumours. Other sites of involvement most frequently identified at operation are the Fallopian tubes and other parts of the female genital tract, the serosa, omentum and mesentery (Monterroso et al 1993).

Histology

It is difficult to evaluate and compare the histopathology of the reported series of ovarian lymphomas because of the different classification systems used. Monterroso et al (1993) used the terminology of the Working Formulation to classify their 39 cases of non-Hodgkin's lymphoma that presented as ovarian tumours: 21 (54%) were small non-cleaved cell (Burkitt and Burkitt-like), 9 (23%) diffuse large cell (high-grade B-cell lymphomas, centroblastic diffuse), 3 (8%) follicular and diffuse large cell (centroblastic, follicular and diffuse), 3 (8%) diffuse, mixed small and large cell (centroblastic/centrocytic diffuse), 2 (5%) large cell immunoblastic (one Richter's syndrome, one anaplastic large cell) and 1 (2%) follicular and diffuse small cleaved cell (centroblastic/centrocytic, follicular and diffuse). There was a large number of Burkitt or Burkitt-like lymphomas in this series (54%), probably related to the referral bias at the National Cancer Institute, USA. The large majority of the lymphomas in this series were of high or intermediate grade; 25 of the 26 (96%) cases on which immunohistochemistry was performed were B-cell tumours and only one was a T-cell lymphoma.

Fox et al (1988) analysed 34 cases of ovarian non-Hodgkin's lymphoma. Twelve were diagnosed as B-cell lymphomas (6 follicle centre cell type and 6 diffuse large cell); 5 were of histiocytic type; 2 were diffuse, undifferentiated large cell lymphomas and 15 were poorly differentiated, lymphocytic/lymphoblastic lymphomas. The latter group included 7 Burkitt's lymphoma, 2 T-cell lymphomas and 6 lymphoblastic lymphomas, 3 of which were leukaemia related.

In the series of 40 patients reported by Osborne & Robboy (1983), 11 cases (27%) were categorised as small non-cleaved cell (Burkitt or Burkitt-like) lymphomas and 6 (15%) as follicular lymphomas (small cleaved cell, mixed small cleaved and large cell, and large cell types). The majority of the cases (58%) were categorised as diffuse large cell or immunoblastic. Rotmensch & Woodruff (1982) used the terminology of the Rappaport classification. This cannot always be easily translated into current terminology. Among the 55 cases of ovarian lymphoma in their series 18 were categorised as nodular histiocytic; 18 as diffuse poorly differentiated; 6 as diffuse well-differentiated lymphocytic; 8 as nodular, mixed lymphocytic and histiocytic; 4 as Hodgkin's disease and one as Burkitt's lymphoma. If one accepts nodularity as indicating follicle centre cell derivation, 47% of the cases in this series were follicle centre cell lymphoma. Well-differentiated lymphocytic lymphoma is usually regarded as the tissue equivalent of chronic lymphocytic leukaemia, not a neoplasm that would be expected to form tumour masses at extranodal sites and a category that does not appear in any of the other series of ovarian lymphomas.

High-grade B-cell (large cell) lymphomas show a range of morphology from centroblastic monomorphic to centroblastic polymorphic (Fig. 28.1) including cells that may be centrocytoid (large cleaved cells) and multilobulated (Hui et al 1988; Lennert & Feller 1990). Admixture with variable numbers of immunoblasts with prominent central nucleoli may be seen. Residual centrocytes (small cleaved cells) may indicate the follicle centre cell origin of some of these neoplasms (Monterroso et al 1993) as may follicular areas. Marked sclerosis may be a feature of these tumours (Monterroso et al 1993). Although mitotic figures are usually easily found, these lymphomas do not show as high a mitotic index as Burkitt-type lymphomas. In addition to high-grade lymphomas with residual features of follicle centre cell origin, occasional ovarian lymphomas of low-grade follicle centre cell origin with a follicular growth pattern have been described (Rotmensch & Woodruff 1982; Monterroso et al 1993; Osborne & Robboy 1983). Monterroso et al (1993) concluded that 10 of 39 ovarian lymphomas were of follicle centre cell origin excluding the large number of cases of Burkitt's lymphoma in their series which some authors believe to be follicle centre cell derived (Mann et al 1976).

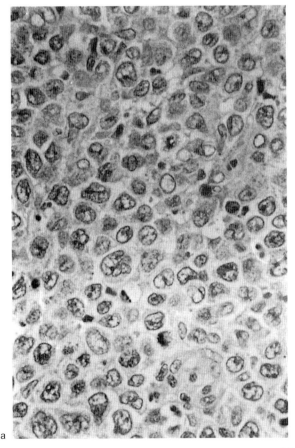
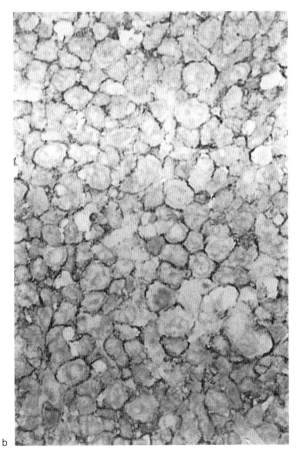

Fig. 28.1 a Ovary replaced by high-grade, centroblastic, B-cell lymphoma. **b** Lymphoma cells immunostain for L26 (CD20) indicating B-cell lineage.

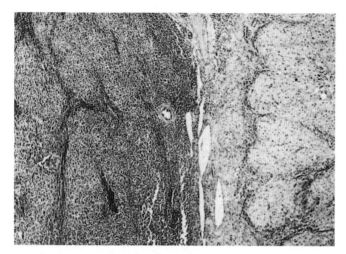

Fig. 28.2 Follicular non-Hodgkin's lymphoma of the ovary with adjacent uninvolved corpus luteum. (From Chorlton et al 1974a.)

Ovarian lymphomas, in common with lymphomas of the female genital tract, may show prominent sclerosis ranging from collagen fibrils between groups of tumour cells to extensive collagen bands in which tumour cell are embedded. Ovarian lymphoma may grow in diffuse sheets (Fig. 28.1) but may also show areas of cord-like growth pattern, particularly in the capsule. Tumour cells tend to encircle residual corpora lutea (Fig. 28.2), corpora albicantes and Graafian follicles rather than to obliterate them. Prominent ovarian stromal luteinization may rarely occur in lymphomas (Ferry & Young 1991; Mittal et al 1992).

Specific subtypes of non-Hodgkin's lymphoma

Plasmacytoma (Bambira et al 1982; Hautzer 1984; Cook & Boylston 1988). Ovarian tumours of this type have

been up to 24 cm in diameter and may be bilateral. Some have occurred in patients with widespread myeloma and others have preceded the diagnosis of myeloma. Plasmacytic tumours, particularly the less well-differentiated ones, may mimic anaplastic carcinoma. If immunohistochemistry is used to resolve this problem it should be borne in mind that plasmacytomas are usually leucocyte common antigen negative, EMA positive and may express cytokeratins (Norton & Isaacson 1989b). The identification of monotypic immunoglobulin production by the tumour cells will establish the diagnosis of plasmacytoma.

T-cell lymphoma Available information suggests that T-cell lymphomas are much less common than B-cell lymphomas in the ovary, but their precise incidence is not known. Monterroso et al (1993) recorded one case of T-cell lymphoma confirmed by immunohistochemistry (see below).

Burkitt's lymphoma Burkitt (1958), working in Uganda, drew attention to the full clinical syndrome of jaw and abdominal tumours now known as Burkitt's lymphoma. The jaw tumours are age related and probably dependent on tooth development, so the proportion of jaw tumours in any series will be dependent on the age of the patients being studied (Burkitt 1970). Burkitt's lymphoma has a predilection for the female genital tract with ovarian lymphomas, usually bilateral, occurring in 75–80% of patients (Fig. 28.3) (O'Conor 1961; Wright 1964). The histopathological features of Burkitt's lymphoma have been well described (Berard et al 1969; Wright 1970), the lymphoma being composed of monomorphic blast cells with a high proliferation index. A WHO-sponsored group defined Burkitt's lymphoma on the basis of its histological features (Berard et al 1969) and, using these histological criteria, cases of Burkitt's

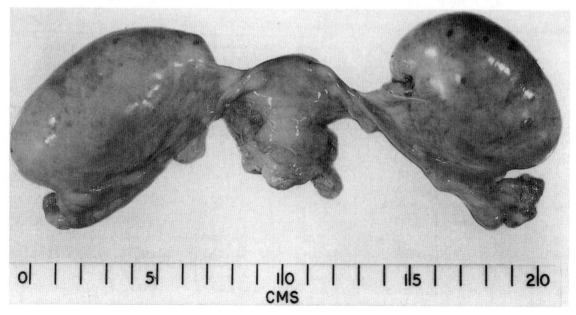

Fig. 28.3 Burkitt's lymphoma producing bilateral ovarian tumours. (From Burkitt & Wright 1980.)

lymphoma have been identified outside the endemic areas of Africa and Papua New Guinea (Wright 1966; Levine et al 1982). These non-endemic cases may have clinical features similar to those of endemic cases but the majority of patients have abdominal tumours in the region of the terminal ileum or tumours of the oropharynx that are not characteristic of the endemic cases (Wright 1966; Grogan et al 1982). Epstein–Barr virus can be found in virtually 100% of cases of endemic Burkitt's lymphoma but in a variable percentage of non-endemic cases. In both the endemic and non-endemic cases translocations involving the immunoglobulin genes and the c-*myc* oncogene are found (Pelicci et al 1986; Neri et al 1988). However, the break points on the immunoglobulin genes differ between the two groups suggesting that they arise at different stages of B-cell differentiation. In both tumours disregulation of the c-*myc* oncogene is probably responsible for both the high rate of proliferation and the undifferentiated nature of the blast cells. While the exact relationship between endemic and non-endemic Burkitt's lymphomas is unclear it is apparent that ovarian and gynaecological tumours are frequent in both groups (Dorfman 1965; Levine et al 1982). Monterroso et al (1993) speculate that possible hormonal influences and growth factors may

lead to localisation in the ovaries and breasts and note the association of tumours at these sites with pregnancy. Magrath (1991) has similarly postulated that growth factors may influence the predilection of Burkitt's lymphoma for the jaws. Wright (1985), however, noting the correspondence between the distribution of Burkitt's lymphoma and lymphoid cells of MALT and the influence of pregnancy on the distribution of these cells (McDermott et al 1980), has postulated that endemic Burkitt's lymphoma is a tumour of mucosa-associated lymphoid tissue.

The tumour cells of Burkitt's lymphoma have rounded, regular nuclei with granular chromatin and 3–4 small nucleoli. The cytoplasm forms a well-defined rim around the nucleus and is amphophilic in H & E-stained sections and deeply basophilic in Giemsa stained preparations. The cytoplasmic lipid vacuoles that form such a prominent feature in imprint preparations can be seen in well-fixed histological preparations with the aid of oil immersion. Burkitt's lymphomas always show a high mitotic index with several mitotic figures visible in a high-power field and the use of proliferation markers will show 100% of tumour cells to be in cycle. Large numbers of apoptotic nuclei are also present and they are frequently engulfed by the abundant 'starry sky' macrophages

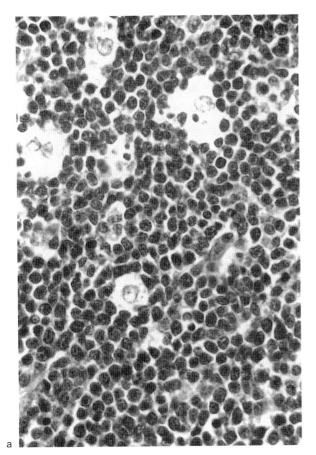 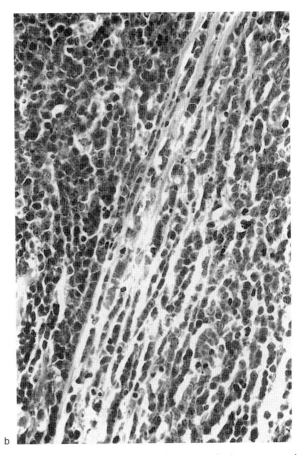

Fig. 28.4 a Burkitt's lymphoma showing a population of monomorphic lymphoid cells and scattered macrophages producing 'a starry sky' appearance. **b** Burkitt's lymphoma of ovary. Tumour cells infiltrate in an 'Indian-file' pattern.

present in the tumour (Fig. 28.4a). In the ovary, the tumour forms a diffuse infiltrate that may surround and eventually infiltrate residual ovarian follicles (Monterroso et al 1993). At the hilum of the ovary and in the capsule, the tumour cells can frequently be seen infiltrating in an Indian-file or cord-like fashion (Fig. 28.4b).

Immunohistochemistry

Immunohistochemistry usually permits the characterisation of non-Hodgkin's lymphoma into B- and T-cell categories. Neoplastic B-cell proliferations may be identified and separated from reactive proliferations by the presence of light chain restriction (Fig. 28.5) which marks a monoclonal proliferation. When this is not possible because of technical or other reasons, evidence for monoclonal B-cell proliferation can be obtained by analysis of tumour DNA for clonal immunoglobulin gene rearrangement using techniques such as Southern blotting and the polymerase chain reaction (Diss et al 1994). In T-cell lymphomas, unlike B-cell lymphomas, there is no consistent method of establishing clonality using immunohistochemistry. Distinguishing between reactive and neoplastic T-cell proliferations depends on the demonstration of T-cell antigens in cells judged to be malignant on morphological grounds (Isaacson 1992). More specific demonstration of

clonal T-cell receptor gene rearrangements is also possible by analysis of tumour DNA using molecular biological techniques (McCarthy et al 1991).

There have been few studies of immunohistochemistry of ovarian lymphomas. Linden et al (1988) performed immunohistochemistry and gene rearrangement studies using Southern blot analysis on three ovarian lymphomas. All three expressed B-cell lineage markers and showed clonal rearrangements of their immunoglobulin genes with germ line T-cell receptor genes. The most comprehensive immunohistochemical study of ovarian lymphomas is that reported by Monterroso et al (1993). They were able to undertake immunophenotypic studies on 26 of their 39 cases. In 25 of the 26 cases (96%) the neoplastic cells were of B-cell phenotype. In 23 of 24 cases studied using paraffin sections the tumour cells were positive for L26 (CD20) and negative with at least one T-cell associated antibody. The T-cell antibodies used in the study were UCHL1 (CD45 RO), MT1 (CD43) and Leu-22(CD43). Five of the B-cell lymphomas reacted with one of these antibodies; however, none of these antibodies is entirely specific for T-cells and may be expressed in cells of other lineages, including B cells (Picker et al 1987; Linden et al 1988; Norton & Isaacson 1989a,b).

One case in the series of Monterroso et al (1993) is particularly instructive. The patient was aged 35 and had

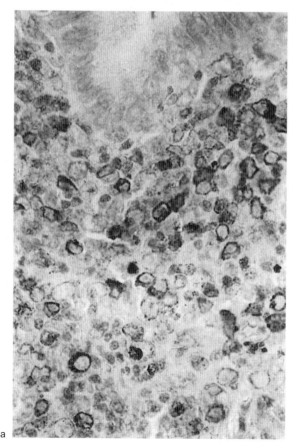
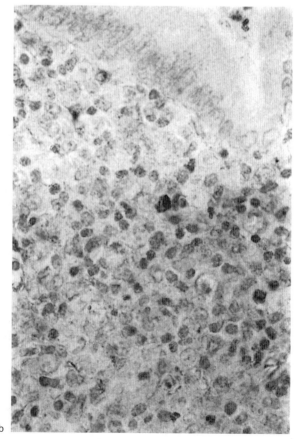

Fig. 28.5 Follicle centre cell, B-cell lymphoma. **a** Tumour cells show kappa immunoglobulin light chain restriction, confirming a monoclonal proliferation. **b** Tumour cells do not immunostain for immunoglobulin lambda light chain.

bilateral ovarian tumours with extensive intra-abdominal disease. Following surgery and chemotherapy the patient was reported to have no evidence of disease after six years. Histologically the tumour was diagnosed as an anaplastic large cell lymphoma of T-cell phenotype (Stein et al 1985; Delsol et al 1988). It was Ber H2 (CD30), epithelial membrane antigen (EMA) and UCHL1 (CD45 RO) positive and negative for leucocyte common antigen (CD45), Leu-M1 (CD15), L26 (CD20), LN1 (CDw75), KP1 (CD68) and lysozyme. In the absence of evidence of CD3 or T-cell receptor expression, this tumour should have been categorised as being of null cell or indeterminate phenotype. The importance of this tumour however is that the leucocyte common antigen negative, epithelial membrane antigen positive phenotype could have led the unwary pathologist into believing that this was an epithelial neoplasm, which would have resulted in inappropriate management. Occasional anaplastic large cell lymphomas can even express cytokeratins, making their distinction from an epithelial neoplasm difficult (Gustmann et al 1991). Pathologists need to be aware of the morphological features of this lymphoma and of its histological and immunophenotypic resemblance to an epithelial neoplasm in some cases.

Differential diagnosis

The two ovarian tumours for which lymphomas are most commonly mistaken are granulosa cell tumour and dysgerminoma (Osborne & Robboy 1983). Granulosa cell tumours account for nearly half the misdiagnoses of ovarian lymphoma at all ages; misdiagnoses are made most often when patients have Burkitt-type lymphoma. In these patients the 'starry sky' macrophages surrounded by tumour cells are frequently misinterpreted as Call–Exner bodies. Osborne & Robboy (1983) attribute these errors, in part, to poor fixation and processing of tissues, a factor aggravated by the frequent large size of the ovarian tumours and consequent slow penetration of fixative.

Clinical features may help to distinguish granulosa cell tumours from ovarian lymphomas. Endocrine manifestations such as breast enlargement, growth of pubic and axillary hair and onset of menses indicative of oestrogen secretion have been observed in three-quarters of patients with juvenile granulosa cell tumours, but were not encountered in any of the patients with lymphoma. Many patients of reproductive age with granulosa cell tumours have disturbances in their menstrual patterns due to oestogenic effects on the endometrium. Older patients often complain of postmenopausal bleeding. In contrast Osborne & Robboy (1983) found that only two of the 19 patients aged 11–44 years with ovarian lymphomas complained of irregular menses or amenorrhoea and that only one of 16 women older than 45 years had postmenopausal bleeding, and in this patient the lymphoma infiltrated the myometrium and endometrium.

Osborne & Robboy (1983) found that large cell lymphomas were frequently misdiagnosed as dysgerminomas, despite the fact that this tumour is uncommonly bilateral. Notwithstanding the fact that dysgerminoma is uncommon after the age of 30, the diagnosis was considered in 28% of the patients above this age. The presence of stromal lymphocytes and epithelioid granulomas, together with the occasional presence of syncytiotrophoblast-like cells, are histological features that aid the diagnosis of dysgerminoma. Metastatic carcinoma, particularly from the breast, undifferentiated and primary small cell carcinomas also need to be considered in the differential diagnosis of lymphomas of the ovary (Chorlton 1987). Fortunately these problems of differential diagnosis can usually easily be resolved by application of immunohistochemistry in difficult cases. What remains is the need for pathologists to be aware of the differential diagnosis of undifferentiated ovarian neoplasms so that the appropriate investigations are undertaken.

Prognosis and survival

The interpretation of survival data for ovarian lymphomas must take into account advances in staging and treatment that have occurred in recent years and the increasing use of chemotherapy either as first line or adjunctive therapy. In the large series of cases reported from the National Cancer Institute (Monterroso et al 1993), 4 patients were stage 1E, 4 patients stage 2E, and 25 patients stage 4 using the Ann Arbor system. Thirty-two patients, of 39 reported cases, received chemotherapy. Forty seven per cent were alive between 15 and 16.5 years following treatment and 53% had died between one week and 9 years from the time of diagnosis. In a further recent series of 14 patients (4 with Ann Arbor stage 1 disease and 10 with stage 4) treated with aggressive chemotherapy the 5-year survival was 57% (Dimopoulos et al 1997). These results are less dismal than the 7% survival reported by Rotmensch & Woodruff (1982) in a series of patients, most of whom had been treated with surgery alone or in combination with radiotherapy. Osborne & Robboy (1983) reported an actuarial survival at five years of 35%; low stage and follicular growth pattern were good prognostic features. Fifteen of the 34 patients (44%) reported by Fox et al (1988) survived between one and more than five years following diagnosis. These authors found that a history of rapid onset of symptoms and advanced stage were poor prognostic features. Association with pregnancy was stated to be a bad prognostic feature (Rotmensch & Woodruff 1982), although some long-term survivors have now been reported (Monterroso et al 1993).

HODGKIN'S DISEASE

Hodgkin's disease has rarely been reported to involve the ovary. In three patients the disease was apparently localised to the ovaries (Bare & McCloskey 1961; Long &

Patchefsky 1971; Khan et al 1986); in the others ovarian involvement was part of more widespread disease (Heller & Palin 1946; Nelson et al 1958). In their review of 55 ovarian lymphomas from the Ovarian Tumour Registry, Rotmensch & Woodruff (1982) include four cases of Hodgkin's disease but details of individual patients are not given. We support the scepticism expressed by Monterroso et al (1993) who noted that some of the published cases of Hodgkin's disease of the ovary were poorly documented and that most were reported before the availability of immunophenotypic analysis. Primary Hodgkin's disease of the ovary is extremely rare if it occurs at all.

LEUKAEMIA

In the huge autopsy study of 1206 cases of acute and chronic leukaemia, Barcos et al (1987) found ovarian involvement of 11% of patients with acute granulocytic leukaemia, 9% with chronic granulocytic leukaemia, 21% with acute lymphoblastic leukaemia and 22% with chronic lymphocytic leukaemia (Fig. 28.6). Involvement of the ovary in lymphoblastic leukaemia (21%) is less frequent than involvement of the testes (40%) and the incidence of ovarian deposits fell during the period of the study (1958–1982), presumably as a result of improvements in therapy. Leukaemic relapse in the ovaries during bone marrow remission (Obeid et al 1979; Chu et al 1981; Cecalupo et al 1982; Wyld & Lilleyman 1983; Heaton & Duff 1989) may occur several years after treatment and may produce tumours up to 15 cm in diameter. It has been postulated that ovarian and central nervous system relapse are associated (Case Records of the Massachusetts General Hospital 1981). The tumours have the typical morphology of lymphoblastic lymphomas, being composed of blast cells with delicate

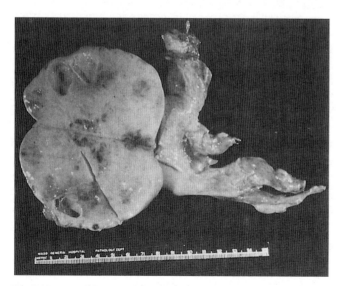

Fig. 28.6 Acute lymphoblastic leukaemia involving the ovary. (Reprinted with permission from Ferry & Young 1991.)

nuclear chromatin, small nucleoli and inconspicuous cytoplasm. These cells expand the ovarian stroma and infiltrate in an Indian-file fashion. If immunohistochemistry is used to confirm the diagnosis, it should be borne in mind that lymphoblastic lymphomas may be negative for leucocyte common antigen and may not express T- or B-cell lineage markers (null or indeterminate phenotype) (Norton & Isaccson 1989b).

GRANULOCYTIC SARCOMA

The term chloroma (Hindkamp & Szanto 1959) has been largely replaced by granulocytic sarcoma (Rappaport 1956). Neither term is strictly appropriate since the majority of tumours do not have a green colour and many show little granulocytic differentiation. Myelosarcoma or extramedullary myeloid tumours are probably more appropriate terms. Granulocytic sarcoma may occur in patients with no leukaemia, or during remission, or may precede the diagnosis of leukaemia by months or years (Rappaport 1966; Neiman et al 1981; Meis et al 1986). In the two largest published series of granulocytic sarcoma, involvement of the genital tract was observed in only one of 30 females (Neiman et al 1981; Meis et al 1986). Nevertheless, although rare, involvement of the ovaries does appear to be a characteristic feature of granulocytic sarcoma. In a review of 29 patients with granulocytic sarcoma of the female genital tract Friedman et al (1992) noted that 13 (45%) had ovarian involvement, whilst 7 of the 11 patients with granulocytic sarcoma of the female genital tract described by Oliva et al (1997) had ovarian lesions. Ovarian granulocytic sarcomas may be unilateral or bilateral and have been recorded as up to 19 cm in diameter. They form solid tumours though cystic degeneration or entrapped serous cysts may occur (Hindkamp & Szanto 1959; Gralnick & Dittmark 1969; Ballon et al 1978; Morgan et al 1981; PreBler et al 1992; Oliva et al 1997). The tumours are composed of blastic cells with delicate nuclear chromatin and inconspicuous cytoplasm (Fig. 28.7). They are most likely to be misdiagnosed as malignant lymphomas and therefore to receive inappropriate therapy. The finding of granulated myelocytes is diagnostic of granulocytic sarcoma. However, such cells may be scanty and are unlikely to be found unless carefully sought. Eosinophilic myelocytes are the cells most easily seen in haematoxylin and eosin-stained sections, but in general granulation is best observed in Giemsa-stained preparations.

In view of the therapeutic implications of the diagnosis of granulocytic sarcoma, the diagnosis should be confirmed using immunohistochemistry. The tumour cells are leucocyte common antigen positive. They are negative with most B- and T-cell lineage markers but usually express CD43 (MT1, DFT1, Leu-22) and may express UCHL1 (CD45 RO) (PreBler et al 1992). Among the B-cell markers, they may express MB2 and KiB3 (PreBler

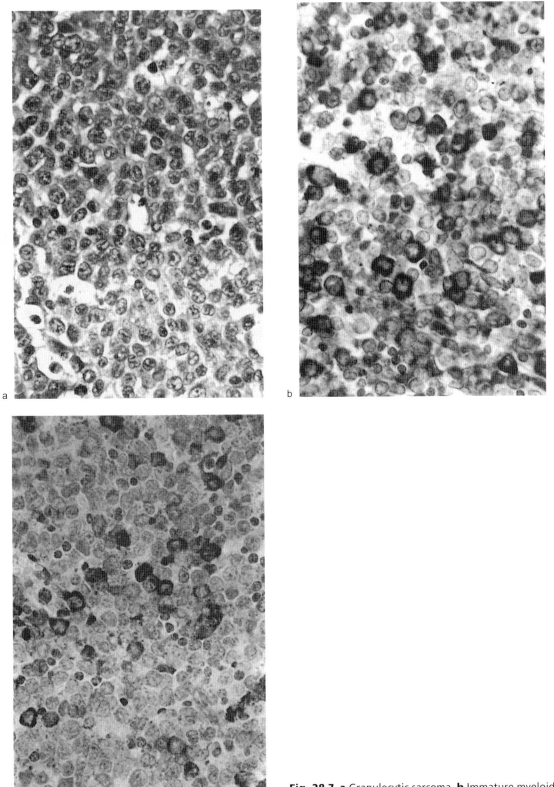

Fig. 28.7 a Granulocytic sarcoma. **b** Immature myeloid cell immunostain for muramidase. **c** CD68 positivity in tumour cells.

et al 1992). Granulocytic sarcomas usually express muramidase and alpha-1-antitrypsin (Muller et al 1986). The staining should be cytoplasmic, granular and accentuated in the Golgi region; diffuse non-granular staining is due to non-specific uptake and is particularly likely to be seen in poorly fixed tissues. CD68 (KP1, PG-M1) staining is seen in most granulocytic sarcomas. KP1 stains myelomonocytic cells, although it is not a specific haematological marker. PG-M1 (Falini et al 1993) stains cells at the monocyte end of the myelomonocyte spectrum and, in the absence of KP1 staining, is a marker of monocyte differentiation. CD15 (Leu-M1) and antibodies to neutrophil elastase identify granulocytic differentiation. The naphthol AS-D chloro-acetate esterase stain (Leder 1964), although widely used for the identification of granulocytic sarcoma, is only of value in those cases showing granulocytic differentiation and is unhelpful in those tumours showing predominantly monocytic differentiation. Megakaryocyte differentiation can be identified by staining for factor VIII-related antigen (PreBler et al 1992).

FALLOPIAN TUBE

The Fallopian tubes are frequently infiltrated by tumour in patients with ovarian lymphomas, particularly those of the small non-cleaved cell, i.e. Burkitt and Burkitt-like type (Osborne & Robboy 1983; Ferry & Young 1991). Primary lymphoma of the Fallopian tube has been reported only twice. Ferry & Young (1991) reported a 68-year-old patient who had previously undergone hysterectomy. At the time of bilateral salpingo-oophorectomy she had a left hydrosalpinx and tubo-ovarian adhesions. The tubal walls were fleshy and studded with nodules, no other abnormality was found in the abdomen. Histology showed a follicle centre cell lymphoma (follicular mixed small cleaved and large cell type) (Fig. 28.8). Isaacson & Norton (1994) reported a case of MALT lymphoma of the Fallopian tube and questioned whether the case reported by Ferry & Young might also be a MALT lymphoma.

UTERUS AND CERVIX

NON-HODGKIN'S LYMPHOMA

Incidence

Lymphomas presenting in the uterus are uncommon; when they do so, they more frequently involve the cervix than the uterine corpus (Ferry & Young 1991). Vang et al (2000a) reported 26 non-Hodgkin's lymphomas of the uterus and cervix. Ten of these were stage 1E or 2E and were considered to be primary tumours. None of these involved the cervix. Twelve cases were stage 3E or 4 and considered to be systemic disease, two of these involved the cervix alone and six the body and cervix. Only 2 malignant lymphomas were identified in a series of 25 000 primary cervical neoplasms (Carr et al 1976). In a review of 12 447 malignant lymphomas, 1467 presented at an extranodal site without evidence of disseminated disease and of these only 3 presented in the cervix, 3 in the body of the uterus and 2 in unspecified sites in the uterus (Freeman et al 1972). In a series of 9500 women with haematological malignancies reported from the Armed Forces Institute of Pathology, 13 cases of malignant lymphoma and 2 cases of granulocytic sarcoma presented in the body of the uterus, cervix or vagina (Chorlton et al 1974b). These tumours can present at any age and may mimic squamous cell carcinoma of the cervix clinically and histologically (Perren et al 1992), but treatment of the two conditions is fundamentally different. Synchronous and metachronous occurrence of lymphoma of the genital tract and endometrial carcinoma has been recorded in three cases (Vang et al 2000b). This is

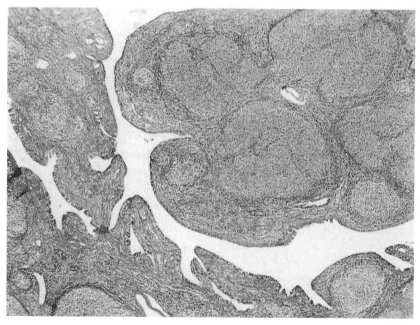

Fig. 28.8 Fallopian tube involved by a follicular lymphoma. (Reprinted with permission from Ferry & Young 1991.)

presumably due to chance rather than to common aetiology. A single instance of endometrial involvement in multiple myeloma has been described (Smith et al 1997).

Clinical features

The reported age range for lymphoma of the uterus is 20–80 years with a median age of presentation of 43 years (Harris & Scully 1984; Muntz et al 1991; Perren et al 1992). Seventy seven per cent of patients are premenopausal at presentation (Muntz et al 1991). The most common presenting symptom is with abnormal bleeding, postcoital or postmenopausal, although 20% were asymptomatic (Muntz et al 1991).

Variable success has been reported in the detection of uterine lymphomas and leukaemias on cervical smears (Ferry & Young 1991). This is in part due to misinterpretation of abnormal cells found in smears (Katayama et al 1973), a factor that my be rectified by greater awareness amongst, and improved training of, screeners and cytopathologists (Ceden & Sakurai 1962; Colmenares & Zuker 1965; Whitaker 1976; Krumerman & Chung 1978; Mikhail et al 1989). It appears however that the failure of cervical cytology to detect leukaemia and lymphoma is partly due to the fact that only 10–40% of cervical lymphomas yield a positive smear (Andrews et al 1988). This is because lymphomas often infiltrate beneath an intact cervical epithelium and sparing of a narrow zone deep to the squamous epithelium in contrast to carcinoma of the cervix where the surface epithelium itself is abnormal (Harris & Scully 1984).

Gross appearance

The most common recorded appearance of cervical lymphomas is a diffuse, barrel-shaped enlargement of the cervix without mucosal abnormality (Fig. 28.9). Other appearances recorded are of multinodular masses, poly-

poid masses protruding through the cervical os or discrete submucosal masses. Ulceration due to lymphoma is distinctly uncommon (Harris & Scully 1984). Extension into the body of the uterus, the vagina, parametrium and pelvic side walls may occur (Harris & Scully 1984; Ferry & Young 1991; Perren et al 1992) making the exact origin of the lymphoma difficult to ascertain in some cases. Most cervical lymphomas are large tumours, half being over 4 cm in diameter. In two patients, lymphoma originated from an endocervical polyp (Muntz et al 1991). Of the 21 cases reported by Harris & Scully (1984) 19 presented in the cervix and 2 in the endometrium. The endometrial lymphomas formed polypoid masses within the uterus. In the case reported by Maeda et al (1988) lymphoma was only found in endometrial curettings but not in the subsequent hysterectomy specimen.

Histology

Harris & Scully (1984) categorised 21 cases of lymphoma of the uterus using both the Rappaport and the Kiel classification. Using the latter, 16 cases were considered to be of follicle centre cell derivation: 6 centroblastic/

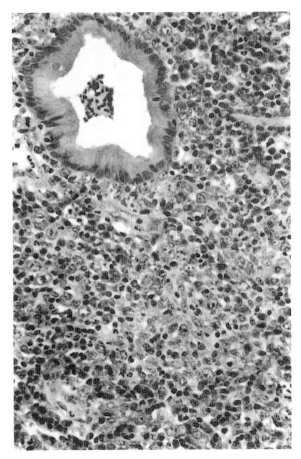

Fig. 28.10 High-grade, B-cell centroblastic lymphoma, arising in the cervix. Tumour cells infiltrate around endocervical glands.

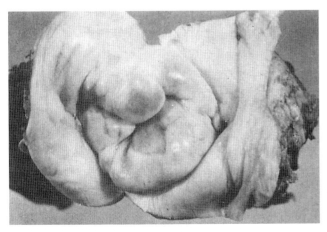

Fig. 28.9 Uterine cervix enlarged by malignant lymphoma producing a barrel-shaped cervix. The overlying mucosa is intact. (Reprinted with permission from Ferry & Young 1991.)

centrocytic follicular; 7 centroblastic/centrocytic diffuse and 3 centroblastic (Fig. 28.10). The remainder included immunoblastic lymphoma (2), lymphoplasmacytic lymphoma (1), Burkitt's lymphoma (1) and unclassified lymphoma (1). Muntz et al (1991) categorised 43 primary malignant lymphomas of the cervix, using the Working Formulation, and categorised 5 as low grade, 36 as intermediate grade and 2 as high grade. Eight (19%) of the patients in this pooled series of cases had tumours with a follicular growth pattern, 5 of low grade and 3 of intermediate grade. Thirty (70%) were diffuse large cell malignant lymphomas; 3 diffuse small cleaved cell lymphomas; 2 mixed small and large cell lymphomas; all of intermediate grade. The high-grade tumours included a large cell immunoblastic lymphoma and a small non-cleaved cell lymphoma.

In the few cases where immunohistochemistry has been performed (Ferry & Young 1991; Muntz et al 1991), nearly all tumours were of B-cell lineage. However, Jack & Lee (1986), in an immunohistochemical study of T-cell lymphomas at various sites, found 2 cases involving the uterus; one was a 25-year-old female with endometrial involvement and the other had cervical involvement. In both cases there was a uniform population of tumour cells with high mitotic rate and a starry sky pattern. Both patients had stage 4 disease and died at 1 and 6 months after diagnosis.

A case of MALT lymphoma of the cervix has been reported by Pelstring et al (1991) (see below). The authors have also seen another case where a 29-year-old woman presented with complaints of a vaginal discharge; she had a total hysterectomy and bilateral salpingo-oophorectomy before the correct diagnosis of MALT lymphoma was established. Following clinical staging, it was found that the disease had been present only in the cervix (stage 1E). Phenotypically this was a B-cell tumour in which there was transformation to a high-grade lymphoma of multilobated type together with residual low-grade areas with infiltration of residual endocervical glands by small lymphoid cells to form the characteristic lymphoepithelial lesions (Fig. 28.11). van de Rijn et al (1997) described three low-grade B-cell lymphomas of the endometrium that did not form tumour masses and were incidental findings, one following currettage and two following hysterectomy. These tumours were composed of centrocyte like cells but showed none of the other

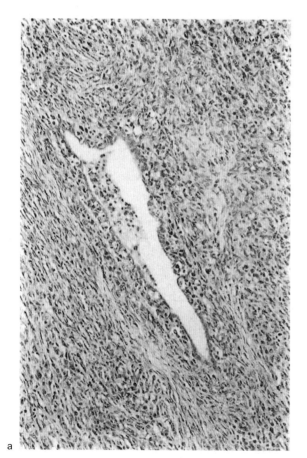

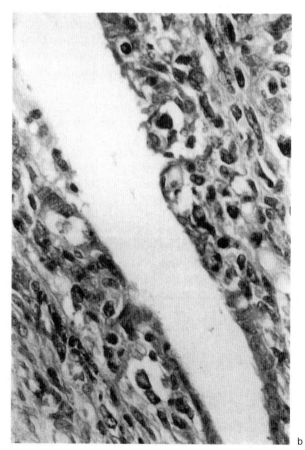

Fig. 28.11 a Uterine cervix infiltrated by malignant lymphoma of 'MALT' type. Lymphoid cells infiltrate endocervical gland epithelium. **b** Higher magnification shows formation of lymphoepithelial lesions within the glandular epithelium. (Courtesy of Dr A Norton, St Bartholomew's Hospital.)

charactreristics of MALT lymphomas. The relationship of these tumours to MALT lymphomas is uncertain.

Sclerosis may be a prominent feature of both cervical and vaginal lymphomas. Traction artefact can present diagnostic problems with cervical biopsies, making differentiation from carcinomas or inflammatory infiltrates difficult. In such cases immunohistochemistry may be of considerable value and techniques such as polymerase chain reaction (PCR) may be used to determine the clonality of the infiltrate (McCarthy et al 1991; Diss et al 1994). The endometrial lymphomas reported by Harris & Scully (1984) were devoid of sclerosis and were sharply demarcated from underlying myometrium.

STAGE AND SURVIVAL

In the series of 25 cases of malignant lymphoma of the uterus and vagina reported by Harris & Scully (1984), 21 were in Ann Arbor stage 1E. The overall actuarial survival of all patients was 73% but with stage 1E tumours it was 89% compared with 20% for patients with lymph node or ovarian involvement. Muntz et al (1991) reported 5 patients with Ann Arbor stage 1E lymphoma of the cervix and reviewed 38 previously reported stage 1E patients. Using the FIGO system for staging cervical carcinoma, 44% were stage 1, 42% stage 2, 12% stage 3 and 2% stage 4. Most of the patients had been treated by a combination of surgery and radiotherapy. Among 28 patients so treated and followed for at least two years there was only one treatment failure. Muntz et al (1991) conclude that 'most cases of primary lymphoma of the uterine cervix are Ann Arbor stage 1E and can be cured with traditional combination of surgery and radiation therapy after careful evaluation'. They do however acknowledge that chemotherapy may be the preferred option in young patients in whom preservation of fertility is important (Johnston et al 1989; Sandvei et al 1990). The patient reported by Sandvei et al (1990) was free of disease after chemotherapy for a large cell lymphoma of the cervix, having had one termination of pregnancy and one full-term pregnancy following treatment. Perren et al (1992) reported 5 patients with non-Hodgkin's lymphoma of the cervix and upper vagina seen at the Royal Marsden Hospital over a period of 20 years and they reviewed a further 72 cases reported in the literature. Seventy-three per cent of patients were Ann Arbor stage 1E and 25% stage 2E. According to the FIGO stage, 40% were stage 1, 38% stage 2, 11% stage 3 and 11% stage 4. In a selected group of 37 of these patients, the survival rate was 76% with only a weak association with stage but a stronger association with grade.

It is apparent from the foregoing data that non-Hodgkin's lymphomas of the uterus and vagina are more frequently of a lower grade and lower stage than ovarian lymphomas and have a better prognosis. An apparent paradox is the association of low-grade and follicular tumours with low stage and with long-term survival following surgery alone (Perren et al 1992). This raises the possibility that some of these patients may have had MALT lymphomas, possibly showing follicular colonisation. In the case of MALT lymphoma of the cervix reported by Pelstring et al (1991), the patient aged 40 years experienced dysfunctional uterine bleeding and underwent a vaginal hysterectomy for presumed uterine fibroids. A 2 cm leiomyoma was identified but sections of the cervix revealed a diffuse infiltrate of marginal zone and lymphoplasmacytoid cells forming lymphoepithelial lesions within the endocervical glands. The lymphoplasmacytic cells showed kappa light chain restriction. The resection margins were involved by lymphoma and computed tomography showed pelvic lymphadenopathy. The patient was given local radiation therapy and had no evidence of disease at three months follow-up.

HODGKIN'S DISEASE

Several cases interpreted as primary Hodgkin's disease of the cervix have been reported (Ferry & Young 1991). All these, however, date back to the 1960s before the advent of modern immunohistochemistry and it must be questioned whether critical review would sustain these diagnoses. Hung & Kurtz (1985) reported a case of Hodgkin's disease of the endometrium in a patient who had been treated three years earlier for stage 4 Hodgkin's disease. It is possible that endometrial involvement may have resulted from retrograde lymphatic flow from involved pelvic lymph nodes. This type of spread may be equivalent to the apparent retrograde flow of Hodgkin's cells into skin, which has occurred in patients with advanced Hodgkin's disease (Benninghoff et al 1970).

GRANULOCYTIC SARCOMA (MYELOSARCOMA)

We have already discussed the diagnosis of granulocytic sarcoma in the ovary. This tumour may accompany, precede or signal relapse of acute myelogenous leukaemia. In a report of a case and review of the literature, Friedman et al (1992) identified 29 cases, including their own, that involved the female genital tract: 15 cases occurred in the cervix (Fig. 28.12). This tendency to involve the cervix was also noted by Oliva et al (1997). Grossly the tumour forms nodules, ulcers or large infiltrating masses extending into adjacent tissues (Chorlton et al 1974b; Kapadia et al 1978). Histologically, granulocytic precursor cells (Fig. 28.12) infiltrate the tissue and immunohistochemistry is useful in confirming the diagnosis, as discussed above.

Other uterine tumours may occur as a manifestation of relapse of leukaemia. The importance of making the correct diagnosis in these rare cases, particularly those without overt leukaemia, is that current opinion indicates that they should be treated as for acute myelogenous

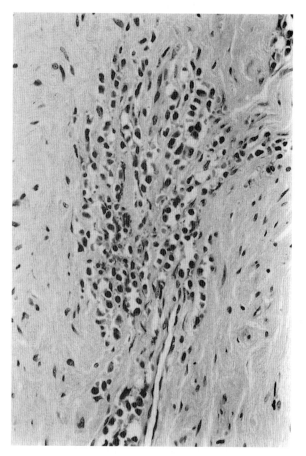

Fig. 28.12 Focus of granulocytic sarcoma in the uterine cervix.

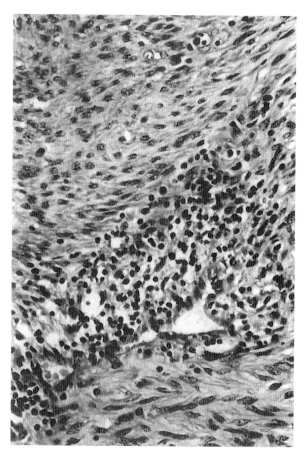

Fig. 28.13 Uterine leiomyoma showing prominent lymphoid infiltration.

leukaemia despite the absence of blood or bone marrow disease (Eshghabadi et al 1986; Banik et al 1989; Hutchinson et al 1990).

Foci of extramedullary haematopoiesis have rarely been detected in the endometrium (Sirgi et al 1994) in the absence of a known haematopoietic disorder. A full histological work-up is nevertheless desirable in these patients to exclude leukaemia.

Differential diagnosis

Undifferentiated neoplasms of the uterus and cervix might enter into the differential diagnosis of malignant lymphomas at this site. These would include lymphoepithelial like carcinoma (lymphoepithelioma) of the cervix which resembles nasopharyngeal carcinoma (Hamazaki et al 1968; Hasumi et al 1977; Hafiz et al 1985; Mills et al 1985; Halpin et al 1989), and small cell (neuroendocrine) carcinoma of the cervix (Ueda et al 1988). However, the judicious use of lymphocyte and epithelial markers should readily identify the nature of these tumours.

A range of inflammatory lesions may be observed in the uterus and cervix (Ferry & Young 1991), sometimes associated with chlamydial infections (Winkler et al 1984). The polymorphous nature of these reactions should make confusion with lymphomas rare. Young et al (1985) studied 16 reactive lymphoma-like lesions involving the cervix (10), endometrum (5) and vulva (1). The reactive lesions were often superficial, involving the overlying epithelium, polymorphous in nature and lacked tumour masses in contrast to lymphomas which usually spared the surface epithelium, were monomorphous and were usually associated with gross tumour masses.

Two examples of so-called inflammatory pseudotumour of the uterus have been described, in a 6-year-old girl and a 30-year-old woman (Gilks et al 1987). A further case was described in a child (Scott et al 1988) and more recently an inflammatory pseudotumour of the cervix has been described (Abenoza et al 1994). These were similar to those described in the lung and elsewhere. They are composed of spindle cells with characteristics of myofibroblasts with a mixed inflammatory infiltrate rich in plasma cells. Such lesions are unlikely to be confused with malignant lymphomas.

Ferry et al (1989) described 7 patients aged 35–50 years with leiomyomas containing a lymphoid infiltrate of sufficient intensity to simulate lymphoma. The distinction from lymphoma could be made by the polymorphous nature of the infiltrate and by the fact that it was confined to the leiomyoma and present only to a minor extent in the adjacent myometrium (Fig. 28.13).

A case of Rosai–Dorfman disease of the cervix (sinus histiocytosis with massive lymphadenopathy) has been reported in a 37-year-old woman (Murray & Fox 1991). The lesion was confined to the cervix and consisted of large histiocytic cells containing engulfed lymphocytes admixed with other inflammatory cells. Apart from malignant lymphoma, this lesion also needs to be distinguished from Langerhans' cell histiocytosis which may rarely affect the cervix.

VAGINA

NON-HODGKIN'S LYMPHOMA

Malignant lymphoma of the vagina is rare and vaginal involvement is more commonly a manifestation of disseminated disease. In some cases, however, the vagina does appear to have been the primary site of origin (Chorlton et al 1974b; Castaldo et al 1979; Harris & Scully 1984; Perren et al 1992; Prevot et al 1992; Clow et al 1995; Skinnider et al 1999; Vang et al 2000c). In the series of 9500 women with lymphoma from the Armed Forces Institute of Pathology, there were 4 cases originat-

ing in the vagina (Chorlton et al 1974b). Prevot et al (1992) reviewed 17 cases of primary non-Hodgkin's lymphoma of the vagina, in the literature, and added 3 cases of their own. Perren et al (1992) described a further 3 primary cases of vaginal lymphoma. Vang et al (2000c) reported 14 cases of non-Hodgkin's lymphoma involving the vagina of which 8 appeared to be primary at that site. The tumours occurred in the fourth to sixth decades with an age range of 19–79 years. Presentation of vaginal lymphoma has been as a vaginal mass or induration, with vaginal bleeding or discharge and, occasionally, urinary symptoms such as frequency or recurrent cystitis.

A total of 23 cases of primary vaginal lymphoma (Perren et al 1992; Prevot et al 1992) were categorised using the Kiel classification or the Working Formulation. Using the Kiel classification, 6 were from the older literature and could only be categorised as large cell malignant lymphoma (high grade); 2 were lymphocytic; 6 follicular or diffuse centroblastic/centrocytic; 2 immunoblastic; 5 centroblastic; 1 anaplastic large cell and 1 angiocentric, pleomorphic T-cell lymphoma. The vast majority of vaginal lymphomas are of B-cell lineage and in the 10 cases of vaginal lymphoma reported in recent series (Harris & Scully 1984; Perren et al 1992; Prevot et al

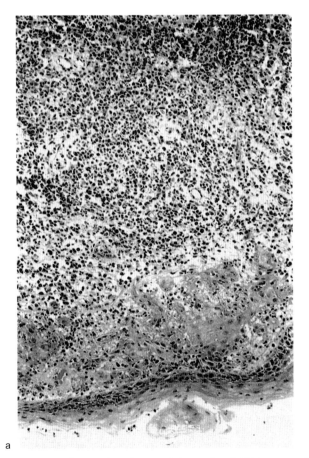
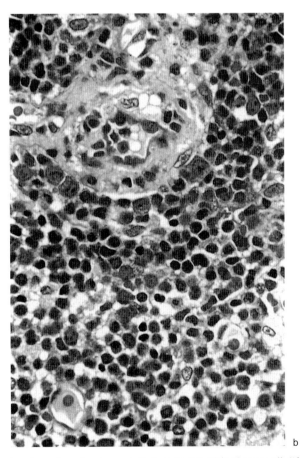

Fig. 28.14 a Malignant lymphoma of the vagina. **b** Higher magnification showing a lymphoplasmacytic lymphoma with plasma cell differentiation.

1992) 9 were follicle centre cell-derived B-cell tumours and 1 was of T-cell lineage. In 8 cases of primary vaginal lymphoma reported by Vang et al (2000c) all were classed, using the Working Formulation, as diffuse large B-cell lymphomas. We have seen a case of lymphoplasmacytic lymphoma, confirmed by immunophenotyping, in the vagina of a female aged 77 who presented with post-menopausal bleeding and had a narrow stenosed vagina (Fig. 28.14). Histologically, vaginal lymphomas, like cervical lymphomas, may show sclerosis ranging from fine fibrils to prominent dense bands of collagen. Traction or crush artefacts often obscure the histology in small biopsies.

In 19 cases of vaginal lymphomas reviewed by Perren et al (1992) and Prevot et al (1992) staging information was available. Of those, 15 cases were Ann Arbor stage 1E, two were stage 2E (with inguinal lymph node involvement) and two were stage 4. In the 8 cases reported by Vang et al (2000c) 4 were stage 1E and 4 were stage 2E. Prognosis of primary vaginal lymphomas, although unpredictable in the individual case, is generally favourable, even with high-grade or extensive disease. Full staging is essential to avoid inappropriate treatment. Radical surgery is considered unnecessary and most localised cases have been treated by radiotherapy, combination chemotherapy and, in some cases, limited surgery. Of the 19 patients reviewed or reported by Prevot et al (1992), 6 patients died of lymphoma within 17 months of diagnosis and 2 died later of unrelated causes. The remainder were alive at follow-up periods ranging from 2 months to over 11 years, the mean follow-up period being 75 months. In a recent series of 8 primary lymphomas of the vagina, 6 patients were alive and well at between 28 and 18 years, 1 died of unrelated causes 9 years after diagnosis and only 1 patient died of the disease (Vang et al 2000c).

Other tumours

Vaginal involvement by Burkitt-type lymphoma has been reported (Castaldo et al 1979). Six cases of plasmacytoma involving the vagina have also been described (Doss 1978; Osanto et al 1981) in women aged between 34 and 78 years. One patient subsequently developed lytic bone lesions but no bone involvement was noted in the others. Rare cases of granulocytic sarcoma and leukaemic vaginal deposits in patients with acute myeloid leukaemia have also been reported (Oliva et al 1997).

Differential diagnosis

A lymphoepithelioma-like carcinoma of the vagina has been described (Dietl et al 1994) similar to those reported in the cervix. Immunohistochemistry of the lymphoid infiltrate within the tumour showed a predominant T-cell and macrophage population but with scanty numbers of B lymphocytes. The polymorphous nature of the inflammatory infiltrate will aid in distinguishing this condition from a true vaginal lymphoma.

VULVA

NON-HODGKIN'S LYMPHOMA

Most lymphomas presenting in the vulva are a manifestation of more widespread disease (Schiller & Madge 1970; Egwuatu et al 1980). Lathrop (1967) noted 4% of cases of vulvar involvement among an autopsy series of lymphomas involving the female genital tract. Cases of apparent primary lymphomas of the vulva are rare and some pre-date the use of critical staging procedures (Buckingham & McClure 1955; Hahn 1958; Iliya et al 1968; Taussig 1973; Wishart 1973; Swanson et al 1987; Bagella et al 1990; Fernando-Manco et al 1992; Marcos et al 1992; Nam et al 1992; Tuder 1992; Kaplan et al 1993, 1996; Vang et al 2000d). The reported patients have had an age range of 25–76 years and most presented with indurated or ulcerated vulval lesions. The vulva may also be involved by Burkitt's lymphoma (Egwuatu et al 1980). Involvement of Bartholin's gland by lymphoma has also been reported (Plouffe et al 1984). We have seen a low-grade MALT lymphoma of the urethral meatus presenting as a vulvar tumour in a 23-year-old woman (Fig. 28.15).

Delayed diagnosis and inappropriate management of lymphomas in the vulva may lead to widely destructive disease of the perineum. Tuder (1992) reported two cases of vulvar lymphoma presenting as progressive non-healing vulval ulcers. One case was a lymphoplasmacytic lymphoma that was untreated and resulted in the patient's death after four years, and the second was an angiocentric, mixed cell lymphoma, the immunophenotype of which was not characterised. Nevertheless amongst the 10 patients with primary lymphoma of the vulva reviewed by Vang et al (2000d) only two died of the disease.

One patient alleged to have Hodgkin's disease was treated with radical vulvectomy and nitrogen mustard and was reported to be well 22 months after presentation (Hahn 1958). It is unlikely that Hodgkin's disease would present as a primary lesion in the vulva, although anaplastic large cell lymphoma may present as a cutaneous tumour (De Bruin et al 1993) and may histologically resemble Hodgkin's disease. We have also seen an anaplastic (Ki-1-positive) large cell lymphoma of T-cell phenotype that presented as a vulvar tumour in a 25-year-old woman with a presenting complaint of pruritis vulvae (Fig. 28.16).

Inflammatory lesions mimicking lymphoma

Inflammatory lesions of the vulva may sometimes simulate malignant lymphoma. The one condition worthy of special consideration is infectious mononucleosis which

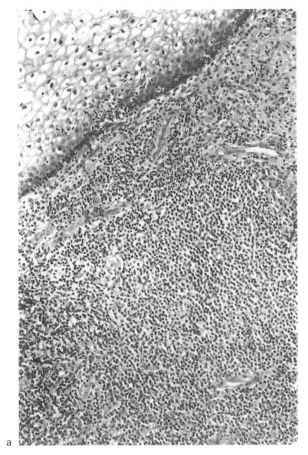

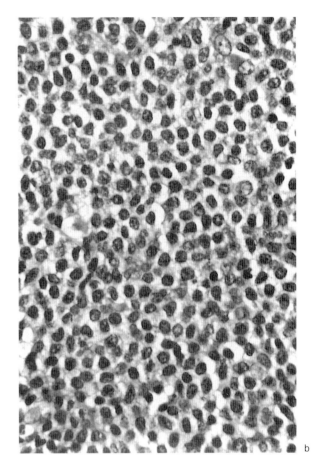

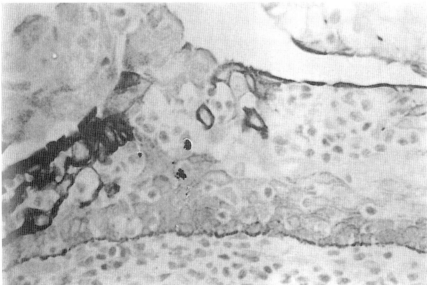

Fig. 28.15 a Vulva: low-grade B-cell lymphoma of 'MALT' type involving the urethral meatus. **b** Higher magnification showing a monomorphic population of centrocyte-like cells.
c Immunostaining for cytokeratin delineates surface epithelium, within which are collections of lymphoid cells forming a lymphoepithelial lesion. CAM 5.2.

may cause vulval ulceration and inguinal lymphadenopathy. The cervix is a recognised site of shedding of the EB virus and ulceration of the lower genital tract is a feature of infectious mononucleosis. It is fortunate that these lesions are rarely biopsied since the blastic proliferation can appear alarming. Biopsy of these lesions reveals a diffuse lymphoid infiltrate with a proliferation of large blastic cells (Fig. 28.17) that might well trap the unwary into making a diagnosis of high-grade lymphoma (Brown & Stenchever 1977; Portnoy et al 1984a; Young et al 1985). In small biopsies it may be impossible to distinguish this blastic proliferation from high-grade lymphoma on morphology alone. Immunohistochemistry may be of help in resolving the problem of identifying both T and B

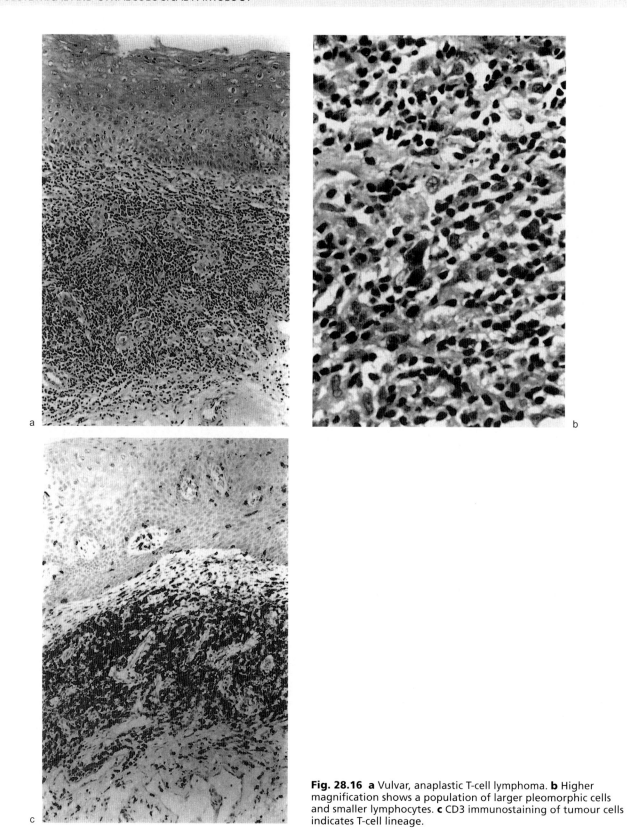

Fig. 28.16 a Vulvar, anaplastic T-cell lymphoma. **b** Higher magnification shows a population of larger pleomorphic cells and smaller lymphocytes. **c** CD3 immunostaining of tumour cells indicates T-cell lineage.

blasts and showing polytypic immunoglobulin in the B cells (Young et al 1985). In most cases, serological tests will confirm Epstein–Barr virus infection. A consideration of the histology in the context of the clinical history should, however, prevent such lesions from being diagnosed as lymphomas.

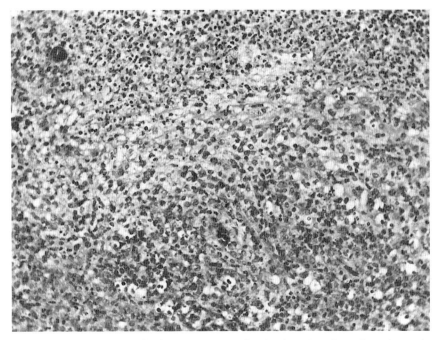

Fig. 28.17 Vulvar lesion of infectious mononucleosis. There is surface ulceration and an underlying infiltrate of large and small lymphoid cells. (Reprinted with permission of Ferry & Young 1991.)

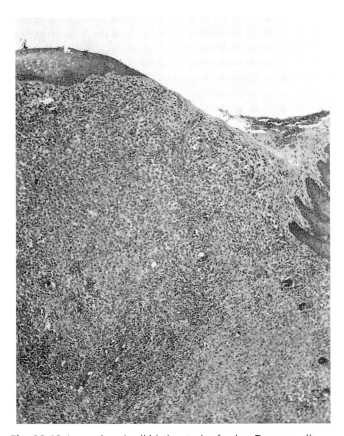

Fig. 28.18 Langerhans' cell histiocytosis of vulva. Tumour cells have abundant cytoplasm and are admixed with eosinophils and lymphocytes. (Reprinted with permission from Ferry & Young 1991.)

LANGERHANS' CELL HISTIOCYTOSIS

The female genital tract may rarely be involved by Langerhans' cell histiocytosis (histiocytosis X) (Dupree & Lee 1973; Issa et al 1980; Lechner et al 1983). Lesions occur most frequently in the vagina and vulva and, rarely, in the cervix and uterus. Lesions are usually part of a more widespread disease involving the lungs and/or the skeleton. With vulvar involvement, patients usually present with one or more painful or itching papules or nodules or ulcers; the clitoris is often involved. Histologically, there is an admixture of Langerhans' cells and eosinophils (Fig. 28.18). The presence of eosinophils, often in clusters, may alert the pathologist to the correct diagnosis. However, eosinophils are not always prominent in Langerhans' cell histiocytosis and the diagnosis rests on the recognition of the characteristic grooved, 'coffee bean' nuclei of the Langerhans' cells and their abundant pale staining cytoplasm. In the vagina and vulva these cells infiltrate immediately below the mucosa. Langerhans' cells stain weakly and patchily for many histiocyte markers but strongly express S-100 protein and more specifically CD1a. The lesions have been treated by local excision, radiation therapy and, rarely, chemotherapy for recurrence (Dupree & Lee 1973; Issa et al 1980).

LYMPHOMA AND PREGNANCY

The occurrence of genital tract lymphomas in pregnancy is well recognised (Armon 1976; Rotmensch & Woodruff 1982; Monterroso et al 1993). Some of the recorded cases are Burkitt's and Burkitt-like lymphomas of the ovary (Finkle & Goldman 1974; Armon 1976). Lymphoma associated with pregnancy was reported to be a bad prognostic feature by Rotmensch & Woodruff (1982), although Monterroso et al (1993) recorded long-term survivors. Successful pregnancy has also been reported after treatment of ovarian and cervical lymphomas by chemotherapy alone or chemotherapy and surgery (Clifford 1968; Sandvei et al 1990).

Non-Hodgkin's lymphomas at all sites may occur during pregnancy and present clinicians with a dilemma of achieving optimum maternal survival without impairing the welfare of the fetus (Steiner-Salz et al 1985; Pejovic et al 2001). The use of chemotherapy in the first trimester of pregnancy, with its potential for causing congenital malformations, is a matter of particular concern. Aviles et al (1990) record the chemotherapy and obstetric care of 16 pregnant patients with non-Hodgkin's lymphomas, mostly of high grade and high stage, seen between 1975 and 1986. Of these, 8 were large cell lymphoma; 2 diffuse, mixed cell lymphoma; 3 diffuse, small non-cleaved cell; 2 lymphoblastic and 1 immunoblastic cell type. Lymphomas occurring in pregnancy are likely to be in younger rather than older women and low-grade follic-

ular lymphomas are, therefore, less likely to be encountered. All patients received chemotherapy, including 8 patients in the first trimester. At the time of birth, 12 mothers were in remission and there were no congenital defects. Fifteen babies were alive and well 3–11 years after birth and 8 mothers who achieved complete remission were alive and free of disease 4–9 years after delivery. Pregnancy is not therefore a contraindication to the treatment of non-Hodgkin's lymphoma with chemotherapy and long-term remissions can be obtained in the mothers.

CONCLUSIONS

Malignant lymphomas of the female genital tract are rare. Their recognition is, however, important, since the treatment of these neoplasms is different from that of epithelial malignancies and may result in long-term survival. Most lymphomas that present in the female genital tract will be found to be part of more widespread disease. However, primary lymphomas at this site undoubtedly occur. These primary tumours often have a good prognosis. Their nature and their relationship to physiological or reactive lymphoid infiltrates at this site merit further study.

REFERENCES

Abenoza P, Shek Y H, Perrone T 1994 Inflammatory pseudotumors of the cervix. International Journal of Gynecological Pathology 13: 80–86

Andrews S J, Hernandez E, Woods J, Cook B 1988 Burkitt's like lymphoma presenting as a gynecologic tumor. Gynecologic Oncology 30: 131–136

Armon P J 1976 Burkitt's lymphoma of the ovary in association with pregnancy: two case reports. British Journal of Obstetrics and Gynaecology 83: 169–172

Aviles A, Diaz-Maques J C, Torras V, Garcia E L, Guzman R 1990 Non-Hodgkin's lymphomas and pregnancy: presentation of 16 cases. Gynecologic Oncology 37: 335–337

Bagella M P, Fadoa C, Cherchi P L 1990 Non-Hodgkin's lymphoma: a rare primary vulvar localization. European Journal of Gynaecological Oncology 11: 153–156

Ballon S C, Donaldson R C, Berman M L, Swanson G A, Byron R L 1978 Myeloblastoma (granulocytic sarcoma) of the ovary. Achives of Pathology and Laboratory Medicine 102: 474–476

Bambira E A, Miranda D, Mugalhaes G M C 1982 Plasma cell myeloma simulating Krukenberg's tumor. Southern Medical Journal 75: 511–512

Banik S, Borg Grech A, Eyden B P 1989 Granulocytic sarcomas of the cervix: an immunohistochemical, histochemical and ultrastructural study. Journal of Clinical Pathology 42: 483–488

Barcos M, Lane W, Gomez G A et al 1987 An autopsy study of 1206 acute and chronic leukemias (1958–1982). Cancer 60: 827–837

Bare W W, McCloskey J F 1961 Primary Hodgkin's disease of the ovary: report of a case. Obstetrics and Gynecology 17: 477–480

Benninghoff D L, Medina A, Alexander L L, Camiel M R 1970 The mode of spread of Hodgkin's disease to the skin. Cancer 26: 1135–1140

Berard C, O'Conor G T, Thomas L B, Torloni H 1969 Histopathological definition of Burkitt's tumour. Bulletin of the World Health Organization 40: 601–607

Brown Z A, Stenchever M A 1977 Genital ulceration and infectious mononucleosis: report of a case. American Journal of Obstetrics and Gynecology 127: 673–674

Buckingham J C, McClure J H 1955 Reticulum cell sarcoma of the vulva. Obstetrics and Gynecology 6: 138–143

Burkitt D 1958 A sarcoma involving the jaws in African children. British Journal of Surgery 46: 218–233

Burkitt D P 1970 General features and facial tumours in Burkitt's lymphoma. In: Burkitt D P, Wright D H (eds) Burkitt's lymphoma. Livingstone, Edinburgh, pp 6–15

Burkitt D P, Wright D H (eds) 1980 Burkitt's lymphoma. Livingstone, Edinburgh

Carbone P P, Kaplan H S, Musshoff K, Smithers D W, Tubiana M 1971 Report of the committee on Hodgkin's disease staging classification. Cancer Research 31: 1860–1861

Carr I, Hill A S, Hancock B, Neal F E 1976 Malignant lymphoma of the cervix uteri: histology and ultrastructure. Journal of Clinical Pathology 29: 680–686

Case Records of the Massachusetts General Hospital (case 45, 1981) 1981 New England Journal of Medicine 305: 1135–1146

Castaldo T W, Ballon S C, Lagasse L D, Petrilli E S 1979 Reticuloendothelial neoplasia of the female genital tract. Obstetrics and Gynecology 54: 167–170

Cattoretti G, Pileri S, Paravicini C et al 1993 Antigen unmasking in formalin fixed paraffin embedded tissue sections. Journal of Pathology 171: 83–98

Cecalupo A J, Frankel L S, Sullivan M P 1982 Pelvic and ovarian extramedullary leukemia relapse in young girls. Cancer 50: 587–593

Ceden G H, Sakurai M 1962 Vaginal cytology in leukemia. Acta Cytologica 6: 379–391

Chan J K C, Ng C S, Isaacson P G 1990 Relationship between high grade lymphoma and low grade B cell mucosa associated lymphoid tissue lymphoma (MALToma) of the stomach. American Journal of Pathology 136: 1153–1164

Chorlton I 1987 Malignant lymphoma of the female genital tract and ovaries. In: Fox H (ed) Haines and Taylor's textbook of obstetrical and gynaecological pathology, 3rd edn. Churchill Livingstone, Edinburgh, pp 737–762

Chorlton I, Norris H J, King F M 1974a Malignant reticuloendothelial disease involving the ovary as a primary manifestation: a series of 19 lymphomas and 1 granulocytic sarcoma. Cancer 34: 397–407

Chorlton I, Kamei R F, King F M, Norris H J 1974b Primary malignant reticuloendothelial disease involving the vagina, cervix and corpus uteri. Obstetrics and Gynecology 44: 735–748

Chu J-Y, Cardock T V, Davis R K, Tennant N E 1981 Ovarian tumor as manifestation of relapse in acute lymphoblastic leukemia. Cancer 48: 377–379

Clifford P 1968 Treatment of Burkitt's lymphoma. Lancet I: 559

Clow W M, Joannides T, Saleem A K, Melville-Jones G R, Martin J 1995 An unusual cause of postmenopausal bleeding and incontinence of urine: primary lymphoma of the vagina. British Journal of Obstetrics and Gynaecology 102: 164–165

Cogliatti S B, Schusia K, Shumaacher K et al 1991 Primary B cell gastric lymphoma: a clinicopathological study of 145 patients. Gastroenterology 101: 1159–1170

Colmenares R F, Zuker M N 1965 Significance of lymphocytic pools in the routine vaginal smear. Obstetrics and Gynecology 26: 909–912

Cook H T, Boylston A W 1988 Plasmacytoma of the ovary. Gynecologic Oncology 29: 378–381

Cuevas E C, Bateman A C, Wilkins B S et al 1994 Microwave antigen retrieval in immunocytochemistry: a study of 80 antibodies. Journal of Clinical Pathology 47: 448–452

De Bruin P, Beljaards R, van Heerde P et al 1993 Differences in clinical behaviour and immunophenotype between primary cutaneous and primary nodlar anaplastic large cell lymphoma of T-cell or null cell phenotype. Histopathology 23: 127–136

Delsol G, Al Saate T, Gatter K et al 1988 Co-expression of epithelial membrane antigen (EMA), Ki-1 and interleukin 2 receptor by anaplastic large cell lymphomas: diagnostic value in so-called malignant histiocytosis. American Journal of Pathology 130: 59–70

Dietl J, Horny H P, Kaiserling E 1994 Lymphoepithelioma-like carcinoma of the vagina: a case report with special reference to the immunophenotype of the tumor cells and tumor infiltrating lymphoreticular cells. International Journal of Gynecological Pathology 13: 186–189

Dimopoulos M A, Daliani D, Pugh W, Gershenson D, Cadanillas F, Sarris A H 1997 Primary ovarian non-Hodgkin's lymphoma: outcome after treatment with combination chemotherapy. Gynaecologic Oncology 64: 446–450

Diss T C, Pan L, Peng H, Wotherspoon A C, Isaacson P G 1994 Sources of DNA for detecting B cell monoclonality using PCR. Journal of Clinical Pathology 47: 493–396

Dorfman R 1965 Childhood lymphoma in St Louis, Missouri, clinically and histologically resembling Burkitt's tumour. Cancer 18: 418–430

Doss L L 1978 Simultaneous extramedullary plasmacytomas of the vagina and vulva: a case report and review of the literature. Cancer 41: 2468–2474

Dupree E L, Lee R A 1973 Histiocytosis X in the female genital tract. Obstetrics and Gynecology 42: 201–204

Durfee H A, Clark B F, Peers J H 1937 Primary lymphosarcoma of the ovary: report of a case. American Journal of Cancer 30: 567–573

Egwuatu V E, Ejeckam G C, Okaro J M 1980 Burkitt's lymphoma of the vulva: case report. British Journal of Obstetrics and Gynaecology 87: 827–830

Eshghabadi M, Shojania A M, Carr I 1986 Isolated granulocytic sarcoma: report of a case and review of the literature. Journal of Clinical Oncology 4: 912–917

Falini B, Flenghi L, Pileri S et al 1993 PGM-I: A new monoclonal antibody directed against a fixative-resistant epitope on the macrophage-restricted form of CD68 molecule. American Journal of Pathology 142: 1359–1372

Federation Internationale of Gynaecologists and Obstetricians (FIGO) Cancer Committee: Annual report on the results of treatment in gynecological cancer, Vol 17. Stockholm 1979

Fernando-Marco J, Mantorell M A, Carrato A, Navanno J T 1992 Primary vulvar lymphoma presenting as a clitoral tumor. Acta Obstericia et Gynecologica Scandinavica 71: 543–546

Ferry J A, Young R H 1991 Malignant lymphoma, pseudolymphoma and hematopoietic disorders of the femal genital tract. In: Rosen P P, Fechner R E (eds) Pathology Annual Part 1 26: 227–263

Ferry J A, Harris N L, Scully R E 1989 Uterine leiomyomas with lymphoid infiltration simulating lymphoma: a report of seven cases. International Journal of Gynecological Pathology 8: 263–270

Finkle H I, Goldman R L 1974 Burkitt's lymphoma: gynecological considerations. Obstetrics and Gynecology 43: 281–284

Fox H, Langley F A 1976 Tumours of the ovary. Heinemann, London

Fox H, Langley F A, Govan A D T, Hill S A, Bennett M H 1988 Malignant lymphoma presenting as an ovarian tumour: a clinicopathological analysis of 34 cases. British Journal of Obstetrics and Gynaecology 95: 386–390

Freeman C, Berg J W, Cutler S J 1972 Occurrence and prognosis of extranodal lymphomas. Cancer 29: 252–260

Friedman H D, Adelson M D, Eider R C, Lemke S M 1992 Case report. Granulocytic sarcoma of the uterine cervix — literature review of granulocytic sarcoma of the female genital tract. Gynecologic Oncology 46: 128–137

Gilks C B, Taylor G P, Clement P B 1987 Inflammatory pseudotumor of the uterus. International Journal of Gynecological Pathology 6: 275–286

Gralnick H R, Dittmark K 1969 Development of meyloblastoma with massive breast and ovarian involvement during remission in acute leukemia. Cancer 24: 746–749

Grogan T, Warnke R, Kaplan H 1982 A comparative study of Burkitt's and non Burkitt's 'undifferentiated' malignant lymphoma: immunological, cytochemical, ultrastructural, cytologic, histopathologic, clinical and cell culture features. Cancer 49: 1817–1828

Gustmann C M A, Osborn M, Griesser H, Feller A C 1991 Cytokeratin expression and vimentin content in anaplastic large cell lympomas and other non-Hodgkin's lymphomas. American Journal of Pathology 138: 1413–1422

Hafiz M A, Kragel P J, Toker C 1985 Carcinoma of the uterine cervix resembling lymphoepithelioma. Obstetrics and Gynecology 66: 829–831

Hahn G A 1958 Gynecological considerations in malignant lymphomas. American Journal of Obstetrics and Gynecology 75: 673–683

Halpin T F, Hunter R E, Cohen M B 1989 Lymphoepithelioma of the uterine cervix. Gynecologic Oncology 34: 101–105

Hamazaki M, Fujita H, Ara T et al 1968 Medullary carcinoma with marked lymphoid infiltration of the uterine cervix. Japanese Journal of Clinical Oncology 4: 787–790

Harris N L, Scully R E 1984 Malignant lymphoma and granulocytic sarcoma of the uterus and vagina: a clinicopathologic analysis of 27 cases. Cancer 53: 2530–2545

Harris N L, Jaffe E S, Stein H et al 1994 A revised European–North American classification of lymphoid neoplasms: a proposal from the International Lymphoma Study Group. Blood 84: 1361–1392

Harris N L, Jaffe E S, Diebold J et al 2000 The World Health Organization classification of neoplastic diseases of the haematopoietic and lymphoid tissues: report of the Clinical Advisory Committee Meeting, Airlie House, Virginia, November 1997. Histopathology 36, 69–87

Hasumi K, Sugano H, Sakamoto G et al 1977 Circumscribed carcinomas of the uterine cervix with marked lymphocytic infiltration. Cancer 39: 2503–2508

Hautzer N W 1984 Primary plasmacytoma of the ovary. Gynecologic Oncology 18: 115–118

Heaton D C, Duff G B 1989 Ovarian relapse in a young woman with acute lymphoblastic leukemia. American Journal of Hematology 30: 42–43

Heller E L, Palin W 1946 Ovarian involvement in Hodgkin's disease. Archives of Pathology 41: 282–289

Hindkamp J F, Szanto P B 1959 Chloroma of the ovary. American Journal of Obstetrics and Gynecology 78: 812–816

Hui P K, Feller A C, Lennert K 1988 High grade non-Hodgkin's lymphoma of B-cell type. 1 Histopathology. Histopathology 12: 127–143

Hung L H Y, Kurtz D M 1985 Hodgkin's disease of the endometrium. Archives of Pathology and Laboratory Medicine 109: 952–953

Hutchinson R E, Kuree A S, Davey F R 1990. Granulocytic sarcoma. Clinics in Laboratory Medicine 10: 889–901

Iliya F A, Muggia F M, O'Leary J A, King T M 1968 Gynecologic manifestations of reticulum cell sarcoma. Obstetrics and Gynecology 31: 266–269

Isaacson P G 1992 The non-Hodgkin's lymphomas. In: McGee J O D, Isaacson P G, Wright N A (eds) Oxford textbook of pathology. Oxford University Press, Oxford, pp 1775–1787

Isaacson P G, Norton A J (eds) 1994 Malignant lymphoma of the urogenital tract. In: Extranodal lymphomas. Churchill Livingstone, Edinburgh, pp 273–280

Isaacson P, Spencer J 1987 Malignant lymphoma of mucosa associated lymphoid tissue. Histopathology 11: 445–462

Isaacson P, Wright D H 1983 Malignant lymphoma of mucosa associated lymphoid tissue: a distinctive type of B-cell lymphoma. Cancer 52: 1410–1416

Isaacson P, Wright D H 1984 Extranodal malignant lymphoma rising from mucosa associated lymphoid tissue. Cancer 53: 2512–2542

Issa P Y, Salem P A, Brihi E, Azoury R S 1980 Eosinophilic granuloma with involvement of the female genitalia. American Journal of Obstetrics and Gynecology 137: 608–612

Jack A S, Lee F D 1986 Morphological and immunohistochemical characteristics of T-cell malignant lymphomas in the West of Scotland. Histopathology 10: 223–234

Johnston C, Senckjiam E, Ratain M, Talerman A 1989 Conservative management of primary cervical lymphoma using combination chemotherapy: a case report. Gynecologic Oncology 35: 391–394

Kapadia S B, Krause J R, Kabour A I, Hartsock J R 1978 Granulocytic sarcoma of the uterus. Cancer 41: 687–691

Kaplan E G, Chadburn A, Caputo T A 1996 HIV-related primary non-Hodgkin's lymphoma of the vulva. Gynecologic Oncology 61: 131–138

Kaplan M A, Jacobson M O, Ferry J A, Harris N L 1993 T-cell lymphoma of the vulva in a renal allograft recipient with associated hemophagocytosis. American Journal of Surgical Pathology 17: 842–849

Katayama I, Hajian G, Enjy J T 1973 Cytological diagnosis of reticulum cell sarcoma of the uterine cervix. Acta Cytologica 17: 498–501

Khan M A T, Dahill S W, Stewart K S 1986 Primary Hodgkin's disease of the ovary: case report. British Journal of Obstetrics and Gynaecology 93: 1300–1301

Koo C H, Reifel J, Kogut N, Cove J K, Rappaport H 1992 True histiocytic malignancy associated with a malignant teratoma in a patient with 46XY gonadal dysgenesis. American Journal of Surgical Pathology 16: 175–183

Krumerman M S, Chung A 1978 Solitary reticulum cell sarcoma of the uterine cervix with initial cytodiagnosis. Acta Cytologica 22: 46–50

Lathrop J C 1967 Views and reviews: malignant pelvic lymphomas. Obstetrics and Gynecology 30: 137–145

Lechner W, Ortner A, Thoni A et al 1983 Histiocytosis X in gynecology. Gynecologic Oncology 15: 253

Leder L D 1964 Uber die selective fermentcytochemische Darstellung von neutrophilen myeloischen Zellen und Gewebmastzellen im paraffin-schmitt. Klinische Wochenschrift 42: 553

Lennert K, Feller A 1990 Histopathology of non-Hodgkin's lymphomas, 2nd edn. Springer-Verlag, New York, pp 53–162

Levine P H, Kamaraju L S, Connelly R P et al 1982 The American Burkitt's Lymphoma Registry: eight years experience. Cancer 49: 1016–1022

Linden M D, Tubbs R R, Fishleder A F, Hart W R 1988 Immunotypic and genotypic characterisation of non-Hodgkin's lymphomas of the ovary. American Journal of Clinical Pathology 89: 156–162

Linder J, Ye Y, Harrington D S, Armitage J O, Weisenberger D D 1987 Monoclonal antibodies marking T-lymphocytes in paraffin-embedded tissue. American Journal of Pathology 127: 1–8

Long H P, Patchefsky A S 1971 Primary Hodgkin's disease of the ovary: a case report. Obstetrics and Gynecology 38: 680–681

Lucia S P, Mills H, Lowenhaup E, Hunt M L 1952 Visceral involvement in primary neoplastic diseases of the reticuloendothelial system. Cancer 5: 1193–1200

McCarthy K P, Sloane J P, Kabarowski J H S, Matutes E, Weidemann L M 1991 The rapid detection of clonal T-cell proliferations in patients with lymphoid disorders. American Journal of Pathology 138: 821–829

McDermott M R, Clark D A, Bienenstock J 1980 Evidence for a common mucosal immunologic system II. Influence of the estrous cycle on B immunoblast migration into genital and intestinal tissues. Journal of Immunology 124: 2536–2539

Maeda T, Komegai H, Mori H 1988 Malignant lymphoma presenting as initial symptom in the uterus: case report. British Journal of Obstetrics and Gynaecology 95: 1195–1197

Magrath I T 1991 African Burkitt's lymphoma: history, biology, clinical features and treatment. American Journal of Pediatric Hematological Oncology 13: 222–246

Mann R B, Jaffe E S, Braylan R C et al 1976 Non-endemic Burkitt's lymphoma: a B-cell tumor related to germinal centers. New England Journal of Medicine 295: 685–691

Marcos C, Martinez L, Esquivias J J, Rosales M A, Khoury J, Herruzo A 1992 Primary non-Hogkin's lymphoma of the vulva. Acta Obstetricia et Gynecologica Scandinavica 71: 298–300

Meis J M, Butler J J, Osborne B M Manning J T 1986 Granulocytic sarcoma in non-leukemic patients. Cancer 58: 2697–2709

Mikhail M S Runowicz C D, Kadish A S, Romney S L 1989 Colposcopic and cytologic detection of chronic lymphocytic leukemia. Gynecologic Oncology 34: 106–108

Mills S E, Austin M B, Randall M E 1985 Lymphoepithelioma-like carcinoma of the uterine cervix. American Journal of Surgical Pathology 9: 883–889

Mittal K R, Blechman A, Alba Greco M, Alfonso F, Demopoulos R 1992 Lymphoma of the ovary with stromal luteinization, presenting as secondary amenorrhoea. Gynecologic Oncology 45: 69–75

Monterroso V, Jaffe E S, Merino M J, Medeiros J 1993 Malignant lymphomas involving the ovary: a clinicopathological analysis of 39 cases. American Journal of Surgical Pathology 17: 154–170

Morgan E R, Labotka R J, Gonzalez-Crussi F, Niaderhold M, Sherman J O 1981 Ovarian granulocytic sarcoma as the primary manifestation of acute infantile myelomonocytic leukemia. Cancer 48: 1819–1824

Muller S, Sangster G, Crocker J et al 1986 An immunohistochemical and clinicopathological study of granulocytic sarcoma ('chloroma'). Hematological Oncology 4: 101–102

Muntz H G, Ferry J A, Flynn D, Fuller A F, Tarraza H M 1991 Stage 1E primary malignant lymphomas of the uterine cervix. Cancer 66: 2023–2032

Murray J, Fox H 1991 Rosai Dorfman disease of the uterine cervix. International Journal of Gynecological Pathology 10: 209–213

Nam J-H, Park M-C, Lee K-M, Yoon C, Park H-R, Chun B-K 1992 Primary Non-Hodgkin's malignant lymphoma of the vulva: a case report. Journal of Korean Medical Sciences 7: 271–275

Neiman R S, Barcos M, Berard C, Mann R, Rydell R E, Bennett J M 1981 Granulocytic sarcoma: a clinicopathologic study of 61 biopsied cases. Cancer 48: 1426–1437

Nelson G A, Docherty M B, Pratt J H, Remine W H 1958 Malignant lymphoma involving the ovaries. American Journal of Obstetrics and Gynecology 76: 861–871

Neri A, Barriga F, Knowles D, Magrath I, Dalla-Favera R 1988 Different regions of the immunoglobulin heavy chain locus are involved in chromosomal translocations in distinct pathogenetic forms of Burkitt's lymphoma. Proceedings of the National Academy of Sciences USA 85: 2748–2752

Norris H J, Jensen R D 1972 Relative frequency of ovarian neoplasms in children and adolescents. Cancer 30: 713–719

Norton A J, Isaacson P G 1989a Lymphoma phenotyping in formalin-fixed and paraffin-wax embedded tissues: I. Range of antibodies and staining patterns. Histopathology 14: 437–446

Norton A J, Isaacson P G 1989b Lymphoma phenotyping in formalin-fixed and paraffin-wax embedded tissue: II. Profiles of reactivity in the various tumour types. Histopathology 14: 557–579

Obeid D, Cotter P, Sturdee D W 1979 Acute leukaemia relapse presenting as ovarian tumour. British Journal of Obstetrics and Gynaecology 86: 578–580

O'Conor G T 1961 Malignant lymphoma in African children II. A pathological entity. Cancer 14: 270–283

Oliva E, Ferry J A, Young R H, Prat J, Srigley J R, Scully R E 1997 Granulocytic sarcoma of the female genital tract: a clinicopathologic study of 11 cases. American Journal of Surgical Pathology 21: 1156–1165

Osanto S, Valk P, Meijer C J L M et al 1981 Solitary plasmacytoma of the vagina. Acta Haematologica 66: 140

Osborne B M, Robboy S J 1983 Lymphomas and leukaemia presenting as ovarian tumors: an analysis of 42 cases. Cancer 52: 1933–1943

Paladugu R R, Bearman R M, Rappaport H 1980 Malignant lymphoma with primary manifestation in the gonad: a clinicopathological study of 38 patients. Cancer 45: 561–571

Pejovic T, Schwartz P E, Mari G 2001 Hematologic malignancies in pregnancy. In: Barnea E R, Schwartz P E, Jauniaux E (eds) Cancer and pregnancy. Springer, London, pp 50–53

Pelicci P, Knowles D, Magrath I, Dalla-Favera R 1986 Chromosomal breakpoints and structural alterations of the C-myc locus differ in endemic and sporadic forms of Burkitt lymphomas. Proceedings of the National Academy of Sciences USA 83: 2984–2988

Pelstring R J, Essell J H, Kurtin P J, Cohen A R, Banks P M 1991 Diversity of organ site involvement among malignant lymphomas of mucosa associated tissues. American Journal of Clinical Pathology 93: 738–745

Perren T, Farrant M, McCarthy K, Harper P, Wiltshaw E 1992 Lymphomas of the cervix and upper vagina: a report of five cases and a review of the literature. Gynecologic Oncology 44: 87–95

Picker L J, Weiss L M, Medeiros C J, Wood G S, Warnke R A 1987 Immunophenotypic criteria for the diagnosis of non-Hodgkin's lymphoma. American Journal of Pathology 128: 181–201

Plouffe L, Tulandi T, Rosenberg A, Ferenczy A 1984 Non-Hodgkin's lymphoma in Bartholin's gland: case report and review of the literature. American Journal of Obstetrics and Gynecology 148: 608–609

Portnoy J, Ahronheim G A, Ghibu F et al 1984 Recovery of Epstein Barr virus from genital ulcers. New England Journal of Medicine 311: 966–968

PreBler H, Horny H-P, Wolf A, Kaiserling E 1992 Isolated granulocytic sarcoma of the ovary: histologic, electron microscopic and immunohistochemical findings. International Journal of Gynecological Pathology 11: 68–74

Prevot S, Hugol D, Andouin J, Diebold J, Truc J B, Decroix Y, Poitout P 1992 Primary non-Hodgkin's malignant lymphoma of the vagina: report of 3 cases with review of the literature. Pathology Research and Practice 188: 78–85

Rappaport H 1966 Tumors of the hematopoietic system. Atlas of tumor pathology, section III, fascicle 8. Armed Forces Institute of Pathology, Washington, DC, pp 97–161

Rotmensch J, Woodruff J D 1982 Lymphoma of the ovary: report of twenty new cases and update of previous series. American Journal of Obstetrics and Gynecology 143: 870–875

Sandvei R, Lote K, Svendsen E, Thunold S 1990 Case report: successful pregnancy following treatment of primary malignant lymphoma of the uterine cervix. Gynecologic Oncology 38: 128–131

Schiller H M, Madge G E 1970 Reticulum cell sarcoma presenting as a vulvar lesion. Southern Medical Journal 63: 471–472

Scott L, Blair G, Taylor G, Dimmick J, Fraser G 1988 Inflammatory pseudotumors in children. Journal of Pediatric Surgery 23: 755–758

Seifer D B, Weiss L M, Kempson R L 1986 Malignant lymphoma arising within thyroid tissue in a mature cystic teratoma. Cancer 58: 2459–2461

Sirgi K E, Swanson P E, Gershell D J 1994 Extramedullary hematopoiesis in the endometrium. American Journal of Clinical Pathology 101: 643–646

Skinnider B F, Clement P B, MacPherson N, Gascoyne R D, Viswanatha D S 1999 Primary non-Hodgkin's lymphoma and malakoplakia of the vagina: a case report. Human Pathology 30: 871–872

Smith J L, Baird D B, Stausbach P M 1997 Endometrial involvement by multiple myeloma. International Journal of Gynecological Pathology 16: 173–175

Staging announcement: FIGO Cancer Committee 1986 Gynecologic Oncology 25: 383–385

Stansfeld A G, D'Ardenne A J (eds) 1992 Lymph node biopsy interpretation. Churchill Livingstone, Edinburgh

Stansfeld A, Diebold J, Kapanci Y et al 1988 Updated Kiel classification for lymphomas. Lancet I: 292–293 (corrected table as p 603).

Stein H, Mason D, Gerdes J et al 1985 The expression of the Hodgkin's disease associated antigen Ki-I in reactive and neoplastic lymphoid tissue: evidence that Reed-Sternberg cells and histiocytic malignancies are derived from activated lymphoid cells. Blood 66: 848–858

Steiner-Salz D, Yahalom J, Samnelov A, Pollack A 1985 Non-Hodgkin's lymphoma associated with pregnancy. Cancer 56: 2087–2091

Swanson S, Innes D J, Frierson H F, Hess C E 1987 T-immunoblastic lymphoma mimicking B-immunoblastic lymphoma. Archives of Pathology and Laboratory Medicine. 111: 1077–1080

Taussig F J 1937 Sarcoma of the vulva. American Journal of Obstetrics and Gynecology 33: 1017–1026

Tuder R M 1992 Vulvar destruction by malignant lymphoma. Gynecologic Oncology 45: 52–57

Ueda G, Shimizu H et al 1988 An immunohistochemical study of small cell and poorly differentiated carcinomas of the cervix using neuroendocrine markers. Gynecologic Oncology 54: 164–169

Ulfelder H 1981 Classification systems. International Journal of Radiation, Oncology, Biology, Physics 7: 1083–1086

van de Rijn M, Kamel O W, Chang P P, Lee A, Warnke R A, Salhany K E, 1997 Primary low-grade endometrial B-cell lymphoma. American Journal of Surgical Pathology 21: 187–194

Vang R, Medeiros L J, Ha C S, Deavers M 2000a Non-Hodgkin's lymphomas involving the uterus: a clinicopathological analysis of 26 cases. Modern Pathology 13: 19–28

Vang R, Silva E G, Medeiros L J, Deavers M 2000b. Endometrial carcinoma and non-Hodgkin's lymphoma involving the female genital tract: a report of three cases. International Journal of Gynecological Pathology 19: 133–138

Vang R, Medeiros J, Silva E G, Gershenson D M, Deavers M 2000c Non-Hodgkin's lymphoma involving the vagina: a clinicopathologic analysis of 14 patients. American Journal of Surgical Pathology 24: 719–725

Vang R, Medeiros L J, Malpica A, Levenback C, Deavers M 2000d Non-Hodgkin's lymphoma involving the vulva. International Journal of Gynecological Pathology 19: 236–242

Walther G 1934 Uber die Lymphosarkomatose der weiblichen Genitalorgane. Archiv fur Gynakologie 157: 44–64

Whitaker D 1976 The role of cytology in the detection of malignant lymphoma of the uterine cervix. Acta Cytologica 20: 510–513

Winkler B, Reumann W, Mitao M et al 1984 Chlamydial endometritis: histological and immunohistochemical analysis. American Journal of Surgical Pathology 8: 771–778

Wishart J 1973 Reticulosarcoma of the vulva complicating azathioprine-treated dermatomyositis. Archives of Dermatology 108: 563–564

Woodruff J D, Noli Castillo R D, Novak E R 1963 Lymphoma of the ovary — a study of 35 cases from the Ovarian Tumor Registry of the American Gynecological Society. American Journal of Obstetrics and Gynecology 85: 912–918

Wright D H 1964 Burkitt's tumour: a post-mortem study of 50 cases. British Journal of Surgery 51: 245–251

Wright D H 1966 Burkitt's tumour in England: a comparison with childhood lymphosarcoma. International Journal of Cancer 1: 503–514

Wright D H 1970 Microscopic features, histochemistry, histogenesis and diagnosis in Burkitt's lymphoma. In: Burkitt D P, Wright D H (eds) Burkitt's lymphoma. Livingstone, Edinburgh, pp 92–103

Wright D H 1985 Histogenesis of Burkitt's lymphoma: a B-cell tumour of mucosa-associated lymphoid tissue. In: Lenoir G, O'Conor G, Olweny C L M (eds) Burkitt's lymphoma: a human cancer model. ARC Scientific Publications, Lyons, no. 60, pp 37–45

Wyld P J, Lilleyman J S 1983 Ovarian disease in childhood lymphoblastic leukaemia. Acta Haematologica 69: 278–280

Young R H, Harris N L, Scully R E 1985 Lymphoma-like lesions of the lower female genital tract: a report of 16 cases. International Journal of Gynecological Pathology 4: 289–299

Ziegler J L 1981 Burkitt's lymphoma. New England Journal of Medicine 305: 735–745

Ziegler J L, Magrath I T 1974 Burkitt's lymphoma. Pathobiology Annual 4: 129–142

29

Endometriosis

B. Czernobilsky   H. Fox

Introduction   963

Aetiology and pathogenesis   963

Epidemiology   966

Classification   967

Gross and microscopic appearances   967

Relationship to neoplasia   974

Clinical aspects   979

INTRODUCTION

Endometriosis can be defined as the presence of ectopic foci of endometrial-type glands and stroma which tend to respond to ovarian hormones in a manner similar to that of the mucosa which lines the uterine body. This response, however, is often variable and incomplete (Metzger et al 1988). Foci of endometrial mucosa within the myometrium, which are sometimes designated as 'internal endometriosis', do not constitute endometriosis and represent adenomyosis, which is a different entity. On the other hand, endometrial tissue situated on the uterine serosa is truly ectopic and therefore represents endometriosis. According to Ranney (1980a), the various sites of endometriosis in order of frequency are as follows: ovary, cul-de-sac, uterosacral ligaments, the anterior wall of the rectosigmoid bowel, bladder peritoneum, round ligaments, appendix, small bowel, umbilicus, abdominal scars and, rarely, pleura, lungs and extremities.

AETIOLOGY AND PATHOGENESIS

The occurrence of endometriosis during the reproductive years and its not uncommon association with uterine leiomyomata, ovarian follicular cysts and endometrial polyps suggests that a disturbance of ovarian hormonal function may play a rôle in its aetiology (Fox 1983). Scott & Wharton (1957) have shown that oestrogen was indeed necessary for the maintenance of endometriotic implants. On the other hand, the experimental studies of Dizerega et al (1980) indicate that ovarian steroids are not necessary for the growth of endometrial implants, a point also supported by clinical observations of endometriosis in postmenopausal women in whom there is no evidence of oestrogenic activity (Toki et al 1996) and in women who have had a previous bilateral oophorectomy (Spence 1992; Redwine 1994).

There are numerous hypotheses concerning the pathogenesis of endometriosis. These have been reviewed by, among others, Javert (1949), Gardner et al (1953), Ridley

(1968), Lauchlan (1972), Ranney (1980a,b), Haney (1990, 1991), Thomas (1993), Oral & Arici (1997), Witz (1999) and Vinatier et al (2001). Endometriosis was first believed to originate in either Wolffian (von Recklinghausen 1885) or Müllerian rests (Cullen 1925). This latter phenomenon is referred to as 'müllerianosis' and implies an embryonic origin of certain forms of endometriosis, a view which, though often thought to be only of historical interest, has nevertheless won some more recent, though limited, support (Batt & Smith 1989; Batt et al 1990; Mai et al 1998).

In 1921 Sampson advanced the theory that abnormally sited endometrium in the pelvis is due to regurgitation of endometrial fragments through the Fallopian tube as a result of retrograde menstruation. The evidence in favour of this hypothesis included:

a. demonstration of tubal menstrual regurgitation when the normal exit through the cervix was blocked
b. a distribution of pelvic endometriosis which corresponds to that which one might expect from tubal regurgitation
c. a patent tubal lumen in patients with endometriosis, and
d. animal experiments in which endometrium grew when implanted in the peritoneal cavity.

Retrograde menstruation is in fact a virtually universal phenomenon (Halme et al 1984), even in the absence of cervical blockage, and endometrial cells are present in the peritoneal fluid of more than 70% of menstruating women (Kruitwagen et al 1991). However, the viability of sloughed endometrial cells and their capacity to implant at ectopic sites is of course crucial for the validity of the regurgitation/implantation theory. In this respect the experiments of Te Linde & Scott (1950), Ridley & Edwards (1958) and D'Hooghe et al (1995), which consisted of injecting and/or diverting menstrual blood into the peritoneal cavity with resultant development of endometriosis in humans and monkeys, have strengthened Sampson's theory. A 'natural' equivalent of these experiments is the high incidence of severe endometriosis that is found in association with congenital uterine abnormalities in which there is obstruction to menstrual outflow (Shifrin et al 1973; Olive & Henderson 1987; Fedele et al 1992).

The coelomic metaplastic theory, first proposed by Robert Meyer, is a plausible hypothesis, at least for endometriosis situated in the ovary and other pelvic organs (Novak & de Lima 1948; Hertig & Gore 1961; Fujii 1991; Suginami 1991; Nakamura et al 1993) and has won recent support from experimental studies (Matsuura et al 1999). The striking metaplastic potential of the pelvic mesothelium in the female is a well-known fact. This mesothelium, which also covers the ovary where it is designated as 'surface epithelium', is of coelomic origin. In the embryo it gives rise to the Müllerian duct

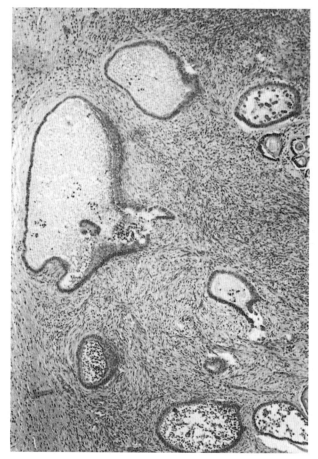

Fig. 29.1 Ovarian surface epithelium inclusion cysts partly lined by endometrial-type cells.

and consequently to the epithelium and stroma of the various organs derived from it such as the uterus, Fallopian tubes and, possibly, part of the vagina. It is this epithelium which is now considered to constitute the source of the common epithelial tumours of the ovary including endometrioid carcinoma (Czernobilsky 1982). The appearance of endometrial-type cells in ovarian surface epithelium as well as the presence of such cells in ovarian inclusion cysts is commonplace and supports the coelomic metaplastic theory of endometriosis (Fig. 29.1). In spite of the attractiveness of the coelomic theory, the validity of this concept has been questioned and the arguments against the metaplasia hypothesis have been summarized by Haney (1990). These include the extreme rarity of endometriosis in males and in peritoneal surfaces other than that of the pelvic cavity, its predominance in reproductive-aged women and the apparent necessity of the presence of the uterus in cases of endometriosis.

Levander & Norman (1955) have attempted to reconcile the reflux and metaplastic theories by suggesting that the menstrual endometrium which is being regurgitated through the Fallopian tube does not itself implant and grow, but rather induces endometrial metaplasia of the serosa. This induction theory is supported by the experimental study of Merrill (1966) who introduced endometrial tissue within millipore filters into the peritoneal cavity and was able to induce endometrial metaplasia within the peritoneum by this technique.

Halban (1925) and, later, Javert (1951) suggested a lymphatic pathway for the dissemination of endometriotic tissue, a view based on the finding of endometriotic tissue in lymphatic channels (Ichimiya et al 1998) and in lymph nodes; Ueki (1991) has argued cogently in support of this concept. Haematogenous spread has also been suggested, especially for the rare extra-abdominal endometriosis, such as that occurring in the brain (Thibodeau et al 1987), skin (Tidman & MacDonald 1988; Naseman 1990), extremities (Gupta 1985; Giangarra et al 1987), pleura or lungs (Charles 1957; Di Palo et al 1989; Espaulella et al 1991; Svendstrup & Husby 1991; Flieder et al 1998). In these locations the haematogenous pathway appears to be the only plausible explanation for the presence of endometriosis.

The not infrequent occurrence of endometriosis in laparotomy scars following a variety of gynaecological procedures involving the uterine lumen points to yet another possible pathogenetic mechanism, namely, that of direct transplantation of endometrial tissue (Steck & Helwig 1965). The presence of endometrium within the scar tissue and in the actual tract made at the operation supports such a mechanism in these cases (Kale et al 1971).

It is quite possible, indeed highly probable, that there may be multiple histogenetic mechanisms for this complex entity and this is emphasised by the recent division of endometriosis into three entities, namely peritoneal, ovarian and rectovaginal-septal by Nisolle & Donnez (1997). Most of the above described pathogenetic mechanisms, and especially the implantation theory, relate mostly to peritoneal endometriosis, whilst coelomic metaplasia of invaginated epithelial inclusions could be responsible for the development of at least some forms of ovarian endometriosis. As to rectovaginal endometriotic nodules, these are considered to represent adenomyotic nodules related to metaplasia of Müllerian remnants situated in the rectovaginal-septum. The metaplastic changes in this location are responsible for the proliferation of smooth muscle, creating an appearance which is similar to that of adenomyosis of the uterus (Donnez et al 1995, 1996). It is also possible that some forms of ovarian endometriosis have a quite different pathogenesis for it has been demonstrated that many ovarian endometriotic cysts are monoclonal in nature (Nilbert et al 1995; Jimbo et al 1997a; Tamura et al 1998; Yano et al 1999): this raises the possibility that such cysts are neoplastic in nature and represent the benign counterpart of an endometrioid adenocarcinoma thus being, in reality, endometrioid cystadenomas (Czernobilsky 1982, 1987).

Despite this plethora of theories it is widely held that retrograde menstruation and implantation of endometrial fragments is the primary mode of development of endometriosis in the peritoneal cavity (Witz 1999). The question arises therefore why, if retrograde menstruation is universal, endometriosis does not arise in all women: the answer is that it probably does at some time in a woman's reproductive life (Evers 1994; Koninckx 1994) but that the early superficial non-invasive lesions of pelvic endometriosis are unstable and most will regress, only a minority progressing to an invasive lesion. The natural history of peritoneal endometriotic lesions is for them to regress and peritoneal macrophages play an important rôle in their destruction and removal. Persistence and progression of endometriotic foci may therefore be taken as a failure of peritoneal cleansing mechanisms and it is thought that both genetic and immunological factors may be involved in this failure.

In terms of possible genetic factors, familial endometriosis has been reported (Ridley 1968; Lamb et al 1986; Moen & Magnus 1993), and in these cases the disease appears to be more severe (Malinak et al 1980; Simpson et al 1980). There is also an increased prevalence of endometriosis in first degree relatives of affected women compared with the general population (Moen & Magnus 1993; Kennedy et al 1995) and it has been estimated that a family history of endometriosis in a primary relative increases the risk for the disease to about 10 times that of women lacking a familial history. The risk of endometriosis appears to follow a maternal inheritance pattern of polygenetic or multifactorial type (Haney et al 1981). A study of 16 pairs of monozygotic twins found that 14 were concordant for endometriosis (Hadfield et al 1997) and this high level of concordance was confirmed in a subsequent Australian study (Treloar et al 1999) which suggested that about 50% of the variance in the liability to develop endometriosis is due to genetic factors.

The possible immunological factors involved in the persistence of endometriotic foci are complex (Dmowski et al 1981, 1990, 1991; D'Hooge & Hill 1995, 1996; Lebovic et al 2001) but emphasis has been placed upon a diminished peritoneal macrophage response (Dmowski et al 1991; Evers 1994) and on decreased natural killer (NK) cell mediated cytotoxicity (Oosterlynck et al 1991, 1992; Hill 1992; Garzetti et al 1993; Wilson et al 1994; Wu et al 1996, 2000) as key factors with various cytokines, such as interleukins 1 and 6 (IL-1, IL-6), also playing a significant rôle (Mazzeo et al 1998; Barcz et al 2000). Alterations in humoral and cell mediated immunity and in soluble products such as complement and immunoglobulins may also be involved but it has to be emphasised, that the rôle of immunological factors is still speculative and that more work is required in this area

The ability of an endometriotic implant to establish itself depends on multiple interrelated factors. Regurgitated endometrial cells express cell adhesion molecules, such as integrins and E-cadherin (van der Linden et al 1994), and these molecules, which are also expressed in endometriotic tissues (Bridges et al 1994; Beliard et al 1997), probably play an important rôle in the attachment of shed endometrial tissue to the peritoneum: their activity in this respect is enhanced by cytokines such as tumour necrosis factor alpha (TNF-alpha) and interleukin-1 (IL-1) which have a greater effect on endometrial cell adhesiveness from women with endometriosis than they do on similar cells from women without the disease (Sillem et al 1999). Early endometriotic lesions invade the peritoneal extracellular matrix and products of local proteolysis and tissue recycling, such as the amino-terminal propeptide of type III collagen, accumulate in the peritoneal fluid of women with early active lesions (Spuijbroek et al 1992): endometriotic foci express high levels of matrix metalloproteinases (Kokerine et al 1997; Osteen et al 1997; Chung et al 2001) and plasminogen activator (Kobayashi 2000) and this increased proteolytic activity is probably of considerable importance in the invasiveness of the early implant. Subsequent development of the endometrial implant depends upon its ability to establish a blood supply. Angiogenic factors are present at a higher concentration in the peritoneal fluid of women with endometriosis than in the fluid of women without the disease (Oosterlynck et al 1993) and it has been suggested that women with endometriosis have increased endometrial angiogenesis (Healy et al 1998): vascular endothelial growth factor, which is present in high concentration in endometriotic lesions, has emerged as the principal angiogenic factor in early endometriosis (Fujimoto et al 1999; Fasciani et al 2000; McLaren 2000). Having acquired a blood supply the implant will subsequently grow and epidermal growth factor (EGF) is thought to be a major growth stimulus, being produced in endometriotic tissue (Haining et al 1991) and EGF receptors being present in such tissue (Prentice et al 1992). Other cytokines, particularly tumour necrosis factor-alpha (TNF-alpha), hepatocyte growth factor (HGF) and interleukin-8 (IL-8), also play significant rôles in promoting the growth of ectopic endometrial tissue (Ryan et al 1995; Fukaya et al 1999; Harada et al 1999; Lebovic et al 2001). Growth of the endometriotic implant may be accentuated by the high proliferative activity (Li et al 1993; Nicolle et al 1997; Khan et al 1999) and reduced level of apoptosis (Dmowski et al 1998; Imai et al 2000; Lebovic et al 2001) in endometriotic foci.

Continued growth of the ectopic areas of endometrial tissue, which contain oestrogen and progesterone receptors (Bergquist 1991; Bergquist et al 1993), is stimulated by cyclic oestrogen while subsequent progesterone will produce a secretory response. As in normal endometrium, withdrawal of these hormones causes bleeding which, in cases of cystic endometriosis, may result in intraluminal haemorrhage (Scott & Wharton 1957). After months of repeated haemorrhage an inflammatory reaction followed by a scar develops in the surrounding tissue

which, according to Sturgis & Call (1954), may interfere with subsequent blood supply and thus gradually decrease the response of the endometriosis to hormonal stimulation.

Some endometriotic lesions become invasive and there is an increasing tendency to distinguish non-invasive endometriotic foci from those which are invasive, the latter often being classed as 'endometriotic disease' rather than endometriosis. It has been suggested that progression from endometriosis to endometriotic disease is due to genetic cellular changes which allow the endometriotic cells to escape from the influence of regulatory factors in the peritoneal fluid (Koninckx et al 1999). Genetic changes certainly have been shown to occur in endometriosis: thus Gogusev et al (1999) found recurrent copy losses on several chromosomes in 15 of 18 cases, the most common being loss of 1p and 22q whilst Jiang et al (1996) found loss of heterozygosity at 9p, 11q or 22q in 28% of cases of endometriosis. How important these genetic alterations are in the progression of endometriosis remains, however, to be determined.

Throughout this discussion of the aetiology and pathogenesis of endometriosis it has been assumed that the disease is due, in the peritoneal cavity at least, to an altered environmental response to regurgitated but normal endometrial tissue. Recently, a strikingly different concept has been proposed, namely that endometriosis is due to the regurgitation of abnormal endometrium and that the basic abnormality lies within the uterus (Kunz et al 2000; Leyendecker 2000; Vinatier et al 2000). This view is based on two findings. Firstly, the normally sited uterine endometrium of women with endometriosis differs from that of women without endometriosis by showing increased proliferation (Wingfield et al 1995), increased expression of monocyte-chemotactic protein-1 (Jolicoeur et al 1998), increased expression of *P*450 aromatase (Noble et al 1996), dysregulated IL-6 production (Tseng et al 1996), increased angiogenic activity (Healy et al 1998), diminished apoptosis (Dmowski et al 1998; Imai et al 2000; Meresman et al 2000) and impaired expression of *HOX* gene (Taylor et al 1999). Secondly, women with endometriosis show increased uterine peristaltic activity (Leyendecker et al 1996, 1998). This intriguing concept clearly needs further consideration and study but the possibility also exists that endometriosis provokes changes in regulatory mechanisms that affect both ectopic and normally sited endometrium.

EPIDEMIOLOGY

Incidence data on endometriosis is limited and variable. Houston et al (1987) reported an incidence ratio of 2.5 cases per 1000 woman-years based on clinically diagnosed disease in Minnesota. When the cases were restricted to histologically confirmed or surgically visualised cases, the incidence was 1.6. Since prevalence is equal to incidence multiplied by the average duration of the disease, which is 40 years, the prevalence of endometriosis in the general United States population, based on an incidence of 2.5, would be 10% (Goldman & Cramer 1990). Rawson (1991) has suggested that the true prevalence, even in asymptomatic fertile women, may be very much higher.

According to Houston et al (1987), the peak incidence is in women aged 35–44. In the United States the disease appears to be most common among middle-class white patients (Novak & Woodruff 1979b). The risk of endometriosis among Orientals appears to be as high or even higher than that in whites (Miyazawa 1976). It is of interest to note that endometriosis appears to be less frequent in Jewish women in Israel as compared to other non-Jewish Western populations (Brzezinki & Koren 1962; Lancet Rotenstreich and Czernobilsky, unpublished data), a phenomenon which remains unexplained.

CLASSIFICATION

Classifications of endometriosis have been of two types. The first type of classification is basically surgico-pathological and has as its aim the forecasting of the prognosis for the patient in terms of either achieving pregnancy or relief of pain. Since the original studies of Sampson (1921) a number of classifications of this type have been suggested. Wicks & Lapson in 1949 proposed histological criteria only as the basis of their classification with a grading system similar to that used for malignant tumours. In Huffman's (1951) classification patients were staged at laparotomy into four groups based on the amount and spread of the disease. Novak & Woodruff (1979a) classified endometriosis according to its location, its macroscopic appearance and/or its severity. A more comprehensive classification was proposed by Acosta et al (1973) and by Cohen (1980) who divided the disease into mild, moderate and severe categories based on surgical findings: site of lesions, presence of adhesions, presence of scarring or retraction were used to distinguish these stages with the presence of small endometriomas or the presence of minimal peritubal or periovarian adhesions distinguishing moderate from mild disease. Using this staging system a weak inverse relationship between stage of disease and pregnancy rates could be shown. Kistner et al (1977) classified adnexal adhesions in a progressive fashion and included for the first time assessment of the potential for endoscopic adhesiolysis in the classification. In 1979 the American Fertility Society (AFS) published its classification system dividing endometriosis into mild, moderate, severe and extensive disease including assessment of the extent of the disease and the presence of adhesions. However, pregnancy after treatment according to extent of the disease could not be predicted by this scheme. A revised American Fertility Society classification was presented in 1985 in which a separate category of minimal disease was created and the extensive disease category eliminated: superficial disease was differentiated from invasive disease, adhesions around the tubes or ovaries were quantitated and a distinction made between filmy and dense adhesions. This classification was revised and refined in 1996 with more emphasis being placed on the morphology of the disease (American Society for Reproductive Medicine 1997). Despite the plethora of classifications proposed so far, none has been reliable for those features which are of critical importance to the patient, the prediction of pregnancy outcome and the assessment and management of pain (Hoeger & Guzick 1999).

The other type of classification of endometriosis has been purely pathological. In the 1973 World Health Organization (WHO) classification (Serov et al 1973) ovarian endometriosis was divided into 'tumours' and 'tumour-like conditions'. Benign endometrioid 'tumours' in this classification included adenoma, cystadenoma, adenofibroma and cystadenofibroma. In the later WHO classification (Scully 1999) endometriosis is simply classed as a tumour-like condition and benign ovarian endometrioid tumours are not included under this heading. It is, however, often difficult, and sometimes impossible, to draw a sharp line between these two categories. This, together with the occurrence of polypoid, hyperplastic and atypical changes in endometriosis (Scully et al 1966; Cantor et al 1979; Czernobilsky & Morris 1979), the not uncommon actual transformation of various types of endometriosis to carcinoma (Brooks & Wheeler 1977; Mostoufizadeh & Scully 1980) and the monoclonal nature of endometriotic cysts (discussed above) may favour the classification of all forms of intra-abdominal, certainly ovarian, endometriosis under one heading, possibly that of 'endometrioid neoplasia'.

GROSS AND MICROSCOPIC APPEARANCES

Endometriosis may appear as tiny foci or as large cystic masses. Because of the frequent bleeding which occurs in endometriosis, as a result of its response to the rise and fall of ovarian hormones, these foci are often dome shaped, of dark bluish coloration with tan to brownish staining of adjacent tissues. Although the latter is the classic description given to endometriotic lesions, the macroscopic appearance of peritoneal endometriosis has been classified as red, black and white in accordance with the age of the lesion (Nisolle & Donnez 1997). Thus red lesions are characteristic of recently implanted endometrial cells and histologically resemble eutopic endometrium. Black lesions appear after menstrual shedding induces an inflammatory reaction provoking a scarification process that encloses the implant and contains intraluminal debris. The white lesion is due to devascularisation of the endometriotic foci, leaving white inactive plaques of collagen at the site. In early stages of the disease, however, the endometriotic lesions may, as has been pointed out by Jansen & Russell (1986), be non-pigmented. Endometriotic cysts are usually well encapsulated and with increasing age of the lesion develop a thick, fibrotic capsule with numerous adhesions (Novak 1931). They can reach dimensions of up to 20 cm in diameter. The lumen of these cysts contains dark brown fluid ranging in consistency from watery to syrupy, hence the term 'chocolate cysts'. It should be emphasised, however, that haemorrhage occurs in a variety of ovarian cysts and neoplasms, and not exclusively in endometriosis. Thus, although haemorrhagic ovarian cysts are certainly suggestive of endometriosis, the exact diagnosis of such cysts can only be established by histological examination. The cyst wall is usually shaggy with dark brown deposits (Figs 29.2, 29.3). In addition to ample sampling

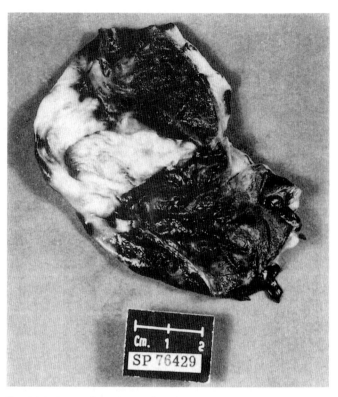

Fig. 29.3 Opened ovarian endometriotic cyst with haemorrhagic lining and thick fibrous wall. (Courtesy of Dr L M Roth, Indianapolis, Indiana, USA.)

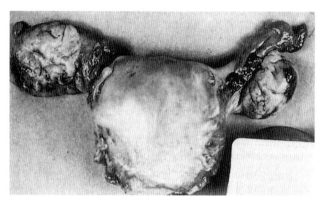

Fig. 29.2 Uterus with both adnexae showing scattered haemorrhagic foci representing endometriosis, especially on right Fallopian tube and adjacent ovary. (Courtesy of Dr H T Enterline, Philadelphia, USA.)

for histological examination from the cyst wall, any thickened or protruding intraluminal areas should be sectioned for microscopic examination. Occasionally, ovarian or extraovarian pelvic endometriosis presents as polypoid masses of soft grey tissue which may simulate a malignant tumour and have been designated as 'polypoid

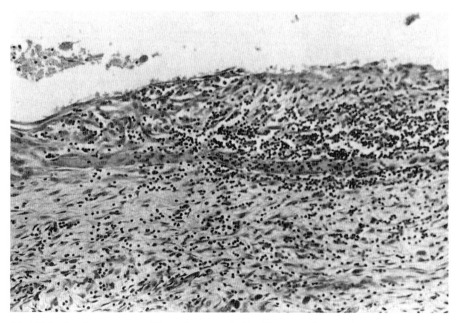

Fig. 29.4 Ovarian cyst, probably endometriosis, lined by granulation tissue.

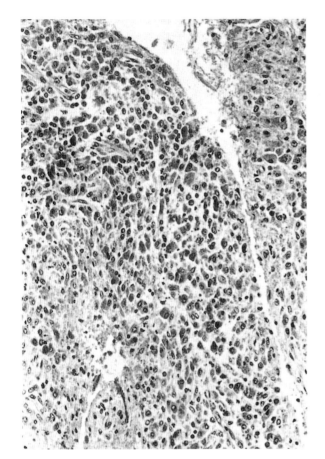

Fig. 29.5 Cyst lining, probably endometriosis, with numerous haemosiderin-laden macrophages.

endometriosis' (Scully et al 1998; Chang & Natarajan 2001).

The histological diagnosis of endometriosis may prove difficult because of the secondary changes occurring in the lesions due to bleeding and fibrosis. These latter may transform the areas of endometriosis, including the lining of large cysts, into granulation tissue, with numerous histiocytes, or so-called 'pseudoxanthoma' cells, and fibrosis. In such circumstances, the pathologist can only reach the diagnosis of 'consistent with endometriosis' (Figs 29.4, 29.5). The pseudoxanthoma cells contain degradation products of blood, especially ceroid (lipofuscin, haemofuchsin), and thus stain positively with periodic acid–Schiff, Ziehl–Neelsen and oil Red-0 stains (Clement et al 1988). These cells also exhibit autofluorescence, which is one of the properties of ceroid (Fig. 29.6). Haemosiderin is much less conspicuous than ceroid in these cells, a fact which does not seem to be generally known (Clement 1990). Rarely granulomatous nodules, characterised by a central zone of necrosis surrounded by pseudoxanthoma cells, often in a palisaded arrangement, referred to as 'necrotic pseudoxanthomatous nodules', have been observed in endometriosis (Clement et al 1988) (Fig. 29.7).

A definite histological diagnosis of endometriosis can be established only when both endometrial-type glands and stroma are evident in ectopic sites (Fig. 29.8). However, because of the great metaplastic potential of mesothelial cells, which are capable of forming inclusions and cysts partially or completely lined by endometrial-type epithelium but lacking endometrial stroma, the latter is more characteristic of endometriosis than the mere presence of endometrial-type glands. It has also been stated that bleeding in endometriosis originates from stromal blood vessels (Hertig & Gore 1961). Thus ovarian surface epithelial inclusion cysts lined by endometrial-type epithelium or endometrial-type glandular inclusions in pelvic lymph nodes, which also originate in mesothelial cells (Karp & Czernobilsky 1969), do not

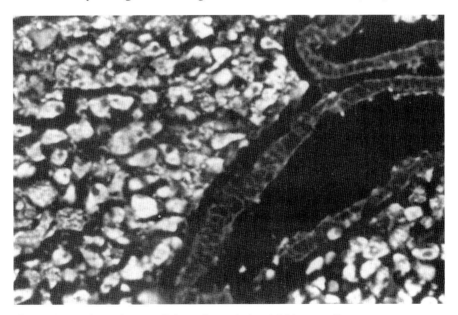

Fig. 29.6 Pseudoxanthoma cells in endometriosis exhibiting autofluorescence (unstained section photographed with fluorescent light). (Reprinted with permission from Clement 1990.)

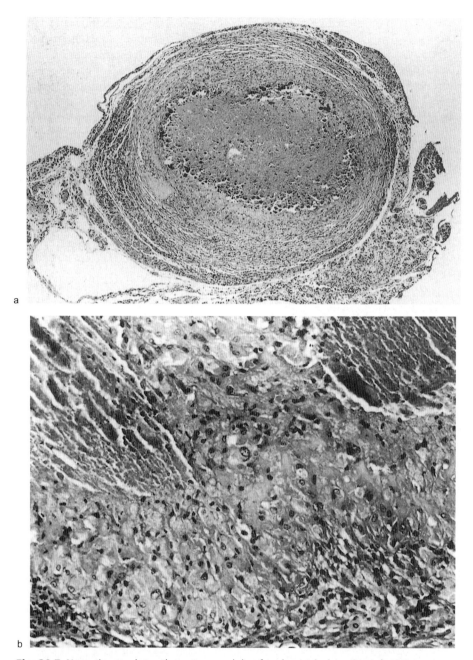

Fig. 29.7 Necrotic pseudoxanthomatous nodule of endometriosis. **a** Granulomatous peritoneal nodule with central necrosis and calcified material. **b** The necrotic centre is surrounded by pseudoxanthoma cells. (Reprinted with permission from Clement et al 1988.)

constitute endometriosis since they are lacking endometrial-type stroma (Fig. 29.9). This is more than of semantic importance because these inclusions without stroma do not respond to ovarian hormones, do not bleed and are therefore usually asymptomatic. When found incidentally at laparotomy, they must be differentiated from metastatic adenocarcinoma especially when the operation was performed for ovarian or endometrial carcinoma. True endometriosis within pelvic lymph nodes exists but is a rare phenomenon.

An interesting observation is the presence of mesothelial inclusions in ovaries which are the site of endometriosis (Kerner et al 1981) (Figs 29.10, 29.11). Since the endometriosis in these cases is always located at a distance from the mesothelial inclusions, it is unlikely that the endometriotic foci act as a non-specific stimulus to the surface epithelium. It appears more likely that a common, possibly hormonal, stimulus is responsible for the development of both the endometriosis and the mesothelial inclusions in these cases.

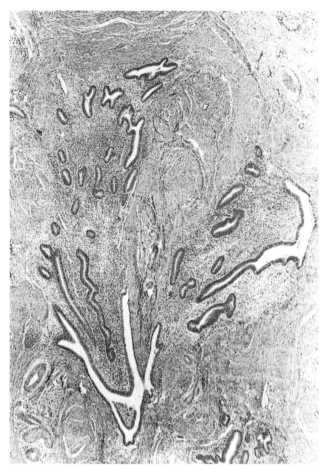

Fig. 29.8 Endometriosis in wall of Fallopian tube showing well-formed endometrial glands with surrounding endometrial stroma.

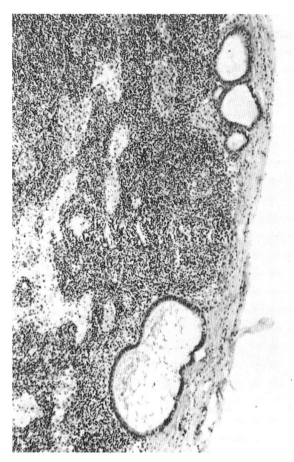

Fig. 29.9 Abdominal lymph node with glandular endometrial-like inclusions in cortical portion. Note absence of surrounding endometrial stroma and of haemorrhage.

The distinction between non-specific fibrous, ovarian and endometrial-type stroma can be difficult. The problem becomes even more complex because of the presence of haemorrhage, inflammatory cells, macrophages and fibrosis in the stroma of endometriosis. In the absence of progestational effect the stroma of endometriosis is characterised by its dense cellularity and is composed of cells with large hyperchromatic round or elongated nuclei, blunted edges and little cytoplasm. These stromal cells closely surround, and adhere to, the endometrial epithelium. By contrast, non-specific fibrous stroma or ovarian stroma in which glandular inclusions are present does not show such an intimate relationship to the epithelial components. In some instances the stroma of endometriosis shows a decidual change due to pregnancy. Predecidual changes have also been observed in endometriosis secondary to intrinsic or extrinsic hormonal effects (Fig. 29.12). Although, as mentioned above, the endometrial stroma constitutes the most specific element in endometriosis, it is not advisable to reach a diagnosis of endometriosis in the presence of nodules composed solely of endometrial-type stroma which lack haemorrhage and/or haemosiderin-laden macrophages

(Fig. 29.13). Rather than endometriosis such foci may represent a low-grade stromal sarcoma (Kempson 1973) which by its very nature may be present in various sites outside the uterus. Even nodules made up of decidual tissue without glandular elements cannot be safely diagnosed as endometriosis since pelvic ectopic decidual reactions also occur, probably as a result of stimulation by progesterone and, possibly, adrenal or pituitary hormones (Bassis 1956). Thus, whilst in ectopic sites the endometrial stromal component in the presence of endometrial glands is, with one proviso, diagnostic of endometriosis, the latter diagnosis cannot be reached when the stromal component alone is present, especially in the absence of evidence of repeated bleeding. The one proviso to the presence of both ectopic endometrial stroma and glands being diagnostic of endometriosis is that, very rarely, an extrauterine stromal sarcoma may show extensive endometrial-type glandular differentiation (Levine et al 2001); the variable distribution of the glands in such a lesion and the presence of vascular invasion help to distinguish it from endometriosis.

The epithelial component of endometriosis may be part of a cyst lining, or represent glandular structures, or

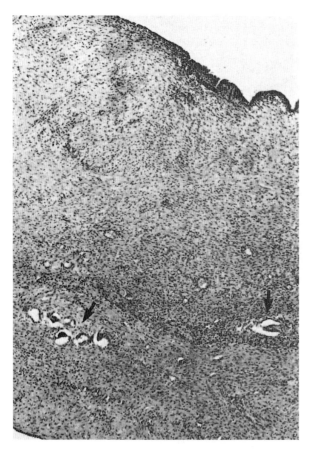

Fig. 29.10 Ovary with endometriotic cyst lining (above) and mesothelial inclusions in opposite area (arrow).

both (Figs 29.8, 29.14). In a study of 194 cases of ovarian endometriosis the epithelium presented as a cyst lining in 89, as glandular structures in 28, while in 77 cases both features were evident; papillary formations lined by endometrial-type epithelium were also observed (Czernobilsky & Morris 1979) (Fig. 29.15). Histological examination of the epithelial elements showed a variety of features such as typical endometrial glands which, although occasionally secretory, were most often of the inactive or proliferative type, as well as simple or complex hyperplasia (Fig. 29.16), hobnail cells and tubal-type epithelium (Fig. 29.17) (Czernobilsky & Morris 1979). 'Endosalpingiosis' which has been defined as ectopic tubal epithelium and which, according to Tutschka & Lauchlan (1980), is 'homologous' with endometriosis, is a confusing term and should not be used as synonymous with endometriosis. The presence of tubal-type epithelium merely reflects the metaplastic potential of Müllerian tissues as does also the presence, in occasional cases, of mucinous epithelium in endometriotic foci (Fukunaga & Ushigome 1998). Indeed endometriotic epithelium may exhibit the full range of metaplastic changes found in eutopic endometrium.

Czernobilsky & Morris (1979) described severe epithelial atypia in ovarian endometriosis in 3.6% of their cases. This was characterised by pleomorphic, often hyperchromatic, nuclei, eosinophilic cytoplasm, squamoid features, tufting and stratification which were present in the lining of endometriotic cysts (Figs 29.18, 29.19). Although some of these changes may be of reactive origin, one should also consider the possibility that, in some instances, these atypical changes may be neoplastic with malignant potential. This latter hypothesis is borne out by the fact that not infrequently the epithelium of endometriotic cysts adjacent to endometrioid carcinomas shows similar changes. The neoplastic transformation of endometriosis is discussed in more detail below.

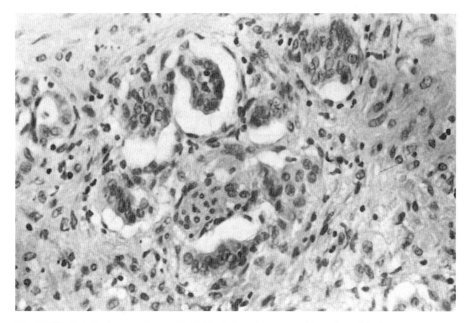

Fig. 29.11 Detail of unusual mesothelial inclusions in ovary with endometriosis.

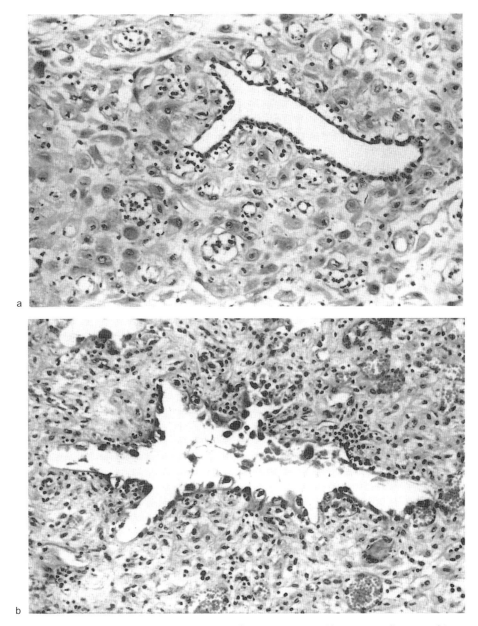

Fig. 29.12 Pregnancy-induced changes in endometriosis. **a** Decidua surrounding atrophic gland. **b** Arias-Stella reaction in endometriotic gland. (Reprinted with permission from Clement 1990.)

Other histological features of endometriosis include the presence of smooth muscle fibres (Rolfing et al 1981; Anaf et al 2000; Fukunaga 2000), calcification, ossification or myxoid change (Gerbie et al 1958). The uterus-like masses in various pelvic sites (Clement 1990) may constitute a special morphological form of endometriosis, although a congenital basis has also been suggested for these structures (Cozzutto 1981; Pueblitz-Peredo et al 1985; Pai et al 1998). A rare finding is that of acellular, ring-like structures or Liesegang rings encountered in debris or in the cyst wall of endometriosis. These probably represent zones of periodic precipitation of supersaturated colloid solutions and can be confused with

organisms or foreign material (Clement et al 1989; Perrotta et al 1998) (Fig. 29.20).

In summary, the definite histological diagnosis of endometriosis can be a difficult one. It depends on the presence of both endometrial glands and stroma, often showing evidence of repeated haemorrhage. In addition, in some instances morphological features can be traced to oestrogenic (Kapadia et al 1984) or progestational influences (Andrews et al 1959) as well as to pregnancy (Moller 1959). These hormonal responses however are often incomplete and variable, a fact which is also supported by ultrastructural (Schweppe et al 1984), histochemical (Prakash et al 1965) and steroid receptor

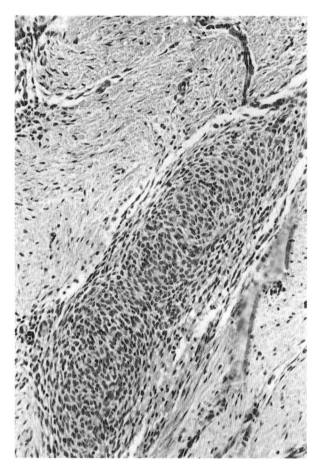

Fig. 29.13 Endometrial-type stroma in abdominal wall without haemorrhage or haemosiderin-laden cells.

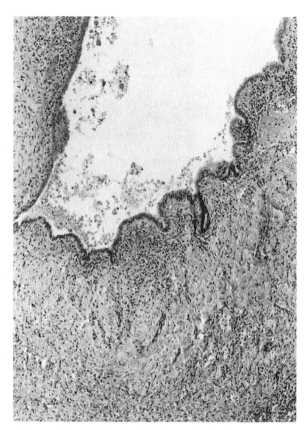

Fig. 29.14 Endometriotic cyst lined by endometrial epithelium with adjacent stromal cells.

studies (Lyndrup et al 1987). Ectopic endometrial-type glands without stroma, or endometrial-type stroma without glands, do not enable the pathologist to reach a diagnosis of endometriosis since these structures can be representative of other pathological entities. If, however, ectopic endometrial glands devoid of endometrial-type stroma or endometrial type stroma devoid of glands show in their respective immediate vicinity evidence of repeated haemorrhage, such as free haemosiderin pigment and pigment-laden macrophages with or without fibrosis, a presumptive diagnosis of endometriosis can be made. Such a presumptive diagnosis can also be made, although with less assurance, in cases of ovarian or pelvic haemorrhagic cysts in which, because of the haemorrhagic episodes, both epithelial and stromal elements have been destroyed.

RELATIONSHIP TO NEOPLASIA

The relationship of endometriosis to ovarian malignancy was first documented by Sampson in 1925, and was reappraised by Czernobilsky (1982). In order to prove that a tumour indeed originated in endometriosis Sampson (1925) required a demonstration of the direct

origin of the carcinoma from the endometriotic tissue (Fig. 29.21). These rigid criteria have by now been abandoned and it was Sampson himself who, in his article in 1925, speculated that ovarian endometrial-type carcinomas might arise de novo from the surface epithelium of the ovary.

The precancerous significance of atypical endometriosis (Czernobilsky & Morris 1979) is not clear since after resection of the lesion follow-up data cannot be obtained. Seidman (1996) followed up 62 women in whom a diagnosis of atypical ovarian endometriosis had been made and found only one case of endometrioid adenocarcinoma at the vaginal apex 8 years later: however, in this case the degree of abnormality within the endometriotic lesion was such that it had been classified as an early carcinoma. However, Fukunaga et al (1997) found that 15% of ovarian epithelial malignancies (23% of which were endometrioid carcinomas) were associated with ipsilateral atypical endometriosis and that 63% of endometriosis associated with carcinomas was atypical: by contrast, ovarian endometriosis not associated with a carcinoma showed atypical features in only 2% of cases, this suggesting that atypical endometriosis does indeed play a rôle in the development of ovarian cancer. Ogawa et al (2000) found a direct transition from ovarian atypical endometriosis to carcinoma in 23 cases and further showed that the proliferative activity of atypical endometriosis was

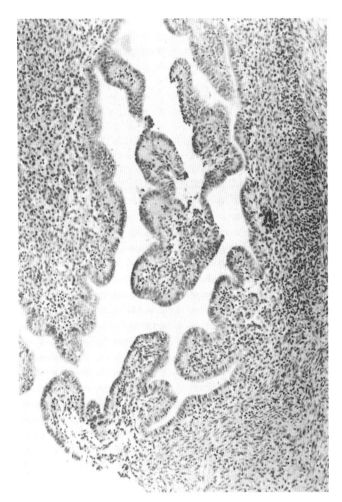

Fig. 29.15 Endometriosis showing papillary formation.

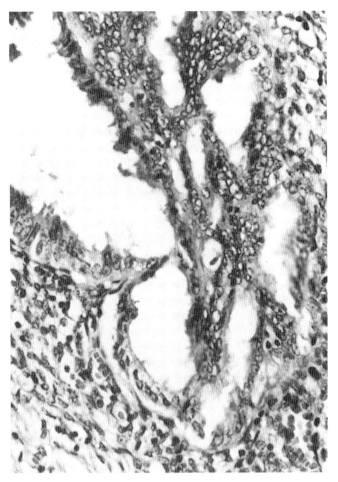

Fig. 29.16 Endometriosis showing evidence of atypical hyperplasia. (Reprinted with permission from Czernobilsky & Morris 1979, and from the American College of Obstetricians and Gynecologists.)

intermediate between the relatively low rate of typical endometriosis and the very high rate of ovarian carcinoma. It is findings such as these that led Feeley & Wells (2001) to suggest that atypical endometriosis should be regarded and classed as ovarian intraepithelial neoplasia.

Studies of the genetic changes in endometriosis may cast more light on its nature as a pre-malignant lesion than do those based solely on morphology. Ballouk et al (1994) showed that atypical ovarian endometriosis was associated with DNA aneuploidy, this suggesting genetic abnormalities whilst, as discussed previously, Jiang et al (1996) demonstrated loss of heterozygosity on chromosomes 9p, 11q or 22q in nearly 30% of cases of endometriosis unassociated with carcinoma and in nearly 75% of cases of endometriosis associated with a carcinoma. The application of molecular genetic techniques coupled with microdissection allowed these workers to subsequently demonstrate that in endometriotic foci adjacent to, or in direct contiguity with, an ovarian carcinoma there were identical genetic lesions in the endometriosis and the carcinoma, thus indicating a common lineage (Jiang et al 1998). Gogusev et al (1999)

demonstrated multiple copy losses on several chromosomes in 15 out of 18 cases of endometriosis, most commonly of 1p and 22q whilst Obata & Hoshiai (2000) found loss of heterozygosity on chromosome 6q and/or chromosome 10q in a high proportion of cases of atypical endometriosis: interestingly, *PTEN* mutations, a common feature of ovarian endometrioid carcinomas, were not detected in atypical endometriosis. There may be overexpression of wild type *p53* in some, but by no means all, cases of atypical endometriosis but mutation of the *p53* gene does not appear to occur (Vercellini et al 1994; Jiang et al 1996; Schneider et al 1998; Bayramoglu & Duzcan 2001; Nakayama et al 2001). This is, however, hardly suprising for *p53* mutation is not a feature of those types of carcinoma most commonly arising from endometriosis, namely early endometrioid and clear cell carcinoma.

The classic example of a malignant tumour arising from endometriosis is the ovarian endometrioid carcinoma which histologically mimics adenocarcinoma of the endometrium (Figs 29.22, 29.23): Toki et al (1996b) thought that approximately 30% of ovarian endometrioid carcinomas were derived from pre-existing

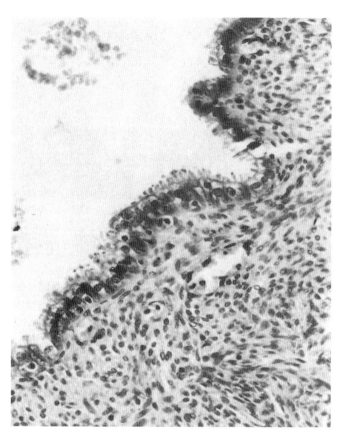

Fig. 29.17 Ovarian endometriosis lined by ciliated oviduct-like epithelium. (Reprinted with permission from Czernobilsky & Morris 1979, and from the American College of Obstetricians and Gynecologists.)

endometriosis. However, since, as mentioned above, endometrioid carcinomas can arise de novo from the ovarian surface epithelium and since even in these cases where the tumour originates from pre-existing endometriosis, it may overgrow the benign process, an actual transition between endometriosis and endometrioid carcinoma can only be demonstrated in relatively few cases. In the series of Czernobilsky et al (1970a,b), this was demonstrated in 4% of the patients. According to Scully (1977) such a continuity between benign endometriosis and endometrioid carcinoma can be shown in 5–10% of cases. Two of four proliferating endometrioid adeno- and cystadeno-fibromatous tumours reported by Roth et al (1981) arose in ovarian endometriosis. As has been mentioned before, the adjacent endometriosis may show atypical changes (Czernobilsky & Morris 1979; LaGrenade & Silverberg 1988). Sainz de la Cuesta et al (1996) have found evidence of endometriosis in 28% of Stage I epithelial ovarian cancer. In 32% of these cases the carcinoma actually arose in endometriosis which showed a spectrum of benign to atypical changes: most of the carcinomas associated and/or arising in endometriosis were of endometrioid or clear cell type. Stern et al (2001) found 8 endometrioid carcinomas and 9 clear cell carcinomas in a review of 484 cases of ovarian endometriosis: about one-third of these tumours were contiguous with a focus of endometriosis and two-thirds were adjacent to such a focus. Endometriosis in the ipsi- or contralateral ovary not showing continuity with endometrioid carcinoma has been reported in 9–17% of cases (Czernobilsky et al

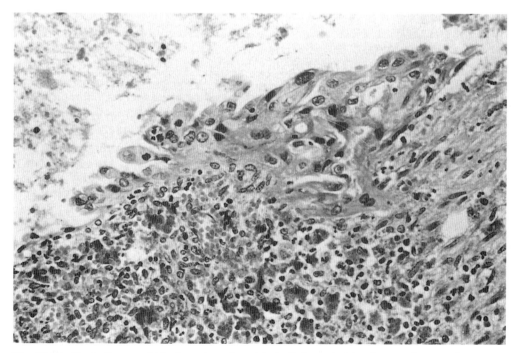

Fig. 29.18 Atypical squamoid features in endometriosis. Note underlying haemorrhage and haemosiderin-laden macrophages.

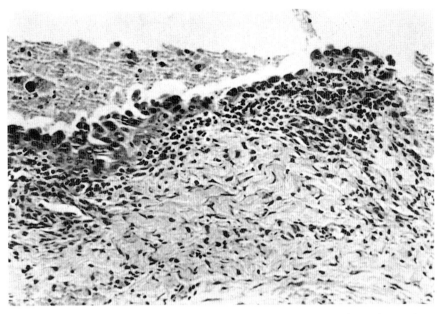

Fig. 29.19 Atypical epithelial lining of endometriotic cyst with large hyperchromatic nuclei.

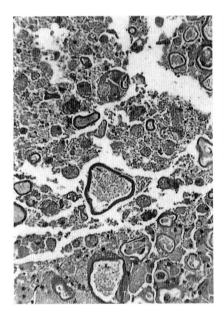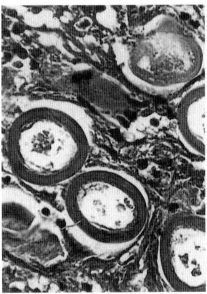

Fig. 29.20 Liesegang rings in endometriosis, admixed with debris within lumen of cyst (left); and embedded within cyst wall (right). (Reprinted with permission from Clement 1990.)

1970a; Aure et al 1971), whereas pelvic extraovarian endometriosis was present in 11–28% of patients with endometrioid carcinoma (Czernobilsky et al 1970a; Kurman & Craig 1972; Curling & Hudson 1975; Russell 1979).

Scully et al (1966) showed that four of 17 cases of ovarian clear cell carcinoma actually arose in endometriosis and in a number of more recent series of ovarian malignancy in endometriosis, clear cell carcinomas have outnumbered endometrioid carcinomas (Vercellini et al 1993; Toki et al 1996; Chew et al 1997; Jimbo et al 1997b; Ogawa et al 2000; Yoshikawa et al 2000; Stern et al 2001). Toki et al (1966a) considered that

approximately 50% of ovarian clear cell carcinomas arose from endometriosis and this close relationship of endometriosis to ovarian clear cell tumours was, in fact, advanced as one of the original arguments in favour of a Müllerian rather than mesonephric origin of clear cell neoplasms (Scully & Barlow 1967).

Although some other common epithelial tumours of the ovary have also been shown to be occasionally associated with endometriosis, the frequency of this association is much lower than that seen in endometrioid and clear cell carcinomas. According to Russell (1979), pelvic endometriosis is present in 3% of patients with serous and 4% of patients with ovarian mucinous carcinomas.

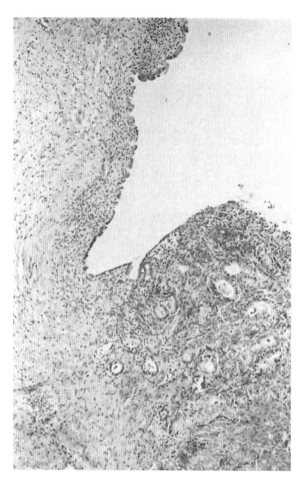

Fig. 29.21 Endometriotic cyst with endometrioid adenocarcinoma directly arising from it.

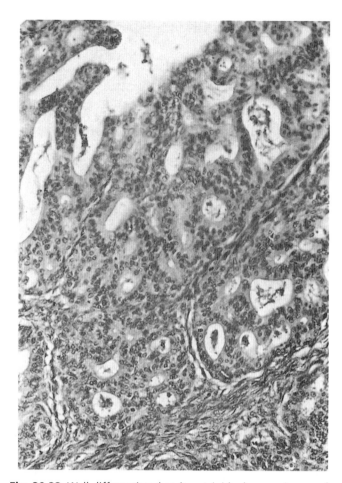

Fig. 29.22 Well-differentiated endometrioid adenocarcinoma of ovary.

There is, however, a high incidence of associated endometriosis in women with mucinous bordeline tumours of Müllerian type (Rutgers & Scully 1988). In addition there have been reports of mixed mesodermal (Müllerian) tumours which arose in endometriosis (Cooper 1978; Marchevsky & Kaneko 1978).

Of about 45 cases of ovarian endometrioid stromal sarcomas reported, at least 40% have been contiguous with endometriosis (Palladino & Trousdell 1969; Gruskin et al 1970; Young et al 1984; Shakfeh & Woodruff 1987; Kavanagh & Wharton 1990; Young & Scully 1990; Baiocchi et al 1990; Shiraki et al 1991; Chang et al 1993). Since in about 30% of these cases there were also sarcomas in the uterus, the question has been raised whether some of the ovarian sarcomas were metastatic from the latter (Young & Scully 1990).

Squamous cell carcinoma arising in ovarian endometriosis is rare and only 12 cases have been reported so far (McCullough et al 1946; Lele et al 1978; Tetu et al 1987; Naresh et al 1991; Pins et al 1996). It should be stressed, however, that in these instances endometrioid adenocarcinoma with extensive squamous differentiation and secondary squamous tumours must be excluded.

Malignant tumours also arise in extraovarian endometriosis, albeit with considerable rarity (Brooks & Wheeler 1977; Heaps et al 1990). In most series two-thirds of these have been endometrioid carcinomas, one-third of which have been situated in the rectovaginal septum (Mostoufizadeh & Scully 1980; Heaps et al 1990). Clear cell carcinomas also develop in extragonadal endometriosis (Brooks & Wheeler 1977; Goldberg et al 1978; Mesko et al 1988; Hitti et al 1990; Balat et al 1996; Bolis & Maccio 2000; McCluggage et al 2001) and in one recent series this was the tumour type most commonly associated with extraovarian endometriosis (Stern et al 2001). Other types of carcinoma, endometrial stromal sarcomas and adenosarcomas have also been reported to arise in extraovarian endometriosis in sites such as the Fallopian tube, rectovaginal septum, vagina, vulva, the colon, rectum, small intestine, urinary bladder, omentum and pleura (La Pava et al 1963; Scully et al 1966; Palladino & Trousdell 1969; Labay & Feiner 1971; Brooks & Wheeler 1977; Persad & Anderson 1977; Berkowitz et al 1978; Brunson et al 1988; Baiocchi et al 1990; Kavanagh & Wharton 1990; Vierhout et al 1992; Bishara & Scapa 1997; Kondi-Paphitis et al 1998; Judson

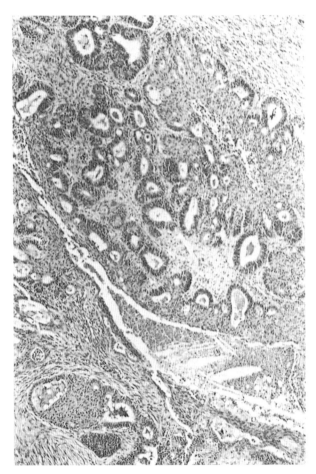

Fig. 29.23 Endometrioid adenocarcinoma with benign squamous differentiation.

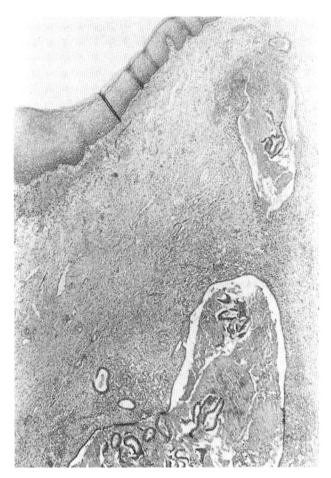

Fig. 29.24 Vagina with endometriosis in wall.

et al 2000; Slavin et al 2000; Yantiss et al 2000; Bosincu et al 2001; Mourra et al 2001). A transition from benign endometriosis to the malignant neoplasm could only be demonstrated in some of these cases but, in general, an endometrioid adenocarcinoma occurring in a site where endometriosis is likely to occur can often be presumed to be derived from endometriosis. Within the bowel the cytokeratin (CK) staining pattern of an adenocarcinoma derived from endometriosis will be similar to that of an ovarian carcinoma (CK7+ CK20–) and unlike that of a gastrointestinal neoplasm (Han et al 1998; McCluggage et al 2001).

CLINICAL ASPECTS

The symptomatology of endometriosis varies considerably from patient to patient and depends, at least to some degree, on the extent of the disease as well as on the location of the endometriotic lesions. Furthermore, about 25% of patients with endometriosis have no symptoms at all (Parsons & Sommers 1978). In the remaining patients there is, in order of decreasing frequency, pelvic pain or discomfort, dyspareunia and irregular uterine bleeding (Ranney 1980b). In those patients in whom endometrio

sis involves the vagina (Fig. 29.24), uterine cervix (Fig. 29.25), intestinal tract (Fig. 29.26), urinary bladder or ureter, the symptomatology is frequently related to the specific areas involved. Thus, with endometriosis of the large intestine it is not unusual for obstruction or tenesmus to develop, whereas patients with endometriosis of the small intestine may suffer from volvulus or intussusception and can even develop a protein-losing enteropathy (Henley et al 1993). Endometriosis of the urinary tract may result in dysuria, haematuria or obstructive phenomena (Honoré 1999).

One of the most significant features of endometriosis is the often associated infertility. The true incidence of infertility is difficult to determine accurately for widely quoted figures of about 40% of patients with endometriosis suffering from this complication (Parsons & Sommers 1978) are mainly based on studies which predate the widespread use of laparoscopy and thus weight the study population disproportionately with patients with severe endometriosis, in whom mechanical damage can clearly cause infertility. It has been much debated as to whether or not reduced fertility is a feature of patients with only minimal or mild endometriosis. Thomas (1991) critically reviewed the literature and came to the conclusion that, in the

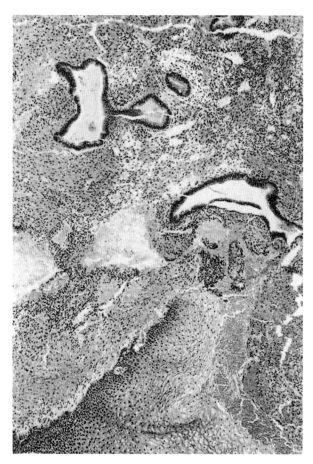

Fig. 29.25 Cervical endometriosis showing endometrial glands surrounded by stroma and haemorrhage causing ulceration of overlying exocervical epithelium.

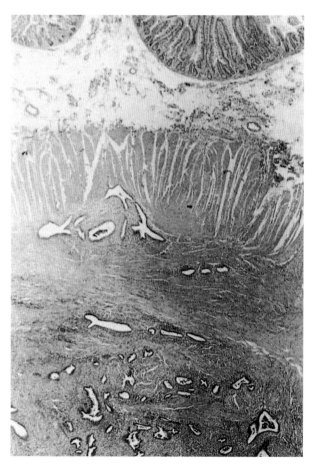

Fig. 29.26 Extensive endometriosis in serosa and muscularis of small intestine.

absence of mechanical damage, endometriosis does not cause infertility. Two recent reviews, both basing their conclusions largely upon studies of women with mild or minimal disease being treated with assisted reproductive techniques, have not fully resolved this problem though Burns & Schenken (1999) pointed out that the one prospective study (Jansen 1986) documented a significant decrease in fecundity in women with minimal endometriosis whilst Wingfield (2000) concluded that in studies involving infertile couples minimal or mild endometriosis did seem to be an added negative fertility factor.

Although the exact mechanism of the infertility in these patients remains unknown, the relatively good results following a variety of surgical procedures indicate that mechanical factors, particularly involving ovaries and oviducts such as fibrosis, adhesions, tubal obstruction (Fig. 29.27) and a retroverted uterus, play a rôle in at least a number of these patients with severe or extensive endometriosis (Kistner 1975; Weed & Holland 1977; Napolitano et al 1994). It has also been suggested that altered tubal secretion due to chronic salpingitis may be instrumental in infertility associated with endometriosis. Some support for this may be found in the surprisingly

high incidence (33%) of chronic salpingitis without obstruction in patients with ovarian endometriosis (Czernobilsky & Silverstein 1978) (Fig. 29.28). To this should also be added other possible factors such as ovarian dysfunction, anovulatory bleeding, and an increase in the incidence of underdeveloped uteri (Parsons & Sommers 1978). Kistner (1975) claimed that if other pathological conditions are excluded, the most important factor responsible for infertility in endometriosis is an inadequacy of tubo-ovarian motility secondary to fibrosis and scarring resulting in imperfect ovum acceptance by the fimbriae.

Other theories which attempt to explain the infertility associated with endometriosis include an autoimmune mechanism. Weed & Arquembourg (1980) suggested that endometriosis stimulates an immune response to the host's own endometrial proteins which are recognised by the host as 'foreign' and that this immune response may result in the rejection of early implantation of embryos or interfere with sperm passage. Anti-endometrial antibodies certainly occur in endometriosis but evidence that such antibodies are not epiphenomenal and play a rôle in the infertility associated with endometriosis is lacking (Halme & Surrey 1990; Burns & Schenken 1999). Yet another

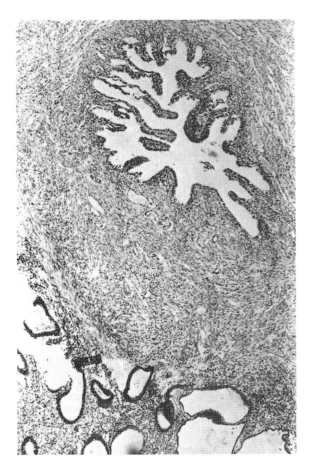

Fig. 29.27 Fallopian tube with endometriosis in wall.

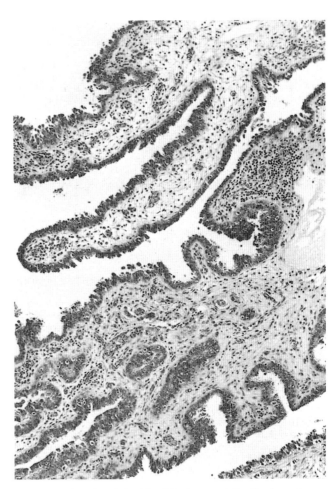

Fig. 29.28 Chronic salpingitis with abnormal distribution of ciliated and secretory cells in a case of ovarian endometriosis. (Reprinted with permission from Czernobilsky & Silverstein 1978, and from the American Fertility Society.)

hypothesis concerns the rôle of prostaglandins in the infertility of these women. Young et al (1981) demonstrated that under in vivo and in vitro conditions ectopically situated endometrium produced larger quantities of prostaglandin F, which affects tubal motility, than in normal conditions, whilst there is also evidence that prostacyclin (PGI_2), which causes relaxation of tubal musculature, is produced in excess by the peritoneal epithelium in women with endometriosis (Drake et al 1981). Although much attention has been lavished upon the putative rôle of prostanoids in endometriosis-related infertility, their significance in this respect is currently out of favour (Hurst & Rock 1991). It has also been shown that peritoneal macrophages in women with endometriosis are unusually numerous and have an enhanced capacity for phagocytosing sperm (Muscato et al 1982); it has therefore been thought that entry of such cells into the tube could lead to excessive engulfment of sperm and hence to infertility. The many studies of peritoneal macrophages in endometriosis have, however, yielded inconsistent results and are open to considerable methodological criticism (Hurst & Rock 1991) and this theory therefore remains to be validated (Burns & Schenken 1999). Infertility in women with mild endometriosis has been attributed to the luteinized unruptured follicle syndrome in

which there is a failure of follicular rupture and retention of the oocyte within the ovary (Brosens et al 1978) and in a definitive study of this relationship Mio et al (1992) found unruptured follicles in nearly 25% of infertile women with minimal or mild endometriosis. It has been commented that 'the luteinized unruptured follicle syndrome could contribute to endometriosis-associated subfertility but does not plausibly qualify as the usual, predominant or exclusive cause of such infertility' (Burns & Schenken 1999).

Recent findings suggest that despite all these various pathophysiological hypotheses, infertility in women with minimal or mild endometriosis may, as with severe disease, also be due to mechanical factors for new techniques of transvaginal laparoscopy and inspection of the ovaries by hydroflotation have shown that even mild cases of endometriosis are very frequently associated with peri-ovarian adhesions (Campo et al 1999).

In addition to surgical management, hormonal therapy plays an important rôle in the control of this disease. This includes oestrogen–progestagen or so-called pseudopregnancy therapy which transforms functioning endometriosis into decidua with subsequent necrosis and healing (Kistner 1958), or the administration of Danazol (Danocrine) to produce a temporary menopausal state. This latter drug is an orally active gonadotrophin inhibitory agent devoid of oestrogenic and progestational activity (Dmowski et al 1971). More recently, LH-releasing hormone analogues, which decrease pituitary sensitivity to LH-releasing hormone, have also been used successfully for the treatment of endometriosis (Shaw 1991). While the advantages of surgical and/or medical therapy for endometriosis are still being debated it appears that surgery still remains the principal means of treatment. According to Puolakka et al (1980), who evaluated the results of operative treatment of pelvic endometriosis, 30% of the patients became symptomless, 41% estimated the overall result as good, and 19% as moderate, whereas only 10% experienced deterioration or had no help from the operation. Eight per cent of the patients had recurrence of the disease that demanded re-operation. Since infertility constitutes one of the major complications of pelvic endometriosis, it is important to note that in Puolakka et al's series (1980) a 63% pregnancy rate was achieved following surgical therapy in 32 patients.

REFERENCES

Acosta A A, Buttram V C Jr, Besch P K, Malinak L R, Franklin R R, Vanderheyden J D 1973 A proposed classification of pelvic endometriosis. Obstetrics and Gynecology 42: 19–25

American Fertility Society 1979 Classification of endometriosis. Fertility and Sterility 32: 631–634

American Fertility Society 1985 Revised American Fertility Society classifications of endometriosis. Fertility and Sterility 43: 351–352

American Society for Reproductive Medicine 1997 Revised American Society for Reproductive Medicine classification of endometriosis: 1996. Fertility and Sterility 65: 817–821

Anaf V, Simon P, Fayt I, Noel J 2000 Smooth muscles are frequent components of endometriotic lesions. Human Reproduction 15: 767–771

Andrews M C, Andrews W C, Strauss A F 1959 Effects of progestin-induced pseudopregnancy on endometriosis: clinical and microscopic studies. American Journal of Obstetrics and Gynecology 78: 776–785

Aure J C, Loeg K, Kolstadt P 1971 Carcinoma of the ovary and endometriosis. Acta Obstetricia et Gynecologica Scandinavica 50: 63–67

Baiocchi G, Kavanagh J J, Wharton J T 1990 Endometrioid stromal sarcomas arising from ovarian and extraovarian endometriosis: report of two cases and review of the literature. Gynecologic Oncology 36: 147–151

Balat O, Kudelka A P, Edwards C L, Silva E, Kavanagh J J 1996 Malignant transformation in endometriosis of the urinary bladder: a case report of clear cell adenocarcinoma. European Journal of Gynaecological Oncology 17: 13–16

Ballouk F, Ross J S, Wolf B C 1994 Ovarian endometriotic cysts: an analysis of cytologic atypia and DNA ploidy. American Journal of Clinical Pathology 102: 415–419

Barcz E, Kaminski P, Marianowski L 2000 Role of cytokines in pathogenesis of endometriosis. Medical Science Monitors 6: 1042–1046

Bassis M L 1956 Pseudodeciduosis. American Journal of Obstetrics and Gynecology 72: 1029–1037

Batt R E, Smith R A 1989 Embryologic theory of histogenesis of endometriosis in peritoneal pockets. Obstetrical and Gynecologic Clinics of North America 16: 15–28

Batt R E, Smith R A, Buck G M, Severino M F, Naples J D 1990 Mullerianosis. In: Chadha D R, Buttram V C (eds) Current concepts in endometriosis. Alan R Liss, New York, pp 413–426

Bayramoglu H, Duzcan E 2001 Atypical epithelial changes and mutant p53 gene expression in ovarian endometriosis. Pathology Oncology Research 7: 33–38

Beliard A, Donnez J, Nisolle M, Foidart J M 1997 Localization of laminin, fibronectin, E-cadherin, and integrins in endometrium and endometriosis. Fertility and Sterility 67: 266–272

Bergquist A 1991 Steroid receptors in endometriosis. In: Thomas E J, Rock J A (eds) Modern approaches to endometriosis. Kluwer Academic Press, Dordecht, pp 33–55

Bergquist A, Ljungberg O, Skoog L 1993 Immunohistochemical analysis of oestrogen and progesterone receptors in endometriotic tissue and endometrium. Human Reproduction 8: 1915–1922

Berkowitz R S, Ehrmann R, Knapp R C 1978 Endometrial stromal sarcoma arising from vaginal endometriosis. Obstetrics and Gynecology 51: 34S–37S

Bishara M, Scapa E 1997 Stromal uterine sarcoma arising from intestinal endometriosis after abdominal hysterectomy and salpingo-oophorectomy. Harefuah 133: 353–355

Bolis G B, Maccio T 2000 Clear cell adenocarcinoma of the vulva arising in endometriosis: a case report. European Journal of Gynaecological Oncology 21: 416–417

Bosincu L, Massarelli G, Cossu-Rocca P, Isaac M A, Nogales F F 2001 Rectal endometrial stromal sarcoma arising in endometriosis: report of a case. Diseases of the Colon and Rectum 44: 890–892

Bridges J E, Prentice A, Roche W et al 1994 Expression of integrin adhesion molecules in endometrium and endometriosis. British Journal of Obstetrics and Gynaecology 101: 696–700

Brooks J J, Wheeler J E 1977 Malignancy arising in extragonadal endometriosis: a case report and summary of the world literature. Cancer 40: 3065–3073

Brosens I A, Koninckx P R, Corveleyn P A 1978 A study of plasma progesterone, oestradiol-17beta, prolactin and LH levels and of the luteal phase appearance of the ovaries in patients with endometriosis and infertility. British Journal of Obstetrics and Gynaecology 85: 246–250

Brunson G L, Barclay D L, Sanders M, Araoz C A 1988 Malignant extraovarian endometriosis: two case reports and review of the literature. Gynecologic Oncology 30: 125–130

Brzezinski A, Koren Z 1962 Endometriosis in Israel. American Journal of Obstetrics and Gynecology 83: 414–416

Burns W N, Schenken R S 1999 Pathophysiology of endometriosis-associated infertility. Clinical Obstetrics and Gynecology 42: 596–610

Campo R, Gordts S, Rombauts L, Brosens I 1999 Diagnostic accuracy of transvaginal hydrolaparoscopy in infertility. Fertility and Sterility 71: 1157–1160

Cantor J O, Fenoglio C M, Richart R M 1979 A case of extensive endometriosis. American Journal of Obstetrics and Gynecology 134: 846–847

Chang A, Natarajan S 2001 Polypoid endometriosis. Archives of Pathology and Laboratory Medicine 125: 1257

Chang K L, Crabtree G S, Li,-Tan S K, Kempson R L, Hendrickson M R 1993 Primary extrauterine endometrial stromal neoplasms: a clinicopathologic study of 20 cases and a review of the literature. International Journal of Gynecological Pathology 12: 282–296

Charles D 1957 Endometriosis and hemorrhagic pleural effusion. Obstetrics and Gynecology 10: 309–312

Chew S, Tham K F, Ratnam S S 1997 A series of ovarian clear cell and endometrioid carcinoma and their association with endometriosis. Singapore Medical Journal 38: 289–291

Chung H W, Wen Y, Chun S H, Nezhat C, Woo B H, Lake-Polan M 2001 Matrix metalloproteinase-9 and tissue inhibitor of metalloproteinase-3 mRNA expression in ectopic and eutopic endometrium in women with endometriosis: a rationale for endometriotic invasiveness. Fertility and Sterility 75: 152–159

Clement P B 1990 Pathology of endometriosis. In: Rosen P R, Fechner R E (eds) Pathology annual, part 1, vol 25. Appleton & Lange, Norwalk, pp 245–295

Clement P V, Young R H, Scully R E 1988 Necrotic pseudoxanthomatous nodules of ovary and peritoneum in endometriosis. American Journal of Surgical Pathology 12: 390–397

Clement P B, Young R H, Scully R E 1989 Liesengang rings in the female genital tract: a report of three cases. International Journal of Gynecological Pathology 8: 271–276

Cohen M R 1980 Laparoscopic diagnosis and pseudomenopause treatment of endometriosis cysts with danazol. Clinical Obstetrics and Gynecology 23: 901–915

Cooper P 1978 Mixed mesodermal tumor and clear cell carcinoma arising in ovarian endometriosis. Cancer 42: 2827–2831

Cozzutto C 1981 Uterus-like mass replacing ovary: report of a new entity. Archives of Pathology and Laboratory Medicine 105: 508–511

Cullen T S 1925 Discussion: Symposium on misplaced endometrial tissue. American Journal of Obstetrics and Gynecology 10: 732–733

Curling O M, Hudson C N 1975 Endometrioid tumours of the ovary. British Journal of Obstetrics and Gynaecology 82: 405–411

Czernobilsky B 1982 Endometrioid neoplasia of the ovary: a reappraisal. International Journal of Gynecological Pathology 1: 203–210

Czernobilsky B 1987 Primary epithelial tumors of the ovary. In: Kurman R J (ed) Blaustein's pathology of the female genital tract, 3rd edn. Springer-Verlag, New York, pp 560–606

Czernobilsky B, Morris W J 1979 A histologic study of ovarian endometriosis with emphasis on hyperplastic and atypical changes. Obstetrics and Gynecology 53: 318–323

Czernobilsky B, Silverstein A 1978 Salpingitis in ovarian endometriosis. Fertility and Sterility 30: 45–49

Czernobilsky B, Silverman B B, Mikuta J J 1970a Endometrioid carcinoma of the ovary: a clinicopathologic study of 75 cases. Cancer 26: 1141–1152

Czernobilsky B, Silverman B B, Enterline H T 1970b Clear cell carcinoma of the ovary: a clinicopathologic analysis of pure and mixed forms and comparison with endometrioid carcinoma. Cancer 25: 762–772

D'Hooghe T M, Hill J A 1995 Autoantibodies in endometriosis. In: Kurpisz M, Fernandez N (eds) Immunobiology of human reproduction. BIOS Scientific Publishers, Oxford, pp 133–162

D'Hooghe T M, Hill J A 1996 Immunobiology of endometriosis. In: Bronson R A, Alexander N Y, Anderson D Y (eds) Reproductive immunology. Blackwell, Cambridge MA, pp 322–356

D'Hooghe T M, Raeymaekers B M, De Jonge I, Lauweryns J M, Koninckx P R 1995 Intrapelvic injection of menstrual endometrium causes endometriosis in baboons (Papio cynocephalus and Papio anubis). American Journal of Obstetrics and Gynecology 173: 125–134

Di Palo S, Mari G, Castolda R et al 1989 Endometriosis of the lung. Respiratory Medicine 83: 255–258

Dizerega G S, Barber D L, Hodgen G D 1980 Endometriosis: role of ovarian steroids in initiation, maintenance and suppression. Fertility and Sterility 33: 649–653

Dmowski W P, Scholer H F, Mahesch V B, Greenblatt R B 1971 Danazol: a synthetic steroid derivative with interesting physiologic properties. Fertility and Sterility 22: 9–18

Dmowski W P, Steele R W, Baker G F 1981 Deficient cellular immunity in endometriosis. American Journal of Obstetrics and Gynecology 141: 377–383

Dmowski W P, Braun D, Gebel H 1990 Endometriosis: genetic and immunologic aspects. In: Chadha D R, Buttram V C (eds) Current concepts in endometriosis. Proceedings of the second international symposium on endometriosis. Alan R Liss, New York, pp 99–122

Dmowski W P, Braun D, Gebel H 1991 The immune system in endometriosis. In: Thomas E J, Rock J A (eds) Modern approaches to endometriosis. Kluwer, Dordrecht, pp 97–111

Dmowski W P, Gebel H, Braun D P 1998 Decreased apoptosis and sensitivity to macrophage mediated cytolysis of endometrial cells in endometriosis. Human Reproduction Update 4: 696–701

Donnez J, Nisolle M, Casanas-Roux F et al 1995 Rectovaginal septum, endometriosis or adenomyosis: laparoscopic management in a series of 231 patients. Human Reproduction 10: 630–635

Donnez J, Nisolle M, Smoes P, Gillet N, Beguin S, Casanas-Roux F 1996 Peritoneal endometriosis and 'endometriotic' nodules of the rectovaginal septum are two different entities. Fertility and Sterility 66: 362–368

Drake T S, O'Brien W F, Ramwell P W, Metz S A 1981 Peritoneal fluid thromboxane B2 and 6-keto-prostaglandin Fla in endometriosis. American Journal of Obstetrics and Gynecology 140: 401–404

Espaulella J, Armengol J, Bella F, Lain J M, Calaf J 1991 Pulmonary endometriosis: conservative treatment with GnRH agonists. Obstetrics and Gynecology 78: 535–537

Evers J L H 1994 Endometriosis does not exist: all women have endometriosis. Human Reproduction 9: 2206–2211

Fasciani A, D'Ambrogio G, Bocci G, Monti M, Genazzani A R, Artini P G 2000 High concentration of the vascular endothelial growth factor and interleukin-8 in ovarian endometriomata. Molecular Human Reproduction 6: 50–54

Fedele L, Bianchi S, Di-Nola G et al 1992 Endometriosis and non-obstructive mullerian anomalies. Obstetrics and Gynecology 79: 515–517

Feeley K M, Wells M 2001 Precursor lesions of ovarian epithelial malignancy. Histopathology 38: 87–95

Flieder D B, Moran C A, Travis W, Koss M N, Mark E J 1998 Pleuro-pulmonary endometriosis and pulmonary ectopic deciduosis: a clinicopathologic and immunohistochemical study of 10 cases with emphasis on diagnostic pitfalls. Human Pathology 29: 1495–1503

Fox H 1983 The pathology of endometriosis. Irish Journal of Medical Sciences 152 (suppl 2): 9–13

Fox H, Buckley C H 1984 Current concepts of endometriosis. Clinics in Obstetrics and Gynaecology 11: 279–287

Fujimoto J, Sakaguchi H, Hirose R, Wen H, Tamaya T 1999 Angiogenesis in endometriosis and angiogenic factors. Gynecologic and Obstetric Investigation 48 (supplement): 114–120

Fujii S 1991 Secondary mullerian system and endometriosis. American Journal of Obstetrics and Gynecology 165: 219–225

Fukaya T, Sugawara J, Yoshida H, Murakami T, Yajima A 1999 Intercellular adhesion molecule-1 and hepatocyte growth factor in human endometriosis: original investigation and a review of the literature. Gynecologic and Obstetric Investigation 47 (Supplement): 16–17

Fukunaga M 2000 Smooth muscle metaplasia in ovarian endometriosis. Histopathology 36: 348–352

Fukunaga M, Ushigome S 1998 Epithelial metaplastic changes in ovarian endometriosis. Modern Pathology 11: 784–788

Fukunaga M, Nomura K, Ishikawa E, Ushigome S 1997 Ovarian atypical endometriosis: its close association with malignant epithelial tumours. Histopathology 30: 249–255

Gardner G H, Greene R R, Ranney B 1953 The histogenesis of endometriosis — recent contributions. Obstetrics and Gynecology 1: 615–637

Garzetti G G, Ciavattini A, Provincial I M et al 1993 Natural killer cell activity in endometriosis: correlation between serum estradiol levels and cytotoxicity. Obstetrics and Gynecology 81: 685–688

Gerbie A B, Green R R, Reis R A 1958 Heteroplastic bone and cartilage in the female genital tract. Obstetrics and Gynecology 11: 573–578

Giangarra C, Gallo G, Newman R, Dorfman H 1987 Endometriosis in the biceps femoris: a case report and review of the literature. Journal of Bone and Joint Surgery 69: 290–292

Gogusev J, Bouquet de Joliniere J, Telvi L et al 1999 Detection of DNA copy number changes in human endometriosis by comparative genomic hybridization. Human Genetics 105: 444–451

Goldberg M I, Ng A B P, Belinson J L, Hutson E D, Nordquist S R B 1978 Clear cell adenocarcinoma arising in endometriosis of the rectovaginal septum. Obstetrics and Gynecology 51: 38S–40S

Goldman M B, Cramer D W 1990 The epidemiology of endometriosis. In: Chadha D R, Buttram V C (eds) Current concepts in endometriosis. Proceedings of the second international symposium on endometriosis. Alan R Liss, New York, pp 15–31

Gruskin P, Osborne N G, Morley G W, Abell M R 1970 Primary endometrial stromatosis of ovary: report of a case. Obstetrics and Gynecology 36: 702–707

Gupta S D 1985 Endometriosis in the thumb. Journal of the Indian Medical Association 83: 122–124

Hadfield R M, Mardon H J, Barlow D H, Kennedy S H 1997 Endometriosis in monozygotic twins. Fertility and Sterility 68: 941–942

Haining R E, Cameron I T, van Papendorp C et al 1991 Epidermal growth factor in human endometrium: proliferative effects in culture and immunocytochemical localization in normal and endometriotic tissues. Human Reproduction 6: 1200–1205

Halban Y 1925 Hysteroadenosis metastatica. Archive fur Gynakologie 124: 457–482

Halme J, Surrey J S 1990 Endometriosis and infertility: the mechanisms invovled. In: Chadha D R, Buttram V C (eds) Current concepts in endometriosis. Alan R Liss, New York, pp 157–178

Halme J, Hammond M G, Hulka J F et al 1984 Retrograde menstruation in healthy women and in patients with endometriosis. Obstetrics and Gynecology 64: 151–154

Han A C, Hovenden S, Rosenblum N G, Salazar H 1998 Adenocarcinoma arising in extragonadal endometriosis: an immunohistochemical study. Cancer 83: 1163–1169

Haney A F 1990 Etiology and histogenesis of endometriosis. In: Chadha D R, Buttram V C (eds) Current concepts in endometriosis. Alan R Liss, New York, pp 1–14

Haney A F 1991 The pathogenesis and aetiology of endometriosis. In: Thomas E J, Rock J A (eds) Modern approaches to endometriosis. Kluwer Academic Press, Dordrecht, pp 3–19

Harada T, Enatsu A, Mitsunari M et al 1999 Role of cytokines in progression of endometriosis. Gynecologic and Obstetric Investigation 47 (Supplement): 141–145

Healy D L, Rogers P A, Hii L, Wingfield M 1998 Angiogenesis: a new theory for endometriosis. Human Reproduction Update 4: 736–740

Heaps J M, Nieberg R K, Berek J S 1990 Malignant neoplasms arising in endometriosis. Obstetrics and Gynecology 75: 1023–1028

Henley J D, Kratzer S S, Seo I S et al 1993 Endometriosis of the small intestine presenting as a protein-losing enteropathy. American Journal of Gastroenterology 88: 130–133

Hertig A T, Gore H 1961 Tumors of female sex organs. Part 3 Tumors of the ovary and fallopian tube. In: Atlas of tumor pathology, section IX, fascicle 33. Armed Forces Institute of Pathology, Washington, DC, pp 106–108

Hill J A 1992 Immunology and endometriosis. Fertility and Sterility 58: 262–264

Hitti I F, Glasberg S S, Lubicz S 1990 Clear cell carcinoma arising in extraovarian endometriosis: report of three cases and review of the literature. Gynecologic Oncology 39: 314–320

Hoeger K M, Guzick D S 1999 An update on the classification of endometriosis. Clinical Obstetrics and Gynecology 42: 611–619

Honoré G M 1999 Extrapelvic endometriosis. Clinical Obstetrics and Gynecology 42: 699–711

Houston D E, Noller K L, Melton L Y, Selwyn B J, Hardy R J 1987 Incidence of pelvic endometriosis in Rochester, Minnesota, 1970–1979. American Journal of Epidemiology 125: 959–969

Huffman J W 1951 External endometriosis. American Journal of Obstetrics and Gynecology 62: 1243–1252

Hurst B S, Rock J A 1991 The peritoneal environment in endometriosis. In: Thomas E J, Rock J A (eds) Modern approaches to endometriosis. Kluwer Academic Press, Dordrecht, pp 79–96

Ichimiya M, Hirota T, Muto M 1998 Intralymphatic embolic cells with cutaneous endometriosis in the umbilicus. Journal of Dermatology 25: 333–336

Imai A, Takagi A, Tamaya T 2000 Gonadotropin-releasing hormone agonist repairs reduced endometrial cell apoptosis in endometriosis in vitro. American Journal of Obstetrics and Gynecology 182: 1142–1146

Jansen R P S 1986 Minimal endometriosis and reduced fecundibility: evidence from an artificial insemination by a donor programme. Fertility and Sterility 46: 141–143

Jansen R P S, Russell P 1986 Non-pigmented endometriosis: clinical, laparoscopic and pathologic definition. American Journal of Obstetrics and Gynecology 155: 1154–1159

Javert C T 1949 Pathogenesis of endometriosis based upon endometrial homeoplasia, direct extension, exfoliation and implantation, lymphatic and hematogenous metastasis (including five case reports of endometrial tissue in pelvic lymph nodes). Cancer 2: 399–410

Javert C T 1951 Observations on the pathology and spread of endometriosis based on the theory of benign metastases. American Journal of Obstetrics and Gynecology 62: 477–487

Jiang X, Hitchcock A, Bryan E J et al 1996 Microsatellite analysis of endometriosis reveals loss of heterozygosity at candidate ovarian tumor suppressor gene loci. Cancer Research 56: 3534–3539

Jiang X, Morland S J, Hitchcock A, Thomas E J, Campbell I G 1998 Allelotyping of endometriosis with adjacent ovarian carcinoma reveals evidence of a common lineage. Cancer Research 58: 1707–1712

Jimbo H, Hitomi Y, Yoshikawa H et al 1997a Evidence for monoclonal expansion of epithelial cells in ovarian endometrial cysts. American Journal of Pathology 150: 1173–1178

Jimbo H, Yoshikawa H, Onda T, Yasugi T, Sakamoto A, Taketani I 1997b Prevalence of ovarian endometriosis in epithelial ovarian cancer. International Journal of Gynaecology and Obstetrics 59: 245–250

Jolicoeur C, Boutouil M, Drouin R et al 1998 Increased expression of monocyte chemotactic protein-1 in the endometrium of women with endometriosis. American Journal of Pathology 152: 125–133

Judson P L, Temple A M, Fowler W C, Novotny D B, Funkhouser W K 2000 Vaginal adenosarcoma arising from endometriosis. Gynecologic Oncology 76: 123–125

Kale S, Shuster M, Shangold J 1971 Endometrioma in cesarian scar: case report and review of the literature. American Journal of Obstetrics and Gynecology 111: 596–597

Kapadia S B, Russak R R, O'Donnell W F, Harris R N, Lecky J W 1984 Postmenopausal ureteral endometriosis with atypical adenomatous hyperplasia following hysterectomy, bilateral oophorectomy and long-term estrogen therapy. Obstetrics and Gynecology 64: 60S–63S

Karp L A, Czernobilsky B 1969 Glandular inclusions in pelvic and abdominal para-aortic lymph nodes: a study of autopsy and surgical material in males and females. American Journal of Clinical Pathology 52: 212–218

Kavanagh J J, Wharton J T 1990 Endometrioid stromal sarcomas arising from ovarian and extraovarian endometriosis: report of two cases and review of the literature. Gynecologic Oncology 36: 147–151

Kempson R K 1973 Sarcomas and related neoplasms. In: Norris H G, Hertig A T, Abell M R (eds) The uterus. Williams & Wilkins, Baltimore, pp 298–319

Kennedy S, Mardon H, Barlow D 1995 Familial endometriosis. Journal of Assisted Reproduction and Genetics 12: 32–34

Kerner H, Gaton E, Czernobilsky B 1981 Unusual ovarian, tubal and pelvic mesothelial inclusions in patients with endometriosis. Histopathology 5: 277–283

Khan M S, Dodson A R, Heatley M K 1999 Ki-67, oestrogen receptor, and progesterone receptor proteins in the human *rete ovarii* and in endometriosis. Journal of Clinical Pathology 52: 517–520

Kistner R W 1958 The use of newer progestins in the treatment of endometriosis. American Journal of Obstetrics and Gynecology 75: 264–278

Kistner R W 1975 Management of endometriosis in the infertile patient. Fertility and Sterility 26: 1151–1166

Kistner R W, Siegler A, Berhman S J 1977 Suggested classification for endometriosis: relationship to infertility. Fertility and Sterility 28: 1008–1010

Kobayashi H 2000 Invasive capacity of heterotopic endometrium. Gynecologic and Obstetric Investigation 50 (Supplement): 126–132

Kokerine I, Nisolle M, Donnez J et al 1997 Expression of interstitial collagenase (matrix metalloproteinase-1) is related to the activity of human endometriotic lesions. Fertility and Sterility 68: 246–251

Kondi-Paphitis A, Smyrniotis B, Liapis A, Kontoyanni A, Deligeorgi H 1998 Stromal sarcoma arising in endometriosis: a clinicopathological and immunohistochemical study of 4 cases. European Journal of Gynaecological Oncology 19: 588–590

Koninckx P R 1994 Is mild endometriosis a disease? Is mild endometriosis a condition occurring intermittently in all women? Human Reproduction 9: 2202–2211

Koninckx P R, Barlow D, Kennedy S 1999 Implantation versus infiltration: the Sampson versus the endometriotic disease theory. Gynecologic and Obstetric Investigation 47 (Supplement): 13–19

Kruitwagen R F P M, Poels L G, Willemsen W N P et al 1991 Endometrial epithelial cells in peritoneal fluid during the early follicular phase. Fertility and Sterility 55: 297–303

Kunz G, Beil D, Huppert P, Leyendecker G 2000 Structural abnormalities of the uterine wall in women with endometriosis and infertility visualized by vaginal sonography and magnetic resonance imaging. Human Reproduction 15: 76–82

Kurman R J, Craig J M 1972 Endometrioid and clear cell carcinoma in the ovary. Cancer 29: 1653–1664

Labay G R, Feiner F 1971 Malignant pleural endometriosis. American Journal of Obstetrics and Gynecology 110: 478–480

LaGrenade A, Silverberg S G 1988 Ovarian tumor associated with atypical endometriosis. Human Pathology 19: 1080–1084

Lamb K, Hoffman R G, Nichols T R 1986 Family trait analysis: a case control study of 43 women with endometriosis and their best friends. American Journal of Obstetrics and Gynecology 154: 596–601

La Pava S, Nigogosyan G, Pickren J W 1963 Sarcomatous transformation of 'true' endometriosis. New York State Journal of Medicine 63: 2548–2553

Lauchlan S C 1972 The secondary Mullerian system. Obstetrical and Gynecological Survey 27: 133–146

Lebovic D I, Mueller M D, Taylor R N 2001 Immunobiology of endometriosis. Fertility and Sterility 75: 1–10

Lele S B, Piver M S, Barlow J J, Tsukada Y 1978 Squamous cell carcinomas arising in ovarian endometriosis. Gynecologic Oncology 6: 290–293

Levander G, Norman P 1955 The pathogenesis of endometriosis: an experimental study. Acta Obstetricia et Gynecologica Scandinavica 34: 366–398

Levine P H, Abou-Nassar S, Mittal K 2001 Extrauterine low-grade endometrial stromal sarcoma with florid endometrioid glandular differentiation. International Journal of Gynecological Pathology 20: 395–398

Leyendecker G 2000 Endometriosis is an entity with an extreme pleomorphism. Human Reproduction 15: 4–7

Leyendecker G, Kunz G, Wildt L et al 1996 Uterine hyperperistalsis and dysperistalsis as dysfunctions of the mechanism of rapid sperm transport in patients with endometriosis and infertility. Human Reproduction 11: 1542–1551

Leyendecker G, Kunz G, Noe M et al 1998 Endometriosis: a dysfunction and disease of the archimetra. Human Reproduction Update 4: 752–762

Li S F, Nakayama K, Masuzawa H, Fujii S 1993 The number of proliferating cell nuclear antigen positive cells in endometriotic lesions differs from that in the endometrium: analysis of PCNA positive cells during the menstrual cycle and in post menopause, Virchows Archiv A Pathological Anatomy and Histopathology 423: 257–263

Lyndrup J, Thorpe S, Glenthoj A, Obel E, Sele V 1987 Altered progesterone/estrogen receptor ratios in endometriosis: a comparative study of steroid receptors and morphology in endometriosis and endometrium. Acta Obstetricia et Gynecologica Scandinavica 66: 625–629

Mai K T, Yazdi H M, Perkind D G, Parks W 1998 Development of endometriosis from embryonic duct remnants. Human Pathology 29: 319–322

Malinak L R, Buttram V C, Elias S, Simpson J L 1980 Heritable aspects of endometriosis. II. Clinical characteristics of familial endometriosis. American Journal of Obstetrics and Gynecology 137: 322–327

Marchevsky A M, Kaneko M 1978 Bilateral ovarian endometriosis associated with carcinosarcoma of the right ovary and endometrioid carcinoma of the left ovary. American Journal of Clinical Pathology 70: 709–712

Matsuura K, Ohtake H, Katabuchi H, Okamura H 1999 Coelomic metaplasia theory of endometriosis: evidence from in vivo studies and an in vitro experimental model. Gynecologic and Obstetric Investigation 47 (Supplement): 118–120

Mazzeo D, Vigano P, Di Blasio A M, Sinigaglia F, Vignali M, Panina-Bordignon P 1998 Interleukin-12 and its free p40 subunit regulate immune recognition of endometrial cells: potential role in endometriosis. Journal of Clinical Endocrinology and Metabolism 83: 911–916

McClaren J 2000 Vascular endothelial growth factor and endometriotic angiogenesis. Human Reproduction Update 6: 45–55

McCluggage W G, Desai V, Toner P G, Calvert C H 2001 Clear cell adenocarcinoma of the colon arising in endometriosis: a rare variant of primary colonic adenocarcinoma. Journal of Clinical Pathology 54: 76–77

McCullough K, Froats E R, Falk H C 1946 Epidermoid carcinoma arising in an endometrial cyst of the ovary. Archives of Pathology and Laboratory Medicine 41: 335–337

Meresman G F, Vighi S, Buquet R A, Contreras-Ortiz O, Tesone M, Rumi L S 2000 Apoptosis and expression of Bcl-2 and Bax in eutopic endometrium from women with endometriosis. Fertility and Sterility 74: 760–766

Merrill J A 1966 Endometrial induction of endometriosis across millipore filters. American Journal of Obstetrics and Gynecology 94: 780–790

Mesko J D, Gates H, McDonald T W, Youmans R, Lewis J 1988 Clear cell ('mesonephroid') adenocarcinoma of the vulva arising in endometriosis: a case report. Gynecologic Oncology 29: 385–391

Metzger D A, Olive D L, Haney A F 1988 Limited hormonal responsiveness of ectopic endometrium: histologic correlation with intrauterine endometrium. Human Pathology 19: 1417–1424

Mio Y, Toda T, Harada T, Terakawa N 1992 Luteinized unruptured follicle in the early stages of endometriosis as a cause of unexplained infertility. American Journal of Obstetrics and Gynecology 167: 271–273

Miyazawa K 1976 Incidence of endometriosis among Japanese women. Obstetrics and Gynecology 48: 407–409

Moen M H, Magnus P 1993 The familial risk of endometriosis. Acta Obstetricia et Gynecologica Scandinavica 72: 560–564

Moller N E 1959 The Arias-Stella phenomenon in endometriosis. Acta Obstetricia et Gynecologica Scandinavica 38: 271–274

Mostoufizadeh G H M, Scully R E 1980 Malignant tumors arising in endometriosis. Clinical Obstetrics and Gynecology 23: 951–963

Mourra N, Tiret E, Parc Y, de Saint Maur P, Parc R, Flejou J F 2001 Endometrial stromal sarcoma of the rectosigmoid colon arising in extragonadal endometriosis and revealed by portal vein thrombosis. Archives of Pathology and Laboratory Medicine 125: 1088–1090

Muscato J J, Haney A F, Weinberg J B 1982 Sperm phagocytosis by human peritoneal macrophages: a possible cause of infertility in endometriosis. American Journal of Obstetrics and Gynecology 144: 503–510

Nakamura M, Katabuchi H, Tohya T et al 1993 Scanning electron microscopic and immunohistochemical studies of pelvic endometriosis. Human Reproduction 8: 2218–2226

Nakayama K, Toki T, Zhai Y L et al 2001 Demonstration of focal p53 expression without genetic alterations in endometriotic lesions. International Journal of Gynecological Pathology 20: 227–231

Napolitano C, Marziani R, Mossa B, Perniola L, Benagiano G 1994 Management of Stage III and IV endometriosis: a 10 year experience. European Journal of Obstetrics, Gynecology and Reproductive Biology 53: 199–204

Naresh K N, Ahuja V K, Rao C R, Mukherjee G, Bhargava M K 1991 Squamous cell carcinoma arising in endometriosis of the ovary. Journal of Clinical Pathology 44: 958–959

Naseman T R 1990 Zur Endometriose der Haut. Zeitschrift fur Hautkrangungen 65: 117–119

Nilbert M, Pejovic T, Mandahl N et al 1995 Monoclonal origin of endometriotic cysts. International Journal of Gynecological Cancer 5: 61–63

Nisolle M, Donnez J 1997 Peritoneal endometriosis, ovarian endometriosis and adenomyotic nodules of the rectovaginal septum are three different entities. Fertility and Sterility 68: 585–596

Nisolle M, Casanas-Roux F Donnez J 1997 Immunohistochemical analysis of proliferative activity and steroid receptor expression in peritoneal and ovarian endometriosis. Fertility and Sterility 68: 912–919

Noble L S, Simpson E R, Johns A, Bulun S E 1996 Aromatase expression in endometriosis. Journal of Clinical Endocrinology and Metabolism 81: 174–179

Novak E 1931 Pelvic endometriosis: spontaneous rupture of endometrial cysts, with a report of three cases. American Journal of Obstetrics and Gynecology 22: 326–335

Novak E, de Lima A 1948 Correlative study of adenomyosis and pelvic endometriosis, with special reference to the hormonal reaction of ectopic endometrium. American Journal of Obstetrics and Gynecology 56: 634–644

Novak E R, Woodruff J D 1979a Novak's gynecologic and obstetric pathology with clinical and endocrine relations, 8th edn. W B Saunders, Philadelphia, p 578

Novak E R, Woodruff J D 1979b Novak's gynecologic and obstetric pathology with clinical and endocrine relations, 8th edn. W B Saunders, Philadelphia, pp 561–584

Obata K, Hoshiai H 2000 Common genetic changes between endometriosis and ovarian cancer. Gynecologic and Obstetric Investigation 50 (Supplement): 139–143

Ogawa S, Kaku T, Amada S et al 2000 Ovarian endometriosis associated with ovarian carcinoma: a clinicopathological and immunohistochemical study. Gynecologic Oncology 77: 298–304

Olive D L, Henderson D Y 1987 Endometriosis and Mullerian anomalies. Obstetrics and Gynecology 69: 412–415

Oosterlynck D J, Cornillie F J, Waer M, Vanderputte M, Koninckx P R 1991 Women with endometriosis show a defect in natural killer activity resulting in a decreased cytotoxicity to autologous endometrium. Fertility and Sterility 56: 45–51

Oosterlynck D J, Meuleman C, Waer M, Vanderputte M, Koninckx P R 1992 The natural killer activity of peritoneal fluid lymphocytes in women with endometriosis. Fertility and Sterility 58: 292–295

Oral O, Arici A 1997 Pathogenesis of endometriosis. Obstetrics and Gynecology Clinics of North America 24: 219–233

Osteen K G, Bruner K L, Sharpe-Timms K L 1997 Steroid and growth factor regulation of matrix metalloproteinase expression and endometriosis. Seminars in Reproductive Endocrinology 14: 247–255

Pai S A, Desai S B, Borges A M 1998 Uterus-like masses of the ovary associated with breast cancer and raised serum CA 125. American Journal of Surgical Pathology 22: 333–337

Palladino V S, Trousdell M 1969 Extra-uterine Mullerian tumors. Cancer 23: 1413–1422

Parsons L, Sommers S C 1978 Gynecology, 2nd edn. W B Saunders, Philadelphia, pp 957–997

Perrotta P L, Ginsburg F W, Siderides C I, Parkash V 1998 Liesegang rings in endometriosis. International Journal of Gynecological Pathology 17: 358–362

Persad V, Anderson M F 1977 Endometrial stromal sarcoma of the broad ligament arising in area of endometriosis in a paramesonephric cyst: case report. British Journal of Obstetrics and Gynaecology 87: 149–152

Pins M R, Young R H, Daly W J, Scully R E 1996 Primary squamous cell carcinomas of the ovary: a report of 37 cases. American Journal of Surgical Pathology 20: 823–833

Prakash S, Ulfelder H, Cohen R B 1965 Enzyme-histochemical observations on endometriosis. American Journal of Obstetrics and Gynecology 91: 990–997

Prentice A, Thomas E J, Weddell A et al 1992 Epidermal growth factor receptor expression in normal endometrium and endometriosis. British Journal of Obstetrics and Gynaecology 99: 395–398

Pueblitz-Peredo S, Luevano-Flores E, Rincon-Taracena R, Ochoa-Carrillo F J 1985. Uterus like mass of the ovary: endometriosis or congenital malformation? A case with a discussion of histogenesis. Archives of Pathology and Laboratory Medicine 109: 361–364

Puolakka Y, Kauppila A, Ronnenberg L 1980 Results in the operative treatment of pelvic endometriosis. Acta Obstetricia et Gynecologica Scandinavica 59: 429–431

Ranney B 1980a Endometriosis: pathogenesis, symptoms and findings. Clinical Obstetrics and Gynecology 23: 865–874

Ranney B 1980b Etiology, prevention and inhibition of endometriosis. Clinical Obstetrics and Gynecology 23: 875–883

Rawson J M 1991 Prevalence of endometriosis in asymptomatic women. Journal of Reproductive Medicine 36: 513–515

Redwine D B 1994 Endometriosis persisting after castration: clinical characteristics and results of surgical management. Obstetrics and Gynecology 83: 405–413

Ridley J H 1968 The histogenesis of endometriosis: a review of facts and fancies. Obstetrical and Gynecological Survey 23: 1–35.

Ridley J H, Edwards I K 1958 Experimental endometriosis in the human. American Journal of Obstetrics and Gynecology 76: 783–790

Rolfing M B, Kao K Y, Woodard B H 1981 Endomyometriosis: possible association with leiomyomatosis disseminata and endometriosis. Archives of Pathology and Laboratory Medicine 105: 556–557

Roth L M, Czernobilsky B, Langley F A 1981 Endometrioid adenofibromatous and cystadenofibromatous tumours: benign, proliferating and malignant. Cancer 48: 1838–1845

Russell P 1979 The pathological assessment of ovarian neoplasms: I. Introduction to the common 'epithelial' tumours and analysis of benign, 'epithelial' tumours. Pathology 11: 5–26

Rutgers J L, Scully R E 1988 Ovarian Mullerian mucinous papillary cystadenomas of borderline malignancy: a clinicopathologic analysis. Cancer 61: 34–38

Ryan I P, Tseng J F, Schriock E D et al 1995 Interleukin-8 concentrations are elevated in peritoneal fluid of women with endometriosis. Fertility and Sterility 63: 929–932

Sainz de la Cuesta R, Eichhorn J H, Rice L W et al 1996 Histologic transformation of benign endometriosis to early epithelial ovarian cancer. Gynecologic Oncology 60: 238–239

Sampson J A 1921 Perforating hemorrhagic (chocolate) cysts of the ovary, their importance and especially their relation to pelvic adenomas of the endometrial type. Archives of Surgery 3: 245–323

Sampson J A 1925 Endometrial carcinoma of ovary, arising in endometrial tissue in that organ. Archives of Surgery 10: 1–72

Schneider J, Jimenez E, Rodriguez F, del Tanago J G 1998 c-myc, c-erb-B2, nm23 and p53 expression in human endometriosis. Oncology Reports 5: 49–52

Schweppe K W, Wynn R W, Beller F K 1984 Ultrastructure comparison of endometriotic implants and ectopic endometrium. American Journal of Obstetrics and Gynecology 148: 1024–1039

Scott R B, Wharton L R Jr 1957 The effect of estrone and progesterone on the growth of experimental endometriosis in Rhesus monkeys. American Journal of Obstetrics and Gynecology 74: 852–865

Scully R E 1977 Ovarian tumors: a review. American Journal of Pathology 87: 686–720

Scully R E 1999 Histological typing of ovarian tumours. Springer, Berlin

Scully R E, Barlow J F 1967 'Mesonephroma' of ovary: tumor of Mullerian nature related to the endometrioid carcinoma. Cancer 20: 1405–1417

Scully R E, Richardson G S, Barlow J F 1966 The development of malignancy in endometriosis. Clinical Obstetrics and Gynecology 9: 384–411

Scully R E, Young R H, Clement P B 1998 Atlas of tumor pathology. Tumors of the ovary, maldeveloped gonads, fallopian tube, and broad ligament, Third Series. Armed Forces Institute of Pathology, Washington

Seidman J D 1996 Prognostic importance of hyperplasia and atypia in endometriosis. International Journal of Gynecological Pathology 15: 1–9

Serov S F, Scully R E, Sobin L H 1973 International histological classification of tumours, no. 9. Histological typing of ovarian tumours. World Health Organization, Geneva, pp 17–21

Shakfeh S M, Woodruff J D 1987 Primary ovarian sarcomas: report of 46 cases and review of the literature. Obstetrical and Gynecological Survey 42: 331–349

Shaw R W 1991 GnRH analogues in the treatment of endometriosis — rationale and efficacy. In: Thomas E J, Rock J A (eds) Modern approaches to endometriosis. Kluwer Academic Publishers, Dordrecht, pp 257–274

Shifrin B S, Erez S, Moore J G 1973 Teen-age endometriosis. American Journal of Obstetrics and Gynecology 116: 973–980

Shiraki M, Otis C N, Powell J L 1991 Endometrial stromal sarcoma arising from ovarian and extraovarian endometriosis — report of two cases and review of the literature. Surgical Pathology 4: 333–343

Sillem M, Prifti S, Monga B, Arslic T, Runnebaum B 1999 Integrin-mediated adhesion of uterine endometrial cells from endometriosis patients to extracellular matrix proteins is enhanced by tumor necrosis factor alpha (TNF alpha) and interleukin-1 (IL-1). European Journal of Obstetrics, Gynecology and Reproductive Biology 87: 123–127

Simpson J L, Elias S, Malinak L R 1980 Heritable aspects of endometriosis. I. Genetic studies. American Journal of Obstetrics and Gynecology 137: 327–331

Slavin R E, Krum R, van Dinh T 2000 Endometriosis-associated intestinal tumors: a clinical and pathological study of 6 cases with a review of the literature. Human Pathology 31: 456–463

Spence M R 1992 Endometriosis occurring eight years after total abdominal hysterectomy and bilateral salpingo-oophorectomy. American Journal of Gynecological Health 6: 22–25

Spuijbroeck M D E H, Dunselman G A J, Menheere P P C A et al 1992 Early endometriosis invades the extracellular matrix. Fertility and Sterility 58: 929–933

Steck W D, Helwig E B 1965 Cutaneous endometriosis. Journal of the American Medical Association 191: 167–170

Stern R C, Dash R, Bentley R C, Snyder M J, Haney A F, Robboy S J 2001 Malignancy in endometriosis: frequency and comparison of ovarian and extraovarian types. International Journal of Gynecological Pathology 20: 133–139

Sturgis S H, Call B J 1954 Endometriosis peritonei: relationship of pain to functional activity. American Journal of Obstetrics and Gynecology 68: 1421–1431

Suginami H 1991 A reappraisal of the coelomic metaplasia theory by reviewing endometriosis occurring in unusual sites and instances. American Journal of Obstetrics and Gynecology 165: 214–218

Svendstrup F, Husby H 1991 Parenchymal pulmonary endometriosis. Journal of Laryngology and Otology 105: 235–236

Tamura M, Fukaya T, Murakami T, Uehara S, Yajima A 1998 Analysis of clonality in human endometriotic cysts based on evaluation of X chromosome inactivation in archival formalin-fixed, paraffin-embedded tissue. Laboratory Investigation 78: 213–218

Taylor H S, Bagot C, Kardana A et al 1999 *HOX* gene expression is altered in the endometrium of women with endometriosis. Human Reproduction 14: 1328–1331

Te Linde R W, Scott R B 1950 Experimental endometriosis. American Journal of Obstetrics and Gynecology 60: 1147–1173

Tetu B, Silva E G, Gershenson D M 1987 Squamous cell carcinoma of the ovary. Archives of Pathology and Laboratory Medicine 111: 864–866

Thibodeau L L, Pridleau G R, Manuelidis E E, Merino M J, Heafner M D 1987 Cerebral endometriosis: case report. Journal of Neurosurgery 66: 609–610

Thomas E J 1991 Endometriosis and infertility. In: Thomas E J, Rock J A (eds) Modern approaches to endometriosis. Kluwer Academic Publishers, Dordrecht, pp 113–128

Thomas E J 1993 Endometriosis: still an enigma. British Journal of Obstetrics and Gynaecology 100: 615–617

Tidman M J, MacDonald D M 1988 Cutaneous endometriosis: a histopathologic study. Journal of the American Academy of Dermatology 18: 373–377

Toki T, Fujii S, Silverberg S G 1996a A clinicopathologic study on the association of endometriosis and carcinoma of the ovary using a scoring system. International Journal of Gynecological Cancer 6: 68–75

Toki T, Horiuchi A, Li S, Nakayama K, Silverberg S G, Fujii S 1996b Proliferative activity of postmenopausal endometriosis: a histopathologic and immunocytochemical study. International Journal of Gynecological Pathology 15: 45–53

Treloar S A, O'Connor D T, O'Connor V M, Martin N G 1999 Genetic influences on endometriosis in an Australian twin sample. Fertility and Sterility 71: 701–710

Tseng J F, Ryan I P, Milam T D et al 1996 Interleukin-6 secretion in vitro is upregulated in ectopic and eutopic endometrial stromal cells from women with endometriosis. Journal of Clinical Endocrinology and Metabolism 81: 1118–1122

Tutschka B G, Lauchlan S C 1980 Endosalpingiosis. Obstetrics and Gynecology 55: 57S–60S

Ueki M 1991 Histologic study of endometriosis and examination of lymphatic drainage in and from the uterus. American Journal of Obstetrics and Gynecology 165: 201–209

van der Linden P J Q, van der Linden E P M, de Goeij A F P M et al 1994 Expression of integrins and E-cadherin in cells from menstrual effluent, endometrium, peritoneal fluid, peritoneum and endometriosis. Fertility and Sterility 61: 85–90

Vercellini P, Parazzini F, Bolis G et al 1993 Endometriosis and ovarian cancer. American Journal of Obstetrics and Gynecology 169: 181–182

Vercellini P, Trecca D, Oldani S, Fracchiolla N S, Neri A, Crosignani P G 1994 Analysis of p53 and ras gene mutations in endometriosis. Gynecologic and Obstetric Investigation 38: 70–71

Vierhout M E, Chadha-Ajwani S, Wijner J A et al 1992 Extra-uterine endometrial stromal sarcoma with DNA flow cytometric analysis. European Journal of Obstetrics, Gynecology and Reproductive Biology 43: 157–161

Vinatier D, Cosson M, Dufour P 2000 Is endometriosis an endometrial disease? European Journal of Obstetrics, Gynecology and Reproductive Biology 91: 113–125

Vinatier D, Orazi G, Cosson M, Dufour P 2001 Theories of endometriosis. European Journal of Obstetrics, Gynecology and Reproductive Biology 96: 21–34

von Recklinghausen F 1885 Uber die venose Embolie und den retrograden Transport in den Venen und in den Lymphgefassen. Virchows Archiv A 100: 503–539

Weed J C, Arquembourg P C 1980 Endometriosis: can it produce an autoimmune response resulting in infertility? Clinical Obstetrics and Gynecology 23: 885–895

Weed J C, Holland J B 1977 Endometriosis and infertility: an enigma. Fertility and Sterility 28: 135–140

Wicks M J, Larson C P 1949 Histologic criteria for evaluating endometriosis. Northwestern Medicine 48: 611–613

Wilson T J, Hertzog P J, Angus D, Munnery L, Wood E C, Kola I 1994 Decreased natural killer cell activity in endometriosis patients: relationship to disease pathogenesis. Fertility and Sterility 62: 1086–1088

Wingfield M 2000 Minimal/mild endometriosis and infertility. The Obstetrician and Gynaecologist 2: 21–24

Wingfield M, Macpherson A, Healy D L, Rogers P A W 1995 Cell proliferation is increased in the endometrium of women with endometriosis. Fertility and Sterility 64: 340–346

Witz C A 1999 Current concepts in the pathogenesis of endometriosis. Clinical Obstetrics and Gynecology 42: 566–585

Wu M Y, Chao K H, Chen S U et al 1996 The suppression of peritoneal cellular immunity in women with endometriosis could be restored after gonadotropin releasing hormone agonist treatment. American Journal of Reproductive Immunology 35: 510–516

Wu M Y, Yang J H, Chao K H, Hwang J L, Yang Y S, Ho H N 2000 Increase in the expression of killer cell inhibitory receptors on peritoneal natural killer cells in women with endometriosis. Fertility and Sterility 74: 1187–1191

Yano T, Jimbo H, Yoshikawa H, Tsutsumi O, Taketani Y 1999 Molecular analysis of clonality in ovarian endometrial cysts. Gynecologic and Obstetric Investigation 47 (Supplement): 141–145

Yantiss R K, Clement P B, Young R H 2000 Neoplastic and preneoplastic changes in gastrointestinal endometriosis: a study of 17 cases. American Journal of Surgical Pathology 24: 513–524

Yoshikawa H, Jimbo H, Okada S et al 2000 Prevalence of endometriosis in ovarian cancer. Gynecologic and Obstetric Investigation 50 (Supplement): 111–117

Young R H, Scully R E 1990 Sarcomas metastatic to the ovary: a report of 21 cases. International Journal of Gynecological Pathology 9: 231–252

Young R H, Prat J, Scully R E 1984 Endometrioid stromal sarcomas of the ovary: a clinicopathologic analysis of 23 cases. Cancer 53: 1143–1155

Young S, Moon D V M, Leung P C S, Yuen B H, Gomel V 1981 Prostaglandin F in human endometriosis tissue. American Journal of Obstetrics and Gynecology 141: 344–346

30

Pathology of infertility

L. H. Honoré

Introduction   989

Definition and prevalence   990

Male infertility   990

Interactive infertility   991
Age   991
Physical factors   991
Psychological factors   991
Genetic factors   992
Immunological factors   992
Microbiological factors   993
Biophysical factors   994
Biochemical factors   994

Female infertility: organ related causes   995
Vulva and vagina   995
Uterine cervix   996
Corpus uteri   998
The Fallopian tube   1006
Ovary   1013
Peritoneum   1018
Disturbances of the hypothalamo-hypophysial system   1020
Systemic diseases and female infertility   1025

Complications of infertility diagnosis and treatment   1026
Complications of infertility investigations   1027
Complications of infertility therapy   1027

INTRODUCTION

Fertility is defined as the ability to procreate, i.e. to achieve a live birth following successful fusion of male and female gametes (fertilisation). Human fertility is the result of two interacting sets of factors: behavioural and biological (Leridon 1977; Weinstein & Stark 1994).

The behavioural factors comprise:

1. Sexual behaviour. Among married couples the peak coital rate occurs on the day of the LH surge indicating a positive influence of the female sex hormones in favour of conception (Hedricks et al 1987) but there is still a strong idiosyncratic element that determines coital frequency in relationships (Rao & Demaris 1995).
2. The duration of postpartum infertility related to breast feeding varies from culture to culture. It has a physiological basis and in some societies it is reinforced by a voluntary (Visness & Kennedy 1997) or taboo-related drop in coital activity.
3. The deliberate control of fertility by voluntary infertility, delayed child-bearing and contraception (affecting fecundability), induced abortion (affecting intrauterine mortality) and sterilisation (affecting the overall level of fertility). These methods of fertility control also have negative short-term or long-term effects on fertility following cessation or reversal. Post-pill usage there is short-term depression of fecundability depending on the patient's age and the oestrogen dose (Bracken et al 1990) but long-term fertility is restored or even enhanced, especially in young women taking the combined monophasic pill (Bagwell et al 1995). The significance of an increased risk of post-pill endometriosis (Italian Endometriosis Study Group 1999) remains uncertain. After removal of an intrauterine contraceptive device there is a definite increase in the prevalence of infertility (Eschenbach 1992). There are conflicting data on the effects of induced abortion on fertility and the risk of miscarriage but the balance of evidence argues against

any significant impact (Parazzini et al 1998). After reversal of tubal sterilisation the intrauterine pregnancy rate is 64% and the ectopic pregnancy rate is 4% with age <30 years and tubal length >4 cm being significant indicators of successful outcome (Rouzi et al 1995).

4. Nuptiality (marital customs), as determined socially by the types of union (stable marriage, common law and successive relationships), age at marriage, conditions or obligations of remarriage following widowhood and consequences of marital infidelity. It has been shown that the level of fertility of a population is greatly affected by these practices (Leridon 1977) with the final number of offspring depending on the number of years a woman has lived 'in unions' and on the nature of these unions. Consanguinity reduces the net fertility of women (Yasim & Mascie-Taylor 1997).

5. Lifestyle, especially in affluent societies, has a considerable influence on fertility. Economic prosperity favours contraception over conception (Evans 1996; Shah 1997) for the following reasons:
   - emancipation of women and greater involvement in the work force;
   - conflicting choices for the advantages of a higher standard of living;
   - high costs of child care and education;
   - the quality/quantity fertility trade-off with reduction in family size in favour of greater involvement with a smaller number of children.

Fertility is improved by better nutrition (Scott & Duncan 1999) but is reduced by heavy exercise (Chen & Brzyski 1999), smoking (Hughes & Brennan 1996), alcohol and caffeine (Hakim et al 1998) and environmental toxicants (Sharara et al 1998).

The biological factors include:

1. Fecundability or the monthly fecundity rate is the probability of achieving pregnancy during a particular month and ranges from 15–20% (Collins et al 1995). It depends on the woman's month of birth (Smits et al 1997); on her cycle length and variability (Kolstad et al 1999); on her rate of reproductive and systemic aging (Miller & Soules 1997) and her own genetically determined trade-off between reproductive success and longevity (Westendorf & Kirkwood 1998). Reproductive aging, which has little impact on males, is typical of females of many species and reflects evolutionary pressure for reproductive altruism that spares the middle-aged the risks and energy costs of pregnancy and increases their chances of survival to protect extant offspring (Keefe 1998).

2. Permanent sterility is imposed by the menopause, which has developed uniquely in humans as the species with the longest period of child rearing: it confers on the aging mother the evolutionary advantage of improving the fitness of her juvenile and adolescent offspring without the burden and risk of a late gestation (Peccei 1995). Age at the menopause is set by the timing of follicular exhaustion that is the result of a genetically determined oocyte stock and a variable oocyte depletion rate, which is reduced by oocyte-sparing factors, i.e. parity, lactation, oral contraceptive use and high socioeconomic status, and enhanced by oocyte-depleting factors, i.e. smoking and low socioeconomic status (van Noord et al 1997). The menopause is preceded by a long period of sub-fertility (Seifer & Naftolin 1998).

3. Intrauterine mortality, subclinical and clinical, is very common in humans (Edmonds et al 1982) and accounts for our low fecundability as compared with domestic animals. In fact, menstruation may have evolved in women, whose sexual activity is not tightly linked to oestrus and ovulation, as a mechanism of early loss of defective embryos produced by the fusion of aged gametes (Clarke 1994).

DEFINITION AND PREVALENCE

Involuntary infertility is defined as the inability to achieve a live birth after a year of regular unprotected coitus. The prevalence of infertility varies widely depending on the definition, the age of the couples examined and the population studied. In the West it is estimated to be 13% (Page 1989). In the US a slight increase is predicted over the next 20 years (Stephen 1996). Clearly, infertility is a 'couple problem' and should be conceptualised, investigated and treated as such. The cause may lie with one of the partners, with both partners to a variable extent (Dunphy et al 1990) or with neither, at least as far as can be determined by modern methods (Jaffe & Jewelewicz 1991). For didactic reasons the subject will be discussed under the following three headings:

1. Male infertility: for the sake of completeness the contribution of the male to human infertility will be briefly mentioned.
2. Interactive infertility: this important aspect covers the negative fertility-depressing factors related to the biological, physical and psychological components of the coital act.
3. Female infertility: this facet of the problem will be discussed in detail.

MALE INFERTILITY

It is estimated that 20% of cases of infertility are due to the male factor and 27% are due to a combination of male and female factors. Thus the overall male contribution to infertility is close to 50%. Male infertility, whether congenital or acquired, is the result of inadequate functioning of testicular tissue, impaired sperm production and function, failure of sperm delivery and transport and disturbances in sperm–oocyte interaction (de Kretzer et al 1998; Chia et al 2000; Gazvani et al 2000; Wong et al 2000).

INTERACTIVE INFERTILITY

This form of infertility, which can be transient or permanent, is related to the following factors acting singly or in concert:

AGE

In humans fertility peaks in the third decade. 'Adolescent sterility' (Montagu 1946) is a well-recognised entity supported by the relatively rare occurrence of illegitimate births in the populations where premarital sex is tolerated and even encouraged. It is largely due to immaturity of the reproductive system in both sexes, reflected in the female by significantly lower fecundity (Jain 1969). In addition there is some evidence, still inconclusive, that young maternal and paternal age predisposes to an increased incidence of lethal heteroploidy in the conceptus, i.e. monosomy X (Warburton et al 1980) and triploidy (Hassold et al 1980), respectively.

The reproductive capacity of the human couple is limited in time by progressive, age-dependent subfertility and eventually by the menopause, which imposes absolute sterility (Leridon 1977). This age-dependent subfertility is multifactorial. Decreased coital frequency, especially after the age of 35 (Leridon 1977), reduces the statistical probability of mid-cycle fertilisation and increases the possibility of fusion of gametes which are defective as a result of prolonged prefertilisation sojourn in the female reproductive tract (Guerrero & Rojas 1975; Bomsel-Helmreich 1976).

In women there is a sharp decline in fecundity after age 40 with a higher spontaneous miscarriage rate and a higher rate of fetal aneuploidy (Feinman 1997). The critical underlying factor is declining ovarian function owing to oocyte deterioration (Lim & Tsakok 1997) and endocrine failure with dwindling ovarian reserve (Danforth et al 1998). Loss of oocyte competency is due to chromosome breakage and replacement of the whole chromosome by single chromatids caused by precocious division of chromosome univalents at anaphase (Angell et al 1993), mitochondrial DNA deletions (Keefe et al 1995) and increased trinucleotide repeat instability (Kaytor et al 1997). Endocrine failure could result from:

- progressive ischaemia due to increased coiling and intimal thickening of the hilar and medullary spiral arteries (Shimada et al 1993);
- decrease in ovarian antioxidants with an increase in lipid peroxides inhibiting aromatase activity and

reducing oestrogen synthesis (Okatani et al 1993);
- mitochondrial DNA deletion in stromal cells due to cumulative exposure to oxygen radicals and resulting in decreased oxidative phosphorylation and steroid synthesis (Suganuma et al 1993);
- disturbed follicular recruitment (Batista et al 1995);
- abnormal inhibin and activin A production by the ovaries (Santoro et al 1999).

The rôle of uterine senescence is controversial with evidence for (Cano et al 1995) and against (Borini et al 1995).

There is no comparable age-dependent decrease in male fertility but men show a variable degree of progressive sexual dysfunction, increasing erectile dysfunction and decreasing libido and sexual activity (Vermeulen 2000).

PHYSICAL FACTORS

Since ovulation occurs once a month at mid-cycle and the shed gametes have a short fertile life span, successful fertilisation depends critically on the timing of intercourse, its frequency and its nature. Mistiming is often due to ignorance of reproductive physiology but can result from avoidance of the fertile period by collusion on the part of an infertile couple with an unconscious aversion to parenthood (Abse 1966). A low coital frequency (Freeman et al 1983) reduces the chance of gamete fusion and enhances the probability of fusion of defective ageing gametes; a high coital frequency gives rise to deficient seminal fluid and oligospermia (Schwartz et al 1983). The physical effectiveness of coitus can also be impaired by:

1. The excessive practice of coital variations with the avoidance of penovaginal intercourse, essential for optimal insemination. Sperm deposition in the female alimentary canal does not produce sperm isoimmunity (Chacho et al 1991).
2. Inadequate or absent vaginal penetration resulting from organic or psychogenic dyspareunia or vaginismus (Fordney 1978) or from male erectile dysfunction (Wong et al 2000).
3. Inadequate vaginal insemination may be due to ejaculatory dysfunction, i.e. premature, sham or retrograde ejaculation (Master & Turek 2001). Moreover, the quantitative efficiency of the emission reflex can be impaired by feelings of guilt and anxiety (Abse 1966) and enhanced by pleasurable foreplay, which releases oxytocin and potentiates the contractility of the excurrent ducts (Amann 1981).

PSYCHOLOGICAL FACTORS

The notion that infertility has psychological causes (the psychogenic hypothesis) is not favoured by most researchers but there is strong evidence that infertility generates considerable psychosocial distress, which is more marked in women regardless of which partner is impaired (Greil 1997). The stress of infertility leads to higher levels of suspicion, guilt, hostility and anxiety and compounds the problem by adversely affecting the success of IVF treatment (Csemiczky et al 2000). Psychological distress reduces fecundability in first-pregnancy planners with long menstrual cycles (Hjøllund et al 1999). Two recent studies report conflicting results on the effects of stress and anxiety on recurrent miscarriage (Aoki et al 1998; Mild et al 1998).

GENETIC FACTORS

Genetic factors are critical in setting the fertility potential of an individual by qualitatively and/or quantitatively affecting gonadal endocrine activity and gametogenesis and conditioning the structural development of genital ducts. They also directly influence the product of interaction, i.e. the zygote/embryo/fetus and depress fertility by influencing intrauterine survival rate. Major genetic differences between mother and father, expressed as ABO (Schaap et al 1984) and P system (Rock & Zacur 1983) incompatibility between mother and fetus, can lead to subfertility and recurrent miscarriages.

The prevalence of detectable chromosomal abnormalities in couples with recurrent spontaneous miscarriages is about 5% (Coulam 1991) but it is much lower (<1%) in couples experiencing only recurrent miscarriages without any other form of reproductive failure (Simpson et al 1996). The chromosomal abnormalities fall into three groups:

1. Structural rearrangements

The commonest form is the non-homologous balanced reciprocal (Fortuny et al 1988) or Robertsonian translocation. Less common forms include: inversions and polymorphisms, balanced homologous translocations (Sudha & Gopinath 1990), intra- or inter-chromosomal insertional translocations (Abuelo et al 1988), familial or de novo complex rearrangements (Timar et al 1991) and maternal gonosomal mosaicism (Holzgreve et al 1984).

2. Abnormal chromosomal behaviour

- Premature or delayed centromere separation leading to non-disjunctional aneuploidy in the offspring (Mehes & Kosztolanyi 1992)
- Increased chromosomal instability detected as increased numbers of aphidicolin; induced fragile sites (Schlegelberger et al *1989*)
- Increased chromosome breaks and acentric fragments in sperm chromosomes of male partners (Rosenbusch & Sterzik 1991).

3. Submicroscopic genetic mutations

These are inferred from circumstantial evidence and also contribute to pregnancy loss. They include:

- familial recessive lethal genes linked to the major histocompatibility complex (Mowbray et al 1991);
- autosomal lethal genes apparently arising de novo (McDonough 1987);
- X-linked lethal syndromes, i.e. focal dermal hypoplasia, incontinentia pigmenti, oral–facial–digital I syndrome (McDonough 1987) and the lethal multiple pterygium syndrome (Lockwood et al 1988).

It is worth noting that recurrent spontaneous miscarriage is not an absolute cause of infertility. Even after three consecutive losses the chances of having a normal pregnancy are close to 60% (Smith & Gaba 1990) but these couples are still more prone to other forms of reproductive failure, e.g. ectopic pregnancy, stillbirth, preterm birth, congenital malformation, intrauterine growth retardation and placenta praevia (Coulam et al 1991; Thom et al 1992).

IMMUNOLOGICAL FACTORS

Immunological infertility is now a recognised entity but the magnitude of its contribution to human infertility is unknown. The immunogenic potential of sperm and seminal fluid is well established and yet male autoimmunisation and female isoimmunisation are relatively rare. The protective mechanisms essential for successful impregnation include sharing of antigens produced by the homologous male and female genital tracts (De Fazio & Ketchel 1971) and the presence of potent immunosuppressive agents present in semen and in the genital tracts and active at multiple levels of the immune response (Alexander & Anderson 1987; Quan et al 1990).

Male autoimmunisation (Mazumdar & Levine 1998) results from mechanical obstruction of the excurrent ducts (congenital anomalies, cystic fibrosis, vasectomy and trauma), clinical and subclinical genital infections, especially with *Chlamydia trachomatis*; T-cell dysfunction reflected by increased CD4/CD8 ratio and from a genetic predisposition associated with the HLA-B7 antigen (Mathur et al 1983a). Female isoimmunisation correlates strongly with sperm autoimmunity in the male (Mathur et al 1981) and in infertile couples antibody titres are higher against the husband's sperms than against sperms from controls (Mathur et al 1983b). It can result from abnormally immunogenic sperms (Mathur et al 1988), from excessive autoimmune sperm destruction (Mathur et al 1981), from deficiency of immune inhibitors (Prakash 1981), and from trauma, e.g., large loop excision of transformation zone of the cervix for intraepithelial neoplasia (Nicholson et al 1996). There is also a genetic predisposition to isoimmunisation, as suggested by the high frequency of HLA-BW35 in women with sperm isoantibodies and the sharing of HLA-B7, HLA-B8 and HLA-BW35 in infertile couples with sperm immunity (Mathur et al 1983a). One mechanism of sperm immunogenicity in the female and male genital tracts is the presence of immunostimulators, e.g. autoantibodies coating the sperm surface, and the secondary induction of interferon production by T cells and the release of macrophage chemotactic factor. Normally macrophages phagocytose and display processed sperm antigens on their surfaces in the absence of Ia antigens; locally produced interferon induces Ia expression on the macrophages and the concurrent display of sperm antigens and Ia antigens leads to immune system activation (Witkin 1988).

The causal link between sperm antibodies and human infertility is well established. Circulating serum antibodies are not directly involved and the local antibodies in the genital tract are only effective if they bind to the head or tail of the sperm and to at least 60% of the sperms (Wolf et al 1995; Francavilla et al 1997). There is no convincing evidence that sperm antibodies cause recurrent clinical miscarriages (Simpson et al 1996).

Four types of immune reactions to constituents of the ejaculate may occur:

1. Allergy to seminal fluid, manifested as immediate or delayed, localised or systemic, hypersensitivity reactions (Jones 1991) and rarely as fixed cutaneous eruptions (Best et al 1988). In the case of reaginic immunity to seminal fluid the severe systemic anaphylactic reaction and the local painful sterile vulvovaginitis can lead to avoidance of coitus and infertility by default. These couples show a high degree of sharing of HLA antigens but the significance of this finding is unclear (Jones 1991).
2. Cell-mediated response to sperm antigens, which is a universal response to repeated exposure to sperms without any impact on fertility (Mettler 1980).
3. Systemic response to sperm antigens: circulating antisperm antibodies are seen in similar frequency in fertile and infertile couples and do not cause infertility (Critser et al 1989).
4. Local immune response in the female and male genital tracts is considered to be the underlying mechanism of immunological infertility. The modes of action of antisperm antibodies remain controversial but may include (Mahony & Alexander 1991; Mazumder & Levine 1998):
   (i) Adverse effects on sperm numbers and forward motility;
   (ii) Disturbed sperm–cervical mucus interaction reflected as a poor postcoital test and leading to impaired sperm motility;
   (iii) Abnormal sperm–oocyte interaction: impaired sperm capacitation, zona-induced acrosome reaction and binding to zona pellucida and oolemma;
   (iv) compromised postfertilisation embryonic development leading to subclinical pregnancy loss and possible to recurrent clinical miscarriage.

MICROBIOLOGICAL FACTORS

The association of infertility with sexually transmitted disease (STD) is firmly established and the prevalence of STD-related infertility (tubal infertility) varies geographically with the highest frequency found in Africa and the lowest in the developed countries (Cates & Brunham 1999). STD is often polymicrobial. The dominant organisms include *Neisseria gonorrhoeae* and *Chlamydia trachomatis* and the less common organisms include endogenous vaginal flora, particularly those involved in bacterial vaginosis (Gram-negative anaerobes and *Mycoplasma hominis*) and even respiratory pathogens, i.e. *Hemophilus influenzae*, *Streptococcus pneumoniae* and Group A Streptococcus. The role of *Ureaplasma urealyticum* in pelvic inflammatory disease (PID) is minimal, if any at all. In 20–30% of women with PID no micro-organisms are isolated (Weström & Eschenbach 1999).

The risk factors for PID (Weström & Eschenbach 1999) include:

1. genetic susceptibility, probably HLA-linked (Kuberski 1980);
2. young age due to greater penetrability of oestrogen-dominant cervical mucus in adolescence (Holmes et al 1980);
3. coitus around the time of menstruation (Holmes et al 1980);
4. type of contraception: the risk is increased with the IUCD and decreased with barrier methods, particularly the combination of condoms and spermicides and the contraceptive pill;
5. therapeutic or diagnostic instrumentation of the cervix, especially if Chlamydia is present (MacMillan & Templeton 1999);
6. smoking, especially with the IUCD in place;
7. concurrent HIV infection (Barbosa et al 1997).

The mechanisms of underlying PID-related infertility are complex. Tubal damage includes distal or proximal occlusion, hydrosalpinx, peritubal adhesions and endosalpingeal disorganisation with loss of secretory cells and deciliation. Chlamydial injury is due to the prolonged salpingitis, often untreated, that results from a poor IgM response and to a chronic delayed hypersensitivity reaction to Chlamydial heat shock protein 60 (Weström & Eschenbach 1999). Chlamydial endometritis may contribute to infertility by secondary damage to sperms and conceptus by local leucocyte release of cytokines and reactive nitrogen intermediates (Tomlinson et al 1992).

Asymptomatic chronic endometritis due to *Ureaplasma urealyticum* (Fahmy et al 1987) may cause direct infection of the implanted conceptus or depression of sperm motility and sperm–egg interaction (Styler & Shapiro 1985). Subclinical ovarian infection by Chlamydia (Toth et al 2000) can lead to infertility by restriction of follicular development secondary to periovarian adhesions and loss of ovarian reserve due to direct follicular damage (Keay et al 1998).

Infections of the lower genital tract can also cause infertility. Bacterial cervicitis impairs sperm motility, survival and penetration (Odeblad 1978) and reduces implantation rates with IVF (Fanchin et al 1998). Cervico-vaginal viral infections may also be implicated. The presence of adeno-associated virus in semen is associated with asthenospermia and male infertility (Rohde et al 1999); its presence in female genital tissues (Walz et al 1998) and its positive interaction with HPV (Walz et al 1997) suggest a possible female contribution to the asthenospermia. Similarly HPV-related asthenospermia may be due to a combination of seminal and cervico-vaginal infections (Lai et al 1997). Trichomonas vaginalis can also cause infertility (el-Sharkawy et al 2000).

BIOPHYSICAL FACTORS

Sperm transport, essential for intratubal fertilisation, is the result of a finely tuned dynamic interaction between semen and female genital tract tissues (Barratt & Cooke 1991; Kunz et al 1997; Wildt et al 1998)). There is a high rate of loss in the vagina with only about 0.05% of ejaculated sperms entering the cervix (Fordney-Settlage et al 1973). After cervical rescue there is an early rapid phase of transport due to contraction of the uterotubal musculature, stimulated by seminal prostaglandins (Jaszczak et al 1980), with oxytocin released at orgasm acting as a potentiator. It is uncertain whether infertility can result from failure of this mechanism, secondary to seminal prostaglandin deficiency (Bygdeman 1970) or stressful intercourse associated with suppression of oxytocin release and neural inhibition of uterotubal activity.

The later and more important phase of sperm transport, which may last up to two days, is due to the storage and release function of the cervix (Zinamen et al 1989). The cervix eliminates abnormal sperms (Katz et al 1990) and may initiate capacitation, which is a prerequisite for the acrosome reaction. There is rapid transit through the uterine cavity where massive sperm phagocytosis occurs. The survivors reaching the tubes, estimated at one per every 14 million ejaculated, are then nurtured by tubal epithelium and tubal fluid as discussed later in the section on Fallopian tube.

There are four subtle biophysical sperm abnormalities that cause infertility. The first is associated with unexplained infertility, i.e. failure of the fertilising sperm to undergo activation inside the egg in preparation for the first meiotic division of the zygote (Brown et al 1995). The second is a sperm membrane abnormality that can be detected by an in vitro hypo-osmotic swelling test and is associated with unexplained recurrent miscarriage (Buckett et al 1997).

The third is abnormal sperm chromatin stability. Chromatin compactness is essential for sperm penetration of oocyte investments but chromatin decondensation and nuclear swelling occur during penetration of the ooplasm. Both decreased and increased sperm chromatin stability impair fertility, the former by causing premature chromatin decondensation and nuclear swelling before fertilisation (Kjellberg et al 1992) and the latter by preventing these processes from occurring (Gonzales & Villena 1997).

The fourth is a sperm defect that interferes with the zona pellucida-induced acrosome reaction and zona penetration (Liu & Baker 1994).

BIOCHEMICAL FACTORS

Biochemical interaction between the ejaculate and the female genital tract is not widely appreciated. Despite the abundance of fructose in semen, glucose is the preferential substrate and is critical for sperm viability and motility (Martikainen et al 1980). Because of the normally low levels of glucose in semen, an alternative source of supply is provided by cervical mucus, and infertility can result when the cervical supply of glucose is reduced (Weed & Carrera 1970). The physiological significance of glucose and fructose in cervical mucus is still unclear, especially as peak values occur only after ovulation (Van der Linden et al 1992). The seminal fluid has a higher pH than the vaginal secretions and its buffering capacity is critical for initial sperm survival. Some patients with oligospermia have significantly depressed levels of seminal free amino acids associated with reduced buffering capacity, a factor which may contribute to their infertility (Silvestroni et al 1979). Low levels of bicarbonate in seminal fluid contribute to infertility by decreasing buffering capacity and sperm motility (Okamura et al 1986).

Sperms stimulate the endometrium by direct cell-to-cell contact causing stimulation of carbonic anhydrase (Collado et al 1979) and increased incorporation of labelled precursors into endometrial macromolecules (Hicks et al 1980). This increased carbonic anhydrase activity, also stimulated by progesterone (Falk & Hodgen 1972), is important in regulating pH and bicarbonate levels, which are critical for fertilisation (Stambaugh et al 1969) and implantation (Friedley & Rosen 1975). This interaction between endometrium and sperms may partly explain the dose-relationship between sperm concentrations $<40 \times 10^6$/ml and the probability of conception (Bonde et al 1998).

Sperms are highly sensitive to oxidative stress because of their high polyunsaturated fatty acid content and any imbalance between the levels of reactive oxygen species (ROS) and antioxidants in semen can lead to sperm dysfunction and infertility. Thus infertility can be related to increased ROS levels, i.e. in leucocytospermia (Rajasekaran et al 1995) and after vasectomy reversal (Kolettis et al 1999) or to reduced antioxidant activity (Lewis et al 1997). Lipid peroxidation reduces sperm motility, capacitation and zona pellucida binding; DNA oxidation may cause sperm degeneration and mutations leading to early pregnancy loss (Kodama et al 1997). Other seminal abnormalities causing sperm dysfunction include a concomitant increase in cadmium and decrease in zinc in varicocele (Benoff et al 1997), decreased α-glycosidase activity (Spiessens et al 1998), disturbed concentrations of proinflammatory cytokines and their soluble receptors (Huleihel et al 1996) and functionally inactive protein C inhibitor that fails to protect sperms from proteolytic damage (He et al 1999).

The number of sperms reaching the fallopian tubes is very low (average 250; range 80–1400) and the probability of successful sperm–oocyte interaction is increased by sperm chemotaxis induced only by released follicular fluids with potentially fertilisable eggs. Positive chemotaxis increases the number of sperms in the ovulatory tubes and preferentially directs capacitated sperms towards the oocyte; negative chemotaxis signals oocyte activation by one sperm and prevents the arrival of others. It is thus possible that infertility may be due to defective precontact sperm–oocyte communication (Eisenbach 1999).

FEMALE INFERTILITY: ORGAN-RELATED CAUSES (Honoré 1994, 1997)

The female contribution to human infertility varies from population to population but in the West a fair estimate would be 40–50%. Often the reproductive system is involved at multiple levels but, for didactic purposes, the infertility-producing lesions will be discussed organ by organ.

Before discussing organ-related causes it is necessary to summarise recent findings concerning genetic causes of female infertility:

1. *Developmental disorders* include abnormal sexual differentiation and maturation due to gonadal dysgenesis, genetically determined gonadotrophin insufficiency, gonadotrophin inactivity due to receptor failure, genetic disorders of sex steroid synthesis and sensitivity, autosomal aneuploidy, syndromal and non-syndromal sexual maldevelopment (Layman 1999a,b; Pinsky et al 1999; Simpson & Rajkovic 1999).
2. *Genomic instability.* Chromosomal instability due to an increased chromosomal breakage rate can lead to streak gonads and female infertility (Duba et al 1997). Subfertility due to male and female hypogonadism can

be seen in trichothiodystrophy which is one of the defective nucleotide excision repair syndromes (de Boer & Hoeijmakers 2000).
3. *Implantation failure* due to abnormal *HOX A10* and *HOX A11* expression (Taylor 2000), inactivating mutations in the leukaemia inhibitory factor gene (Giess et al 1999) and deficient HLA-G expression in implanting blastocysts (Jurisicova et al 1996).
4. *Recurrent pregnancy loss* due to familial skewed X inactivation (Pegoraro 1997), inherited thrombophilic disorders (Blumenfeld & Brenner 1999), hyperhomocysteinaemia due to mutations in the cystathionine β synthase and in the methylene-tetrahydrofolate reductase genes (Obwegeser et al 1999), altered frequencies of certain DQ and DR haplotypes predisposing to anticardiolipin antibody formation (Hataya et al 1998) and genomic instability manifest as increased chromosomal breakage rates in lymphocytes of recurrent miscarriage after exposure to methotrexate (Velissariou et al 1993). Sperm aneuploidy may also cause recurrent miscarriages (Giorlandino et al 1998).
5. *Increased susceptibility to fertility-depressing diseases*:
   a) Increased predisposition to endometriosis due to inheritance of unknown susceptibility genes (Treloar et al 1999), oestrogen receptor gene polymorphisms (Georgiou et al 1999) and altered expression of *HOX A10* and *HOX A11* genes (Taylor 2000).
   b) Predisposition to polycystic ovarian disease due to a polymorphism in the gene *CYP17* promoter (Diamanti-Kandarakis et al 1999).
   c) Predisposition to ovarian and endometrial cancer whose treatment may further reduce fertility potential. It is unclear whether this increased incidence of ovarian and endometrial cancer in the infertile is due to inheritance of susceptibility to infertility and cancer or due to hormonal disturbances related to infertility (Duckitt & Templeton 1998).

VULVA AND VAGINA

By impeding or preventing normal penovaginal intercourse and vaginal insemination, congenital and acquired abnormalities of these structures can lead to infertility in a small proportion of potentially fertile couples. Congenital malformations causing permanent infertility are rare (Simpson et al 1993) and include:

1. Complete transverse vaginal septum, resulting from failure of canalisation of the solid vaginal plate, causes infertility indirectly. The imperforate septum leads to haematometrocolpos after puberty and secondary transtubal reflux with chronic tubal damage and endometriosis; these adverse sequelae can be

prevented by early diagnosis and treatment. The perforate septum only causes infertility after treatment if it is located high in the vagina and has led to secondary endometriosis.

2. Vaginal atresia/agenesis/aplasia in the presence of normal external and internal genitalia and upper vagina can occur singly or as part of complex malformation syndromes. Surgical intervention allows satisfactory sexual activity but has little impact on the improvement of fertility (Mobus et al 1996).

3. Chronic vulvovaginitis (Friedrich 1976) and asymptomatic infections of the vaginal fornices and ectocervix can cause infertility, the latter by decreasing sperm survival and motility (Wah et al 1990). The commonest vaginal infection of relevance is bacterial vaginosis due to a complex change in the vaginal flora with reduced prevalence and concentration of lactobacilli and increased prevalence and concentration of Gram-negative rods, *Gardnerella vaginalis* and *Mycoplasma hominis*. It is associated with genitourinary infections (Harmanli et al 2000), i.e. PID, postabortal PID, mucopurulent cervicitis and urinary tract infections, and with obstetrical complications, i.e. preterm labour, preterm rupture of the membranes, chorioamnionitis, postpartum endometritis and increased first trimester pregnancy loss after IVF (Ralph et al 1999).

4. Vulvar atrophy with introital stenosis (Friedrich 1976).

5. Mechanical disorders, e.g. scars secondary to childbirth, episiotomy, introital injury and paravaginal lesions such as uterine prolapse, ovarian fixation to vaginal vault or cervix, endometriosis of uterosacral ligaments, broad ligament varicosities and the Allen–Masters syndrome (Fordney 1978), and endometriosis of the uterosacral ligaments and rectovaginal septum (Donnez et al 1997). Organic dyspareunia can lead to vaginismus, which usually has psychological causes, e.g. severe penetration phobia (Drenth et al 1996; Jacob et al 1997).

6. Drug-induced dysfunction seen with amphetamines and cocaine (Gay & Shepard 1972).

UTERINE CERVIX

The cervix plays a critical rôle in reproduction by controlling sperm transport and by protecting the intrauterine conceptus from premature expulsion and ascending infection (Chretien 1978). Impediment to sperm ascent can be due to mechanical or biophysical abnormalities. Mechanical lesions of the cervix constitute a rare cause of infertility and include:

1. Malposition of the cervix due to severe anteflexion of the cervix, fixed retroversion of the uterus or uterine prolapse. The significant spatial dissociation between the external os and the vaginal pool, aggravated by oligospermia, can seriously curtail upward sperm migration (Moghissi 1979).

2. The effect of ablative therapy for cervical intraepithelial neoplasia on fertility remains controversial because of the limited and contradictory nature of the available data but the general conclusion stands that stenosis leading to infertility can follow cold knife conisation but not cryotherapy, laser vaporisation, electrocoagulation diathermy or the loop electrical excision procedure (Montz 1996). The data are also contradictory on the impact of the large loop excision of the transformation zone (LLETZ) procedure (Cruickshank et al 1995). Laparoscopic vaginal radical trachelectomy for early invasive cervical carcinoma has an increased risk of infertility and late miscarriage (Dargent et al 2000). Stenosis reduces the capacity to conceive directly by impeding the passage of sperms and indirectly by promoting retrograde menstruation and endometriosis (Barbieri 1998).

3. Congenital aplasia of the cervix (Niver et al 1980) is rare and is often associated with absence of the vagina and/or of the uterine isthmus, i.e. the Rokitansky–Küstner–Hauser syndrome (Golan et al 1989), which rarely may be caused by maternal galactosaemia (Cramer et al 1987). Pure cervical aplasia leads to haematometra with reflux menstruation and tubo-ovarian endometriosis. When combined with isthmic atresia there is reflex suppression of menstruation and no ensuing haematometra (Musset et al 1978). As a rule, cervical aplasia presents with painful or painless amenorrhoea fairly early in adolescence but, unless successfully treated (Edmonds 2000), it can be a cause of permanent sterility.

4. Ligneous (pseudomembranous) inflammation of the genital tract from vulva to tubes with preferential localisation in the cervicovaginal area (Scurry et al 1993) is a non-infectious treatment-resistant inflammatory process of unknown aetiology. It is related to ligneous conjunctivitis, and is characterised grossly by formation of indurated plaques or ulcerated firm polyps and microscopically by subepithelial deposition of dense amorphous hypocellular avascular eosinophilic material associated with secondary ulceration and nonspecific inflammation. These deposits stain positively for fibrin, IgG, IgA but negatively for IgM, IgD, C-reactive protein and amyloid. The infertility is due to widespread mucosal involvement of cervix, endometrium and tubes.

Mucus is fundamental to cervical function (Morales et al 1993). The cervix can be viewed as a biological valve which is closed to spermatozoal penetration for most of the cycle and allows entry only in the periovulatory period. The valve is controlled by hormone-induced variations in the physical properties of cervical mucus with its highly organised infrastructure. Its glycoprotein solid phase is disposed as a meshwork of fibrils cross-linked by oblique or transverse bonds, i.e. a 'tricot-like macromolecular arrangement' (Odeblad 1968; Cazabat et al 1982; Barros et al 1985). At mid-cycle, with rising oestrogen levels, endocervical secretions increase in amount with higher levels of sialomucin (Gaton et al 1982) and a higher content of water and salt (Gould & Ansari 1983) causing viscosity to drop, stretchability (spinnbarkeit) to increase and characteristic fern patterns to appear on air drying. This mucoid hydrogel (E-type mucus) is organised into fibrils to form a meshwork large enough to allow sperm passage and these fibrillar 'micelles' act as harmonic oscillators promoting onward progress of sperms through the intermicellar spaces by 'thermal modulations' which can cause the cavities to expand and contract rhythmically (Odeblad 1962). With low levels of oestrogen in the early part of the cycle and after the menopause and with high levels of progesterone in the luteal phase and in pregnancy (Chretien 1978), the glycoprotein chains assume greater autonomy and form tighter cross-linkages to produce an obstructive meshwork (G-type mucus). Postpartum mucus (Vigil et al 1991) from amenorrhoeic breast-feeding women is predominantly of the dense obstructive pattern but some samples are of the penetrable spongy periovulatory type, which probably accounts for the occasional 'contraceptive failure' of lactational infertility.

Another important periovulatory change in cervical mucus is chemical and consists of a significant decrease in the content of C, immunoglobulins, proteinase inhibitors and lysozyme, substances potentially harmful to sperm viability and motility (Schumacher et al 1977). The fertility promoting effects of these periovulatory alterations in cervical mucus include (Moghissi 1979):

1. Rapid sequestration of viable sperms from the lethal vaginal acidic milieu
2. Storage and preservation of actively motile sperms, particularly in the large and giant crypts of the endocervix (Insler et al 1980)
3. Sustained and prolonged postcoital release of sperms into the uterine cavity thus enhancing the probability of successful fertilisation.

Interaction between cervical mucus and sperms is critical for their survival and ability to reach and fertilise the ovum and can be studied clinically with the use of the postcoital test (Overstreet 1986). Abnormalities of cervical mucus, i.e. the cervical factor (Lunenfeld et al 1993), can be a cause of infertility in 15% of women and include:

1. Inadequate mucus secretion due to surgical removal or electrical destruction of the endocervical glands, endorgan insensitivity to oestrogen due to hypoplasia or receptor deficiency (Abuzeid et al 1987) and

oestrogen deficiency (Roumen et al 1982), which also produces viscid impenetrable mucus (Sher & Katz 1976; Morales et al 1993).
2. Changes in composition resulting from chronic cervicitis or cervicovaginitis. Depending on the type, duration and severity of the inflammation the secretory cells lose their sensitivity to oestrogen and start to secrete autonomously E- or G-type mucus and a third type (Q-type) of mucus, which is variable in constitution and is made up of subunits or partial components. This viscid mucus, consisting of a mixture of E-, G- and Q-types of mucus, is impenetrable to sperms (Odeblad 1978). Penetrability is also reduced by increasing acidity with inflammation (Ansari et al 1980). Finally, inflammation increases cervical levels of immunoglobulins and inflammatory mediators (Wah et al 1990), which are potentially toxic to sperms (Tomlinson et al 1992).
3. The presence of sperm-coating autoantibodies or isoantibodies on the sperm surface decreases mucus penetration by entangling the Fc portion in the glycoprotein matrix of the mucus (Jager et al 1978). The immunological reaction also causes mucus hypersecretion and intraluminal exudation of active leucocytes (Nicosia & Johnson 1983) with acidification of the mucus (Parish & Ward 1968).
4. Non-inflammatory mucus hyperacidity present in women taking dexamethasone, clomiphene citrate and bromocriptine synergises with oligospermia to produce infertility by depressing sperm viability and motility (Eggert-Kruse et al 1993). It is the most likely link between subfertility and a high waist–hip ratio associated with high serum androgen levels (Jenkins et al 1995). It may also contribute to mucus hostility after treatment with clomiphene citrate, which induces abnormally high levels of testosterone in the mid-follicular periovulatory periods (Langer et al 1990) and is antroestrogenic in the cervix (Gelety & Buyalos 1993).
5. Specific incompatibility of sperm and mucus in some infertile couples for unknown reasons (Overstreet 1986).

Cervical incompetence

The cervix plays a critical rôle in pregnancy by mechanically supporting the enlarging conceptus and preventing its premature expulsion. It is not surprising therefore that cervical incompetence can lead to repeated pregnancy loss in the second trimester. An aetiological classification of cervical incompetence includes four types (Shortle & Jewelewicz 1989):

1. Acquired: a gross defect is visible in the cervix. This follows traumatic deliveries with inadequately repaired

lacerations or may be iatrogenic, i.e. produced by diagnostic and therapeutic procedures. Excessive and rapid cervical dilatation during dilatation and curettage is the commonest causative factor but there is no consensus about the rôle of the more gradual and gentler dilatation achieved by laminaria tents during induced second-trimester abortions. Conisation can cause incompetence depending on cone size and depth but cryotherapy and shallow laser surgery are harmless.

2. Congenital: the cervix is grossly normal but there is a histological defect which compromises its ability to resist pressure during pregnancy. This can be due to an abnormally high ratio of smooth muscle to collagen, a deficiency of elastin or a biochemical abnormality in the collagen, as in the Ehlers–Danlos syndrome (Leduc & Wasserstrum 1992). Primary incompetence is also common with prenatal exposure to diethylstilboestrol (Goldberg & Falcone 1999) and in association with uterine anomalies.

3. Physiological or dysfunctional: early effacement and dilatation of the cervix follow subclinical inappropriate uterine irritability.

4. Anatomical: the normal cervico-isthmic region is distorted by local lesions, e.g. low-lying leiomyomas.

The diagnosis of cervical incompetence is suggested by recurrent second-trimester spontaneous miscarriages in the absence of uterine contractions, especially if the fetus is fresh and not macerated or survives briefly after expulsion. During pregnancy, symptoms include a sense of pressure in the lower abdomen or in the upper vagina, watery or mucoid vaginal discharge and urinary frequency and urgency without dysuria. The diagnostic sign is the palpation or visualisation of bulging membranes in the second trimester without evidence of premature labour. Diagnosis is more difficult in the non-pregnant state and relies on the use of dilators, hysterosalpingography and ultrasonography (Guzman et al 1994). Cervical incompetence is now considered to be not an all-or-none phenomenon but a continuum related to pregnancy loss or premature labour (Iams et al 1995).

CORPUS UTERI

The corpus uteri plays a vital rôle in reproduction by providing a free passageway to the sperms in their ascent from cervix to tube and by harbouring the conceptus from implantation to delivery. Its function depends on normal structural development, its position relative to the cervix and the structural and functional integrity of its blood supply and its two components, i.e. endometrium and myometrium. Corporeal abnormalities, causing infertility by interfering with pre- and postfertilisation events, can be classified as structural, positional, vascular, myometrial and endometrial.

Structural abnormalities

These lesions, whether arising spontaneously or after intrauterine exposure to diethylstilboestrol (DES), are an uncommon cause of female infertility by preventing conception and increasing pregnancy loss. They are discussed in Chapter 2.

Positional disturbances

There is little evidence to suggest that infertility can result from abnormal positions of the uterus per se. For instance, fixed retroversion is due to concomitant pelvic disease, e.g. endometriosis or salpingitis, which is more likely to underlie the infertility (Wallach 1972). Uterine hyperflexion has been implicated in infertility and recurrent miscarriages (Liliequist & Lindgren 1964).

Vascular abnormalities

Anatomical variations of blood vessels are usually harmless but in the uterus a simple variation of arterial supply can lead to a significant increase in the incidence of low birth weight infants and of early sporadic, but not necessarily recurrent, miscarriages. Normally the uterine artery gives off a single ascending branch from which all the arcuate arteries arise. In some patients the ascending artery divides into two separate branches which give rise to the anterior and posterior arcuate arteries and this arterial configuration is associated with reproductive dysfunction (Burchell et al 1978). An adequate blood supply is essential for successful pregnancy and this effect depends on the appropriate development of endometrial receptivity (Steer et al 1994).

The role of uterine vascular insufficiency in infertility and early pregnancy loss is gaining support from Doppler studies of uterine blood flow (Goswany et al 1988; Kurjak et al 1991; Steer et al 1994). Postpubertal uterine growth is also critically dependent on adequate perfusion and uterine hypoplasia can be produced experimentally by devascularisation (Gardey et al 1975a) or prevented by combining devascularisation with beta-adrenergic drug therapy (Gardey et al 1975b). It is likely, although unproven, that the hypoplastic or infantile uterus, seen in endocrinologically normal adults and characterised by a small uterus with a disproportionately long, narrow, poorly vascularised cervix with a pinhole os, is the result of congenital hypovascularity. The associated infertility (Field-Richards 1954) is due to a combination of factors, i.e. the hypoplastic endometrium and myometrium, the poorly developed cervix, the associated shallow vaginal fornix and retroflexion or acute anteflexion of the uterus.

Myometrial abnormalities

Current evidence favours a causal relationship between adenomyosis and infertility, which is probably the result of associated immunological disturbances similar to those seen with endometriosis (Ota et al 1998). The connection between adenomyoma and infertility is less certain (Honoré et al 1988a; Fedele et al 1993). The critical infertility-related myometrial lesion is the leiomyoma; which can be confused clinically with the adenomatoid tumour (Honoré unpublished observations) or with the rare leiomyosarcoma (Hitti et al 1991). This common benign tumour, much more common in black than in white women, usually occurs in perimenopausal women and is thus an infrequent cause of infertility (Buttram & Reiter 1981). The mechanisms underlying the infertility include:

1. Interference with sperm transport. The tumour may mechanically obstruct sperm passage through the cervix and the uterotubal junction or it may distort the uterine cavity, thus increasing the distance to be covered by the sperms (Hunt & Wallach 1974). It may also interfere with sperm transport facilitation by rhythmic myometrial contraction induced by seminal prostaglandins (Coutinho & Maia 1971).

2. Myometrial irritation and hyperactivity due to degeneration or torsion of the tumour.
3. Atrophy or alteration of the endometrium overlying a submucous leiomyoma (Fig. 30.1), if extensive, can prevent successful nidation.
4. Vascular disturbances in the endometrium may interfere with implantation. A leiomyoma may compress endometrial and myometrial venous plexuses to cause venous ectasia and congestion or hypoperfusion of the endometrium (Farrer-Brown et al 1971). There is also a significant reduction in the blood flow through the leiomyoma and adjacent uterus (Forssman 1976).
5. Failure of blastocyst retention. It has been suggested that the biological function of endometrial thickening in the luteal phase, produced by tissue increase, stromal oedema and particularly by occlusion and distension of the secretory glands, is to obliterate the lumen and retain the blastocyst (Datnow 1973). Another mechanism favouring blastocyst retention in the upper corpus is the presence of unidirectional cervix-to-fundus periovulatory endometrial waves generated by contraction of the submucosal myometrium and associated with a change in uterine shape from cylindrical to piriform, i.e. a narrow cervico-isthmic region and a spheroid corpus (Ijland et al 1999).
6. Associated salpingitis (Mitami et al 1959).
7. Bilateral cornual obstruction by multiple leiomyomas which can be successfully treated by a GnRH agonist (Gardner & Shaw 1989).

The hormone-sensitive leiomyoma can be treated by myomectomy or with a gonadotrophin-releasing hormone agonist prior to removal. There is no consensus on the pathology of the post-medical treatment leiomyoma: some authors report no specific changes (Sreenan et al 1996) while others describe blood vessel wall thickening, thrombosis, infarctive necrosis, hydropic change, hyalinisation, dehydration of the extracellular matrix and cellular atrophy without reduction in cell numbers (Colgan et al 1993; Rein et al 1993; Deligdisch et al 1997; Demopoulos et al 1997). A rare finding is the development of severe vasculitis with fibrinoid necrosis, atherosis and thrombosis with IgG, IgM, and IgA deposition (Mesia et al 1997). An unfortunate side effect of treatment is loss of the cleavage plane between myoma and myometrium making enucleation more difficult (Deligdisch et al 1997). The most likely mechanism of shrinkage is oestrogen deprivation with reduced blood flow, detected ultrasonically by increased arterial resistance index (Spong et al 1995) and related pathologically to a decrease in the diameter of small intratumoral arteries with non-occlusive intimal and medial fibrosis (Rutgers et al 1995). The degree of myoma shrinkage after treatment can be predicted from the extent of hyaline change and the amount of collagen

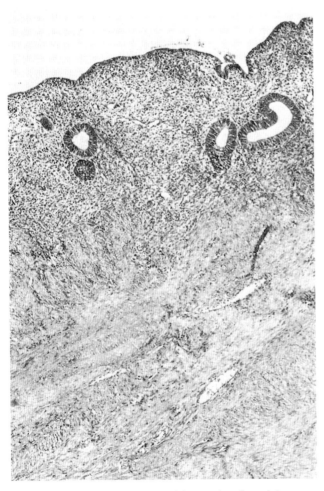

Fig. 30.1 Submucous leiomyoma with atrophy of overlying endometrium.

present in the pre-treatment needle biopsy of the tumor (Kawamura et al 1997).

A potentially serious problem with medical treatment of leiomyomas is the risk of missing a leiomyosarcoma that can grow and kill the patient (Murphy & Wallace 1993); fortunately leiomyosarcoma in premenopasual patients with presumed leiomyomas is quite rare (Parker et al 1994).

Endometrial abnormalities

The endometrium, which is the site of implantation, undergoes an orderly series of hormonally controlled structural, histochemical, biochemical and vascular changes (see Chapter 11). These cyclical changes, i.e. proliferation, secretory transformation and gestational decidualisation or menstruation, affect principally the anterior and posterior walls of the corpus with the isthmus and cornua exhibiting lesser degrees of proliferation (Ferenczy et al 1979) and secretory alterations. It is tempting to suggest that such geographical disparities underlie nature's way of preventing isthmic or cornual implantation with its attendant complications.

Unlike the proliferative phase, the secretory or luteal phase is more constant in duration and the tissue changes follow a fairly uniform schedule, which allows accurate day dating of the secretory endometrium (Noyes et al 1950). Despite early warnings (Noyes & Haman 1954) the accuracy of endometrial dating and the ability of the endometrium to reflect corpus luteum function has been taken for granted and the clinical diagnosis of luteal phase deficiency is now based on at least two sequential endometrial biopsies showing a lag of > 2 days between histological dating and chronological dating and other qualitative abnormalities (Zaino 1996; Deligdisch 2000). This simplistic equation between endometrial dating and corpus luteum dysfunction is now under attack on multiple fronts, as follows:

1. The accuracy of histological day dating is affected by subjectivity of interpretation (Scott et al 1993) and by regional endometrial variability. The overall error (Gibson et al 1991) is due to inconsistencies between evaluators (65%), intra-observer discrepancies (27%) and regional differences in the endometrium (8%). This lack of precision of endometrial dating (Li et al 1989) has raised serious doubts about its value in the diagnosis of luteal phase defects and it has been estimated that a false positive diagnosis may be made in 22–39% of patients, depending on the clinical setting (Scott et al 1988). Hence the need to devise other methods of endometrial evaluation, e.g. morphometric (Kim-Bjorklund et al 1991; Li et al 1991), immunocytochemical (Self et al 1989; Tabibzadeh 1990) and biochemical (Giudice 1999).

2. The timing of the endometrial biopsy can influence the accuracy of histological dating. Most authors have recommended a late luteal biopsy, i.e. about 2 days before the expected menses, but recent studies claim that accuracy of dating is better when the biopsy is taken on luteal day 9–10 (Lessey et al 2000), i.e. at the end of the implantation window (Bergh & Navot 1992).

3. The classical method for chronological dating of the cycle uses the first day of the post-biopsy menstruation to define day 14 postovulatory (retrospective dating) but recent evidence suggests that greater accuracy is achieved when the dating is prospective using the day of LH surge as the critical landmark (Li et al 1991; Lessey et al 2000).

4. The type of biopsy instrument, i.e. the stainless steel Novak curette or the polypropylene cannula ('Pipelle'), can significantly affect the frequency of out of phase endometrial biopsies, raising the possibility that the diagnosis of an inadequate luteal phase can be influenced by a purely technical factor (Honoré et al 1988b).

5. The incidence of luteal phase defect, as determined by serial endometrial biopsies, was found not to be significantly different between a fertile and an infertile population (Davis et al 1989); this casts some doubt on the standard criteria for diagnosing luteal defect but the study was small and uncontrolled. Nonetheless, histological dating remains the gold standard for endometrial assessment with additional information provided by morphometry (Li et al 1988), electron microscopy (Kolb et al 1997) and molecular studies (Tabizadeh et al 1999; Lessey et al 2000). It is unlikely that Doppler ultrasonography will replace the endometrial biopsy (Sterzik et al 2000).

Despite these criticisms luteal phase deficiency is still recognised as a cause of reproductive dysfunction, i.e. infertility, recurrent miscarriage and tubal ectopic pregnancy (Guillaume et al 1995) and the endometrial biopsy remains the most practical test of corpus luteum function (Li & Cooke 1991), despite its insensitivity (Blacker et al 1997). As diagnosed by endometrial biopsy luteal phase deficiency can be due to deficient endometrial response to normal progesterone levels (Cumming et al 1985; Li et al 1991; Hirama & Ochiai 1995). It is more common after ovulation induced by clomiphene citrate as a result of defective follicular maturation (Keenan et al 1989) or a direct endometrial antioestrogenic effect without steroid receptor disruption (Fritz et al 1991).

The diagnosis of luteal phase deficiency is based on the following abnormalities detected in at least two sequential biopsies (Zaino 1996; Deligdisch 2000):

a) Delay of more than 2 days in histological dating as compared with chronological dating based on the LH surge or post-biopsy menstruation.

b) Glandular stromal asynchrony with a maturational disparity of at least 2 days between glands and stroma; as a rule, the stroma shows advanced maturation.

c) Uneven maturation characterised by normal synchronous maturation of glands and stroma varying by at least 2 days in different areas.

d) Underdeveloped endometrium with straight tubular glands, scanty glycogen and thin arterioles.

e) Mixed endometrium with persistent mitoses in secretory glands.

Despite the fact that gestational hyperplasia has been beautifully described and illustrated by Hertig (1954), it regularly goes unrecognised in endometrial biopsies taken during the luteal phase of the cycle of conception (Karrow et al 1971; Rosenfeld & Garcia 1975; Mazur et al 1989). In the sterile cycle the phase of active glandular secretions peaks around day 6 postovulatory and is followed by progressive epithelial exhaustion; the stromal phase, typified by condensation of stroma with loss of oedema, vascular development and stromal growth and differentiation (Fig. 30.2), starts after the ninth postovulatory day. With early pregnancy there is overlapping and exaggeration of the glandular and stromal phases (Hertig 1954). I have found the following criteria (Honoré & Scott 1982) useful in the diagnosis of a concurrent undisturbed pregnancy from a late luteal phase endometrial biopsy:

1. Focal resurgence of sub-nuclear vacuolisation in the surface epithelium and in the subsurface glands, seen only in early or midluteal biopsies.

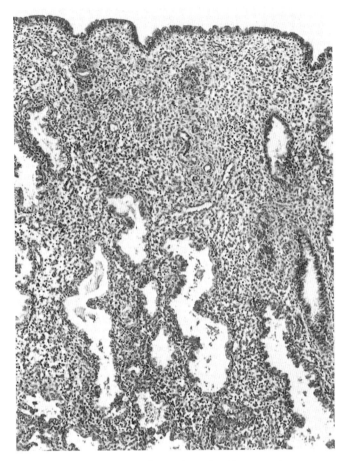

Fig. 30.2 Late secretory endometrium, day 11 postovulatory.

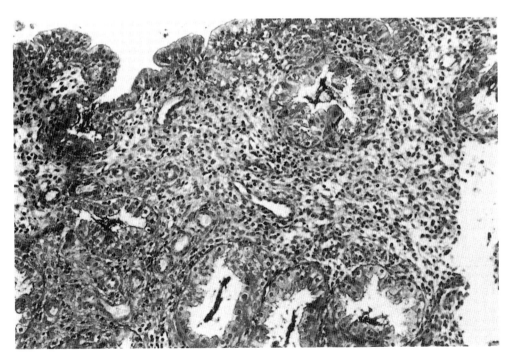

Fig. 30.3 'Secretory' endometrium with viable undisturbed intrauterine pregnancy: persistent and enhanced glandular secretion in presence of arterial fields and stromal decidualisation. PAS–Alcian Blue.

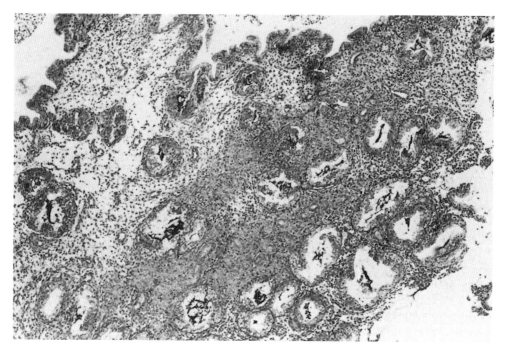

Fig. 30.4 'Secretory' endometrium with viable undisturbed intrauterine pregnancy: coexistence of stromal oedema, well-developed arterial fields, perivascular decidualisation and persistent glandular secretion. PAS–Alcian Blue.

2. Persistence and exaggeration of glandular secretion in the presence of well-developed arterial fields and decidualisation (Fig. 30.3).
3. Coexistence of patchy oedema with well-established vascular and predecidual changes (Fig. 30.4).
4. Dilatation and congestion of the superficial blood vessels.
5. Reduced 'leucocytic' infiltration of the premenstrual stroma (Daly et al 1982). These 'leucocytes' are stromal granulocytes, which become degranulated and apparently more prominent as the premenstrual endometrium dehydrates and the stromal cells shrink. The early gestational endometrium does not undergo premenstrual collapse and the stromal granulocytes appear less prominent, without any decrease in numbers (Mazur et al 1989).

The diagnosis of an undisturbed concurrent pregnancy was followed in some cases by a successful pregnancy and in others by delayed heavy menstruation, which is in effect an early subclinical miscarriage. The prevalence of early implantation failure (biochemical pregnancy) detected by intensive daily monitoring of β-hCG levels, is about 20% in healthy fertile women (Ellish et al 1996) and 80–85% in infertile women undergoing assisted conception (Edwards 1995). This early pregnancy loss is supported by the detection of a degenerating conceptus (Fig. 30.5) in curettings obtained from an infertile patient.

Endometrial disturbances often passively reflect ovarian dysfunction but there are primary endometrial lesions, which can be the dominant cause of infertility. These include:

1. Endometrial unresponsiveness to oestrogen, partial or complete: the partial variant is detected ultrasonically as a thin endometrium and responds poorly to controlled ovarian hyperstimulation (Hassan & Saleh 1996); the complete variant is characterised by absent ultrasonic visualisation, the sensation of absence of tissue on biopsy or curettage, lack of endometrial tissue after these procedures and failure to respond to large doses of steroids (Ruiz-Velasco et al 1997).
2. Acquired uterine adhesions (Asherman's syndrome). This endometrial lesion is discussed in detail in Chapter 11.
3. Endometrial polyps have been described in patients with primary and secondary infertility (Valle 1980) but their aetiological significance must be viewed with caution, as suggested by a study showing a 15% incidence of polyps in women with no apparent cause of infertility except voluntary tubal sterilisation (Goerzen et al 1983). There is some evidence that fertility impairment may be due to a higher propensity to spontaneous miscarriage (Overstreet 1959). Hypertrophic endometrium, represented by polyps and polypoid endometrium, is significantly associated with pelvic or peritoneal endometriosis and may partly account for the associated infertility and abnormal uterine bleeding (McBean et al 1996).
4. Chronic endometritis is a rare cause of infertility (Czernobilsky 1978) and can be subdivided

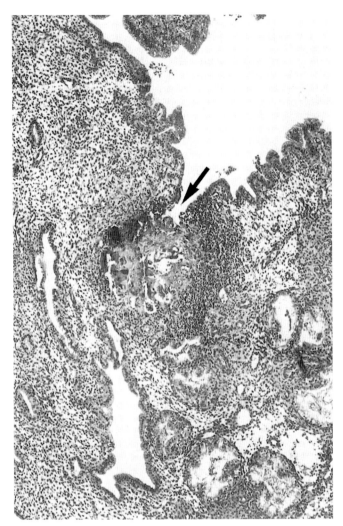

Fig. 30.5 Late 'secretory' endometrium with early postimplantation failure: 'ulceration' of endometrial surface epithelium, degenerating trophoblast (arrow) and lymphoid infiltration of adjacent stroma.

into tuberculous or non-tuberculous, as follows:

A. Tuberculous endometritis is a rare cause of infertility in the West but has a significantly higher prevalence in developing countries (Bazak-Malik et al 1983). The lesion, typically involving the spongiosa and the compacta and less commonly the basalis and the myometrium, consists in most cases of single or coalescent granulomas with absent, minimal or rarely extensive caseation (Fig. 30.6), epithelioid cells, lymphocytes, scanty plasma cells and a variable number of Langhans giant cells. In some cases tubercles are not seen and the focal or diffuse infiltration is made up of lymphocytes, plasma cells and a few eosinophils, but the presence of dilated glands with or without intraluminal exudate or glands with microabscesses should alert the pathologist to the fact that tuberculous endometritis can masquerade

as a non-specific non-granulomatous lesion (Govan 1962; Bazak-Malik et al 1983). Acid-fast bacilli are rarely detected in excised tissue but guinea pig inoculations are consistently positive (Nogales-Ortiz et al 1979). Endometrial tuberculosis is usually secondary to descending infection from the infected tubes and tuberculous infertility can be due to a combination of endometrial and tubal damage. Despite intensive therapy the reproductive prognosis is poor (Schaeffer 1976).

B. Non-tuberculous chronic endometritis can be further broken down into non-specific and specific:

   i.   The non-specific form is due to ascending infection from the lower tract and can be part of a generalised genital infection or can follow miscarriage or delivery, usually complicated by retention of decidua and/or fetal tissue, or can result from stagnation of menstrual flow due to outflow obstruction by isthmic or cervical stenosis, polyps or neoplasms. The inflammatory infiltrate contains plasma cells, lymphocytes, macrophages, neutrophils and rarely eosinophils but the diagnosis rests on the presence of plasma cells (Rotterdam 1978) which can be difficult to differentiate from lymphocytes or stromal cells and may need the methyl pyronin stain or immunoglobulin immunostaining. Plasma cells can be scanty, especially in endometrial biopsies, and useful diagnostic clues include peri-glandular pinwheel arrangement of fusiform stromal cells and irregular secretory maturation of the glands and stroma. The luminal epithelium may show regeneration or squamous metaplasia.

   ii.   Chlamydial endometritis resembles non-specific chronic endometritis but it shows a higher percentage of plasma cells, peri-glandular lymphoid follicles with transformed lymphocytes, intracellular inclusions detected by immunofluorescence or immunohistochemistry and loss of glandular response to progesterone (Winkler & Crum 1987; Kiviat et al 1990).

   iii.   Gonococcal endometritis differs from chlamydial endometritis in showing fewer plasma cells, no lymphoid follicles and more extensive tissue fragmentation (Kiviat et al 1990).

   iv.   Mycoplasmal endometritis has been described in patients investigated for infertility (Horne et al 1973; Cumming et al 1984) but the actual rôle of *Ureaplasma urealyticum* in the causation of infertility is still unsettled. The

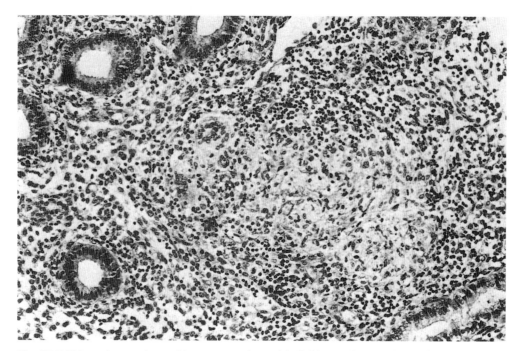

Fig. 30.6 Tuberculous endometritis: non-caseating epithelioid granuloma with Langhans giant cells. (Courtesy of Dr R. Hodkinson, Edmonton.)

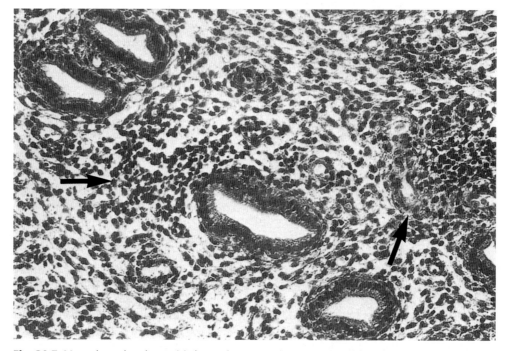

Fig. 30.7 Mycoplasmal endometritis (*Ureaplasma urealyticum* isolated from endometrial biopsy sample): patchy discrete paraglandular and paravascular lymphocytic clusters (arrows).

lesion, as a rule asymptomatic, consists of a non-granulomatous non-necrotising subacute inflammation featuring a variable number of small discrete clusters of lymphocytes lying under the surface epithelium or flanking the occasional gland or blood vessel (Fig. 30.7). The lymphocytes often infiltrate the glandular epithelium without causing necrosis. This inflammatory reaction, typically focal, discrete and centred on anatomical structures, differs from the commonly encountered lymphoid follicles in perimenopausal women (Sen & Fox 1967) which lie in the deep stroma without any glandular or vascular relationship, and also from the premenstrual leucocyte infiltration of the stroma (Daly et al 1982), which is diffuse and bears no relationship to blood vessels, glands or surface epithelium. The significance of this subacute focal endometritis is still undefined but we find it more commonly in biopsies obtained from infertile patients (Honoré personal observations). Some authors have claimed that subacute focal endometritis is a significant indicator of pelvic adhesions and endometriosis (Burke et al 1985); we have failed to confirm this and we have found that this lesion does not interfere with normal secretory maturation of the endometrium (Fahmy et al 1987).

The mechanisms underlying human infertility related to chronic endometritis are unknown but they include the toxic effects of leucocytic extracts on ascending spermatozoa (Tredway et al 1975) and on the preimplantation zygote (Parr & Shirley 1976).

v. Squamous metaplasia of the endometrial epithelium and smooth muscle metaplasia of the stroma are rare causes of infertility and they can be misinterpreted as endometrial ossification on ultrasound (Ruiz-Velasco et al 1997).

vi. Endometrial osseous metaplasia is another rare cause of infertility and recurrent pregnancy loss. It can be due to chronic endometritis or retention of fetal bones after an induced or spontaneous miscarriage (Bahceci & Demirel 1996; Feyles et al 2000; Graham et al 2000).

vii. Biochemical defects have been sporadically identified in the endometria of infertile women but there has been no controlled systematic study of endometrial biochemistry in infertility. Hughes et al (1963) showed that endometria obtained from women with infertility and repeated miscarriage were deficient in RNA and DNA, glycogen, alkaline phosphatase, glucose-6-phosphatase, isocitric dehydrogenase and malic dehydrogenase; without concurrent hormone studies they were unable to determine if these deficiencies were primary or secondary. Disturbances in glycogen metabolism (Mimori et al 1981), e.g. significantly reduced levels of glycogen, glycogen synthetase and glycogen phosphorylase, were detected in endometria of patients with unexplained infertility in the presence of normal progesterone levels; the authors could not establish whether these deficiencies were due to an abnormal endometrial response or reflected inadequate oestrogenic stimulation in the follicular phase. In some patients with unexplained infertility, there is defective biosynthesis and distribution of glycoconjugates in the glandular epithelium, as determined by lectin histochemistry; as these substances play a significant rôle in recognition and attachment (the 'sugar language'), their deficiency and maldistribution may lead to implantation failure (Klentzeris et al 1991). Finally, a deficiency of the oestrogen and progesterone sensitive endometrial RNA polymerase has been reported in women with persistent unexplained infertility (Soutter et al 1979). The role of primary biochemical or molecular aberrations of the endometrium in infertility remains uncharted territory.

viii. Abnormal ciliary structure in the endometrial surface epithelium was reported in a 29-year-old woman with primary infertility and Kartagener's syndrome (Marchini et al 1992). The cilia lacked the central pair of microtubules and one of the outer doublets was transposed, while the dynein arms were unaffected. It was suggested that ciliary immotility or dyskinesia altered the flow of endometrial secretions and interfered with the upstream migration of spermatozoa.

ix. Molecular defects: it is now clear that endometrial receptivity is the critical determinant of successful implantation and that endometrial histology, which can be normal in infertile patients (Saleh et al 1995), is only a crude functional indicator. Hence the search for subtle molecular defects in infertile endometria. The most critical integrin for receptivity is $\alpha V\beta 3$ (vitronectin receptor), which is normally upregulated during the implantation window; failure of upregulation is associated with unexplained infertility, luteal phase defect, endometriosis and hydrosalpinx (Lessey et al 1995; Meyer et al 1997; Sueoka et al 1997). Deficiency of endometrial secretion of leukaemia inhibitory factor (LIF), essential for murine implantation, is observed in women with recurrent IVF-embryo transfer failure or idiopathic infertility (Hambartsoumian 1998).

Homeobox genes *HOXA 10* and *HOXA 11* regulate endometrial development during the menstrual cycle and patients with endometriosis-related infertility fail to upregulate the midluteal expression of these genes (Taylor et al 1999). Aromatase cytochrome P450, absent in the endometrium of healthy women, is abnormally expressed in the eutopic endometrium of women with endometriosis, adenomyosis and leiomyomas. Its immunohistochemical detection with a sensitivity of 91% and a specificity of 100% offers a simple screening test for these diseases in infertile women (Kitawaki et al 1999).

During and after implantation tolerance of the semi-allogeneic conceptus is achieved by a complex 'double-jointed' interaction between trophoblast and endometrium. Isolated defects of the endometrial component can lead to infertility due to subclinical or clinical miscarriage. These include:

a) reduced levels of decay accelerating factor in out of phase endometrium with luteal phase defect causing inadequate suppression of complement and embryo toxicity (Kaul et al 1995);

b) decreased production of immunosuppressive factors like MUC1 and PP14 (glycodelin) in recurrent miscarriage (Aplin et al 1996; Okon et al 1998);

c) inappropriate setting at the time of implantation of the T-helper balance favouring the production of TH-1 over TH-2 cytokines with conceptus rejection (Lim et al 2000);

d) increase of cytotoxic natural killer (NK) cells in the peripheral blood and in the endometrium of patients with IVF failure (Fukui et al 1999);

e) increased endometrial leucocytes and disturbed cytokine profile, i.e. increased IFN-γ and decreased IL-4 and IL-10, in women with implantation defects related to autoimmune thyroid disease (Stewart-Akers et al 1998).

THE FALLOPIAN TUBE

The tube plays a pivotal rôle in reproduction by regulating bidirectional gamete transport, providing the site for fertilisation, supporting the newly fertilised zygote and releasing it after a physiologically timed delay (Harper 1988). As the tube is geographically specialised it is tempting to ascribe unique functions to these individual segments but experience with clinical and experimental ablative surgery has shown that appreciable functional compensation occurs when isolated segments are missing. Thus in rabbits selective microsurgical resection of the fimbria, ampulla, ampulloisthmic junction (AIJ) and uteroisthmic junction (UIJ) has failed to significantly impair fertility but excision of the fimbria along with the distal ampulla (Halbert & McComb 1981) and of the entire isthmus including the AIJ and UIJ (McComb et al 1981) causes sterility. In women successful pregnancy occurs, although at a variably reduced rate, after selective segmental loss (Gomel 1983). Aside from patency the crucial factor for maintenance of fertility is tubal length (McComb et al 1981); in humans, following microsurgical reversal of tubal sterilisation, the critical length is 5 cm and the pregnancy rate drops from 100% to 18% as tubal

length decreases to below 3 cm (Rock et al 1987). Experimental tubal lengthening in rabbits reduces fertility (Bateman et al 1983) but it is not clear whether human infertility can result from excessively long tubes, as seen in some women with idiopathic infertility after intrauterine exposure to diethylstilboestrol. Dependency on the tube is not absolute as evidenced by the low but far from negligible pregnancy rate after the Estes operation, i.e. intrauterine ovarian implantation (Adams 1979) and the occurrence of spontaneous pregnancies in women with bilateral tubal occlusion (Gomel & McComb 1981).

The tubal mechanisms ensuring gamete transport are not fully understood (Jansen 1984). In women the ovum reaches the fimbria seven hours after ovulation, stays in the ampulla for 72 hours and traverses the isthmus rapidly to reach the uterine cavity after 80 hours (Croxatto et al 1978; Harper 1988). Ovum pick-up is achieved by increased periovulatory contractility of the ovary, mesotubarium ovaricum and adnexal ligaments (Morikawa et al 1980); as a result, the fimbriae sweep the ovarian surface and directly contact the ovum as it emerges through the ovulation stigma.

This contact between ovum and tubal fimbriae is enhanced by the presence of a sticky gelatinous matrix on the outer aspect of the cumulus oophorus. The fimbrial cilia, stuck to the outer cumulus, pull it out into long streamers as they move the ovum towards the tubal ostium, a process aided by rhythmic contractions of the fimbriae and adjacent broad ligament (Harper 1988). This anatomical and functional co-operation between tube and ovary is important (Ahmad-Thabet 2000) but not essential for ovum capture as pregnancy occurs after salpingoneostomy (Gomel 1983), microsurgical dissociation of ovary and fimbria (Eddy & Laufe 1983) and when the patient has one functional tube and ovary on opposite sides (First 1954). In the ampulla the ovum is conveyed ad uterum by to-and-fro pendular motions caused by alternating peristaltic waves propagated for short distances in the tubal muscle. This random Brownian movement of the ovum has a definite aduterine bias provided for by at least three possible mechanisms, i.e. aduterine ciliary action (Verdugo et al 1980), asymmetry of muscular contraction with statistical preponderance ad uterum (Chatkoff 1975) and the peculiar tubal anatomy with a reflecting barrier at the fimbria and an absorbing barrier at the isthmus (Portnow et al 1977). A three-dimensional anatomical study (Vizza et al 1995) has challenged this concept by showing that the human ampullary myosalpinx is organised not into defined longitudinal circular or spiral layers capable of generating unidirectional peristalsis like the gut but as an anastomosing intermingling and continuous network of muscle fibres designed to produce a random pendulous movement for stirring and mixing rather than propelling luminal controls; other factors, i.e. ciliary action, tubal fluid flow, paracrine secretions from the ovum, etc., are needed to derandomise this pendulous motion and produce aduterine movement. The compensatory synergism between ciliary and muscular action in the ampulla is shown by the occasional pregnancy after surgical reversal of an ampullary segment in rabbits (McComb et al 1980) and the occurrence of fertility (Jean et al 1979) or infertility (McComb et al 1986) in women with defective cilia depending on the degree of ciliary dyskinesia.

The transient hold-up followed by eventual release of the ovum at the ampulloisthmic junction is a consistent phenomenon but its modus operandi is uncertain (Sayegh & Mastroianni 1991). The following mechanisms have been proposed:

1. The ampulloisthmic junction, which displays periodic electrical activity, dilates for a brief period after ovulation and allows passage of the ovum (Anand & Guha 1982). This process is probably facilitated by ovum size reduction, achieved by stripping of the cumulus and corona cells by locally secreted acid phosphatase (Gupta et al 1970).
2. The periovulatory rise in oestrogen levels leads to the production of tenacious mucus in the isthmus and to ciliary immobilisation; postovulatory progesterone disperses the mucus and frees the cilia for ovum carriage (Jansen 1980).
3. Modulation of adrenoreceptor activity of the isthmic muscle: alpha-activity and muscle contraction are promoted by high periovulatory oestrogen levels; beta-activity and muscle relaxation are enhanced by rising postovulatory progesterone levels (Korenaga & Kadota 1981). This shift in adrenoreceptor function is favoured by the higher concentration of postovulatory progesterone in isthmic than in ampullary tissues (De Voto et al 1980) and the predominance of beta receptors in the inner longitudinal and circular coats of the isthmus (Wilhelmsson & Lindblom 1980). Vasoactive intestinal polypeptide may also contribute to the postovulatory relaxation of the isthmic sphincter (Harper 1988; Sayegh & Mastroianni 1991).

Finally, isthmic transport of the ovum is rapid (Croxatto et al 1978) and is due to ciliary action (Jansen 1980) or, more likely, to periodic to-and-fro muscular contractions resulting in forward motion through the uteroisthmic junction (McComb et al 1981). Transport of the bulky immotile ovum is absolutely dependent on tubal activity but migration of sperms to and through the tube is largely contingent on their morphology and motility with only 'normal' motile sperms reaching the ampulla (Fordney-Settlage et al 1973) but there is also mechanical sperm transport by the uterus and tubes functioning together as a peristaltic pump biased towards the tube ipsilateral to the dominant follicle and augmented by oxytocin (Kunz et al 1997; Wildt et al 1998). Sperm passage through the isthmus is facilitated around the time of ovulation by the thick intraluminal mucus, which provides a three-dimensional meshwork for upstream sperm migration and also reduces antagonistic downstream ciliary action and fluid flow. With its mucus plug the isthmus resembles the cervix and exerts an additional 'purifying' effect (Jansen 1980). The isthmus is also critical in preventing polyspermy (Hunter & Leglise 1971) by reducing the number of sperms entering the ampulla. Since the number of sperms reaching the tube is directly proportional to the sperm density of the ejaculate (Fordney-Settlage et al 1973) it is possible that the isthmic filter is overwhelmed in cases of polyzoospermia (Glezerman et al 1982) resulting in polyspermy and embryonic loss. In the ampulla the vastly reduced numbers of motile sperms, i.e. probably less than 200, swim up the tube to reach the peritoneal cavity for macrophagic disposal and they only accumulate in the ampulla when the ostium is closed (Ahlgren 1975).

The tube plays an active role in supporting perifertilisation events (Gandolfi 1995), which include:

1. Sperm preparation for oocyte penetration. Metabolic support depends on glucose and other energy substrates secreted by the tubal epithelium (Vandewoort & Overstreet 1995). In humans, the loss of the exquisite synchronisation of ovulation and insemination typical of reflex ovulators, the highly variable coital frequency, the probable absence of preovulatory sperm storage in the proximal tube and the short life span of capacitated sperm require tubal compensation designed to maximize sperm survival and function and optimise sperm–oocyte interaction. This is orchestrated by sperm interaction with tubal epithelium, oviductal secretions and follicular fluid released at ovulation. Thus cell-to-cell interaction between sperm and apical membrane of tubal epithelium increases motility but delays capacitation (Murray & Smith 1997); oviductal secretions increase sperm survival by DNA stabilisation (Ellington et al 1998) and enhance capacitation and the acrosome reaction while suppressing binding to the zona pellucida and fusion with the oocyte (Yao et al 1999); follicular fluid augments sperm motility, capacitation and the acrosome reaction (Yao et al 2000).
2. Preparation of ovum for sperm penetration. Partial zona exposure is achieved by stripping the corona cells surrounding the ovum; bicarbonate, which increases in concentration after ovulation, is one of the mediators. The highly glycosylated and charged oviduct-specific mucins with lubricant and antiadhesive properties may facilitate intratubal transport of ovum and prevent ectopic implantation (Malette et al 1995).
3. The embryotrophic role of the tube is indirectly supported by the failure of most mammalian preimplantation embryos to sustain prolonged normal growth and development even in the best in vitro

culture media, by the higher pregnancy rate after tubal transfer and by improved pregnancy rates following transfer of embryos grown in human tubal cell coculture (Bongso et al 1992). The factors underlying this effect are unknown but include a chemically ideal medium supplemented by appropriate levels of peptide growth factors (Sayegh & Mastroianni 1991; Maguiness et al 1992).

4. The tubal contribution to the immune protection of early preimplantation embryos includes the production of a glycoprotein with anticomplement activity (Sayegh & Mastroianni 1991), the postovulatory hormone-dependent downregulation of major histocompatibility complex class II antigen expression in the endosalpinx (Edelstam et al 1992) and secretion of the immunosuppressive placental protein 14 or glycocodelin (Saridogan et al 1997).

Pregnancy can occur without tubal contribution under special circumstances, i.e. in vitro fertilisation and embryo transfer, and after intrauterine ovarian implantation (the Estes procedure), but in nature the tube is the physiological regulator of perifertilisation events and it is not surprising that tubal disease is the single commonest cause of female infertility. Tubal lesions can be primarily functional or anatomical. Functional lesions, considered as biophysical and biochemical derangements, are probably common but have not been intensively studied because of technical problems. Nine such lesions deserve comment:

1. Chronic tubal spasm, manifested as proximal obstruction seen at salpingography, is an uncommon cause of infertility (Mendel 1964) and of ectopic pregnancy (Grant 1962), which can resolve spontaneously or respond to antispasmodics (Thurmond et al 1998). It is psychogenic in origin and its pathogenesis undoubtedly involves disturbed interaction among catecholamines, prostaglandins, sex steroids and substance P (Skrabanek & Powell 1983). It has been suggested (Honoré 1978b) that chronic tubal spasm leads to salpingitis isthmica nodosa (SIN), a lesion discussed more fully in Chapter 15. How SIN causes infertility and ectopic pregnancy remains speculative but the following mechanisms may contribute: narrowing of the isthmic lumen, resulting from spasm and secondary myohypertrophy, may accentuate the filtering effect of the isthmus and reduce the available number of sperms for fertilisation; it is also possible that the sperms may be 'lost' in the diverticula. Incomplete relaxation may interfere with downstream release of the zygote, which may be trapped and implant in the ampulla or may degenerate on its way through a 'tight' isthmus.

2. Hyperactive tubal macrophages (Haney et al 1983) compete with the ovum for sperm availability and reduce the probability of fertilisation. These phagocytes, which normally come from the peritoneal cavity, are increased in numbers and activity in endometriosis, probably as a result of peritoneal irritation from recurrent menstrual reflux. This phenomenon may account for infertility in women who have normal ovaries and tubes.

3. 'Tubo-ovarian interference' across the midline. Normally the ovulating ovary is in close contact with the fimbria, ovum pick-up occurs within seven hours of ovulation (Croxatto et al 1978) and fertilisation takes place in the ampulla. In a small percentage of women one tube may be non-functional while the ipsilateral ovary and the contralateral adnexa are normal; this disturbed anatomy leads to infertility, which responds to excision of the diseased tube and the normal ipsilateral ovary, i.e. the so-called paradoxical oophorectomy (Trimbos-Kemper et al 1982). The mechanisms underlying the infertility are unknown but ectopic pregnancy, which can follow ovum transmigration (Honoré 1978a), is not a major factor.

4. Depressed ciliary activity in the distal tube caused by oedema and vasocongestion related to Chlamydial infection (Leng et al 1998).

5. Inhibition of tubal pick-up of the oocyte–cumulus complex on exposure to cigarette smoke, as demonstrated in vitro (Knoll & Talbot 1998). This may explain why cigarette smoking is a risk fact or for primary tubal infertility (Buck et al 1997).

6. Impaired tubal transportation capacity without anatomical block, demonstrated by radionuclide hysterosalpingography in some women with endometriosis (McQueen et al 1993) and unexplained infertility (Brundon et al 1993).

7. Elevated tubal perfusion pressure demonstrated by selective salpingography and considered to be due to reduced tubal compliance from endometriotic involvement of the wall (Karande et al 1995).

8. Environmental xeno-oestrogens, i.e. polychlorinated biphenyls (PCB), and phyto-oestrogens, i.e. gennistein, induce LIF secretion by tubal epithelium and may disrupt the normal cyclicity of tubal LIF secretion in vivo leading to tubal infertility (Reinhart et al 1999). Abnormally high levels of LIF, due to increased stromal secretion induced by inflammatory cytokines, i.e. IL-1α, TNF-α and TGF-β1, may be one of the links between salpingitis and ectopic pregnancy (Keltz et al 1996).

9. Depressing effect of hydrosalpinx on pregnancy rates in in vitro fertilisation-embryo transfer cycles. This non-mechanical effect is due to leakage of hydrosalpinx contents into the uterine cavity and compromise of endometrial receptivity, embryo–endometrial interaction and embryogenesis, leading to reduced implantation rates and increased

rates of miscarriage and ectopic pregnancy (Camus et al 1999).

The morbid anatomy of the tube is discussed in detail in Chapter 15 and the anatomical lesions associated with infertility will be briefly reviewed. Tubal disease is the most important single factor in female infertility and is often unsuspected clinically (Rosenfeld et al 1983); some of the lesions are endosalpingeal and undetectable by palpation or laparoscopy but can be diagnosed histologically (Cumming et al 1988), and by transvaginal falloposcopy and transfimbrial salpingoscopy using advanced fibre optic technology (Surrey 1999). The mucosal lesions include chronic endosalpingitis, mucosal adhesions, frondal distortion, luminal dilatation and vascular disturbances. The infertility-causing anatomical lesions of the tube include:

1. Congenital defects are rare and include segmental atresia (Richardson et al 1982; Wanerman et al 1986), hypoplasia (Aronnet et al 1969), excessive convolution associated with elongated ovarian and tubal ligaments (Cohen & Katz 1978), ostial phimosis, segmental sacculation or diverticula and accessory tubes or ostia (Yablonski et al 1990). Unique structural defects, related to infertility and ectopic pregnancy, are seen in women exposed in utero to diethylstilboestrol, e.g. foreshortening and convolution of the tube, 'withered' fimbria and a pinpoint ostium (De Cherney et al 1981). Bilateral tubo-ovarian absence is a rare cause of primary infertility associated with primary amenorrhoea and sexual infantilism (Gold et al 1997).

Congenital absence of the tubes can be mimicked by autoamputation following torsion (Beyth & Bar-On 1984).

2. Mucosal polyps of the intramural portion of the tube, especially if bilateral, are a rare cause of infertility (David et al 1981; Wansaicheong & Ong 1998). These benign lesions of unknown causation are sessile or polypoid masses with a fibrous or a loose vascular stroma and canalicular or adenoid structures lined by tubal epithelium (Fig. 30.8). Another rare type is the falloscopically retrieved inflammatory polyp causing reversible isthmic construction and deemed to result from treated endometriosis. Grossly the plug is a pale yellow irregular mass espousing the shape of the lumen and histologically it consists of chronic inflammatory cells, thin-walled blood vessels, fibroblasts, collagen and calcific bodies (Kinderman et al 1993). In contrast, the tubal ostial membrane, hysteroscopically visible at the uterotubal ostium, is not related to infection and appears to be due to congenital elevation of the endometrium, particularly in the infertility-related unilateral type (Coeman et al 1995).

3. Tubal infection is the single most important cause of female infertility and its incidence has risen dramatically in recent decades. Non-granulomatous salpingitis is an ascending infection and the risk factors include sexual activity, puerperal or postabortal endometritis, therapeutic or diagnostic manipulations of the cervix, and the use of the intrauterine contraceptive device (Eschenbach 1992;

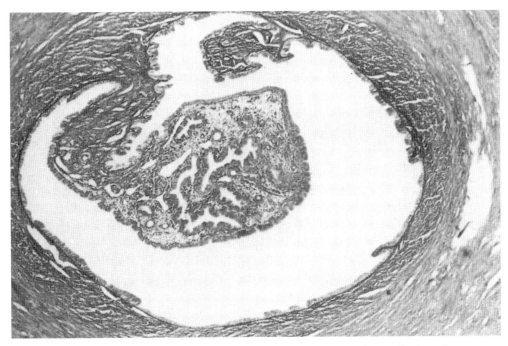

Fig. 30.8 Benign adenofibromatous polyp of the intramural segment of the Fallopian tube.

Bahamondes et al 1994). The organisms involved include: *Neisseria gonorrhoeae*, anaerobic organisms, *Mycoplasma hominis*, *Ureaplasma urealyticum* and *Chlamydia trachomatis* (Shafrin et al 1992). In the West, the major pathogen responsible for tubal infertility is *Chlamydia trachomatis*, as demonstrated indirectly by positive serology (Ault et al 1998) or directly by tubal tissue examination using culture (Marana et al 1990), the direct fluorescent antibody test for the major outer-membrane protein of *C. trachomatis* (Dieterle et al 1998) and the polymerase chain reaction (PCR) to detect chlamydial DNA (Hinton et al 2000). There is also convincing experimental evidence of its rôle in causing tubal damage and infertility (Zana et al 1990). In Chlamydial salpingitis tubal damage is caused by the host immune response to chlamydial heat shock protein 60 (La Verda et al 1999); in gonococcal salpingitis tubal damage results from local over-production of TNFα, leading to inflammation and sloughing of the ciliated cells (McGee et al 1999). Salpingitis causes infertility by the following mechanisms:

i.   Fimbrial agglutination with ostial phimosis or occlusion, secondary hydrosalpinx (Fig. 30.9) and loss of the fimbria ovarica. The net result is failure of ovum pick-up (Bateman et al 1987).

ii. Midtubal occlusion due to tuberculosis, arrested tubal pregnancy, endometriosis or surgical damage during inguinal herniorrhaphy (Urman et al 1992). It is now recognised that some tubal pregnancies may arrest with spontaneous subsidence of symptoms and progressive tubal damage leading to occlusion and secondary infertility (Gomel & Filmar 1987). Post-methotrexate persistence of chorionic villi with endosalpingeal necrosis and widespread myosalpingeal fibrosis is followed by infertility (Klinkert et al 1993).

iii. Proximal tubal blockage, located in the isthmic or intramural (cornual) segment, can be due to time-limited and potentially reversible obstruction or permanent organic occlusion (Honoré et al 1999). Obliterative fibrosis (Fig. 30.10) and interfrondal adhesions (Fortier & Haney 1985; Letterie & Sakas 1991) usually follow infectious salpingitis. Reversible obstruction results from spasm (Thurmond et al 1988), dislodgeable intraluminal casts containing mucin, collagen and calcium (Sulak et al 1987), or oestrogen-sensitive anatomic lesions, i.e. adenomyosis, endometriosis, endosalpingiosis and leiomyomata, which can be successfully treated with GnRH agonists (Surrey et al 2000).

iv. Mesh-like adhesions at the uterotubal ostium, visualised hysteroscopically (Daly et al 1986).

v.   Follicular salpingitis in the ampulla.

vi. Perisalpingeal (Fig. 30.11), tubo-ovarian, uterotubal and periovarian adhesions interfering with ovum pick-up and transport.

vii. Constrictive perisalpingitis with obstruction of the proximal third of the tube (Resnick 1962).

Granulomatous salpingitis is largely due to *Mycobacterium tuberculosis*. It is rare in the West but remains one of the major causes of tubal infertility in India (Schaefer 1976; Parikh et al 1997). It carries a

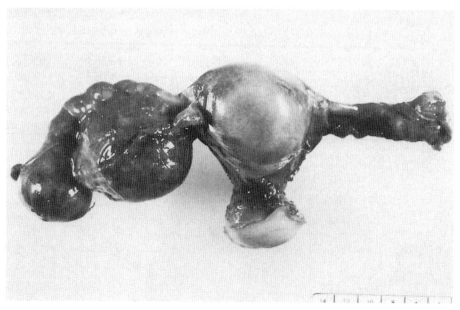

Fig. 30.9 Postinflammatory bilateral fimbrial occlusion with hydrosalpinx and tubo-ovarian adhesions (right).

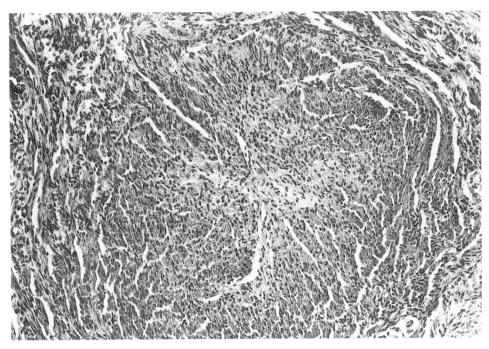

Fig. 30.10 Isthmic occlusion: loss of endosalpinx and replacement by fibrous tissue.

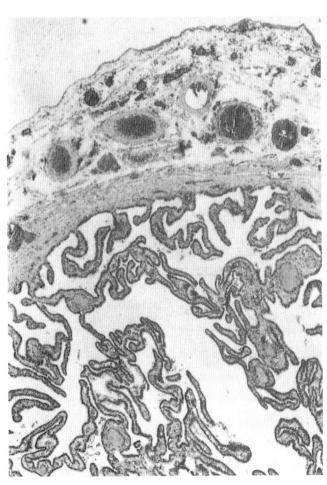

Fig. 30.11 Perisalpingeal adhesion: vascular stage.

poor prognosis and a higher risk of ectopic pregnancy (Durukan et al 1990). As a rule, the tubal lesions are typical with a diffuse infiltration of the endosalpinx in particular by lymphocytes, histiocytes and giant cells (Fig. 30.12) together with a variable degree of caseating necrosis, ulceration and fibrosis. Occasionally the pattern is atypical and may mimic a non-specific salpingitis or even sarcoidosis (De Brux & Dupre-Froment 1965). Tuberculosis can occasionally be associated with chronic lipoid salpingitis (Fig. 30.13) secondary to salpingography. A rare cause of tubal infertility, likely to increase in the West as a result of expanding air travel, is schistosomiasis (Balasch et al 1995).

4. Postoperative adhesions (di Zerega 1994) are the bête noire of infertility surgery and can occur following the most meticulous operation. They result from trauma to the peritoneum, particularly the visceral layer (Wallwiener et al 1998), followed by local production of cytokines and growth factors and the development of a sterile reaction with fibrin deposition, formation of a fibrin bridge between the apposed surfaces, consolidation of this bridge by organisation of the exudate and finally reactive fibrosis with scar contraction. The aberrant expression of oestrogen and progesterone receptors in the traumatised peritoneum in some women may predispose to adhesions and may provide the rationale for hypo-oestrogenic therapy (Wiczyk et al 1998). They can also be produced by a granulomatous reaction to cornstarch powder present in surgical gloves (Yaffe et al 1980), and can also

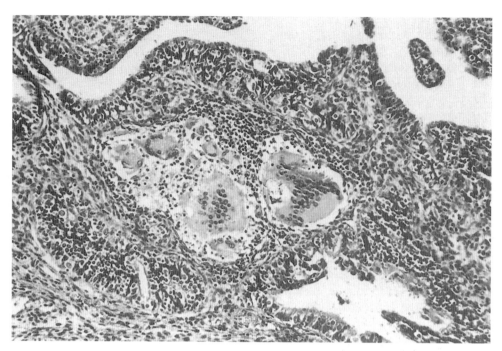

Fig. 30.12 Tuberculous salpingitis: non-caseating granuloma with Langhans giant cells and lymphocytes.

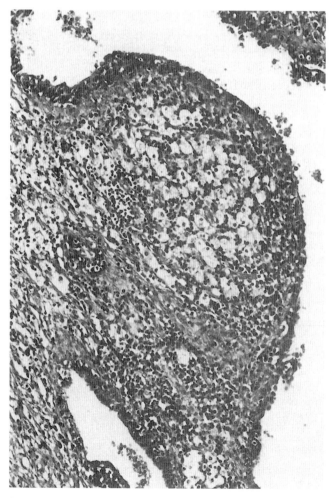

Fig. 30.13 Lipoid salpingitis following salpingography: lymphocytes and foamy macrophages.

occur after pelvic surgery, especially caesarean section (Stovall et al 1989) or after appendectomy, even when a normal appendix is removed (Lehmann-Willenbrock et al 1990). Such adhesions, causing mechanical infertility, are an important reason for the failure of reconstructive surgery. Immune mechanisms may also contribute to tubal infertility in the presence of pelvic adhesions. Normal fimbrial epithelium shows patchy HLA-DR positivity and contains a few CD4+ (helper/inducer) T cells, whereas fimbrial tissue from infertile women exhibits persistently high HLA-DR expression and increased numbers of CD4+ T cells; such changes reflect an active immune reaction potentially detrimental to gametes and/or embryos (Edelstam & Karlsson-Parra 1996).

5. Tubal lesions causing infertility after attempts at sterilisation reversal include adhesions, re-occlusion, excessively short tubes and more subtle changes in the presence of grossly normal and patent tubes, i.e. loss and distortion of mucosal folds, epithelial deciliation, intraluminal polyp formation (Vasquez et al 1980), development of intramural epithelial inclusions and endometriosis (Donnez et al 1984). Pregnancy outcome has improved with laparoscopic microsurgery (Yoon et al 1999).

6. Tubointestinal fistulas are a rare cause of infertility. They arise as a complication of tuberculosis, pelvic inflammatory disease, diverticulitis, Crohn's disease, lymphogranuloma venereum and appendicitis and they can develop between the tube and the sigmoid colon, rectum, appendix, caecum and ileum (Locher & Maroulis 1983).

7. Tubal endometriosis is an important cause of infertility. The lesion is discussed in Chapter 29.

OVARY

Unlike the testis, which is continuously active in adult life, the cyclic ovary is critical in regulating the pattern and efficiency of human fertility by determining the monthly occurrence of ovulation and hence of the fertile period in women, the refractory period in pregnancy and postpartum and the onset of premenopausal subfertility and postmenopausal sterility. Ovulation integrates the endocrine and 'exocrine' (ovum release) functions of the ovary and is thus the pivot of ovarian activity. Ovarian infertility is intimately related to ovulatory dysfunction and can only be understood in terms of disturbances of the normal process of ovulation.

Ovulation, culminating in ovum release and corpus luteum formation, is a complex event comprising four interdependent components, i.e. feedback interactions in the hypothalamus–pituitary–ovary (HPO) axis, structural and functional intra-ovarian events, mechanical release of the ovum, and the development of the corpus luteum. These components will be discussed separately.

Hypothalamus–pituitary–ovary (HPO) axis: feedback mechanisms (Carr 1998)

The hypothalamus is the master regulator of the reproductive system and is directly connected to the pituitary by a bidirectional vascular system that exploits the pituitary as an amplifier of hypothalamic activity and provides for a short feedback loop from pituitary to hypothalamus. The pulsatile release of gonadotrophin-releasing hormone (GnRH) in the arcuate nucleus is locally modulated by stimulatory (adrenaline and noradrenaline) and inhibitory inputs (dopamine, serotonin and endogenous opioid peptides). GnRH binds to high-affinity receptors on the gonadotrophs and regulates gonadotrophin synthesis and storage, transfer from storage pool to secretory pool and acute release. FSH and LH are secreted by the gonadotroph in a coordinated fashion to stimulate the peripheral amplifier (the ovary) and promote follicle growth, ovulation and corpus luteum support.

Negative and positive feedback loops underlie the function of the HPO axis. Oestrogen is the dominant negative inhibitor of hypothalamus and pituitary while high concentrations of progesterone inhibit the hypothalamus. Inhibin and folliculostatin produced by the preovulatory follicle inhibit FSH secretion. Positive feedback, crucial to the midcycle ovulatory LH surge, is triggered by secretions from the preovulatory follicle: rapidly escalating plasma oestrogen levels trigger the LH surge; low levels of progesterone at midcycle are synergistic favouring the FSH surge, which is also augmented by activin.

The feedback loop of the HPO axis is not normally affected by the negligible amounts of oestrogen produced by the adrenals and by the low levels of extraglandular formation of oestrogen from ovarian and adrenal androgenic precursors.

Preovulatory intraovarian events

These occur throughout the follicular phase of the cycle, and are critical for ovulation and the development of an adequate corpus luteum (Jones 1990). In the luteal phase, follicular growth is arrested but further follicular recruitment starts a few days before the end of the cycle and continues during the first 5 or 6 days of the new cycle under the influence of rising levels of FSH brought about by decreasing levels of oestradiol, inhibin and progesterone from the dying corpus luteum. This causes a shift from preantral to antral follicles and by day 4–5 the follicle destined to ovulate is selected by mechanisms as yet not fully understood. The process appears to be stochastic and the choice of the dominant follicle depends on a delicate balance between progressive oestrogenisation and androgenisation of the intrafollicular milieu. As a rule, one follicle (with the largest complement of FSH-sensitive granulosa cells) is at the right stage to be able to establish a rapidly progressive oestrogenic environment essential for development. This dominance is due to local positive feedback synergism between E_2 and FSH, achieved by three mechanisms:

1. FSH induces and stimulates aromatase in granulosa cells thus increasing local E_2 production from thecal androgenic precursors.
2. E_2 increases FSH receptors in granulosa cells thus potentiating its stimulatory effect.
3. Thecal vascularity in the dominant follicle increases significantly causing preferential FSH delivery to the follicle with the highest density of FSH receptors.

Meanwhile, increasing levels of E_2 and inhibin produced by the developing follicles suppress FSH, which is preferentially shunted to the dominant follicle. The other follicles, deprived of FSH, show a decline in aromatase and a rise in the activity of 5alpha-reductase resulting in a progressively androgenic milieu and follicular atresia. Under the influence of FSH the preovulatory follicle develops LH and prolactin receptors and is able to produce escalating levels of E_2 needed for the LH surge and also small sensitising amounts of progesterone. Additional autocrine and paracrine factors involved in follicle growth include a complex system of stimulatory and inhibitory molecules, e.g. inhibin, activin, follistatin, TGFα, TGFβ, cytokines, nitric oxide, insulin-like growth factors, GnRH and VEGF (Kol & Adashi 1995; Taylor 1996; Giudice 1999).

Mechanics of ovulation

The LH surge is essential for ovulation, which is estimated to occur 10–12 hours after the LH peak,

28–32 hours after the onset of the LH surge and 24–36 hours after the E_2 peak (Fritz & Speroff 1982). Rising levels of LH induce the formation of cAMP, which mediates the resumption of oocyte meiosis, granulosa cell luteinization and synthesis of prostaglandins and proteolytic enzymes. At the same time these high LH levels suppress thecal steroidogenesis in other antral follicles, further asserting the dominance of the chosen follicle. The more modest concurrent FSH surge also plays a role in ovulation: LH receptor development in granulosa cells is enhanced, plasminogen activator is induced and detachment of the oocyte-bearing cumulus is elicited by mucification of the cumulus matrix. It is not clear whether the ovulatory follicle actively migrates to the ovarian surface or whether the ovulatory cone approaches the ovarian capsule as a result of follicular expansion due to increased wall compliance and a rapid accumulation of follicular fluid. Softening of the follicular wall and stigma formation are caused by locally generated proteolytic enzymes, such as plasmin, peptidases and a specific collagenase, which is rate-limiting (Fukumoto et al 1981; Yoshimura & Wallach 1987). The prostaglandins are critical in the ovulation process: they stimulate intrafollicular progesterone synthesis and they participate in ovum expulsion by promoting the activity of collagenolytic enzymes and stimulating the contraction of perifollicular smooth muscle cells in the theca externa (Kohda et al 1983). The role of ovarian nerves in ovulation is still undefined (Weiner et al 1977). The physical act of ovulation culminates in the gentle non-explosive extrusion of the oocyte cum cumulo onto the ovarian surface for pick-up by the sweeping action of the tubal fimbria. Since ovulation resembles an inflammatory process, it is not surprising that chemokines play a critical role (Garcia-Velasco & Arici 1999).

Exposure to the synergistic effect of high levels of LH and steroids in the preovulatory follicle leads to coordinated nuclear and cytoplasmic maturation of the oocyte. Before release the oocyte completes the first meiotic division and is primed for the fertilisation-induced second meiotic division and the formation of a haploid female pronucleus; the critical event in cytoplasmic maturation is the production of proteins needed for mRNA synthesis, which will help the oocyte through fertilisation and the first four mitotic divisions (Jones 1990).

Corpus luteum (CL) formation (Jones 1990)

After ovum escape the follicle collapses and the antrum fills with lymph and blood, which then stimulates the centripetal growth of blood vessels from the theca, a process enhanced by theca cell production of angiogenetic factors related to angiotensin II. Granulosal vascularisation is essential for luteal function as progesterone synthesis (Hansen et al 1991) is critically dependent on a supply of blood-borne cholesterol, which is avidly picked up by spe-

cific receptors induced by LH and prolactin. At the time of the LH surge and at ovulation the granulosa and theca cells luteinize forming two functional compartments. The granulosa cells stop dividing and acquire LH neoreceptors, which when occupied do not internalise and thus limit LH sensitivity and progesterone synthesis in time. After 10 days the cells run out of stable mRNA species and they stop producing progesterone while becoming refractory to LH or hCG stimulation. In contrast, the endogenous LH receptors of luteinized theca cells are normally internalised and these cells respond to LH by proliferation and secretion of oestrogen and progesterone. In the absence of pregnancy the corpus luteum involutes as a result of E_2-induced luteolysis, mediated by reduced LH binding capacity and sensitivity of the luteal cells and by a rise in the $PGF_{2\alpha}/PGE_2$ (Vijayakumar & Walters 1983).

If pregnancy occurs, trophoblastic hCG rescues the corpus luteum by stimulating the luteinized thecal cells to produce increasing amounts of oestrogen and progesterone. Early pregnancy, up to 7 weeks, is absolutely dependent on steroids produced by the corpus luteum and lutectomy causes miscarriages; thereafter a luteoplacental shift takes place with corpus luteum involution and placental takeover. Recent work clashes with this classic concept of the luteal–placental shift, which implies corpus luteum failure followed by transfer of steroid production to the placenta (Nakajima et al 1991). What happens in the first and early second trimesters is a puzzling dose–response relationship between the corpus luteum and exponentially rising hCG levels: progesterone secretion by the corpus luteum is clamped at a steady level without decline while placental secretion keeps rising and in effect takes over pregnancy maintenance. This explains why there is still hCG-dependent steroid production by the corpus luteum at term. Postpartum luteolysis occurs rapidly but at a slower rate in nursing mothers (Fritz & Speroff 1982).

Ovulatory disorders

Ovulation is not an all-or-none event but constitutes a spectrum characterised by 'normal' ovulation at the one end and anovulation at the other with intermediate grades of suboptimal quantity and quality. Infertility can thus result from anovulation, oligo-ovulation or dysovulation. These ovulatory disturbances will be discussed under the following headings.

1. Absent or reduced follicular pool

Ovulation, a highly selective process, requires a grossly superfluous follicular pool for recruitment, and anovulation or oligo-ovulation can result from:
(i) Congenital anomalies of the ovary, which are discussed in detail in Chapter 36. Only a few relevant

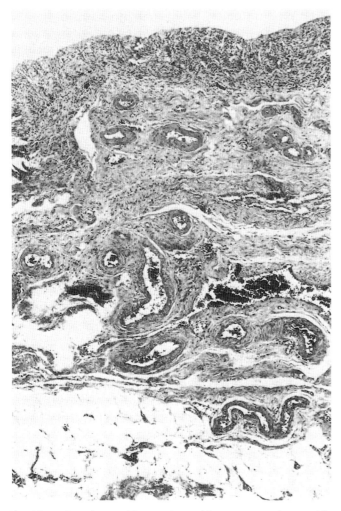

Fig. 30.14 Streak gonad in a patient with Turner's syndrome: thin ovarian cortex with wavy stromal cells and no follicles.

comments are included here. The streak gonad (Fig. 30.14), seen with chromosomal anomalies, or with a 46,XX and 46,XY constitution, is usually afollicular and absolutely sterile but rarely follicles persist into adult life (Coulam 1982). Such patients can become pregnant but their gestational outcome is poor with an increased incidence of spontaneous miscarriage, stillbirth and abnormal offspring (Reyes et al 1976; Wray et al 1981). Rare causes of chromosome-related ovarian failure include the triple X syndrome (Itu et al 1990), X-autosome translocation (Katayama et al 1991), familial terminal deletion of the long arm of X (Veneman et al 1991) and 45X/46XX mosaicism (Devi et al 1998). Two other inherited conditions due to genetic mutations cause premature ovarian failure. Blepharophimosis type I is an autosomal dominant syndrome associated with hypergonadotrophic hypogonadism due to follicular gonadotrophin resistance or premature follicular depletion (Fraser et al 1988). Ovarian hypoplasia, associated with

primary amenorrhoea, can be due to subtle abnormalities of the D chromosomes and is characterised by small shrunken ovaries containing closely packed inactive primordial follicles in a fibrous cortex (Lazlo et al 1976).

(ii) Acquired lesions resulting in severe follicular damage are relatively uncommon. Mumps oophoritis, which affects 5% of patients with mumps parotitis, can cause extensive follicular damage followed by cortical fibrosis, and pubescent females are more sensitive (Prinz & Taubert 1968). The late sequelae include infertility, menstrual disturbances and premature menopause (Morrison et al 1975). Ovarian failure with subfertility, infertility or premature menopause often follows chemotherapy or the various modalities of radiotherapy (Byrne et al 1992; Levitt & Jenney 1998; Bath et al 1999). Chemotherapy has been shown by electron microscopy to damage, and thus reduce, the number of follicles and to cause diffuse stromal damage with fibrosis, hyalinisation, calcification and vascular sclerosis (Marcello et al 1990; Familiari et al 1993). These deleterious effects depend on the dose used, the type of treatment (alkylating agents being particularly harmful) and the age of the patient (older patients being more sensitive).

2. Anatomical or functional folliculopathy

This includes the following four unrelated conditions:

(i) The recurrent empty follicle syndrome, first described by Coulam et al (1986), is seen in cases of unexplained infertility and of infertility related to endometriosis or the tubal factor and after treatment with pure FSH preparations (Ashkenazi et al 1987). It is diagnosed by follicular aspiration, which yields only follicular fluid and granulosa cells (La Scala et al 1991). Its aetiology is unknown and, since it is unpredictable and since fertilisation occurs in 70% of women with later successful cycles, it is probably a sporadic event rather than a syndrome and may or may not be aetiologically related to infertility (Ben-Shlomo et al 1991). In fact, it may be an artifact produced by some batches of commercial hCG with abnormally rapid clearance and no bioactivity (Zegers-Hochschild et al 1995).

(ii) Defective oocytes (Ezra et al 1992). Diagnosis of this condition is based on circumstantial evidence provided by the significantly greater in vitro failure rates of oocytes retrieved from women with unexplained infertility as compared to those with tuboperitoneal infertility. Possible mechanisms for this oocyte defect include defective zona pellucida sperm receptor, antizona antibody and failure of maternal pronucleus formation or syngamy.

(iii) Diminished ovarian reserve, as detected by increased serum FSH levels and decreased inhibin-a and inhibin-b levels, is typical of premenopausal women (Danforth et al 1998) and may contribute to their subfertility. It has also been reported in younger women with unexplained infertility (Leach et al 1997).

(iv) Congenital increase in aromatase activity of ovarian follicles and peripheral tissues is associated with elevated serum oestrogen and progesterone levels, hyperprolactinaemia, menometrorrhagia due to endometrial hyperplasia and infertility (Odell & Meikle 1986).

3. Premature ovarian failure (POF)

This, defined as cessation of ovarian activity before age 40 and supranormal basal FSH and LH levels, is a misnomer since it is in fact a state of variably reversible intermittent activity (Conway 1997; Anasti 1998). Clinical diagnosis is difficult since pelvic ultrasound, ovarian biopsy (Fig. 30.15) and detection of circulating antiovarian antibodies are not entirely reliable. It can result from an inadequate initial follicular endowment, accelerated follicular depletion or follicular dysfunction, as follows:

(i) In humans factors controlling germ cell migration, proliferation and incorporation into primordial follicles are unknown. In accordance with the essential prenatal role of the thymus in establishing the critical follicular complement, thymic hypoplasia or aplasia in women is associated with POF.

(ii) Accelerated follicular depletion is due to X chromosome abnormalities (single X, mosaicism and deletions), galactosaemia and excessive follicular destruction from infections, cancer therapy and autoimmune oophoritis.

(iii) Follicular dysfunction can be due to enzymatic deficiencies, defective follicle-gonadotrophin interaction and autoimmunity. Deficiencies of certain steroidogenic enzymes, in particular 17α-hydroxylase, lead to local oestrogen deficiency and severe follicular disorganization (Coulam 1982; Araki et al 1987). Defective follicle-gonadotrophin interaction can result from abnormal forms of FSH and LH due to gene mutations or polymorphisms; inadequate gonadotrophin synthesis due to GnRH deficiency with the KAL mutation (Kallman syndrome) and the DAX-1 mutation (X-linked adrenal hypoplasia); abnormal FSH and LH receptors and a postreceptor defect with an unresponsive cAMP second messenger system (pseudohypoparathyroidism).

Autoimmunity (Sedmak et al 1987; Hoek et al 1997) is a recognised cause of POF and may be associated with other autoimmune diseases, i.e. myasthenia gravis and

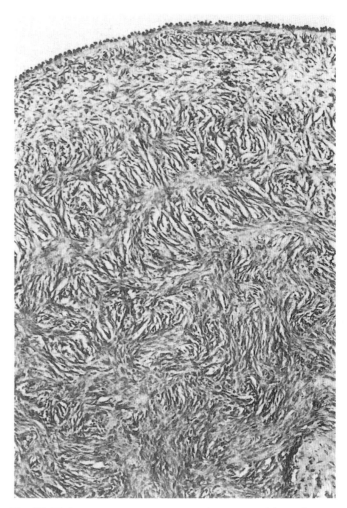

Fig. 30.15 Premature menopause: ovarian cortex with patchy stromal fibrosis and no follicles.

the polyglandular syndrome. The ovarian antigens triggering this combined humoral and cell-mediated response are unknown and the significance of circulating antiovarian antibodies is uncertain, except for the specific antibodies against the gonadotrophin receptors and the steroidogenic cells of the follicle that are associated with endocrine failure. Information on the pathology of autoimmune oophoritis is limited, largely because of the paucity of biopsy material. The ovaries are often enlarged with palpable tender cysts because of deranged feedback caused by follicular steroidogenesis suppression by locally released lymphokines. Histologically, the mononuclear infiltrate favours the developing and spares the primordial follicles and is concentrated in the theca interna and externa with initial sparing of the granulosa until corpus luteum formation, a response pattern consistent with the notion that the steroidogenic cells are the main targets. Two rare pathologic variants include: (a) eosinophilic perifolliculitis (Lewis 1993) and (b) widespread oocyte degeneration in primary and secondary follicles with dystrophic calcification, loss of antral follicles and corpora lutea/albicantia and ovarian hypoplasia (Biberoglu et al 1988).

Immunotyping has shown that the inflammatory cells are mostly T lymphocytes (CD4+ and CD8+) and plasma cells with a few B cells, natural killer (NK) cells and macrophages. There is also inappropriate expression of MHC Class II antigens on granulosa cells spontaneously or after induction with gonadotrophins and interferon-gamma (Sedmak et al 1987).

4. The 'hyper-responsive' ovary

This is a rare and poorly defined entity characterised by the recurrence of painful functional ovarian cysts and reproductive difficulties in young women. There is no direct evidence of ovarian hypersensitivity to gonadotrophins (Stone & Swartz 1979).

5. Abnormal hypothalamo-hypophysio-ovarian relationships

These will be discussed under the rubrics of hypothalamic and pituitary disturbances. To complete the picture abnormal feedback mechanisms are presented here. The normal feedback loop depends on a well-defined pattern of oestrogen and progesterone secretion by the ovary and the loop can be opened by an uncontrolled extraovarian supply of sex steroids. This can result from:

(i) The combined contraceptive pill, which suppresses tonic secretion of gonadotrophins and inhibits the mid-cycle surge. Normal ovarian function and fertility usually return after cessation of contraception but in about 1 in 1000 users post-pill amenorrhoea ensues as a result of a cycle initiation defect (Hull et al 1981). These women respond well to ovulation induction and their prognosis is excellent (Soltan & Hancock 1982).
(ii) In obesity abnormally high acyclic oestrogen levels, resulting from excessive extraovarian oestrogen production from androgenic precursors (Bates & Whetworth 1982) and through decreased binding capacity of sex-hormone binding globulin (Siiteri 1981), can lead to anovulatory infertility.
(iii) Increased supply of androgenic precursors with extraglandular conversion to oestrogen arises from adrenal hypersecretion (Lobo et al 1983) and/or overproduction by the ovaries as a result of polycystic ovarian disease, hyperthecosis or an androgen/oestrogen secreting tumour (Insler & Lunenfeld 1991).
(iv) A unique ovarian fibrothecoma with inhibin-B production and selective FSH suppression causing secondary amenorrhoea and infertility (Meyer et al 2000).

6. Dysovulation

This can result from dissociation of the physical and endocrine components of ovulation, i.e. pseudo-ovulation, luteal insufficiency and disturbances in ovum pick-up.

(i) The luteinized unruptured follicle (LUF) syndrome is now a recognised cause of infertility in some women with no detectable male or female factors and may contribute to infertility in some women with pelvic adhesions or endometriosis, especially if the ovaries are involved (Katz 1988; Kaya & Oral 1999). It may be induced by ovulation induction with clomiphene citrate, menotropin and chorionic gonadotrophin (Coetsiert & Dhont 1996) and by non-steroidal anti-inflammatory drugs in the treatment of arthritis (Smith et al 1996). It may be due to a primary granulosa cell defect leading to reduced follicle growth and blood flow and an absent primary progesterone rise (Zaidi et al 1995). It reflects a dissociation between the mechanical (follicle rupture and ovum release) and the endocrine (luteinization of the dominant follicle) components of ovulation and may be due to disturbed prostaglandin activity, since its incidence is significantly increased in normally cycling women treated with prostaglandin synthetase inhibitors (Killick & Elstein 1987). The unruptured luteinized follicle becomes transformed into a luteal cyst, which produces subnormal levels of progesterone (Hamilton et al 1990).
(ii) Follicular rupture with failure of ovum release or ovum retention can be seen in spontaneous and induced ovulations (Stanger & Yovich 1984). It may differ from the luteinized unruptured follicle only in degree (Hamilton et al 1990); it is followed by luteal cyst formation and marginal progesterone deficiency, indicating the importance of follicular rupture for efficient progesterone synthesis. It is characterised by failure of dispersal of the cumulus oophorus and ovum release, possibly due to inhibition of LH-induced hyaluronic acid synthesis caused by excessive production of FSH-stimulated glycosaminoglycan (Katz 1988).
(iii) Premature luteinization is diagnosed if serum progesterone levels greater than 1.5 ng/ml are associated with an LH surge before serum oestradiol levels reach 100 pg/ml and before the follicle is fully mature. It is a cause of pregnancy failure in anovulatory women treated with human menopausal gonadotrophin and clomiphene citrate and also in a small subset of untreated infertile women (Check et al 1991) and it may result from augmented FSH-induced sensitivity of granulosa cells to the LH surge (Ubaldi et al 1996). Its adverse effect on pregnancy rates may be due to poor quality cervical

mucus (Taney et al 1991), dyssynchrony between endometrium and implanted embryo as a result of advanced endometrial secretory maturation (Chetkowski et al 1997) or decreased ovarian reserve (Younis et al 1998).

(iv) Luteal phase defect is now a recognised entity associated with infertility, early recurrent miscarriage and tubal ectopic pregnancy (McNeely & Soules 1988; Guillaume et al 1995; Blacker et al 1997), despite problems inherent in its diagnosis (Davis et al 1989; Li & Cooke 1991). It is a common sporadic event in normal women, occurring in about 30% of random cycles but it is less common as a recurrent event with a frequency of 3–24% in the infertile. It is a multifactorial disease (Kusuhara 1992; Dawood 1994; Hinney et al 1996) with dysfunction at three levels:

1. *hypothalamus-pituitary*: low basal LH levels without pulsality, imbalance between FSH and LH levels in the follicular phase, thyroid dysfunction and hyperprolactinaemia.

2. *Ovary*: inadequate granulosa cell development and response, possibly related to abnormal LH/hCG receptors and IGF-1 receptors.

3. *Endometrium*: inadequate response due to deficient oestrogen and progesterone receptors.

The net effect is inadequate endometrial preparation leading to implantation failure.

7. Disturbed tubo-ovarian relationships

These interefere with the passage of the ovum from ovary to tube (Fig 30.16). In women ovum pick-up is normally achieved by direct contact of the cilia with the ovarian

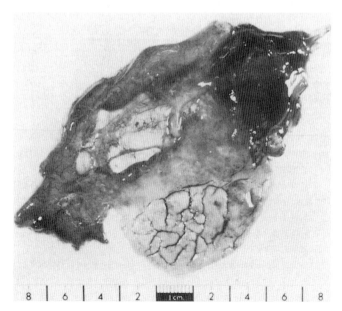

Fig. 30.16 Normal tubo-ovarian relationship: freely mobile tube and ovary with no adhesions.

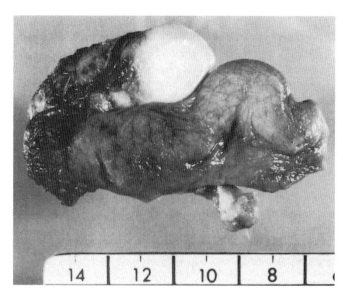

Fig. 30.17 Extensive tubo-ovarian adhesions.

surface (Ahmad-Thabet 2000). This close apposition is brought about by coordinate movements of the fimbria ovarica, ovarian ligament, mesovarium and mesosalpinx. Such contact can be prevented by an excessively long fimbria ovarica and surgical shortening by plication leads to pregnancy in some infertile women (Cohen 1980). This contact can also fail to occur if the ligaments are shortened and fixed by fibrosis or if the ovaries and tubes are bound down by adhesions to each other (Fig 30.17) and to the ligaments (Fig 30.18). Unilateral or bilateral malposition of the ovary above the pelvic brim due to an unusually long utero-ovarian ligament is a rare contributor to infertility in women with associated Müllerian and renal anomalies (Rock et al 1986). Periovarian adhesions, which can be localised or diffuse, filmy and avascular or coarse, vascular and fibrous (Fig 30.19), cause infertility depending on their severity (Hulka 1982) and it is presumed that they interfere with ovum release from the ovary. In addition these adhesions appear to block ovulation (Quan et al 1963), as ovaries surrounded by adhesions show fewer corpora lutea and corpora albicantia and a micropolycystic pattern commonly seen with chronic anovulation.

Bychkov (1990) has failed to confirm ovulatory failure in chronic pelvic inflammatory disease; there was an increase in both follicular and corpus luteum cysts, presumably due to alterations in the ovarian supply.

PERITONEUM

The peritoneum is critically located with respect to the female genitalia and peritoneal fluid, which is an ovarian exudate influenced by follicular activity, corpus luteum vascularity and hormone production (Syrop & Halme 1987), conditions the microenvironment of fertilisation and early embryonic development. Infertility often results

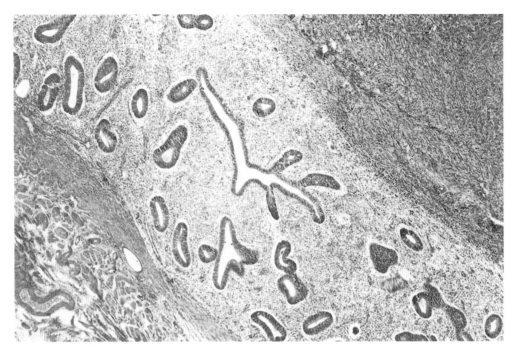

Fig. 30.18 Ovarioligamentous adhesions with a surface endometriotic bridge.

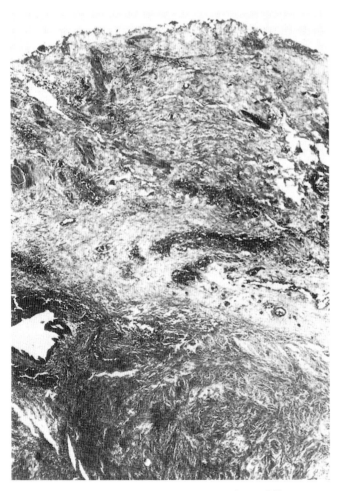

Fig. 30.19 Periovarian adhesion: coarse, vascular and fibrous. Masson trichrome.

from gross mechanical disturbances of the peritoneum, in particular post-inflammatory or post-operative adnexal adhesions (Drolette & Badawy 1992; Tulandi 1997). Aberrant development of oestrogen and progesterone receptors in the peritoneum may predispose to adhesion formation (Wiczyk et al 1998).

Infertility can also be caused by functional disorders of the peritoneum (Syrop & Halme 1987). In some patients with idiopathic infertility the peritoneal fluid contains increased levels of reactive oxygen species that may interfere with sperm motility and sperm–oocyte fusion (Wang et al 1997). In endometriosis the over-abundant peritoneal fluid has been shown to exhibit multiple abnormalities including:

1. increased sperm phagocytosis by activated macrophages (Martinez-Roman et al 1997);
2. antibodies to transferrin and alpha 2-HS glycoprotein adversely affecting post-coital sperm motility and survival in vitro (Pillai et al 1998);
3. increased levels of inflammatory cytokines, i.e. TNFα, IL-8 and IL-10 (Rana et al 1996);
4. increased proteolytic activity due to reduced levels of tissue inhibitor of metalloproteinase and possibly related to ovulatory dysfunction (Sharpe-Timms et al 1998);
5. substances that reduce implantation in a mouse model by decreasing levels of leukaemia inhibitory factor and αVβ integrin (Illera et al 2000).

DISTURBANCES OF THE HYPOTHALAMO-HYPOPHYSIAL SYSTEM

Despite their embryological and anatomical distinctness the hypothalamus and the anterior pituitary constitute a single functional unit crucial in reproductive control. This functional unity is largely achieved by structural contiguity and the hypothalamo-hypophysial portal venous system, which links the median eminence and the pituitary and funnels the hypophysiotrophic factors at high concentrations into the gland. The hypothalamus can thus be viewed as the noise generator in the system and the pituitary as a multichannel amplifier. The system is stabilised and integrated with the nervous system and the soma via negative or positive long, short and ultra-short feedback loops (Locke 1978). Reproductive dysfunction can be caused by anatomical or functional lesions of the hypothalamus or pituitary and by vascular disconnection of these two elements.

Hypothalamic disorders

These can be subdivided into anatomical and functional. *Anatomical:* These rare lesions consist of:

1. Intrinsic hypothalamic tumours, e.g. gliomas, especially the juvenile astrocytomas, and parahypophysial tumours that compress the hypothalamus or the portal venous system. These latter include pituitary neoplasms, ectopic pinealomas or germinomas, dural meningiomas and posterior pituitary tumours (Landholt 1975).
2. Selective dysgenesis of the medial basal hypothalamus due to failure of migration of GnRH neurones from the olfactory placode to the arcuate nucleus whence they send their terminals to the median eminence (Schwanzel-Fukuda et al 1989). This rare condition, which can be familial and affects females only rarely, is characterised by primary isolated gonadotrophin deficiency, hypogonadism and hyposmia or anosmia (Kallman syndrome). The anatomical lesions are variable, and include defective development of the olfactory area, the anterior hypothalamus and the lateral tuberal nuclei (Kovacs & Sheehan 1982).
3. Damage to the arcuate nucleus and the GnRH neurones caused by infectious (tuberculosis) and noninfectious (sarcoidosis) granulomas, histiocytosis X and primary or secondary neoplasms (Kovacs & Horvath 1987).

Functional: These disturbances, which can be transient or permanent, often afflict young women and arise from malfunction of the hypothalamic neurotransmitter network. They can be subdivided into the following categories:

1. Subclinical relative growth hormone (GH) deficiency has been detected in some patients with primary infertility, anovulation and regular menses (Ovesen et al 1992). These patients have normal basal GH levels but show a significantly reduced response to an arginine challenge, which would indicate reduced GH secretory capacity and lack of synergism with gonadotrophins to induce mid-cycle ovulation. It is worth noting that GH activity is not absolutely essential for ovulation as spontaneous pregnancies can occur in women with Laron-type dwarfism which is due to lack of GH receptor activity (Menashe et al 1991).
2. Stress-induced amenorrhoea/anovulation. These disturbances constitute a spectrum of hypothalamic response to sustained emotional stress depending on the subject's sensitivity to stressful stimuli (Gallinelli et al 2000). Initially stress inhibits only the cyclic centre causing anovulation, i.e. the responsive phase; if anovulation persists for over a year, ovarian function deteriorates by mechanisms similar to those operative in the premenopausal state, oestrogen production drops and there is a secondary rise in gonadotrophin secretion, i.e. the refractory phase (Yaginuma 1979). Exactly how stress inhibits gonadotrophin secretion is not fully known but the following mechanisms are considered contributory (Seibel & Taymor 1982):
   (i) Increased dopaminergic and opioid activity in the hypothalamus (Quigley et al 1980); stress activates the corticotrophs with release of ACTH and β-endorphin and GnRH inhibition is caused by the increased levels of cortisol and β-endorphin (Seifer & Collins 1990).
   (ii) Increased production of catecholoestrogens, i.e. 2-hydroxy-oestrone, causing suppression of LH and FSH release.
   (iii) Hyperprolactinaemia.
   (iv) Adrenocortical hyperactivity causing hirsutism and acne in susceptible patients.
3. Exercise-related reproductive dysfunction ranges from delayed menarche to luteal phase deficiency, oligomenorrhoea, amenorrhoea and anovulation with its prevalence depending on the intensity of the athletic activity. The underlying mechanisms are unclear but a primary hypothalamic defect is indicated. Changes in the pulsatile release of GnRH leading to reduced frequency of gonadotrophin secretory pulses and ovarian dysfunction. Increased levels of opioid peptides and of corticotropin-releasing factor (CRF) are probably responsible for the hypothalamic inhibition while increased levels of cortisol may further suppress pituitary gonadotrophin secretion (De Souza & Metzger 1991; Chen & Brzyski 1999).
4. Food intake and reproductive dysfunction. In female mammals reproduction and sexual behaviour are exquisitely sensitive to availability of oxizable metabolic fuels and are shut down whenever food

intake is inadequate or an inordinate fraction is channelled into other uses, i.e. exercise or fattening. These nutritional effects on reproduction occur via alterations in the activity of GnRH neurones and the dampening of sexual activity is mediated at least partly by reduced oestrogen receptor activity in the ventromedial hypothalamus. Any changes in glucose and fatty acid oxidation are recognised in the viscera (mostly the liver) and in the caudal hindbrain (most likely the area postema) and the message is then relayed to the GnRH secreting neurones and the oestradiol-binding effector neurones in the forebrain (Wade et al 1996). How the hypothalamus is suppressed is not clear but it may involve complex interactions among galanin, opioids and neuropeptide Y (Kalra & Horvath 1998). Severe under-nutrition, including its extreme variant, i.e. anorexia nervosa, and obesity are associated with oligo-ovulation, oligomenorrhoea, amenorrhoea and infertility (Eisenberg 1981; Bray 1997).

5. Hypothalamic dysfunction secondary to diseases of other systems. Anovulatory infertility can result from deranged pineal function with abnormal patterns of melatonin secretion but the pathogenetic link is unknown (Turi & Garzetti 1993). Chronic renal failure is often followed by menstrual disturbances, anovulation and infertility, possibly related, as demonstrated in experimental animals, to GnRH secretion inhibition, hypersensitivity to negative feedback and naloxone resistance (Handelsman & Dong 1993). In multiple sclerosis menstrual disorders and infertility are common and are due to abnormal central regulation with increased serum levels of prolactin, LH, FSH and free testosterone and reduced levels of oestrone sulphate (Grinsted et al 1989).

Pituitary disorders

Mammalian reproduction is critically dependent on the hypothalamo-hypophysial complex, which is not only the vital link between the nervous system and the reproductive tract but also an indispensable controller of the tonic and phasic activity of the female gonads. The pituitary plays a key role as an endocrine transducer and amplifier of neural microsignals and it has an enormous reserve capacity that ensures functional compensation until over 90% of the gland is destroyed. Pituitary failure of relevance to female infertility is caused by anatomical and functional lesions interfering with the secretion of gonadotrophins and prolactin.

Anatomical lesions include:

1. Infarction due to postpartum haemorrhage (Sheehan & Summers 1949).
2. Inflammatory processes include abscess formation or chronic infections, e.g. tuberculosis (Sharma et al

2000), syphilis, fungal (Heary et al 1995) and parasitic (Reincke et al 1998) infections. Non-infectious lesions include giant cell granulomas, sarcoidosis, histiocytosis X, xanthomatous hypophysitis (Folkerth et al 1998) and granulomatous inflammation secondary to a ruptured Rathke's cleft cyst (Roncaroli et al 1998). Lymphocytic hypophysitis, which can mimic an adenoma (Saiwai et al 1998), is autoimmune (Stromberg et al 1998) and can cause amenorrhoea and anovulatory infertility. The inflammatory infiltrate consists predominantly of activated CD4+ T lymphocytes with MHC class I and class II antigens and IL-2 receptors expressed on the lymphocytes and macrophages (McCutcheon & Oldfield 1991).

3. Systemic diseases. Secondary pituitary amyloidosis is a rare cause of hypogonadism (Las & Surks 1983). With the progressive deposition of amyloid fibres between the pituitary cells and the blood vessels there is ischaemic atrophy, failure of delivery of GnRH to the gonadotrophs and failure of release of FSH and LH into the circulation. In haemosiderosis or haemochromatosis the excess iron is deposited in many tissues including the pituitary, and the gonadotrophs are the most prone of the pituitary cells to the effects of iron storage. Hence hypogonadotrophic hypogonadism is the earliest sign of pituitary involvement (Kovacs & Horvath 1987; Meyer et al 1990).

4. The empty sella mimics a pituitary adenoma radiologically and the differentiation is made by the demonstration of air entering the sella during pneumoencephalography. The cause of this peculiar anatomical aberration is unclear but theories of causation include rupture of an intra- or parasellar cyst, infarction of normal or abnormal (neoplastic) sellar contents, pituitary hypertrophy followed by atrophy and transmission of cerebrospinal fluid pressure through a congenitally deficient sellar diaphragm (Ho 1996). As a result, the pituitary is flattened and distorted but maintains its vascular link with the hypothalamus (Neelon et al 1973). The lesion is rarely associated with significant endocrinopathy (Futterweit et al 1984) but occasionally it may be found with myxoedema, hypogonadotrophic hypogonadism and hyperprolactinameia (Archer et al 1978).

5. Neoplastic disorders of the pituitary include:
   (i) Extrapituitary intrasellar and parasellar tumours which can cause hypogonadotrophic hypogonadism by direct destruction of the gland, obstruction of the portal circulation with reduced GnRH delivery or ischaemic necrosis, and damage to the median eminence or hypothalamus. They include primary tumours, e.g. craniopharyngiomas, meningiomas and malignant

lymphomas, and the even rare metastatic carcinomas, especially from breast (Kovacs & Horvath 1987). There is often associated diabetes insipidus from neurohypophysial damage.

(ii) Primary pituitary tumours, which are predominantly adenomas, can now be accurately classified into distinct morphological entities on the basis of their cellular composition, hormone content and their immunocytochemical and ultrastructural features (Kovacs & Horvath 1987). Any pituitary adenoma can cause hypogonadism by directly or indirectly compromising FSH and LH secretion but there are two adenomas, which are particularly associated with hypogonadism — the prolactinoma and the gonadotroph cell adenoma.

Pathologically the prolactinoma can be a microadenoma (Serri et al 1987), a circumscribed non-encapsulated macroadenoma or a locally invasive tumour extending through the dura and the bone of the sellar

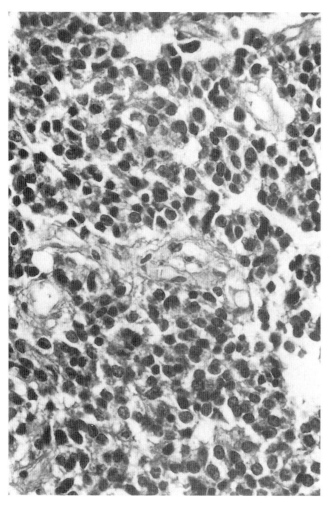

Fig. 30.20 Prolactin cell pituitary adenoma: sheets of polygonal cells with scanty granular cytoplasm and dark ovoid nuclei.

floor to invade the sphenoid sinus. Usually the prolactinoma is a solitary lesion of the pituitary but rarely the microprolactinoma with hyperprolactinaemic secondary amenorrhoea can be the initial finding in patients with familial multiple endocrine neoplasia syndrome type 1 (Lucas et al 1988). When small, the tumour is often deeply set and lies posteriorly within the lateral wing of the pituitary; when larger, it often lies in one of the lateral wings. Grossly it is soft grey, creamy white or purple and histologically it consists of solid epithelial sheets and strands often arranged concentrically around small simple capillaries (Fig 30.20); the cells are small and polygonal with an ovoid central nucleus. Mitotic figures and multinucleated cells are rare (Robert & Hardy 1975). The immunoperoxidase technique, using specific antisera, is reliable and sensitive (Mukai 1983). Electronmicroscopy is also important in the morphological diagnosis of a prolactinoma (Kovacs & Horvath 1987). Typically the well-granulated 'acidophilic' cell contains an ovoid, often pleomorphic, nucleus, parallel stacks of well-developed RER usually located at the periphery, a prominent Golgi apparatus with few dense immature secretory granules and well-formed electron-dense secretory granules with characteristic size and morphology (Fig 30.21). The granules, averaging 600 nm in diameter, are oval or pleomorphic with a loosely arranged limiting membrane and an irregular electronlucent halo between the membrane and the dark core. The sparsely granulated 'chromophobe' cell contains extensively developed RER with concentric whorls and free ribosomes; a prominent Golgi complex occupying almost a third of the cytoplasmic area and variably filled with immature granules; and sparse dense spherical or pleomorphic granules with an average diameter of 250 nm. Some granules are often seen being extruded on the lateral cell membranes into the intercellular space away from the perivascular spaces and the intercellular extensions of basement membrane — a phenomenon called misplaced exocytosis (Horvath & Kovacs 1976).

Touch preparations using routine staining and immunocytochemistry can also be useful in the diagnosis of pituitary adenomas: the prolactinoma displays recognisable features, i.e. microcalcifications, small size of cell and nucleus and the 'Golgi' pattern of prolactin immunopositivity (Kontogeorgos et al 1995).

Macroprolactinomas respond to medical treatment. Bromocriptine, a dopamine agonist, directly inhibits prolactin synthesis and secretion leading to secondary cellular atrophy with reduction in cell size, nuclear shrinkage and marked involution of the rough endoplasmic reticulum and Golgi system. This cellular collapse underlies the tumour shrinkage following bromocriptine therapy (Bassetti et al 1984).

1. Neoplastic hypersecretion of ACTH related to a benign ACTH or ACTH-MSH adenoma or rarely to a carcinoma associated with extracranial metastases. These

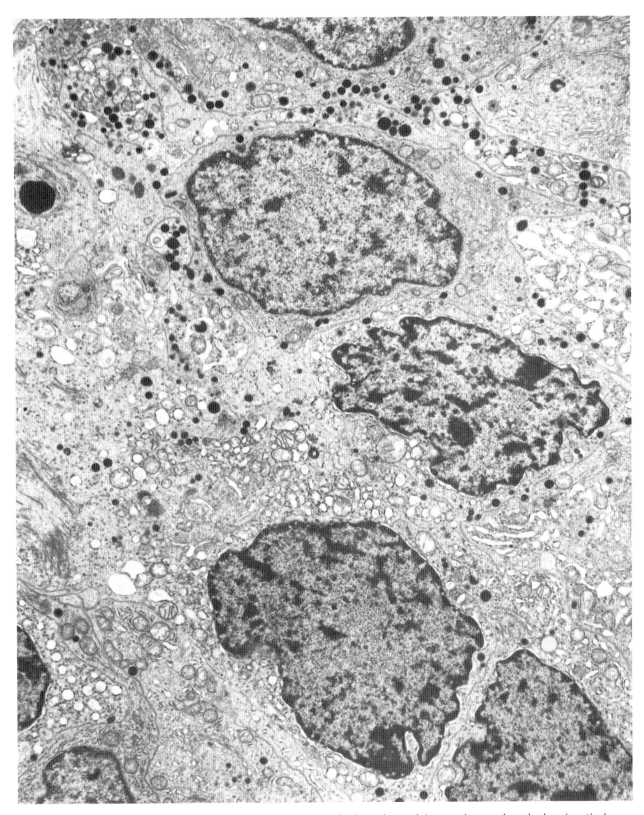

Fig. 30.21 Sparsely granulated prolactin cell pituitary adenoma. Note the irregular nuclei, extensive rough endoplasmic reticulum, scattered Golgi areas, and dense spherical or pleomorphic secretory granules, ranging in diameter from 130 to 400 nm. (Courtesy of Dr T K Shnitka, Edmonton.)

rare tumours, comprising about 10% of all pituitary adenomas, give rise to secondary hypercorticism (Cushing's disease) and derangements of the reproductive axis (Berry & Caplan 1979).

2. Silent corticotroph adenoma (Serri et al 1987), without manifestations of Cushing's disease, can present with infertility, amenorrhoea, galactorrhoea and hyperprolactinaemia. These microadenomas, secreting ACTH β-lipotrophin and β-endorphin, probably cause hyperprolactinaemia either by compressing the pituitary stalk or because of the high intrahypothalamic levels of ACTH or β-endorphin.

3. The newly recognised gonadotroph cell adenomas secrete a variable excess of complete FSH or LH or of molecular fragments or subunits with apparently no biological activity (Ho et al 1997). Many patients with these tumours are hypogonadal, probably as a result of inappropriate occupancy of ovarian receptors by tumour-derived inactive gonadotrophin molecules (Kovacs & Horvath 1987).

4. A rare cause of infertility is TSH-secreting macroadenoma (Caron et al 1996).

There are two aspects of pituitary adenoma vasculature worth mentioning. The first is the unexpectedly low vascularity, far inferior to that of the normal gland, suggesting the presence of angiogenetic inhibitors (Turner et al 2000). The second is the direct arterial supply of prolactin adenomas bypassing the hypothalamo-hypophysial portal system and thus evading dopamine-induced inhibition of prolactin secretion; this finding in the rat (Elias & Weiner 1984) has not been confirmed in humans but indirect evidence is provided by the presence of arteries in human prolactinomas (Schechter et al 1988).

There is intense interest in the cytogenetic and molecular aspects of pituitary adenomas (Kovacs 1996; Osamura et al 2000). Flow cytometry has shown the common occurrence of aneuploidy in these benign tumours (Garcia et al 1997); cytogenetic studies have confirmed that aneuploidy is associated with chromosomal rearrangements and numerical abnormalities (Kontogeorgos et al 1999; Finelli et al 2000) and comparative genomic hybridisation has identified losses and gains of specific chromosomal regions (Daniely et al 1998). Molecular data on pituitary adenomas are already quite extensive and only selected aspects will be presented. These tumours are clonal (Boggild et al 1994) and rarely show microsatellite instability (Zhu et al 1996) or *p53* mutations (Levy et al 1994). Since the behaviour of pituitary adenomas, as with most other endocrine tumours, cannot be reliably predicted on the usual histological criteria, molecular markers of aggressiveness are being sought and the following have been identified: tenascin (Ikeda et al 1995), type IV collagenase activity (Kawamoto et al 1996) and the heparin-binding secretory transforming gene (hst) protein product (Shimon et al 1998).

One of the major complications of pituitary adenomas is apoplexy or haemorrhagic infarction, possibly related to the local secretion of tissue factor by the tumour cells (Nishi et al 1999). It can occur spontaneously, as a result of a tumour-to-tumour metastasis, from an extracranial malignancy (Hanna et al 1999), after adenomectomy (Berthelot & Rey 1995), or cardiac surgery (Pilam et al 1995) and after a stimulation test (Otsuka et al 1998). It is worth noting that the incidence of cerebrovascular accidents is significantly higher in patients treated with surgery or radiotherapy (Brada et al 1999). Silent infarction or haemorrhage can rarely lead to spontaneous regression (Van Zandijcke & Casselman 1994). Another rare serious complication is the secondary development of a sarcoma after irradiation (Niwa et al 1996) and bromocriptine therapy (Nagasaka et al 1998).

Functional hypothalamo-hypophysial disorders include:

1. Hyperprolactinaemia, unrelated to a secreting pituitary adenoma, can result from (Yazigi et al 1997; Luciano 1999):
   i. Hypothalamic and pituitary stalk diseases: granulomatous inflammation, lymphocytic hypophysitis, craniopharyngiomas and other tumors, cranial irradiation, stalk section, vascular anomalies including carotid aneurysms, metastatic carcinoma. These conditions reverse the tonic dopamine-mediated hypothalamic suppression of prolactin secretion.
   ii. Systemic disorders: primary hypothyroidism, chronic renal failure, cirrhosis, and epilepsy.
   iii. Traumatic or inflammatory diseases of the chest wall.
   iv. Lesions of the upper spinal cord: ependymoma.
   v. Polycystic ovarian disease (PCO): the association between PCO and hyperprolactinaemia is not clear.
   vi. Drug-induced: dopamine-receptor agonists (phenothiazines, etc.), dopamine-depleting agents (α-methyldopa and reserpine) and hormones (oestrogens, contraceptive pill, androgens).
   vii. Ectopic production by renal cell carcinoma, gonadoblastoma, ectopic pituitary tissue in ovarian teratomas.

The clinical presentation is variable ranging from galactorrhoea, oligomenorrhoea, hirsutism, chronic anovulation and infertility. The association of hyperprolactinaemia and recurrent miscarriage is still debatable (Dlugi 1998; Hirahara et al 1998). The mechanisms of prolactin-associated reproductive dysfunction include inhibition of GnRH pulsatility and suppression of the mid-cycle gonadotrophin surge induced by oestrogen positive feedback. Some hyperprolactinaemic patients have a high level of anxiety but it is unclear whether psychological stress contributes to the antifertility effects of hyperprolactinaemia (Reavley et al 1997).

2. Hypoprolactinaemia is much less common and is seen as absence of the mid-cycle prolactin rise in some women with unexplained infertility (Subramanian et al 1997). In transgenic mice over-expressing the bovine growth hormone gene the neuroendocrine control of prolactin secretion is disrupted in early pregnancy leading to luteal failure, early loss of embryos and infertility (Cecim et al 1995).

Hypothalamo-hypophysial disconnection

This process is an uncommon cause of pituitary failure with decreased or increased prolactin secretion. It is achieved by interruption of the crucial hypothalamo-hypophysial portal system by surgery or by space-occupying lesions, e.g. parahypophysial tumours, suprasellar tumours like craniopharyngioma or Rathke cleft cyst and non-functioning pituitary macroadenoma (Berry & Caplan 1979; Young et al 1996; Hansen et al 1999). If the disconnection is coupled with pituitary destruction progressive panhypopituitarism results; if the disconnection occurs with preservation of the pituitary cells, the lactotrophs are released from their blood-borne inhibitor (dopamine) and over-secrete prolactin, i.e. dissociated hypopituitarism (McCarty & Dobson 1980).

SYSTEMIC DISEASES AND FEMALE INFERTILITY

Systemic diseases cause infertility by reducing fecundability and increasing pregnancy loss; they include congenital heart disease (McAnulty et al 1982), chronic renal disease (Katz et al 1980; Cochrane & Regan 1997), inflammatory bowel disease (Weber et al 1995), eating disorders (Morgan 1999), epilepsy (Schupf & Ottman 1996), first-onset schizophrenia (Hutchinson et al 1999), myeloproliferative disorders (Griesshammer et al 1998), chronic musculoskeletal disorders (Skomsvoll et al 2000), β-thalassaemia major (Reubinoff et al 1994), neurofibromatosis (Blickstein & Lurie 1990) and Wilson's disease (Kaushansky et al 1987; van Leeuwen et al 1991). It is worth noting that fertility can also be impaired by immunosuppressive, anti-inflammatory and neuroleptic drugs (Dickson et al 2000; Janssen & Genta 2000).

The greater prevalence of autoimmune diseases in women reflects the sex hormone dimorphism: experimentally, autoimmune processes are suppressed by androgens and enhanced by oestrogens, presumably via their direct interaction with specific receptors on CD8+ T cells and CD5+ B cells. Autoantibodies play a special rôle in female infertility as their clinical or subclinical presence is associated with a wide range of reproductive dysfunction, i.e. unexplained infertility, IVF failure, premature ovarian failure, endometriosis and recurrent pregnancy loss (Geva et al 1997). Some of the mechanisms underlying the reproductive failure include:

1. associated T-cell function which may be the real culprit (Stagnaro-Green et al 1992);
2. defective decidual response in early pregnancy due to antiphospholipid inhibition of decidual cell phospholipase A2 and reduced availability of local prostaglandin formation (Pierro et al 1999);
3. placental dysfunction due to excessive thrombosis associated with antibodies to phospholipids, β2-glycoprotein 1 and prothrombin (Ailus et al 1996) and by placental damage by chronic villitis and deciduitis, haemorrhagic endovasculitis, infarction and basal decidual arterial lesions (Labarrere et al 1986).

Endocrine diseases depress fertility by decreasing a woman's fecundability or ability to give birth to a live infant. The effects of pituitary dysfunction have already been described and the discussion here will be confined to the peripheral endocrine organs. In the pre-insulin era, young diabetics had a 5% chance of conceiving as compared with non-diabetics and their pregnancies often came to grief. Insulin has greatly improved their prognosis but the incidence of dysovulation and infertility is still higher in diabetics. Anovulation occurs with normal prolactin levels and a reduced LH:FSH ratio. The mechanism underlying this hypothalamic defect is unknown but it may be related to an increased dopaminergic activity in the hypothalamus with a normal dopamine–prolactin system (Djursing et al 1982). Insulin therapy and tighter metabolic control have greatly improved the prognosis for diabetic women. Their ability to conceive is now normal though they still have fewer pregnancies and fewer births than non-diabetics. This is due to a higher rate of voluntary infertility, pregnancy complications and late intrauterine and neonatal death (Kjaer et al 1992). There is no evidence that well-controlled diabetics are unduly prone to recurrent spontaneous miscarriage (Crane & Wahl 1981) but some women who develop gestational diabetes have recurrent losses due to the presence of β2-glycoprotein 1 and prothrombin antibodies (Ailus et al 1996).

Chronic reactive hyperinsulinaemia, which is the opposite of the hypoinsulinaemia of juvenile diabetes, results from impaired peripheral insulin action caused by intrinsic abnormalities in the insulin receptor, circulating antibodies to the receptor and inappropriate levels of physiological insulin antagonists, as in acromegaly and Cushing's syndrome (Buyalos et al 1992). While insulin action on glucose disposal is reduced, its action on the ovarian thecal and stromal cells, largely dependent on the IGF-1 receptor–effector mechanism, remains unaffected. Thus the excess insulin synergises with LH to increase intraovarian androstenedione and testosterone production, which leads to secondary derangements in gonadotrophin secretion and the development of polycystic ovaries with anovulation and infertility (Barbieri et al 1988). A rare but serious complication of untreated polycystic ovarian syndrome is endometrial carcinoma (Honoré & Davey 1989).

In women and adolescents primary hypothyroidism, usually of the autoimmune type, can cause menstrual irregularities, anovulation and infertility, disturbances readily reversed by substitution therapy. Ovarian enlargement that may cause torsion normally results from persistence of partially luteinized follicular cysts (van Voorhis et al 1994) and rarely from myxoedematous stromal infiltration and formation of non-luteinized cysts (Hansen et al 1997). Occult hypothyroidism may lead to the polycystic ovarian syndrome and infertility (Insler & Lunenfeld 1991). The mechanism whereby decreased thyroid function disturbs the hypothalamic–pituitary–gonadal axis is unclear but abnormal responses to TRH, LH and bromocriptine have been described, suggesting a central defect (Muechler & Huang 1982). It is possible that sellar enlargement due to secondary thyrotroph hypertrophy interferes with gonadotroph function resulting in a failure of LH surge and an acyclic secretory pattern often associated with polycystic ovaries (Lindsay et al 1983). In hypothyroidism there is also an increased rate of spontaneous miscarriage, stillbirth and fetal anomalies which may be related to decreased availability of maternal thyroxine to the developing embryo before fetal thyroid ontogenesis and to maternal deficiencies in some thyroxine-dependent crucial enzymes, i.e. Na^+-K^+ adenosine triphosphatase, critical in the membrane transport of glucose (Potter 1980). Hyperthyroidism is also associated with primary and secondary infertility. (Joshi et al 1993).

Hyperparathyroidism in pregnancy is associated with a significant increase in spontaneous miscarriage, fetal death, premature labour and neonatal hypocalcaemia and tetany (Ludwig 1962; Delmonico et al 1976). The disease can present insidiously (Shangold et al 1982) or acutely with pancreatitis (Hess et al 1980). A significant association between nephrolithiasis and spontaneous miscarriage has been noted; it is possible that these stone-formers had subclinical hyperparathyroidism (Honoré 1980).

Severe hypofunction or hyperfunction of the adrenal cortex causes widespread systemic disturbances that reduce fertility but these problems as a rule present to the internist. There is a more subtle and selective form of adrenal dysfunction with direct reproductive impact, i.e. adrenal hyperandrogenism. This condition, often coexisting with ovarian hyperandrogenism, is associated with infertility, anovulation, oligomenorrhoea and somatic manifestations, i.e. hirsutism, acne, clitoromegaly, etc. It can be diagnosed by measurements of serum androgens, including dehydroepiandrosterone sulphate, and by the dexamethasone suppression test. Excessive androgen

secretion by the adrenals can result from (Maroulis 1981):

1. Benign or malignant tumours with excessive production of adrenal androgens and/or testosterone.
2. Non-classic late-onset adrenal hyperplasia due to partial deficiency of 11- or 21-hydroxylase or 3β-hydroxysteroid dehydrogenase (Azziz et al 1996). Late-onset 21-hydroxylase deficiency, considered to be an allelic variant of virilising congenital adrenal hyperplasia, can mimic polycystic ovarian disease (Chrousos et al 1982).
3. Selective androgen hypersecretion in the presence of normal levels of cortisol and ACTH and normal appearing adrenal glands with slight widening of the zona fasciculata and the zona reticularis (Benedict et al 1962). The functional defect appears to be due to an 'exaggerated adrenarche' with a higher than normal setting for androgen secretion, resulting not from primary enzyme deficiency and feedback-related ACTH hypersecretion but from dysregulation of one critical enzyme, i.e. cytochrome P450C 17β-hydroxylase in the adrenal cortex and ovaries (Rosenfield et al 1990).
4. Chronic stress may activate the adrenals and account for the raised serum androgens detected in some infertile women (Lobo et al 1983).

The mechanisms whereby hyperandrogenism cause infertility include (Maroulis 1981):

i. Anovulation with or without polycystic ovaries
ii. Corpus luteum deficiency due to depression of progesterone secretion by testosterone (Rodriguez-Rigau et al 1979)
iii. Interference with fertilisation or nidation, as indirectly suggested by the failure of pregnancy to occur despite clomiphene-induced ovulation (Dupon et al 1973) and an increased rate of recurrent miscarriage (Okon et al 1998)
iv. Possible interference with oestrogen-induced changes in the cervical mucus (Langer et al 1990).

COMPLICATIONS OF INFERTILITY DIAGNOSIS AND TREATMENT

Infertility is now a recognised affliction that demands action and infertile couples are automatically exposed to an ever-increasing list of investigations and therapeutic modalities. It is salutary to pause and reflect that these patients can develop life-threatening, crippling or infertility-enhancing complications, which, although admittedly infrequent, arise in young healthy 'normal' people and thus assume greater clinical and personal significance. Moreover, since these patients are often emotionally distressed and frustrated (Menning 1980), such complications can be perceived with hostility and lead to litigation. For these reasons the significant complications of infertility diagnosis and treatment in women will be briefly discussed.

COMPLICATIONS OF INFERTILITY INVESTIGATIONS

These are uncommon and are best discussed in relation to the four primary forms of investigation performed:

Endometrial sampling

Excepting the rare complication of uterine perforation requiring emergency hysterectomy, the time-honoured diagnostic curettage is safe and widely used in gynaecology but serious doubt has been cast on its safety and advisability in infertility investigation. It can give rise to intrauterine adhesions (Taylor et al 1981) and to chronic pelvic inflammatory disease with its usual sequelae, i.e. tubal adhesions, hydrosalpinx, proximal tubal occlusion and distal phimosis (Taylor & Graham 1982). Hence curettage has been replaced by endometrial biopsy, which is less traumatic and can be performed on an outpatient basis. Its complications are minimal and include inadequate sampling due to cervical stenosis, excessive hemorrhage, excessive discomfort, fever, vasovagal reaction, uterine perforation and interruption of pregnancy. The chances of biopsying the endometrium during a cycle of conception are 3–5%; the overall risk of interrupting a pregnancy is 0.06% and about 2% if the implantation site is biopsied (Jaffe & Jewelewicz 1991). It would appear that endometrial biopsy has a detrimental effect on pregnancies following gonadotrophin therapy (Jacobson & Marshall 1980).

Laparoscopy

Laparoscopy is extensively used to assess ovulation, tubal patency and normalcy or otherwise of tubo-ovarian anatomy. Significant complications of gynaecological laparoscopy are rare, with a total rate of 3.6/1000 procedures and a rate of 1.4/1000 for major complications (Häarki-Siren & Kurki 1997). The most serious complication is death from cardiac arrest, which occurs in about one to three patients per 10 000. Other non-lethal complications include: cardiac arrest and arrhythmia with survival; vascular disturbances, i.e. deep vein thrombosis and pulmonary embolism, hypertension and gas embolism; bleeding arising at the site of abdominal puncture or at the site of biopsy; bowel burn or trauma (Loffer & Pent 1975; Carron Brown et al 1978); subcutaneous emphysema, gas extravasation into the mesentery, mediastinum or pleural sacs and anaesthetic complications (Loffer & Pent 1975; Carron Brown et al 1978; Ohlgisser et al 1985). Rarely bowel injuries may not be recognised at the time of direct vision laparoscopy and fragments of small intestine are only detected pathologically (Gentile & Siegler 1981); direct traumatic injury to bowel can be distinguished pathologically from injury caused by electrocoagulation (Levy et al 1985). Small bowel obstruction due to herniation through an incisional defect following laparoscopy is a rare complication (Sauer & Jarrett 1984). Significant infections, i.e. infection of pelvic haematoma or pelvic inflammatory disease, rarely follow investigative laparoscopy.

Hysteroscopy

Hysteroscopy is now a well-established procedure with negligible risks in experienced hands (Siegler & Valle 1988). Its complications include cervical laceration, uterine perforation, especially when therapeutic manoeuvres are performed, uterine bleeding rarely needing transfusion, ascending genital infection, which so far appears to be a theoretical rather than a real danger, gas embolism, bowel burn and perforation (Sugimoto 1978). Additional complications related to the use of dextran as a distending medium include cardiovascular overload, allergic reactions (Trimbos-Kemper & Veering 1990) and non-cardiogenic pulmonary oedema (Leake et al 1987). Severe haemorrhage after hysteroscopic division of a uterine septum is rare (Kazer et al 1992).

Hysterosalpingography

Hysterosalpingography is widely used to evaluate the uterine cavity and the tubes. Adverse reactions, occurring in 2% of cases, include: mechanical complications, i.e. cervical laceration, uterine perforation, tubal rupture; chemical complications, i.e. acute allergic reactions (Schwitemaker et al 1990), slight and transient thyroid dysfunction, and lipoid granulomas of the tube; vascular complications, i.e. pulmonary oil embolism; infective complications, i.e. usually due to exacerbation of chronic pelvic infection giving rise to acute salpingitis and peritonitis. The most serious complication is death occurring during the procedure or within two weeks as a result of peritonitis, pulmonary embolism or lipoid pneumonia (Jaffe & Jewelewicz 1991).

Hysterosalpingography increases the pregnancy rate in some women and its therapeutic effect is due to the bacteriostatic effect of iodine, enhancement of ciliary action, hydrotubation effect with mechanical lavage and adhesiolysis and decreased spermiophagy (Jaffe & Jewelewicz 1991).

COMPLICATIONS OF INFERTILITY THERAPY

These complications, arising from deliberate interventions in the female, are variably inherent in the methods and secondary to extraneous factors, such as patient selection, the skill of the operator and the efficiency of patient monitoring during and after treatment. A brief review is included in terms of the three major therapeutic modalities, i.e. surgery, medical therapy and transfer methods.

Surgery

Surgery plays an important role in infertility therapy and recent advances in anaesthesia, surgical technique, postoperative support and a better understanding of reproductive anatomy and physiology have greatly improved the success rate. The complications will be discussed in relation to the organ operated upon.

Tubal surgery has changed drastically with the introduction of microsurgery and the results are significantly better than those obtained by conventional macrosurgery (Posaci et al 1999). Lysis of tubal or tubo-ovarian adhesions, with or without associated uterine suspension, has no significant complication (Gomel 1983). A higher rate of ectopic pregnancy, the major complication of tubal surgery, is associated with fimbrioplasty (the surgical correction of partial fimbrial occlusion), salpingoneostomy (the surgical repair of a totally occluded distal tube) and tubotubal or tubocornual anastomosis (De Cherney et al 1983; Gomel 1983). There is also an increased incidence of spontaneous miscarriage, especially after uterotubal implantation (Jansen 1982). Rare complications of tuboplasty include traumatic femoral neuropathy (Hassan et al 1986) and intercornual bridging by a swollen blocked tube showing haematosalpinx, chronic salpingitis and perisalpingeal endometriosis (Honoré & Scott 1992).

Postoperative adhesions, whether as de novo or as reformed adhesions, remain a significant surgical and economic problem with no improvement in outcome with the use of corticosteroids, anti-inflammatory drugs, crystalloids or barrier agents (di Zerega 1994). There is a definite predisposition to adhesion formation and one possible marker is the ability of the normally negative peritoneum to express oestrogen and progesterone receptors, which may explain the suppression of adhesion enlargement in hypo-oestrogenic animals (Wiczyk et al 1998). Laparoscopic surgery has also reduced the incidence of postoperative adhesions (Lundorff et al 1991).

Ovarian surgery, confined to bilateral wedge resection in drug-resistant cases of polycystic ovarian disease, is followed by significant pelvic adhesions in at least 8% of cases (Adashi et al 1981). These adhesions, constituting an iatrogenically induced mechanical cause of infertility (Weinstein & Polishuk 1975), account in large measure for the discrepancy between the rate of postoperative ovulation and the crude pregnancy rate. Microsurgery appears to reduce the chances of postoperative adhesions. Another complication is the significantly increased incidence of ectopic pregnancy after wedge resection (Adashi et al 1981).

Uterine surgery involves intervention at the level of the cervix, myometrium and endometrium. Cervical cerclage, done for incompetence, can be associated with premature rupture of membranes, ascending chorioamnionitis, prematurity and uterine rupture requiring hysterectomy (Peters et al 1979). Myomectomy, despite its variable success in correcting infertility (Bernard et al 2000; Dubuisson et al 2000;), is not followed by obstetrical problems, except for the occasional rupture of the pregnant uterus (Dubuisson et al 1995). Lysis of intrauterine adhesions by conventional methods is complicated by a high rate of pregnancy loss, prematurity, placenta accreta and placenta praevia (Schenker & Margalioth 1982); these complications are significantly reduced by hysteroscopic lysis (March & Israel 1981).

Pituitary surgery by the trans-sphenoidal route is a safe and highly successful form of treatment for hyperprolactinaemia due to a pituitary adenoma with a low mortality and complication rate (Oruckaptan et al 2000).

Medical therapy

Medical therapy is widely used and its complications can be reproductive or systemic depending on the drug used. The reports of the adverse effects of clomiphene citrate, used to stimulate ovulation, are so discrepant that no meaningful conclusions can be drawn (Adashi et al 1979). It is still unclear whether the drug is associated with a higher incidence of spontaneous miscarriage, ectopic pregnancy, hydatidiform mole, prematurity and preeclampsia (Correy et al 1982; Shoham et al 1991; Bateman et al 1992). There is, however, good evidence that such treatment is followed by multiple gestations including superfetation (Bsat & Seoud 1987) but there is no increase in congenital malformations (Shoham et al 1991). Clomiphene often causes cystic enlargement of the ovaries (Farrari et al 1969), which is rarely symptomatic (Chow & Choo 1984); bilateral adnexal torsion is exceptional (Bider et al 1991).

The antigonadotrophin drug, danazol, is widely used in the conservative management of endometriosis, particularly in the young infertile patient, and its side effects are relatively minor (Dmowski 1979) including carpal tunnel syndrome (Sikka et al 1983), sensorineural hearing loss (Ennyeart & Price 1984), post-therapy amenorrhoea (Peress 1984) and reversible elevation of serum enzymes (Holt & Keller 1984). There is surprisingly little information regarding its possible effects on pregnancy. The rate of spontaneous miscarriage is reported as increased or unchanged after cessation of therapy (Dmowski & Cohen 1978; Barbieri et al 1982) and there are no teratological consequences when the drug is taken in early pregnancy. Two cases of female pseudohermaphroditism with intrauterine danazol exposure are on record (Duck & Katayama 1981; Peress et al 1982). A rare complication is the combination of toxic dermatitis, fulminant hepatic failure and aplastic anaemia (Nakajima et al 1986).

Bromocriptine, a dopaminergic agonist used in the treatment of hyperprolactinaemia, has no adverse effects on the pregnancy or the fetus (Dewit et al 1984) and the only 'complication' of bromocriptine-induced pregnancy is symptomatic growth of a prolactinoma (Dommerholt et al 1981). Rarely, low dose treatment of infertile hyperprolactinaemic patients can cause cold-induced vasospasm or Raynaud's phenomenon (Quagliarello & Barakat 1987).

Prednisone, used for the treatment of anovulation due to adrenal hyperandrogenism, has a variable effect on pregnancy depending on the dose and the length of administration during pregnancy. Large doses and prolonged administration can cause increased fetal wastage, adrenal atrophy, congenital malformations and intrauterine growth retardation; low-dose therapy has no ill effects (Lee et al 1982). Intramuscular injections rarely cause local complications but progesterone, administered as part of an IVF treatment schedule, can rarely provoke severe thigh myositis (Phipps et al 1988).

Assisted reproductive technology (ART)

The complications of ART include ectopic pregnancy, heterotopic (combined intrauterine and extrauterine) pregnancy, spontaneous miscarriage, multiple fetuses, pregnancy-induced hypertension, prematurity, low birth weight and intrauterine death (Serour et al 1998) with heterotopic pregnancy carrying a high morbidity (Habana et al 2000). Micro-manipulative methods, i.e. assisted hatching and intracytoplasmic sperm injection (ICSI) are quite safe with an increase in mono-amniotic twinning (Wright et al 1998) but, when used in cases of severe oligospermia and non-obstructive azospermia, ICSI is associated with an increased risk of sex chromosome aneuploidy in the offspring (Johnson 1998). In general, infertility treatment has little impact on the newborn except for an increased incidence of multiplicity and prematurity (Addor et al 1998) and it is reassuring that children born after in vitro fertilisation are not more prone to cancer (Bruinsma et al 2000). Multifetal pregnancy reduction may be a further risk factor for periventricular leukomalacia in premature infants (Geva et al 1998).

Rare complications of ART include metastatic strumosis in an in vitro fertilisation (Balasch et al 1993), ruptured tubo-ovarian abscesses after transcervical embryo transfer (Friedler et al 1996), recurrent cervical pregnancy after assisted reproduction by intrafallopian transfer (Qasim et al 1996) and exacerbation of recurrent leiomyomatosis peritonealis disseminata by in vitro fertilisation (Deering et al 2000).

The major complication of gonadotrophin-induced ovarian hyperstimulation is the ovarian hyperstimulation syndrome variably associated with ovarian enlargement, adnexal torsion, ascites, hydrothorax, anasarca, oliguric renal failure, liver dysfunction, venous thrombosis, pulmonary thromboembolism and infection, adult respiratory distress syndrome and death (Navot et al 1992; Abramov et al 1999). Pregnancies thus complicated have higher rates of early and late miscarriage (Abramov et al 1998). The other potentially serious complication of gonadotrophin treatment is ovarian and breast cancer. This topic remains controversial but the evidence points to two conclusions: (1) women with refractory infertility constitute a high-risk group for ovarian cancer, and (2) ovulation induction by gonadotrophin and/or clomiphene citrate does not increase the risk of ovarian or breast cancer (Bristow & Karlan 1996; Mosgaard et al 1998; Potashnik et al 1999; Wakeley & Grendys 2000).

Acknowledgements

I would like to express my sincere thanks to Ms Lynda Harrison for her patience and unfailing support during the typing of the updated manuscript and to Mr Tom Turner for the excellent photographs.

REFERENCES

Abramov Y, Elchalal U, Schenker J G 1998 Obstetric outcome of in vitro fertilized pregnancies complicated by severe ovarian hyperstimulation syndrome: a multicenter study. Fertility and Sterility 70: 1070–1076

Abramov Y, Elchalal U, Schenker J G 1999 Pulmonary manifestations of severe ovarian hyperstimulation syndrome: a multicenter study. Fertility and Sterility 71: 645–651

Abse D W 1966 Psychiatric aspects of human male infertility. Fertility and Sterility 17: 133–139

Abuelo D N, Barsel-Powers G, Richardson A 1988 Insertional translocations: report of two new families and review of the literature. American Journal of Medical Genetics 31: 319–329

Abuzeid M I, Weibe R H, Askel S, Shepherd J, Yeoman R R 1987 Evidence of a possible cytosol estrogen receptor deficiency in endocervical glands of infertile women with poor cervical mucus. Fertility and Sterility 47: 101–107

Adams C E 1979 Consequences of accelerated ovum transport, including a reevaluation of Estes' operation. Journal of Reproduction and Fertility 55: 239–246

Adashi E Y, Rock J A, Sapp K C, Martin E J, Wentz A C, Seegar-Jones G A 1979 Gestational outcome of clomiphene-related conceptions. Fertility and Sterility 31: 620–626

Adashi E Y, Rock J A, Guzick D, Wentz A C, Seegar-Jones G A, Jones J W Jr 1981 Fertility following bilateral ovarian wedge resection: a critical analysis of 90 consecutive cases of the polycystic ovary syndrome. Fertility and Sterility 36: 320–325

Addor V, Santos-Eggimann B, Fawer C-L, Paccaud F, Calame A 1998 Impact of infertility treatments on the health of new borns. Fertility and Sterility 69: 210–217

Ahlgren M 1975 Sperm transport to and survival in the human fallopian tube. Gynecologic Investigation 6: 206–214

Ahmad-Thabet 2000 The fimbrio-ovarian relation and its role on ovum picking in unexplained infertility: the fimbrio-ovarian accessibility tests. Journal of Obstetrical and Gynaecological Research 26: 65–70

Ailus K, Tulppala M, Palosuo T, Ylikorkala O, Vaarala O 1996 Antibodies to β2-glycoprotein 1 and prothrombin in habitual abortion. Fertility and Sterility 66: 937–941

Alexander N J, Anderson D J 1987 Immunology of semen. Fertility and Sterility 47: 192–205

Amann R P 1981 A critical review of methods of evaluation of spermatogenesis from seminal characteristics. Journal of Andrology 2: 37–58

Anand S, Guha S K 1982 Dynamics of the ampullary-isthmic junction in rabbit oviduct. Gynecologic and Obstetrical Investigation 14: 39–46

Anasti J N 1998 Premature ovarian failure: an update. Fertility and Sterility 70: 1–15

Anestad G, Lunde O, Moen M, Dalaker K 1987 Infertility and Chlamydial infection. Fertility and Sterility 48: 787–790

Angell R R, Xian J, Keith J 1993 Chromosome anomalies in human oocytes in relation to age. Human Reproduction 8: 1047–1052

Ansari A H, Gould K G, Ansari V M 1980 Sodium bicarbonate douching for improvement of the postcoital test. Fertility and Sterility 33: 608–612

Aoki K, Furukawa T, Ogasawara M, Hori S, Kitamura T 1998 Psychological factors in recurrent miscarriages. Acta Obstetricia et Gynecologica Scandinavica 77: 572–573

Aplin J D, Hey N A, Li T L 1996 MUC1 as a cell surface and secretory component of the endometrial epithelium: reduced levels in recurrent miscarriage. American Journal of Reproductive Immunology 35: 261–266

Araki S, Chikazawa K, Sekiguchi I, Yamauchi H, Motoyama M, Tamada T 1987 Arrest of follicular development in a patient with 17β-hydroxylase deficiency: folliculogenesis in association with a lack of estrogen synthesis in the ovaries. Fertility and Sterility 47: 169–172

Archer D F, Maroon J C, Dubois P J 1978: Galactorrhoea, amenorrhoea, hyper-prolactinemia and an empty sella. Obstetrics and Gynecology 52: 23S–27S

Aronnet G H, Eduljee S Y, O'Brien J R 1969 A nine-year survey of fallopian tube dysfunction in human infertility. Fertility and Sterility 20: 903–908

Ashkenazi J, Feldberg D, Shelef M, Dicker D, Goldman J A 1987 Empty follicle syndrome: an entity in the etiology of infertility of unknown origin or a phenomenon associated with purified follicle-stimulating hormone therapy. Fertility and Sterility 48: 152–154

Ault K A, Statland B D, King M M, Dozier D I, Joachims M L, Gunter J 1998 Antibodies to the chlamydial 60 kilodalton heat shock protein in women with tubal factor infertility. Infectious Diseases in Obstetrics and Gynecology 6: 163–167

Azziz R, Dewailly D, Owerbach D 1996 Nonclassic adrenal hyperplasia: current concepts. Clinical Review 56. Journal of Clinical Endocrinology and Metabolism 78: 810–815

Bagwell M A, Thompson S J, Addy C L, Coker A L, Baker E R 1995 Primary infertility and oral contraceptive steroid use. Fertility and Sterility 63: 1161–1166

Bahamondes L, Bueno J G R, Hardy E, Vera S, Pimentel E, Ramos M 1994 Identification of main risk factors for tubal infertility. Fertility and Sterility 61: 478–482

Bahceci M, Demirel L C 1996 Osseous metaplasia of the endometrium: a rare cause of infertility and its hysteroscopic management. Human Reproduction 11: 2537–2539

Balasch J, Martinez-Roman S, Creus M, Campo E, Fortuny A, Vanrell J A 1995 Schistosomiasis: an unusual cause of tubal infertility. Human Reproduction 10: 1725–1727

Balasch J, Pahisa J, Marquez M, Ordi J, Fabregues F, Puerto B, Vanrell J A 1998 Metastatic ovarian strumosis in an in-vitro fertilization. Human Reproduction 12: 2075–2079

Barbieri R L 1998 Stenosis of the external cervical os: an association with endometriosis in women with chronic pelvic pain. Fertility and Sterility 70: 571–573

Barbieri R L, Evans S, Kistner R W 1982 Danazol in the treatment of endometriosis: analysis of 100 cases with a 4-year follow-up. Fertility and Sterility 37: 737–746

Barbieri R L, Smith S, Ryan K J 1988 The role of hyperinsulinemia in the pathogenesis of ovarian hyperandrogenism. Fertility and Sterility 50: 197–212

Barbosa C, Malasaet M, Brockmann S, Sierra M F, Xia Z, Duerr A 1997 Pelvic inflammatory disease and human immunodeficiency virus infection. Obstetrics and Gynecology 89: 65–70

Barmat L I, Worrilow K C, Paynton B V 1997 Growth factor expression by human oviduct and buffalo rat-liver coculture cells. Fertility and Sterility 67: 775–779

Barratt C L R, Cooke I D 1991 Sperm transport in the human female reproductive tract: a dynamic interaction. International Journal of Andrology 14: 394–411

Barros C, Arguello B, Jedlicki A, Vigil P, Herrea E 1985 Scanning electron microscopy study of human cervical mucus. Gamete Research 12: 85–89

Bassetti M, Spada A, Pezzo G, Giannattasio G 1984 Bromocriptine treatment reduces cell size in human macroprolactinomas: a morphometric study. Journal of Clinical Endocrinology and Metabolism 58: 268–273

Bateman B G, Eddy C A, Kitchin J D III 1983 Effect of lengthening the fallopin tube on fertility in the rabbit. American Journal of Obstetrics and Gynecology 147: 569–573

Bateman B G, Nonley S C Jr, Kitchen J D III 1987 Surgical management of distal tubal obstruction — are we making progress? Fertility and Sterility 48: 523–542

Bateman B G, Kolp L A, Nunley W C Jr, Felder R, Burkett B 1992: Subclinical pregnancy loss in clomiphene citrate-treated women. Fertility and Sterility 57: 25–27

Bates G W, Whitworth N S 1982 Effect of body weight reduction on plasma androgen in obese infertile women. Fertility and Sterility 38: 406–309

Bath L E, Critchley H O D, Chambers S E, Anderson R A, Kelnar C J H, Wallace W H B 1999 Ovarian and uterine characteristics after total body irradiation in childhood and adolescence: response to sex steroid replacement. British Journal of Obstetrics and Gynaecology 106: 1265–1272

Batista M C, Cartledge T P, Zellmer A W, Merino N J, Axiotis C, Bremner W J, Nieman C K 1995 Effects of aging on menstrual cycle hormones and endometrial maturation. Fertility and Sterility 64: 492–499

Bazak-Malik G, Mashewari B, Lan N 1983 Tuberculous endometritis: a clinicopathological study of 100 cases. British Journal of Obstetrics and Gynaecology 90: 84–86

Benedict P H, Cohen R, Cope O, Scully R E 1962: Ovarian and adrenal morphology in cases of hirsutism or virilism and the Stein–Leventhal syndrome. Fertility and Sterility 13: 380–395

Benoff S, Hurley I R, Barcia M, Mandel F S, Cooper G W, Hershlag A 1997 A potential role for cadmium in the etiology of varicocele-associated infertility. Fertility and Sterility 67: 336–347

Ben-Shlomo I, Schiff E, Levran D, Ben-Rafael Z, Maschiach S, Dor J 1991 Failure of oocyte retrieval during in vitro fertilization: a sporadic event rather than a syndrome. Fertility and Sterility 55: 324–327

Bergh P A, Navot D 1992 The impact of embryonic development and endometrial maturity on the timing of implantation. Fertility and Sterility 58: 537–542

Bernard G, Darai E, Poncelet C, Benifla J Z, Madelenat P 2000 Fertility after hysteroscopic myomectomy: effect of intramural myomas associated. European Journal of Obstetrics, Gynecology and Reproductive Biology 88: 85–90

Berry R G, Caplan H J 1979 An overview of pituitary tumors. Annals of Clinical and Laboratory Science 9: 94–102

Berthelot J L Rey A 1995 Pituitary apoplexy. Presse Médicale 24: 501–503

Best C L, Walters G, Adelman D C 1988 Fixed cutaneous eruptions to seminal-plasma challenge: a case report. Fertility and Sterility 50: 532–534

Beyth Y, Bar-On E 1984 Tubo-ovarian amputation and infertility. Fertility and Sterility 42: 932–934

Biberoglu K O, Damewood M D, Parmley T, Rock J A 1988 Insensitive ovary syndrome with a unique process of follicular degeneration. Fertility and Sterility 49: 367–369

Bider D, Goldenberg M, Ben-Rafael Z, Oelsner G 1991 Bilateral adnexal torsion after clomiphene citrate therapy. Human Reproduction 6: 1443–1444

Blacker C M, Ginsburg K A, Leach R E, Randolph J, Moghissi K S 1997 Unexplained infertility: evaluation of the luteal phase: results of the National Center for Infertility Research at Michigan. Fertility and Sterility 67: 437–442

Blickstein I, Lurie S 1990 The gynaecological problems of neurofibromatosis. Australian and New Zealand Journal of Obstetrics and Gynaecology 30: 380–382

Blumenfeld Z, Brenner B 1999 Thrombophilia-associated pregnancy wastage. Fertility and Sterility 72: 765–774

Boggild M D, Jenkinson S, Pistorello M et al 1994 Molecular genetic studies of sporadic pituitary tumors. Journal of Clinical Endocrinology and Metabolism 78: 387–392

Bomsel-Helmreich O 1976 The aging of gametes, heteroploidy and embryonic death. International Journal of Gynaecology and Obstetrics 14: 98–104

Bonde J P E, Ernst E, Jensen T K, Hjollund N H I, Kolstad H, Henriksen T B 1998 Relation between semen quality and fertility: a population-based study of 430 first-pregnancy planners. Lancet 352: 1172–1177

Bongso A, Ng S-C, Fong C Y et al 1992 Improved pregnancy rate after transfer of embryos grown in human fallopian tubal cell coculture. Fertility and Sterility 58: 569–574

Borini A, Bafaro G, Violini F, Bianchi L, Casadio V, Flamigni C 1995 Pregnancies in postmenopausal women over 50 years old in an oocyte donation program. Fertility and Sterility 63: 258–261

Bracken M B, Hellenbrand K G, Holford T R 1990 Conception delay after oral contraceptive use: the effect of estrogen dose. Fertility and Sterility 53: 21–27

Brada M, Burchell L, Ashley S, Traish D 1999 The incidence of cerebrovascular accidents in patients with pituitary adenoma. International Journal of Radiation Oncology, Biology and Physics 45: 693–398

Bray G A 1997 Obesity and reproduction. Human Reproduction 12 (supplement 1): 26–32

Bristow R E, Karlan B Y 1996 The risk of ovarian cancer after treatment for infertility. Current Opinion in Obstetrics and Gynaecology 8: 32–37

Brown W M, Hayes E J, Uchida T, Nagamannni M 1995 Some cases of human male infertility are explained by abnormal in vitro human sperm activation. Fertility and Sterility 64: 612–622

Bruinsma F, Venn A, Lancaster P, Spiers A, Healy D 2000 Incidence of cancer in children born after in-vitro fertilization. Human Reproduction 15: 604–607

Brundon J, Bremmer S, Grundstrom H, Lundberg H J, Lundberg S, Asard P E 1993 Developmental steps for radionuclide hysterosalpingography. Gynecologic and Obstetric Investigation 36: 34–38

Bsat F A, Senud M A F 1987 Superfetation secondary to ovulation induction with clomiphene citrate: a case report. Fertility and Sterility 47: 516–518

Buck G M, Sever L E, Batt R E, Mendola P 1997 Life-style factors and female infertility. Epidemiology 8: 435–441

Buckett W M, Luckas M J J, Aird I A, Farquaharson R G, Kingsland C R, Lewis-Jones D I 1997 The hypo-osmotic swelling test in recurrent miscarriage. Fertility and Sterility 68: 506–509

Burchell R C, Creed F, Rasoulpour M, Whitcomb M 1978 Vascular anatomy of the human uterus and pregnancy wastage. British Journal of Obstetrics and Gynaecology 85: 698–706

Burke K, Hertig A T, Miele A 1985 Diagnostic value of subacute focal inflammation of the endometrium, with special reference to pelvic adhesions as observed on laparoscopic examination: an eight year review. Journal of Reproductive Medicine 30: 646–649

Buttram V C Jr, Reiter R C 1981 Uterine leiomyomata: etiology, symptomatology and management. Fertility and Sterility 36: 433–445

Buyalos R P, Geffner M E, Bersch N et al 1992 Insulin and insulin-like growth factor-1 responsiveness in polycystic ovarian syndrome. Fertility and Sterility 57: 796–803

Bychkov V 1990 Ovarian pathology in chronic pelvic inflammatory disease. Gynecologic and Obstetric Investigation 30: 31–33

Bygdeman M 1970 The relation between fertility and prostaglandin content of seminal fluid in man. Fertility and Sterility 21: 622–629

Byrne J, Mulvihill J J, Myers M H et al 1992 Early menopause in long-term survivors of cancer during adolescence. American Journal of Obstetrics and Gynecology 166: 788–793

Camus E, Poncelet C, Goffinet F et al 1999 Pregnancy rates after in-vitro fertilization in cases of tubal infertility with and without hydrosalpinx: a meta-analysis of published comparative studies. Human Reproduction 14: 1243–1249

Cano F, Simon C, Remohi J, Pellicer A 1995 Effect of aging on the female reproductive system: evidence for a role of uterine senescence in the decline of female fecundity. Fertility and Sterility 64: 584–589

Caron P, Gerbeau C, Pradayrol L, Simonetta C, Bayard F 1996 Successful pregnancy in an infertile woman with a thyrotropin-secreting macroadenoma treated with somatostatin analog (octreotide). Journal of Clinical Endocrinology and Metabolism: 81: 1164–1168

Carr B R 1998 Disorders of the ovaries and female reproductive tract. In: Wilson J D, Foster D W, Kronenberg H M, Larsen P R (eds) Williams' Textbook of Endocrinology, edn. 9th W B Saunders Company, Philadelphia, London, p 761

Carron Brown J A, Chamberlain G V P, Jordan J A et al 1978: Gynaecological laparoscopy. The report of the working party of the confidential inquiry into gynaecological laparoscopy. British Journal of Obstetrics and Gynaecology 85: 401–403

Cates W Jr, Brunham R C 1999 Sexually transmitted diseases and infertility. In: Holmes K K, Sparling P F, Mårdh P-A, Lemon S M, Estamm W, Piot P, Wasserheit J M (eds) Sexually transmitted diseases, 3rd edn. McGraw-Hill, New York, pp 1079–1088

Cazabat A M, Volochine B, Kuntsmann J M, Chretien F C 1982 Human cervical mucus. Acta Obstetricia et Gynecologica Scandinavica 61: 385–392

Cecim M, Fadden C, Kerr J, Sieger R W, Bartke A 1995 Infertility in transgenic mice overexpressing the bovine growth hormone gene: disruption of the neuroendocrine control of prolactin secretion during pregnancy. Biology of Reproduction 52: 1187–1192

Chacho K J, Hage C W, Shulman S 1991 The relationship between female sexual practices and the development of antisperm antibodies. Fertility and Sterility 56: 461–464

Chatkoff M L 1975 A biophysicist's view of ovum transport. Gynecologic Investigation 6: 105–122

Check J H, Chase J S, Nowroozi K, Dietterich C J 1991 Premature luteinization: treatment and incidence in natural cycles. Human Reproduction 6: 190–193

Chen E C, Brzyski R G 1999 Exercise and reproductive dysfunction. Fertility and Sterility 71: 1–6

Chetkowski R J, Kiltz R J, Salyer W R 1997 In premature luteinization, progesterone induces secretory transformation of the endometrium without impairment of embryo viability. Fertility and Sterility 68: 292–297

Chia S-E, Lim S T A, Tay S-K, Lim S-T 2000 Factors associated with male infertility: a case control study of 218 infertile and 240 fertile men. British Journal of Obstetrics and Gynaecology 107: 55–61

Chow K K, Choo H T 1984: Ovarian hyperstimulation syndrome with clomiphene citrate: case report. British Journal of Obstetrics and Gynaecology 91: 1051–1052

Chretien F C 1978 Ultrastructure and variations of human cervical mucus during pregnancy and the menopause. Acta Obstetricia et Gynecologica Scandinavica 57: 337–348

Chrousos G P, Loriaux D L, Mann D L, Cutler B 1982 Late onset 21-hydroxylase deficiency mimicking idiopathic hirsutism or polycystic ovarian disease. Annals of Internal Medicine 96: 143–148

Clarke J 1994 The meaning of menstruation in the elimination of abnormal embryos. Human Reproduction 9: 1204–1206

Cochrane R, Regan L 1997 Undetected gynaecological disorders in women with renal disease. Human Reproduction 12: 667–670

Coeman D, Van Belle Y, Vanderick G 1995 Tubal ostium membranes and their relation to infertility. Fertility and Sterility 63: 666–668

Coetsiert T, Dhont 1996 Complete and partial luteinized unruptured follicle syndrome after ovulation with clomiphene citrate/human menopausal gonadotrophin/human chorionic gonadotrophin. Human Reproduction 11: 583–587

Cohen B M 1980 Surgical repair and abnormal fimbrial gonadal relationships in the human female. Journal of Reproductive Medicine 25: 33–37

Cohen B M, Katz M 1978 The significance of the convoluted oviduct in the infertile woman. Journal of Reproductive Medicine 21: 31–35

Colgan T L, Pendergast S, Leblanc M 1993 The histopathology of uterine leiomyomas following treatment with gonadotrophin-releasing hormone analogues. Human Pathology 24: 1073–1077

Collado M L, Castro G, Hicks J J 1979 Effect of spermatozoa upon carbonic anhydrase activity of rabbit endometrium. Biology of Reproduction 20: 747–750

Collins J A, Burrow E A, Wilanar 1995 The prognosis of live birth among untreated infertile couples. Fertility and Sterility 64: 22–28

Conway G S 1997 Premature ovarian failure. Current Opinion on Obstetrics and Gynaecology 9: 202–206

Corbetta S, Pizzocaro A, Peracchi M, Beck-Peccoz P, Faglia G, Spada A 1997 Multiple endocrine neoplasia type I in patients with recognized pituitary tumours of different types. Clinical Endocrinology 47: 507–512

Correy J F, Marsden D E, Schokman F M C 1982 The outcome of pregnancies resulting from clomiphene-induced ovulation. Australian and New Zealand Journal of Obstetrics and Gynaeology 22: 18–21

Coulam C B 1982 Premature gonadal failure. Fertility and Sterility 38: 645–655

Coulam C B 1991 Epidemiology of recurrent spontaneous abortion. American Journal of Reproductive Immunology 26: 23–27

Coulam C B, Annegers J F, Krantz J S 1982 The association between pituitary adenomas and chronic anovulation syndrome. American Journal of Obstetrics and Gynecology 143: 319–322

Coulam C B, Bustilloa M, Schulman J D 1986 Empty follicle syndrome. Fertility and Sterility 46: 1153–1155

Coulam C B, Wagenknecht D, McIntyre J A, Faulk W P, Annegers J F 1991 Occurrence of other reproductive failures among women with recurrent spontaneous abortion. American Journal of Reproductive Immunology 25: 96–98

Coutinho E M, Maia H S 1971 The contractile response of the human uterus, fallopian tubes and ovary to prostaglandins in vivo. Fertility and Sterility 15: 367–372

Cramer D W, Ravnikar V A, Craighill M, Ng W G, Goldstein D P, Reilly R 1987 Mullerian aplasia associated with maternal deficiency of galactose-1-phosphate uridyl transferase. Fertility and Sterility 47: 930–934

Crane J P, Wahl N 1981 The role of maternal diabetes in repetitive spontaneous abortion. Fertility and Sterility 36: 477–479

Critser J K, Villines P M, Coulam C B, Critser E S 1989 Evaluation of circulating anti-sperm antibodies in fertile and infertile patient populations. American Journal of Reproductive Immunology 21: 137–142

Croxatto H B, Ortiz M E, Diaz S, Hess R, Balmaceda J, Croxatto H-D 1978 Studies on the duration of egg transport by the human oviduct II Ovum location at various intervals following luteinizing hormone peak. American Journal of Obstetrics and Gynecology 132: 629–634

Cruickshank M E, Flannelly G, Campbell D M, Kitchener H C 1995 Fertility and pregnancy outcome following large loop excision of the cervical transformation zone. British Journal of Obstetrics and Gynaecology 102: 467–470

Csemiczky G, Landgren B-M, Collins A 2000 The influence of stress and state anxiety on the outcome of IVF treatment: psychological and endocrinological assessment of Swedish women entering IVF treatment. Acta Obstetricia et Gynecologica Scandinavica 79: 113–118

Cumming D C, Honoré L H, Scott J Z 1984 Mycoplasmal endometritis: correlation with cervical and endometrial bacteriology. Infertility 7: 203–214

Cumming D C, Honoré L H, Scott J Z, Williams K E 1985 The late luteal phase in infertile women: comparison of simultaneous endometrial biopsy and progesterone levels. Fertility and Sterility 43: 715–719

Cumming D C, Honoré L H, Scott J Z, Williams K E 1988 Microscopic evidence of silent inflammation in grossly normal fallopian tubes with ectopic pregnancy. International Journal of Infertility 33: 324–328

Czernobilsky B 1978 Endometritis and infertility. Fertility and Sterility 30: 119–130

Daly D C, Tohan N, Doney T J, Masler I A, Riddick D H 1982 The significance of lymphocytic-leukocytic infiltrates in interpreting late luteal phase endometrial biopsies. Fertility and Sterility 37: 786–791

Daly D C, Soto-Albers C E, Aversa M A 1986 Hysteroscopic detection and treatment of adhesions at the tubal ostium/uterine junction in infertile patients. Fertility and Sterility 46: 138–140

Danforth D R, Arbogast L K, Mroueh J et al 1998 Dimeric inhibin: a direct marker of ovarian aging. Fertility and Sterility 70: 119–123

Daniely M, Aviram A, Adams E F et al 1998 Comparative genomic hybridization analysis of non-functioning pituitary tumors. Journal of Clinical Endocrinology and Metabolism 83: 1801–1805

Dargent D, Martin X, Saccheion T A, Mateievet P 2000 Laparoscopic vaginal radical trachelectomy. A treatment to preserve the fertility of cervical carcinoma patients. Cancer 88: 1877–1882

Datnow A D 1973 A reconsideration of the secretory function of the human endometrium. Journal of Obstetrics and Gynaecology of the British Commonwealth 80: 865–871

David M P, Ben-Zwi D, Langer L 1981 Tubal intramural polyps and their relationship to infertility. Fertility and Sterility 35: 526–531

Davis O K, Berkeley A S, Naus G J, Cholst I N, Freedman K S 1989 The incidence of luteal phase defect in normal fertile women determined by serial endometrial biopsies. Fertility and Sterility 51: 582–586

Dawood M Y 1994 Corpus luteal insufficiency. Current Opinion in Obstetrics and Gynecology 6: 121–127

de Boer J, Hoeijmakers J H J 2000 Nucleotide excision repair and human syndromes. Carcinogenesis 21: 453–460

De Brux J, Dupré-Froment J 1965 Etude anatomo-pathologique de la tuberculose génitale féminine cliniquement 'latente'. Revue Française de Gynécologie 60: 57–88

De Cherney A H, Cholst I, Naftolin F 1981 Structure and function of the fallopian tubes following exposure to diethylstilbestrol (DES) during gestation. Fertility and Sterility 36: 741–745

De Fazio S R, Ketchel M M 1971 Immuno-electrophoretic analysis of human cervical mucus and seminal plasma with an antiserum of cervical mucus. Journal of Reproduction and Fertility 25: 11–19

de Kretzer D M, Huidobro C, Southwick G J, Temple-Smith P D 1998 The role of the epididymis in human infertility. Journal of Reproductive Fertility Supplement 53: 271–275

De Souza M J, Metzger D A 1991 Reproductive dysfunction in amenorrheic athletes and anorexic patients: a review. Medicine and Science in Sports and Exercise 23: 995–1007

De Voto L, Soto E, Majofke A M, Sierralta W 1980 Unconjugated steroids in the fallopian tube and peripheral blood during the normal menstrual cycle. Fertility and Sterility 33: 613–617

Deering S, Miller B, Kopelman J N, Reed M 2000 Recurrent leiomyomatosis peritonealis disseminata exacerbated by in vitro fertilization. American Journal of Obstetrics and Gynecology 182: 725–726

Deligdisch L 2000 Hormonal pathology of the endometrium. Modern Pathology 13: 285–294

Deligdisch L, Hirschmann S, Altchek A 1997 Pathologic changes in gonadotrophin releasing hormone agonist analogue treated uterine leiomyomata. Fertility and Sterility 67: 837–841

Delmonico F L, Neer R M, Cosimi A B, Barnes A B, Russell P S 1976 Hyperparathyroidism during pregnancy. American Journal of Surgery 131: 328–337

Demopoulos R I, Jones K Y, Mittal K R, Vamvakas E C 1997 Histology of leiomyomata in patients treated with leuprolide acetate. International Journal of Gynecological Pathology 16: 131–137

Devi A S, Metzger D A, Luciano A A, Benn P A 1998 45X/46XX mosaicism in patients with idiopathic premature ovarian failure. Fertility and Sterility 70: 89–93

di Zerega 1994 Contemporary adhesion prevention. Fertility and Sterility 61: 219–235

Dewit W, Bennink H J T, Gerards L J 1984 Prophylactic bromocriptine treatment during pregnancy in women with macroprolactinomas: report of 13 pregnancies. British Journal of Obstetrics and Gynaecology 91: 1059–1069

Diamanti-Kandarakis E, Bartzis M I, Zapanti E D et al 1999 Polymorphism T → C (-34 bp) of gene CYP17 promoter in Greek patients with polycystic ovarian syndrome. Fertility and Sterility 71: 431–435

Dickson R A, Seeman M V, Corenblum B 2000 Hormonal side effects in women: typical versus atypical antipsychotic treatment. Journal of Clinical Psychiatry 61 (supplement 3): 10–15

Dieterle S, Rummel C, Bader L W, Petersen H, Fenner T 1998 Presence of the major outermembrane protein of Chlamydia trachomatis in patients with chronic salpingitis and salpingitis isthmica nodosa with tubal occlusion. Fertility and Sterility 70: 774–776

Djursing H, Nyholm H Chr, Hagen G, Molsted-Pedersen L 1982 Depressed prolactin levels in diabetic women with anovulation. Acta Obstetricia et Gynecologica Scandinavica 61: 403–406

Dlugi A M 1998 Hyperprolactinemic recurrent spontaneous pregnancy loss: a true clinical entity or a spurious finding? Fertility and Sterility 70: 253–255

Dmowski W B 1979 Endocrine properties and clinical application of danazol. Fertility and Sterility 31: 237–251

Dmowski W B, Cohen M R 1978 Antigonadotropin (damazol) in the treatment of endometriosis: evaluation of posttreatment fertility and three-year follow up data. American Journal of Obstetrics and Gynecology 130: 41–45

Dommerholt H B R, Assies J, Van der Werf, A J M 1981 Growth of a prolactinoma during pregnancy: case report and review. British Journal of Obstetrics and Gynecology 88: 62–70

Donnez J, Casanas-Roux F, Ferin J, Thomas K 1984 Tubal polyps, epithelial inclusions and endometriosis after tubal sterilization. Fertility and Sterility 41: 564–568

Donnez J, Nisolle M, Gillerot S, Smets M, Bassil S, Casanas-Roux F 1997 Rectovaginal septum adenomyotic nodules: a series of 500 cases. British Journal of Obstetrics and Gynecology 104: 1014–1018

Drenth J J, Andriessen S, Heringa M P, Mourits M J, van de Wiel H B, Weijmar Schultz W C 1996 Connections between primary vaginismus and procreation: some observations from clinical practice. Journal of Psychosomatic Obstetrics and Gynecology 17: 195–201

Drolette C M, Badawy S Z 1992 Pathophysiology of pelvic adhesions. Modern trends in preventing infertility. Journal of Reproductive Medicine 37: 107–121

Duba H C, Weirich H G, Weirich-Schwaiger H et al 1997 Chromosomal instability in a woman with infertility and two unaffected brothers: a new familial chromosomal breakage syndrome? Human Genetics 100: 431–440

Dubuisson J B, Chavet X, Chapron C, Gregorakis S S, Morice P 1995 Uterine rupture during pregnancy after laparoscopic myomectomy. Human Reproduction 10: 1475–1477

Dubuisson J B, Fauconnier A, Chapron C, Kreiker G, Norgaard C 2000 Reproductive outcome after laparoscopic myomectomy in infertile women. Journal of Reproductive Medicine 45: 23–30

Duck S C, Katayama K P 1981 Danazol may cause female pseudohermaphroditism. Fertility and Sterility 35: 230–231

Duckitt K, Templeton A A 1998 Cancer in women with infertility. Current Opinion in Obstetrics and Gynecology 10: 199–203

Dunphy B C, Li T C, McLeod I C, Barratt C L R, Lenton E A, Cooke I D 1990 The interaction of parameters of male and female infertility in couples with previously unexplained infertility. Fertility and Sterility 54: 824–827

Dupon C, Rosenfeld R L, Cleary R E 1973 Sequential changes in total and free testosterone and androstenediol in plasma during spontaneous and clomid-induced ovulatory cycles. American Journal of Obstetrics and Gynecology 115: 478–482

Durukan T, Urman B, Yarali H, Arikan U, Beykal O 1990 An abdominal pregnancy 10 years after treatment for pelvic tuberculosis. American Journal of Obstetrics and Gynecology 163: 594–595

Eddy C J, Laufe L E 1983 Fertility following microsurgical dissociation of the ovary and fimbria in the rhesus monkey. Fertility and Sterility 39: 566–568

Edelstam G A, Lundkvist O E, Klaresko G L, Larsson-Parra A 1992 Cyclic variation of major histocompatibility complex class II antigen expression in the human fallopian tube epithelium. Fertility and Sterility 57: 1225–1229

Edelstam G A B, Karlsson-Parra A 1996 The human leucocyte antigen (HLA) DR expression and the distribution of T-lymphocytes in the fimbriae of the normal fallopian tube and during pelvic adhesion disease. Journal of Reproductive Immunology 35: 471–476

Edmonds D K 2000 Congenital malformations of the genital tract. Obstetrics and Gynecology Clinics of North America 27: 49–62

Edmonds D K, Kindsay K S, Miller J F, Williamson E, Wood P J 1982 Early embryonic mortality in women. Fertility and Sterility 38: 447–453

Edwards R G 1995 Clinical approaches to increasing uterine receptivity during human implantation. Human Reproduction 10 (Supplement 2): 60–66

Eggert-Kruse W, Köhler A, Rohr G, Runnebaum B 1993 The pH as an important determinant of sperm-mucus interaction. Fertility and Sterility 59: 617–628

Eisenman M 1999 Mammalian sperm chemotaxis and its association with capacitation. Developmental Genetics 25: 87–94

Eisenberg E 1981 Toward an understanding of reproductive function in anorexia nervosa. Fertility and Sterility 36: 543–550

Elias K A, Weiner R I 1984 Direct arterial vascularization of estrogen-induced prolactin-secreting anterior pituitary tumors. Proceedings of the National Academy of Sciences USA 81: 4549–4553

Ellington J E, Evenson D P, Fleming J E et al 1998 Coculture of human sperm with bovine oviduct-epithelial cells decreases sperm chromatin structural changes seen during culture in media alone. Fertility and Sterility 69: 643–649

Ellish N J, Saboda K, O'Connor J, Nasca P C, Stanek E J, Boyle C 1996 A prospective study of early pregnancy loss. Human Reproduction 11: 406–412

el-Sharkawy I M, Hamza S M, el-Sayed M K 2000 Correlation between trichomoniasis vaginalis and female infertility. Journal of the Egyptian Society of Parasitology 30: 287–294

Ennyeart J J, Price W A 1984 Bilateral sensorineural hearing loss from danazol therapy: a case report. Journal of Reproductive Medicine 29: 351–353

Eschenbach D A 1992 Earth, motherhood and the intrauterine device. Fertility and Sterility 57: 1177–1179

Evans V J 1996 Fertility: past, present and future. American Journal of Reproductive Immunology 35: 131–139

Ezra Y, Simon A, Laufer N 1992 Defective oocytes: a new subgroup of unexplained infertility. Fertility and Sterility 58: 24–27

Fahmy N W, Honoré L H, Cumming D C 1987 Subacute focal endometritis: association with cervical colonization with ureaplasma urealyticum, pelvic pathology and endometrial maturation. Journal of Reproductive Medicine 32: 685–687

Falk R K, Hodgen G D 1972 Carbonic anhydrase isoenzymes in normal human endometrium and erythrocytes. American Journal of Obstetrics and Gynecology 112: 1047–1051

Familiari G, Gaggiati A, Nottola S et al 1993 Ultrastructure of human ovarian primordial follicles after combination therapy for Hodgkin's disease. Human Reproduction 8: 2020–2087

Fanchin R, Harmas A, Benaoudia F, Lundkvist U, Olivennes F, Frydman R 1998 Microbial flora of the cervix assessed at the time of embryo transfer adversely affects in vitro fertilization outcome. Fertility and Sterility 70: 866–870

Farrari A N, Russowsky M, Wanderley C de B 1969 Morphology of ovaries treated with Clomiphene citrate. International Journal of Fertility 14: 289–294

Farrer-Brown G, Bellby J O W, Tarbit M H 1971 Venous changes in the endometrium of myomatous uteri. Obstetrics and Gynecology 38: 743–746

Fedele L, Bianchi S, Zanotti F, Marchini M, Candiani G B 1993 Fertility after conservative surgery for adenomyomas. Human Reproduction 8: 1708–1710

Feichtinger W 1991 Environmental factors and fertility. Human Reproduction 6: 1170–1175

Feinman M A 1997 Infertility treatment in women over 40 years of age. Current Opinion in Obstetrics and Gynaecology 9: 165–168

Ferenczy A, Bertrand G, Gelfand M M 1979 Proliferation kinetics of human endometrium during the normal menstrual cycle. American Journal of Obstetrics and Gynecology 133: 859–867

Feyles V, Moyana T N, Pierson R A 2000 Recurrent pregnancy loss associated with endometrial hyperechoic areas (endometrial calcifications): a case report and review of the literature. Clinical and Experimental Obstetrics and Gynecology 27: 5–8

Field-Richards S 1954 A preliminary series of cases of uterine hypoplasia treated by local injection of an oestrogenic emulsion. Journal of Obstetrics and Gynaecology of the British Empire 62: 205–213

Finelli P, Giardino D, Rizzi N et al 2000 Non-random trisomies of chromosomes 5, 8 and 12 in the prolactinemia subtype of pituitary adenomas: conventional cytogenetics and interphase FISH study. International Journal of Cancer 86: 344–350

First A 1954 Transperitoneal migration of ovum or spermatozoon. Obstetrics and Gynecology 4: 431–433

Folkerth R D, Price D L, Schwartz M, Black P M, DeGirolami U 1998 Xanthomatous hypophysitis. American Journal of Surgical Pathology 22: 736–741

Fordney D S 1978 Dyspareunia and vaginismus. Clinical Obstetrics and Gynecology 21: 205–221

Fordney-Settlage D S, Motoshima M, Tredway D R 1973 Sperm transport from the external cervical os to the fallopian tubes in women: a time and quantitation study. Fertility and Sterility 24: 655–661

Forssman L 1976 Distribution of blood flow in myomatous uteri as measured by locally injected[133] Xenon. Acta Obstetricia et Gynecologica Scandinavica 5: 101–105

Fortier K J, Haney A F 1985 The pathologic spectrum of uterotubal junction obstruction. Obstetrics and Gynecology 65: 93–98

Fortuny A, Carrio A, Soler A, Cararach J, Fuster J, Salami C 1988 Detection of balanced chromosome rearrangements in 445 couples with repeated abortion and cytogenetic prenatal testing in carriers. Fertility and Sterility 49: 774–778

Francavilla F, Romano R, Santucci R, Marrone V, Properzi G, Ruvolo G 1997 Interference of antisperm antibodies with the induction of the acrosome reaction by zona pellucida (ZP) and its relationship with the inhibition of ZP binding. Fertility and Sterility 67: 1128–1133

Fraser I S, Shearman R P, Smith A, Russell P 1988 An association among blepharophimosis, resistant ovary syndrome, and true premature menopause. Fertility and Sterility 50: 747–751

Freeman E W, Garcia C-R, Rickels K 1983 Behavioural and emotional factors: comparisons of an ovulatory infertile woman with fertile and other infertile women. Fertility and Sterility 40; 195–201

Friedler S, Ben-Schachar I, Abramov Y, Schenker J G, Lewin A 1996 Ruptured tubo-ovarian abscess complicating transcervical embryo transfer. Fertility and Sterility 65: 1065–1066

Friedley N J, Rosen S 1975 Carbonic anhydrase activity in mammalian ovary, fallopian tube and uterus. Histochemical and biochemical studies. Biology and Reproduction 12: 293–304

Friedrich E G Jr 1976 Vulvar disease. Major problems in obstetrics and gynecology, vol 9. Saunders, Philadelphia

Fritz M A, Speroff L 1982 The endocrinology of the menstrual cycle: the interaction of folliculogenesis and neuroendocrine mechanisms. Fertility and Sterility 38: 509–529

Fritz M A, Holmes R T, Keenan E J 1991 Effect of clomiphene citrate on endometrial estrogen and progesterone receptor induction in women. American Journal of Obstetrics and Gynecology 165: 177–185

Fukui A, Fuju S, Yamaguchi E, Kimura H, Sato S, Saito Y 1999 Natural killer cell subpopulations and cytotoxicity for infertile patients undergoing in vitro fertilization. American Journal of Reproductive Immunology 41: 413–422

Fukumoto M, Yajima Y, Oakamura H, Midorikawa O 1981 Collagenolytic enzyme activity in the human ovary: an ovulatory enzyme system. Fertility and Sterility 36: 746–750

Futterweit W, Smith H Jr, Holt J E 1984 Dissociation of serum prolactin response to sequential thyrotropin-releasing hormone and chlorpromazine stimulation in patients with primary empty sella syndrome. Fertility and Sterility 42: 573–578

Gallinelli A, Matteo M, Volpe A, Facchinetti F 2000 Autonomic and neuroendocrine responses to stress in patients with functional hypothalamic secondary amenorrhea. Fertility and Sterility 73: 812–816

Gandolfi F 1995 Functions of proteins secreted by oviduct epithelial cells. Microscopy Research and Technique 32: 1–12

Garcia R, Bueno A, Castanon S et al 1997 Study of the DNA content by flow cytometry and proliferation in 281 brain tumors. Oncology 54: 112–117

Garcia-Velasco J A, Arici A 1999 Chemokines and human reproduction. Fertility and Sterility 71: 983–993

Gardey G, Viala J L, Caderas de Kerleau J, Serrano J S, Lalaurie M, Boucard M 1975a Etude experimentale de l'hypoplasie uterine I — influence du facteur vasculaire. Journal de Gynecologie, Obstetrique et de Biologie de la Reproduction 4: 43–49

Gardey G, Viala J L, Caderas de Kerleau J, Serrano J J, Lalaurie M, Boucard M 1975b Etude experimentale de l'hypoplasie uterine II — influence du traitement par un beta-mimetique. Journal de Gynecologie, Obstetrique et de Biologie de la Reproduction 4: 177–182

Gardner R L, Shaw R W 1989 Cornual fibroids: a conservative approach to restoring tubal patency using a gonadotropin-releasing hormone agonist (goserelin) with successful pregnancy. Fertility and Sterility 52: 332–334

Gaton E, Seidel L, Bernstein D, Glezerman M, Czernobilsky B, Insler V 1982. The effects of estrogen and gestagen on the mucus production of endocervical cells: a histochemical study. Fertility and Sterility 29: 257–265

Gay G, Shepard C 1972 Sex in the 'drug culture'. Medical Aspects of Human Sexuality, 6: 28–33

Gazvani M R, Wilson D A, Richmond D H, Howard P J, Kingsland C R, Lewis-Jones D I 2000 Evaluation of the role of mitotic instability in karyotypically normal men with oligozoospermia. Fertility and Sterility 73: 51–55

Gelety T J, Buyalos R P 1993 The effect of clomiphene citrate and menopausal gonadotropins on cervical mucus in ovulatory cycles. Fertility and Sterility 60: 471–476

Gentile G P, Siegler A M 1981 Inadvertent intestinal biopsy during laparoscopy and hysteroscopy: a report of two cases. Fertility and Sterility 36: 402–404

Georgiou I, Syrrou M, Bouba et al 1999 Association of estrogen receptor gene polymorphisms with endometriosis. Fertility and Sterility 72: 164–166

Geva E, Amit A, Lerner-Geva L, Lessing J B 1997 Autoimmunity and reproduction. Fertility and Sterility 67: 599–611

Geva E, Lerner-Geva L, Stavorosky Z et al 1998 Multifetal pregnancy reduction: a possible risk factor for periventricular leukomalacia in premature infants. Fertility and Sterility 69: 845–850

Gibson M, Badger G J, Byrn F, Lee K R, Korson R, Trainer T D 1991 Error in histologic dating of secretory endometrium: variance component analysis. Fertility and Sterility 56: 242–247

Giess R, Tanasescu I, Steck T, Sendtner M 1999 Leukemia inhibitory factor gene mutations in infertile women. Molecular Human Reproduction 5: 581–586

Giorlandino C, Calugi G, Iaconiani L, Santoro M L, Lippa A 1998 Spermatozoa with chromosomal abnormalities may result in a higher rate of recurrent abortion. Fertility and Sterility 70: 576–577

Giudice L C 1999 Potential biochemical markers of uterine receptivity. Human Reproduction 14 Supplement 2: 3–16

Glezerman M, Bernstein D, Zakut C, Misgav N, Insler V 1982 Polyzoospermia: a definite pathologic entity. Fertility and Sterility 38: 605–608

Goerzen J L, Leader A, Taylor P J 1983 Hysteroscopic findings in 100 women requesting reversal of a previously performed voluntary tubal sterilization. Fertility and Sterility 39: 103–104

Golan, Langer R, Bukovsky I, Caspi E 1989 Congenital anomalies of the Mullerian system. Fertility and Sterility 51: 747–755

Gold M A, Schmidt R R, Parks N, Trauma R E 1997 Bilateral absence of the ovaries and distal fallopian tubes. Journal of Reproductive Medicine 42: 375–377

Goldberg J M, Falcone T 1999 Effect of diethylbestrol on reproductive function. Fertility and Sterility 72: 1–7

Gomel V 1983 An odyssey through the oviduct. Fertility and Sterility 39: 144–156

Gomel V, Filmar S 1987 Arrested tubal pregnancy. Fertility and Sterility 48: 1043–1047

Gomel V, McComb P 1981 Unexpected pregnancies in women afflicted by occlusive tubal disease. Fertility and Sterility 36: 529–530

Gonzales G F, Villena A 1997 Influence of low corrected seminal fructose levels on sperm chromatin stability in semen from men attending an infertility service. Fertility and Sterility 67: 763–768

Goswany R K, Williams G, Steptoe P C 1988 Decreased uterine perfusion — a cause of infertility. Human Reproduction 3: 955–958

Gould K G, Ansari A H 1983 Chemical alteration of cervical mucus by electrolytes. American Journal of Obstetrics and Gynecology 145: 92–99

Govan A D T 1962 Tuberculous endometritis. Journal of Pathology and Bacteriology 83: 363–372

Graham O, Cheng L C, Parsons J H 2000 The ultrasound diagnosis of retained fetal bones in West African patients complaining of infertility. British Journal of Obstetrics and Gynaecology 107: 122–124

Grant A 1962 The effect of ectopic pregnancy on fertility. Clinics in Obstetrics and Gynecology 5: 861–874

Greil A L 1997 Infertility and psychological distress: a critical review of the literature. Social Science in Medicine 45: 1679–1704

Griesshammer, Bergmann L, Pearson T 1998 Fertility, pregnancy and the management of myeloproliferative disorders. Bailliere's Clinical Haematology 11: 859–874

Grinsted L, Heltberg A, Hagen C, Djursing H 1989 Serum sex hormones and gonadotropin concentrations in premenopausal women with multiple sclerosis. Journal of Internal Medicine 226: 241–244

Guerrero R, Rojas O I 1975 Spontaneous abortion and aging of human ova and spermatozoa. New England Journal of Medicine 293: 573–575

Guillaume A J, Benjamin F, Sicuranza B, Deutsch S, Spitzer M 1995 Luteal phase defects and ectopic pregnancy. Fertility and Sterility 63: 30–33

Gupta D M, Karkun J N, Kar A B 1970 Biochemical changes in different parts of the rabbit fallopian tube during passage of ova. American Journal of Obstetrics and Gynecology 106: 833–837

Guzman E R, Rosenberg J C, Houlihan C et al 1994 A new method using vaginal ultrasound and transfundal pressure to evaluate the asymptomatic incompetent cervix. Obstetrics and Gynecology 83: 248–252

Häarki-Siren P, Kurki T 1997 A nationwide analysis of laparoscopic complications. Obstetrics and Gynecology 89: 108–112

Habana A, Dokras A, Giraldo J L, Jones E E 2000 Cornual heterotopic pregnancy: contemporary management options. American Journal of Obstetrics and Gynecology 182: 1264–1270

Hakim R B, Gray R H, Zacur H 1998 Alcohol and caffeine consumption and decreased fertility. Fertility and Sterility 70: 632–637

Halbert S A, McComb P F 1981 Function and structure of the rabbit oviduct after fimbriectomy II Proximal ampullary salpingostomy. Fertility and Sterility 35: 355–358

Hambartsoumian E 1998 Endometrial leukemia inhibitory factor (LIF) as a possible cause of unexplained infertility and multiple failures of implantation. American Journal of Reproductive Immunology 39: 137–143

Hamilton M P R, Fleming R, Coutts J R T, MacNaughton M C, Whitfield C R 1990 Luteal cysts and unexplained infertility: biochemical and ultrasonic evaluation. Fertility and Sterility 54: 32–37

Handelsman D J, Dong Q 1993 Hypothalamus-pituitary-gonadal axis in chronic renal failure. Endocrinology and Metabolism Clinics of North America 22: 145–161

Haney A F, Musukonis M A, Weinberg J B 1983 Macrophages and infertility: oviductal macrophages as potential mediators of infertility. Fertility and Sterility 39: 310–315

Hanna F W, Williams C M, Davies J S, Dawson T, Neal J, Scanlon M F 1999 Pituitary apoplexy following metastasis of bronchogenic adenocarcinoma to a prolactinoma. Clinical Endocrinology 51: 377–381

Hansen K A, Tho S P T, Hanly M, Moretuzzo R W, McDonough P G 1997 Massive ovarian enlargement in primary hypothyroidism. Fertility and Sterility 67: 169–171

Hansen K K, Knopp R H, Soules M R 1991 Lipoprotein-cholesterol levels in infertile women with luteal phase deficiency. Fertility and Sterility 55: 916–921

Harmanli O H, Cheng G Y, Nyirjesy P, Chatwani A, Gaughan J P 2000 Urinary tract infections in women with bacterial vaginosis. Obstetrics and Gynecology 95: 710–712

Harper M J K 1988 Gamete and zygote transport. In: Knobil E, Neill J (eds) The physiology of reproduction. Raven Press, New York, p 103

Hassan A A, Reiff R H, Fayez J A 1986 Femoral neuropathy following microscopical tuboplasty. Fertility and Sterility 45: 889–891

Hassan H A, Saleh H A 1996 Endometrial unresponsiveness: a novel approach to assessment and prognosis in in vitro fertilization cycles. Fertility and Sterility 66: 604–607

Hassold T, Jacobs P, Kline J, Stein Z, Warburton D 1980 Effect of maternal age on autosomal trisomies. Annals of Human Genetics 44: 29–36

Hataya I, Takakuwa K, Tanaka K 1998 Human leukocyte antigen class II genotype in patients with recurrent fetal miscarriage who are positive for anti-cardiolipin antibody. Fertility and Sterility 70: 919–923

He S, Lin Y-L, Liu Y-X 1999 Functionally inactive protein C inhibitor in seminal plasma may be associated with infertility. Molecular Human Reproduction 5: 513–519

Heary R F, Maniker A H, Wolansky L J 1995 Candidal pituitary abscess: case report. Neurosurgery 36: 1009–1012

Hedricks C, Piccino L J, Udry J R, Chimbria T H K 1987 Peak coital rate coincides with onset of luteinizing hormone surge. Fertility and Sterility 48: 234–238

Hertig A T 1954 Gestational hyperplasia of endometrium. Laboratory Investigation 13: 1153–1191

Hess H M, Dickson J, Fox H E 1980 Hyperfunctioning parathyroid carcinoma presenting as acute pancreatitis in pregnancy. Journal of Reproductive Medicine 25: 83–87

Hicks J J, Callado M L, Castro-Osuna G 1980 Effect of rabbit spermatozoa on the incorporation of labeled precursors into endometrial marcomolecules. Archives of Andrology 5: 349–354

Hinney B, Henze C, Kuhn W, Wuttke W 1996 The corpus luteal insufficiency: a multifactorial disease. Journal of Clinical Endocrinology and Metabolism 81: 565–570

Hinton E L, Bobo L D, Wu T-C, Kurman R J, Viscidi R P 2000 Detection of Chlamydia trachomatis DNA in archival paraffinized specimens from chronic salpingitis cases using the polymerase chain reaction. Fertility and Sterility 74: 152–157

Hirahara F, Andoh N, Sawai K, Hirabuki T, Demura T, Minaguchi H 1998 Hyperprolactinaemic recurrent miscarriage and results of randomized bromocriptine treatment trials. Fertility and Sterility 70: 246–252

Hirama Y, Ochiai K 1995 Estrogen and progesterone receptors of the out-of-phase endometrium in female infertile patients. Fertility and Sterility 63: 984–988

Hitti I F, Glasberg S S, McKenzie C, Meltzer B A 1991 Uterine leiomyosarcoma with massive necrosis diagnosed during gonadotropin-releasing hormone analog therapy for presumed uterine fibroid. Fertility and Sterility 56: 778–780

Hjøllund N H I, Jensen T K, Bonde J P E et al 1999 Distress and reduced fertility: a follow-up study of first-pregnancy planners. Fertility and Sterility 72: 47–53

Ho D M, Hsu C Y, Ting L T, Chiang H 1997 The clinicopathological characteristics of gonadotroph cell adenoma: a study 118 cases. Human Pathology 28: 905–911

Ho K-L 1996 Coexistence of primary empty sella and silent corticotrophic adenoma. Modern Pathology 9: 521–525

Hoek A, Schoemaker, Drexhage H A 1997 Premature ovarian failure: ovarian autoimmunity. Endocrine Reviews 18: 107–134

Holmes K K, Eschenbach D A, Knapp J S 1980 Salpingitis: overview of etiology and epidemiology. American Journal of Obstetrics and Gynecology 138: 893–900

Holt J P, Keller D 1984 Danazol treatment increases serum enzyme levels. Fertility and Sterility 41: 70–74

Holzgreve W, Schonberg S A, Douglas B G, Golbus M S 1984 N-chromosome hyperploidy in couples with multiple spontaneous abortions. Obstetrics and Gynecology 63: 237–240

Honoré L H 1978a Tubal ectopic pregnancy with contralateral corpus luteum: a report of 5 cases. Journal of Reproductive Medicine 21: 269–271

Honoré L H 1978b Salpingitis isthmica nodosa in female infertility and ectopic tubal pregnancy. Fertility and Sterility 29: 164–168

Honoré L H 1980 The increased incidence of renal stones in women with spontaneous abortion: a retrospective study. American Journal of Obstetrics and Gynecology 137: 145–146

Honoré L H 1994 Pathology of female infertility. Current Opinion in Obstetrics and Gynecology 6: 364–371

Honoré L H 1997 Pathology of female infertility. Current Opinion in Obstetrics and Gynecology 9: 37–43

Honoré L H, Cumming D C, Scott J Z 1985 Mycoplasmal endometritis in female infertility. Infertility 7: 203–208

Honoré L H, Davey S J 1989 Endometrial carcinoma in young women: a report of four cases. Journal of Reproductive Medicine 34: 845–849

Honoré L H, Scott J Z 1982 Human infertility: the histologic diagnosis of pregnancy from endometrial biopsies. Presented at the Poster Session of the Meeting of Canadian Investigators in Reproduction, Toronto, June 1982

Honoré L H, Scott J Z 1992 An unusual acquired lesion: post-salpingostomy intercornual bridging with hematosalpinx, chronic salpingitis and perisalpingeal endometriosis. Journal of Reproductive Medicine 37: 221–222

Honoré L H, Cumming D C, Dunlop D L, Scott J Z 1988a Uterine adenomyoma associated with infertility: report of three cases. Journal of Reproductive Medicine 33: 331–335

Honoré L H, Cumming D C, Fahmy N 1988b Significant difference in the frequency of out-of-phase endometrial biopsies depending on the use of the Novak curette or the flexible polypropylene endometrial biopsy cannula ('Pipelle'). Gynecologic and Obstetric Investigation 26: 338–340

Honoré G M, Holden A E C, Schenken R S 1999 Pathophysiology and management of proximal tubal blockage. Fertility and Sterility 71: 785–795

Horne H W, Hertig A T, Knudsin R B, Kosasa T S 1973 Subclinical endometrial inflammation and T-mycoplasma. International Journal of Fertility 18: 226–231

Horvath E, Kovacs K 1976 Ultrastructural classification of pituitary adenomas. Canadian Journal of Neurological Sciences 3: 9–21

Hughes E G, Brennan B G 1996 Does cigarette smoking impair natural or assisted fertility? Fertility and Sterility 66: 679–689

Hughes E G, Jacobs R D, Rubulis A, Husney R M 1963 Carbohydrate pathways of the endometrium. American Journal of Obstetrics and Gynecology 85: 594–608

Huleihel M, Lunenfeld E, Levy A, Potashnik G, Glezerman M 1996 Distinct expression levels of cytokines and soluble cytokine receptors in seminal plasma of fertile and infertile men. Fertility and Sterility 66: 135–139

Hulka J F 1982 Adnexal adhesions: a prognostic staging and classification system based on a five year survey of results at Chapel Hill, North Carolina. American Journal of Obstetrics and Gynecology 144: 141–147

Hull M G R, Bromham D R, Savage P E, Barlow T M, Hughes A O, Jacobs H S 1981 Postpill amenorrhea: a causal study. Fertility and Sterility 36: 472–476

Hunt J E, Wallach E E 1974 Uterine factors in infertility – an overview. Clinical Obstetrics and Gynecology 17: 44–59

Hunter R H F, Leglise P C 1971 Polyspermic fertilization following tubal surgery in pigs, with particular reference to the role of the isthmus. Journal of Reproduction and Fertility 24: 233–246

Hutchinson G, Bhugra D, Mallett R, Burnett R, Corridan B, Leff J 1999 Fertility and marital rates in first-onset schizoprenia. Social Psychiatry and Psychiatric Epidemiology 34: 617–621

Iams J D, Johnson F F, Snoek J, Sachs L, Gebauer C, Samuels P 1995 Cervical incompetence as a continuum: a study of ultrasonographic cervical length and obstetric performance. American Journal of Obstetrics and Gynecology 172: 1097–1106

Ijland M M, Hoogland H J, Dunselman G A J, Lo C R, Evers J L H 1999 Endometrial wave direction switch and the outcome of in vitro fertilization. Fertility and Sterility 71: 476–481

Ikeda H, Yoshimoto T, Fujiwara K, Ogawa Y 1995 Immunohistochemical demonstration of tenascin in human pituitary glands and adenomas. Acta Histochemica 97: 273–280

Illera M J, Juan L, Stewart C L, Cullinan S E, Roman J, Lessey B A 2000 Effect of peritoneal fluid from women with endometriosis on implantation in the mouse model. Fertility and Sterility 74: 41–48

Insler V, Lunenfeld B 1991 Pathophysiology of polycystic ovarian disease: new insights. Human Reproduction 6: 1025–1029

Insler V, Glezerman M, Zeidel L, Bernstein D, Misgav N 1980 Sperm storage in the human cervix: a quantitative study. Fertility and Sterility 33: 288–293

Italian Endometriosis Study Group, 1999 Oral contraceptive use and risk of endometriosis. British Journal of Obstetrics and Gynaecology 106: 695–699

Itu M, Neelam T, Ammini A C, Kucheria K 1990 Primary amenorrhea in a triple X female. Australian and New Zealand Journal of Obstetrics and Gynaecology 30: 286–288

Jacob S, Leveque J, Dugast J, Minoui P, Delavel M, Grail Y 1997 Gynecologic allergy to spermatic fluid. A case report. Journal de Gynécologie, Obstétique et de Biologie de la Reproduction 26: 825–827

Jacobson A, Marshall J R 1980 Detrimental effect of endometrial biopsies on pregnancy rate following human menopausal gonadotropin/human chorionic gonadotropin-induced ovulation. Fertility and Sterility 33: 602–604

Jaffe R B, Jewelewicz R 1991 The basic infertility investigation. Fertility and Sterility 56: 599–613

Jager S, Kremer J, Van Slockteren-Draaisma T 1978 A simple method of spermatozoal surface IgG with the direct mixed antiglobulin reaction carried out on undiluted fresh human semen. International Journal of Fertility 23: 12–21

Jain A K 1969 Fecundability and its relation to age in a sample of Taiwanese women. Population Studies 23: 69–85

Jansen R P 1980 Cyclic changes in the human fallopian tube isthmus and their functional significance. American Journal of Obstetrics and Gynecology 136: 292–308

Jansen R P S 1984 Endocrine response in the fallopian tube. Endocrine Reviews 5: 525–551

Janssen N M, Genta M S 2000 The effects of immunosuppressive and anti-inflammatory medications on fertility, pregnancy and lactation. Archives of Internal Medicine 160: 610–619

Jaszczak S, Moghissi K S, Hafez E S E 1980 Effect of prostaglandin F2 alpha on sperm transport in the reproductive tract of female macaques (Macaca fascicularis). Archives of Andrology 4: 17–27

Jean Y, Langlais J, Roberts K D, Chapdelain A, Bleau G 1979 Fertility of a woman with nonfunctional ciliated cells in the fallopian tubes. Fertility and Sterility 31: 349–350

Jenkins J M, Brook P F, Sargeant S, Cooke I D 1995 Endocervical mucus pH is inversely related to serum androgen levels and waist to hip ratio. Fertility and Sterility 63: 1005–1008

Johnson M D 1998 Genetic risks of intracytoplasmic sperm injection in the treatment of male infertility: recommendations for genetic counselling and screening. Fertility and Sterility 70: 397–411

Jones G S 1990 Corpus luteum: composition and function. Fertility and Sterility 54: 1–18

Jones W R 1991 Allergy to coitus. Australian and New Zealand Journal of Obstetrics and Gynaecology 31: 137–141

Joshi J V, Bhandakar S D, Chadha M, Balaiah D, Shah R 1993 Menstrual irregularities and lactation failure may precede thyroid dysfunction or goitre. Journal of Postgraduate Medicine 39: 137–141

Jurisicova A, Casper R F, MacLusky N J, Librach C L 1996 Embryonic human leukocyte antigen-G expression: possible implications for human preimplantation development. Fertility and Sterility 65: 997–1002

Kalra S P, Horvath T L 1998 Neuroendocrine interactions between galanin, opioids and neuropeptide Y in the control of reproduction and appetite. Annals of the New York Academy of Sciences 863: 236–240

Karande V C, Pratt D E, Rao R, Balin M, Gleicher N 1995 Elevated tubal perfusion pressures during selective salpingography are highly suggestive of tubal endometriosis. Fertility and Sterility 64: 1070–1073

Karrow W G, Gentry W C, Skeels R F, Payne S A 1971 Endometrial biopsy in the luteal phase of the cycle of conception. Fertility and Sterility 22: 482–495

Katayama K P, Valencia A L, Wise L, Stehlik E 1991 Pregnancy with X-autosome translocation. Fertility and Sterility 55: 438–439

Katz A I, Davidson J M, Hayslett J P, Singson E, Lindheimer M D 1980 Pregnancy in women with kidney disease. Kidney International 18: 192–198

Katz D F, Morales P, Samuels S J, Overstreet J W 1990 Mechanisms of filtration of morphologically abnormal human sperm by cervical mucus. Fertility and Sterility 54: 513–516

Katz E 1988 The luteinized unruptured follicle and other ovulatory dysfunctions. Fertility and Sterility 50: 839–850

Kaul A, Nagamanni M, Nowicki B 1995 Decreased expression of endometrial decay accelerating factor (DAF), a complement regulating protein, in patients with luteal phase defect. American Journal of Reproductive Immunology 34: 236–240

Kaushansky A, Frydman M, Kaufman H, Homburg R 1987 Endocrine studies of the ovulatory disturbances in Wilson's disease (hepatolenticular degeneration). Fertility and Sterility 47: 270–273

Kawamoto H, Uozumi T, Kawamoto K, Arita K, Yano T, Hirohata T 1996 Type IV collagenase activity and cavernous sinus invasion in human pituitary adenomas. Acta Neurochirurgica (Wien) 138: 390–395

Kawamura N, Ito F, Ichimura T, Shibata S, Umesaki N, Ogita S 1997 Correlation between shrinkage of uterine leiomyoma treated with buserelin acetate and histopathologic findings of biopsy specimens before treatment. Fertility and Sterility 68: 632–636

Kaya H, Oral B 1999 Effect of ovarian involvement on the frequency of luteinized unruptured follicle in endometriosis. Gynecologic and Obstetric Investigation 48: 123–126

Kaytor M D, Burright E N, Duvick L A, Zoghai H Y, Orr H T 1997 Increased trinucleotide repeat instability with advanced maternal age. Human Molecular Genetics 6: 2135–2139

Kazer R R, Meyer K, Valle R F 1992 Late hemorrhage after transcervical division of a uterine septum: a report of two cases. Fertility and Sterility 57: 930–932

Keay S D, Liversedge N H, Jenkins J M 1998 Could ovarian infection impair ovarian response to gonadotrophin stimulation? British Journal of Obstetrics and Gynaecology 105: 252–254

Keefe D L 1998 Reproductive aging is an evolutionarily programmed strategy that no longer provides adaptive value. Fertility and Sterility 70: 204–206

Keefe D L, Niven-Fairchild T, Powell S, Buradagunta S 1995 Mitochondrial deoxynucleic acid deletions in oocytes and reproductive aging in women. Fertility and Sterility 64: 577–583

Keenan J A, Herbert C M, Bush J R, Wentz A C 1989 Diagnosis and management of out-of-phase endometrial biopsies among patients receiving clomiphene citrate for ovulation induction. Fertility and Sterility 51: 964–967

Keltz M D, Attar E, Buradagunta S, Olive D L, Kliman H J, Arici A 1996 Modulation of leukemia inhibitory factor gene expression and protein biosynthesis in the human fallopian tube. American Journal of Obstetrics and Gynecology 175: 1611–1619

Killick S, Elstein M 1987 Pharmacologic production of luteinized unruptured follicles by prostaglandin synthetase inhibitors. Fertility and Sterility 47: 773–777

Kim-Bjorklund T, Landeren B M, Hamberger L, Johannison E 1991 Comparative morphometric study of the endometrium, fallopian tube and the corpus luteum during the post-ovulatory phase in normally menstruating women. Fertility and Sterility 56: 842–850

Kinderman D, Bauer D, Fischer J P, Dietrich K 1993 Histological findings in a falloscopically retrieved isthmic plug causing reversible proximal tubal obstruction. Human Reproduction 9: 1429–1434

Kitawaki J, Kusuki I, Koshiba H, Tsukamoto K, Fushiki S, Honjo H 1999 Detection of aromatase cytochrome P-450 in endometrial biopsy specimens as a diagnostic test for endometriosis. Fertility and Sterility 72: 1100–1106

Kiviat N B, Wølner-Hanssen P, Eschenbach D A et al 1990 Endometrial histopathology in patients with culture-proved upper genital tract infection and laparoscopically diagnosed acute salpingitis. American Journal of Surgical Pathology 14: 167–175

Kjaer K, Hagen C, Sando S H, Eshoj O 1992 Infertility and pregnancy outcome in an unselected group of women with insulin-dependent diabetes mellitus. American Journal of Obstetrics and Gynecology 166: 1412–1418

Kjellberg S, Bjorndahl L, Kvist U 1992 Sperm chromatin stability and zinc binding properties in semen from men in barren unions. International Journal of Andrology 15: 103–113

Klentzeris L D, Bulmer J N, Li T C, Morrison L, Warren A, Cooke I D 1991 Lectin binding of endometrium in women with unexplained infertility. Fertility and Sterility 56: 660–667

Klinkert J, Van Geldrop H J, Chadha-Ajwani S, Huikeshoven F J M 1993 Tubal damage after intratubal methotrexate treatment. Fertility and Sterility 59: 926–927

Knoll M, Talbot P 1998 Cigarette smoke inhibits oocyte-cumulus complex pick-up by the oviduct in vitro independent of ciliary beat frequency. Reproductive Toxicology 12: 57–68

Kodama H, Yamaguchi R, Fukuda J, Kasai H, Tanaka T 1997 Increased oxidative deoxynucleic acid damage in the spermatozoa of infertile male patients. Fertility and Sterility 68: 519–524

Kohda H, Mori T, Nishimura T, Kambegawa A 1983 Cooperation of progesterone and prostaglandins in ovulation induced by human chorionic gonadotrophin in immature rats primed with pregnant mare serum gonadotrophin. Journal of Endocrinology 96: 387–393

Kol S, Adashi E Y 1995 Intraovarian factors regulating ovarian function. Current Opinion in Obstetrics and Gynaecology 7: 209–213

Kolb B A, Najmabadi S, Paulson R J 1997 Ultrastructural characteristics of the luteal phase endometrium in patients undergoing controlled ovarian hyperstimulation. Fertility and Sterility 67: 625–630

Kolettis P N, Sharma R K, Pasqualotto F F, Nelson D, Thomas A J, Agarwal A 1999 Effect of seminal oxidative stress on fertility after vasectomy reversal. Fertility and Sterility 71: 249–255

Kolstad H A, Bonde J P, Hjollund N H et al 1999 Menstrual cycle pattern and fertility: a prospective follow-up study of pregnancy and early embryonal loss in 295 couples who were planning their first pregnancy. Fertility and Sterility 71: 490–496

Kontogeorgos G, Bassiouka I, Giannou P, Vamvassakis E, Rologis D, Orphanidis G 1995 Diagnosis of pituitary adenomas on touch preparations assisted by immunocytochemistry. Acta Cytologica 39: 141–152

Kontogeorgos G, Kapranos N, Orphanidis G, Rologis D, Kokka E 1999 Molecular cytogenetics of chromosome 11 in pituitary adenomas: a comparison of fluorescence in situ hybridization and DNA ploidy study. Human Pathology 30: 1377–1382

Korenaga M, Kadota T 1981 Changes in the mechanical properties of the circular muscle of the isthmus of the human fallopian tube in relation to hormonal domination and postovulatory time. Fertility and Sterility 36: 343–350

Kovacs K 1996 Molecular biological research in pituitary adenomas from the pathologists' view. Acta Neurochirugia Supplement (Wien) 65: 4–6

Kovacs K, Horvath E 1987 Hypothalamic-pituitary abnormalities in ovulatory disorders. In: Gondos B, Riddick D H (eds) Pathology of infertility. Thieme Medical Publishers, New York, p 185

Kovacs K, Sheehan H L 1982 Pituitary changes in Kallmann's syndrome: a histologic, immunocytologic, ultrastructural and immunoelectron-microscopic study. Fertility and Sterility 37: 83–89

Kuberski T 1980 Histocompatibility antigens and the sexually transmitted diseases. Sexually Transmitted Diseases 7: 203–205

Kunz G, Bell D, Deniger H, Einspanier A, Mall G, Legendecker G 1997 The uterine peristaltic pump. Normal and impeded sperm transport within the female genital tract. Advances in Experimental Medicine and Biology 424: 267–277

Kurjak A S, Kupesic-Urek S, Schulman H, Zalud I 1991 Transvaginal color flow Doppler in the assessment of ovarian and uterine blood flow in infertile women. Fertility and Sterility 56: 870–873

Kusuhara K 1992 Clinical importance of endometrial histology and progesterone level assessment in luteal-phase defect. Hormone Research 37 (supplement 1): 53–58

La Scala G B, Ghirardini G, Cantarelli M, Dotti C, Cavalieri S, Torelli M G 1991 Recurrent empty follicle syndrome. Human Reproduction 6: 651–652

La Verda D, Kalayoglu M V, Byrne G I 1999 Chlamydial heat shock proteins and disease pathology: new paradigms for old problems? Infectious Disease in Obstetrics and Gynaecology 7: 64–71

Labarrere C A, Catoggio L J, Mullen E G, Althabe O H 1986 Placental lesions in maternal autoimmune disease. American Journal of Reproductive Immunology 12: 78–86

Lai J M, Lee J F, Huong H Y, Soong Y K, Yang F-P, Pao C C 1997 The effect of human papilloma virus infection on sperm cell motility. Fertility and Sterility 67: 1152–1155

Landholt A M 1975 Ultrastructure of human sella tumors: correlation of clinical findings and morphology. Acta Neurochirurgica (Wien) 22: 1–67

Langer R, Golan A, Ron-El R, Pansky M, Neuman M, Caspi E 1990 Hormonal changes related to impairment of cervical mucus in cycles stimulated by Clomiphene citrate. Australian and New Zealand Journal of Obstetrics and Gynaecology 30: 254–256

Las M S, Surks M I 1983 Hypopituitarism associated with systemic amyloidosis. New York State Journal of Medicine 83: 1183–1185

Laurent S L, Thompson S J, Addy C, Garrison C Z, Moore E E 1992 An epidemiologic study of smoking and primary infertility in women. Fertility and Sterility 57: 565–572

Layman L C 1999a Genetics of human hypogonadotrophic hypogonadism. American Journal of Medical Genetics (Seminars in Medical Genetics) 89: 240–248

Layman L C 1999b Mutations in human gonadotrophin genes and their physiologic significance in puberty and reproduction. Fertility and Sterility 71: 201–218

Lazlo J, Gaal M, Bosze P 1976 Chromosome studies in ovarian hypoplasia. Clinical Genetics 9: 61–70

Leach R E, Moghissi K S, Randolph J F et al 1997 Intensive hormone monitoring in women with unexplained infertility: evidence for subtle abnormalities suggestive of diminished ovarian reserve. Fertility and Sterility 68: 413–420

Leake J F, Murphy A A, Zacur H A 1987 Noncardiogenic pulmonary edema: a complication of operative hysteroscopy. Fertility and Sterility 48: 497–499

Leduc L, Wasserstrum N 1992 Successful treatment with the Smith–Hodge pessary of cervical incompetence due to defective connective tissue in Ehlers–Danlos syndrome. American Journal of Perinatology 9: 25–27

Lee F, Nelson N, Faiman C, Choi N W, Reyes F I 1982 Low-dose corticoid therapy for anovulation: effect upon fetal weight. Obstetrics and Gynecology 60: 314–317

Lehmann-Willenbrock E, Mecke H, Riedel H-H 1990 Sequelae of appendectomy, with special reference to intraabdominal adhesions, chronic abdominal pain and infertility. Gynecologic and Obstetric Investigation 29: 241–245

Leng Z, Moore D E, Mueller B A et al 1998 Characterization of ciliary activity in distal fallopian tube biopsies of women with obstructive tubal infertility. Human Reproduction 13: 3121–3127

Leridon H 1977 Human fertility. The University of Chicago Press, Chicago

Lessey B A, Castelbaum A J, Sawin S W, Sun J 1995 Integrins as markers of uterine receptivity in women with primary unexplained infertility. Fertility and Sterility 63: 535–542

Lessey B A, Castelbaum A J, Wolf L et al 2000 Use of integrins to date the endometrium. Fertility and Sterility 73: 779–787

Letterie G S, Sakas E L 1991 Histology of proximal tubal obstruction in cases of unsuccessful tubal canalization. Fertility and Sterility 56: 831–835

Levitt G A, Jenney M E M 1998 The reproductive system after childhood cancer. British Journal of Obstetrics and Gynaecology 105: 946–953

Levy A, Hall L, Yeu Dall W A, Lightman S L 1994 p53 gene mutations in pituitary adenomas: rare events. Clinical Endocrinology 41: 809–814

Levy B S, Soderstrom R M, Dail D M 1985 Bowel injuries during laparoscopy: gross anatomy and histology. Journal of Reproductive Medicine 30: 168–172

Lewis J 1993 Eosinophilic perifolliculitis: a variant of autoimmune oophoritis. International Journal of Gynecological Pathology 6: 73–81

Lewis S E M, Sterling E S L, Young I S, Thompson W 1997 Comparison of individual antioxidants of sperm and seminal plasma in fertile and infertile men. Fertility and Sterility 67: 142–147

Li T-C, Cooke I D 1991 Evaluation of the luteal phase. Human Reproduction 6: 484–499

Li T-C, Rogers W, Dockery P, Lenton E A, Cooke I D 1988 A new method of histologic dating of human endometrium in the luteal phase. Fertility and Sterility 50: 52–60

Li T-C, Dockery P, Rogers A W, Cooke I D 1989 How precise is histologic dating of endometrium using the standard dating criteria? Fertility and Sterility 51: 759–763

Li T-C, Dockery P, Cooke I D 1991 Endometrial development in the luteal phase of women with various types of infertility: comparison with women of normal fertility. Human Reproduction 6: 325–330

Lilequist B, Lindgren L 1964 Hyperflexion of the uterus and infertility. Acta Obstetricia et Gynecologica Scandinavica 43: 240–254

Lim A S T, Tsakok M F H 1997 Age-related decline in fertility: a link to degenerative oocytes. Fertility and Sterility 68: 265–271

Lim K J H, Odukoya O A, Ajjan R A, Li T-C, Weetman A P, Cooke I D 2000 The role of T-helper cytokines in human reproduction. Fertility and Sterility 73: 136–142

Lindsay A H, Voorhess M L, MacGillivray M H 1983 Multicystic ovaries in primary hypothyroidism. Obstetrics and Gynecology 61: 433–437

Liu D Y, Baker H W G 1994 Disordered acrosome reaction of spermatozoa bound to the zona pellucida: a newly discovered sperm defect causing infertility with reduced sperm-zona pellucida penetration and reduced fertilization in vitro. Human Reproduction 9: 1694–1700

Lobo R G, Granger L R, Paul W L, Goebelsmann U, Mishell D R Jr 1983 Psychological stress and increases in urinary norepinephrine metabolites, platelet serotonin, and adrenal androgens in women with polycystic ovary syndrome. American Journal of Obstetrics and Gynecology 145: 496–503

Locher E W, Maroulis G B 1983 Tubointestinal fistula. Fertility and Sterility 39: 235–237

Locke W 1978 Control of anterior pituitary function. Archives of Internal Medicine 138: 1541–1545

Lockwood C, Irons M, Troiani T, Kawada C, Chaudhury A, Cetrulo C 1988 The prenatal sonographic diagnosis of lethal multiple pterygium syndrome: a heritable cause of recurrent abortion. American Journal of Obstetrics and Gynecology 159: 474–476

Loffer F D, Pent D 1975 Indications, contraindications and complications of laparoscopy. Obstetrical and Gynecological Survey 30: 407–427

Lucas J A Kahlstorf J H, Cowan B D 1988 Multiple endocrine neoplasia — type I syndrome and hyperprolactinaemia. Fertility and Sterility 50: 514–515

Luciano A A 1999 Clinical presentation of hyperprolactinaemia. Journal of Reproductive Medicine 44: 1085–1090

Ludwig G D 1962 Hyperparathyroidism in relation to pregnancy. New England Journal of Medicine 267: 637–640

Lundorff P, Hahlin M, Kallfelt B, Thorburn J, Lindblom B 1991 Adhesion formation after laparoscopic surgery in tubal surgery: a randomized trial versus laparotomy. Fertility and Sterility 55: 911–915

Lunenfeld B, Insler V, Glezerman M 1993 The cervical factor. In: Diagnosis and treatment of functional infertility 3rd Revised Edition. Blackwell Wissenschaft, Berlin, pp 104–119

MacMillan S, Templeton A 1999 Screening for Chlamydia trachomatis in subfertile women. Human Reproduction 14: 3009–3012

Maguiness S D, Shrimank E R, Djahanbaruch O, Grudzinskas J G 1992 Oviduct proteins. Contemporary Review of Obstetrics and Gynecology 4: 42–50

Mahony M C, Alexander N J 1991 Sites of antisperm antibody action. Human Reproduction 6: 1426–1430

Malette B, Paquette Y, Merlen Y, Bleau G 1995 Oviductins possess chitinase and mucin-like domains: a lead in the search for the biological function of these oviduct-specific ZP-associating glycoproteins [review]. Molecular Reproduction and Development 41: 384–397

Marana R, Lucisano A, Leone F, Sanna A, Dell'Acqua S, Mancuso S 1990 High prevalence of silent Chlamydial colonization of the tubal mucosa in infertile women. Fertility and Sterility 53: 354–356

Marcello M F, Nuciforo G, Romeo R et al 1990 Structural and ultrastructural study of the ovary in childhood leukemia after successful treatment. Cancer 66: 2099–2104

March C M, Israel R 1981 Gestational outcome following hysteroscopic lysis of adhesions. Fertility and Sterility 36: 455–459

Marchini M, Losa G A, Mava S, Di Nola G, Fedele L 1992 Ultrastructural aspects of endometrial surface in Kartegener's syndrome. Fertility and Sterility 57: 461–463

Maroulis G H 1981 Evaluation of hirsutism and hyperandrogenemia. Fertility and Sterility 36: 273–305

Martikainen P, Sanikaa E, Suominen J, Santti R 1980 Glucose content as a parameter of semen quality. Archives of Andrology 5: 337–343

Martinez-Roman S, Balasch J, Creus M et al 1997 Immunological factors in endometriosis-associated reproductive failure: studies in fertile and infertile women with and without endometriosis. Human Reproduction 12: 1794–1799

Master V A, Turek P J 2001 Ejaculatory physiology and dysfunction. Urology Clinics of North America 28: 363–375

Mathur S, Williamson H O, Baker E R, Fudenberg H H 1981 Immunoglobulin E levels and antisperm antibody titers in infertile couples. American Journal of Obstetrics and Gynecology 140: 923–930

Mathur S, Williamson H O, Genes P V et al 1983a Association of human leukocytic antigens B7 and BW35 with sperm antibodies. Fertility and Sterility 39: 343–349

Mathur S, Williamson H O, Genco P V, Koopmann W R, Rust P F, Fudenberg H H 1983b Sperm immunity in fertile couples: antibody titers are higher against husband's sperm than to sperm from controls. American Journal of Reproductive Immunology 3: 18–27

Mathur S, Chao L, Goust J M et al 1988 Special antigens on sperm from autoimmune infertile men. American Journal of Reproductive Immunology 17: 5–13

Mazumdar S, Levine A 1998 Antisperm antibodies: etiology, pathogenesis, diagnosis and treatment. Fertility and Sterility 70: 799–810

Mazur M T, Duncan D A, Younger I B 1989 Endometrial biopsy in the cycle of conception: histologic and lectin histochemical evaluation. Fertility and Sterility 51: 764–769

McAnulty J H, Metcalfe T, Veland K 1982 Cardiovascular disease. In: Burrow G N, Ferris T F (eds) Medical complications during pregnancy. W B Saunders, Philadelphia, pp 145–168

McBean J H, Gibson M, Brumsted J R 1996 The association of intrauterine filling defects on hysterosalpingogram with endometriosis. Fertility and Sterility 66: 522–526

McCarty K S Jr, Dobson C E II 1980 Pituitary pathology associated with abnormalities of prolactin secretion. Clinical Obstetrics and Gynecology 23: 367–384

McComb P F, Halbert S A, Gomel V 1980 Pregnancy, ciliary transport and the reversed ampullary segment of the rabbit fallopian tube. Fertility and Sterility 34: 386–390

McComb P F, Newman H, Halbert S A 1981 Reproduction in rabbits after excision of the oviductal isthmus, ampullary-isthmic junction and uteroisthmic junction. Fertility and Sterility 36: 669–677

McComb P, Langley L, Villalon M, Verdugo P 1986 The oviductal cilia and Kartagener's syndrome. Fertility and Sterility 46: 412–416

McCutcheon I E, Oldfield E H 1991 Lymphocytic adenohypophysitis presenting as infertility. Case report. Journal of Neurosurgery 74: 821–826

McDonough P G 1987 Recurrent aneuploidic and euploidic abortion. Obstetrics and Gynecology Clinics of North America 14(4): 1099–1113

McGee Z A, Jensen R L, Clemens C M, Taylor-Robinson D, Johnson A P, Gregg C R 1999 Gonococcal infection of human fallopian tube mucosa in organ culture: relationship of mucosal tissue TNF-alpha concentration to sloughing of ciliated cells. Sexually Transmitted Diseases 26: 160–165

McNeely M J, Soules M R 1988 The diagnosis of luteal phase deficiency: a critical review. Fertility and Sterility 50: 1–15

McQueen D, McKillop J H, Gray H W, Callaghan M, Monoghan C, Bessent R G 1993 Radionuclide migration through the genital tract in infertile women with endometriosis. Human Reproduction 8: 1910–1914

Mehes K, Kosztolanyi G 1992 A possible mosaic form for delayed centromere separation and aneuploidy. Human Genetics 88: 477–478

Menashe Y, Sack J, Mashiach S 1991 Spontaneous pregnancies in two women with Laron-type dwarfism: are growth hormone and circulating insulin-like growth factor mandatory for induction of ovulation? Human Reproduction 6: 670–671

Mendel E B 1964 Chronic tubal spasm. International Journal of Fertility 9: 383–389

Menning B B 1980 The emotional needs of infertile couples. Fertility and Sterility 34: 313–319

Mesia A F, Gahr D, Wild M, Mittak K R, Demopoulos R I 1997 Immunohistochemistry of vascular changes in leuprolide acetate-treated leiomyomas. Obstetrics and Gynecology 176: 1026–1029

Mettler L 1980 Immunology and reproduction. I. Sterility immunology. Gynecologic and Obstetrical Investigation 11: 129–160

Meyer W R, Papadimitriou J C, Silverberg S G, Sharara F I 2000 Secondary amenorrhea and infertility caused by an inhibin-B producing ovarian fibrothecoma. Fertility and Sterility 73: 258–260

Meyer A R, Hutchinson-Williams K A, Jones E E, De Cherney A H 1990 Secondary hypogonadism in hemochromatosis. Fertility and Sterility 54: 740–742

Meyer W R, Castelbaum A J, Somkuti S, Sagoskin A W, Doyle M, Harris J E 1997 Hydrosalpinges adversely affect markers of endometrial receptivity. Human Reproduction 12: 1393–1398

Mild M P, Klock S C, Moses S, Chatterton R 1998 Stress and anxiety do not result in pregnancy wastage. Human Reproduction 13: 2296–2300

Miller P B, Soules M R 1997 Correlation of reproductive aging with function in selected organ systems. Fertility and Sterility 68: 443–448

Mimori H, Fukuma K, Matsuo I, Nakahara K, Maeyama M 1981 Effect of progesterone on glycogen metabolism in the endometrium of infertile patients during the menstrual cycle. Fertility and Sterility 35: 289–295

Mitami Y, Takaki C H, Iwasaki H 1959 Myoma of the uterus and sterility with particular reference to the tubal pathology. Journal of the Japanese Obstetrical and Gynecological Society 6: 347–352

Mobus V J, Kortenhorn K, Kreienberg R, Friedberg V 1996 Long-term results after operative correction of vaginal aplasia. American Journal of Obstetrics and Gynecology 175: 617–624

Moghissi K S 1979 The cervix in infertility. Clinical Obstetrics and Gynecology 22: 27–42

Montagu M F A 1946 Adolescent sterility. Thomas, Springfield, Illinois

Montz F J 1996 Impact of therapy for cervical intraepithelial neoplasia on fertility. American Journal of Obstetrics and Gynecology 175: 1129–1136

Morales P, Roco M, Vigil P 1993 Human cervical mucus: relationship between biochemical characteristics and ability to allow migration of spermatozoa. Human Reproduction 8: 78–83

Morgan J F 1999 Eating disorders and reproduction. Australian and New Zealand Journal of Obstetrics and Gynaecology 39: 167–173

Morikawa H, Okamura H, Takenaka A, Morimoto K, Nishimura T 1980 Physiological study of the human mesotubarium ovarica. Obstetrics and Gynecology 55: 493–496

Morrison J C, Givens J R, Wiser W L, Fish S A 1975 Mumps oophoritis: a cause of premature menopause. Fertility and Sterility 26: 655–659

Mosgaard B J, Lidegaardø, Krüger Kjaer S, Schou G, Andersen A N 1998 Ovarian stimulation and borderline ovarian tumors: a case-control study. Fertility and Sterility 70: 1049–1055

Mowbray J F, Underwood J, Gill T J III 1991 Familial recurrent spontaneous abortions. American Journal of Reproductive Immunology 26: 17–18

Muechler E K, Huang K-E 1982 Paradoxical pituitary hormone response in a case of primary hypothyroidism and Hashimoto's thyroiditis. Fertility and Sterility 38: 423–426

Mukai K 1983 Pituitary adenomas: immunocytochemical study of 150 tumors with clinicopathologic correlation. Cancer 52: 648–653

Murphy N J, Wallace D L 1993 Gonadotropin-releasing hormone (GnRH) agonist therapy for reduction of leiomyoma volume. Gynecologic Oncology 49: 266–267

Murray S C, Smith T T 1997 Sperm interaction with fallopian tube apical membrane enhances sperm motility and delays capacitation. Fertility and Sterility 68: 351–357

Musset R, Poitout P L, Truc J B, Paniel B J 1978 Aplasie vaginale avec uterus fonctionnel: resultats operatoires et commentaires. Journal de Gynecologie, Obstetrique et Biologie de la Reproduction 7: 316–333

Nagasaka T, Nakashima N, Furui A, Wakabayashi Y, Yoshida J 1998 Sarcomatous transformation of pituitary adenoma after bromocriptine therapy. Human Pathology 29: 190–193

Nakajima I, Mizushima N, Matsuda H et al 1986 Fulminant hepatic failure associated with aplastic anemia after treatment with Danazol. British Journal of Obstetrics and Gynaecology 93: 1013–1015

Nakajima S T, Nason F G, Badger G J, Gibson M 1991 Progesterone production in early pregnancy. Fertility and Sterility 55: 516–521

Navot D, Bergh P A, Laufer N 1992 Ovarian hyperstimulation syndrome in novel reproductive technologies: prevention and treatment. Fertility and Sterility 58: 249–261

Neelon F A, Goree J A, Lebowitz H E 1973 The primary empty sella: clinical and radiographic characteristics and endocrine function. Medicine 52: 72–92

Nicholson S C, Robinson J N, Sargent I L, Hallam N F, Charnock F M L, Barlow D H 1996 Does large loop excision of the transformation zone of the cervix predispose to the development of antisperm antibodies in women. Fertility and Sterility 65: 871–873

Nicosia S V, Johnson J H 1983 Histochemistry and ultrastructure of the rabbit endocervical mucosa after intravaginal antigen administration. Fertility and Sterility 39: 408–409

Nishi T, Goto T, Takeshima H et al 1999 Tissue factor expressed in pituitary adenoma cells contributes to the development of vascular events in pituitary adenomas. Cancer 86: 1354–1361

Niver D H, Barrett G, Jewelewicz R 1980 Congenital atresia of the uterine cervix and vagina: three cases. Fertility and Sterility 33: 25–29

Niwa J, Hashi K, Minase T 1996 Radiation induced intracranial leiomyosarcoma: its histopathological features. Acta Neurochirugica (Wien) 138: 1470–1471

Nogales-Ortiz F, Tarancon I, Nogales F F Jr 1979 The pathology of female genital tuberculosis. Obstetrics and Gynecology 53: 422–428

Noyes R W, Haman J O 1954 Accuracy of endometrial dating. Fertility and Sterility 4: 504–508

Noyes R W, Hertig A T, Rock J 1950 Dating the endometrial biopsy. Fertility and Sterility 1: 3–25

Obwegeser R, Hochlag Schwandtner M, Sinzinger H 1999 Homocysteine — a pathophysiological cornerstone in obstetrical and gynaecological disorders? Human Reproduction Update 5: 64–72

Odeblad E 1962 Undulations of macromolecules in cervical mucus. International Journal of Fertility 7: 313–318

Odeblad E 1968 The functional structure of human cervical mucus. Acta Obstetricia et Gynecologica Scandinavica 47 (suppl 1): 59–70

Odeblad E 1978 Cervical factors. Contributions to Obstetrics and Gynecology 4: 132–142

Odell W D, Meikle A W 1986 Menorrhagia, infertility, elevated serum estradiol, and hyperprolactinemia resulting from increased aromatase activity (MIEHA syndrome). Fertility and Sterility 46: 321–324

Ohlgisser M, Sorokin Y, Heifetz M 1985 Gynecologic laparoscopy: a review article. Obstetrical and Gynecological Survey 40: 385–396

Okamura N, Tajima Y, Ishikawa H, Yoshi I S, Koiso K, Sugita Y 1986 Lowered bicarbonate levels in seminal plasma cause the poor sperm motility in human infertile patients. Fertility and Sterility 45: 265–272

Okatani Y, Morioka N, Wakatsuki A, Nakano Y, Sagara Y 1993 Role of the free radical-scavenger system in aromatase activity of the human ovary. Hormone Research 39 (Supplement 1): 22–27

Okon M A, Laird S M, Tuckerman E M, Li T-C 1998 Serum androgen levels in women who have recurrent miscarriages and their correlation with markers of endometrial function. Fertility and Sterility 69: 682–690

Oruckaptan H H, Drnmrbdim O, Ozcan O E, Ozgen T 2000 Pituitary adenoma: results of 684 surgically treated patients and review of the literature. Surgical Neurology 53: 211–219

Osamura R Y, Tahara S, Kurotani R, Sanno N, Matsuno A, Teramoto S 2000 Contributions of immunohistochemistry and in situ hybridization to the functional analysis of pituitary adenomas. Journal of Histochemistry and Cytochemistry 48: 445–458

Ota H, Igarashi S, Hatazawa J, Tanaka T 1998 Is adenomyosis an immune disease? Human Reproduction Update 4: 360–367

Otsuka F, Kageyama J, Ogura T, Makino H 1998 Pituitary apoplexy induced by a combined anterior pituitary test: case report and literature review. Endocrinology Journal 45: 393–398

Overstreet E W 1959 Endometrial polyps: their relationship to fertility and abortion. International Journal of Fertility 4: 263–267

Overstreet J W 1986 Evaluation of sperm-cervical mucus interactions. Fertility and Sterility 45: 324–326

Ovesen P, Moller J, Moller N, Christiansen D S, Orskov H, Jorgensen J O L 1992 Growth hormone secretory capacity and serum insulin-like growth factor I levels in primary infertile anovulatory women with regular menses. Fertility and Sterility 57: 97–101

Page H 1989 Estimation of the prevalence and incidence of infertility in a population: a pilot study. Fertility and Sterility 51: 571–577

Parazzini F, Chatenoud L, Tozzi L, Di Cintio E, Benzi G, Fedele L 1998 Induced abortion in the first trimester of pregnancy and risk of miscarriage. British Journal of Obstetrics and Gynaecology 105: 418–421

Parikh F R, Nadkarni S G, Kamat S A, Naik N, Soonawala S B, Parikh R M 1997 Genital tuberculosis — a major pelvic factor causing infertility in Indian women. Fertility and Sterility 67: 497–500

Parish W E, Ward A 1968 Studies of cervical mucus and serum from infertile women. Journal of Obstetrics and Gynaecology of the British Commonwealth 75: 1089–1092

Parker W H, Fu Y S, Berek J S 1994 Uterine sarcoma in patients operated on for presumed leiomyoma and rapidly growing leiomyomas. Obstetrics and Gynecology 83: 414–418

Parr E L, Shirley R L 1976 Embryotoxicity of leukocyte extracts and its relationship to intrauterine contraception in humans. Fertility and Sterility 27: 1067–1077

Peccei J S 1995 A hypothesis for the origin and evolution of menopause. Maturitas 21: 83–89

Pegoraro E, Whitaker J, Mowery-Rushton P, Surti U, Lanasa M, Hoffman E P 1997 Familial skewed X inactivation: a molecular trait associated with high spontaneous abortion rate maps to Xq28. American Journal of Human Genetics 61: 160–170

Peress M R 1984 Persistent amenorrhea following discontinuation of danazol therapy. Fertility and Sterility 41: 322–323

Peress M R, Kreutner A K, Mathur R S, Williamson H O 1982 Female pseudohermaphroditism with somatic chromosomal anomaly in association with in utero exposure to danazol. American Journal of Obstetrics and Gynecology 142: 708–709

Peters W A 3rd, Thiagarajah S, Harbert G M Jr 1979 Cervical cerclage: Twenty years' experience. Southern Medical Journal 72: 933–937

Phipps W R, Benson C B, McShane P M 1988 Severe thigh myositis following intramuscular progesterone injections in an in vitro fertilization patient. Fertility and Sterility 49: 536–537

Pierro E, Cirino G, Bucci M R et al 1999 Antiphospholipid antibodies inhibit prostaglandin release by decidual cells of early pregnancy: possible involvement of extracellular secretory phospholipase A2. Fertility and Sterility 71: 342–346

Pilam M B, Cohen M, Cheng L, Spaenle M, Bronstein M H, Atkin T W 1995 Pituitary adenomas complicating cardiac surgery: summary and review of 11 cases. Journal of Cardiac Surgery 10: 125–132

Pillai S, Rust P F, Howard L 1998 Effects of antibodies to transferrin and alpha 2-HS glycoprotein on in vitro sperm motion: implication in infertility associated with endometriosis. American Journal of Reproductive Immunology 39: 235–242

Pinsky L, Erickson R P, Schimke R N 1999 Genetic disorders of human sexual development. Oxford University Press, New York

Portnow J, Talo A, Hodgson B J 1977 A random walk model of ovum transport. Bulletin of Mathematical Biology 39: 349–357

Posaci C, Camus M, Osmanaoglu K, Devroey P 1999 Tubal surgery in the era of assisted reproductive technology: clinical options. Human Reproduction 14, Supplement 1: 120–136

Potashnik G, Lerner-Geva L, Genkin L, Chetrit A, Lunenfeld E, Porath A 1999 Fertility drugs and the risk of breast and ovarian cancers: results of a long-term follow-up study. Fertility and Sterility 71: 853–859

Potter J D 1980 Hypothyroidism and reproductive failure. Surgery Gynecology and Obstetrics 150: 251–255

Prakash C 1981 Etiology of immune infertility. In: Gleicher N (ed) Reproductive immunology, progress in clinical and biological research, vol. 70. Liss, New York, pp. 403–412

Prinz W, Taubert H-D 1968 Mumps in pubescent females and its effect on later reproductive function. Gynaecology 167: 23–27

Qasim S M, Bohrer M K, Kemmann E 1996 Recurrent cervical pregnancy after assisted reproduction by intrafallopian transfer. Obstetrics and Gynecology 87: 831–832

Quagliarello J, Barakat R 1987 Raynaud's phenomenon in infertile women treated with bromocriptine. Fertility and Sterility 48: 877–879

Quan A, Charles D, Craig J M 1963 Histologic and functional consequences of periovarian adhesions. Obstetrics and Gynecology 22: 96–101

Quan C P, Roux C, Rillot J, Bouvet J-P 1990 Delineation of T and B suppressive molecules from human seminal plasma II spermine is the major suppressor of T-lymphocytes in vitro. American Journal of Reproductive Immunology 22: 64–69

Quigley M E, Sheehan K L, Casper R F, Yen S S C 1980 Evidence for increased dopaminergic and opioid activity in patients with hypothalamic hypogonadotropic amenorrhea. Journal of Clinical Endocrinology and Metabolism 50: 949–954

Rabinowe S L, Ravnilcar V A, Dib S A, George K L, Dluhy R G 1989 Premature menopause: monoclonal antibody defines T-lymphocyte abnormalities and antiovarian antibodies. Fertility and Sterility 51: 450–454

Rajasekaran M, Hellstrom W J G, Naz R K, Sikka S C 1995 Oxidative stress and interleukins in seminal plasma during leukocytospermia. Fertility and Sterility 64: 166–171

Ralph S G, Rutherford A-J, Wilson J D 1999 Influence of bacterial vaginosis on conception and miscarriage in the first trimester. Cohort study. British Medical Journal 319 (7204): 220–223

Rana N, Braun D P, House R, Gebel H, Rotman C, Dmowski W P 1996 Basal and stimulated secretion of cytokines by peritoneal macrophages in women with endometriosis. Fertility and Sterility 65: 925–930

Rao K V, Demaris A 1995 Coital frequency among married and cohabiting couples in the United States. Journal of Biosocial Science 27: 135–150

Reavley A, Fisher A D, Owen D, Creed F H, Dais R 1997 Psychological distress in patients with hyperprolactinaemia. Clinical Endocrinology 47: 343–348

Rein M S, Barbieri R L, Welch N, Gleason R E, Caulfield J P, Friedman A J 1993 The concentrations of collagen associated with amino acids are higher in GnRH agonist treated uterine myomas. Obstetrics and Gynecology 82: 901–905

Reincke M, Arlt W, Heppnet C, Petzke F, Chrousos G B, Allolio B 1998 Neuroendocrine dysfunction in African trypanosomiasis. The role of cytokines. Annals of the New York Academy of Sciences 840: 809–821

Reinhardt K C, Dubey R K, Keller P J, Lauper U, Rosselli M 1999 Xeno-oestrogen and phyto-oestrogens induce the synthesis of leukemia inhibitory factor by human and bovine oviduct cells. Molecular Human Reproduction 5: 899–907

Resnick L 1962 Constrictive perisalpingitis. South African Journal of Medicine 2: 769–772

Reubinoff B E, Simon A, Friedler S, Schenker J G, Lewin A 1994 Defective oocytes as a possible cause of infertility in a β-thalassaemia major patient. Human Reproduction 9: 1143–1145

Reyes F I, Kohn S, Faiman C 1976 Fertility in women with gonadal dysgenesis. American Journal of Obstetrics and Gynecology 126: 668–670

Richardson D A, Evans M I, Talerman A, Maroulis G B 1982 Segmental absence of the mid-portion of the fallopian tube. Fertility and Sterility 37: 577–578

Robert F, Hardy J 1975 Prolactin-secreting adenomas. Archives of Pathology 99: 625–633

Rock J A, Zacur H A 1983 The clinical management of repeated early pregnancy wastage. Fertility and Sterility 39: 123–140

Rock J A, Parmley T, Murphy A A, Jones H W Jr 1986 Malposition of the ovary associated with uterine anomalies. Fertility and Sterility 45: 561–563

Rock J A, Guzick D S, Katz E, Zacur H A, King T M 1987 Tubal anastomosis: pregnancy success following reversal of Fallopian or monopolar cautery sterilization. Fertility and Sterility 48: 13–17

Rodriguez-Rigau L J, Steinberger E, Atkins B J, Lucci J A 1979 Effect of testosterone on human corpus luteum steroidogenesis in vitro. Fertility and Sterility 31: 448–450

Rohde V, Erles K, Sattler H P, Derouet H, Wullich B, Schlehofer J R 1999 Detection of adeno-associated virus in human semen: does viral infection play a role in the pathogenesis of male infertility. Fertility and Sterility 72: 814–816

Roncaroli F, Baci A, Frank G, Calbucci F 1998 Granulomatous hypophysitis caused by a ruptured intrasellar Rathke's cleft cyst: report of a case and review of the literature. Neurosurgery 43: 146–149

Rosenbusch B, Sterzik K 1991 Sperm chromosomes and habitual abortion. Fertility and Sterility 56: 370–372

Rosenfeld D L, Garcia C-R 1975 Endometrial biopsy in the cycle of conception. Fertility and Sterility 26: 1088–1093

Rosenfeld D L, Seidman S M, Bronson R A, Scholl G M 1983 Unsuspected chronic pelvic inflammatory disease in the infertile female. Fertility and Sterility 39: 44–48

Rosenfield R L, Barnes R B, Cara J F, Lucky A W 1990 Dysregulation of cytochrome P450C 17α as the cause of polycystic ovarian syndrome. Fertility and Sterility 53: 785–791

Rotterdam H 1978 Chronic endometritis: a clinicopathologic study. Pathology Annual 13: 209–225

Roumen F J M E, Doesburg W H, Rolland R 1982 Hormonal patterns in infertile women with a deficient postcoital test. Fertility and Sterility 38: 42–47

Rouzi A A, MacKinnon M, McComb P F 1995 Predictors of success of reversal of sterilization. Fertility and Sterility 64: 29–36

Ruiz-Velasco V, Alfani G G, Sanchez L P, Vera M A 1997 Endometrial pathology and infertility. Fertility and Sterility 67: 687–692

Rutgers J L, Spong C Y, Sinow R, Heiner J 1995 Leuprolide acetate treatment and myoma arterial size. Obstetrics and Gynecology 86: 386–388

Saiwai S, Inoue Y, Ishihara T et al 1998 Lymphocytic adenohypophysitis: skull radiographs and MRI. Neuroradiology 40: 114–120

Saleh M I, Warren M A, Li T-C, Cooke I D 1995 A light microscopical morphometric study of the luminal epithelium of the human endometrium during the peri-implantation period. Human Reproduction 10: 1828–1832

Santoro N, Adel T, Skurnick J H 1999 Decreased inhibin and increased activin A secretion characterize reproductive aging in women. Fertility and Sterility 71: 658–662

Saridogan E, Djahandakhch O, Kervancioglu M E, Kahyaogly F, Shrimanker K, Grudzinkas J G 1997 Placental protein 14 production by human fallopian tube epithelial cells. Human Reproduction 12: 1500–1507

Sauer M, Jarrett J C II 1984 Small bowel obstruction following diagnostic laparoscopy. Fertility and Sterility 42: 653–654

Sayegh R, Mastroianni L Jr 1991 Recent advances in our understanding of tubal function. Annals of the New York Academy of Sciences 626: 266–275

Schaap T, Shemer R, Palti Z, Sharon R 1984 ABO incompatibility and reproductive failure. I. Prenatal selection. American Journal of Human Genetics 36: 143–151

Schaeffer G 1976 Female genital tuberculosis. Clinical Obstetrics and Gynecology 19: 223–239

Schechter J, Goldsmith P, Wilson C, Weiner R 1998 Morphological evidence for the presence of arteries in human prolactinomas. Journal of Clinical Endocrinology and Metabolism 67: 713–719

Schenker J G, Margalioth E J 1982 Intrauterine adhesions: an updated appraisal. Fertility and Sterility 37: 593–610

Schlegelberger B, Gripp K, Grote W 1989 Common fragile sites in couples with recurrent spontaneous abortions. American Journal of Medical Genetics 32: 45–51

Schumacher G F S, Kim M H, Hossienian A H, Dupon C 1977 Immunoglobulins, proteinase inhibitors, albumin and lysozymes in human cervical mucus. I. Communication: hormonal profiles and cervical mucus changes – methods and results. American Journal of Obstetrics and Gynecology 129: 629–636

Schupf N, Ottman R 1996 Reproduction among individuals with idiopathic cryptogenic epilepsy: risk factors for reduced fertility in marriage. Epilepsia 37: 833–840

Schwanzel-Fukuda M, Bick D, Pfaff D W 1989 Luteinizing hormone-releasing hormone (LHRH)-expressing cells do not migrate normally in an inherited hypogonadal (Kallmann) syndrome. Brain Research and Molecular Brain Research 6: 311–326

Schwartz D, Mayaux M-J, Spira A et al 1983 Semen characteristics as a function of age in 833 fertile men. Fertility and Sterility 39: 530–535

Schwitemaker N W E, Helderhorst F M, Tjontham R T O, van Saase J L C 1990 Late anaphylactic shock after hysterosalpingography. Fertility and Sterility 54: 535–536

Scott R T, Snyder R R, Bagnall J W et al 1993 Evaluation of the impact of intra-observer variability on endometrial dating and the diagnosis of luteal phase defects. Fertility and Sterility 80: 652–657

Scott S, Duncan C J 1999 Nutrition, fertility and steady-state dynamics in a pre-industrial community in Penrith, Northern England. Journal of Biosocial Sciences 31: 505–523

Scurry J, Planner R, Fortune D F, Lee C S, Rode J 1993 Ligneous (pseudomembranous) inflammation of the female genital tract. A report of two cases. Journal of Reproductive Medicine 38: 407–412

Sedmak D D, Hart W R, Tubbs R R 1987 Autoimmune oophoritis: a histopathologic study of involved ovaries with immunologic characterization of the mononuclear cell infiltrate. International Journal of Gynecological Pathology 6: 73–81

Seibel M M, Taymor M L 1982 Emotional aspects of infertility. Fertility and Sterility 37: 137–145

Seifer D B, Collins R L 1990 Current concepts of β-endorphin physiology in female reproduction dysfunction. Fertility and Sterility 54: 757–771

Seifer D B, Naftolin F 1998 Moving toward an earlier and better under-standing of perimenopause. Fertility and Sterility 69: 387–388

Self M N, Aplin J D, Buckley C H 1989 Luteal phase defect: the possibility of an immunohistochemical diagnosis. Fertility and Sterility 51: 273–279

Sen D K, Fox H 1967 The lymphoid tissue of the endometrium. Gynaecologica 163: 371–378

Serour G I, Aboulchar M, Mansour R, Sattar M, Min Y, Aboulghar H 1998 Complications of medically assisted conception in 3,500 cycles. Fertility and Sterility 70: 638–642

Serri O, Robert F, Pelletier G, Beauregard H, Hardy J 1987 Hyperprolactinemia associated with clinically silent adenomas: endocrinologic and pathologic studies; a report of two cases. Fertility and Sterility 47: 792–796

Shafrin S, Schachter J, Dahrouge D, Sweet R L 1992 Long term sequelae of acute pelvic inflammatory disease. American Journal of Obstetrics and Gynecology 166: 1300–1305

Shah I 1997 Fertility and contraception in Europe: the case of low fertility in Southern Europe. European Journal of Contraception and Reproductive Health 2: 53–61

Shangold M M, Dor N, Welt S I, Fleischman A R, Crenshaw M C 1982 Hyperparathyroidism and pregnancy: a review. Obstetrical and Gynecological Survey 37: 217–228

Sharara F I, Seifer D B, Flaws J A 1998 Environmental toxicants and female reproduction. Fertility and Sterility 70: 613–622

Sharma M C, Arora R, Mohapatra A K, Sarat-Chandra P, Galkwad S B, Sarkar C 2000 Intrasellar tuberculoma – an enigmatic infection: a series of 18 cases. Clinical Neurology and Neurosurgery 102: 72–77

Sharpe-Timms K L, Keisler L W, McIntosh E W, Keisler D H 1998 Tissue inhibitor of metalloproteinase-1 concentrations are attenuated in peritoneal fluid and sera of women with endometriosis and restored in sera by gonadotropin-releasing hormone agonist therapy. Fertility and Sterility 69: 1128–1134

Sheehan H L, Summers V K 1949 The syndrome of hypopituitarism. Quarterly Journal of Medicine 72: 319–378

Sher G, Katz M 1976 Inadequate cervical mucus — a cause of 'idiopathic' infertility. Fertility and Sterility 27: 886–889

Shimada T, Norita T, Nagai M, Sato S, Mori K, Campbell G R 1993 Morphological changes in spiral artery of the mammalian ovary with age. Hormone Research 39 (Supplement 1): 9–15

Shimon I, Hinton D R, Weiss M H, Meimed S 1998 Prolactinomas express human heparin-binding secretory transforming gene (hst) protein product: marker of tumor invasiveness. Clinical Endocrinology 48: 23–29

Shoham Z, Zosmer A, Insler V 1991 Early miscarriage and fetal malformations after induction of ovulation (by clomiphene citrate and/or human menotropins), in vitro fertilization and gamete intrafallopian transfer. Fertility and Sterility 55: 1–11

Shortle B, Jewelewicz R 1989 Cervical incompetence. Fertility and Sterility 52: 181–188

Siegler A M, Valle R F 1988 Therapeutic hysteroscopic procedures. Fertility and Sterility 50: 685–701

Siiteri P K 1981 Extragonadal oestrogen formation and serum binding of oestradiol: relationship to cancer. Journal of Endocrinology 89: 119P–129P

Sikka A, Kemmann E, Vrablik R M, Grossman L 1983 Carpal tunnel syndrome associated with danazol therapy. American Journal of Obstetrics and Gynecology 147: 102–103

Silverman A Y, Greenberg E I 1983 Absence of a segment of the proximal portion of a fallopian tube. Obstetrics and Gynecology (suppl) 62: 90–91

Silvestroni L, Morisi G, Malandrino F, Frajese G 1979 Free amino acids in semen: measurement and significance in normal and oligozoospermic men. Archives of Andrology 2: 257–261

Simpson J L, Rajkovic A 1999 Ovarian differentiation and gonadal failure. American Journal of Medical Genetics 89: 186–200

Simpson J L, Verp M S, Plouffe L Jr 1993 Female genital system. In: Stevenson R E, Hall J G, Goodman R M (eds) Human malformations and related anomalies. Oxford University Press, New York, pp 575–578

Simpson J L, Carson S A, Mills J L et al 1996 Prospective study showing that antisperm antibodies are not associated with pregnancy losses. Fertility and Sterility 66: 36–42

Skomsvoll J F, Ostensen M, Schei B 2000 Reproduction in women reporting chronic musculoskeletal disorders. Scandinavian Journal of Rheumatology 29: 103–107

Skrabanek P, Powell D 1983 Substance P in obstetrics and gynecology. Obstetrics and Gynecology 61: 641–646

Smith A, Gaba T J 1990 Data on families of chromosome translocation car-riers because of habitual spontaneous abortion. Australian and New Zealand Journal of Obstetrics and Gynaecology 30: 57–62

Smith G, Roberts R, Hall C, Nuki G 1996 Reversible ovulatory failure associated with the development of luteinized unruptured follicles in women with inflammatory arthritis taking non-steroidal anti-inflammatory drugs. British Journal of Rheumatology 35: 458–462

Smits L J, Van Poppel F W, Verduin J A, Jongbloft P H, Straatman H, Zielhuis G A 1997 Is fecundability associated with month of birth? An analysis of 19th and early 20th century family reconstruction data from the Netherlands. Human Reproduction 12: 2572–2578

Soltan M H, Hancock K W 1982 Outcome in patients with postpill amenorrhoea. British Journal of Obstetrics and Gynaecology 89: 745–748

Soutter W P, Allan H, Cowan S, Aitchison T C, Leake R E 1979 A study of endometrial RNA polymerase activity in infertile women. Journal of Reproduction and Fertility 55: 45–52

Spiessens C, D'Hooghe T, Wouters E, Meuleman C, Vanderschuerend D 1998 α-glycosidase activity in seminal plasma: predictive value for outcome in intrauterine insemination and in vitro fertilization. Fertility and Sterility 69: 735–739

Spong C, Sinow R, Renslo R, Cabus E, Rutgers J, Kletsky O A 1995 Induced hypoestrogenism increases the arterial resistance index of leiomyomata without affecting uterine or carotid arteries. Journal of Assisted Reproduction and Genetics 12: 338–340

Sreenan J J, Prayson R A, Biscotti C V, Thornton M H, Easley K A, Hart W R 1996 Histopathologic findings in 107 uterine leiomyomas treated with leuprolide acetate compared with 126 controls. American Journal of Surgical Pathology 20: 427–432

Stagnaro-Green A, Roman S H, Cobin R H, el-Harazy E, Wallenstein S, Davies T F 1992 A prospective study of lymphocyte-mediated immunosuppression in normal pregnancy: evidence of a T-cell etiology for postpartum thyroid dysfunction. Journal of Clinical Endocrinology and Metabolism 74: 645–653

Stambaugh R, Noriega C, Mastroianni L 1969 Bicarbonate ion; the coronal cell dispersing factor of rabbit tubal fluid. Journal of Reproduction and Fertility 18: 51–58

Stanger J D, Yovich J L 1984 Failure of human oocyte release at ovulation. Fertility and Sterility 41: 827–832

Steer C V, Tan S L, Mason B A, Campbell S 1994 Midluteal phase vaginal color Doppler assessment of uterine artery impedance in a subfertile population. Fertility and Sterility 61: 53–58

Stephen E H 1996 Projections of impaired fecundity among women in the United States: 1995 to 2020. Fertility and Sterility 66: 205–209

Sterzik K, Abt M, Grab D, Schneider V, Strehler E 2000 Predicting the histologic dating of an endometrial biopsy with the use of Doppler ultrasonography and hormone measurements in patients undergoing spontaneous ovulatory cycles. Fertility and Sterility 73: 94–98

Stewart-Akers A M, Krasnow J S, Brekosky J, De Loia J A 1998 Endometrial leukocytes are altered numerically and functionally in women with implantation defects. American Journal of Reproductive Immunology 39: 1–11

Stone S G, Swartz W J 1979 A syndrome characterized by recurrent symptomatic ovarian cysts in young women. American Journal of Obstetrics and Gynecology 134: 310–314

Stovall T G, Elder R F, Ling F W 1989 Predictors of pelvic adhesions. Journal of Reproductive Medicine 34: 345–348

Stromberg S, Crock P, Lernmark A, Hutting A L 1998 Pituitary autoantibodies in patients with hypopituitarism and their relatives. Journal of Endocrinology 157: 475–480

Styler M, Shapiro S S 1985 Mollicutes (mycoplasma) in infertility. Fertility and Sterility 44: 1–11

Subramanian M G, Kowalczk C L, Leach R E, et al 1997 Midcycle increase of prolactin seen in normal women is absent in subjects with unexplained infertility. Fertility and Sterility 67: 644–647

Sudha T, Gopinath P M 1990 Homologous Robertsonian translocation (21q21q) and abortions. Human Genetics 85: 253–255

Sueoka K, Shiokawa S, Miyazaki T, Kuji N, Tanaka M, Yoshimura Y 1997 Integrins and reproductive physiology: expression and modulation in fertilization, embryogenesis and implantation. Fertility and Sterility 67: 799–811

Suganuma N, Kitagawa T, Nawa A, Tomoda Y 1993 Human ovarian aging and mitochondrial DNA deletion. Hormone Research 39 (Supplement 1): 16–21

Sugimoto O 1978 Diagnostic and therapeutic hysteroscopy. Igaku-Shoin, Tokyo, pp 27–28

Sulak P J, Letterie G S, Coddington C C, Hayslip C C, Woodward J E, Klein T A 1987 Histology of proximal tubal occlusion. Fertility and Sterility 48: 437–440

Surrey E S 1999 Microendoscopy of the human fallopian tube. Journal of the American Association of Gynecologic Laparoscopy 6: 383–389

Surrey E S, Bishop J A, Surrey M W 2000 Role of GnRH agonists in managing proximal fallopian tube obstruction. Journal of Reproductive Medicine 45: 126–130

Syrop C H, Halme J 1987 Peritoneal fluid environment and infertility. Fertility and Sterility 48: 1–9

Tabibzadeh S 1990 Immunoreactivity of human endometrium: correlations with endometrial dating. Fertility and Sterility 54: 624–631

Tabibzadeh S, Shea W, Lessey B A, Broome J 1999 From endometrial receptivity to infertility. Seminars in Reproductive Endocrinology 17: 197–203

Taney F H, Grazi R V, Weiss G, Schmidt C L 1991 Detection of premature luteinization with serum progesterone levels at the time of the postcoital test. Fertility and Sterility 55: 513–515

Taylor H S 2000 The role of HOX genes in human implantation. Human Reproduction Update 6: 75–79

Taylor H S, Bagot C, Kardana A, Olive D, Aricia 1999 HOX gene expression is altered in the endometrium of women with endometriosis. Human Reproduction 14: 1328–1331

Taylor M L 1996 The regulation of follicle growth: some clinical implications in reproductive endocrinology. Fertility and Sterility 65: 235–247

Taylor P J, Graham G 1982 Is diagnostic curettage harmful in women with unexplained infertility? British Journal of Obstetrics and Gynaecology 89: 296–298

Taylor P J, Cumming D C, Hill P 1981 The significance of hysteroscopically detected intrauterine adhesions in eumenorrheic infertile women and the role of antecedent curettage in their formation. American Journal of Obstetrics and Gynecology 139: 239–242

Thom D H, Nelson L M, Vaughan T L 1992 Spontaneous abortion and subsequent adverse birth outcomes. American Journal of Obstetrics and Gynecology 166: 111–116

Thurmond A S, Novy M, Rosch J 1988 Terbutaline in diagnosis of interstitial fallopian tube obstruction. Investigative Radiology 23: 209–210

Timar L, Beres J, Kosztolanyi G, Nemeth I 1991 De novo complex chromosomal rearrangement in a woman with recurrent spontaneous abortion and one healthy daughter. Human Genetics 86: 421

Tomlinson M J, East S J, Barratt C L R, Bolton A E, Cooke I D 1992 Preliminary communication: possible role of reactive nitrogen intermediates in leucocyte-mediated sperm dysfunction. American Journal of Reproductive Immunology 27: 89–92

Toth M, Patton D L, Campbell A et al 2000 Detection of Chlamydial antigenic material in ovarian, prostatic, ectopic pregnancy and semen sample of culture-negative subjects. American Journal of Reproductive Immunology 43: 218–222

Treadwell M C, Bronsteen R A, Bottoms S F 1991 Prognostic factors and complication rates for cervical cerclage: A review of 482 cases. American Journal of Obstetrics and Gynecology 165: 555–558

Tredway D R, Umezaki C U, Mishell D Jr, Germanowski J 1975 Effect of intrauterine devices on sperm transport in the human being. American Journal of Obstetrics and Gynecology 123: 734–735

Treloar S A, O'Connor D T, O'Connor V M, Martin N G 1999 Genetic influences on endometriosis in an Australian twin sample. Fertility and Sterility 71: 701–710

Trimbos-Kemper T C M, Veering B T 1990 Anaphylactic shock from intracavitary 32% Dextran-70 during hysteroscopy. Fertility and Sterility 51: 1053–1054

Trimbos-Kemper T C M, Trimbos J V, Van Hall E 1982 Management of infertile patients with unilateral tubal pathology by paradoxical oophorectomy. Fertility and Sterility 37: 623–626

Tulandi T 1997 How can we avoid adhesions after laparoscopic surgery? Current Opinion in Obstetrics and Gynaecology 9: 239–243

Turi A, Garzetti G G 1993 The pattern of melatonin in amenorrhoeic women affected by sterility. Acta European Fertilitalis 24: 71–74

Turner H E, Nagy Z, Gatter K C, Esiri M M, Harris A L, Wass J A 2000 Angiogenesis in pituitary adenomas and the normal pituitary. Journal of Clinical Endocrinology and Metabolism 85: 1159–1162

Ubaldi F, Camus M, Smitz J, Bennink H C, Van Steirteghem A, Devroey P 1996 Premature luteinization in in vitro fertilization cycles using gonadotrophin-releasing hormone agonist (GnRH-a) and recombinant follicle-stimulating hormone (FSH) and GnRH-a and urinary FSH. Fertility and Sterility 66: 275–280

Urman B, Gomel V, McComb P, Lee N 1992 Midtubal occlusion: etiology, management and outcome. Fertility and Sterility 57: 747–750

Valle R 1980 Hysteroscopy and evaluation of female infertility. American Journal of Obstetrics and Gynecology 137: 425–429

Van der Linden P J Q, Kets M, Gimpel J A, Wiegerinck M A H M 1992 Cyclic changes in the concentration of glucose and fructose in human cervical mucus. Fertility and Sterility 57: 573–577

Van Leeuwen J H S, Christiaens G M L, Hoogenraad T U 1991 Recurrent abortion and the diagnosis of Wilson's disease. Obstetrics and Gynecology 78: 547–549

van Noord P A H, Dubas J S, Dorland M, Boersma H, te Velde E 1997 Age at natural menopause in a population-based screening cohort: the role of menarche, fecundity and lifestyle factors. Fertility and Sterility 68: 95–102

van Voorhis B J, Neff T W, Syrop C H, Chapler F K 1994 Primary hypothyroidism associated with mylticystic ovaries and ovarian torsion in an adult. Obstetrics and Gynecology 83: 885–887

Van Zandijcke M, Casselman J 1994 The vanishing pituitary adenoma. Acta Neurologica Belgica 94: 256–258

Vanderwoort C A, Overstreet J W 1995 Effects of glucose and other energy substrates on the hyperactivated motility of macaque sperm and the zona pellucida-induced acrosome reaction. Journal of Andrology 16: 327–333

Vasquez G, Winston R M L, Boeckx W D, Brosens I 1980 Tubal lesions subsequent to sterilization and their relationship to fertility after attempts at reversal. American Journal of Obstetrics and Gynecology 138: 86–92

Velissariou V, Lyberatou E, Antonopoulou E, Polymilis C 1993 Chromosome breakage in individuals with single-cell structural aberrations and habitual abortions. Gynecologic and Obstetric Investigation 36: 71–74

Veneman T F, Beverstock G C, Exalto N, Mollevenger P 1991 Premature menopause because of an inherited deletion of the long arm of the X-chromosome. Fertility and Sterility 55: 631–633

Verdugo P, Lee W I, Halbert S A, Blandau R J, Tam P Y 1980 A stochastic model for oviductal egg transport. Biophysical Journal 29: 257–270

Vermeulen A 2000 Andropause. Maturitas 34: 5–15

Vigil P, Perez A, Neira J, Morales P 1991 Postpartum cervical mucus: biological and rheological properties. Human Reproduction 6: 475–479

Vijayakumar R, Walters W A W 1983 Human luteal tissue prostaglandins, 17β-estradiol, and progesterone in relation to the growth and senescence of the corpus luteum. Fertility and Sterility 39: 298–303

Visness C M, Kennedy K I 1997 The frequency of coitus during breastfeeding. Birth 24: 253–257

Vizza E, Correr S, Muglia U, Marchiolli F, Motta P M 1995 The three-dimensional organization of the smooth musculature in the ampulla of the human fallopian tube: a new morpho-functional model. Human Reproduction 10: 2400–2405

Wade G N, Schneider J E, Li H Y 1996 Control of fertility by metabolic cues. American Journal of Physiology 270 (1 Part 1): E1–E19

Wah P M, Anderson D J, Hill J A 1990 Asymptomatic cervicovaginal leukocytosis in infertile women. Fertility and Sterility 54: 445–450

Wakeley K E, Grendys E C 2000 Reproductive technologies and risk of ovarian cancer. Current Opinion in Obstetrics and Gynaecology 12: 43–47

Wallach E E 1972 The uterine factor in infertility. Fertility and Sterility 23: 138–158

Wallweiner D, Meyer A, Bastert G 1998 Adhesion formation of the parietal and visceral peritoneum: an explanation for the controversy on the use of autologous and alloplastic barriers? Fertility and Sterility 68: 132–137

Walz C, Deprez A, Dupressoir T, Dürst M, Rabreau M, Schlehofer J R 1997 Interaction of human papilloma virus 16 and adeno-associated virus type 2 co-infecting human cervical epithelium. Journal of General Virology 78: 1441–1452

Walz C, Anisi T R, Schlehofer J R, Gissmann L, Schneider A, Müller M 1998 Detection of infectious adeno-associated virus particles in human cervical biopsies. Virology 247: 97–105

Wanerman J, Wolwick R, Brenner S 1986 Segmental absence of the fallopian tube. Fertility and Sterility 46: 525–527

Wang Y, Sharma R K, Falcone J, Goldberg J, Agarwal A 1997 Importance of reactive oxygen species in the peritoneal fluid of women with endometriosis or idiopathic infertility. Fertility and Sterility 68: 826–830

Wansaicheong G K, Ong C L 1998 Intramural tubal polyps — a villain in the shadows? Singapore Medical Journal 39: 97–100

Warburton D, Kline J, Stein Z, Susser M 1980 Monosomy X: a chromosomal anomaly associated with young maternal age. Lancet 1: 167–169

Weber A A, Ziegler C, Belinson J L, Mitchinson A R, Widrich T, Fazio V 1995 Gynecologic history of women with inflammatory bowel disease. Obstetrics and Gynecology 86: 843–847

Weed J C, Carrera A E 1970 Glucose content of cervical mucus. Fertility and Sterility 21: 866–872

Weiner S, Wright K H, Wallach E E 1977 The influence of ovarian denervation and nerve stimulation on ovarian contractions. American Journal of Obstetrics and Gynecology 128: 154–160

Weinstein D, Polishuk W Z 1975 The role of wedge resection of the ovary as a cause of mechanical infertility. Surgery Gynecology and Obstetrics 141: 417–418

Weinstein M, Stark M 1994 Behavioral and biological determinants of fecundability. Annals of the New York Academy of Sciences 709: 128–144

Westendorf R G J, Kirkwood T B L 1998 Human longevity at the cost of reproductive success. Nature 396: 743–746

Weström L, Eschenbach D, 1999 Pelvic inflammatory disease. In: Holmes K K, Sparling P F, Mårdh P-A et al (eds) Sexually transmitted diseases, 3rd edn. McGraw-Hill, New York, p 783

Wiczyk H P, Grow D R, Adams L A, O'Shea D L, Reece M T 1998 Pelvic adhesions contain sex steroid receptors and produce angiogenesis factors. Fertility and Sterility 69: 511–516

Wildt L, Kissler S, Licht P, Becker W 1998 Sperm transport in the human female genital tract and its modulation by hysterosalpingo-scintigraphy, hysterosonography, electrohysterography and Doppler sonography. Human Reproduction Update 4: 655–666

Wilhelmsson L, Lindblom B 1980 Adrenergic responses of the various smooth muscle layers at the human uterotubal junction. Fertility and Sterility 33: 280–282

Winkler B, Crum C P 1987 Chlamydia trachomatis infection of the female genital tract: pathogenetic and clinicopathologic correlations. Pathology Annual 22(1): 193–223

Witkin S S 1988 Production of interferon gamma by lymphocytes exposed to antibody-coated spermatozoa: a mechanism for sperm antibody production in females. Fertility and Sterility 50: 498–502

Wolf J P, DeAlmeida M, Ducot B, Rodrigues D, Jouannet P 1995 High levels of sperm-associated antibodies impair human sperm-oolemma interaction after subzonal insemination. Fertility and Sterility 63: 584–590

Wong W Y, Thomas C M G, Merkkus J M W M, Zielhuis G A, Steegers-Theunissen R P M 2000 Male factor subfertility: possible causes and impact of nutritional factors. Fertility and Sterility 73: 435–442

Wray H L, Freeman M V R, Ming P M L 1981 Pregnancy in the Turner syndrome with only 45, X chromosome constitution. Fertility and Sterility 35: 509–514

Wright G, Tucker M J, Morton P C, Sweltzer-Yoder C L, Smith S E 1998 Micromanipulation in assisted reproduction: a review of current technology. Current Opinion in Obstetrics and Gynaecology 10: 221–226

Yablonski M, Sarge T, Wild R A 1990 Subtle variations in tubal anatomy in infertile women. Fertility and Sterility 54: 455–458

Yaffe H, Beyth J, Reinhartz T, Levi J 1980 Foreign body granulomas in peritubal and periovarian adhesions: a possible cause for unsuccessful reconstructive surgery in infertility. Fertility and Sterility 33: 277–279

Yaginuma T 1979 Progress and therapy of stress amenorrhea. Fertility and Sterility 32: 36–39

Yao Y-Q, Ho P-C, Yeung WS-B 1999 Effects of human oviductal cell coculture on various functional parameters of human spermatozoa. Fertility and Sterility 71: 232–239

Yao Y-Q, Ho P-C, Yeung WS-B 2000 Effects of human follicular fluid on the capacitation and motility of human spermatozoa. Fertility and Sterility 73: 680–686

Yasim N J M, Mascie-Taylor C G 1997 Consanguinity and its relationships to differential fertility and mortality in the Koha: a tribal population of Andra Pradesh. Journal of Biosocial Sciences 29: 171–180

Yazigi R A, Quintero C H, Salameh W A 1997 Prolactin disorders. Fertility and Sterility 67: 215–222

Yoon T K, Sung H R, Kang H G, Cha S H, Lee C N, Cha K Y 1999 Laparoscopic tubal anastomosis: fertility outcome in 202 cases. Fertility and Sterility 72: 1121–1126

Yoshimura Y, Wallach E E 1987 Studies of the mechanisms of mammalian ovulation. Fertility and Sterility 47: 22–34

Young W F, Scheithauer B W, Kovacs K T, Horvath E, Davis D H, Randall R V 1996 Gonadotropin adenoma of the pituitary gland: a clinicopathologic analysis of 100 cases. Mayo Clinical Proceedings 71: 649–656

Younis J S, Haddad S, Matilsky M, Ben-Ami M 1998 Premature luteinization: could it be an early manifestation of low ovarian reserve. Fertility and Sterility 69: 461–465

Zaidi J, Jurkovic D, Campbell S, Collins W, McGregor A, Tan S L 1995 Luteinized unruptured follicle: morphology, endocrine function and blood flow during the menstrual cycle. Human Reproduction 10: 14–19

Zaino R J 1996 Infertility and dysfunctional bleeding associated with hormonal imbalance. In: Interpretation of endometrial biopsies and curettings. Lippincott-Raven, Philadelphia, p 125

Zana J, Thomas D, Muffat-Joly M et al 1990 An experimental model for salpingitis due to Chlamydia trachomatis and residual tubal infertility in the mouse. Human Reproduction 5: 274–278

Zegers-Hochschild F, Fernandez E, MacKenna A, Fabres C, Altieri E, Lopez T 1995 The empty follicle syndrome: a pharmaceutical industry syndrome. Human Reproduction 10: 2262–2265

Zhu J, Guos Z, Beggs A H et al 1996 Microsatellite instability analysis in primary human brain tumors. Oncogene 12: 1417–1423

Zinamen M et al 1989 The physiology of sperm recovered from the human cervix: acrosomal status and response to inducers of the acrosome reaction. Biology of Reproduction 41: 790–797

31

Ectopic pregnancy

H. Fox

Introduction   1045

Incidence   1045

Demography   1046

Aetiology and pathogenesis   1046
Tubal factors   1046
Extratubal factors   1049
Cause of increasing incidence   1051

Tubal pregnancy   1051
Implantation and placentation in the tube   1051
Morphology of placental villi in tubal pregnancy   1053
Immunological and immunohistochemical features of
   trophoblast in tubal pregnancy   1055
Tubal response to pregnancy   1055
Uterine response to tubal pregnancy   1056
Natural history of tubal pregnancies   1058
Pathological findings   1059
Effects and complications of treatment   1060

Ovarian pregnancy   1061

Cervical pregnancy   1062

Abdominal pregnancy   1062

Post-hysterectomy pregnancy   1063

INTRODUCTION

An ectopic pregnancy is one in which the conceptus implants either outside the uterus or in an abnormal position within the uterus. In practice, between 95 and 98% of ectopic pregnancies occur in the Fallopian tube, other sites, in probable descending order of frequency, being the ovary, cervix and abdominal cavity with occasional instances being reported in such exotic locations as the vagina, liver or spleen.

Studies of the incidence, epidemiology and aetiology of ectopic gestation almost invariably consider all varieties of ectopic implantation as a single entity and this practice will, of necessity, be followed in this chapter even though it is recognised that this 'blunderbuss' approach may well conceal subtle differences in the aetiological factors which are of particular importance for each different site.

INCIDENCE

The incidence of ectopic pregnancies within any given institution or centre is commonly expressed as a proportion of the number of live births, e.g. from 1 ectopic pregnancy per 32 live births to 1 ectopic pregnancy per 300 live births (Macafee 1982; Weinstein et al 1983). Figures such as these do not, however, yield any valid information about the proportion of conceptions which implant ectopically for they take no account of those pregnancies which are terminated by either miscarriage or medical intervention (Beral 1975; Cuckle & Murray 1997).

Optimally the incidence of ectopic gestation should be defined in terms of the population at risk and the incidence in any given area or country should be quoted as the number of ectopic pregnancies per 100 000 women in the population aged between 14 and 44 years (Barnes et al 1983; Cuckle & Murray 1997). Community based data of this type have rarely been reported but nevertheless it is clear that there has been, over the last two or three decades, at least a doubling, and in some areas a trebling or quadrupling, of the incidence of tubal pregnancies (Chow et al 1987; Drife 1990a; Stabile & Grudzinskas 1990; Doyle et al 1991; Cartwright 1993; Goldner et al 1993), to the extent that the usage of the term 'epidemic' (Weinstein et al 1983; Coupet 1989; Maymon et al 1992) does not appear unduly hyperbolic. There is some evidence that the incidence is now stabilising at a plateau (Centers for Disease Control 1992; Rajkhowa et al 2000) or even, in some areas, decreasing (Kamwendo et al 2000) but the level of this plateau remains disturbingly high, probably at between 14 and 20 per 1000 reported pregnancies in North America and Western Europe.

DEMOGRAPHY

It is usually stated that ectopic pregnancies occur more commonly in urban than in rural populations, are encountered most often in women of low socioeconomic status and occur more frequently in black than in white women (Kallenberger et al 1978; Helvacioglu et al 1979; Gonzalez & Waxman 1981; Goldner et al 1993; Zhang et al 1994). These factors are, rather obviously, interrelated but there has been no real attempt to determine which is the key one or whether these social and ethnic differences are independent of confounding factors, such as the incidence of pelvic inflammatory disease or the rate of cigarette smoking.

The increased frequency of ectopic pregnancy in women of African descent in North America mirrors the high incidence of this condition in the West Indies and in many African countries (Douglas 1963; Van Iddekinge 1972; Dow et al 1975; Baffoe & Nkyekyer 1999) and it is of note that in Trinidad ectopic gestations occur much more frequently in women of African descent than in those of Indian origin (Daisley 1989). Any assumption that international variations in the incidence of ectopic pregnancy are related principally to the proportion of the population that are of African origin is, however, dispelled by the high incidence of this condition in Spain (Cagliero 1961) and, most strikingly, in Greenland (Johnsen et al 1990); there is, interestingly and in contrast, an unusually low incidence of ectopic pregnancy in Malaysia (Sambhi 1967) and a relatively low incidence in both Nigeria (Makinde & Ogguniyi 1990) and Ethiopia (Yoseph 1990).

The incidence of ectopic pregnancy increases with advancing maternal age (Beral 1975; Westrom et al 1981; Rubin et al 1983; Skjeldestad & Backe 1990; Doyle et al 1991; Goldner et al 1993; Cuckle & Murray 1997), the highest incidence being in women aged between 35 and 44 years. In view of this age distribution it is not surprising that most women suffering an ectopic gestation are parous, the highest incidence being in those having two or three children (Hlavin et al 1978; De Cherney et al 1981a; Skjeldstad et al 1997). The reported proportion of primigravida amongst women with an ectopic pregnancy has ranged from 11 to 32% (Johnson 1952; Kleiner & Roberts 1967; Franklin et al 1973; Helvacioglu et al 1979; Randall 1983)

with the figure, in most series, being towards the lower, rather than the higher, extreme of this range.

Despite the fact that women with an ectopic gestation are generally parous, many have a history of diminished reproductive capacity. The incidence of antecedent infertility has been quoted as being between 19 and 37% (Swolin & Fall 1972; Hughes 1980; Li et al 1990; Parazzini et al 1992) but these figures do not adequately take into account the rather high frequency of one child infertility, or the incidence of three or more years preceding infertility, often either unrecognised or not complained of, in multiparous women. If all these patients are grouped together the incidence of antecedent infertility in patients with an ectopic pregnancy is very high, probably between 55 and 80% (Bobrow & Bell 1962; Tancer et al 1981). It should be noted that infertility persists as a strong independent risk factor for ectopic pregnancy even after elimination of confounding factors such as pelvic inflammatory disease, anovulation, drug therapy and pelvic surgery (Marchbanks et al 1988; Coulam & Wells 1992; Ankum et al 1996). Furthermore, a high proportion of patients have suffered one or more spontaneous miscarriages (Honoré 1978; Hughes 1980; Fedele et al 1989; Coulam et al 1989), many give a history of pelvic inflammatory disease (see later) and a significant proportion, between 6 and 16% have had a previous ectopic pregnancy (De Cherney et al 1981; Alsuleiman & Grimes 1982; Coste et al 1991; Nlome-Nzear et al 1992).

The overall picture which emerges is that the women most likely to have an ectopic pregnancy are those who are relatively elderly and who, despite being parous, have a poor reproductive history, women of African descent being particularly at risk.

AETIOLOGY AND PATHOGENESIS

It is certain that no single factor is responsible for all ectopic gestations and probable that most cases are multifactorial in origin. Nevertheless each proposed aetiological factor is dealt with here independently and it will be appreciated that most apply principally, and often only, to tubal pregnancies though some are of equal importance in ovarian gestations.

TUBAL FACTORS

Congenital abnormalities

A number of congenital abnormalities of the tube have been implicated in the causation of tubal pregnancy: these include diverticula, accessory ostia, hypoplasia and focal aplasia (Oscakina-Rojdestvenskaia 1938; Szlachter & Weiss 1979; Beyth & Kopolovic 1982) but claims that such abnormalities account for approximately 20% of tubal gestations (Oscakina-Rojdestvenskaia 1938) would be generally considered as exaggerated.

The incidence and significance of congenital tubal diverticula in tubal pregnancies is a matter of some dispute. Niles & Clark (1969) found such lesions to be extremely rare in tubes harbouring a gestation but Persaud (1970) is often quoted as having demonstrated that diverticula are present in 49% of gravid tubes: it is in fact clear that the vast majority of the lesions described by Persaud were examples of salpingitis isthmica nodosa and were not spatially related to the site of implantation.

Women who have been prenatally exposed to diethylstilboestrol suffer a considerable excess of ectopic pregnancies (Barnes et al 1980; Schmidt et al 1980; Pons et al 1988; Ankum et al 1996) and this may be related to the fact that a proportion of such women have foreshortened, convoluted, 'withered' tubes with minimal fimbrial tissue and a pin-hole os (De Cherney et al 1981b).

Tubal neoplasms

These are commonly listed as a possible cause of an ectopic pregnancy but, in reality, there have been only a few recorded instances of a tubal gestation complicating either an intrinsic tubal neoplasm or an extrinsic paraovarian tumour Honoré & Korn 1976; Casapeto et al 1978; Gray et al 1983; Kutteh & Albert 1991).

Salpingitis isthmica nodosa

There is a probable, though not fully proven, association between this condition and ectopic pregnancy (Honoré 1978; Green & Kott 1989; Saracoglu et al 1992). Gonzalez & Waxman (1981), studying a largely black population, noted salpingitis isthmica nodosa in 9.9% of patients with an ectopic pregnancy but in our own series in Manchester, in which a careful search was made for this lesion, it was found in only 3.3% of gravid tubes (Randall 1983). Persaud (1970) and Majmudar et al (1983) have, by contrast, quoted incidences of 49% and 57%, respectively, of salpingitis isthmica nodosa in tubal pregnancies. Two points should be noted, however, about these latter studies: firstly, the populations studied were almost entirely black and, secondly, both have broadened the concept of salpingitis isthmica nodosa in that over a third of the diverticular lesions were ampullary rather than isthmic and were not necessarily associated with visible nodularity. There is a consensus that salpingitis isthmica nodosa is found unduly commonly in black women but there would be less agreement as to whether all the lesions described in these two studies as salpingitis isthmica nodosa truly merit this designation.

Even the strongest proponents of the association between salpingitis isthmica nodosa and tubal pregnancy admit that implantation of the conceptus is rarely into a diverticulum in such cases and have noted the discrepancy between the site of the diverticula and that of tubal pregnancy. It has been suggested that the hypertrophied muscle which is a characteristic feature of salpingitis isthmica nodosa may either undergo spasm and thus obstruct the tubal lumen or, by its presence, disturb tubal motility.

Tubal endometriosis

Endometriosis of the tube is often cited as a risk factor for tubal pregnancy, it being argued that endometrial tissue in this site confers an increased 'receptivity' of the tube for a fertilised ovum. Nevertheless, Gonzalez & Waxman (1981) found endometriosis in only 1.2% of gravid tubes, a figure virtually identical to that (1.1%) in our own series (Randall 1983) and very similar to the incidence (1.5%) noted by Kleiner & Roberts (1967). Women with endometriosis do not, as a group, have any excess risk of suffering an ectopic gestation (Marchbanks et al 1988).

Tubal sterilisation

A significant proportion, variously estimated at between 10 and 15%, of pregnancies which occur after a failed tubal sterilisation are ectopic (Chakravarti & Shardlow 1975; Tatum & Schmidt 1977; Wright & Stadel 1981; WHO 1985; Makar et al 1990; Falfoul et al 1993; Peterson et al 1997). The proportion of pregnancies which are ectopic varies with the type of procedure employed being 4.4% after clipping, 19.5% after ligation, 43–51% following laparoscopic diathermy and 60% after application of Falope rings (Tatum & Schmidt 1977). If laparoscopic diathermy is accompanied by tubal transection the proportion of ectopic pregnancies falls to 14.5% (McCausland 1982) whilst if Haulker clips are used instead of Falope rings only 4.4% of subsequent gestations are ectopically sited (Hughes 1980). It is possible that these differing rates of ectopic pregnancy following different forms of tubal sterilisation are simply a reflection, in part at least, of the efficiency of each particular technique in preventing *intrauterine* pregnancies (Chow et al 1987). It has been claimed that there is a particularly high risk of later ectopic implantation if sterilisation is performed during the postpartum or postabortal period (Sivanesaratnam & Ng 1975; Honoré & O'Hara 1978) but in more recent carefully controlled studies it has been shown that postpartum sterilisation is associated with a lower risk of subsequent tubal gestation than is interval sterilization (Holt et al 1991).

The actual mechanisms by which tubal implantation occurs following tubal sterilisation are somewhat uncertain but both recanalisation and the formation of tuboperitoneal fistulas, of sufficient size to allow for the passage of a sperm but not of an embryo, have been proposed as possible factors (Chakravarti & Shardlow 1975; McCausland 1982). The ability of tubal epithelium to recanalise an occluded segment has not, however, been conclusively established.

With the increasing number of women being subjected to tubal sterilisation this factor is of increasing importance in the aetiology of ectopic pregnancy. Badawy et al (1979) noted that in the United States between 1947 and 1967 only 0.6% of patients with an ectopic pregnancy had been previously sterilised but that this proportion had risen to 4.2% by 1972 and to 7% by 1977. In Canada the proportion of patients who had been previously sterilised was 7.6% in a study of cases of tubal pregnancy reported in 1991 (Greisman 1991).

It should be noted that although a greater proportion of pregnancies after failed sterilisation are ectopic, tubal sterilisation actually decreases the absolute risk of ectopic implantations and diminishes an individual woman's risk of future ectopic pregnancy when compared with all women who have not undergone sterilisation or women using no contraceptives (de Stefano et al 1982; WHO 1985; Kjer & Knudsen 1989).

Reconstructive tubal surgery

Approximately 5–10% of pregnancies which follow reconstructive operations, of all types and including reversal of sterilisation, on the tube are ectopically sited (Rock et al 1979; Hulka & Halme 1988; Singhal et al 1991; Tomazevic & Ribic-Pucelj 1992); the incidence of tubal pregnancy is strikingly high after repeated tuboplasties (Lauritsen et al 1982).

Tubal deciliation

Vasquez et al (1983) have shown, with the aid of the scanning electronmicroscope, a marked deficiency of epithelial cilia in the tubes of women currently suffering from, or having a history of, a tubal pregnancy. They suggest that diminished ampullary cilial action lessens the efficiency of ovum transport and that delayed entry into the isthmus will result in tubal implantation.

Granulomatous salpingitis

Women with tubal tuberculosis rarely conceive but patients treated for this disease have a high risk of an ectopic pregnancy (Halbrecht 1957; Varela-Nunez 1961) this being attributed to residual tubal scarring with narrowing and distortion of the lumen.

Bilharzial salpingitis, relatively common in some areas of the world, results in marked tubal deformity and is associated with a significant risk of an ectopic gestation (Rosen & Kim 1974; Okonofua et al 1990; Picaud et al 1990; Ville et al 1991a).

Non-granulomatous salpingitis

It is usually taken as axiomatic that pelvic inflammatory disease and tubal infection are major risk factors for tubal

pregnancy, it being assumed that postinflammatory damage, in the form of scarring together with deciliation and plical fusion, predisposes to arrest of the fertilised ovum in the tube. It has, however, been rather difficult to establish the true rôle of tubal inflammatory disease in the aetiology of tubal pregnancy for the following reasons:

1. In most studies of ectopic pregnancy there has been a very poor correlation between a history of pelvic inflammatory disease, macroscopic evidence of postinflammatory damage and histological evidence of a tubal inflammatory process (Kleiner & Roberts 1967; Helvacioglu et al 1979; Gonzalez & Waxman 1981; Cumming et al 1988).
2. Amongst women with a tubal pregnancy the reported incidence of a history of previous pelvic inflammatory disease has varied from 6% to 58%, that of macroscopically evident postinflammatory damage from 21% to 72% and that of histologically proven salpingitis from 18% to 55% (Bone & Greene 1961; Kleiner & Roberts 1967; Brenner et al 1975; Helvacioglu et al 1979; Gonzalez & Waxman 1981; Alsuleiman & Grimes 1982; Cole & Corlett 1982; Weinstein et al 1983; Krantz et al 1990).
3. Case-control studies showing an association between ectopic pregnancy and a history of either pelvic inflammatory disease or sexually transmitted disease (World Health Organization 1985; Coste et al 1991) have used control groups consisting of women with normal pregnancies; this latter group may have been less likely than the general population to have had pelvic infections since their fertility was unimpaired.

Quite apart from the methodological difficulties encountered in trying to prove an association between tubal inflammatory disease and ectopic pregnancy it has to be pointed out that historically there has been only a weak association between the incidences of hospitalisation for ectopic gestations and pelvic inflammatory disease (Beral 1975; Westrom et al 1981; Shiono et al 1982) and that during a decade when, in the United States, there was a huge increase in the incidence of tubal pregnancies the annual rate of pelvic inflammatory disease increased only moderately (Chow et al 1987). However, by contrast, in two recent studies it was shown that a reduced incidence of pelvic inflammatory disease correlated with a decrease in the number of ectopic pregnancies (Bjartling et al 2000; Kamwendo et al 2000).

Despite these discrepancies and inconsistencies it remains true that inflammation is present in areas remote from the implantation site in nearly 40% of tubes containing an ectopic gestation (Bone & Greene 1961; Randall 1983). Even, however, if it is accepted that about 40% of tubes in which a conceptus is lodged show evidence of salpingitis this does not, in itself, prove an association unless the incidence of tubal inflammation in the overall population of women of reproductive age is known. This particular difficulty has, to some extent, been overcome by a prospective cohort study which has shown that women with laparoscopically proven salpingitis have a much greater risk of eventually having an ectopic gestation than do those with laparoscopically normal tubes (Westrom 1975; 1985; Westrom et al 1992).

It is now recognised that *Chlamydia trachomatis* is the most important cause of pelvic inflammatory disease and that infection of this type is often asymptomatic. It is therefore of particular note that there has been, during the last decade, a considerable number of reports that women who are seropositive for antibodies to *Chlamydia* have a markedly increased risk of ectopic pregnancy and that patients with such antibodies form a high proportion (40–50%) of cases of tubal pregnancy (Chow et al 1990; De Muylder et al 1990; Hodgson et al 1990; Kihlstrom et al 1990; Miettenen et al 1990; Sherman et al 1990; Coste et al 1991; Picaud et al 1991; Ville et al 1991b; Chrysostomou et al 1992). The particular importance of this observation, which has admittedly not been totally unanimous (Phillips et al 1992), is that it circumvents the discrepancies between clinical history and pathological findings and provides an objective criterion of past or current tubal infection. In fact, plasma cell infiltration of tubes harbouring a gestation in women seropositive for Chlamydia is not always present (Brunham et al 1992) whilst cultures of the tube for the organism are usually negative (Berenson et al 1991; Neiger & Croom 1991; Maccato et al 1992) and chlamydial DNA was not detected by the polymerase chain reaction in an admittedly small study of tubes harbouring a gestation (Osser & Persson 1992). Despite these caveats it has been shown that a decrease in the incidence of chlamydial infection, as diagnosed by cervical cultures, is accompanied by a decline in the incidence of ectopic pregnancies (Egger et al 1998).

Women with antibodies to *Mycoplasma hominis* also are at increased risk of an ectopic gestation (Miettenen et al 1990) but the proportion of women with a tubal pregnancy who are seropositive for antibodies to *Neisseria gonorrhoea* is low (Miettenen et al 1990; Ville et al 1991b).

EXTRATUBAL FACTORS

Ovulatory dysfunction

Iffy (1963) noted that the fetus in a tubal gestation often appeared to be three to four weeks older than would be expected from the period of amenorrhoea, this suggesting that conception had actually occurred before the bleeding episode which the patient considered as her last menstrual period. He therefore proposed that a conception leading to a tubal pregnancy occurred during a cycle in which there was delayed ovulation and a short, inadequate luteal phase. Hence, at the time of corpus luteum decay the conceptus would not have reached the stage when it was producing sufficient human chorionic gonadotrophin to prevent luteolysis and subsequent menstruation. During the subsequent menstrual bleeding the fertilised ovum could be arrested in its transit through the tube by a reflux of menstrual blood or, if it had already reached the uterine cavity, flushed back into the tube by menstrual regurgitation. Iffy's hypothesis is supported by the frequency, between 10 and 50% of cases, with which the corpus luteum of pregnancy is on the opposite side to a tube containing a gestation (Kleiner & Roberts 1967; Honoré 1978; Kitchin et al 1979; Pauerstein et al 1986) and by the fact that ectopic pregnancy is virtually confined to humans and those primates which menstruate (McElin & Iffy 1976).

The presence of a corpus luteum of pregnancy in the gonad contralateral to the gravid tube could, of course, also be due to transuterine migration of the fertilised ovum into the opposite tube (Honoré 1978).

Contraceptive factors

Intrauterine contraceptive device

If a pregnancy occurs in a woman wearing an intrauterine contraceptive device (IUCD) it will be ectopically sited in about 4–8% of cases, an incidence much in excess of that found in non-contraceptive users (Tatum & Schmidt 1977; Vessey et al 1979): furthermore, about 10% of the ectopic pregnancies will be ovarian (Herbertsson et al 1987; Sandvei et al 1987). It should not, however, be thought that IUCDs actually *cause* ectopic implantation for the absolute risk of an ectopic pregnancy is, with one exception, markedly reduced in women wearing an IUCD relative to that for women using no contraception (Ory 1981; Sivin 1991; Skjeldestad 1997): the one exception to this general rule are those devices which are progesterone coated and releasing 65 micrograms, or more, of progesterone per day (Sivin 1991).

The cause of the high incidence of ectopic pregnancies in IUCD users is far from being fully understood. It is tempting to attribute the high proportion of such pregnancies to IUCD-induced tubal inflammation but this appears unlikely as there is now wide, though perhaps not universal, agreement that, with the exception of those who had used a Dalkon shield, former IUCD wearers are not at any significantly increased risk of suffering a tubal pregnancy (Vessey et al 1979; WHO 1985; Chow et al 1986; Marchbanks et al 1988; Edelman & Van-Os 1990; Pouly et al 1991a,b; Randic & Haller 1992): further, tubal damage could not account for the high proportion of ovarian pregnancies. A more plausible explanation is that IUCDs are much more effective in inhibiting uterine implantation than they are in inhibiting either tubal or ovarian implantation (Lehfeldt et al 1970). A further possibility is that IUCDs reduce the number of ciliated cells in the tube and thus hamper ovum transport (Vasquez et al 1983; Wollen et al 1984), a view supported by the much lower incidence of ectopic gestations in the proximal third of the tube in IUCD users than in non-users (WHO 1985; Pouly et al 1991 a,b).

Oral steroid contraception

Prior use of combined oral steroid contraception is not associated with either an excess or a deficit of ectopic pregnancies (Vessey et al 1979) and there is no tendency for pregnancies occurring in current users of combined oral steroid contraceptives to be ectopically sited (Vessey et al 1976, 1979); indeed, as would perhaps be expected, combined oral contraceptive usage reduces the absolute risk of an ectopic pregnancy in any individual woman (WHO 1985; Drife 1990b), largely by preventing pregnancy in the first place. An increased incidence of tubal gestation has, however, been noted in women who became pregnant whilst using low-dose progestagen-only oral contraception (Liukko & Erkkola 1976; Tatum & Schmidt 1977), possibly because of the inhibitory effect of progesterone on tubal peristalsis.

Barrier contraception

Condom usage is associated with a reduced risk of ectopic pregnancy (Li et al 1990), this probably being due to the decreased risk of pelvic inflammatory disease.

Ovulatory agents

It has been claimed that pregnancies resulting from ovulation induction by either clomiphene or gonadotrophins are more likely to be ectopic than are those derived from a spontaneous ovulation (Chow et al 1987), though Grab et al (1992) found that this risk is confined to the use of gonadotrophins. The reasons for this association are far from clear for many of the ectopic pregnancies have occurred in patients without any evidence of pelvic disease and with normal hysterosalpingograms (Cartwright 1993).

Prior pregnancy loss

There has been much debate in the past as to whether or not previous pregnancy loss, either spontaneous or induced, is a risk factor for ectopic pregnancy. The meta-analysis of Ankum et al (1996) and the subsequent studies of Skjeldestad et al (1997) and Atrash et al (1997) have, however, resolved this dispute by clearly showing that there is either no increase or, at most, only a very slight increase in the risk of ectopic pregnancy in women who had suffered a previous pregnancy loss whether this

was spontaneous or induced, this negative effect also extending to multiple miscarriages.

Abdominal surgery

The role of previous abdominal surgery, particularly of appendicectomy, as a risk factor for ectopic pregnancy has been, and indeed still is, the subject of a contradictory literature. Thus in the meta-analysis of Ankum et al (1996) previous abdominal surgery was associated with only a slightly increased risk of tubal gestation but in a subsequent study (Bastianelli et al 1998) prior abdominal surgery was found to be associated with a doubling of the risk of ectopic pregnancy. In a later review Urbach & Cohen (1999) could not confirm that perforation of the appendix was associated with a subsequently increased risk of ectopic pregnancy.

Assisted reproduction

Historically, a quite high proportion of pregnancies (between 2 and 10%) resulting from assisted reproductive techniques occurred in the tube (Yuzpe et al 1989; Formigli et al 1990; Jansen et al 1990; Dubuisson et al 1991; Herman et al 1990; Karande et al 1991; Nygren et al 1991; Wennerholm et al 1991; Yang et al 1992), the incidence being somewhat higher with in vitro fertilisation and embryo transfer (IVF) than with gamete intra-Fallopian transfer (GIFT). Currently, the incidence of tubal gestations is still higher than in unassisted pregnancies (Koudstaal et al 1999; Abusheikha et al 2000) but is progressively declining (Bachelot et al 1996). Amongst women undergoing IVF the incidence of ectopic gestation is much higher in those with tubal infertility than in those who are infertile from other causes (Lesny et al 1999). A possible explanation for this is that many transferred embryos reflux into the tube and are then later regurgitated to the uterus: it has been suggested that the embryos may fail to be returned to the uterus if there is tubal dysfunction (Cartwright 1993).

Cigarette smoking

A meta-analysis by Ankum et al (1996) showed that women who currently smoke, or had ever smoked, cigarettes are at slightly increased risk of a tubal gestation. Subsequent studies have, however, laid greater stress on cigarette smoking as an independent dose-related risk factor for ectopic pregnancy (Saraiya et al 1998; Bastianelli et al 1998; Bouyer et al 1998; Castles et al 1999). Proffered explanations for the association between smoking and ectopic gestation include impaired tubal motility, decreased ciliary action and abnormal blastocyst implantation, all possibly related to the reduced oestrogen levels found in smokers (Cartwright 1993).

Abnormal conceptus

It has intermittently been suggested that an abnormal conceptus is more likely to implant in the tube than is a normal one (Carr 1969; Emmrich & Kopping 1981). Phillipe et al (1970) and Elias et al (1981) examined the chromosomal constitution of ectopic embryos, the latter combining their results with those of two other studies (Busch & Benirschke 1974; Poland et al 1976): it was clearly shown that ectopic conceptuses do not have a higher frequency of chromosomal abnormalities than do intrauterine embryos of comparable gestational age. Nevertheless flow cytometric analysis of tissue from tubal conceptuses has shown a surprisingly high incidence of fetal aneuploidy (Karikoski et al 1993), a finding that awaits further investigation.

CAUSE OF INCREASING INCIDENCE

The increased incidence of ectopic pregnancy during the last three decades is usually attributed principally to an increased incidence of sexually transmitted disease and the introduction of the IUCD. Other factors do, however, need to be considered such as the fact that attempts to preserve, or restore, fertility may well increase the incidence of ectopic gestations; thus antibiotic treatment of salpingitis will result in a scarred, rather than a blocked, tube, as will many instances of tubal surgery whilst the use of ovulatory agents and of assisted reproductive techniques also increase the risk of an ectopic pregnancy. An increased ability to diagnose ectopic pregnancy at an early stage in its evolution probably also plays a rôle in the apparent increased incidence of tubal pregnancies (Ong & Wingfield 1999). Quite apart from these iatrogenic factors is the change in lifestyle amongst many women: increased cigarette smoking will increase the incidence of ectopic pregnancies whilst it has been suggested that both dieting and exercise may have a similar effect (James 1989), the common factor linking these activities being reduced oestrogen levels with possible consequent impairment in tubal motility. None of these factors appears, however, to afford a complete answer and it has been suggested that the increasing incidence of ectopic pregnancies is largely a cohort phenomenon (Makinen 1989; Makinen et al 1998)

TUBAL PREGNANCY

Over 50% of tubal pregnancies are situated in the ampulla whilst approximately 20% occur in the isthmus: around 12% are fimbrial whilst about 10% are interstitial. The pregnancy is usually unilateral and singleton but bilateral tubal pregnancies (Falk & Lackritz 1977; Robertson 1980; Sherman et al 1991; Adair et al 1994; Abramovici et al 1995; Marcovici & Scoccia 1997; De Graaf & Demetroulis 1997) and twins within a single tube (Storch & Petrie 1976; Misra et al 1992) can occur, albeit rarely. In bilateral tubal pregnancies the two fetuses may be of the same or different age (Hakim-Elahi 1965) whilst tubal twin pregnancies, though usually monozygotic, may be dizygotic (Neuman et al 1990). Triplet tubal pregnancies have been recorded (Forbes & Natale 1968; Singhal & Chin 1992).

Combined tubal and intrauterine (heterotopic) pregnancies are distinctly uncommon, though probably less rare than was previously thought (Keskes et al 1989). Such pregnancies have been noted with increased frequency after administration of ovulatory agents (Eckshtein et al 1978; Glassner et al 1990; Dietz et al 1993) and after both IVF and GIFT (Dimitry et al 1990; Molloy et al 1990; Dor et al 1991; Lewin et al 1991; Rizk et al 1991; Tanbo et al 1991; Chang et al 1992; Goldman et al 1992; Svare et al 1993; Johnson et al 1998; Diallo et al 2000): whether this is simply a reflection of the high incidence of multiple gestations following these procedures is a moot point.

IMPLANTATION AND PLACENTATION IN THE TUBE

Implantation in the tube may be fimbrial, plical, mural or muro-plical (Schumann 1921). In a plical implantation the conceptus implants on the tip of a mucosal fold and although it may subsequently embed into the plical tissues it does not establish contact with the wall of the tube (Fig. 31.1). This is a rare form of tubal implantation and, indeed, doubts have been expressed as to its existence: scepticism on this point has, however, been dispelled by Falk et al (1975) who described and fully illustrated an undoubted example of plical implantation and this form of implantation was noted in 11% of our cases (Randall et al 1987).

Mural implantation occurs when the conceptus is in direct contact with the lumenal surface of the tubal wall between the plicae whilst in a muro-plical implantation the fertilised ovum embeds between adjacent plical folds and trophoblast invades both the plicae and the tubal wall. Fimbrial implantation occurs in about 7% of cases and in these it may be difficult to know whether one is dealing with a tubal or an ovarian pregnancy, it not uncommonly being necessary to resort to the somewhat noncommittal and unsatisfactory diagnosis of 'tubo-ovarian' pregnancy.

In mural implantations the process is very similar to that which occurs in an intrauterine gestation for the conceptus penetrates the tubal mucosa and becomes embedded in the tissues of the tubal wall. In a plical implantation the situation is different for here there is, of course, little volume of tissue in which the conceptus can embed and early rupture of the involved plical fold, usually after its almost complete replacement by trophoblast, is the rule. It is not known if, after implantation, the trophoblast becomes orientated at one pole of the

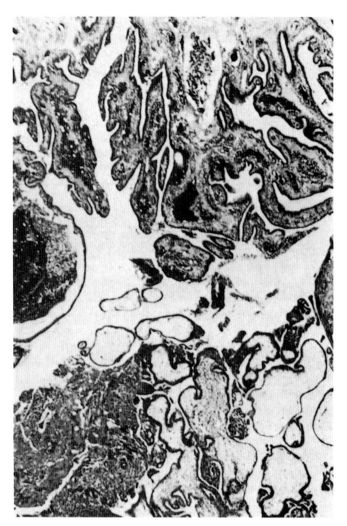

Fig. 31.1 Plical implantation in the tube.

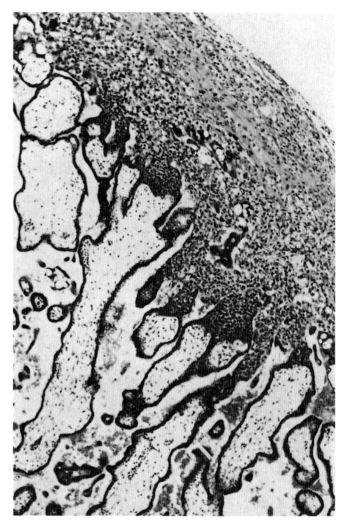

Fig. 31.2 Tubal mural implantation. Anchoring villi, cytotrophoblastic cell columns and trophoblastic shell are all apparent.

conceptus to form a definitive placenta: certainly in some tubal pregnancies the trophoblast does appear to penetrate a localised area of the tubal wall to form an approximation of a discoid placenta but in most cases all the trophoblast surrounding the blastocyst develops to form a circumferential placental attachment, one almost akin to a placenta membranacea in an intrauterine pregnancy.

Following implantation the two layers of trophoblast, the inner cytotrophoblast and the outer syncytiotrophoblast, can be identified and if implantation has occurred into a site which offers a sufficient area for placentation to occur, as in mural and muro-plical implantations, then the process of placentation will ensue in a manner which is virtually identical to that occurring in an intrauterine site (Randall et al 1987). Thus, anchoring villi, cytotrophoblastic cell columns and a trophoblastic shell all develop (Fig. 31.2) and extravillous cytotrophoblast streams out from the tips of the cytotrophoblastic cell columns to infiltrate, and extensively colonise, the adjacent tubal tissues. Extravillous interstitial trophoblast, sometimes known as intermediate trophoblast, grows into the mural tissue

in a fashion akin to that seen in the penetration of the decidua and inner myometrium in an intrauterine gestation (Fig. 31.3) and infiltrates between the muscle cells of the tubal wall as it does between the myometrial fibres (Fig. 31.4). The invading interstitial cytotrophoblast fans out towards the serosal surface, not infrequently penetrating the full thickness of the muscular layer to reach the subserosa. There may be relatively little lateral spread of these interstitial cytotrophoblastic cells but in some tubes there is a considerable spread laterally, in the longitudinal axis of the tube, either in the muscle coat (Fig. 31.5) or in the subserosa. Overall, the degree and extent of invasion of the muscle coat of the tube is often more exuberant than is the similar invasion of the myometrium in an intrauterine pregnancy and this may be indicative of an absence of regulating factors at this site. Very few multinucleated cells are seen in this interstitial population but the invading trophoblastic cells do tend to aggregate around vessels in the tubal wall.

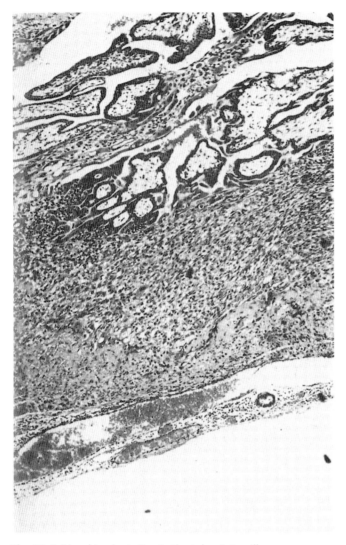

Fig. 31.3 Mural implantation in the tube. Extravillous cytotrophoblast is colonising the 'decidua' at the site of placental attachment.

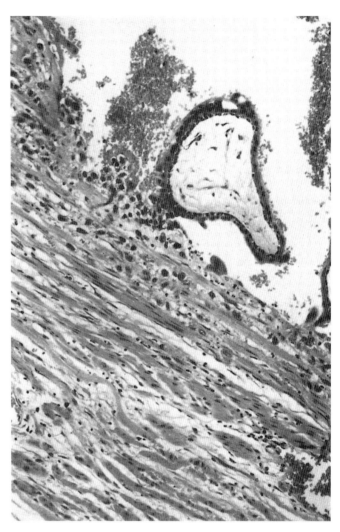

Fig. 31.4 Tubal mural implantation. Extravillous cytotrophoblast cells are infiltrating between muscle fibres in the tubal wall at a point immediately adjacent to the site of placental attachment.

Extravillous cytotrophoblast, from the cytotrophoblastic cell columns, also grows directly into the lumens of the arteries of the tube (Fig. 31.6), destroys the endothelium, invades the vessel wall and destroys the medial musculo-elastic tissue, the wall being eventually replaced by fibrinoid material (Fig. 31.7). Changes in the tubal vessels usually extend through the full thickness of the muscular coat of the tubal wall and, exceptionally, may extend into vessels outside the serosa.

Although it is true that tubal placentation occurs in a less consistent and more erratic pattern than it does in the uterus the overall pattern of placentation is the same in the two sites and, in particular, the vascular changes are identical to those which occur in an intrauterine pregnancy during the transformation of the spiral arteries into uteroplacental vessels.

This description of tubal placentation is based on our own observations (Randall et al 1987) which are broadly in accord with those of Stock (1991, 1993). A different

version was, however, suggested by Budowick et al (1980) who maintained that trophoblast rapidly penetrates the tube wall to grow principally, together with the embryo, in an extratubal site, invading the retroperitoneal space and growing circumferentially around the outside of the tube. Stock (1993) has, however, provided good evidence that this concept of primary extratubal growth is based upon misinterpretation of an artefact caused by convolution of the tube.

MORPHOLOGY OF PLACENTAL VILLI IN TUBAL PREGNANCY

The appearances of the placental villi in tubal gestations have received little attention. Laufer et al (1962) found that in most cases the placental villous morphology resembled that found in an intrauterine miscarriage but noted that in 12% of cases the villous appearances were suggestive of a 'blighted ovum'. Emmrich & Kopping

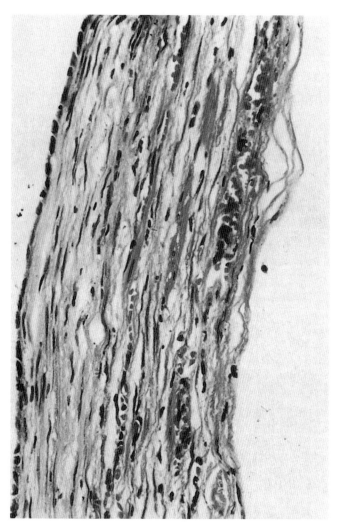

Fig. 31.5 Tubal pregnancy. At a site some distance from the area of placental attachment there is longitudinal spread of extravillous cytotrophoblast between the muscle fibres of the tubal wall.

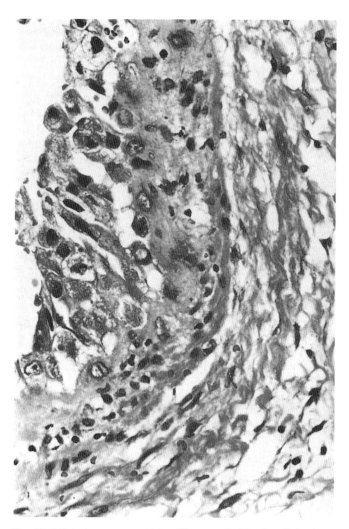

Fig. 31.6 Tubal pregnancy. Extravillous trophoblastic cells in the lumen of a mural artery at the site of placental implantation.

(1981) thought that the placental villi showed changes suggestive of a 'blighted ovum' in a very high proportion of tubal pregnancies, attributing this phenomenon to the effects of the unfavourable environment on the fertilised ovum. When considering these reports it is necessary to bear in mind that these authors are equating hydropic change in the villi with a 'blighted ovum' (by which is presumably meant an anembryonic pregnancy); in reality, hydropic change can occur in miscarriages of any type after long-standing fetal death and is by no means an absolute indication of an anembryonic gestation.

Approximately a third of placentas from tubal pregnancies have a fully normal first trimester appearance (Fig. 31.8), this usually being in cases in which tubal rupture has been rapidly followed by operative removal. In the remaining two-thirds of cases the villi show no abnormality apart from those changes which normally follow fetal death, whether this be in an intrauterine or

extrauterine site, i.e. stromal fibrosis and sclerosis of the villous fetal vessels. Amongst the placentas showing post-mortem changes a minor degree of hydropic change is common (Fig. 31.9) but this is rarely a conspicuous feature. Occasionally hydropic change is marked and this can lead to a mistaken diagnosis of a partial mole (Burton et al 2001): rare authentic examples of a tubal partial mole have, however, been described (Newcomer 1998). The placental tissue may show areas of infarction or perivillous fibrin deposition as may placentas of similar gestational age from intrauterine pregnancies.

It is probable, however, that placental growth is diminished in tubal pregnancies: thus there is a lesser degree of proliferative activity in the trophoblast of tubally sited placental villi than there is in intrauterine placentas (Klein et al 1995) whilst scanning electron microscopy of tubal placentas has revealed decreased trophoblastic sprouting and diminished transformation into primary, secondary and tertiary villous trees (Demir et al 1995).

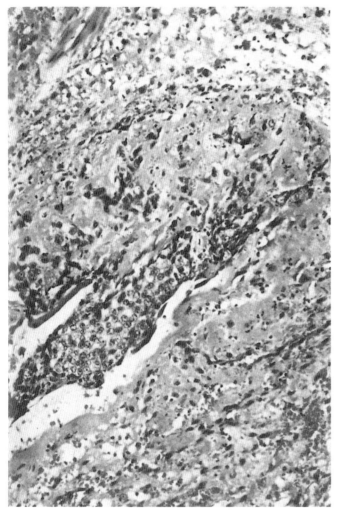

Fig. 31.7 Tubal pregnancy. The wall of a mural artery at the site of placental implantation is infiltrated by trophoblastic cells and shows fibrinoid necrosis.

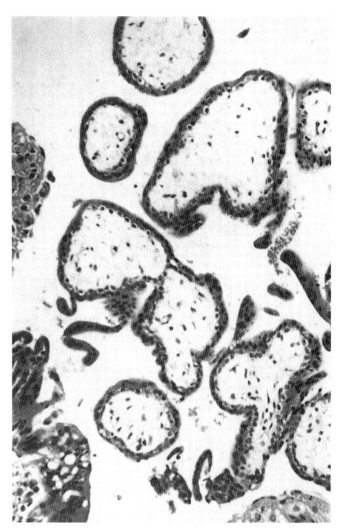

Fig. 31.8 Normal first-trimester villi in a placenta from a tubal pregnancy.

IMMUNOLOGICAL AND IMMUNOHISTOCHEMICAL FEATURES OF TROPHOBLAST IN TUBAL PREGNANCY

The distribution of major histocompatibility antigens in the villous and extravillous trophoblast in tubal gestations is identical to that noted in the trophoblast populations of an intrauterine pregnancy (Earl et al 1986). Similarly, the distribution of trophoblastic membrane antigens, hCG, human placental lactogen (hPL) and Schwangerschafts protein 1 (SP1) in a tubal pregnancy is similar to that described in normal early intrauterine placentas (Earl et al 1985). Immunohistochemical studies have also shown that the distribution of proteinases and proteinase inhibitors in trophoblast is identical in intrauterine and tubal pregnancies (Earl et al 1989). The only disparity that has been shown between intrauterine and extrauterine trophoblast is that pregnancy-associated plasma protein A (PAPP-A) can be demonstrated in the former but not in the latter (Chemnitz et al 1984).

TUBAL RESPONSE TO PREGNANCY

The tube can show a decidual response in a tubal pregnancy (Randall et al 1987; Green & Kott 1989): whether this is, in fact, a direct response to the tubal implantation is a moot point for a degree of decidual change is not uncommonly seen in tubes removed during the immediately postpartum period following an intrauterine gestation and there is little or no information as to whether the degree of decidual change in a gravid tube exceeds that normally occurring in association with an intrauterine gestation. Be that as it may, any decidual response seen in a tube containing a pregnancy tends to be patchy and relatively inconspicuous, possibly because gravid tubes appear to lack progesterone receptors (Land & Arends 1992): in our own series a decidual change was, in fact, seen in only 25% of gravid tubes (Fig. 31.10) and this was patchy in 11%, involved only scattered cells in 10% and was extensive in only 4%. The degree and extent of decidual

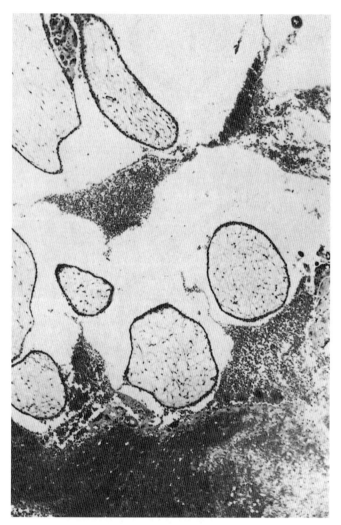

Fig. 31.9 A minor degree of placental villous hydropic change following fetal death in a tubal pregnancy.

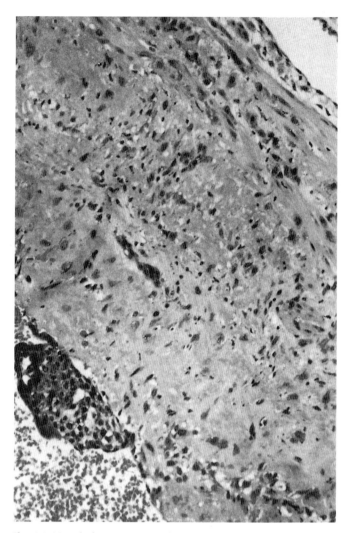

Fig. 31.10 Tubal pregnancy. A decidual reaction in the wall of the tube.

change in the tube is unrelated to the site of implantation, the duration of the pregnancy or the size of the implantation site; even in those few tubes showing extensive decidual change the 'decidua' is, of course, very much thinner than that found in the gravid uterus. A non-specific mixed acute and chronic inflammatory cell infiltration, which includes T lymphocytes and macrophages but not large granular lymphocytes (Earl et al 1987; Stewart-Akers et al 1997; Marx et al 1999), of the tubal wall and plicae at the site of implantation is a common, but not invariable, feature (Fig. 31.11); this localised inflammatory/immunological response is sometimes mistakenly considered as evidence of prior tubal inflammatory disease but is, in fact, very similar in nature to that found in the decidua of intrauterine pregnancies (Stewart-Akers et al 1997).

Focal endosalpingeal hyperplasia has been noted in association with a tubal pregnancy and the hyperplastic epithelium can occasionally show, in some areas, appearances reminiscent of an Arias-Stella reaction (Mikhael et al 1977).

UTERINE RESPONSE TO TUBAL PREGNANCY

In an ectopic gestation the endometrium usually, though far from invariably, responds to the hormonal changes of pregnancy and undergoes decidual change (Fig. 31.12); the degree and extent of the decidual change is somewhat variable but is not uncommonly quantitatively comparable to that found in an intrauterine gestation. The endometrial glands also commonly undergo a typical pregnancy change and are hypersecretory with a markedly scalloped outline. An Arias-Stella reaction (Fig. 31.13) is seen focally in a proportion, variably reported as between 2.9 and 100% of cases, with a majority of authors agreeing that this change can be found in between 60 and 70% of endometria from women with a tubal pregnancy (Birch & Collins 1961; Charles 1962; Laluppa & Cavanagh 1963; Lloyd & Feinberg 1965; Bernhardt et al 1966; Ollendorf et al 1987): our own experience would be that this figure is too high. The Arias-Stella reaction is invariably focal and involves only one gland or a group of glands which show

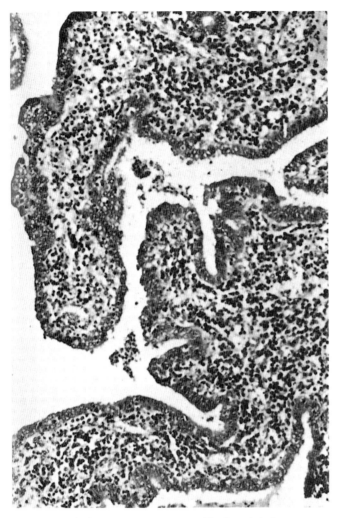

Fig. 31.11 Tubal pregnancy. A non-specific chronic inflammatory cell infiltration in plicae immediately adjacent to the site of placental implantation.

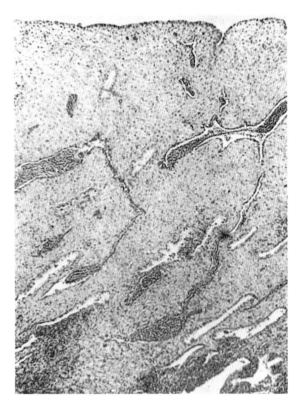

Fig. 31.12 Endometrium in a case of tubal pregnancy. There is a well-marked decidual change but no placental site reaction is seen.

a variable degree of epithelial multilayering and papillary infolding: the cells in these glands lose their polarity, have enlarged, pleomorphic, hyperchromatic nuclei and vacuolated clear cytoplasm (Arias-Stella 1954): mitotic figures are present in a small proportion of Arias-Stella reactions and these may, rarely, have a tripolar form (Arias-Stella 1994). The Arias-Stella change is not specific to an ectopic pregnancy and can occur in association with any pregnancy, either normal or abnormal, in either an intrauterine or an extrauterine site: there is no doubt that an Arias-Stella reaction can occur in a normal, fully viable intrauterine gestation (Silverberg 1972; Oertel 1978). Furthermore, an Arias-Stella reaction may occasionally be seen in non-pregnant women who are receiving exogenous progestins or gonadotrophins (Huettner & Gersel 1994).

A significant proportion of endometria from women with an ectopic pregnancy show, however, neither a decidual change nor a hypersecretory pattern, a normal proliferative or secretory phase appearance being found in almost one-third of cases (Lopez et al 1994).

If the ectopically sited fetus dies the uterine decidua may slough off as a cast (Fig. 31.14) but more commonly crumbles, fragments and is irregularly shed. If there is a long interval between fetal death and endometrial sampling the original decidua may be completely lost and replaced by a proliferative endometrium which, because the first few cycles after an ectopic gestation tend to be anovulatory, may be mildly hyperplastic (Robertson 1981).

The findings in uterine curettings from a woman with a tubal pregnancy vary considerably therefore with the progestational response of the endometrium, the viability or otherwise of the conceptus and with the time interval between fetal demise and endometrial sampling. In some instances the endometrium may show no pregnancy-related changes and a normal secretory or proliferative endometrium is found (Ollendorf et al 1987; Lopez et al 1994). The most characteristic appearances are, however, seen in a continuing viable gestation when curettage produces decidua and pregnancy-type endometrial glands, with or without an Arias-Stella change: there is typically little necrosis or inflammation and, most importantly, there is an absence not only of placental villi but also of a placental site reaction in the decidual tissue. The mere absence of placental villi does not necessarily indicate an ectopic pregnancy for they may be lacking in samples obtained after a miscarriage from an undoubted intrauterine site. Conversely, the presence of placental villi does not invalidate completely a diagnosis of tubal

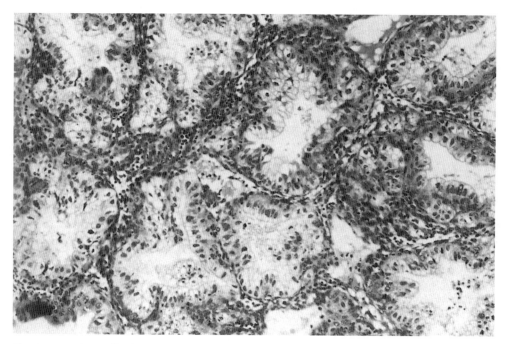

Fig. 31.13 Arias-Stella change in the endometrium. From a case of tubal pregnancy.

pregnancy for a tubal gestation may abort into the uterine cavity with subsequent retrieval of placental tissue on curettage (Gruber et al 1997); only the finding of a placental site reaction offers absolute proof of an intrauterine gestation. If the clinical picture of an ectopic pregnancy is associated with clear-cut histological evidence of an intrauterine gestation the possibility of a heterotopic pregnancy should be borne in mind.

NATURAL HISTORY OF TUBAL PREGNANCIES

Tubal pregnancies may terminate in a number of ways:

1. Miscarriage without tubal rupture

A high proportion of tubal pregnancies spontaneously miscarry during the early stages of gestation. This is invariably the rule in cases of plical and fimbrial implantation, simply because these sites offer insufficient tissue to allow for adequate placentation, but is also common with mural implantations. There is usually intramural and intralumenal haemorrhage with subsequent fetal death and it is assumed that this bleeding is largely a consequence of trophoblastic invasion of the tubal wall and vasculature. It has to be borne in mind that the haemostatic mechanisms which are operative in the uterus are lacking in the tube and that minor degrees of bleeding from eroded vessels, during the process of placentation, which are easily controlled in the uterus may, in the tube, assume a magnitude sufficient to endanger the continuing viability of the fetus.

Following miscarriage the products of conception may persist for a considerable period of time within the tube,

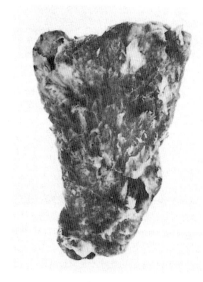

Fig 31.14 A uterine decidual cast in a case of ectopic pregnancy.

as one form of 'chronic ectopic pregnancy', or be gradually absorbed, this latter event probably occurring with a greater frequency than is realised (Atri et al 1993) and often escaping clinical diagnosis. Absorption of trophoblastic tissue after a clinically silent ectopic gestation may be less than complete and placental site nodules or ghost villi can be unexpected histological findings in the tubes of women who have no history of an ectopic pregnancy (Nayar et al 1996; Jacques et al 1997). As an alternative to absorption the dead fetus, with or without associated blood clot, may be expelled into the abdominal cavity via the ostium or can pass through the isthmus to enter the uterus from whence it is expelled via the cervix.

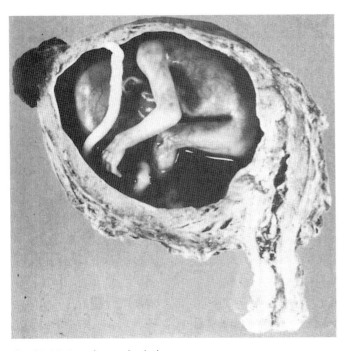

Fig. 31.15 An advanced tubal pregnancy.

It is assumed that the extremely rare apparently primary tubal hydatidiform moles (Diouf et al 1995) and choriocarcinomas (Madden 1950) represent, or follow, a tubal miscarriage.

2. Tubal rupture

At least 60% of tubal pregnancies result in rupture of the tube. This is due largely to the limited distensibility of the tube which is unable to dilate adequately to accommodate the developing conceptus; whether the deep trophoblastic penetration of the wall contributes to a liability to rupture is a debateable point but Stock (1991, 1993) has pointed out that the site of rupture does not necessarily correspond with the site of mural implantation. In at least some cases the tubal rupture appears to be a consequence of the intratubal placental tissue acting as a placenta percreta: we have observed a number of examples of deep villous penetration of the wall (Randall et al 1987) with the villous tissue penetrating the tubal wall in the same fashion as an intrauterine placenta percreta penetrates the myometrium. This invasiveness may be secondary to the failure of the tube to mount a decidual reaction, for lack of decidualisation is considered to be an aetiological factor in intrauterine placenta percreta.

Tubal rupture is usually acute, macroscopically obvious and associated with a dramatic clinical picture. Less commonly, however, there is a slow leakage of tubal contents and blood into the abdominal cavity. The clinical features are, in these circumstances, far less striking and the slow seepage of blood results in a gradually enlarging haematoma and causes dense adhesions between the ruptured tube and adjacent structures: not uncommonly the tube is bound down to omentum, small and large bowel, pelvic wall and, occasionally, the contralateral adnexae (Johnson 1952; Parker & Parker 1957; Cole & Corlett 1982). The ureters may be obstructed as a result of entrapment in this paratubal mass (Hovadhanakul et al 1971).

Although tubal rupture is usually accompanied by fetal death it is occasionally the case that the fetus, following the rupture, retains sufficient attachment to its blood supply to maintain its viability: the trophoblast grows out from the rupture site and forms a secondary placental site on the tubal serosa, in the broad ligament or in the abdomen (Pauerstein et al 1986; Randall et al 1987). A secondary abdominal pregnancy of this type can proceed to term (Clark & Jones 1975; Paterson & Grant 1975).

3. Unruptured term pregnancy

There have been many reports of term, or third trimester, pregnancies (Fig. 31.15) in unruptured tubes (Deopuria 1970; Clark & Jones 1975; Augensen 1983). In theory the following criteria, suggested by McElin & Randall (1951), should be met for the establishment of a diagnosis of term tubal pregnancy:

a. Complete extirpation of the fetal sac and products of conception is achieved by salpingectomy.
b. There is no evidence of tubal rupture.
c. Ciliated columnar epithelium is demonstrable at some point in the inner lining of the sac.
d. Smooth muscle is present in the cyst wall.

In practice the meeting of the first of these criteria is usually accepted as sufficient proof of a tubal gestation at term. The reasons why some tubal pregnancies are capable of progressing to term without rupture of the tube are unknown and no studies have been made of the vascular supply of the placenta and fetus in such pregnancies.

PATHOLOGICAL FINDINGS

From what has been said above it will be clear that the operative specimen received by the pathologist after surgical treatment of a tubal pregnancy, usually a salpingectomy specimen, will show a range of appearances which vary with the site of nidation within the tube, the viability or otherwise of the fetus, the duration of the pregnancy and whether or not tubal rupture has occurred. In a 'typical' case the tube is focally or generally distended to a variable degree whilst the peritoneal surface is congested and sometimes inflamed (Fig. 31.16). The fimbrial ostium may be occluded by blood clot but if it is still patent blood may be seen oozing from the fimbrial end of the tube. If rupture has occurred blood clot and placental tissue may be seen protruding through the rupture site and blood clot may envelop the tube. On opening the tube a complete amniotic sac and fetus is sometimes seen

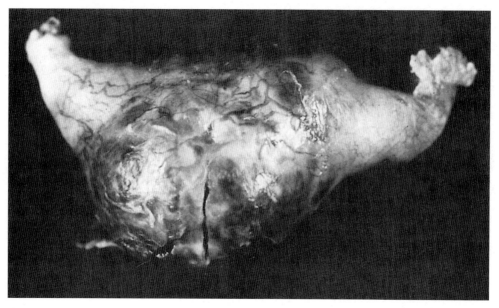

Fig. 31.16 External appearances of a tube containing an ectopic gestation. The tube is focally distended and congested.

(Fig. 31.17) but more commonly the lumen appears to contain only fresh and old blood clot: the accumulation of blood clot may be sausage shaped and sufficiently large to distend the tube (Fig. 31.18).

If a recognisable fetus is not present the diagnosis of a tubal gestation can only be confirmed by histological examination. Usually a few placental villi will be found either embedded within the blood clot or attached to the tubal wall whilst, occasionally, fragments of fetal tissue are seen. In some cases many sections have to be examined before placental tissue is detected whilst in some cases of abortion or tubal rupture no residual fetal or placental tissue is present: even in such circumstances, however, an implantation site can often be identified by the presence of extravillous trophoblastic tissue which is infiltrating the wall and invading its vessels.

EFFECTS AND COMPLICATIONS OF TREATMENT

Tubal pregnancies have traditionally been treated by laparotomy and salpingectomy and this is still often the preferred treatment for a ruptured tubal pregnancy. Increasingly, however, laparoscopic salpingectomy or salpingostomy are the surgical treatments of choice whilst many cases of unruptured tubal pregnancy are being treated nonsurgically with methotrexate which can be administered systematically or locally. Methotrexate inhibits trophoblastic growth and spread in the tube (Floridan et al 1999) but has no adverse effects on the tube itself (Lecuru et al 1999).

Following laparoscopic or medical treatment residual trophoblastic tissue may be retained within the tube with resulting continued elevation of the patient's hCG levels: the elevated levels usually fall spontaneously but may require treatment with methotrexate. It is possible that

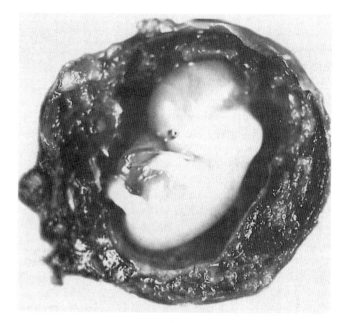

Fig. 31.17 A tube containing a clearly recognisable fetus.

unrecognised persistent trophoblatic tissue is the source of the very rare post-ectopic-pregnancy choriocarcinoma (Horn et al 1994; Terada et al 1994; Logani et al 1995).

Laparoscopic treatment of a tubal gestation may be complicated by implantation of trophoblastic tissue on to the peritoneum (Foulot et al 1994): the implants appear macroscopically as small (30 mm diameter) red–black nodules which are seen histologically to consist of degenerating chorionic villi with implantation changes in the surrounding tissue (Doss et al 1998). These peritoneal implants of trophoblastic tissue can be complicated by severe bleeding (Giuliani et al 1998).

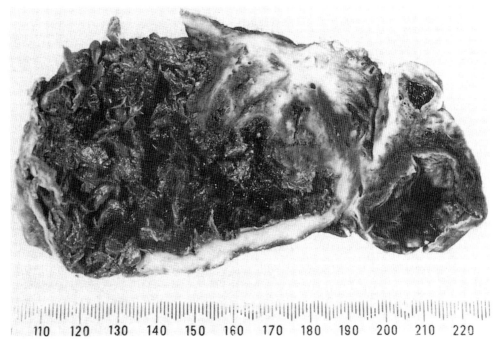

Fig. 31.18 A tubal pregnancy. The tube is distended with old and fresh blood clot.

OVARIAN PREGNANCY

Less than 1% of ectopic pregnancies in women not using an IUCD are found in an ovarian site (Lehfeldt et al 1970); in women using an IUCD the proportion of ovarian to tubal gestations is much higher and has been variously reported as 1 to 9 (Lehfeldt et al 1970; 1 to 7 (Tietze 1968) and 1 to 3 (Gray & Ruffolo 1978). There is, however, some evidence that the incidence of ovarian pregnancy is increasing both in IUCD wearers and non-wearers (Grimes et al 1983; Schwartz et al 1993).

Criteria for the recognition of an ovarian pregnancy (Fig. 31.19) were first formulated by Spiegelberg in 1878 and have not been improved on since that date (Speigelberg 1878):

1. The Fallopian tube on the affected side must be mor-phologically normal, clearly separated from the ovary and devoid of any evidence of a tubal gestation.
2. The gestational sac must occupy the normal position of the ovary.
3. The gestational sac must be connected to the uterus by the ovarian ligament.
4. Ovarian tissue must be histologically demonstrable in the wall of the gestational sac.

Ovarian pregnancy may be primary or secondary. A primary ovarian pregnancy occurs if the ovum is fertilised whilst still within the follicle or if an ovum, fertilised outside the tube, primarily implants in the ovary. A sec-ondary ovarian pregnancy occurs when fertilisation takes place in the tube and the conceptus is regurgitated to implant on the ovary: a secondary ovarian pregnancy may

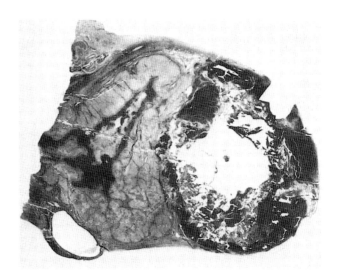

Fig. 31.19 Ovarian pregnancy. Chorionic villi can be seen in the blood clot (right) attached to a corpus luteum.

also occur as a consequence of tubal rupture though this is distinctly uncommon. An ovarian gestation may be intrafollicular or extrafollicular and it will be appreciated that Spiegelberg's criteria apply particularly to an intrafol-licular pregnancy, which is presumed to be invariably primary. Many extrafollicular ovarian pregnancies, whether they be primary or secondary, do not fulfil the criteria in so far as ovarian tissue is not necessarily present in the wall of the gestational sac.

It is assumed that an intrafollicular ovarian pregnancy is due to fertilisation of the ovum whilst it is still retained within the follicle and this phenomenon is postulated to be a consequence of ovulatory dysfunction (Boronow et al 1965; Procope & Vesanto 1966). There is a clear association between ovarian pregnancy and IUCD usage (Lehfeldt et al 1970; Hallatt 1976; Grimes et al 1983; Rivera et al 1988; Raziel et al 1990; Xie et al 1991) but, as previously pointed out, this does not mean that an IUCD causes an ovarian pregnancy but that it simply fails to prevent such a gestation: hence IUCD usage is not associated with any absolute increase in the incidence of ovarian pregnancy. There have been several reports of ovarian pregnancy following in vitro fertilisation and embryo transfer (Carter & Jacobson 1986; Rizk et al 1990) and GIFT (Lehmann et al 1991) whilst ovarian pregnancy combined with an intrauterine gestation (heterotopic pregnancy) has occurred following the use of an ovulatory agent (McLain & Kirkwood 1987). A single instance of a twin ovarian pregnancy has been recorded (Tuncer et al 1994).

Ovarian pregnancies usually miscarry during the first trimester but there have been a number of such gestations which have proceeded to term or into the third trimester (Nicholls 1941; Pratt-Thomas et al 1974; Williams et al 1982; Belfar et al 1991; Kosovski et al 1992; Aligbe et al 1999).

CERVICAL PREGNANCY

Ectopic pregnancies located in the uterine cervix are rare, probably accounting for only 1% of ectopic gestations (Kouyoundjian 1984). The aetiology and pathogenesis of cervical pregnancy clearly differ from those of a tubal pregnancy and Studdiford (1945) suggested that unusually rapid transport of the fertilised ovum was an important aetiological factor, this resulting in it having reached the endocervical canal before reaching a stage of development compatible with nidation. Schneider & Dreizin (1957) suggested, as an alternative view that, whilst ovum transport was normal, maturation of the conceptus was delayed, this again allowing it to enter the endocervical canal before having reached a stage at which it could implant. These are, however, hypothetical concepts and, in more practical terms, a correlation has been reported between induction of miscarriage by sharp curettage and subsequent cervical pregnancy (Shinagawa & Nagayama 1969; Parente et al 1983) whilst Dicker et al (1985) noted an association of cervical pregnancy with Asherman's syndrome. It is reports such as these that have led to a growing agreement that adverse endometrial factors ('endometrial hostility') are probably the most important aetiological factors in cervical implantation (Yankowitz et al 1990; Casson 1993).

Cervical pregnancy has also been reported after IVF (Weyerman et al 1989), possibly because of unusually low placement of the embryo within the endocervical canal.

Women with a cervical pregnancy usually present as an apparent spontaneous miscarriage and a clinical suspicion of a cervical pregnancy may be raised by the finding of an expanded cervix in association with a normally-sized uterine body. Proof of a cervical pregnancy, as distinct from the cervical stage of an abortion from an intrauterine site, rests solely, however, on pathological examination and the criteria, laid down almost a century ago, for this by Rubin (1911) are:

1. Cervical crypts must be in close approximation to placental tissue.
2. There must be an intimate attachment between the placenta and the cervix.
3. The entire placenta must lie below the entry point of the uterine vessels or below the site of peritoneal reflection on the anterior and posterior uterine surfaces.
4. Fetal tissue must not be present in the uterine cavity.

It is rare for cervical pregnancies to progress beyond the first trimester though occasional third trimester live births have been documented (Pisarki 1960; Mitrani 1973; Jelsema & Zuidema 1992; Casson 1993). Miscarriage of a cervical pregnancy is often accompanied by severe bleeding which has, in the past, led to a high maternal mortality rate. With current therapeutic measures, which include treatment with methotrexate, the maternal death rate is, however, now extremely low (Pretzsch et al 1997).

ABDOMINAL PREGNANCY

The incidence of abdominal pregnancy in the United States has been estimated to be just over 1 in 10 000 deliveries (Atrash et al 1987), a figure that probably applies to other Western countries. Abdominal implantation may be either primary or secondary and it is highly probable that most cases are of the secondary type and are a consequence of tubal rupture: even those which are apparently primary probably result from regurgitation of an ovum which has been fertilised in the tube. The criteria, laid down many years ago but still valid, for the diagnosis of a primary abdominal pregnancy (Studdiford 1942) are:

1. Both tubes and ovaries must be normal.
2. There must be no evidence of a uteroperitoneal fistula.
3. The pregnancy must be related principally to the peritoneum.

An abdominal gestation may implant anywhere within the peritoneal cavity and reported sites include the broad ligament, colonic mesentery, lumbar gutter, mesentery of the small bowel, omentum, ileum and lesser peritoneal cavity (Friedrich 1968). Cases have also been described in which the conceptus has implanted onto the liver (Mear et al 1965; Kirkby 1969; Harris et al 1989; Delabrousse et al 1999), spleen (Yackel 1988; Kahn et al

1989) or diaphragm (Norenberg et al 1977). A particular form of abdominal pregnancy is an intraligamentous gestation (Cordero et al 1994): this may be due to rupture of a tubal pregnancy at the mesosalpingeal margin of the tube or to a gestation primarily implanted on the surface of the broad ligament burrowing into the ligament.

Despite this availability of possible sites most early abdominal pregnancies are located in the cul-de-sac and involve either the posterior surface of the uterus or the anterior aspect of the rectosigmoid colon. In advanced gestations the placenta has a broad base of attachment and it may be extremely difficult to localise the site of implantation (Dehner 1972).

A gestation situated within the abdominal cavity is not subject to the same restraints of space as is a pregnancy within a tube and the limiting factor determining whether the pregnancy aborts or continues is the ability of the placenta to establish an adequate blood supply. Surprisingly, as many as 25% of abdominal pregnancies do achieve adequate placentation and progress to an advanced stage (Hlavin et al 1978; Golan et al 1985; White et al 1989; Diouf et al 1996). It has to be said, however, that the mechanism of placentation within the abdominal cavity remains obscure.

The term abdominal pregnancy presents a surgical challenge for attempts at removing the placenta, though often successful, may be complicated by severe haemorrhage. The placenta can, however, be left in the abdominal cavity and its presence there does not usually appear to cause any signs or symptoms (Petrie & Duchin 1980) though instances have been noted of sepsis, abscess formation, intestinal obstruction and fistula formation (Casson 1993).

POST-HYSTERECTOMY PREGNANCY

There have been a considerable number of reports of post-hysterectomy ectopic pregnancy (Cooks 1980; Zolli & Rocko 1982; Nehra & Loginsky 1984; Salmi et al 1984; Reese et al 1989). In most cases the woman had conceived immediately prior to the hysterectomy and the fertilised ovum had been trapped in the tube. Some gestations have, however, occurred many years after removal of the uterus and it is thought that under such circumstances fertilisation had occurred as a result of sperm passage through a fistulous track in the vaginal vault.

REFERENCES

Abramovici D, Morfesis F A, Ally S, Bathija N R 1995 Bilateral ectopic pregnancy: a case report. Journal of the Kentucky Medical Association 93: 295

Abusheikha N, Salha O, Brinsden P 2000 Extra-uterine pregnancy following assisted conception treatment. Human Reproduction Update 6: 80–92

Adair C D, Benrubi G I, Sanchez-Ramos L, Rhatigan R 1994 Bilateral tubal ectopic pregnancies after bilateral partial salpingectomy: a case report. Journal of Reproductive Medicine 39: 131–133

Aligbe J U, Igbokwe U O, Kpolugbo J 1999 Ovarian ectopic gestation carried to term. International Journal of Gynaecology and Obstetrics 67: 191–192

Alsuleiman S A, Grimes T 1982 Ectopic pregnancy: a review of 147 cases. Journal of Reproductive Medicine 27: 101–106

Ankum W M, Mol B W J, van der Veen F, Bossuyt P M M 1996 Risk factors for ectopic pregnancy — a metaanalysis. Fertility and Sterility 65: 1093–1099

Arias-Stella J 1954 Atypical endometrial changes associated with the presence of chorionic tissue. Archives of Pathology 58: 112–128

Arias-Stella J 1994 Normal and abnormal mitoses in the atypical endometrial change associated with chorionic tissue effect. American Journal of Surgical Pathology 18: 694–701

Atrash H K, Friede A, Hogue C J R 1987 Abdominal pregnancy in the United States: frequency and maternal mortality. Obstetrics and Gynecology 69: 333–337

Atrash H K, Strauss L T, Kendrick J S, Skjeldestad F E, Ahn Y W 1997 The relation between induced abortion and ectopic pregnancy. Obstetrics and Gynecology 89: 512–518

Atri M, Bret P M, Tulandi T 1993 Spontaneous resolution of ectopic pregnancy: initial appearance and evolution at transvaginal US. Radiology 186: 83–86

Augensen K 1983 Unruptured tubal pregnancy with survival of mother and child. Obstetrics and Gynecology 61: 259–261

Bachelot A, Rossinamar B, Logerot-Lebrun H, Demouzon J 1996 French IVF registry FIVNAT 1995 report. Contraception Fertility and Sex 24: 694–699

Badawy S, Gilman T, Mroziewicz E 1979 The role of recanalization in tubal pregnancy after sterilization. International Surgery 64: 49–51

Baffoe S, Nkyekyer K 1999 Ectopic pregnancy in Korie Bu Teaching Hospital, Ghana: a three-year review. Tropical Doctor 29: 18–22

Barnes A B, Colton T, Gunderson J et al 1980 Fertility and outcome of pregnancy in women exposed in utero to diethylstilbestrol. New England Journal of Medicine 302: 609–613

Barnes A B, Wennberg C N, Barnes B A 1983 Ectopic pregnancy: incidence and review of determinant factors. Obstetrical and Gynecological Survey 38: 345–356

Bastianelli C, Lucantoni V, Valente A, Farris M, Lippa A, Dionisi B 1998 Fattori di rischio per la gravidanza ectopica: studio caso-controllo. Minerva Ginecologica 50: 469–473

Belfar H, Heller K, Edelstone D I, Hill L M, Martin J G 1991 Ovarian pregnancy resulting in a surviving neonate: ultrasound findings. Journal of Ultrasound Medicine 10: 465–467

Beral V 1975 An epidemiological study of recent trends in ectopic pregnancy. British Journal of Obstetrics and Gynaecology 82: 775–782

Berenson A, Hammill H, Martens M, Faro S 1991 Bacteriologic findings with ectopic pregnancy. Journal of Reproductive Medicine 36: 118–120

Berger M J, Taymor M L 1972 Simultaneous intrauterine and tubal pregnancies following ovulation induction. American Journal of Obstetrics and Gynecology 113: 812–813

Bernhardt R N, Bruns D P, Drose V E 1966 Atypical endometrium associated with ectopic pregnancy. Obstetrics and Gynecology 28: 849–853

Beyth Y, Kopolovic J 1982 Accessory tubes: a possible contributing factor in infertility. Fertility and Sterility 38: 382–383

Birch H W, Collins C G 1961 Atypical changes in genital epithelium associated with ectopic pregnancy. American Journal of Obstetrics and Gynecology 82: 1198–1208

Bjartling C, Osser S, Persson K 2000 The frequency of salpingitis and ectopic pregnancy as epidemiologic markers of Chlamydia trachomatis. Acta Obstetricia et Gynecologica Scandinavica 79: 123–128

Bobrow M L, Bell H G 1962 Ectopic pregnancy: a 16 year survey of 905 cases. Obstetrics and Gynecology 60: 500–502

Bone N L, Greene R R 1961 Histologic study of uterine tubes with tubal pregnancy. American Journal of Obstetrics and Gynecology 82: 1166–1171

Boronow R C, McElin T W, West R H, Buckingham J C 1965 Ovarian pregnancy. American Journal of Obstetrics and Gynecology 91: 1096–1106

Bouyer J, Coste J, Fernandez H, Job-Spira N 1998 Tabac et grossesse extrauterine: argument en faveur d'une relation causale. Revue d'Epidemiologie et Sante Publique 46: 93–99

Brenner P F, Roy S, Mishell D R 1975 Ectopic pregnancy: a study of 300 surgically treated cases. Journal of the American Medical Association 243: 673–676

Brunham R C, Binns B, McDowell J, Paraskevas M 1986 Chlamydia trachomatis infection in women with ectopic pregnancy. Obstetrics and Gynecology 67: 722–736

Brunham R C, Peeling R, McLean I, Kosseim M L, Oaraskevas M 1992 Chlamydia trachomatis-associated ectopic pregnancy: serologic and histologic correlates. Journal of Infectious Diseases 165: 1076–1081

Budowick M, Johnson T R B, Genadry R, Parmley T H, Woodruff J D 1980 The histopathology of the developing tubal ectopic pregnancy. Fertility and Sterility 34: 1169–1171

Burton J L, Lidbury A E, Gillespie A M et al 2001 Over-diagnosis of hydatidiform mole in early tubal ectopic pregnancy. Histopathology 38: 409–417.

Busch D H, Benirschke K 1974 Cytogenetic studies of ectopic pregnancies. Virchows Archiv B Cell Pathology 16: 319–330

Cagliero L 1961 Fertilita nella donne gravidanza extra uterina. Minerva Ginecologica 13: 10–13

Carr D H 1969 Cytogenetics and the pathology of hydatidiform degeneration. Obstetrics and Gynecology 33: 333–341

Carter J E, Jacobsen A 1986 Reimplantation of a human embryo with subsequent ovarian pregnancy. American Journal of Obstetrics and Gynecology 155: 282–283

Cartwright P S 1993 Incidence, epidemiology, risk factors, and etiology. In: Stovall T G, Ling F W (eds) Extrauterine pregnancy. McGraw-Hill, New York, pp 27–63

Casapeto R, Nogales F F, Matilla A 1978 Ectopic pregnancy coexisting with a primary carcinoma of the Fallopian tube: a case report. International Journal of Gynaecology and Obstetrics 16: 263–264

Casson P R 1993 The non-tubal ectopic pregnancy: cervical, abdominal, and ovarian. In: Stovall T G, Ling F W (eds) Extrauterine pregnancy. McGraw-Hill, New York, pp 287–303

Castles A, Adama E K, Melvin C L, Keisch C Boulton M L 1999 Effects of smoking during pregnancy; five meta-analyses. American Journal of Preventive Medicine 16: 208–215

Centers for Disease Control 1992 Ectopic pregnancy in the USA. CDC surveillance summary

Chaim W, Sarov B, Sarov I, Piura B, Cohen A Insler V 1989 Serum IgG and IgA antibodies to Chlamydia in ectopic pregnancies. Contraception 40: 59–71

Chang J C, Sun T T, Li Y C 1992 Simultaneous ectopic pregnancy with intrauterine gestation after in vitro fertilization and embryo transfer. European Journal of Obstetrics, Gynecology and Reproductive Biology 44: 157–160

Chakravarti S, Shardlow J 1975 Tubal pregnancy after sterilization. British Journal of Obstetrics and Gynaecology 82: 58–60

Charles D 1962 The Arias-Stella reaction. Journal of Obstetrics and Gynaecology of the British Commonwealth 69: 1006–1010

Chemnitz J, Tornehave D, Teisner B, Poulsen H K, Westergaard J G 1984 The localization of pregnancy proteins (hPL, SP1 and PAPP-A) in intra- and extrauterine pregnancies. Placenta 5: 489–494

Chow J M, Yonekura M L, Richwald G A, Greenland S, Sweet R L, Schachter J 1990 The association between Chlamydia trachomatis and ectopic pregnancy: a matched pair, case control study. Journal of the American Medical Association 263: 3164–3167

Chow W H, Daling J R, Cates W Jr, Greenberg R S 1987 Epidemiology of ectopic pregnancy. Epidemiologic Reviews 9: 70–94

Chrysostomou M, Karafyllidi P, Papadimitriou V, Bassiotou V, Mayakos G 1992 Serum antibodies to Chlamydia trachomatis in women with ectopic pregnancy, normal pregnancy or salpingitis. European Journal of Obstetrics, Gynecology and Reproductive Biology 44: 101–105

Clark J F, Jones S A 1975 Advanced ectopic pregnancy. Journal of Reproductive Medicine 14: 30–33

Cole T, Corlett R C 1982 Chronic ectopic pregnancy. Obstetrics and Gynecology 59: 63–68

Cooks P S 1980 Early ectopic pregnancy after vaginal hysterectomy. British Journal of Obstetrics and Gynaecology 87: 363–365

Cordero D R, Adra A, Yasin S, O'Sullivan M J 1994 Intraligamentous pregnancy. Obstetrical and Gynecological Survey 49: 206–209

Coste J, Job-Spira N, Fernandez H, Papiernik E, Spira A 1991 Risk factors for ectopic pregnancy: a case control study in France with special focus on infectious factors. American Journal of Epidemiology 133: 839–849

Coulam C B, Wells M 1992 Ectopic pregnancy loss. In: Coulam C B, Faulk W P, McIntyre J A (eds) Immunological obstetrics. Norton, New York, pp 464–478

Coulam C B, Johnson P M, Ramsden P H et al 1989 Occurrence of ectopic pregnancy among women with recurrent spontaneous abortion. American Journal of Reproductive Immunology 21: 105–107

Coupet E 1989 Ectopic pregnancy: the surgical epidemic. Journal of the National Medical Association 81: 567–572

Cuckle H S, Murray J 1997 Epidemiology of ectopic pregnancy. In: Grudzinskas J G, O'Brien P M S (eds.) Problems in early pregnancy: advances in diagnosis and management. RCOG Press, London, pp 65–76

Cumming D C, Honoré L H, Scott J Z, Williams K E 1988 Microscopic evidence of silent inflammation in grossly normal fallopian tubes with ectopic pregnancies. International Journal of Fertility 33: 324–328

Daisley H 1989 Ectopic pregnancies in Trinidad: a clinico-pathological study of 154 consecutive surgically treated cases. West Indian Medical Journal 38: 222–227

De Cherney A H, Minkin M J, Spangler S 1981a Contemporary management of ectopic pregnancy. Journal of Reproductive Medicine 26: 519–523

De Cherney A H, Cholst I, Naftolin F 1981b Structure and functions of the Fallopian tubes following exposure to diethylstilbestrol (DES) during gestation. Fertility and Sterility 36: 741–745

De Graaf F L, Demetroulis C 1997 Bilateral tubal ectopic pregnancy: diagnostic pitfalls. British Journal of Clinical Practice 51: 56–58

Dehner L P 1972 Advanced extra-uterine pregnancy and the fetal death syndrome. Obstetrics and Gynecology 40: 525–534

Delabrousse E, Site O, Le Mouel A, Riethmuller D, Kastler B 1999 Intrahepatic pregnancy: sonography and CT findings. American Journal of Roentgenology 173: 1377–1378

Demir R, Demir N, Ustunel I, Erbengi T, Trak I, Kaufmann P 1995 The fine structure of normal and ectopic (tubal) human placental villi as revealed by scanning and transmission electron microscopy. Zentralblatt fur Pathologie 140: 427–442

De Muylder X, Laga M, Tennstedt C, Van Dyck E, Aelbers G H, Plot P 1990 The role of *Neisseria gonorrhoeae* and *Chlamydia trachomatis* in pelvic inflammatory disease and its sequelae in Zimbabwe. Journal of Infectious Diseases 162: 501–505

Deopuria R H 1970 Full term, unruptured, intratubal pregnancy. Journal of Obstetrics and Gynaecology of India 566–571

De Stefano F, Peterson H B, Layde P, Rubin G L 1982 Risk of ectopic pregnancy following tubal sterilization. Obstetrics and Gynecology 60: 326–330

Diallo D, Aubard Y, Piver P, Baudet J H 2000 Grossesse heterotopique: a propos de 5 cas et revue de la litterature. Journal de Gynecologie, d'Obstetrique et Biologie de la Reproduction 29: 131–134

Dicker D, Feldberg D, Samuel N, Goldman J 1985 Etiology of cervical pregnancy: association with abortion, pelvic pathology, IUDs and Asherman's syndrome. Journal of Reproductive Medicine 30: 25–27

Dietz T U, Haenggi W, Birkhaeuser M, Gyr T, Dreher T 1993 Combined bilateral tubal and multiple intrauterine pregnancy after ovulation induction. European Journal of Obstetrics, Gynecology and Reproductive Biology 48: 69–71

Dimitry E S, Subak-Sharpe R, Mills M, Margara R, Winston R 1990 Nine cases of heterotopic pregnancies in 4 years of in vitro fertilization. Fertilty and Sterility 53: 107–110

Diouf A, Camara A, Mendez V, Rupari L, Diadhiou F 1995 Grossesse molaire ectopique: a propos deux observations en 16 ans, Contraception Fertilite Sexologie 23: 674–676

Diouf A, Diouf F, Cisse C T, Diallo D, Gaye T, Diadhiou F 1996 La grossesse abdominale a terme avec enfant vivant. Journal de Gynecologie, Obstetrique et Biologie de la Reproduction, Paris 25: 212–215

Dor J, Seidman D S, Levran D, Ben-Rafael Z, Ben-Shlomo I, Mashiach S 1991 The incidence of combined intrauterine and extrauterine pregnancy after in vitro fertilization and embryo transfer. Fertility and Sterility 55: 833–834

Doss B J, Jacques S M, Qureshi F, Ramirez N C, Lawrence W D 1998 Extratubal secondary trophoblastic implants: clinicopathologic correlation and review of the literature. Human Pathology 29: 184–187

Douglas C P 1963 Tubal ectopic pregnancy. British Medical Journal 2: 838–841

Dow E K, Wilson J B, Klufio C A 1975 Tubal pregnancy: a review of 404 cases. Ghana Medical Journal 14: 232–237

Doyle M B, De Cherney A H, Diamond M P 1991 Epidemiology and etiology of ectopic pregnancy. Obstetrics and Gynecology Clinics of North America 18: 1–17

Drife J 1990a Tubal pregnancy. British Medical Journal 301: 1057–1058

Drife J 1990b Benefits and risks of oral contraceptives. Advances in Contraception 6 (Supplement): 15–25

Dubuisson J B, Aubriot F X, Mathieu L, Foulot H, Mandelbrot L, de Joliere J B 1991 Risk factors for ectopic pregnancy in 556 pregnancies after in vitro fertilization: implications for preventive management. Fertility and Sterility 56: 686–690

Earl U, Wells M, Bulmer J N 1985 The expression of major histocompatibility antigens by trophoblast in ectopic tubal pregnancy. Journal of Reproductive Immunology 8: 13–24

Earl U, Wells M, Bulmer J N 1986 Immunohistochemical characterization of trophoblast antigens and secretory products in ectopic tubal pregnancy. International Journal of Gynecological Pathology 5: 132–142

Earl U, Lunny D P, Bulmer J N 1987 Leukocyte populations in ectopic tubal pregnancy. Journal of Clinical Pathology 40: 901–905

Earl U, Morrison L, Gray C, Bulmer J N 1989 Proteinase and proteinase inhibitor localization in the human placenta. International Journal of Gynecological Pathology 8: 114–124

Eckshtein N, Ismajowich B, Yedwab G, David M P 1978 Combined tubal and multiple intrauterine pregnancies following ovulation induction. Fertility and Sterility 30: 707–709

Edelman D A, Van-Os W A 1990 Safety of intrauterine contraception. Advances in Contraception 6: 207–217

Egger M, Low N, Smith G D, Lindblom B, Herrmann B 1998 Screening for chlamydial infections and the risk of ectopic pregnancy in a county in Sweden: ecological analysis. British Medical Journal 316: 1776–1780

Elias S, LeBeau M, Simpson J L, Martin A D 1981 Chromosome analysis of ectopic human conceptuses. American Journal of Obstetrics and Gynecology 141: 698–703

Emmrich P, Kopping H 1981 A study of placental villi in extrauterine gestation: a guide to the frequency of blighted ova. Placenta 2: 63–70

Falfoul A, Friaa R, Chelli M, Kharouf M 1993 Grossesses survenues apres sterilisation chirurgicale feminine: etude apropos de 30 cas. Journal de Gynecologie, Obstetrique et Biologie de Reproduction (Paris) 22: 23–25

Falk H C, Hassid R, Dazo E P 1975 Tubal pregnancy: a report of a very early luminal form of embedding. Obstetrics and Gynecology 45: 215–216

Falk R J, Lackritz R M 1977 Bilateral simultaneous tubal pregnancy after ovulation induction with clomiphene-menotrophin combination. Fertility and Sterility 28: 32–34

Fedele L, Acria B, Parazzini F, Ricciardiello O, Candiani C-B 1989 Ectopic pregnancy and recurrent spontaneous abortion: two associated reproductive failures. Obstetrics and Gynecology 73: 206–208

Floridan C, Nielson O, Byrjalsen C et al 1999 Ectopic pregnancy: histopathology and assessment of cell proliferation with and without methotrexate treatment. Fertility and Sterility 65: 730–738

Forbes D A, Natale A 1968 Unilteral triplet tubal pregnancy: report of a case. Obstetrics and Gynecology 31: 360–362

Formigli L, Coglitore M T, Roccio C, Belotti G, Stangalini A. Formigli G 1990 One-hundred-and-six gamete intra-fallopian transfer procedures with donor semen. Human Reproduction 5: 549–552

Foulot H, Chapron C, Morice P, Mouly M, Aubriot F X, Dubuisson J B 1994 Failure of laparoscopic treatment for peritoneal trophoblastic implants. Human Reproduction 9: 92–93

Franklin E W, Zeiderman A M, Laemmle P 1973 Tubal ectopic pregnancy: etiology and obstetric and gynecologic sequelae. American Journal of Obstetrics and Gynecology 117: 220–225

Friedrich M A 1968 Primary omental pregnancy. Obstetrics and Gynecology 31: 104–109

Golan A, Sandbank O, Adrowskou A, Rubin A 1985 Advanced extrauterine pregnancy. Acta Obstetricia et Gynecologia Scandinavica 64: 21–25

Giuliani A, Panzitt T, Schoell W, Urdi W 1998 Severe bleeding from peritoneal implants of trophoblastic tissue after laparoscopic salpingostomy for ectopic pregnancy. Fertility and Sterility 70: 369–370

Glassner M J, Aron E, Eskin B A 1990 Ovulation induction with clomiphene and the rise in heterotopic pregnancies: a report of two cases. Journal of Reproductive Medicine 35: 175–178

Goldman G A, Fisch B, Ovadia J, Tadir Y 1992 Heterotopic pregnancy after assisted reproductive technologies. Obstetrical and Gynecological Survey 47: 217–221

Goldner T E, Lawson H W, Zia Z, Atrash H K 1993 Surveillance for ectopic pregnancy — United States, 1975–1989. Maternal Mortality Weekly Reports 42: 73–85

Gonzalez F A, Waxman M 1981 Ectopic pregnancy: a retrospective study of 501 consecutive patients. Diagnostic Gynecology and Obstetrics 3: 181–186

Grab D, Wolf A, Kunzel H, Sterzik K 1992 Die ovarielle Stimulation mit Clomifen stelt keinen Riskfaktor fur eine Extrauteringravidatat dar. Zentralblatt fur Gynakologie 114: 289–291

Gray C L, Ruffolo E H 1978 Ovarian pregnancy associated with intrauterine contraceptive device. American Journal of Obstetrics and Gynecology 132: 134–139

Gray C, Wells M, Kingston R 1983 Tubal pregnancy associated with a papillary serous neoplasm arising in a paraovarian cyst. Journal of Obstetrics and Gynaecology 4: 61–62

Green L K, Kott M L 1989 Histopathologic findings in ectopic tubal pregnancy. International Journal of Gynecological Pathology 8: 255–262

Greisman B 1991 Ectopic pregnancy in women with previous tubal sterilization at a Canadian community hospital. Journal of Reproductive Medicine 36: 206–209

Grimes H C, Nosal R A, Gallagher J C 1983 Ovarian pregnancy: a review of 24 cases. Obstetrics and Gynecology 61: 174–180

Gruber K, Gelven P L, Austin R M 1997 Chorionic villi or trophoblastic tissue in uterine samples of four women with ectopic pregnancies. International Journal of Gynecological Pathology 16: 28–32

Guirgis R R 1990 Simultaneous intrauterine and ectopic pregnancies following in-vitro fertilization and gamete intra-fallopian transfer: a review of nine cases. Human Reproduction 5: 484–486

Hakim-Elahi E 1965 Unruptured bilateral tubal pregnancy: report of a case. Obstetrics and Gynecology 26: 763–766

Halbrecht G 1957 Healed genital tuberculosis. Obstetrics and Gynecology 10: 73–76

Hallatt J G 1976 Ectopic pregnancy associated with the intrauterine device: a study of seventy cases. American Journal of Obstetrics and Gynecology 125: 754–758

Harris G J, Al-Jurf A S, Yuh W T, Abu-Yousef M M 1989 Intrahepatic pregnancy: a unique opportunity for evaluation with sonography, computed tomography, and magnetic resonance imaging. Journal of the American Medical Association 261: 902–904

Helvacioglu A, Long A M Jr, Yang S 1979 Ectopic pregnancy: an eight-year review. Journal of Reproductive Medicine 22: 87–92

Herbertsson G, Magnusson S S, Bendiktsdottir K 1987 Ovarian pregnancy and IUCD use in a defined complete population. Acta Obstetricia et Gynecologica Scandinavica 66: 607–610

Herman A, Ron-El R, Golan A, Weinraub Z, Bukovsky I, Caspi E 1990 Role of tubal pathology and other parameters in ectopic pregnancies occurring in in-vitro fertilization and embryo transfer. Fertility and Sterility 54: 864–868

Hlavin G E, Ladoski L T, Breen J L 1978 Ectopic pregnancy: an analysis of 153 patients. International Journal of Gynaecology and Obstetrics 16: 42–47

Hodgson R, Driscoll G I, Dodd J K, Tyler J P 1990 Chlamydia trachomatis: the prevalence, trend and importance in initial infertility management. Australian and New Zealand Journal of Obstetrics and Gynaecology 30: 251–254

Holt V L, Chu J, Daling J R, Stergachis A S, Weiss N S 1991 Tubal sterilization and subsequent ectopic pregnancy: a case control study. Journal of the American Medical Association 266: 242–246

Honoré L H 1978a Tubal ectopic pregnancy with contra lateral corpus luteum: A report of five cases. Journal of Reproictive Medicine 21: 269–271

Honoré L H 1978b Salpingitis isthmica nodosa in female fertility and ectopic tubal pregnancy. Fertility and Sterility 29: 164–168

Honoré L M 1979a A significant association between spontaneous abortion and ectopic tubal pregnancy. Fertility and Sterility 32: 401–402

Honoré L H, Korn G W 1976 Coexistence of tubal ectopic pregnancy and adenomatoid tumor. Journal of Reproductive Medicine 17: 342–344

Honoré L H, O'Hara K E 1978 Failed tubal sterilization as an etiologic factor in ectopic pregnancy. Fertility and Sterility 29: 509–511

Horn L C, Bilek K, Pretzsch G, Baier D 1994 Chorionkarzinom bei tubarer Extrauteringravidat. Geburtshilfe und Frauenheilkunde 54: 375–377

Hovadhanakul P, Eachempati U, Cavanagh D 1971 Ureteral obstruction in chronic ectopic pregnancy. American Journal of Obstetrics and Gynecology 110: 311–313

Huettner P C, Gersel D J 1994 Arias-Stella reaction in nonpregnant women: a clinicopathologic study of nine cases. International Journal of Gynecological Pathology 13: 241–247

Hughes G J 1980 Fertility and ectopic pregnancy. European Journal of Obstetrics, Gynecology and Reproductive Biology 10: 361–365

Hulka J F, Halme J 1988 Sterilization reversal: results of 101 attempts. American Journal of Obstetrics and Gynecology 159: 767–774

Iffy 1963 The role of premenstrual, post mid-cycle conception in the aetiology of ectopic gestation. Journal of Obstetrics and Gynaecology of the British Commonwealth 70: 996–1000

Jacques S M, Qureshi F, Ramirez N C, Lawrence W D 1997 Retained trophoblastic tissue in fallopian tubes: consequence of unsuspected ectopic pregnancies. International Journal of Gynecological Pathology 16: 219–224

James W H 1989 A hypothesis on the increasing rates of ectopic pregnancy. Paediatric and Perinatal Epidemiology 3: 189–193

Jansen R P, Anderson J C, Birrell W S et al 1990 Outpatient gamete intrafallopian transfer: a clinical analysis of 710 cases. Medical Journal of Australia 153: 182–188

Jelsema R D, Zuidema L 1992 First-trimester diagnosed cervicoisthmic pregnancy resulting in term delivery. Obstetrics and Gynecology 80: 517–519

Johnsen H M, Becker-Christensen F 1990 Ectopic pregnancy in Greenland: an epidemiological study. Arctic Medical Research 49: 43–47

Johnson N, McComb P, Gudex G 1998 Heterotopic pregnancy complicating in vitro fertilization. Australian and New Zealand Journal of Obstetrics and Gynaecology 38: 151–155

Johnson W O 1952 A study of 245 cases of ruptured ectopic pregnancy. American Journal of Obstetrics and Gynecology 64: 1102–1110

Kahn J A, Skjeldestad F E, During V et al 1989 A spleen pregnancy. Acta Obstetricia et Gynecologica Scandinavica 68: 83–84

Kalandidi A, Doulgerakis M, Tzonou A, Hsieh C C, Aravandinos D, Trichopoulos D 1991 Induced abortions, contraceptive practices, and tobacco smoking as risk factors for ectopic pregnancy in Athens, Greece. British Journal of Obstetrics and Gynaecology 98: 207–213

Kallenberger D A, Ronk D A, Kimerson G K 1978 Ectopic pregnancy: 15-year review of 160 cases. Southern Medical Journal 71: 758–765

Kamwendo F, Forslin L, Bodin L, Danielsson D 2000 Epidemiology of ectopic pregnancy during a 28 year period and the role of pelvic inflammatory disease. Sexually Transmitted Infections 76: 28–32

Karande V C, Flood J T, Heard N, Veeck L, Muasher S J 1991 Analysis of ectopic pregnancies resulting from in-vitro fertilization and embryo transfer. Human Reproduction 6: 446–449

Karikoski P, Aine R, Heinonen P K 1993 Abnormal embryogenesis in the etiology of ectopic pregnancy. Gynecologic and Obstetric Investigation 36: 158–162

Keskes J, Ben Siad A, Khairi H, Hidar M 1989 Simultaneous intra- and extra-uterine pregnancy: a report of six cases. Journal de Gynecologie, d'Obstetrique et de la Biologie de Reproduction 18: 181–184

Kihlstrom E, Lindgren R, Ryden G 1990 Antibodies to Chlamydia trachomatis in women with infertility, pelvic inflammatory disease and ectopic pregnancy. European Journal of Obstetrics, Gynecology and Reproductive Biology 35: 199–204

Kirkby N G 1969 Primary hepatic pregnancy. British Medical Journal 1: 296

Kitchen J D, Wein R M, Nunley W C, Thiagarajan S, Thornton W N 1979 Ectopic pregnancy: current clinical trends. American Journal of Obstetrics and Gynecology 134: 870–876

Kjer J J, Knudsen L B 1989 Ectopic pregnancy subsequent to laparoscopic sterilization. American Journal of Obstetrics and Gynecology 160: 1202–1204

Klein M, Graf A H, Hutter W et al 1995 Proliferative activity in ectopic trophoblastic tissue. Human Reproduction 10: 2441–2444

Kleiner G J, Roberts T W 1967 Current factors in causation of tubal pregnancy: a prospective clinicopathologic study. Journal of the National Medical Association 99: 21–28

Kosovski I, Schopova P, Skotschev S 1992 Ein Fall einer ausgetragenen Ovarialschwangerschaft. Zentralblatt fur Gynakologie 114: 316–317

Koudstaal J, van Dop P A, Hogerzeil H V et al 1999 Beloop en uitkomst van 2956 zwangerschappen na in-vitrofertilisatie in Nederland. Nederlandsche Tijdschrift voor Geneeskunde 143: 2375–2380

Kouyoundjian A J 1984 Cervical pregnancy: case report and literature review. Journal of the National Medical Association 76: 791–796

Krantz S G, Gray R H, Damewood M D, Wallach E E 1990 Time trends in risk factors and clinical outcome of ectopic pregnancy. Fertilty and Sterility 54: 42–46

Kutteh W H, Albert T 1991 Mature cystic teratoma of the fallopian tube associated with an ectopic pregnancy. Obstetrics and Gynecology 78: 984–986

Laluppa M A, Cavanagh D 1963 The endometrium in ectopic pregnancy: a study based on 35 patients by hysterectomy. Obstetrics and Gynecology 21: 155–164

Land J A, Arends J W 1992 Immunohistochemical analysis of estrogen and progesterone receptors in fallopian tubes during ectopic pregnancy. Fertility and Sterility 58: 335–337

Laufer A, Sadovsky A, Sadovsky E E 1962 Histologic appearance of the placenta in ectopic pregnancy. Obstetrics and Gynecology 20: 350–353

Lauritsen J G, Pagel V D, Vangstedt P, Starup J 1982 Results of repeated tuboplasties. Fertility and Sterility 37: 68–72

Lecuru F, Robin F, Taurelle R, Bernard J P, Vilde F 1999 Effect of methotrexate on tubal epithelium: a report of three cases. Journal of Reproductive Medicine 44: 46–48

Lehfeldt H, Tietze G, Gorstein F 1970 Ovarian pregnancy and the intrauterine device. American Journal of Obstetrics and Gynecology 108: 1005–1009

Lehmann F, Baban N, Harms B, Gethmann U, Krech R 1991 Ovargraviditat nach Gametentransfer (GIFT); ein Fallbericht. Geburtshilfe und Frauenheilkunde 51: 945–947

Lesny P, Killick S R, Robinson J, Maguiness S D 1999 Transcervical embryo transfer as a risk factor for ectopic pregnancy. Fertility and Sterility 72: 305–309

Lewin A, Simon A, Rabinowitz R, Schenker J G 1991 Second trimester heterotopic pregnancy after in-vitro fertilization and embryo transfer: a case report and review of the literature. International Journal of Fertility 36: 227–230

Li D K, Daling J P, Stergachis A S, Chu J, Weiss N S 1990 Prior condom use and the risk of tubal pregnancy. American Journal of Public Health 80: 964–966

Liukko P, Erkkola R 1976 Low dose progestogens and ectopic pregnancy. British Medical Journal 2: 1257–1258

Lloyd H E D, Feinberg R 1965 The Arias-Stella reaction: a nonspecific involutional phenomenon in intra- as well as extrauterine pregnancy. American Journal of Clinical Pathology 43: 428–432

Logani K B, Sharma S, Kohli T P, Khemani M, Prakash N 1995 Gestational choriocarcinoma of the fallopian tube — a case report. Indian Journal of Cancer 32: 183–185

Lopez H B, Micheelsen U, Berendtsen H, Kock K 1994 Ectopic pregnancy and its associated endometrial changes. Gynecologic and Obstetric Investigation 38: 104–106

Lower A M, Tyack A J 1989 Heterotopic pregnancy following in-vitro fertilization and embryo transfer: two case reports and a review of the literature. Human Reproduction 4: 126–128

Macafee C A J 1982 Ectopic pregnancy. British Journal of Hospital Medicine 28: 246–249

Maccato M, Estrada H, Hammill H, Faro S 1992 Prevalence of active Chlamydia trachomatis at the time of exploratory laparotomy for ectopic pregnancy. Obstetrics and Gynecology 79: 211–213

McCausland A 1982 Endosalpingosis (endosalpingoblastosis) following laparoscopic tubal coagulation as an etiological factor of ectopic pregnancy. American Journal of Obstetrics and Gynecology 143: 12–21

McElin T W, Iffy L 1976 Ectopic gestation: a consideration of new and controversial issues relating to pathogenesis and management. Obstetrics and Gynecology Annual 61: 130–138

McElin T W, Randall L M 1951 Intratubal term pregnancy without rupture: review of the literature and presentation of diagnostic criteria. American Journal of Obstetrics and Gynecology 61: 130–138

McLain P L, Kirkwood C R 1987 Ovarian and heterotopic pregnancy following clomiphene ovulation induction: report of a healthy live birth. Journal of Family Practice 24: 76–79

Madden S 1950 Chorioepithelioma of the fallopian tube. Journal of Obstetrics and Gynaecology of the British Empire 57: 68–70

Majmudar B, Henderson P H, Semple E 1983 Salpingitis isthmica nodosa: a high risk factor for tubal pregnancy. Obstetrics and Gynecology 62: 73–78

Makar A P, Vanderheyden J S, Schatteman E A, Albertyn G P, Verkinderen J J, Van Marck E A 1990 Female sterilization failure after bipolar electrocoagulation: a 6 year retrospective study. European Journal of Obstetrics, Gynecology and Reproductive Biology 37: 237–246

Makinde O O, Ogunniyi S O 1990 Ectopic pregnancy in a defined Nigerian population. International Journal of Gynaecology and Obstetrics 33: 239–241

Makinen J I 1989 Increase of ectopic pregnancy in Finland — combination of time and cohort effects. Obstetrics and Gynecology 73: 21–24

Makinen J, Rantala M, Vanha-Kamppa O 1998 A link between the epidemic of ectopic pregnancy and the 'baby-boom' cohort. American Journal of Epidemiology 148: 369–374

Marchbanks P A, Annegers J F, Coulam C B, Strathy J H, Kurland L T 1988 Risk factors for ectopic pregnancy: a population based study. Journal of the American Medical Association 259: 1823–1827

Marcovici I, Scoccia B 1997 Spontaneous bilateral tubal pregnancy and failed methotrexate therapy: a case report. American Journal of Obstetrics and Gynecology 177: 1545–1546

Marx L, Arck P, Kapp M, Kieslich C, Dietl J 1999 Leukocyte populations, hormone receptors and apoptosis in eutopic and ectopic first trimester human pregnancies. Human Reproduction 14: 1111–1117

Maymon R, Shulman A, Maymon B B, Bar-Levy F, Lotan M, Bahary C 1992 Ectopic pregnancy, the new gynaecological epidemic disease: review of the modern work-up and the non-surgical treatment option. International Journal of Fertility 37: 146–164

Mear Y, Ekra J B, Raoelison S 1965 Un cas de grossesse a implantation hepatique avec enfant. Semaine des Hopitaux de Paris 41: 1430–1433

Miettinen A, Heinonen P K, Teisala K, Hakkarainen K, Punnonen R 1990 Serologic evidence for the role of Chlamydia trachomatis, Neisseria gonorrhoeae, and Mycoplasma hominis in the etiology of tubal factor infertility and ectopic pregnancy. Sexually Transmitted Diseases 17: 10–14

Mikhael N Z, Campbell J S, Lee S Y, Acharya V C, Hurteau G D 1977 Tubal Arias-Stella atypia. European Journal of Obstetrics, Gynecology and Reproductive Biology 7: 13–15

Misra R, Misra K, Agrawal D 1992 Bilateral ectopic pregnancy. International Journal of Fertility 37: 24–25

Mitrani A 1973 Cervical pregnancy ending in a live birth. Journal of Obstetrics and Gynaecology of the British Commonwealth 80: 761–763

Molloy D, Deambrosis W, Keeping D, Hynes J, Harrison K, Hennessy J 1990 Multiple-sited (heterotopic) pregnancy after in vitro fertilization and gamete intrafallopian transfer. Fertility and Sterility 53: 1068–1071

Nayar R, Snell J, Silverberg S G, Lage J M 1996 Placental site nodule occurring in a fallopian tube. Human Pathology 27: 1243–1245

Nehra P C, Loginsky S J 1984 Pregnancy after vaginal hysterectomy. Obstetrics and Gynecology 64: 735–737

Neiger R, Croom C S 1991 Culturing tubal pregnancies for Chlamydia trachomatis: is it beneficial? International Journal of Fertility 36: 215–218

Neuman W L, Ponto K, Farber R A, Shangold G A 1990 DNA analysis of unilateral twin ectopic gestation. Obstetrics and Gynecology 75: 479–483

Newcomer J R 1998 Ampullary tubal hydatidiform mole treated with linear salpingotomy: a case report. Journal of Reproductive Medicine 43: 913–915

Nicholls R R 1941 Ovarian pregnancy with living child and mother. American Journal of Obstetrics and Gynecology 42: 341

Niles J H, Clark J J 1969 Pathogenesis of tubal pregnancy. American Journal of Obstetrics and Gynecology 105: 1230–1234

Nlome-Nzear A R, Picaud A, Ogowet-Igumu N Faye A, Ella-Ekogha R 1992 Recurrent extra-uterine pregnancies: 63 cases treated at the Hospital Center Libreville from 1985 to 1989. Revue Francaise de Gynecologie et d'Obstetrique 87: 12–16

Norenberg D D, Gundersson J H, Janis J F et al 1977 Early pregnancy on the diaphragm with endometriosis. Obstetrics and Gynecology 49: 620–624

Nygren K G, Bergh T, Nylund L, Wramsby H 1991 Nordic in vitro fertilization embryo transfer (IVF/ET) treatment outcomes 1982–1989. Acta Obstetricia et Gynecologica Scandinavica 70: 561–563

Oertel Y C 1978 The Arias-Stella reaction revisited. Archives of Pathology and Laboratory Medicine 102: 651–654

Okonofua F E, Ojo O S, Odunsi O A, Odesanmi W O 1990 Ectopic pregnancy associated with schistosomiasis in a Nigerian woman. International Journal of Gynaecology and Obstetrics 32: 281–284

Ollendorf D A, Fejgin M D, Barzilai M, Ben-Noon I, Gerbie A B 1987 The value of curettage in the diagnosis of ectopic pregnancy. American Journal of Obstetrics and Gynecology 157: 71–72

Ong S, Wingfield M 1999 Increasing incidence of ectopic pregnancy: is it iatrogenic? Irish Medical Journal 92: 364–365

Ory W H 1981 Ectopic pregnancy and intrauterine contraceptive device: new perspectives. Obstetrics and Gynecology 57: 137–143

Oscakina-Rojdestvenskaia A J 1935 Etiology of extrauterine pregnancy. Surgery Gynecology and Obstetrics 67: 308–311

Osser S, Persson K 1992 Chlamydial antibodies and deoxyribonucleic acid in patients with ectopic pregnancy. Fertility and Sterilty 57: 578–582

Paldi E, Gergely R Z, Abramavici H, Rimor-Tritsch I 1975 Clomiphene-citrate induced simultaneous intra- and extrauterine pregnancy. Fertility and Sterility 26: 1140

Parazzini F, Tozzi L, Ferraroni M, Bocciolone L, La-Vecchia C, Fedele L 1992 Risk factors for ectopic pregnancy: an Italian case control study. Obstetrics and Gynecology 80: 821–826

Parente J T, Ou C, Levy J, Legatt E 1983 Cervical pregnancy analysis: a review and report of five cases. Obstetrics and Gynecology 62: 79–83

Parker S L, Parker R T 1957 'Chronic' ectopic tubal pregnancy. American Journal of Obstetrics and Gynecology 74: 1174–1179

Paterson W G, Grant K A 1975 Advanced intraligamentous pregnancy: report of a case, review of the literature and a discussion of the biological implications. Obstetrical and Gynecological Survey 30: 715–726

Pauerstein C J, Croxatto H B, Eddy C A, Ramzy I, Walters M P 1986 Anatomy and pathology of tubal pregnancy. Obstetrics and Gynecology 67: 301–308

Persaud V 1970 Etiology of tubal ectopic pregnancy: radiologic and pathologic studies. Obstetrics and Gynecology 36: 257–263

Peterson H B, Xia Z, Hughes J M, Wilcox L S, Tylor L R, Trussell J 1997 The risk of ectopic pregnancy after tubal sterilization: U. S. Collaborative Review of Sterilization Working Group. New England Journal of Medicine 336: 796–797

Petrie R H, Duchin S 1980 Diagnosis and placental management of a viable term abdominal gestation. Diagnostic Gynecology and Obstetrics 2: 299–301

Phillipe E, Ritter J, Lefakis D 1970 Grossesse tubulaire, ovulation tardive et anomalie de nidation. Gynecologie et Obstetrique 69: 617–621

Phillips R S, Tuomala R E, Feldblum P J, Schachter J, Rosenberg M J, Aronson M D 1992 The effect of cigarette smoking, Chlamydia trachomatis infection, and vaginal douching on ectopic pregnancy. Obstetrics and Gynecology 79: 85–90

Picaud A, Walter P, Bennani S, Minko-Mi-Etoua D, Nlome-Nze AR 1990 Bilharziose tubaire a Schistosoma intercalatum revelee par un hemoperitoine. Archives d'Anatomie, Cytologie et Pathologie 38: 208–211

Picaud A, Berthonneau J P, Nlome-Nze A R, Ogowet-Igumu H, Engomgah-Beka T 1991 Serologie des Chlamydiae et grossesse extra-uterine; frequence du syndrome Fitz-Hugh-Curtis, Journal de Gynecologie, Obstetrique et Biologie de la Reproduction (Paris) 20: 209–215

Pisarki T S 1960 Cervical pregnancy. Journal of Obstetrics and Gynaecology of the British Empire 67: 759–762

Poland B J, Dill F J, Styblo C 1976 Embryonic development in ectopic human pregnancy. Teratology 14: 315–321

Pons J C, Goujard J, Derbanne C, Tournaire M 1988 Devenir des grossesses des patientes exposees in utero au diethylstilbeostrol. Journal de Gynecologie, Obstetrique et Biologie de la Reproduction (Paris) 17: 307–316

Pouly J L, Chapron C, Canis M et al 1991a Grossesses extra-uterines sur sterilet: caracteristiques et fertilite ulterieurs. Journal de Gynecologie, Obstetrique et Biologie de la Reproduction (Paris) 20: 1069–1073

Pouly J L, Chapron C, Canis M, Mage G et al 1991b Subsequent fertility for patients presenting with an ectopic pregnancy and having an intra-uterine device in situ. Human Reproduction 6: 999–1001

Pratt-Thomas H R, White L, Messka H H 1974 Primary ovarian pregnancy: presentations of three cases including one full term pregnancy. Southern Medical Journal 67: 920–925

Pretzsch G, Einenkel J, Baier D, Horn L C, Alexander H 1997 Zervikale Graviditat: Kasuistik und Literaturubersicht. Zentralblatt fur Gynakologie 119: 25–34

Procope B-J, Vesanto T 1966 Primary ovarian pregnancy. Acta Obstetricia et Gynecologica Scandinavica 44: 534–542

Rajkhowa M, Glass M R, Rutherford A J, Balen A H, Sharma V, Cuckle H S 2000 Trends in the incidence of ectopic pregnancy in England and Wales from 1966 to 1996. British Journal of Obstetrics and Gynecology 107: 369–374

Randall S 1983 A clinico-pathological study of ectopic pregnancy. MD Thesis, University of Manchester

Randall S, Buckley C H, Fox H 1987 Placentation in the Fallopian tube. International Journal of Gynecological Pathology 6: 132–139

Randic L, Haller H 1992 Ectopic pregnancy amongst past IUD users. International Journal of Gynaecology and Obstetrics 58: 299–304

Raziel A, Golan A, Neuman M, Ron-El R, Bukovsky I, Caspi E 1990 Ovarian pregnancy: a report of twenty cases in one institution. American Journal of Obstetrics and Gynecology 163: 1182–1185

Reese W A, O'Connor R, Bouzoukis J K, Sutherland S F 1989 Tubal pregnancy after total vaginal hysterectomy. Annals of Emergency Medicine 18: 1107–1110

Rivera F H, Torres F J, Rodriguez A F 1988 Ovarian pregnancy: a clinicopathological study of eight cases. European Journal of Obstetrics, Gynecology and Reproductive Biology 29: 339–345

Rizk B, Tan S I, Morcos S et al 1991 Heterotopic pregnancies after in vitro fertilization and embryo transfer. American Journal of Obstetrics and Gynecology 164: 161–164

Robertson J N, Hogston P, Ward H E 1988 Gonococcal and chlamydial antibodies in ectopic and intrauterine pregnancy. British Journal of Obstetrics and Gynaecology 95: 711–716

Robertson W B 1981 The endometrium. Butterworths, London

Robertson W H 1980 Bilateral Fallopian tube pregnancy. Fertility and Sterility 33: 86–87

Rock J A Katayama K P, Martin E J, Rock B M, Woodruff J D, Jones W H 1979 Pregnancy outcome following utero-tubal implantation: a comparison of the reamer and sharp cornual wedge excision techniques. Fertility and Sterility 31: 634–640

Rosen Y, Kim B 1974 Tubal gestation associated with Schistosoma mansoni salpingitis. Obstetrics and Gynecology 43: 413–417

Rubin G L, Peterson H B, Forfman S F et al 1983 Ectopic pregnancy in the United States: 1970–1978. Journal of the American Medical Association 249; 1725–1729

Rubin I C 1911 Cervical pregnancy. Surgery, Gynecology and Obstetrics 13: 625–627

Salmi T, Punnonen R, Gronroos M 1984 Tubal pregnancy after vaginal hysterectomy. Obstetrics and Gynecology 64: 826

Sambhi J S 1967 Ectopic pregnancy in Malaya. Medical Journal of Malaya 21: 344–351

Sandvei R, Sandstad E, Steier J A, Ulstein M 1987 Ovarian pregnancy associated with the intra-uterine contraceptive device. Acta Obstetricia et Gynecologica Scandinavica 66: 137–141

Saracoglu F O, Mungan T, Tanzer F 1992 Salpingitis isthmica nodosa in infertility and ectopic pregnancy. Gynecologic and Obstetric Investigation 34: 202–205

Saraiya M, Berg C J, Kendrick J S, Strauss L T, Atrash A K, Ahn Y W 1998 Cigarette smoking as a risk factor for ectopic pregnancy. American Journal of Obstetrics and Gynecology 178: 493–498

Schmidt G, Fowler W C, Talbert L M, Edelman D A 1980 Reproductive history of women exposed to diethylstilbestrol in utero. Fertility and Sterility 33: 21–24

Schneider P, Dreizin D H 1957 Cervical pregnancy. American Journal of Surgery 93: 27

Schumann E A 1921 Extra-uterine pregnancy. Appleton, New York

Schwartz L B, Carcangiu M L, DeCherney A H 1993 Primary ovarian pregnancy: a case report. Journal of Reproductive Medicine 38: 155–158

Sherman K J, Daling J R, Stergachis A et al 1990 Sexually transmitted diseases and tubal pregnancy. Sexually Transmitted Diseases 17: 115–121

Sherman S J, Werner H, Husain M 1991 Bilateral ectopic gestations. International Journal of Gynaecology and Obstetrics 35: 255–257

Shinagawa S, Nagayama M 1969 Cervical pregnancy as a possible sequela of abortion: report of 19 cases: American Journal of Obstetrics and Gynecology 105: 282–284

Shiono P H, Harlap S, Pellegrin F 1982 Ectopic pregnancies: rising incidence rates in northern California. American Journal of Public Health 72: 173–175

Silverberg S G 1972 Arias-Stella phenomenon in spontaneous and therapeutic abortion. American Journal of Obstetrics and Gynecology 112: 777–780

Singhal A M, Chin V P 1992 Unilateral triplet ectopic pregnancy: a case report. Journal of Reproductive Medicine 37: 187–188

Singhal V, Li T C, Cooke I D 1991 An analysis of factors influencing the outcome of 232 consecutive tubal microsurgery cases. British Journal of Obstetrics and Gynecology 98: 628–636

Sivanesaratnam V, Ng K H 1975 Tubal pregnancy following pospartum sterilization. Fertility and Sterility 26: 945–946

Sivin J 1991 Dose- and age- dependent ectopic pregnancy risks with intrauterine contraception. Obstetrics and Gynecology 78: 291–298

Skjeldestad F E 1997 How effectively do copper intrauterine devices prevent ectopic pregnancy? Acta Obstetricia et Gynecologica Scandinavica 76: 684–690

Skjeldestad F E, Backe B 1990 Incidence of extrauterine pregnancy in Norway in 1986: a population based overview from 15 counties. Tidsskrift Norwege for Laegeforen 110: 470–473

Skjeldestad F E, Gargiullo P M, Kendrick J S 1997 Multiple induced abortions as risk factor for ectopic pregnancy: a prospective study. Acta Obstetricia et Gynecologica Scandinavica 76: 691–696

Skjeldestad F E, Kendrick J S, Atrash H K, Daltveit A K 1997 Increasing incidence of ectopic pregnancy in one Norwegian county — a population based study, 1975–1993. Acta Obstetricia et Gynecologica Scandinavica 76: 159–165

Spiegelberg O 1878 Zur Casuistik der Ovarialschwangerschaft. Archiv fur Gynakologie 13: 73–79

Stabile I, Grudzinskas J G 1990 Ectopic pregnancy: a review of incidence, etiology and diagnostic aspects. Obstetrical and Gynecological Survey 45: 335–347

Stewart-Akers A M, Krasnow J S, Deloia J A 1997 Decidual leukocyte populations in ectopic pregnancies. Fertility and Sterility 68: 1103–1107

Stock R J 1991 Tubal pregnancy: associated histopathology. Obstetrics and Gynecology Clinics of North America 18: 73–94

Stock R J 1993 Gross pathology and microscopic histopathology. In: Stovall T G, Ling F W (eds) Extrauterine pregnancy. McGraw-Hill, New York, pp 65–96

Storch M P, Petrie R H 1976 Unusual tubal twin gestation. American Journal of Obstetrics and Gynecology 125: 1148

Studdiford W E 1942 Primary peritoneal pregnancy. American Journal of Obstetrics and Gynecology 44: 487–491

Studdiford W E 1945 Cervical pregnancy. American Journal of Obstetrics and Gynecology 49: 169–174

Svare J, Norup P, Grove-Thomsen S et al 1993 Heterotopic pregnancies after in-vitro fertilization and embryo transfer — a Danish survey. Human Reproduction 8: 116–118

Swolin K, Fall M 1972 Ectopic pregnancy: recurrence, postoperative fertility and aspects of treatment based on 192 patients. Acta Europaea Fertilitas 3: 147–157

Szlachter N, Weiss G 1979 Distal tubal pregnancy in a patient with a bicornuate uterus and segmental absence of the Fallopian tube. Fertility and Sterility 32: 602–603

Tanbo T, Dale P O, Lunde O, Abyholm T 1991 Heterotopic pregnancy following in vitro fertilization. Acta Obstetricia et Gynecologica Scandinavica 70: 335–338

Tancer M L, Delke I, Veridiano L 1981 A fifteen year experience with ectopic pregnancy. Surgery Gynecology and Obstetrics 152: 179–182

Tatum H G, Schmidt F H 1977 Contraceptive and sterilization practices and extrauterine pregnancy: a realistic perspective. Fertility and Sterility 28: 407–421

Terada S, Uchide K, Suzuki N, Ueno H, Akasofu K 1994 Choriocarcinoma secondary to isthmic tubal pregnancy. Gynecological and Obstetric Investigation 37: 69–72

Tietze C 1968 Wanted: ovarian pregnancies. American Journal of Obstetrics and Gynecology 101: 275

Tomazevic T, Ribic-Pucelj M 1992 Ectopic pregnancy following the treatment of tubal infertility. Journal of Reproductive Medicine 37: 611–614

Tuncer R, Sipahi T, Erkaya S, Akar N K, Baysar N S, Ercevik S 1994 Primary twin ovarian pregnancy. International Journal of Gynaecology and Obstetrics 46: 57–59

Urbach D R, Cohen M M 1999 Is perforation of the appendix a risk factor for tubal infertility and ectopic pregnancy? An appraisal of the evidence. Canadian Journal of Surgery 42: 101–108

van Iddekinge B 1972 Ectopic pregnancy: a review. South African Medical Journal 46: 1844

Varela-Nunez A 1961 Tubal pregnancy following treated genital tuberculosis: report of 2 cases and review of the literature. American Journal of Obstetrics and Gynecology 82: 1162–1165

Vasquez G, Winston R M L, Brosens I A 1983 Tubal mucosa and ectopic pregnancy. British Journal of Obstetrics and Gynaecology 90: 468–474

Vessey M P, Doll R, Petro R, Johnson B, Wiggins P 1976 A long-term follow-up study of women using different methods of contraception. Journal of Biosocial Science 8: 373–427

Vessey M P, Yeates D, Flavel R 1979 Risk of ectopic pregnancy and duration of use of an intrauterine device. Lancet i: 501–502

Ville Y, Leruez M, Picaud A, Walter P, Fernandez H 1991a Tubal schistosomiasis as a cause of ectopic pregnancy in endemic areas: a report of three cases. European Journal of Obstetrics, Gynecology and Reproductive Biology 42: 77–79

Ville Y, Leruez M, Glowaczower E, Robertson J N, Ward M E 1991b The role of Chlamydia trachomatis and Neisseria gonorrhoeae in the aetiology of ectopic pregnancy in Gabon. British Journal of Obstetrics and Gynaecology 98: 1260–1266

Weinstein L, Morris M B, Dotters D, Christian C D 1983 Ectopic pregnancy: a new surgical epidemic. Obstetrics and Gynecology 61: 698–701

Wennerholm U B, Janson P O, Wennergren M, Kjellmer I 1991 Pregnancy complications and short term follow up of infants born after in vitro fertilization and embryo transfer (IVF/ET). Acta Obstetricia et Gynecologica Scandinavica 70: 565–573

Westrom L 1975 Effect of pelvic inflammatory disease on fertilty. American Journal of Obstetrics and Gynecology 121: 707–713

Westrom L 1985 Influence of sexually transmitted diseases on sterility and ectopic pregnancy. Acta Europaea Fertilitas 16: 21–24

Westrom L, Bengtsson L P H, Mardh P-A 1981 Incidence, trends and risks of etopic pregnancy in a population of women. British Medical Journal 282: 15–18

Westrom L, Joesoef R, Reynolds G, Hagdu A, Thompson S E 1992 Pelvic inflammatory disease and fertility: a cohort study of 1,844 women with laparoscopically verified disease and 657 control women with normal laparoscopic results. Sexually Transmitted Diseases 19: 185–192

Weyerman P C, Verhoeven A T M, Alberda A T 1989 Cervical pregnancy after in vitro fertilization and embryo transfer. American Journal of Obstetrics and Gynecology 161: 1145–1146

White R G 1989 Advanced abdominal pregnancy: a review of 23 cases. Irish Journal of Medical Sciences 158: 77–78

Williams P C, Malvar T C, Kraft J R 1982 Term ovarian pregnancy with delivery of a live female infant. American Journal of Obstetrics and Gynecology 142: 589–591

Wollen A L, Flood P R, Sandvei R et al 1984 Morphological changes in tubal mucosa associated with the use of intrauterine contraceptive devices. British Journal of Obstetrics and Gynaecology 91: 1123–1128

World Health Organization 1985 WHO Task Force on Intrauterine Devices for Fertility Regulation: a multinational case control study of ectopic pregnancy. Clinical Reproduction and Fertility 3: 131–143

Wright N H, Stadel B V 1981 Ectopic pregnancy and tubal ligation. American Journal of Obstetrics and Gynecology 139: 611–612

Xie P Z, Feng Y Z, Zhao B H 1991 Primary ovarian pregnancy: report of fifteen cases. Chinese Medical Journal 104: 217–220

Yackel D B, Panton O M N, Martin D J, Lee D 1988 Splenic pregnancy — case report. Obstetrics and Gynecology 71: 471–473

Yang M H, Ng S C, Ratnam S S, et al, 1992 Outcome of 143 pregnancies conceived by assisted reproductive techniques. Asia Oceania Journal of Obstetrics and Gynaecology 18: 299–307

Yankowitz J, Leake J, Huggins G, Gazaway P, Gates E 1990 Cervical ectopic pregnancy: review of the literature and report of a case treated by single-dose methotrexate therapy. Obstetrical and Gynecological Survey 45: 405–414

Yoseph S 1990 Ectopic pregnancy at Tikur Anbessa Hospital, Addis Ababa, Ethiopia, 1981–1987: a review of 176 cases. Ethiopian Medical Journal 28: 113–118

Yuzpe A A, Brown S E, Casper R F, Nisker J A, Graves G 1989 Rates and outcomes of pregnancies achieved in the first 4 years of an in-vitro fertilization program. Canadian Medical Association Journal 140: 167–172

Zhang Z M, Weng L J, Zhang Z Y et al 1994 An epidemiologic study on the relationship of ectopic pregnancy and the use of contraceptives in Beijing — the incidence of ectopic pregnancy in the Beijing area. Contraception 50: 263–262

Zelinger B B, Grinvalsky H T, Fields C 1960 Simultaneous dermoid cyst of the tube and ectopic pregnancy. Obstetrics and Gynecology 15: 340–343

Zolli A, Rocko J M 1982 Ectopic pregnancy months and years after hysterectomy. Archives of Surgery 117: 962–964

32

Pathology of contraception and hormonal therapy

C. H. Buckley   S. M. Ismail

Introduction   1071

The pathology of hormonal therapy   1071
Oestrogens   1071
Diethylstilboestrol   1074
Anti-oestrogens (clomiphene and tamoxifen)   1075
Progestagens   1082
Antiprogestins   1086
Gonadotrophin-releasing hormone agonists:gonadorelin analogues (e.g. Goserelin, Zoladex)   1087

The pathology of hormone replacement therapy (HRT)   1087
Combined hormones   1087
Tibolone   1090

Hormones in the treatment of infertility   1090

The pathology of contraception   1090
Introduction   1090
Steroid contraception   1091
Intrauterine contraceptive devices   1106

INTRODUCTION

A wide variety of progestational and oestrogenic compounds is used for therapeutic and contraceptive purposes in gynaecological practice, synthetic products often being preferred to their natural counterparts because of their potency and efficacy. The hormones may be given orally, vaginally, systemically, by means of depot injections or implants, topically, by skin patches, in intrauterine devices or by a combination of these methods. The therapeutic effects are, to a large extent, independent of their mode of administration.

A range of other drugs, such as antiprogestins, gonadotrophin-releasing hormone agonists, Tamoxifen and Tibolone is also used therapeutically to modulate progesterone mediated endometrial changes, suppress ovulatory function, modulate oestrogen-induced activity and to act as hormone replacement, respectively. In addition to their desired clinical effect these products may induce changes in both the target organs and other tissues.

THE PATHOLOGY OF HORMONAL THERAPY

OESTROGENS

The oestrogens used therapeutically are of three main types, the conjugated and esterified naturally occurring hormones, such as that found in mare's urine, the non-steroidal stereochemical mimics of oestrogen, such as diethylstilboestrol, and non-conjugated steroids derived from oestrogen, such as ethinyloestradiol and its 3-methyl ether mestranol.

Oestrogens may be given alone, but it is more usual and prudent to use a regimen combining them with a progestagen, particularly in those women retaining their uterus. They have a wide variety of therapeutic indications, which, broadly, include replacement or supplement of an endogenous deficit or correction of an endogenous imbalance.

Effects on the endometrium

Oestrogens are responsible, in the normal proliferative phase, for the synchronous growth of the glands, stroma and vasculature of the endometrium and the induction of progesterone receptors. Following ovulation, they cause the oedema characteristic of the mid-secretory phase and promote the growth of the spiral arteries in the late secretory phase, following their differentiation by progesterone.

Withdrawal of oestrogen after prolonged use results in withdrawal bleeding, but this can be distinguished, in curettings, from menstruation by the absence of secretory glands. Bleeding may also occur spontaneously if small doses of oestrogen are given continuously.

If oestrogens are given to a patient early in the normal proliferative phase, endometrial growth is prolonged and the endometrium may exhibit features of a prolonged proliferative phase: ovulation is suppressed due to gonadotrophin inhibition and the secretory phase is delayed or absent (Dallenbach-Hellweg 1981). If oestrogen is given to a patient already in the secretory phase, there may be severe stromal oedema, a delay in the secretory transformation of the glands and retarded maturation of the stroma (Egger & Kindermann 1980).

More commonly, however, oestrogens are used in patients in whom there is a paucity of endogenous hormone and thus an absence of normal cyclical changes. The appearance of the endometrium in these women is due, therefore, entirely to the exogenous hormone. The morphological pattern most commonly encountered in the postmenopausal patient receiving small doses of oestrogen, or absorbing oestrogen from vaginal pessaries given to relieve dryness and soreness, is that of a weakly proliferative endometrium (Fig. 32.1). This is characterised by the presence of glands lined by single-layered or, occasionally, focally multilayered, epithelium containing only infrequent mitoses, and a densely cellular inactive stroma. There is little thickening of the endometrium and the functionalis is poorly defined. In some patients, the appearances, at least initially, may resemble those seen in the normal proliferative phase. Gradually, however, or sometimes ab initio, the picture becomes that of 'disordered proliferative endometrium' (Hendrickson & Kempson 1980) (Fig. 32.2) or mild complex hyperplasia. The endometrial stroma is abundant and of normal structure whilst the glands show varying degrees of architectural atypia and dilatation; there is no evidence of cytological atypia.

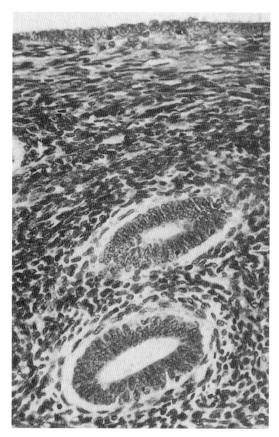

Fig. 32.1 The endometrium from a postmenopausal patient who has been using oestrogens. The glandular epithelium is multilayered but the stroma is compact.

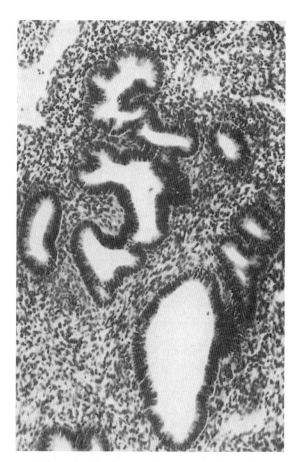

Fig. 32.2 The endometrium from a postmenopausal woman who had been given small cyclical doses of oestrogen. There is a minor degree of complex hyperplasia characterised by invaginations and outpouchings of the glands. The epithelium lining the glands is multilayered but there is no evidence of cytological atypia.

Metaplastic squamous epithelium develops in the endometrium of experimental animals given large doses of oestrogen (Baggish & Woodruff 1967) and is not uncommonly seen in the endometrium of postmenopausal women receiving oestrogen-only hormone replacement therapy (Hendrickson & Kempson 1980) and in women whose endometrium has been subject to unopposed endogenous oestrogen. Tubal (serous) metaplasia is also common under such circumstances and mucinous metaplasia and ciliated cell metaplasia are occasionally seen. A significant proportion of women who are given continuous or cyclical unopposed oestrogen for menopausal symptoms (Schiff et al 1982) or for primary hypo-oestrogenic amenorrhoea (Van Campenhout et al 1980) develop a hyperplastic endometrium. Whilst this may have a simple pattern (Fig. 32.3), in some cases it may be complex (Fig. 32.4) or atypical (Fig. 32.5) (Whitehead et al 1977; Fox & Buckley 1982; Buckley & Fox 2002). Hyperplasia may occur soon after therapy commences or be delayed for up to two years. The administration of progestagens alone or in combination with an oestrogen in sequential or continuous pattern has been observed to reverse hyperplasia (Whitehead et al 1977) or protect against its development (Sturdee et al 1978; Whitehead et al 1981).

It is widely accepted that the use of unopposed oestrogens is an important aetiological factor in the development of endometrial carcinoma (Antunes et al 1979; Brinton & Hoover 1993) in postmenopausal women, in women with polycystic ovary syndrome and in younger women with dysgenetic gonads (McCarty et al 1978) who have been given unopposed oestrogen. It makes no difference whether the oestrogen used is conjugated or unconjugated, low dose or high dose (Cushing et al 1998), nor whether it is used continuously or cyclically (Shapiro et al 1980) and this form of therapy is, therefore, seldom recommended. There is also some evidence that the risk of developing carcinoma persists after the cessation of therapy and that it may be related to the total dose of oestrogen given (Rosenwaks et al 1979; Brinton & Hoover 1993). There are reports that women who smoke or are thin are most adversely affected (Brinton & Hoover 1993). The tumours which arise following oestrogen therapy are generally lower staged, better differentiated and occur in younger women than do those occurring in non-hormone users (Robboy & Bradley 1979; Elwood & Boyes 1980) (Fig. 32.6). Histologically, they comprise a greater proportion of well-differentiated (histological grade 1) endometrioid adenocarcinomas with squamous metaplasia than do tumours from oestrogen non-users, whilst the proportion of prognostically unfavourable subtypes, such as

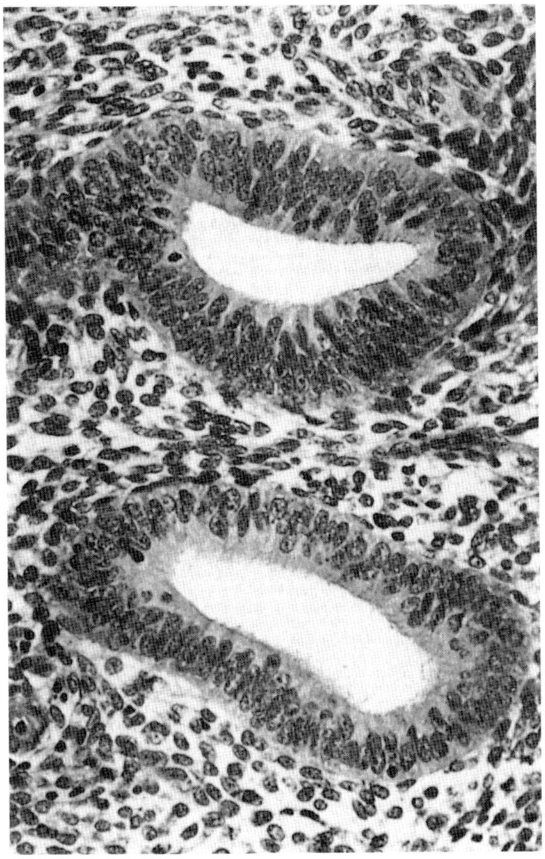

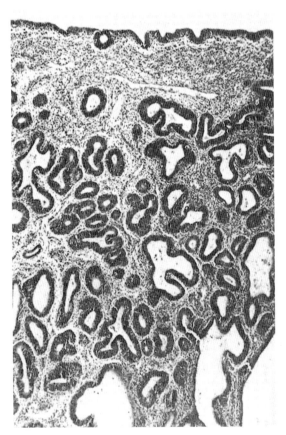

Fig. 32.3 Simple endometrial hyperplasia. The glands are smooth contoured and their epithelium multilayered but there is no loss of nuclear polarity.

Fig. 32.4 Complex endometrial hyperplasia. Variably sized, irregularly shaped glands lined by a multilayered epithelium lie closely packed; the intervening stroma is rather sparse.

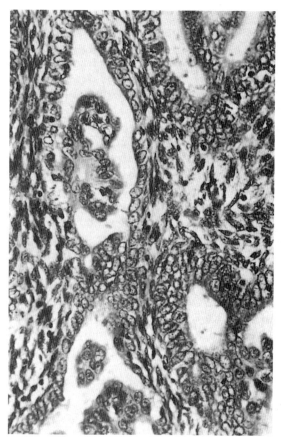

Fig. 32.5 Atypical endometrial hyperplasia. The glandular epithelium is irregularly invaginated and there is loss of nuclear polarity.

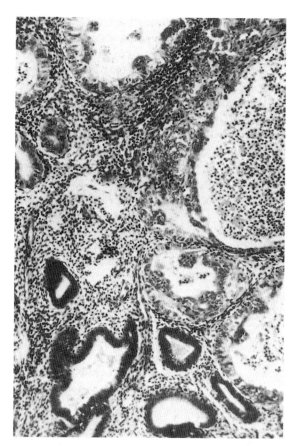

Fig. 32.6 Well-differentiated endometrioid endometrial adenocarcinoma in the right of the field arising in a patient with endometrial hyperplasia.

adenosquamous carcinoma, serous carcinoma and clear cell carcinoma, occur less frequently (Silverberg et al 1982). If, however, the woman has taken oestrogens for 3 or more years, the tumours are likely to have invaded the myometrium at the time of diagnosis (Shapiro et al 1998). The use of a progestagen for at least ten days per month (Paterson et al 1980) or, alternatively, the use of a combined oestrogen/progestagen preparation, in no way appears to affect adversely the therapeutic effect of the oestrogen but does appear to protect the patient from the risk of carcinoma.

A rare association between atypical polypoid adenomyoma of the uterus and oestrogen therapy has been described (Clement & Young 1987) and it is now also apparent that women who are given unopposed oestrogen for long periods of time are at increased risk of developing endometrial carcinosarcomas (malignant mixed Müllerian tumours) (Schwartz et al 1996).

Effect on other tissues

The cervical smear of women using oestrogens characteristically has a superficial pattern whilst histologically the squamous epithelium is mature, thickened and contains glycogen (Hammond & Maxson 1982).

The epithelium of the Fallopian tube is hormone responsive (Fig. 32.7) and there may be general hyperplasia or multiple hyperplastic foci which may be remarkably localised (Fox & Buckley 1983). In the postmenopausal woman, the tubal epithelium may recover the form it had in the reproductive years with an increase in ciliated cells.

Hypercellular leiomyomas, which also grow rapidly, are encountered in some women receiving oestrogens (Dallenbach-Hellweg 1980a).

Foci of endometriosis, being sensitive to oestrogenic stimulation, may undergo proliferative activity or become hyperplastic when oestrogen therapy is given and endometrial stromal sarcoma has been reported in such foci (McCluggage et al 1996a).

The risk of breast carcinoma does not appear to be increased when unopposed oestrogen is used for hormone replacement (Kaufman et al 1991).

DIETHYLSTILBOESTROL

Twenty per cent of women exposed to Diethylstilboestrol (DES) in utero exhibit a range of genital tract abnormalities rarely encountered in non-exposed women (Herbst et al 1975). The features are also discussed in Chapter 36 and will be only summarised here.

Between 34 and 45% of such women have vaginal adenosis (Kurman & Scully 1974; Hart et al 1976; Robboy et al 1979; Ostergard 1981). The condition affects 73% of the women who were exposed before the eighth week of gestation (Herbst et al 1975), but after the 20th week of intrauterine life the effect is much reduced (Robboy et al 1979), although there is some evidence that the total dose of DES that the fetus receives may be significant (Robboy et al 1982).

Vaginal adenosis is not limited to women exposed to DES; it also occurs in 4% of fetuses and neonates exposed in utero to progestagens and oestrogens other than DES (Johnson et al 1979) and in women with no history of exposure to hormone therapy.

Cervical and vaginal deformities are also described (Herbst et al 1972; O'Brien et al 1979; Antonioli et al 1980). In addition, hysterosalpingograms may demonstrate small T-shaped uterine cavities with dilatation of the interstitial and proximal isthmic portions of the Fallopian tubes (Kaufman et al 1977; Haney et al 1979; DeCherney et al 1981). The tubes may also be foreshortened and convoluted and have 'withered' fimbria (DeCherney et al 1981).

Functional uterine problems arise as a consequence of these structural anomalies. These women have an increased

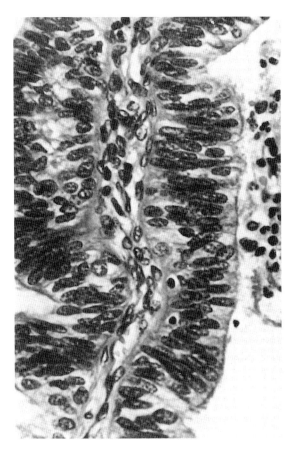

Fig. 32.7 The epithelium of the Fallopian tube in a patient subjected to prolonged high levels of oestrogenic stimulation from a granulosa cell tumour. The epithelium is multilayered and contains few secretory cells.

number of spontaneous miscarriages, ectopic pregnancies and premature deliveries and their children are more likely to die in the perinatal period than are children of normal women (Herbst 1981a; Stillman 1982).

Probably the most serious complication developing in the young DES-exposed woman is clear cell carcinoma of the cervix or vagina (Herbst & Scully 1970; Herbst et al 1974; Herbst et al 1981b). Fortunately, it occurs in only 0.014 to 0.14% of affected women (Herbst et al 1977) a much lower incidence than was originally feared. Very few cases have occurred in the United Kingdom (Buckley et al 1982). The pathology of these tumours is described in Chapter 36. Invasive neoplasms other than clear cell carcinoma appear to be very rare. As the cohort of DES-exposed women age, however, the position may be changing. A single case of cervical adenosquamous carcinoma has been reported (Vandrie et al 1983) and more recently, attention has been drawn to the development, in older DES-exposed women, of non-clear cell, mucin-secreting adenocarcinoma of the cervix (DeMars et al 1995).

Cytological surveillance has accurately predicted the development of clear cell carcinoma in patients with DES-associated adenosis (Taft et al 1974; Anderson et al 1979; Kaufman et al 1982; Ghosh & Cera 1983). Cytological atypia, in the areas of adenosis, has been described and almost certainly represents a precursor of the carcinoma (Antonioli et al 1979).

Fowler et al (1981) hold the view that there is an increased risk of squamous intraepithelial neoplasia in the large metaplastic transformation zone of women with cervical ectopy and adenosis but Herbst (1981b) and Robboy et al (1981) could find no evidence to support this and, indeed, intraepithelial neoplasia may be less frequent in DES-exposed individuals than in matched controls (Robboy et al 1982).

ANTI-OESTROGENS (CLOMIPHENE AND TAMOXIFEN)

Clomiphene

Clomiphene (clomifene citrate) is used in the treatment of infertility associated with hyperprolactinaemia, oligomenorrhoea or secondary amenorrhoea. The drug occupies the oestrogen receptors in the hypothalamus and thereby interferes with the feedback mechanism of ovarian oestrogen on the hypothalamus. As a consequence, gonadotrophins are released by the anterior pituitary.

Clomiphene may result in ovarian hyperstimulation, superovulation, intermenstrual spotting and menorrhagia. The appearance of the endometrium in women who are given clomiphene depends upon whether they are normally cycling or have already experienced ovulatory dysfunction. Clomiphene tends to impair the development of a normal secretory endometrium because its anti-oestrogenic effect causes deficient oestrogen priming of the endometrium

(Dallenbach-Hellweg 1988). In normal, regularly cycling women, therefore, it results in maturation and developmental delay, which may at first glance not be readily apparent. There are, however, subtle changes such as a reduction in the number of glands per unit volume and a reduction in mean gland diameter whilst the number of vacuolated cells per thousand in the glandular epithelium is increased (Sereepapong et al 2000). In women with pre-existing luteal phase defect, treatment with clomiphene corrects the luteal phase in those in whom the defect is preceded by excessive oestrogen, for example, polycystic ovary syndrome (Cook et al 1984; Dallenbach-Hellweg 1988) and in the majority of women who develop more than one pre-ovulatory follicle following treatment, but only occasionally in those who have only one pre-ovulatory follicle (Guzick & Zeleznik 1990). In women who have polycystic ovary syndrome, and anovulation, luteal phase defect does not develop after treatment with clomiphene; on the contrary, a normal endometrial pattern may emerge (Cook et al 1984).

Tamoxifen

Tamoxifen is a non-steroidal triphenylethylene derivative (Furr & Jordan 1984) which has proved useful in the management of established breast cancer. Breast cancer patients treated with tamoxifen have a lower mortality from their tumour (Early Breast Cancer Triallists' Collaborative Group 1988, 1992), longer tumour-free survival (Early Breast Cancer Triallists' Collaborative Group 1988, 1992), and a lower risk of contralateral breast cancer when compared to non-tamoxifen treated controls (Early Breast Cancer Triallists' Collaborative Group 1988, 1992; Fisher et al 1989; Fornander et al 1989). The value of tamoxifen in breast cancer prevention among women at increased risk of breast cancer is still not clear. Although the British (Powles et al 1998a) and Italian (Veronesi et al 1998) studies were unable to show a definite beneficial effect, the American NSABP-P1 study found a 49% reduction in invasive breast cancer among tamoxifen-treated versus placebo-treated women (Fisher et al 1998).

Prolonged tamoxifen treatment affects all parts of the female genital tract. The effects of tamoxifen on postmenopausal endometrial and cervical epithelia tend to be predominantly oestrogen-like, but the drug also has stromal effects which are unlike those seen in unopposed oestrogen treatment. It is strongly polypogenic in the postmenopausal endometrium and early reports suggest that it has a similar effect on endometriotic foci occurring in postmenopausal women.

Tamoxifen and the endometrium

As tamoxifen has been used predominantly in the management of established breast cancer, a disease which affects mainly postmenopausal women, much of the information about the endometrial side effects of long term treatment pertains to such women. In this age group, prolonged treatment is associated with an increased incidence of endometrial hyperplasia, endometrial polyps and malignant endometrial neoplasms. Much less information is available about the effects, if any, on the endometrium of premenopausal women. The ensuing discussion is therefore confined to the postmenopausal endometrium.

Endometrial hyperplasia. Modern imaging techniques allow in vivo measurements of endometrial thickness in asymptomatic women. A series of studies using transvaginal ultrasonography have conclusively demonstrated that the endometrium of tamoxifen-treated postmenopausal breast cancer patients is significantly thicker than that of comparable women not treated with tamoxifen (Lahti et al 1993; Cohen et al 1994b; Bese et al 1996), that the endometrium becomes thicker during treatment with tamoxifen but not with other modalities (Lindahl et al 1997) and that there is a significant correlation between increased endometrial thickness and tamoxifen treatment for longer than 5 years (Hann et al 1997).

Attempts to investigate the pathological basis of these ultrasonographic changes have been hampered because it is difficult to obtain adequate biopsies for tamoxifen-treated endometrium. In one study, investigators attempted to biopsy the endometrium of 77 asymptomatic tamoxifen-treated postmenopausal women, 76 of whom had an ultrasonographic thickness >5 mm. Despite the ultrasonographic abnormality, endometrial tissue was unobtainable in 55 cases (Cohen et al 1993). In another study, no endometrial tissue was obtained in 30 out of 48 tamoxifen-treated women even though the mean endometrial thickness in this group was twice that of comparable women not treated with tamoxifen. Eight tamoxifen-treated women in this study had cystic endometrial thickening >10 mm, but endometrial tissue was unobtainable in 5 of these patients (Bese et al 1996).

Because of the difficulties of obtaining adequate biopsy material from tamoxifen-thickened endometrium, information about its pathological features is relatively limited. However, a number of investigators have reported an increased incidence of proliferative activity in the biopsied endometrium of tamoxifen-treated postmenopausal breast cancer patients (Neven et al 1989, 1990; De Muylder et al 1991; Cohen et al 1993; Kedar et al 1994).

Hysterectomy specimens from tamoxifen-treated women with gynaecological symptoms show diffuse endometrial thickening. The cut surface of the endometrium has a characteristic 'Swiss cheese' appearance caused by cystic dilatation of endometrial glands. On microscopic examination, some endometrial glands show complex branching and there may be focal glandular crowding. A range of epithelial metaplasias may be seen. Endometrial stroma is abundant and stromal cells are separated by interstitial collagen bundles and fibrils. In the majority of cases, both the epithelial and stromal components of the endometrium show mitotic activity (Ismail 1994).

There has been some debate on the nature of these morphological findings (Ismail 1998; Neven et al 1998). It has been assumed by some authors that tamoxifen-induced endometrial thickening represents cystic endometrial atrophy (Touraine et al 1995; McGonigle et al 1998; Neven et al 1998). This view is based partly on the assumption, in general gynaecological practice, that a poor or inadequate yield of endometrial tissue on attempted biopsy equates with endometrial atrophy. It is also contributed to by the peculiar hysteroscopic appearances of tamoxifen-treated endometrium which differs from that of endometrial hyperplasia occurring in a non-tamoxifen setting. Moreover, many women who develop ultrasonographic endometrial thickening while receiving tamoxifen have no gynaecological symptoms and pose a management dilemma, particularly if labelled as having endometrial hyperplasia.

Despite the weight of these arguments, it is questionable whether the term atrophy is applicable to tamoxifen-thickened endometria. Atrophy as a pathological term denotes lack of growth and reduction in the amount of affected tissue; it is normal in the endometrium of postmenopausal women. Thus, the term atrophy may be appropriate when applied to the few postmenopausal endometria that do not increase in thickness in response to tamoxifen treatment. It is, however, inappropriate when applied to the endometrium of most tamoxifen-treated postmenopausal women which demonstrably increases in thickness during tamoxifen treatment and which shows proliferative activity in both its epithelial and stromal components. These endometria are demonstrating excessive growth and the pathological process involved would be more correctly regarded as hyperplasia than atrophy.

Endometrial polyps. Postmenopausal women who receive prolonged treatment with tamoxifen have an increased prevalence of endometrial polyps (Neven et al 1989; Lahti et al 1993; Silva et al 1994; Powles et al 1998b). In a study of 103 postmenopausal breast cancer patients without gynaecological symptoms, endometrial polyps were present in 36% of the 51 tamoxifen-treated women as compared to 10% of untreated controls (Lahti et al 1993). The Royal Marsden tamoxifen chemoprevention trial detected endometrial polyps in 11% of women randomised to receive tamoxifen 20 mg/day while less than 1% of the placebo group had endometrial polyps (Powles et al 1998b); the subjects in this trial were also asymptomatic. The prevalence of tamoxifen-associated polyps would be expected to be higher in women with gynaecological symptoms and to increase with increasing duration of treatment.

Tamoxifen-associated endometrial polyps usually occur on a background of endometrial hyperplasia and are often multiple (Ismail 1994). They may recur after polypectomy. They are considerably larger than polyps which develop sporadically in untreated women (Ismail 1994; Schlesinger et al 1998). Their large size combined with the frequent finding of ulceration and infarction may lead to a clinical suspicion of malignancy. On microscopic examination, the polyps are composed of glandular structures in abundant fibromyxoid connective tissue. Focally, there is alteration in polarity of periglandular stromal cells which gives rise to an appearance of periglandular stromal condensation (Figs 32.8, 32.9). The glands are elongated, often branching or budding and occasionally cystic. There may be focal glandular crowding. The

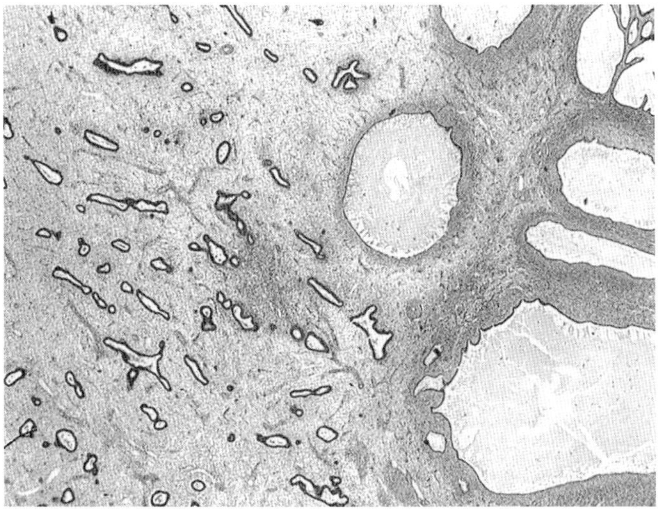

Fig. 32.8 Low-power view of a tamoxifen-associated endometrial polyp showing focal periglandular stromal condensation.

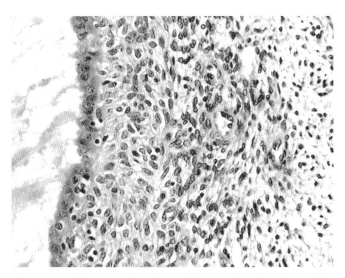

Fig. 32.9 High power view of tamoxifen-associated endometrial polyp showing part of a glandular structure and surrounding stroma. There is alteration in the polarity of periglandular stromal cells but no mitoses are seen in this field and there is no significant cytological atypia.

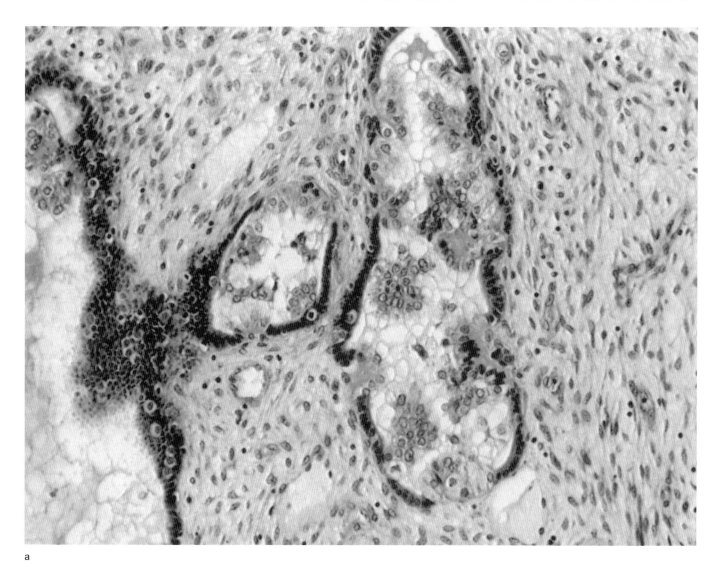

a

Fig. 32.10 a The epithelial component of a tamoxifen-associated endometrial polyp: Tubal and papillary oxyphil metaplasia.

epithelial cells lining the glands are predominantly of endometrioid type but show a range of metaplasias including apocrine, squamoid, mucinous, clear cell and papillary oxyphil cell metaplasia (Fig. 32.10a–c). Proliferative activity is common in both the epithelial and stromal elements (Ismail 1994).

The presence of mitotic activity and periglandular condensation within the stroma of tamoxifen-associated polyps may lead to a suspicion of Müllerian adenosarcoma. Tamoxifen-associated polyps can be distinguished from adenosarcomas by the focal nature of periglandular stromal changes, relatively low mitotic activity within the stroma and lack of significant stromal atypia (Fig. 32.8). In contrast, Müllerian adenosarcomas have overt features of malignancy in stromal cells with frequent atypical mitoses, a high mitotic rate ranging from 1/10 high-power fields to 40/10 high-power fields and generalised periglandular stromal condensation.

Another characteristic feature of tamoxifen-associated endometrial polyps is the relatively high prevalence of endometrial carcinoma developing within them (Ismail 1994; Schlesinger et al 1998; Cohen et al 1999a). This is a rare phenomenon in sporadic endometrial polyps. An early study carried out prior to the introduction of tamoxifen found 4 instances in 1100 endometrial polyps while a more recent study reported 5 cases in 1034 polyps occurring in otherwise healthy postmenopausal women (Cohen et al 1999a). The precise risk of endometrial carcinoma developing in tamoxifen-associated polyps remains uncertain as many studies are relatively small. Cohen et al (1999b) found 2 endometrial polyp-cancers in 67 tamoxifen-associated endometrial polyps while Schlesinger et al (1998) reported 2 cases in 28 tamoxifen-associated polyps studied.

Endometrial carcinoma. In 1989 Fornander et al reported an increased risk of uterine corpus cancer among tamoxifen-treated postmenopausal breast cancer

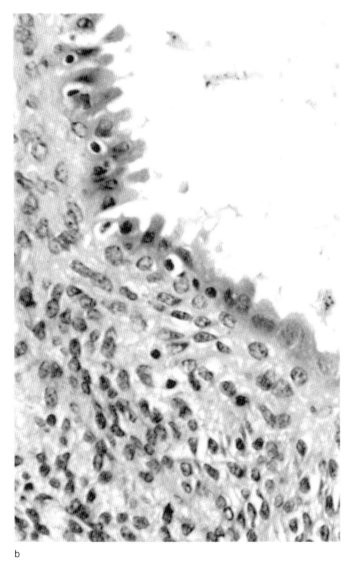

b

Fig. 32.10 b The epithelial component of a tamoxifen-associated endometrial polyp: Apocrine metaplasia.

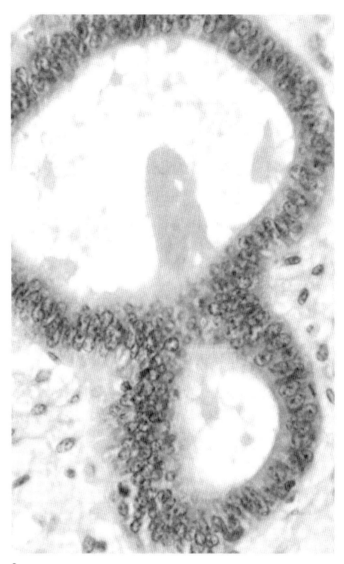

c

Fig. 32.10 c The epithelial component of a tamoxifen-associated endometrial polyp: A gland lined by endometrioid epithelium.

patients when compared to similar women randomised to receive placebo (risk ratio 6.4, 95% confidence interval 1.4–28). The findings of these investigators have since been confirmed by a series of large, well-designed studies all of which found that women with breast cancer who are treated with tamoxifen are at increased risk of endometrial carcinoma when compared to breast cancer patients who are not receiving tamoxifen (Fisher et al 1994; Van Leeuwen et al 1994; Rutqvist et al 1995; Early Breast Cancer Triallists' Collaborative Group 1998; Fisher et al 1998). Reported risk ratios have ranged from 1.3 (Van Leeuwen et al 1994) to 7.5 (Fisher et al 1994). In the American Breast Cancer Prevention Trial NSABP P-1, there were 36 invasive endometrial cancers among the tamoxifen group (n=6681) and 15 in the placebo group (n=6707). The risk ratio for endometrial cancer was 2.53 (95% CI 1.35–4.97). The increased risk was confined to women aged 50 and over (Fisher et al 1998).

The risk of endometrial carcinoma in tamoxifen-treated women increases with increasing cumulative dose of tamoxifen. In the study of Fornander et al (1989), women who received tamoxifen for 5 years had a significantly greater cumulative frequency of uterine cancer than women who received tamoxifen for 2 years. Another study found a significant trend of increasing endometrial cancer risk with increasing duration of treatment and cumulative dose of tamoxifen (Van Leeuwen et al 1994). More recently, an overview of the randomised tamoxifen trials noted that the incidence of endometrial cancer doubled in trials lasting one or two years and quadrupled in trials of five years (Early Breast Cancer Triallists' Collaborative Group 1998). Thus, the causal relationship between prolonged tamoxifen treatment and endometrial cancer is now well established. The increased risk of endometrial carcinoma among tamoxifen-treated breast cancer patients has been regarded as a relatively minor side effect since, unlike breast cancer, the majority of endometrial cancers are low grade and early stage at presentation and highly amenable to treatment. Given the beneficial effects of tamoxifen, this cost-benefit analysis is clearly acceptable in the setting of breast cancer. It is, however, open to question in the context of breast cancer prevention particularly in the light of suggestions that tamoxifen-associated endometrial cancer may have a poorer prognosis than non-tamoxifen associated endometrial cancer (Magriples et al 1993; Silva et al 1994; Bergman et al 2000).

Magriples et al (1993) compared endometrial cancers occurring in 15 tamoxifen-treated breast cancer patients with those found in 38 breast cancer patients not treated with this drug. Sixty-seven per cent of the tamoxifen group had poorly differentiated or poor prognosis variants of endometrial carcinoma (e.g. serous carcinoma, clear cell carcinoma or malignant mixed Müllerian tumour) compared to 24% of the untreated group. Moreover, 33% of tamoxifen patients and 2.6% of the untreated patients died of endometrial cancer. They concluded that tamoxifen-treated women have a predilection to poor prognosis endometrial carcinomas. In a similar study from another institution, Silva et al (1994) reported a statistically significant excess of serous type endometrial carcinoma in tamoxifen-treated women, but were unable to demonstrate a clear difference between treated and untreated women with regard to other histological subtypes, tumour stage at presentation or clinical outcome.

Other investigators have reported contradictory findings. Barakat et al (1994) and van Leeuwen et al (1994) found no difference in stage, grade or histological subtype of endometrial carcinoma which could be attributed to tamoxifen use. In the NSABP P-1 study 36 women developed invasive endometrial cancer; all the cancers were FIGO stage I, but no information is provided about the pathological subtype of the tumours (Fisher et al 1998).

It has been difficult to draw definite conclusions from these studies as all have been relatively small and some have lacked important pathological detail. A recent study from Holland which tried to address both these criticisms has added weight to suggestions that tamoxifen-associated endometrial cancers may have a relatively poor prognosis (Bergman et al 2000). The authors compared 309 women who developed endometrial cancer after a diagnosis of breast cancer with 860 matched controls with breast cancer but without endometrial cancer. The study included 108 women with endometrial cancer who had been treated with tamoxifen. Women treated with tamoxifen for 2 or more years were more likely to develop mixed Müllerian tumours or sarcomas and more likely to present in FIGO stage III or IV than untreated women. Tamoxifen users had a worse endometrial-cancer-specific survival at 3 years than non-users and there was a tendency for endometrial-cancer-specific survival to decrease with increasing duration of tamoxifen use. Although this is the largest and most authoritative study to date of tamoxifen-associated endometrial cancer, it is important to emphasise that the number of cases in some groups is very small. In order to enable significance testing, the authors combined malignant mixed Müllerian tumours, usually regarded as a variant of endometrial carcinoma, and pure uterine sarcomas. Combining unrelated entities in this way raises questions about the validity of the analyses. Nevertheless, this is the most substantial study currently available on the subject and, although not conclusive, its findings are impossible to dismiss.

Uterine stromal tumours

Uterine sarcomas reported in association with tamoxifen use have, so far, been confined to case reports and small series. They have included one rhabdomyosarcoma (Okada et al 1999), six leiomyosarcomas (Silva et al 1994; Gillett 1995; Chew et al 1996; McCluggage et al 1996b; Sabatini et al 1999), three endometrial stromal sarcomas (Beer et al 1995; Eddy & Mazur 1997; Pang 1998) and 13 adenosarcomas (Bocklage et al 1992; Clement et al 1996; Mourits et al 1998; Jessop & Roberts 2000).

A substantial recent study (Bergman et al 2000) reported that long-term tamoxifen users 'were more likely than non-users to have had malignant mixed mesodermal tumours or sarcomas of the endometrium'. As this study combined mixed Müllerian tumours with sarcomas for purposes of statistical analysis, it is impossible to determine the number of cases of sarcoma in tamoxifen users versus non-users. The type of sarcoma involved is not specified. Thus, evidence implicating tamoxifen as a cause of uterine sarcoma is so far anecdotal and incomplete. Bearing in mind that women with breast cancer may have a predisposition to some types of uterine sarcoma whether they are treated with tamoxifen or not (Silva et al 1994), it is not yet certain whether treatment with tamoxifen confers an increased risk of uterine sarcoma.

Other uterine effects

Cohen et al (1995) noted adenomyosis in the uterus of 8 out of 14 tamoxifen-treated postmenopausal breast cancer patients. As adenomyosis is otherwise rare in postmenopausal women, the authors suggested a causal link between tamoxifen and adenomyosis.

Effects on the ovary

In premenopausal women, prolonged use of tamoxifen is associated with development of bilateral ovarian cysts (Barbieri et al 1993; Cohen et al 1994c; Hochner-Celnikier et al 1995; Shushan et al 1996; Cohen et al 1999b; Mourits et al 1999) which are oestrogen-secreting

(Cohen et al 1994c; Mourits et al 1999). Shushan et al (1996) found ultrasonographically detectable ovarian cysts in 37.5% of their premenopausal tamoxifen-treated breast cancer patients. In the study of Mourits et al (1999) 81% of women with menstrual periods developed ovarian cysts while receiving tamoxifen for breast cancer. Cohen et al (1999b) reported that ovarian cysts occurred in 80% of tamoxifen-treated premenopausal breast cancer patients, but only in 8.3% of comparable patients not treated with tamoxifen.

During ultrasonographic follow-up Mourits et al (1999) found that 32% of ovarian cysts continued to grow, 36% became smaller and 32% disappeared altogether. New cysts developed in the opposite ovary in 41% of patients. Others have noted that tamoxifen-induced ovarian cysts regress when tamoxifen is discontinued (Cohen et al 1994c; Shushan et al 1996).

The pathology of these cysts is poorly documented but they have been variously described as luteinized follicle cysts (Barbieri et al 1993), simple functional cysts (Cohen et al 1994c) and corpus luteum cysts (Hochner-Celnikier et al 1995).

The mechanisms by which tamoxifen induces ovarian cysts remain unclear. It has been postulated that the anti-oestrogenic effects of tamoxifen on the hypothalamus result in increased secretion of gonadotrophin releasing hormone with consequent increase in FSH and LH secretion by pituitary gonadotrophs, followed by ovarian follicle development and possible superovulation. However, tamoxifen administration has not been shown to induce a significant rise in FSH and LH levels (Sherman et al 1979). An alternative hypothesis raises the possibility that tamoxifen induces ovarian follicle development by direct effects on local growth control mechanisms.

Ovarian cysts have also been reported, albeit less frequently, in postmenopausal breast cancer patients receiving tamoxifen. Shushan et al (1996) detected ovarian cysts in 6.3% of postmenopausal breast cancer patients receiving tamoxifen. Pathologically, these are much more heterogeneous than tamoxifen-associated cysts occurring in premenopausal women. Those reported to date have included cystic ovarian tumours (Cohen et al 1996a) and endometriotic cysts.

Cohen et al (1996b) documented ovarian neoplasms in 10 of 16 tamoxifen-treated women who underwent total abdominal hysterectomy and bilateral salpingo-oophorectomy for various indications. Six of these patients had benign serous neoplasms which were bilateral in five. Other tumours detected included an endometrioid adenocarcinoma, a Brenner tumour, a thecoma and bilateral ovarian fibromas. However, women with breast cancer are at increased risk of developing ovarian neoplasms irrespective of tamoxifen treatment and McGonigle et al (1999) found that tamoxifen-treated breast cancer patients were less likely to have ovarian tumours than breast cancer patients not receiving tamoxifen. In the American Breast Cancer Prevention Study no excess of ovarian tumours was noted in the tamoxifen group. Thus, the balance of available evidence does not confirm a causal link between tamoxifen treatment and ovarian neoplasia.

Tamoxifen and the cervix

It has been repeatedly demonstrated that squamous epithelial cells in cervical smears from postmenopausal women treated with tamoxifen show oestrogenic changes which regress when tamoxifen is discontinued (Ferrazzi et al 1977; Boccardo et al 1981; Eells et al 1990; Lahti et al 1994). Eighty-nine per cent of postmenopausal breast cancer patients treated with tamoxifen develop oestrogenised cervical smears even though their serum oestradiol levels are within the normal postmenopausal range (Lahti et al 1994). Oestrogenisation of cervical squamous epithelium is a consistent feature in sections of the cervix from hysterectomy specimens of tamoxifen-treated postmenopausal women.

Effects of tamoxifen on endometriosis

The incidence of endometriosis in tamoxifen-treated women is unknown, but 10 cases of tamoxifen-associated endometriosis have so far been reported in the English language literature. In five cases the patients were pre- or perimenopausal. As endometriosis is common in this age group, its association with tamoxifen could be due to chance. However, endometriosis is uncommon in post-menopausal women and the occurrence of this oestrogen-driven disease in postmenopausal women treated with tamoxifen suggests a causal link between the drug and endometriosis in this age group. It is not known if tamoxifen activates pre-existing foci of endometriosis or stimulates the development of endometriosis in previously unaffected women.

Of the five postmenopausal patients with tamoxifen-associated endometriosis, one presented with pelvic pain (Hajjar et al 1993), two with postmenopausal bleeding (Ismail & Maulik 1997; Schlesinger & Silverberg 1999) and two with ultrasonographic abnormalities during surveillance (Bardi et al 1994; Cohen et al 1994a). The pathological features reported have included atypical glandular hyperplasia (Ismail & Maulik 1997), epithelial metaplasias (Ismail & Maulik 1997), mixed epithelial–stromal polyps similar to endometrial polyps (Ismail & Maulik 1997; Schlesinger & Silverberg 1999) and endometrioid carcinomas arising in endometriotic foci (Bardi et al 1994; Cohen et al 1994a).

Thus, prolonged treatment with tamoxifen appears to have effects on endometriotic foci that are very similar to its effects on the endometrium. This raises important questions about the safety of long-term tamoxifen in hysterectomised women, particularly those with a history of endometriosis.

PROGESTAGENS

The synthetic progestagens used therapeutically, which are preferred to their natural counterparts for their more sustained action when given orally, are derived either from 17-alpha-hydroxy-progesterone or 19-nortestosterone. A variety of progestagens, which have fewer undesirable side effects, have been developed in recent years.

Progestagens may be given alone, systemically or in intrauterine devices, for the treatment of dysfunctional uterine bleeding, endometriosis or neoplasms and as contraceptives; in intrauterine devices, they also directly counteract the effects, on the endometrium, of oestrogen (Suvanto-Luukkonen et al 1998) and tamoxifen (Gardner et al 2000). They are, however, more commonly used in combination with oestrogens for contraception and as part of the programme of hormone replacement therapy at, or after, the menopause.

Effects on the endometrium

Progestagens will act only upon an endometrium in which progesterone receptors have been induced by prior exposure to oestrogen or tamoxifen (Cohen et al 1996b). They cause cellular differentiation and inhibit the effects of oestrogen. When they are given in the proliferative phase, ovarian follicular development is depressed, ovulation is postponed or prevented, and endometrial growth ceases (Dallenbach-Hellweg 1980b). Even if given only briefly, the cycle will be prolonged (Carter et al 1964). Withdrawal of the hormone will produce bleeding in a few days and if it is given continuously irregular spontaneous breakthrough bleeding will occur.

The effect which high doses of progestagen have depends upon the extent to which the endometrium has been previously stimulated by endogenous or exogenous oestrogen and upon the properties of the particular hormone.

If the hormone is given early in the proliferative phase, there is little stromal pseudodecidualisation and there may be only minimal abortive glandular secretory change. Spiral artery differentiation does not occur. Similar doses of hormone given in the late secretory phase induce marked stromal pseudodecidualisation (Fig. 32.11), a granulated lymphocytic infiltrate and transitory glandular secretory activity. As the glands are more sensitive to progestagens than is the stroma, however, they rapidly become refractory to stimulation and cease functioning (Dallenbach-Hellweg 1980b) becoming small and inactive though occasional glands may retain a secretory, or even hypersecretory appearance (Fig. 32.12). The picture

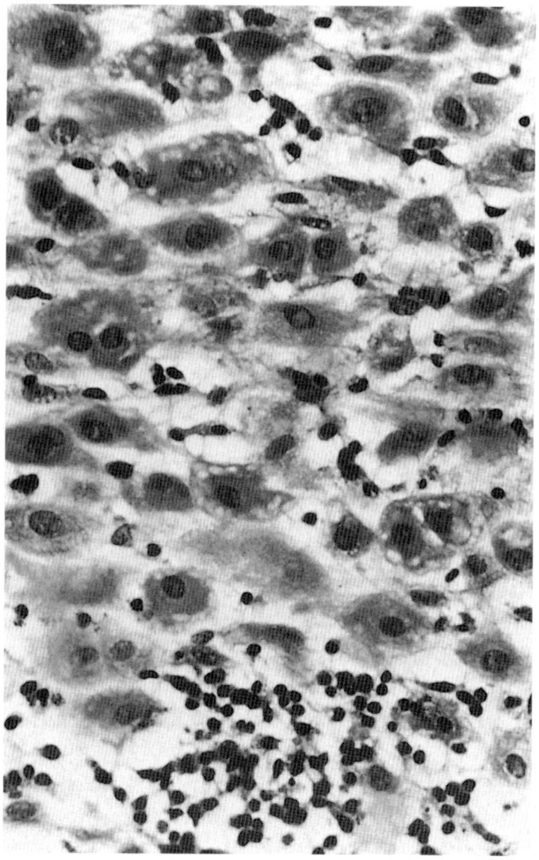

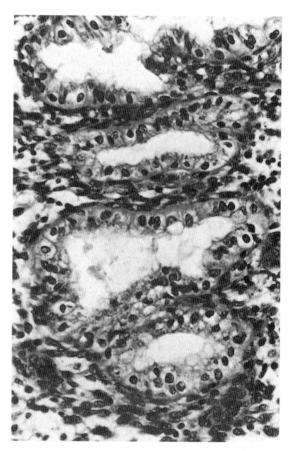

Fig. 32.11 The stroma of the functional layer of the endometrium in a patient given norethisterone. The individual cells have copious densely staining cytoplasm and are interspersed with granulated lymphocytes.

Fig. 32.12 An endometrial gland in a patient given norethisterone. This particular gland has a hypersecretory appearance. Elsewhere secretion was less well developed.

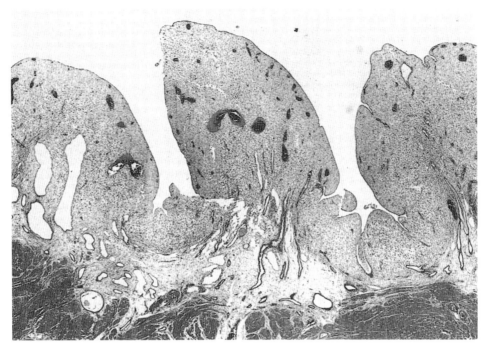

Fig. 32.13 Progestagen therapy. The polypoidal appearance which the endometrium assumes following treatment with norethisterone. The superficial part of the stroma is markedly pseudodecidualised and contains congested, thin-walled blood vessels: there is no spiral artery development. The glands are sparse and inactive. (From C H Buckley & H Fox *Biopsy Pathology of the Endometrium* reproduced by permission of Edward Arnold Limited.)

of small, inactive glands set in a pseudodecidualised stroma with little or no spiral artery growth (Fig 32.13) contrasts with the well-developed spiral arteries and glandular hypersecretion seen in both early intrauterine and ectopic pregnancy.

The prolonged use of progestagens produces an atrophic endometrium with sparse, uncoiled glands set in a shallow, compact, sometimes weakly pseudodecidualised stroma (Fig 32.14). Although the glands are inactive their epithelium may remain columnar rather than becoming cuboidal. It is usual for the granulated lymphocytic infiltrate to persist, whilst thin-walled vascular channels are a conspicuous feature (Fig 32.13). Spiral artery growth is absent. In some cases more marked atrophy may develop (Figure 32.15). Atrophy of this type, which is due to the anti-oestrogenic effect of the progestagen, persists as long as the therapy continues but usually recovers rapidly after withdrawal of the exogenous hormone. An irreversible atrophy with stromal hyalinisation has also been described (Dallenbach-Hellweg 1980b) but is rarely encountered in practice.

The appearances described above are seen most markedly in women receiving 19-nortestosterone-derived progestagens. In women using some of the modern progestagens and the weakly progestagenic, synthetic antigonadotrophic androgen Danazol (Fig. 32.16), a moderately atrophic endometrium, lacking stromal decidualisation and secretory activity develops rapidly ab initio. This effect is utilised in the thinning of the endometrium prior to endometrial resection (Rai et al 2000).

The appearance of the endometrium in patients given progestagens for the treatment of dysfunctional uterine bleeding is extremely varied and depends upon the nature of the underlying hormonal abnormality and the stage of the cycle at which therapy was commenced. Commonly, the appearances resemble those which have already been described. When the patient is anovulatory, however, secretory changes may be superimposed upon a hyperplastic endometrium (Fig. 32.17). This is indistinguishable from the appearance which is seen if such a patient ovulates. With continued therapy simple and mild complex hyperplasia may regress completely, but atypical hyperplasia may regress only partly leaving islands of architecturally atypical glands set in an endometrium which is otherwise normal in appearance, pseudodecidualised or atrophic. The failure of an atypical hyperplasia to respond to progestagen therapy is usually regarded as an indication for surgical treatment. Sometimes, when metaplastic squamous epithelium has been absent from a hyperplastic endometrium, it may develop following progestagen therapy (Miranda & Mazur 1995).

Hormonally responsive endometrial adenocarcinomas, which are usually well differentiated (Histological Grade 1), may show glandular secretory changes within 10 to 14 days of administering progestagens (Figs 32.18, 32.19), and the stromal cells may resemble those of the late secretory phase, normal pregnancy, or those seen in

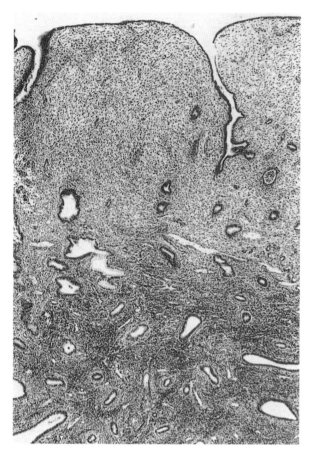

Fig. 32.14 Moderate endometrial atrophy, the result of prolonged progestagen therapy. The endometrial depth is reduced, there is weak stromal pseudodecidualisation and the glands are uncoiled and inactive. (From C H Buckley & H Fox 2002 *Biopsy Pathology of the Endometrium* reproduced by permission of Edward Arnold Limited.)

the endometrium of other exogenous hormone users (Ferenczy 1980). In addition, there is often focal cellular degeneration, growth of the tumour may be suppressed and the tumour may regress (Anderson 1972; Rozsier & Underwood 1974; Dallenbach-Hellweg 1980b; Ferenczy 1980; Randall & Kurman 1997).

There is evidence that progestagens protect against the development of endometrial carcinoma in women who receive oestrogen replacement therapy (vide supra). This is thought to be due to their interrupting endometrial growth by lowering the concentration of oestradiol receptors, promoting endometrial shedding and inducing the formation of endometrial 17-beta-dehydrogenase which converts oestradiol to the less potent oestrone (Judd 1980).

Effects on the myometrium

Leiomyomas may enlarge and show mitotic activity, increased cellularity and cellular atypia (Prakash & Scully 1964; Fechner 1968) when large doses of progestagen are given continuously for a prolonged period, but there is no risk of malignant change. Occasionally, leiomyomas may undergo degeneration, such as that seen in pregnancy, or may diminish in size and appear highly cellular due to cytoplasmic shrinkage.

Effects on the cervix

Distension of the cervical crypts by mucus and microglandular hyperplasia of the cervix are concomitants of progestagen therapy. Microglandular hyperplasia is described more fully below.

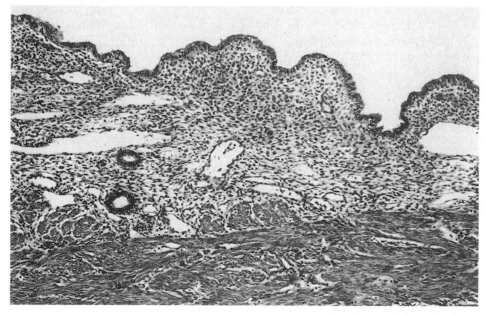

Fig. 32.15 Endometrial atrophy resulting from prolonged progestagen therapy. (From C H Buckley & H Fox 2002 *Biopsy Pathology of the Endometrium* reproduced by permission of Edward Arnold Limited.)

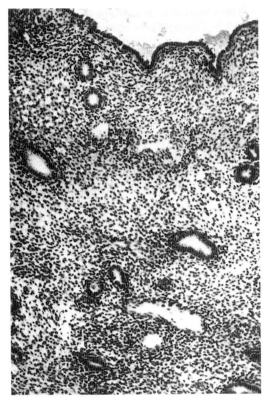

Fig. 32.16 Endometrium after the administration of Danazol. The glands are small and there is neither secretory nor proliferative activity. The stroma is immature.

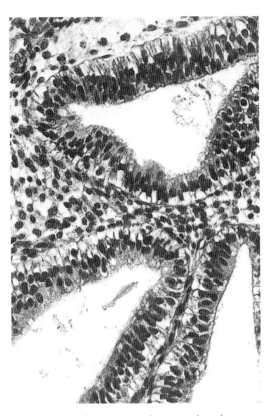

Fig. 32.17 Secretory changes, seen here as subnuclear vacuolation of the glandular epithelium, superimposed upon a simple endometrial hyperplasia by the administration of norethisterone.

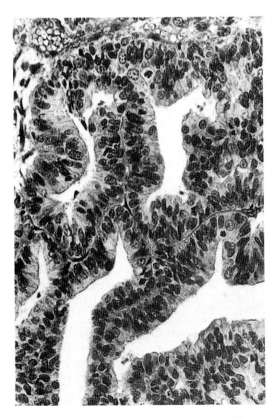

Fig. 32.18 An endometrial biopsy from a women with a well-differentiated endometrioid adenocarcinoma of the corpus uteri.

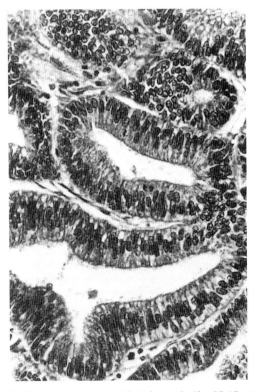

Fig. 32.19 The same tumour as that shown in Fig. 35.15 at the time of the hysterectomy when progestagens had been given for three weeks. Vacuolation of the epithelium is indicative of secretory change.

Effects on the ovary

With high doses of exogenous progestagen, just as in normal pregnancy, there may be multifocal decidualisation of the subepithelial stroma of the ovary (Figs 32.20, 32.21).

Effects on endometriosis

In the treatment of endometriosis, the inhibition of proliferation and induction of atrophy in the endometrium consequent to progestagen therapy is used to advantage. The progestagen acts both directly on the endometriotic foci and indirectly by suppression of ovulation. Initially, the stroma of the endometriotic foci may become pseudo-decidualised (Fig. 32.22) and increasingly vascular but later, focal necrobiosis of the individual cells indicates the commencement of degeneration (Gunning & Moyer 1967). Eventually, the foci may consist only of inactive glands set in an atrophic stroma and care should be taken to distinguish such foci histologically from endosalpingiosis. In addition to systemic progestagen therapy, progestagen-impregnated intrauterine contraceptive devices have been used to treat endometriosis with similar inactivation of such foci (Fedele et al 2001).

Effects in other extragenital sites

A progestagenic effect may also be manifest in decidualised foci in subperitoneal stroma, in the great omentum and in pelvic lymph nodes. Such foci are sometimes biopsied at laparotomy in the mistaken belief that they may be foci of metastatic carcinoma.

A statistically significant increase in thromboembolism, but not stroke or myocardial infarction, has been reported in women using therapeutic progestagen (Poulter et al 1999a; Vasilakis et al 1999).

ANTIPROGESTINS

Onapristone (ZK98299) and Mifepristone (RU486) are antiprogestins, that is, they bind to, and inhibit the transcriptional activity of, progesterone receptors. Altered conformation is central to the antagonist inhibition of the transcriptional activity of progesterone receptors. Antagonists also promote inappropriate association of progesterone receptors with corepressors (Edwards et al 2000). They are said, in the majority of women, to hinder these progesterone-induced changes in the endometrium without upsetting ovarian function. They have, therefore, been considered as potential contraceptives. When

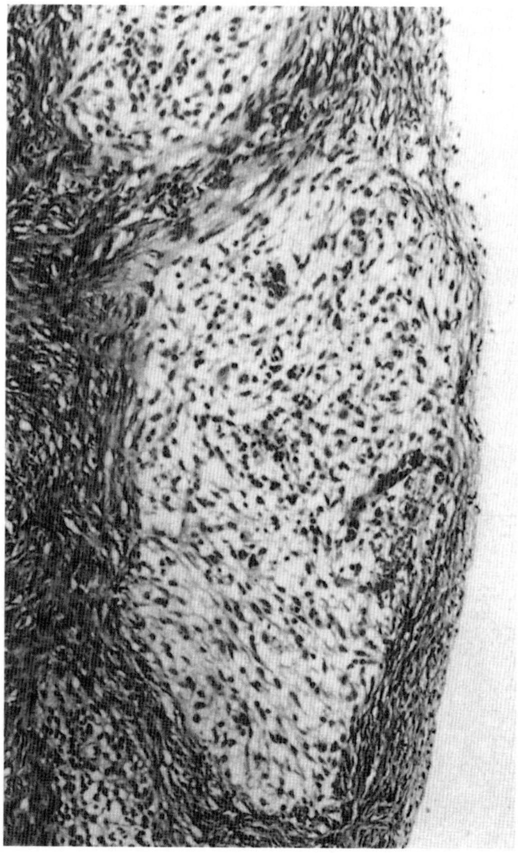

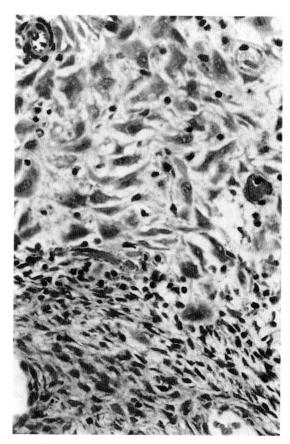

Fig. 32.20 The surface of the ovary in a patient given norethisterone. Many nodules of similar decidua-like tissue were present in both ovaries.

Fig. 32.21 A detail from an area similar to those seen in Fig. 32.20, showing the somewhat spindle-celled shape of the individually decidualised cells.

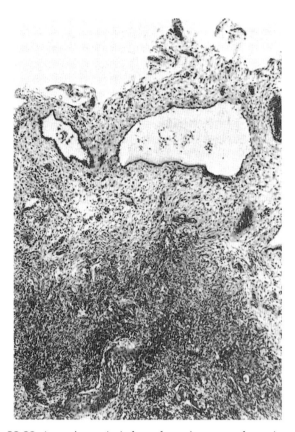

Fig. 32.22 An endometriotic focus from the ovary of a patient treated with norethisterone. The glands are dilated and there is neither secretory nor proliferative activity: the stroma is pseudodecidualised.

antiprogestins are given after the mid-cycle LH surge, they cause retardation of secretory changes in the endometrium but do not alter the length of the secretory phase (Cameron et al 1996a; Cameron et al 1996b; Cameron et al 1997). It is likely, therefore, that they alter the receptivity of the endometrium to the conceptus. In some women, however, there may also be inhibition of ovulation, and in these circumstances, some authors have reported oestrogenic effects, including increased endometrial thickness, irregularly shaped endometrial glands of varying size, many of which are dilated, lined by epithelium of varying appearance, some of which appears to be secretory, dense cellular stroma with mitoses and increased oestrogen receptor staining (Murphy et al 1995; Croxatto et al 1998). Others have found that despite the exposure of the endometrium to unopposed oestrogens, there is no significant morphological change, mitoses are absent and there is significantly less oestrogen receptor staining, although Ki-67 and PCNA are present throughout the cycle (Cameron et al 1996b). In rats, the anovulatory effect of Onapristone is thought to be due to a reduction in preovulatory progesterone production and progesterone receptor expression in the ovary and also the down-regulation of progesterone receptors in the anterior pituitary and hypothalamus (Donath et al 2000).

GONADOTROPHIN-RELEASING HORMONE AGONISTS: GONADORELIN ANALOGUES (e.g. GOSERELIN, ZOLADEX)

The prolonged use of luteinizing hormone releasing hormone (LHRH) agonists has the effect of suppressing ovulatory function. They are used for this purpose prior to the induction of superovulation in women being treated by in vitro fertilisation (IVF) or gamete intrafallopian transfer (GIFT). They have also been used to treat menorrhagia, endometrial hyperplasia (Agorastos et al 1997) and endometriosis and to produce endometrial atrophy prior to transcervical resection of the endometrium. Although the endometrium becomes atrophic, there is no increase in microvascular density (Hickey et al 1996a). A suspected rebound phenomenon has been observed when multiple vascular endometrial polyps developed in foci of endometriosis in the pelvis, vagina and cervix as well as in the endometrium following the withdrawal of Zoladex given for the treatment of endometriosis (Othman et al 1996).

Uterine leiomyomas may shrink, assume a markedly cellular appearance (Crow et al 1995), sufficient to superficially mimic endometrial stromal sarcoma (McCluggage & Bharucha 1999), become infiltrated by T-lymphocytes (Bardsley et al 1998; Laforga & Aranda 1999), plasma cells and B-lymphocytes (Crow et al 1995), and sometimes contain areas of necrosis. Once treatment is suspended, however, regrowth occurs rapidly. Hypo-oestrogenic effects such as vaginal dryness and a decrease in trabecular bone density also occur (Bianchi et al 1995).

THE PATHOLOGY OF HORMONE REPLACEMENT THERAPY (HRT)

COMBINED HORMONES

Hormone replacement therapy is used in young women who are hypogonadal, such as those with gonadal dysgenesis, and in postmenopausal women. It is also used, in a more precise way to provide a suitable environment in which to replace previously frozen or donated pre-embryos in infertile women (Critchley et al 1990).

It is generally considered unwise to use oestrogen alone as hormone replacement therapy when the uterus is in situ. Nonetheless, this sometimes occurs and the appearance of the endometrium varies according to the dose and duration of therapy (vide supra).

More commonly, oestrogen is given in combination with a progestagen, there being variation in the method of administration. The hormones may be given orally or by skin patches. Sometimes, whilst oestrogen is taken orally or administered by skin patch, the progestagen is provided by a progestagen-impregnated intrauterine contraceptive device.

Hormone may be given in a sequential pattern, with, for example, oestrogen alone given for between 10 and 15 days, on average, and then a progestagen added to the regimen for the next 10 to 14 days to allow monthly bleeding when oestrogen alone is re-started. Other regimens provide for the progestagen to be given only in alternate months (Lingren et al 1995) or three-monthly (Boerrigter et al 1996) to reduce the number of episodes of bleeding. An oestrogen and progestagen may also be given in combination every day. The combined hormone may be given continuously or may be interrupted to allow hormone withdrawal bleeding. These patterns of treatment eliminate the risk that iatrogenic endometrial carcinoma may be induced (Whitehead et al 1981). This does not, however, mean that carcinoma cannot develop spontaneously in the endometrium of a woman taking hormone replacement therapy.

Effects on the endometrium

In women receiving a sequential pattern of hormonal therapy, the oestrogen in the first part of the cycle causes endometrial growth and, after the introduction of progestagen, there is a brief, poorly developed, variably delayed secretory phase which may not appear until shortly before hormone withdrawal bleeding. There is little or no stromal pseudodecidualisation, though there may be marked stromal oedema, a reflection of the dominant oestrogenic activity (Fig. 32.23): granulated lymphocytes are sparse or absent. In some women the endometrial appearances are apparently inconsistent with the pattern of hormone administration and may appear proliferative or inactive following progestagen (Habiba et al 1998). Compared to the corresponding phase of the physiological cycle, sequential HRT-treated endometrium exhibits an increase in total leucocytes, proliferating leucocytes, granulated lymphocytes, and T cells. There is a non-statistically significant drop in the number of macrophages (Habiba et al 1999). Endometrial atrophy does not usually occur with sequential hormone replacement.

When combined oestrogen and progestagen are given continuously, as for example in Kliofem, usually the endometrium gradually becomes shallow and atrophic, the glands sparse, narrow and inactive and the stroma spindle-celled (Fig. 32.24) whilst in other cases, a weak pseudodecidualised appearance may develop (AinMelk 1996; Piegsa et al 1997; Sturdee et al 2000).

In some women, particularly those being prepared for pre-embryo transfer, an endometrial appearance approximating to the normal may be achieved (Fig. 32.25) (Critchley et al 1990), although the induction of an endometrium of fully normal appearance is not a necessary prerequisite to successful pregnancy.

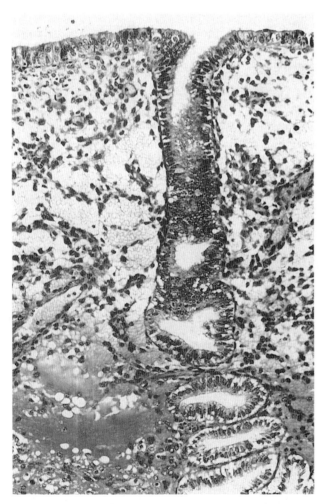

Fig. 32.23 Hormone replacement therapy, sequential pattern. The sample was taken on the 23rd day of an artificial 28 day cycle. The endometrium is well grown and there is subnuclear vacuolation of the glandular epithelium. Stromal oedema is marked and spiral artery differentiation has not yet occurred. (From C H Buckley & H Fox 2002 *Biopsy Pathology of the Endometrium* reproduced by permission of Edward Arnold Limited.)

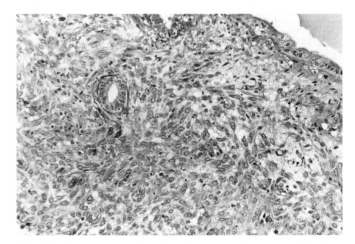

Fig. 32.24 Hormone replacement therapy, continuous combined pattern. The endometrial glands are sparse, narrow and inactive and the stroma cellular and compact in a woman taking 2 mg oestradiol combined with 1 mg norethisterone acetate daily. (From C H Buckley & H Fox 2002 *Biopsy Pathology of the Endometrium* reproduced by permission of Edward Arnold Limited.)

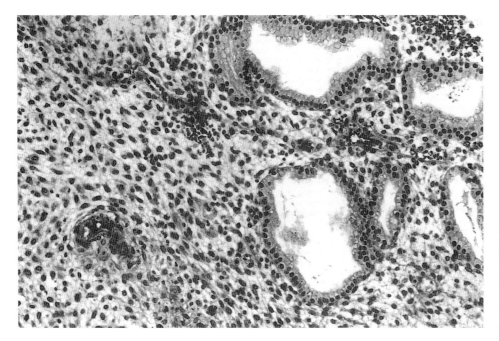

Fig. 32.25 Hormone replacement therapy. The glands are well grown, secretory activity is present, spiral artery differentiation has occurred and mild stromal pseudodecidualisation has developed. (From C H Buckley & H Fox 2002 *Biopsy Pathology of the Endometrium* reproduced by permission of Edward Arnold Limited.)

It is generally agreed that prolonged, balanced hormone replacement therapy has few serious adverse effects on the endometrium. A regular bleeding pattern cannot, however, be taken to indicate that there will be no pathological findings in the endometrium because in a multicentre study (Sturdee 1996), 2.7% of hormone replacement users were found to have complex hyperplasia. Polyps, with accompanying irregular bleeding, may develop despite regular hormone withdrawal bleeding (Maia et al 1996) and this is thought to be due to the fact that the stromal cells of the polyps contain fewer oestrogen and progesterone receptors than the non-polyoidal endometrium making them relatively insensitive to cyclical hormonal changes (Mittal et al 1996). In practice, endometrial abnormalities are most likely to be found when the endometrial depth, as measured on ultrasound, is more than 8 mm and the risk of an abnormality increases with increasing endometrial thickness (Granberg et al 1997). There is no increased risk of endometrial carcinoma in women using an oestrogen/progestagen combination (Persson et al 1996). Care has to be exercised, however, in the use of oestrogen-only HRT, in women who have had a hysterectomy for endometrial carcinoma (Carr et al 1996) as recurrence has been reported in such cases.

Other target organs

A small increase in the risk of breast carcinoma, with a relative risk of around 1.5, which seems to increase with duration of use, has been reported (Persson et al 1996; Hankinson & Stampfer 1997; Winther et al 1997) but HRT does not appear to adversely affect the course of the disease (Verheul et al 2000). As there may be confounding factors, however, these data need to be interpreted with caution, and balanced against the advantages of the therapy. For example, a publication from the Royal College of General Practitioners Oral Contraceptive Study emphasises the problems in obtaining accurate, long-term follow-up data on HRT use and the individual's previous use of steroid contraceptives. It may also be that women who use HRT do not have the same clinical and social characteristics as those that do not (Moorhead et al 1997). A recurrent question from women who have had breast carcinoma is whether it is safe to use HRT. There appears to be no contraindication to oestrogen/progestagen combinations in women who have had an oestrogen-receptor-negative tumour (Birkhauser 1994) or for those with a family history of breast carcinoma; indeed there may be survival advantages (Sellers et al 1998). The recurrence rate for breast carcinoma in women using HRT is 17/1000/year compared with 30/1000/year whilst death rates for users is 5/1000/year and for non-users 15/1000/year (O'Meara et al 2001).

There are indications that the number of ovarian cysts is reduced in the early years of the menopause in women who use HRT (Bar-Hava et al 1997).

Systemic effects

Hormone replacement therapy protects, to some extent, against osteoporosis and myocardial ischaemia (Knopp 1990; La Vecchia 1992; Speroff et al 1996) and it may suppress disease activity in rheumatoid arthritis. There is some indication that colonic carcinoma risk may be reduced in recent, postmenopausal users of HRT, and that the risk of death from disease may also be reduced (Nanda et al 1999).

TIBOLONE

Tibolone is a drug combining oestrogenic and progestagenic activity with weak androgenic activity. The progestagenic metabolites are said to predominate at the level of the endometrium (Rymer 1998). It is given continuously for the treatment of the vasomotor symptoms of the menopause and can be used to treat the hypo-oestrogenic symptoms in women given luteinizing hormone releasing hormone (LHRH) agonists for the treatment of endometriosis (Taskin et al 1997). Its effect on the endometrium may vary. It may be predominantly oestrogenic, and it is not uncommon to find a proliferative endometrium in women using the drug. In others, the endometrium may be moderately well grown with the development of a shallow functionalis in which there is weak, irregular secretory activity, indicative of the progestagenic effect, or it may be shallow and inactive. The suppressive effect on endometrial growth has sometimes been used in women who require HRT, but who have endometriosis, and in women who have had a hormone-dependent tumour. Polyps, simple hyperplasia and early carcinoma have also been reported (Ginsburg & Prelevic 1996).

The effect of Tibolone on the vaginal epithelium is predominantly oestrogenic (Rymer et al 1994) with an increase in the karyopyknotic index and clinical improvement in vaginal dryness and dyspareunia.

The hormone is also said to have a protective effect as regards bone loss (Gambacciani & Ciaponi 2000) even in the absence of additional physical exercise (Brooke-Wavell et al 2000).

As Tibolone and its oestrogenic metabolites exert direct actions on the vascular wall and decrease the expression of endothelial-leukocyte adhesion molecules, it has been suggested that it may have a direct anti-atherogenic effect (Simoncini et al 2000). Winkler et al (2000) have also shown that Tibolone changes haemostasis parameters toward a more fibrinolytic profile, which may diminish the risk of venous thrombosis. Both Tibolone and combined HRT tend to lower total serum cholesterol and HDL-C (Al-Azzawi et al 1999) whilst continuous combined HRT significantly reduces LDL-C but Tibolone does not.

HORMONES IN THE TREATMENT OF INFERTILITY

Down regulation of the ovulatory cycle, by an LHRH agonist, is frequently used prior to the harvesting of ova in assisted reproduction, that is, in vitro fertilisation (IVF) and gamete intrafallopian transfer (GIFT)(vide supra). Ovulation is subsequently induced by the administration of human chorionic gonadotrophin (hCG). Studies of the endometrial changes following ovulation in such patients reveal glandular maturation which corresponds with that

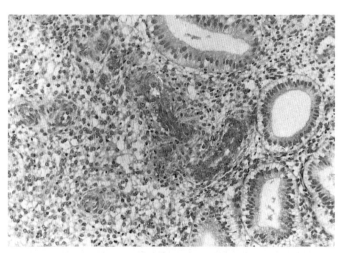

Fig. 32.26 Assisted reproduction. Premature spiral artery development consistent in appearance with the 9th to 10th post-ovulatory day contrasts with the subnuclear secretory vacuoles in the glands which are characteristic of the early secretory phase. H & E (From C H Buckley & H Fox 2002 *Biopsy Pathology of the Endometrium* reproduced by permission of Edward Arnold Limited.)

which would have been expected had ovulation occurred naturally, but there is premature differentiation of the spiral arteries (Fig. 32.26) (Seif et al 1992; Koib & Paulson 1997). Noci et al (1997) have also reported precocious endometrial stromal development in women undergoing ovarian hyperstimulation and in some of these women the serum progesterone level and endometrial oestrogen and progesterone receptor content has been higher than normal. It is possible, therefore, that local and systemic factors may play a part in the development of the abnormal endometrial pattern. Further, in women being prepared for embryo transfer by the therapeutic use of oestrogen and progesterone, the administration of progesterone too early in the artificial follicular phase produces an impairment of endometrial development that cannot be corrected by progesterone supplements later in the cycle (Ezra et al 1994).

THE PATHOLOGY OF CONTRACEPTION

INTRODUCTION

In any reasoned account of the pathology of contraceptive methods, the morbidity, mortality and minor pathological manifestations resulting from their use must be compared with the morbidity and mortality of the 80 pregnancies per 100 women-years, and their sequelae, which, it is estimated, would have occurred had contraception not been practiced. Examined in these terms, the majority of modern contraceptives are not only highly effective, but are also extremely safe. Furthermore, in addition to their prime purpose, the prevention of unwanted pregnancy, a number of desirable 'side effects' result from the use of steroid contraceptives and these

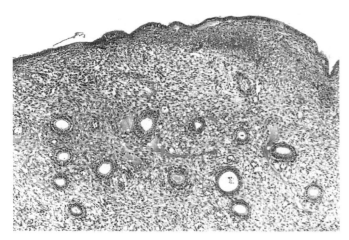

Fig. 32.27 Anti-androgenic hormone contraception. The narrow glands and cellular stroma seen in a women taking 35 μg ethinyloestradiol in combination with 2 mg cyproterone for 21 days out of 28. H & E (From C H Buckley & H Fox 2002 *Biopsy Pathology of the Endometrium* reproduced by permission of Edward Arnold Limited.)

must be considered in any balanced view of the pros and cons of this form of contraception. Nonetheless, such lesions and complications that do develop, occur, for the most part, in a population of healthy women and an understanding and recognition of the more serious side effects is a prerequisite to the identification of the individuals at greatest risk.

The majority of simple contraceptives are virtually devoid of risk although occasionally local irritation and eczematous lesions may accompany the use of spermicides whilst cystitis may occur, if, in addition, a diaphragm is used (Vessey et al 1976). Problems most commonly occur with steroid contraceptives and intrauterine contraceptive devices (IUCDs) and whilst the undesirable effects of the IUCD usually remain local, widespread systemic disturbances may accompany steroid contraception.

STEROID CONTRACEPTION

Steroid contraceptives fall into two main groups, those in which an oestrogen and progestagen are given in combination and those composed entirely of progestagen. The term 'pill' is often used colloquially to encompass all such preparations.

The majority of women follow a regimen in which a combination of between 20 and 50 μg of oestrogen, usually ethinyloestradiol, and a progestagen is given for 21 days out of 28 with seven hormone-free days which are either pill-free or a placebo is taken. This is the monophasic pattern. Alternatively a phased formulation is given in which the proportions of hormone differ in different phases of the cycle. This may be biphasic in which the proportion of oestrogen and progestagen given in the first seven days of the cycle is different from that given in

the next 14 days (e.g. Binovum) or triphasic when three different combinations may be given (e.g. Logynon). A small number of women also use combined, monthly injectable steroid contraceptives (Thomas et al 1989). In women being treated for acne, a preparation containing 35 μg ethinyloestradiol combined with 2 mg of the anti-androgen cyproterone acetate (Dianette) both acts as a contraceptive and treats the acne (Fig. 32.27).

The quantity of hormone in the early steroid contraceptives is now known to have been unnecessarily high, simply to inhibit ovulation. As a consequence, there were undesirable systemic side effects and bizarre morphological abnormalities in the target organs. The present low-dose steroid contraceptives, with newer generations of synthetic gestagens (second generation, levonorgestrel, and third generation Gestodene, Desogestrel and Norgestimate), produce fewer systemic side effects and the changes in the target organs are less dramatic. Patients included in the current follow-up series may, however, in their early days, have taken high doses of hormones and data collected from these women may not be applicable to patients who have used only the more modern low-dose preparations.

Not only have the quantities of hormone in the preparations been altered in the light of experience, but so too have the patterns of administration. It was recognised some time ago, for example, that some of the sequential patterns of administration, in which relatively large doses of oestrogen alone were given from day 5 to day 15 to 20 of the cycle followed by a progestagen–oestrogen combination for the following 10 or 5 days, were associated with the development of endometrial carcinoma in some women.

The reporting of abnormalities identified in steroid contraceptive users has followed trends, and anecdotal case reports have created the impression that certain problems may be more common than they in fact are. This is clearly seen in the clustering of reports concerning certain topics which is apparent in this review. It is important, therefore, that when we consider the pathology of contraception that we allow sufficient time to permit placing of the problems in perspective.

Combined steroid contraceptives prevent ovulation by their negative feedback effect on pituitary gonadotrophin secretion, acting via the hypothalamus (Bye 1982; Fay 1982) to diminish FSH secretion and the mid-cycle LH surge (Mishell 1976). There is no evidence that this function is less effective with the newer, low-dose combinations and those using the second and third generation gestagens (Rossmanith et al 1997; Spona et al 1997; Coney & DelConte 1999).

The progestagen-only 'mini-pill', which is taken every day, suppresses ovulation in only about 50% of cycles. It depends for its contraceptive effect not only upon the suppression of ovulation but also upon changes in the quality of cervical mucus which impedes sperm transport, upon modification of endometrial maturation rendering it unsuitable for nidation (Hawkins & Elder 1979), and upon alterations in tubal motility and secretion. It is used by a smaller proportion of women, particularly those over the age of 35 years, heavy smokers and those in whom oestrogen induces severe side effects. Progestagens may also be given as a depot injection of medroxyprogesterone acetate (DMPA) or in subcutaneous, etonogestrel-containing silicone capsule implants (e.g. Implanon). Unusual complications of progestagen implants and their removal are the development of site-related neuropathy involving the ulnar nerve, lateral cutaneous nerve and antebrachial cutaneous nerve, expulsion of the implants and infection (Alfa et al 1995; Marin & McMillian 1998). There may also be some delay in the return of fertility following discontinuation of DMPA (Kauntiz 2000).

Combined steroid contraceptives have a very low failure rate, estimated as 0.2%, if they are taken regularly, though poor patient compliance reduces this considerably (Hillard 1992). The failure rate for the progestagen-only pill is somewhat higher. The efficacy of the combined steroid contraceptives may be diminished, or even abolished, if they are taken simultaneously with a wide variety of commonly used drugs such as barbiturates, phenytoin, rifampicin, ampicillin, griseofulvin (Weaver & Glasier 1999) and phenylbutazone, which accelerate their metabolism. Rifampicin also accelerates the metabolism of progestagen-only contraceptives.

Steroid contraceptives are sometimes accompanied by a number of undesirable local and systemic effects such as breakthrough bleeding, headache, nausea, hirsutes, acne, chloasma and increases in body weight (Berger & Talwar 1978; Speroff 1982; London 1992; Rosenberg & Long 1992). These are, however, less common with the modern generation of low-dose preparations and the newer gestagens. Progestagen-only regimens are particularly associated with disturbances of the bleeding pattern (Chi 1993) but are the treatment of choice for women who are breastfeeding, the older woman, smokers and hypertensive women.

Basal levels of serum cholecystokinin are reduced in steroid contraceptive users and this has been correlated with the increase in body fat which is reported in some women using monophasic steroid contraceptives (Hirschberg et al 1996). Simultaneously, serum levels of gastrin and insulin remain unchanged, low-density lipoprotein levels are reduced and triglycerides and post-prandial glucose levels are elevated. Impairment of the glucose tolerance test was a fairly constant finding when older high-dose oral contraceptives were in vogue but the introduction of the newer low-dose pill, and new gestagens have reduced this risk. These newer contraceptives are even regarded as suitable for women at high risk of developing diabetes mellitus, for example, those with a history of gestational diabetes and those having a first degree relative with diabetes (Harvengt 1992), and there

is no evidence that diabetic patients are more difficult to control when using third generation gestagens (Petersen et al 1996).

It has been reported that persistent trophoblastic disease is more common in women using contraceptive steroids than other forms of contraception (Stone et al 1976; Palmer 1991).

Effects on the endometrium

The appearance of the endometrium depends upon the potency, quantity and proportion of the constituent hormones in the pill and their pattern of administration. The changes currently seen are far more subtle than those which related to high-dose hormone preparations.

Combined steroid contraceptives

In the first few months of use, a discernible cyclical pattern can be recognised and with the newer low-dose preparations this may persist for as long as the product is used. With the higher-dose formulations the regenerative capacity of the endometrium may be diminished due to progestagen predominance and there is variable, though rarely profound, atrophy.

The morphological effects of combined steroid contraceptives, whilst being generally similar whatever the precise hormone combination and dosage, show sufficient variation for the relative importance of the oestrogen and progestagen in the combination to be recognised (Buckley & Fox 2002). Following withdrawal bleeding (Fig. 32.28), at the end of each cycle, the endometrium proliferates. This phase is short because of the inhibiting effect of the progestagen on the oestrogen-stimulated growth, and the endometrium, therefore, remains shallow. The glands at this stage are narrow, tubular and lined by a single layer of cubo-columnar cells or, much less commonly, by pseudostratified epithelium. Scanty mitoses can be seen in both the stroma and epithelium. The stromal cells remain spindled and have the so-called 'bare-nucleus' appearance.

At about the eighth day of the cycle, the progestagen effect becomes apparent, with the appearance, in the glandular epithelium, of subnuclear vacuoles. However, because of the brief, inadequate oestrogenic priming in the early part of the cycle, progesterone receptors are few and glandular secretory changes are weak and poorly developed. By day 10, the subnuclear vacuoles move into the supranuclear cytoplasm and there is a brief, premature secretory phase lasting only until day 14 or 15. The glands remain narrow, or only minimally dilated, and straight or only gently convoluted. The apices of the cells remain, for the most part, intact and there is only a trace of secretion within the lumena. There may be a little stromal oedema. In the latter half of the cycle there is regression of the secretory changes and the endometrium

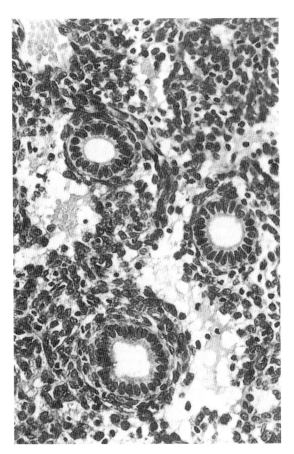

Fig. 32.28 Hormone withdrawal bleeding in a patient using a combined steroid contraceptive containing 50 μg ethinyloestradiol and 1 mg norethisterone acetate. The glands are small and inactive and there is no stromal decidualization-contrast with menstrual endometrium.

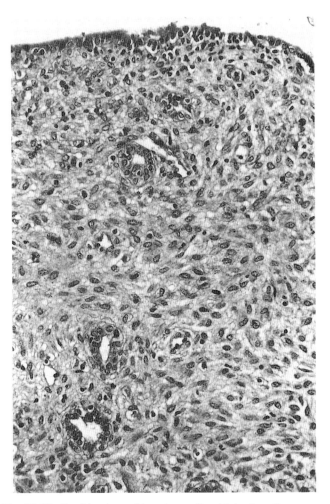

Fig. 32.29 Combined steroid contraceptive, biphasic pattern, 50 μg ethinyloestradiol, 250 mg levonorgestrel, 26th day of the cycle. The glands are extremely narrow and inactive, the stroma is markedly pseudodecidualised, forming a compacta and there is a granulated lymphocyte infiltrate. (From C H Buckley & H Fox 2002 *Biopsy Pathology of the Endometrium* reproduced by permission of Edward Arnold Limited.)

becomes inactive. The degree of spiral artery differentiation and growth, the quality of the stromal pseudodecidualisation and the extent of the glandular secretory transformation vary according to the relative potency of the oestrogen and progestagen in the combination (Figs 32.26 to 32.32).

With high doses of progestagen and oestrogen there is stromal pseudodecidualisation and the glands are narrow and inactive (Fig. 32.29). When the same dose of progestagen is combined with a lower dose of oestrogen there is no stromal decidualisation, the glands are atrophic and the stroma is immature (Fig. 32.30). In other cases the stroma contains many thin-walled vascular channels (Fig. 32.31) and in yet other cases the endometrium may contain well-developed secretory glands and the stroma may contain differentiated spiral arteries (Fig. 32.32).

The effects of phased steroid contraceptives are very variable even in women using the same hormone preparation. Sometimes the appearances, in the later part of the cycle, are indistinguishable from those seen in the monophasic contraceptives users whilst in others the appearances are those of a weakly secretory endometrium (Figs 32.33, 32.34) that persists to the time of hormone withdrawal bleeding. In those preparations with increased mid-cycle oestrogen, perhaps as a consequence of more adequate progesterone receptor induction, there is better growth and muscularisation of the spiral arteries (Buckley & Fox 2002). This correlates well with the clinical observation of a reduced incidence of mid-cycle breakthrough bleeding (Elder 1982).

The alternating nodules of stromal hyperplasia and oedema described by Dallenbach-Hellweg (1981) are not, in our experience, a feature of modern steroid contraceptives, nor are the bizarre stromal pseudosarcomatous changes described by Dockerty et al (1959). It is most important to note that profound irreversible endometrial atrophy (Fig. 32.35) resulting from prolonged high-dose contraception no longer appears to occur.

In a proportion of women who have stopped taking steroid contraceptives in the previous month or so, there is a mild to moderate, non-specific chronic endometritis

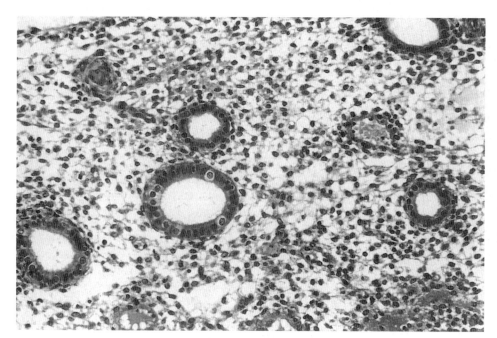

Fig. 32.30 Combined steroid contraceptive, biphasic pattern, 30 μg ethinyloestradiol, 250 mg levonorgestrel, three weeks since hormone withdrawal bleed. In comparison with Fig. 32.29, the glands are less atrophic and the stroma is immature; there is no decidualisation. (From C H Buckley & H Fox 2002 *Biopsy Pathology of the Endometrium* reproduced by permission of Edward Arnold Limited.)

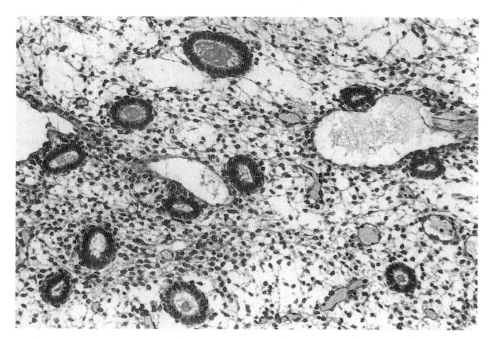

Fig. 32.31 Combined steroid contraceptive, biphasic pattern, 35 μg ethinyloestradiol, 1 mg norethisterone. The glands are small and inactive, the stroma is immature and there is no spiral artery differentiation; thin-walled vascular channels are present. The appearances are similar to those seen in Fig. 32.33. (From C H Buckley & H Fox 2002 *Biopsy Pathology of the Endometrium* reproduced by permission of Edward Arnold Limited.)

which is probably due to a low-grade infection (Buckley & Fox 2002). Alterations in the quality of the cervical mucus may render it less able to provide a satisfactory barrier to ascending infection and shedding of the endometrium may have been inadequate when the pill was used.

Early reports of an increased risk of endometrial adenocarcinoma in women using steroid contraceptives are now known to have been limited, almost entirely, to a particular 100 μg oestrogen pill (Cohen & Deppe 1977; Blythe & Ali 1979; Weiss & Sayvetz 1980). More recent studies show that the current, low-dose combined steroid contraceptives halve the risk of endometrial carcinoma (Huggins & Giuntoli 1979; Kaufman et al

1980; Hulka et al 1982; Jick et al 1993). In the WHO Collaborative study (WHO 1988a) ever-users of combined steroid contraceptives had a relative risk of developing endometrial carcinoma of 0.55, whilst those in the Oxford Family Planning Association contraceptive study had a relative risk of 0.1 for ever-users compared with never-users (Vessey & Painter 1995). This represents a significant reduction in risk. Maximum protection is given to those who are nulliparous and have used the pill for more than one year. There is also, as might be expected, a negative correlation between the use of depot medroxyprogesterone acetate and the development of endometrial carcinoma (WHO 1991a). When,

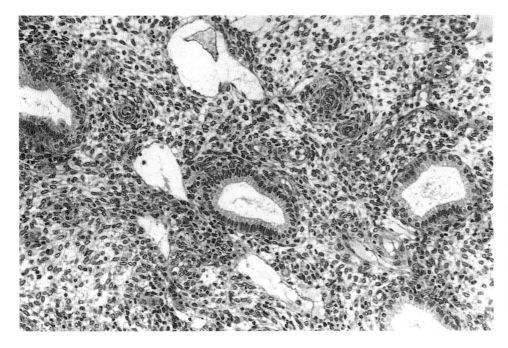

Fig. 32.32 Combined steroid contraceptive, biphasic pattern, 30 µg ethinyloestradiol, 150 mg levonorgestrel, three weeks since hormone withdrawal bleed. In contrast to the three preceding illustrations, the glands are moderately well grown, exhibit secretory activity and spiral artery differentiation has occurred. A granulated lymphocyte infiltrate is present. (From C H Buckley & H Fox 2002 *Biopsy Pathology of the Endometrium* reproduced by permission of Edward Arnold Limited.)

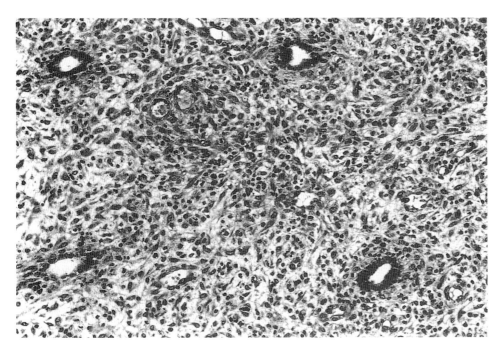

Fig. 32.33 Phased steroid contraceptive. The glands are small, narrow, tubular and devoid of secretion. The stroma is pseudodecidualised and infiltrated by granulated lymphocytes. The degree of glandular regression is similar to that seen in Fig. 32.29. (From C H Buckley & H Fox 2002 *Biopsy Pathology of the Endometrium* reproduced by permission of Edward Arnold Limited.)

however, the past history of women with newly diagnosed uterine sarcomas was investigated (Schwartz et al 1996), a positive correlation was found between the use of oral contraceptives prior to 1980 and leiomyosarcoma. The long-term follow-up of women who used the older high-dose formulations may, therefore, need to be life long.

The beneficial effect of the use of steroid contraception on the endometrium persists after the menopause providing that the woman is not subsequently given sequential or unopposed oestrogen hormone replacement therapy.

Progestagen-only contraceptives

The so-called 'mini-pill' or progestagen-only pill produces a much more variable picture in the endometrium than that which is seen in patients using combined regimens, the appearances often resembling those seen in spontaneously occurring luteal phase defect (Fig. 32.36) following an inadequate follicular phase. The variability of the appearance depends on a number of factors. Firstly, ovulation is not consistently inhibited. Secondly, bleeding occurs somewhat erratically and is followed by a healing rather than a true proliferative phase, unless there is

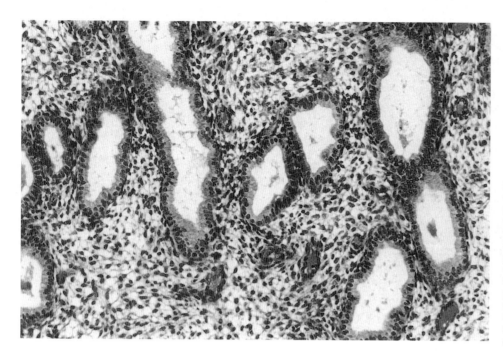

Fig. 32.34 Phased steroid contraceptive. This biopsy was from a patient receiving a hormone combination identical to that given to the women whose biopsy appears in Fig. 32.33. In striking contrast glandular growth and secretion are much better developed, there is a minor degree of spiral artery differentiation and granulated lymphocyte infiltration is absent. (From C H Buckley & H Fox 2002 *Biopsy Pathology of the Endometrium* reproduced by permission of Edward Arnold Limited.)

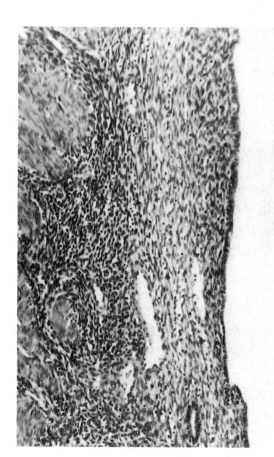

Fig. 32.35 Endometrial atrophy following the prolonged use of high-dose steroid contraceptives.

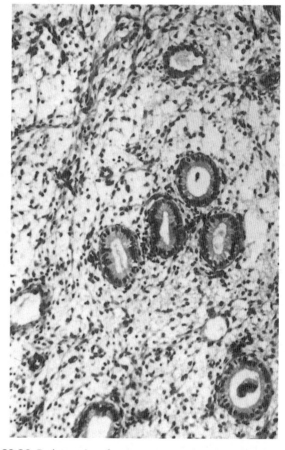

Fig. 32.36 Endometrium from a woman using a continuous progestagen contraceptive (0.35 mg norethisterone daily). The glands are small and there is variable secretory activity. Vascular and stromal development is poor.

ovarian follicular activity, when a more adequate proliferative phase may be observed. Most commonly the endometrium is shallow, proliferative activity somewhat limited and occasional mitoses may be observed at almost any time, whilst mature glands or glands showing variable secretory activity coexist. Stromal decidualisation is poorly developed because of the low oestrogen levels and the failure of progesterone receptor induction. Occasional granulated lymphocytes may be seen and there are changes in the lymphomyeloid cell subsets in the endometrium (Clark et al 1996).

In patients who have been given depot progestagens for contraceptive purposes, and particularly in those taking progestagens over a long period of time, there may be a marked degree of endometrial atrophy (Hadisaputra et al 1996) and this may take many months to recover (Dallenbach-Hellweg 1980b). It may be difficult in such cases to obtain an endometrial biopsy whether hysteroscopic directed biopsy is used or suction curettage (Hadisaputra et al 1996). Sufficient material for examination is obtained in only about half the cases and these tend to be the women with the highest endogenous oestrogen levels in the two weeks preceding the biopsy. The endometrium in these cases resembles basalis only, lacking spiral arteries and with thin-walled lymphovascular channels which may be numerous (Fig. 32.37) (Rogers 1996), and which are more fragile than in women with dysfunctional uterine bleeding (Hickey et al 2000); superficial petechiae and haemorrhages are also frequently observed (Hickey et al 2000). There are also larger numbers of blood vessels with endothelial gaps and haemostatic plugs than normal (Hourihan et al 1991).

Endometrial microvascular density is increased in women using Norplant (Hickey et al 1996b) and matrix metalloproteinase-1 and -9 (MMP-1 and MMP-9) may be involved in the irregular endometrial breakdown of the vessels which characterised its use in some women (Vincent et al 1999; Vincent et al 2000) and was one of the reasons for its discontinuation. In this respect, it is interesting to note that MMP-1, MMP-3 and mast cells have a similar distribution in the endometrium of women using progestagen-only contraception and in menstrual endometrium and that these vary with different progestagens (Vincent et al 2000). This disturbance in the angiogenic process may be caused by an imbalance of pro- and antioxidant processes in the endometrium of Norplant users. In the endometrium from Norplant users with bleeding problems, in vitro supplementation of vitamin E results in a significantly higher angiogenic score than placebo, and women given vitamin E have significantly fewer bleeding days than those given a placebo (Subakir et al 2000).

Effects on the myometrium

The effect of steroid contraceptives on the myometrium is usually ignored but contraceptives may stimulate or

maintain leiomyomas as shrinkage after cessation of steroid contraceptives has been reported (Barbieri 1997).

Effects on the cervix

The older high-dose combined hormone preparations were frequently associated with the development of cervical oedema, congestion and, in the majority of cases, a large ectopy. An ectopy is still common but generally less florid. Reserve cell hyperplasia is observed more frequently in the cervices of pill users (Schaude et al 1980), probably a natural consequence of squamous metaplasia of the columnar epithelium of the ectopy.

It is often accepted, although the view has been challenged (Greeley et al 1995), that the progestagen in the combined pill, or in the mini-pill, induces minor degrees of microglandular hyperplasia (Kyriakos et al 1968), often detectable only microscopically, on the surface of the endocervical canal or on an ectopy. Less commonly, it forms a sessile or polypoidal mass in the endocervix (Govan et al 1969; Tsukada et al 1977), on an ectopy or in areas of vaginal adenosis (Robboy & Welch 1977).

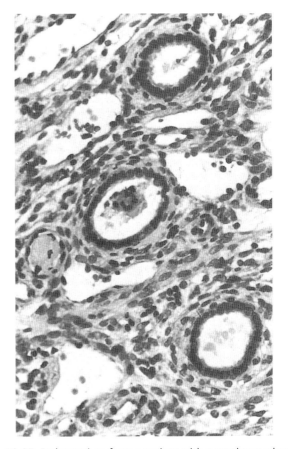

Fig. 32.37 Endometrium from a patient with a renal transplant, given 0.35 mg norethisterone daily as a contraceptive. Her clinical complaint of repeated, prolonged bleeding can possibly be explained on the basis of the numerous thin-walled blood vessels in the endometrial stroma.

There is no evidence that microglandular hyperplasia is associated with, or is a precursor of carcinoma of the cervix (Jones & Silverberg 1989). Histologically, microglandular hyperplasia consists of closely packed glandular acini lined by flattened or cuboidal epithelium poor in mucin (Fig. 32.38). Foci of reserve cell hyperplasia, squamous metaplasia and an inflammatory cell infiltrate are often present. Usually the cells lining the acini are regular, and their nuclear chromatin uniformly dispersed. Sometimes, however, the lesion is particularly florid (Fig. 32.39) and the glandular component arranged in a reticulated or solid pattern (Taylor et al 1967). In these cases the cells may have pleomorphic, hyperchromatic nuclei and the solid areas appear vacuolated due to cystic dilatation of the intercellular spaces: there can therefore be a resemblance to clear cell carcinoma (Fox & Buckley 1983) or microglandular hyperplasia of this type may be mimicked by carcinoma (Young & Scully 1992).

Arguments have been put forward linking the use of steroid contraceptives with the development of squamous intraepithelial neoplasia of the cervix (CIN) (Joswig-Priewe & Schlüster 1980) and invasive carcinoma. Doubts have been expressed, however, as to whether this is a cause and effect relationship (Boyce et al 1977) or might not be explained simply by taking sexual factors (Swan & Brown 1981), the pattern of sexual activity, the time since the last cervical smear and the absence of a barrier contraceptive into consideration (Vessey 1979). Further analyses, taking these confounding factors into consideration, initially failed to provide incontrovertible evidence concerning the relationship of CIN and the use of steroid contraceptives (Ebeling et al 1987; Cuzick et al 1990; Coker et al 1992; Delgado Rodriguez et al 1992). Population studies (Gram et al 1992), however, which looked at women who used steroid contraceptives in 1979 and 1980, and which adjusted the results for confounding factors such as smoking, age, marital status and frequency of alcoholic intoxication continue to indicate a relative risk of 1.5 for current steroid contraceptive users and 1.4 for past users compared with those who have not used steroid contraceptives (see also Chapter 8).

The positive relationship between steroid contraceptive use and the development of invasive cervical carcinoma becomes statistically significant when steroid contraceptives have been used for more than 7 years and use commenced before the age of 24 years, the relative risks being 1.8 and 3.0 respectively (Ebeling et al 1987). The WHO Collaborative Study (WHO 1985a) found similar results with ever-users having a relative risk of developing cervical carcinoma of 1.19 compared with non-users, the

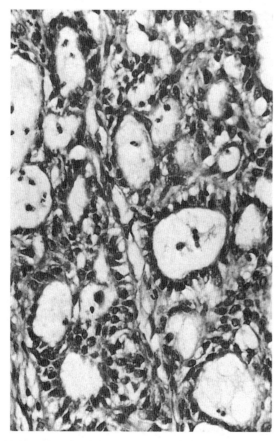

Fig. 32.38 Microglandular hyperplasia of the cervix in a combined steroid contraceptive user.

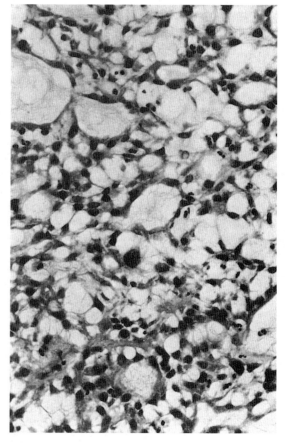

Fig. 32.39 Microglandular hyperplasia of the cervix with an atypical reticulated pattern.

relative risk rising to 1.53 after 5 years of use. The Royal College of General Practitioners' Study (Hannaford 1991) also reported a possible increased risk of cervical carcinoma in women using steroid contraceptives and a review of the literature from 1990 onwards (La Vecchia et al 1996) confirms a moderate increase in cervical carcinoma. The risk of developing carcinoma does not appear to apply to women who have used depot-medroxyprogesterone acetate (WHO 1992; Thomas & Ray 1995). There may also be differences in the risk of developing different forms of carcinoma. A possible association with, in particular, well-differentiated villoglandular adenocarcinoma has been described (Jones et al 1993) and there is a suggestion that the risk of developing adenocarcinoma may be even greater than that of developing squamous carcinoma (relative risk 2.2 compared with 1.1) (Brinton et al 1990) although this has been refuted by others (Honoré et al 1991): it is probable that the risk of adenocarcinoma and adenosquamous carcinoma is similar to that for squamous carcinoma (Thomas & Ray 1996) (see also Chapters 8 & 9).

Effects on the vagina

In women who have used a combined contraceptive with a low oestrogen content or a relatively potent progestagen, the vaginal epithelium may be atrophic (Joswig-Priewe & Schluster 1980) and this may be of sufficient severity as to produce symptoms. There is some evidence that Chlamydial infection is twice as common in steroid contraceptive users (Cottingham & Hunter 1992) but that they are at decreased risk of developing bacterial vaginosis and Trichomonal infection compared with users of other forms of contraception (Roy 1991).

Pelvic inflammatory disease (PID)

After stratification for age, number of pregnancies and lifetime sexual partners, women using steroid contraceptives, or ever-users, have lower rates of Chlamydial pelvic inflammatory disease than those who do not use birth control methods (Spinillo et al 1996). Steroid contraceptive users are, however, more likely to have asymptomatic endometritis, that is, endometritis without associated clinical features of PID, than non-users (Ness et al 1997).

Effects on the ovary

Steroid contraceptives do not inhibit ovulation in every cycle (Hawkins & Elder 1979) nor do they alter the process of normal follicular atresia. Indeed, tertiary follicles, varying greatly in size and development, can be found even after many years of combined steroid contraceptive use (Mestwerdt & Kranzfelder 1980), although with prolonged use there is usually a reduction in the number of developing follicles and ovarian volume is

consistently lower in these women compared with those who use no contraception or have an IUCD in situ (Christensen et al 1997). On the other hand, whilst early studies from the Boston Collaborative Drug Surveillance Program (Ory 1974) revealed a reduction in the number of functional ovarian cysts more recent studies on the effects of the modern lower-dose preparations suggest that these do not substantially reduce the risk of a woman's developing functional ovarian cysts (Holt et al 1992). A feature not usually observed in the normal ovary is a thickening of the basement membrane of primary follicles which may be seen on light microscopy (Mestwerdt & Kranzfelder 1980).

Studies have shown a reduced incidence of malignant epithelial tumours of the ovary in steroid contraceptive users (McGowan et al 1979; Weiss et al 1981; Cramer et al 1982; Rosenberg et al 1982; WHO 1988b). Protection appears to increase with duration of use, starting after three years (Weiss et al 1981; Cramer et al 1982; Rosenberg et al 1982) and persisting for at least 10 years after cessation of use (Rosenberg et al 1982). The greatest reduction is variously quoted as occurring in women between the ages of 35 years and 55 years (Weiss et al 1981) and between 40 and 59 years (Cramer et al 1982). This advantageous effect can still be demonstrated even when allowances are made for age and parity. An explanation of these findings has been provided by observations that ovarian carcinoma occurs most frequently in those women who ovulate incessantly (Casagrande et al 1979). The implication is either that the surface epithelium, which is in a constant state of repair, is particularly susceptible to carcinogens, a finding corresponding with the finding of a reduced number of epithelial tumours in parous patients (Newhouse et al 1977; McGowan et al 1979), or that there is more chance of surface epithelial cysts forming from which carcinomas may develop (Fathalla 1972). A retrospective case-control study of the occurrence of benign epithelial tumours of the ovary in steroid contraceptive users, however, found that there was no reduction in their incidence, a finding that tends to refute the view that benign epithelial tumours are the precursors of carcinomas (personal communication, Fox H).

The relative risk of an ever-user of steroid contraceptives developing carcinoma of the ovary is 0.75 (WHO 1988b) after allowing for the confounding effect of pregnancy. The reduction of risk is most marked in nulliparous women and is reduced for all epithelial types except mucinous. This last observation may, perhaps, be explained by the possibility that some mucinous tumours are of germ cell origin and the aetiological factors may differ from those which are of surface epithelial origin.

There is also, as would be expected, a reduced risk of steroid contraceptive users dying of ovarian carcinoma. The Oxford Study found that the relative risk was only 0.4 compared with never-users of steroid contraceptives (Vessey et al 1989a).

An as yet unexplained finding has been that of Cramer et al (1982) who observed that pill users under the age of 40 years had an increased risk of developing epithelial tumours of borderline malignancy.

Effects on the breast

It is generally accepted that steroid contraceptives are associated with a decreased risk of benign breast disease (Ory et al 1976; LiVolsi et al 1978; Huggins & Giuntoli 1979; Brinton et al 1981; Huggins & Zucker 1987; Vessey 1989; Tzingounis et al 1996) and that the overall risk of a woman developing breast carcinoma is not increased by the use of combined or progestagen-only steroid contraceptives (Royal College of General Practitioners' Study 1981a; UK National Case-Control 1989; Olsson 1989; Paul et al 1989; Romieu et al 1989; Stanford et al 1989; WHO 1991b). Further, there is no increased risk for the woman over the age of 40 years (Vessey et al 1989b; Harlap 1991), for those taking contraceptives around the time of the menopause (Romieu et al 1990; Thomas & Noonan 1991) or for those who stopped steroid contraception 10 or more years previously (Westhoff 1999). There is, however, a slight increase for current or recent users (Chilvers 1996; Collaborative Group on Hormonal Factors in Breast Cancer 1996; Kaunitz 1996) which declines with time since last use regardless of the duration of use (WHO 1990) and some studies report an increased risk of breast carcinoma in younger women (Chilvers & Deacon 1990; Rosenberg et al 1992; Wingo et al 1993). The increased risk is variably reported as affecting those who have used steroid contraceptives for a long time (Miller et al 1989a; UK National Case-Control Study 1989), those who started the pill at an early age (Johnson 1989; Olsson et al 1989), those who are nulliparous (Meirik et al 1989; Rushton & Jones 1992), and those who used the pill before the first pregnancy (Lund et al 1989). A similar, but not statistically significant trend was reported by the WHO (WHO 1990) in 2116 cases of newly diagnosed carcinoma of the breast when compared with 12 077 controls. Ever-users of combined steroid contraceptives were found to have a relative risk of 1.15 of developing carcinoma. Women under the age of 35 years had a relative risk of 1.26 and those over 35 years had a relative risk of 1.12 but neither of these figures reached statistical significance. The risk was not found to increase with use of the pill before the age of 25 years or before the first pregnancy but there was a borderline statistically significant relative risk of 1.5 in women who had used the pill for more than 2 years before the age of 25 years.

Two factors may have an impact on the apparently contradictory evidence that cases of breast carcinoma may be increased in younger women whilst the total number of cases has not increased. Firstly, oral contraceptives with less than 50 μg of oestrogen have a lower risk of causing carcinoma and progestagen-only contraceptives may even be protective (UK National Case-Control Study 1989). Secondly, the pill may accelerate the presentation of carcinoma rather than cause it because fewer cases are found as the cohort ages (Schlesselman 1990).

The relative risk of dying from breast carcinoma in steroid contraceptive users is 0.9 (Vessey et al 1989a).

The histological type of carcinoma is not affected by the use of oral contraceptives (Miller et al 1989b). The carcinomas diagnosed in these women tend, however, to be less advanced clinically and this suggests that there may be a screening bias (Plu Bureau & Le 1997).

Effects on the liver

A variety of functional and morphological changes have been described in the livers of hormone contraceptive users. Transient small rises in serum bilirubin (Orellana-Alcade & Dominguez 1966) and transaminases are recorded in the first few cycles of usage. Changes recorded in women with implants of etonogestrel (the biologically active metabolite of desogestrel) or levonorgestrel include an increase in total bilirubin and gamma-glutamyl transferase and a decrease in alanine aminotransferase and aspartate aminotransferase (Egberg et al 1998). Women who have a pre-existing hepatic disorder, such as Dubin–Johnson or Rotor syndrome, or who have had idiopathic jaundice of pregnancy may become jaundiced on the pill and should not use this form of contraception. The histological features are of a bland hepatocellular and canalicular cholestasis with no evident liver cell necrosis or inflammation (Fig. 32.40). Steroid contraceptives are also contraindicated in patients with acute or severe chronic hepatocellular disease because, occasionally, severe cholestatic jaundice may develop in these patients. Generally, cholestasis resolves when the hormone is stopped but occasionally the condition may persist (Weden et al 1992).

The older literature contains reports of sinusoidal dilatation in periportal areas (Figs 32.41, 32.42) and hepatomegaly, in both high-dose steroid contraceptive and androgen users, which recedes after withdrawal of the drugs (Winkler & Poulsen 1975; Spellberg et al 1979). The liver function tests in these cases show only minor changes and electronmicroscopic studies show dilatation of the endoplasmic reticulum in the liver cells (Spellberg et al 1979). Peliosis, an extreme form of vascular dilatation with large blood-filled cysts or lacunae was also reported in these patients and sinusoidal dilatation was often present elsewhere in the liver (Wight 1982). Peliosis also occurs within and around steroid contraceptive induced hepatic neoplasms (Taxy 1978; Williams & Neuberger 1981) and is believed to be due to a direct effect of the steroids (Editorial 1973).

Rarely, Budd–Chiari syndrome has been described after prolonged use of contraceptive steroids with a latent period of about 20 months (Wu et al 1977). It may be

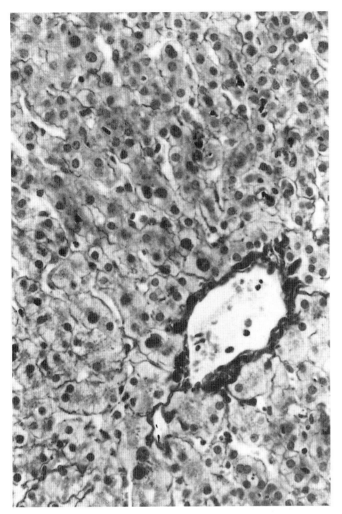

Fig. 32.40 Intrahepatic cholestasis in a steroid contraceptive user: canalicular bile retention is present but no liver cell swelling and no inflammatory reaction. Van Gieson. (Courtesy of Professor R. N. M. MacSween.)

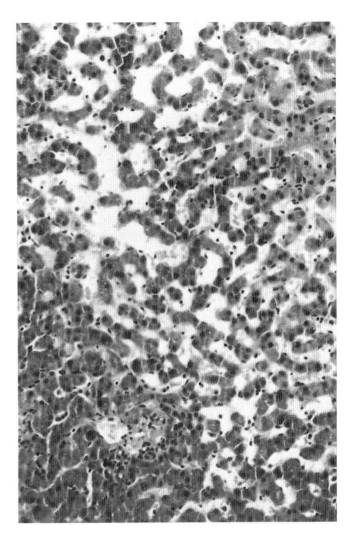

Fig. 32.41 Contraceptive steroid-induced hepatic sinusoidal dilatation: this is periportal in distribution and of a mild degree — compare with Fig. 32.42. (Courtesy of Professor R. N. M. McSween.)

due to obliteration of the central and sublobular hepatic veins by a process of intimal cell proliferation and fibrosis (Alpert 1976) or hepatic vein thrombosis which appears to develop over a period of time and may or may not extend into the inferior vena cava (Ecker et al 1966; Sterup & Mosbech 1967; Irey et al 1970; Hoyumpa et al 1971; Barnet & Joffe 1991). In many cases the condition has been fatal but recovery may occur after stopping the steroids (Hoyumpa et al 1971). It is difficult to place this information in context as it appears likely that the problem was another aspect of the high oestrogen content of the earlier pills although occasional cases are still reported in women in whom there is already some defect of the clotting mechanism (Simsek et al 2000).

Earlier reports that the development of hepatic adenoma was causally related to the use of steroid contraceptives have, to some extent, been substantiated (Horvath et al 1972; Baum et al 1973; Contostavlos 1973; Edmondson et al 1976; Christopherson & Mays

1977; Fechner 1977; Klatskin 1977; Rooks et al 1979; Kerlin et al 1983). Reports of an association continue to appear in the literature (Tao 1992) and case-control studies provide evidence that the risk is greatest, but not limited to, those who have used steroid contraceptives for a long time (Rosenberg 1991; Shortell & Schwartz 1991). There have been reports that adenomata in which there is dysplasia may be the precursors of hepatocellular carcinoma in some steroid contraceptive users (Tao et al 1991) and some authors report the finding of focal carcinoma in such adenomas (Perret et al 1996).

Hepatocellular carcinoma, (Christopherson & Mays 1979; Ishak 1979; Neuberger et al 1980), hepatoblastoma (Klatskin 1977), rhabdomyosarcoma (Coté & Urmacher 1990) and cholangiocarcinoma (Klatskin 1977; Ellis et al 1978) have been reported in steroid contraceptive users. There has been considerable debate as to whether there is a causal relationship or not, and opinions differ. A positive association between oral contraceptive use and

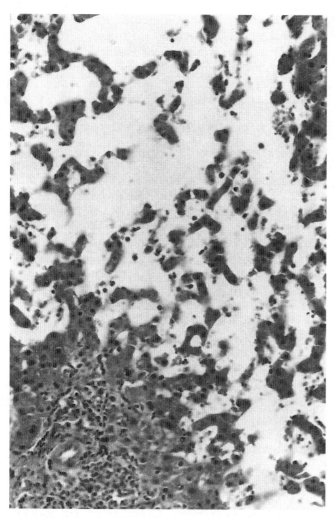

Fig. 32.42 Contraceptive steroid-induced hepatic sinusoidal dilatation: there is more marked atrophy and disruption of the liver cell plates than in Fig. 32.41. H & E. (Courtesy of Professor R. N. M. McSween.)

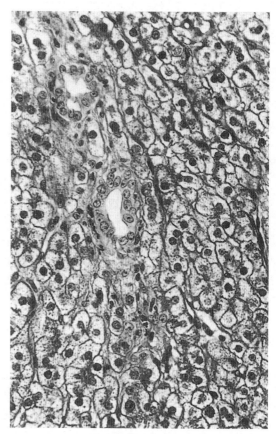

Fig. 32.43 Focal nodular hyperplasia of the liver showing hepatocytes and bile ducts of normal form. Masson Trichrome.

hepatocellular carcinoma (Palmer et al 1989; Prentice 1991; Rosenberg 1991; Hsing et al 1992; Tavani et al 1993) is reported in countries where hepatocellular carcinoma is uncommon. Steroid contraceptive ever-users are reported to have a relative risk of developing hepatocellular carcinoma of 1.6 compared with never-users, and for those who have used steroid contraceptives for more than 10 years, the odds ratio is 2.0 (Hsing et al 1992). The WHO Collaborative Study of Neoplasia and Steroid Contraceptives (WHO 1989a), on the other hand, based upon the examination of 122 newly reported cases of hepatocellular carcinoma and 802 controls from countries in which hepatitis B is endemic, found no evidence that short-term use of combined steroid contraceptives increases the risk of either hepatocellular carcinoma or cholangiocarcinoma: the relative risk in ever-users is 0.71. In addition, depot-medroxyprogesterone acetate when used as a contraceptive in a population in which hepatitis B is endemic (WHO 1991c) does not increase the risk of

hepatoma or cholangiocarcinoma. Nonetheless, hepatocellular carcinoma is still reported in women in whom there is no other apparent risk factor (Fiel et al 1996).

Focal nodular hyperplasia of the liver occurs in the absence of steroid contraceptive use (Ishak & Rabin 1975; Kerlin et al 1983; Shortell & Schwartz 1991) but case reports indicate that following the use of steroid contraceptives, and in pregnancy, focal nodular hyperplasia and, more commonly, hepatic adenoma may enlarge, undergo necrosis and rupture (Mays et al 1974; Knowles & Wolff 1976; Kent et al 1977; Kinch & Lough 1978; Buckley & Lewis 1982; Leborgne et al 1990; Chiappa et al 1999). The mortality associated with rupture of such hepatic lesions is around 5 to 10% (Brady & Coit 1990). On the other hand, complete regression of focal nodular hyperplasia 5 years after stopping steroid contraceptives has been reported (Meunier et al 1998). The behaviour of focal nodular hyperplasia in pregnancy is considered in Chapter 43.

Focal nodular hyperplasia forms a well-circumscribed, often lobulated mass of morphologically normal hepatocytes. A fibrous core may be present from which bands radiate between the lobules; bile ducts and thick-walled arteries within fibrous septa (Fig. 32.43) help to distinguish the lesion from an adenoma (Knowles & Wolff

1976). An adenoma is a completely or partially encapsulated cellular mass of hepatocytes showing only minimal cellular atypia and lacking a normal lobular architecture and bile ducts (Fig. 32.44). These lesions may be multiple (Mdel et al 1975). Hepatocellular carcinoma occurring in pill takers is similar to that seen under other conditions.

Steroid contraceptives are not a significant aetiological factor in the development of gall stones (Kay 1984; van Beek et al 1991; La Vecchia et al 1992). There is no evidence that steroid contraceptives affect the risk of individuals developing carcinoma of the gall bladder (WHO 1989b).

Effects on the cardiovascular system

It can be difficult to evaluate fully the effects of contraceptive hormones on the cardiovascular system as there are so many confounding factors. These difficulties are

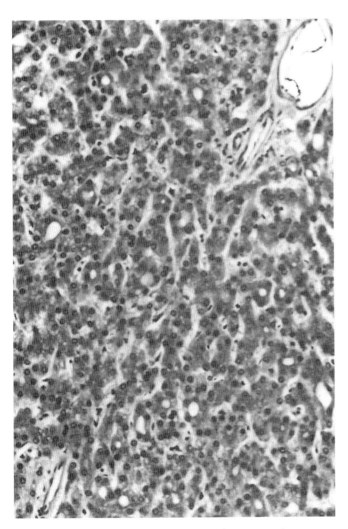

Fig. 32.44 A liver cell adenoma in a steroid contraceptive user. The tumour cells resemble normal hepatocytes but with irregular plate formation and some acinar development. There are no portal tracts: two thin-walled vessels are seen. (Courtesy of Professor R. N. M. McSween.)

well illustrated by a Norwegian study (Graff-Iversen et al 1996) in which it was revealed that women between the ages of 20 and 39 years were more likely to have used low-dose preparations, have lower body masses, less often have relatives with coronary heart disease and less often eat saturated fats than women over the age of 40; the latter were more likely to have smoked.

The majority of early studies found that combined steroid contraceptive users had an increased risk of death from a variety of cardiovascular diseases when compared with non-users (Inman et al 1970; Collaborative Group for the Study of Stroke 1973; Royal College of General Practitioners' 1981b; Vessey et al 1981a; Wingrave 1982). The early report from the Royal College of General Practitioners' Study (Beral 1977), however, suggesting that death rate from circulatory disease increased with duration of pill use, was later shown to have been fallacious (Royal College of General Practitioners 1981b).

Thromboembolic disease

The oestrogen in combined steroid contraceptives is responsible for a dose-related increase in serum levels of fibrinogen (Ernst 1992), factors VIIc and XIIc (Kelleher 1990), triglycerides and HDL-cholesterol (HDL-C) and a decrease in LDL-cholesterol (LDL-C). The progestagen is associated with a decrease in HDL-C and an increase in LDL-C (Mishell 1992; Diab & Zaki, 2000). The latter is most marked, as might be expected, in women using progestagen-only contraceptives such as medroxyprogesterone acetate. Whilst modifications in the hormone content of the pill and the use of some new progestagens have diminished these changes (Janaud et al 1992), the formulation of the oral contraceptive, the relative potency of the progestagen and the oestrogen/progestagen balance continue to have an impact on cardiovascular disease (Godsland 1991).

In some women, steroid contraceptives act synergistically with inherited thrombophilic defects to increase the risk of venous thromboembolism. These include a congenital deficiency of Protein C, which normally inhibits coagulation and promotes fibrinolysis (Trauscht van Horn et al 1992), G20120A mutation of the prothrombin gene (Martinelli et al 1999) and a mutation in factor V (Factor V Leiden) which results in resistance to the anticoagulant action of activated Protein C (APC-resistance). APC-resistance occurs in 3 to 5% of the general population and increases the risk of thrombosis in affected individuals using oral contraceptives by 35 times. Protein C deficiency increases the risk by 15 times. Differences have been shown in the sensitivity to activated Protein C in women using the second and third generations of gestagens, those using the third generation preparations being more resistant than those using the second generation gestagens (Rosing et al 1997; Vandenbroucke & Shelton

1997). This is seen particularly in those who are using the new gestagens for the first time and in young users (Vandenbroucke & Shelton 1997).

In general, oral contraceptives increase the risk of venous thrombosis 3- to 4-fold. The use of second and third generation gestagens appears to have further increased this risk (Bauersachs et al 1996; Douketis et al 1997) and third generation gestagens carry a greater risk than second (Spitzer et al 1996; Jick et al 2000), although others have disputed this (Speroff 1996; Suissa et al 1997; Winkler 1998; Lewis et al 1999; Todd et al 1999).

The relative risk of thrombosis in users of second and third generation gestagens continues to be the subject of debate in the medical literature. The possibility of bias in observational research (Lewis et al 1996b) has been suggested and attention has been drawn to possible discrepancies between drug company sponsored publications and those published by independent workers, all of the latter having demonstrated a significant increase in the risk of thromboembolism (van Heteren 2001).

In 1995, the UK Committee on the Safety of Medicines drew attention to a 2- to 3-fold increase in thromboembolic episodes in users of combined steroid contraceptives containing the third generation gestagens such as Desonorgestrel and Gestodene, compared with those containing Levonorgestrel. As a consequence the UK Committee on Safety of Medicines advised that whilst there may be an excess risk of thromboembolism in women using preparations containing levonorgestrel, norethisterone or ethynodiol of 5 to 10 cases per 100 000 women per annum, the risk with desogestrel and gestodene is about twice this (Kemmeren et al 2001). Weiss (1999) writing on behalf of the American College of Obstetrics and Gynecology endorsed this view. The use of third generation gestagens has not, therefore, been recommended in women with known risk factors and following the publication of these data, the proportion of women prescribed third generation-containing contraceptives fell (van Heteren 2001) as people reverted to the second generation combinations.

The pattern of thromboembolic disease has, to some extent, changed over the years. Early investigations identified oestrogen as an aetiological factor in thromboembolic disease (Vessey & Doll 1969) and a reduction in oestrogen content of the pill was accompanied by the expected reduction in the number of general thromboembolic episodes (Böttiger et al 1980). Superficial venous thrombosis had been linked to both the oestrogen and progestagen content of the pill whilst no link had been demonstrated with deep vein thrombosis (Royal College of General Practitioners' Study 1978). The high hormone content of the early pill was almost certainly also the cause of the fatal proliferative endothelial lesions with intravascular thrombosis in both arteries and veins which were reported by Irey (1970). In some cases the pulmonary vasculature was affected and in others the

hepatic veins: other authors described mesenteric vascular occlusion (Nothmann et al 1973). Despite the reduction in hormone levels in contraceptive pills, women remain at risk of venous thromboembolic disease (WHO 1989c; Katerndahl et al 1992) and cerebral thrombosis (Thorogood et al 1992). There is also a statistically non-significant increase in thromboembolism in users of progestagen-only contraception (WHO 1998; Vasilakis et al 1999). Although relatively rare, many thrombotic episodes give rise to serious clinical problems; for example, there are recent reports of mesenteric thrombosis with intestinal infarction (Engelke et al 1995), coeliac axis thrombosis with splenic infarction (Arul et al 1998; Gould et al 1998), and retinal vein thrombosis (Kirwan et al 1997). The latter is regarded as a contraindication to the use of steroid contraceptives.

Ischaemic heart disease

In the 1970s and 1980s, deaths due to coronary artery disease (Inman et al 1970) were found to occur more frequently in current contraceptive users (Royal College of General Practitioners' 1981b, 1983) (relative risk 4.2) and were related to the dose of oestrogen in the combination (Meade et al 1980). By 1991, however, the relative risk had fallen to between 1.5 (Vessey et al 1989a) and 1.9 (Thorogood et al 1991) for current and past users of oral contraceptives and previous use of steroid contraceptives carried no increased risk of myocardial infarction (Stampfer et al 1990). This was almost certainly a reflection of the reduction in the oestrogen content of the pill because in those women who continued to use preparations with 50 μg of oestrogen the relative risk remained at 4.2 (Thorogood et al 1991). Smoking counteracts the effects of oestrogen reduction, with heavy smokers having a relative risk of dying from myocardial infarction of 20.8 (Croft & Hannaford 1989). A similar high risk has also been identified by the WHO Collaborative Study of Cardiovascular Disease and Steroid Hormone Contraception (1997) in smokers and hypertensive women. Progestagen-only, or non-hormonal contraceptives are, therefore, recommended for women over the age of 35 years who continue to smoke (Burkman 1997).

The mechanism by which the combined steroid contraceptives affect the incidence of ischaemic heart disease is believed to be related to the effect of the progestagen component in lowering HDL-C (Kremer et al 1980) a reduction in which, it is generally accepted, is associated with an increased incidence of arterial disease, especially ischaemic heart disease (Miller et al 1977; Yaari et al 1981; Kay 1982). The second and third generation progestagens used in many of the current combined steroid contraceptives have, however, much less effect on the HDL-C (Janaud et al 1992) and it might be expected, therefore, that the incidence of ischaemic heart disease might fall even further in women who have used only these newer preparations. The reduced risk of myocardial infarction (Rosenberg et al 1997) may, however, have to be balanced against the increased risk of thromboembolism in those who use the third generation gestagens (Lewis et al 1996a; Schwingl & Shelton, 1997), the risk of thromboembolism being three- to four-fold (Mishell 1999) (see above).

Cerebrovascular disease

The Royal College of General Practitioners' study (1981b) found a statistically significant increased risk of subarachnoid haemorrhage in women using the pill. Vessey et al (1981a), reporting data from the Oxford Study, found only a slight increase which was not of statistical significance and was confined to women with systemic hypertension. A later report from the Oxford Study confirms this slight increase in subarachnoid haemorrhage (Thorogood et al 1992). Recent reports have raised the possibility that current users of low-dose combined steroid contraceptives containing second generation gestagens may have an increased risk of both haemorrhagic stroke and aneurysmal bleeding (Schwartz et al 1997).

The WHO (1998) found that systemic hypertension played a part in strokes of all types in progestagen-only contraceptive users, when compared with non-users, raising the odds ratio from 7.2 for non-hypertensive women to 12.4 for hypertensive women.

The 1983 report of the Royal College of General Practitioners' Study (Royal College of General Practitioners' Study 1983) described a significantly increased risk of cerebrovascular disease in both current users and former steroid contraceptive users, particularly for cerebral thrombosis and transient ischaemic attacks. The risk remained elevated for more than six years after stopping the pill and may have been related to the duration of oral contraceptive use. Analysis of the Oxford data (Thorogood et al 1992) confirmed a substantial risk of veno-occlusive stroke. There does not, however, seem to have been an increase in strokes with the introduction of the second and third generation gestagens (Jick et al 1999; Poulter et al 1999b). These latter two reports analyse data from the RCGP database and the WHO Collaborative Case-Control Study, respectively. The WHO Collaborative Study of Cardiovascular disease and Steroid Hormone Contraception further emphasises that the increased risk of ischaemic stroke could be reduced further if women with hypertension and those who smoke are treated with caution. Migraine sufferers with aura may have an increased risk of ischaemic stroke and this risk may be further increased with the use of steroid contraceptives (Becker 1997).

Hypertension

The 1974 report of the Royal College of General Practitioners' Oral Contraceptive Study notes a small reversible elevation in the systemic blood pressure of oral contraceptive users. This amounts to between 3.6 and 5.0 mm of mercury in systolic pressure and between 1.9 and 2.7 mm of mercury in diastolic pressure (WHO 1989d; Leaf et al 1991). This may be due to an increase in renin substrate through increased generation of either angiotensin (Laragh 1976) or an unusually potent renin substrate (Eggena et al 1978). The report further suggests that hypertensive changes might be related to the potency of the progestagen (Royal College of General Practitioners 1974). These observations have been confirmed (Meade et al 1977; Andrew 1979; Kay 1982; Khaw & Peart 1982), but it is apparent that the effect depends not only on the progestagen content of the pill, but also upon the oestrogen–progestagen balance (Edgren & Sturtevant 1976) and on the duration of contraceptive use (Khaw & Peart 1982).

Effects on other tissues

The general suppressive effect of steroid contraceptives on endometrial growth and development results in an improvement of the clinical symptoms in some cases of endometriosis (Crosignani et al 1997).

The Royal College of General Practitioners' Oral Contraception Study has shown that, contrary to earlier reports, the use of steroid contraceptives might reduce the risk of fracture from osteoporosis later in life, they significantly increase the risk (Cooper et al 1993). Depot medroxyprogesterone acetate, used as a contraceptive, has also been shown, in some studies, to reduce bone densities with the development of fractures, because of the associated reduction in oestrogen levels (Cundy et al 1991; Harkins et al 1999; Scholes et al 1999) whilst others (Gbolade et al 1998) report that, despite the low serum oestradiol, bone densities are only minimally reduced below that of the normal population, that any loss of spinal bone density is reversible (Kaunitz 1999) and that previous use is not detrimental to bone density (Orr-Walker et al 1998). Depot levonorgestrel does not appear to be associated with loss of bone density (Intaraprasert et al 1997). A small study of women using etonogestrel (Implanon) also found little change in bone densities but also noted that oestradiol levels were not significantly changed compared with controls which may explain these apparently contradictory findings (Beerthuizen et al 2000).

Steroid contraceptives are said to reduce the severity of rheumatoid arthritis (Jorgensen et al 1996).

There have been three reported cases of thrombocytopaenic purpura developing in women using implants of levonorgestrel (Fraser et al 1996) but no causal relationship has been established.

Earlier reports that women using steroid contraceptives were at increased risk of developing malignant melanoma have not been substantiated (Grimes 1991; Hannaford et al 1991; La Vecchia et al 1996).

There are differences of opinion as to whether the use of combined steroid contraceptives improves or worsens Crohn's disease and ulcerative colitis. Lashner et al in the USA found no increased risk in either Crohn's disease (Lashner et al 1989) or ulcerative colitis (Lashner et al 1990) whilst Logan & Kay (1989) using data from the Royal College of General Practitioners' Study found that both Crohn's disease and ulcerative colitis are more common in oral contraceptive users. On the other hand, use of steroid contraceptives does not affect either the symptomatic or operative recurrence of Crohn's disease following intestinal resection (Moskovitz et al 1999).

There has been a report of the worsening of porphyria cutanea tarda in a woman taking steroid contraceptives although she did not have an exacerbation in pregnancy (Urbanek & Cohen 1994).

INTRAUTERINE CONTRACEPTIVE DEVICES

The composition and structure of intrauterine contraceptive devices (IUCDs) has changed over the years and thus data relating to women in the 1970s or early 1980s is almost certainly inapplicable to current users.

Current IUCDs are made of plastic partly covered by coils of closely wound copper wire or are made of progestagen-impregnated polymer covered by a release rate-controlling membranelastic. Although inert, non-medicated plastic devices are no longer inserted, women who have worn them for many years may still have them in situ and it is appropriate, when considering the pathology of IUCDs, to include data relating to these devices.

The uterus may be perforated or lacerated when the IUCD is inserted. Perforation of the uterus is said to occur, at the time of insertion, in between 0.012 and 0.29% of insertions (Key & Kreutner 1980; Van Os & Edelman 1989), the variation being mainly due to differences in operative skill and training (Craig 1975). The hazard of perforation is said to be greatest in the postpartum and post-miscarriage states when the tissues are soft (Heinonen et al 1984; Kiilholma et al 1990) but this claim has not always been substantiated (Mishell & Roy 1982) unless the patient is lactating (Heartwell & Schlesselman 1983). Cervical laceration is a rare complication of IUCD insertion which happens most commonly in nulliparous women. The accident occurs in 1.8% of insertions (Chi et al 1989) and is more common with a copper or multiload device than with a loop.

Studies of the forces required to perforate the uterus suggest that the majority of perforations may, initially, be partial (Goldstuck 1987) and that the device gradually works its way through the uterine wall. Perforation may occur in the corpus uteri or in the cervix (Rienprayura et al 1973). If the perforation is partial, the tail of the IUCD may remain palpable at the external cervical os and the operator may not be aware of the fact that the uterus has been perforated unless the patient complains

of abnormal bleeding (Tadesse & Wamsteker 1985) or until attempts are made to remove the device, when great difficulty may be encountered.

When the perforation is partial, the IUCD is usually found lying malaligned partly within the uterine cavity and partly embedded in the myometrium. When a complete perforation has occurred, or a partial perforation has become complete due to migration of the IUCD through the uterine wall, a complication perhaps more likely to occur if the patient is breastfeeding (Mittal et al 1986), the device may be found in the broad ligament, peritoneal cavity (Gorsline & Osborne 1985; Ohana et al 2000), bladder (Hefnawi et al 1975; Thomalla 1986; Kiilholma et al 1989; Khan & Wilkinson 1990; Dietrick et al 1992; Caspi et al 1996; Bjornerem & Tollan 1997; Yalcin et al 1998), where it may be a nidus for a calculus (Reyes-Acededo et al 1995; Cumming et al 1997; Hermida-Perez et al 1997; Maskey et al 1997; Yalcin et al 1998), adjacent to the ureter (Timonen & Kurppa 1987), in the small intestine (Chen et al 1998), in the large bowel (Key & Kreutner 1980; Hays et al 1986; Browning & Bigrigg 1988) or in the rectum (Sepulveda 1990; Ramsewak et al 1991; Sogaard 1993). Cases of iliac vein obstruction (Ibghi et al 1995), vesico-uterine fistulae (Schwartzwald et al 1986; Szabo et al 1997) and colo-colic fistula (Pirwany & Boddy 1997) have also been reported in association with ectopic IUCDs. Those devices containing copper are a particular hazard as the copper may elicit a brisk inflammatory response (Fig. 32.45) and if this occurs in the peritoneal cavity it may cause adhesions leading to intestinal obstruction (Osborne & Bennett 1978; Mittal et al 1986; Adoni & Ben Chetrit 1991). In one patient, two devices which had penetrated the uterine wall were retrieved from the pelvis (Gruber et al 1996). There has even been a report of a device expelled via the Fallopian tube (Burkhonov & Bozorov 1993). It is important to remember that the perforation may not be detected until the woman is postmenopausal (Phupong et al 2000).

Multiple device insertion is usually found when a woman believes, erroneously, that her previous device has been expelled (Porges 1973; Nanda & Rathee 1992) or there may be a complaint of infertility when the presence of a device has been forgotten (Olson & Jones 1967; Abramovici et al 1987).

A transient bacteraemia can be detected in 13% of women within a few minutes of replacing an IUCD (Murray et al 1987). This clearly has implications for the patient at risk of developing endocarditis (Smith et al 1983).

Some devices are spontaneously expelled, the proportion depending upon the type of device, the duration of the study and on the patient. The expulsion rate for copper devices ranges from approximately 5.0% (19 821 treatment cycles) within 36 months of use (Fylling 1987) to 1.8% (1038 women, 66% of whom were in the

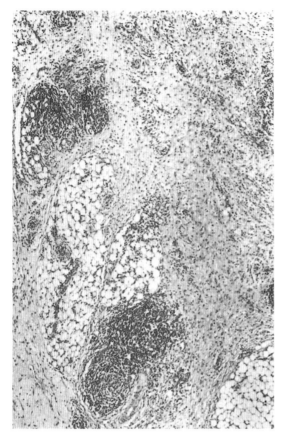

Fig. 32.45 The omentum from a patient in whom a copper-containing IUCD had perforated the uterus and entered the peritoneal cavity. There is extensive fibrosis and a non-specific chronic inflammatory cell infiltrate.

postpartum or post-miscarriage state) within 2 years (Tsalikis et al 1986). Expulsion rates are not affected by the timing of insertion in relation to the menstrual cycle

(Otolorin & Ladipo 1985). There is, however, an increased rate of expulsion if the device is fitted immediately following second trimester miscarriage (Grimes et al 2000) or delivery of the placenta in full term pregnancy (Thiery et al 1985) and this risk can be reduced if insertion is delayed for between 2 and 72 hours (Chi et al 1985).

On rare occasions the device may fracture in utero and this may hinder removal (Custo et al 1986; Blaauwhof & Goldstuck 1988). Fragmentation of the copper on the device increases with duration of use but in only 0.1% of cases is this of sufficient degree as to impair future fertility (Edelman & Van Os 1990).

Death seldom occurs as a direct consequence of IUCD use but occasional deaths from septic miscarriage are well documented (Christian 1974; Preston et al 1975; Cates et al 1976; Foreman et al 1981). These were almost entirely confined to one particular device, a fact that prompted its withdrawal from the market (Cates et al 1976) (see below).

Effects on the endometrium

Morphological changes in the endometrium, although often subtle, are an almost invariable accompaniment of the IUCD. In most IUCD wearers, the changes are limited to the contact sites of the IUCD, are relatively minor and are the result of irritation and pressure. In the majority of cases, the changes affect only the superficial layers of the endometrium and, on removal of the device, the abnormal tissue is shed in the next menstrual cycle (Badrawi et al 1988).

At the contact sites, there is compression of the tissue, pseudodecidualisation of the stroma and, almost invariably, an inflammatory cell response (Fig. 32.46). Although the inflammatory infiltrate may persist for some

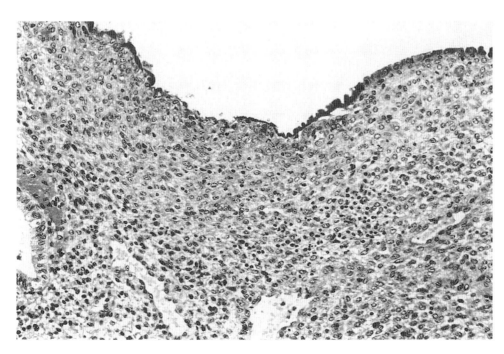

Fig. 32.46 Inert intrauterine contraceptive device contact site. The surface of the endometrium is depressed, the epithelium flattened and the underlying stroma pseudodecidualised and infiltrated by a round cell population. (From C H Buckley & H Fox 2002 *Biopsy Pathology of the Endometrium* reproduced by permission of Edward Arnold Limited.)

time after removal of the device (Moyer & Mishell 1971) there is little doubt that it is the consequence of irritation and not infection, as an infiltrate is seen in experimental animals kept in a germ-free environment (Davis 1972). An inflammatory infiltrate extending beyond the contact site, however, suggests an infectious rather than an irritative aetiology.

In the period immediately following insertion of the device, the inflammatory infiltrate is composed entirely of polymorphonuclear leucocytes but with time, in the absence of infection, polymorphs become scanty and limited to the surface epithelium, to the immediate subepithelial stroma and to the lumina of the superficial stromal capillaries. Gradually, the infiltrate, which is most marked with copper-covered devices (Moyer et al 1970; Sheppard 1987), becomes plasma-lymphocytic (Figs 32.47, 32.48). Lymphocytes are generally increased throughout the tissue, beyond the contact sites, but this may not be apparent on routine histological examination (Mishell & Moyer 1969).

At the contact sites of the IUCD, the compression artefact may accurately reflect the surface contours of the device (Fig. 32.49). The surface epithelium may be flattened or there may be reactive cellular atypia (Fig. 32.50) with some loss of nuclear polarity, mild nuclear pleomorphism, increased nucleo-cytoplasmic ratios, the development of nucleoli and cytoplasmic vacuolation. Much less commonly these days, there is ulceration of the surface epithelium (Moyer & Mishell 1971), sometimes with preservation of the underlying basement membrane, the formation of non-specific granulation tissue and stromal fibrosis (Fig. 32.51) (Bonney et al 1966; Shaw et al 1979a). These features are more typically associated with the presence of an inert IUCD. Rarely there is squamous metaplasia (Tamada et al 1967) or the development of foreign body granulomata (Fig. 32.52) (Ragni et al 1977).

In addition to the local irritative effects, there are, with progestagen-impregnated devices, changes which are attributable to the progestagen and are dose dependent. Initially, in the tissue immediately adjacent to the device (Dallenbach-Hellweg 1981; Ermini et al 1989), there is pseudodecidualisation of the stroma and the cells in the glandular and surface epithelium gradually become cuboidal. The glands become fewer, smaller in calibre and inactive whilst the stroma becomes less mature, losing its decidualised appearance and appearing spindle-celled (Fig. 32.53) (Critchley et al 1998). Over a period, which may be as long as 6 to 12 months, if the amount of progestagen liberated is sufficient, these appearances may

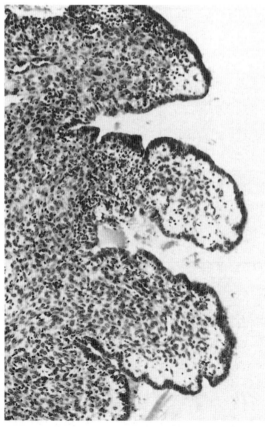

Fig. 32.47 An endometrial IUCD contact site. In addition to the copper wire imprint, there is a scattering of intrastromal and intraepithelial inflammatory cells.

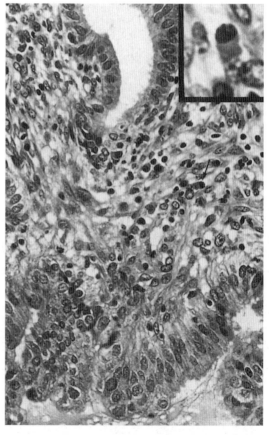

Fig. 32.48 A detail from the endometrium shown in Fig. 32.41, showing the scanty nature of the inflammatory cell infiltrate. Insert of cell group indicated by the arrow.

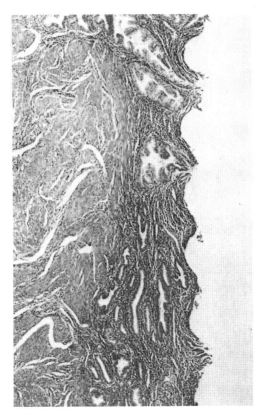

Fig. 32.49 The endometrium in a copper IUCD wearer. The imprint of the copper wire can be clearly seen on the endometrial surface. Loss of surface epithelium is artifactual, having occurred as the device was removed after tissue fixation.

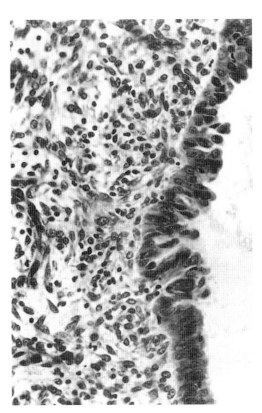

Fig. 32.50 The endometrial surface epithelium at an IUCD contact site. There is irregularity of the epithelium with nuclear enlargement, an increase in nucleocytoplasmic ratios and some loss of cellular polarity. Nuclear chromatin dispersion is, however, normal.

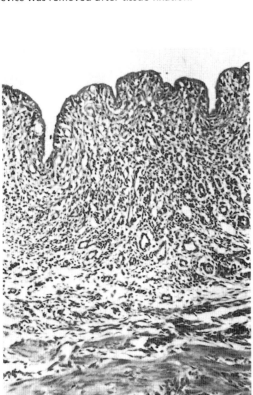

Fig. 32.51 Postinflammatory fibrosis in an endometrium from a patient wearing an inert IUCD and in whom there had been sepsis.

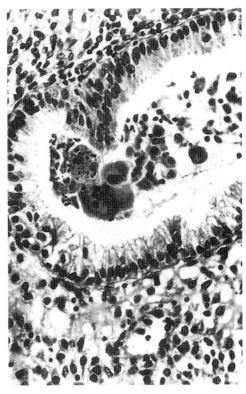

Fig. 32.52 Intraglandular giant cells in an endometrium from an IUCD wearer.

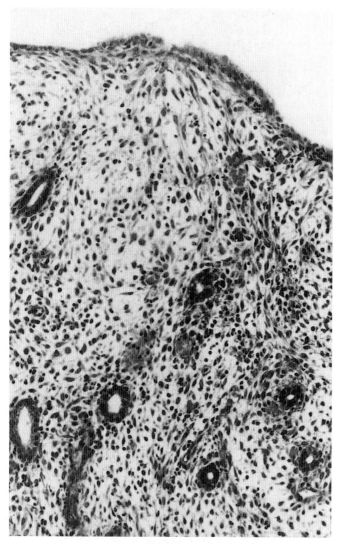

Fig. 32.53 Endometrium from a woman wearing a progestagen-impregnated intrauterine contraceptive device. The glands are narrow and inactive and the stroma is weakly pseudodecidualised and spindle-celled. (From C H Buckley & H Fox 2002 *Biopsy Pathology of the Endometrium* reproduced by permission of Edward Arnold Limited.)

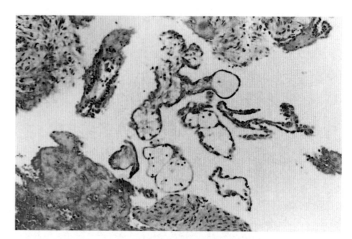

Fig. 32.54 Micropapillae which have formed on the surface of the endometrium in a progestagen-impregnated IUCD user. (From C H Buckley & H Fox 2002 *Biopsy Pathology of the Endometrium* reproduced by permission of Edward Arnold Limited.)

spread to the whole of the endometrium. The functionalis thus becomes thin and there are no cyclical changes (El-Mahgoub 1980; Silverberg et al 1986). The appearances may closely resemble those seen in systemic progestagen users (Buckley & Fox 2002). With devices delivering only a small dose, the changes may remain limited to the tissue adjacent to the contact site and the stroma may remain focally pseudodecidualised (Shaw 1985). With devices delivering 20–30 μg of progestagen (Sheppard 1987) profound atrophy develops within a month of insertion of the device. Stromal calcification, microscopic polyps (Fig. 32.54) (Critchley et al 1998) and thick-walled fibrotic blood vessels, similar to those seen in endometrial polyps, may develop after several years of use (Silverberg et al 1986). Ulceration of the surface epithelium is less common with progestagen-impregnated

devices than with either inert or copper-covered devices (Sheppard & Bonnar 1985).

Between the contact sites, particularly of inert and large devices, there is oedema (Fig. 32.55) and vascular congestion whilst at the contact sites there is vascular blanching (Shaw 1985). Both beneath and adjacent to the device there are microvascular defects with endothelial damage. Particularly in some women who experience menorrhagia whilst wearing an IUCD, there are degenerative changes in the spiral arteries with dilatation of the lumena, particularly in the stratum spongiosum (Pan et al 1994). With progestagen-impregnated devices vascular damage also occurs but there is a reduction in the vascularity of the tissues commensurate with the reduction in bleeding experienced by these women (Shaw et al 1979b; Shaw et al 1981). Oestrogen and progesterone receptors are decreased in proportion to the amount of copper in the device (de Castro et al 1986). However, as copper concentration becomes lower towards the end of the first year, the endometrium, more consistently, shows secretory changes indicating a return of steroid receptors. With devices having a surface area of 375 mm², and hence delivering a larger concentration of copper, however, the endometrium remains shallow.

Sometimes, the glands immediately deep to the contact site have a pattern of maturation which differs slightly from that in the adjacent areas; there may be delayed maturation, premature secretory maturation or, rarely, the glands may be inactive (Buckley & Fox 2002). Even when the endometrium is of apparently normal morphology, and ovarian function is normal, there is a reduction in the binding of D9B1, a monoclonal antibody binding to a polypeptide-associated oligosaccharide epitope that is secreted by endometrial epithelium in the luteal phase (Seif et al 1989). Another feature suggesting a luteal phase-like defect in the endometrium of women wearing copper-covered devices is an increased glandular

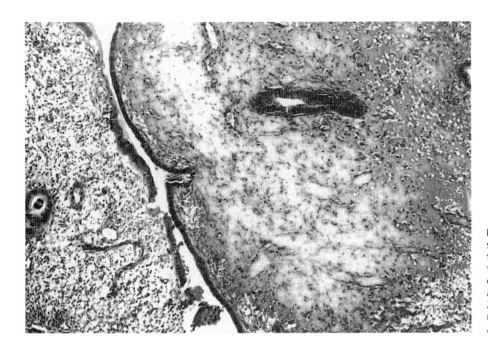

Fig. 32.55 The marked oedema, which sometimes develops in the stroma between the contact sites of an IUCD, is seen in the fragment of endometrium to the right; the endometrium on the left is of more normal appearance. (From C H Buckley & H Fox 2002 *Biopsy Pathology of the Endometrium* reproduced by permission of Edward Arnold Limited.)

epithelial height in the secretory phase, compared to that in controls (Wang et al 1995). This, it is suggested, may correlate with the menorrhagia that is sometimes experienced by these women.

Infection is less common with modern copper-covered than with earlier inert devices. When it occurs, it is associated with a widespread inflammatory cell infiltrate which may extend into the myometrium and persist after removal of the device. Extension of infection into the myometrium has led to an anecdotal report of severe postmenopausal bleeding from an arteriovenous malformation in a woman in whom an IUCD was still present (Busmanis et al 2000). Usually, when endometrial inflammation is severe, it interferes with the development or function of hormone receptors and the endometrium fails to show normal cyclical changes. It is characterised by intraglandular polymorphonuclear leucocytes and a stromal infiltrate of polymorphonuclear leucocytes, plasma cells and lymphocytes (Fig. 32.56). The plasma cells are often predominantly periglandular whilst the lymphocytes may be diffuse or form aggregates or lymphoid follicles. The irritative cytological atypia in the epithelial cells (Fig. 32.57) may be so severe that the detection of these cells in a cervical smear may give rise to a suspicion of malignancy (Gupta et al 1978a). Low-grade inflammation (Fig. 32.58) does not significantly disturb the cyclical changes.

In addition to morphological changes in the endometrium, there are, in women wearing a levonorgestrel releasing device, functional changes. These include a significant increase in granulocyte-macrophage colony stimulating factor immunoreactivity in decidualised stromal cells, glandular and stromal prolactin receptor expression and an infiltrate of CD56+, large granular lymphocytes and CD38+ macrophages (Critchley et al 1998). There is also down-regulation of

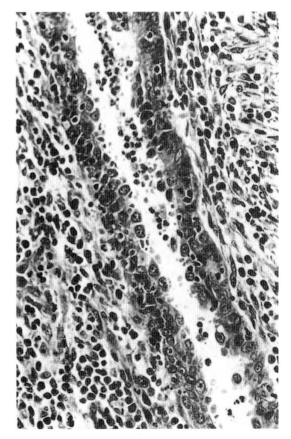

Fig. 32.56 Intrauterine infection in an inert IUCD wearer. The glands contain polymorphonuclear leucocytes and cellular debris and the stroma is infiltrated by plasma cells and lymphocytes. Note the reactive cellular atypia and the absence of hormonal changes in the epithelium.

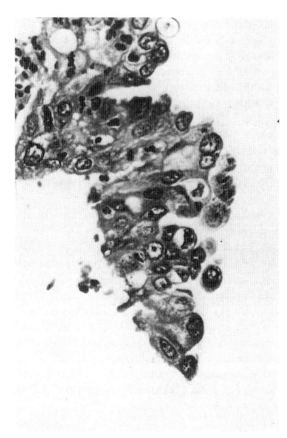

Fig. 32.57 A cluster of highly atypical endometrial epithelial cells from an IUCD wearer with endometritis. There is nuclear pleomorphism, cytoplasmic vacuolation, an increased nucleocytoplasmic ratio in many cells and a complete loss of cellular polarity.

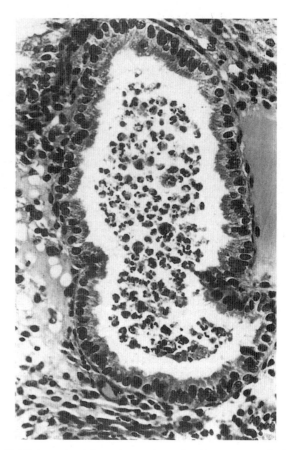

Fig. 32.58 Intraglandular polymorphonuclear leucocytes and cellular debris in an endometrium from an IUCD wearer.

oestrogen and progesterone receptors which gradually recover in the six months after removal of the device (Jones & Critchley 2000).

Uterine malignancy has developed in association with long-term use of an IUCD but no causal relationship has been demonstrated (Hsu et al 1989; Rosenblatt & Thomas 1996). On the contrary, Pike suggested in 1990 that a progestagen-containing IUCD could reduce the incidence of endometrial carcinoma and Parazzini et al (1994) and Hill et al (1997) have data which suggest that any inert or copper-covered device could have a protective effect against carcinoma.

Effects on the cervix and vagina

Non-specific, non-infectious cervicitis occurs more often in both copper-containing and progestagen-releasing IUCD wearers (Winkler & Richart 1985; Fahmy et al 1990) than in women using other forms of contraception. This is associated with cytological atypia in both the squamous and the columnar epithelium of the cervix (Gupta et al 1978a) and is more severe with copper than inert devices (Misra et al 1977). In the squamous epithelium the nuclear atypia is usually mild, but in the

columnar epithelium it may be so severe as to suggest the presence of an adenocarcinoma or adenocarcinoma in situ.

In asymptomatic, sexually active healthy women using an IUCD or steroid contraceptives, the vaginal flora is more likely to contain anaerobes than that from a barrier contraceptive user (Haukkamaa et al 1986) and IUCD wearers are more likely to develop bacterial vaginosis than are steroid contraceptive users (Roy 1991). There are no significant differences between users of copper-containing devices and progestagen-containing devices (Ulstein et al 1987).

An increased prevalence of various strains of Candida in the vagina of women, in whom there are no factors predisposing to infection, occurs in 20% of IUCD wearers compared with 6% of controls. In some the fungus is also found on the tail of the device (Parewijck et al 1988).

Actinomyces-like organisms are reported in between 14.3 and 2.8% (Nayar et al 1985; Mali et al 1986; Cleghorn & Wilkinson 1989; Chatwani et al 1994) of cervical smears depending, to some extent, on the type of device being used. The rate of colonisation, as judged by the presence of Actinomyces-like organisms in the cervical smear, and which increased with time, is reported as 14.3% for a progestagen impregnated device, 10.8% for inert devices and only 6.6% for copper-covered devices (Chatwani et al 1994). In a small series of women, some of whom had worn the device for as little as nine months, colonisation was reported to be greater in copper-covered device wearers than in levonorgestrel impregnated devices (Merki-Feld et al 2000). The majority of these women are asymptomatic. Indeed many of these organisms have neither the immunological nor cultural characteristics of Actinomyces (Gupta et al 1978b; Valicenti et al 1982) (Fig. 32.59). Proven *Actinomyces israelii* may, however, be found in women using copper covered or inert plastic devices and they tend to be more common when the device has been in place for several years (Cleghorn & Wilkinson 1989). Actinomycosis of the cervix may result in the formation of a cervical mass which may mimic a cervical carcinoma (Snowman et al 1989). In the absence of inflammation or pelvic inflammatory disease, Actinomyces can be regarded as saprophytic but in the presence of inflammation an aetiological role should be assumed and the device removed (Grimes 1981; Lippes 1999).

Coexistent Actinomyces and amoebae have been identified in the cervical smear of an IUCD wearer (Arroyo & Quinn 1989). Colonisation of the uterus by *Entamoeba gingivalis*, usually an inhabitant of the mouth (Clark & Diamond 1992), has also led to their detection in the cervical smear.

Over a period of time, material collects on the surface of IUCDs of all types and is amorphous or filamentous, eosinophilic, often partly calcified and resembles dental plaque. It is composed of a mixture of leucocytes, erythrocytes, epithelial cells, sperm and bacteria, fibrillary material, which is mainly fibrin, and amorphous acellular material consisting mainly of calcite (calcium carbonate) (Patai et al 1998), calcium phosphate (Khan & Wilkinson 1985) and magnesium phosphate (Rizk et al 1990). In patients in whom there has been heavy bleeding there is often a very thick layer of amorphous deposits. In a histological or cytological preparation it forms so-called 'pseudo-sulphur granules' (O'Brien et al 1981; O'Brien et al 1985) which may be confused with bacterial colonies (Fig. 32.60).

In women wearing copper-covered devices, immunoglobulin levels (IgG, IgA and IgM) in the serum and in the mucus on the tail of the device are significantly higher than in women using steroid contraception or no contraceptive (Eissa et al 1985). It is uncertain whether this represents a response to the bacteria that are present in these patients or is a form of foreign body response to the device.

Changes in the fatty acid composition of mid-cycle lecithin in the cervical mucus, which is similar to that detected in women with unexplained primary infertility, suggests that part of the contraceptive effect of copper IUCDs may be due to changes in the cervical mucus (Pschera et al 1988).

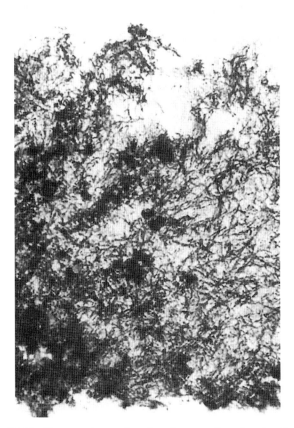

Fig. 32.59 Clusters of organisms in a tissue section showing the pseudofilamentous arrangement that may be mistaken for *Actinomyces*. Gram stain.

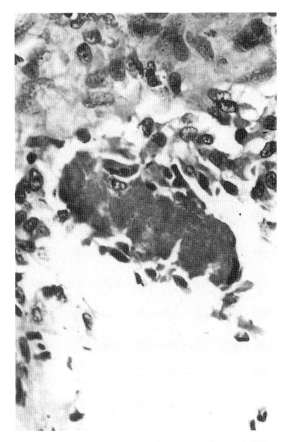

Fig. 32.60 A pseudo-sulphur granule in an endometrial biopsy from a patient wearing an inert intrauterine device.

In a comparison between IUCD users and combined steroid contraceptive users, Fiore (1986) found that mild dyskaryosis was more likely to be found in the cervical smears from IUCD users (17.6%) when compared with steroid contraceptive users (10.53%). A more recent study from New Zealand, however, showed no difference in risk between women using IUCDs, oral contraceptives and depot medroxyprogesterone acetate if confounding factors were taken into consideration (The New Zealand Contraception and Health Study Group 1994).

Effects on the Fallopian tube, ovary and pelvic organs

The incidence of pelvic inflammatory disease (PID) in IUCD wearers, that is, infection centred on the Fallopian tube and adjacent structures, varies according to the population studied and the criteria used for its diagnosis. Early reports indicated that IUCD wearers had a 1.6 to 3 times increased risk of developing PID when compared with an otherwise similar group of non-users (Flesh et al 1979; Burkman 1981). More recent reports (Lee et al 1988; Kessel 1989; Kronmal et al 1991; Odlind 1996) have questioned the interpretation of the original data and have evaluated the more modern copper-covered and progestagen-releasing devices.

Case-control studies which have been widely used to evaluate the risk of PID are vulnerable to bias even when carefully conducted (Edelman & Porter 1986a; Mumford & Kessel 1992). Firstly, most series are hospital based and as women with acute PID, who use an IUCD, are more likely to be admitted to hospital than are women with PID, who are not wearing an IUCD, the apparent risk of acute PID in IUCD wearers may appear higher than it really is. Secondly, case-control studies only provide a comparison between the two chosen groups of women so that if there is a reduced risk of PID in women forming the control group, the risk of PID in IUCD wearers will appear relatively higher though the rate of infection may actually be similar to that of the general population. Most case-control studies have not considered the contraceptive methods of their control patients (Edelman 1985) yet there is evidence that methods of contraception, other than the IUCD, in particular steroid contraceptives and barrier methods, provide some protection from PID (Keith & Berger 1985; Wolner-Hanssen et al 1985; Buchan et al 1990). Finally, whilst case-control studies almost invariably reveal an increased risk of PID in IUCD wearers, cohort studies usually reveal an increase in only certain groups of IUCD wearers (Edelman & Porter 1986a).

Undoubtedly, certain groups of IUCD wearers are at increased risk of developing PID (Daling et al 1985). There is, for example, a transient increased risk in the first few months after insertion (Mishell et al 1966; Vessey et al 1981b; Wright & Aisien 1989; Lovset 1990;

Beerthuizen 1996). The incidence then declines the longer the device remains in place (Vessey et al 1981b). Cautious interpretation of these data is required, however, as it is only in asymptomatic women that the device is left, whilst in women with PID the device has often been removed. The risk of PID is also computed to be greater for IUCD-wearing women with multiple sexual partners who would have been at risk of contracting sexually transmitted disease whether they used an IUCD or not (Burkman 1981; Cramer et al 1985; Huggins & Cullins 1990; Farley et al 1992). The Oxford Family Planning Study (Buchan et al 1990) also identified an increased risk of PID for non-medicated (inert) IUCD users (with 95% CI) of 3.3 (2.3–5.0). This compares with those wearing medicated devices where the relative risk is 1.8 (0.8–4.0) and for ex-users 1.3 (0.7–2.3). In considering these data, however, it should be remembered that inert devices are no longer inserted. Nowadays, many believe that there is little risk of infection for women in a monogamous relationship who are not at risk of sexually transmitted disease and who are parous at the time of insertion (Cramer et al 1985; Lee et al 1988; Burkman 1990; Lovset 1990).

Some of this change in opinion may be the result of the changes in the composition of IUCDs. Toivonen and colleagues (1991), for example, found that PID is less likely to develop with a device releasing 20 μg of levonorgestrel per day than with a standard copper device.

In fact, the presence of an intrauterine device of any type may compromise the sterility of the uterine cavity (Hill et al 1986). Bacteria are introduced into the uterus when the device is inserted (Mishell et al 1966) and small numbers of bacteria ascend from the vagina and cervix into the cavity of both mono- and multi-filamentous tailed device wearers (Sparks et al 1977; Sparks et al 1981). The debate as to whether the presence of a tail string is necessary for colonisation of the uterine cavity by bacteria continues. Whilst devices which are tailless, or ones in which the tail no longer lies in the endocervical canal, will be sterile in 50% of cases (Wolf & Kriegler 1986), and infection may be reduced by placing the tail of the device within the uterine cavity at the time of insertion (Akeson et al 1992), a more recent meta-analysis of 22 studies revealed no increase in pelvic inflammatory disease in those wearing a tailed device compared with those wearing a tailless device (Ebi et al 1996).

PID in IUCD users may be caused by a variety of organisms, including pneumococcus (Goldman et al 1986), but is frequently polymicrobiol with a preponderance of anaerobic organisms (Landers & Sweet 1985). PID can range from minor, asymptomatic episodes of endosalpingitis to major pelvic sepsis with tubo-ovarian abscess, which may be unilateral or bilateral (Landers & Sweet 1985), and has been reported as leading to rectal stenosis (Girardot et al 1990), local or generalised peritonitis (Brinson et al 1986), hepatic phlebitis and intrahepatic or subphrenic abscess formation. Such complications are, however, rare and reports frequently pre-date the introduction of copper-containing devices.

Tubal damage, as determined histologically, may be minimal but often, in those patients in whom pelvic infection requires surgery, it is extensive and severe. The histopathologist's view is, therefore, somewhat biased. Smith & Soderstrom (1976), for example, reported a 47% incidence of salpingitis in tubal sterilisation specimens from IUCD users, and in our own series an incidence of approximately 30% was seen. The majority of women included in these data, however, wore only inert devices and the current figures can be expected to be lower.

The endosalpingitis which occurs in IUCD wearers is histologically characteristic of infection ascending from the uterine cavity. In the acute stage there is a polymorphonuclear leucocyte infiltrate in the tubal mucosa and with more severe infection this may extend through the tube wall with the subsequent development of local peritonitis. Active chronic inflammation is characterised by the presence of an infiltrate of polymorphonuclear leucocytes, plasma cells and lymphocytes which may be limited to the mucosa or involve the deeper tissues (Fig. 32.61); there may be

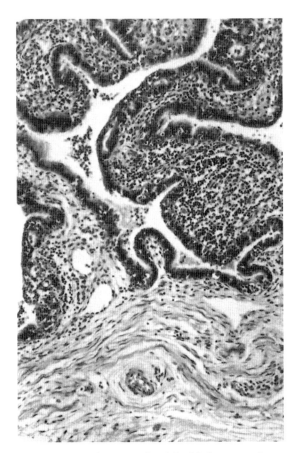

Fig. 32.61 An active chronic endosalpingitis from a patient wearing an IUCD. Inflammation is almost entirely limited to the mucosa in this example with minimal mural involvement.

collections of macrophages in the mucosal stroma. In extreme cases, there may be xanthogranulomatous endosalpingitis (Gray & Libbey 2001). More commonly, at the time of surgery, the tubes show evidence of chronic inflammation, previous inflammatory episodes or acute on chronic inflammation. There may, therefore, be active chronic endosalpingitis, hydrosalpinx follicularis, salpingitis isthmica nodosa (diverticular disease of the tube), mural scarring, local chronic peritonitis with peritoneal adhesions or a pyosalpinx lined only by non-specific granulation tissue. Inflammation may be limited to the tube but more commonly there is also evidence of inflammation of the ovary. This may take the form of an acute on chronic peri-oophoritis, an intraovarian abscess or a tubo-ovarian abscess.

Exceptionally, infection may be due to Actinomyces and there may be an endometritis, endocervicitis, salpingitis (Hansen 1989; Phupong et al 2000), ovarian abscess (Maroni & Genton 1986; de Clercq et al 1987), tubo-ovarian abscess (Schmidt et al 1980; Müller-Holzner et al 1995; Kirova et al 1997), which may be bilateral (Chang et al 1996), abdomino-pelvic abscess (O'Brien 1975; Yoonessi et al 1985: Maenpaa et al 1988; Laurent et al 1996; Atad et al 1999; Kurz et al 2000), which may extend to the bladder (Franz et al 1992), acute peritonitis (Dawson et al 1992) or an abdominal wall abscess (Adachi et al 1985). On rare occasions disseminated infection (Fisher 1980), infection in the chest wall (McBride et al 1995) or hepatic abscess has occurred secondary to the pelvic infection (Shurbaji et al 1987; Hochsztein et al 1996). Infection associated with IUCDs usually occurs in the reproductive years but it is worth noting that an actinomycotic pyometra has been reported in a woman 13 years after the menopause in whom an IUCD remained in situ (Kriplani et al 1994) and that perforation of the uterus associated with actinomycotic infection and IUCD has also been reported in a 67-year-old (Phupong et al 2000). Clinically, the firm masses created by actinomycosis may be mistaken for carcinoma, particularly in the cervix, ovaries and pelvis, and this impression is enhanced if there are intrahepatic metastatic abscesses (Antonelli & Kustrup 1999).

Inflammation, sufficient to cause structural or functional damage to the Fallopian tubes, may occur in the absence of symptoms. Asymptomatic sterile, histologically proven endosalpingitis may also be detected more often in IUCD wearers than never-wearers or former wearers during hysterectomy for non-IUCD-associated disease (Kajanoja et al 1987; Vanlancker et al 1987; Ghosh et al 1989) and is more frequent in copper-device users (Vanlancker et al 1987). At an ultrastructural level, in a small series, Wollen et al (1990) have described a reduction in tubal epithelial cilial length, less well-orientated cilia and a reduction in the proportion of cilia with a ciliary crown.

Pregnancy and the IUCD

Pregnancy may occur in an intrauterine or ectopic site in a current IUCD user and occasionally it occurs in both simultaneously (Clausen et al 1990). Between 5 and 7.8% of accidental pregnancies in IUCD wearers are ectopic compared with 0.5 to 1.3% in non-users (Dommisse 1977; Snowden et al 1977; Tatum & Schmidt 1977; WHO 1985b; Skjeldestad et al 1988).

Intrauterine pregnancy occurs in less than 1 woman per 100 wearing a copper impregnated device in the first year of use (Sivin 1985a). The risk is similar with inert and low-dose copper devices but is lower with both modern high-dose copper devices and those delivering 20 μg/day of levonorgestrel (Sivin & Schmidt 1987; Lovsett 1990; Toivonen et al 1991). The cumulative gross pregnancy rate at 5 years of use is 1.1 +/– 0.5 with levonorgestrel-releasing devices and 1.4 +/–0.4 for copper-device users (Sivin et al 1990). The reason for the lower rate with progestagen-releasing devices is that they act not only locally but that the amount of progestagen absorbed, although small, may be sufficient to impair ovarian follicular development by disturbing the pituitary–ovarian axis (Barbosa et al 1990).

Up to 50% of pregnancies that occur in IUCD wearers end in spontaneous miscarriage (Dommisse 1977) although this figure has been modified in recent years by termination of pregnancy on request. It is said that of women who conceive with an IUCD in situ up to three-quarters (n=154) will request a termination of pregnancy (Tews et al 1988) and of the patients reported to the University of Exeter, Family Planning Research Unit, in whom the outcome of the pregnancy was known, 41% were terminated and 26% miscarried spontaneously (Snowden et al 1977). There has been an anecdotal report of miscarriage associated with Candida infection in an IUCD wearer (Marelli et al 1996).

Early removal of the device can reduce the spontaneous miscarriage rate to approximately 25% (Alvior 1973), although miscarriage during removal may occur if the device lies lateral to the fetus or nearer the uterine fundus than the implantation site (Serr & Shalev 1985). A comparison of women with and without IUCDs who presented for termination of pregnancy in Tronsheim, Norway, (n=962) (Skjeldestad et al 1988) revealed that, despite removal of the device in the first trimester, women who had an IUCD in place when they became pregnant were more likely to experience a spontaneous miscarriage (15.6% compared with 7.0%, P =0.05). In the 1970s, mid-trimester miscarriage accompanied by pyrexia was frequently reported (Kim-Farley et al 1978). This seems to have been a hazard with a particular inert device and is no longer a problem. The adverse publicity associated with this was largely responsible for the withdrawal of the IUCD from the American market.

Of pregnancies going to term, in 28% of those reported to the Exeter Family Planning Research Unit (Snowden et al 1977), there is no evidence of an increased risk of fetal abnormality and the device is usually found embedded in the placenta where, if copper-covered, it elicits a minor degree of focal inflammation: occasionally, intrauterine monilial infection of the fetus and placenta have occurred (Spaun & Klunder 1986; Smith et al 1988; Michaud et al 1989). There have, however, been reports that women with an IUCD in situ have an increased risk of pre-term labour (Chaim & Mazor 1992).

There is a statistically significant negative relationship between the IUCD and complete molar pregnancies (Honoré 1986) and a reduced risk of having a spontaneous miscarriage with morphological evidence suggestive of heteroploidy (Honoré 1985). It has been suggested that the IUCD may selectively inhibit chromosomally abnormal conceptuses.

The reason that some women with an IUCD become pregnant whilst others do not has lead to speculation as to the reason but few data are available. It is known, however, that in women who become pregnant the percentage of CD3+ mature T lymphocytes is fewer in the cells adherent to the device than in non-pregnant women. CD4+ cells are increased and CD8+ cells are decreased. This raises the possibility that immunological factors may play a part. The percentage of B lymphocytes is similar in pregnant and non-pregnant IUCD wearers (Randic et al 1990).

Ectopic pregnancy

It is generally reported that the proportion of ectopic pregnancies occurring in the Fallopian tube and ovary is greater in IUCD wearers than in women using other forms of contraception (Paavonen et al 1985). This view is not, however, universally held. A statistically insignificant number also occur in other sites (Muzsnai et al 1980; Goldman et al 1988).

The WHO (WHO 1985b) multinational case-control study describes an increased relative risk of ectopic pregnancy of 6.4 for IUCD wearers compared with pregnant non-users matched for parity and marital status. Edelman & Porter (1986b), on the other hand, analysing published data reached the conclusion that there is no increased risk of ectopic pregnancy in current and past users of the IUCD. Those reporting an increased risk, however, find that the risk is different for different types of device and the series examined by Edelman & Porter may not be comparing like with like.

The lowest rate of ectopic pregnancy is found in copper device users and the highest rate in those using low dose (2 μg/24 h) progestagen-releasing devices (WHO 1987; Sivin 1991). There is also some evidence of an increased risk of ectopic pregnancy for users of progestagen-impregnated devices delivering high doses, up to 65 μg per day (Fylling & Fagerhol 1979; Larsen et al 1981), but the risk for those using devices delivering between 20 and 30 μg of progestagen daily (Sivin 1985b) is similar to that found in wearers of copper-covered or inert devices.

Sivin (1991) analysed randomised trials of copper IUCDs and confirmed that the ectopic pregnancy rate varied, not only according to the dose of progestagen, but also inversely with the surface area of the copper on the device.

The incidence of ectopic pregnancy doubled between the 8th and 9th decades of the 20th century and there is a consensus that the increase was related to the increased incidence of tubal damage secondary to sexually transmitted disease (Sivin 1985b). This increase coincided with a time when the IUCD had been more widely used (Tuomivaara et al 1986; Thorburn et al 1987). It is important, therefore, to distinguish between an increased incidence of ectopic pregnancy in the population as a whole and that which might be attributable to the use of the IUCD. Evaluation of the role of the IUCD in the increased reporting of ectopic gestation is complex, although multivariate analysis (Makinen et al 1989) indicates that it plays an aetiological role.

Tubal damage is a potent and well-recognised cause of tubal ectopic pregnancy and this may be a factor in the development of ectopic pregnancy in IUCD wearers. This presupposes, however, that conception regularly occurs in IUCD users, that there is sufficient tubal damage in IUCD users to account for the increased incidence of tubal ectopic pregnancy and that it is the tubal damage, together with the greater protection against intrauterine compared with extrauterine pregnancy afforded to IUCD wearers, which determines the tubal implantation site. This is not, however, supported by the evidence.

Firstly, in women wearing the newer, high-dose copper and progestagen releasing IUCDs, monitoring of hCG in the latter part of the menstrual cycle indicates that covert pregnancies do not routinely occur (Segal et al 1985; Wilcox et al 1987; Sivin 1989). Indeed recovery of ova flushed from the Fallopian tubes also shows that conception rates are lower than would be expected in normally ovulating women having unprotected coitus (Alvarez et al 1988). It may be, however, that in the past, frequent conception did play an important part in the development of ectopic pregnancies because, in women wearing an inert IUCD, conception occurs in about 20% of cycles (Videla-Rivero et al 1987) and in those wearing the older copper-containing devices in up to 50% of cycles (Capitanio et al 1978).

Secondly, the ratio of ovarian to all ectopic pregnancies in IUCD wearers lies between 1:10 and 1:13 compared with 1:78 to 1:111 in a group of non-IUCD wearers (Herbertsson et al 1987; Sandvei et al 1987) and it seems unlikely that tubal damage alone would cause this.

Thirdly, it is only in women who are at risk of developing sexually transmitted PID that the tubes are likely to

be damaged and they constitute a small proportion of wearers (see above).

The single most important clinical correlate remains the history of PID which increases the risk of subsequent ectopic pregnancy in both pregnant and non-pregnant controls (2.8 and 2.0 relative risk, respectively) and the risk may be increased with multiple episodes of PID (Herbertsson et al 1987). It may be that the reported incidence of ectopic gestation in IUCD wearers represents simply a combination of an increased risk, in certain users, of tubal damage secondary to PID, the device's somewhat reduced efficiency in preventing tubal implantation and its inefficiency in preventing ovarian implantation. It remains a fact that current IUCD wearers have a lower rate of ectopic pregnancy than women not using any form of contraception (Rossing et al 1993).

Systemic effects

Systemic effects are much less common in women wearing IUCDs than they are in women using steroid contraceptives.

Menstrual blood loss tends to be increased in women wearing a copper-covered IUCD (Christiaens et al 1981) and this may be sufficient to require removal of the device. Rarely does haemorrhage, in the presence of an IUCD, reach life-threatening proportions (Glew & Singh 1989) but it is, on average, increased by about 50% compared with non-users (Odlind 1996). In contrast, amenorrhoea, scanty regular or scanty infrequent menstrual loss occurs with the levonorgestrel releasing intrauterine system (Luukkainen & Toivonen 1995; Ronnerdag & Odlind 1999) and the irregular intermenstrual spotting which may also occur with progestagen containing devices may also be grounds for removal (Sivin 1985a; Scholten et al 1987; Sivin et al 1990). Whilst prolonged menstrual bleeding may lead to depletion of body iron stores, the scanty menstrual loss resulting from most progestagen-releasing devices enhances the body's iron stores (Haukkamaa et al 1985; Andrade & Pizarro-Orchard 1987; Luukkainen et al 1987; Faundes et al 1988; Ronnerdag & Odlind 1999). This advantageous effect does not, however, apply to devices delivering only 2 μg levonorgestrel which are less effective in reducing bleeding (WHO 1987).

There is no evidence that copper absorbed from the device results in increased serum copper levels even after 12 months of continuous use (Arowojolu et al 1989), although there has been a report of interstitial nephritis which resolved when a copper-containing IUCD was removed (Hocher et al 1992).

Effects on fertility

In the absence of significant PID, removal of the device, in asymptomatic women, is accompanied by the return of normal fertility, as measured by the pregnancy rate, and this is independent of the type of device (Rioux et al 1986). The relative risk of primary tubal infertility in nulligravid women who have ever used an IUCD lies between 2.0 and 2.6 times that in women who have never used one (Cramer et al 1985; Daling et al 1985). In an examination of the results following the use of inert devices, the risk was greater for those using the Dalkon Shield (6.8 to 3.3) and lower for Lippes loop and Saf-T-coil (3.2 to 2.9). The smallest risk is for those using copper-covered devices (1.9 to 1.6) and if they have used only a copper-covered device it is 1.3. These latter figures are the ones that are applicable nowadays to women using only medicated devices.

In the short term, there is no significant difference in the pregnancy rate in previous IUCD wearers and non-wearers although IUCD wearers have a higher rate of miscarriage (Bernoux et al 2000). Within 3 months of removal, in women wishing to conceive, Randic et al (1985) found that 55.9% of women became pregnant and, in longer-term follow-up, 86% (Tadesse 1996) to 94.3% (Randic et al 1985) conceived. In India, Gupta et al (1989) reported a pregnancy rate of 96.7% in the 18 months following the removal of an IUCD. Recent work by Doll et al (2001), however, has demonstrated that the duration of use affects pregnancy rates. Whilst nulliparous women using an IUCD for less than 42 months have a better pregnancy rate (39%) than those stopping steroid contraceptives (32%), those who wear an IUCD for more than 78 months have the greatest impairment of fertility. Only 28% delivered a child at 12 months compared with 46% in those wearing a device for less than 42 months. The corresponding figures at 36 months are 79% and 91%, respectively. The timing of the insertion and the type of IUCD, however, do not appear to affect fertility. Pregnancy rates are similar even for the progestagen impregnated devices delivering 20 μg of levonorgestrel and which are associated with a marked degree of endometrial atrophy (Andersson et al 1992). Older age at removal is, however, associated with a reduced conception rate which is probably a consequence of the natural decline in fertility with age.

REFERENCES

Abramovici H, Faktor J H, Bornstein J, Sorokin Y 1987 The 'forgotten' intrauterine device. Fertility and Sterility 47: 519–521

Adachi A, Kleiner G J, Bezahler G H, Greston W M, Friedland G H 1985 Abdominal wall actinomycosis with an IUD. A case report. Journal of Reproductive Medicine 30: 145–148

Adoni A, Ben Chetrit A 1991 The management of intrauterine devices following uterine perforation. Contraception 43: 77–81

Agorastos T, Bontis J, Vakiani A, Vavilis D, Constantinidis T 1997 Treatment of endometrial hyperplasias with gonadotropin-releasing hormone agonists: pathological, clinical, morphometric, and DNA-cytometric data. Gynecologic Oncology 65: 102–114

AinMelk Y 1996 Comparison of two combined estrogen and progestogen regimens in postmenopausal women: a randomized trial. Fertility and Sterility 66: 962–968

Akeson M, Solheim F, Thorbert G, Akerlund M 1992 Genital tract infections associated with the intrauterine contraceptive device can be reduced by inserting the threads into the uterine cavity. British Journal of Obstetrics and Gynaecology 99: 676–679

Al-Azzawi F, Wahab M, Habiba M, Akkad A, Mason T 1999 Continuous combined hormone replacement therapy compared with tibolone. Obstetrics and Gynecology 93: 258–264

Alfa M J, Sisler J J, Hardin G K 1995 Mycobacterium abscessus infection of a Norplant contraceptive implant site. Canadian Medical Association Journal 153: 1293–1296

Alpert L I 1976 Veno-occlusive disease of the liver associated with oral contraceptives: case report and review of the literature. Human Pathology 7: 709–718

Alvarez F, Brache V, Fernandez E et al 1988 New insights on the mode of action of intrauterine contraceptive devices in women. Fertility and Sterility 49: 768–773

Alvior G T Jr 1973 Pregnancy outcome with removal of intrauterine device. Obstetrics and Gynecology 41: 894–896

Anderson B, Watring W G, Edinger D D Jr, Small E C, Netland A T, Safaii H 1979 Development of DES-associated clear-cell carcinoma: the importance of regular screening. Obstetrics and Gynecology 53: 293–299

Anderson D G 1972 The possible mechanisms of action of progestins on endometrial adenocarcinoma. American Journal of Obstetrics and Gynecology 113: 195–211

Andersson K, Batar I, Rybo G 1992 Return to fertility after removal of a levonorgestrel-releasing intrauterine device and Nova-T. Contraception 46: 575–584

Andrade A T, Pizarro-Orchard E 1987 Quantitative studies on menstrual blood loss in IUD users. Contraception 36: 129–144

Andrew W C 1979 Oral contraception. Clinics in Obstetrics and Gynaecology 6: 3–26

Antonelli D, Kustrup J F Jr 1999 Large bowel obstruction due to intrauterine device: associated pelvic inflammatory disease. The American Surgeon 65: 1165–1166

Antonioli D A, Rosen S, Burke L, Donahue V 1979 Glandular dysplasia in diethylstilbestrol-associated vaginal adenosis. A case report and review of the literature. American Journal of Clinical Pathology 71: 715–721

Antonioli D A, Burke L, Friedman E A 1980 Natural history of diethylstilbestrol-associated genital tract lesions: cervical ectopy and cervicovaginal hood. American Journal of Obstetrics and Gynecology 137: 847–853

Antunes C M F, Strolley P D, Rosenshein N B et al 1979 Endometrial cancer and estrogen use. Report of a large case-control study. New England Journal of Medicine 300: 9–13

Arowojolu A O, Otolorin E O, Ladipo O A 1989 Serum copper levels in users of multiload intrauterine contraceptive devices. African Journal of Medical Science 18: 295–299

Arroyo G, Quinn J A Jr 1989 Association of amoebae and actinomyces in an intrauterine contraceptive device user. Acta Cytologica 33: 298–300

Arul G S, Dolan G, Rance C H, Singh S J, Sommers J 1998 Coeliac axis thrombosis associated with the combined oral contraceptive pill: a rare cause of an acute abdomen. Pediatric Surgery International 13: 285–287

Atad J, Hallak M, Sharon A, Kitzes R, Kelner Y, Abramovici H 1999 Pelvic actinomycosis. Is long-term antibiotic therapy necessary? Journal of Reproductive Medicine 44: 939–944

Badrawi H H, van Os W A, Edelman D A, Rhemrev P E 1988 Effects of intrauterine devices on the surface ultrastructure of human endometrium before and after removal. Advances in Contraception 4: 295–305

Baggish M S, Woodruff J D 1967 The occurrence of squamous epithelium in the endometrium. Obstetrical and Gynecological Survey 22: 69–115

Barakat R R, Wong G, Curtin J P, Vlamis V, Hoskins W J 1994 Tamoxifen use in breast cancer patients who subsequently develop corpus cancer is not associated with a higher incidence of adverse histologic features. Gynecologic Oncology 55: 164–168

Barbieri R L 1997 Reduction in the size of a uterine leiomyoma following discontinuation of an estrogen-progestin contraceptive. Gynecologic and Obstetric Investigation 43: 276–277

Barbieri R L, Ferracci A I, Droesch J N, Rochelson B L 1993 Ovarian torsion in a premenopausal woman treated with tamoxifen for breast cancer. Fertility and Sterility 59: 459–460

Barbosa I, Bakos O, Olsson S E, Odlind V, Johansson E D 1990 Ovarian function during use of a levonorgestrel-releasing IUD. Contraception 42: 51–66

Bardi M, Arnoldi E, Pizzocchero G, Pezzica E, Mattioni D, Perotti M 1994 Endometrioid carcinoma in pelvic endometriosis in a post-menopausal woman with tamoxifen adjuvant therapy for breast cancer: a case report. European Journal of Gynaecological Oncology 15: 393–395

Bardsley V, Cooper P, Peat D S 1998 Massive lymphocytic infiltration of uterine leiomyomas associated with GnRH agonist treatment. Histopathology 33: 80–82

Bar-Hava I, Orvieto R, Vardimon D et al 1997 Ovarian cysts and cyclic hormone replacement therapy: is there an association? Acta Obstetricia et Gynecologica Scandinavica 76: 563–566

Barnet B, Joffe A 1991 Hepatic vein thrombosis in a teenager: a case report. Journal of Adolescent Health 12: 60–62

Bauersachs R, Kuhl H, Lindhoff-Last E, Ehrly A M 1996 [Risk of thrombosis with oral contraceptives: value of thrombophilia screening test] Thromboserisiko bei oralen Kontrazeptiva: Stellenwert eines Thrombophilie-Screenings. Vasa 25: 209–220

Baum J K, Bookstein J J, Holtz F, Klein E W 1973 Possible association between benign hepatomas and oral contraceptives. Lancet 2: 926–929

Becker W J 1997 Migraine and oral contraceptives. Canadian Journal of Neurological Sciences 24: 16–21

Beer T W, Buchanan R, Buckley C H 1995 Uterine stromal sarcoma following tamoxifen treatment. Journal of Clinical Pathology 48: 596

Beerthuizen R J 1996 Pelvic inflammatory disease in intrauterine device users. European Journal of Contraception and Reproductive Health Care 1: 237–243

Beerthuizen R, van-Beek A, Massai R, Makarainen L, Hout J, Bennink H C 2000 Bone mineral density during long-term use of the progestagen contraceptive implant Implanon compared to a non-hormonal method of contraception. Human Reproduction 15: 118–122

Beral V 1977 Royal College of General Practitioners Oral Contraception Study. Mortality among oral-contraceptive users. Lancet ii: 727–731

Berger G S, Talwar P P 1978 Oral contraceptive potencies and side effects. Obstetrics and Gynecology 51: 545–547

Bergman L, Beelen M L R, Gallee M P, Hollema H, Benraadt J, van Leeuwen F E 2000 Risk and prognosis of endometrial cancer after tamoxifen for breast cancer. Comprehensive Cancer Centres' ALERT Group. Assessment of Liver and Endometrial cancer Risk following Tamoxifen. Lancet 356: 881–887

Bernoux A, Job-Spira N, Germain E, Coste J, Bouyer J 2000 Fertility outcome after ectopic pregnancy and use of an intrauterine device at the time of the index ectopic pregnancy. Human Reproduction 15: 1173–1177

Bese T, Kösebay D, Demirkiran F, Arvas M, Bese N, Mandel N 1996 Ultrasonographic appearance of endometrium in postmenopausal breast cancer patients receiving tamoxifen. European Journal of Obstetrics, Gynecology and Reproductive Biology 67: 157–162

Bianchi S, Fedele L, Vignali M, Galbiati E, Cherubini R, Ortolani S 1995 Effects on bone mineral density of 12-month goserelin treatment in over 40-year-old women with uterine myomas. Calcified Tissue International 57: 78–80

Birkhauser M 1994 Hormone replacement therapy and estrogen-dependent cancers. International Journal of Fertility and Menopausal Studies 39 (Suppl 2): 99–114

Bjornerem A, Tollan A 1997 Intrauterine device–primary and secondary perforation of the urinary bladder. Acta Obstetricia et Gynecologica Scandinavica 76: 383–385

Blaauwhof P C, Goldstuck N D 1988 Intrauterine breakage of a Multiload Cu250 intrauterine device: report of a case. Advances in Contraception 4: 217–220

Blythe J G, Ali Z 1979 Endometrial adenocarcinoma: in estrogen, oral contraceptive and non-hormone users. Gynecologic Oncology 7: 199–205

Boccardo F, Bruzzi P, Rubagotti A, Nicolo G U, Rosso R 1981 Estrogen-like action of tamoxifen on vaginal epithelium of breast cancer patients. Oncology 30: 281–285

Bocklage T, Lee K R, Belinson J L 1992 Uterine müllerian adenosarcoma following adenomyoma in a woman on tamoxifen therapy. Gynecologic Oncology 44: 104–109

Boerrigter P J, van de Weijer P H, Baak J P, Fox H, Haspels A A, Kenemans P 1996 Endometrial response in estrogen replacement therapy quarterly combined with a progestogen. Maturitas 24: 63–71

Bonney W A Jr, Glasser S R, Clewe T H, Noyes R W, Cooper C L 1966 Endometrial response to the intrauterine device. American Journal of Obstetrics and Gynecology 96: 101–113

Böttiger L E, Boman G, Eklund G, Westerholm B 1980 Oral contraceptives and thromboembolic disease: effects of lowering oestrogen content. Lancet 1: 1097–1101

Boyce J G, Lu T, Nelson J H Jr, Fruchter R G 1977 Oral contraceptives and cervical carcinoma. American Journal of Obstetrics and Gynecology 128: 761–766

Brady M S, Coit D G 1990 Focal nodular hyperplasia of the liver. Surgery, Gynecology and Obstetrics 171: 377–381

Brinson R R, Kolts B E, Monif G R 1986 Spontaneous bacterial peritonitis associated with an intrauterine device. Journal of Clinical Gastroenterology 8: 82–84

Brinton L A, Hoover R N 1993 Estrogen replacement therapy and endometrial cancer risk: unresolved issues. Obstetrics and Gynecology 81: 265–271

Brinton L A, Vessey M P, Flavel R, Yeates D 1981 Risk factors for benign breast disease. American Journal of Epidemiology 113: 203–214

Brinton L A, Reeves W C, Brenes M M et al 1990 Oral contraceptive use and risk of invasive cervical cancer. International Journal of Epidemiology 19: 4–11

Brooke-Wavell K, Prelevic G M, Bartram C, Ginsburg J 2000 The influence of physical activity on the response of bone mineral density to 5 years tibolone. Maturitas 35: 229–235

Browning J J, Bigrigg M A 1988 Recovery of the intrauterine contraceptive device from the sigmoid colon. Three case reports. British Journal of Obstetrics and Gynaecology 95: 530–532

Buchan H, Villard-Mackintosh L, Vessey M, Yeates D, McPherson K 1990 Epidemiology of pelvic inflammatory disease in parous women with special reference to intrauterine device use. British Journal of Obstetrics and Gynaecology 97: 780–788

Buckley C H, Fox H 2002 Biopsy pathology of the endometrium, 2nd edn. Edward Arnold, London

Buckley C H, Lewis G J 1982 Focal nodular hyperplasia of the liver presenting as a postpartum abdominal mass. Journal of Obstetrics and Gynaecology 2: 173–174

Buckley C H, Butler E B, Donnai P, Fouracres M, Fox H, Stanbridge C M 1982 A fatal case of DES-associated clear cell adenocarcinoma of the vagina. Journal of Obstetrics and Gynaecology 3: 126–127

Burkhonov K B, Bozorov A Sh 1993 Vykhozhdenie vnutrimatochnoi spirali cherez matochnuiu trubu. [The expulsion of an intrauterine coil via the fallopian tube]. Vestnik Khirurgii Imeni I I Grekova 150: 126

Burkman R T 1990 Modern trends in contraception. Obstetrics and Gynecology Clinics of North America 17: 759–774

Burkman R T 1997 The estrogen component of OCs: cardiovascular benefits and risks. International Journal of Fertility and Womens Medicine Suppl 1: 145–157

Burkman R T and the Women's Health Study 1981 Association between intrauterine device and pelvic inflammatory disease. Obstetrics and Gynecology 57: 269–276

Busmanis I, Ong C L, Tan A C 2000 Uterine haemorrhage in a menopausal female–associated with an arteriovenous malformation and myometritis. Pathology 32: 220–222

Bye P 1982 Failure with the new triphasic oral contraceptive Logynon. British Medical Journal 284: 422–423

Cameron S T, Critchley H O D, Buckley C H, Chard T, Kelly R W, Baird D T 1996a The effects of post-ovulatory administration of onapristone on the development of a secretory endometrium. Human Reproduction 11: 40–49

Cameron S T, Critchley H O D, Thong K J, Buckley C H, Williams A R, Baird D T 1996b Effects of daily low dose mifepristone on endometrial maturation and proliferation. Human Reproduction 11: 2518–2526

Cameron S T, Critchley H O D, Buckley C H, Kelly R W, Baird D T 1997 Effect of two antiprogestins (mifepristone and onapristone) on endometrial factors of potential importance for implantation. Fertility and Sterility 67: 1046–1053

Capitanio G L, Conte N, Ragni N, Rossato P, Pedretti E 1978 Demonstration of human chorionic gonadotropin during the second half of the menstrual cycle in plasma of regularly menstruating women users of copper IUDs. Acta Europaea Fertilitatis 9: 11–19

Carr J A, Schoon P A, Look K Y 1996 An atypical recurrence of endometrial carcinoma following estrogen replacement therapy. Gynecologic Oncology 60: 498–499

Carter E R, Faucher G L, Greenblatt R B 1964 Evaluation of a new progestational agent, 6, 17alpha-dimethyl-6-dehydro-progesterone. American Journal of Obstetrics and Gynecology 89: 635–641

Casagrande J T, Louie E W, Pike M C, Roy S, Ross R K, Henderson B E 1979 'Incessant ovulation' and ovarian cancer. Lancet 2: 170–173

Caspi B, Rabinerson D, Appelman Z, Kaplan B 1996 Penetration of the bladder by a perforating intrauterine contraceptive device: a sonographic diagnosis. Ultrasound in Obstetrics and Gynecology 7: 458–460

Cates W Jr, Ory H W, Rochat R W, Tyler C W Jr 1976 The intrauterine device and deaths from spontaneous abortion. New England Journal of Medicine 295: 1155–1159

Chaim W, Mazor M 1992 Pregnancy with an intrauterine device in situ and preterm delivery. Archives of Gynecology and Obstetrics 252: 21–24

Chang B C, Lee H S, Liou S M, Liu J Y, Lee W H 1996 Bilateral tubo-ovarian actinomycosis in the presence of an intrauterine device: a case report. Chung Hua I Hsueh Tsa Chih (Taipei) (Chinese Medical Journal) 57: 228–231

Chatwani A, Amin-Hanjani S 1994 Incidence of actinomycosis associated with intrauterine devices. Journal of Reproductive Medicine 39: 585–587

Chen C P, Hsu T C, Wang W 1998 Ileal penetration by a Multiload-Cu 375 intrauterine contraceptive device. A case report with review of the literature. Contraception 58: 295–304

Chew S B, Carmalt H, Gillett D 1996 Leiomyosarcoma of the uterus in a woman on adjuvant tamoxifen therapy. Breast 5: 429–431

Chi I 1993 The safety and efficacy issues of progestin-only contraceptives – an epidemiological perspective. Contraception 47: 1–21

Chi I C, Wilkens L, Rogers S 1985 Expulsions in immediate postpartum insertions of Lippes Loop D and Copper T IUDs and their counterpart Delta devices – an epidemiological analysis. Contraception 32: 119–134

Chi I C, Wilkens L R, Robinson N, Dominik R 1989 Cervical laceration at IUD insertion – incidence and risk factors. Contraception 39: 507–518

Chiappa A, Zbar A, Audisio R, Di-Palo S, Bertani E, Staudacher C 1999 Ruptured hepatic adenoma in liver adenomatosis: a case report of emergency surgical management. Hepatogastroenterology 46: 1942–1943

Chilvers C E 1996 Depot medroxyprogesterone acetate and breast cancer. A review of current knowledge. Drug Safety 15: 212–218

Chilvers C E D, Deacon J M 1990 Oral contraceptives and breast cancer. British Journal of Cancer 61: 1–4

Christensen J T, Boldsen J, Westergaard J G 1997 Ovarian volume in gynecologically healthy young women using no contraception or using IUD or oral contraception. Acta Obstetricia et Gynecologica Scandinavica 76: 784–789

Christiaens G C M L, Sixma J J, Haspels A A 1981 Haemostasis in menstrual endometrium in the presence of an intrauterine device. British Journal of Obstetrics and Gynaecology 88: 825–837

Christian C D 1974 Maternal deaths associated with an intrauterine device. American Journal of Obstetrics and Gynecology 119: 441–444

Christopherson W M, Mays E T 1979 Relation of steroids to liver oncogenesis. In: Lupis W, Johanessen J (eds) Liver carcinogenesis. Hemisphere Publishing Corporation, Washington, p 207

Clark C G, Diamond L S 1992 Colonization of the uterus by the oral protozoan Entamoeba gingivalis. American Journal of Tropical Medicine and Hygiene 46: 158–160

Clark D A, Wang S, Rogers P, Vince G, Affandi B 1996 Endometrial lymphomyeloid cells in abnormal uterine bleeding due to levonorgestrel (Norplant). Human Reproduction 11: 1438–1444

Clausen I, Borium K G, Frost L 1990 Heterotopic pregnancy. The first case with an IUD in situ. Zentralblatt für Gynäkologie 112: 45–47

Cleghorn A G, Wilkinson R G 1989 The IUCD-associated incidence of Actinomyces israelii in the female genital tract. Australian and New Zealand Journal of Obstetrics and Gynaecology 29: 445–449

Clement P B, Young R H 1987 Atypical polypoid adenomyoma of the uterus associated with Turner's syndrome. A report of three cases, including a review of estrogen-associated neoplasms and neoplasms associated with Turner's syndrome. International Journal of Gynecological Pathology 6: 104–113

Clement P B, Oliva E, Young R H 1996 Müllerian adenosarcoma of the uterine corpus associated with tamoxifen therapy: a report of six cases and a review of tamoxifen-associated endometrial lesions. International Journal of Gynecological Pathology 15: 222–229

Cohen C J, Deppe G 1977 Endometrial carcinoma and oral contraceptive agents. Obstetrics and Gynecology 49: 390–392

Cohen I, Rosen D J D, Shapira J et al 1993 Endometrial changes in postmenopausal women treated with tamoxifen for breast cancer. British Journal of Obstetrics and Gynaecology 100: 567–570

Cohen I, Altaras M M, Lew S, Tepper R, Beyth Y, Ben-Baruch G 1994a Ovarian endometrioid carcinoma and endometriosis developing in a postmenopausal breast cancer patient during tamoxifen therapy: a case report and review of the literature. Gynecologic Oncology 55; 443–447

Cohen I, Rosen D J D, Shapira J et al 1994b Endometrial changes with tamoxifen: comparison between tamoxifen-treated and nontreated asymptomatic, postmenopausal breast cancer patients. Gynecologic Oncology 52: 185–190

Cohen I, Rosen D J D, Altaras M, Beyth Y, Shapira J, Yigael D 1994c Tamoxifen treatment in premenopausal breast cancer patients may be associated with ovarian overstimulation, cystic formation and fibroid overgrowth. British Journal of Cancer 69: 620–621

Cohen I, Beyth Y, Tepper R et al 1995 Adenomyosis in postmenopausal breast cancer patients treated with tamoxifen — a new entity. Gynecologic Oncology 58: 86–91

Cohen I, Beyth Y, Tepper R et al 1996a Ovarian tumors in postmenopausal breast cancer patients treated with tamoxifen. Gynecologic Oncology 60: 54–58

Cohen I, Figer A, Altaras M M et al 1996b Common endometrial decidual reaction in postmenopausal breast cancer patients treated with tamoxifen and progestogens. International Journal of Gynecological Pathology 15: 17–22

Cohen I, Bernheim J, Azaria R, Tepper R, Sharony R, Beyth Y 1999a Malignant endometrial polyps in postmenopausal breast cancer tamoxifen-treated patients. Gynecologic Oncology 75: 136–141

Cohen I, Figer A, Tepper R et al 1999b Ovarian overstimulation and cystic formation in premenopausal tamoxifen exposure: comparison between tamoxifen-treated and nontreated breast cancer patients. Gynecologic Oncology 72: 202–207

Coker A L, McCann M F, Hulka B S, Walton L A 1992 Oral contraceptive use and cervical intraepithelial neoplasia. Journal of Clinical Epidemiology 45: 1111–1118

Collaborative Group on Hormonal Factors in Breast Cancer 1996 Breast cancer and hormonal contraceptives: collaborative reanalysis of individual data on 53 297 women with breast cancer and 100 239 women without breast cancer from 54 epidemiological studies. Lancet 347: 1713–1727

Collaborative Group for the Study of Stroke in Young Women 1973 Oral contraception and increased risk of cerebral ischemia or thrombosis. New England Journal of Medicine 288: 871–878

Coney P, DelConte A 1999 The effects on ovarian activity of a monophasic oral contraceptive with 100 microg levonorgestrel and 20 microg ethinyl estradiol. American Journal of Obstetrics and Gynecology 181: 53–58

Contostavlos D L 1973 Benign hepatomas and oral contraceptives. Lancet 2: 1200

Cook C L, Schroeder J A, Yussman M A, Sanfilippo J S 1984 Induction of luteal phase defect with clomiphene citrate. American Journal of Obstetrics and Gynecology 149: 613–616

Cooper C, Hannaford P, Croft P, Kat C R 1993 Oral contraceptive pill use and fractures in women: a prospective study. Bone 14: 41–45

Coté R J, Urmacher C 1990 Rhabdomyosarcoma of the liver associated with long-term oral contraceptive use. Possible role of estrogens in the genesis of embryologically distinct liver tumors. American Journal of Surgical Pathology 14: 784–790

Cottingham J, Hunter D 1992 Chlamydia trachomatis and oral contraceptive use: a quantitative review. Genitourinary Medicine 68: 209–216

Craig J M 1975 The pathology of birth control. Archives of Pathology 99: 233–236

Cramer D W, Hutchison G B, Welch W R, Scully R E, Knapp R C 1982 Factors affecting the association of oral contraceptives and ovarian cancer. New England Journal of Medicine 307: 1047–1051

Cramer D W, Schiff I, Schoenbaum S C et al 1985 Tubal infertility and the intrauterine contraceptive device. New England Journal of Medicine 312: 941–947

Critchley H O D, Buckley C H, Anderson D C 1990 Experience with a 'physiological' steroid replacement regimen for the establishment of a receptive endometrium in women with premature ovarian failure. British Journal of Obstetrics and Gynaecology 97: 804–810

Critchley H O D, Wang H, Jones R L et al 1998 Morphological and functional features of endometrial decidualization following long-term intrauterine levonorgestrel delivery. Human Reproduction 13: 1218–1224

Croft P, Hannaford P C 1989 Risk factors for acute myocardial infarction in women: evidence from the Royal College of General Practitioners' oral contraception study. British Medical Journal 298: 165–168

Crosignani P G, Vegetti W, Bianchedi D 1997 Hormonal contraception and ovarian pathology. European Journal of Contraception and Reproductive Health Care 2: 207–211

Crow J, Gardner R L, McSweeney G, Shaw R W 1995 Morphological changes in uterine leiomyomas treated by GnRH agonist goserelin. International Journal of Gynecological Pathology 14: 235–242

Croxatto H B, Kovacs L, Massai R et al 1998 Effects of long-term low-dose mifepristone on reproductive function in women. Human Reproduction 13: 793–798

Cumming G P, Bramwell S P, Lees D A 1997 An unusual case of cystolithiasis: a urological lesson for gynaecologists. British Journal of Obstetrics and Gynaecology 104: 117–118

Cundy T, Evans M, Roberts H, Wattie D, Ames R, Reid I R 1991 Bone density in women receiving depot medroxyprogesterone acetate for contraception. British Medical Journal 303: 13–16

Cushing K L, Weiss N S, Voigt L F, McKnight B, Beresford S A 1998 Risk of endometrial cancer in relation to use of low-dose, unopposed estrogens. Obstetrics and Gynecology 91: 35–39

Custo G, Saitto C, Cerza S, Cosmi E V 1986 Intrauterine rupture of the intrauterine device 'ML Cu 250': an uncommon complication: presentation of a case. Fertility and Sterility 45: 130–131

Cuzick J, Singer A, De Stavola B L, Chomet J 1990 Case-control study of risk factors for cervical intraepithelial neoplasia in young women. European Journal of Cancer 26: 684–690

Daling J R, Weiss N S, Metch B J, Chow W H, Soderstrom R M, Moore D E 1985 Primary tubal infertility in relation to the use of an intrauterine device. New England Journal of Medicine 312: 937–941

Dallenbach-Hellweg G 1980a Morphological changes induced in the human uterus and Fallopian tube by exogenous estrogens. In: Dallenbach-Hellweg G (ed) Functional morphologic changes in the female sex organs induced by exogenous hormones. Springer-Verlag, Berlin, pp 39–44

Dallenbach-Hellweg G 1980b Morphological changes induced by exogenous gestagens in normal human endometrium. In: Dallenbach-Hellweg G (ed) Functional morphologic changes in the female sex organs induced by exogenous hormones. Springer-Verlag, Berlin, pp 95–100

Dallenbach-Hellweg G 1981 Histopathology of the endometrium, 3rd edn. Springer-Verlag, Berlin, pp 126–256

Dallenbach-Hellweg G 1988 The endometrium in natural and artificial luteal phases. Human Reproduction 3: 165–168

Davis H J 1972 Intrauterine contraceptive devices: present status and future prospects. American Journal of Obstetrics and Gynecology 114: 134–151

Dawson J M, O'Riordan B, Chopra S 1992 Ovarian actinomycosis presenting as acute peritonitis. Australian and New Zealand Journal of Surgery 62: 161–163

de Castro A, Gonzalez-Gancedo P, Contreras F, Lapena G 1986 The effect of copper ions in vivo on specific hormonal endometrial receptors. Advances in Contraception 2: 399–404

DeCherney A H, Cholst I, Naftolin F 1981 Structure and function of the fallopian tubes following exposure to diethylstilbestrol (DES) during gestation. Fertility and Sterility 36: 741–745

de Clercq A G, Bogaerts J, Thiery M, Claeys G 1987 Ovarian actinomycosis during first-trimester pregnancy. Advances in Contraception 3: 167–171

Delgado-Rodriguez M, Sillero-Arenas M, Martin-Moreno J M, Galvez-Vargas R 1992 Oral contraceptives and cancer of the cervix uteri. A meta-analysis. Acta Obstetricia et Gynecologica Scandinavica 71: 368–376

DeMars L R, Van-Le L, Huang I, Fowler W C 1995 Primary non-clear cell adenocarcinoma of the vagina in older DES-exposed women. Gynecologic Oncology 58: 389–392

De Muylder X, Neven P, De Somer M, Van Belle Y, Vanderick G, De Muylder E 1991 Endometrial lesions in patients undergoing tamoxifen therapy. International Journal of Gynaecology and Obstetrics 36: 127–130

Diab K M, Zaki M M 2000 Contraception in diabetic women: comparative metabolic study of Norplant, depot medroxyprogesterone acetate, low dose oral contraceptive pill and CuT380A. Journal of Obstetrics and Gynaecology Research 26: 17–26

Dietrick D D, Issa M M, Kabalin J N, Bassett J B 1992 Intravesical migration of intrauterine device. Journal of Urology 147: 132–134

Dockerty M B, Smith R A, Symmonds R E 1959 Pseudomalignant endometrial changes induced by administration of new synthetic progestins. Proceedings of the Mayo Clinic 34: 321–328

Doll H, Vessey M, Painter R 2001 Return of fertility in nulliparous women after discontinuation of the intrauterine device: comparison with women discontinuing other methods of contraception. British Journal of Obstetrics and Gynaecology 108: 304–314

Dommisse J 1977 Intra-uterine contraceptive devices. South African Medical Journal 52: 495–496

Donath J, Nishino Y, Schulz T, Michna H 2000 The antiovulatory potential of progesterone antagonists correlates with a down-regulation of progesterone receptors in the hypothalamus, pituitary and ovaries. Anatomischer Anzeiger (Jena) 182: 143–150

Douketis J D, Ginsberg J S, Holbrook A, Crowther M, Duku E K, Burrows R F 1997 A re-evaluation of the risk for venous thromboembolism with the use of oral contraceptives and hormone replacement therapy. Archives of Internal Medicine 157: 1522–1530

Early Breast Cancer Triallists' Collaborative Group 1988 Effects of adjuvant tamoxifen and of cytotoxic therapy on mortality in early breast cancer: an overview of 61 randomized trials among 28,896 women. New England Journal of Medicine 319: 1681–1692

Early Breast Cancer Triallists' Collaborative Group 1992 Systemic treatment of early breast cancer by hormonal, cytotoxic or immune therapy. 133 randomized trials involving 31,000 recurrences and 24,000 deaths among 75,000 women. Lancet 339: 1–15

Early Breast Cancer Triallists' Collaborative Group 1998 Tamoxifen for early breast cancer: an overview of the randomised trials. Lancet 351: 1451–1467

Ebeling K, Nischan P, Schwindler C 1987 Use of contraceptives and risk of invasive cervical cancer in previously screened women. International Journal of Cancer 39: 427–430

Ebi K L, Piziali R L, Rosenberg M, Wachob H F 1996 Evidence against tailstrings increasing the rate of pelvic inflammatory disease among IUD users. Contraception 53: 25–32

Ecker J A, McKittrick J E, Failing R M 1966 Thrombosis of the hepatic veins. 'The Budd-Chiari syndrome' — a possible link between oral contraceptives and thrombosis formation. American Journal of Gastroenterology 45: 429–443

Eddy G L, Mazur M T 1997 Endolymphatic stromal myosis associated with tamoxifen use. Gynecologic Oncology 64: 262–264

Edelman D A 1985 Selection of appropriate comparison groups to evaluate PID risk in IUD users. In: Zatuchni G I, Goldsmith A, Sciarra J J (eds) Intrauterine contraception. Advances and future prospects. Harper & Row, Philadelphia, pp 412–419

Edelman D A, Van Os W A 1990 Duration of use of copper releasing IUDs and the incidence of copper wire breakage. European Journal of Obstetrics, Gynecology and Reproductive Biology 34: 267–272

Edelman D A, Porter C W Jr 1986a Pelvic inflammatory disease and the IUD. Advances in Contraception 2: 313–325

Edelman D A, Porter C W Jr 1986b The intrauterine device and ectopic pregnancy. Advances in Contraception 2: 55–63

Edgren R A, Sturtevant F M 1976 Potencies of oral contraceptives. American Journal of Obstetrics and Gynecology 125: 1029–1038

Editorial 1973 Liver tumours and steroid hormones. Lancet 2: 1481

Edmondson H A, Henderson B, Benton B 1976 Liver cell adenomas associated with use of oral contraceptives. New England Journal of Medicine 294: 470–472

Edwards D P, Leonhardt S A, Gass-Handel E 2000 Novel mechanisms of progesterone antagonists and progesterone receptor. Journal of the Society for Gynecologic Investigation 7(1 Suppl): s22–s24

Eells T P, Alpern H D, Grzywacz C, MacMillan R W, Olson J E 1990 The effect of tamoxifen on cervical squamous maturation in Papanicolaou stained cervical smears of post-menopausal women. Cytopathology 1: 263–268

Egberg N, van Beek A, Gunnervik C et al 1998 Effects on the hemostatic system and liver function in relation to Implanon and Norplant. A prospective randomized clinical trial. Contraception 58: 93–98

Eggena P, Hidaka H, Barrett J D, Sambhi M P 1978 Multiple forms of human plasma renin substrate. Journal of Clinical Investigation 26: 367–372

Egger H, Kindermann 1980 Effects of high estrogen doses on the endometrium. In: Dallenbach-Hellweg G (ed) Functional morphologic changes in the female sex organs induced by exogenous hormones. Springer-Verlag, Heidelberg, pp 51–53

Eissa M K, Sparks R A, Newton J R 1985 Immunoglobulin levels in the serum and cervical mucus of tailed copper IUD users. Contraception 32: 87–95

Elder M G 1982 New hormone contraceptives: injectable preparations. Journal of Obstetrics and Gynaecology 3 (suppl): s21–s24

Ellis E F, Gordon P R, Gottlieb L S 1978 Oral contraceptives and cholangiocarcinoma. Lancet 1: 207

El-Mahgoub S 1980 The Norgestrel-T IUD. Contraception 22: 271–286

Elwood J M, Boyes D A 1980 Clinical and pathological features and survival of endometrial cancer patients in relation to prior use of estrogens. Gynecologic Oncology 10: 173–187

Engelke C, Bittscheidt H, Poley F 1995 Mesenterialvenenthrombose mit hamorrhagischem Dunndarminfarkt als Komplikation oraler Contraeptiva. (Mesenteric vein thrombosis with haemorrhagic infarct of the small intestine as a complication of oral contraceptives). Chirurgie 66: 634–637

Ermini M, Carpino F, Petrozza V, Benagiano G 1989 Distribution and effect on the endometrium of progesterone released from a progestasert device. Human Reproduction 4: 221–228

Ernst E 1992 Oral contraceptives, fibrinogen and cardiovascular risk. Atherosclerosis 93: 1–5

Ezra Y, Simon A, Sherman Y, Benshushan A, Younis J S, Laufer N 1994 The effect of progesterone administration in the follicular phase of an artificial cycle on endometrial morphology: a model of premature luteinization. Fertility and Sterility 62: 108–112

Fahmy K, Ismail H, Sammour M, el Tawil A, Ibrahim M 1990 Cervical pathology with intrauterine contraceptive devices – a cyto-colpo-pathological study. Contraception 41: 317–322

Farley T M, Rosenberg M J, Rowe P J, Chen J H, Meirik O 1992 Intrauterine devices and pelvic inflammatory disease: an international perspective. Special Programme of Research, Development, and Research Training in Human Reproduction, World Health Organization. Lancet 339: 785–788

Fathalla M F 1972 Factors in the causation and incidence of ovarian cancer. Obstetrical and Gynecological Survey 27: 751–768

Faundes A, Alvarez F, Brache V, Tejada A S 1988 The role of the levonorgestrel intrauterine device in the prevention and treatment of iron deficiency anemia during fertility regulation. International Journal of Gynaecology and Obstetrics 26: 429–433

Fay R A 1982 Failure with the new triphasic oral contraceptive Logynon. British Medical Journal 284: 17–18

Fechner R E 1968 Atypical leiomyomas and synthetic progestin therapy. American Journal of Clinical Pathology 49: 697–703

Fechner R E 1977 Benign hepatic lesions and orally administered contraceptives. A report of seven cases and a critical analysis of the literature. Human Pathology 8: 255–268

Fedele L, Bianchi S, Zanconato G, Portuese A, Raffaelli R 2001 Use of levonorgestrel-releasing intrauterine device in the treatment of rectovaginal endometriosis. Fertility and Sterility 75: 485–488

Ferenczy A 1980 Morphological effects of exogenous gestagens on abnormal human endometrium. In: Dallenbach-Hellweg G (ed), Functional morphologic changes in the female sex organs induced by exogenous hormones. Springer-Verlag, Heidelberg, pp 101–110

Ferrazzi E, Cartei G, Mattarazzo R, Fiorentino M 1977 Oestrogen-like effect of tamoxifen on vaginal epithelium. British Medical Journal 1(6072): 1351–1352

Fiel M I, Min A, Gerber M A, Faire B, Schwartz M, Thung S N 1996 Hepatocellular carcinoma in long-term oral contraceptive use. Liver 16: 372–376

Fiore N 1986 Epidemiological data, cytology and colposcopy in IUD (intrauterine device), E-P (estro-progestogens) and diaphragm users. Study of cytological changes of endometrium IUD related. Clinical and Experimental Obstetrics and Gynecology 13: 34–42

Fisher B, Costantino J P, Redmond C et al 1989 A randomised clinical trial evaluating tamoxifen in the treatment of patients with node negative breast cancer who have oestrogen-receptor-positive tumors. New England Journal of Medicine 320: 479–484

Fisher B, Costantino J P, Redmond C K, Fisher E R, Wickerham D L, Cronin W M 1994 Endometrial cancer in tamoxifen-treated breast cancer patients: findings from the National Surgical Adjuvant Breast and Bowel Project (NSABP) B-14. Journal of the National Cancer Institute 86: 527–537

Fisher B, Costantino J P, Wickerham D L et al 1998 Tamoxifen for prevention of breast cancer: report of the National Surgical Adjuvant Breast and Bowel Project P-1 study. Journal of the National Cancer Institute 90: 1371–1388

Fisher M S 1980 'Miliary' actinomycosis. Journal of the Canadian Radiology Association 31: 149–150

Flesh G, Weiner J M, Corlett R C, Boice C, Mishell D R Jr, Wolf R M 1979 The intrauterine contraceptive device and acute salpingitis: a multifactor analysis. American Journal of Obstetrics and Gynecology 135: 402–408

Foreman H, Stadel B V, Schlesselman S 1981 Intrauterine device usage and fetal loss. Obstetrics and Gynecology 58: 669–677

Fornander T, Rutqvist L E, Cedermark B et al 1989 Adjuvant tamoxifen in early breast cancer: occurrence of new primary cancers. Lancet 1 (8630): 117–120

Fowler W C Jr, Schmidt G, Edelman D A, Kaufman D G, Fenoglio C M 1981 Risks of cervical intraepithelial neoplasia among DES-exposed women. Obstetrics and Gynecology 58: 720–724

Fox H, Buckley C H 1982 The endometrial hyperplasias and their relationship to neoplasia. Histopathology 6: 493–510

Fox H, Buckley C H 1983 Atlas of gynaecological pathology, vol 5 of Current histopathology. MTP Press, Lancaster

Franz H B, Strohmaier W L, Geppert M, Wechsel H 1992 Infiltrierender Tuboovarialabszess bei IUP-assoziierter Aktinomykose. Geburtshilfe und Frauenheilkunde 52: 496–498

Fraser J L, Millenson M, Malynn E R, Uhl L, Kruskall M S 1996 Possible association between the Norplant contraceptive system and thrombotic thrombocytopenic purpura. Obstetrics and Gynecology 87: 860–863

Furr B J A, Jordan V C 1984 The pharmacology and clinical uses of tamoxifen. Pharmacology and Therapeutics 25: 127–205

Fylling P 1987 Clinical performance of Copper T 200, Multiload 250 and Nova-T: a comparative multicentre study. Contraception 35: 439–446

Fylling P, Fagerhol M 1979 Experience with two different medicated intrauterine devices: a comparative study of the Progestasert and Nova T. Fertility and Sterility 31: 138–141

Gambacciani M, Ciaponi M 2000 Postmenopausal osteoporosis management. Current Opinion in Obstetrics and Gynecology 12: 189–197

Gardner F J, Konje J C, Abrams K R et al 2000 Endometrial protection from Tamoxifen-stimulated changes by a levonorgestrel-releasing intrauterine system: a randomised controlled trial. Lancet 356: 1711–1717

Gbolade B, Ellis S, Murby B, Randall S, Kirkman R 1998 Bone density in long term users of depot medroxyprogesterone acetate. British Journal of Obstetrics and Gynaecology 105: 790–794

Ghosh K, Gupta I, Gupta S K 1989 Asymptomatic salpingitis in intrauterine contraceptive device users. Asia-Oceania Journal of Obstetrics and Gynaecology 15: 37–40

Ghosh T K, Cera P J 1983 Transition of benign vaginal adenosis to clear cell carcinoma. Obstetrics and Gynecology 61: 126–130

Gillett D 1995 Leiomyosarcoma of the uterus in a woman taking adjuvant tamoxifen therapy. Medical Journal of Australia 163: 160–161

Ginsburg J, Prelevic G M 1996 Cause of vaginal bleeding in postmenopausal women taking tibolone. Maturitas 24: 107–110

Girardot C, Legman P, Le Goff J Y 1990 La stenose rectale. Une complication rare des salpingites chroniques sur dispositifs intra-uterins. Journal de Radiologie 71: 23–26

Glew S, Singh A 1989 Uterine bleeding with an IUD requiring emergency hysterectomy. Advances in Contraception 5: 51–53

Godsland I F, Crook D, Wynn V 1991 Coronary heart disease risk markers in users of low-dose oral contraceptives. Journal of Reproductive Medicine 36(3 Suppl): 226–237

Goldman G A, Dicker D, Ovadia J 1988 Primary abdominal pregnancy: can artificial abortion, endometriosis and IUD be etiological factors. European Journal of Obstetrics, Gynecology and Reproductive Biology 27: 139–143

Goldman J A, Yeshaya A, Peleg D, Dekel A, Dicker D 1986 Severe pneumococcal peritonitis complicating IUD: case report and review of the literature. Obstetrics and Gynecology 41: 672–674

Goldstuck N D 1987 Insertion forces with intrauterine devices: implications for uterine perforation. European Journal of Obstetrics, Gynecology and Reproductive Biology 25: 315–323

Gorsline J C, Osborne N G 1985 Management of the missing intrauterine contraceptive device: report of a case. American Journal of Obstetrics and Gynecology 153: 228–229

Gould J, Deam S, Dolan G 1998 Prothrombin 20210A polymorphism and third generation oral contraceptives — a case report of coeliac axis thrombosis and splenic infarct (Letter). Thrombosis and Haemostasis 79: 1214–1215

Govan A D T, Black W P, Sharp J L 1969 Aberrant glandular polypi of the uterine cervix associated with contraceptive pills: pathology and pathogenesis. Journal of Clinical Pathology 22: 84–89

Graff-Iversen S, Tverdal A, Stensvold I 1996 Cardiovascular risk factors in Norwegian women using contraceptives: results from a cardiovascular health screening 1985–1988 Contraception 53: 337–344

Gram I T, Macaluso M, Stalsberg H 1992 Oral contraceptive use and the incidence of cervical intraepithelial neoplasia. American Journal of Obstetrics and Gynecology 167: 40–44

Granberg S, Ylostalo P, Wikland M, Karlsson B 1997 Endometrial sonographic and histologic findings in women with and without hormonal replacement therapy suffering from postmenopausal bleeding. Maturitas 27: 35–40

Gray Y, Libbey N P 2001 Xanthogranulomatous salpingitis and oophoritis: a case report and review of the literature. Archives of Pathology and Laboratory Medicine 125: 260–263

Greeley C, Schroeder S, Silverberg S G 1995 Microglandular hyperplasia of the cervix: a true 'pill' lesion? International Journal of Gynecological Pathology 14: 50–54

Grimes D A 1981 Nongonococcal pelvic inflammatory disease. Clinical Obstetrics and Gynecology 24: 1227–1243

Grimes D A 1991 Neoplastic effects of oral contraceptives. International Journal of Fertility 36 Suppl 1: 19–24

Grimes D A, Schulz K F 2000 Antibiotic prophylaxis for intrauterine contraceptive device insertion. Cochrane Database Systematic Reviews 2000: CD001327

Gruber A, Rabinerson D, Kaplan B, Pardo J, Neri A 1996 The missing forgotten intrauterine contraceptive device. Contraception 54: 117–119

Gunning J E, Moyer D 1967 The effect of medroxyprogesterone acetate on endometriosis in the human female. Fertility and Sterility 18: 759–774

Gupta B K, Gupta A N, Lyall S 1989 Return of fertility in various types of IUD users. International Journal of Fertility 34: 123–125

Gupta P K, Burroughs F, Luff R D, Frost J K, Erozan Y S 1978a Epithelial atypias associated with intrauterine contraceptive devices (IUD). Acta Cytologica 22: 286–291

Gupta P K, Erozan Y S, Frost J K 1978b Actinomycetes and the IUD: an update. Acta Cytologica 22: 281–282

Guzick D S, Zeleznik A 1990 Efficacy of clomiphene citrate in the treatment of luteal phase deficiency: quantity versus quality of preovulatory follicles. Fertility and Sterility 54: 206–210

Habiba M A, Bell S C, Al-Azzawi F 1998 Endometrial responses to hormone replacement therapy: histological features compared with those of late luteal phase endometrium. Human Reproduction 13: 1674–1682

Habiba M A, Bell S C, Al-Azzawi F 1999 The effect of hormone replacement therapy on the number and the proliferation index of endometrial leukocytes. Human Reproduction 14: 3088–3094

Hadisaputra W, Affandi B, Witjaksono J, Rogers P A 1996 Endometrial biopsy collection from women receiving Norplant. Human Reproduction 11(Suppl 2): 31–34

Hajjar L R, Kim W S, Nolan G H, Turner S, Raju U R 1993 Intestinal and pelvic endometriosis presenting as a tumor and associated with tamoxifen therapy: report of a case. Obstetrics and Gynecology 82: 642–644

Hammond C B, Maxson W S 1982 Current status of estrogen therapy for the menopause. Fertility and Sterility 37: 5–25

Haney A F, Hammond C B, Soules M R, Creasman W T 1979 Diethylstilbestrol-induced upper genital tract abnormalities. Fertility and Sterility 31: 142–146

Hankinson S E, Stampfer M J 1997 Estrogens and breast cancer. Salud Publica de Mexico 39: 370–378

Hann L E, Giess C S, Bach A M, Tao Y, Baum H J, Barakat R R 1997 Endometrial thickness in tamoxifen-treated patients: correlation with clinical and pathologic findings. American Journal of Roentgenology 168: 657–661

Hannaford P C 1991 Cervical cancer and methods of contraception. Advances in Contraception 7: 317–324

Hannaford P C, Villard-Mackintosh L, Vessey M P, Kay C R 1991 Oral contraceptives and malignant melanoma. British Journal of Cancer 63: 430–433

Hansen L K 1989 Bilateral female pelvic actinomycosis. Acta Obstetricia et Gynecologica Scandinavica 68: 189–190

Harkins G J, Davis G D, Dettori J, Hibbert M L, Hoyt R A 1999 Decline in bone mineral density with stress fracture in a woman on depot medroxyprogesterone acetate. A case report. Journal of Reproductive Medicine 44: 309–312

Harlap S 1991 Oral contraceptives and breast cancer. Cause and effect? Journal of Reproductive Medicine 36: 374–395

Hart W R, Townsend D E, Aldrich J O, Henderson B E, Roy M, Benton B 1976 Histopathologic spectrum of vaginal adenosis and related changes in stilbestrol-exposed females. Cancer 37: 763–775

Harvengt C 1992 Effect of oral contraceptive use on the incidence of impaired glucose tolerance and diabetes mellitus. Diabetes/Metabolism Reviews 18: 71–77

Haukkamaa M, Allonen H, Heikkilä M et al 1985 Long-term clinical experience with Levonorgestrel-releasing IUD. In: Zatuchni G I, Goldsmith A, Sciarra J J (eds) Intrauterine contraception. Advances and future prospects. Harper & Row, Philadelphia, pp 232–237

Haukkamaa M, Stranden P, Jousimies-Somer H, Siitonen A 1986 Bacterial flora of the cervix in women using different methods of contraception. American Journal of Obstetrics and Gynecology 154: 520–524

Hawkins D F, Elder M G 1979 Human fertility control. Butterworth, London

Hays D, Edelstein J A, Ahmad M M 1986 Perforation of the sigmoid colon by an intrauterine contraceptive device. Contraception 34: 413–416

Heartwell S F, Schlesselman S 1983 Risk of uterine perforation among users of intrauterine devices. Obstetrics and Gynecology 61: 31–36

Hefnawi F, Hosni M, El-Shiekha Z, Serour G I, Hasseeb F 1975 Perforation of the uterine wall by Lippes loop in postpartum women. In: Hefnawi F, Segal S J (eds) Analysis of intrauterine contraception. North-Holland, Amsterdam, pp 469–476

Heinonen P K, Merikari M, Paavonen J 1984 Uterine perforation by copper intrauterine device. European Journal of Obstetrics, Gynecology and Reproductive Biology 17: 257–261

Hendrickson M R, Kempson R L 1980 Surgical pathology of the uterine corpus. W B Saunders, Philadelphia

Herbertsson G, Magnusson S S, Benediktsdottir K 1987 Ovarian pregnancy and IUCD use in a defined complete population. Acta Obstetricia et Gynecologica Scandinavica 66: 607–610

Herbst A L 1981a Diethylstilbestrol and other sex hormones during pregnancy. Obstetrics and Gynecology 58 (suppl): 35s–40s

Herbst A L 1981b Clear cell adenocarcinoma and the current status of DES-exposed females. Cancer 48 (suppl): 484–488

Herbst A L, Scully R E 1970 Adenocarcinoma of the vagina in adolescence: a report of 7 cases including 6 clear-cell carcinomas (so-called mesonephromas). Cancer 25: 745–757

Herbst A L, Kurman R J, Scully R E 1972 Vaginal and cervical abnormalities after exposure to stilbestrol in utero. Obstetrics and Gynecology 40: 287–298

Herbst A L, Robboy S J, Scully R E, Poskanzer D C 1974 Clear-cell adenocarcinoma of the vagina and cervix in girls: analysis of 170 reported cases. American Journal of Obstetrics and Gynecology 119: 713–724

Herbst A L, Poskanzer D C, Robboy S J, Friedlander L, Scully R E 1975 Prenatal exposure to stilbestrol: a prospective comparison of exposed female offspring with unexposed control. New England Journal of Medicine 292: 334–339

Herbst A L, Cole P, Colton T, Robboy S J, Scully R E 1977 Age-incidence and risk of diethylstilbestrol-related clear cell adenocarcinoma of the vagina and cervix. American Journal of Obstetrics and Gynecology 128: 43–50

Hermida-Perez J A, del Corral-Suarez T, Cerdeiras-Martinez G, Aguero-Gomez J L, Machado V 1997 Litiasis vesical formada a partir de un DIU (dispositivo intrauterino). Un caso raro. Archivos Espanoles de Urologia 50: 808–809

Hickey M, Lau T M, Russell P, Fraser I S, Rogers P A 1996a Microvascular density in conditions of endometrial atrophy. Human Reproduction 11: 2009–2013

Hickey M, Fraser I, Dwarte D, Graham S 1996b Endometrial vasculature in Norplant users: preliminary results from a hysteroscopic study. Human Reproduction 11 (Suppl 2): 35–44

Hickey M, Dwarte D, Fraser I S 2000 Superficial endometrial vascular fragility in Norplant users and in women with ovulatory dysfunctional uterine bleeding. Human Reproduction 15: 1509–1514

Hill D A, Weiss N S, Voigt L F, Beresford S A 1997 Endometrial cancer in relation to intra-uterine device use. International Journal of Cancer 70: 278–281

Hill J A, Talledo E, Steele J 1986 Quantitative transcervical uterine cultures in asymptomatic women using an intrauterine contraceptive device. Obstetrics and Gynecology 68: 700–704

Hillard P J 1992 Oral contraceptive noncompliance: the extent of the problem. Advances in Contraception 8(suppl): 13–20

Hirschberg A L, Bystrom B, Carlstrom K, von Schoultz B 1996 Reduced serum cholecystokinin and increase in body fat during oral contraception. Contraception 53: 109–113

Hocher B, Keller F, Krause PH, Gollnick H, Oelkers W 1992 Interstitial nephritis with reversible renal failure due to a copper-containing intrauterine contraceptive device. Nephron 61: 111–113

Hochner-Celnikier D, Anteby E, Yagel S 1995 Ovarian cysts in tamoxifen-treated premenopausal women with breast cancer — a management dilemma. American Journal of Obstetrics and Gynecology 172: 1323–1324

Hochsztein J G, Koenigsberg M, Green D A 1996 US case of the day. Actinomycotic pelvic abscess secondary to an IUD with involvement of the bladder, sigmoid colon, left ureter, liver and upper abdominal wall. Radiographics 16: 713–716

Holt V L, Daling J R, McKnight B, Moore D, Stergachis A, Weiss N S 1992 Functional ovarian cysts in relation to the use of monophasic and triphasic oral contraceptives. Obstetrics and Gynecology 79: 529–533

Honoré L H 1985 The negative effect of the IUCD on the occurrence of heteroploidy-correlated abnormalities in spontaneous abortions: an update. Contraception 31: 253–260

Honoré L H 1986 The intrauterine contraceptive device and hydatidiform mole: a negative association. Contraception 34: 213–219

Honoré L H, Koch M, Brown L B 1991 Comparison of oral contraceptive use in women with adenocarcinoma and squamous cell carcinoma of the uterine cervix. Gynecologic and Obstetric Investigation 32: 98–101

Horvath E, Kovacs K, Ross R C 1972 Ultrastructural findings in a well-differentiated hepatoma. Digestion 7: 74–82

Hourihan H M, Sheppard B L, Belsey E M, Brosens I A 1991 Endometrial vascular features prior to and following exposure to levonorgestrel. Contraception 43: 375–385

Hoyumpa A M Jr, Schiff L, Helfman E L 1971 Budd-Chiari syndrome in women taking oral contraceptives. American Journal of Medicine 50: 137–140

Hsing A W, Hoover R N, McLaughlin J K et al 1992 Oral contraceptives and primary liver cancer among young women. Cancer Causes and Control 3: 43–48

Hsu C T, Hsu M L, Hsieh T M, Lin C T, Wang T T, Lin Y N 1989 Uterine malignancy developing after long term use of IUCD additional report of 2 cases: endometrial stromal sarcoma and leiomyosarcoma. Asia-Oceania Journal of Obstetrics and Gynaecology 15: 237–243

Huggins G R, Cullins V E 1990 Fertility after contraception or abortion. Fertility and Sterility 54: 559–573

Huggins G R, Giuntoli R L 1979 Oral contraceptives and neoplasia. Fertility and Sterility 32: 1–23

Huggins G R, Zucker P K 1987 Oral contraceptives and neoplasia: 1987 update. Fertility and Sterility 47: 733–761

Hulka B S, Chambless L E, Kaufman D G, Fowler W C Jr, Greenberg B G 1982 Protection against endometrial carcinoma by combination-product oral contraceptives. Journal of the American Medical Association 247: 475–477

Ibghi W, Batt M, Bongain A et al 1995 Stenose de la veine iliaque par migration d'un dispositif intra-uterin (Iliac vein stenosis caused by intrauterine device migration) Journal de Gynecologie, Obstetrique et Biologie de la Reproduction (Paris) 24: 273–275

Inman W H W, Vessey M P, Westerholm B, Engelund A 1970 Thromboembolic disease and the steroidal content of oral contraceptives. A report to the Committee on Safety of Drugs. British Medical Journal 2: 203–209

Intaraprasert S, Taneepanichskul S, Theppisai U, Chaturachinda K 1997 Bone density in women receiving Norplants for contraception. Journal of the Medical Association of Thailand 80: 738–741

Irey N S, Manion W C, Taylor H B 1970 Vascular lesions in women taking oral contraceptives. Archives of Pathology 89: 1–8

Ishak K G 1979 Morphologic hepatic lesions associated with oral contraceptives (OC) and anabolic steroids (AS). In: Olive G (ed) Advances in pharmacology and therapeutics, vol 8. Pergamon Press, Oxford, p 185

Ishak K G, Rabin L 1975 Benign tumors of the liver. Medical Clinics of North America 59: 995–1013

Ismail S M 1994 Pathology of endometrium treated with tamoxifen. Journal of Clinical Pathology 47: 827–833

Ismail S M 1998 Endometrial changes during tamoxifen treatment. Lancet 351: 838

Ismail S M, Maulik T G 1997 Tamoxifen-associated postmenopausal endometriosis. Histopathology 30: 187–191

Janaud A, Rouffy J, Upmalis D, Dain M P 1992 A comparison study of lipid and androgen metabolism with triphasic oral contraceptive formulations containing norgestimate or levonorgestrel. Acta Obstetricia et Gynecologica Scandinavica 156(Suppl): 33–38

Jessop F A, Roberts P F 2000 Müllerian adenosarcoma of the uterus in association with tamoxifen therapy. Histopathology 36: 91–92

Jick H, Kaye J A, Vasilakis-Scaramozza C, Jick S S 2000 Risk of venous thromboembolism among users of third generation oral contraceptives compared with users of oral contraceptives with levonorgestrel before and after 1995: cohort and case-control analysis. British Medical Journal 321: 1190–1195

Jick S S, Walker A M, Jick H 1993 Oral contraceptives and endometrial cancer. Obstetrics and Gynecology 82: 931–935

Jick S S, Myers M W, Jick H 1999 Risk of idiopathic haemorrhage in women on oral contraceptives with differing progestagen components (Letter). Lancet 354: 302–303

Johnson J H 1989 Weighing the evidence on the pill and breast cancer. Family Planning Perspectives 21: 89–92

Johnson L D, Driscoll S G, Hertig A T, Cole P T, Nickerson R J 1979 Vaginal adenosis in stillborns and neonates exposed to diethylstilbestrol and steroidal estrogens and progestins. Obstetrical and Gynecological Survey 34: 845–846

Jones M W, Silverberg S G 1989 Cervical adenocarcinoma in young women: possible relationship to microglandular hyperplasia and use of oral contraceptives. Obstetrics and Gynecology 73: 984–989

Jones M W, Silverberg S G, Kurman R J 1993 Well-differentiated villoglandular adenocarcinoma of the uterine cervix: a clinicopathological study of 24 cases. International Journal of Gynecological Pathology 12: 1–7

Jones R L, Critchley H O D 2000 Morphological and functional changes in human endometrium following intrauterine levonorgestrel delivery. Human Reproduction 15(suppl 3): 162–172

Jorgensen C, Picot M C, Bologna C, Sany J 1996 Oral contraception, parity, breast feeding, and severity of rheumatoid arthritis. Annals of Rheumatic Diseases 55: 94–98

Joswig-Priewe H, Schlüster K 1980 Comparative study of vaginal cytology involving controls and patients receiving oral contraceptive agents. In: Dallenbach-Hellweg G (ed) Functional morphologic changes in female sex organs induced by exogenous hormones. Springer-Verlag, Berlin, p 199

Judd H L 1980 Menopause and postmenopause. In: Benson R C (ed) Current obstetrics and gynecologic diagnosis and treatment. Large Medical Publications, Los Altos, California, USA, pp 510–529

Kajanoja P, Lang B, Wahlstrom T 1987 Intra-uterine contraceptive devices (IUDs) in relation to uterine histology and microbiology. Acta Obstetricia et Gynecologica Scandinavica 66: 445–449

Katerndahl D A, Realini J P, Cohen P A 1992 Oral contraceptive use and cardiovascular disease: is the relationship real or due to study bias? Journal of Family Practice 35: 147–157

Kaufman D W, Shapiro S, Slone D et al 1980 Decreased risk of endometrial cancer among oral contraceptive users. New England Journal of Medicine 303: 1045–1047

Kaufman D W, Palmer J R, de Mouzon J et al 1991 Estrogen replacement therapy and the risk of breast cancer: results from the case-control surveillance study. American Journal of Epidemiology 134: 1375–1385

Kaufman R H, Binder G L, Gray P M Jr, Adam E 1977 Upper genital tract changes associated with exposure in utero to diethylstilbestrol. American Journal of Obstetrics and Gynecology 128: 51–59

Kaufman R H, Korhonen M O, Strama T, Adam E, Kaplan A 1982 Development of clear cell adenocarcinoma in DES-exposed offspring under observation. Obstetrics and Gynecology 59 (suppl): suppl 68s–72s

Kaunitz A M 1996 Depot medroxyprogesterone acetate contraception and the risk of breast and gynecologic cancer. Journal of Reproductive Medicine 41: 419–427

Kaunitz A M 1999 Long-acting hormonal contraception: assessing impact on bone density, weight, and mood. International Journal of Fertility and Women's Medicine 44: 110–117

Kauntiz A M 2000 Injectable contraception. New and existing options. Obstetric and Gynecology Clinics of North America 27: 741–780

Kay C R 1982 Progestogens and arterial disease – evidence from the Royal College of General Practitioners' Study. American Journal of Obstetrics and Gynecology 142: 762–765

Kay C R 1984 The Royal College of General Practitioners' Oral Contraception Study some recent observations. Clinics in Obstetrics and Gynaecology 11: 759–786

Kedar R P, Bourne T H, Powles T J et al 1994 Effects of tamoxifen on the uterus and ovaries of postmenopausal women in a randomised breast cancer prevention trial. Lancet 343: 1318–1321

Keith L G, Berger G S 1985 The pathogenic mechanisms of pelvic infection. In: Zatuchni G I, Goldsmith A, Sciarra J J (eds) Intrauterine contraception. Advances and future prospects. Harper & Row, Philadelphia, pp 232–237

Kelleher C C 1990 Clinical aspects of the relationship between oral contraceptives and abnormalities of the hemostatic system: relation to the development of cardiovascular disease. American Journal of Obstetrics and Gynecology 163: 392–395

Kemmeren J M, Algra A, Grobbee D E 2001 Third generation oral contraceptives and the risk of venous thrombosis: meta-analysis. British Medical Journal 323: 131–134

Kent D R, Nissen E D, Nissen S E, Chambers C 1977 Maternal death resulting from rupture of liver adenoma associated with oral contraceptives. Obstetrics and Gynecology 50 (suppl): 5s–6s

Kerlin P, Davis G L, McGill D B et al 1983 Hepatic adenoma and focal nodular hyperplasia: clinical, pathologic, and radiologic features. Gastroenterology 84: 994–1002

Kessel E 1989 Pelvic inflammatory disease with intrauterine device use: a reassessment. Fertility and Sterility 51: 1–11

Key T C, Kreutner A K 1980 Gastrointestinal complications of modern intrauterine devices. Obstetrics and Gynecology 55: 239–244

Khan S R, Wilkinson E J 1985 Scanning electron microscopy, X-ray diffraction, and electron microprobe analysis of calcific deposits on intrauterine contraceptive devices. Human Pathology 16: 732–738

Khan S R, Wilkinson E J 1990 Bladder stone in a human female: the case of an abnormally located intrauterine contraceptive device. Scanning Microscopy 4: 395–398

Khaw K T Peart W S 1982 Blood pressure and contraceptive use. British Medical Journal 285: 403–407

Kiilholma P, Makinen J, Vuori J 1989 Bladder perforation: uncommon complication with a misplaced IUD. Advances in Contraception 5: 47–49

Kiilholma P, Makinen J, Maenpaa J 1990 Perforation of the uterus following IUD insertion in the puerperium. Advances in Contraception 6: 57–61

Killackey M A, Hakes T B, Pierce V K 1985 Endometrial adenocarcinoma in breast cancer patients receiving antiestrogens. Cancer Treatment Reviews 69: 237–238

Kim-Farley R J, Cates W Jr, Ory H W, Hatcher R A 1978 Febrile spontaneous abortion and the IUD. Contraception 18: 561–570

Kinch R, Lough J 1978 Focal nodular hyperplasia of the liver and oral contraceptives. American Journal of Obstetrics and Gynecology 132: 717–727

Kirova Y M, Feuilhade F, Belda-Lefrere M A, Le Bourgeois J P 1997 Intrauterine device-associated pelvic actinomycosis: a rare disease mimicking advanced ovarian cancer: a case report. European Journal of Gynaecological Oncology 18: 502–503

Kirwan J F, Tsaloumas M D, Vinall H, Prior P, Kritzinger E E, Dodson P M 1997 Sex hormone preparations and retinal vein occlusion. Eye 11: 53–56

Klatskin G 1977 Hepatic tumors: possible relationship to use of oral contraceptives. Gastroenterology 73: 386–394

Knopp R H 1990 Effects of sex steroid hormones on lipoprotein levels in pre- and post menopausal women. Canadian Journal of Cardiology 6 Suppl B: 31B–35B

Knowles D M, Wolff M 1976 Focal nodular hyperplasia of the liver. Human Pathology 7: 533–545

Koib B A, Paulson R J 1997 The luteal phase of cycles utilizing controlled ovarian hyperstimulation and the possible impact of this hyperstimulation on embryo implantation. American Journal of Obstetrics and Gynecology 176: 1262–1267 (discussion 1267–1269)

Kremer J, de Bruijn H W A, Hindriks F R 1980 Serum high density lipoprotein cholesterol levels in women using a contraceptive injection of depot-medroxy-progesterone acetate. Contraception 22: 359–367

Kriplani A, Buckshee K, Relan S, Kapila K 1994 'Forgotten' intrauterine device leading to actinomycotic pyometra — 13 years after menopause. European Journal of Obstetrics, Gynecology and Reproductive Biology 53: 215–216

Kronmal R A, Whitney C W, Mumford S D 1991 The intrauterine device and pelvic inflammatory disease: the Women's Health Study reanalysed. Journal of Clinical Epidemiology 44: 109–122

Kurman R J, Scully R E 1974 The incidence and histogenesis of vaginal adenosis. An autopsy study. Human Pathology 5: 265–276

Kurz R, Amon K, Laqua D, Fischbach F, Buck J, Heinkelein J 2000 [Actinomycosis of the pelvis with an indwelling IUD] Aktinomykose des Beckens bei liegendem IUP. Zeitschrift für Gastroenterologie 38: 375–379

Kyriakos M, Kempson R L, Konikov N F 1968 A clinical and pathologic study of endocervical lesions associated with oral contraceptives. Cancer 22: 99–110

Laforga J B, Aranda F I 1999 Uterine leiomyomas with T-cell infiltration associated with GnRH agonist goserelin. Histopathology 33: 80–82

Lahti E, Blanco G, Kauppila A, Apaja-Sarkkinen M, Taskinen P J, Laatikainen T 1993 Endometrial changes in postmenopausal breast cancer patients receiving tamoxifen. Obstetrics and Gynecology 81: 660–664

Lahti E, Vuopala S, Kauppila A, Kauppila A J, Apaja-Sarkkinen M A, Laatikainen T J 1994 Maturation of vaginal and endometrial epithelium in postmenopausal breast cancer patients receiving long-term tamoxifen. Gynecologic Oncology 55: 410–414

Landers D V, Sweet R L 1985 Current trends in the diagnosis and treatment of tuboovarian abscess. American Journal of Obstetrics and Gynecology 151: 1098–1110

Laragh J H 1976 Oral contraceptives — induced hypertension — nine years later. American Journal of Obstetrics and Gynecology 126: 141–147

Larsen S, Hansen M K, Jacobsen J C, Ladehoff P, Sorensen T, Westergaard J G 1981 Comparison between two IUDs: Progestasert and CuT 200. Contraception Delivery Systems 2: 281–286

Lashner B A, Kane S V, Hanauer S B 1989 Lack of association between oral contraceptive use and Crohn's disease: a community-based matched case-control study. Gastroenterology 97: 1442–1447

Lashner B A, Kane S V, Hanauer S B 1990 Lack of association between oral contraceptive use and ulcerative colitis. Gastroenterology 99: 1032–1036

Laurent T, de Grandi P, Schnyder P 1996 Abdominal actinomycosis associated with intrauterine device: CT features. European Radiology 6: 670–673

La Vecchia C 1992 Sex hormones and cardiovascular risk. Human Reproduction 7: 162–167

La Vecchia C, Negri E, D'Avanzo B, Parazzini F, Gentile A, Franceschi S 1992 Oral contraceptives and non-contraceptive oestrogens in the risk of gallstone disease requiring surgery. Journal of Epidemiology and Community Health 46: 234–236

La Vecchia C, Tavani A, Franceschi S, Parazinni F 1996 Oral contraceptives and cancer: a review of the evidence. Drug Safety 14: 260–272

Leaf D A, Bland D, Schaad D, Neighbor W E, Scott C S 1991 Oral contraceptive use and coronary risk factors in women. American Journal of the Medical Sciences 301: 365–368

Leborgne J, Lehur P A, Horeau J M et al 1990 Problemes therapeutiques lies aux ruptures de volumineux adenomes hepatiques de siege central. A propos de 3 observations. Chirurgie 116: 454–460

Lee N C, Rubin G L, Borucki R 1988 The intrauterine device and pelvic inflammatory disease revisited: new results from the Women's Health Study. Obstetrics and Gynecology 72: 1–6

Lewis M A, MacRae K D, Kuhl-Habichi D, Bruppacher R, Heinemann L A, Thorogood M 1996a Transnational Research Group on Oral Contraceptives and the Health of Young Women. Third generation oral contraceptives and risk of myocardial infarction: an international case-control study. British Medical Journal 312: 88–90

Lewis M A, Heinemann L A, MacCrae K D, Bruppacher R, Spitzer W O 1996b The increased risk of venous thromboembolism and the use of third generation progestagens: role of bias in observational research. The Transnational Research Group on Oral Contraceptives and the Health of Young Women. Contraception 54: 5–13

Lewis M A, Spitzer W O, Heinemann L A, MacRae K D, Bruppacher R, Spitzer W O 1999 The differential risk of oral contraceptives: the impact of full exposure history. Human Reproduction 14: 1493–1499

Lindahl B, Andolf E, Ingvar C, Liedman R, Ranstam J, Willen R 1997 Endometrial thickness and ovarian cysts as measured by ultrasound in asymptomatic postmenopausal breast cancer patients on various adjuvant treatments including tamoxifen. Anticancer Research 17: 3821–3824

Lindgren R, Risberg B, Hammar M, Berg G 1995 Transdermal hormonal replacement therapy with transdermal progestin every second month. Maturitas 22: 25–30

Lippes J 1999 Pelvic actinomycosis: a review and preliminary look at prevalence. American Journal of Obstetrics and Gynecology 180: 265–269

LiVolsi V A, Stadel B V, Kelsey J L, Holford T R, White C 1978 Fibrocystic breast disease in oral contraceptive users. A histopathological evaluation of epithelial atypia. New England Journal of Medicine 299: 381–385

Logan R F, Kay C R 1989 Oral contraception, smoking and inflammatory bowel disease — findings in the Royal College of General Practitioners' Oral Contraception Study. International Journal of Epidemiology 18: 105–107

London R S 1992 The new era in oral contraception: pills containing gestodene, norgestimate and desogestrel. Obstetrical and Gynecological Survey 47: 777–782

Lovset T 1990 A comparative evaluation of the Multiload 250 and Multiload 375 intra-uterine devices. Acta Obstetricia et Gynecologica Scandinavica 69: 521–526

Lund E, Meirik O, Adami H O, Bergstrom R, Christoffersen T, Bergsjo P 1989 Oral contraceptive use and premenopausal breast cancer in Sweden and Norway: possible effects of different pattern of use. International Journal of Epidemiology 18: 527–532

Luukkainen T, Toivonen J 1995 Levonorgestrel-releasing IUD as a method of contraception with therapeutic properties. Contraception 52: 269–276

Luukkainen T, Allonen H, Haukkamaa M et al 1987 Effective contraception with the levonorgestrel-releasing intrauterine device: 12-month report of a European multicenter study. Contraception 36: 169–179

McBride W J, Hill D R, Gordon D L 1995 Chest wall actinomycosis in association with the use of an intra-uterine device. Australian and New Zealand Journal of Surgery 65: 141–143

McCarty K S Jr, Barton T K, Peete C H Jr, Creasman W T 1978 Gonadal dysgenesis with adenocarcinoma of the endometrium: an electron microscopic and steroid receptor analyses with a review of the literature. Cancer 42: 512–520

McCluggage W G, Bharucha H 1999 Cellular leiomyoma mimicking endometrial stromal neoplasm in association with GnRH agonist goserelin. Histopathology 34: 184–186

McCluggage W G, Bailie C, Weir P, Bharucha H 1996a Endometrial stromal sarcoma arising in pelvic endometriosis in a patient receiving unopposed oestrogen therapy. British Journal of Obstetrics and Gynaecology 103: 1252–1254

McCluggage W G, Varma M, Weir P, Bharucha H 1996b Uterine leiomyosarcoma in a patient receiving tamoxifen therapy. Acta Obstetricia et Gynecologica Scandinavica 75: 593–595

McGonigle K F, Shaw S L, Vasilev S A, Odom-Maryon T, Roy S, Simpson J F 1998 Abnormalities detected on transvaginal ultrasonography in tamoxifen-treated postmenopausal women may represent cystic atrophy. American Journal of Obstetrics and Gynecology 178: 1145–1150

McGonigle K F, Vasilev S A, Odom Maryon T, Simpson J F 1999 Ovarian histopathology in breast cancer patients receiving tamoxifen. Gynecologic Oncology 73: 402–406

McGowan L, Parent L, Lednar W, Norris H J 1979 The woman at risk for developing ovarian cancer. Gynecologic Oncology 7: 325–344

Maenpaa J, Taina E, Gronroos M, Soderstrom K O, Ristmaki T, Narhinen L 1988 Abdominopelvic actinomycosis associated with intrauterine devices. Two case reports. Archives of Gynecology and Obstetrics 243: 237–241

Magriples U, Naftolin F, Schwartz P E, Carcangiu M L 1993 High grade endometrial carcinoma in tamoxifen-treated breast cancer patients. Journal of Clinical Oncology 11: 485–490

Maia H Jr, Barbosa I C, Marques D, Calmon L C, Lapido O A, Coutinho E M 1996 Hysteroscopic and transvaginal sonography in menopausal women receiving hormone replacement therapy. Journal of the American Association of Gynecologic Laparoscopists 4: 13–18

Makinen J I, Erkkola R U, Laippala P J 1989 Causes of the increase in the incidence of ectopic pregnancy. A study on 1017 patients from 1966 to 1985 in Turku, Finland. American Journal of Obstetrics and Gynecology 160: 642–646

Mali B, Joshi J V, Wagle U et al 1986 Actinomyces in cervical smears of women using intrauterine contraceptive devices. Acta Cytologica 30: 367–371

Marelli G, Mariani A, Frigerio L, Leone E, Ferrari A 1996 Fetal Candida infection associated with an intrauterine contraceptive device. European Journal of Obstetrics, Gynecology and Reproductive Biology 68: 209–212

Marin R, McMillian D 1998 Ulnar neuropathy associated with subdermal contraceptive implant. Southern Medical Journal 91: 875–878

Maroni E S, Genton C Y 1986 IUD-associated ovarian actinomycosis causing bowel obstruction. Archives of Gynecology and Obstetrics 239: 59–62

Martinelli I, Taioli E, Bucciarelli P, Akvahan S, Mannucci P M 1999 Interaction between the G20120A mutation of the prothrombin gene and oral contraceptive use in deep vein thrombosis. Arteriosclerosis, Thrombosis, and Vascular Biology 19: 700–703

Maskey C P, Rahman M, Sigdar T K, Johnsen R 1997 Vesical calculus around an intrauterine device. British Journal of Urology 79: 654–655

Mays E T, Christopherson W M, Barrows G H 1974 Focal nodular hyperplasia of the liver. Possible relationship to oral contraceptives. American Journal of Clinical Pathology 61: 735–746

Mdel D G, Fox J A, Jones R W 1975 Multiple hepatic adenomas associated with an oral contraceptive. Lancet 1: 865

Meade T W, Haines A P, North W R S, Chakrabarti R, Stirling Y, Howarth D J 1977 Haemostatic, lipid, and blood pressure profiles of women on oral contraceptives, containing 50 μg or 30 μg oestrogen. Lancet 2: 948–951

Meade T W, Greenberg G, Thompson S G 1980 Progestogens and cardiovascular reactions associated with oral contraceptives and a comparison of the safety of 50 and 30 μg oestrogen preparations. British Medical Journal 280: 1157–1161

Meirik O, Farley T M, Lund E, Adami H O, Christoffersen T, Bergsjo P 1989 Breast cancer and oral contraceptives: patterns of risk among parous and nulliparous women — further analysis of the Swedish-Norwegian material. Contraception 39: 471–475

Merki-Feld G S, Lebeda E, Hogg B, Keller P J 2000 The incidence of actinomyces-like organisms in Papanicolou-stained smears of copper- and levonorgestrel-releasing intrauterine devices. Contraception 61: 365–368

Mestwerdt W, Kranzfelder D 1980 Morphological findings in the human ovary under physiologic conditions and after contraceptive use. In: Dallenbach-Hellweg G (ed) Functional and morphologic changes in female sex organs induced by exogenous hormones. Springer- Verlag, Berlin, pp 168–179

Meunier F, Boyer L, Abergel A, Perez N, Ravel A, Lhopital F, Viallet J F 1998 Regression d'une hyperplasie nodulaire focale apres arret d'une contraception orale. Journal de Radiologie 79: 341–343

Michaud P, Lemaire B, Tescher M 1989 Avortement spontane d'une grossesse sur DIU par chorioamniotite a Candida. Revue Francaise de Gynecologie et d'Obstetrique 84: 45–46

Miller D R, Rosenberg L, Kaufman D W, Stolley P, Warshauer M E, Shapiro S 1989a Breast cancer before age 45 and oral contraceptive use: new findings. American Journal of Epidemiology 129: 269–280

Miller N, McPherson K, Jones L, Vessey M 1989b Histopathology of breast cancer in young women in relation to use of oral contraceptives. Journal of Clinical Pathology 42: 387–390

Miller N E, Thelle D S, Førde O H, Mjøs O D 1977 The Tromso heart-study. High density lipoprotein and coronary heart disease: a prospective case control study. Lancet 1: 965–968

Miranda M C, Mazur M T 1995 Endometrial squamous metaplasia. An unusual response to progestin therapy of hyperplasia. Archives of Pathology and Laboratory Medicine 119: 458–460

Mishell D R Jr 1976 Current status of oral contraceptive steroids. Clinical Obstetrics and Gynecology 19: 743–764

Mishell D R Jr 1992 Oral contraception: past, present, and future perspectives. International Journal of Fertility 37 Suppl 1: 7–18

Mishell D R Jr 1999 Cardiovascular risks: perceptions versus reality. Contraception 59 (1 Suppl): 21S–24S

Mishell D R Jr, Moyer D L 1969 Association of pelvic inflammatory disease with the intrauterine device. Clinical Obstetrics and Gynecology 12: 179–197

Mishell D R Jr, Roy S 1982 Copper intrauterine contraceptive device event rates following insertion 4 to 8 weeks post partum. Obstetrics and Gynecology 143: 29–35

Mishell D R Jr, Bell J H, Good R G, Moyer D L 1966 The intrauterine device: A bacteriologic study of the endometrial cavity. American Journal of Obstetrics and Gynecology 96: 119–126

Misra J S, Engineer A D, Tandon P 1977 Cytological studies in women using copper intrauterine devices. Acta Cytologica 21: 514–518

Mittal K, Schwartz L, Goswami S, Demopoulos R 1996 Estrogen and progesterone receptor expression in endometrial polyps. International Journal of Gynecological Pathology 15: 345–348

Mittal S, Gupta I, Lata P, Mahajan U, Gupta A N 1986 Management of translocated and incarcerated intrauterine contraceptive devices. Australian and New Zealand Journal of Obstetrics and Gynaecology 26: 232–234

Moorhead T, Hannaford P, Warskyj M 1997 Prevalence and characteristics associated with use of hormone replacement therapy in Britain. British Journal of Obstetrics and Gynaecology 104: 290–297

Moskovitz D, McCleod R S, Greenberg G R, Cohen Z 1999 Operative and environmental risk factors for recurrence of Crohn's disease. International Journal of Colorectal Disease 14: 224–226

Mourits M J E, Hollema H, Willemse P H B, De Vries E G E, Aalders J G, Van der Zee A G J 1998 Adenosarcoma of the uterus following tamoxifen treatment for breast cancer. International Journal of Gynecological Cancer 8: 168–171

Mourits M J E, de Vries E G E, Willemse P H B et al 1999 Ovarian cysts in women receiving tamoxifen for breast cancer. British Journal of Cancer 79: 1761–1764

Moyer D L, Mishell D R Jr, Bell J 1970 Reactions of human endometrium to the intrauterine device. I. Correlation of the endometrial histology with the bacterial environment of the uterus following short-term insertion of the IUD. American Journal of Obstetrics and Gynecology 106: 799–809

Moyer D L, Mishell D R Jr 1971 Reactions of human endometrium to the intrauterine foreign body. II. Long term effects on the endometrial histology and cytology. American Journal of Obstetrics and Gynecology 111: 66–80

Müller-Holzner E, Ruth N R, Abfalter E et al 1995 IUD-associated pelvic actinomycosis: a report of five cases. International Journal of Gynecological Pathology 14: 70–74

Mumford S D, Kessel E 1992 Was the Dalkon Shield a safe and effective intrauterine device? The conflict between the case-control and clinical trial study findings. Fertility and Sterility 57: 1151–1176

Murphy A A, Kettel L M, Morales A J, Roberts V, Parmley T, Yen S S 1995 Endometrial effects of long-term low-dose administration of RU486. Fertility and Sterility 63: 761–766

Murray S, Hickey J B, Houang E 1987 Significant bacteremia associated with replacement of intrauterine contraceptive device. American Journal of Obstetrics and Gynecology 156: 698–700

Muzsnai D, Hughes T, Price M, Bruksch L 1980 Primary abdominal pregnancy associated with the IUD (2 case reports). European Journal of Obstetrics, Gynecology and Reproductive Biology 10: 275–278

Nanda K, Bastian L A, Hasselblad V, Simel D L 1999 Hormone replacement therapy and the risk of colorectal cancer: a meta-analysis. Obstetrics and Gynecology 93: 880–888

Nanda S, Rathee S 1992 Three intrauterine contraceptive devices in a single uterus. Tropical Doctor 22: 33–44

Nayar M, Chandra M, Chitraratha K, Kumari-Das S, Rai-Chowdhary G 1985 Incidence of actinomycetes infection in women using intrauterine contraceptive devices. Acta Cytologica 29: 111–116

Ness R B, Keder L M, Soper D E et al 1997 Oral contraceptives and the recognition of endometritis. American Journal of Obstetrics and Gynecology 176: 580–585

Neuberger J, Portmann B, Nunnerley H B, Laws J W, Davis M, Wiliams R 1980 Oral contraceptive-associated liver tumours: occurrence of malignancy and difficulties in diagnosis. Lancet i: 273–276

Neven P, De Muylder X, Van Belle Y et al 1989 Tamoxifen and the uterus and endometrium. Lancet i: 375

Neven P, De Muylder X, Van Belle Y, Vanderick G, De Muylder E 1990 Hysteroscopic follow-up during tamoxifen treatment. European Journal of Obstetrics, Gynecology and Reproductive Biology 35: 235–238

Neven P, De Muylder X, Van Belle Y, Van Hooff I, Vanderick G 1998 Longitudinal hysteroscopic follow-up during tamoxifen treatment. Lancet 351: 36

Newhouse M L, Pearson R M, Fullerton J M, Boesen E A M, Shannon H S 1977 A case control study of carcinoma of the ovary. British Journal of Preventative and Social Medicine 31: 148–153

Noci I, Borri P, Coccia M E et al 1997 Hormonal patterns, steroid receptors and morphological pictures of endometrium in hyperstimulated IVF cycles. European Journal of Obstetrics, Gynecology and Reproductive Biology 75(2): 215–20

Nothmann B J, Chittinand S, Schuster M M 1973 Reversible mesenteric vascular occlusion associated with oral contraceptives. American Journal of Digestive Diseases 18: 361–368

O'Brien P C, Noller K L, Robboy S J et al 1979 Vaginal epithelial changes in young women enrolled in the National Comparative Diethylstilbestrol Adenosis (DESAD) Project. Obstetrics and Gynecology 53: 300–308

O'Brien P K 1975 Abdominal and endometrial actinomycosis associated with an intrauterine device. Canadian Medical Association Journal 112: 596–597

O'Brien P K, Roth-Moyo L A, Davis B A 1981 Pseudo-sulfur granules associated with intrauterine contraceptive devices. American Journal of Clinical Pathology 75: 822–825

O'Brien P K, Lea P J, Roth-Moyo L A 1985 Structure of a radiate pseudocolony associated with an intrauterine contraceptive device. Human Pathology 16: 1153–1156

Odlind V 1996 Modern intra-uterine devices. Bailliere's Clinical Obstetrics and Gynaecology 10: 55–67

Ohana E, Sheiner E, Leron E, Mazor M 2000 Appendix perforation by an intrauterine contraceptive device. European Journal of Obstetrics, Gynecology and Reproductive Biology 88: 129–131

Okada D H, Rowland J B, Petrovic L M 1999 Uterine pleomorphic rhabdomyosarcoma in a patient receiving tamoxifen therapy. Gynecologic Oncology 75: 509–513

Olson R O, Jones S 1967 The forgotten IUD as a cause of infertility. Review of world literature and report of a case. Obstetrics and Gynecology 29: 579–580

Olsson H 1989 Oral contraceptives and breast cancer. A review. Acta Oncologica 28: 849–863

Olsson H, Moller T R, Ranstam J 1989 Early oral contraceptive use and breast cancer among premenopausal women: final report from a study in southern Sweden. Journal of the National Cancer Institute 81: 1000–1004

O'Meara E S, Rossing M A, Daling J R, Elmore J G, Barlow W E, Weiss N S 2001 Hormone replacement therapy after a diagnosis of breast cancer in relation to recurrence and mortality. Journal of the National Cancer Institute 93: 754–761

Orellana-Alcalde J M, Dominguez J P 1966 Jaundice and oral contraceptives. Lancet 2: 1279–1280

Orr-Walker B J, Evans M C, Ames R W, Clearwater J M, Cundy T, Reid I R 1998 The effect of past use of the injectable contraceptive depot medroxyprogesterone acetate on bone mineral density in normal post-menopausal women. Clinical Endocrinology 49: 615–618

Ory H W, Boston Collaborative Drug Surveillance Program 1974 Functional ovarian cysts and oral contraceptives. Negative association confirmed surgically. Journal of American Medical Association 228: 68–69

Ory H W, Cole P, MacMahon B, Hoover R 1976 Oral contraceptives and reduced risk of benign breast diseases. New England Journal of Medicine 294: 419–422

Osborne J L, Bennett M J 1978 Removal of intra-abdominal intrauterine contraceptive devices. British Journal of Obstetrics and Gynaecology 85: 868–871

Ostergard D R 1981 DES-related vaginal lesions. Clinical Obstetrics and Gynecology 24: 379–394

Othman N H, Othman M S, Ismail A N, Mohammad N Z, Ismail Z 1996 Multiple polypoid endometriosis — a rare complication following withdrawal of gonadotrophin releasing hormone (GnRH) agonist for severe endometriosis: a case report. Australian and New Zealand Journal of Obstetrics and Gynaecology 36: 216–218

Otolorin E O, Ladipo O A 1985 Comparison of intramenstrual IUD insertion with insertion following menstrual regulation. Advances in Contraception 1: 45–49

Paavonen J, Varjonen-Toivonen M, Komulainen M, Heinonen P K 1985 Diagnosis and management of tubal pregnancy: effect on fertility. International Journal of Gynaecology and Obstetrics 23: 129–133

Palmer J R 1991 Oral contraceptive use and gestational choriocarcinoma. Cancer Detection and Prevention 15: 45–48

Palmer J R, Rosenberg L, Kaufman D W, Warshauer M E, Stolley P, Shapiro S 1989 Oral contraceptive use and liver cancer. American Journal of Epidemiology 130: 878–882

Pan J F, Yu Y L, Wang L J, Yan Q H 1994 The morphologic changes of endometrial spiral arterioles in IUD-induced menorrhagia. Advances in Contraception 10: 213–222

Pang L C 1998 Endometrial stromal sarcoma with sex cord-like differentiation associated with tamoxifen therapy. Southern Medical Journal 91: 592–594

Parazzini F, La Vecchia C, Moroni S 1994 Intrauterine device use and risk of endometrial cancer. British Journal of Cancer 70: 672–673

Parewijck W, Claeys G, Thiery M, van Kets H 1988 Candidiasis in women fitted with an intrauterine contraceptive device. British Journal of Obstetrics and Gynaecology 95: 408–410

Patai K, Berenyi M, Sipos M, Noszal B 1998 Characterization of calcified deposits on contraceptive intrauterine devices. Contraception 58: 305–308

Paterson M E L, Wade-Evans T, Sturdee D W, Thom M H, Studd J W W 1980 Endometrial disease after treatment with oestrogens and progestogens in the climacteric. British Medical Journal 1: 822–824

Paul C, Skegg D C, Spears G F 1989 Depot medroxyprogesterone (Depo-Provera) and risk of breast cancer. British Medical Journal 299: 759–762

Perret A G, Mosnier J F, Porcheron J et al 1996 Role of oral contraceptives in the growth of multilobular adenoma associated with hepatocellular carcinoma in a young woman. Journal of Hepatology 25: 976–979

Persson I, Yuen J, Bergkvist L, Schairer C 1996 Cancer incidence and mortality in women receiving estrogen and estrogen-progestin replacement therapy — long-term follow-up of a Swedish cohort. International Journal of Cancer 67: 327–332

Petersen K R, Skouby S O, Jepsen P V, Haaber A B 1996 Diabetesregulering og p-piller. Lipoproteinomsaetnig hos kvinder med insulinkraevende diabetes mellitus i p-pillebehandling. (Diabetes regulation and oral contraceptives. Lipoprotein metabolism in women with insulin dependent diabetes mellitus using oral contraceptives). Ugeskrift for Laeger 158: 2388–2392

Phupong V, Sueblinvong T, Pruksananonda K, Taneepanichskul S, Triratanachat S 2000 Uterine perforation with Lippes loop intrauterine device-associated actinomycosis: a case report and review of the literature. Contraception 61: 347–350

Piegsa K, Calder A, Davis J A, McKay-Hart D, Wells M, Bryden F 1997 Endometrial status in post-menopausal women on long-term continuous combined hormone replacement therapy (Kliofem). A comparative study of endometrial biopsy, outpatient hysteroscopy and intravaginal ultrasound. European Journal of Obstetrics, Gynecology and Reproductive Biology 72: 175–180

Pike M C 1990 Reducing cancer risk in women through lifestyle-mediated changes in hormone levels. Cancer Detection and Prevention 14: 595–607

Pirwany I R, Boddy K 1997 Colocolic fistula caused by a previously inserted intrauterine device. Case report. Contraception 56: 337–339

Plu Bureau G, Le M G 1997 Oral contraception and the risk of breast cancer. Contraception Fertilite Sexualite 25: 301–305

Porges R F 1973 Complications associated with the unsuspected presence of intrauterine contraceptive devices. American Journal of Obstetrics and Gynecology 116: 579–580

Poulter N R, Chang C L, Farley T M, Meirik O 1999a Risk of cardiovascular diseases in association with oral progestagen preparations with therapeutic indications (Letter). Lancet 354: 1610

Poulter N R, Chang C L, Farley T M, Marmot M G, Meirik O 1999b Effect on stroke of different progestagens in low oestrogen dose oral contraception. WHO Collaborative Study of Cardiovascular Disease and Steroid Hormone Contraception (Letter). Lancet 354: 301–302

Powles T, Eeles R, Ashley S et al 1998a Interim analysis of the incidence of breast cancer in the Royal Marsden Hospital tamoxifen randomised chemoprevention trial. Lancet 352: 98–101

Powles T J, Bourne T, Athanasiou S et al 1998b The effects of orethisterone on endometrial abnormalities identified by transvaginal ultrasound screening of healthy post-menopausal women on tamoxifen or placebo. British Journal of Cancer 78: 272–275

Prakash S, Scully R E 1964 Sarcoma-like pseudopregnancy changes in uterine leiomyomas. Obstetrics and Gynecology 24: 106–110

Prentice R L 1991 Epidemiologic data on exogenous hormones and hepatocellular carcinoma and selected other cancers. Preventive Medicine 20: 38–46

Preston E J, Ervin D K, McMichael A O, Preston L W 1975 Septic spontaneous abortion associated with the Dalkon Shield. In: Hefnawi F, Segal S J (eds) Analysis of intrauterine contraception. North Holland, Biomedical Press, Amsterdam, pp 417–428

Pschera H, Larsson B, Lindhe B A, Kjaeldgaard A 1988 The influence of copper intrauterine device on fatty acid composition of cervical mucus lecithin. Contraception 38: 341–348

Ragni N, Rugiati S, Rossato P, Venturini P L, Foglia G, Capitanio G L 1977 Modificazioni istologiche ed ultrastrutturali dell' endometrio in portatrici di iud e di iud potenziati al rame. Acta Europaea Fertilitatis (Roma) 18: 193–210

Rai V S, Gillmer M D, Gray W 2000 Is endometrial pre-treatment of value in improving the outcome of transcervical resection of the endometrium? Human Reproduction 15: 1989–1992

Ramsewak S, Rahaman J, Persad P, Narayansingh G 1991 Missing intrauterine contraceptive device presenting with strings at the anus. West Indian Medical Journal 40: 185–186

Randall T C, Kurman R J 1997 Progestin treatment of atypical hyperplasia and well-differentiated carcinoma of the endometrium in women under age 40. Obstetrics and Gynecology 90: 434–440

Randic L, Vlasic S, Matrljan I, Waszak C S 1985 Return to fertility after IUCD removal for planned pregnancy. Contraception 32: 253–259

Randic L, Haller H, Susa M, Rukavina D 1990 Cells adherent to copper-bearing intrauterine contraceptive devices determined by monoclonal antibodies. Contraception 42: 35–42

Reyes-Acevedo J, Bustamante-Sarabia J, Galindo-Martinez D F 1995 [Uterine perforation and localization of an IUD in the bladder associated with bladder calculosis. Report of a case and review of the literature] Perforacion uterina y localizacion vesical de un dispositivo intrauterino y cistolitiasis. Comunicacion de un caso y revision de la literatura. Ginecologia y Obstetricia de Mexico 63: 407–409

Rienprayura D, Phaosavasdi S, Semboonsuk S 1973 Cervical perforation by the copper-T intrauterine device. Contraception 7: 515–521

Rioux J E, Cloutier D, Dupont P, Lamonde D 1986 Pregnancy after IUD use. Advances in Contraception 2: 185–192

Rizk M, Shaban N, Medhat I, Moby el Dien Y, Ollo M A 1990 Electron microscopic and chemical study of the deposits formed on the copper and inert IUCDs. Contraception 42: 643–653

Robboy S J, Bradley R 1979 Changing trends and prognostic features in endometrial cancer associated with exogenous estrogen therapy. Obstetrics and Gynecology 54: 269–277

Robboy S J, Welch W R 1977 Microglandular hyperplasia in vaginal adenosis associated with oral contraceptives and prenatal diethylstilbestrol exposure. Obstetrics and Gynecology 49: 430–434

Robboy S J, Kaufman R H, Prat J et al 1979 Pathologic findings in young women enrolled in the National Cooperative Diethylstilbestrol Adenosis (DESAD) Project. Obstetrics and Gynecology 53: 309–317

Robboy S J, Truslow G Y, Anton J, Richart R M 1981 Role of hormones including diethylstilbestrol (DES) in the pathogenesis of cervical and vaginal intraepithelial neoplasia. Gynecologic Oncology 12: 98–110

Robboy S J, Young R H, Herbst A L 1982 Female genital tract changes related to prenatal diethylstilbestrol exposure. In: Blaustein A (ed) Pathology of the female genital tract, 2nd edn. Springer-Verlag, New York, pp 99–118

Rogers P A 1996 Endometrial vasculature in Norplant users. Human Reproduction 11 Suppl 2: 45–50

Romieu I, Willett W C, Colditz G A 1989 Prospective study of oral contraceptive use and risk of breast cancer in women. Journal of the National Cancer Institute 81: 1313–1321

Romieu I, Berlin J A, Colditz G 1990 Oral contraceptives and breast cancer. Review and meta-analysis. Cancer 66: 2253–2263

Ronnerdag M, Odlind V 1999 Health effects of long-term use of the intrauterine levonorgestrel-releasing system. A follow-up study over 12 years of continuous use. Acta Obstetricia et Gynecologica Scandinavica 78: 716–721

Rooks J B, Oray H W, Ishak K G et al 1979 Epidemiology of hepatocellular adenoma. The role of oral contraceptive use. Journal of the American Medical Association 242: 644–648

Rosenberg L 1991 The risk of liver neoplasia in relation to combined oral contraceptive use. Contraception 43: 643–652

Rosenberg M J, Long S C 1992 Oral contraceptives and cycle control: a critical review of the literature. Advances in Contraception 8(Suppl) 1: 35–45

Rosenberg L, Shapiro S, Slone D et al 1982 Epithelial ovarian cancer and combination oral contraceptives. Journal of the American Medical Association 247: 3210–3212

Rosenberg L, Palmer J R, Clarke E A, Shapiro S 1992 A case-control study of the risk of breast cancer in relation to oral contraceptive use. American Journal of Epidemiology 136: 1437–1444

Rosenberg L, Palmer J R, Sands M I et al 1997 Modern oral contraceptives and cardiovascular disease. American Journal of Obstetrics and Gynecology 177: 707–715

Rosenblatt K A, Thomas D B 1996 Intrauterine devices and endometrial cancer. The WHO Collaborative Study of Neoplasia and Steroid Contraceptives. Contraception 54: 329–332

Rosenwaks Z, Wentz A C, Jones G S et al 1979 Endometrial pathology and estrogens. Obstetrics and Gynecology 53: 403–410

Rosing J, Tans G, Nicolaes G A et al 1997 Oral contraceptives and venous thrombosis: different sensitivities to activated protein C in women using second- and third-generation oral contraceptives. British Journal of Haematology 97: 233–238

Rossing M A, Daling J R, Voigt L F, Stergachis A S, Weiss N S 1993 Current use of an intrauterine device and risk of tubal pregnancy. Epidemiology 4: 252–258

Rossmanith W G, Steffens D, Schramm G 1997 A comparative randomised trial on the impact of two low-dose oral contraceptives on ovarian activity, cervical permeability, and endometrial receptivity. Contraception 56: 23–30

Roy S 1991 Nonbarrier contraceptives and vaginitis and vaginosis. American Journal of Obstetrics and Gynecology 165: 1240–1244

Royal College of General Practitioners 1974 Oral Contraceptives and health. Pitman Medical, London

Royal College of General Practitioners' Oral Contraceptive Study 1978 Oral contraceptives, venous thrombosis and varicose veins. Journal of the Royal College of General Practitioners 28: 393–399

Royal College of General Practitioners' Oral Contraceptive Study 1981a Breast cancer and oral contraceptives: findings in Royal College of General Practitioners' Study. British Medical Journal 282: 2089–2093

Royal College of General Practitioners' Oral Contraceptive Study 1981b Further analyses of mortality in oral contraceptive users. Lancet 1: 541–546

Royal College of General Practitioners' Oral Contraception Study 1983 Incidence of arterial disease among oral contraceptive users. Journal of the Royal College of General Practitioners 33: 75–82

Rozsier J G Jr, Underwood P B 1974 Use of progestational agents in endometrial adenocarcinoma. Obstetrics and Gynecology 44: 60–64

Rushton L, Jones D R 1992 Oral contraceptive use and breast cancer risk: a meta-analysis of variations with age at diagnosis, parity and total duration of oral contraceptive use. British Journal of Obstetrics and Gynaecology 99: 239–246

Rutqvist L E, Johansson H, Signomklao T, Johansson U, Fornander T, Wilking N 1995 Adjuvant tamoxifen therapy for early stage breast cancer and second primary malignancies. Journal of the National Cancer Institute 87: 645–651

Rymer J M 1998 The effects of tibolone. Gynecologic Endocrinology 12: 213–220

Rymer J, Chapman M G, Fogelman I, Wilson P O 1994 A study of the effect of tibolone on the vagina in postmenopausal women. Maturitas 18: 127–133

Sabatini R, Di Fazio F, Loizzi P 1999 Uterine leiomyosarcoma in a postmenopausal woman treated with tamoxifen: case report. European Journal of Gynaecological Oncology 20: 327–328

Sandvei R, Sandstad E, Steier J A, Ulstein M 1987 Ovarian pregnancy associated with the intra-uterine contraceptive device. A survey of two decades. Acta Obstetricia et Gynecologica Scandinavica 66: 137–141

Schaude H, Dallenbach-Hellweg G, Schlaefer K 1980 Histologic changes of the cervix uteri following contraceptive use. In: Dallenbach-Hellweg G (ed) Functional morphologic changes in the female sex organs induced by exogenous hormones. Springer-Verlag, Heidelberg, pp 191–198

Schiff I, Sela H K, Cramer D, Tulchinsky D, Ryan K J 1982 Endometrial hyperplasia in women on cyclic or continuous estrogen regimens. Fertility and Sterility 37: 79–82

Schlesinger C, Silverberg S G 1999 Tamoxifen-associated polyps (basalomas) arising in multiple endometriotic foci: a case report and review of the literature. Gynecologic Oncology 73: 305–311

Schlesinger C, Kamoi S, Ascher S M, Kendell M, Lage J M, Silverberg S G 1998 Endometrial polyps: a comparison study of patients receiving tamoxifen with two control groups. International Journal of Gynecological Pathology 17: 302–311

Schlesselman J J 1990 Oral contraceptives and breast cancer. American Journal of Obstetrics and Gynecology 163: 1379–1387

Schmidt W A, Bedrossian C W, Ali V, Webb J A, Bastian F O 1980 Actinomycosis and intrauterine contraceptive devices — the clinicopathologic entity. Diagnostic Gynecology and Obstetrics 2: 165–177

Scholes D, Lacroix A Z, Ott S M, Ichikawa L E, Barlow W E 1999 Bone mineral density in women using depot medroxyprogesterone acetate for contraception. Obstetrics and Gynecology 93: 233–238

Scholten P C, Christaens G C, Haspels A A 1987 Intrauterine steroid contraceptives. Wiener Medizinische Wochenschrift 137: 479–483

Schwartz S M, Weiss N S, Daling J R et al 1996 Exogenous sex hormone use, correlates of endogenous hormone levels, and the incidence of histologic types of sarcoma of the uterus. Cancer 77: 717–724

Schwartz S M, Siscovick D S, Lonstreth W T Jr et al 1997 Use of low-dose oral contraceptives and stroke in young women. Annals of Internal Medicine 127: 596–603

Schwartzwald D, Mooppan U M, Tancer M L, Gomez-Leon G, Kim H 1986 Vesicouterine fistula with menouria: a complication from an intrauterine contraceptive device. Journal of Urology 136: 1066–1067

Schwingl P J, Shelton J 1997 Modelled estimates of myocardial infarction and venous thromboembolic disease in users of second and third generation oral contraceptives. Contraception 55: 125–129

Segal S J, Alvarez-Sanchez F, Adejuwon C A, Brache-de-Mejia V, Leon P, Faundes A 1985 Absence of chorionic gonadotropin in sera of women who use intrauterine devices. Fertility and Sterility 44: 214–218

Seif M W, Aplin J D, Awad H, Wells D 1989 The effect of the intrauterine contraceptive device on endometrial secretory function: a possible mode of action. Contraception 40: 81–89

Seif M W, Pearson J M, Ibrahim Z H Z et al 1992 Endometrium in in-vitro fertilization cycles: morphological and functional differentiation in the implantation phase. Human Reproduction 7: 6–11

Sellers T A, Mink P J, Cerhan J R et al 1998 The role of hormone replacement therapy in the risk for breast cancer and total mortality in women with a family history of breast cancer. Annals of Internal Medicine 127: 973–980

Sepulveda W H 1990 Perforation of the rectum by a Copper-T intra-uterine contraceptive device: a case report. European Journal of Obstetrics, Gynecology and Reproductive Biology 35: 275–278

Sereepapong W, Suwajanakorn S, Triratanachat S 2000 Effects of clomiphene citrate on the endometrium of regularly cycling women. Fertility and Sterility 73: 287–291

Serr D M, Shalev J 1985 Ultrasound guidance for IUD removal in pregnancy. In: Zatuchni G I, Goldsmith A, Sciarra J J (eds) Intrauterine contraception. Advances and future prospects. Harper & Row, Philadelphia, pp 194–197

Shapiro J A, Weiss N S, Beresford S A, Voigt L F 1998 Menopausal hormone use and endometrial cancer, by tumor grade and invasion. Epidemiology 9: 99–101

Shapiro S, Kaufman D W, Slone D et al 1980 Recent and past use of conjugated estrogens in relation to adenocarcinoma of the endometrium. New England Journal of Medicine 303: 485–489

Shaw S T 1985 Endometrial histopathology and ultrastructural changes with IUD use. In: Zatuchni G I, Goldsmith A, Sciarra J J (eds) Intrauterine contraception. Advances and future prospects. Harper & Row, Philadelphia, pp 276–296

Shaw S T Jr, Macaulay L K, Hohman W R 1979a Vessel density in endometrium of women with and without intrauterine contraceptive devices: a morphometric evaluation. American Journal of Obstetrics and Gynecology 135: 202–206

Shaw S T Jr, Macaulay L K, Hohman W R 1979b Morphologic studies on IUD-induced metrorrhagia. I. Endometrial changes and clinical correlations. Contraception 19: 47–61

Shaw S T Jr, Macaulay L K, Aznar R, Gonzalez-Angulo A, Roy S 1981 Effects of a progesterone-releasing intrauterine contraceptive device on the endometrial blood vessels: a morphometric study. American Journal of Obstetrics and Gynecology 141: 821–827

Sheppard B L 1987 Endometrial morphological changes in IUD users: a review. Contraception 36: 1–10

Sheppard B L, Bonnar J 1985 Endometrial morphology and IUD-induced bleeding. In: Zatuchni G I, Goldsmith A, Sciarra J J (eds) Intrauterine contraception. Advances and future prospects. Harper & Row, Philadelphia, p 297–306

Sherman B M, Chapler F K, Crickard K, Wycoff D 1979 Endocrine consequences of continuous antiestrogen therapy with tamoxifen in premenopausal women. Journal of Clinical Investigation 64: 398–404

Shortell C K, Schwartz S I 1991 Hepatic adenoma and focal nodular hyperplasia. Surgery Gynecology and Obstetrics 173: 426–431

Shurbaji M S, Gupta P K, Newman M M 1987 Hepatic actinomycosis diagnosed by fine needle aspiration. A case report. Acta Cytologica 31: 751–755

Shushan A, Peretz T, Uziely B, Lewin A, Mor-Yosef S 1996 Ovarian cysts in premenopausal and postmenopausal tamoxifen-treated women with breast cancer. American Journal of Obstetrics and Gynecology 174: 141–144

Silva E G, Tornos C S, Follen-Mitchell M 1994 Malignant neoplasms of the uterine corpus in patients treated for breast carcinoma: the effects of tamoxifen. International Journal of Gynecological Pathology 13: 248–258

Silverberg S G, Mullen D, Faraci J A et al 1982 Endometrial carcinoma: clinical-pathologic comparison of cases in post-menopausal women receiving and not receiving exogenous estrogens. Cancer 45: 3018–3026

Silverberg S G, Haukkamaa M, Arko H, Nilsson C G, Luukkainen T 1986 Endometrial morphology during long-term use of Levonorgestrel-releasing intrauterine devices. International Journal of Gynecological Pathology 5: 235–241

Simoncini T, Genazzani A R 2000 Tibolone inhibits leukocyte adhesion molecule expression in human endothelial cells. Molecular and Cellular Endocrinology 162: 87–94

Simsek S, Verheesen R V, Haagsma E B, Lourens J 2000 Subacute Budd–Chiari syndrome associated with polycythemia vera and factor V Leiden mutation. The Netherlands Journal of Medicine 57: 62–67

Sivin I 1985a Recent studies of more effective copper-T devices. In: Zatuchni G I, Goldsmith A, Sciarra J J (eds) Intrauterine contraception. Advances and future prospects. Harper & Row, Philadelphia, pp 70–78

Sivin I 1985b IUD-associated ectopic pregnancies, 1974 to 1984. In: Zatuchni G I, Goldsmith A, Sciarra J J (eds) Intrauterine contraception. Advances and future prospects. Harper & Row, Philadelphia, pp 340–353

Sivin I 1989 IUDs are contraceptives, not abortifacients: a comment on research and belief. Studies in Family Planning 20: 355–359

Sivin I 1991 Dose- and age-dependent ectopic pregnancy risks with intrauterine contraception. Obstetrics and Gynecology 78: 291–298

Sivin I, Schmidt F 1987 Effectiveness of IUDs: a review. Contraception 36: 55–84

Sivin I, el Mahgoub S, McCarthy T, Mishell D R R Jr, Shoupe D, Alvarez F 1990 Long-term contraception with the levonorgestrel 20 mcg/day (LNg 20) and the copper T 380Ag intrauterine devices: a five-year randomized study. Contraception 42: 361–378

Skjeldestad F E, Hammervold R, Peterson D R 1988 Outcomes of pregnancy with an IUD in situ-a population based case-control study. Advances in Contraception 4: 265–270

Smith C V, Horenstein J, Platt L D 1988 Intramniotic infection with Candida albicans associated with a retained intrauterine contraceptive device: a case report. American Journal of Obstetrics and Gynecology 159: 123–124

Smith M R, Soderstrom R 1976 Salpingitis: a frequent response to intrauterine contraception. Journal of Reproductive Medicine 16: 159–162

Smith P A, Ellis C J, Sparks R A, Guillebaud J 1983 Deaths associated with intrauterine contraceptive devices in the United Kingdom between 1973 and 1983. British Medical Journal 287: 1537–1538

Snowden R, Williams M, Hawkins D 1977 The IUD: a practical guide. Croom Helm, London, p 38

Snowman B A, Malviya V K, Brown W, Malone J M Jr, Deppe G 1989 Actinomycosis mimicking pelvic malignancy. International Journal of Gynaecology and Obstetrics 30: 283–286

Sogaard K 1993 Unrecognized perforation of the uterine and rectal walls by an intrauterine contraceptive device. Acta Obstetricia et Gynecologica Scandinavica 72: 55–56

Sparks R A, Purrier B G A, Watt P J, Elstein M 1977 The bacteriology of the cervix and uterus. British Journal of Obstetrics and Gynaecology 84: 701–704

Sparks R A, Purrier B G A, Watt P J, Elstein M 1981 Bacteriological colonisation of the uterine cavity: role of tailed intrauterine contraceptive device. British Medical Journal 282: 1189–1191

Spaun E, Klunder K 1986 Candida chorioamnionitis and intra-uterine contraceptive device. Acta Obstetricia et Gynecologica Scandinavica 65: 183–184

Spellberg M A, Mirro J, Chowdhury L 1979 Hepatic sinusoidal dilatation related to oral contraceptives. A study of two patients showing ultrastructural changes. American Journal of Gastroenterology 72: 248–252

Speroff L 1982 The formulation of oral contraceptives: does the amount of estrogen make any clinical difference? Johns Hopkins Medical Journal 150: 170–176

Speroff L 1996 Oral contraceptives and venous thromboembolism. International Journal of Gynaecology and Obstetrics 54: 45–50

Speroff L, Rowan J, Symons J, Genant H, Wilborn W 1996 The comparative effect on bone density, endometrium, and lipids of continuous hormones as replacement therapy (CHART study). A randomized controlled trial. Journal of the American Medical Association 276: 1397–1403

Spinillo A, Gorini G, Piazzi G, Baltaro F, Monaco A, Zara F 1996 The impact of oral contraception on chlamydial infection among patients with pelvic inflammatory disease. Contraception 54: 163–168

Spitzer W O, Lewis M A, Heinemann L A, Thorogood M, MacRae K D 1996 Third generation oral contraceptives and risk of venous thromboembolic disorders: an international case-control study. Transnational Research Group on Oral Contraceptives and the Health of Young Women. British Medical Journal 312: 83–88

Spona J, Feichtinger W, Kindermann C et al 1997 Modulation of ovarian function by oral contraceptive containing 30 micrograms ethinyl estradiol in combination with 2.00 mg dienogest. Contraception 56: 185–191

Stampfer M J, Willett W C, Colditz G A, Speizer F E, Hennekens C H 1990 Past use of oral contraceptives and cardiovascular disease: a meta-analysis in the context of the Nurses' Health Study. American Journal of Obstetrics and Gynecology 163: 285–291

Stanford J L, Brinton L A, Hoover R N 1989 Oral contraceptives and breast cancer: results from an expanded case-control study. British Journal of Cancer 60: 375–381

Sterup K, Mosbech J 1967 Budd-Chiari syndrome after taking oral contraceptives. British Medical Journal 4: 660

Stillman R J 1982 In utero exposure to diethylstilbestrol: adverse effects on the reproductive tract and reproductive performance in male and female offspring. American Journal of Obstetrics and Gynecology 142: 905–921

Stone M, Dent J, Kardana A, Bagshawe K D 1976 Relationship of oral contraception to development of trophoblastic tumour after evacuation of a hydatidiform mole. British Journal of Obstetrics and Gynaecology 83: 913–916

Sturdee D W 1996 Endometrial morphology and bleeding patterns as a function of progestogen supplementation. International Journal of Fertility and Menopausal Studies 41: 22–28

Sturdee D W, Wade-Evans T, Paterson M E L, Thom M, Studd J W 1978 Relations between the bleeding pattern, endometrial histology and oestrogen treatment in menopausal women. British Medical Journal 1: 1575–1577

Sturdee D W, Ulrich L G, Barlow D H et al 2000 The endometrial response to sequential and continuous combined oestrogen-progestogen replacement therapy. British Journal of Obstetrics and Gynaecology 107: 1392–1400

Subakir S B, Setiadi E, Affandi B, Pringgoutomo S, Freisleben H J 2000 Benefits of vitamin E supplementation to Norplant users — in vitro and in vivo studies. Toxicology 148: 173–178

Suissa S, Blais L, Spitzer W O, Cusson J, Lewis M, Heinemann L 1997 First-time use of newer oral contraceptives and the risk of venous thromboembolism. Contraception 56: 141–146

Suvanto-Luukkonen E, Malinen H, Sundstrom H, Penttinen J, Kauppila A 1998 Endometrial morphology during hormone replacement therapy with estradiol gel combined to levonorgestrel-releasing intrauterine device or natural progesterone. Acta Obstetricia et Gynecologica Scandinavica 77: 758–763

Swan S H, Brown W L 1981 Oral contraceptive use, sexual activity, and cervical carcinoma. American Journal of Obstetrics and Gynecology 139: 52–57

Szabo Z, Ficsor E, Nyiradi J et al 1997 Rare case of the utero-vesical fistula caused by intrauterine contraceptive device. Acta Chirurgica Hungarica 36: 337–339

Tadesse E 1996 Return of fertility after IUD removal for planned pregnancy: a six year prospective study. East African Medical Journal 73: 169–171

Tadesse E, Wamsteker K 1985 Evaluation of 24 patients with IUD-related problems: hysteroscopic findings. European Journal of Obstetrics, Gynecology and Reproductive Biology 19: 37–41

Taft P D, Robboy S J, Herbst A L, Scully R E 1974 Cytology of clear cell adenocarcinoma of genital tract in young females: review of 95 cases from the registry. Acta Cytologica 19: 279–290

Tamada T, Okagaki T, Maruyama M, Matsumoto S 1967 Endometrial histology associated with an intrauterine contraceptive device. American Journal of Obstetrics and Gynecology 98: 811–817

Tao L C 1991 Oral contraceptive-associated liver cell adenoma and hepatocellular carcinoma. Cytomorphology and mechanism of malignant transformation. Cancer 68: 341–347

Tao L C 1992 Are oral contraceptive-associated liver cell adenomas premalignant? Acta Cytologica 36: 338–344

Taskin O, Yalcinoglu A I, Kucuk S, Uryan I, Buhur A, Burak F 1997 Effectiveness of tibolone on hypoestrogenic symptoms induced by goserelin treatment in patients with endometriosis. Fertility and Sterility 67: 40–45

Tatum H J, Schmidt F H 1977 Contraceptive and sterilization practices and extrauterine pregnancy: a realistic perspective. Fertility and Sterility 28: 407–421

Tavani A, Negri E, Parazzini F, Franceschi S, La Vecchia C 1993 Female hormone utilization and risk of hepatocellular carcinoma. British Journal of Cancer 67: 635–637

Taxy J B 1978 Peliosis: a morphologic curiosity becomes an iatrogenic problem. Human Pathology 9: 331–340

Taylor H B, Irey N S, Norris H J 1967 Atypical endocervical hyperplasia in women taking oral contraceptives. Journal of the American Medical Association 202: 637–639

Tews G, Arzi W, Stoger H 1988 74 Schwangerschaften trotz liegendem IUD. Geburtshilfe und Frauenheilkunde 48: 349–351

The New Zealand Contraception and Health Study Group 1994 Risk of cervical dysplasia in users of oral contraceptives, intrauterine devices or depot-medroxyprogesterone acetate. Contraception 50: 431–441

Thiery M, Van Kets H, Van der Pas H 1985 Immediate post-placental IUD insertion: the expulsion problem. Contraception 31: 331–349

Thomalla J V 1986 Perforation of urinary bladder by intrauterine device. Urology 27: 260–264

Thomas D B, Noonan E A 1991 Risk of breast cancer in relation to use of combined oral contraceptives near the age of menopause. WHO Collaborative Study of Neoplasia and Steroid Contraceptives. Cancer Causes and Control 2: 389–394

Thomas D B, Ray R M 1995 Depot-medroxyprogesterone acetate (DMPA) and risk of invasive adenocarcinomas and adenosquamous carcinomas of the uterine cervix. WHO Collaborative Study of Neoplasia and Steroid Contraceptives. Contraception 52: 307–312

Thomas D B, Ray R M 1996 Oral contraceptives and invasive adenocarcinomas and adenosquamous carcinomas of the uterine cervix. The World Health Organization Collaborative Study of Neoplasia and Steroid Contraceptives. American Journal of Epidemiology 144: 281–289

Thomas D B, Molina R, Rodriguez-Cuevas H et al 1989 Monthly injectable steroid contraceptives and cervical carcinoma. American Journal of Epidemiology 130: 237–247

Thorburn J, Friberg B, Schubert W, Wassen A C, Lindblom B 1987 Background factors and management of ectopic pregnancy in Sweden. Changes over a decade. Acta Obstetricia et Gynecologica Scandinavica 66: 597–602

Thorogood M, Mann J, Murphy M, Vessey M 1991 Is oral contraceptive use still associated with an increased risk of fatal myocardial infarction? Report of a case-control study. British Journal of Obstetrics and Gynaecology 98: 1245–1253

Thorogood M, Mann J, Murphy M, Vessey M 1992 Fatal stroke and use of oral contraceptives: findings from a case-control study. American Journal of Epidemiology 136: 35–45

Timonen H, Kurppa K 1987 IUD perforation leading to obstructive nephropathy necessitating nephrectomy: a rare complication. Advances in Contraception 3: 71–75

Todd J, Lawrenson R, Farmer R D, Williams T J, Leydon G M 1999 Venous thromboembolic disease and combined oral contraceptives: a re-analysis of the MediPlus database. Human Reproduction 14: 1500–1505

Toivonen J, Luukkainen T, Allonen H 1991 Protective effect of intrauterine release of levonorgestrel on pelvic infection: three years' comparative experience of levonorgestrel- and copper-releasing intrauterine devices. Obstetrics and Gynecology 77: 261–264

Touraine P, Driguex P, Cartier I, Yaneva H, Kuttenn F, Mauvais-Jarvis P 1995 Lack of induction of endometrial hyperplasia with tamoxifen. Lancet 345: 254–255

Trauscht Van Horn J J, Capeless E L, Easterling T R, Bovill E G 1992 Pregnancy loss and thrombosis with protein C deficiency. American Journal of Obstetrics and Gynecology 167: 968–972

Tsalikis T, Stamatopoulos P, Kalachanis J, Mantalenakis S 1986 Experience with the MLCu250 IUD. Advances in Contraception 2: 393–398

Tsukada Y, Piver M S, Barlow J J 1977 Microglandular hyperplasia of the endocervix following long-term estrogen treatment. American Journal of Obstetrics and Gynecology 127: 888–889

Tuomivaara L, Kauppila A, Puolakka J 1986 Ectopic pregnancy – an analysis of the etiology, diagnosis and treatment in 552 cases. Archives of Gynecology and Obstetrics 237: 135–147

Tzingounis V, Cardamakis E, Ginpoulos P, Argiropoulos G 1996 Incidence of benign and malignant breast disorders in women taking hormones (contraceptive pill or hormonal replacement therapy). Anticancer Research 16: 3997–4000

UK National Case-Control Study Group 1989 Oral contraceptive use and breast cancer risk in young women. Lancet 1: 973–982

Ulstein M, Steier A J, Hofstad T, Digranes A, Sandvei R 1987 Microflora of cervical and vaginal secretion in women using copper- and norgestrel-releasing IUCDs. Acta Obstetricia et Gynecologica Scandinavica 66: 321–322

Urbanek R W, Cohen D J 1994 Porphyria cutanea tarda: pregnancy versus estrogen effect. Journal of the American Academy of Dermatology 31: 390–392

Valicenti J F, Pappas A A, Graber C D, Williamson H O, Willis N F 1982 Detection and prevalence of IUD-associated *Actinomyces* colonization and related morbidity. A prospective study of 69,925 cervical smears. Journal of the American Medical Association 247: 1149–1152

van Beek E J, Farmer K C, Millar D M, Brummelkamp W H 1991 Gallstone disease in women younger than 30 years. Netherlands Journal of Surgery 43: 60–62

Van Campenhout J, Choquette P, Vauclair R 1980 Endometrial pattern in patients with primary hypoestrogenic amenorrhoea receiving estrogen replacement therapy. Obstetrics and Gynecology 56: 349–355

Vandenbroucke P J, Shelton J 1997 Modeled estimates of myocardial infarction and venous thromboembolic disease in users of second and third generation oral contraceptives. Contraception 55: 125–129

Vandrie D M, Puri S, Upton R T, DeMeester L J 1983 Adenosquamous carcinoma of the cervix in a woman exposed to diethylstilbestrol in utero. Obstetrics and Gynecology 61(suppl): 84s–87s

van Heteren G 2001 Wyeth suppresses research on pill, programme claims. British Medical Journal 322: 571

Vanlancker M, Dierick A M, Thiery M, Claeys G 1987 Histologic and microbiologic findings in the fallopian tubes of IUD users. Advances in Contraception 3: 147–157

Van Leeuwen F E, Benraadt J, Coebergh J W W et al 1994 Risk of endometrial cancer after tamoxifen treatment of breast cancer. Lancet 343: 448–452

Van Os W A, Edelman D A 1989 Uterine perforation and use of the Multiload IUD. Advances in Contraception 5: 121–126

Vasilakis C, Jick H, del Mar-Melero-Montes M 1999 Risk of venous thromboembolism in users of progestagens alone (Letter). Lancet 354: 1610–1611

Verheul H A, Coelingh-Bennink H J, Kenemans P et al 2000 Effects of estrogens and hormone replacement therapy on breast cancer risk and efficacy of breast cancer therapies. Maturitas 36: 1–17

Veronesi U, Maisonneuve P, Costa A et al 1998 Prevention of breast cancer with tamoxifen: preliminary findings from the Italian randomised trial among hysterectomised women. Italian Tamoxifen Prevention Study. Lancet 352: 93–97

Vessey M P 1979 Oral contraception and neoplasia. British Journal of Family Planning 4: 65–71

Vessey M P 1989 Epidemiologic studies of oral contraception. International Journal of Fertility 34 Suppl: 64–70

Vessey M P, Doll R 1969 Investigation of relation between use of oral contraceptives and thromboembolic disease. A further report. British Medical Journal ii: 651–657

Vessey M P, Painter R 1995 Endometrial and ovarian cancer and oral contraceptives — findings in a large cohort study. British Journal of Cancer 71: 1340–1342

Vessey M P, Doll R, Peto R, Johnson B, Wiggins P 1976 Long-term follow-up of women using different methods of contraception – an interim report. Journal of Biosocial Science 8: 373–427

Vessey M P, McPherson K, Yeates D 1981a Mortality in oral contraceptive users. Lancet 1: 549–550

Vessey M P, Yeates D, Flavel R, McPherson K 1981b Pelvic inflammatory disease and the intrauterine device: findings in a large cohort study. British Medical Journal 282: 855–857

Vessey M P, Villard-Mackintosh L, McPherson K, Yeates D 1989a Mortality among oral contraceptive users: 20 year follow up of women in a cohort study. British Medical Journal 299: 1487–1491

Vessey M P, McPherson K, Villard-Mackintosh L, Yeates D 1989b Oral contraceptives and breast cancer: latest findings in a large cohort study. British Journal of Cancer 59: 613–617

Videla-Rivero L, Etchepareborda J J, Kesseru E 1987 Early chorionic activity in women bearing inert IUD, copper IUD and levonorgestrel-releasing IUD. Contraception 36: 217–226

Vincent A J, Malakooti N, Zhang J, Rogers P A, Affandi B, Salamonsen L A 1999 Endometrial breakdown in women using Norplant is associated with migratory cells secreting metalloproteinase-9 (gelatinase B). Human Reproduction 14: 807–815

Vincent A J, Zhang J, Östör A et al 2000 Matrix metalloproteinase-1 and -3 and mast cells are present in the endometrium of women using progestin-only contraceptives. Human Reproduction 15: 123–130

Wang I Y, Russell P, Fraser I S 1995 Endometrial morphometry in users of intrauterine contraceptive devices and women with ovulatory dysfunctional uterine bleeding: a comparison with normal endometrium. Contraception 51: 243–248

Weaver K, Glasier A 1999 Interaction between broad-spectrum antibiotics and the combined oral contraceptive pill. A literature review. Contraception 59: 71–78

Weden M, Glaumann H, Einarsson K 1992 Protracted cholestasis probably induced by oral contraceptive. Journal of Internal Medicine 231: 561–565

Weiss G 1999 Risk of venous thromboembolism with third generation oral contraceptives: a review. American Journal of Obstetrics and Gynecology 180: 295–301

Weiss N S, Sayvetz T A 1980 Incidence of endometrial cancer in relation to the use of oral contraceptives. New England Journal of Medicine 302: 551–554

Weiss N S, Lyon J L, Liff J M, Vollmer W M, Daling J R 1981 Incidence of ovarian cancer in relation to the use of oral contraceptives. International Journal of Cancer 28: 669–671

Westhoff C L 1999 Breast cancer risk: perception versus reality. Contraception 59 (Suppl 1): 25s–28s

Whitehead M I, McQueen J, Beard R J, Minardi J, Campbell S 1977 The effects of cyclical oestrogen therapy and sequential oestrogen/progestogen therapy on the endometrium of post-menopausal women. Acta Obstetricia et Gynecologica Scandinavica (suppl) 65: 91–101

Whitehead M I, Townsend P T, Pryse-Davies J, Ryder T A, King R J B 1981 Effects of estrogens and progestins on the biochemistry and morphology of the post-menopausal endometrium. New England Journal of Medicine 305: 1599–1605

Wight D G D 1982 Atlas of liver pathology. MTP Press, Lancaster

Wilcox A J, Weinberg C R, Armstrong E G, Canfield R E 1987 Urinary human chorionic gonadotropin among intrauterine device users: detection with a highly specific and sensitive assay. Fertility and Sterility 47: 265–269

Williams R, Neuberger J 1981 Occurrence, frequency and management of oral contraceptive associated liver tumours. British Journal of Family Planning 7: 35–41

Wingo P A, Lee N C, Ory H W, Beral V, Peterson H B, Rhodes P 1993 Age-specific differences in the relationship between oral contraceptive use and breast cancer. Cancer 71(4 Suppl): 1506–1517

Wingrave S 1982 Progestogen effects and their relationship to lipoprotein changes. A report from the Oral Contraception Study of the Royal College of General Practitioners. Acta Obstetricia et Gynecologica Scandinavica 105(Suppl): 33–36

Winkler B, Richart R M 1985 Cervical/uterine pathologic considerations in pelvic infection. In: Zatuchni G I, Goldsmith A, Sciarra J J (eds) Intrauterine contraception. Advances and future prospects. Harper & Row, Philadelphia, pp 438–449

Winkler K, Poulsen H 1975 Liver disease with periportal sinusoidal dilatation. A possible complication to contraceptive steroids. Scandinavian Journal of Gastroenterology 10: 699–704

Winkler U H 1998 Effects on hemostatic variables of desogestrel- and gestodene-containing oral contraceptives in comparison with lev-onorgestrel-containing oral contraceptives: a review. American Journal of Obstetrics and Gynecology 179: s51–s61

Winkler U H, Altkemper R, Kwee B, Helmond F A, Coelingh-Bennink H J 2000 Effects of tibolone and continuous combined hormone replacement therapy on parameters in the clotting cascade: a multicenter, double-blind, randomized study. Fertility and Sterility 74: 10–19

Winther J F, Dreyer L, Tryggvadottir L 1997 Avoidable cancers in the Nordic countries. Exogenous hormones. Acta Pathologica, Microbiologica, et Immunologica Scandinavica Suppl 76: 132–140

Wolf A S, Kriegler D 1986 Bacterial colonization of intrauterine devices (IUDs). Archives of Gynecology and Obstetrics 239: 31–37

Wollen A L, Flood P R, Sanvei R 1990 Altered ciliary substructure in the endosalpinx in women using an IUCD. Acta Obstetricia et Gynecologica Scandinavica 69: 307–312

Wolner-Hanssen P, Svensson L, Mårdh P A, Westrom L 1985 Laparoscopic findings and contraceptive use in women with signs and symptoms suggestive of acute salpingitis. Obstetrics and Gynecology 66: 233–238

World Health Organization Collaborative Study of Neoplasia and Steroid Contraceptives 1985a Invasive cervical cancer and combined oral contraceptives. British Medical Journal 290: 961–965

World Health Organization's Special Programme of Research, Development and Research Training in Human Reproduction. 1985b Task Force on Intrauterine Devices for Fertility Regulation. A multinational case-

control study of ectopic pregnancy. Clinical Reproduction and Fertility 3: 131–143

World Health Organization Special Programme of Research, Development and Research Training in Human Reproduction. 1987 Task Force on Intrauterine Devices for Fertility Regulation. Microdose intrauterine levonorgestrel for contraception. Contraception 35: 363–79

World Health Organization Collaborative Study of Cardiovascular Disease and Steroid Hormone Contraception. 1998 Cardiovascular disease and use of oral and injectable progestogen-only contraceptives and combined injectable contraceptives. Results of an international, multicenter, case-control study. Contraception 57: 315–324

World Health Organization Collaborative Study of Neoplasia and Steroid Contraceptives 1988a Endometrial cancer and combined oral contraceptives. International Journal of Epidemiology 17: 263–269

World Health Organization Collaborative Study of Neoplasia and Steroid Contraceptives 1988b Epithelial ovarian cancer and combined oral contraceptives. International Journal of Epidemiology 18: 538–545

World Health Organization Collaborative Study of Neoplasia and Steroid Contraceptives. 1989a Combined oral contraceptives and liver cancer. International Journal of Cancer 43: 254–259

World Health Organization Collaborative Study of Neoplasia and Steroid Contraceptives. 1989b Combined oral contraceptives and gallbladder cancer. International Journal of Epidemiology 18: 309–314

World Health Organization Collaborative Study of Cardiovascular Disease and use of oral contraceptives. 1989c Bulletin of the World Health Organization 67: 417–423

World Health Organization multicentre trial of the vasopressor effects of combined oral contraceptives: 1. Comparisons with IUD. Task Force on Oral Contraceptives. 1989d WHO Special Programme of Research, Development and Research Training in Human Reproduction. Contraception 40: 129–145

World Health Organization Collaborative Study of Neoplasia and Steroid Contraceptives. 1990 Breast cancer and combined oral contraceptives: results from a multinational study. British Journal of Cancer 61: 110–119

World Health Organization Collaborative Study of Neoplasia and Steroid Contraceptives 1991a Depot-medroxyprogesterone acetate (DMPA) and risk of endometrial cancer. International Journal of Cancer 49: 186–190

World Health Organization Collaborative Study of Neoplasia and Steroid Contraceptives 1991b Breast cancer and depot-medroxyprogesterone acetate: a multinational study. Lancet 338: 833–838

World Health Organization Collaborative Study of Neoplasia and Steroid Contraceptives 1991c Depot-medroxyprogesterone acetate (DMPA) and risk of liver cancer. International Journal Cancer 49: 182–185

World Health Organization Collaborative Study of Neoplasia and Steroid Contraceptives 1992 Depot-medroxyprogesterone acetate (DMPA) and risk of invasive squamous cell cervical cancer. Contraception 45: 299–312

World Health Organization Collaborative Study of Cardiovascular Disease and Steroid Hormone Contraception. 1996 Ischaemic stroke and combined oral contraceptives: results of an international, multicentre, case-control study. Lancet 348: 498–505

World Health Organization Collaborative Study of Cardiovascular Disease and Steroid Hormone Contraception 1997 Acute myocardial infarction and combined oral contraceptives: result of an international multicentre case-control study. Lancet 349: 1202–1209

Wright E A, Aisien A O 1989 Pelvic inflammatory disease and the intrauterine contraceptive device. International Journal of Gynaecology and Obstetrics 28: 133–136

Wu S M, Spurny O M, Klotz A P 1977 Budd-Chiari syndrome after taking oral contraceptives. A case report and review of 14 reported cases. American Journal of Digestive Disease 22: 623–628

Yaari S, Goldbourt U, Even-Zohar S, Neufeld H N 1981 Associations of serum high density lipoprotein and total cholesterol with total, cardiovascular, and cancer mortality in a 7-year prospective study of 10,000 men. Lancet 1: 1001–1015

Yalcin V, Demirkesen O, Alici B, Onol B, Solok V 1998 An unusual presentation of a foreign body in the urinary bladder. A migrant intrauterine device. Urologia Internationalis 61: 240–242

Yoonessi M, Crickard K, Cellino I S, Satchidanand S K, Fett W 1985 Association of actinomyces and intrauterine contraceptive devices. Journal of Reproductive Medicine 30: 48–52

Young R H, Scully R E 1992 Uterine carcinomas simulating microglandular hyperplasia. A report of six cases. American Journal of Surgical Pathology 16: 1092–1097

33

Tropical pathology of the female genital tract and ovaries

S. B. Lucas

Introduction   1133

Infections   1134
Bacterial infections   1134
Fungal infections   1140
Protozoal infections   1140
Helminth infections   1141

Neoplastic diseases   1148
Carcinoma of the cervix   1149
Carcinoma of the endometrium   1149
Tumours of the ovary   1149
Burkitt's lymphoma   1150
Gestational trophoblastic tumours   1150

Other diseases of the female genital tract   1151
Ectopic pregnancy   1151
Female circumcision   1151
Postpartum fistulae   1151
Adenomyosis and endometriosis   1151

HIV, AIDS and gynaecological diseases   1151
Epidemiology   1151
Pathology   1152
Vulvo-vaginal ulceration and fistula formation   1153
HIV, HPV and cervical neoplasia   1153

INTRODUCTION

By tradition, 'tropical pathology' implies exotic parasitic diseases (protozoal and helminthic) endemic in poor countries in hot climates. In practice, two overlapping topics are included. First, 'developing countries in the tropics' are those in warm climates where health is affected by mass poverty, poor sanitation, poor provision of clean water, poor access to medical care, poor provision of pathology services, and low per capita expenditure on health (World Bank 1993): in other words, resource-poor countries. Such countries are characterised by high transmission rates of infectious diseases, high infant and maternal mortalities, and by having up to half the population under 16 years of age (Mahler 1987; Parkin et al 1988a). Maternal mortality is probably the single biggest global differential in health statistics: in eastern Africa one in eleven women suffer a lifetime risk of such mortality compared with one in 4000 in western Europe (WHO 2000). Secondly, there is the vast range of infectious diseases. Some are ecologically restricted to warm climates (such as filariasis and schistosomiasis), some are global but more common in warm climates. However, with modern international travel, a patient with any infectious disease may present anywhere in the world.

Since the first editions of this book, the most significant change in world health has been the pandemic of infection with human immunodeficiency virus (HIV) and consequent acquired immunodeficiency syndrome (AIDS). The impact of HIV on gynaecological disease is summarised below.

A large part of the pathologist's work in the tropics — in the post-mortem room as in the biopsy reporting room — is concerned with gynaecological and obstetric pathology. In this chapter, the emphasis is on gynaecological conditions that pathologists encounter in resource-poor countries, plus some unusual infections that are not covered elsewhere in this book. The standard encyclopaedia of infectious diseases, particularly microbial, is by Mandell et al (2000). For the parasitic infections discussed, no details of life cycles are given: these can be found in Lucas (1992). An account of all parasitic (and other infectious disease) pathology is in Connor & Chandler (1996). Helminthic infections, including those affecting the female genital tract, are comprehensively covered in Meyers et al (2000).

INFECTIONS

BACTERIAL INFECTIONS

These include pelvic inflammatory diseases and genital ulcer diseases. The highest rates are found in the tropics (Bang et al 1989; Laga et al 1991). Sexually transmitted diseases (STD) with genital ulcers are not only numerically important in the resource-poor regions of the tropics, they are contributing significantly to the spread of HIV infection (Grosskurth et al 2000). When receiving biopsy material from vulval and vaginal ulcers, typical specific infections that may be encountered are herpes (prevalence in STD clinics 10–20%), syphilis (10–20%), chancroid (10–15%), lymphogranuloma venereum (5%) and granuloma inguinale (3–6%) (Braithwaite et al 1997). In Africa, chancroid, caused by *Haemophilus ducreyi*, is a common identifiable genital ulcer disease, and gonorrhoea (*Neisseria gonorrhei*) is ubiquitous (Muir & Belsey 1980).

Pelvic inflammatory disease

Acute and chronic inflammatory disease is common in the lower socioeconomic groups of the tropics not only because of the high prevalence of sexually transmitted diseases and post-abortion or postpartum sepsis but also because therapy is often delayed (Muir & Belsey 1980; Bang et al 1989). Early age of first intercourse — in some regions, before the menarche — is associated with increased risk of sexually transmitted diseases (Duncan et al 1990). The sequelae of criminal abortion, a common practice in many developing countries through lack of access to safe abortion, are particularly demanding of hospital resources (Liskin 1980; Kulczycki & Potts 1996) and are a major septic cause of maternal mortality in the tropics (Graham 1991). An analysis of gynaecological admissions to a major hospital in Uganda showed that 30% were for pelvic inflammatory disease. This is associated with a high rate of sterility (26%) and ectopic gestation (Grech et al 1973).

For the practising histopathologist, acute and chronic salpingitis, tubo-ovarian abscess, ectopic pregnancy and 'non-specific chronic endometritis' account for a large proportion of gynaecological pathology. In the main pathology laboratory in Nairobi in the early 1980s, receiving specimens from all around Kenya, one-quarter of submitted histology specimens were endometrial curettings with a clinical label of infertility (personal observations).

This comes as an initial surprise considering the high population growth rate, but reflects the social pressures to bear children, coupled with the high prevalence of pelvic inflammatory disease. The logistical consequence for resource-poor laboratories is that unless a clinical indication of carcinoma, tuberculosis, or trophoblastic disease in the lower genital tract is present, analysis of endometrial curettings is not productive of clinically useful results (personal observations).

The late effects of untreated pelvic sepsis present problems to both clinicians and pathologists. The pelvis may be filled with a mass of proliferating vascular fibrous tissue — the 'plaster of Paris' pelvis — which is often mistaken for a diffusely invasive cancer. Proliferation of entrapped mesothelial cells may also mimic carcinoma.

Chronic endometritis and tuberculosis

Plasma cell infiltration of the endometrial stroma is the morphological hallmark of chronic endometritis, and may be focal or diffuse (see also Chapter 11). In many resource-poor countries, 'routinely' submitted endometrial curettings show this in up to 20% of specimens (Farooki 1967; Liomba et al 1982), associated with infertility in up to one-third of patients. The distribution of the main aetiological agents — chlamydial infection and gonorrhoea — is inadequately documented for poor tropical countries (Muir & Belsey 1980; Laga et al 1991), and the histological appearances are non-specific. Histologically identifiable forms of chronic endometritis include donovanosis and tuberculosis (see below). Endometrial actinomycete infections, associated with intrauterine contraceptive devices, and artefactual pseudoactinomycotic granules occur globally (Bhagavan et al 1982; Arroyo & Quinn 1989).

Infection by *Mycobacterium tuberculosis* has always been one of the most important causes of morbidity and mortality in the tropics. In a typical resource-poor country in the tropics, the annual rate of acquisition of tuberculous infection is 1–2.5% per annum from birth, so that the majority of adults harbour infection which can reactivate to produce disease. The incidence of female genital tract tuberculosis parallels closely the overall prevalence of tuberculosis. Its spread to the genital tract is predominantly haematogenous from a pulmonary lesion. In a large series from India of non-pregnancy related endometrial curettings examined up to 1980, tuberculosis was diagnosed in 2.3% (Bazaz-Malik et al 1983). During an 11-year period of routine diagnostic histopathology from Malawi, female genital tuberculosis was found in 90 patients: 59 endometrial curettings, 17 tubes, 9 cervical biopsies, and two cases of ovarian tuberculosis (Liomba & Chiphangwi 1982). Up to 6% of infertility has been attributed to pelvic tuberculosis in resource-poor countries (Muir & Belsey 1980).

The histological diagnosis of genital tuberculosis presents no problems when the typical caseating epithelioid and giant cell granulomas are present in tissues from any site. However, in curettings this well-developed picture is often lacking and the lesions are focal and scanty. Tuberculous endometritis has to be diagnosed as an occasional finding in a sea of non-specific endometritis. Focal lymphocytic and plasma cell infiltration are seen in both. Most tuberculous granulomas start in the stroma adjacent to a gland. The early lesions are mainly composed of lymphocytes with only an occasional macrophage, and necrosis may be minimal (Fig. 33.1). The wall of the gland is involved and the lumen filled with exudate, often eosinophilic, and inflammatory cells including polymorphs, lymphocytes and macrophages. The residual epithelial lining of these glands may be stratified with some papillary infoldings and show nuclear pleomorphism. Dissociation between the glandular and stromal appearances causes difficulty in dating the endometrium (Liomba & Chiphangwi 1982). In proliferative endometrium, the glands are often angulated, and in the secretory phase the affected glands may be non-secretory. In more advanced cases, granulomas are seen in the stroma although caseation is usually minimal unless the patient has amenorrhoea (Fig. 33.2). Glands may then be very scanty. In such advanced disease, cervical, vaginal and vulvar tuberculous lesions occur (Fig. 33.3). Acid-fast bacilli are usually difficult to detect in endometrial tuberculosis. The exception to this is non-reactive tuberculosis in immunosuppressed patients where abundant bacilli are seen in necrotic tissue that has a poor cellular reaction and no giant cells.

Although tuberculosis of the Fallopian tubes is almost always the primary site of infection of the female genital tract, tuberculous salpingitis will not commonly be encountered by the pathologist (see also Chapter 15). The macroscopic appearances may be indistinguishable from those of chronic non-specific salpingitis, unless there is extensive caseation or a tuberculous pyosalpinx. In advanced cases, typical coalescing granulomas are present in the tubal folds and may involve the muscularis and serosa (Fig. 33.4). In early cases the diagnosis may be more difficult. The appearances are those of chronic salpingitis, often the follicular type, with only occasional non-necrotic granulomas. In tubes containing predominantly noncaseating granulomas, laminated haematoxyphilic

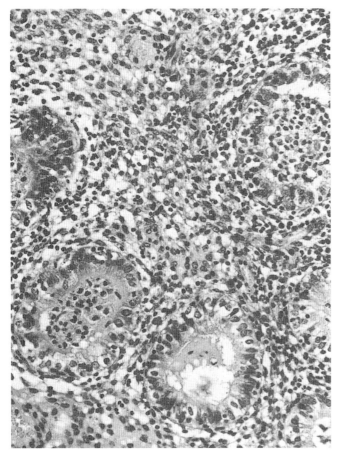

Fig. 33.1 Tuberculous endometritis. Note glands full of exudate with blurring of epithelial outlines. No granulomas are seen.

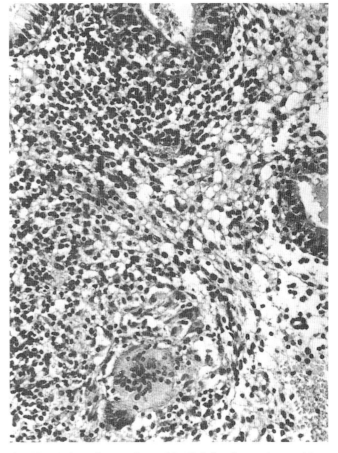

Fig. 33.2 Tuberculous endometritis. Ill-defined granuloma with giant cell (bottom), non-specific infiltrate of stroma and extension of these cells (lymphocytes) into glandular epithelium.

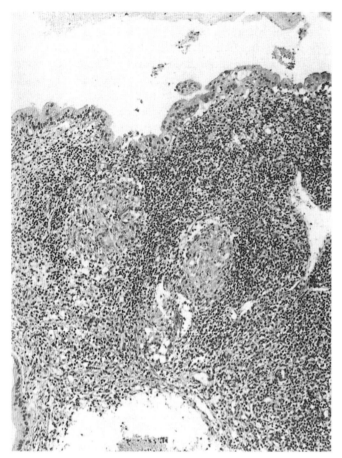

Fig. 33.3 Non-caseating tuberculous granulomas in endocervical tissues.

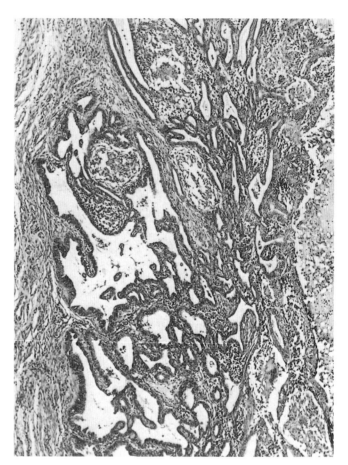

Fig. 33.4 Tuberculous salpingitis with plical adhesions giving appearance of follicular salpingitis and scattered epithelioid cell granulomas.

bodies indistinguishable from Schaumann bodies of sarcoidosis may be seen. Superficially these resemble dead and calcified schistosome eggs.

Syphilis

Infection with *Treponema pallidum* is widely associated with poverty. Within Africa, prevalence rates of positive syphilis serology among pregnant women range from 1–17%, and among female prostitutes from 18–38% (Laga et al 1991). Consequently congenital syphilis is an important cause of neonatal death (Lucas et al 1983).

Primary and secondary syphilis lesions (see also Chapter 3) are not always easy to specify amidst the inflow of vulvar inflammatory lesions that are biopsied. The condyloma latum of secondary syphilis has an oedematous hyperplastic epithelium diffusely infiltrated by polymorphs, and an underlying chronic inflammatory infiltrate that includes variable numbers of plasma cells. The oft-mentioned hypertrophy of endothelial cells in small vessels ('endarteritis obliterans') may not be seen. However, a silver stain such as Dieterle or Warthin–Starry usually demonstrates spirochaetes within the epithelium (Fig. 33.5) (Freinkel 1987). Serological evidence and

empirical chemotherapy may be required to prove the diagnosis of syphilis.

Granuloma inguinale (donovanosis)

Donovanosis is a sexually transmitted disease caused by the Gram-negative bacillus *Calymmatobacterium granulomatis*, and is found throughout the tropics.

In the female the initial lesion is a papule which then ulcerates. The vulva and perineum are the commonest sites, but vaginal and cervical ulcers also occur (Fig. 33.6). The ulcer enlarges, has a thick rolled edge and a beefy, red granulation tissue base. Satellite lesions are frequent, but inguinal node involvement is uncommon (Freinkel 1988). Left untreated, donovanosis has a relapsing course and may heal with an atrophic scar. It may spread upwards to involve the endometrium, tubes, ovaries and adnexae, causing a frozen pelvis (Bhagwandeen & Mottiar 1972; Sengupta & Das 1984). Cases of psoas abscess are recorded (Mein et al 1999). Secondary fusospirochaetal infection of the ulcer produces widespread mutilation of the external genitalia. Occasionally the inflammation with fibrosis results in vulvar elephantiasis and urethral stricture. Clinically, the ulcerated lesion resembles diverse other conditions such as carcinoma

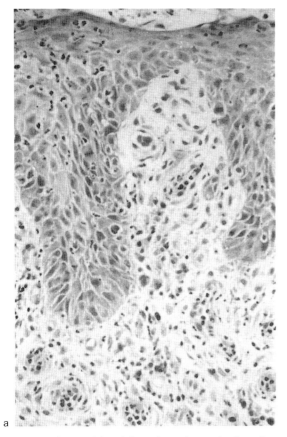
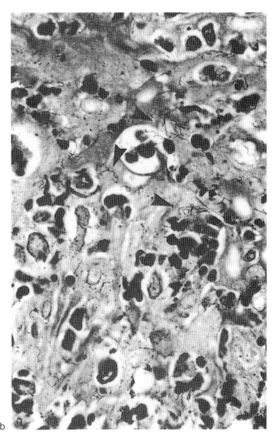

a   b

Fig. 33.5 Secondary syphilis of the vulva. **a** hyperplastic oedematous epithelium containing scattered polymorphs; the dermis is vascular and the endothelial cells are hypertrophied. **b** Warthin–Starry stain of the epithelium with several spirochaetes (arrowheads).

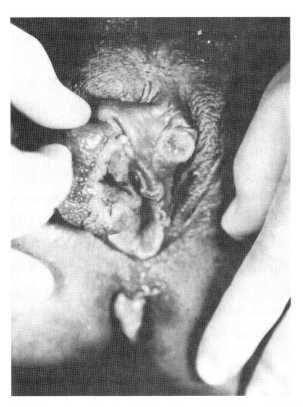

Fig. 33.6 Granuloma inguinale. Ulceration of the labia, resembling carcinoma. (Reproduced by kind permission of Mr J B Lawson.)

and amoebiasis (Bhagwandeen & Naik 1977). There is some evidence that in women with HIV infection, the lesions of donovanosis take longer to heal and are more destructive (Jamkhedkar et al 1998).

Histologically, donovanosis may seem non-specific, forming papules, nodules verrucous and ulcerative lesions. The overlying epithelium is hyperplastic (Fig. 33.7). The inflammatory tissue comprises microabscesses, vascular proliferation and variable numbers of macrophages and plasma cells (Fig. 33.8). The characteristic feature is the presence of large macrophages with clear or foamy cytoplasm; these may be so numerous as to produce a starry-sky appearance. In their cytoplasm are the Donovan bodies (Fig. 33.9); these are the bacilli of *C. granulomatis* which, faintly seen on H & E and PAS stains, are well shown by the Giemsa, Dieterle or Warthin–Starry method. They measure $1–1.5 \times 0.6$ μm, and are also seen within polymorphs and in the extracellular matrix. This histology is similar to that of rhinoscleroma of the upper respiratory tract. Transepithelial elimination of free and intra-macrophage bacilli occurs with organisms on the epithelial surface (Ramdial et al 2000). A smear of fresh tissue, air-dried and stained with a Romanovsky stain, will demonstrate the typical macrophages and organisms. The term 'Donovan body' should not be confused with 'Leishman–Donovan body' which is the old term for a *Leishmania* amastigote.

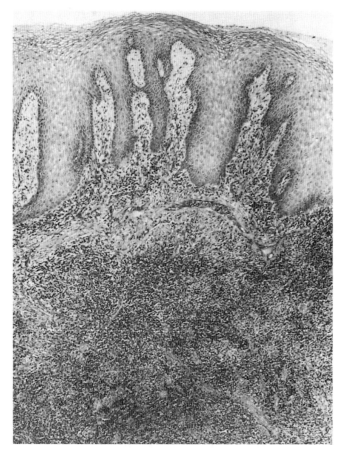

Fig. 33.7 Granuloma inguinale of the vagina. Granulation tissue beneath acanthotic epithelium.

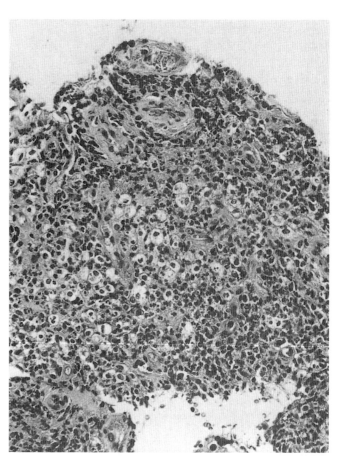

Fig. 33.8 Granuloma inguinale. Within the granulation tissue are large, empty-looking macrophages.

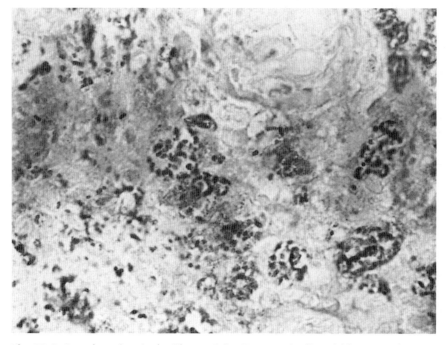

Fig. 33.9 Granuloma inguinale. Silver-staining Donovan bodies within macrophages. Dieterle.

Lymphogranuloma venereum (LGV)

This disease is distinct from granuloma inguinale. It is caused by *Chlamydia trachomatis*, is transmitted sexually, and is most prevalent in the tropics (Braithwaite et al 1997).

The vulva, vagina and cervix are the sites of infection and the earliest lesion is a vesicle which breaks down to form a punched-out painless ulcer. This may heal and the primary lesion is often unnoticed. Histologically, it has a non-specific appearance of granulation tissue.

Instead of healing, the primary lesion may become secondarily infected and persist. Involvement of the inguinal lymph nodes is less common in females than in males. It occurs within a month of the primary lesion and buboes may develop. Their histology shows the familiar stellate abscess with surrounding epithelioid cell reaction (Fig. 33.10). This is similar to the nodal lesions of cat scratch disease and of *Yersinia enterocolitica* intestinal infection. The bubo may discharge with sinus formation.

The later response to LGV infection is abundant granulation tissue with scarring. This cicatrisation around both an unhealed primary lesion and pelvic nodes causes the chronic form of the disease. The urethra may be destroyed (Fig. 33.11) or undergo stricture (as occurs in the rectum). Multiple labial ulcers, recto-vaginal fistula and vaginal fibrosis can occur. Lymphatic obstruction may result in vulvar swelling or elephantiasis (so-called 'esthiomène'). At this stage, the histology is non-specific. Serology and culture of tissue are important aids to the diagnosis.

Clinically, LGV can mimic vulvar carcinoma; subsequent development of vulvar and anal malignancy is held to be a true aetiological association.

Other bacterial genital ulcer diseases

The histological features of gonorrhoeal ulcers are non-specific — acute inflammation and much exudate. Chancroid (*Haemophilus ducreyi*) may show a characteristic vertical pattern of three zones: superficial necrotic exudate (in which short Gram-negative bacilli may be visible on Gram stain), a broad layer of oedematous granulation tissue and a deep zone with many plasma cells and lymphocytes (Freinkel 1987).

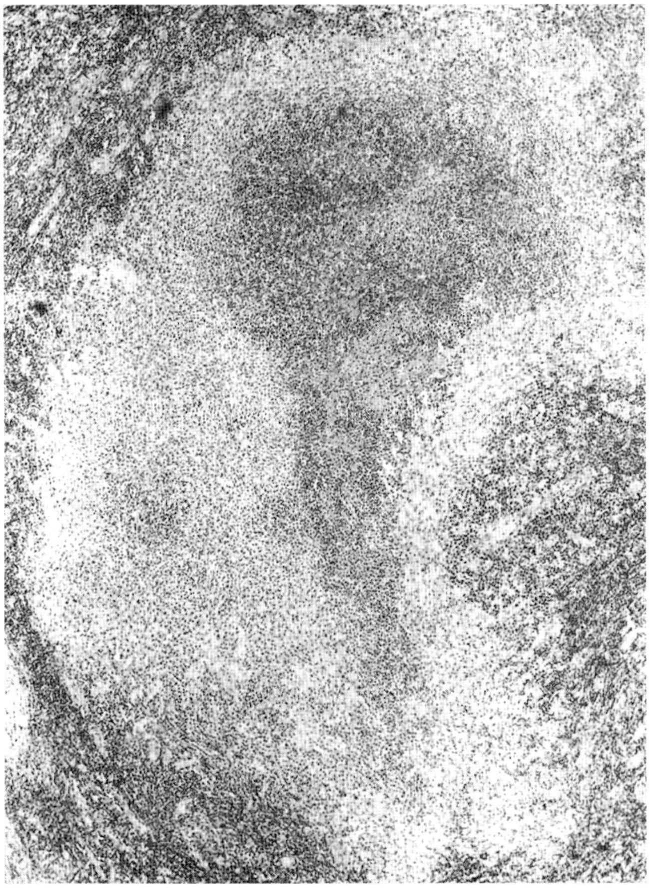

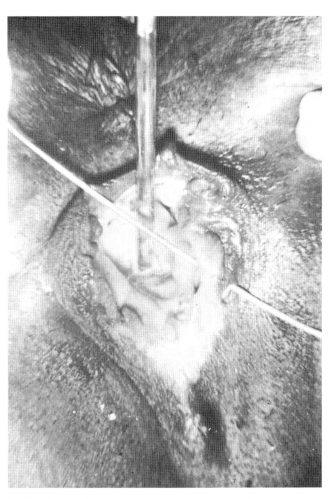

Fig. 33.10 Lymphogranuloma venereum. Inguinal node with a necrotic granuloma.

Fig. 33.11 Lymphogranuloma venereum. Gross vulval damage with ulceration and destruction of the urethra — the catheter is entering the base of the bladder. (Reproduced by kind permission of Mr J B Lawson.)

FUNGAL INFECTIONS

Candida infections of the vagina are ubiquitous (see also below in 'HIV and AIDS'). Disseminated fungal infections in immunocompromised patients (e.g. systemic candidiasis and aspergillosis) or apparently immunocompetent patients (e.g. coccidioidomycosis and histoplasmosis) may involve the female genital tract, but are unlikely to present a primary diagnostic problem (Chandler et al 1980). In contrast, subcutaneous zygomycosis (ex 'phycomycosis') may present as a vulvar lesion, although it usually affects the thighs and buttocks. Seen in Central America, Africa and Asia, this disease follows traumatic implantation of *Basidiobolus haptosporus*. It causes a diffuse subcutaneous panniculitis which forms a woody hard plaque and may ulcerate (Scott et al 1985). Histologically, the fungal hyphae are seen as circular holes or clefts on H & E stain (Fig. 33.12). A PAS or Grocott stain demonstrates non-septate, irregularly branching hyphae of variable width — up to 30 *µm*. Initially, the host reaction is granulomatous with abundant eosinophils, and a Hoeppli–Splendore reaction around the hyphae is typical. With chronicity, extensive fibrosis develops.

PROTOZOAL INFECTIONS

Amoebiasis

Carriage of *Entamoeba histolytica* and *E. dispar* infections in the large bowel are ubiquitous, with about 10% of the global population infected. *Entamoeba* cysts may be encountered as faecal contaminants in cervical smears. However, invasive amoebic disease is more common in the tropics with poor socioeconomic conditions and sanitation. Also it is now clear that only *Entamoeba histolytica* species is pathogenic (Spice & Ackers 1992; Ravdin 2000); the morphologically identical *E. dispar* causes non-invasive bowel infection only. Whilst the classical patterns of amoebiasis are of colo-rectal ulceration and liver abscess, amoebiasis of the perineum and male and female genitalia may occur. This follows either direct spread from rectal lesions or is due to homosexual or heterosexual intercourse (Mylius & Ten Seldam 1962; Phillips et al 1981).

Perianal amoebiasis presents with raised irregularly ulcerated lesions. As shown in Fig. 33.13, similar ulcerated destructive lesions may occur on the clitoris,

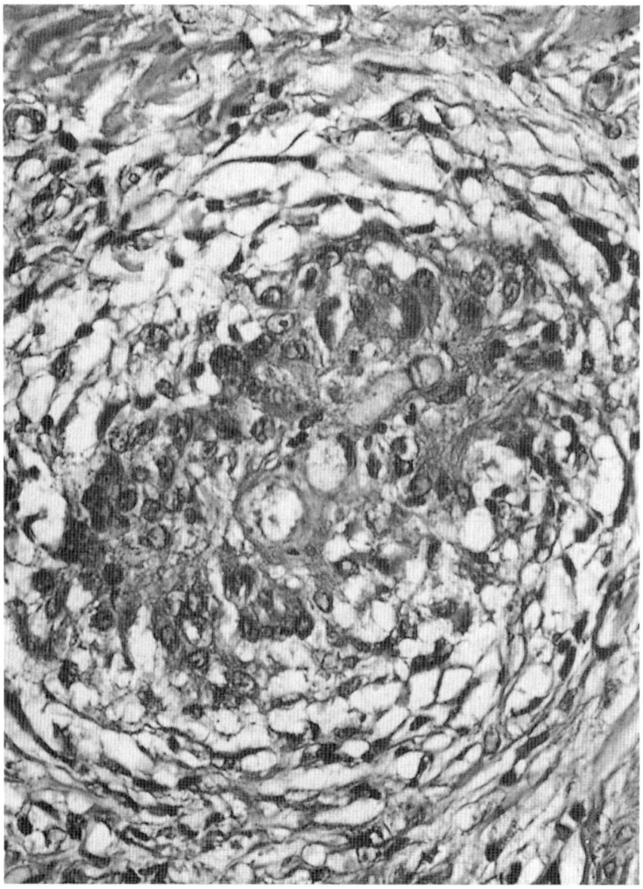

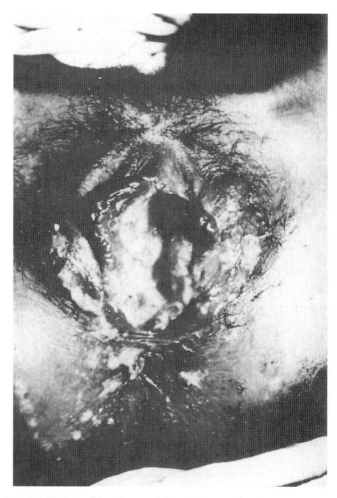

Fig. 33.12 Zygomycosis. Within the granuloma are broad hyphae, seen in cross and longitudinal section.

Fig. 33.13 Amoebic vulvo-vaginitis with extensive tissue destruction. (Reproduced by kind permission of Mr J B Lawson.)

urethra, labia, vagina and cervix following sexual trans- mission (Agranal & Bausal 1981; Nopdonrattakon 1996). In all these sites, the clinical impression is frequently that of carcinoma; there are also occasional reports of carcinoma of the cervix associated with concurrent or treated amoebic cervicitis (Haibach et al 1985; Arroyo & Elgueta 1989).

Histopathologically, these lesions are characterised by epithelial necrosis, reactive epithelial hyperplasia, which may simulate carcinoma, and a variable inflammatory response. Amoebic trophozoites are seen on the superficial parts of the epithelium as well as in the ulcer slough (Figs 33.14–16). In H & E stains they are large cells (15–30 μm in diameter) with pale grey to mauve cytoplasm, a well-defined round purple nucleus, and, often, phagocytosed erythrocytes. Viable amoebae are strongly PAS positive. Once secondary infection has occurred, widespread non-specific inflammatory changes may complicate the lesion and dominate the overall picture.

Leishmaniasis

Cutaneous leishmaniasis due to various species of *Leishmania* is endemic in the tropics, Mediterranean basin, the Middle East and Indian subcontinent. Transmission is via the bite of an infected sandfly, hence genital lesions are rare (Blickstein et al 1993). A case of vulvar leishmaniasis by sexual transmission from a man with visceral leishmaniasis is recorded (Symmers 1960). The histopathology shows the typical amastigotes within macrophages in the dermis.

Mucocutaneous leishmaniasis is caused by *L. brasiliensis* infection in South America. Lesions at mucocutaneous junctions ('espundia') occasionally involve the vulva as well as the more frequent facial and pharyngeal locations. They are ulcerative and widely destructive; histopathology usually does not reveal parasites but may include granulomas as a diagnostic clue (Connor & Chandler 1996).

HELMINTH INFECTIONS

Nematode infections

Filariasis

Chronic lymphoedema of the vulva, usually associated with elephantiasis of the legs, may be due to filariasis. *Wuchereria bancrofti* is endemic in South and Central

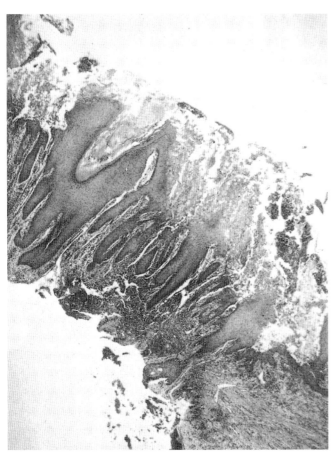

Fig. 33.14 Vulvar amoebiasis. Pseudoepitheliomatous hyperplasia and necrotic inflammatory slough.

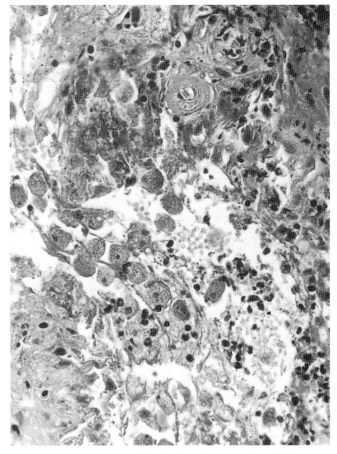

Fig. 33.15 Numerous amoebae in slough over perianal lesions.

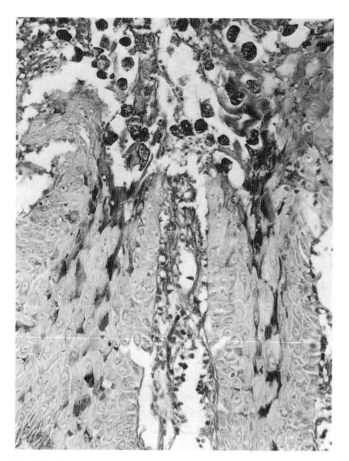

Fig. 33.16 Amoebae in slough over vulvar skin. PAS.

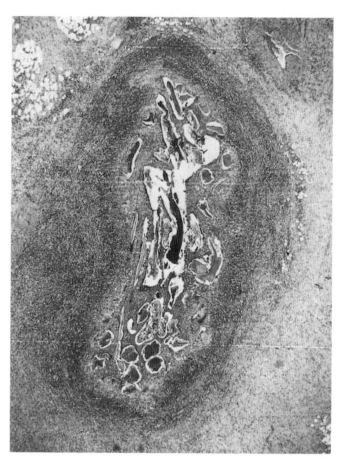

Fig. 33.17 Bancroftian filariasis. A degenerating female worm; the inflammation has obliterated the lymph node and there is surrounding fibrosis.

America and Africa. Filariasis in south-east Asia is caused by *Brugia malayi*: both worms cause similar clinical features.

Adult male and female worms inhabit the large lymphatic vessels, most frequently adjacent to the large lymph nodes in the inguinal region.

Clinical disease usually develops months or years after infection and is due to repeated episodes of lymphangitis caused by the reaction to worms in the lymphatics. Blockage of lymphatics may lead to lymphoedema of the vulva. The vulva may be grossly distorted by warty fibrous masses with a crusted surface. There may be associated chyluria and ascites. Histologically, the features in vulvar skin are of chronic lymphoedema: epithelial hyperplasia, dermal oedema and fibrosis, and dilated lymphatics. The amount of inflammation is variable. A specific histological diagnosis can only be made if a worm or fragments of worm are found in the deeper tissues. They are easily recognisable when viable, and the gravid female contains embryonic microfilariae in the uterine cavity (Figs 33.17, 33.18). More frequently the worms are degenerate with some loss of internal structures, and may calcify. Later a giant cell granulomatous reaction develops. An aetiological association of filariasis with pelvic inflammatory disease and tubal occlusion is unlikely (Muir & Belsey 1980).

Enterobiasis

This is a common large bowel and appendiceal infection by the nematode *Enterobius vermicularis* (the pin-worm). It is usually found in younger people and is more a disease of temperate than tropical zones (Sinniah et al 1991). That there may be an ethnic susceptibility to infection is suggested by studies in the USA which detected a lower infection prevalence in Puerto Rican and black children compared with Caucasian controls (Most et al 1963).

Usually symptoms arise from deposition of eggs on the perineum. During their nocturnal perineal perambulations, the gravid female worms may enter the vagina and ascend the female genital tract. A worm lodging on the hymen may cause pain. Both deposited eggs, and the worm as it degenerates, elicit a host reaction, resulting in inflammatory lesions of the vulva, vagina, endometrium, myometrium, tubes, ovaries and peritoneum (Sinniah et al 1991; Sun et al 1991). The commonest lesions are serosal nodules on the uterus and mesosalpinx. Pyosalpinx and tubo-ovarian abscess may occur. One patient with a tubo-ovarian abscess that had ruptured and caused generalised peritonitis had had a hysterectomy four years earlier (Khan & Stell 1981). Despite the abscess formation evident in *Enterobius* lesions, cultures for bacteria are negative. Rarely, an adult worm

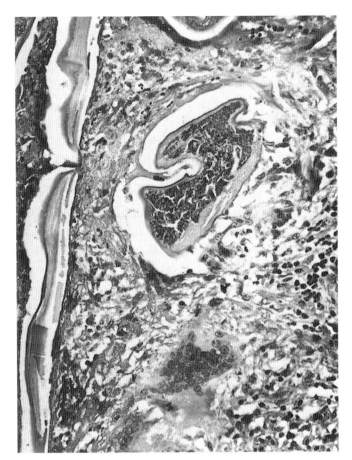

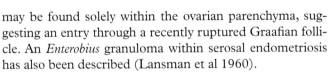

Fig. 33.18 Bancroftian filariasis. Parts of a degenerating female adult worm. Note the dark-staining microfilariae within a uterus, and the giant cell inflammatory reaction.

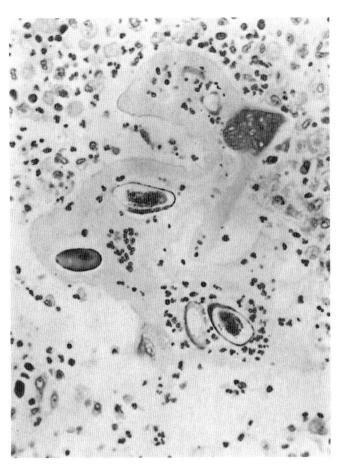

Fig. 33.19 Ova of *Enterobius vermicularis* within a degenerate adult.

may be found solely within the ovarian parenchyma, suggesting an entry through a recently ruptured Graafian follicle. An *Enterobius* granuloma within serosal endometriosis has also been described (Lansman et al 1960).

The lesion around a worm is characteristically a 1–3 cm nodule with a central yellow necrotic core. Histologically, within a fibrous capsule there is granulation tissue and variable amounts of eosinophilic necrosis, admixed with tuberculoid granulomas. In lesions with no worm residue evident, eggs are seen within non-necrotic granulomas. Occasionally, the eggs have a Hoeppli–Splendore reaction around the shells. The eggs are unilaterally flat, measure 50–60 × 20–30 μm and have a thick shell (Fig. 33.19); recently laid specimens contain a coiled larva. A degenerate *Enterobius* worm is 0.5 mm in diameter and, apart from the characteristic internal structure of uterine tubes and gut, the lateral paired triangular alae on the cuticle are distinctive (Fig. 33.20).

Other nematode infections

Calcospherites are to be distinguished from helminth eggs. The main differential diagnosis of invasive female genital enterobiasis is schistosomiasis (see below). *Ascaris*

eggs are occasionally found in granulomatous peritoneal and adnexal lesions. *Gnathostoma* is a cause of visceral larva migrans, and may result in abscesses in the upper female genital tract, containing a larval worm.

Cestode infections

Hydatid disease of the female genital tract

Hydatid disease is acquired by ingestion of eggs of *Echinococcus granulosus* tapeworm in the faeces of infected canines. It is prevalent in the Middle East and Africa, but is also endemic in South America, Australia and Europe. The liver and peritoneal cavity are the most frequent locations of cysts. The female genital tract thus occasionally becomes involved secondarily, with the ovary most often affected (Hiller et al 2000). A study in Lebanon of 532 patients with hydatidosis found ovarian involvement in 0.75% and uterine cysts in 0.4% (Bickers 1970). Rarely, the ovary is the site of primary cyst formation (Hangval et al 1979). Cysts may be located in the pouch of Douglas and adnexae (Rahman et al 1982), and there are frequently adhesions between the cyst and adjacent omentum, bowel, bladder and other pelvic structures. Cyst size may reach 15 cm.

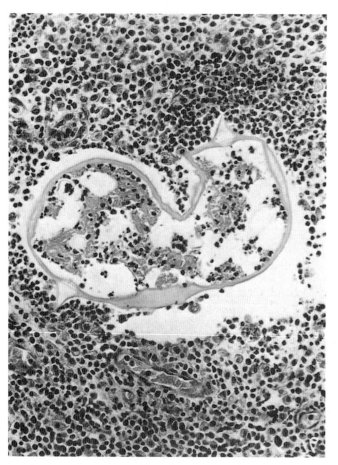

Fig. 33.20 *Enterobius* abscess in adnexae. Transverse section of an adult female showing the paired, pyramidal lateral alae.

Histologically, gynaecological hydatid cysts have the usual structure of laminated membrane and germinal layer with internal daughter cysts containing protoscolices. Externally, there is a host fibrous capsule of variable thickness, which may calcify. Clinical effects include a pelvic mass and obstructed labour. Occasionally cysts are passed per vaginam from the uterus.

Other cestode infections

Spirometra is a cause of visceral larva migrans and may present as an abscess, containing a worm, in the upper female genital tract and adnexae.

Trematode infections

Schistosomiasis

Some 200 million people in tropical zones of Asia, Africa and South America are infected with schistosome worms. The major species affecting the female genital tract is *Schistosoma haematobium*, but *S. mansoni* is also found in some lesions. *S. japonicum* infection in China seems to be associated with no specific gynaecological lesions apart

from menstrual disorders (Qunhua et al 2000). *Schistosoma haematobium* is endemic in 54 countries in Africa and the Middle East (WHO 1993). Prevalence of infection varies widely, but in some communities in Africa nearly 100% of children and adolescent females are infected, infection rates declining thereafter. A major review of female genital tract schistosomiaisis is provided by Poggensee & Feldmeier (2001).

The dioecious *S. haematobium* worms (i.e. male and female) locate and move in the pelvic veins, and cause no direct pathology. The main exit for their eggs — laid at the rate of 200–400 per worm pair per day — is the bladder mucosa and urine. The inflammatory reaction around eggs deposited in the small veins disrupts the vessels, enabling the eggs to enter tissues. There they induce a mixed eosinophil and granulomatous host response; with time, and particularly with anti-schistosomal therapy, the eosinophilia goes, the granulomas become more compact around the eggs, and there may be a central fibrinoid necrotic reaction. Eventually, there is fibrosis around the eggs and granulomas, the latter being reduced to giant cell clusters. About half of the eggs deposited in the bladder are excreted; the rest remain, die, and calcify or are destroyed by macrophages. Eggs formed in extravesical organs thus form chronic inflammatory masses. Often a worm pair remains in one location and cumulatively lays vast numbers of eggs to produce a large tumour mass ('bilharzioma'). Autopsy studies find that about 10% of eggs retained in the body are deposited in the internal genitalia (Cheever et al 1977).

The prevalence of schistosomal lesions of the genitalia reflects the prevalence of urinary schistosomiasis in the population. The lower female organs — vagina, vulva and cervix — are involved more often than the uterus, ovary and tubes. In terms of sensitivity, tissue digestion for eggs provides the highest estimates of prevalence and histology the lowest; examination of compressed fresh tissues provides an intermediate level; Pap smears notably underdiagnose the presence of schistosomal eggs (Poggensee & Feldmeier 2000). Cervical lesions are most commonly encountered in all series (Table 33.1), though a distinction has to be made as to whether the schistosomal

Table 33.1 The distribution of lesions in gynaecological schistosomiasis in three African countries, using histological examinations — % prevalence data

Organ	Egypt	Malawi	South Africa
Vulva	17	9	9
Vagina	26	10	3
Cervix	31	60	67
Uterus	4	0.1	4
Fallopian tube	7	16	10
Ovary	16	10	5

Reference sources: Egypt — Youssef et al 1970; Malawi — Wright et al 1982; South Africa — Berry 1966.

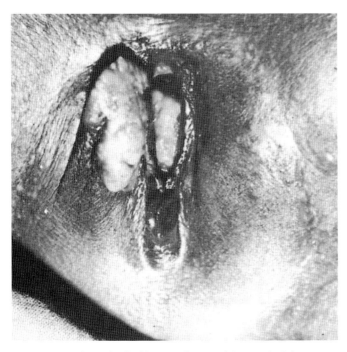

Fig. 33.21 Polypoid vulval lesions due to schistosomiasis in an 11-year-old girl. (Reproduced by kind permission of Mr J B Lawson.)

pathology is an incidental finding or is the prime cause of the clinical lesion and hence of the biopsy. For example, blind biopsy of the vagina in a population heavily infected with *S. haematobium* found a 75% prevalence of eggs in the vagina among women with proven urinary schistosomiasis, but most of the lesions were subclinical (Renaud et al 1989).

Vulvar lesions are typically encountered in girls and adults under 20 years. They are warty or nodular masses on any part such as the clitoris, labia minora and majora (Fig. 33.21). They may be ulcerated or have an intact surface, and sizes up to 5 cm are noted (Attili et al 1983; Mawad et al 1992). Histologically, paired worms may be seen in veins (Fig. 33.22). In the earlier stages of infection, large numbers of eggs are present in subepidermal tissues. These are viable, with brown chitinous shells, and have an internal miracidium with haematoxyphilic nuclei and deeply eosinophilic cytoplasm. The eggs are surrounded by a granulomatous reaction with giant cells, and eosinophils and plasma cells (Fig. 33.23). Sometimes eggs are seen within an eosinophil abscess. *S. haematobium* eggs have a terminal spine (those of *S. mansoni* have a lateral spine), but malorientation within the section and

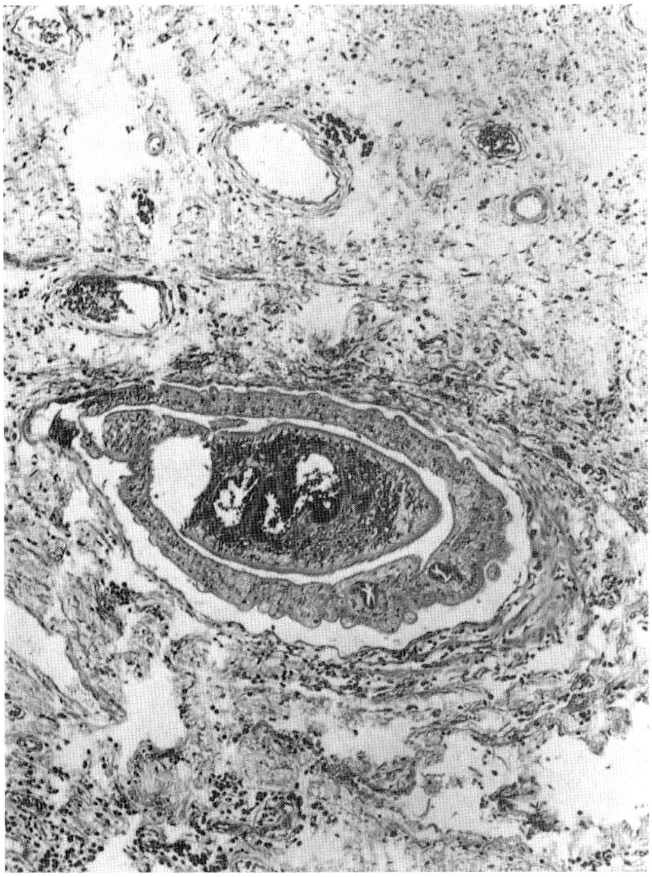

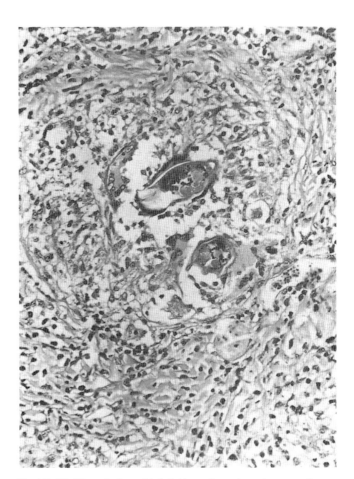

Fig. 33.22 Paired schistosome worms in vein from polypoid vulval lesion. The female is embraced by the male.

Fig. 33.23 Warty lesion of left labium. Granulomatous reaction around schistosomal ova in subepidermal tissues. Non-specific inflammation and fibrosis around the granuloma.

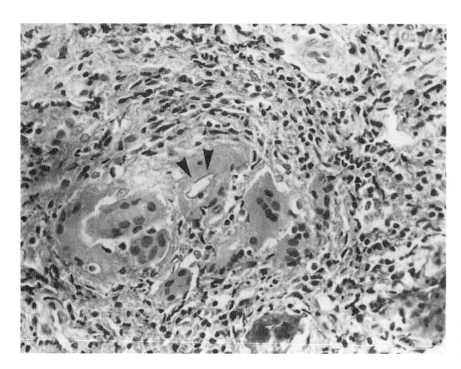

Fig. 33.24 Foreign body giant cell reaction around degenerate and distorted schistosomal ova (arrow) from biopsy of cervix.

the crushing effect of the microtome blade often preclude precise speciation of *Schistosoma* on histology. The eggs die after three weeks, the internal nuclei shrink, the cytoplasm vanishes, and the eggshell becomes distorted. The tissue eosinophilia diminishes and fibrosis increases. Finally the shells disintegrate and many are engulfed by macrophage giant cells (Fig. 33.24). These stages are common to the natural history of all schistosomal urinary and gynaecological lesions, but the early stage is more frequently seen in vulvar lesions, probably because the clinical features are external and therefore biopsies are taken early in the course of infection. Because reinfection is common in endemic areas, the different stages often coexist in the same tissue. In vulvar lesions, the majority of eggs are deposited near the surface, and this induces pseudoepitheliomatous hyperplasia of the epidermis (Fig. 33.25). Florid lesions are to be distinguished from condylomata acuminata which coincidentally contain a few eggs. There is no indication that vulvar schistosomiasis is a premalignant condition.

Vaginal and cervical schistosomiasis may present clinically as nodules, polyps or warty tumours. These may be mistaken for neoplasms. Large numbers of eggs are deposited in the immediate subepithelial tissues and associated, as in the vulva, with a diffuse and granulomatous inflammatory reaction (Figs 33.26, 33.27). In Malawi, 25 of the 793 cases of squamous cervical carcinoma had associated schistosomal eggs (Lowe et al 1981). There is no definite epidemiological evidence that cancer of the cervix is associated with schistosomiasis. However, it has been suggested that schistosomiasis interferes with the mechanisms of clearing human papillomavirus infection in the cervix, thereby augmenting viral load. Moreover, in

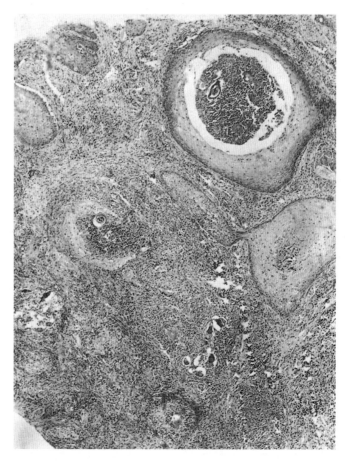

Fig. 33.25 Warty polyp of vulva. Widespread inflammation and pseudoepitheliomatous hyperplasia are present. Schistosomal ova (black) are scattered through the tissues.

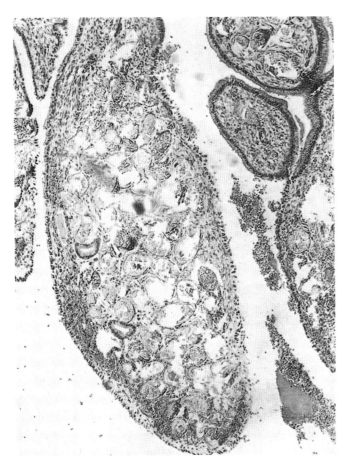

Fig. 33.26 Endocervical schistosomal polyp containing large numbers of dead ova, many of which are 'empty' and only recognisable by their shells.

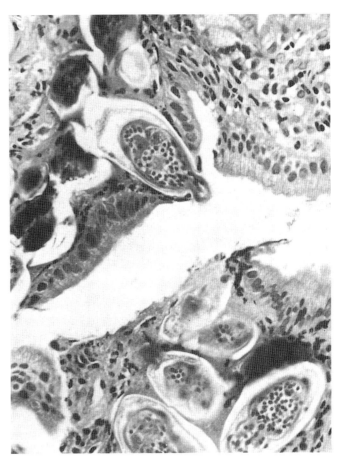

Fig. 33.27 Schistosomal cervicitis with many ova in the tissues. Most of these ova are viable with well-developed internal structure (miracidium). One is being extruded through a cervical gland.

Tanzania the presence of genital schistosomiasis was associated with younger age at presentation of cervical carcinoma (Moubayed et al 1995).

Endometrial and myometrial schistosomiasis is uncommon, fewer than 1% of specimens received from Malawi being affected (Wright et al 1982). This is possibly because the tortuous venules of the uterine wall prevent access by the worms, and the endometrium is regularly shed. Occasionally, ova are seen in endometrial curettings with little or no inflammatory reaction but in postmenopausal women the characteristic tissue histology is present. Eggs are sometimes found in leiomyomas.

Schistosomiasis of the ovary and tube often coexist, sometimes with involvement of the adnexae. Ovarian schistosomiasis is comprehensively reviewed by Tiboldi (1978); its prevalence varies widely. In spite of case reports, there is no good evidence of hormonal dysfunction of the ovaries (Chen & Mott 1989). Eggs are usually an incidental finding, as for example in resected cystic teratomas which can also contain adult worms. Adnexal lesions, fibrous 'sandy patches' and nodules less than 1 cm in size are seen (El-Mahgoub 1982). Laparoscopically these can look similar to tuberculous lesions. Larger bilharziomas in the pelvis may mimic

neoplasms because of the fibrous tissue that develops around the egg-granulomas (Fig. 33.28). A 10 cm diameter parauterine inflammatory mass of schistosomiasis that also contained the tube and ovary is reported (Bac et al 1987).

Tubal schistosomiasis has been implicated in infertility and tubal pregnancy (El-Mahgoub 1982). Given that an inflammatory mass may obstruct the lumen this is reasonable, but again, there is no good epidemiological evidence of an aetiological association (Chen & Mott 1989) and bacterial pelvic inflammatory disease is far more important. Egg densities in tubal resections for infertility are generally small when estimated by histology. However, systematic evaluation of autopsy and surgical biopsy material using the more sensitive technique of tissue digestion for schistosome eggs has shown that 10–30% of female genital organs can contain eggs without any being identified in standard tissue sections (Edington et al 1975; Frost 1975).

The eggshell of *S. haematobium* is not acid-fast with carbol fuchsin stains whereas that of *S. mansoni* is. This is a useful empirical method of distinguishing species in histological sections and can highlight mixed infections.

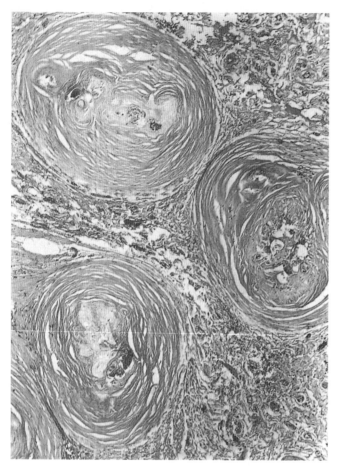

Fig. 33.28 Schistosomal hyaline nodules found on the external aspects of a Fallopian tube. A few degenerate ova are present in the centre of each nodule.

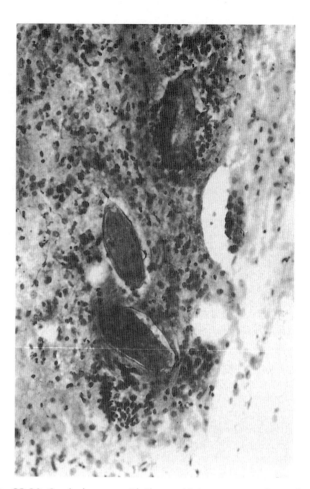

Fig. 33.29 Cervical smear with three schistosome eggs. A terminal spine is barely visible in the central egg. Papanicolaou stain.

Schistosomiasis may rarely affect the placenta. Worms are seen in decidual vessels and lying free in the maternal sinus. The eggs may be found in the intervillous space and also within villi, accompanied by a variable inflammatory reaction. Fetal infection does not occur and the functional effect of the schistosomal infection on the placental unit appears to be minimal (Bittencourt et al 1980).

Cytology. As might be expected (Fig. 33.27), schistosome eggs emerge from cervical glands and may be detected in cervical smears. High numbers, up to 250 per smear, may be encountered although the usual is 1–2 per smear (Fig. 33.29) (Berry 1966). If the egg is orientated appropriately, the terminal spine of *S. haematobium* is visible.

Other trematode infections

Extrapulmonary *Paragonimus* and ectopic *Fasciola* worms are uncommon; they may be found within abscesses in the uterus and Fallopian tube. Pentastomiasis, caused by worm-like parasites (*Armillifer*) in Africa and the Far East, can also involve the upper female genital tract with inflammatory lesions containing nymphs (Ong 1974).

Parasites in cervical smears

Cervical smears may contain parasites. In addition to schistosomiasis, discussed above, eggs of *Enterobius* are noted from invasive infection. *Ascaris* eggs in smears arise from faecal contamination rather than genital tract infection. Larvae of *Strongyloides* (a rare occurrence) must be distinguished from free-living nematodes that contaminate laboratory water supplies. Various protozoa are encountered in smears. *Trichomonas* is well known. *Entamoeba histolytica* trophozoites are uncommon but can be confused with a variety of contaminant free-living protozoa and the commensal *Entamoeba gingivalis*.

NEOPLASTIC DISEASES

The world over, there is an approximately four-fold variation in estimated female mortality rates due to all non-skin cancers, the highest rates occurring in industrialised countries, the lowest in poor countries in the tropics (Parkin et al 1988a). These differences may in reality be less, given the difficulties of accurate diagnosis and consequent under-registration in poor countries, and it is unfortunate that the cancer registries in Africa that, in the past, provided excellent data for epidemiological studies have found it nearly impossible to continue (Wabinga et al 1993). Gynaecological malignancies, particularly cancer of the cervix, contribute importantly to cancer in the tropics (Table 33.2).

CARCINOMA OF THE CERVIX

In most populations in the tropics, cervical carcinoma is the commonest malignant tumour of women (Parkin et al 1988a). Clinically, cervical carcinoma tends to present at a relatively early age in the tropics, though many cases are seen at a late stage because medical facilities (including cervical cytology) are scarce, particularly in rural and poor urban areas (Rogo & Kavoo-Linge 1990). In Malawi and Kenya, over 55% of newly diagnosed patients are stage 3 or 4. The histopathological features of cervical carcinoma are similar to those reported from other parts of the world, and massive eosinophilia is occasionally seen, as elsewhere (Ojwang & Mati 1978; Lowe et al 1981). Adenocarcinoma accounts for 4–5% of cases in Africa as it does in India (Kushtagi & Rao 1991).

The types of human papillomavirus (HPV) associated with carcinoma of the cervix in industrialised countries — HPV 16 and 18 — are also found infecting patients in Africa, South America and India (Das et al 1989; Reeves et al 1989; Schmauz et al 1989). Early age at onset of sexual activity is also a risk factor for cervical cancer (Duncan et al 1990). The association of HIV infection with cervical neoplasia is discussed below.

CARCINOMA OF THE ENDOMETRIUM

In industrialised countries, the ratio of endometrial carcinoma to cervical carcinoma has changed greatly in the last 60 years. In earlier times cervical cancer was 6–8 times more frequent than endometrial cancer, but now the ratios approach unity or are even inverted (Table 33.2). By contrast, in tropical countries the cervical/endometrial cancer ratios are 5–15 to 1. In many African countries, choriocarcinoma is more frequent than endometrial cancer (James et al 1973). These differences are not mainly attributable to age since they remain after age-standardisation of incidence rates. Overall in 'developing countries', whilst cancer of the cervix is the commonest non-skin malignancy, endometrial cancer ranks sixteenth; in 'developed countries' the respective rankings are tenth and ninth (Parkin et al 1988a).

As might be expected from the age structure of populations in poor countries, with many fewer old people, patients with endometrial cancer present at a lower mean age than elsewhere. In India, the mean age at presentation is 51 years, with postmenopausal bleeding in 56% of patients (Kapila & Verma 1981). Infertility was not a major factor.

Table 33.2 Incidences of cancer of cervix, endometrium (corpus uteri) and ovary in various regions of the world: estimated crude rates in 1980, per 100 000 women. Data from Parkin et al (1988a).

Region	Cervix	Corpus uteri	Ovary
Western Europe	19	20	16
North America	11	26	14
Japan	16	3	5
Tropical South America	32	7	6
East Africa	23	2	4
Caribbean	24	5	5
China	27	3	4
India	20	1	4

In industrialised countries, many studies have noted the association of endometrial cancer with diabetes, hypertension and obesity. This elderly archetype is less common in the tropics, though hypertension is common among some black populations. The important rôle of dietary factors, particularly the consumption of fats, in predisposing to endometrial cancer is suggested by the low incidence in Japan (Table 33.2) (Gusberg & Mulvihill 1986).

TUMOURS OF THE OVARY

In resource-poor countries in the tropics the whole range of ovarian tumours is seen, but the frequency and patterns differ from those in Europe and North America. The incidence of primary ovarian cancer is less, as is the total proportion of cancer among women that is ovarian (Table 33.2). This also applies to metastatic tumours, because of the lower incidence of gastrointestinal tract and breast cancers in these populations.

Ovarian tumours in blacks in Africa present a distinctive spectrum. Compared with the USA and Europe, epithelial tumours form a smaller proportion overall. Of these the proportion that are malignant (i.e. invasive plus borderline tumours) is greater, at around half of cases. Sex-cord and stromal tumours are more frequent (Dennis et al 1980; Lucas & Vella 1983). Germ cell tumours are more frequent, the great majority being mature cystic treatomas (Akang et al 1992). This frequency of cystic teratomas is probably a reflection of demography. Everywhere they are the commonest ovarian tumour in children and adolescents. Thus in African countries where half the population is 15 years or younger, their reported prevalence of about 40% of all ovarian tumours is hardly surprising.

In Asian countries, the data suggest that the patterns of ovarian tumours more resemble those found in industrialised countries (Ramachandran et al 1972; Verma & Bhatia 1980; Gatphoh & Darnal 1990) although the overall incidence of ovarian cancer is significantly less (Parkin et al 1988a).

In the USA, Caucasian females have a higher incidence of ovarian cancer than blacks, and reproductive factors do not account for this difference, suggesting there may be genetic factors (John et al 1993). Certain risk factors for ovarian cancer may explain some of the geographical variation: multiple pregnancies and interventions to reduce the number of ovulations protect against cancer, and everywhere the age-specific incidence increases to a peak in the sixth to eighth decades. Regarding the apparently different histogenetic patterns, the age-specific decline in incidence of sex-cord stromal and germ cell tumours with increasing age may be important (Yancik 1993). However, we await studies of ovarian tumours from different geographical centres, which stratify comparably according to histological type as well as for age, to provide further epidemiological evidence.

BURKITT'S LYMPHOMA (see also Chapter 28 for pathological description)

Prior to the classical account of Burkitt's lymphoma which described ovarian involvement as a common clinical feature (Burkitt 1958), there had been many reports of children with ovarian lymphosarcoma in several countries in Africa; in retrospect these were recognised to be the same tumour. Aetiologically, the predisposing factors for endemic Burkitt's lymphoma are early infection with Epstein–Barr virus and holoendemic falciparum malaria.

This lymphoma accounts for 68% of all childhood malignancies in the West Nile District of Uganda and for 47% in Ibadan, Nigeria (Parkin et al 1988b). Clinically, ovarian tumours are the commonest presenting feature in girls over the age of five years in endemic areas (Burkitt 1970). In Nigeria, in females under 20 years, Burkitt's lymphoma is the commonest neoplasm (55%) of the ovary (Junaid 1981).

GESTATIONAL TROPHOBLASTIC TUMOURS

The received wisdom is that the incidence of trophoblastic tumours — hydatidiform mole and choriocarcinoma — is greater in Africa and Asia (particularly among the Chinese) than in Caucasian populations. For example, choriocarcinoma comprised 2% of female cancers in Uganda (James et al 1973). However, there are considerable methodological problems in determining the population incidences of these tumours (Grimes 1984) and it is currently unclear whether there really are large regional differences. What is undoubted is that pathologists in resource-poor countries see more trophoblastic tumours than their counterparts in industrialised countries; their submitted specimens come from a larger population base and women there have more pregnancies.

Histologically, these tumours are no different from those in industrialised countries, except that the host inflammatory reaction to choriocarcinoma may be less marked. The types of pregnancy antecedent to choriocar-

cinoma and the time intervals before presentation with it appear to be similar everywhere. However, the mode of presentation of choriocarcinoma is more varied than in industrialised countries. Although vaginal bleeding is the commonest presenting sign (Makokha & Mati 1982), a tumour nodule in the vagina or vulva, or a haemorrhagic carcinoma anywhere in the body of a woman during reproductive life should be considered a choriocarcinoma until proved otherwise.

Autopsy series indicate the wide distribution of choriocarcinoma metastases, with lung, liver and brain as the commonest sites (Chapter 40). However, in the tropics, a metastasis is often the presenting feature. A clinical stroke, meningoencephalitis or cauda equina lesion may result from a deposit (Bahemuka 1981). Haematemesis and melaena from gastric or ileal metastases may be the first indication of tumour (Villet et al 1979). Other unusual presentations include a polyp in the finger (Fig. 33.30) and ejection of a tooth from the mandible by a deposit of choriocarcinoma (personal observations).

It is an impression that tubal mole and choriocarcinoma, very rare tumours in industrialised countries, are more common in the tropics, probably due to the high incidence of ectopic pregnancy.

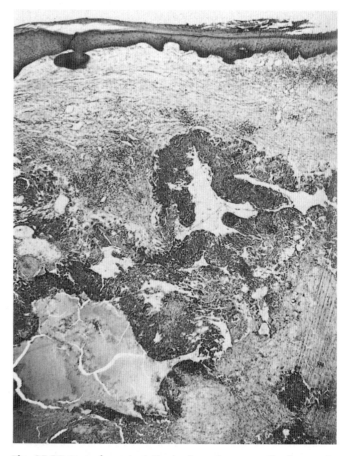

Fig. 33.30 Part of a metastatic choriocarcinoma on the finger of a 19-year-old female; it formed a polyp 4 cm in diameter.

OTHER DISEASE OF THE FEMALE GENITAL TRACT

ECTOPIC PREGNANCY

The incidence of ectopic pregnancy — whether expressed per total deliveries or pregnancies or per gynaecological admissions or per female surgical emergencies — is higher (up to three-fold) in resource-poor countries than in industrialised countries (Muir & Belsey 1980; Oronsaye & Odiase 1981). A recent survey in Ghana noted an ectopic pregnancy rate of 40/1000 deliveries; 98% presented with rupture and haemoperitoneum, and a high proportion had pelvic inflammatory disease and previous salpingitis; the mortality rate was 3% (Baffoe & Nkyekyer 1999). The high prevalence of unsafe abortion undoubtedly contributes (Kulczycki & Potts 1996).

Over 95% of these ectopic pregnancies are tubal; the proportion of abdominal pregnancies amongst total ectopic pregnancies appears to be similar in the USA and Africa at 1.5%. Thus 1 in 4000–5000 pregnancies in African women is abdominal (Paes 1981). Patients in the tropics with ectopic pregnancy are half as likely to be nulliparous compared with their counterparts in industrialised countries.

FEMALE CIRCUMCISION

The major form of female circumcision — infibulation — is practised in some Islamic cultures, and has many late complications in addition to the immediate sequelae of an unhygienically practised mutilating operation. Keloid scarring, abscess formation, implantation dermoid cysts and traumatic neuroma of the vulva are common. Haematocolpos and chronic urinary fistula also occur (McLean & Graham 1983; Dirie & Lindmark 1992). The complications during the delivery of babies are well known.

POSTPARTUM FISTULAE

A frequent complication of childbirth in resource-poor countries is fistula formation between the vagina and the bladder, and the vagina and the rectum. This results from compression necrosis when the fetus' head impacts against the symphysis pubis or the sacrum. Often the mother is a young teenager with immature pelvic proportions. The fistulae are permanent until effective surgery is performed. The pathology is of a chronically inflamed sinus tract with partial epithelialisation (Steiner 1996).

ADENOMYOSIS AND ENDOMETRIOSIS

Adenomyosis is only diagnosable after hysterectomy. Its prevalence among hysterectomy specimens in resource-poor countries (11–57%) appears similar to that in industrialised countries (Pendse 1981; Daisley 1987; Shaikh & Khan 1990).

For endometriosis, on the other hand, there are held to be significant ethnic and regional differences in its frequency. Reports from Jamaica, India and Nigeria all indicate that the prevalence of endometriosis at gynaecological laparoscopic or operative procedures is considerably less than that seen in industrialised countries (Pendse 1981; Rao & Persaud 1984; Osefo & Okele 1989). Personal experience of gynaecological material from Africa supports this impression, although rare cases of skin endometriosis are reported (Fahal & Yagi 1987). In contrast, endometriosis is more common in Asian women in Kuala Lumpur than in Caucasian women in the UK (Arumugam & Templeton 1992).

In fact, the descriptive epidemiology of endometriosis is unclear, due to the methodological problems of case definition and study populations (Mangtani & Booth 1993). Whether black women are genuinely less prone to endometriosis than Caucasian (a phenomenon not observed in private practice in the USA) or whether socioeconomic conditions may account for any real observed differences remain to be proved. The implication of immunological factors in the pathogenesis of endometriosis (Rock & Markham 1992), may also help to explain the apparent infrequency of the disease in Africa and other areas where the populations are subject to multiple chronic infections.

HIV, AIDS AND GYNAECOLOGICAL DISEASES

EPIDEMIOLOGY

Of the global total of more than 40 million adults and children infected with the human immunodeficiency viruses (HIV-1 and/or HIV-2), the great majority reside in resource-poor countries, half the adults are women, and most of them are of reproductive age (UNAIDS 2001). The modes of HIV transmission vary from country to country, but in poor countries in the tropics, it is overwhelmingly by heterosexual intercourse (Ancelle-Park & De Vincenzi 1993). Genital ulcer disease certainly predisposes to HIV infection (Grosskurth et al 2000), and it is possible that genital schistosomiasis also enhances male to female transmission (Poggensee & Feldmeier 2001).

Africa has borne the major brunt of this pandemic, and in some cities HIV prevalence among women of reproductive age is up to 32% (Allen et al 1991; UNAIDS 2001). Countries in Asia such as India, China, Burma, Vietnam and Thailand are now experiencing increasing transmission of HIV (Mann et al 1992, UNAIDS 2001). Through the development of acquired immunodeficiency syndrome (AIDS) with the large range of serious opportunistic infections and tumours, HIV infection contributes to premature mortality in women. Combined with the already high rate of maternal mortality in poor countries, it means that disease related to sexual behaviour is by far the major cause of adult female mortality in many tropical countries (De Cock et al 1990).

In Africa, women acquire HIV infection earlier than men, and the modal age at presentation with AIDS is the third decade (Mann et al 1992). Epidemiological studies have shown that in asymptomatic women who are not significantly immunocompromised, HIV infection has no consistent effect on the menstrual cycle or on fertility (Carpenter et al 1991; Ryder et al 1991). There appears to be a slight effect on the outcome of pregnancy, with increased frequency of spontaneous miscarriage, preterm labour and low birth weight among HIV-positive compared with HIV-negative women (Gichangi et al 1993; Johnstone 1993). Some of this may relate to the increased frequency of chorioamnionitis in HIV-positive women; this lesion is also associated with a greater likelihood of HIV-1 transmission to the fetus (St Louis et al 1993). There is no good evidence that pregnancy per se accelerates the course of HIV disease (Mandlebrot & Henrion 1993).

PATHOLOGY

The impact of HIV/AIDS on the pathology of the female genital tract is through the predisposition to, and worsening of, certain diseases of the female genital tract (Table 33.3) (Korn & Landers 1995).

Pelvic inflammatory disease is expected to be more frequent and more severe in HIV-positive women, given the bi-directional positive interactions of STDs and HIV infection (Laga et al 1991). Studies to prove this are still awaited (McCarthy & Norman 1993), and practical experience of African patients in the UK does not indicate a major problem. Genital ulcer diseases are more prevalent among HIV-positive than HIV-negative women. This is mainly due to herpes simplex and chancroid; in Africa, granuloma inguinale and lymphogranuloma venereum do not appear to contribute to the increase. HIV itself has been demonstrated in endometrial macrophages in an HIV-positive woman with chronic endometritis (Peuchmaur et al 1989); nonetheless endometritis is not a major problem, and endometrial atrophy is the norm in women dying of advanced HIV disease. Menstrual irregularity and amenorrhoea are frequent towards the end of the course of HIV disease.

Table 33.3 Associations of gynaecological disease with HIV infection; lesions known to be, or probably, more prevalent and severe in HIV-infected than in non-infected women

1. Fungal infections: vulvo-vaginal candidiasis
2. Viral infections: herpes simplex and zoster virus; human papillomaviruses
3. Bacterial infections: pelvic inflammatory disease; chorioamnionitis
4. Tumours: Kaposi's sarcoma; lymphoma; cervical neoplasia
5. Ulcers: vulvo-vaginal ulceration and fistula formation
6. Menstrual irregularity and endometritis

HIV infection is the most significant risk factor for the development of tuberculosis (De Cock et al 1992), and in countries in Africa where both infections are endemic, tuberculosis is the cause of death in more than 30% of HIV-positive adults (Lucas et al 1993). The adnexae are involved as part of miliary tuberculosis in HIV-positive women (personal observations), but there are no data demonstrating an increase in clinically significant gynaecological tuberculosis because of HIV infection.

Herpes zoster is reactivated by HIV infection, usually before an AIDS-defining diagnosis has occurred. It often affects multiple dermatomes and can involve the female genital area, producing painful ulceration which heals with a scar. Herpes simplex ulceration of more than one month's duration is an AIDS-defining disease and vulvar ulceration is seen among older children and adults with HIV infection (Fig. 33.31).

Vulvo-vaginal candidiasis is more frequent among HIV-positive compared with HIV-negative women, and may be more refractory to treatment. The severity appears to be inversely related to the patient's degree of immunocompetence as measured by blood CD4+ T-lymphocyte count (McCarthy & Norman 1993).

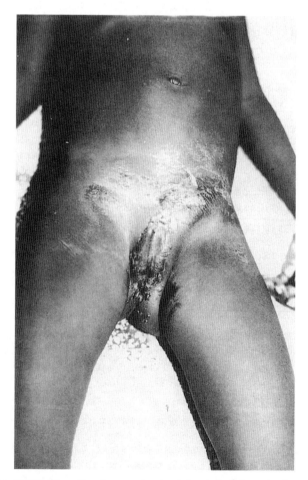

Fig. 33.31 Ulcerating herpes simplex infection of the vulva in a 6-year-old girl who died of HIV-associated disseminated herpes infection.

Although non-Hodgkin's lymphoma has a greatly augmented incidence in HIV-positive patients and tends to be extranodal, pelvic lymphoma has only occasionally been reported in HIV-positive women (Fineberg & Schinella 1990). In Africa, Burkitt's lymphoma of the ovary is not more frequent in HIV-positive children than in HIV-negative, probably because children who are infected with HIV perinatally do not usually survive beyond five years in resource-poor countries (Lucas et al 1994). The advent, since 1996, of powerful anti-retroviral therapy is prolonging the life of adults and perinatally infected children in industrialised countries, and therefore the pattern of opportunistic diseases including tumours; what impact if any this will have in poor countries remains to be seen. Kaposi's sarcoma can involve the epithelium of the lower genital tract and the adnexal surfaces.

VULVO-VAGINAL ULCERATION AND FISTULA FORMATION

Women and children with advanced HIV infection frequently develop ulceration of the vulva and vagina without definable cause (Andersen et al 1996; Bankole et al 1997). In addition to herpes infection, the differential diagnosis includes drug-related allergy, lymphoproliferative disease and lymphoma. Microbiology and serology are also helpful in excluding the standard bacterial genital ulcer diseases. The idiopathic ulcers are analogous to the aphthous oro-oesophageal ulcers encountered in HIV patients. However, they may progress to the formation of recto-vaginal and perineal–vaginal fistulae; steroid therapy has proved beneficial (Schuman et al 1996).

HIV, HPV AND CERVICAL NEOPLASIA

In 1993 the Centers for Disease Control and Prevention modified the surveillance case definition for AIDS in adolescents and adults. For HIV-positive women, the criteria for AIDS now include invasive carcinoma of the cervix. It should be noted that HIV-infected women who are asymptomatic, or who have persistent vulvo-vaginal candidiasis or pelvic inflammatory disease or cervical dysplasia, are also counted as having AIDS if the CD4+ T-lymphocyte count in the blood is $<200 \times 10^6/l$ (Centers for Disease Control and Prevention 1992). In the USA the addition of cervical cancer resulted in less than 1% of extra reported cases of AIDS in 1993 (Centers for Disease Control and Prevention 1993).

The associations of HIV with cervical neoplasia and HPVs are complex and are still being evaluated. There is no doubt that in both industrialised nations and countries in Africa, HIV seropositivity is associated with an increased prevalence of HPV infection (Kreiss et al 1992; Hankins et al 1994). The prevalence of HPV infection increases as the CD4+ T-lymphocyte count declines. In most, but not all, studies HIV-positive women have a higher prevalence of cervical intraepithelial neoplasia (CIN), with odds ratios of up to 14 (Laga et al 1992; Mandelblatt et al 1992). The prevalence of CIN also increases as CD4+ T-lymphocyte counts drop (LaGuardia 1993).

Cases of carcinoma of the cervix that progress with greater rapidity in HIV-positive patients are reported (Maiman et al 1990; Schwartz et al 1991). Experience in South Africa shows that HIV-infected patients with invasive cervical carcinoma present 10 years earlier than HIV-ve patients, and that those with CD4+ T-cell counts $<200 \times 10^6/l$ are more likely to have advanced stage disease at initial diagnosis (Lomalisa et al 2000).

What is not yet clear is whether HIV-positive women have a significantly higher incidence of invasive carcinoma compared with HIV-negative women; the epidemiological problem is that many of the risk factors for CIN are also risk factors for HIV infection. If the incidence of invasive disease is not greatly increased by HIV infection, it may be because the patients with CIN tend to die of other HIV-related disease before the tumour spreads. In USA there is evidence that the prevalence of invasive carcinoma is higher in those with HIV infection (Chin et al 1998), but information from tropical countries is less clear.

A recent autopsy study in Côte d'Ivoire found no invasive cervical cancer in HIV-positive or HIV-negative women (Lucas et al 1993). Cancer registry data from Uganda show a progressive increase in the incidence of cancer of the cervix since the 1950s, but a causative association with HIV infection has not been found (Wabinga et al 1993; Newton et al 2001). In Zambia, where HIV infection is also epidemic, there has been no change in the incidence or age distribution of cervical cancer over the decade since 1980 (Rabkin & Blattner 1991). A study of cervical cancer patients in Kenya, performed early on in the epidemic, found no increased prevalence of HIV infection compared with the non-cancer female population (Rogo & Kavoo-Linge 1990). The Zimbabwe cancer registry does not indicate an increased incidence in cervical cancer up to 1995 (Chokunonga et al 2000). However, in South Africa a small relative risk of cervical carcinoma associated with HIV (relative risk = 1.2) has been documented (Sitas et al 2000).

Natural history studies of HIV infection and cervical neoplasia in tropical resource-poor countries are being done, and if the length of survival with HIV infection increases, cervical cancer may become more prominent. At present, however, there seems little prospect of the universal availability of cervical screening that is advocated for HIV-positive women in industrialised countries (Hankins et al 1994).

Acknowledgements

The late Professor Michael Hutt co-authored the earliest edition of this chapter. Much of his years of experience of pathology in Africa and his wisdom has been retained in the later versions.

REFERENCES

Agranal S, Bausal M P 1981 Amoebiasis of the uterine cervix and vagina mimicking carcinoma. Journal of Obstetrics and Gynaecology of India 31: 153–154

Akang E E, Odunfa A O, Aghadiuno P U 1992 Childhood teratomas in Ibadan, Nigeria. Human Pathology 23: 449–453

Al-Adnani M S, Saleh K M 1982 Extraurinary schistosomiasis in Southern Iraq. Histopathology 6: 747–752

Allen S, Lindan C P, Serufilira A et al 1991 Human immunodeficiency virus infection in urban Rwanda. Journal of the American Medical Association 266: 1657–1663

Ancelle-Park R, De Vincenzi I 1993 Epidemiology and natural history of HIV/AIDS in women. In: Johnson M A, Johnstone F D (eds) HIV infection in women. Churchill Livingstone, Edinburgh, pp 1–15

Anderson J, Clark R A, Watts D H et al 1996 Idiopathic genital ulcers in women infected with HIV. Journal of the Acquired Immune Deficiency Syndrome 13: 343–347

Arroyo G, Elgueta R 1989 Squamous cell carcinoma associated with amoebic cervicitis. Acta Cytologica 33: 301–304

Arroyo G, Quinn J A 1989 Association of amoebae and *Actinomyces* in an intrauterine contraceptive device user. Acta Cytologica 3: 298–300

Arumugam K, Templeton A A 1992 Endometriosis and race. Australian and New Zealand Journal of Obstetrics and Gynaecology 32: 164–165

Attili V R, Hira S K, Dube M K 1983 Schistosomal genital granulomas: a report of 10 cases. British Journal of Venereal Diseases 59: 269–272

Bac D J, Teichler M J, Jonker L C, van der Merwe C F 1987 Schistosomiasis in ectopic or unusual sites, a report of 5 cases. South African Medical Journal 72: 717–718

Baffoe S, Nkyekyer K 1999 Ectopic pregnancy in Korle Bu Teaching Hospital, Ghana: a 3 year review. Tropical Doctor 29: 18–22

Bahemuka M 1981 Neurological complications of choriocarcinoma at Kenyatta National Hospital. East African Medical Journal 58: 117–123

Bang R A, Bang A T, Baitule M, Choudhary Y, Sarmukaddam S, Tale O 1989 High prevalence of gynaecological diseases in rural Indian women. Lancet 1: 85–88

Bankole Sanni R, Denoulet C, Coulibaly B, Mobiot M L, Anglaret X, Sylla-Koko F 1997 Acquired recto-vaginal fistula in children: is HIV infection a cause? Bulletin de la Societé de Pathologie Exotique 90: 111–112

Bazaz-Malik G, Maheshwari B, Lal N 1983 Tuberculous endometritis: a clinicopathological study of 1000 cases. British Journal of Obstetrics and Gynaecology 90: 84–86

Berry A 1966 A cytopathological and histopathological study of bilharziasis of the female genital tract. Journal of Pathology and Bacteriology 91: 325–338

Bhagavan B S, Ruffier J, Shinn B 1982 Pseudoactinomycotic radiate granules in the lower female genital tract: relationship to Splendore-Hoeppli phenomenon. Human Pathology 13: 898–904

Bhagwandeen S B, Mottiar Y A 1972 Granuloma venereum. Journal of Clinical Pathology 25: 812–816

Bhagwandeen S B, Naik K G 1977 Granuloma venereum (granuloma inguinale) in Zambia. East African Medical Journal 54: 637–642

Bickers W M 1970 Hydatid disease of the female pelvis. American Journal of Obstetrics and Gynecology 107: 477–483

Bittencourt A L, de Almeida M A C, Junes M A F, da Motta L D C 1980 Placental involvement in schistosomiasis mansoni: report of four cases. American Journal of Tropical Medicine and Hygiene 29: 571–575

Blickstein I, Dgani R, Lifschitz-Mercer B 1993 Cutaneous leishmaniasis of the vulva. International Journal of Obstetrics & Gynaecology 42: 46–47

Braithwaite A R, Figueroa J P, Ward E 1997 A comparison of prevalence rates of genital ulcers among persons attending a sexually transmitted disease clinic in Jamaica. West Indian Medical 46: 67–71

Burkitt D P 1958 A sarcoma involving the jaws in African children. British Journal of Surgery 46: 218–223

Burkitt D P 1970 General features and facial tumours: lesions outside the jaws. In: Burkitt D P, Wright D H (eds) Burkitt's lymphoma. Livingstone, Edinburgh, pp 6–16

Carpenter C C J, Mayer K H, Stein M D, Leibman B D, Fisher A, Fiore T C 1991 Human immunodeficiency virus infection in North American women: experience with 200 cases and a review of the literature. Medicine 70: 307–325

Centers for Disease Control and Prevention 1992–1993 revised classification system for HIV infection and expanded surveillance case definition for AIDS among adolescents and adults. Morbidity and Mortality Weekly Report 41 [RR-17]: 1–19

Centers for Disease Control and Prevention 1993 Impact of the expanded AIDS surveillance case definition on AIDS case reporting — United States, First Quarter, 1993. Morbidity and Mortality Weekly Report 42: 308–310

Chandler F W, Kaplan W, Ajello L 1980 A color atlas and text of the histopathology of mycotic diseases. Wolfe Medical, London

Cheever A W, Kamel I A, Elwi A M, Mosimann J E, Danner R 1977 *Schistosoma mansoni* and *Schistosoma haematobium* infections in Egypt. II. Quantitative parasitological findings at necropsy. American Journal of Tropical Medicine and Hygiene 26: 702–716

Chen M G, Mott K E 1989 Progress in assessment of morbidity due to *Schistosoma haematobium* infection: a review of recent literature. Tropical Diseases Bulletin 86: R1–R36

Chin K M, Sidhu J S, Janssen R S, Weber J T 1998 Invasive cervical cancer in HIV-infected and uninfected hospital patients. Obstetrics and Gynecology 92: 83–85

Chokunonga E, Levy L M, Bassett M T, Mauchaza B G, Thomas D B, Parkin D M 2000 Cancer incidence in the African population of Harare, Zimbabwe: second results from the cancer registry 1993–1995. International Journal of Cancer 85: 54–59

Connor D H, Chandler F W 1996 Pathology of infectious diseases. Appleton & Lange, New York

Daisley H 1987 Adenomyosis uteri: a prospective study in Trinidad & Tobago (January–May 1986) West Indian Medical Journal 36: 166–173

Das B C, Murthy N S, Sharma J K et al 1989 Human papillomavirus and cervical cancer in Indian women. Lancet 2: 1271

De Cock K M, Barrere B, Diaby et al 1990 AIDS — the leading cause of adult death in the West African city of Abidjan, Côte d'Ivoire. Science 249: 793–796

De Cock K M, Soro B, Coulibaly I-M, Lucas S B 1992 Tuberculosis and HIV infection in sub-Saharan Africa. Journal of the American Medical Association 268: 1581–1587

Dennis P M, Coode P E, Hulewicz B S F, Kung'u A 1980 Comparative study of ovarian neoplasms in Kenya and Britain. East African Medical Journal 57: 562–565

Dirie M A, Lindmark G 1992 The risk of medical complications after female circumcision. East African Medical Journal 69: 479–482

Duncan M E, Tibaux G, Pelzer A et al 1990 First coitus before menarche and risk of sexually transmitted disease. Lancet 335: 338–340

Edington G M, Nwabuebo I, Junaid T A 1975 The pathology of schistosomiasis in Ibadan, Nigeria with special reference to the appendix, brain, pancreas and genital organs. Transactions of the Royal Society of Tropical Medicine and Hygiene 69: 153–162

El-Mahgoub S 1982 Pelvic schistosomiasis and infertility. International Journal of Gynaecology and Obstetrics 20: 201–206

Fahal A H, Yagi K I 1987 Skin endometriosis in Sudan. Tropical and Geographical Medicine 39: 383–384

Farooki M A 1967 Epidemiology and pathology of chronic endometritis. International Surgery 48: 566–573

Fineberg S A, Schinella R 1990 Human immunodeficiency virus infection in women: report of 102 cases. Modern Pathology 3: 575–580

Freinkel A L 1987 Histological aspects of sexually transmitted genital lesions. Histopathology 11: 819–831

Freinkel A L 1988 Granuloma inguinale of cervical lymph nodes simulating tuberculous lymphadenitis: two case reports and review of the literature. Genitourinary Medicine 64: 339–343

Frost O 1975 Bilharziasis of the Fallopian tube. South African Medical Journal 49: 1201–1203

Gatphoh E D, Darnal H K 1990 Pattern of ovarian neoplasm in Manipur. Journal of the Indian Medical Association 88: 338–339

Gichangi P B, Nyongo A O, Temmerman M 1993 Pregnancy outcome and placental weights: their relationship to HIV-1 infection. East African Medical Journal 70: 85–89

Graham W J 1991 Maternal mortality: levels, trends, and data deficiencies. In: Feachem R G, Jamison D T (eds) Disease and mortality in sub-Saharan Africa. World Bank/OUP, Oxford, pp 101–116

Grech E S, Everett J V, Mukasa F 1973 Epidemiological aspects of acute pelvic inflammatory disease in Uganda. Tropical Doctor 3: 123–127

Grimes D A 1984 Epidemiology of gestational trophoblastic disease. American Journal of Obstetrics and Gynecology 150: 309–318

Grosskurth H, Gray R, Hayes R, Mabey D, Mawer D 2000 Control of sexually transmitted diseases for HIV-1 prevention. Lancet 355: 1981–1987

Gusberg S B, Mulvihill M N 1986 Epidemiology [endometrial cancer]. Clinics in Obstetrics and Gynecology 13: 665–672

Haibach H, Bickel J T, Podrecca G I, Llorens A S 1985 Squamous cell carcinoma of the uterine cervix subsequent to amebiasis. Archives of Pathology and Laboratory Medicine 109: 1121–1123

Hangval H, Habibi H, Moshref A, Rahimi A 1979 Case report of an ovarian hydatid cyst. Journal of Tropical Medicine & Hygiene 82: 34–35

Hankins C A, Lamont J A, Handley M A 1994 Cervicovaginal screening in women with HIV infection: a need for increased vigilance? Canadian Medical Association Journal 150: 681–686

Hiller N, Zagal I, Hadas-Halpern I 2000 Echinococcal ovarian cyst. A case report. Journal of Reproductive Medicine 45: 224–226

James P D, Taylor C W, Templeton A C 1973 Tumours of the female genitalia. In: Templeton A C (ed) Tumours in a tropical country. Heinemann, London, pp 101–131

Jamkhedkar P P, Hira S K, Shroff H J, Lanjewar D N 1998 Clinico-epidemiologic features of granuloma inguinale in the era of AIDS. Sexually Transmitted Infections 25: 196–200

John E M, Whittemore A S, Harris R, Itnyre J, Collaborative Ovarian Cancer Group 1993 Characteristics relating to ovarian cancer risk: collaborative analysis of seven US case control studies. Epithelial cancer in black women. Journal of the National Cancer Institute 85: 142–146

Johnstone F D 1993 Pregnancy outcome and pregnancy management in HIV-infected women. In: Johnson M A, Johnstone F D (eds) HIV infection in women. Churchill Livingstone, Edinburgh, pp 187–199

Junaid T A 1981 Ovarian neoplasms in children and adolescents in Ibadan. Cancer 47: 610–614

Kapila K, Verma K 1981 Adenocarcinoma of the endometrium — a clinicopathological study. Journal of Obstetrics and Gynaecology of India 31: 538–542

Khan J S, Stell R J C 1981 *Enterobius vermicularis* infestation of the female genital tract causing generalised peritonitis. British Journal of Obstetrics and Gynaecology 88: 681–683

Korn A P, Landers D V 1995 Gynecologic disease in women infected with HIV-1. Journal of Acquired Immune Deficiency Syndromes and Human Retrovirology 9: 361–367

Kreiss J K, Kiviat N B, Plummer F A et al 1992 Human immunodeficiency virus, human papilloma virus, and cervical intraepithelial neoplasia in Nairobi prostitutes. Sexually Transmitted Diseases 19: 54–59

Kulczycki A, Potts M 1996 Abortion and fertility regulation. Lancet 347: 1663–1668

Kushtagi P, Rao K 1991 Primary adenocarcinoma of the uterine cervix: changing clinical profile. Australian and New Zealand Journal of Obstetrics and Gynaecology 31: 86

Laga M, Nzila N, Goeman J 1991 The interrelationship of sexually transmitted diseases and HIV infection: implications for the control of both epidemics in Africa. AIDS 5 (suppl 1): S55–S63

Laga M, Icenogle J P, Marsella R et al 1992 Genital papillomavirus infection and cervical dysplasia — opportunistic complications of HIV infection. International Journal of Cancer 50: 45–48

LaGuardia K D 1993 Other sexually transmitted disease: cervical intraepithelial neoplasia. In: Johnson M A, Johnstone F D (eds) HIV infection in women. Churchill Livingstone, Edinburgh, pp 247–261

Lansman H H, Lapin A, Blaustein A 1960 Pelvic *Oxyuris* granuloma associated with endometriosis. American Journal of Obstetrics and Gynecology 79: 1178–1180

Liomba N G, Chiphangwi J D 1982 Female genital tuberculosis in Malawi: a report of 90 cases. Journal of Obstetrics and Gynaecology of Eastern and Central Africa 1: 69–72

Liomba N G, Castro F, Chiphangwi J D 1982 Chronic endometritis in Malawi: a report of 112 cases. Journal of Obstetrics and Gynaecology of Eastern and Central Africa 1: 117–120

Liskin L S 1980 Complications of abortion in developing countries. Population Reports 8. Johns Hopkins University, Baltimore, pp 105–155

Lomalisa P, Smith T, Guidozzi F 2000 HIV infection and invasive cervical cancer in South Africa. Gynecologic Oncology 77: 460–463

Lowe D, Jorizzo J, Chiphangwi J D, Hutt M S R 1981 Cervical carcinoma in Malawi: a histopathologic study of 460 cases. Cancer 47: 2493–2495

Lucas S B 1992 Pathology of tropical infections. In: McGee J O'D, Isaacson P G, Wright N A (eds) Oxford textbook of pathology. OUP, Oxford, pp 2187–2266

Lucas S B, Vella E J 1983 Ovarian tumours in Malawi — a histopathological study. Journal of Obstetrics and Gynaecology of Eastern and Central Africa 2: 97–101

Lucas S B, Mati J K G, Aggarwal V P, Sanghvi H C G 1983 The pathology of perinatal mortality in Nairobi, Kenya. Bulletin de la Societe de Pathologie Exotique 76: 579–583

Lucas S B, Hounnou A, Peacock C S et al 1993 The mortality and pathology of HIV disease in a West African city. AIDS 7: 1569–1579

Lucas S B, Diomande M, Honnou A et al 1994 HIV-associated lymphoma in Africa: an autopsy study in Côte d'Ivoire. International Journal of Cancer 59: 20–24

McCarthy K H, Norman S G 1993 Gynaecological problems in women infected with the human immunodeficiency virus. In: Johnson M A, Johnstone F D (eds) HIV infection in women. Churchill Livingstone, Edinburgh, pp 263–268

McLean S, Graham S E 1983 Female circumcision, excision and infibulation: the facts and proposals for change. Report No. 47, Minority Rights Group Ltd, London

Mahler H 1987 The safe motherhood initiative: a call to action. Lancet 1: 668–670

Maiman M, Fruchter R G, Serur E, Remy J C, Feuer G, Boyce J 1990 Human immunodeficiency virus infection and cervical neoplasia. Gynecologic Oncology 38: 377–382

Makokha A E, Mati J K G 1982 Choriocarcinoma at Kenyatta National Hospital 1973–79. Journal of Obstetrics and Gynaecology of Eastern and Central Africa 1: 27–31

Mandelblatt J S, Fahs M, Garibaldi K, Senie R T, Peterson H B 1992 Association between HIV infection and cervical neoplasia: implications for clinical care of women at risk for both conditions. AIDS 6: 173–178

Mandell G L, Bennett J E, Dolin R 2000 Principles and practice of infectious diseases, 5th edn. Churchill Livingstone, New York

Mandlebrot L, Henrion R 1993 Does pregnancy accelerate disease progression in HIV-infected women? In: Johnson M A, Johnstone F D (eds) HIV infection in women. Churchill Livingstone, Edinburgh, pp 157–171

Mangtani P, Booth M 1993 Epidemiology of endometriosis. Journal of Epidemiology and Community Health 47: 84–88

Mann J M, Tarantola D J M, Netter T W 1992 AIDS in the world. Harvard University Press, Cambridge, Mass

Mawad N M, Hassanein O M, Mahmoud O M, Taylor M G 1992 Schistosomal vulval granuloma in a 12 years old Sudanese girl. Transactions of the Royal Society of Tropical Medicine and Hygiene 86: 644

Mein J, Russell C, Knox J, Coppola A, Bowden F K 1999 Intrapelvic donovanosis presenting as a psoas abcess in two patients. Sexually Transmitted Infections 75: 75–76

Meyers W M, Neafie R C, Marty A M, Wear D J (eds) 2000 Pathology of Infectious Diseases, vol 1 Helminthiases. Armed Forces Institute of Pathology, Washington DC

Most H, Gellin G A, yager R, Aron B, Friedlander M, Quarfordt S 1963 Enterobiasis (pinworm infection): a study of 951 Puerto Rican and 315 non-Puerto Rican children in New York City. American Journal of Tropical Medicine and Hygiene 12: 65–68

Moubayed P, Ziehe A, Peters J, Mwakhyoma H, Schmidt D 1995 Carcinoma of the uterine cervix associated with schistosomiasis and induced by human papillomaviruses. International Journal of Obstetrics & Gynaecology 49: 175–179

Muir D G, Belsey M A 1980 Pelvic inflammatory disease and its consequences in the developing world. American Journal of Obstetrics and Gynecology 138: 913–928

Mylius R E, Ten Seldam R E 1962 Venereal infection by *Entamoeba histolytica* in a New Guinea native couple. Tropical and Geographical Medicine 14: 20–26

Newton R, Ziegler J, Beral V et al 2001 A case-control study of HIV infection and cancer in adults and children residing in Kampala, Uganda. International Journal of Cancer 92: 622–627

Nopdonrattakon L 1996 Amoebiasis of the female genital tract: a case report. Journal of Obstetrics & Gynaecology Research 22: 235–238

Ojwang S B O, Mati J K G 1978 Carcinoma of the cervix in Kenya. East African Medical Journal 55: 194–198

Ong H C 1974 An unusual case of pentastomiasis of the Fallopian tube in an Aborigine woman. Journal of Tropical Medicine and Hygiene 77: 187–189

Oronsaye A U, Odiase G I 1981 Incidence of ectopic pregnancy in Benin City, Nigeria. Tropical Doctor 11: 160–163

Osefo N J, Okele B C 1989 Endometriosis: incidence among the Igbos of Nigeria. International Journal of Gynecology and Obstetrics 30: 349–353

Paes E H J 1981 Advanced abdominal pregnancy: case report and review of the recent literature. East African Medical Journal 58: 142–147

Parkin D M, Läärä E, Muir C S 1988a Estimates of the worldwide frequency of sixteen major cancers in 1980. International Journal of Cancer 41: 184–197

Parkin D M, Stiller C A, Draper G J, Bieber C A 1988b The international incidence of childhood cancer. International Journal of Cancer 42: 511–520

Pendse V 1981 Adenomyosis uteri. Journal of the Indian Medical Association 76: 75–77

Peuchmaur M, Emilie D, Vazeux R et al 1989 HIV-associated endometritis. AIDS 3: 239–241

Phillips S C, Mildran D, William D C 1981 Sexual transmission of enteric protozoa and helminths in a venereal disease clinic population. New England Journal of Medicine 305: 603–605

Poggensee G, Feldmeier H 2001 Female genital schistosomiasis: facts and hypotheses. Acta Tropica 79: 193–210

Qunhua L, Jiaven Z, Bozhao L et al 2000 Investigation of association between female genital tract diseases and schistosomiasis japonicum infection. Acta Tropica 77: 179–183

Rabkin C S, Blattner W A 1991 HIV infection and cancers other than non-Hodgkin lymphoma and Kaposi's sarcoma. In: Beral V, Jaffe H W, Weiss R A (eds) Cancer, HIV and AIDS. Cold Spring Harbour Laboratory Press, New York, pp 151–160

Rahman M S, Rahman J, Lysikiewicz A 1982 Obstetric and gynaecological presentations of hydatid disease. British Journal of Obstetrics and Gynaecology 89: 665–670

Ramachandran G, Harilal K R, Chinnamma K K, Thangavelu H 1972 Ovarian neoplasms — a study of 903 cases. Journal of Obstetrics and Gynaecology of India 22: 309–315

Ramdial P K, Kharsany A B, Reddy R, Chetty R 2000 Transepithelial elimination of cutaneous granuloma inguinale. Journal of Cutaneous Pathology 27: 493–499

Rao B N, Persaud V 1984 Endometriosis in Jamaica: report on a 15-year study at the University Hospital of the West Indies (1968–1982). West Indian Medical Journal 33: 36–44

Ravdin J I (ed) 2000 Amebiasis. Tropical medicine, Science and practice, vol 2. Imperial College Press, London

Reeves W C, Brinton L A, Garcia M et al 1989 Human papilloma virus infection and cervical cancer in Latin America. New England Journal of Medicine 320: 1437–1441

Renaud G, Devidas A, Develoux M, Lamothe F, Bianchi G 1989 Prevalence of vaginal schistosomiasis caused by *Schistosoma haematobium* in an endemic village in Niger. Transactions of the Royal Society of Tropical Medicine and Hygiene 83: 797

Rock J A, Markham S M 1992 Pathogenesis of endometriosis. Lancet 340: 1264–1267

Rogo K O, Kavoo-Linge 1990 Human immunodeficiency virus seroprevalence among cervical cancer patients. Gynecologic Oncology 37: 87–92

Ryder R W, Batter V L, Nsuami M et al 1991 Fertility rates in 238 HIV-1-seropositive women in Zaire followed for 3 years post-partum. AIDS 5: 1521–1527

St Louis M E, Kamenga M, Brown C et al 1993 Risk for perinatal HIV-1 transmission according to maternal, immunologic, virologic, and placental factors. Journal of the American Medical Association 269: 2853–2859

Schmauz R, Okong R, de Villiers E-M et al 1989 Multiple infections in cases of cervical cancer from a high incidence area in tropical Africa.

International Journal of Cancer 43: 805–809

Schuman P, Christensen, Sobel J D 1996 Aphthous vaginal ulceration in two women with AIDS. American Journal of Obstetrics & Gynecology 174: 1660–1663

Schwartz L B, Carcangiu M L, Bradham L, Schwartz P E 1991 Rapidly progressive squamous cell carcinoma of the cervix coexisting with human immunodeficiency virus infection: clinical opinion. Gynecologic Oncology 41: 255–258

Scott R A, Gallis H A, Livengood C H 1985 Phycomycosis of the vulva. American Journal of Obstetrics & Gynecology 153: 675–676

Sengupta S K, Das N 1984 Donovanosis affected cervix, uterus, and adnexae. American Journal of Tropical Medicine and Hygiene 33: 632–636

Shaikh H, Khan K S 1990 Adenomyosis in Pakistani women: four year experience at the Aga Khan University Medical Centre, Karachi. Journal of Clinical Pathology 43: 817–819

Sinniah B, Leopairut J, Neafie R C, Connor D H, Voge M 1991 Enterobiasis: a histopathological study of 259 patients. Annals of Tropical Medicine and Parasitology 85: 625–635

Sitas F, Pacella-Norman B, Carrara H et al 2000 The spectrum of HIV-1 related cancers in South Africa. International Journal of Cancer 88: 489–492

Spice W M, Ackers J P 1992 The amoeba enigma. Parasitology Today 8: 402–406

Steiner A K 1996 The problems of post-partum fistulas in developing countries. Acta Tropica 62: 217–223

Sun T, Schwartz N S, Sewell C, Lieberman P, Gross S 1991 Enterobius egg granuloma of the vulva and peritoneum; review of the literature. American Journal of Tropical Medicine and Hygiene 45: 249–253

Symmers W St C 1960 Leishmaniasis acquired by contagion: a case of marital infection in Britain. Lancet i: 127–132

Tiboldi T 1978 Involvement of human and primate ovaries in schistosomiasis: a review of the literature. Annales de la Societé Belge de Medecine Tropicale 58: 9–20

UNAIDS 2001 AIDS Epidemic Update. Updated every six months on website www.unaids.org

Verma K, Bhatia A 1980 Ovarian neoplasm: a study of 403 tumours. Journal of Obstetrics and Gynaecology of India 30: 106–111

Villet W T, du Toit D F, Conroy C 1979 Unusual presentation of choriocarcinoma. South African Medical Journal 55: 96–98

Wabinga H R, Parkin D M, Wabwire-Mangen F, Mugerwa J W 1993 Cancer in Kampala, Uganda, in 1989–91; changes in incidence in the era of AIDS. International Journal of Cancer 54: 26–36

WHO 1993 The control of schistosomiasis. Second report of the WHO expert committee. WHO, Geneva

WHO 2000 World Health Organisation, Geneva: data on website *www.who.org*

World Bank 1993 World development report 1993. Investing in Health. Oxford University Press, Oxford

Wright E D, Chiphangwi J D, Hutt M S R 1982 Schistosomiasis of the female genital tract: a histopathological study of 176 cases from Malawi. Transactions of the Royal Society of Tropical Medicine and Hygiene 76: 822–829

Yancik R 1993 Ovarian cancer: age contrasts in incidence, histology, disease stage at diagnosis, and mortality. Cancer 71 (suppl 2): 517–523

Youssef A F, Fayad M M, Shafeek M A 1970 Bilharziasis of the cervix uteri. Journal of Obstetrics & Gynaecology of the British Commonwealth. 19: 669–671

34

Pathology of the female genital tract and ovaries in childhood and adolescence

A. M. Kelsey   M. J. Newbould

Introduction   1157

Developmental disorders of the gonads and genital tract   1157
Development of the gonads, urogenital tract and perineum   1157
Anomalies of the genital tract and perineum   1158
Sexual ambiguity in the newborn child   1158

Non-neoplastic lesions of the ovary in childhood   1162
Torsion of the uterine adnexa where there is no tumour   1163

Miscellaneous, non-neoplastic disease of the genital tract in childhood and adolescence   1163

Pregnancy in childhood and adolescence   1163

Neoplasms of the female genital tract and ovaries in childhood and adolescence   1163
The pattern of disease   1163
Germ cell tumours   1164
Sex cord–stromal tumours of the ovary   1169
Mixed germ cell sex cord–stromal tumours   1172
Mesenchymal neoplasms   1172
Epithelial tumours   1174
Miscellaneous neoplasms   1175

INTRODUCTION

Most of the information in this chapter can be found scattered throughout the rest of this volume. The aim of this chapter is, however, to collect together these widely disseminated pieces of information so as to give an indication of how gynaecological disorders present to pathologists working in a children's hospital and to give non-paediatric pathologists, who may well encounter a gynaecological lesion in an unexpectedly young patient, a concise overview of gynaecological disease in childhood and adolescence.

DEVELOPMENTAL DISORDERS OF THE GONADS AND GENITAL TRACT

DEVELOPMENT OF THE GONADS, UROGENITAL TRACT AND PERINEUM

Initially both genders share a common genital development and a common undifferentiated gonad (Lauchlan & Pinar 1998). Germ cells migrate to the gonad from the yolk sac and this has the effect of inducing formation of genital ridges by the metanephroi and adjacent coelomic epithelium. The coelomic mesothelium proliferates and projections grow into the developing gonadal ridges to form sex cords. At 44 days following ovulation the gonads show divergent differentiation into either ovary or testis (Lauchlan & Pinar 1998). Male gonadal sex is governed by the presence of the Y chromosome which contains a gene which determines testis development, previously known as the testis-determining factor (TDF) and now known as the *SRY* gene, which encodes a testis-specific transcript highly conserved within mammals (Berta et al 1990; Gubbay et al 1990; Sinclair et al 1990). The male phenotypic gender develops under the influence of hormones produced by the gonad (Lauchlan & Pinar 1998).

Traditionally, it was thought that female gender differentiation was an essentially passive process mediated by the absence of androgens and Müllerian inhibitory substance, but the demonstration that some 46,XY individuals with male to female sex reversal have duplication of a locus on the short arm of the X chromosome — called the *DSS* (dosage-sensitive sex reversal) gene (Lauchlan & Pinar 1998), suggests otherwise. In the absence of the *SRY* gene and the presence of the *DSS* gene, paired structures, the para-mesonephric (Müllerian) ducts, form the lining of the Fallopian tubes, the endometrium, the endocervical epithelium and, possibly, part of the vagina. By the eighth to ninth week, the caudal parts of the ducts lie in close apposition and fuse to form a uterovaginal canal. The fusion is initially partial with a dividing septum. The smooth muscle of these structures differentiates from the urogenital ridge and the serosa from the coelomic epithelium. The vagina develops as a solid cord initially, and results from the fusion of cells growing downwards from the tip of the uterovaginal canal with a cord of endodermal cells growing upwards from the urogenital sinus. The cord is canalised, with the hymen representing the site of fusion between the two cell cords (Huffman et al 1981; Lauchlan & Pinar 1998).

Many of the Müllerian anomalies encountered can be explained in terms of different degrees of failure of fusion or canalisation of the Müllerian ducts. For example, persistence of the septum between the ducts or atresia of the lower part of one or other ducts or of the urogenital endoderm results in duplications, unilateral or bilateral developmental failure, respectively.

In early embryonic development, the ducts from the primitive kidney and the hindgut open into a common channel, the cloaca. Further development requires septation of the cloaca into an anterior urogenital sinus and a posterior anorectum. Caudally, the fusion of endoderm and ectoderm without the interposition of mesoderm results in the formation of the cloacal membrane, which later perforates to form the perineum and anal openings. There is a wide range of possible malformations.

ANOMALIES OF THE GENITAL TRACT AND PERINEUM

Many anomalies present during the reproductive years with obstetric problems. Disorders presenting during the perinatal period or childhood are amongst the more severe or form one part of a lethal malformation syndrome or sequence.

Imperforate hymen

This may present in the neonate with hydrometrocolpos, in which the vagina above the obstruction and the uterus become severely distended due to the presence of mucoid secretions, or it may present during adolescence with haematocolpos (Huffman et al 1981).

Vaginal atresia

This occurs in one in approximately 4000–5000 births (Lauchlan & Pinar 1998). It can present in a similar way to imperforate hymen, but may also be one of a lethal constellation of malformations.

Perineal abnormalities

The most severe of these is cloacal dysgenesis sequence in which the usual fusion of endoderm and ectoderm at the caudal end of the embryo is prevented by the interposition of mesoderm. In its most complete form there is a complete absence of anal, genital and urinary orifices in the perineum (Liang et al 1998). This results in dilatation of the viscera that usually open into the perineum and there may be megacolon, hydrometrocolpos, megacystis, megaureter, renal dysplasia and prune belly (Lauchlan & Pinar 1998).

There are a large number of possible varieties of malformations which represent lesser degrees of cloacal membrane and cloacal anomalies; anovestibular fistula in which the anal opening is absent but the distal large bowel opens into the lower vagina is said to be the commonest of these in the female (DeSa 1998).

The vagina and uterus may also be the site into which an ectopic ureter drains and this anomaly may present during childhood with incontinence (Huffman et al 1981).

Genital tract anomalies associated with malformation syndromes

Genital tract abnormalities are closely associated with anomalies of the renal tract. Any form of complete lower renal tract obstruction, which, as explained above, can often be associated with generalised perineal anomalies, will almost certainly be associated with renal dysplasia. There is a familial form of renal agenesis, inherited as an autosomal dominant, in which Müllerian abnormalities form an integral part (Biedel et al 1984). However, genital tract malformations may also be seen in non-familial renal agenesis (Duncan et al 1979) so that family studies are often required to distinguish the familial form.

Vaginal atresia and hydrometrocolpos may be seen in association with cryptophthalmos, syndactyly and multiple organ atresia in the autosomal recessive Fraser's syndrome (Gilbert-Barness & Opitz 1998a).

Chromosomal anomalies, such as trisomy 18 or trisomy 13, often include Müllerian abnormalities as one of the features (Gilbert-Barness & Opitz 1998b).

SEXUAL AMBIGUITY IN THE NEWBORN CHILD

The commonest cause in the newborn is congenital adrenal hyperplasia. In this condition, the genotype is 46, XX and the gonads are ovaries. There is a deficiency of one of the several enzymes involved in cortisol synthesis with resulting accumulation of androgenic intermediate metabolites. In the female the increased androgen to which the fetus is exposed results in varying degrees of masculinisation of the external genitalia, though not the internal organs (Scully 1991). Several functional maternal ovarian lesions, such as pregnancy luteoma, may also lead to masculinisation of a female fetus (Scully 1991). Other disorders associated with sexual ambiguity are considered below with other developmental disorders of the gonads.

Developmental abnormalities of the ovary

Very rarely, there may be bilateral or unilateral agonadism or accessory gonads due to abnormalities of germ cell migration (Kini et al 1998; Lauchlan & Pinar 1998).

Turner's syndrome

This condition results from a variety of abnormalities in one or more areas on the X chromosome which are necessary for the development and function of normal ovaries. The most common karyotype is 45,XO (Fig. 34.1), but some cases are mosaics, for example 45, XO/46,XX or other forms with additional X-chromosomes or ring and dicentric chromosomes. The majority of 45,XO fetuses, probably more than 95%, are aborted early in pregnancy and only 1 in 2500 female live births have this karyotype (Gilbert-Barness & Opitz 1998b). Only 50% of patients with Turner's syndrome surviving beyond infancy have a 45,XO genotype. These patients have no increased risk of gonadal germ cell neoplasia, but any genotype that includes Y chromosome material confers a 15–20% risk of developing a gonadoblastoma. The availability of specific DNA probes allows identification of these individuals (Cooper et al 1991).

In those fetuses which survive, the ovaries are normal until the second trimester in utero when ova begin to undergo atresia, a process which is commonly complete before puberty so that primary amenorrhoea is a common finding (Scully 1991). However, cases are reported in which girls with Turner's syndrome, usually those with a mosaic genotype, have borne normal children.

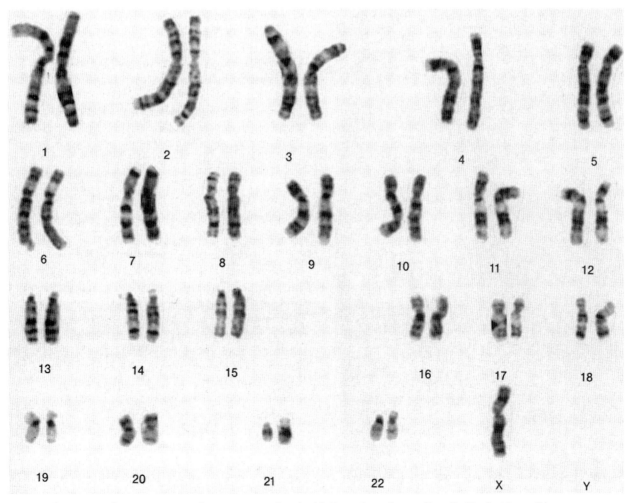

Fig. 34.1 45,X karyotype: the most common karyotype associated with Turner's syndrome. (Supplied by Dr J Fennell.)

The phenotype is characterised by short stature, broad chest, lymphoedema with puffy fingers and toes, anomalous ears, webbed posterior neck, cubitus valgus and an excessive number of pigmented naevi (Gilbert-Barness & Opitz 1998b). Marked nuchal oedema is common in fetuses (Fig. 34.2), probably due to a partial agenesis of the lymphatic system. Renal tract anomalies are found in three-quarters of cases and include horseshoe kidney, duplex systems, agenesis or hypoplasia (Gilbert-Barness & Opitz 1998b). Common cardiac malformations include atrial septal defect, patent ductus, transposition and coarctation of the aorta (Gilbert-Barness & Opitz 1998b).

The mature gonads are streak-shaped structures composed entirely of ovarian-type stroma in which the hilar areas are normal, with a normal rete ovarii and hilar cells (Scully 1991).

Streak gonads may also be seen in isolation from abnormalities of other organ systems (pure gonadal dysgenesis). The genotype of these patients may be 46, XX, in which case there is no association with an increased incidence of gonadal germ cell neoplasia.

Mixed gonadal dysgenesis and other intersex disorders with abnormal gonads

Mixed gonadal dysgenesis (MGD) is characterised by a unilateral testis, usually abdominal, with a contralateral streak gonad and persistent Müllerian structures (Davidoff & Federman 1973); in some cases there may be bilateral abdominal streak-testes. It is the second commonest cause of ambiguous genitalia in the newborn (Scully 1991). Phenotypic sex is commonly female (Wallace & Levin 1990) but there is usually some degree of masculinisation and one-third are phenotypic males. Most individuals are genotypically 45,XO/46,XY mosaics and stigmata of Turner's syndrome, such as congenital heart disease, may be present (Wallace & Levin 1990). In one series one-third of patients with mixed gonadal dysgenesis had a gonadoblastoma (discussed below) and this was bilateral in over half of them (Wallace & Levin 1990). The dysgenetic testes in this condition may be involved in other forms of neoplasia including intratubular germ cell neoplasia (Müller et al 1985; Wallace & Levin 1990), sex cord–stromal tumour of undefined type (Wallace & Levin 1990) and juvenile granulosa cell tumour (Young et al 1985). Clear cell adenocarcinoma of the cervix and vagina has been recorded in mixed gonadal dysgenesis (Resnik et al 1989) and there are a few reports of endometrial adenocarcinoma (Wallace & Levin 1990). There is also an association with Wilms' tumour and abnormalities of renal function (Scully 1991). In the small number of cases studied the *SRY* gene appears to be normal (Lauchlan & Pinar 1998).

46,XY pure gonadal dysgenesis (Swyer syndrome) is characterised by persistent internal Müllerian structures, bilateral streak gonads and a female phenotype (Olsen et al 1988; Wallace & Levin 1990). Approximately 30% of patients develop a gonadoblastoma (Rutgers & Scully 1987). At least some patients have mutations of the *SRY* gene (Lauchlan & Pinar 1998).

In dysgenetic male pseudohermaphroditism the characteristic features are bilateral cryptorchid testes accompanied by persistent Müllerian structures and a 46,XY genotype (Mandell et al 1977). There is considerable clinical and pathological overlap between this disorder and mixed gonadal dysgenesis and it may well represent one variant (Scully 1991). Again, approximately 30% develop a gonadoblastoma.

Androgen resistance syndromes

These may present to gynaecologists as a cause of primary amenorrhoea. Patients have a 46,XY genotype and tests but due to failure to produce active androgens or a failure to respond to them they fail to develop a male

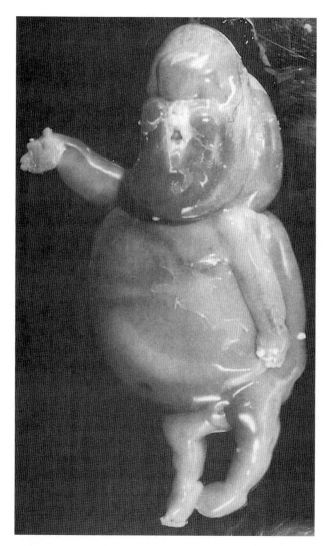

Fig. 34.2 Fetus with nuchal and generalised oedema: Turner's syndrome.

phenotype and express a complete or partial female phenotype with very occasional cases presenting as phenotypically normal males with azoospermia (Ahmed et al 2000). The androgen receptor is a nuclear protein, the gene coding for which is located on the long arm of the X chromosome (Ahmed et al 2000). Both point mutations and deletions in this region have been demonstrated to result in a proportion of the cases of the complete androgen insensitivity syndrome (Ahmed et al 2000). In the presence of defects in androgen synthesis, such as 5α-reductase deficiency, which is the enzyme involved in the conversion of testosterone to dihydrotestosterone, the complete male phenotype may also fail to develop. In this case the condition has an autosomal recessive inheritance (Scully 1991). In its fully expressed form, male pseudohermaphroditism is characterised by unambiguously female external genitalia, breast development at puberty, poorly formed Wolffian structures and the persistence of Müllerian structures. The Fallopian tubes may be well developed (Rutgers & Scully 1987). The testes can be sited anywhere along the normal path of testicular descent.

The microscopic appearance of the testes is characteristic. There are immature seminiferous tubules containing only a few germ cells, abundant Leydig cells and multiple hamartomatous nodules. The latter are more common in adults and, microscopically, nodules consist of tightly packed tubules containing Sertoli cells with only a few germ cells (Fig. 34.3); other elements, such as Leydig cells, ovarian stroma and smooth muscle may be present (Rutgers & Scully 1987).

Approximately 10% of those affected have an incomplete form of the disorder in which the genitalia are ambiguous, often within the same kindred as those with the complete form (Lauchlan & Pinar 1998). At puberty there is a degree of virilisation.

Five to 10 per cent of cases of male pseudohermaphroditism develop malignant germ cell tumours, almost always post-pubertally, in contrast to mixed gonadal dysgenesis and related conditions. Seminoma is the most common malignant neoplasm (Rutgers & Scully 1987). There may be associated intratubular germ cell neoplasia (ITGCN) (Müller & Skakkebaek 1984) (Fig. 34.4a). Placental alkaline phosphatase can be of great assistance in diagnosing this lesion (Fig. 34.4b). Though it can be demonstrated in normal fetal germ cells, this marker is largely lost by eight months of age in both normal boys and patients with testicular feminisation and therefore provides a specific marker of ITGCN beyond this age (Armstrong et al 1991). In one series, two of 14 patients with male pseudohermaphroditism had evidence of ITGCN (Armstrong et al 1991).

There are a few reports of sex cord–stromal tumours occurring in testes in patients with the androgen insensitivity syndrome, some of which have the appearance of large cell calcifying Sertoli cell tumours (Scully 1991). In

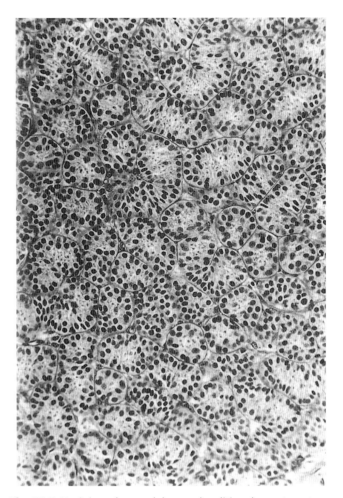

Fig. 34.3 Testis in male pseudohermaphroditism: hamartomatous nodule.

some patients malignant sex cord–stromal tumours of the testes have been recorded (O'Dowd et al 1990; Scully 1991).

True hermaphroditism

In this condition, both ovarian and testicular tissue is present, either contralaterally or joined in the form of bilateral or unilateral ovotestes. The condition can be easily missed by gonadal biopsy for obvious reasons. The phenotype ranges from normal female to normal male but there is commonly sexual ambiguity. The condition is genetically heterogeneous; most commonly (in 60%) the genotype is 46,XX but 46,XY and mosaics have been recorded (Scully 1991). Some (but not all) 46,XX individuals have been demonstrated to carry the Y-chromosomal material, including the *SRY* gene, possibly resulting from paternal meiotic exchange of chromosomal material (Hadjiathanasiou et al 1994). Epithelial neoplasms of both ovary and breast, in addition to gonadoblastoma and germ cell neoplasms have been reported in true hermaphrodites (Talerman et al 1990; Scully 1991).

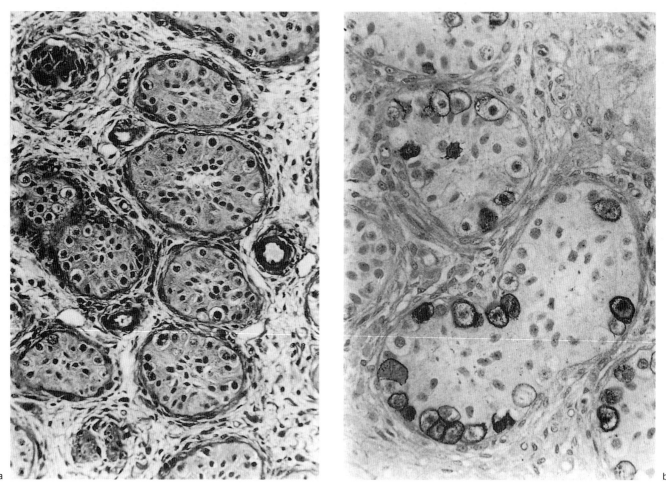

Fig. 34.4 Testis in male pseudohermaphroditism: intratubular germ cell neoplasia. **a** Characteristic large atypical germ cells within seminiferous tubules. **b** Abnormal germ cells stain positively with immunostains for PLAP.

However, germ cell neoplasia is much less common than in mixed gonadal dysgenesis and has a slightly higher incidence in those patients whose genotype includes a Y chromosome (Talerman et al 1990).

Since not all true hermaphrodites have been shown to possess the *SRY* gene, it has been suggested that in some cases the gonadal differentiation may be controlled by a more primitive evolutionary mechanism whereby the direction of differentiation is controlled by gonadal growth rate. When a certain threshold is exceeded, a testis results even in the absence of the *SRY* gene (Blyth & Duckett 1991).

NON-NEOPLASTIC LESIONS OF THE OVARY IN CHILDHOOD

Multiple cysts of follicular origin are extremely common in the neonate and in the immediate postmenarchal years though these lesions commonly regress and are asymptomatic. Marked enlargement of both ovaries due to massive multiple follicular cysts has been reported in an infant with the autosomal recessive Donahue syndrome

(Lauchlan & Pinar 1998). This condition is associated with a defect in the insulin receptor (Gilbert-Barness & Opitz 1998a). Large follicular cysts have also been noted in the infants of diabetic mothers (Huffman et al 1981).

Symptomatic follicular cysts are less common. They are often solitary and form a substantial proportion of surgically treated ovarian lesions in infants and prepubertal children, accounting for 36% of such cases in one review (Breen & Maxson 1977). Neonatal cysts may be diagnosed antenatally and may occasionally require surgical intervention as a result of rupture, haemorrhage, and bowel occlusion due to compression or adhesions (Luzzatto et al 2000). Later in childhood, cysts may become symptomatic because of hormone production, usually resulting in isosexual precocious puberty, or because of abdominal pain resulting from torsion or haemoperitoneum consequent upon bleeding (Breen & Maxson 1977; Schwöbel & Stauffer 1991). Multiple luteinized follicular cysts are found in the ovaries of girls with the McCune–Albright syndrome, where they are functional and associated with sexual precocity. This disorder is characterised by polyostotic fibrous dysplasia of bone, cafe-au-lait spots and sexual precocity.

Hyperthyroidism, acromegaly, hyperparathyroidism and Cushing's syndrome are other recorded associations. It appears therefore that there is hyperplasia of multiple endocrine organs (Danon et al 1975).

Cysts originating in the corpus luteum may be found in postmenarchal girls, though, rarely, female neonates may have this type of lesion. Paraovarian cysts are also reported but are more commonly found in young women after the menarche.

Ovarian fibromatosis, described by Young & Scully (1984), affects women from the teenage years to the fourth decade. Patients present with menstrual irregularities, excessive bleeding or androgenic symptoms. The condition may involve both ovaries and microscopically part or all of the ovary may be expanded by a spindle cell stroma with varying amounts of associated collagen. Nests of cells of sex-cord type may be found within the stroma (Young & Scully 1984). Massive ovarian oedema involves a similar age group and may also involve both ovaries. It is, according to the World Health Organisation definition, a tumour-like condition in which there is ovarian enlargement due to accumulation of oedema fluid. Modes of presentation are similar to those for fibromatosis and in the prepubertal girl there may be sexual precocity. In some cases there is acute abdominal pain due to torsion (Heiss et al 1994; Nogales et al 1996) and one theory as to its cause is that fluid accumulates as a result of intermittent torsion (Nogales et al 1996). It has been suggested that the two conditions may be related and that massive oedema results when the stroma in fibromatosis accumulates a large amount of tissue fluid (Young & Scully 1984).

TORSION OF THE UTERINE ADNEXA WHERE THERE IS NO TUMOUR

This uncommon (though not excessively rare) condition, which more usually involves the right side, clinically very closely mimics acute appendicitis (Huffman et al 1981). It is most common in the first three decades of life (Meyer et al 1995) and may occur prenatally (Mordehai et al 1991). The involved ovary may be completely normal or follicular cysts may be present. Occasionally the condition may present not acutely but as a wandering calcified pelvic mass (Keshtgar & Turnock 1997).

MISCELLANEOUS, NON-NEOPLASTIC DISEASE OF THE GENITAL TRACT IN CHILDHOOD AND ADOLESCENCE

The vulva may be involved in inflammatory conditions not specific to childhood or to this site, such as, for example, lichen sclerosus, Behçet's syndrome or ulceration associated with malnutrition (Huffman et al 1981). Vulvovaginitis may be associated with poor perineal hygiene, it may be secondary to intestinal parasites, such as *Enterobius vermicularis*, or to foreign bodies or it may be caused by an infection usually transmitted venereally in the sexually active. The latter include gonorrhoea, Herpes simplex and Trichomonas. Gonorrhoeal vulvovaginitis was formerly a very common infection in children brought up in crowded conditions and, though some cases were sexually transmitted, others appear to have been infected by close non-sexual family contact and via fomites (Huffman et al 1981).

Epithelial inclusion cysts, paraurethral cysts, and cysts of the canal of Nuck may all rarely occur during childhood. Cysts of the mesonephric (Gartner's) duct remnants are the commonest benign vaginal swellings in infancy and childhood. Occasionally, hymenal cysts may be present in the neonate (Garden 1998). Cystic remnants of unfused segments of Müllerian ducts may also be found at any age and if lined with endometrial-type epithelium they may become blood filled at the menarche (Huffman et al 1981).

PREGNANCY IN CHILDHOOD AND ADOLESCENCE

Pregnancies have been well documented in girls as young as 5 years though this is clearly a most exceptional occurrence (Huffman et al 1981). Teenage pregnancies are associated with an increased incidence of complications such as pre-eclampsia and eclampsia, anaemia, low birthweight babies, perinatal mortality, cephalopelvic disproportion and prolonged labour (Huffman et al 1981).

NEOPLASMS OF THE FEMALE GENITAL TRACT AND OVARIES IN CHILDHOOD AND ADOLESCENCE

THE PATTERN OF DISEASE

Considering childhood to span an age range of 0–14 years, childhood cancers comprise only 0.5–3% of all neoplastic disease, depending on population structure (Parkin et al 1988). In the Manchester series this amounts to a total incidence of 122.5 tumours per 10^6 child-years, of which leukaemia, lymphoma and central nervous system tumours account for almost 80%. In the same series, germ cell and other gonadal neoplasms have a total incidence of only 2.3 per 10^6 years (Birch 1990). Of all ovarian tumours, only 0.2–0.3% occur in girls aged less than 15 years (La Vecchia et al 1983) and the proportion of genital tract neoplasms occurring in this age group is very much lower.

Since its foundation in 1953, the Manchester Children's Tumour Registry has recorded all cases of malignant neoplasms and all germ cell neoplasms occurring in children aged 15 years or less from a defined geographical area. Data regarding the occurrence of non-germ cell benign neoplasms, which are not commonly subject to registration, are unavailable. Statistics collected by the registry are population based and avoid the bias introduced by patterns of referral which are inherent in data generated from hospitals. It originally drew from a child population of one million but boundary and demographic changes (Birch 1988) have since resulted in a fall so that the population served is now 850,000. Over the 46 years between 1954 and 2000 less than 100 neoplasms of the ovary and female genital tract were recorded in this population; that is approximately two cases each year. Table 34.1 illustrates the tumour types, site and relative frequency. The ovary is the most common site and germ cell tumours form the most common type of neoplasm. Other studies, which were concerned with only ovarian tumours, have generated similar data regarding the relative frequency of tumour types (Norris & Jensen 1972; Breen & Maxson 1977; La Vecchia et al 1983; Gribbon et al 1992).

It is evident from Table 34.1 that genital tract neoplasms are largely tumours of the first decade, that mature ovarian teratomas and sex cord–stromal tumours occur throughout childhood and that malignant ovarian germ cell neoplasms increase in frequency from the end of the first decade. There are few tumours that occur exclusively in the paediatric age group. In almost all cases, the age range of neoplasms listed in Table 34.1 extends into the second, third or subsequent decades.

GERM CELL TUMOURS

Epidemiology

Paediatric germ cell tumours have a bimodal age distribution with the first peak (involving extragonadal and testicular tumours) occurring before three years of age and the second peak beginning during puberty and involving gonadal neoplasms (Silver et al 1994).

Over the past 30 years the incidence of germ cell tumours has risen. This has been noted in series that have examined all germ cell neoplasms (Birch et al 1982) and also more specifically in studies examining the incidence of malignant gonadal neoplasms (Walker et al 1984; Senturia 1987). This is particularly due to a rising incidence of testicular cancer, but there is evidence that at least some groups of ovarian malignant germ cell neoplasms may be subject to a similar trend (Walker et al 1984), for example yolk sac tumours (La Vecchia 1983).

The aetiological factors associated with the development of most germ cell tumours are poorly understood, though there is some evidence that there is an increased risk in the child where there has been in utero exposure to excess oestrogens, maternal exposure to solvents, plastics or resin fumes during pregnancy and where there is a history of maternal urinary infection during pregnancy (Shu et al 1995).

Ovarian germ cell tumours

The ovary is usually considered to be the second commonest site of origin in the paediatric age group after

Table 34.1 Gynaecological tumours collected by Manchester Children's Tumour Registry 1954–2000

Ovarian tumours (n=82)	Number	Age range (years)
Germ cell tumours	69	
Mature teratomas	36	2–15
Malignant germ cell tumours comprising:	33	4–14
— dysgerminoma	14	4–13
— immature teratoma	8	7–14
— endodermal sinus tumour	7	6–14
— embryonal carcinoma	2	12–14
— choriocarcinoma	1	10
— other	1	7
Sex cord–stromal tumours comprising:	9	2–14
— juvenile granulosa cell tumour	4	2–10
— Sertoli–Leydig cell tumour	2	9–13
— sex-cord tumour with annular tubules	2	6–12
— fibroma	1	14
Other ovarian tumours comprising:	4	
— small cell carcinoma	1	12
— other malignant neoplasms	3	2–13
Genital tract tumours (n=12)		
Malignant germ cell tumours comprising:	5	1–8
— vaginal endodermal sinus tumour	4	1–3
— embryonal carcinoma of the uterine corpus	1	8
Sarcomas comprising:	5	1–4
— vaginal rhabdomyosarcoma	4	1–4
— cervical rhabdomyosarcoma	1	2
Others comprising:	2	
— small cell malignant tumour of the vulva	1	6
— malignant lymphoma of the genital tract	1	4

the sacrococcygeal region (Dehner 1983). However, in one population-based study (Marsden et al 1981) and in one large series from a children's hospital (Malogolowkin et al 1990), ovarian tumours were the most common. The incidence of female gonadal germ cell tumours for 1954–1998 in the Manchester Children's Tumour Registry was low, with only 1.3 such tumours per million person-years; this figure includes only malignant neoplasms since it is not possible to be certain that all benign tumours were reported.

Mature teratomas

Overall, at least 90% of ovarian germ cell tumours are mature teratomas and two types are described: the mature cystic teratoma (dermoid cyst) and the mature solid teratoma. The former accounts for over 20% of all ovarian neoplasms, affects women in all age groups from childhood to old age and forms over half of all ovarian tumours in the first two decades (Scully 1979). In the Manchester series (Table 34.1), 53% of tumours in girls aged 15 years or less were mature cystic teratomas. This could represent an underestimate; whilst it is probable that all malignant neoplasms were recorded, it is possible that some benign tumours escaped registration.

Mature solid teratoma is a tumour of the first two decades. The diagnosis should be made only after careful sampling to exclude the presence of immature tissues or other malignant germ cell elements. At least one block per centimetre of tumour is recommended (Norris et al 1976).

Dysgerminoma

Germinoma is the general designation for the neoplasm that is known as seminoma in the testis and dysgerminoma in the ovary (Fig. 34.5). It is the commonest malignant germ cell tumour, comprising almost half of those collected in Manchester. Overall survival is high. In one series, no patient had died since the introduction of megavoltage radiotherapy in 1963 (Björkholm et al

1990), though this treatment almost invariably results in the loss of fertility (Mitchell et al 1991). In the series of children aged 15 years or less from Manchester, all 10 patients with dysgerminoma (three of whom had bilateral disease) have survived for more than 10 years to date.

Immature teratoma

This is the third most common malignant germ cell neoplasm and accounted for 8% of all ovarian tumours in patients aged less than 15 years in Manchester (Fig. 34.6). The proportion of immature tissue present determines grading though the exact criteria used have varied from series to series (Thurlbeck & Scully 1960; Nogales et al 1976; Norris et al 1976; O'Connor & Norris 1994). It has recently been suggested that the presence of abundant immature neuroepithelium is important only in that it signals that yolk sac elements are more likely to be present within the tumour and it is this latter feature which is considered by some to be the only significant predictor of recurrent/metastatic disease in immature teratomas (Heifetz et al 1998). However, this is disputed and at least one series includes cases of

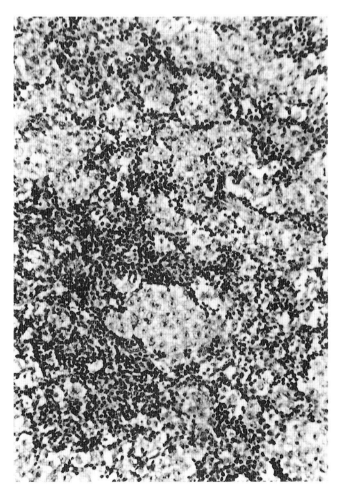

Fig. 34.5 Dysgerminoma: groups of neoplastic germ cells within a sea of lymphocytes.

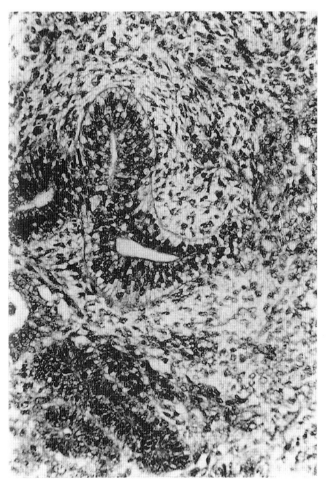

Fig. 34.6 Ovarian immature teratoma.

recurrence of tumours considered to be pure immature teratomas without yolk sac elements (Norris 1999). It should be noted that this does apply specifically to ovarian teratomas. Tumours at other sites, such as the sacrococcygeal region or the mediastinum, frequently contain immature elements which are of no prognostic significance in neoplasms occurring in children in the first three months of life (Carter et al 1982; Dehner 1983), though they may indicate malignancy beyond infancy.

A high proportion of immature and mature solid ovarian teratomas, a third in one series (Norris et al 1976), are associated with extraovarian disease. However, the factors determining prognosis are the grade of the primary tumour and the grade of tumour deposits in extraovarian sites rather than the stage per se. The presence of fully mature glial implants on the peritoneum increases stage but is not an adverse prognostic factor (Nogales et al 1976; Truong et al 1982). Therefore, pathological assessment demands adequate sampling of both the primary tumour and extraovarian deposits to disclose the extent of immature tissues or the presence of other malignant germ cell elements. Tumours containing a small proportion of immature tissue have always been associated with an excellent prognosis, but, prior to the

advent of modern combination chemotherapy in the 1970s, only 30% of patients with high-grade neoplasms survived (Norris et al 1976). Therapeutic advances have resulted in significant improvements (Taylor et al 1985; O'Connor & Norris 1994).

Yolk sac tumour

This is the second most frequent form of malignant ovarian germ cell tumour in many series (Kurman & Norris 1977). Numerous histological patterns have been described (Fig. 34.7a–c). Patients commonly present with an abdominal mass, fever and pain rather than with hormonal effects (Kurman & Norris 1976a). Though yolk sac tumour was originally regarded as a highly malignant neoplasm with a 13% three-year survival (Kurman & Norris 1976a), modern chemotherapy has reduced mortality considerably and now over 80% of patients have a long-term survival (Gershenson et al 1983; Taylor et al 1985). One series, considering yolk sac tumours at all sites, found a survival rate of 99% (Mann et al 1989). Furthermore, the combination of conservative surgery and chemotherapy offers the option of preservation of fertility (Wu et al 1991).

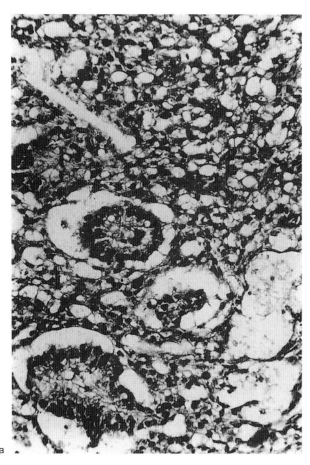

Fig. 34.7 Yolk sac tumour. **a** Endodermal sinus pattern with Schiller–Duval body.

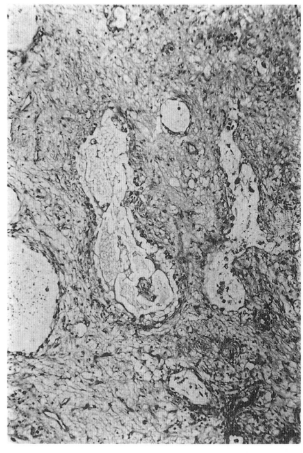

Fig. 34.7 Yolk sac tumour. **b** Polyvesicular pattern.

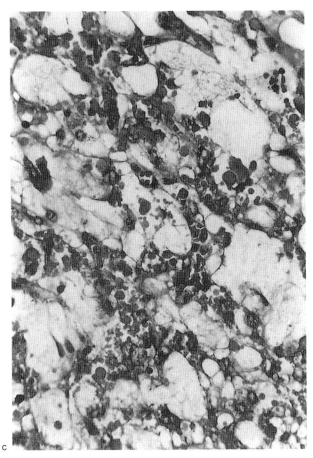

Fig. 34.7 Yolk sac tumour. **c** Hyaline globules, both intracellular and extracellular.

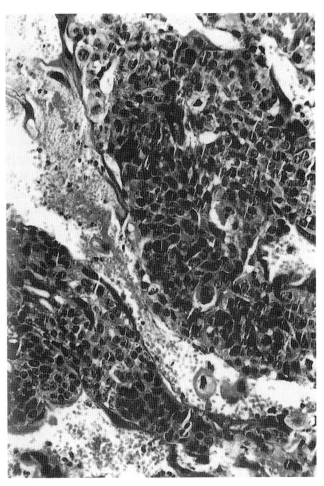

Fig. 34.8 Choriocarcinoma: solid islands of cytotrophoblast covered by a layer of syncytiotrophoblast.

The introduction of serum tumour markers, such as alpha-fetoprotein (and hCG in the case of certain other germ cell neoplasms) and the development of better imaging techniques have also considerably facilitated follow-up of patients with malignant germ cell neoplasms (Mann et al 1989; Gribbon et al 1992).

Other malignant germ cell tumours of the ovary

Embryonal carcinoma resembles the tumour of the same name in the adult testis, but it is much less common in the ovary. Its distinct clinicopathological features were described by Kurman & Norris (1976b). Unlike yolk sac tumours, 60% of embryonal carcinomas present with hormonal manifestations (Kurman & Norris 1976b).

Pure non-gestational choriocarcinoma is very rare in the ovary (Fig. 34.8). In an infant with multiple visceral lesions or in a post-pubertal female, the possibility of metastatic gestational choriocarcinoma should be considered (Kurman & Norris 1977; Dehner 1983; Flam et al 1989).

Malignant neuroectodermal tumours resembling those of the central nervous system have been described in the ovary (Aguirre & Scully 1982). Since some of these neoplasms contained areas of mature teratoma, it seems probable that these are germ cell neoplasms.

Cytogenetics

Testicular germ cell tumours characteristically carry multiple copies of isochromosome 12p (Atkin & Baker 1983), this abnormality being present in more than 80% of cases and found in neoplasms of most histological types (Geurts van Kessel et al 1991). This anomaly has also been reported in at least some malignant ovarian germ cell tumours (Dal Cin & Van Den Berghe 1991; Rodriguez et al 1995).

Lesions associated with the development of germ cell neoplasms

Gonadoblastoma

This is one tumour within the group of mixed germ cell sex cord–stromal neoplasms. Gonadoblastoma has been reported in patients aged from infancy through to the fourth decade (Rutgers & Scully 1987).

In 50% of cases an associated malignant germ cell tumour develops either in the same or the contralateral gonad. This is most commonly a germinoma but in some cases another malignant neoplasm such as a yolk sac tumour, embryonal carcinoma, choriocarcinoma or immature teratoma may develop (Rutgers & Scully 1987). Gonadoblastoma has a characteristic insular structure (Fig. 34.9). The lesions are frequently calcified and may be visible radiologically (Rutgers & Scully 1987). They can be microscopic in size or may form a sizeable ovarian mass.

Ninety-five per cent of tumours occur in patients with a Y chromosome, though 80% of them are phenotypic females (Scully 1970). Usually, the tumour occurs within the dysgenetic gonads of one of three syndromes, discussed earlier: mixed gonadal dysgenesis, pure XY gonadal dysgenesis or dysgenetic male pseudohermaphroditism. The risk of prepubertal germ cell malignancy is sufficiently high in these disorders to warrant gonadectomy at diagnosis. Twenty per cent of gonadoblastomas occur in a streak gonad, 20% in a testis and in most of the other cases the underlying gonad is of indeterminate

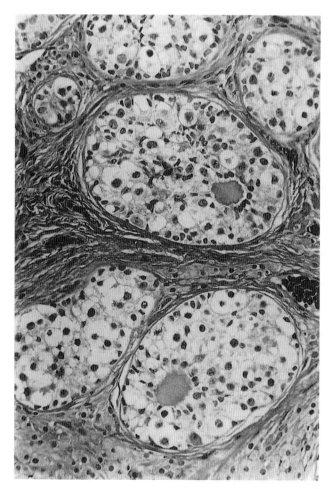

Fig. 34.9 Gonadoblastoma: islands of cells composed of both sex cord and germ cell elements. (Case provided by Dr D L Bisset.)

type. There are a very few instances of the tumour occurring in the ovary of an apparently normal fertile woman (Scully 1970). One example has been recorded in a 46,XX infant with the autosomal recessive Fraser's (cryptophthalmos) syndrome (Greenberg et al 1986).

Familial cancer syndromes

Familial cancer syndromes are characterised by malignancies in more than two generations of one family. Often, age at presentation is young, the pattern of organ involvement is distinctive and a high proportion of siblings is affected.

There are several recorded instances of germ cell neoplasms occurring in several members of one family (La Vecchia et al 1983; Dahl et al 1990; Stettner et al 1999) in the absence of other types of tumour. In other examples, germ cell neoplasms have been recorded in association with tumours of different histogenesis. For example, there is a report of one kindred in which ovarian germ cell neoplasms occurred in patients from two generations and one sibling in the second generation developed a rhabdomyosarcoma (Weinblatt & Kochen 1991).

It has been suggested that the incidence of gonadal germ cell tumours may be increased in the Li-Fraumeni cancer family syndrome (Hartley et al 1987, 1989, 1993), though one recent study has implied that this may not be the case (Birch et al 2001).

The syndrome was first described in 1969 on the basis of familial clusters of cancers in association with childhood soft tissue sarcomas in other family members (Li & Fraumeni 1969). Though constitutional mutation of the tumour suppressor gene *TP53* was demonstrated in six Li-Fraumeni families (Malkin et al 1990; Srivastava et al 1990) subsequent studies have shown that this is not the case in all such families (Birch et al 1994; Evans et al 1998). It has also become clear that families with patterns of cancer outside the strict Li-Fraumeni criteria may carry germline *TP53* mutations (Birch et al 1998).

Germ cell tumours occurring in the female genital tract

Endodermal sinus tumour of the vagina is the only neoplasm of this type to occur with any frequency in the female genital tract. It characteristically involves a younger age group than its ovarian counterpart and patients are usually in the first decade of life (Brown & Langley 1976; Kohorn et al 1985; Clement & Young 1993). Classically, it was described as an aggressive neoplasm metastasising to lymph nodes, liver and lungs (Kohorn et al 1985) with a mean survival of less than a year (Dehner 1987). Most series include only a few cases so that the impact of modern chemotherapy is somewhat difficult to assess. However, it is notable that in the Manchester series there have been no deaths in the children with ovarian or genital tract malignant germ cell neoplasms who received combination chemotherapy since the mid-1970s.

SEX CORD–STROMAL TUMOURS OF THE OVARY

Juvenile granulosa cell tumour

Less than 5% of all granulosa cell tumours occur in premenarchal girls but approximately 90% of those that do have distinct clinicopathological and microscopic features. The age range affected is from infancy onwards. The characteristic appearance of the juvenile granulosa cell tumour is well documented (Young et al 1984) (Fig. 34.10) (see Chapter 20). In the prepubertal girl presentation is typically with isosexual precocious pseudopuberty (Lack et al 1981; Young et al 1984; Biscotti & Hart 1989). In one large series survival was 92% with an average of five years follow-up; extraovarian disease at diagnosis was the most significant factor

in predicting an adverse prognosis (Young et al 1984), though there is some suggestion that a high mitotic index may also be of some significance (Calaminus et al 1997). In contrast to adult-type granulosa cell tumour, in which late recurrences occur (Young & Scully 1982), the patients succumbing to juvenile granulosa cell tumour do so within three years of diagnosis (Young et al 1984). In most patients surgery alone is curative and the rarity of this tumour means that the rôle of chemotherapy in advanced disease is unclear, though there is some evidence that some patients may respond (Calaminus et al 1997).

Sertoli–Leydig cell tumours

The histological and clinical features of the neoplasms are well documented (Young & Scully 1982). Approximately half of all Sertoli–Leydig cell tumours (SLCT) (Fig. 34.11) are hormonally active with patients showing virilisation, hirsutism, menstrual irregularities or occasionally oestrogenic effects (Young & Scully 1982). Other patients present with non-specific features

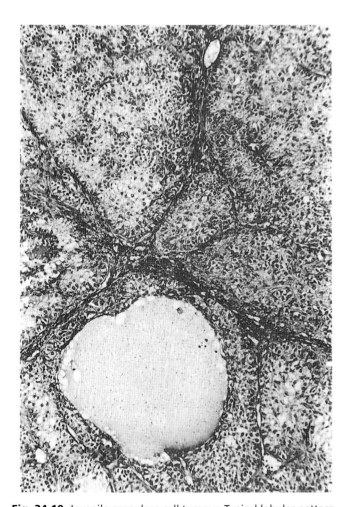

Fig. 34.10 Juvenile granulosa cell tumour. Typical lobular pattern with luteinized granulosa cells surrounding follicular spaces.

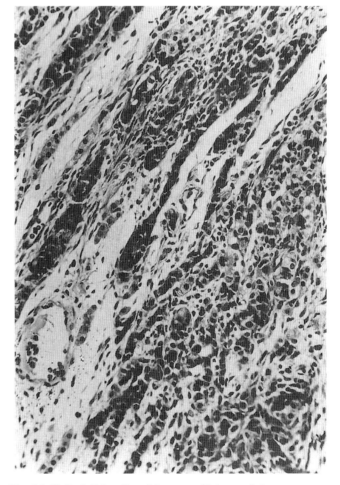

Fig. 34.11 Sertoli–Leydig cell tumour of intermediate differentiation.

such as an abdominal mass (Zaloudek & Norris 1984). These tumours do occur during the paediatric years (Young & Scully 1985) with the exception of the well-differentiated subtype which is more commonly seen in patients aged 35 years or older. Ten to fifteen per cent of Sertoli–Leydig cell tumours contain a prominent retiform component (Young & Scully 1983) (Fig. 34.12). This subtype has a particular propensity to affect adolescents and young adults, with a mean age at diagnosis of 15 years, 10 years younger than the mean for Sertoli–Leydig cell tumours in general (Young & Scully 1983). This histological variant is open to misinterpretation, particularly if it is the predominant feature in a tumour.

Prognosis depends upon stage and differentiation (Young & Scully 1985). Overall, 12% of tumours behave in a malignant fashion and approximately 20% of those with a prominent retiform component are malignant, reflecting the fact that retiform areas are commonly associated with the less well-differentiated neoplasms (Young & Scully 1983).

Ovarian sex-cord tumour with annular tubules

This sex-cord tumour has a distinctive microscopic appearance (Fig. 34.13) and up to 40% may present with symptoms of oestrogen excess (Young & Scully 1982).

A third of the cases are associated with the rare Peutz–Jeghers syndrome (PJS). This condition, inherited as an autosomal dominant with variable penetrance, is characterised by mucocutaneous pigmentation and hamartomas of the gastrointestinal tract. It is associated with a significantly increased risk of death from cancer at an early age (Spigelman et al 1989). The principal sites affected are: breast, where bilateral tumours are characteristic (Trau et al 1982); cervix, in which the well-differentiated adenocarcinoma, adenoma malignum, is the distinctive associated tumour (Young et al 1982); and the gastrointestinal tract, where there is evidence for a hamartoma-carcinoma sequence (Spigelman et al 1989). The predisposing locus is sited on the short arm of chromosome 19 and appears to involve the gene for a serine/threonine kinase (Hemminki 1999).

Probably all females with the syndrome have ovarian SCTAT and the tumours are characteristically small,

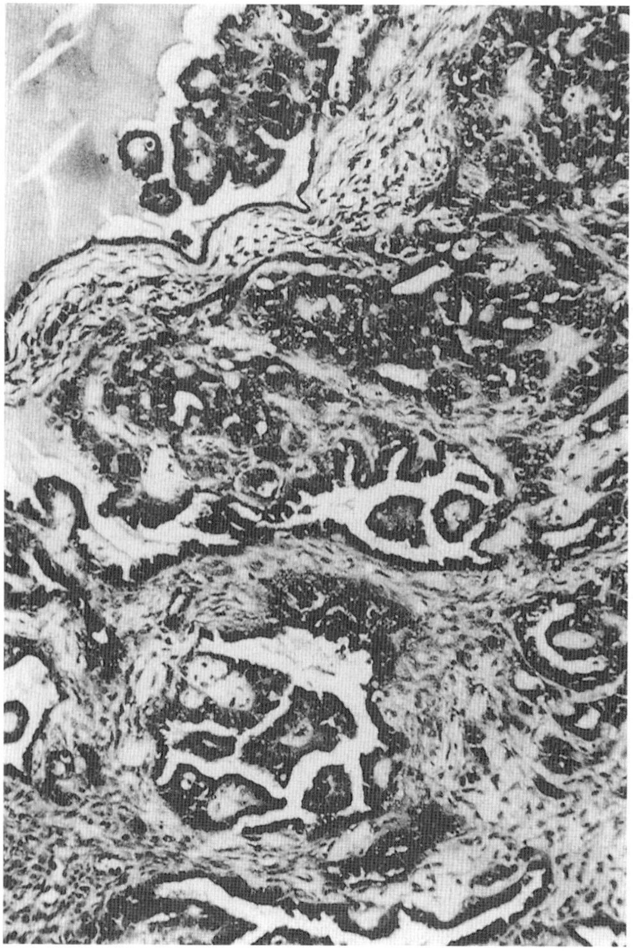

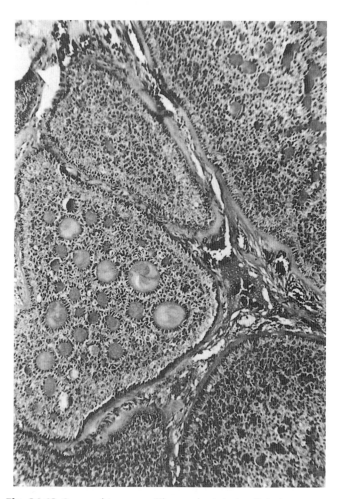

Fig. 34.12 Retiform differentiation in a Sertoli–Leydig cell tumour; blunt papillae are covered by low cuboidal epithelium.

Fig. 34.13 Sex-cord tumour with annular tubules. Tubules encircling nodules of hyaline material.

often microscopic, multifocal, bilateral, calcified and benign (Young et al 1982). Other, unclassified sex-cord tumours may also occur in prepubertal girls with PJS (Young et al 1983). Sertoli cell tumours have been reported in affected boys (Cantu et al 1980).

The remaining two-thirds of cases of sex-cord tumour with annular tubules (SCTAT) are unassociated with PJS. Here the tumours are large and unilateral, and up to 20% are clinically malignant (Young & Scully 1982). Rarely SCTAT has been reported in streak gonads, associated with germinoma in the same or contralateral gonad (Young et al 1982).

Other disorders associated with sex cord–stromal tumours

Gorlin's syndrome. The disorder is characterised by multicentric, early-appearing basal cell carcinomas (Fig. 34.14), often involving non-sun-exposed skin, odontogenic keratocysts, pits of the palms and soles,

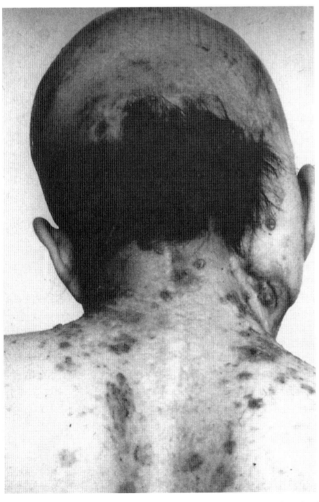

Fig. 34.14 Patient with Gorlin's syndrome. Following craniospinal irradiation for medulloblastoma, multiple basal cell carcinomas developed in the radiation field.

strabismus, dysgenesis of the corpus callosum, spina bifida occulta, ectopic calcifications, hypogonadism and bifid ribs. It is inherited as an autosomal dominant disorder with variable to high penetrance. The gene responsible is located on chromosome 9 (Bale et al 1998) and is a member of the Hedgehog signalling pathway, important in embryological development; inherited mutations of the Patched gene, part of this pathway are associated with Gorlin's syndrome (Saldanha 2001). In addition to basal cell carcinomas, cerebellar medulloblastomas are also associated neoplasms (Kraemer et al 1984). Female patients with the syndrome are prone to develop bilateral calcified multinodular ovarian fibromas (Young & Scully 1982) and these tumours may form the first stigmata of the syndrome. Similar ovarian tumours have rarely been recorded in children showing no other evidence of the syndrome (Howell et al 1990). In some cases the tumours show metaplastic stromal bone formation (Bosch-Banyeras et al 1989). In Gorlin's syndrome, recurrences of the ovarian tumours have been recorded (Howell et al 1990) and in one case, in which the presence of focal mitotically active areas in the tumour was in keeping with a diagnosis of low-grade fibrosarcoma, an adnexal metastasis developed two years following initial salpingo-oophorectomy (Kraemer et al 1984).

Ollier's disease. Ollier's disease is a non-hereditary mesodermal dysplasia, affecting the metaphyseal ends of long bones, which predisposes to the formation of multiple enchondromas. There is often an asymmetrical hemiskeletal distribution (Velasco-Oses et al 1988). Maffucci's syndrome is the association of subcutaneous haemangiomas with enchondromas (Weyl-Ben & Oslander 1991). The development of chondrosarcoma is a well-recognised complication of both disorders. Juvenile granulosa cell tumour of the ovary may also occur in both conditions (Tamimi & Bolen 1984; Young et al 1984; Velasco-Oses et al 1988; Gell et al 1998) and, interestingly, the ovarian tumours appear to involve the same side as the skeletal lesions (Velasco-Oses et al 1988). There is one report of a poorly differentiated Sertoli–Leydig cell tumour in a girl with Ollier's disease (Weyl-Ben & Oslander 1991).

Juvenile granulosa cell tumour in dysmorphic infants. Bilateral juvenile granulosa cell tumours have occurred in a female infant with bilateral renal agenesis and other features of the oligohydramnios sequence (Roth et al 1979). In another case an infant, also with bilateral tumours, was the product of a consanguineous (brother– sister) pregnancy and manifested poor growth, microcephaly, facial asymmetry and a malformed left ear (Pysher et al 1981). On the evidence of these cases, bilateral tumours appear to represent a distinct subset of this neoplasm.

Other stromal neoplasms

Less than 10% of fibrothecomas occur in patients below 30 years of age (Young & Scully 1982). Steroid cell neoplasms, previously called lipid cell tumours, are predominantly neoplasms of the reproductive years (Scully 1979), but cases have occurred in prepubertal girls in association with virilisation (Harris et al 1991; Snyder & La Franchi 1999).

The sclerosing stromal tumour is a neoplasm with a characteristic pseudolobular pattern on microscopic examination. It tends to occur in women in the third and fourth decades but has been recorded in patients less than 15 years of age (Chalvardjian & Scully 1973). Interestingly, bilateral tumours with this histological appearance have been reported in a pregnant adult female with Gorlin's syndrome, raising the possibility that this type of tumour and the fibroma may have a common pathogenesis (Ismail & Walker 1990).

The ovarian myxoma is a neoplasm, which mainly affects women in the reproductive years, but it has occurred in teenage patients (Eichorn & Scully 1991).

Bilateral thecomatous ovarian neoplasms have been reported in children taking anticonvulsant therapy. Though usually benign (Faber 1962; Schweisguth et al 1971), at least one case of bilateral clinically and pathologically malignant thecomatous tumours has been noted in a child on anticonvulsants (Dudzinski et al 1989).

MIXED GERM CELL SEX CORD–STROMAL TUMOURS

Gonadoblastoma, described above, is the best-known neoplasm in this group. In contrast to gonadoblastoma, the other tumour types tend to occur in the normal gonads of genotypically normal individuals of both sexes; affected females are most commonly in the prepubertal years but in males the tumours are more common in adults (Talerman 1972; Bolen 1981). A mixed tumour which included epithelial elements in addition to germ cells and sex-cord structures has been described in a female infant (Tavassoli 1983). Mixed germ cell sex cord–stromal neoplasms are usually benign, but malignant tumours are described (Lacson et al 1988).

MESENCHYMAL NEOPLASMS

Rhabdomyosarcoma is the most common soft tissue sarcoma of childhood (Miller 1969). Thirty to thirty five per cent are sited in the genitourinary tract or pelvic region (Clatworthy et al 1973; Kilman et al 1973).

Historically, survival has been poor, but it has improved significantly with the implementation of combined modality therapy employing surgery, radiotherapy and chemotherapy (Pizzo & Triche 1987). There are striking differences in outcome, however, between the two major forms of childhood rhabdomyosarcoma — embryonal and alveolar — which also show differences in their site of origin and mean age of patient at presentation.

There are biological differences between the tumour types; alveolar rhabdomyosarcoma is characterised by a t(2;13)(q37;q14) translocation (Turc-Carel et al 1986). This or its variant t(1;13)(p36;q14) (Biegel et al 1991) are found in over 80% of cases (Barr et al 1996) and its recognition has prognostic significance.

Rhabdomyosarcoma in the female genital tract occurs most commonly in the vagina (Hilgers et al 1970; Davos & Abell 1976). Grossly, most tumours originate in the anterior vaginal wall and may extend into the introitus and bladder (Fig. 34.15a,b). The Intergroup Rhabdomyosarcoma Study (IRS I–II), the results of which were published in 1988 (Hays et al 1988), revealed that children with primary vaginal tumours were, on average, less than two years of age and histology was uniformly of embryonal type. Vulvar neoplasms occurred over a wider age range (from one to 19 years) and both embryonal and alveolar patterns occurred. Uterine sarcomas involved patients in the teenage years and often, but not always, consisted of a single polyp.

In the IRS study, overall survival following a combination of surgery and chemotherapy was over 80%, though the number of patients studied was small (only 47 collected over 12 years).

The entity called sarcoma botryoides of the uterine cervix by Daya & Scully appears to be a different tumour to classical rhabdomyosarcoma. The patients are older, with a mean age of 18 years, loci of cartilage are often present within the tumour and prognosis appears to be good (Daya & Scully 1988).

Primary rhabdomyosarcoma of the ovary is rare but there are occasional case reports (Nunez et al 1983; Akhtar et al 1989; Chan et al 1989; Nielson et al 1998).

Other soft tissue tumours

Rare cases of neurofibroma of the clitoral region have been described in children with neurofibromatosis (Schepel & Tolhurst 1981; Ravikumar & Lakshmanan 1983; Rink & Mitchell 1983). Malignant nerve sheath tumour of the clitoris has been reported in an infant (Thomas et al 1989). A few examples of leiomyomas of the uterine corpus have been recorded during childhood (Huffman et al 1981).

Aggressive angiomyxoma is a soft tissue tumour in which the bland histological appearance (Fig. 34.16) belies a tendency towards multiple local recurrences (Steeper & Rosai 1983). Cases have been reported in the teenage years (Begin et al 1985).

Though mixed Müllerian tumours occur almost exclusively in postmenopausal women, occasional examples have been described in children (Chumas et al 1983; Amr et al 1986). Congenital infantile haemangioendothelioma of the ovary has been reported (Prus et al 1997).

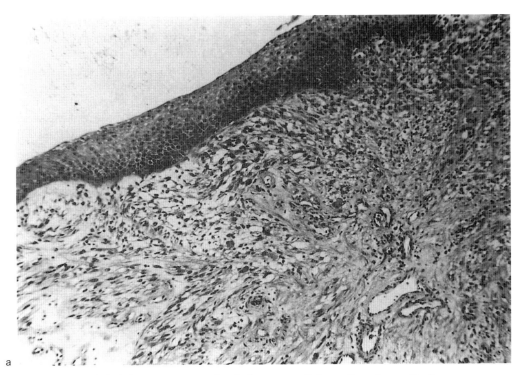

a

Fig. 34.15 Vaginal rhabdomyosarcoma. **a** Band of tumour cells beneath surface epithelium.

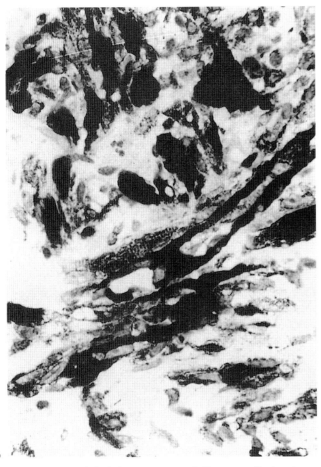

b

Fig. 34.15 Vaginal rhabdomyosarcoma. **b** Tumour cells showing cross-striations. Immunostain for desmin.

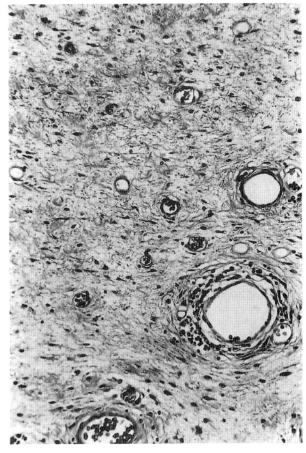

Fig. 34.16 Aggressive angiomyxoma. Prominent blood vessels within hypocellular tissue composed of spindle cells. (Case supplied by Dr M Harris.)

EPITHELIAL TUMOURS

In the 36-years series from the Manchester Children's Tumour Registry there were no cases of malignant epithelial tumours at any site within the female genital tract (Table 34.1), but this is probably not unexpected in view of the upper age limit of 15 years.

Epithelial neoplasms of the ovary, both benign and malignant, are rare below 15 years of age (Norris & Jensen 1972; La Vecchia et al 1983). Occasional cases of epithelial tumours of borderline malignancy have been reported in girls under 17 years of age (Gribbon et al 1992). In prepubertal children malignant epithelial tumours are virtually unknown, though isolated case reports do exist (Blom & Torkildsen 1982; Akinola et al 1988).

In the world literature there are no undisputed examples of endometrial carcinoma occurring in patients less than 15 years of age. An extensive review covering the period 1929–1976 identified five possible cases (Huffman et al 1981) but their validity has been questioned (Lee & Scully 1989). One study included 10 patients under 21 years of age with complex endometrial hyperplasia or well-differentiated adenocarcinoma but there were none aged less than 15 years (Lee & Scully 1989).

Cervical and vaginal adenocarcinoma

Spontaneous vaginal adenocarcinoma is primarily a disease of women in the late reproductive and peri-menopausal years (Herbst et al 1970) but cases have been reported in teenage patients and infants (Drogemueller et al 1970; Norris et al 1970; Kaminski & Maier 1983).

Consequences of intrauterine diethylstilboestrol (DES) exposure. DES was introduced in the late 1940s as a treatment for recurrent miscarriage (Herbst & Anderson 1990) and several million women received it before it was officially banned for use during pregnancy by the US Food and Drug Administration. By this time the association between intrauterine DES exposure and subsequent development of clear cell adenocarcinoma of the vagina and cervix had been recognised (Herbst et al 1971). It has now been out of use for over 20 years. However, clear cell carcinoma is a very infrequent consequence of exposure, the risk being of the order of 1 in 1000 (Herbst 1981; Herbst & Anderson 1990). Furthermore, in the registry set up in 1971 to study the outcome, histopathology and epidemiology of clear cell adenocarcinoma in women born after 1940, in only 60% of the cases was there definite evidence of DES exposure (Herbst & Anderson 1990). DES-associated adenocarcinoma is predominantly a disease of the late teens and twenties, with a few cases occurring in the latter half of the first decade (Dehner 1987; Herbst & Anderson 1990) and some women presenting during their thirties (Herbst & Anderson 1990). Histologically,

the tumour is predominantly clear celled and is composed of cells with a characteristic 'hobnail' appearance which form papillae, cysts and tubules (Fig. 34.17).

Factors commensurate with a good prognosis are low stage, small size, predominant tubulocystic pattern and a low grade of nuclear atypia (Herbst & Anderson 1990; Hanselaar et al 1991). Overall, between 80 and 90% of patients survive five years (Dehner 1987; Hanselaar et al 1991), but most patients have low-stage disease at diagnosis. Late recurrences, up to 20 years after initial therapy, are reported and metastases seem frequently to involve the lungs and supraclavicular lymph nodes (Herbst & Anderson 1990).

Developmental abnormalities of the cervix and vagina are far more commonly associated with maternal DES exposure. An extensive cervical ectropion is the most common finding, occurring in 95%. Though a few glands may be found in the vaginas of normal women, extensive adenosis is very rare in unexposed women, but occurs in at least one-third of young women who were exposed to DES in utero (Scully & Welch 1981). Clear cell adenocarcinoma is often found in close apposition to vaginal

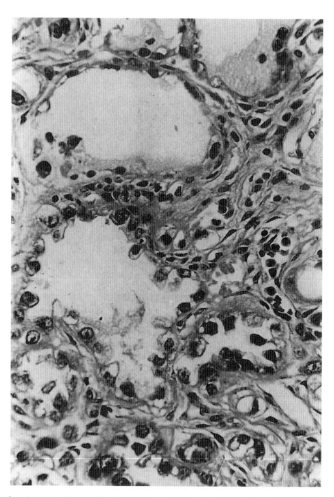

Fig. 34.17 Clear cell adenocarcinoma of the cervix. (Case supplied by Dr C H Buckley.)

adenosis (Scully & Welch 1981). Gross anomalies of the cervix, such as cervical peaks, collars and hoods, are found in at least 20% of exposed girls (Scully & Welch 1981; Coleman & Evans 1988).

Squamous neoplasia of the genital tract and related lesions

Condyloma acuminata and human papillomavirus (HPV) infection. Genital warts are caused mostly by HPV types 6 and 11 and have increased in incidence in all age groups, including children, over the past two decades (Bender 1986; Cripe 1990).

The occurrence of carcinoma of the cervix in adolescent females is rare (Cario et al 1984; Dehner 1987, Tscherne 1997), though there is a significant incidence of HPV infection and intraepithelial disease (Sadeghi et al 1988). Few data are available on the prevalence of each of these parameters in strictly defined groups of adolescents. Most studies either combine adolescents with women in their early twenties or exclude women aged less than 16 years. Prevalence rates for human papillomavirus infection are between 13 and 38% (Moscicki 1996). The rates of cervical intraepithelial neoplasia are up to 3% for high-grade lesions and 10% for low-grade lesions (Moscicki 1996). Sexual activity is the principle risk factor. Most studies on young women use under 35, 40 or even 45 years of age as their reference point and some studies do not include females under the age of 18 years. The National Health Service Cervical Screening Programme in the United Kingdom does not recommend routine cervical smears under the age of 20 years. There appears to be a relationship between high-risk HPV infection and cervical intraepithelial neoplasia in adolescent females and immunosuppression particularly associated with HIV infection and AIDS (Moscicki et al 2000).

In young women (aged 20 +/− 3 years) HPV infection is highly prevalent in sexually active young women and the risk of cervical intraepithelial neoplasia increases with persistent HPV infection indicated by repeatedly positive tests (Ho et al 1998; Moscicki 1998). Woodman and colleagues have recently reported on the findings in 2011 women aged 15–19 years. In women who were negative for HPV at the outset of the study the cumulative risk of detecting HPV at three years was 44% with HPV 16 being the most common type. Two hundred and forty-six women had an abnormal smear and 28 progressed to high-grade cervical intraepithelial neoplasia. The risk of high-grade disease was greatest in women who tested positive for HPV 16; this risk was maximum 6–12 months after first detection of HPV 16. The evaluation of risk of development of cervical neoplasia, however, is made difficult by the 'limited inferences that can be drawn from the characterisation of a woman's HPV status at a single point in time and the short lead time gained by its detection' (Woodman et al 2001).

At least one case of vulvar carcinoma in a teenager was associated with a history of anogenital warts since infancy (Bender 1986).

In prepubertal children, the infection implies the possibility of sexual abuse (Bender 1986; Rock et al 1986; Hanson et al 1989; Cripe 1990). Not surprisingly, in view of the controversial nature of this subject, estimates as to the proportion of cases transmitted sexually vary from virtually all (Gutman 1990), to less than one-third of cases (Cripe 1990). However, there are reports of congenital condylomata acuminata (Shelton et al 1986) and in a high proportion of cases of affected infants maternal condylomata are present (Shelton et al 1986; Cripe 1990) so that at least some infantile lesions may be transmitted vertically or during close physical, but not sexual, contact.

MISCELLANEOUS NEOPLASMS

Ovarian small cell carcinoma, hypercalcaemic type

This neoplasm was originally described in 1982 as a tumour frequently, though not invariably, associated with hypercalcaemia (Dickersin et al 1982) (Fig. 34.18).

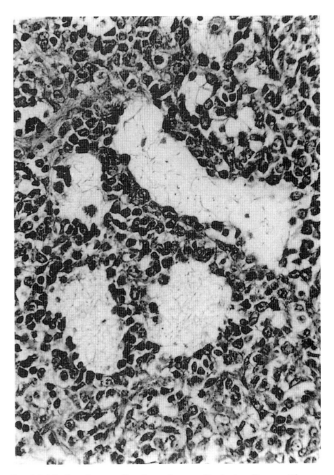

Fig. 34.18 Ovarian small cell carcinoma. Typical pattern with follicle-like spaces. (Case supplied by Dr R Williams.)

Though described as 'small cell' many tumours contain foci of large cells and this pattern may be the predominant one (Young et al 1994). Published cases range in age from the first decade (Malfetano et al 1990) to the fifth with a mean of around 23 years (Dickersin et al 1982; Young et al 1987, 1994). Familial occurrence has been recorded (Young et al 1994). The tumour characteristically has an aggressive clinical course. In one series mortality was 88%, with most fatalities occurring in the first year. Only 12% were free of disease after four years follow-up (Young et al 1987). Extensive intra-abdominal spread is characteristic (Dickersin et al 1982).

The histogenesis of this tumour is unknown (Scully 1993), but it clearly bears no histogenetic relationship to the small cell carcinoma of neuroendocrine origin. In view of the age range and pathological features a germ cell origin (Ulbright et al 1987) or sex-cord origin (Young et al 1994) have been considered, but there are histopathological and immunocytochemical differences between small cell carcinoma and other primary ovarian neoplasms (Young et al 1994).

Lymphoma and leukaemia

Though ovarian infiltration is present at 35–50% of autopsies performed on girls dying of acute lymphoblastic leukaemia, clinical ovarian disease is rare (Heaton & Duff 1989; Pais et al 1991). It can be bilateral and is most frequently seen as recurrent disease with relapse occurring some years after initial diagnosis. Treatment is with systemic chemotherapy rather than surgery (Pais et al 1991).

Primary lymphoma of the female genital tract presenting in childhood is rare, but has been reported (Egwuata 1989).

Non-lymphomatous, non-leukaemic metastatic ovarian tumours in childhood

These are rare, partly because the common neoplasms that spread to the ovary, such as carcinomas of breast and gastrointestinal tract, are unusual in children, but also because the ovary of the child lacks the vascularity of the adult structure. Occasional cases do occur, however, and may prove difficult diagnostically. One review cites examples of neuroblastoma, rhabdomyosarcoma, Ewing's sarcoma, renal rhabdoid tumour and carcinoid tumour, all of which presented initially as ovarian neoplasms and some of which were initially misdiagnosed as primary ovarian tumours (Young et al 1993).

Müllerian papilloma

This is a benign neoplasm that occurs exclusively in children. It involves the cervix or, more rarely, the vagina. Patients are usually aged between two and five years and

present with vaginal bleeding. The tumour is a small polypoid or papillary lesion involving the cervical lip or the endocervical canal. Microscopically, it consists of oedematous fibrovascular papillae, in which there may be metaplastic bone (Ulbright et al 1981). The overlying epithelium is single-layered and varies from flat to columnar (Fig. 34.19). Some cases have recurred locally (Clement 1990). The stroma is uniformly bland in appearance, so that the lesion is easily distinguished from embryonal rhabdomyosarcoma (Lawrence 1991).

Other neoplasms

Extrarenal Wilms' tumours are uncommon, and appear to be least rare in the retroperitoneal site (Wakely et al 1989) but examples have occurred adjacent to the ovary or within the female genital tract (Bell et al 1985; Wakely et al 1989; Pereira et al 2000). Cases reported in the literature have closely resembled the more common renal tumours, giving rise to the theory that they originate from heterotopic rests of renal tissue. The

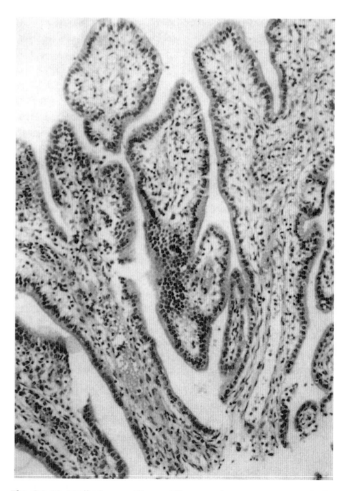

Fig. 34.19 Müllerian papilloma. Fibrovascular cores composed of bland spindle cells covered by a single layer of cuboidal epithelium. (Photograph supplied by Dr W D Lawrence and reproduced with kind permission from W B Saunders Company.)

clinical course and prognosis seem similar to that of the renal tumour.

The vulva may be the site of several entities presenting during childhood which are not specific to this region or age group, including haemangioma (Levin & Selbst 1988), granular cell tumour (Brooks 1985), Langherhans' cell histiocytosis (Otis et al 1990), localised mastocytosis (Wells & Jenkins 1999), lymphangioma, lipoma and teratoma (Huffman et al 1981). Malignant melanoma is rare at all sites during childhood, but has been reported involving the vulva (Egan et al 1997).

REFERENCES

Aguirre P, Scully R E 1982 Malignant neuroectodermal tumor of the ovary: a distinctive form of monodermal teratoma: report of five cases. American Journal of Surgical Pathology 6: 283–292

Ahmed S F, Cheng L, Dovey J R, et al 2000 Phenotypic features, androgen receptor binding, and mutational analysis in 278 clinical cases reported as androgen insensitivity syndrome. Journal of Clinical Endocrinology and Metabolism 85: 658–665

Akhtar M, Bakri Y, Rank F 1989 Dysgerminoma of the ovary with rhabdomyosarcoma. Cancer 64: 2309–2312

Akinola O, Okonofua F E, Odesanmi W O, Oshinaike A I 1988 Serous papillary adenocarcinoma of the ovary in a Nigerian child. Tropical and Geographical Medicine 40: 251–253

Amr S S, Tavassoli F A, Hassan A A, Issa A A, Madanat F F 1986 Mixed mesodermal tumor of the uterus in a 4 year old girl. International Journal of Gynecological Pathology 5: 371–378

Armstrong G R, Buckley C H, Kelsey A M 1991 Germ cell expression of placental alkaline phosphatase in male pseudohermaphroditism. Histopathology 18: 541–547

Atkin N B, Baker M C 1983 i(12p): specific chromosomal marker in seminoma and malignant teratoma of the testis? Cancer Genetics and Cytogenetics 10: 199–204

Bale S J, Falk R T, Rogers G R 1998 Patching together the genetics of Gorlin syndrome. Journal of Cutaneous Medicine and Surgery 3: 31–43

Barr F G, Nauta L E, Davis R J, Schäfer B W, Nycum L M, Biegel J A 1996 In vivo amplification of the PAX3-FKHR and PAX7-FKHR fusion genes in alveolar rhabdomyosarcoma. Human Molecular Genetics 5: 15–21

Begin L R, Clement P B, Kirk M E et al 1985 Aggressive angiomyxoma of pelvic soft parts: a clinicopathologic study of nine cases. Human Pathology 16: 621–628

Bell D A, Shimm D S, Gang D L 1985 Wilms' tumor of the endocervix. Archives of Pathology and Laboratory Medicine 109: 371–373

Bender M E 1986 New concepts of condyloma acuminata in children. Archives of Dermatology 122: 1121–1124

Berta P, Hawkins J R, Sinclair A H et al 1990 Genetic evidence equating SRY and the testis-determining factor. Nature 348: 448–450

Biedel C W, Pagon R A, Zapata J O 1984 Müllerian anomalies and renal agenesis: autosomal dominant urogenital adysplasia. Journal of Pediatrics 104: 861–864

Biegel J A, Meek R S, Parmiter A H, Conrad K, Emanuel B S 1991 Chromosomal translocation t(1;13)(p36;q14) in a case of rhabdomyosarcoma. Genes, Chromosomes & Cancer 3: 483–484

Birch J M 1988 Manchester Children's Tumour Registry 1954–1970 and 1971–1983. In: Parkin D M, Stiller C A, Draper G J, Bieber C A, Terracini B, Young J L (eds) International agency for incidence of childhood cancer. International Agency for Research on Cancer Publications, no 87, Lyon, pp 299–304

Birch J M 1990 Epidemiology of childhood cancer. Annales Nestlé 3 (Childhood oncology), Nestec Ltd., Vevey, Switzerland, pp 105–116

Birch J M, Marsden H B, Swindell R 1982 Pre-natal factors in the origin of germ cell tumours of children. Carcinogenesis 3: 75–80

Birch J M, Hartley A L, Tricker K J et al 1994 Prevalence and diversity of constitutional mutations in the p53 gene among 21 Li-Fraumeni families. Cancer Research 54: 1298–1304

Birch J M, Blair V, Kelsey A M et al 1998 Cancer phenotype correlates with constitutional TP53 genotype in families with the Li-Fraumeni syndrome. Oncogene 17: 1061–1068

Birch J M, Alston R D, McNally R J Q et al 2001 Relative frequency and morphology of cancers in carriers of germline TP53 mutations. Oncogene 20: 4621–4628

Biscotti C V, Hart W R 1989 Juvenile granulosa cell tumors of the ovary. Archives of Pathology and Laboratory Medicine 113: 40–46

Björkholm E, Lundell M, Gyftodimas A, Silfverswärd C 1990 Dysgerminoma: the Radiumhemmet series 1927–1984. Cancer 65: 38–44

Blom G P, Torkildsen E M 1982 Ovarian cystadenocarcinoma in a 4-year-old girl: report of a case and review of the literature. Gynecologic Oncology 13: 242–246

Blyth B, Duckett J W 1991 Gonadal differentiation: a review of the physiological process and influencing factors based on recent experimental evidence. Journal of Urology 145: 689–694

Bolen J W 1981 Mixed germ cell-sex cord-stromal tumor: a gonadal tumor distinct from gonadoblastoma. American Journal of Clinical Pathology 75: 565–573

Bosch-Banyeras J M, Lucaya X, Bernet M et al 1989 Calcified ovarian fibromas in prepubertal girls. European Journal of Pediatrics 148: 749–750

Breen J L, Maxson W S 1977 Ovarian tumors in children and adolescents. Clinical Obstetrics and Gynecology 20: 607–623

Brooks G G 1985 Granular cell myoblastoma of the vulva in a 6-year-old girl. American Journal of Obstetrics and Gynecology 153: 897–898

Brown N J, Langley F A 1976 Teratomas and other genital tumours. In: Marsden H B, Steward J K (eds) Tumours in children. Springer-Verlag, Berlin, pp 362–402

Calaminus G, Wessalowski R, Harms D, Göbel U 1997 Juvenile granulosa cell tumors of the ovary in children and adolescents: results from 33 patients registered in a prospective cooperative study. Gynecologic Oncology 65: 447–452

Cantu J M, Rivera H, Ocampo-Campos R et al 1980 Peutz-Jeghers syndrome with feminizing Sertoli cell tumor. Cancer 46: 223–228

Cario G M, House M J, Paradinas F J 1984 Squamous cell carcinoma of the vulva in association with mixed vulval dystrophy in an 18-year-old girl. British Journal of Obstetrics and Gynaecology 91: 87–90

Carter D, Bibro M C, Touloukin R J 1982 Benign clinical behaviour of immature mediastinal teratoma in infancy and childhood: report of two cases and review of the literature. Cancer 49: 398–402

Chalvardjian A, Scully R E 1973 Sclerosing stromal tumors of the ovary. Cancer 31: 664–670

Chan Y F, Leung C S, Ma L 1989 Primary embryonal rhabdomyosarcoma of the ovary in a 4-year-old girl. Histopathology 15: 309–311

Chumas J C, Mann W J, Tseng L 1983 Malignant mixed Müllerian tumor of the endometrium in a young woman with polycystic ovaries. Cancer 52: 1478–1481

Clatworthy H W, Braden M, Smith J P 1973 Surgery of bladder and prostatic neoplasms in children. Cancer 32: 1157–1160

Clement P B 1990 Miscellaneous primary and metastatic tumors of the uterine cervix. Seminars in Diagnostic Pathology 7: 228–247

Clement P B, Young R H 1993 Pathology of extragonadal yolk sac tumors. In: Nogales F F (ed) The human yolk sac. Springer, Berlin, pp 295–308

Coleman D V, Evans D M D 1988 Biopsy pathology and cytology of the cervix. Chapman & Hall Medical, London, pp 181–188

Cooper C, Crolla J A, Laister C, Johnson D I, Cooke P 1991 An investigation of ring and dicentric chromosomes found in three Turner's syndrome patients using DNA analysis and in situ hybridization with X and Y chromosome specific probes. Journal of Medical Genetics 28: 6–9

Cripe T P 1990 Human papillomaviruses: pediatric perspectives on a family of multifaceted tumorigenic pathogens. Pediatric Infectious Disease Journal 9: 836–844

Dahl N, Gustav K-H, Rune C, Gustavsson I, Pettersson U 1990 Benign ovarian teratomas: an analysis of their cellular origin. Cancer Genetics and Cytogenetics 46: 115–123

Dal Cin P, Van Den Berghe H 1991 Isochromosome (12p) in germ cell tumors. In: Oosterhuis J W, Walt H, Damjanov I (eds) Pathobiology of germ cell neoplasia. Springer-Verlag, Berlin, pp 105–111

Danon M, Robboy S J, Kim S, Scully R, Crawford J D 1975 Cushing syndrome, sexual precosity and polyostotic fibrous dysplasia (Albright syndrome) in infancy. Journal of Pediatrics 87: 917–921

Davidoff F, Federman D D 1973 Mixed gonadal dysgenesis. Pediatrics 52: 725–742

Davos I, Abell M R 1976 Sarcomas of the vagina. Obstetrics and Gynecology 47: 342–350

Daya D A, Scully R E 1988 Sarcoma botryoides of the uterine cervix in young women: a clinicopathological study of 13 cases. Gynecologic Oncology 29: 290–304

Dehner L P 1983 Gonadal and extragonadal germ cell neoplasia of childhood. Human Pathology 14: 493–511

Dehner L P 1987 Female reproductive system. In: Dehner L P (ed) Pediatric surgical pathology. Williams & Wilkins, Baltimore, pp 743–791

DeSa D J 1998 The alimentary tract. In: Wigglesworth J S, Singer D B (eds) Textbook of fetal and perinatal pathology, 2nd edn. Blackwell Scientific Publications, Boston, pp 799–864

Dickersin G R, Kline I W, Scully R E 1982 Small cell carcinoma of the ovary with hypercalcemia: a report of 11 cases. Cancer 49: 188–197

Drogemueller W, Makowski E L, Taylor E S 1970 Vaginal mesonephric adenocarcinoma in two prepubertal children. American Journal of Diseases of Children 119: 168–170

Dudzinski M, Cohen M, Ducatman B 1989 Ovarian malignant luteinized thecoma — an unusual tumor in an adolescent. Gynecologic Oncology 35: 104–109

Duncan P A, Shapiro L R, Stangel J J, Klein R M, Addonizio 1979 The MURCS association: Müllerian duct aplasia, renal aplasia and cervicothoracic somite dysplasia. Journal of Pediatrics 95: 399–402

Egan C A, Bradley R R, Logsdon V K, Summers B K, Hunter G R, Vanderhooft S L 1997 Vulvar melanoma in childhood. Archives of Dermatology 133: 345–348

Egwuata V E 1989 Non-Hodgkin's lymphoma of the uterus in a child. Journal of Pediatric Surgery 24: 220–222

Eichorn J H, Scully R E 1991 Ovarian myxoma: clinicopathologic and immunocytologic analysis of five cases and a review of the literature. International Journal of Gynecological Pathology 10: 156–169

Evans S C, Mims B, McMasters K M et al 1998 Exclusion of a p53 germline mutation in a classic Li-Fraumeni family. Human Genetics 102: 681–686

Faber H K 1962 Meig's syndrome with thecomas of both ovaries in a 4 year old girl. Journal of Pediatrics 61: 769–773

Flam F, Lundstrom V, Silfersward C 1989 Choriocarcinoma in mother and child: case report. British Journal of Obstetrics and Gynaecology 96: 241–244

Garden A S 1998 Gynaecological tumours. In: Garden A S (ed) Paediatric & adolescent gynaecology Arnold, London, pp 242–271

Gell J S, Stannard M W, Ramnani D M, Bradshaw K D 1998 Juvenile granulosa cell tumor in a 13-year-old girl with enchondromatosis (Ollier's disease): a case report. Journal of Pediatric and Adolescent Gynecology 11: 147–150

Gershenson D M, Del Junco G, Herson J, Rutledge F N 1983 Endodermal sinus tumor of the ovary: the M D Anderson experience. Obstetrics and Gynecology 61: 194–202

Geurts van Kessel A, Suijkerbuijk R, de Jong B, Oosterhuis J W 1991 Molecular analysis of isochromosome 12p in testicular germ cell tumors. In: Oosterhuis J W, Walt H, Damjanov I (eds) Pathobiology of germ cell neoplasia. Springer-Verlag, Berlin, pp 105–111

Gilbert-Barness E F, Opitz J M 1998a Congenital anomalies: malformation syndromes. In: Wigglesworth J S, Singer D B (eds) Textbook of fetal and perinatal pathology, 2nd edn. Blackwell Scientific Publications, Boston, pp 323–357

Gilbert-Barness E F, Opitz J M 1998b Chromosomal abnormalities. In: Wigglesworth J S, Singer D B (eds) Textbook of fetal and perinatal pathology, 2nd edn. Blackwell Scientific Publications, Boston, pp 291–322

Greenberg F, Keenan B, DeYanis V, Finegold M 1986 Gonadal dysgenesis and gonadoblastoma in situ in a female with Fraser (cryptophthalmos) syndrome. Journal of Pediatrics 108: 952–954

Gribbon M, Ein S H, Mancer K 1992 Pediatric malignant ovarian tumors: a 43-year review. Journal of Pediatric Surgery 27: 480–484

Gubbay J, Collignon J, Koopman P et al 1990 A gene mapping to the sex determining region of the mouse Y chromosome is a member of a novel family of embryonically expressed genes. Nature 346: 345–350

Gutman L T 1990 Sexual abuse and human papilloma virus infection. Journal of Pediatrics 116: 495–496

Hadjiathanasiou C G, Brauner R, Lortat-Jacob S et al 1994 True hermaphroditism: genetic variants and clinical management. Journal of Pediatrics 125: 738–744

Hanselaar A G J M, Van Leusen N D M, De Wilde P C M, Vooijs G P 1991 Clear cell adenocarcinoma of the vagina and cervix: a report of the central Netherlands with emphasis on early detection and prognosis. Cancer 67: 1971–1978

Hanson R M, Glasson M, McCrssin I, Rogers M 1989 Anogenital warts in childhood. Child Abuse and Neglect 13: 225–233

Harris A C, Wakely P E, Kaplowitz P B, Loringer R D 1991 Steroid cell tumor of the ovary in a child. Archives of Pathology and Laboratory Medicine 115: 150–154

Hartley A L, Birch J M, Marsden H B, Harris M 1987 Malignant melanoma in families of children with osteosarcoma, chondrosarcoma and adrenal cortical carcinoma. Journal of Medical Genetics 24: 664–668

Hartley A L, Birch J M, Kelsey A M, Marsden H B, Harris M, Teare M D 1989 Are germ cell tumors part of the Li-Fraumeni cancer family syndrome? Cancer Genetics and Cytogenetics 42: 221–226

Hartley A L, Birch J M, Tricker K et al 1993 Wilms' tumor in the Li-Fraumeni cancer family syndrome. Cancer Genetics and Cytogenetics 67: 133–135

Hays D M, Shimada H, Raney R B et al 1988 Clinical staging and treatment results in rhabdomyosarcoma of the female genital tract among children and adolescents. Cancer 61: 1893–1903

Heaton D C, Duff G B 1989 Ovarian relapse in a young woman with acute lymphoblastic leukemia. American Journal of Hematology 30: 42–43

Heifetz S A, Cushing B, Giller R et al 1998 Immature teratomas in children: pathologic considerations: from the combined Pediatric Oncology Group/Children's Cancer Group. American Journal of Surgical Pathology 22: 1115–1124

Heiss K F, Zwiren G T, Winn K 1994 Massive ovarian edema in the pediatric patient: a rare solid tumor. Journal of Pediatric Surgery 29: 1392–1394

Hemminki A 1999 The molecular basis and clinical aspects of Peutz-Jeghers syndrome. Cellular and Molecular Life Sciences 55: 735–750

Herbst A L 1981 Clear cell adenocarcinoma and current status of DES exposed females. Cancer 48: 484–488

Herbst A L, Anderson D 1990 Clear cell adenocarcinoma of the vagina and cervix secondary to intrauterine exposure to stilbestrol. Seminars in Surgical Oncology 6: 343–346

Herbst A L, Green T H, Ulfelder R H 1970 Primary carcinoma of the vagina: an analysis of 68 cases. American Journal of Obstetrics and Gynecology 106: 210–218

Herbst A L, Ulfelder R H, Poskanzer D C 1971 Adenocarcinoma of vagina: association of maternal stilbestrol therapy with tumor appearance in young women. New England Journal of Medicine 284: 878–881

Hilgers R D, Malkasian G D, Soule E D 1970 Embryonal rhabdomyosarcoma (botryoid type) of the vagina: a clinicopathological review. American Journal of Obstetrics and Gynecology 107: 484–502

Ho G Y, Bierman R, Beardsley L, Chang C J, Burk R D 1989 Natural history of cervicovaginal papillomavirus infection in young women. New England Journal of Medicine 338: 423–428

Howell C G, Rogers D A, Gable D S, Falls G D 1990 Bilateral ovarian fibromas in children. Journal of Pediatric Surgery 25: 690–691

Huffman J W, Dewhurst J C, Copraro V J 1981 The gynecology of childhood and adolescence, 2nd edn. W B Saunders, Philadelphia, pp 270–272

Ismail S M, Walker S M 1990 Bilateral virilizing sclerosing stromal tumours of the ovary in a pregnant woman with Gorlin's syndrome: implications for pathogenesis of ovarian stromal neoplasms. Histopathology 17: 159–163

Kaminski P F, Maier R C 1983 Clear cell adenocarcinoma of cervix unrelated to diethylstilbestrol exposure. Obstetrics and Gynecology 62: 720–727

Kilman J W, Clatworthy H W, Newton W A, Grosfield J L 1973 Reasonable surgery for rhabdomyosarcoma. Annals of Surgery 178: 346–351

Kini H, Baliga P B, Pai K G 1998 Supernumerary ovary associated with Wilms' tumor. Pediatric Surgery International 13: 67–69

Keshtgar A S and Turnock R R 1997 Wandering calcified ovary in children. Pediatric Surgery International 12: 215–216

Kohorn E I, McIntosh S, Lytton B, Knowlton A H, Merino M 1985 Endodermal sinus tumor of the infant vagina. Gynecologic Oncology 20: 196–203

Kraemer B B, Silva E G, Sneige N 1984 Fibrosarcoma of ovary: a new component in the nevoid basal-cell carcinoma syndrome. American Journal of Surgical Pathology 8: 231–236

Kurman R J, Norris H J 1976a Endodermal sinus tumor of the ovary: a clinical and pathological analysis of 71 cases. Cancer 38: 2402–2419

Kurman R J, Norris H J 1976b Embryonal carcinoma of the ovary: a clinicopathological entity distinct from endodermal sinus tumor resembling embryonal carcinoma of the adult testis. Cancer 38: 2420–2433

Kurman R J, Norris H J 1977 Malignant germ cell tumors of the ovary. Human Pathology 8: 551–562

Lack E E, Perez-Atayde A R, Murthy A S K, Goldstein D P, Crigler J F, Vawter G F 1981 Granulosa theca cell tumors in premenarchal girls: a clinical and pathological study of 10 cases. Cancer 48: 1846–1854

Lacson A G, Gillis D A, Shawwa A 1988 Malignant mixed germ cell-sex cord-stromal tumors of the ovary associated with isosexual precocious puberty. Cancer 61: 2122–2133

Lauchlan S C, Pinar H 1998 The reproductive system. In: Wigglesworth J S, Singer D B (eds) Text book of fetal and perinatal pathology, 2nd edn. Blackwell Scientific Publications, Boston, pp 1013–1038

La Vecchia C, Morris H B, Draper G J 1983 Malignant ovarian tumours in childhood in Britain 1962–78. British Journal of Cancer 48: 363–374

Lawrence W D 1991 Advances in the pathology of the uterine cervix. Human Pathology 22: 792–806

Lee K R, Scully R E 1989 Complex endometrial hyperplasia and carcinoma in adolescents and young women 15–20 years of age. International Journal of Gynecological Pathology 8: 201–213

Levin A V, Selbst S M 1988 Vulvar hemangioma simulating child abuse. Clinical Pediatrics 27: 213–215

Li F P, Fraumeni J F 1969 Soft tissue sarcomas, breast cancer and other neoplasms. Annals of Internal Medicine 71: 747–752

Liang X, Ioffe O B, Chen-Chih J S 1998 Cloacal dysgenesis sequence: observations in four patients including three fetuses of second trimester gestation. Pediatric and Developmental Pathology 1: 281–288

Luzzatto C, Midrio P, Toffolutti T, Suma V 2000 Neonatal Ovarian cysts: management and follow-up. Pediatric Surgery International 16: 56–59

Malfetano J H, Degnan E, Florentin R 1990 Para-endocrine hypercalcemia and ovarian small cell carcinoma. New York State Journal of Medicine 90: 206–207

Malkin D, Li F P, Strong L C et al 1990 Germline p53 mutations in a familial syndrome of breast cancer, sarcomas, and other neoplasms. Science 250: 1233–1238

Malogolowkin M H, Mahour G H, Krailo M, Ortega J A 1990 Germ cell tumors in infancy and childhood: a 45 year experience. In: Jaffe R, Dahms B B, Krous H F, Lieberman E, Triche T J (eds) Forefront of pediatric pathology. Hemisphere Publishing Corporation, New York, pp 231–241

Mandell J, Stevens P S, Fried F A 1977 Childhood gonadoblastoma and seminoma in a dysgenetic cryptorchid gonad. Journal of Urology 117: 674–675

Mann J R, Pearson D, Barett A, Raafat F, Barnes J M, Wallendszus K R 1989 Results of the United Kingdom Children's Cancer Study Group's malignant germ cell tumor studies. Cancer 63: 1657–1667

Marsden H B, Birch J M, Swindell R 1981 Germ cell tumours of childhood: A review of 137 cases. Journal of Clinical Pathology 34: 879–883

Meyer J S, Harmon C M, Harty H P, Markowitz R I, Hubbard A M, Bellah R D 1995 Ovarian torsion: clinical and imaging presentation in children. Journal of Pediatric Surgery 30: 1433–1436

Miller R W 1969 Fifty-two forms of childhood cancer: United States mortality experience 1960–1966. Journal of Pediatrics 75: 685–689

Mitchell M F, Gershenson D M, Soeters R P, Eifel P J, Delclos L, Wharton J T 1991 The long-term effects of radiotherapy on patients with ovarian dysgerminoma. Cancer 67: 1084–1090

Mordehai J, Mares A J, Barki R, Finaly R, Meizner I 1991 Torsion of uterine adnexa in neonates and children: a report of 20 cases. Journal of Pediatric Surgery 26: 1195–1199

Moscicki A B 1996 Genital HPV infections in children and adolescents. Obstetric and Gynecology Clinics of North America 23: 675–697

Moscicki A B, Shiboski S, Broering J et al 1998 The natural history of human papillomavirus infection as measured by repeated DNA testing in adolescent and young women. Journal of Pediatrics 132: 277–284

Moscicki A B, Ellenberg J H, Vermund S H et al 2000 Prevalence of and risk for cervical human papillomavirus infection and squamous intra-epithelial lesions in adolescent girls: impact of infection with human immunodeficiency virus. Archives of Pediatric and Adolescent Medicine 154: 127–134

Müller J, Skakkebaek N E 1984 Testicular carcinoma in situ in children with the androgen insensitivity syndrome. British Medical Journal 288: 1419–1420

Müller J, Skakkebaek N E, Ritzen M, Plöen L, Petersen K E 1985 Carcinoma in situ of the testis in children with 45X/46XY gonadal dysgenesis. Journal of Pediatrics 106: 431–436

Neilson G P, Oliva E, Young R H, Rosenberg A E, Prat J, Scully R E 1998 Primary ovarian rhabdomyosarcoma: a report of 13 cases. International Journal of Gynecological Pathology 17: 113–119

Nogales F F, Favara B E, Major F J, Silverberg S G 1976 Immature teratoma of the ovary with a neural component ('solid' teratoma): a clinicopathologic study of 20 cases. Human Pathology 7: 625–642

Nogales F F, Martin-Sances L, Mendoza-Garcia E, Salamanca A, Gonzalez-Nunez M A, Pardo Mindan F J 1996 Massive ovarian oedema. Histopathology 28: 229–234

Norris H J 1999 Immature teratomas in children. American Journal of Surgical Pathology 23: 1160–1161

Norris H J, Jensen R D 1972 Relative frequency of ovarian neoplasms in children and adolescents. Cancer 30: 713–719

Norris H J, Bagley G P, Taylor H B 1970 Carcinoma of the infant vagina: a distinctive tumor. Archives of Pathology 90: 473–479

Norris H J, Zirkin H J, Benson W L 1976 Immature (malignant) teratoma of the ovary: a clinical and pathological study of 58 cases. Cancer 37: 2359–2372

Nunez C, Abboud S L, Lemon N C, Kemp J A 1983 Ovarian rhabdomyosarcoma presenting as leukemia. Cancer 52: 297–300

O'Connor D M, Norris H J 1994 The influence of grade on the outcome of stage 1 ovarian immature (malignant) teratomas and the reproducibility of grading. International Journal of Gynecological Pathology 13: 283–289

O'Dowd J, Gaffney E F, Young R H 1990 Malignant sex cord-stromal tumour in a patient with the androgen insensitivity syndrome. Histopathology 16: 279–282

Olsen M M, Caldamone A A, Jackson C L, Zinn A 1988 Gonadoblastoma in infancy: indications for early gonadectomy in 46, XY gonadal dysgenesis. Journal of Pediatric Surgery 23: 270–271

Otis C N, Fischer R A, Johnson N, Kelleher J F, Powell J L 1990 Histiocytosis X of the vulva: a case report and review of the literature. Obstetrics and Gynecology 75: 555–558

Pais R C, Kim T H, Zwiren G T, Ragab A H 1991 Ovarian tumors in relapsing acute lymphoblastic leukemia: a review of 23 cases. Journal of Pediatric Surgery 26: 70–74

Parkin D M, Stiller C A, Draper G J, Bieber C A, Terracini B, Young J L 1988 International incidence of childhood cancer. International Agency for Research on Cancer Publications, no 87, Lyon

Pereira F, Carrascal E, Canas C, Florez L 2000 Extrarenal Wilms tumor of the left ovary: a case report. Journal of Pediatric Hematology and Oncology 22: 88–89

Pizzo P A, Triche T J 1987 Clinical staging in rhabdomyosarcoma: current limitations and future prospects. Journal of Clinical Oncology 5: 8–9

Prus D, Rosenberg A E, Blumenfeld A et al 1997 Infantile hemangioendothelioma of the ovary: a monodermal teratoma or a neoplasm of ovarian somatic cells? American Journal of Surgical Pathology 21: 1231–1235

Pysher T J, Hitch D C, Krous H F 1981 Bilateral juvenile granulosa cell tumors in a 4-month-old dysmorphic infant: a clinical, histologic and ultrastructural study. American Journal of Surgical Pathology 5: 789–794

Ravikumar V R, Lakshmanan D 1983 Solitary neurofibroma of the clitoris masquerading as intersex. Journal of Pediatric Surgery 18: 617

Resnik E, Christopherson W A, Stock R 1989 Clear cell adenocarcinoma of the cervix and vagina in a woman with mixed gonadal dysgenesis: a case report. Journal of Reproductive Medicine 34: 981–984

Rink R C, Mitchell M E 1983 Genitourinary neurofibromatosis in childhood. Journal of Urology 130: 1176–1179

Rock B, Naghashfar Z, Barnett N, Buscema J, Woodruff J D, Shah K 1986 Genital tract papillomavirus infection in children. Archives of Dermatology 122: 1129–1132

Rodriguez E, Melamed J, Reuter V, Chaganti R S K 1995 Chromosome 12 abnormalities in malignant ovarian germ cell tumors. Cancer Genetics and Cytogenetics 82: 62–66

Roth L M, Nicholas T R, Ehrlich C E 1979 Juvenile granulosa cell tumor: a clinicopathologic study of three cases with ultrastructural observations. Cancer 44: 2194–2205

Rutgers J L, Scully R E 1987 Pathology of the testis in intersex syndromes. Seminars in Diagnostic Pathology 4: 275–291

Sadeghi S B, Sadeghi A, Cosby M, Olincy A, Robboy S J 1988 Human papillomavirus infection: frequency and association with cervical neoplasia in a young population. Acta Cytologica 33: 319–323

Saldanha G 2001 The Hedgehog signalling pathway and cancer. Journal of Pathology 193: 427–432

Schepel S J, Tolhurst D E 1981 Neurofibroma of clitoris and labium majus simulating a penis and testicle. British Journal of Plastic Surgery 34: 221–223

Schweisguth O, Gerard-Marchant R, Plainfosse B, Lemerle J, Watchi J M, Seringe P 1971 Bilateral non-functioning thecoma of the ovary in epileptic children under anticonvulsant therapy. Acta Paediatrica Scandinavica 60: 6–10

Schwöbel M G, Stauffer U G 1991 Surgical treatment of ovarian tumors in childhood. Progress in Pediatric Surgery 26: 112–123

Scully R E 1970 Gonadoblastoma; a review of 74 cases. Cancer 25: 1340–1356

Scully R E 1979 Tumors of the ovary and maldeveloped gonads. Atlas of tumor pathology, fascicle 16. Armed Forces Institute of Pathology, Washington, DC

Scully R E 1991 Gonadal pathology of genetically determined disease. In: Kraus F T, Damjanov I, Kaufman N (eds) Pathology of reproductive failure. Williams & Wilkins, Baltimore, pp 257–285

Scully R E 1993 Small cell carcinoma of hypercalcemic type. International Journal of Gynecological Pathology 12: 148–152

Scully R E, Welch W R 1981 Pathology of the female genital tract after prenatal exposure to diethylstilbestrol. In: Herbst A L, Bern H A (eds) Developmental effects of diethylstilbestrol (DES) in pregnancy. Thieme-Stratton, New York, pp 26–45

Senturia Y D 1987 The epidemiology of testicular cancer. British Journal of Urology 60: 285–291

Shelton T B, Jerkins G R, Noe H N 1986 Condylomata acuminata in the pediatric patient. Journal of Urology 135: 548–549

Shu X O, Nesbit M E, Buckley J D, Krailo M D, Robison L L 1995 An exploratory analysis of risk factors for childhood malignant germ-cell tumors: report from the Children's Cancer Group (Canada, United States). Cancer Causes and Control 6: 187–198

Silver S A, Wiley J M, Perlman E J 1994 DNA ploidy analysis of pediatric germ cell tumors. Modern Pathology 7: 951–955

Sinclair A H, Berta P, Palmer M S et al 1990 A gene for the human sex determining region encodes a protein with homology to a conserved DNA binding motif. Nature 346: 240–244

Srivastava S, Zou Z, Pirollo K, Blattner W, Chang E H 1990 Germline transmission of a mutated p53 gene in a cancer prone family with Li-Fraumeni syndrome. Nature 348: 747–749

Snyder D, La Franchi S 1999 Severe virilization in a girl with a steroid cell tumor of the ovary. Journal of Pediatric Endocrinology & Metabolism 12: 221–224

Spigelman A D, Muriday V, Philips R K S 1989 Cancer and the Peutz-Jeghers syndrome. Gut 30: 1588–1590

Steeper T A, Rosai J 1983 Aggressive angiomyxoma of the female pelvis and perineum: report of nine cases of a distinctive type of gynecologic soft-tissue neoplasm. American Journal of Surgical Pathology 7: 463–475

Stettner A R, Hartenbach E M, Schink J C et al 1999 Familial ovarian germ cell cancer: report and review. American Journal of Medical Genetics 84: 43–46

Talerman A A 1972 A mixed germ cell-sex cord tumor of the ovary in a normal female infant. Obstetrics and Gynecology 40: 473–478

Talerman A, Verp M S, Senekjian E, Gilewski T, Vogelzang N 1990 True hermaphrodite with bilateral ovotestes, bilateral gonadoblastomas and dysgerminomas, 46,XX/46,XY karyotype and a successful pregnancy. Cancer 66: 2668–2672

Tamimi H K, Bolen J W 1984 Enchondromatosis (Ollier's disease) and ovarian juvenile granulosa cell tumor: a case report and review of the literature. Cancer 53: 1605–1608

Tavassoli F A 1983 A combined germ cell-gonadal stromal-epithelial tumor of the ovary. American Journal of Surgical Pathology 7: 73–84

Taylor M H, DePetrillo A D, Turner A R 1985 Vinblastine, bleomycin and cisplatin in malignant germ cell tumors of the ovary. Cancer 56: 1341–1349

Thomas W J, Bevan H E, Hooper D G, Downey E J 1989 Malignant schwannoma of the clitoris in a 1-year-old child. Cancer 63: 2216–2219

Thurlbeck W M, Scully R E 1960 Solid teratoma of the ovary: a clinicopathological analysis of 9 cases. Cancer 13: 804–811

Trau H, Schewach-Millet M, Fisher B K, Tsur H 1982 Peutz-Jeghers syndrome and bilateral breast carcinoma. Cancer 50: 788–792

Truong L D, Jurco S, McGavran M H 1982 Gliomatosis peritonei: report of two cases and review of the literature. American Journal of Surgical Pathology 6: 443–449

Tscherne G 1997 Female genital tract malignancies during puberty. Uterine and cervical malignancies. Annals of the New York Academy of Sciences 816: 331–337

Turc-Carel C, Lizard-Nacol S, Justrabo E et al 1986 Consistent chromosomal translocation in alveolar rhabdomyosarcoma. Cancer Genetics and Cytogenetics 19: 361–362

Ulbright T M, Alexander R W, Kraus F T 1981 Intramural papilloma of the vagina: evidence of Müllerian histogenesis. Cancer 48: 2260–2266

Ulbright T M, Roth L M, Stehman F B, Talerman A, Senekjian E K 1987 Poorly differentiated (small cell) carcinoma of the ovary in young women: evidence supporting a germ cell origin. Human Pathology 18: 175–184

Velasco-Oses A, Alanso-Alvaro A, Blanco-Pozo A, Nogales F F 1988 Ollier's disease associated with ovarian juvenile granulosa cell tumor. Cancer 62: 222–225

Wakely P E, Sprague R I, Kornstein M J 1989 Extrarenal Wilms' tumor: an analysis of four cases. Human Pathology 20: 691–695

Walker A H, Ross R K, Pike M C, Henderson B E 1984 A possible rising incidence of malignant germ cell tumours in young women. British Journal of Cancer 49: 669–672

Walker A H, Ross R K, Haile R W C, Henderson B E 1988 Hormonal factors and risk of ovarian germ cell cancer in young women. British Journal of Cancer 57: 418–422

Wallace T M, Levin H S 1990 Mixed gonadal dysgenesis: a review of 15 patients reporting single cases of malignant intratubular germ cell neoplasia of the testis, endometrial adenocarcinoma and a complex vascular anomaly. Archives of Pathology and Laboratory Medicine 114: 679–688

Weinblatt M, Kochen J 1991 An unusual family cancer syndrome manifested in young siblings. Cancer 68: 1068–1070

Wells M, Jenkins M 1994 Selected topics in the histopathology of the vulva. Current Diagnostic Pathology 1: 41–47

Weyl-Ben M, Oslander L 1991 Ollier's disease associated with ovarian Sertoli-Leydig cell tumor and breast adenoma. American Journal of Pediatric Hematology/Oncology 13: 49–51

Woodman C B, Collins S, Winter H et al 2001 Natural history of cervical human papillomavirus infection in young women: a longitudinal cohort study. Lancet 357: 1831–1836

Wu P O, Huang R L, Lang J H et al 1991 Treatment of malignant ovarian germ cell tumors with preservation of fertility: a report of 28 cases. Gynecologic Oncology 40: 2–6

Young R H, Scully R E 1982 Ovarian sex cord-stromal tumors: recent progress. International Journal of Gynecological Pathology 1: 101–123

Young R H, Scully R E 1983 Sertoli-Leydig tumors with a retiform pattern: a problem in histopathologic diagnosis. American Journal of Surgical Pathology 7: 755–771

Young R H, Scully R E 1984 Fibromatosis and massive edema of the ovary; possibly related entities: a report of 14 cases of fibromatosis and 11 cases of massive edema. International Journal of Gynecological Pathology 3: 153–178

Young R H, Scully R E 1985 Ovarian Sertoli-Leydig cell tumors: a clinicopathologic study of 207 cases. American Journal of Surgical Pathology 9: 543–569

Young R H, Welch W R, Dickerson G R, Scully R E 1982 Ovarian sex cord tumor with annular tubules: review of 74 cases including 27 with Peutz-Jeghers syndrome and four with adenoma malignum of the cervix. Cancer 50: 1384–1402

Young R H, Dickersin G R, Scully R E 1983 A distinctive ovarian sex cord-stromal tumor causing sexual precocity in the Peutz-Jeghers syndrome. American Journal of Surgical Pathology 7: 233–243

Young R H, Dickersin G R, Scully R E 1984 Juvenile granulosa cell tumor of the ovary: a clinicopathological analysis of 125 cases. American Journal of Surgical Pathology 8: 575–596

Young R H, Lawrence W D, Scully R E 1985 Juvenile granulosa cell tumor — another neoplasm associated with abnormal chromosomes and ambiguous genitalia: a report of three cases. American Journal of Surgical Pathology 10: 737–743

Young R H, Dickersin G R, Scully R E 1987 Small cell carcinoma: an analysis of 75 cases of a distinctive ovarian tumor commonly associated with hypercalcemia. Laboratory Investigation 56: 89A

Young R H, Kozakewich H P W, Scully R E 1993 Metastatic ovarian tumors in children: a report of 14 cases and review of the literature. International Journal of Gynecological Pathology 12: 8–19

Young R H, Oliva E, Scully R E 1994 Small cell carcinoma of the ovary, hypercalcaemic type. A clinicopathological analysis of 150 cases. American Journal of Surgical Pathology 18: 1102–1116

Zaloudek C, Norris H J 1984 Sertoli-Leydig tumors of the ovary: a clinicopathological study of 64 intermediate and poorly differentiated neoplasms. American Journal of Surgical Pathology 8: 405–418

35

Interrelationships of non-gynaecological and gynaecological disease

C. H. Buckley

Introduction   1181

Non-gynaecological conditions presenting as a
gynaecological problem or associated with gynaecological
disorders   1181

Non-gynaecological conditions incidentally affecting the
genital tract   1192

The gynaecological consequences of the treatment of
non-gynaecological disease   1192

The non-gynaecological consequences of gynaecological
disease and treatment   1193

INTRODUCTION

It is important in specialised texts such as this not to overlook the impact which systemic disease may have on the practice of gynaecology, and to see gynaecological disorders in their wider context. The gynaecologist or gynaecological pathologist may encounter systemic disease in a variety of guises and should also be aware of the systemic impact of gynaecological disease.

The relationship between gynaecological practice and non-gynaecological disease has many facets. There are congenital and acquired biochemical and haematological conditions which may affect case management, systemic or local non-gynaecological abnormalities which may present as gynaecological problems or affect the genital tract fortuitously, non-gynaecological disease which may affect the morphology and function of the genital tract and, finally, gynaecological disorders which may have local or systemic non-gynaecological complications.

NON-GYNAECOLOGICAL CONDITIONS PRESENTING AS A GYNAECOLOGICAL PROBLEM OR ASSOCIATED WITH GYNAECOLOGICAL DISORDERS

In some instances a patient with a non-gynaecological disease may present with symptoms referable to the genital tract, or histopathological examination of biopsy or surgical resection material from the female genital tract may reveal a systemic disorder.

Achlorhydria

Some patients with achlorhydria are found to have a vulvar dermatosis (Jeffcoate 1962) and a possible causal relationship between the two conditions has been postulated (Lavery 1984).

Acromegaly

Menstrual irregularities, which are common in women with acromegaly, are usually attributed to gonadotrophin deficiency or hyperprolactinaemia (Kaltsas et al 1999). There is also a reduction in sex hormone binding protein and hyperinsulinaemia and these too may play a part.

Amyloidosis

Systemic amyloid has, rarely, presented as a vulvar nodule (Taylor et al 1991). Localised deposition of amyloid in the cervix (Yamada et al 1988; Gibbons et al 1998) has also been reported in the absence of systemic disease.

Ataxia-telangiectasia

Ataxia-telangiectasia is an autosomal recessive inherited disorder characterised by immunodeficiency, progressive cerebellar ataxia and cutaneous telangiectases. Malignant neoplasms develop in 10–15% of patients (Gatti & Good 1971) and in a small proportion the tumour is a dysgerminoma of the ovary (Goldsmith & Hart 1975; Narita & Takagi 1984), which may be bilateral (Dunn et al 1964). Gonadoblastoma (Goldsmith & Hart 1975) and yolk sac tumour of the ovary have also been described (Pecorelli et al 1988). Care should be taken in interpreting a raised alpha-fetoprotein in these latter patients as it may also be raised as a consequence of chronic hepatitis, vascular abnormalities and an embryonic thymus. Neoplasms are not limited to the ovary, for uterine leiomyoma, smooth muscle tumour of uncertain malignancy and leiomyosarcoma have also been recorded (Gatti et al 1989). Premature ovarian failure may also occur in this group of women (Friedman et al 1984).

Blepharophimosis (Blepharophimosis, ptosis and epicanthus inversus syndrome)

Blepharophimosis syndrome is an autosomal dominant disorder in which resistant ovary (Fraser et al 1988; Panidis et al 1994), gonadal dysgenesis (Nicolino et al 1995; Ogata et al 1998) premature menopause, due to increased follicular apoptosis (Christin-Maitre 1999), and bilateral granulosa cell tumours (Maede et al 1999) have been reported.

Carney complex

Carney complex (CNC) is a syndrome characterised by familial multiple neoplasia and lentiginosis with features overlapping those of other similar syndromes, in particular Peutz–Jeghers syndrome. The ovarian tumours in Carney complex are, however, not the same as those in Peutz–Jeghers syndrome. The tumours that have been described include bilateral asynchronous serous cystadenomas, unilateral serous cystadenoma, endometrioid adenocarcinoma and mucinous adenocarcinoma. The chromosome 2p16 CNC locus is involved in the ovarian pathology with apparent copy number gain, suggesting that at the molecular level there is some involvement of the *CNC* gene(s) in these lesions (Stratakis et al 2000).

Chédiak-Higashi syndrome

In individuals with this syndrome, a defect in microtubule polymerisation leads to defective leucocyte function. A sclerosing stromal tumour of the ovary has been reported in an affected patient (Inoue et al 1991).

Cowden's disease

Cowden's disease (multiple hamartoma syndrome) is a rare autosomal dominant condition first described by Lloyd & Dennis (1963). It is characterised by the presence of facial trichilemmomas, acral keratoses, cutaneous horns, oral mucosal papillomas, colorectal polyposis, thyroid tumours, diffuse nodular goitre, lipomas, punctate keratoses on palms and soles and angiomas: in some patients malignant changes have been reported in the hamartomatous lesions (Carlson et al 1984; Starink 1984). Breast lesions, including carcinoma and fibrocystic disease, are reported in 76% of female patients (Starink 1984). In addition, endometrial and ovarian carcinoma has been described at a somewhat earlier age than would usually be expected, in a 35-year-old woman (Carlson et al 1984). Carcinoma of the cervix has also been recorded. A further series of gynaecological neoplasms and developmental cysts have also been reported in patients with this condition: they include benign ovarian cysts of unspecified type (Walton et al 1986), serous cystadenoma of the ovary, immature ovarian teratoma, granulosa cell tumour, uterine leiomyomas, Gartner's cyst of the vagina, apocrine hydrocytoma of the vulva, sebaceous cyst of the vulva and urethral polyps (Starink 1984; Grattan & Hamburger 1987; Neumann 1991). In many instances the association could have been fortuitous but some of these lesions may represent further potential problems for these patients.

Cytogenetic disorders

Cytogenetic disorders affecting the sex chromosomes (Chapter 36) may be manifest as gynaecological disorders but more commonly it is their systemic features which are first identified, although, as for example in ovarian dysgenesis, some of those systemic abnormalities, such as the failure of secondary sexual characteristics, are a consequence of the failure of ovarian development and are not primary components of the disorder. There is, however, an association between Hashimoto's thyroiditis and Turner's syndrome and a case has been reported in which there was, in addition, sarcoidosis (Tsuji et al 1992).

Dermatological disorders

Dermatological diseases that affect the vulva are described in detail in Chapter 3 but it is important to recognise that gynaecological problems may be the first indication that the patient has a systemic dermatological problem and that the presentation may not be typical of that seen elsewhere in the body.

Pemphigus vulgaris, for example, may persist or recur in the vagina even when the skin lesions have responded to treatment (Zosmer et al 1992).

Previously unrecognised **Darier's disease** of the cervix has been the cause of a misleading abnormal cervical smear (Adam 1996).

Diabetes mellitus

The first indication of diabetes mellitus, particularly in elderly women, may be the development of a vulvovaginitis due to infection with *Candida albicans*. This condition is also a problem in the poorly controlled diabetic patient whilst pyogenic infection of the perineum may follow a more aggressive course than in the non-diabetic woman. Delayed menarche or, more commonly, secondary amenorrhoea may also occur in diabetics.

Type II insulin resistant diabetes with hyperinsulinaemia is a feature of some cases of polycystic ovary syndrome although polycystic ovaries do not develop in all such cases (Conn et al 2000). Therapeutic reduction in insulin levels in these patients is associated with a decrease in androgen levels (Taylor 2000). An association between diabetes and endometrial carcinoma, with a relative risk of 4.1, has been reported (Maatela et al 1994).

Down's syndrome

A case of ovarian dysgerminoma has been reported in a patient with Down's syndrome (Gesmundo et al 1988).

Enchondromatosis (Ollier's disease and Maffucci's syndrome)

Ollier's disease is a non-hereditary mesodermal dysplasia that affects the metaphyses of long bones. When there are, in addition, subcutaneous haemangiomas, it is known as Maffucci's syndrome. Both syndromes may be complicated by the development of ovarian neoplasms. Kuzma & King (1948) first described this association and reported an atypical granulosa cell tumour of the ovary in a patient with Maffucci's syndrome. Lewis & Ketcham (1973) subsequently described a malignant tumour of sex-cord origin. When Tamimi & Bolen (1984) described a further case, they took the opportunity of re-examining the data from the previous descriptions and suggested that all three were similar and were in fact examples of juvenile granulosa cell tumours. Since then, there have been other reports describing juvenile granulosa cell tumours in individuals with Ollier's disease (Young et al 1984; Vaz & Turner 1986; Velasco-Oses et al 1988; Plantaz et al 1992; Tanaka et al 1992; Gell et al 1998). In one case, the condition was associated with precocious pseudopuberty (Vaz & Turner 1986).

It should not, however, be assumed that the development of a juvenile granulosa cell tumour necessarily indicates the presence of Ollier's disease, bilateral juvenile granulosa cell tumours having also been described in patients with other abnormalities. They have been found, for example, in a poorly growing 4-month-old dysmorphic infant (Pysher et al 1981), in a newborn with Potter's syndrome (Roth et al 1979), in a child with leprechaunism (Brisigotti et al 1993) and in a 14-week-old child with poor weight gain (Zemke & Herrel 1941). Other gynaecological neoplasms reported in patients with enchondromatosis include thecoma (Hamdoun et al 1993), Sertoli–Leydig cell tumour (Weyl-Ben Arush & Oslander 1991), steroid cell tumour (Fristachi et al 1991), and fibrosarcoma (Christman & Ballon 1990).

Fraser syndrome (Cryptophthalmos)

Gonadal dysgenesis and gonadoblastoma have been described in a child with cryptophthalmos (Greenberg et al 1986).

Galactosaemia

Galactosaemia may result in premature ovarian failure (Russell et al 1982; Fraser et al 1986; Kaufman et al 1986; Cramer et al 1987; Hagenfeldt et al 1989). Despite a low galactose diet, the follicles are damaged. This contrasts with the condition in males in whom normal gonadal function is preserved. The risk of premature menopause can be predicted by analysing the patient's molecular genotype for galactose-1-phosphate uridyltransferase (GALT) and examining alternative pathways for galactose metabolism. The development of premature ovarian failure is more likely if the patient's genotype is Q188R/Q188R, if the mean erythrocyte galactose-1-phosphate is more than 3.5 mg/ml during therapy, and if the whole body oxidation of galactose is less than 5% (Guerrero et al 2000). It has been noted that the mutations in GALT detected in Japanese and Caucasian subjects differ (Hirokawa et al 1999).

Müllerian aplasia has been described in the offspring of a woman with GALT levels below the normal range (Cramer et al 1987).

Gaucher's disease

The association of Gaucher's disease and malignant tumours is very rare, but Kojiro et al (1983) reviewed the literature and described an example of dysgerminoma developing in a 22-year-old woman with Gaucher's disease; it is thought likely that the association was fortuitous.

Goldberg–Maxwell–Morris syndrome (testicular feminisation)

Sertoli cell tumours have been described in a patient with the Goldberg–Maxwell–Morris syndrome (Moneta et al 1981).

Gorlin's syndrome (basal cell naevus syndrome: naevoid basal cell carcinoma syndrome)

Gorlin's syndrome is an autosomal dominant inherited disorder characterised by the presence of basal cell naevi and carcinomas, dental cysts, dural calcification, ocular hypertelorism, and various skeletal abnormalities. Ovarian calcification and ovarian fibromas have been described in many adults (Clendenning et al 1963; Raggio et al 1983; Evans et al 1993) and indeed fibromas are said to occur in up to 75% of female patients (Gorlin & Sedano 1971). They are, however, rare in adolescents (Burket & Rauh 1976) and children (Rater et al 1968; Raggio et al 1983; Bosch-Banyeras et al 1989; Howell et al 1990). Bilateral sclerosing stromal tumours (Ismail & Walker 1990), renin-secreting fibrothecoma (Fox et al 1994), and fibrosarcoma (Kraemer et al 1984) of the ovary have also been described. Endometrial adeno-carcinoma has been reported in a woman with an ovarian fibroma (Khalifa et al 1997).

Grzybowski's generalised eruptive keratoacanthoma

Grzybowski's generalised eruptive keratoacanthoma is a disorder in which pruritic papules appear as crops which heal leaving pitted scars. They have, rarely, been described on the vulva (Yell 1991) in association with carcinoma of the Fallopian tube (Weber et al 1970) and ovary (Snider & Benjamin 1981; Fathizadeh et al 1982).

Hereditary Non-Polyposis colorectal cancer (HNPCC)

This term is used to encompass individuals with Lynch type II syndrome and Torre–Muir or Muir–Torre syndrome.

Lynch type II syndrome

This is an autosomal dominant disease characterised by the development of colorectal and small intestinal carci-noma and is due to a germline mutation in one of a family of mismatch repair genes. Endometrial and ovarian carcinomas are reported in these women (Lynch et al 1989; Hakala et al 1991; Lynch et al 1993). The endome-trial carcinomas tend to occur at an earlier age than in the general population (Vasen et al 1994), in 22% to up to 60% of affected individuals in their lifetimes (Watson et al 1994; Berends et al 1999; Millar et al 1999; Brown et al 2001): one case has been reported in a woman who had an otherwise normal secretory endometrium (Scurry et al 1996). Ovarian carcinoma is reported in up to 12% of the affected population (Brown et al 2001).

Torre-Muir syndrome

This differs from Lynch type II only in the additional presence of multiple cutaneous sebaceous neoplasms and keratoacanthomas (Weitzer et al 1995). The most common visceral neoplasms are colonic, but tumours in other areas of the gastrointestinal tract and urinary tract also occur. Female patients are prone to develop endome-trial carcinomas (41% in one series) but tumours of the vulva and ovary have also been described (Bitran & Pellettiere 1974; Leonard & Deaton 1974; Rulon & Helwig 1974; Tschang et al 1976; Householder & Zeligman 1980; Lynch et al 1981; Graham et al 1985).

Hypothyroidism

Polycystic ovaries have been reported in cases of primary hypothyroidism (van Voorhis et al 1994).

Intestinal inflammatory disease

The intrapelvic location of the genital tract renders it inevitable that it will become involved in any inflamma-tory process which affects the other pelvic organs or pelvic peritoneum whether this is a pyogenic infection, such as that seen following non-specific appendicitis, or a specific infection.

Diverticular disease

Diverticular disease of the large bowel, particularly if complicated by infection, may result in the formation of intestino-vaginal fistula and the patient may pass flatus per vaginam; the passage of faeces is, however, uncom-mon because the fistula is usually small and the contents of the bowel solid at this level. Tubo-intestinal fistula (Rohatgi & Mukherjee 1973) may also complicate diver-ticular disease of the large intestine and intestinal tuber-culosis. Lymphogranuloma venereum and endometriosis should be considered in the differential diagnosis.

Crohn's disease

Crohn's disease is a chronic noncaseating granulomatous disease of unknown aetiology which typically involves one or more segments of the gastrointestinal tract but which may also affect other organs. There is a marked tendency for internal and external fistulae to form and the disease is often progressive.

A suspicion of Crohn's disease may be raised by the finding in patients with anal disease, both adults and children (Tuffnell & Buchan 1991), of perineal and perianal oedema, fissures, fistulae, fenestrations or ulcers (Parks et al 1965; Lockart-Mummery, 1972; Morson 1972; Kao et al 1975; Levine et al 1982) although more commonly such lesions occur in patients in whom the condition has already been recognised. Crohn's disease may also affect the vulva and the resulting lesions (Ansell & Hogbin 1973; Ridley 1975; Levine et al 1982; Kremer et al 1984; Schulman et al 1987; Kingsland & Alderman 1991; Tuffnell & Buchan 1991) may present as diffuse reddening of the skin or as 'metastatic' ulcers, that is, normal skin lies between the ulcers and there is no link to the gastrointestinal lesions by a fistulous communication. These ulcers are often secondarily infected and surrounded by a marked granulomatous response. Prezyna & Kalyanaraman (1977) described a patient in whom 'Bowen's carcinoma' complicated vulvo-vaginal Crohn's disease. Hidradenitis suppurativa (Attanoos et al 1993; Roy et al 1997) and lymphangiectasia of the vulva have also been reported in patients with Crohn's disease (Handfield-Jones et al 1989). Persistent, unhealed perineal operative wounds may be complicated by the development of squamous cell carcinoma (Sarani & Orkin 1997).

Crohn's disease may also affect other areas of the genital tract, for example, presenting rarely as an ileo-vaginal fistula (Crohn & Yarnis 1958; Atwell et al 1965; Kyle & Sinclair 1969; Hudson 1970; Geurkink et al 1983), ileo-uterine fistula (Crohn & Yarnis 1958), ileo-tubal fistula (Crohn & Yarnis 1958), recto-vaginal fistula (Cornes & Stecher 1961; Beecham 1972; Steinberg et al 1973; Levine et al 1982; Henrich et al 2000), oophoro-vesicular-colonic fistula (Goldberg et al 1988), tubo-cutaneous fistula (Palnaes-Hansen et al 1987), ano-vestibular fistula to Bartholin's gland (Cripps & Northover 1998), or as disease in the Fallopian tube (Atwell et al 1965; Brooks & Wheeler 1977) where it may, rarely, produce bilateral obstruction (Zetzel 1980) and hence infertility (Weber & Belinson 1997): granulomas can be found in the tubal mucosa or muscularis (Fig. 35.1) and the tubal epithelium may show severe, non-specific reactive changes (Wheeler 1982). A granulomatous tubo-ovarian mass may result when tubo-ovarian adhesions are dense and granulomas may be seen within the ovarian substance (Fig. 35.2), these indicating the presence of a granulomatous oophoritis (Wlodarski & Trainer 1975; Allen & Calvert 1995; Savoye et al 2000). It should not be presumed that ovarian granulomas are necessarily due to Crohn's disease, however, as they may also be caused by a reaction to suture material, previous diathermy, tuberculosis, endometriosis and infection (McCluggage & Allen 1997). A most unusual complication of Crohn's disease in pregnancy has been reported with perforation of the terminal ileum when contraction of the uterus postpartum avulsed an area of small intestine to which it had previously been adherent and where it had previously plugged a small perforation (Solomon et al 1996).

As with any granulomatous disorder, the condition must be distinguished from tuberculosis, a complicating factor in this distinction being the occurrence within the female genital tract of non-caseating tuberculosis (Haines & Stallworthy 1952).

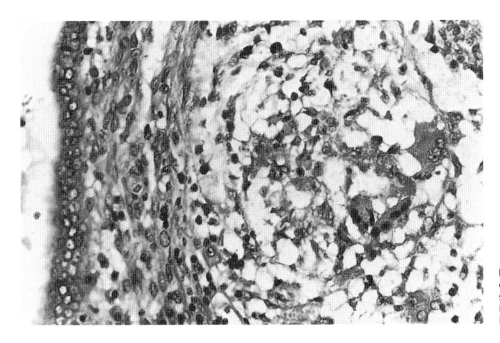

Fig. 35.1 Crohn's disease. A non-caseating tuberculoid granuloma is seen within the mucosa of the Fallopian tube: the lumen lies to the left.

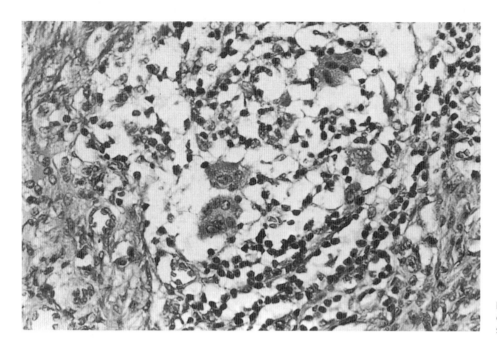

Fig. 35.2 Crohn's disease. A non-caseating tuberculoid granuloma is seen within the ovarian stroma.

The fistulae of Crohn's disease are lined by non-specific granulation tissue and contain pus, but often, deep to the tract wall, it may be possible to identify the non-caseating granulomas which are typical of the condition. The granulomas may be set in fibrous tissue and, not uncommonly, lie adjacent to a lymphatic channel into which they may protrude. In the absence of fistulae the granulomas may be associated with remarkably little tissue destruction and this, in itself, should raise the possibility of Crohn's disease. In vulvar lesions, particularly when the skin is ulcerated, there may also be pseudoepitheliomatous hyperplasia of the epidermis (Kingsland & Alderman 1991).

It has been suggested that steroid contraceptives may play an aetiological rôle in intestinal Crohn's disease (Sandler et al 1992) but other workers have found no evidence that this is so (Lashner et al 1989). On the other hand, there is some agreement that smoking and steroid contraceptives may act synergistically to exacerbate the activity of intestinal Crohn's disease (Wakefield et al 1991; Sandler et al 1992; Wright 1992).

Ulcerative colitis

Unlike Crohn's disease, ulcerative colitis does not directly affect the genital tract but, rarely, may be complicated by the development in the groins of a pustular vegetating lesion which resembles pemphigus vegetans (Ridley 1975).

Complications may also arise as a consequence of the necessity for surgical intervention in severe episodes of ulcerative colitis. Wittich et al (1982) reported the occurrence of a tubo-cutaneous fistula between the right Fallopian tube and the perineum in a young woman six months after a panproctocolectomy which had been carried out for the treatment of 'toxic megacolon'. It was thought probable that a drainage track in the perineal wound had provided the basis of the fistula. The histological features of ulcerative colitis may also develop in a segment of sigmoid colon used to create a neovagina (Froese et al 1991).

Tuberculosis

Tuberculosis may spread to the genital tract, usually the Fallopian tube, via the lymphatics from an intestinal primary site (Wheeler 1982) or may spread directly from the intestine or bladder (Rohatgi & Mukherjee 1973).

Actinomycosis

Actinomycosis may spread directly from the intestine to the genital tract although this mode of transmission is rare.

Haemochromatosis

Selective impairment of anterior pituitary function due to the deposition of iron in the gonadotrophs of the anterior pituitary is typical of haemochromatosis in young females who present with hypogonadotrophic hypogonadism (Herick et al 1989). Amenorrhoea persists despite the lowering of body iron.

Human immunodeficiency virus (HIV/AIDS)

Immunosuppression, whether due to HIV infection or immunosuppressive therapy, appears to act as a co-factor in the development of neoplastic human papillomavirus

(HPV) lesions in both the cervix and the vulva (Petry et al 1996). Even within these groups, however, the risk varies, perhaps according to the degree of immunosuppression (Abercrombie & Korn 1998) and the risk of contracting HPV infection (Mandelblatt et al 1999). Whilst the pattern of disease may be similar to that in women with an apparently normal immunological state, there is a tendency for CIN to progress more rapidly and recur more frequently in HIV-positive women (Palefsky 1995). HIV-infected women are also likely to have larger cervical lesions and be more at risk of coexisting vulvo-vaginal lesions (Fruchter et al 1994). Should they develop cervical carcinoma, their disease tends to follow a more aggressive course (Amit et al 2001).

Hydatid disease

Hydatid cysts of the ovary are rare lesions which usually develop secondary to the rupture of a hepatic cyst. They may remain asymptomatic for long periods of time and may be discovered incidentally but they can cause irritation or compression symptoms (Solidoro & Del Gaudio 1991).

Klippel–Trenaunay–Weber syndrome

In Klippel–Trenaunay–Weber syndrome there are cutaneous vascular naevi extending in a segmental distribution with associated varicosities limited to the same side of the body. It is usually recognised in infancy and is associated with hypertrophy of both soft tissue and bones (Klippel & Trenaunay 1900). Arterial abnormalities range from small malformations to large arterio-vascular fistulae.

Uterine haemangiomas with multiple feeding arteries have been described in a 25-year-old woman with this syndrome who had experienced catastrophic bleeding, requiring transfusion, since the onset of menstruation (Lawlor & Charles-Holmes 1988).

Langerhans' cell histiocytosis

Langerhans' cell histiocytosis, previously included under the generic designation 'histiocytosis X' to indicate its unknown aetiology, may occur as a single osteolytic lesion in bone which has a relatively benign course. It may also be multifocal with a more variable and generally less favourable outcome; in such patients, the lower genital tract may be affected (McKay et al 1953; Borglin et al 1966; Lieberman 1979; Blaauwgeers et al 1993; Savell et al 1995). For a fuller review of vulvar involvement see Chapter 3.

Patients complain of vulvar itching, irritation and pain, and may develop ulcers (Otis et al 1990). Within the vagina, elevated dark yellow–brown mucosal papular lesions are found and similar, though paler, lesions are seen in the cervix (Issa et al 1980).

Histologically, sheets of histiocytes interspersed with eosinophils, lymphocytes and plasma cells characterise the papular and ulcerated lesions. When there are areas of necrosis they are often surrounded by a rim of polymorphonuclear leucocytes. Within the endometrium there may be an eosinophilic infiltrate.

The prognosis is worst in children, particularly neonates, when the lesions are widespread and the histiocytes less well differentiated. The multifocal form of the condition is often associated with diabetes insipidus (Issa et al 1980), and in adults the disease tends to be progressive over a period of time and may recur after treatment.

The aetiology is uncertain although in some cases it is thought to represent an abnormal immunological response to an infective agent; atypical mycobacteria have been isolated in some cases, but in others no agent has been detected. It would appear that there is some genetic predisposition to the condition (Zinkham 1976). Further, there has been a report of a clustering of malignant germ cell tumours and Langerhans' histiocytosis (Mandel et al 1994).

Leprechaunism

Congenital bilateral juvenile granulosa cell tumours of the ovaries have been reported in an individual with the biochemical and clinical features of leprechaunism (Brisigotti et al 1993).

Li-Fraumeni syndrome

In addition to breast carcinoma, soft tissue sarcoma, brain tumours and osteosarcoma, there is a family history of ovarian carcinoma in women with Li-Fraumeni syndrome (Sobol et al 1993).

Ligneous (pseudomembranous) conjunctivitis

Ligneous conjunctivitis is a rare form of idiopathic chronic membranous conjunctivitis which is refractory to all forms of therapy. In the chronic phase there may be associated lesions in the endometrium and Fallopian tube (Scurry et al 1993), whilst lesions in the cervix and vagina may give rise to abnormal cervical smears (Hidayat & Riddle 1987). Histologically, these lesions are similar to those in the conjunctiva. There are subepithelial deposits of amorphous eosinophilic material superficially resembling amyloid and containing albumin, fibrin and immunoglobulin which is thought to have leaked from the local blood vessels. The amount of this material is very variable and small foci of granulation tissue, which in some cases may be a major feature, may also be present. The surface of the epithelium may ulcerate or may be hyperplastic. The presence of lesions in the uterus and tube may be the cause of infertility and dysmenorrhoea which has been reported in some cases.

Lipodystrophy

The presence of polycystic ovaries has been described in individuals with lipodystrophy (Huseman et al 1979; Penney et al 1981).

Malaria

In some parts of the world, falciparum malaria is a potent cause of miscarriages, stillbirths, intrauterine growth retardation (IUGR) and premature labour. The death rate, and anaemia rate, is significantly greater than in non-pregnant women (Kochar et al 1999). Malaria and the placenta is discussed in more detail in Chapter 38.

Malouf syndrome

An association between dilated cardiomyopathy and ovarian dysgenesis has been reported (Malouf et al 1985; Narahara et al 1992).

Megaloblastic anaemia

In patients with both vitamin B_{12} and folate deficiency, there may be changes in the squamous epithelium of the cervix which are characterised by the formation of 'megaloblasts' (see Chapter 7).

Melkersson–Rosenthal syndrome

Vulvitis granulomatosa is the vulvar variant of Melkersson–Rosenthal syndrome and its clinical and histological similarity to Crohn's disease (Lloyd et al 1994) has led to suggestions that the two diseases may be related. Squamous carcinoma of the vulva may occur in this condition (Samaratunga et al 1991).

Metastatic tumour in the female genital tract

The female genital tract and, particularly, the ovaries can be involved by metastatic tumour from primary neoplasms elsewhere, not only in the abdomen and pelvis but also in extra-abdominal sites. It is vitally important that the possibility of a metastatic lesion be considered in every case of apparently primary tumour of the genital tract and ovaries (see Chapter 25). Leukaemia and lymphoma may also involve the female genital tract and ovaries (see Chapter 28).

Multiple endocrine neoplasia type 1

Very rarely, multiple endocrine neoplasia type 1 syndrome may present with amenorrhoea (Lucas et al 1988) and both ovarian carcinoma and ovarian strumal carcinoid have been reported in patients with this syndrome (Frilling et al 1992; Tamsen & Mazur 1992).

Organ transplantation

There is an increased incidence of ano-rectal and vulvar intraepithelial and invasive neoplasia in patients in receipt of immunosuppressive treatment following organ transplantation (Penn 1986). Some women develop a field change in the lower genital tract involving the vulva, vagina and cervix; this is usually HPV-associated and may represent a considerable clinical problem. Other neoplasms, such as endometrial carcinoma, have also been reported following a successful renal transplant (Husslein et al 1978) and infections, such as tuberculosis, may present an atypical picture — for example, vulvar tuberculosis has been reported (Tham & Choong 1992).

Osteogenesis imperfecta

Serous adenocarcinoma of the ovary and osteogenesis imperfecta have been reported as coexisting in a patient (Nishida et al 1993).

Peutz–Jeghers syndrome

Peutz–Jeghers syndrome is a non-sex-linked, autosomal dominant inherited disorder characterised by hamartomatous polyposis of the entire gastrointestinal tract (Bartholomew et al 1957) and melanin pigmentation of the buccal mucosa, lips and digits. It may come to the attention of the gynaecological pathologist because some patients develop ovarian sex cord–stromal tumours with annular tubules (Scully 1970; Young et al 1982; Herruzo et al 1990; Podczaski et al 1991). Such neoplasms are not limited to patients with Peutz–Jeghers syndrome, but when they are associated with the syndrome they tend to be in the form of multiple tumourlets which undergo calcification rather than in the form of a single large mass (Scully 1982) which suggests that they too may represent hamartomatous malformations in these patients rather than true neoplasms. A second, as yet incompletely understood, ovarian sex cord–stromal neoplasm has also been described (Young et al 1983) in two young girls with Peutz–Jeghers syndrome: its microscopic appearance suggests that it may well have been a Sertoli cell neoplasm. A feminising Sertoli cell tumour has also been described by Cantu et al (1980). Peutz–Jeghers syndrome is also associated with the rare, well-differentiated minimal deviation adenocarcinoma of the endocervix, so-called adenoma malignum (McGowan et al 1980; Young et al 1982; Young & Scully 1988; Gilks et al 1989). Tumour in the Fallopian tube has also been documented (Spigelman et al 1989).

Pituitary disease

Normal fertility may be impaired in patients who have ovarian dysfunction secondary to pituitary neoplasms (Fisken et al 1989) (see acromegaly above), pituitary infarction (McAlpine & Thomson 1989) or pituitary ablation and in those suffering from anorexia nervosa and organic endocrine disorders such as myxoedema and thyrotoxicosis. The latter probably exert their effects via disturbances to the hypothalamic–pituitary–ovarian axis.

Polycystic kidney disease

The presence of hepatic cysts is well recognised in polycystic renal disease and whilst ovarian cysts have been reported in as many as a quarter of affected individuals, a recent prospective study revealed no statistically significant increase in affected women (Stamm et al 1999).

Polyostotic fibrous dysplasia (Albright's syndrome; McCune–Albright's syndrome)

The association of skin pigmentations, precocious sexual development and polyostotic fibrous dysplasia is referred to as Albright's syndrome. These individuals may also have hyperthyroidism, Cushing's disease, acromegaly, hyperparathyroidism and adenomas of various endocrine glands. In the ovaries, there may be granulosa lutein cysts (Danon et al 1975).

Prader–Willi syndrome

Individuals with Prader–Willi syndrome suffer from neonatal hypotonia and feeding difficulties, excessive appetite and obesity in early childhood, short stature and cognitive impairment. Dysmorphic features include small hands and feet, almond-shaped eyes and a triangular mouth. The syndrome may be complicated by diabetes, scoliosis and cor pulmonale. There is hypogonadism but approximately half the females with the condition menstruate, although menstruation is usually of short duration or irregular (Clarke et al 1989).

Precocious puberty

Precocious puberty has been reported in association with hepatoblastoma (Navarro et al 1985) and as a consequence of the hCG produced by an ectopic pinealoma (Kubo et al 1977). It has also been reported in a child with a hypothalamic hamartoma. The possibility that the associated juvenile granulosa cell tumour was due to the presence of the raised luteinizing hormone levels was postulated (Feilberg-Jorgensen et al 1998).

Retroperitoneal fibrosis

Retroperitoneal fibrosis is an infiltrative fibromatosis characterised by ill-defined masses of fibrous tissue which encircle the lower abdominal aorta and the ureters, giving rise to ureteric narrowing or obstruction. Histologically, the fibrous tissue is infiltrated by lymphocytes, plasma cells

and eosinophils and there may be foci of necrosis, phlebitis and arteritis (Mitchinson 1970; Simon et al 1985). It is this appearance which has led to the suggestion that the process is inflammatory rather than neoplastic, although its aetiology is uncertain.

The process may, in rare circumstances, extend down to the bladder and vagina (Heah 1979; Manetta et al 1987) where it may cause dysuria and abnormal bleeding per vaginam. Fibromatosis has also been reported to form a mass on the posterior wall of the uterus (Tamaya et al 1986).

Rheumatoid arthritis

An elderly woman with an ulcerated rheumatoid nodule on the vulva and inguinal lymphadenopathy presented with a clinical picture resembling carcinoma (Appleton & Ismail 1996).

Sarcoidosis

Non-caseating epithelioid granulomas of the female genital tract are, as a matter or course, regarded as tuberculous until otherwise proven but, on rare occasions, sarcoidosis of the uterus, Fallopian tubes and ovary has been described in the course of systemic disease (Garland & Thomson 1933; Longcope & Freiman 1952; Cowdell 1954; Altchek et al 1955; Castolidi & Giudici 1955; Kay 1956; Zachwiej et al 1956; Taylor 1960; Maycock et al 1963; Ho 1979; Honoré 1981; Rosenfeld et al 1989; White et al 1990; Romer et al 2001). There is a reported association between polyglandular autoimmune syndrome type II and sarcoidosis and premature ovarian failure has been found in occasional patients with the disorder (Papadopoulos et al 1996). A raised CA125 level has also been noted in a woman with an adnexal mass and peritoneal disease due to sarcoidosis (Trimble et al 1991).

Occasionally the histological diagnosis of sarcoidosis in endometrial curettings (Fig. 35.3) has pre-dated the development of systemic disease (Elstein et al 1994). Disease has sometimes been limited to the endometrium (Sandvei & Bang 1991) and, rarely, it may present with postmenopausal bleeding (Pearce & Nolan 1996). Endometrial biopsy in such patients may reveal a picture quite indistinguishable from non-caseating tuberculosis (Taylor 1960). Whilst caseation is absent in the granulomas of sarcoidosis, the central area may develop acellular fibrinoid necrosis in which Schaumann bodies, asteroids and irregular crystals may be identified. Microbiological investigations fail to reveal *Mycobacterium tuberculosis* and, unlike women with pelvic tuberculosis, the patients are often parous. Sarcoidosis of the Fallopian tube (Kay 1956) and ovary (Winslow & Funkhouser 1968) has been described but the disease in the pelvis is self-limiting (Blaustein 1982) and does not cause the degree of tubal damage seen in tuberculosis.

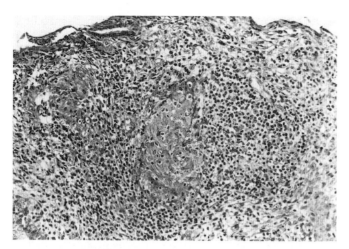

Fig. 35.3 Sarcoidosis. A granuloma in the endometrium of a woman who presented with menorrhagia and whose systemic symptoms of sarcoidosis did not develop for several months. (From C H Buckley & H Fox 2002 *Biopsy Pathology of the Endometrium* by permission of Edward Arnold Ltd.)

Sensorineural deafness (Perrault syndrome)

Autosomal recessive ovarian dysgenesis may develop with facultative, non-sex-limited sensorineural deafness (Pallister & Opitz 1979).

Situs inversus totalis

A variety of ovarian neoplasms have been reported in individuals with situs inversus totalis. These include embryonal carcinoma, yolk sac tumour and mucinous cystadenoma (Rao et al 1977; Abdel-Dayem et al 1984; Ibrahim et al 1984; Talerman 1984).

Smith–Lemli–Opitz syndrome

This is a rare autosomal recessive disorder with a mixture of neurological and somatic disorders including mental and growth retardation, hypotonia, seizures, abnormalities of the face, palate, torso and extremities. Gonadal dysgenesis has also been described in the syndrome (Fukuzawa et al 1992). A malignant mixed ovarian germ cell tumour with elements of yolk sac tumour, embryonal carcinoma and dysgerminoma has been described in a 19-year-old patient who had a contralateral streak gonad (Patsner et al 1989).

Systemic hypertension

Twenty per cent of hypertensive postmenopausal women have increased endometrial thickness even after allowances have been made for such confounding factors as diabetes, abnormal fasting blood glucose level, obesity, hormonal medication and hormone replacement therapy in the previous 6 months: they also have a history of hormonal disturbances, infertility, or polycystic ovary syndrome (Bornstein et al 2000). There is an increased risk of these women developing endometrial carcinoma (Maatela et al 1994).

Systemic lupus erythematosus (SLE)

Women with SLE are reported to be at increased risk of having an abnormal cervical smear whether or not they have been treated with cytotoxic drugs for their disease (Blumenfeld et al 1994). Menses are frequently heavy and irregular in patients with systemic lupus, in whom there are circulating anticoagulants; bleeding may be profound (Schur 1979). In contrast, there is a tendency to vascular thrombosis, including arterial thrombosis, and high titres of antiphospholipid antibody reflect a high risk for spontaneous miscarriage (Harris et al 1988). Remission of systemic lupus erythematosus has been reported (Kahn et al 1966) following the removal of an ovarian dysgerminoma. Serum levels of CA125 and hCG are said to be elevated in nearly one-third of patients with the disease (Moncayo & Moncayo 1995).

Thyroid adenoma and ovarian neoplasms

A familial association between thyroid adenomas and Sertoli–Leydig cell tumours (Jensen et al 1974; O'Brien & Wilansky 1981) has been described and there is a possibility that other ovarian neoplasms may also arise in these families as both a sex cord–stromal tumour and a mucinous cystoma were removed from a sibling of one of the patients with a Sertoli–Leydig cell tumour.

Tuberous sclerosis

A case has been reported in which the typical lesions of tuberous sclerosis, intracranial calcification and renal angiomyolipoma, were present together with pulmonary lymphangiomyomatosis and low-grade endometrial stromal sarcoma (Kuramoto et al 1996). Uterine lymphangiomyomatosis (lymphangioleiomyomatosis) has also been reported in conjunction with high-grade papillary adenocarcinoma of mixed epithelial type in the ovary (Gyure et al 1995). In a further case, lymphangioleiomyomatosis affected the uterus, ovaries and liver (Lack et al 1986).

Vasculitis

Granulomatous vasculitis

Granulomatous vasculitis may be a local, asymptomatic condition limited to the vasculature of part or all of the genital tract (Pirozynski 1976; Summers et al 1991), a local asymptomatic condition (Crow & McWhinney 1979), or may be part of a systemic disease. In the latter case, an association with polymyalgia rheumatica and temporal arteritis (Polasky et al 1965; Petrides et al 1979) is well recognised.

The affected vessels, usually small muscular arteries, are cuffed by lymphocytes and epithelioid macrophages with or without giant cells (Fig. 35.4). The vessel wall may show signs of necrosis but even when the destructive process is well advanced, elastic stains will usually reveal fragments of elastin in the inflammatory focus (Fig. 35.5) and, in minimally affected vessels, small defects may be revealed in the elastic lamina.

The presence of epithelioid granulomas related to spiral arteries in the endometrium may give rise to a suspicion of tuberculosis but the total absence of caseation together with negative cultures and the presence of vascular damage should be sufficient to confirm the diagnosis. The morphological changes are consistent with an immunological response to a vascular wall component and this concept is supported by the finding of cell-mediated immunity to arterial antigen in some people (Hazleman et al 1975) and the rapid response to corticosteroids.

Necrotising arteritis

The medium and small arteries of the uterus may be involved by an intramural non-specific inflammatory infiltrate associated with vessel necrosis (Pirozynski 1976); isolated arteritis of the cervix, which is identical histologically with polyarteritis nodosa, has also been reported (Crow & McWhinney 1979; Padwell 1986; Ganesan et al 2000). This latter arteritis may be asymptomatic but can also be associated with bleeding. Involvement of the ovaries in polyarteritis nodosa is frequent but usually asymptomatic (Austen 1971) and such a vasculitis in the uterus and cervix is usually overshadowed by the systemic component of the disease. It should not be assumed, however, that the histological detection of polyarteritis in the ovary is necessarily indicative of systemic disease as isolated involvement of the ovarian vasculature has been reported (Kaya et al 1994).

A somewhat similar necrotising vasculitis, which caused massive intra-abdominal haemorrhage, has also been described in the ovary of a woman undergoing in vitro fertilisation (Ilbery et al 1991).

Von Hippel–Lindau disease

This is a rare autosomal disorder characterised by the development of benign and malignant neoplasms widely dispersed throughout the body. Many of these are angiomatous, the most serious being the haemangioblastomas of the central nervous system. Of much less significance is the almost incidental but common occurrence of intraovarian haemangiomas (Horton et al 1976).

A papillary cystadenoma of the mesosalpinx which was multicystic, and in which the walls were locally calcified has also been described in a patient with this syndrome. It was believed to be of mesonephric origin and the epithelium was cuboidal with central round nuclei and clear cytoplasm: ciliated and secretory cells were not seen. Electronoptically the cells were said to be similar to those of the adnexal tumour of Wolffian origin (Gersell & King 1988).

Von Recklinghausen's syndrome (Neurofibromatosis 1)

Von Recklinghausen's disease (neurofibromatosis 1) is characterised by the presence of multiple neural tumours and pigmented skin lesions, some of which are café au lait

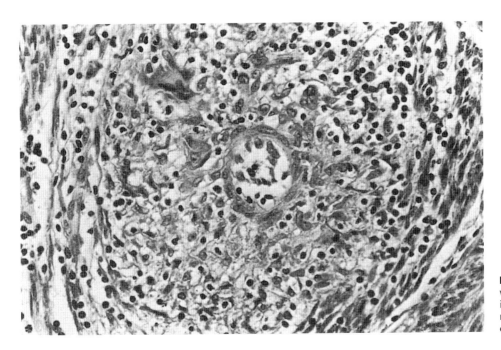

Fig. 35.4 Granulomatous arteritis. The wall of a small muscular uterine artery is infiltrated by epithelioid macrophages and lymphocytes: a giant cell lies in the upper left of the field.

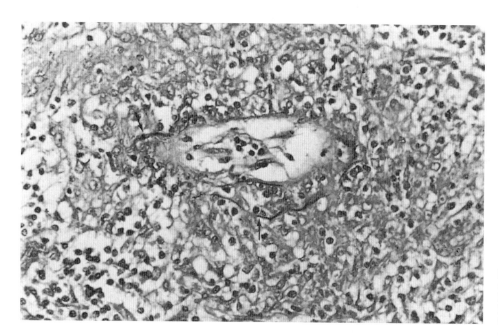

Fig. 35.5 Granulomatous arteritis. The elastic lamina, which appears as a fine black line, is fragmented and disrupted by the inflammatory infiltrate. Elastic van Gieson.

spots, plexiform neurofibromas and Lisch nodules. In about half the patients there is a family history consistent with an autosomal dominant pattern of inheritance but, in the other half, there is no family history. Eighteen per cent of women with the disorder have vulvar neurofibromas (Schreiber 1963) and in children, the presenting sign may be clitoromegaly (Sutphen et al 1995). Rarely, a malignant peripheral nerve sheath tumour has been reported (Lee et al 1997). An ovarian neurofibroma (Smith 1931) and a neurofibrosarcoma (Dover 1950) have been reported in affected individuals and diffuse plexiform neurofibromatosis affecting the cervix, endometrium, myometrium, ovarian cortex, and peritoneum has been recorded (Gordon et al 1996) with, in one case, extension to the vagina, urinary bladder, urethra and ureter (Gersell & Fulling 1989).

Wilson's disease

Wilson's disease is an autosomal recessive disorder in which copper accumulates in many tissues. Resistant ovary syndrome has been recorded in affected individuals (Hartemann et al 1983).

NON-GYNAECOLOGICAL CONDITIONS INCIDENTALLY AFFECTING THE GENITAL TRACT

In many cases the involvement of the genital tract is largely fortuitous and in fact may be detected only if it is specifically sought. This applies to the situation in which the vulva may be involved in the systemic rashes of chickenpox, scarlet fever, drug eruptions and the prodroma of measles. It also applies to a large number of dermatological disorders such as pellagra, vitiligo, albinism and alopecia

and to the petechial rashes which are found in patients with bleeding disorders. There are, however, a number of circumstances when the systemic disorder shows a predilection for the genital tract or ovary, such as the ovary in mumps or the vulva in psoriasis and cicatricial pemphigoid.

THE GYNAECOLOGICAL CONSEQUENCES OF THE TREATMENT OF NON-GYNAECOLOGICAL DISEASE

Whether or not a non-gynaecological disease affects the genital tract, its treatment may have a profound effect on the morphology or function of the genital tract and ovary. Such changes may be perplexing for the histopathologist or cytopathologist, particularly if the history of the systemic disease has not been provided.

In patients receiving hormone therapy for the treatment of non-gynaecological disease, for example, for the treatment of breast carcinoma, both the cervical cytology and the endometrial appearances may be abnormal. Tamoxifen, a partial oestrogen agonist, is widely used in the treatment of breast carcinoma and its oestrogenic effect may be manifest in the form of vaginal bleeding from proliferative or hyperplastic endometrium, occasionally from endometrial carcinoma and in the recrudescence of endometriotic foci (Buckley 1990) (see Chapter 32). If progestagens are used the endometrium may show inappropriate secretory activity and pseudodecidualisation (Chapter 32) or there may be endometrial atrophy. In the cervix, there may be a degree of cervical microglandular hyperplasia and the cervical smear may show inappropriate progestational effects.

It is well recognised that the metabolism of steroid contraceptives is accelerated by a variety of commonly used drugs such as, for example, antimicrobial agents and antiepileptics. Other drugs, such as Misoprostol (Cytotec), a selective orally active prostaglandin that has been used in women with peptic ulceration, may cause menorrhagia, intermenstrual bleeding, postmenopausal bleeding and, in young women, miscarriage (Committee on Safety of Medicines 1989). It also increases uterine tone and should be avoided in pregnancy. Many other drugs need to be avoided in pregnancy because of their potential teratogenic or abortifacient properties.

The use of some non-hormone preparations such as the antidepressive, antipsychotic (Dickson et al 2000) and anti-inflammatory drugs may exert an influence on the ovary by virtue of their interference with the control of prolactin secretion. There may subsequently be sequential changes in the Fallopian tube, cervix, vagina and endometrium.

Problems may be encountered in the interpretation of cervical and vaginal smear material in patients who have been treated either by radiotherapy locally or have received chemotherapy. It may be difficult to distinguish the observed changes from those which are the result of a neoplastic process. Opportunistic infections too may afflict patients receiving cytotoxic drugs or immunosuppressives, and those patients in whom immunosuppression is part of the disease process. They may thus present to the gynaecologist with Candida infection or condylomas. Disseminated granulomatous disease (BCGosis) has also been reported following chemoimmunotherapy for ovarian carcinoma (Kelleher et al 1988).

THE NON-GYNAECOLOGICAL CONSEQUENCES OF GYNAECOLOGICAL DISEASE AND TREATMENT

Amyloidosis secondary to gynaecological malignancy

Systemic amyloidosis, with renal involvement, has been attributed to the presence of an ovarian carcinoma (Fernandez-Miranda et al 1994) and a cervical carcinoma (Sakemi et al 1992).

Arthritis

The patient who presents with acute arthritis may have gonorrhoea and this may be the first indication that something is wrong because the local disease in the cervix may be entirely asymptomatic.

Congenital malformations

The association of congenital anomalies of the Müllerian system with systemic structural abnormalities is well recognised (see Chapter 2). The most common non-gynaecological anomalies associated with Müllerian tract anomalies lie in the renal tract, and of these renal agenesis

is the most common (Golan et al 1989), being most frequently associated with unicornuate uterus (70–80% of cases). Rarely duplication of the whole urinary collecting system has been reported. Between 10% and 12% of women with Müllerian malformations also have anomalies in the musculo-skeletal system (Siegler 1983; Bernhisel et al 1985), 12% have imperforate anus and 6% have cardiac abnormalities and anomalies of the ear and eye (Pinsonneault & Goldstein 1985).

Dermatological disorders

Acanthosis nigricans

The development of acanthosis nigricans may be the first intimation that a patient has ovarian carcinoma (Dingley & Marten 1957), this being particularly mentioned in relation to serous carcinoma (Curth et al 1962). Acanthosis nigricans has also been noted in association with a mature cystic teratoma of the ovary (Imperato-McGinley et al 1978) in a patient in whom there was also primary amenorrhoea, hirsutism and insulin resistance.

Benign lymphangiomatous papules

This pseudosarcomatous vascular proliferation in the skin may occur at the site of radiotherapy following surgery for carcinoma of the endometrium (Diaz-Cascajo et al 1999). The lesions form solitary or multiple papules or vesicles localised to the field of radiation. Microscopically, the lesions are composed of vascular spaces that exhibit atypical features without qualifying for a diagnosis of angiosarcoma.

Linear IgA disease

Linear IgA disease is an uncommon autoimmune dermatosis with subepidermal blistering, diagnosed by demonstrating a band-like deposition of IgA in the basement membrane of non-blistered areas. Circulating IgA autoantibodies are thought to be pathogenic. It has been described in a woman with a molar pregnancy and it is suggested that the mole triggered the abnormal immune response by expressing the linear IgA antigen (Kelly & Wojnarowska 1989).

Pemphigoid gestationis

Pemphigoid gestationis may occur in normal pregnancy (Kelly et al 1988), where the placenta expresses a pemphigoid gestationis related antigen, and in association with hydatidiform mole (Tindall et al 1981).

Dermatomyositis

Dermatomyositis/polymyositis may be associated with serous carcinoma of the ovary (Peters et al 1983; Verducci et al 1984) dysgerminoma (Solomon & Maurer 1983) and with other ovarian carcinomas (Cortes et al 1962; Chamberlain & Whittaker 1963).

Endocrine disorders

A variety of systemic endocrine disturbances accompany gynaecological disorders (Shane & Naftolin 1975; Clement et al 1991).

Carcinoid syndrome

Carcinoid syndrome develops in approximately one-third of patients with an ovarian carcinoid tumour even in the absence of metastases (Qizilbash et al 1974; Robboy et al 1975) because secretions from such neoplasms pass, via the venous drainage, directly into the systemic circulation and are not inactivated by the liver. Carcinoid syndrome has also been reported in association with carcinoid tumour (small cell carcinoma) of the uterine cervix (Brown & Lane 1965; Stockdale et al 1986) (see also Chapter 10).

Cushing's syndrome

Cushing's syndrome has been reported as resulting from the ectopic production of cortisol in patients with steroid cell tumours of the ovary (Kepler et al 1944; Deaton & Freedman 1957; Rosner et al 1964; Osborn et al 1969; Motlik & Starka 1973; Marieb et al 1983; Adeyemi et al 1986; Hayes & Scully 1987; Young & Scully 1987; Donovan et al 1993; Elhadd et al 1996) and by a pituitary cell adenoma within an ovarian teratoma (Axiotis et al 1987). Cushing's syndrome has been described as a result of ectopic production of ACTH by a Sertoli cell tumour of the ovary (Nichols et al 1962), by Sertoli–Leydig cell tumour (Canelo & Lisser 1939; Kasperlik-Zaluska et al 1993), by a carcinoid tumour of the ovary (Brown & Lane 1965; Schlaghecke et al 1989), by ovarian carcinoma (Crawford et al 1994; Orbetzova et al 1997), by other ovarian neoplasms (Parsons & Rigby 1958; Lipsett et al 1964; Odell et al 1977; Baylin & Mendelsohn 1980) and by small cell endocrine tumours of the uterine cervix (Berthelot et al 1961; Jones et al 1976; Matsuyama et al 1979; Lojek et al 1980; Iemura et al 1991; Hashi et al 1996).

Hyperaldosteronism

Hyperaldosteronism associated with isosexual precocious puberty has been reported in a 9-year-old girl who had a Sertoli cell tumour of the ovary (Erlich et al 1963). The child had an elevated systemic blood pressure, hypokalaemia and a high urinary secretion of aldosterone. Hyperaldosteronism has also been recorded in other patients with sex cord–stromal tumours (Jackson et al

1986; Tetu et al 1988), Sertoli–Leydig cell tumours (Todesco et al 1975) and in a patient with a steroid cell tumour of the ovary (Kulkarni et al 1990).

Hypercalcaemia

Hypercalcaemia may develop in patients with a variety of gynaecological tumours, probably due to the production of more than one humoral substance; in some cases, a parathyroid hormone-like substance has been identified (Allan et al 1984; Takeuchi et al 2000). Hypercalcaemia has been reported, for example, in association with a variety of ovarian neoplasms, these including squamous carcinoma arising in ovarian teratomas (Kim et al 1981; Ribeiro et al 1988; Takeuchi et al 2000), papillary serous cystadenocarcinoma (Ferenczy et al 1971; Rivett & Robinson 1972; Josse et al 1981), clear cell carcinoma (Powell et al 1973; Biron et al 1977; Skrabanck et al 1980; Tsunematsu et al 2000), endometrioid carcinoma (Stewart et al 1982), mucinous adenocarcinoma (Boyer et al 1989), steroid (lipid) cell tumour (Abouav et al 1959), small cell carcinoma, both small cell and large cell variants (Dickersin et al 1982; Taraszewski et al 1991; Di Vagno et al 2000), undifferentiated sex cord–stromal tumour (Holtz et al 1979), juvenile granulosa cell tumour (Daubenton & Sinclair-Smith 2000), granulosa cell tumour (Cannon et al 1975) and dysgerminoma (Stewart et al 1982; Anstey et al 1990; Fleischhacker & Young 1994; Allbery & Swischuk 1998). Hypercalcaemia has also been described in a patient with a malignant paraovarian tumour of probable Wolffian origin (Abbot et al 1981) and may also develop in patients with adenocarcinoma or adenosquamous carcinoma of the endometrium (Stewart et al 1982), squamous carcinoma of the vulva (Shane & Naftolin 1975; Stewart et al 1982) and squamous carcinoma of the cervix uteri (Lacey & Morrow 1979).

Hyperchorionic gonadotrophinism

It is well recognised that very high concentrations of hCG have a thyroid-stimulating effect (Cave & Dunn 1976; Davies et al 1979) and thus symptoms of thyrotoxicosis or high output cardiac failure (French et al 1977; Twiggs et al 1979; Soutter et al 1981) may occur in patients with trophoblastic disease (Higgins & Herschman 1978). This is seen both in patients with choriocarcinoma (Cohen & Utiger 1970; Cave & Dunn 1976; Morley et al 1976) and in those with hydatidiform mole (Herschman & Higgins 1971; Kim et al 1976; Osathanondh et al 1976; French et al 1977).

Human chorionic gonadotrophin may also be secreted by other ovarian carcinomas without the development of clinical symptoms (Montiero et al 1983; Vaitukaitis 1974), and more specifically by serous carcinoma of the ovary (Civantos & Rywlin 1972; Samaan et al 1976), mucinous carcinoma (Civantos & Rywlin 1972; Samaan et al 1976), endometrioid carcinoma (Samaan et al 1976), dysgerminoma (Gough 1939; Kapp et al 1985), mixed germ cell tumour which includes choriocarcinoma (O'Reilly et al 1993) and mature cystic teratoma (Downey et al 1989). In some cases, human placental lactogen can also be identified (Samaan et al 1976; Montiero et al 1983).

Hyperprolactinaemia

On rare occasions, ovarian teratomas have produced sufficient prolactin as to cause hyperprolactinaemia (Kallenberg et al 1990; Palmer et al 1990).

Hyperthyroidism

In addition to the thyroid stimulating effect of hCG (see above) hyperthyroidism has also been reported in women with ovarian teratomas (Lipsett et al 1964; Kempers et al 1970), struma ovarii (Young 1993; Grandet & Remi 2000) and malignant struma ovarii (Devaney et al 1993; Kano et al 2000).

Hypoglycaemia

Hypoglycaemia has been described as a consequence of ectopic insulin production by a primary ovarian carcinoid (Morgello et al 1988) and as a consequence of the production of an insulin-like substance by an ovarian serous cystadenocarcinoma of the ovary (O'Neill & Mikuta 1970), an ovarian fibroma (Michael 1967), a dysgerminoma (Von Meyer-Hofmann et al 1960) and a malignant schwannoma (Shetty et al 1982).

Inappropriate antidiuretic hormone (ADH) secretion

Inappropriate antidiuretic hormone secretion has been described in a patient with an endometrial adenocarcinoma (Fung & Lee 1985).

Masculinisation

Masculinisation may occur as a consequence of hormones secreted by a variety of ovarian neoplasms. These include Leydig cell tumours and other lipid cell tumours, granulosa cell tumour (usually the cystic variant), thecoma, Sertoli–Leydig cell tumours and non-neoplastic conditions such as polycystic ovary syndrome, luteoma of pregnancy and massive oedema of the ovary (see Chapters 17, 20, 23).

Zollinger–Ellison syndrome

Zollinger–Ellison syndrome may develop in patients with gastrin-secreting mucinous cystadenomas (Julkunen et al 1983; Morgan et al 1985; Primrose et al 1988), ovarian mucinous tumours of borderline malignancy (Garcia-Villaneuva et al 1990) and mucinous cystadeno-carcinoma (Cocco & Conway 1975; Long et al 1980; Bollen et al 1981; Connell et al 1993; Hirasawa et al 2000).

Endometriosis

Endometriosis is discussed fully in Chapter 29 and it is only its non-gynaecological aspects that will be mentioned here. Pelvic endometriosis not uncommonly affects the serosa of the bowel where its tendency to undergo cyclical breakdown and bleeding may cause symptoms referable to the gastrointestinal tract. Endometriosis of the vermiform appendix may present as right iliac fossa pain mimicking acute appendicitis, whilst in the sigmoid colon its presence may elicit a fibroblastic and muscular hypertrophic response which may be so severe as to produce a segmental stenosis. The symptoms of large bowel obstruction may then closely mimic carcinoma, inflammatory bowel disease or diverticular disease. The resected specimen usually reveals an excentric mural thickening which has a dense, grey–white fibrous appearance and within which small haemorrhagic foci may be apparent. Histological examination demonstrates functional endometriotic foci set in fibrous tissue in which there are haemosiderin-containing macrophages, surrounded by hypertrophied smooth muscle. Occasionally the overlying bowel mucosa may become ulcerated, but more commonly it is of normal appearance and the lesion is limited to the serosa, sub-serosa and musculature of the bowel wall. These foci of endometriosis may, in rare circumstances, undergo a range of neoplastic changes similar to those which occur in the endometrium (Yantiss et al 2000). Foci of endometriosis in the rectus abdominis muscle may, on occasion, form a tender anterior abdominal wall mass and there is usually a history of previous uterine surgery (Roberge et al 1999).

Haematological disorders

Erythrocytosis

The development of erythrocytosis in patients with uterine leiomyomas (Menzies 1965; Fried et al 1968; Wrigley et al 1971; Ossias et al 1973; Weiss et al 1975; LevGur & Levie 1995), mature cystic teratoma (Ghio et al 1981), mucinous adenocarcinoma (Hudson et al 1993), endometrioid adenocarcinoma (Girsh et al 2001) and steroid (lipid) cell tumour of the ovary (Montag et al 1984; Stephen & Lindop 1998) is attributed to the production, by these tumours, of erythropoietin (Suzuki et al 2001), or factors that stimulate erythropoietin production (Fried et al 1968).

Haemolytic anaemia

Autoimmune haemolytic anaemia has been reported in patients with ovarian teratomas (Barry & Crosby 1957; McAndrew 1964; Davidsohn et al 1968; Bernstein et al 1974; Payne et al 1981), with granulosa-theca cell tumour (Dawson et al 1971), serous cystadenoma (Blau & Kaplinsky 1982) and mucinous carcinoma of the ovary (André et al 1969) and with uterine non-Hodgkin's lymphoma (Bär et al 1986).

Hypercoagulability

In common with other systemic neoplasms, ovarian carcinoma may be associated with thrombophlebitis migrans (Henderson 1955; Lieberman et al 1961) or deep vein thrombosis (Adamson et al 1988). Reports have also been published giving further evidence of a state of hypercoagulability in women with a variety of ovarian malignancies including serous carcinoma, mucinous carcinoma and endometrioid carcinoma (Mosesson et al 1968; Siegman-Igra et al 1977; Scully et al 1978; Landolfi et al 1984). The reports have included non-bacterial thrombotic endocarditis (Delgado & Smith 1975).

Pancytopaenia

Pancytopaenia is an unusual finding in gynaecological malignancy but it has been described in association with a granulosa cell tumour (Napoli & Wallach 1976).

Thrombocytopaenia

Thrombocytopaenia may occur in patients with haemangiomas but the association of bilateral ovarian haemangiomas and diffuse abdominopelvic haemangiomatosis is exceptionally rare (Lawhead et al 1985).

Hormone therapy and contraception

In patients using steroid contraceptives there may be widespread systemic consequences and abnormalities may develop in the cardiovascular system, liver, breast or nervous systems (Chapter 32). In certain groups of women using depot medroxyprogesterone acetate as a contraceptive there is a decrease in spinal bone density and an increased risk of fracture which appears to be reversible after cessation of treatment (Harkins et al 1999; Kaunitz 1999). Patients wearing an intrauterine contraceptive device may, in the first instance, develop pelvic sepsis and subsequently develop pelvic and subphrenic abscess, portal pyaemia or thoracic actinomycosis (Witwer et al 1977; Anteby et al 1991) although fortunately such occurrences are nowadays rare. As the patient will often present not to the gynaecologist but to the general surgeon, the possibility must always be borne in mind.

A further, rare, complication of the use of steroid contraceptives has been reported in a woman with McCune–Albright syndrome who suffered a pathological fracture (Maccari et al 1989). In this syndrome the bone lesions contain oestrogen and progesterone receptors and their progression in pregnancy is also well recognised.

Retinal vein occlusion has been related to the use of steroid contraceptives (Kirwan et al 1997) but not to hormone replacement therapy.

On the positive side, it has been suggested that women who use hormone replacement therapy after the menopause are at reduced risk of developing colonic carcinoma (Gerhardsson de Verdier & London 1992).

Hyperamylasaemia

A raised serum amylase has been described in many patients with ovarian neoplasms. They include a patient with a mucinous tumour which had benign, borderline and malignant areas (Teshima et al 1988), a patient with a low-grade serous papillary neoplasm (Cramer & Bruns 1979), women with serous surface papillary carcinoma and conventional serous carcinoma (Hayakawa et al 1984; Hodes et al 1985; O'Riordan et al 1990), endometrioid carcinoma (Yagi et al 1986) and adenosquamous carcinoma (Norwood et al 1981).

Hypertrophic pulmonary osteoarthropathy

Hypertrophic pulmonary osteoarthropathy may develop in association with ovarian carcinoma (Lester & Robertson 1981).

Malacoplakia

Malacoplakia rarely affects the female genital tract but a case has been described in which primary malacoplakia of the female genital tract led to urethral and ureteral obstruction (Bessim et al 1991).

Meigs' syndrome

The association of ascites and hydrothorax (Meigs' syndrome) with ovarian fibromas is well recognised and familiar (Salmon 1934; Meigs & Cass 1937; Rhoads & Terrell 1937). The recognition that CA125 may be elevated in such cases has, however, only recently been recognised (Siddiqui & Toub 1995; Dunn et al 1998; Abad et al 1999). Perhaps less familiar too is the association of ascites and hydrothorax, so-called Meigs-like or pseudo-Meigs' syndrome, with uterine leiomyomas (O'Flanagan et al 1987), some with elevated CA125 (Migishima et al 2000), leiomyoma in the broad ligament (Brown et al 1998), paraovarian fibroma (Giannacopoulos et al 1998), ovarian tumours and non-neoplastic conditions including serous tumours (Fox & Langley 1976), benign mucinous tumours (Brenner & Scott 1986; Jimerson 1973), malignant mucinous tumours (Jimerson 1973), endometrioid adenocarcinoma (Yin et al 1999), Brenner tumour (Pratt-Thomas et al 1976), granulosa cell tumour (Meigs 1954), thecoma (Faber 1962), fibrothecoma (Koussidis et al 1984), dysgerminoma (Simon & Delavierre 1981), mature cystic teratoma (Mantouvalos et al 1982), struma ovarii with elevated CA125 (Bethune et al 1996), lymphoma (Yutani et al 1982), massive oedema of the ovary (Slotky et al 1982; Fukuda et al 1984) and adeno-carcinoma of the Fallopian tube (Chen et al 1995). A similar clinical picture has also been reported in a patient with colon carcinoma metastatic to the ovaries (Nagakura et al 2000). The combination of chylous and serous pleural effusions with ovarian cancer is sometimes termed Contarini's syndrome (Lawton et al 1985). Chylothorax, spontaneous pneumothorax, haemoptysis and slowly progressive dyspnoea may also occur in women with lymphangiomyomatosis (lymphangioleiomyomatosis) (Gyure et al 1995).

Direct spread and metastases from gynaecological cancer

Neoplasms of the genital tract and ovary may directly involve the adjacent bowel and intestinal obstruction may herald residual carcinoma (Christopherson et al 1985). Primary intestinal adenocarcinoma may also develop in a segment of large intestine used to create a neovagina (Munkarah et al 1994).

Metastases from gynaecological neoplasms may produce symptoms which may be clinically 'misleading'. Amin (1986) described a case of classical Horner's syndrome and Pancoast's syndrome in a woman with metastatic cervical carcinoma in the lung apex. She also had ipsilateral vocal cord and phrenic nerve palsies. This particular combination of symptoms has been described as a syndrome (Rowland Payne 1981). Superior vena cava syndrome has been reported secondary to mediastinal metastases from endometrial carcinoma and uterine leiomyosarcoma (Puleo et al 1986). A malignant pericardial effusion has been described in a woman with metastatic squamous cell carcinoma of the uterine cervix (Rieke & Kapp 1988). Cervical carcinoma is an important cause of cavitating metastases in the lung and these have a tendency to give rise to pneumothorax (Lane et al 1986). Metastases from cervical carcinoma also occur in other unusual sites, for example, the tongue (personal observation). The presence of raised intracranial pressure was the first sign that a woman had ovarian carcinoma when a cerebral metastasis was found (Matsunami et al 1999). Ileo-rectal fistula has been reported as complicating advanced ovarian carcinoma (Jeon et al 1999).

Nephrotic syndrome

Nephrotic syndrome, which is attributed to the glomerular deposition of immune complexes, has been described in women with metastatic epithelial malignancy of the ovary (Hoyt & Hamilton 1987) and is a not uncommon feature in patients with a placental site tumour (see Chapter 40).

Neuropathy and neuromyopathy

Paraneoplastic neuropathies and neuromyopathies are not uncommon in patients with malignant disease and these have been reported in patients with gynaecological malignancy (Croft & Wilkinson 1965). Reflex sympathetic dystrophy (shoulder-hand syndrome) has been reported to pre-date the clinical recognition of endometrial carcinoma (Hudson et al 1993). It has also been described in patients with tubo-ovarian carcinoma (Taggart et al 1984).

Palmar fasciitis and polyarthritis

Palmar fasciitis and polyarthritis have been described in patients with serous carcinoma of the ovary, endometrioid carcinoma of the ovary and in patients with ovarian cancer of unspecified types (Medsger et al 1982; Shiel et al 1985).

Premature menopause

Rosenberg et al (1981) have shown that a premature menopause, in particular removal of the ovaries during a gynaecological procedure in a woman under the age of 35 years, significantly increases the risk of non-fatal myocardial infarct, the factor being 7.2 times. After the menopause too, at whatever age it occurs, a woman is susceptible to osteoporosis, its subsequent deformities and the increased risk of fracture.

Pyrexia of unknown origin

Pyrexia may accompany the presence of many neoplasms and ovarian tumours are no exception. Patients with such tumours may, in some instances, present with a fever for which there is no apparent cause (Maestu et al 1979; Schofield et al 1985).

Systemic hypertension

Treatment-resistant systemic hypertension has been described in association with a renin-producing ovarian Sertoli cell tumour (Korzets et al 1986) and with an ovarian stromal tumour (Tetu et al 1988). In the latter case, the hypertension resolved after removal of the neoplasm but returned when the tumour recurred. Intracellular renin granules were demonstrated by electron microscopy in what were thought to be granulosa cells.

Subacute cerebellar degeneration

A description of the paraneoplastic syndromes in women with ovarian neoplasms is provided by Russell & Bannatyne (1989) and by Hudson et al (1993). One of the most striking examples of this is subacute cerebellar degeneration associated with serous carcinoma of the ovary (Steven et al 1982; Greenlee & Brashear 1983; Cocconi et al 1985; Hall et al 1985; McCrystal et al 1995) in which a Purkinje cell antibody can be identified.

Vasculitis

A necrotising vasculitis causing major intra-abdominal haemorrhage has complicated ovarian superovulation carried out for in vitro fertilisation (IVF) (llbery et al 1991). Intra-abdominal haemorrhage is an infrequent but well-recognised complication of IVF. In the immediate postoperative days it is usually the result of trauma to the ovary or periovarian tissues whilst, in the weeks following the procedure, it is usually due to rupture of a corpus luteum cyst or an ectopic pregnancy.

Miscellaneous disorders

Mature cystic teratomas may rupture not only into the peritoneum, giving rise to shock and peritonitis, but may also rupture into the bladder or rectum creating a fistula (Dandia 1967). Fistulae may also develop should carcinoma of the vulva, vagina, cervix or endometrium spread directly to the urethra, a site in which fistulous communications are not uncommon.

Systemic sclerosis and polyarteritis have also been reported in women with ovarian neoplasms (Hudson et al 1993).

Occasionally a gynaecological disease may simulate a systemic disorder. An unusual case is recorded by Nunez et al (1983) in which the disseminated cells from an embryonal rhabdomyosarcoma were mistaken for those of acute lymphoblastic leukaemia in both the blood and bone marrow. After death, bilateral ovarian embryonal rhabdomyosarcomas were discovered and the cellular infiltrate, previously thought to be leukaemic, was correctly identified. Infectious pneumoperitoneum due to gas-forming organisms has been described as an uncommon presentation of endometrial carcinoma (Douvier et al 1989).

REFERENCES

Abad A, Cazorla E, Ruiz F, Aznar I, Asins E, Llixiona J 1999 Meigs' syndrome with elevated CA125: case report and review of the literature. European Journal of Obstetrics, Gynecology and Reproductive Biology 82: 97–99

Abbot R L, Barlogie B, Schmidt W A 1981 Metastasizing malignant juxtaovarian tumor with terminal hypercalcemia: a case report. Cancer 48: 860–865

Abdel-Dayem H M, Motawi S, Jahan S, Kubasik H 1984 Liver metastases from embryonal carcinoma of the ovary with complete situs inversus. First reported case and review of the literature. Clinical Nuclear Medicine 9: 558–560

Abercrombie P D, Korn A P 1998 Lower genital tract neoplasia in women with HIV infection. Oncology 12: 1735–1739. Discussion 1742, 1745, 1747

Abouav J, Berkowitz S B, Kolb F O 1959 Reversible hypercalcemia in masculinizing hypernephroid tumor of the ovary: report of a case. New England Journal of Medicine 260: 1057–1062

Adam A E 1996 Ectopic Darier's disease of the cervix: an extraordinary cause of an abnormal smear. Cytopathology 7: 414–421

Adamson A S, Littlewood T J, Poston G J, Hows J M, Wolfe J N 1988 Malignancy presenting as peripheral venous gangrene. Journal of the Royal Society of Medicine 8: 609–610

Adeyemi S D, Grange A O, Giwa-Osagie O F, Elesha S O 1986 Adrenal rest tumor of the ovary associated with isosexual precocious pseudopuberty and cushingoid features. European Journal of Pediatrics 145: 236–238

Allan S G, Lockhart S P, Leonard R C, Smyth J F 1984 Paraneoplastic hypercalcaemia in ovarian carcinoma. British Medical Journal 228: 1714–1715

Allbery S M, Swischuk L E, John S D 1998 Hypercalcemia associated with dysgerminoma: case report and imaging findings. Pediatric Radiology 28: 183–185

Allen D C, Calvert C H 1995 Crohn's ileitis and salpingo-oophoritis. Ulster Medical Journal 64: 95–97

Altchek A, Gaines J A, Siltzbach L E 1955 Sarcoidosis of the uterus. American Journal of Obstetrics and Gynecology 70: 540–547

Amin R 1986 Bilateral Pancoast's syndrome in a patient with carcinoma of the cervix. Gynecologic Oncology 24: 126–128

Amit A, Edwards C L, Athey P, Kaplan A L 2001 Extensive subcutaneous metastases from squamous cell carcinoma of the cervix in patient with HIV. International Journal of Gynecological Cancer 11: 78–80

André R, Duhamel G, Najman A, Homberg J C, Mawas C, Armangol R 1969 Anemie hemolytique auto-immune et tumeur maligne de l'ovarie. Presse Médicale 77: 2133–2136

Ansell I D, Hogbin B 1973 Crohn's disease of the vulva. Journal of Obstetrics and Gynaecology of the British Commonwealth 80: 376–378

Anstey A, Gowers L, Vass A, Robson A O 1990 Ovarian dysgerminoma presenting with hypercalcaemia. Case report and review of the literature. British Journal of Obstetrics and Gynaecology 97: 641–644

Anteby E, Milvidsky A, Goshen R, Ben Chetrit A, Ron M 1991 IUD-associated abdominopelvic actinomycosis. Harefuah 121: 150–153

Appleton M A, Ismail S M 1996 Ulcerating rheumatoid nodule of the vulva. Journal of Clinical Pathology 49: 85–87

Attanoos R L, Appleton M A, Hughes L E, Ansell I D, Douglas-Jones A G, Williams G T 1993 Granulomatous hidradenitis suppurativa and cutaneous Crohn's disease. Histopathology 23: 111–115

Atwell J D, Duthie H L, Goligher J C 1965 The outcome of Crohn's disease. British Journal of Surgery 52: 966–972

Austen K F 1971 Periarteritis nodosa (polyarteritis nodosa) In: Beeson P B, McDermott W (eds) Cecil Loeb textbook of medicine, 13th edn. Saunders, Philadelphia

Axiotis C A, Lippes H A, Merino M J, deLanerolle N C, Stewart A F, Kinder B 1987 Corticotroph cell pituitary adenoma within an ovarian teratoma: a new cause of Cushing's syndrome. The American Journal of Surgical Pathology 11: 218–224

Bär B M, Reijinders F J, Keuning J J, Bal H, van Beek M 1986 Primary malignant lymphoma of the uterine cervix associated with cold-reacting autoantibody-mediated hemolytic anemia. Acta Haematologica (Basel) 75: 232–235

Barry K G, Crosby W H 1957 Autoimmune hemolytic anemia arrested by removal of ovarian teratoma: review of the literature and report of a case. Annals of Internal Medicine 47: 1002–1007

Bartholomew L G, Dahlin D C, Waugh J M 1957 Intestinal polyposis: association with mucocutaneous melanin pigmentation (Peutz-Jeghers' syndrome). Gastroenterology 32: 434–451

Baylin S B, Mendelsohn G 1980 Ectopic (inappropriate) hormone production by tumors: mechanisms involved and the biological and clinical implications. Endocrine Reviews 1: 45–77

Beecham C T 1972 Recurring rectovaginal fistulas. Obstetrics and Gynecology 40: 323–326

Berends M J, Kleibeuker J H, de-Vries E G et al 1999 The importance of family history in young patients with endometrial cancer. European Journal of Obstetrics, Gynecology and Reproductive Biology 82: 139–141

Bernhisel M A, London S N, Haney A F 1985 Unusual Müllerian anomalies associated with distal extremity abnormalities. Obstetrics and Gynecology 65: 291–294

Bernstein D, Naor S, Rokover M, Manahem H 1974 Hemolytic anemia related to ovarian tumor. Obstetrics and Gynecology 43: 276–280

Berthelot P, Benhamou J P, Fauvert R 1961 Hypercorticisme et cancer de l'uterus. Presse Médicale 69: 1899–1902

Bessim S, Heller D S, Dottino P, Deligdisch L, Gordon R E 1991 Malakoplakia of the female genital tract causing urethral and ureteral obstruction: a case report. Journal of Reproductive Medicine 36: 691–694

Bethune M, Quinn M, Rome R 1996 Struma ovarii presenting as acute pseudo-Meigs syndrome with an elevated CA125 level. Australian and New Zealand Journal of Obstetrics and Gynaecology 36: 372–373

Biron S, Bercovici B, Brufman G 1977 Paraneoplastic hypercalcemic syndrome associated with ovarian cancer. European Journal of Obstetrics, Gynecology and Reproductive Biology 7: 239–242

Bitran J, Pellettiere E V 1974 Multiple sebaceous gland tumors and internal carcinoma: Torre's syndrome. Cancer 33: 835–836

Blaauwgeers J L, Bleker O P, Veltkamp S, Weigel H M 1993 Langerhans cell histiocytosis of the vulva. European Journal of Obstetrics, Gynecology and Reproductive Biology 48: 145–148

Blau A, Kaplinsky J 1982 Microangiopathic haemolytic anaemia associated with recurrent pulmonary emboli and benign pelvic tumours. Postgraduate Medical Journal 58: 362–363

Blaustein A 1982 Inflammatory diseases of the ovary. In: Blaustein A (ed) Pathology of the female genital tract, 2nd edn. Springer-Verlag, New York, p 445

Blumenfeld Z, Lorber M, Yoffe N, Scharf Y 1994 Systemic lupus erythematosus: predisposition for uterine cervical dysplasia. Lupus 3: 59–61

Bollen E C, Lamers C B, Jansen J B, Larsson L I, Joosten H J 1981 Zollinger-Ellison syndrome due to gastrin producing ovarian cystadenocarcinoma. British Journal of Surgery 68: 776–777

Borglin N E, Söderstrom J, Wehlin L 1966 Eosinophilic granuloma (histiocytosis X) of the vulva. Journal of Obstetrics and Gynaecology of the British Commonwealth 73: 478–486

Bornstein J, Auslender R, Goldstein S, Kohan R, Stolar Z, Abramovici H 2000 Increased endometrial thickness in women with hypertension. American Journal of Obstetrics and Gynecology 183: 583–587

Bosch-Banyeras J M, Lucaya X, Bernet M et al 1989 Calcified fibromas in prepubertal girls. European Journal of Pediatrics 148: 749–750

Boyer M, Friedlander M, Bannatyne P, Atkinson K 1989 Hypercalcemia in association with mucinous adenocarcinoma of the ovary: a case report. Gynecologic Oncology 35: 387–390

Brenner W E, Scott R B 1968 Meigs-like syndrome secondary to Krukenberg's tumor. Obstetrics and Gynecology 31: 40–44

Brisigotti M, Fabbretti G, Pesce F et al 1993 Congenital bilateral juvenile granulosa cell tumor of the ovary in leprechaunism: a case report. Pediatric Pathology 13: 549–558

Brooks J J, Wheeler J E 1977 Granulomatous salpingitis secondary to Crohn's disease. Obstetrics and Gynecology 49 (suppl): 31s–33s

Brown G J, St John D J, Macrae F A, Aittomaki K 2001 Cancer risk in young women at risk of nonpolyposis colorectal cancer: implications for gynecologic surveillance. Gynecologic Oncology 80: 346–349

Brown H, Lane M 1965 Cushing's and malignant carcinoid syndromes from ovarian neoplasm. Archives of Internal Medicine 115: 490–494

Brown R S, Marley J L, Cassoni A M 1998 Pseudo-Meigs' syndrome due to broad ligament leiomyoma: a mimic of ovarian carcinoma. Clinical Oncology (Royal College of Radiologists) 10: 198–201

Buckley C H 1990 Tamoxifen and endometriosis: case report. British Journal of Obstetrics and Gynaecology 97: 645–646

Burket R L, Rauh J L 1976 Gorlin's syndrome: ovarian fibromas at adolescence. Obstetrics and Gynecology 47: 43s–46s

Canelo C K, Lisser H 1939 A case of arrhenoblastoma which simulated Cushing's disease. Endocrinology 24: 838–847

Cannon P M, Smart C R, Wilson N M L, Edwards C B 1975 Hypercalcemia with ovarian granulosa cell carcinoma. Rocky Mountain Medical Journal 72: 72–74

Cantu J M, Rivera H, Ocampo-Campos R et al 1980 Peutz-Jeghers syndrome with feminizing Sertoli cell tumor. Cancer 46: 223–228

Carlson G J, Nivatvongs S, Snover D C 1984 Colorectal polyps in Cowden's disease (multiple hamartoma syndrome). American Journal of Surgical Pathology 8: 763–770

Castolidi P, Giudici E 1955 Granuloma di Besnier-Boeck-Schaumann con localizzazioni alle salpingi. Minerva Ginecologica 7: 627–630

Cave W T, Dunn J T 1976 Choriocarcinoma with hyperthyroidism: probable identity of the thyrotropin with human chorionic gonadotropin. Annals of Internal Medicine 85: 60–63

Chamberlain M J, Whittaker S R F 1963 Hashimoto's disease, dermatomyositis and ovarian carcinoma. Lancet 1: 1398–1400

Chen F C, Fink R L, Jolly H 1995 Meigs' syndrome in association with a locally invasive adenocarcinoma of the fallopian tube. Australian and New Zealand Journal of Surgery 65: 761–762

Christin-Maitre S 1999 Premature ovarian insufficiency. La Revue du Praticien 49: 1297–1302

Christman J E, Ballon S C 1990 Ovarian fibrosarcoma associated with Maffucci's syndrome. Gynecologic Oncology 37: 290–291

Christopherson W, Voet R, Buchsbaum H J 1985 Recurrent cervical cancer presenting as small bowel obstruction. Gynecologic Oncology 22: 109–114

Civantos F, Rywlin A M 1972 Carcinomas with trophoblastic differentiation and secretion of chorionic gonadotrophins. Cancer 29: 789–798

Clarke D J, Waters J, Corbett J A 1989 Adults with Prader-Willi syndrome: abnormalities of sleep and behaviour. Journal of the Royal Society of Medicine 82: 21–24

Clement P B, Young R H, Scully R E 1991 Clinical syndromes associated with tumors of the female genital tract. Seminars in Diagnostic Pathology 8: 204–233

Clendenning W E, Herdt J R, Block J B 1963 Ovarian fibromas and mesenteric cysts: their association with hereditary basal cell cancer of the skin. American Journal of Obstetrics and Gynecology 87: 1008

Cocco A E, Conway S J 1975 Zollinger-Ellison syndrome associated with ovarian mucinous cystadenocarcinoma. New England Journal of Medicine 293: 485–486

Cocconi G, Ceci G, Juvarra G et al 1985 Successful treatment of subacute cerebellar degeneration in ovarian carcinoma with plasmapheresis: a case report. Cancer 56: 2318–2320

Cohen J D, Utiger R D 1970 Metastatic choriocarcinoma associated with hyperthyroidism. Journal of Endocrinology and Metabolism 30: 423–429

Committee on Safety of Medicines 1989 Current Problems, no. 27

Conn J J, Jacobs H S, Conway G S 2000 The prevalence of polycystic ovaries in women with type 2 diabetes mellitus. Clinical Endocrinology 52: 81–86

Connell W R, Price J D, Lowe D G, Shepherd J H, Farthing M J 1993 Zollinger-Ellison syndrome caused by a mucinous cystadenocarcinoma of the ovary. Australian and New Zealand Journal of Medicine 23: 520–521

Cornes J S, Stecher M 1961 Primary Crohn's disease of the colon and rectum. Gut 2: 189–201

Cortes F M, Morris C E, Hunter R V P 1962 Polymyositis: observations in three cases. American Journal of Medical Science 243: 77–85

Cowdell R H 1954 Sarcoidosis: with special reference to diagnosis and prognosis. Quarterly Journal of Medicine 23: 29–55

Cramer D W, Ravnikar V A, Craighill M, Ng W G, Goldstein D P, Reilly R 1987 Müllerian aplasia associated with maternal deficiency of galactose-1-phosphate uridyl transferase. Fertility and Sterility 47: 930–934

Cramer S F, Bruns D E 1979 Amylase producing ovarian neoplasm with pseudo-Meigs' syndrome and elevated pleural fluid amylase: case report and ultrastructure. Cancer 44: 1715–1721

Crawford S M, Pyrah R D, Ismail S M 1994 Cushing's syndrome associated with recurrent endometrioid adenocarcinoma of the ovary. Journal of Clinical Pathology 47: 766–768

Cripps N P, Northover J M 1998 Anovestibular fistula to Bartholin's gland. British Journal of Surgery 85: 659–661

Croft P B, Wilkinson M 1965 The incidence of carcinomatous neuromyopathy in patients with various types of carcinoma. Brain 88: 427–434

Crohn B B, Yarnis H 1958 Regional ileitis, 2nd edn. Grune & Stratton, New York, Ch 5

Crow J, McWhinney N 1979 Isolated arteritis of the cervix uteri. British Journal of Obstetrics and Gynaecology 86: 393–398

Curth H O, Hilberg A W, Machacek G F 1962 The site and histology of the cancer associated with malignant acanthosis nigricans. Cancer 15: 364–382

Dandia S D 1967 Rectovesical fistula following an ovarian dermoid with recurrent vesical calculus: a case report. Journal of Urology 97: 85–87

Danon M, Robboy S J, Kim S, Scully R E, Crawford J D 1975 Cushing syndrome sexual precocity and polyostotic fibrous dysplasia (Albright syndrome). Journal of Pediatrics 87: 917–921

Daubenton J D, Sinclair-Smith C 2000 Severe hypercalcemia in association with a juvenile granulosa cell tumor of the ovary. Medical and Pediatric Oncology 34: 301–303

Davidsohn I, Kovarik S, Stejskal R 1968 Immunological aspects. Influence of prognosis and treatment. In: Gentil F, Junqueira A C (eds) Ovarian cancer. UICC monograph series, vol 11. Springer-Verlag, New York, pp 105–121

Davies T F, Taliadouros G S, Catt K J, Nisula B C 1979 Assessment of urinary thyrotropin-competing activity in choriocarcinoma and thyroid disease: further evidence for human chorionic gonadotropin interacting at the thyroid cell membrane. Journal of Clinical Endocrinology and Metabolism 49: 353–357

Dawson M A, Talbert W, Yarbro J W 1971 Hemolytic anemia associated with an ovarian tumor. American Journal of Medicine 50: 552–556

Deaton W R, Freedman A 1957 Cushing's syndrome due to masculinovoblastoma. North Carolina Medical Journal 18: 101–105

Delgado G, Smith J P 1975 Gynecological malignancy associated with nonbacterial thrombotic endocarditis (NBTE). Gynecologic Oncology 3: 205–209

Devaney K, Snyder R, Norris H J, Tavassoli F A 1993 Proliferative and histologically malignant struma ovarii: a clinicopathologic study of 54 cases. International Journal of Gynecological Pathology 12: 333–343

Diaz-Cascajo C, Borghi S, Weyers W, Retzlaff H, Requena L, Metze D 1999 Benign lymphangiomatous papules of the skin following radiotherapy: a report of five new cases and review of the literature. Histopathology 35: 319–327

Dickersin G R, Kline I W, Scully R E 1982 Small cell carcinoma of the ovary with hypercalcemia: a report of eleven cases. Cancer 49: 188–197

Dickson R A, Seeman M V, Corenblum B 2000 Hormonal side effects in women: typical versus atypical antipsychotic treatment. Journal of Clinical Psychiatry 61: 10–15

Dingley E R, Marten R H 1957 Adenocarcinoma of the ovary presenting as acanthosis nigricans. Journal of Obstetrics and Gynaecology of the British Commonwealth 64: 898–900

Di Vagno G, Melilli G A, Cormio G et al 2000 Large-cell variant of small cell carcinoma of the ovary with hypercalcaemia. Archives of Gynecology and Obstetrics 264: 157–158

Donovan J T, Otis C N, Powell J L, Cathcart H K 1993 Cushing's syndrome secondary to malignant lipoid cell tumor of the ovary. Gynecologic Oncology 50: 249–253

Douvier S, Nabholtz J-M, Friedman S, Cougard P, Ferry C, Aupecle P 1989 Infectious pneumoperitoneum as an uncommon presentation of endometrial carcinoma: report of two cases. Gynecologic Oncology 33: 392–394

Dover H 1950 Neurofibrosarcoma of the ovary associated with neurofibromatosis. Canadian Medical Association Journal 63: 488–490

Downey G P, Prentice M, Penna L K, Gleeson R P, Elder M G 1989 Ectopic β-human chorionic gonadotropin production by a dermoid cyst. American Journal of Obstetrics and Gynecology 160: 449–451

Dunn H G, Meuwissen H, Livingstone C S, Pump K K 1964 Ataxiatelangiectasia. Canadian Medical Association Journal 91: 1106–1118

Dunn J S Jr, Anderson C D, Method M W, Brost B C 1998 Hydropic degenerating leiomyoma presenting as pseudo-Meigs syndrome with elevated CA125. Obstetrics and Gynecology 92: 648–649

Elhadd T A, Connolly V, Cruickshank D, Kelly W F 1996 An ovarian lipid cell tumour causing virilization and Cushing's syndrome. Clinical Endocrinology 44: 723–725

Elstein M, Woodcock A J, Buckley C H 1994 An unusual case of sarcoidosis. British Journal of Obstetrics and Gynaecology 101: 452–453

Erlich E N, Dominguez O V, Samuels L T, Lynch D, Oberhelman H, Warner N E 1963 Aldosteronism and precocious puberty due to an ovarian androblastoma (Sertoli cell tumor). Journal of Clinical Endocrinology and Metabolism 23: 358–367

Evans D G, Ladusans E J, Rimmer S, Burnell L D, Thakker N, Farndon P A 1993 Complications of the naevoid basal cell carcinoma syndrome: results of a population based study. Journal of Medical Genetics 30: 460–464

Faber H K 1962 Meigs' syndrome with thecoma of both ovaries in a 4-year-old girl. Journal of Pediatrics 61: 769–773

Fathizadeh A, Medenica M M, Soltani K, Lorincz A L, Griem M L 1982 Aggressive keratoacanthoma and internal malignant neoplasm. Archives of Dermatology 118: 112–114

Feilberg-Jorgensen N, Brosk-Jacobsen B, Ahrons S, Starklint H 1998 An association of hypothalmic hamartoma, central precocious puberty and juvenile granulosa cell tumour in early childhood. Hormone Research 49: 292–294

Ferenczy A, Okagaki T, Richart R M 1971 Para-endocrine hypercalcemia in ovarian neoplasms: report of mesonephroma with hypercalcemia and review of the literature. Cancer 27: 427–433

Fernandez-Miranda C, Mateo S, Gonzalez-Gomez C, Ballestin C 1994 Systemic amyloidosis and ovarian carcinoma. Postgraduate Medical Journal 70: 505–506

Fisken R A, Walker B A, Buxton P H, Jeffreys R V, Hipkin L J, White M C 1989 A pituitary thyrotrophinoma causing thyrotoxicosis and amenorrhoea: studies of α-subunit in the tumour and in blood. Journal of the Royal Society of Medicine 82: 298–299

Fleischhacker D S, Young R H 1994 Dysgerminoma of the ovary associated with hypercalcemia. Gynecologic Oncology 52: 87–90

Fox H, Langley F A 1976 Tumours of the ovary. Heinemann, London

Fox R, Eckford, Hirschowitz L, Browning J, Lindop G 1994 Refractory gestational hypertension due to renin-secreting ovarian fibrothecoma associated with Gorlin's syndrome. British Journal of Obstetrics and Gynaecology 101: 1015–1017

Fraser I S, Russell P, Greco S, Robertson D M 1986 Resistant ovary syndrome and premature ovarian failure in young women with galactosaemia. Clinical Reproduction and Fertility 4: 133–138

Fraser I S, Shearman R P, Smith A, Russell P 1988 An association among blepharophimosis, resistant ovary syndrome, and true premature menopause. Fertility and Sterility 50: 747–751

French W, Freund U, Carlson R W, Weil M H 1977 High output heart failure associated with pulmonary edema complicating hydatidiform mole. Archives of Internal Medicine 137: 367–369

Fried W, Ward H P, Hopeman A R 1968 Leiomyoma and erythrocytosis: a tumor producing a factor which increases erythropoietin production. Report of a case. Blood 31: 813–816

Friedman C I, Neff J, Kim M H 1984 Immunologic parameters in premature ovarian follicular depletion: T and B lymphocytes, T-cell subpopulations, cutaneous reactivity, and serum immunoglobulin concentrations. Diagnostic Immunology 2: 48–52

Frilling A, Becker H, Roeher H D 1992 Unusual features of multiple endocrine neoplasia. Henry Ford Hospital Medical Journal 40: 253–255

Fristachi C E, Santo G C, Pascalicchio J C, Baracat F F 1991 Lipoid cell tumor of the ovary. Revista Paulista de Medicina 109: 88–90

Froese D P, Haggitt R C, Friend W G 1991 Ulcerative colitis in the autotransplanted neovagina. Gastroenterology 100: 1749–1752

Fruchter R G, Maiman M, Sillman F H, Camilien L, Webber C A, Kim D S 1994 Characteristics of cervical intraepithelial neoplasia in women infected with the human immunodeficiency virus. American Journal of Obstetrics and Gynecology 171: 531–537

Fukuda O, Munemura M, Tohya T, Maeyama M, Iwamasa T 1984 Massive edema of the ovary associated with hydrothorax and ascites. Gynecologic Oncology 17: 231–237

Fukuzawa R, Nakahori Y, Kogo T et al 1992 Normal Y sequences in Smith-Lemli-Opitz syndrome with total failure of masculinisation. Acta Paediatrica 81: 570–572

Fung S Y, Lee K W 1985 Inappropriate antidiuretic hormone secretion associated with adenocarcinoma of the endometrium: case report. British Journal of Obstetrics and Gynaecology 92: 423–425

Ganesan R, Ferryman S R, Meier L, Rollason T P 2000 Vasculitis of the female genital tract with clinicopathologic correlation: a study of 46 cases with follow-up. International Journal of Gynecological Pathology 19: 258–265

Garcia-Villanueva M, Badia-Figuerola N, Ruiz-del-Arbol L, Hernandez-Ortiz M J 1990 Zollinger-Ellison syndrome due to a borderline mucinous cystadenoma of the ovary. Obstetrics and Gynecology 75: 549–552

Garland H G, Thomson J G 1933 Uveo-parotid tuberculosis (febris uveo-parotidea of Heerfordt). Quarterly Journal of Medicine 2: 157–177

Gatti R A, Good R A 1971 Occurrence of malignancy in immunodeficiency diseases: a literature review. Cancer 28: 89–98

Gatti R A, Nieberg R, Boder E 1989 Uterine tumors in ataxiatelangiectasia. Gynecologic Oncology 32: 257–260

Gell J S, Stannard M W, Ramani D M, Bradshaw K D 1998 Juvenile granulosa cell tumor in a 13-year-old girl with enchondromatosis (Ollier's disease): a case report. Journal of Pediatric and Adolescent Gynecology 11: 147–150

Gerhardsson de Verdier M, London S 1992 Reproductive factors, exogenous female hormones, and colorectal cancer by subsite. Cancer Causes and Control 3: 355–360

Gersell D J, Fulling K H 1989 Localized neurofibromatosis of the female genitourinary tract. American Journal of Surgical Pathology 13: 873–878

Gersell D J, King T C 1988 Papillary cystadenoma of the mesosalpinx in von Hippel-Lindau disease. American Journal of Surgical Pathology 12: 145–149

Gesmundo R, Bevilacqua A, Gandini R, Maiullari E, Moro G 1988 Su do caso di disgerminoma ovarico in sindrome di Down. Minerva Ginecologica 40: 277–280

Geurkink R E, Rauter M, Bayly M A 1983 Spontaneous ileovaginal fistula caused by Crohn's disease: a case report. American Journal of Obstetrics and Gynecology 145: 107–108

Ghio R, Haupt E, Ratti M, Boccaccio P 1981 Erythrocytosis associated with a dermoid cyst of the ovary and erythropoietic activity of the tumour fluid. Scandinavian Journal of Haematology 27: 70–74

Giannacopoulos K, Giannacopolou C, Matalliotakis I, Neonaki M, Papanicolaou N, Koumantakis E 1998 Pseudo-Meigs' syndrome caused by paraovarian fibroma. European Journal of Gynaecological Oncology 19: 389–390

Gibbons D, Lindberg G M, Ashfaq R, Saboorian M H 1998 Localized amyloidosis of the uterine cervix. International Journal of Gynecological Pathology 17: 368–371

Gilks C B, Young R H, Aguirre P, DeLellis R A, Scully R E 1989 Adenoma malignum (minimal deviation adenocarcinoma) of the uterine cervix: a clinicopathological and immunohistochemical analysis of 26 cases. American Journal of Surgical Pathology 13: 717–729

Girsh T, Lamb M P, Rollason T P, Brown L J 2001 An endometrioid tumour of the ovary presenting with hyperandrogenism, secondary polycythaemia and hypertension. British Journal of Obstetrics and Gynaecology 108: 330–332

Golan A, Langer R, Bukovsky I, Caspi E 1989 Congenital anomalies of the Müllerian system. Fertility and Sterility 51: 747–755

Goldberg S D, Gray R R, Cadesky K I, Mackenzie R L 1988 Oophorovesicular-colonic fistula: a rare complication of Crohn's disease. Canadian Journal of Surgery 31: 427–428

Goldsmith C I, Hart W R 1975 Ataxia telangiectasia with ovarian gonadoblastoma and contralateral dysgerminoma. Cancer 36: 1838–1842

Gordon M D, Weilert M, Ireland K 1996 Plexiform neurofibromatosis involving the uterine cervix, endometrium, myometrium, and ovary. Obstetrics and Gynecology 88: 699–701

Gorlin R J, Sedano H O 1971 The multiple nevoid basal cell carcinoma syndrome revisited. Birth Defects 7: 140–148

Gough A 1939 A case of dysgerminoma of the ovary associated with masculinity. Journal of Obstetrics and Gynaecology of the British Empire 45: 799–801

Graham R, McKee P, McGibbon D, Heyderman E 1985 Torre-Muir syndrome: an association with isolated sebaceous carcinoma. Cancer 55: 2868–2873

Grandet P J, Remi M H 2000 Struma ovarii with hyperthyroidism. Clinical Nuclear Medicine 25: 763–765

Grattan C E, Hamburger J 1987 Cowden's disease in two sisters, one showing partial expression. Clinical and Experimental Dermatology 12: 360–363

Greenberg D, Keenan B, de Yanis V, Finegold M 1986 Gonadal dysgenesis and gonadoblastoma in situ in a female with Fraser (cryptophthalmos) syndrome. Journal of Pediatrics 108: 952–954

Greenlee J E, Brashear H R 1983 Antibodies to cerebellar Purkinje cells in patients with paraneoplastic cerebellar degeneration and ovarian carcinoma. Annals of Neurology 14: 609–613

Guerrero N V, Singh R H, Manatunga A et al 2000 Risk factors for premature ovarian failure in females with galactosemia. Journal of Pediatrics 137: 833–841

Gyure K A, Hart W R, Kennedy A W 1995 Lymphangiomyomatosis of the uterus associated with tuberous sclerosis and malignant neoplasm of the female genital tract: A report of two cases. International Journal of Gynecological Pathology 14: 344–351

Hagenfeldt K, von Dobeln U, Hagenfeldt L 1989 Gonadal failure in young women and galactose-1-phosphate uridyl transferase activity. Fertility and Sterility 51: 177–178

Haines M, Stallworthy J A 1952 Genital tuberculosis in the female. Journal of Obstetrics and Gynaecology of the British Empire 59: 721–747

Hakala T, Mecklin J P, Forss M, Jarvinen H, Lehtovirta P 1991 Endometrial carcinoma in cancer family syndrome. Cancer 68: 1656–1659

Hall D J, Dyer M L, Parker J C Jr 1985 Ovarian cancer complicated by cerebellar degeneration: a paraneoplastic syndrome. Gynecologic Oncology 21: 240–246

Hamdoun L, Mouelhi C, Zhioua F, Jedoui A, Meriah S, Houet S 1993 Syndrome de Maffucci et tumeur ovarienne. Bulletin du Cancer (Paris) 80: 816–819

Handfield-Jones S E, Prendiville W J, Norman S 1989 Vulval lymphangiectasia. Genitourinary Medicine 65: 335–337

Harkins G J, Davis G D, Dettori J, Hibbert M L, Hoyt R A 1999 Decline in bone mineral density with stress fractures in a woman on depot medroxyprogesterone acetate. A case report. Journal of Reproductive Medicine 44: 309–312

Harris E N, Asherson R A, Hughes G R 1988 Antiphospholipid antibodies — autoantibodies with a difference. Annual Review of Medicine 39: 261–271

Hartemann P, Leclere J, Thomas J L, Genton P, Arbogast J 1983 Syndrome des ovaires résistant aux gonadotrophines et maladie de Wilson. Une observation. Revue de Medecine Interne 4: 353–355

Hashi A, Yasumizu T, Yoda I et al 1996 A case of small cell carcinoma of the uterine cervix presenting Cushing's syndrome. Gynecologic Oncology 61: 427–431

Hayakawa T, Kameya A, Mizuno R, Noda A, Kondo T, Hirabayashi N 1984 Hyperamylasemia with papillary serous cystadenocarcinoma of the ovary. Cancer 54: 1662–1665

Hayes M C, Scully R E 1987 Ovarian steroid cell tumors (not otherwise specified): a clinicopathological analysis of 63 cases. American Journal of Surgical Pathology 11: 835–845

Hazleman B L, Maclennan I C, Esiri M M 1975 Lymphocyte proliferation to artery antigen as a positive diagnostic test in polymyalgia rheumatica. Annals of the Rheumatic Diseases 34: 122–127

Heah J T 1979 Idiopathic retroperitoneal fibrosis involving the vagina: case report. British Journal of Obstetrics and Gynaecology 86: 407–410

Henderson P H Jr 1955 Multiple migratory thrombophlebitis associated with ovarian carcinoma. American Journal of Obstetrics and Gynecology 70: 452–453

Henrich W, Meckies J, Friedmann W 2000 Demonstration of a recto-vaginal fistula with ultrasound contrast medium Echivist. Ultrasound Obstetrics and Gynecology 15: 148–149

Herick A L, McInnes G T, MacSween R N M, Goldberg A 1989 Idiopathic haemochromatosis in a young female with amenorrhoea. Journal of the Royal Society of Medicine 82: 556–558

Herruzo A J, Redondo E, Perex de Avila M, Menjon S 1990 Ovarian sex cord tumor with annular tubules and Peutz-Jeghers syndrome. European Journal of Gynaecological Oncology 26: 441–452

Herschman J M, Higgins H P 1971 Hydatidiform mole — a cause of clinical hyperthyroidism: report of two cases with evidence that the molar tissue secreted a thyroid stimulator. New England Journal of Medicine 284: 573–577

Hidayat A A, Riddle P J 1987 Ligneous conjunctivitis: a clinicopathologic study of 17 cases. Ophthalmology 94: 949–959

Higgins H P, Herschman J M 1978 The hyperthyroidism due to trophoblastic hormone. Clinics in Endocrinology and Metabolism 7: 167–175

Hirasawa K, Yamada M, Kitagawa et al 2000 Ovarian mucinous cystadenocarcinoma as a cause of Zollinger-Ellison syndrome: report of a case and review of the literature. American Journal of Gastroenterology 95: 1348–1351

Hirokawa H, Okana Y, Asada M, Fujimoto A, Suyama I, Isshiki G 1999 Molecular basis for phenotypic heterogeneity in galactosaemia: prediction of clinical phenotype from genotype in Japanese patients. European Journal of Human Genetics 7: 757–764

Ho K L 1979 Sarcoidosis of the uterus. Human Pathology 10: 219–222

Hodes M E, Sisk C J, Karn R C et al 1985 An amylase producing serous cystadenocarcinoma of the ovary. Oncology 42: 242–247

Holtz G, Johnson T R Jr, Schrock M E 1979 Paraneoplastic hypercalcemia in ovarian tumors. Obstetrics and Gynecology 5: 483–487

Honoré L H 1981 Asymptomatic genital sarcoidosis. Australian and New Zealand Journal of Obstetrics and Gynecology 21: 188–190

Horton W A, Wong V, Eldridge R 1976 Von Hippel-Lindau disease: clinical and pathological manifestations in nine families with 50 affected members. Archives of Internal Medicine 136: 769–777

Householder M S, Zeligman I 1980 Sebaceous neoplasms associated with visceral carcinomas. Archives of Dermatology 116: 61–64

Howell C G Jr, Rogers D A, Gable D S, Falls G D 1990 Bilateral ovarian fibromas in children. Journal of Pediatric Surgery 25: 690–691

Hoyt R E, Hamilton J F 1987 Ovarian cancer associated with the nephrotic syndrome. Obstetrics and Gynecology 70: 513–514

Hudson C N 1970 Acquired fistulae between the intestine and the vagina. Annals of the Royal College of Surgeons of England 46: 20–40

Hudson C N, Curling M, Potsides P, Lowe D G 1993 Paraneoplastic syndromes in patients with ovarian neoplasia. Journal of the Royal Society of Medicine 86: 202–204

Huseman C A, Johanson A J, Varma M M, Blizzard R M 1979 Congenital lipodystrophy. II: Association with polycystic ovary disease. Journal of Pediatrics 95: 72–74

Husslein H, Breitenecker G, Tatra G 1978 Premalignant and malignant uterine changes in immunosuppressed renal transplant recipients. Acta Obstetricia et Gynaecologica Scandinavica 57: 73

Iemura K, Sonoda T, Hayakawa A et al 1991 Small cell carcinoma of the uterine cervix showing Cushing's syndrome caused by ectopic adrenocorticotropin hormone production. Japanese Journal of Clinical Oncology 21: 293–298

Ibrahim E M, Al-Idrissi H, Al-Farag A, Al-Timimi D, Perry W 1984 Situs inversus totalis with embryonal cell carcinoma of the ovaries. Gynecologic Oncology 18: 270–273

Ilbery M, Lyons B, Sundaresan V 1991 Ovarian necrotizing vasculitis causing major intra-abdominal haemorrhage after IVF: case report and literature review. British Journal of Obstetrics and Gynaecology 98: 596–599

Imperato-McGinley J, Peterson R E, Sturla E, Dawood Y, Bar R S 1978 Primary amenorrhea associated with hirsutism, acanthosis nigricans, dermoid cysts of the ovaries and a new type of insulin resistance. American Journal of Medicine 65: 389–395

Inoue R, Kondo N, Motoyoshi F, Hori Y, Orii T 1991 Chediak-Higashi syndrome: report of a case with an ovarian tumor (letter). Clinical Genetics 39: 316–318

Ismail S, Walker S M 1990 Bilateral virilizing sclerosing stromal tumours of the ovary in a pregnant woman with Gorlin's syndrome: implications for pathogenesis of ovarian stromal neoplasms. Histopathology 17: 159–163

Issa P Y, Salem P A, Brihi E, Azoury R S 1980 Eosinophilic granuloma with involvement of the female genitalia. American Journal of Obstetrics and Gynecology 137: 608–612

Jackson B, Valentine R, Wagner G 1986 Primary aldosteronism due to a malignant ovarian tumour. Australian and New Zealand Journal of Medicine 16: 69–71

Jeffcoate T N A 1962 The dermatology of the vulva. Journal of Obstetrics and Gynaecology of the British Commonwealth 69: 889–890

Jensen R D, Norris H J, Fraumeni J F Jr 1974 Familial arrhenoblastoma and thyroid adenoma. Cancer 33: 218–223

Jeon H M, Kim J S, Oh S T, Kim K H, Ahn B Y, Lee E J 1999 Ileo-rectal fistula complicating advanced ovarian carcinoma. Oncology Reports 6: 1243–1247

Jimerson S D 1973 Pseudo-Meigs' syndrome: an unusual case with analysis of the effusion. Obstetrics and Gynecology 42: 535–537

Jones H W, Plymate S, Gluck F B, Miles P A, Green J F 1976 Small cell nonkeratinising carcinoma of the cervix associated with ACTH production. Cancer 38: 1629–1635

Josse R G, Wilson D R, Heersche J N M, Mills J R F, Murray T M 1981 Hypercalcemia with ovarian carcinoma: evidence of a pathogenetic role for prostaglandins. Cancer 48: 1233–1241

Julkunen R, Partanen S, Salaspuro M et al 1983 Gastrin-producing ovarian mucinous cystadenoma. Journal of Clinical Gastroenterology 5: 67–70

Kahn M F, Ryckewaert A, Cannat A, Solnica J, de Seze S 1966 Systemic lupus erythematosus and ovarian dysgerminoma: remission of the systemic lupus erythematosus after extirpation of the tumour. Clinical and Experimental Immunology 1: 355–359

Kallenberg G A, Pesce C M, Norman B, Ratner R E, Silverberg S G 1990 Ectopic hyperprolactinemia resulting from an ovarian teratoma. Journal of the American Medical Association 263: 2472–2474

Kaltsas G A, Mukherjee J J, Jenkins P J et al 1999 Menstrual irregularity in women with acromegaly. Journal of Clinical Endocrinology and Metabolism 84: 2731–2735

Kano H, Inoue M, Nishino T, Yoshimoto Y, Arima R 2000 Malignant struma ovarii with Graves' disease. Gynecologic Oncology 79: 508–510

Kao M S, Paulson J D, Askin F B 1975 Crohn's disease of the vulva. Obstetrics and Gynecology 46: 329–333

Kapp D S, Kohorn E I, Merino M J, LiVolsi V A 1985 Pure dysgerminoma of the ovary with elevated serum human chorionic gonadotropin: diagnostic and therapeutic considerations. Gynecologic Oncology 20: 234–244

Kasperlik-Zaluska A A, Sikorowa L, Ploch E 1993 Ectopic ACTH syndrome due to bilateral ovarian androblastoma with double, gynandroblastic

differentiation in one ovary. European Journal of Obstetrics, Gynecology and Reproductive Biology 52: 223–228

Kaufman F R, Donnell G N, Roe T F, Kogut M D 1986 Gonadal function in patients with galactosemia. Journal of Inherited Metabolic Disease 9: 140–146

Kaunitz A M 1999 Long-acting hormonal contraception: assessing the impact on bone density, weight and mood. International Journal of Fertility and Women's Medicine 44: 110–117

Kay S 1956 Sarcoidosis of the Fallopian tubes: report of a case. Journal of Obstetrics and Gynaecology of the British Empire 63: 871–874

Kaya E, Utas C, Balkanli S, Basbug M, Onursever A 1994 Isolated ovarian polyarteritis nodosa. Acta Obstetricia et Gynecologica Scandinavica 73: 736–738

Kelleher M B, Christopherson W A, Macpherson T A 1988 Disseminated granulomatous disease (BCGosis) following chemoimmunotherapy for ovarian carcinoma. Gynecologic Oncology 31: 321–326

Kelly S E, Wojnarowska F 1989 Linear IgA disease in association with hydatidiform mole. Journal of the Royal Society of Medicine 82: 438–439

Kelly S E, Bhogal B S, Wojnarowska F, Black M M 1988 Expression of a pemphigoid gestationis related antigen by human placenta. British Journal of Dermatology 118: 605–611

Kempers R D, Dockerty M B, Hoffman D L, Bartholomew L G 1970 Struma ovarii — ascites, hyperthyroid and asymptomatic syndromes. Annals of Internal Medicine 72: 883–893

Kepler E J, Dockerty M B, Priestley J T 1944 Adrenal-like ovarian tumor associated with Cushing's syndrome (so-called masculinovoblastoma, luteoma, hypernephroma, adrenal cortical carcinoma of the ovary). American Journal of Obstetrics and Gynecology 47: 43–62

Khalifa M A, Patterson-Cobbs G, Hansen C H, Hines J F, Johnson J C 1997 The occurrence of endometrial adenocarcinoma in a patient with basal cell nevus syndrome. Journal of the National Medical Association 89: 549–552

Kim J M, Arakawa K, McCann V 1976 Severe hyperthyroidism associated with hydatidiform mole. Anesthesiology 44: 445–448

Kim W, Bockman R, Lemos L, Lewis J L Jr 1981 Hypercalcemia associated with epidermoid carcinoma in ovarian cystic teratoma. Obstetrics and Gynecology 57: 81s–85s

Kingsland C R, Alderman B 1991 Crohn's disease of the vulva. Journal of the Royal Society of Medicine 84: 236–237

Kirwan J F, Tsaloumas M D, Vinall H, Prior P, Kritzinger E E, Dodson P M 1997 Sex hormone preparations and retinal vein occlusion. Eye 11: 53–56

Klippel M, Trenaunay P 1900 Du naevus variqueux osteo hypertrophique. Archive de General Medicine Paris 185: 641–671

Kochar D K, Thanvi I, Joshi A, Shubhakaran, Agarwal N, Jain N 1999 Mortality trends in falciparum malaria — effect of gender difference and pregnancy. Journal of the Association of Physicians of India 47: 774–778

Kojiro M, Kage M, Abe H, Imamura M, Shiraisha K, Mizoguchi M 1983 Association of dysgerminoma and Gaucher's disease. Cancer 51: 712–715

Korzets A, Nouriel H, Steiner Z, Griffel B, Kraus L, Freund U, Klajman A 1986 Resistant hypertension associated with a renin-producing ovarian Sertoli cell tumor. American Journal of Clinical Pathology 85: 242–247

Koussidis A, Koussidou M, Dounabis A, Kiriakou K 1984 Ein Fibrothekom des Ovars mit typischem Meigs Syndrom und tumoroser Kachexie. Zentralblatt für Gynäkologie 106: 341–344

Kraemer B B, Silva E G, Sneige N 1984 Fibrosarcoma of ovary. A new component in the nevoid basal-cell carcinoma syndrome. American Journal of Surgical Pathology 8: 231–236

Kremer M, Nussenson E, Steinfeld M, Zuckerman P 1984 Crohn's disease of the vulva. American Journal of Gastroenterology 79: 376–378

Kubo O, Yamasaki N, Kamijo Y, Amano K, Kitamura K 1977 A case of HCG-producing ectopic pinealoma in a girl with precocious puberty. Neurological Surgery 5: 363–369

Kulkarni J N, Mistry R C, Kamat M R, Chinoy R, Lotlikar R G 1990 Autonomous aldosterone-secreting ovarian tumor. Gynecologic Oncology 107: 538–545

Kuramoto M, Kato M, Inoue Y 1996 Pulmonary lymphangiomyomatosis with tuberous sclerosis and endolymphatic stromal myosis of the uterus. Nippon Kyobu Shikkan Gakkai Zasshi (Japanese Journal of Thoracic Diseases) 34: 322–326

Kuzma J F, King J M 1948 Dyschondroplasia with hemangiomatosis (Maffucci's syndrome) and teratoid tumor of the ovary. Archives of Pathology 46: 74–82

Kyle J, Sinclair W Y 1969 Ileovaginal fistula complicating regional enteritis. British Journal of Surgery 56: 474–475

Lacey C G, Morrow C P 1979 Hypercalcemia in patients with squamous cell carcinoma of the cervix. Gynecologic Oncology 7: 215–222

Lack E E, Dolan M F, Finisio J, Grover G, Singh M, Triche T J 1986 Pulmonary and extrapulmonary lymphangioleiomyomatosis. Report of a case with bilateral renal angiomyolipomas, multifocal lymphangioleiomyomatosis, and a glial polyp of the endocervix. American Journal of Surgical Pathology 10: 650–657

Landolfi R, Storti S, Sacco F, Scribano D, Cudillo L, Leone G 1984 Platelet activation in patients with benign and malignant ovarian diseases. Tumori 70: 459–462

Lane S, Fasano J B, Levitt A B, Brandstetter R D 1986 (letter) Spontaneous bilateral pneumothorax due to metastatic cervical carcinoma. Chest 91: 151–152

Lashner B A, Kane S V, Hanauer S B 1989 Lack of association between oral contraceptive use and Crohn's disease: a community-based matched case-control study. Gastroenterology 97: 1442–1447

Lavery H A 1984 Vulval dystrophies: new approaches. Clinics in Obstetrics and Gynaecology 11: 155–169

Lavery H A, Pinkerton J H, Roberts S D, Sloan J, Walsh M 1985 Dermatomyositis of the vulva — first reported case. British Journal of Dermatology 113: 349–352

Lawhead R A, Copeland L J, Edwards C L 1985 Bilateral ovarian hemangiomas associated with diffuse abdominopelvic hemangiomatosis. Obstetrics and Gynecology 65: 597–599

Lawlor F, Charles-Holmes S 1988 Uterine haemangioma in Klippel-Trenaunay-Weber syndrome. Journal of the Royal Society of Medicine 81: 665–666

Lawton F, Blackledge G, Johnson R 1985 Co-existent chylous and serous pleural effusions associated with ovarian cancer: a case report of Contarini's syndrome. European Journal of Surgical Oncology 11: 177–178

Lee Y S, Choi Y J, Kang C S, Kang S J, Kim B K, Shim S I 1997 Purely epithelioid malignant peripheral nerve sheath tumor of the vulva. Journal of Korean Medical Science 12: 78–81

Leonard D D, Deaton W R Jr 1974 Multiple sebaceous gland tumors and visceral carcinomas. Archives of Dermatology 110: 917–920

Lester W M, Robertson D I 1981 Hypertrophic osteoarthropathy complicating metastatic ovarian adenocarcinoma. Canadian Journal of Surgery 24: 520–521, 523

Lev Gur M, Levie M D 1996 The myomatous erythrocytosis syndrome: a review. Obstetrics and Gynecology 86: 1026–1030

Levine E M, Barton J J, Grier E A 1982 Metastatic Crohn disease of the vulva. Obstetrics and Gynecology 60: 395–397

Lewis R J, Ketcham A S 1973 Maffucci's syndrome: functional and neoplastic significance: case report and review of the literature. Journal of Bone and Joint Surgery American Volume 55(A): 1465–1479

Lieberman J S, Borrero J, Urdaneta E, Wright I S 1961 Thrombophlebitis and cancer. Journal of the American Medical Association 177: 542–545

Lieberman P H 1979 Eosinophilic granuloma and related syndromes. In: Beeson P B, McDermott W, Wyngaarden J B (eds) Cecil-Loeb textbook of medicine, 15th edn. Saunders, Philadelphia, pp 1848–1851

Lipsett M B, Odell W D, Rosenberg L E, Waldman T A 1964 Humoral syndromes associated with nonendocrine tumors. Annals of Internal Medicine 61: 733–756

Lloyd D A, Payton K B, Guenther L, Frydman W 1994 Melkersson-Rosenthal syndrome and Crohn's disease: one disease or two? Report of a case and discussion of the literature. Journal of Clinical Gastroenterology 18: 213–217

Lloyd K M, Dennis M 1963 Cowden's disease: a possible new syndrome complex with multiple system involvement. Annals of Internal Medicine 58: 136–142

Lockart-Mummery H E 1972 Anal lesions of Crohn's disease. In: Clinics in gastroenterology. Saunders, Philadelphia, pp 377–382

Lojek M A, Fer M F, Kasselberg A G et al 1980 Cushing's syndrome with small cell carcinoma of the uterine cervix. American Journal of Medicine 69: 140–144

Long T T III, Barton T K, Draffin R, Reeves W J, McCarty K S Jr 1980 Conservative management of the Zollinger-Ellison syndrome: ectopic gastrin production by an ovarian cystadenoma. Journal of the American Medical Association 243: 1837–1839

Longcope W T, Freiman D G 1952 A study of sarcoidosis. Medicine 31: 1–132

Lucas J A, Kahlstorf J H, Cowan B D 1988 Multiple endocrine neoplasia — type I syndrome and hyperprolactinemia. Fertility and Sterility 50: 514–515

Lynch H T, Lynch P M, Pester J, Fusaro R M 1981 The cancer family syndrome: rare cutaneous phenotypic linkage of Torre's syndrome. Archives of Internal Medicine 141: 607–611

Lynch H T, Smyrk T C, Lynch P M et al 1989 Adenocarcinoma of the small bowel in Lynch syndrome II. Cancer 64: 2178–2183

Lynch H T, Smyrk T C, Watson P et al 1993 Genetics, natural history, tumour spectrum, and pathology of hereditary non-polyposis colorectal cancer: an updated review. Gastroenterology 104: 1535–1549

Maatela J, Aromaa A, Salmi T, Pohja M, Vuento M, Gronroos M 1994 The risk of endometrial cancer in diabetic and hypertensive patients: a nationwide record-linkage study in Finland. Annales Chirurgiae et Gynaecologiae Suppl 208: 20–24

McAlpine J K, Thomson J E 1989 Hypopituitarism and empty sella due to endocarditis. Journal of the Royal Society of Medicine 82: 769–770

McAndrew G M 1964 Haemolytic anaemia associated with ovarian teratoma. British Medical Journal 2: 1307–1308

Maccari S, Fornaciari G, Bassi C, Beltrami M, Tinterri N, Plancher A C 1989 Contraceptive methods in the McCune-Albright syndrome. Clinical and Experimental Obstetrics and Gynecology 16: 129–130

McCluggage W G, Allen D C 1997 Ovarian granulomas: a report of 32 cases. Journal of Clinical Pathology 50: 324–327

McCrystal M, Anderson N E, Jones R W, Evans B D 1995 Paraneoplastic cerebellar degeneration in a patient with chemotherapy-responsive ovarian cancer. International Journal of Gynecological Cancer 5: 396–399

McGowan L, Young R H, Scully R E 1980 Peutz-Jeghers syndrome with 'adenoma malignum' of the cervix: a report of two cases. Gynecologic Oncology 10: 125–133

McKay D G, Street R B Jr, Benirschke K, Duncan C J 1953 Eosinophilic granuloma of the vulva. Surgery, Gynecology and Obstetrics 96: 437–447

Maede Y, Fujiwaki R, Watanabe Y, Hata K, Miyazaki K 1999 Bilateral granulosa cell tumor in a patient with blepharophimosis syndrome. Gynecologic Oncology 73: 335–336

Maestu R P, Buzon L M, Fraile L et al 1979 Carcinoma de ovario como causa de fiebre de origen desconocido: a proposito de un caso. Revista Clinica Espanola 153: 65–67

Malouf J, Alam S, Kanj H, Mufarrij A, Der Kaloustian V M 1985 Hypergonadotropic hypogonadism with congestive cardiomyopathy: an autosomal recessive disorder? American Journal of Medical Genetics 20: 483–492

Mandel M, Toren A, Kende G, Neuman Y, Kenet G, Rechavi G 1994 Familial clustering of malignant germ cell tumors and Langerhans' histiocytosis. Cancer 73: 1980–1983

Mandelblatt J S, Kanetsky P, Eggert L, Gold K 1999 Is HIV infection a cofactor for cervical squamous cell neoplasia? Cancer Epidemiology Biomarkers and Prevention 8: 97–106

Manetta A, Abt A B, Mamourian A C et al 1987 Pelvic fibromatosis: case report and review of the literature. Gynecologic Oncology 32: 91–94

Mantouvalos C, Metallinos C, Gouskos A 1982 Struma ovarii with Meigs' syndrome. Australian and New Zealand Journal of Obstetrics and Gynaecology 22: 101–102

Marieb N J, Spangler S, Kashgarian M et al 1983 Cushing's syndrome secondary to ectopic cortisol production by an ovarian carcinoma. Journal of Clinical Endocrinology and Metabolism 57: 737–740

Matsunami K, Imai A, Tamaya T, Takagi H, Noda K 1999 Brain metastasis as first manifestation of ovarian cancer. European Journal of Obstetrics, Gynecology and Reproductive Biology 82: 81–83

Matsuyama M, Inoue T, Ariyoshi Y et al 1979 Argyrophil cell carcinoma of the uterine cervix with ectopic production of ACTH, beta-MSH, serotonin, histamine and amylase. Cancer 44: 1813–1823

Maycock R L, Bertrand P, Morrison C E, Scott J H 1963 Manifestations of sarcoidosis: analysis of 145 patients with a review of nine series selected from the literature. American Journal of Medicine 35: 67–89

Medsger T A, Dixon J A, Garwood V F 1982 Palmar fasciitis and polyarthritis associated with ovarian carcinoma. Annals of Internal Medicine 96: 424–431

Meigs J V 1954 Pelvic tumors other than fibromas of the ovary with ascites and hydrothorax. Obstetrics and Gynecology 3: 471–486

Meigs J V, Cass J W 1937 Fibroma of the ovary with ascites and hydrothorax. American Journal of Obstetrics and Gynecology 33: 249–267

Menzies D N 1965 Two further cases of erythrocytosis secondary to fibromyomata. Proceedings of the Royal Society of Medicine 58: 239

Michael C A 1967 Pelvic fibroma causing recurrent attacks of hypoglycaemia. Journal of Obstetrics and Gynaecology of the British Commonwealth 74: 301–303

Migishima F, Jobo T, Hata H et al 2000 Uterine leiomyoma causing massive ascites and left pleural effusion with elevated CA 125: a case report. Journal of Obstetrics and Gynecology Research 26: 283–287

Millar A L, Pal T, Madlensky L et al 1999 Mismatch repair gene defects contribute to the genetic basis of double primary cancers of the colorectum and endometrium. Human Molecular Genetics 8: 823–829

Mitchinson M J 1970 The pathology of idiopathic retroperitoneal fibrosis. Journal of Clinical Pathology 23: 681–689

Moncayo R, Moncayo H E 1995 A new endocrinological and immunological syndrome in SLE: elevation of human chorionic gonadotropin and of antibodies directed against ovary and endometrium antigens. Lupus 4: 39–45

Moneta E, Benedetti Panici P L, Sacco F, Pizzolato G P 1981 Sertoli cell adenoma in Morris syndrome. European Journal of Gynaecologic Oncology 2: 48–50

Montag T W, Murphy R E, Belinson J L 1984 Virilizing malignant lipid cell tumor producing erythropoietin. Gynecologic Oncology 19: 98–103

Montiero J C M P, Baker G, Ferguson K M, Wiltshaw E, Munro-Neville A 1983 Ectopic production of human chorionic gonadotrophin (HCG) and human placental lactogen (HPL) by ovarian carcinoma. European Journal of Cancer and Clinical Oncology 19: 173–178

Morgan D R, Wells M, MacDonald R C, Johnston D 1985 Zollinger-Ellison syndrome due to a gastrin secreting ovarian mucinous cystadenoma: case report. British Journal of Obstetrics and Gynaecology 92: 867–869

Morgello S, Schwartz E, Horwith M et al 1988 Ectopic insulin production by a primary ovarian carcinoid. Cancer 61: 800–805

Morley J E, Jacobson R J, Melamed J, Hershman J M 1976 Choriocarcinoma as a cause of thyrotoxicosis. American Journal of Medicine 60: 1036–1040

Morson B C 1972 Pathology of Crohn's disease. In: Clinics in gastroenterology. Saunders, Philadelphia, pp 265–277

Mosesson M W, Colman R W, Sherry S 1968 Chronic intravascular coagulation syndrome: report of a case with special studies of an associated plasma cryoprecipitate ('cryofibrinogen'). New England Journal of Medicine 278: 815–821

Motlik K, Starka L 1973 Adrenocortical tumor of the ovary (a case report with particular stress upon the morphological and biochemical findings). Neoplasma 20: 97–110

Munkarah A, Malone J M, Budev H D, Evans T N 1994 Mucinous adenocarcinoma arising in a neovagina. Gynecologic Oncology 52: 272–275

Nagakura S, Shirai Y, Hatakeyama K 2000 Pseudo-Meigs' syndrome caused by secondary ovarian tumors from gastrointestinal cancer. A case report and review of the literature. Digestive Surgery 17: 418–419

Napoli V M, Wallach H 1976 Pancytopenia associated with a granulosa-cell tumor of the ovary: report of a case. American Journal of Clinical Pathology 65: 344–350

Narahara K, Kamada M, Takahashi Y et al 1992 Case of ovarian dysgenesis and dilated cardiomyopathy supports existence of Malouf syndrome. American Journal of Medical Genetics 44: 369–373

Narita T, Takagi K 1984 Ataxia-telangiectasia with dysgerminoma of right ovary, papillary carcinoma of thyroid and adenocarcinoma of pancreas. Cancer 54: 1113–1116

Navarro C, Corretger J M, Sancho A, Rovira J, Morales L 1985 Paraneoplastic precocious puberty: report of a new case with hepatoblastoma and review of the literature. Cancer 56: 1725–1729

Neumann S 1991 Cowden-Syndrom mit einem Ovarialtumor (Multiple-Hamartome-Syndrom). Chirurgie 62: 629–630

Nichols J, Warren J C, Mantz F A 1962 ACTH-Like excretion from carcinoma of the ovary. Journal of the American Medical Association 182: 713–718

Nicolino M, Bost M, David M, Chaussain J L 1995 Familial blepharophimosis: an uncommon marker of gonadal dysgenesis. Journal of Pediatric Endocrinology and Metabolism 8: 127–133

Nishida T, Oda T, Sugiyama T, Izumi S, Yakashiji M 1993 Concurrent ovarian serous carcinoma and osteogenesis imperfecta. Archives of Gynecology and Obstetrics 253: 153–156

Norwood S H, Torma M J, Fontenelle L J 1981 Hyperamylasemia due to poorly differentiated carcinoma of the ovary. Archives of Surgery 116: 225–226

Nunez C, Abboud S L, Lemon N C, Kemp J A 1983 Ovarian rhabdomyosarcoma presenting as leukemia: case report. Cancer 52: 297–300

O'Brien P K, Wilansky D L 1981 Familial thyroid nodulation and arrhenoblastoma. American Journal of Clinical Pathology 75: 578–581

Odell W D, Wolfsen A, Yoshimoto Y, Weitzman R, Fisher D, Hirose F 1977 Ectopic peptide synthesis: a universal concomitant of neoplasia. Transactions of the Association of American Physicians 90: 204–227

O'Flanagan S J, Tighe B F, Egan T J, Delaney P V 1987 Meigs' syndrome and pseudo-Meigs' syndrome. Journal of the Royal Society of Medicine 80: 252–253

Ogata T, Hasegawa T, Tamai S, Sato S, Hasegawa Y, Matsuo N 1998 Hypergonadotropic hypogonadism in a 3-year-old girl with blepharophimosis, ptosis and epicanthus inversus syndrome. Hormone Research 50: 190–192

O'Neill R T, Mikuta J J 1970 Hypoglycemia associated with serous cystadenocarcinoma of the ovary. Obstetrics and Gynecology 35: 287–289

Orbetzova M, Andreeva M, Zacharieva S, Ivanova R, Dashev G 1997 Ectopic ACTH-syndrome due to ovarian carcinoma. Experimental and Clinical Endocrinology and Diabetes 105: 363–365

O'Reilly S, Lyons D J, Harrison M, Gaffney E, Cullen M, Clancy L 1993 Thyrotoxicosis induced by choriocarcinoma. A report of two cases. Irish Medical Journal 86: 124–127

O'Riordan T, Gaffney E, Tormey V, Daly P 1990 Hyperamylasemia associated with progression of a serous surface papillary carcinoma. Gynecologic Oncology 36: 432–434

Osathanondh R, Tulchinsky D, Chopra I J 1976 Total and free thyroxine and tri-iodothyronine in normal and complicated pregnancy. Journal of Clinical Endocrinology and Metabolism 42: 98–104

Osborn R H, Bradbury J T, Yannone M E 1969 Androgen studies in a patient with lipoid-cell tumor of the ovary. Obstetrics and Gynecology 33: 666–672

Ossias A L, Zanjani E D, Zalusky R, Estren S, Wasserman L R 1973 Case report: studies on the mechanism of erythrocytosis associated with a uterine fibromyoma. British Journal of Haematology 25: 179–185

Otis C N, Fischer R A, Johnson N, Kelleher J F, Powell J L 1990 Histiocytosis X of the vulva: a case report and review of the literature. Obstetrics and Gynecology 75: 555–558

Padwell A 1986 Isolated arteritis of the uterine cervix: three case reports. British Journal of Obstetrics and Gynaecology 93: 1176–1180

Palefsky J 1995 Human papillomavirus-associated malignancies in HIV-positive men and women. Current Opinion in Oncology 7: 437–441

Pallister P D, Opitz J M 1979 The Perrault syndrome: autosomal recessive ovarian dysgenesis with facultative non-sex-linked sensorineural deafness. American Journal of Medical Genetics 4: 239–246

Palmer P E, Bogojavlenski S, Bhan A K, Scully R E 1990 Prolactinoma in wall of ovarian dermoid cyst with hyperprolactinemia. Obstetrics and Gynecology 75: 540–543

Palnaes-Hansen C, Bulow S, Karlsen J 1987 Tubocutaneous fistula. Case report. Acta Chirurgica Scandinavica 153: 465–466

Panidis D, Rousso D, Vavilis D, Skiadopoulos S, Kalogeropoulos A 1994 Familial blepharophimosis with ovarian dysfunction. Human Reproduction 9: 2034–2037

Papadopoulos K I, Hornblad Y, Liljebladh H, Hallengren B 1996 High frequency of endocrine autoimmunity in patients with sarcoidosis. European Journal of Endocrinology 134: 331–336

Parks A G, Morson B C, Pegum J S 1965 Crohn's disease with cutaneous involvement. Proceedings of the Royal Society of Medicine 58: 241–242

Parsons V, Rigby B 1958 Cushing's syndrome associated with adenocarcinoma of the ovary. Lancet 2: 992–994

Patsner B, Mann W J, Chumas J 1989 Malignant mixed germ cell tumor of the ovary in a young woman with Smith-Lemli-Opitz syndrome. Gynecologic Oncology 33: 386–388

Payne D, Muss H B, Homesley H D, Jobson V W, Baird F G 1981 Autoimmune hemolytic anemia and ovarian dermoid cysts: case report and review of the literature. Cancer 48: 721–724

Pearce K F, Nolan T E 1996 Endometrial sarcoidosis as a cause of postmenopausal bleeding. Journal of Reproductive Medicine 41: 878–880

Pecorelli S, Sartori E, Favalli G, Ugazio A G, Gastaldi A 1988 Ataxia-telangiectasia and endodermal sinus tumor of the ovary: report of a case. Gynecologic Oncology 29: 240–244

Penn I 1986 Cancers of the anogenital region in renal transplant recipients: analysis of 65 cases. Cancer 58: 611–616

Penney L L, Ruangwit U, Miles P A 1981 Congenital lipodystrophy and polycystic ovarian disease. Journal of Reproductive Medicine 26: 145–148

Peters W A, Andersen W A, Thornton W N Jr 1983 Dermatomyositis and coexistent ovarian cancer: a review of the compounding clinical problems. Gynecologic Oncology 15: 440–444

Petrides M, Robertson I G, Fox H 1979 Giant cell arteritis of the female genital tract. British Journal of Obstetrics and Gynaecology 86: 148–151

Petry K U, Kochel H, Bode U et al 1996 Human papillomavirus is associated with the frequent detection of warty and basaloid high-grade neoplasia of the vulva and cervical neoplasia among immunocompromised women. Gynecologic Oncology 60: 30–34

Pinsonneault O, Goldstein D P 1985 Obstructing malformations of the uterus and vagina. Fertility and Sterility 44: 241–247

Pirozynski W J 1976 Giant-cell arteritis of the uterus: report of two cases. American Journal of Clinical Pathology 65: 308–313

Plantaz D, Flamant F, Vassal G et al 1992 Granulosa cell tumors of the ovary in children and adolescents. Multicenter retrospective study in 40 patients aged 7 months to 22 years. Archives Francaises Pediatrie 49: 793–798

Podczaski E, Kaminski P F, Pees R C, Singapuri K, Sorosky J I 1991 Peutz-Jeghers syndrome with ovarian sex cord tumor with annular tubules and cervical adenoma malignum. Gynecologic Oncology 42: 74–78

Polasky N, Polasky S H, Magenheim H, Abrams N R 1965 Giant-cell arteritis: review and report of a case. Journal of the American Medical Association 191: 341–343

Powell D, Singer F R, Murray T M, Minkin C, Potts T J Jr 1973 Nonparathyroid humoral hypercalcemia in patients with neoplastic diseases. New England Journal of Medicine 289: 176–181

Pratt-Thomas H R, Kreutner A Jr, Underwood P B, Dowdeswell R H 1976 Proliferative and malignant Brenner tumors of the ovary: report of two cases, one with Meigs' syndrome, review of literature and ultrastructural comparisons. Gynecologic Oncology 4: 176–193

Prezyna A P, Kalyanaraman U 1977 Bowen's carcinoma in vulvovaginal Crohn's disease (regional enterocolitis): report of first case. American Journal of Obstetrics and Gynecology 128: 914–916

Primrose J N, Maloney M, Wells M, Bulgim O, Johnston D 1988 Gastrin-producing ovarian mucinous cystadenomas: a cause of the Zollinger-Ellison syndrome. Surgery 104: 830–833

Puleo J G, Clarke-Pearson D L, Smith E B, Barnard D E, Creasman W T 1986 Superior vena cava syndrome associated with gynecologic malignancy. Gynecologic Oncology 23: 59–64

Pysher T J, Hitch D C, Krous H F 1981 Bilateral juvenile granulosa cell tumors in a 4-month-old dysmorphic infant: a clinical, histologic, and ultrastructural study. American Journal of Surgical Pathology 5: 789–794

Qizilbash A H, Trebilcock R G, Patterson M C, Lamont K G 1974 Functioning primary carcinoid tumor of the ovary: a light-and electron-microscopic study with review of the literature. American Journal of Clinical Pathology 62: 629–638

Raggio M, Kaplan A L, Harberg J F 1983 Recurrent ovarian fibromas with basal cell nevus syndrome (Gorlin syndrome). Obstetrics and Gynecology 61: 95s–96s

Rao P G, Katariya R N, Sood S, Rao P L 1977 Situs inversus totalis with calculus cholecystitis and mucinous cystadenoma of the ovaries. Journal of Postgraduate Medicine (Bombay) 23: 89–90

Rater C J, Selke A C, Van Epps E F 1968 Basal cell nevus syndrome. American Journal of Roentgenology Radium Therapy and Nuclear Medicine 103: 589–594

Rhoads J E, Terrell A W 1937 Ovarian fibroma with ascites and hydrothorax (Meig's syndrome). Journal of the American Medical Association 109: 1684–1687

Ribeiro G, Hughesdon P, Wiltshaw E 1988 Squamous carcinoma arising in dermoid cysts and associated with hypercalcemia: a clinicopathologic study of six cases. Gynecologic Oncology 29: 222–230

Ridley C M 1975 The vulva. Saunders, Philadelphia

Rieke J W, Kapp D S 1988 Successful management of malignant pericardial effusion in metastatic squamous cell carcinoma of the uterine cervix. Gynecologic Oncology 31: 338–351

Rivett J D, Robinson J M 1972 Hypercalcaemia associated with an ovarian carcinoma of mesonephromatous type. Journal of Obstetrics and Gynaecology of the British Commonwealth 79: 1047–1052

Robboy S J, Norris H J, Scully R E 1975 Insular carcinoid primary in the ovary: a clinicopathologic analysis of 48 cases. Cancer 36: 404–418

Roberge R J, Kantor W J, Scorza L 1999 Rectus abdominis endometrioma. American Journal of Emergency Medicine 17: 675–677

Rohatgi M, Mukherjee A K 1973 Tubo-intestinal fistula. Journal of Obstetrics and Gynaecology of the British Commonwealth 80: 379–380

Romer T, Schwesinger G, Foth D 2001 Endometrial sarcoidosis manifesting as recurrent serometra in a postmenopausal woman. Acta Obstetricia et Gynecologica Scandinavica 80: 482–483

Rosenberg L, Hennekens C H, Rosner B, Belanger C, Rothman K J, Speizer F E 1981 Early menopause and the risk of myocardial infarction. American Journal of Obstetrics and Gynecology 139: 47–51

Rosenfeld S I, Steck W, Breen J L 1989 Sarcoidosis of the female genital tract: a case presentation and survey of the world literature. International Journal of Gynaecology and Obstetrics 28: 373–380

Rosner J M, Conte M F, Horita S, Forsham P H 1964 In vivo and in vitro production of testosterone by a lipid cell ovarian tumour. American Journal of Medicine 37: 638–642

Roth L M, Nicholas T R, Ehrlich C E 1979 Juvenile granulosa cell tumor: a clinicopathologic study of three cases with ultrastructural observations. Cancer 44: 2194–2205

Rowland Payne C M E 1981 Newly recognized syndrome in the neck: Horner's syndrome with ipsilateral vocal cord and phrenic nerve. Journal of the Royal Society of Medicine 74: 814–818

Roy M K, Appleton M A, Delicata R J, Sharma A K, Williams G T, Carey P D 1997 Probable association between hidradenitis suppurativa and Crohn's disease: significance of epithelioid granuloma. British Journal of Surgery 84: 375–376

Rulon D B, Helwig E B 1974 Cutaneous sebaceous neoplasms. Cancer 33: 82–102

Russell P, Bannatyne P 1989 Surgical pathology of the ovaries. Churchill Livingstone, Edinburgh

Russell P, Bannatyne P, Shearman R P, Fraser I S, Corbett P 1982 Premature hypergonadotropic ovarian failure: clinicopathologic study of 19 cases. International Journal of Gynecological Pathology 1: 185–201

Sakemi T, Nakamura K, Baba N, Watanabe T 1992 Rapidly progressive renal amyloidosis associated with uterine cervical cancer. Clinical Nephrology 38: 173–174

Salmon U J 1934 Benign pelvic tumors associated with ascites and pleural effusion. Journal of the Mount Sinai Hospital 1: 169–172

Samaan N A, Smith J P, Rutledge F N, Schultz P N 1976 The significance of measurement of human placental lactogen, human chorionic gonadotropin, and carcinoembryonic antigen in patients with ovarian carcinoma. American Journal of Obstetrics and Gynecology 126: 186–189

Samaratunga H, Strutton G, Wright R G et al 1991 Squamous carcinoma arising in a case of vulvitis granulomatosa or vulval variant of Melkersson-Rosenthal syndrome. Gynecologic Oncology 41: 263–269

Sandler R S, Wurzelmann J I, Lyles C M 1992 Oral contraceptive use and the risk of inflammatory bowel disease. Epidemiology 3: 374–378

Sandvei R, Bang G 1991 Sarcoidosis of the uterus. Acta Obstetricia et Gynecologica Scandinavica 70: 165–167

Sarani B, Orkin B A 1997 Squamous cell carcinoma arising in an unhealed wound in Crohn's disease. Southern Medical Journal 90: 940–942

Savell V, Hanna R, Benda J A, Argenyi Z B 1995 Histiocytosis X of the vulva with a confusing clinical and pathologic presentation. A case report. Journal of Reproductive Medicine 40: 323–326

Savoye G, Forestier F, Scotte M, Descargues J, Mace P, Guedon C 2000 Ovarian granulomas associated with Crohn's disease: an unusual location of the disease or a delayed postoperative adverse event? Gastroenterologie Clinique et Biologique 24: 588–589

Schlaghecke R, Kreuzpaintner G, Burrig K F, Juli E, Kley H K 1989 Cushing's syndrome due to ACTH-production of an ovarian carcinoid. Klinische Wochenschrift 67: 640–644

Schofield P M, Kirsop B A, Reginald P, Harington M 1985 Ovarian carcinoma presenting as pyrexia of unknown origin. Postgraduate Medical Journal 61: 177–178

Schreiber M M 1963 Vulvar von Recklinghausen's disease. Archives of Dermatology 88: 320–321

Schulman D, Beck L S, Roberts I M, Schwartz A M 1987 Crohn's disease of the vulva. American Journal of Gastroenterology 82: 1328–1330

Schur P H 1979 Systemic lupus erythematosus. In: Beeson P B, McDermott W Y, Wyngaarden J B (eds) Cecil-Loeb textbook of medicine, 15th edn. Saunders, Philadelphia, pp 174–180

Scully R E 1970 Sex cord tumor with annular tubules: a distinctive ovarian tumor of the Peutz-Jeghers syndrome. Cancer 25: 1107–1121

Scully R E 1982 Sex cord stromal tumors. In: Blaustein A (ed) Pathology of the female genital tract, 2nd edn. Springer-Verlag, New York, pp 598–599

Scully R E, Galdabini J J, McNeely B U 1978 Case records of the Massachusetts General Hospital. Case 13 — 1978. Disseminated intravascular coagulation with endometrioid carcinoma of the ovary. New England Journal of Medicine 298: 786–792

Scurry J, Planner R, Fortune D W, Lee C S, Rode J 1993 Ligneous (pseudomembranous) inflammation of the female genital tract. A report of two cases. Journal of Reproductive Medicine 38: 407–412

Scurry J, Brand A, Sheehan P, Planner R 1996 High-grade endometrial carcinoma in secretory endometrium in young women: a report of five cases. Gynecologic Oncology 60: 224–227

Shane J M, Naftolin F 1975 Aberrant hormone activity by tumors of gynaecologic importance. American Journal of Obstetrics and Gynecology 121: 133–143

Shetty M R, Boghossian H M, Duffell D, Freel R, Gonzales J C 1982 Tumor-induced hypoglycemia: a result of ectopic insulin production. Cancer 49: 1920–1923

Shiel W C Jr, Prete P E, Jason M, Andrews B S 1985 Palmar fasciitis and arthritis with ovarian and non-ovarian carcinomas: new syndrome. American Journal of Medicine 79: 640–644

Siddiqui M, Toub D B 1995 Cellular fibroma of the ovary with Meigs' syndrome and elevated CA-125. A case report. Journal of Reproductive Medicine 40: 817–819

Siegler A M 1983 Hysterosalpingography. Fertility and Sterility 40: 139–158

Siegman-Igra Y, Flatau E, Deligdish L 1977 Chronic diffuse intravascular coagulation (DIC) in nonmetastatic ovarian cancer: report of a case and review of the literature. Gynecologic Oncology 5: 92–100

Simon G C, Delavierre P 1981 Demons-Meigs' syndrome associated with a seminoma of the ovary (Syndrome de Demons-Meigs au cours d'un seminome ovarien). Semaine des Hopitaux de Paris 57: 653–656

Simon N L, Mazur M T, Shingleton H M 1985 Pelvic fibromatosis: an unusual gynecologic tumor. Obstetrics and Gynecology 65: 767–769

Skrabanck P, McParthin J, Powell D 1980 Tumor hypercalcemia and 'ectopic hyperparathyroidism'. Medicine 59: 262–282

Slotky B, Shrivastav R, Lee B M 1982 Massive edema of the ovary. Obstetrics and Gynecology 59: 92s–94s

Smith F R 1931 Neurofibroma of the ovary associated with von Recklinghausen's disease. American Journal of Cancer 15: 859–862

Snider B L, Benjamin D R 1981 Eruptive keratoacanthoma with an internal malignant neoplasm. Archives of Dermatology 117: 788–790

Sobol H, Mazoyer S, Smith S A et al 1993 Familial ovarian carcinoma: pedigree studies and preliminary results from linkage analysis. Bulletin du Cancer (Paris) 80: 121–134

Solidoro G, Del Gaudio G A 1991 Le cisti di echinococco dell'ovario. Descrizione di un caso. Minerva Chirurgica (Torino) 46: 571–575

Solomon M J, Deva A K, Corcoran S J, Gallagher N 1996 Postpartum avulsion of the terminal ileal wall in Crohn's disease. Australian and New Zealand Journal of Surgery 66: 849–851

Solomon S D, Maurer K H 1983 Association of dermatomyositis and dysgerminoma in a 16-year-old patient. Arthritis and Rheumatology 26: 572–573

Soutter W P, Norman R, Green-Thompson R W 1981 The management of choriocarcinoma causing severe thyrotoxicosis: two case reports. British Journal of Obstetrics and Gynaecology 88: 938–943

Spigelman A D, Murday V, Phillips R K 1989 Cancer and the Peutz-Jeghers syndrome. Gut 30: 1588–1590

Stamm E R, Townsend R R, Johnson A M, Garg K, Manco-Johnson M, Gabow P A 1999 Frequency of ovarian cysts in patients with autosomal dominant polycystic kidney disease. American Journal of Kidney Diseases 34: 120–124

Starink T M 1984 Cowden's disease: analysis of fourteen new cases. Journal of the American Academy of Dermatology 11: 1127–1141

Steinberg D M, Cooke W T, Alexander-Williams J 1973 Abscess and fistulae in Crohn's disease. Gut 14: 865–869

Stephen M R, Lindop G B 1998 A renin secreting ovarian steroid cell tumour associated with secondary polycythaemia. Journal of Clinical Pathology 51: 75–77

Steven M M, Mackay I R, Camegie P R, Bhathal P S, Anderson R M 1982 Cerebellar cortical degeneration with ovarian carcinoma. Postgraduate Medical Journal 58: 47–51

Stewart A F, Romero R, Schwartz P E, Kohorn E I, Broadus A E 1982 Hypercalcemia associated with gynaecologic malignancies: biochemical characterization. Cancer 49: 2389–2394

Stockdale A D, Leader M, Phillips R H, Henry K 1986 The carcinoid syndrome and multiple hormone secretion associated with a carcinoid tumour of the uterine cervix: case report. British Journal of Obstetrics and Gynaecology 93: 397–401

Stratakis C A, Papageorgiou T, Premkumar A et al 2000 Ovarian lesions in Carney complex: clinical genetics and possible predisposition to malignancy. Journal of Clinical Endocrinology and Metabolism 85: 4010–4012

Summers P R, Biswas M K, Boulware D W, Green L, Herrera E H, O'Quinn A G 1991 A case report of giant cell arteritis of the uterus and adnexa. American Journal of Obstetrics and Gynecology 164: 540–542

Sutphen R, Galan-Gomez E, Kousseff B G 1995 Clitoromegaly in neurofibromatosis. American Journal of Medical Genetics 55: 325–330

Suzuki M, Takamizawa S, Nomaguchi K et al 2001 Erythropoietin synthesis by tumour tissues in a patient with uterine myoma and erythrocytosis. British Journal of Haematology 113: 49–51

Taggart A J, Iveson J M, Wright V 1984 Shoulder-hand syndrome and symmetrical arthralgia in patients with tubo-ovarian carcinoma. Annals of the Rheumatic Diseases 43: 391–393

Takeuchi K, Murata K, Funaki K, Kitazawa S, Kitazawa R 2000 Immunohistochemical detection of parathyroid hormone-related protein in a squamous cell carcinoma arising from mature cystic teratoma causing humoral hypercalcemia of malignancy. Gynecologic Oncology 79: 504–507

Talerman A 1984 A patient with situs inversus totalis and embryonal carcinoma of the ovary. Gynecologic Oncology 19: 371–372

Tamaya T, Ohno Y, Fujimoto J, Nakata Y, Sato S, Okada H 1986 Huge intraabdominal fibromatosis on the posterior wall of uterus: a case report. Gynecologic Oncology 24: 129–134

Tamimi H K, Bolen J W 1984 Enchondromatosis (Ollier's disease) and ovarian juvenile granulosa cell tumor: a case report and review of the literature. Cancer 53: 1605–1608

Tamsen A, Mazur M T 1992 Ovarian strumal carcinoid in association with multiple endocrine neoplasia type IIA. Archives of Pathology and Laboratory Medicine 116: 200–203

Tanaka Y, Sasaki Y, Nishihara H, Izawa T, Nishi T 1992 Ovarian juvenile granulosa cell tumor associated with Maffucci's syndrome. American Journal of Clinical Pathology 97: 523–527

Taraszewski R, Rosman P M, Knight C A, Cloney D J 1991 Small cell carcinoma of the ovary. Gynecologic Oncology 41: 149–151

Taylor A B 1960 Sarcoidosis of the uterus. Journal of Obstetrics and Gynaecology of the British Empire 67: 32–35

Taylor A E 2000 Insulin-lowering medication in polycystic ovary syndrome. Obstetric and Gynecology Clinics of North America 27: 583–595

Taylor S C, Baker E, Grossman M E 1991 Nodular vulvar amyloid as a presentation of systemic amyloidosis. Journal of the American Academy of Dermatology 24: 139

Teshima H, Kitamura H, Mizoguchi Y et al 1988 Immunohistochemical and immunoelectron microscopic study of an amylase-producing, CA19-9 positive ovarian mucinous cystadenocarcinoma. Gynecologic Oncology 30: 372–380

Tetu B, Lebel M, Camilleri J P 1988 Renin-producing ovarian tumor. A case report with immunohistochemical and electron-microscopic study. American Journal of Surgical Pathology 12: 634–640

Tham S N, Choong H L 1992 Primary tuberculous chancre in a renal transplant patient. Journal of the American Academy of Dermatology 26: 342–344

Tindall J G, Rea T H, Shulman I, Quismorio F P Jr 1981 Herpes gestationis with hydatidiform mole: immunologic studies. Archives of Dermatology 117: 510–512

Todesco S, Terribile V, Borsatti A, Mantero F 1975 Primary aldosteronism due to a malignant ovarian tumor. Journal of Clinical Endocrinology and Metabolism 41: 809–819

Trimble E L, Saigo P E, Freeberg G W, Rubin S C, Hoskins W J 1991 Peritoneal sarcoidosis and elevated CA 125. Obstetrics and Gynecology 78: 976–977

Tschang T P, Poulos P, Ho C K, Kuo T T 1976 Multiple sebaceous adenomas and internal malignant disease: a case report with chromosomal analysis. Human Pathology 7: 589–594

Tsuji S, Matsuoka Y, Suzuki Y et al 1992 Turner's syndrome associated with Hashimoto's thyroiditis and sarcoidosis: a case report. Annals of Internal Medicine 31: 131–133

Tsunematsu R, Saito T, Iguchi H, Fukuda T, Tsukamoto N 2000 Hypercalcemia due to parathyroid hormone-related protein produced by primary ovarian clear cell adenocarcinoma: case report. Gynecologic Oncology 76: 218–222

Tuffnell D Buchan P C 1991 Crohn's disease of the vulva in childhood. British Journal of Clinical Practice 45: 159–160

Twiggs L B, Morrow C P, Schlaerth J B 1979 Acute pulmonary complications of molar pregnancy. American Journal of Obstetrics and Gynecology 135: 189–194

Vaitukaitis J L 1974 Human chorionic gonadotropin as a tumor marker. Annals of Clinical and Laboratory Science 4: 276–280

van Voorhis B J, Neff T W, Syrop C H, Chapler F K 1994 Primary hypothyroidism associated with multicystic ovaries and ovarian torsion in an adult. Obstetrics and Gynecology 83: 885–887

Vasen H F, Watson P, Mecklin J P et al 1994 The epidemiology of endometrial cancer in hereditary nonpolyposis colorectal cancer. Anticancer Research 14: 1675–1678

Vaz R M, Turner C 1986 Ollier's disease (enchondromatosis) associated with ovarian juvenile granulosa cell tumor and precocious pseudopuberty. Journal of Pediatrics 108: 945–947

Velasco-Oses A, Alonso-Alvaro A, Blanco-Pozo A, Nogales F F Jr 1988 Ollier's disease associated with ovarian juvenile granulosa cell tumor. Cancer 62: 222–225

Verducci M A, Malkasian G D Jr, Friedman S J, Winkelmann R K 1984 Gynecologic carcinoma associated with dermatomyositis-polymyositis. Obstetrics and Gynecology 64: 695–698

Von Meyer-Hofmann G, Schwarzhopf H, Hartmann H 1960 Spontaneous hypoglycaemia with extrapancreatic tumours. Deutsche Medizinische Wochenschrift 85: 2106–2112

Wakefield A J, Sawyerr A M, Hudson M, Dhillon A P, Pounder R E 1991 Smoking, the oral contraceptive pill, and Crohn's disease. Digestive Diseases and Sciences 36: 1147–1150

Walton B J, Morain W D, Baughman R D, Jordan A, Crichlow R W 1986 Cowden's disease: a further indication for prophylactic mastectomy. Surgery 99: 82–86

Watson P, Vasen H F, Mecklin J P, Jarvinen H, Lynch H T 1994 The risk of endometrial cancer in hereditary nonpolyposis colorectal cancer. American Journal of Medicine 96: 516–520

Weber A M, Belinson J L 1997 Inflammatory bowel disease — a complicating factor in gynecological disorders? Medscape Women's Health 2: 4

Weber G, Stetter H, Pliess G, Stickl H 1970 Assoziiertes Vorkommen von eruptiven Keratoacanthomen, Tuben carcinom und Paramyeloblasten-leukamie. Archiv für Klinische und Experimentelle Dermatologie 238: 107–119

Weiss D B, Aldor A, Aboulafia Y 1975 Erythrocytosis due to erythropoietin-producing uterine fibromyoma. American Journal of Obstetrics and Gynecology 122: 358–360

Weitzer M, Pokos V, Jeevaratnam P et al 1995 Isolated expression of the Muir-Torre phenotype in a member of a family with hereditary non-polyposis colorectal cancer. Histopathology 27: 573–575

Weyl-Ben Arush M, Oslander L 1991 Ollier's disease associated with ovarian Sertoli–Leydig cell tumor and breast adenoma. American Journal of Pediatric Hematology and Oncology 13: 49–51

Wheeler J E 1982 Pathology of the Fallopian tube. In: Blaustein A (ed) Pathology of the female genital tract, 2nd edn. Springer-Verlag, New York, pp 401–403

White A, Flaris N, Elmer D, Lui R, Fanburg B L 1990 Coexistence of mucinous cystadenocarcinoma of the ovary and ovarian sarcoidosis. American Journal of Obstetrics and Gynecology 162: 1284–1285

Winslow R C, Funkhouser J W 1968 Views and reviews: sarcoidosis of the female reproductive organs: report of a case. Obstetrics and Gynecology 32: 285–289

Wittich A C, Morales H, Braeuer N R 1982 Tubocutaneous fistula. American Journal of Obstetrics and Gynecology 144: 109–110

Witwer M W, Farmer M F, Wand J S, Solomon L S 1977 Extensive actinomycosis associated with an intrauterine contraceptive device. American Journal of Obstetrics and Gynecology 128: 913–914

Wlodarski F M, Trainer T D 1975 Granulomatous oophoritis and salpingitis associated with Crohn's disease of the appendix. American Journal of Obstetrics and Gynecology 122: 527–528

Wright J P 1992 Factors influencing first relapse in patients with Crohn's disease. Journal of Clinical Gastroenterology 15: 12–16

Wrigley P F, Malpas J S, Turnbull A L, Jenkins G C, McArt A 1971 Secondary polycythaemia due to a uterine fibromyoma producing erythropoietin. British Journal of Haematology 21: 551–555

Yagi C, Miyata J, Hanai J, Ogawa M, Ueda G 1986 Hyperamylasemia associated with endometrioid carcinoma of the ovary: case report and immunohistochemical study. Gynecologic Oncology 25: 250–255

Yamada M, Hatakeyama S, Yamamoto E et al 1988 Localized amyloidosis of the uterine cervix. Virchows Archiv. A, Pathological Anatomy and Histopathology 413: 265–268

Yantiss R K, Clement P B, Young R H 2000 Neoplastic and pre-neoplastic changes in gastrointestinal endometriosis: a study of 17 cases. American Journal of Surgical Pathology 24: 513–524

Yell J A 1991 Grzybowski's generalized eruptive keratoacanthoma. Journal of the Royal Society of Medicine 84: 170–171

Yin H, Li X H, Xu H M, Lu Y P 1999 Pseudo-Meigs' syndrome secondary to bilateral endometrioid adenocarcinomas. International Journal of Gynaecology and Obstetrics 66: 293–295

Young R E, Welch W R, Dickersin G R, Scully R E 1982 Ovarian sex cord tumor with annular tubules: review of 74 cases including 27 with Peutz-Jeghers syndrome and 4 with adenoma malignum of the cervix. Cancer 50: 1384–1402

Young R H, Scully R E 1987 Ovarian steroid cell tumors associated with Cushing's syndrome: a report of three cases. International Journal of Gynecological Pathology 6: 40–48

Young R H, Scully R E 1988 Mucinous ovarian tumors associated with mucinous adenocarcinomas of the cervix: a clinicopathological analysis of 16 cases. International Journal of Gynecological Pathology 7: 99–111

Young R H, Dickersin G R, Scully R E 1983 A distinctive ovarian sex cord-stromal tumor causing sexual precosity in the Peutz-Jeghers syndrome. American Journal of Surgical Pathology 7: 233–243

Young R H, Dickersin G R, Scully R E 1984 Juvenile granulosa cell tumor of the ovary. A clinicopathological analysis of 125 cases. American Journal of Surgical Pathology 8: 575–596

Young R R 1993 New and unusual aspects of germ cell tumors. American Journal of Surgical Pathology 17: 1210–1224

Yutani C, Maeda H, Nakajima H, Takeuchi N, Kimura M, Kitamura H 1982 Primary ovarian lymphomas associated with Meigs' syndrome: a case report. Acta Cytologica 26: 44–48

Zachwiej E, Hatys-Skirzynska H, Szamborski J 1956 Sarkoioza macicy. Ginekologia Polska 28: 655 (cited by Ho, 1979)

Zemke E E, Herrel W E 1941 Bilateral granulosa cell tumors: successful removal from a child of fourteen weeks of age. American Journal of Obstetrics and Gynecology 41: 704–707

Zetzel L 1980 Fertility, pregnancy and idiopathic inflammatory bowel disease. In: Kirsner J B, Shorter R G (eds) Inflammatory bowel disease, 2nd edn. Lea & Febiger, Philadelphia, pp 241–253

Zinkham W H 1976 Multifocal eosinophilic granuloma: natural history, etiology and management. American Journal of Medicine 60: 457–463

Zosmer A, Kogan S, Frumkin A, Dagni R, Lifschitz-Mercer B 1992 Unsuspected involvement of the female genitalia in pemphigus vulgaris. European Journal of Obstetrics, Gynecology and Reproductive Biology 47: 260–263

36

Pathology of abnormal sexual development

S. J. Robboy   R. C. Bentley   P. Russell   M. C. Anderson

Introduction   1209

Overview of embryology in abnormal sexual
   development   1209

Gender identification disorders with a normal chromosome
   constitution   1212
Female pseudohermaphroditism (female intersex)   1212
Male pseudohermaphroditism (male intersex)   1214

Gender identification disorders with an abnormal sex
   chromosome constitution   1220
Sexual ambiguity infrequent   1220
Sexual ambiguity frequent   1224

True hermaphroditism   1228

INTRODUCTION

New insights into the biology of sexual development and advances in chromosome analysis have led to early identification and prompt treatment of the intersexual patient which permit the individual to lead a more normal life. Based on these advances, a classification of abnormal sexual development has been developed which correlates the gonadal and genital anatomy with the chromosomal findings and specific genetic or metabolic defects (Robboy et al 2002) (Table 36.1). This permits an integrated approach to this complex group of disorders according to the manner by which patients present as well as on the pathophysiological basis of the defect. The classification also groups patients who are at high risk for development of gonadal neoplasia.

OVERVIEW OF EMBRYOLOGY IN ABNORMAL SEXUAL DEVELOPMENT

In humans and other mammals, the karyotype 'XY' genetically defines the sex as male, while 'XX' defines the female sex. Sex is determined by the presence or absence of a signal from a substance called the testis-determining factor (TDF) found on the Y chromosome. Testes are formed if this gene is expressed by the embryo prior to the differentiation of the urogenital ridge. Further male development occurs under the influence of hormones secreted later by the testes (Fig. 36.1). In the absence of testis-determining factor, the gonads differentiate as ovaries and the embryo develops as a female. The timely expression of testis-determining factor is critical to the development of male sex; in the absence of timely expression of this factor, the embryo develops a female phenotype by 'default', regardless of genetic sex (Hunter 1995d).

Extensive efforts have been expended to identify the testis-determining region. Several candidates have been proposed and discarded in recent years. The candidate now accepted is a gene called *SRY* (sex region 'Y'). It is

Table 36.1 Classification of intersexual disorders

Disorders associated with a normal chromosome constitution
  Female pseudohermaphroditism (Female intersex)
    Fetal defect
      Adrenogenital syndrome (Testosterone overproduction due to adrenocorticoid insufficiency)
        21 α-hydroxylase deficiency
        11 β-hydroxylase deficiency
      Placental aromatase defect
    Maternal influence
      Maternal ingestion of progestins or androgens
      Maternal virilising tumour

  Male pseudohermaphroditism (Male intersex)
    Gonadal defects
      Testicular regression syndrome (Gonadal destruction)
      Leydig cell agenesis
        Defective hCG-LH receptor
      Defects in testosterone synthesis
        Testosterone and adrenocorticoid insufficiency
          20,22-demolase deficiency
          3 β-hydroxylase dehydrogenase deficiency
          17 α-hydroxylase deficiency
        Testosterone insufficiency only
          17-20-desmolase deficiency
          17 β-hydroxysteroid (17-Ketosteroid reductase) dehydrogenase deficiency
      Persistent Müllerian Duct Syndrome (Defect in Müllerian Inhibiting Substance System)

    End-organ defects
      Disordered androgen receptor binding
        Androgen insensitivity syndrome (Testicular feminisation)
        Incomplete androgen insensitivity syndrome (Reifenstein syndrome)
      Disordered testosterone metabolism
        5 α-reductase deficiency

    Defect uncertain
      Smith–Lemli–Opitz syndrome
Disorders associated with an abnormal sex chromosome constitution
  Sexual ambiguity infrequent
    Klinefelter syndrome
    Turner syndrome
    XX male & XY female syndrome (sex reversal)
    Pure gonadal dysgenesis (some forms)
  Sexual ambiguity frequent
    Mixed gonadal dysgenesis (MGD), including
      Pure gonadal dysgenesis (some forms)
      Dysgenetic male pseudohermaphroditism
    True hermaphroditism

'Idiopathic' or 'unclassified' conditions exist within each major category. We assume that each category of male pseudohermaphroditism with defects in specific protein products or receptors has forms where the abnormality is total or partial, or where the defect results from a qualitatively abnormal structure.

located in a region just central to the pseudoautosomal pairing region at the distal end of the short arm of the Y chromosome (Brennan et al 1998). The gene, which has a strongly conserved motif (Hunter 1995c), encodes for a DNA binding protein, the binding activity product (transcriptional switch) of which orchestrates the action of other genes. It does so by initiating a cascade of gene expressions that regulate the development of the testis (MacLean et al 1997; Brennan et al 1998). It has been proposed that *SRY* acts to repress other inhibitory regulators of male development (Vilain & McCabe 1998). Some

of the target genes may also have been identified (Vilain & McCabe 1998).

Evidence supporting this thesis includes:

- the *SRY* gene is absent from the normal X chromosome and somatic chromosomes
- the *SRY* gene is present on the X chromosome of 'sex reversed' XX human males
- the homologous gene in the mouse is initially expressed just before sexual differentiation begins (the genital ridge initially swells)
- *SRY* gene acts in the absence of germ cells
- genetic splicing of the *SRY* gene into the chromosomally female embryo causes it to develop as a male (Hunter 1995c). Single base pair point mutations in the *SRY* gene or in promoter regions essential for gene expression render an XY patient as a phenotypic female (Swain & Lovell-Badge 1997; Veitia et al 1997; Mendez et al 1999).

One role of *SRY*, and possibly the most important, is to initiate the indifferent cells in the genital ridge to differentiate into Sertoli cells. This is the first type of cell required to form in the embryonic testis (Swain & Lovell-Badge 1997). With monoclonal antibodies, a SRY-specific epitope (protein) has been found in the nuclei of Sertoli cells and germ cells (Salas-Cortes et al 1999). Two other genes are thought to be important in Sertoli cell differentiation and function. These include *Sox9*, an SRY-related gene, and *SF-1*, a nuclear hormone receptor. Sox9, which the Sertoli cells express, results in XY females when mutations inactivate the gene. SF-1 is also expressed in Sertoli cells and is believed to activate the *Müllerian Inhibiting Substance* (*MIS*) gene (See Vilain & McCabe 1998 for an in-depth review of the genes involved in male sex determination).

In the event that the embryo does not express SRY on a time sensitive basis as a transcription factor, and therefore does not develop a testis, then other genes activate later that are responsible for the development of the ovary (Hunter 1995c; MacLean et al 1997).

The gene, *DAX1*, the action of which may be to antagonise the *SRY* gene, appears involved in ovarian development (Vilain & McCabe 1998). The *DAX1* gene, thus, may also play a key rôle in sex determination. It is expressed in the genital ridge precisely at the critical time for sex determination. Its expression turns off at the critical moment if the gonad is to become a testis, but remains expressed in females. It has the structural and biochemical properties typical of a transcription factor and seems to be a transcriptional repressor. Mutations of the gene in males are associated with immaturity of Sertoli cells, suggesting a rôle in Sertoli cell function, and an absence of germ cells in the embryonic testis. However, XY patients with mutations in the *DAX1* gene are not sex reversed as females, but rather remain as males.

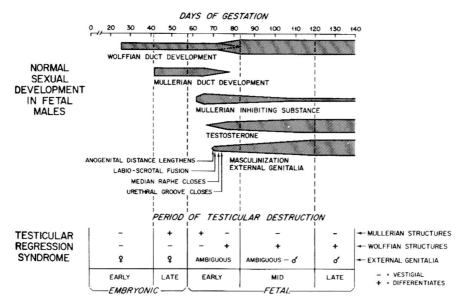

Fig. 36.1 Normal sexual development in the male and application in testicular regression syndrome. (Reprinted from Welch & Robboy 1981, with kind permission of Kluwer Academic Publishers.)

During the development of both male and female human embryos, the primordial germ cells, characterised by large clear cells with vesicular nuclei, migrate from the yolk sac to the urogenital ridges via the hindgut approximately three weeks after fertilisation. The mesodermal epithelium on the medial surface of the urogenital ridge begins to proliferate, resulting in the epithelium of the eventual gonad, while the gonads themselves begin to differentiate. In males, the testis is anatomically distinct with early tubular formation and immature Sertoli cells by day 44. In females, ovarian differentiation, characterised by the development of primordial follicles, begins some five weeks later. The initial stages of both testicular and ovarian development appear independent of whether the primordial germ cells are present or absent in the gonad or have proliferated normally.

Once the male pathway of development has begun, two hormones produced by the fetal testis then control the differentiation of the male phenotype. The first is MIS, a large glycoprotein that Sertoli cells produce early in fetal life (Rey & Josso 1996; Josso et al 1998). The gene responsible for this substance is on chromosome 19 (Lane & Donahoe 1998). MIS is also known as anti-Müllerian hormone (AMH). The primary function of MIS is to cause regression of the Müllerian (paramesonephric) ducts in the male fetus.

MIS is first secreted in effective amounts 56 to 62 days after fertilisation, and the process of Müllerian regression is normally completed by about day 77, after which the Müllerian tissue is no longer sensitive to MIS. During this critical period, even relatively small amounts of MIS given over a short period of time can be effective in

causing irreversible damage to the embryonic Müllerian tract (Hunter 1995b). In the female, MIS is produced in insignificant amounts during fetal life (as there are no Sertoli cells) and the Müllerian ducts develop passively to form the Fallopian tubes, uterus and vaginal wall. Other functions of MIS, secreted later in fetal life, are discussed below.

MIS has a local action, and inhibits development of the ipsilateral Fallopian tube. To prevent development of both the uterus and vagina, both testes must secrete adequate amounts of MIS. Thus, a patient with a testis and a contralateral streak, ovary or ovotestis generally has a uterus and vagina and a single Fallopian tube on the side with the streak or ovary.

Additional functions of MIS have recently been discovered. In the female, ovarian granulosa cells begin producing MIS only after the Müllerian-derived tissues (Fallopian tubes, uterus and vagina) are well developed and no longer susceptible to the regressive effects of MIS. Serum levels of MIS in girls rise slowly after birth from nearly undetectable levels until they reach a plateau after 10 years of life equivalent to the adult male serum concentration. In contrast, the male serum MIS concentration is relatively high at birth, peaks at 4–12 months of age, and then falls progressively to a baseline low adult level by about 10 years of age. A major action of MIS in the young female may be to inhibit oocyte meiosis in the developing follicle. Dramatically high levels of MIS have been found in women with ovarian sex cord tumours, thus serving potentially as a diagnostic marker or method to evaluate the effectiveness of therapy (Lane & Lee 1999). Another important action of MIS in males may be to initiate testicular descent, principally by its postulated regulatory control over the gubernaculum testis (Clarnette et al 1997).

The second hormone the fetal testis secretes is testosterone. This androgenic steroid, which is critical for male development, is required for the Wolffian (mesonephric) duct to differentiate into epididymis, vas deferens and seminal vesicle. Leydig cells appear in the testis circa day 54–64 and shortly thereafter begin to produce testosterone. Leydig cell activity is probably stimulated by increased production of chorionic gonadotrophin by the placenta at that time. Testosterone acts locally on the ipsilateral Wolffian duct by binding to a specific high affinity intracellular receptor protein. This receptor hormone complex binds DNA to regulate transcription of specific genes which govern further development. In the absence of a testis or inability of a testis to produce testosterone in adequate amounts by 10–12 weeks, or insensitivity of the Wolffian duct anlage to testosterone, the epididymis, vas deferens and seminal vesicle do not differentiate. Only rarely are abnormally elevated testosterone levels reached sufficiently early during embryogenesis in a female fetus to cause the Wolffian duct to differentiate into definitive male organs (androgen administration to the mother during pregnancy, or congenital adrenogenital syndrome).

Testosterone also acts as a prohormone for dihydrotestosterone, the substance ultimately responsible for initiating masculinisation of the external genitalia and differentiation of the prostate. The enzyme 5α-reductase, found in the tissues of the external genitalia and urogenital sinus, mediates the conversion of testosterone to dihydrotestosterone. Dihydrotestosterone causes:

1. the genital tubercle to enlarge and form the glans penis
2. the genital folds to enlarge and fuse to form the penile shaft with migration of the urethral orifice along the lower border of the shaft to the tip of the glans
3. the genital swellings to fuse and form a scrotum
4. the urogenital sinus tissues to differentiate into prostate.

Failure of the external genitalia to develop in males in the presence of testes may be due to a lack of adequate testosterone secretion into the systemic circulation, deficient enzyme (5α-reductase) at the end-organ level to convert testosterone to dihydrotestosterone, or complete end-organ insensitivity (testicular feminisation). Lesser degrees of deficiency or end-organ insensitivity may result in partial male development characterised by a small penis, hypospadias, deficient formation of the scrotum, or a persistent urogenital sinus (vaginal opening into urethra). The effects of dihydrotestosterone begin about day 70, with fusion of the labioscrotal folds and closure of the median raphe, and continue at day 74 with closure of the urethral groove. External genital development is complete by day 120–140 (18th–20th week).

Finally, female internal organs and external genitalia develop in the absence of hormones secreted by the fetal ovary, and differentiate even when gonads are absent. Unless interrupted by the regressive influence of Müllerian inhibiting substance, differentiation of the Müllerian ducts proceeds cephalocaudally to form Fallopian tubes, a uterus and a vagina. In the absence of the masculinising effect of dihydrotestosterone, the undifferentiated external genital anlage develops into the vulva. The genital tubercle develops into the clitoris, the genital folds into the labia minora, and the genital swellings into the labia majora. Thus, the infant with ovaries or streak gonads has female internal and external genitalia at birth. Only if a female fetus has systemically elevated levels of androgens prior to the 10th–12th week of gestation does any degree of internal male development occur. In such cases the external genitalia may appear ambiguous or may resemble those of a normal phenotypic male; the vagina in these instances opens into the membranous portion of the urethra. If the androgens are not elevated until after the 20th week, by which time the external genitalia have fully formed, the only virilising effect is an enlarged clitoris.

GENDER IDENTIFICATION DISORDERS WITH A NORMAL CHROMOSOME CONSTITUTION

FEMALE PSEUDOHERMAPHRODITISM (FEMALE INTERSEX)

Female pseudohermaphroditism occurs as a result of relative androgen excess in utero in an individual with two ovaries and two X chromosomes (46,XX). The elevated level of androgen present during embryogenesis usually results in genital ambiguity and may result in the appearance of a phenotypic male.

Fetal defects

Adrenogenital syndrome

Congenital adrenal hyperplasia, unlike all other conditions responsible for the appearance of ambiguous genitalia in the newborn, may be life threatening because of a lack of synthesis of specific adrenal steroids. Prompt diagnosis and institution of appropriate therapy are therefore essential. With early treatment normal external genitalia and fertility can be achieved. The manifestations of the adrenogenital syndrome in the XX individual are most easily summarised through an understanding of the biosynthetic pathways of mineralocorticoid, glucocorticoid, and sex steroids (Fig. 36.2) (New & Newfield 1997; Newfield & New 1997; New 1998; Carlson et al 1999). Two enzymes, 21-hydroxylase and 11-beta-hydroxylase, participate in the formation of the glucocorticoids, des-

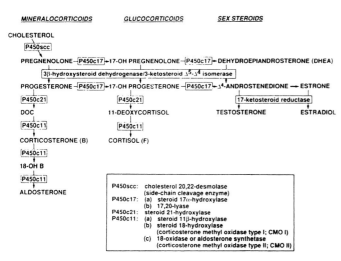

Fig. 36.2 Biosynthesis of mineralocorticoids, glucocorticoids and sex steroids. (Modified from New 1998, with kind permission of Annual Review publishers.)

oxycorticosterone (DOC) and cortisol (F), and the mineralocorticoid, aldosterone, but neither in testosterone nor the oestrogens, oestrone (E) or oestradiol (E_2). Deficiency of either enzyme in the 46,XX female leads to elevated ACTH products and hence elevated levels of testosterone and other strongly androgenic intermediates, which may result in sexual ambiguity or marked virilisation of the newborn's external genitalia (Ferrari et al 1996; Cerame et al 1999). 3β-hydroxysteroid dehydrogenase is required for testosterone formation. In its absence, the principal androgen to form is the weak androgen, dehydroepiandrosterone (DHEA), which has one-twentieth the potency of testosterone. Patients with deficiency of this enzyme, therefore, show only signs of mild virilisation, usually clitoral hypertrophy but with no labial fusion or anterior displacement of the urethral orifice (Mendonca et al 1999).

21-hydroxylase deficiency is inherited as an autosomal recessive trait caused by an abnormal gene on chromosome 6 that encodes for cytochrome P450c21 (i.e. *CYP21*). It accounts for more than 95% of cases of congenital adrenal hyperplasia, occurring once in 15 000 births. It is high especially in Ashkenazi Jews (1:27 live births). The genetic aberrations responsible for expression of the disease are complicated. This gene exists in tandem with a pseudogene, CYP21P, which is believed to be non-transcribable as it contains a high number of documented mutations (Moran et al 1998). The clinical manifestations depend upon the absence of the single active gene (*CYP21*, formerly called CYP21B) that actively expresses the 21-hydroxylase enzyme, or of the rearrangements, deletions or point mutations transferred from the pseudogene present (Ludwig et al 1998; Moran et al 1998; Carlson et al 1999). Approximately a fourth of cases of classical congenital adrenogenital syndrome are due to deletion of the *CYP21* gene. The remainder are due to

non-deleted mutant gene sequences that have been transferred from the pseudogene, rendering the active gene non-functional (Carlson et al 1999). If the allele carries a defect encoding for a mild defect, then the child will develop a non-classical form of adrenal hyperplasia, which by definition occurs after birth and is never associated with genital ambiguity (Moran et al 1998). This latter syndrome is common, occurring in 1% of all women, and is thought to be a major cause of adult-onset virilism.

In the congenital form of the adrenogenital syndrome, the extent of virilisation depends upon which time during fetal life the disease began. If the onset begins after the 16th week of gestation, the clitoris may be enlarged; if androgen excess occurs earlier, the vagina and urethra may open into a common urogenital sinus. More marked clitoral enlargement and an opening of the urogenital sinus at the clitoral base may mimic penile hypospadias and suggest an even earlier temporal effect. On occasion, the changes have been of such severity that the female infants have been misdiagnosed as cryptorchid males with or without hypospadias.

Tumour development in genetic females with this condition is rare. In one unusual case, prostatic adenocarcinoma developed with osteoblastic skeletal metastases. Presumably, the initial development of the prostate itself was based on excessive testosterone formation during embryogenesis, which itself was reflective of 21-hydroxy-

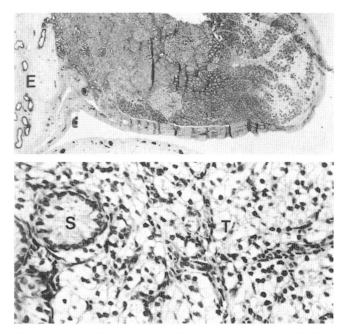

Fig. 36.3 Interstitial cell tumour of the testis in a 4-year-old infant with adrenogenital syndrome. The tumour cells (T), which are illustrated at high magnification adjacent to immature seminiferous tubules (S) in the inset, resemble adrenocortical cells more closely than Leydig cells. The epididymis (E) is adjacent to the testis. (Reprinted from Welch & Robboy 1981, with kind permission of Kluwer Academic Publishers.)

lase deficiency (Winters et al 1996). In addition, the patient subsequently developed clear cell carcinoma of the endometrium.

Males who have the adrenogenital syndrome show no evidence of genital ambiguity, but may have an enlarged phallus and a hyperpigmented rugated scrotum. Clinically detectable bilateral testicular nodules that are composed of interstitial cells resembling Leydig cells or cells of adrenal rest origin occasionally develop during childhood or young adulthood and must be distinguished from true Leydig cell tumors (Fig. 36.3) (Rich et al 1998). Bilaterality and decreasing tumour size after corticosteroid therapy are features indicative that the testicular 'tumour' of the adrenogenital syndrome is hyperplastic rather than neoplastic (Rutgers et al 1988). Screening examinations with ultrasonography and magnetic resonance imaging have shown that intratesticular masses are far more common than expected, being present in 40% of affected males (Avila et al 1999).

Placental aromatase defect

Placental aromatase deficiency is a rare cause of maternal virilisation during pregnancy and pseudohermaphroditism of the female fetus (Shozu et al 1991; MacGillivray et al 1998). Mutations in the aromatase gene, CYP19, which causes abnormally low conversion of androstenedione to 17 beta-oestradiol and estrone, result in virilisation of the mother and her female fetus because of the accumulation of potent androgens that are not converted to oestrogens. The mothers usually show the onset of progressive virilisation during the third trimester. The male fetus has normal genitalia.

Maternal influence

Maternal ingestion of progestins or androgens

Maternal ingestion of synthetic progestins was implicated as a cause of female pseudohermaphroditism in the late 1950s when such treatment was employed for threatened or habitual miscarriage; subsequently, progestins have also been implicated in the development of hypospadias in male offspring. Most cases of female pseudohermaphroditism in this category developed after maternal ingestion of Ethisterone (17α-ethinyl-testosterone) or Norlution (17α-ethinyl-19-nortestosterone), but occasionally after the ingestion of Enovid, diethylstilboestrol, androgens, or after the intramuscular administration of progesterone. Masculinisation usually consists of phallic enlargement and variable degrees of labioscrotal fusion, depending on the time during gestation when the therapy was administered. Although the degree of masculinisation is usually less than that associated with the adrenogenital syndrome, the sexual ambiguity in female infants has been of such severity in some instances as to result in

male sex assignment. The degree of virilisation does not progress with age. The gonads and internal genital organs are unaffected, and ovulation, menstruation and normal secondary female characteristics appear at puberty.

Maternal virilising tumours

A variety of benign and malignant tumours, primary as well as metastatic to the ovary have been associated with virilisation of the mother and her female offspring (Fung et al 1991; Vauthier-Brouzes et al 1997). The luteoma of pregnancy and the probably related hyperreactio luteinalis, are the most common lesions that cause maternal virilisation during pregnancy (Vanslooten et al 1992). The pregnancy luteoma is a benign hyperplastic lesion of the ovary that is most often encountered as an incidental finding at the time of Caesarean section or postpartum sterilisation, usually in women who are multiparous. Elevated levels of hCG are thought to induce hyperplasia of theca-lutein or stroma-lutein cells. A small percentage of the female infants have become masculinised, with mild enlargement of the clitoris and occasionally minimal degrees of labioscrotal fusion or rugate, hyperpigmented ('scrotal') labia. The nature of these changes indicates that the ovarian nodules do not function until the second half of gestation, which is in accord with the occasional onset of masculinisation in the mother during the third trimester.

At operation, one and often both maternal ovaries are enlarged by one or more soft, yellow–brown nodules that are well circumscribed but not encapsulated. Although most are less than 2 cm in diameter, they may be as large as 20 cm in greatest dimension. On microscopical examination, the nodules consist of large, polygonal cells with granular, eosinophilic cytoplasm, which are smaller and more eosinophilic than the luteinized granulosa cells of the corpus luteum but larger than the theca-lutein cells. Intracellular lipid is sparse, if at all present. Mitoses may be observed, but only rarely are they numerous.

Elevated plasma and tissue levels of testosterone, dihydrotestosterone, androstenedione and DHEA have been detected in virilised patients; the plasma levels return to normal once the tumour is extirpated. Even without treatment, the nodules regress and disappear shortly after delivery. Rarely, a functional luteoma may reoccur during a subsequent pregnancy. Other primary functioning tumours of the ovary that may lead to virilisation of the female offspring as well as metastatic tumours to the ovary that induce the stroma to function during pregnancy are discussed elsewhere in this book.

MALE PSEUDOHERMAPHRODITISM (MALE INTERSEX)

Male pseudohermaphroditism defines a heterogeneous group of intersex conditions which are characterised by an intrauterine state of relative functional androgen deficiency, an apparently normal 46,XY karyotype and either identifiable testes or evidence that testes were present during fetal development. The external genitalia are usually female or ambiguous, although in certain categories (e.g. testicular regression syndrome) they may appear as phenotypically male. The responsible defect may be in the gonad, leading to deficiency in androgens, Müllerian inhibiting substance, or both. Alternatively, end organ defects in which developing tissues are unresponsive to androgens or Müllerian inhibiting substance may lead to the abnormal phenotype.

Primary gonadal defects

A primary defect of the gonad in an XY karyotype individual may lead to male pseudohermaphroditism by any one of the following mechanisms: regression (destruction) of the gonads or their anlage during intrauterine life, agenesis of the Leydig cells, a specific enzymatic defect in testosterone synthesis, dihydrotestosterone synthesis or receptors to these hormones, or a defect in elaboration or action of Müllerian inhibiting substance.

Testicular regression syndrome

Testicular regression follows the irreparable destruction of the testes at a critical stage of fetal development in an XY individual. The phenotype of the affected individual reflects the specific stage of fetal development during which the testes were damaged. In general, gonadal regression that occurs during embryonic life, prior to the elaboration of Müllerian inhibiting substance and/or androgenic steroids by the testes, leads to a female phenotype. Regression of the testes during late embryonic through mid-fetal life permits a masculine phenotype (Fig. 36.1). The testicular regression syndrome has a variety of aetiologies, some possibly as diverse as inherited genetic defect, intrauterine infection, or infarction. The heterogeneity of presentation of this syndrome and its relative rarity have led to numerous and sometimes confusing terms for this disorder, including: true agonadism, testicular dysgenesis, rudimentary testis, vanishing testis, and complete bilateral anorchia. The terms pure gonadal dysgenesis and Swyer's syndrome have been used for the testicular regression syndrome by some authors. We avoid these terms so as not to confuse them with other conditions similarly named and discussed below.

At one end of the spectrum of the testicular regression syndrome, the internal genitalia and gonads are absent and the external genitalia are female (Rattanachaiyanont et al 1999). Presumably, the urogenital ridge was destroyed in its entirety during early embryonic life, even before the Müllerian ducts began to differentiate (prior to day 42).

At the other end of the spectrum, which approximates to the end point of normal genital development, the patients are phenotypic males with infantile to nearly normal male external genitalia, normally differentiated Wolffian duct structures and completely inhibited Müllerian duct development. Often in these cases no genital tissue is identified. However, there is sometimes a focus of vascularised fibrosis (85%), haemorrhage or haemosiderin deposition (70%), calcification (60%) or giant cells at the expected site of the gonad, which is near the residual vas deferens or epididymis (Merry et al 1997; Cendron et al 1998; Spires 1999). Occasionally, atrophic seminiferous tubules may be found amidst a fibrous stroma. Testicular regression presumably occurred during the late fetal period (after 120 days) when Müllerian structures had already atrophied under the influence of Müllerian inhibiting substance and testosterone and dihydrotestosterone had exerted a major influence on the normal development of internal and external genitalia. Torsion and infarction of improperly descended testes has been suggested (Smith et al 1991).

Intermediate in the spectrum of these disorders are patients with ambiguous genitalia and various combinations of Wolffian and/or Müllerian duct development. Testes that regressed during the late embryonic period (day 43–59) will have secreted insufficient testosterone to affect the Wolffian duct. The production of Müllerian inhibiting substance will have been variable, resulting in poorly differentiated or rudimentary Müllerian structures (incomplete inhibition). In the absence of systemic androgens, the external genitalia appear female.

Regression of the testes during the early fetal period (day 59–84) after Sertoli cell Müllerian inhibiting substance and Leydig cell (testosterone) function have begun or are about to begin results in an individual with ambiguous external genitalia and various combinations of Wolffian and Müllerian development depending on the duration of androgen secretion and Müllerian inhibition.

Regression of the testes during the mid-fetal period (day 84–120) results in more advanced masculinisation of the external genitalia, although degrees of ambiguity are usually present. Since Müllerian duct inhibition is normally completed by day 80, the Müllerian structures will have been suppressed and Wolffian structures are developed.

Leydig cell agenesis

Leydig cell agenesis is a very rare cause of male pseudohermaphroditism (Arnhold et al 1999). Affected individuals have a 46,XY karyotype and testes with interstitial fibrosis, but no mature Leydig cells. Tubules with Sertoli cells and, sometimes, immature spermatogonia are found. The Müllerian structures are absent, indicating appropriate testicular production of Müllerian inhibiting substance during fetal life. The Wolffian duct system is either partially or fully developed so that identifiable vasa deferentia and epididymides are present. The phenotype varies and is usually female with unremarkable or ambiguous external genitalia, although unambiguous males with evidence of primary hypogonadism have been reported. The presence of Wolffian duct development, and the variable degrees of masculinisation of the external genitalia indicate that some Leydig cells must have differentiated and functioned during early fetal life. Luteinizing hormone levels are elevated in affected individuals. The underlying defect in this disorder is believed to be an absence or defect of the LH-hCG receptor on the Leydig cell or some other, unknown, factor arresting Leydig cell development.

Defects in testosterone synthesis

Congenital deficiency of any enzyme involved in the production of testosterone in the testis or adrenal gland results in a state of androgen deficiency (relative oestrogen excess) (Fig. 36.2). The histological appearance of the testicular tissue is variable. It has been described occasionally as 'normal', but the photomicrographs in some reports have disclosed large clusters of Leydig cells surrounding tubules lined only by Sertoli cells. Spermatogonia are often normal in children, but disappear by puberty (Bale et al 1992). In general, the number of gonads studied for any of the conditions and the range of ages studied (infancy, childhood, adulthood) has been limited. Müllerian structures are absent, but Wolffian duct structures may be present. The degree to which the external genitalia develop depends upon the type and severity of the defect.

Congenital lipoid adrenal hyperplasia

Congenital lipoid adrenal hyperplasia (lipoid CAH), the most severe form of CAH, results from mutations in the steroidogenic acute regulatory (StAR) gene (Korsch et al 1999). This state of hypergonadotropic hypogonadism shows markedly elevated levels of gonadotropic hormones (LH, FSH, ACTH), but markedly impaired synthesis of all gonadal and adrenal cortical steroids, even with trophic stimulation tests. The patients, who have a 46,XY karyotype, are born as phenotypically normal females, but may have a palpable gonad in the inguinal canal. In keeping with the disease affecting the most basic steps in conversion of cholesterol esters into steroids, florid lipid deposits are found in the fetal adrenal cortex.

Few reports describe the testicular findings. Generally, the seminiferous tubules show changes consistent with the age of the patient. Occasional Leydig cells are present. The germ cells may disappear over time resulting in a Sertoli-only syndrome, although this is not inevitable. Germ cells can persist and rarely develop into intratubular germ cell neoplasia (Korsch et al 1999).

Congenital adrenal hyperplasia

Several inherited enzymatic defects involve both the synthesis of adrenal mineralocorticoid and glucocorticoid hormones as well as adrenal and testicular sex hormones. Due to these genetic defects, one or more adrenal cortical enzymes fail to be synthesised or are defective (New 1998). The most severe defect, which involves the conversion of cholesterol intermediates to pregnenolone (20,22-desmolase), almost always ends lethally from a salt-wasting crisis if untreated during infancy. Although the external genitalia in the male are ambiguous or female, sufficient testosterone must be secreted during embryogenesis since the internal genitalia are male. The testes in the infant disclose immature seminiferous tubules with spermatogonia. The germ cells disappear by several years of age.

A deficiency of 3β-hydroxylase dehydrogenase, like a 20,22-desmolase deficiency, results in decreased synthesis of mineralocorticoid and glucocorticoid hormones as well as adrenal and testicular sex hormones, and may lead to life-threatening salt wasting in infancy. DHEA, which is a weak androgen secreted in high amounts, results in slight clitoral enlargement in the female, but rarely completely masculinises the external genitalia in males. Hence, the male may be born with ambiguous genitalia and may resemble a virilised female. Males in whom the defect is partial may be born with hypospadias, but at puberty develop gynaecomastia. The testes in older boys generally are immature, exhibiting seminiferous tubules with spermatogenic arrest and diminished numbers of Leydig cells.

In contrast to the early age of diagnosis in the above two syndromes, the diagnosis in most patients with 17α-hydroxylase deficiency is not suspected until the anticipated time of puberty or later. Detailed steroid analysis of the urine of newborn males presenting with ambiguous genitalia indicates that the correct diagnosis can be made in the young.

Deficiencies of two enzymes, 17,20-desmolase and 17-hydroxysteroid dehydrogenase (17-ketosteroid reductase), result in deficient testosterone synthesis but do not affect the production of either mineralocorticoids or glucocorticoids. The former defect (conversion of 17-hydroxypregnenolone to DHEA) is extremely rare. The patients reported presented with ambiguous external genitalia and inguinal or intra-abdominal testes. Spermatogonia were present in the testis of infants but were absent in the biopsies of their older teenage relatives. All had third-degree hypospadias, but normal male internal ductal differentiation. Genetic males with 17-β-hydroxysteroid dehydrogenase (17β-HSD) deficiency have uniformly been raised as females and have unambiguous female external genitalia. Most are diagnosed at or after puberty when they fail to menstruate and instead show signs of virilisation such as clitoromegaly (enlarged phallus) and hirsutism (Zhu et al 1998). Breast development may or may not take place. At surgery, Müllerian duct derivatives are absent, consistent with normal anti-Müllerian hormone action. Wolffian duct differentiation, indicative of testosterone secretion during embryogenesis, is normal (Andersson & Moghrabi 1997). The testes present in the inguinal canal or labia majora, contain rare to no spermatogonia and may exhibit numerous Leydig cells. Detailed endocrine studies have shown that testicular 17β-HSD is under different genetic control to that in extragonadal tissues, and while affected males lack testicular 17β-HSD, the extragonadal activity is normal or enhanced. More than 15 mutations have been identified in the responsible gene (Andersson & Moghrabi 1997; Bilbao et al 1998; Mendonca et al 1999).

Defect in Müllerian inhibiting system

The persistent Müllerian duct syndrome, also known as 'hernia uteri inguinalis' is a rare form of male pseudohermaphroditism characterised by the presence of Müllerian duct structures in 46,XY phenotypic males. These patients usually present when young with unilateral or bilateral cryptorchid testes, normal or almost normal male external genitalia and an inguinal hernia into which prolapses an infantile uterus and Fallopian tubes (Lima et al 1997; Buchholz et al 1998; Rizk et al 1998). Some patients may be older (Erk et al 1999). The testes are histologically normal, Wolffian duct structures are developed, the pubertal development is normal and a rare patient has been fertile. Treatment is surgical, consisting of orchiopexy and herniorrhaphy with hysterectomy and bilateral salpingectomy. If at operation any patient has a streak gonad or a tumour rather than bilateral testes, the diagnosis of mixed gonadal dysgenesis should be considered. In most cases of persistent Müllerian duct syndrome, the vas deferens is tightly adherent to the residual uterus or upper vagina and in some cases the Müllerian structures must be left intact to preserve the vas. Malignant testicular tumours have been reported in the very rare cases of adult patients with persistent Müllerian duct syndrome and uncorrected cryptorchid testes. The persistent Müllerian duct syndrome currently seems to be a heterogeneous group of disorders, caused by different defects in the Müllerian inhibiting system. Familial cases have been reported. Mutations in the MIS gene are responsible for at least half of the cases with persistent Müllerian ducts. The remainder appear due to mutations in the receptor for the gene products (Imbeaud et al 1996). Several rare types of receptor alterations have been described (Faure et al 1996). The effect of these abnormalities is that some patients produce no biologically functional MIS, whereas the others that produce normal amounts of biologically active MIS have end-organ insensitivity to MIS or an abnormality of the timing of MIS secretion. A model for MIS receptor signaling has been proposed and illustrated elsewhere (Lane & Donahoe 1998).

End-organ defects

The normal development of the Wolffian duct derivatives and the external genitalia requires that these structures be responsive to androgen and that the enzyme, 5α-reductase, be present in the anlage of the prostate and external genitalia to convert testosterone to dihydrotestosterone (DHT). A molecular defect of the androgen receptor system (e.g. unstable androgen receptor or lack of androgen receptor) leads to impaired development of both Wolffian duct structures and external genitalia in 46,XY individuals. If only 5α-reductase is absent or defective, the abnormalities in the reproductive tract are confined to the external genitalia and prostate.

Androgen receptor disorders (androgen insensitivity syndromes)

Disorders of androgen receptor function result in a variety of phenotypes ranging from phenotypic women with intra-abdominal testes to individuals with ambiguous genitalia to phenotypic men with minimal clinical abnormalities. In one classification scheme (McPhaul & Griffin 1999), four categories exist and are in order of increasing virilisation (decreasing feminisation): complete and incomplete testicular feminisation, Reifenstein phenotype, and undervirilised and/or infertile male. All share an X-linked recessive inheritance, the result of a defect in the androgen receptor gene, which has been localised to the long arm of the X chromosome. A variety of different mutations of this gene have been characterised (Quigley et al 1995; Dork et al 1998; Hiort et al 1998; Radmayr et al 1998), many of which are limited to individual families (Kanayama et al 1999). These mutations may lead to functional absence of the androgen receptor because the primary sequences of the gene are affected. These patients generally present as complete testicular feminisation. The more common defect is caused by single amino acid substitutions and is associated with the various other forms of the disease as described below. Rare patients have also been described where the androgen receptor disorder has occurred in combination with other unusual karyotypes; e.g 47,XXY (Uehara et al 1999b) and 47,XYY (Naguib et al 1997).

Complete testicular feminisation. Complete testicular feminisation is the most common form of male pseudohermaphroditism. The external genitalia are phenotypically female and, for this reason, the condition is rarely diagnosed before puberty unless an inguinal hernia or labial mass is encountered or unless the disease is known to be familial (Alvarez-Nava et al 1997; Viner et al 1997). Primary amenorrhoea is the most common complaint leading to evaluation and subsequent diagnosis. The medical history usually reveals that breast development occurred as expected at puberty. Pubic and axillary hair are scant, the vagina is shortened, and the epididymides, vasa deferentia, seminal vesicles and prostate are absent. As a rule, both the cervix and the body of the uterine corpus are absent. A fragment of Fallopian tube may be found in up to one-third of cases (Rutgers & Scully 1991). The testes are cryptorchid and may be located in the inguinal canal, the pelvis or rarely the labia. In the complete or almost complete form of the syndrome, the individual exhibits a truly female consciousness gender identity with normal extragenital erotogenic sensitivity and a normal maternal attitude.

The gonads in infants and young children are relatively normal but by age 5 years they show abnormalities. By young adulthood, the gonad is often involved with benign or malignant tumours as described below. If tumours are not present by this age, the gonad is usually small and on section is tan to brown and traversed by thin white bands. A 1–2 cm firm, white nodule of hyalinised smooth muscle is usually present at one pole of the testis. Theories regarding what this nodule might represent include an abnormally hypertrophied gubernaculum or rudimentary uterine structure. Microscopical examination of the testicular parenchyma discloses immature seminiferous tubules usually sparsely distributed or clustered in small aggregates. Spermatogonia may be present, but spermatogenesis is absent. The number of spermatogonia that are

found is age dependent, diminishing as the patient ages. The interstitium is usually abundant and often resembles ovarian stroma (Fig. 36.4). Fetal-type Leydig cells may be abundant. The findings indicate that Leydig cells are active hormone producers. The Leydig cells in individuals with testicular feminisation have an ultrastructure typical of cells involved in active hormone synthesis, and the systemic androgen levels in these individuals are characteristically elevated. These findings indicate that the pathological defect in the testicular feminisation syndrome is an end-organ defect and not lack of hormone production by the testes.

Most testes of affected individuals contain multiple benign nodules that are discrete, firm, yellow to brown and bulge above the sectioned surface (Fig. 36.4). Hamartomatous nodules have been present, usually bilaterally, in virtually every case the authors have personally examined. The typical size varies from 1 mm to 1 cm, but occasionally up to 4 cm (Rutgers & Scully 1991). The bulk of the nodule is usually composed of seminiferous tubules lacking lumina; spermatogonia may be present. The seminiferous tubules that have a diffuse distribution and are located outside the nodules have a lamina propria that is of normal thickness in prepubertal testes, but thickened and hyalinised in the adult (Regadera et al 1999).

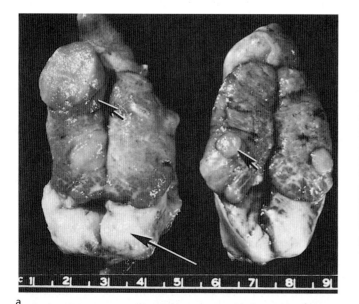

a

b

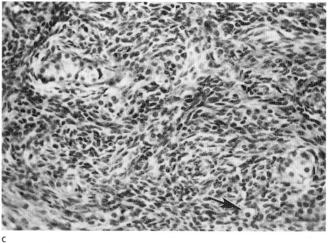

c

Fig. 36.4 a Testis in a 17-year-old with the complete form of androgen insensitivity (testicular feminisation) syndrome. Numerous Sertoli cell adenomas (short arrows) are present in the parenchyma. The mass near one pole (long arrow) may represent an abnormally hypertrophied gubernaculum. **b** Hamartoma with immature seminiferous tubules (s), numerous germ cells (g), and numerous Leydig cells (l) in the interstitium. **c** Contralateral testis with scattered immature seminiferous tubules embedded in a dense ovarian-type cortical stroma. Occasional interstitial cells (arrows) are present. (Reprinted from Welch & Robboy 1981, with kind permission of Kluwer Academic Publishers.)

Sertoli cell adenomas are hamartomas composed predominantly or exclusively of closely packed immature seminiferous tubules lacking lumina and lined by immature, uniform Sertoli cells (Rutgers & Scully, 1991; Hawkyard et al 1999). The adenomas average 3 cm in diameter, ranging up to 25 cm.

The interstitium in the testes of affected patients often resembles ovarian stroma, and frequently contains Leydig cells. On rare occasions, Leydig cell nodules form, and have been considered benign tumours. In summary, the name applied to each type of nodule is somewhat arbitrary and depends largely upon the types of components present as well as their number and size. Most nodules are classified as hamartomas, Sertoli cell adenomas or, rarely, as Leydig cell tumours.

Malignant gonadal tumours develop with increasing frequency with age in patients with testicular feminisation. Seminoma is the most commonly encountered gonadal malignancy in this syndrome. Intratubular germ cell neoplasia is sometimes seen, either independently or in association with seminoma. Other malignant germ cell tumours and malignant sex-cord tumours are also rarely encountered. One malignant sex cord–stromal tumor that was oestrogen secreting has been reported (McNeill et al 1997). Unlike mixed gonadal dysgenesis, in which tumours develop in young individuals, the risk of malignancy in patients with testicular feminisation is only 4% by the age of 25 years, but reaches 33% by 50 years. Since malignant tumours rarely develop before completion of puberty, castration can usually be delayed until after adolescence, thus permitting the patient to undergo a normal pubertal spurt and develop female secondary sex characteristics.

Incomplete testicular feminisation. About 10% of patients with an androgen insensitivity syndrome have incomplete testicular feminisation. The clinical manifestations vary depending on the classification system used. If restricted, it resembles complete testicular feminisation except that there is partial fusion of the labioscrotal folds and usually some clitoromegaly at birth. If inclusive of all forms of the androgen insensitivity syndrome that are not considered *complete* testicular feminisation, then greater percentages of patients will look and be raised as males (Hiort et al 1996; Viner et al 1997). As in the complete form, underdeveloped Wolffian duct derivatives are often present. If the diagnosis is established during childhood, gonadectomy should be performed before puberty, since disfiguring virilisation may accompany breast development at puberty. Estrogen therapy should be given at the appropriate time to initiate feminisation. The pathological findings are similar to those described for the complete form of testicular feminization (Regadera et al 1999).

Other forms. Reifenstein's syndrome, infertile male syndrome, and undervirilised male syndrome are other forms of incomplete androgen insensitivity in which the phenotype is male. There are few reports describing the microscopic findings of the gonads.

Men with Reifenstein's syndrome usually present with gynaecomastia and severe hypospadias, and children or teenagers with perineoscrotal hypospadias. However, the phenotypic spectrum is wide, even within the same affected family with a single androgen receptor abnormality in all affected family members. The usual abnormalities include: hypospadias, breast development at puberty, female habitus, azoospermia, cryptorchidism, and hypoplasia or absence of Wolffian duct structures. The 'infertile male syndrome' is a rare androgen receptor defect characterised by a phenotypically normal man with infertility caused by azoospermia. Finally, in the 'undervirilised male syndrome' the individual is a male with gynaecomastia, a small penis, decreased beard and body hair, a normal male urethra, a normal sperm density and an identifiable androgen receptor defect. The majority of affected individuals are infertile.

Disordered testosterone metabolism

5 α-reductase 2 deficiency

Deficiency of the enzyme 5-α-reductase 2 impairs the conversion of testosterone to DHT, the hormone that masculinises the indifferent urogenital sinus and induces development of the prostate (Mendonca et al 1996; Imperato-McGinley 1997). The disorder, formerly known as 'pseudovaginal perineoscrotal hypospadias', has an autosomal recessive inheritance and is rare. As in other forms of pseudohermaphroditism, some of the abnormality relates to mutations identified in the gene structure (Anwar et al 1997; Ferraz et al 1999). The majority of reported cases have come from family clusters found in a number of relatively isolated geographical locations (Al-Attia 1997). Affected males typically are phenotypically female with female to ambiguous external genitalia at birth (Sinnecker et al 1996). The small clitoris-like phallus lacks a urethral orifice. In most affected individuals the urogenital sinus opens on the perineum and within the sinus an anterior orifice leads to the urethra and a posterior orifice to a blind vaginal pouch. The testes are in the inguinal canals or labia. The Müllerian-derived structures are absent whereas Wolffian-derived structures (vas deferens, epididymis and seminal vesicle), the anlage of which respond to testosterone, are normal.

At puberty, virilisation occurs and the breasts fail to develop. The penis lengthens, the bifid scrotum grows, becomes rugated and hyperpigmented, and the testes enlarge and descend. Testicular biopsy specimens reveal spermatogenesis and tubular atrophy in some individuals, complete spermatogenic arrest and Leydig cell hyperplasia in others. The prostate fails to develop and remains impalpable. Erection, ejaculation and orgasm are possible in some affected individuals; these individuals are not, however, fertile.

Neonates with this disorder frequently go unrecognised and are raised as females. After the virilisation that accompanies puberty, individuals raised as girls sometimes reverse their sex rôles and function as men, often with a stormy period of adjustment. Interestingly, the syndrome was known in New Guinea as 'penis at 12' where a familial clustering of the disorder was predictably seen among a group of pubescent children. Individuals with a male gender identity benefit from surgical correction of hypospadias and cryptorchidism. High doses of testosterone enhance virilisation. Persons raised as females who elect to continue to function as females into adulthood benefit from orchiectomy prior to the onset of puberty to avoid the accompanying virilisation. Oestrogen therapy is useful to promote feminisation. One patient has been described who developed a squamous cell carcinoma of the vagina at age 50 years (Aartsen et al 1994).

Defect uncertain

Smith–Lemli–Opitz syndrome

The Smith–Lemli–Opitz syndrome, inherited as an autosomal recessive trait, shows ambiguous genitalia, mental retardation, small stature, anteverted nostrils, ptosis, holoprosencephaly and syndactyly of the second and third toes. The pathogenesis of the ambiguous genitalia reported in some 46,XY patients as well as the morphogenic abnormalities described in general is uncertain, although the syndrome results from an enzymatic defect in the last step of cholesterol metabolism (reduction of 7-dehydrocholesterol due to mutations in the 7-dehydrocholesterol reductase gene) (Fitzky et al 1999; Nowaczyk et al 1999; Optiz 1999). Studies of testicular function both in vivo and in vitro in a 46,XY patient with ambiguous genitalia and raised as a girl suggested that the fetal testes might have failed to respond to placental hCG at the time of male external genital differentiation (Berensztein et al 1999). The findings suggest an abnormality in the function of the LH receptor or in the postreceptor message. Testicular histology in this patient was normal for age.

GENDER IDENTIFICATION DISORDERS WITH AN ABNORMAL SEX CHROMOSOME CONSTITUTION

Additions, deletions or mosaicism of the sex chromosomes characterise individuals in this category. The appearance of the gonads is variable and ranges from the presence of a streak gonad to a nearly normal female or male gonad on both gross and microscopic examination. These disorders are subdivided into two broad categories depending on the frequency with which sexual ambiguity occurs.

SEXUAL AMBIGUITY INFREQUENT

Klinefelter's syndrome

Klinefelter's syndrome occurs in about one in every 1000 live newborn males. The karyotype is usually 47,XXY which, in most cases, results from non-dysjunction occurring during meiosis of either paternal or maternal gametes. Less frequently, a 47,XXY/46,XY mosaic karyotype is found, caused by non-dysjunction during mitosis of the developing zygote. Other chromosomal anomalies have been described (Bertelloni et al 1999). Molecular probe studies have shown that both parents contribute the extra chromosome in about half of the cases. They result as an error in the first paternal meiotic division, but in the mother over a quarter (28%) occur at the second maternal meiotic division (Hunter 1995a). Unlike trisomy 21, which occurs as a failure of the first maternal meiotic division, the likelihood of Klinefelter's is not increased with advancing maternal age.

The diagnosis is usually first suspected at adolescence when the patient presents with gynaecomastia, obesity or signs of eunuchism. The testes are small. The beard and body hair are frequently sparse. Most patients are tall with long legs, resulting in a diminished upper to lower body segment ratio. Laboratory tests reveal low testosterone levels, elevated gonadotrophic levels (postpuberty) and azoospermia. Frequently associated clinical findings include learning disabilities, behavioural disorders, reduced economic striving and limited sexual drive. The diagnosis may also be established at other stages of life due to evaluation of age-related clinical concerns. Genetic screening programmes identify the fetus with Klinefelter's syndrome. Although infants with Klinefelter's syndrome usually have normal external male genitalia at birth, the syndrome is sometimes discovered during evaluations of newborns with hypospadias, micropenis, and small soft testes or cryptorchidism. In adults, Klinefelter's syndrome may be discovered during an evaluation for infertility or malignancy.

The Klinefelter's testis is morphologically normal at birth in most cases. Primary spermatogonia are already greatly reduced in number by late childhood. Shortly before the expected time of puberty, the seminiferous tubules begin to degenerate. The absence of elastic fibres in the tubular wall indicates that the process of atrophy began prepubertally. The testes in adult 47,XXY individuals are small and rarely exceed 2 cm in maximal dimension (Fig. 36.5). On microscopical examination, they are largely atrophic, have hyalinised seminiferous tubules, and a relative increase in the number of Leydig cells. Some tubules may be preserved, but are lined only by Sertoli cells. Rarely, an occasional seminiferous tubule of the adult testis contains germ cells in varying stages of maturation. If sperm are detected, mosaicism, most likely of the 46,XY/47,XXY pattern, should be suspected. Patients with this mosaic karyotype are sometimes fertile.

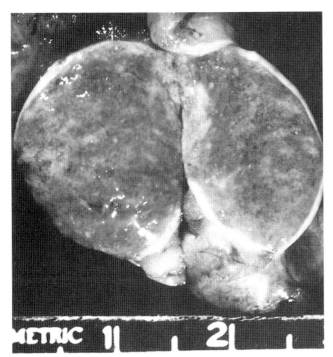

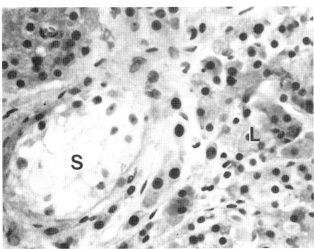

Fig. 36.5 Klinefelter's syndrome. **Top** The parenchyma of the 2 cm testis is golden-yellow to slightly brown. **Bottom** Clusters of Leydig cells (L) surround a seminiferous tubule (S). (Reprinted from Welch & Robboy 1981, with kind permission of Academic Publishers.)

The Leydig cells become pronounced in number some time after puberty. Although they appear hyperplastic relative to the atrophic appearance of the other elements, it is uncertain whether the absolute volume is greater than in normal testes. Functionally, the Leydig cells are abnormal as evidenced by low levels of serum testosterone in the setting of elevated levels of serum LH and FSH and subnormal increase in response to administration of hCG.

A variety of neoplasms have been associated with Klinefelter's syndrome. Both gonadal and extragonadal germ cell tumours develop with increased frequency.

Most extragonadal tumours occur in the mediastinum as teratoma and embryonal cell carcinoma (teratocarcinoma) or choriocarcinoma. In the testis, seminoma, teratoma and embryonal cell carcinoma have been encountered (Matsuki et al 1999). Leydig cell tumors are rare (Okada et al 1994). The risk of breast carcinoma in men with Klinefelter's syndrome may be 20% higher than in normal men. Haematological malignancies have also been reported, including acute leukaemia, Hodgkin's disease, malignant lymphoma, and chronic myelogenous leukaemia.

Turner's syndrome

In the classic form, Turner's syndrome is a disorder in which sexually immature phenotypic females of short stature have various congenital anomalies and streak gonads. The cytogenetic hallmark is the 45,X karyotype with a sporadic, non-familial pattern of inheritance. A critical region is the short arm of the X chromosome (Xp11.2-p22) (Rao et al 1997). Other karyotypes identified less frequently in this syndrome include mosaic 45,X/46,XX and 45,X/47,XXX/46,XX, or additional anomalies of the X chromosome (Jacobs et al 1997). The X chromosome in 75% of cases is maternal in origin (Jacobs et al 1997; Martinez-Pasarell et al 1999). Patients with a 45,X/46,XY mosaic karyotype (considered in mixed gonadal dysgenesis) usually present with obvious sexual ambiguity, but sometimes present as phenotypic females with the clinical stigmata of Turner's syndrome. In several recent studies which by conventional cytogenetic analysis disclosed pure X monosomy but hidden 'Y' mosaicism or cryptic Y chromosomal material was found in 3% (Quilter et al 1998; Vlasak et al 1999) to about 30% (Patsalis et al 1998; Mendes et al 1999; Nazarenko et al 1999) of the patients after the additional testing was performed. The complex nature of karyotyping is expressed in a recent study where the blood from a single adult with Turner syndrome was examined in 287 cytogenetic laboratories with many differing results (Park et al 1999). A significant difference between patients with 45,X/46,XY mosaic karyotype and those with classic 45,X Turner's syndrome is that gonadoblastoma and malignant germ cell tumours are common in patients with the former and rare in those with the latter (Tanaka et al 1994a). Currently, it is common practice to actively exclude Y mosaicism in individuals with Turner syndrome if virilisation or a small marker chromosome is seen (Chu 1999). In an occasional instance, microscopical gonadoblastoma or other germ cell tumour has been found in some of these Turner-like patients with a cryptic Y chromosome (Ito et al 1998; Mendes et al 1999).

About 98% of fetuses with a 45,X karyotype abort; the frequency of Turner's syndrome is about 1:3000 liveborn females. In the newborn, the overt findings are related to lymph stasis, which manifests itself as oedema of the dorsum of the hands or feet or, less frequently, as swellings of the nape of the neck (cystic hygroma). Later in childhood and in adult life, webbing of the neck or elevation of the distal portion of the nails are residua of more marked swellings present during fetal life and may still provide a clue to the correct diagnosis. A rare, but important major presentation is hydronephrosis due to ureteropelvic stenosis; all female neonates with a ureteropelvic obstruction should have a buccal smear. Congenital anomalies of other organ systems are associated with Turner's syndrome and include a short fourth metacarpal, hypoplastic nails, multiple pigmented naevi and coarctation of the aorta. Growth retardation (short stature) is common (Gicquel et al 1998). More than 40 somatic anomalies are associated with this condition.

Spontaneous puberty occurs in 5–10% of women with Turner's syndrome (Hovatta 1999). While most patients will have been diagnosed earlier, those who reach adolescence undiagnosed often present with primary amenorrhoea. Examination reveals underdeveloped secondary sex characteristics and a small uterus. Urinary gonadotrophins are always elevated and the vaginal smear lacks cornified cells. The buccal smear in a 45,X individual reveals few if any Barr bodies; in those 20% of patients with a mosaic karyotype (usually 45,X/46,XX or 45,X/47,XXX, the smear discloses a subnormal number of chromatin-positive cells (about 5–15% for a female). Only rare patients with Turner's syndrome have become pregnant and the majority of these have a 46,XX cell line. Some of these women have mosaic patterns that are

found only after extensive search (Magee et al 1998). Oocyte donation programmes have recently proved effective with one centre recording 20 clinical pregnancies in 18 women, the majority of whom achieved a live birth via Caesarean section (Foudila et al 1999).

At laparotomy, the internal genitalia are female and, although small, are in normal relation to one another. The adult gonads appear as white fibrous streaks, 2–3 cm long and 0.5 cm in diameter and are located in the position normally occupied by the ovary (Fig. 36.6). On microscopical examination a streak consists of an attenuated cortex, a medulla and a hilus. The cortex is composed of characteristic ovarian stroma in which the cells are elongate, wavy and are composed of conspicuous nuclei and scant cytoplasm. Rete tubules (rete ovarii) and hilar cells are typically present in the hilus region. Oocytes are almost always absent in adults with Turner's syndrome. Oocytes are present in normal numbers in 45,X embryos prior to the 12th week of gestation. In older fetuses and young children, the number of oocytes falls progressively relative to the normal number for the age until the number reaches zero, usually before the time of normal menarche, thus leading to primary amenorrhoea. These findings suggest that the second X chromosome is necessary for granulosa cell development and primary follicular formation; in the absence of this X chromosome, granulosa cells fail to differentiate and, as a result, the oocytes degenerate.

Gonadal tumours are exceedingly rare. Tumours of germ cell origin are undoubtedly rare due to the paucity of germ cells. While occasional germ cell tumours have been reported (Pierga et al 1994), care must be exercised as with more sophisticated tools for chromosome analysis, especially using newer molecular biologic techniques, cryptic Y chromosomal fragments have been discovered associated with the tumour tissue (Ito et al 1998; Mendes et al 1999). Most reported cases with a gonadoblastoma component have had a mosaic pattern with a Y chromosome (Vanderbijl et al 1994; Mendes et al 1999), and more appropriately should be considered under the category of mixed gonadal dysgenesis. Development of neoplasms of the so-called 'common epithelial type' suggests that the coelomic epithelium encapsulating the gonad can undergo malignant change even if the gonad is a streak. Endometrial carcinoma may develop occasionally in those patients who have had long-term exogenous oestrogen therapy to foster the appearance of the female secondary sex characteristics. Both natural oestrogens and synthetic non-steroidal oestrogens have been implicated. The duration of usage usually exceeds 3 years. Extragonadal tumours, most often of neurogenic origin, have been reported in children and young adults.

XX male syndrome

The XX male syndrome is a disorder characterised by a nearly normal but infertile phenotypic male with a 46,XX

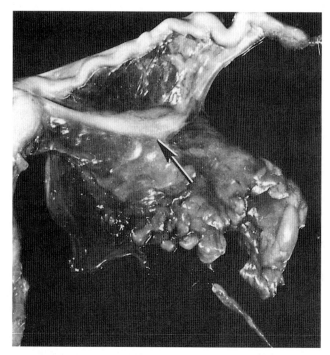

Fig. 36.6 Streak ovary (arrow) in Turner's syndrome. (Reprinted from Welch & Robboy 1981, with kind permission of Kluwer Academic Publishers.)

karyotype. This syndrome, one of the rarest of all sex chromosome anomalies, occurs in about 1 of 24 000 newborn males (Tateno et al 1999). XX males share many characteristics of men with Klinefelter's syndrome. Both have a generally masculine appearance, normal or near normal external genitalia, male psychosexual orientation, normal to weak secondary sexual characteristics, normal to low androgen levels and azoospermia. The testes are small with prominent Leydig cells and tubules lined only by Sertoli cells. The most common reasons for referral are similar to those with Klinefelter's syndrome, namely infertility or abnormal secondary sexual characteristics. XX males also tend to differ clinically from men with Klinefelter's syndrome: the former are generally shorter in height, and the frequency of hypospadias and gynaecomastia is higher. The frequency of impaired intelligence is not increased in XX males relative to the general population. Increasingly, with ultrasonography and genetic analyses being performed during gestation, the XX male syndrome is now being discovered prenatally (Ginsberg et al 1999).

The XX male syndrome potentially results from at least three distinctly different mechanisms. About 70% of these patients have a small portion of paternally derived Y chromosome, which contains the *SRY* gene, the testis-determining factor present abnormally on the X chromosome. The *SRY* gene is normally found on the short arm of the Y chromosome adjacent to the pseudoautosomal pairing region. During meiosis in the father, an abnormal exchange sometimes leads to the transfer onto the X chromosome of the entire pseudoautosomal region plus the adjacent portion of the Y chromosome with the *SRY* gene. Inheritance of such an X chromosome from the father leads to the Y(+) XX male syndrome. The inheritance pattern of this form of the syndrome is sporadic. These patients have normal male external genitalia. Hypospadias and ambiguous genitalia are virtually never found. Apparently, the presence of the *SRY* gene is adequate to lead to normal male phenotype. Azoospermia in these patients results from the lack of other genes normally found on the Y chromosome necessary for sperm development.

Some patients with the XX male syndrome lack Y-derived DNA. Such Y(–) XX males might result from two different mechanisms. The first accounts for the familial transmission of an autosomal dominant or X-linked inheritance of XX maleness. These patients usually have ambiguous genitalia. This indicates that genes exist, probably downstream from the testis-determining factor, which can trigger testis determination when mutated (Kolon et al 1998). Nothing specific is known about these putative genes, but their phenotypic effect seems slightly different from that of testis determining factor. A second potential mechanism that might lead to the Y(–) condition is chromosomal mosaicism with a prevalent XX lineage. In such patients, the Y-containing cell line might simply be techni-

cally too difficult to identify due to the small number of such cells. Alternatively, a 47,XXY zygote might lose its Y chromosome by non-dysjunction early in ontogeny allowing a 46,XX cell line to persist; the 47,XXY cell line may have persisted long enough to induce male gonadal development. Such patients, just as patients with familial Y(–) XX maleness, often present with sexual ambiguity suggesting that patients with Y(–) XX male syndrome are closely related both phenotypically and aetiologically to XX true hermaphrodites, who present with both testicular and ovarian tissue.

Pure gonadal dysgenesis

Pure gonadal dysgenesis is a term that has historically been encompassed in a number of diverse conditions, including testicular regression syndrome. In the context defined herein, pure gonadal dysgenesis refers to a phenotypic female without genetic ambiguity where the internal genitalia include Müllerian structures (uterus and Fallopian tubes) and generally streak gonads, a constellation which still probably encompasses a multitude of diverse conditions. The patients may appear phenotypically normal or have hypoplastic external genitalia. The pure gonadal dysgenesis syndrome occurs with both 46,XX and 46,XY karyotypes and has both familial and sporadic patterns of inheritance.

The 46,XX type pure gonadal dysgenesis is either an autosomal recessive disorder or, possibly as a mosaic 45,X cell line confined to the gonad (Meyers et al 1996). Deletions of the short or long arm of an X chromosome have been identified in some cases. Such patients have greater ovarian development than those with 46,XY pure gonadal dysgenesis or Turner's syndrome and present more often with signs of ovarian dysfunction (secondary amenorrhoea or infertility) rather than primary gonadal failure (primary amenorrhoea). Some patients may also have mosaic cell lines with the SRY gene absent in some tissues (peripheral leucocytes), but present in others (testicular tissue) (Dardis et al 1997).

The 46,XY type pure gonadal dysgenesis is more common than the 46,XX form of the disorder. The syndrome of pure gonadal dysgenesis may be sporadic or familial with either X linked recessive or autosomal recessive patterns of inheritance (Rutgers 1991; Bilbao et al 1996). Some patients have a mosaic 45,X/46,XY karyotype.

Patients with 46,XX pure gonadal dysgenesis, like those with Turner's syndrome, very rarely develop gonadal tumours. Some have had hilus cell hyperplasia and hilus cell tumours with the usual associated virilising effects. Epithelial tumours are extremely rare, but of these mucinous tumours occur more frequently than serous (Lam et al 1996). Rare examples of germ cell tumours have been reported (Morimura et al 1998), and even though no identifiable Y chromosome component could be detected in some, the possibility of a cryptic Y fragment cannot be excluded. Patients with 46,XY pure gonadal dysgenesis are at high risk for gonadoblastoma and other germ cell tumours as is true of all patients with streak gonads and a Y chromosome (Uehara et al 1999a). In one series, 11 of 20 patients had neoplasms in the gonads; 8 patients had gonadoblastomas, half of which were bilateral, and 8 patients had dysgerminomas, all unilateral (Radakovic et al 1999). On this basis, patients with 46,XY pure gonadal

dysgenesis might be considered a subset of the broader condition of mixed gonadal dysgenesis.

SEXUAL AMBIGUITY FREQUENT

Patients in this category exhibit a wide range of phenotypic appearances and internal genitalia. A 'Y' chromosome is often present, usually as part of a mosaic complement. Sexual ambiguity is a common finding.

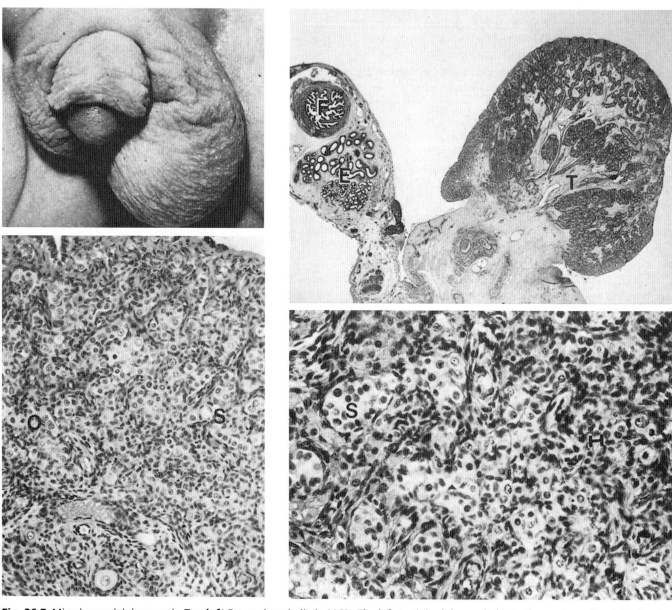

Fig. 36.7 Mixed gonadal dysgenesis. **Top left** External genitalia in MGD. The left testis had descended into the scrotum; the right streak was in the abdominal cavity. Because of this characteristic appearance, some investigators prefer the name 'asymmetric gonadal dysgenesis' rather than mixed gonadal dysgenesis. **Top right** Testis (T) and adjacent Fallopian tube (F) and epididymis (E). The medulla contains immature seminiferous tubules with germ cells and interstitial cells while the region nearer the cortex resembles fetal ovary with immature sex cords and rare primordial follicles. **Bottom left** Cortex of gonad in which testicular seminiferous tubules (S) merge into fetal-type ovary (O). **Bottom right** The medullary parenchyma of the testis is composed of normal immature seminiferous tubules (S) with germ cells and occasional interstitial cells, while the parenchyma in the region of the hilus: (H) near the rete testis appears less committed as testis and is characterised by abnormal, pleomorphic seminiferous tubules. The photograph is taken at the junction of the two zones. (Reprinted from Robboy et al 1982, with permission of Human Pathology.)

Mixed gonadal dysgenesis

Mixed gonadal dysgenesis is a heterogeneous syndrome characterised usually by a 45,X/46,XY or 46,XY karyotype, persistent Müllerian duct structures, an abnormal testis and a contralateral streak gonad (Alvarez-Nava et al 1999a). The functional deficit imposed by the abnormal testis is expressed as incomplete inhibition of Müllerian development, incomplete differentiation of Wolffian duct structures and incomplete male development of the external genitalia. Often, incomplete mediation of the testicular descent occurs, resulting in both internal and external asymmetry of the genitalia and a mixture of male and female features in an individual in whom neither gonad is normal. About two-thirds of the affected individuals are raised as females and the remainder as males. Some patients with mixed gonadal dysgenesis exhibit phenotypic features of Turner's syndrome (Alvarez-Nava et al 1999b; Telvi et al 1999). Elsewhere, we have suggested that the syndrome of mixed gonadal dysgenesis should be enlarged to incorporate some patients with bilateral streak gonads (described above as 46,XY type pure gonadal dysgenesis) or bilateral abnormal testes with mosaic 45,X/46,XY karyotype (dysgenetic male pseudohermaphroditism), since the clinical, pathological and chromosomal features of these syndromes closely resemble each other.

The underlying genetic and karyotype abnormalities leading to the syndrome of mixed gonadal dysgenesis are currently under investigation. A variety of different genetic abnormalities appear to result in mixed gonadal dysgenesis, thus leading to the phenotypic heterogeneity of mixed gonadal dysgenesis. Partial deletions of both the short and long arms of chromosome Y have been detected in these individuals. Most cases where no detectable Y chromosomal anomaly is observed by conventional chromosome analysis have a Y fragment found when additional testing is performed (Gibbons et al 1999).

Clinically, mixed gonadal dysgenesis is usually detected in the neonate because of ambiguity of the external genitalia. Frequently, a palpable testis bulges through an indirect inguinal hernia or descends completely into the labioscrotal fold, resulting in asymmetry of the genital swellings. This clinical appearance has prompted some investigators to name the syndrome 'asymmetric gonadal dysgenesis'. If the gonads are intra-abdominal, the labioscrotal folds may appear as normal labia or as empty scrotal sacs. The condition is likely to go unrecognised unless the clitoris is sufficiently enlarged to mandate investigation, which is common. The gonad that descends is almost always a testis, and the streak gonads are always intra-abdominal unless dragged into a 'hernia uteri inguinale'.

Organs derived from the Müllerian duct persist in 95% of cases (Fig. 36.7) (Robboy et al 1982; Mendez et al 1993). The uterus is usually infantile or rudimentary. The Fallopian tubes are frequently bilateral. If a testis is grossly near normal size and well differentiated, the fimbriated end of the ipsilateral tube may be absent, but in only one-third of cases is the ipsilateral tube entirely absent. Organs of Wolffian duct derivation may also be present, but their frequency is variable. The epididymis is identified in two-thirds of cases and is usually present on the side where there is a testis. The vas deferens is encountered less frequently. The seminal vesicle is only rarely identified, probably because tissue near the bladder/prostate region is not usually removed.

The gonad may be a testis or a streak. Streak gonads may be partially differentiated towards ovary or testis. Bilateral gross testes, frequently of an asynchronous degree of maturity, are found in about 15% of cases while a unilateral gross testis is found in 60%. The testis is consistently abnormal architecturally, its organisation being divided into three zones, each of which reflects the quantity and type of cellular components present. The three zones, which are described below in detail, include:

1. the region of the tunica albuginea or cortex, which exhibits widely spaced seminiferous tubules or differentiation towards ovary
2. the medulla, which is composed of normal or near-normal seminiferous tubules and interstitium
3. a hilar region with poorly differentiated seminiferous tubules that are only partly differentiated towards testis.

The superficial cortex may contain seminiferous tubules that are often widely separated by oedematous, undifferentiated stroma. Sometimes the tubules penetrate the incompletely formed tunica albuginea and open onto the serosa. Occasionally, broad zones of cortex differentiate slightly towards ovary, even displaying rare primordial follicles. Mice that spontaneously develop chromosomal mosaicism as a result of non-dysjunction often show gonads with ovarian tissue at the periphery and seminiferous cords centrally.

The central zone (medulla) of the macroscopic infant testis is architecturally and cytologically normal. Narrow closed seminiferous tubules are lined by Sertoli cells with abundant cytoplasm. The number of spermatogonia varies; advanced forms of spermatogenic maturation are not observed. Leydig cells are present in small clusters of varying size. The nuclei of the Leydig cells contain finely dispersed chromatin, and the cytoplasm varies from minimal and amphophilic or slightly basophilic to abundant and eosinophilic. In older patients, the medulla is atrophic and the tubules are lined only by Sertoli cells (Fig. 36.8). The basement membranes are often thickened. Prominent clusters of Leydig cells fill the interstitium.

The architecturally disorganised hilar region discloses seminiferous tubules that are swollen by increased numbers of Sertoli cells and are lined by indistinct basement membranes. These tubules also merge with the

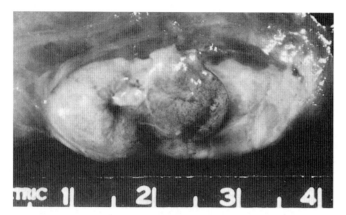

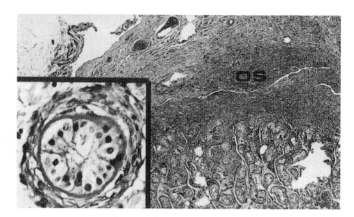

Fig. 36.8 Testis in a 35-year-old phenotypic male with mixed gonadal dysgenesis. **Left** The tunica albuginea is tan and maximally 1 mm thick; the parenchyma is golden yellow. **Right** Cross section of tunica albuginea which is composed of stroma resembling the stroma of ovarian cortex (OS) and medulla with seminiferous tubules. **Insert** Detail of seminiferous tubules lined only by Sertoli cells. The interstitium is filled with Leydig cells. (Reprinted from Robboy et al 1982, with permission of Human Pathology.)

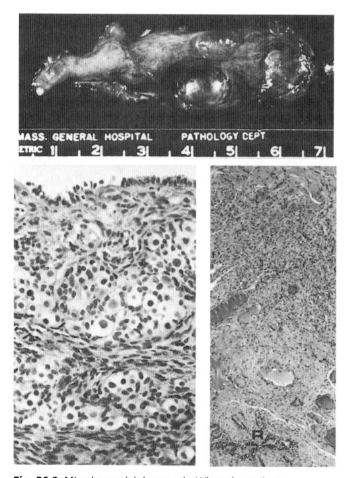

Fig. 36.9 Mixed gonadal dysgenesis. When the patient was an infant the streak gonad resembled a fetal ovary with germ cells and immature sex cords (left lower). When the streak gonad was removed in its entirety 13 years later (top), it existed only as several microscopical areas of whispy ovarian-type cortical stroma and rete ovarii (R). (Reprinted from Robboy et al 1982, with permission of Human Pathology.)

surrounding stroma, imparting the appearance of a homogeneous blend of Leydig cells, germ cells, Sertoli cells, and an indeterminate type of interstitial stroma. The region resembles neither fetal ovary nor testis.

The streak gonads appear similar to those found in Turner's syndrome. We have not observed a gonad that has been identifiable grossly as an ovary or has been shown microscopically to contain Graafian follicles, corpora lutea or corpora albicantia. The presence of rare primordial follicles or, as in the fetal ovary, aggregates of germ cells partially surrounded by immature granulosa cells, is evidence that a streak gonad can differentiate towards ovary. Morphological changes may occur over time in the streak gonads. Myriads of germ cells present in a streak of an infant may degenerate and disappear by puberty, resulting in a gonad composed exclusively of fibrous tissue and a few rete tubules (Fig. 36.9); similar changes occur in the streak gonads of Turner's syndrome (45,X karyotype).

Approximately one-third of patients with mixed gonadal dysgenesis develop gonadoblastoma, a tumour found almost exclusively in patients with an intersex syndrome and a Y chromosome (Scully et al 1998) and one that most likely has its beginnings during prenatal life (Jorgensen et al 1997). Gonadoblastoma accounts for three-quarters of the gonadal tumours arising in dysgenetic gonads and is usually discovered during the first to fourth decades of life. Many of the isolated reports of gonadoblastoma associated with other forms of hermaphroditism described clinically and pathologically may in actuality be examples of mixed gonadal dysgenesis.

The role of the Y chromosome in the development of cancer is a controversial subject. Since the bulk of the Y chromosome (except for the pseudoautosomal regions at both ends of the chromosomes, initialled PAR) neither pairs with nor recombines with the X chromosome during meiosis, it has been difficult to study this chromosome and identify its oncogenic genes and tumour-suppressor genes. Current evidence suggests the gonadoblastoma Y gene locus (GBY) is located on the short or long arm of the Y chromosome near the centromere (Muroya et al 1999).

About 20% of gonadoblastomas arise in a streak gonad and another 20% arise in a dysgenetic testis; in the

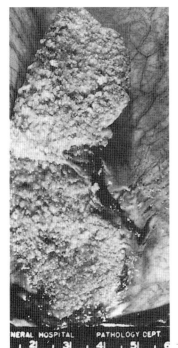
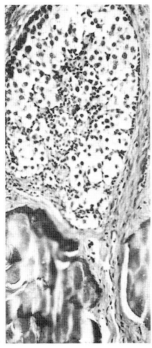
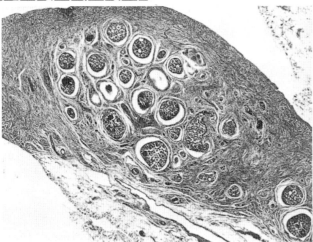

Fig. 36.10 Gonadoblastoma in mixed gonadal dysgenesis. **Top left** 15 cm gonadal tumour composed largely of dysgerminoma. At one pole is a 5 × 2 × 0.5 cm calcified gonadoblastoma. **Top right** Gonadoblastoma. Multiple mulberry-like calcific masses partially replace the tumour nests composed of germ cells surrounded by sex-cord derivatives. **Bottom** Gonadoblastoma occupying a gonadal streak. (Reprinted from Welch & Robboy 1981, with permission of Kluwer Academic Publishers and Scully 1970, with permission of Cancer.)

remaining cases, the nature of the underlying gonad cannot be determined with certainty because it is replaced by tumour. The gross appearance of the gonad with gonadoblastoma varies according to the size of the neoplasm, the presence of calcification and whether the gonadoblastoma has been overgrown by a malignant form of germ cell tumour (usually germinoma) (Fig. 36.10). Approximately one-fifth of gonadoblastomas are discovered solely because a streak gonad was examined microscopically. The contralateral gonad also contains a gonadoblastoma in over one-third of patients.

On microscopical examination, the gonadoblastoma appears as circumscribed nests of neoplastic germ cells having the cytological properties of germinoma (dysgerminoma and seminoma) and which are encompassed individually or in groups by sex-cord derivatives with inconspicuous cytoplasm and small round to oval nuclei resembling immature Sertoli cells.

The malignant germ cells have large, generally centrally placed nuclei in the cell, obvious macronucleoli that are one to several in number, and copious light cytoplasm with usually a distinct cytoplasmic membrane. Carcinoma in situ cells express placental-like alkaline phosphatase and the protooncogene, *c-kit* (CD-117) (Jorgensen et al 1997; Rajpert-De Meyts et al 1998). They also react immunocytochemically with several monoclonal antibodies (Jorgensen et al 1997). Inhibin reactivity is also commonly demonstrable, which is in keeping with the sex-cord cells (immature Sertoli/granulosa cells) being an integral part of the tumour (Kommoss et al 1998).

Hyaline, composed of basement membrane material, is found along the margin or as nodules within the nests of cells. In four-fifths of cases the hyaline material is calcified, initially appearing as small, laminated spheres, which eventually fuse and coalesce into large mulberry-like masses. Not infrequently, the only evidence that a dysgerminoma originated in a gonadoblastoma is the presence focally of mulberry-like calcifications. Hormonally active cells that resemble lutein and Leydig cells are found interspersed among the nests of tumour in about two-thirds of cases. These hormonally active cells are found least frequently in non-virilised phenotypic females, more often in virilised females, and most frequently in phenotypic males. To some degree, their appearance may be related to the postpubertal age of the patient when the gonad is examined.

Approximately 30% of gonadoblastomas are overgrown by a malignant germ cell tumour, usually a germinoma; 8% are overgrown by endodermal sinus tumour, immature teratoma, embryonal carcinoma, or choriocarcinoma. An occasional gonad may also show proliferative sex-cord elements and resemble a Sertoli cell tumour (Nomura et al 1999). Most gonadoblastomas occur in phenotypic females with abnormal gonads (Scully et al 1998). Some occur in phenotypic males, almost all of whom have cryptorchism or abnormal external or abnormal internal genitalia. Only the rare patient is a normal phenotypic male without apparent abnormal genitals (Hatano et al 1999). Although the gonadoblastoma itself does not metastasise and therefore can be considered as an in situ malignancy, the typically malignant behaviour of the other tumours makes early prophylactic removal of the gonads in all patients advisable. Also, to avoid the consequences of onset of virilisation if the patient is to be raised as a female, it is important that gonadectomy be performed before the patient reaches puberty. Patients who have been treated with long-term administration of oestrogen may on occasion develop endometrial carcinoma. Congenital cardiovascular anomalies have also been reported in patients with mixed gonadal dysgenesis.

TRUE HERMAPHRODITISM

True hermaphroditism is defined as the presence of both testicular and ovarian tissue in a patient. True hermaphroditism is a rare condition of intersex both in North America, Europe and Australasia. It is, in contrast, common in Africa, especially in South Africa (van Niekerk & Retief 1981). Clusters in other geographical locations are known (Damiani et al 1997; Guerra Junior et al 1998), some with data differing from the summary given below. Affected individuals may have either a female or male phenotype with a variable degree of sexual ambiguity. Because the wavy, cortical-type stroma typically seen in the female gonad can be found in both female and male gonads and therefore is non-specific, follicular structures must be identified to classify gonadal tissue as ovarian and seminiferous tubules to classify the tissue as testicular. In true hermaphrodites, the gonads may be ovary and testis separately or combined in an ovotestis.

The ovotestis is the most frequently encountered gonad in true hermaphroditism. In four-fifths of cases the ovarian and testicular tissues are arranged in an end-to-end fashion. The ovarian portion of an ovotestis has a convoluted surface while the testicular portion is smooth and glistening. Frequently, a distinct line demarcates the two tissues. The firm nature of the palpable ovarian tissue and the soft texture of the testis are valuable clinical signs when evaluating the nature of a gonad in an infant with ambisexual external genitalia.

An ovary, which preferentially develops on the left side, is the second most common gonad in true hermaphrodites. Every patient over 15 years of age in the series of van Niekerk & Retief (1981) had either a corpus luteum or a corpus albicans. The testis, which is the gonad least often encountered, develops preferentially on the right.

The location of the gonad is influenced by the type and quantity of gonadal tissue present. Increasing amounts of ovarian tissue increase the probability that the gonad will be in an ovarian position. When a gonad with the macroscopic features of an ovary is situated in the inguinal canal or in the labioscrotal fold, the possibility of it being an ovotestis should be seriously considered. The position of the testis is less constant. The majority (63%) reside in the scrotum, 14% in the inguinal region, 1% in the internal inguinal ring, and 22% in a normal ovarian position.

The nature of the genital organ adjacent to a gonad in true hermaphroditism is dependent upon the nature of the gonad, which is in contrast to mixed gonadal dysgenesis, where a Fallopian tube is often adjacent to the gonad, regardless of whether it is a testis or streak. In true hermaphroditism a Fallopian tube is adjacent to an ovary and an epididymis or vas deferens is adjacent to a testis. Either a Müllerian or a Wolffian structure, but not both, is adjacent to an ovotestis. Müllerian inhibiting substance appears to be functional. Ninety-five per cent of Fallopian tubes adjacent to ovotestes have closed ostia. Only 10% of uteri are normal; the other patients have absent uteri (13%), unicornuate uteri (10%), absent cervix (14%) or uterine hypoplasia (46%).

The most common karyotypes in true hermaphroditism are 46,XX (60%), 46,XY (12%), and mosaic (28%), usually 46,XX/46,XY, 46,XY/47,XXY, or least frequently 45,X/46,XY. Patients with a 'Y' chromosome have a 2–3-fold increased frequency of having a testis as opposed to an ovotestis. Nearly 75% of true hermaphrodites with an ovary and ovotestis have a 46,XX karyotype.

As in other subclasses of intersex, the causes of true hermaphroditism at the genetic level are under investigation. Chromosome Y specific genes (e.g. SRY) have been detected in some but not all 46,XX true hermaphrodites, suggesting several potential mechanisms for the development of XX true hermaphroditism, similar to individuals with XX male syndrome. In some series, however, SRY was undetected in the 46,XX patients, (Guerra Junior et al 1998) indicating that other mechanisms may also be important. Mutations that mimic the SRY gene have been suggested as one possibility where the SRY gene was absent (Slaney et al 1998). One explanation proposed for patients with an XY chromosome is the possibility that the SRY gene, if present, may act at a time too late to stimulate the development of a testis, hence permitting ovarian tissue to develop.

The clinical presentations of true hermaphrodites vary to some extent depending upon the patient's age at the time of diagnosis. Until recently, the condition often went undetected until adolescence when phenotypic male patients were evaluated for gynaecomastia and phenotypic female patients were evaluated for amenorrhoea or failure to develop secondary sex changes. Thus, in the series of van Niekerk & Retief (1981), three-quarters of patients were raised as males and one-quarter as females. Many patients, however, menstruated and a few became pregnant. Phenotypic males may experience monthly haematuria due to menstruation into a persistent urogenital sinus. With an increased awareness of intersex states, the condition is more often recognised in infants because of ambiguous genitalia, usually in the form of a small phallus (enlarged clitoris) (Damiani et al 1997). As in mixed gonadal dysgenesis, the scrotum may be asymmetrical, with the larger, more normal-appearing hemiscrotum containing a testis. Among 160 patients the external genitalia were asymmetrical in three-quarters (labioscrotal folds in 63% and hemiscrotums in 13%).

On microscopical examination, the gonadal tissue often appears normal if the patient is young. In infants the ovarian tissue contains numerous follicles, while the testicular parenchyma discloses normal-appearing seminiferous tubules with spermatogonia. Patients in the reproductive years may have ovarian tissue with structures indicative of ovulation, e.g. follicles, corpora lutea, and corpora albicantia, but spermatogenesis is rare in the testicular portion. The testicular portion of an ovotestis is usually abnormal with incomplete development, loss of germ cells, and tubular sclerosis. Scrotal testes in these patients show less severe changes, sometimes showing faulty spermatogenesis.

At times, distinction between true hermaphroditism and mixed gonadal dysgenesis can be difficult. In the newborn, asymmetric ambiguous genitalia may be observed in both conditions. If a streak gonad from a patient with mixed gonadal dysgenesis is serially sectioned, a rare primordial follicle may be encountered in what otherwise appears to be a fetal-type ovary admixed with testis with well-developed seminiferous tubules. If the term 'true hermaphroditism' is restricted to those patients in whom the ovarian and testicular tissue are both apparent grossly, it should be possible to segregate more clearly those individuals in whom the ovarian tissue may be functional.

Gonadal tumours occur in less than 3% of affected individuals. Germinoma is the most common type of tumour, but gonadoblastomas and a variety of other tumours have been reported. One case has been reported where the primitive sex-cord cellular elements adjacent to seminiferous tubules in a testis gave rise to cancer in the form of a juvenile granulosa cell tumour (Tanaka et al 1994b).

REFERENCES

Aartsen E J, Snethlage R A I, Vangeel A N, Gallee M P W 1994 Squamous cell carcinoma of the vagina in a male pseudohermaphrodite with 5 alpha-reductase deficiency. International Journal of Gynecological Cancer 4: 283–287

Al-Attia H M 1997 Male pseudohermaphroditism due to 5 alpha-reductase-2 deficiency in an Arab kindred. Postgraduate Medical Journal 73: 802–807

Alvarez-Nava F, Gonzalez S, Soto M, Martinez C, Prieto M 1997 Complete androgen insensitivity syndrome: clinical and anatomopathological findings in 23 patients. Genetic Counseling 8: 7–12

Alvarez-Nava F, Gonzalez S, Soto M, Pineda L, Morales-Machin A 1999a Mixed gonadal dysgenesis: a syndrome of broad clinical cytogenetic and histopathologic spectrum. Genetic Counseling 10: 233–243

Alvarez-Nava F, Martinez M C, Gonzalez S, Soto M, Borjas L, Rojas A 1999b FISH and PCR analysis of the presence of Y-chromosome sequences in a patient with Xq-isochromosome and testicular tissue. Clinical Genetics 55: 356–361

Andersson S, Moghrabi N 1997 Physiology and molecular genetics of 17 beta-hydroxysteroid dehydrogenases. Steroids 62: 143–147

Anwar R, Gilbey S G, New J P, Markham A F 1997 Male pseudohermaphroditism resulting from a novel mutation in the human steroid 5 alpha-reductase type 2 gene (SRD5A2). Journal of Clinical Pathology-Molecular Pathology 50: 51–52

Arnhold I J, Latronico A C, Batista M C, Mendonca B B 1999 Menstrual disorders and infertility caused by inactivating mutations of the luteinizing hormone receptor gene. Fertility and Sterility 71: 597–601

Avila N A, Premkumar A, Merke D P 1999 Testicular adrenal rest tissue in congenital adrenal hyperplasia: comparison of MR imaging and sonographic findings. American Journal of Roentgenology 172: 1003–1006

Bale P M, Howard N J, Wright J E 1992 Male pseudohermaphroditism in XY children with female phenotype. Pediatric Pathology 12: 29–49

Berensztein E, Torrado M, Belgorosky A, Rivarola M 1999 Smith–Lemli–Opitz syndrome: in vivo and in vitro study of testicular function in a prepubertal patient with ambiguous genitalia. Acta Paediatrica 88: 1229–1232

Bertelloni S, Battini R, Baroncelli G I, et al 1999 Central precocious puberty in 48, XXYY Klinefelter syndrome variant. Journal of Pediatric Endocrinology & Metabolism 12: 459–465

Bilbao J R, Loridan L, Castano L 1996 A novel postzygotic nonsense mutation in SRY in familial XY gonadal dysgenesis. Human Genetics 97: 537–539

Bilbao J R, Loridan L, Audi L, Gonzalo E, Castano L 1998 A novel missense (R80W) mutation in 17-beta-hydroxysteroid dehydrogenase type 3 gene associated with male pseudohermaphroditism. European Journal of Endocrinology 139: 330–333

Brennan J, Karl J, Martineau J et al 1998 Sry and the testis: molecular pathways of organogenesis. Journal of Experimental Zoology 281: 494–500

Buchholz N P, Biyabani R, Herzig M J U et al 1998 Persistent mullerian duct syndrome. European Urology 34: 230–232

Carlson A D, Obeid J S, Kanellopoulou N, Wilson R C, New M I 1999 Congenital adrenal hyperplasia: update on prenatal diagnosis and treatment. Journal of Steroid Biochemistry & Molecular Biology 69: 19–29

Cendron M, Schned A R, Ellsworth P I 1998 Histological evaluation of the testicular nubbin in the vanishing testis syndrome. Journal of Urology 160: 1161–1163

Cerame B I, Newfield R S, Pascoe L et al 1999 Prenatal diagnosis and treatment of 11 beta-hydroxylase deficiency congenital adrenal hyperplasia resulting in normal female genitalia. Journal of Clinical Endocrinology & Metabolism 84: 3129–3134

Chu C 1999 Y-chromosome mosaicism in girls with Turner's syndrome. Clinical Endocrinology 50: 17–18

Clarnette T D, Sugita Y, Hutson J M 1997 Genital anomalies in human and animal models reveal the mechanisms and hormones governing testicular descent. British Journal of Urology 79: 99–112

Damiani D, Fellous M, McElreavey K et al 1997 True hermaphroditism: clinical aspects and molecular studies in 16 cases. European Journal of Endocrinology 136: 201–204

Dardis A, Saraco N, Mendilaharzu H, Rivarola M, Belgorosky A 1997 Report of an XX male with hypospadias and pubertal gynecomastia, SRY gene negative in blood leukocytes but SRY gene positive in testicular cells. Hormone Research 47: 85–88

Dork T, Schnieders F, Jakubiczka S, Wieacker P, Schroeder-Kurth T, Schmidtke J 1998 A new missense substitution at a mutational hot spot of the androgen receptor in siblings with complete androgen insensitivity syndrome. Human Mutation 11: 337–339

Erk A, Ozeren S, Ozbay O, Vural B, Elcioglu N 1999 Persistent mullerian duct syndrome — A case report. Journal of Reproductive Medicine 44: 135–138

Faure E, Gouedard L, Imbeaud S et al 1996 Mutant isoforms of the anti-Mullerian hormone type II receptor are not expressed at the cell membrane. Journal of Biological Chemistry 271: 30571–30575

Ferrari P, Obeyesekere V R, Li K et al 1996 Point mutations abolish 11 beta-hydroxysteroid dehydrogenase type II activity in three families with the congenital syndrome of apparent mineralocorticoid excess. Molecular Cellular Endocrinology 119: 21–24

Ferraz L F C, Baptista M T M, Maciel-Guerra A T, Junior G G, Hackel C 1999 New frameshift mutation in the 5 alpha-reductase type 2 gene in a Brazilian patient with 5 alpha-reductase deficiency. American Journal of Medical Genetics 87: 221–225

Fitzky B U, Glossmann H, Utermann G, Moebius F F 1999 Molecular genetics of the Smith-Lemli-Opitz syndrome and postsqualene sterol metabolism. Current Opinions in Lipidology 10: 123–131

Foudila T, Soderstrom-Anttila V, Hovatta O 1999 Turner's syndrome and pregnancies after oocyte donation. Human Reproduction 14: 532–535

Fung M F, Vadas G, Lotocki R, Heywood M, Krepart G 1991 Tubular Krukenberg tumor in pregnancy with virilization. Gynecologic Oncology 41: 81–84

Gibbons B, Tan S Y, Yu C C, Cheah E, Tan H L 1999 Risk of gonadoblastoma in female patients with Y chromosome abnormalities and dysgenetic gonads. Journal of Paediatric & Child Health 35: 210–213

Gicquel C, Gaston V, Cabrol S, Le Bouc Y 1998 Assessment of Turner's syndrome by molecular analysis of the X chromosome in growth-retarded girls. Journal of Clinical Endocrinology & Metabolism 83: 1472–1476

Ginsberg N A, Cadkin A, Strom C, Bauer-Marsh E, Verlinsky Y 1999 Prenatal diagnosis of 46,XX male fetuses. American Journal of Obstetrics and Gynecology 180: 1006–1007

Guerra Junior G, de Mello M P, Assumpcao J G et al 1998 True hermaphrodites in the southeastern region of Brazil: a different cytogenetic and gonadal profile. Journal of Pediatric Endocrinology & Metabolism 11: 519–524

Hatano T, Yoshino Y, Kawashima Y et al 1999 Case of gonadoblastoma in a 9-year-old boy without physical abnormalities. International Journal of Urology 6: 164–166

Hawkyard S, Poon P, Morgan D R 1999 Sertoli tumour presenting with stress incontinence in a patient with testicular feminization. British Journal of Urology International 84: 382–383

Hiort O, Sinnecker G H, Holterhus P M, Nitsche E M, Kruse K 1996 The clinical and molecular spectrum of androgen insensitivity syndromes. American Journal of Medical Genetics 63: 218–222

Hiort O, Holterhus P M, Nitsche E M 1998 Physiology and pathophysiology of androgen action. Bailliere's Clinical Endocrinology & Metabolism 12: 115–132

Hovatta O 1999 Pregnancies in women with Turner's syndrome. Annals of Medicine 31: 106–110

Hunter R H F 1995a Abnormal sexual development in man. In: Hunter R H F (ed) Sex determination, differentiation and intersexuality in placental mammals. Cambridge University Press, Cambridge. pp 204–238

Hunter R H F 1995b Differentiation of the genital duct system. In: Hunter R H F (ed) Sex determination, differentiation and intersexuality in placental mammals. Cambridge University Press, Cambridge, pp 107–138

Hunter R H F 1995c Mechanisms of sex determination. In: Hunter R H F (ed) Sex determination, differentiation and intersexuality in placental mammals. Cambridge University Press, Cambridge, pp 22–68

Hunter R H F 1995d Sex determination, differentiation and intersexuality in placental mammals. Cambridge University Press, Cambridge, pp 1–310

Imbeaud S, Belville C, Messika-Zeitoun L et al 1996 A 27 base-pair deletion of the anti-mullerian type II receptor gene is the most common cause of the persistent mullerian duct syndrome. Human Molecular Genetics 5: 1269–1277

Imperato-McGinley J 1997 5 alpha-reductase-2 deficiency. Current Therapy in Endocrinology & Metabolism 6: 384–387

Ito K, Kawamata Y, Osada H, Ijichi M, Takano E, Sekiya S 1998 Pure yolk sac tumor of the ovary with mosaic 45X/46X+mar Turner's syndrome with a Y-chromosomal fragment. Archives of Gynecology and Obstetrics 262: 87–90

Jacobs P, Dalton P, James R et al 1997 Turner syndrome: a cytogenetic and molecular study. Annals of Human Genetics 61: 471–483

Jorgensen N, Muller J, Jaubert F, Clausen C P, Skakkebaek N E 1997 Heterogeneity of gonadoblastoma germ cells: similarities with immature germ cells, spermatogonia and testicular carcinoma in situ cells. Histopathology 30: 177–186

Josso N, Racine C, di Clemente N, Rey R, Xavier F 1998 The role of anti-Mullerian hormone in gonadal development. Molecular & Cellular Endocrinology 145: 3–7

Kanayama H, Naroda T, Inoue Y, Kurokawa Y, Kagawa S 1999 A case of complete testicular feminization: laparoscopic orchiectomy and analysis of androgen receptor gene mutation. International Journal of Urology 6: 327–330

Kolon T F, Ferrer F A, McKenna P H 1998 Clinical and molecular analysis of XX sex reversed patients. Journal of Urology 160: 1169–1172

Kommoss F, Oliva E, Bhan A K, Young R H, Scully R E 1998 Inhibin expression in ovarian tumors and tumor-like lesions: an immunohistochemical study. Modern Pathology 11: 656–664

Korsch E, Peter M, Hiort O et al 1999 Gonadal histology with testicular carcinoma in situ in a 15-year-old 46,XY female patient with a premature termination is the steroidogenic acute regulatory protein causing congenital lipoid adrenal hyperplasia. Journal of Clinical Endocrinology & Metabolism 84: 1628–1632

Lam S K, Yu M Y, To K F, Chan M K M, Chun T K H 1996 Ovarian epithelial tumour in gonadal dysgenesis: a case report and literature review. Australian and New Zealand Journal of Obstetrics and Gynaecology 36: 106–109

Lane A H, Donahoe P K 1998 New insights into Mullerian inhibiting substance and its mechanism of action. Journal of Endocrinology 158: 1–6

Lane A H, Lee M M 1999 Clinical applications of Mullerian inhibiting substance in patients with gonadal disorders. Endocrinologist 9: 208–215

Lima M, Domini M, Libri M 1997 Persistent mullerian duct syndrome associated with transverse testicular ectopia: a case report. European Journal of Pediatric Surgery 7: 60–62

Ludwig M, Beck A, Wickert L et al 1998 Female pseudohermaphroditism associated with a novel homozygous G-to-A (V370-to-M) substitution in the P-450 aromatase gene. Journal of Pediatric Endocrinology & Metabolism 11: 657–664

MacGillivray M H, Morishima A, Conte F, Grumbach M, Smith E P 1998 Pediatric endocrinology update: an overview. The essential roles of estrogens in pubertal growth, epiphyseal fusion and bone turnover: lessons from mutations in the genes for aromatase and the estrogen receptor. Hormone Research 49: 2–8

MacLean H E, Warne G L, Zajac J D 1997 Intersex disorders: shedding light on male sexual differentiation beyond SRY. Clinical Endocrinology 46: 101–108

McNeill S A, O'Donnell M, Donat R, Lessells A, Hargreave T B 1997 Estrogen secretion from a malignant sex cord stromal tumor in a patient with complete androgen insensitivity. American Journal of Obstetrics and Gynecology 177: 1541–1542

McPhaul M J, Griffin J E 1999 Male pseudohermaphroditism caused by mutations of the human androgen receptor. Journal of Clinical Endocrinology & Metabolism 84: 3435–3441

Magee A C, Nevin N C, Armstrong M J, McGibbon D, Nevin J 1998 Ullrich-Turner syndrome: seven pregnancies in an apparent 45,X woman. American Journal of Medical Genetics 75: 1–3

Martinez-Pasarell O, Nogues C, Bosch M, Egozcue J, Templado C 1999 Analysis of sex chromosome aneuploidy in sperm from fathers of Turner syndrome patients. Human Genetics 104: 345–349

Matsuki S, Sasagawa I, Kakizaki H, Suzuki Y, Nakada T 1999 Testicular teratoma in a man with XX/XXY mosaic Klinefelter's syndrome. Journal of Urology 161: 1573–1574

Mendez J P, Ulloa-Aguirre A, Kofman-Alfaro S et al 1993 Mixed gonadal dysgenesis: clinical, cytogenetic, endocrinological, and histopathological findings in 16 patients. American Journal of Medical Genetics 46: 263–267

Mendez J P, Canto P, Lopez M et al 1999 Scant XY qh-testicular cells with normal SRY was enough to differentiate bilateral testes in a 45,X/46,XYqh-patient. European Journal of Obstetrics, Gynecology and Reproductive Biology 87: 159–162

Mendes J R T, Strufaldi M W L, Delcelo R et al 1999 Y-chromosome identification by PCR and gonadal histopathology in Turner's syndrome without overt Y-mosaicism. Clinical Endocrinology 50: 19–26

Mendonca B B, Inacio M, Costa E M et al 1996 Male pseudohermaphroditism due to steroid 5alpha-reductase 2 deficiency. Diagnosis, psychological evaluation, and management. Medicine (Baltimore) 75: 64–76

Mendonca B B, Arnhold I J, Bloise W, Andersson S, Russell D W, Wilson J D 1999 17Beta-hydroxysteroid dehydrogenase 3 deficiency in women. Journal of Clinical Endocrinology & Metabolism 84: 802–804

Merry C, Sweeney B, Puri P 1997 The vanishing testis: anatomical and histological findings. European Urology 31: 65–66

Meyers C M, Boughman J A, Rivas M, Wilroy R S, Simpson J L 1996 Gonadal (ovarian) dysgenesis in 46,XX individuals: frequency of the autosomal recessive form. American Journal of Medical Genetics 63: 518–524

Moran C, Knochenhauer E S, Azziz R 1998 Non-classic adrenal hyperplasia in hyperandrogenism: a reappraisal. Journal of Endocrinological Investigation 21: 707–720

Morimura Y, Nishiyama H, Yanagida K, Sato A 1998 Dysgerminoma with syncytiotrophoblastic giant cells arising from 46,xx pure gonadal dysgenesis. Obstetrics and Gynecology 92: 654–656

Muroya K, Ishii T, Nakahori Y et al 1999 Gonadoblastoma, mixed germ cell tumor, and Y chromosomal genotype: molecular analysis in four patients. Genes Chromosomes Cancer 25: 40–45

Naguib K K, Al-Etreibi N N, Al-Awadi S A, El-Harbi M K, Kamal A S 1997 Complete testicular feminization syndrome with 47,XYY karyotype: a double hit phenomenon. Medical Principles & Practice 6: 216–221

Nazarenko S A, Timoshevsky V A, Sukhanova N N 1999 High frequency of tissue-specific mosaicism in Turner syndrome patients. Clinical Genetics 56: 59–65

New M I 1998 Diagnosis and management of congenital adrenal hyperplasia. Annual Review of Medicine 49: 311–328

New M I, Newfield R S 1997 Congenital adrenal hyperplasia. Current Therapy in Endocrinology & Metabolism 6: 179–187

Newfield R S, New M I 1997 21-hydroxylase deficiency. Annals of the New York Academy of Science 816: 219–229

Nomura K, Matsui T, Aizawa S 1999 Gonadoblastoma with proliferation resembling Sertoli cell tumor. International Journal of Gynecological Pathology 18: 91–93

Nowaczyk M J, Whelan D T, Heshka T W, Hill R E 1999 Smith-Lemli-Opitz syndrome: a treatable inherited error of metabolism causing mental retardation. Canadian Medical Association Journal 161: 165–170

Okada H, Gotoh A, Takechi Y, Kamidono S 1994 Leydig cell tumour of the testis associated with Klinefelter's syndrome and Osgood-Schlatter disease. British Journal of Urology 73: 457

Opitz J M 1999 RSH (so-called Smith–Lemli–Opitz) syndrome. Current Opinions in Pediatrics 11: 353–362

Park J P, Brothman A R, Butler M G et al 1999 Extensive analysis of mosaicism in a case of Turner syndrome: the experience of 287 cytogenetic laboratories. College of American Pathologists/American College of Medical Genetics Cytogenetics Resource Committee. Archives of Pathology and Laboratory Medicine 123: 381–385

Patsalis P C, Sismani C, Hadjimarcou M I et al 1998 Detection and incidence of cryptic Y chromosome sequences in Turner syndrome patients. Clinical Genetics 53: 249–257

Pierga J Y, Giacchetti S, Vilain E et al 1994 Dysgerminoma in a pure 45,X Turner syndrome: report of a case and review of the literature. Gynecologic Oncology 55: 459–464

Quigley C A, DeBellis A, Marschke K B, El-Awady M F, Wilson E M, French F S 1995 Androgen receptor defects: historical, clinical, and molecular perspectives. Endocrine Reviews 16: 271–321

Quilter C R, Taylor K, Conway G S, Nathwani N, Delhanty J D 1998 Cytogenetic and molecular investigations of Y chromosome sequences and their role in Turner syndrome. Annals of Human Genetics 62: 99–106

Radakovic B, Jukic S, Bukovic D, Ljubojevic N, Cima I 1999 Morphology of gonads in pure XY gonadal dysgenesis. Collegium Antropologicum 23: 203–211

Radmayr C, Culig Z, Hobisch A, Corvin S, Bartsch G, Klocker H 1998 Analysis of a mutant androgen receptor offers a treatment modality in a patient with partial androgen insensitivity syndrome. European Urology 33: 222–226

Rajpert-De Meyts E, Jorgensen N, Brondum-Nielsen K, Muller J, Skakkebaek N E 1998 Developmental arrest of germ cells in the pathogenesis of germ cell neoplasia. APMIS 106: 198–204

Rao E, Weiss B, Fukami M et al 1997 Pseudoautosomal deletions encompassing a novel homeobox gene cause growth failure in idiopathic short stature and Turner syndrome. Nature Genetics 16: 54–63

Rattanachaiyanont M, Phophong P, Techatraisak K, Charoenpanich P, Jitpraphai P 1999 Embryonic testicular regression syndrome: a case report. Journal of Medical Association of Thailand 82: 506–510

Regadera J, Martinez-Garcia F, Paniagua R, Nistal M 1999 Androgen insensitivity syndrome — an immunohistochemical, ultrastructural, and morphometric study. Archives of Pathology and Laboratory Medicine 123: 225–234

Rey R, Josso N 1996 Regulation of testicular anti-Mullerian hormone secretion. European Journal of Endocrinology 135: 144–152

Rich M A, Keating M A, Levin H S, Kay R 1998 Tumors of the adrenogenital syndrome: an aggressive conservative approach. Journal of Urology 160: 1838–1841

Rizk D E E, Ezimokhai M, Hussein A S, Gerami S, Deb P 1998 Persistent Mullerian duct syndrome. Archives of Gynecology and Obstetrics 261: 105–107

Robboy S J, Miller T, Donahoe P K et al 1982 Dysgenesis of testicular and streak gonads in the syndrome of mixed gonadal dysgenesis: perspective derived from a clinicopathologic analysis of twenty-one cases. Human Pathology 13: 700–716

Robboy S J, Anderson M C, Russell P 2002 Pathology of the female reproductive tract. Churchill Livingstone, London

Rutgers J L 1991 Advances in the pathology of intersex conditions. Human Pathology 22: 884–891

Rutgers J L, Scully R E 1991 The androgen insensitivity syndrome (testicular feminization): a clinicopathologic study of 43 cases. International Journal of Gynecological Pathology 10: 126–144

Rutgers J L, Young R H, Scully R E 1988 The testicular 'tumor' of the adrenogenital syndrome. A report of six cases and review of the literature on testicular masses in patients with adrenocortical disorders. American Journal of Surgical Pathology 12: 503–513

Salas-present in fetal and adult Sertoli cells and germ cells. International Journal of Developmental Biology 43: 135–140

Scully R E, Young R H, Clement R B 1998 Tumors of the ovary, maldeveloped gonads, Fallopian tube, and broad ligament. Armed Forces Institute of Pathology, Washington DC, pp 1–527

Shozu M, Akasofu K, Harada T, Kubota Y 1991 A new cause of female pseudohermaphroditism: placental aromatase deficiency. Journal of Clinical Endocrinology & Metabolism 72: 560–566

Sinnecker G H, Hiort O, Dibbelt L et al 1996 Phenotypic classification of male pseudohermaphroditism due to steroid 5 alpha-reductase 2 deficiency. American Journal of Medical Genetics 63: 223–230

Slaney S F, Chalmers J, Affara N A, Chitty L S 1998 An autosomal or X linked mutation results in true hermaphrodites and 46,XX males in the same family. Journal of Medical Genetics 35: 17–22

Smith N M, Byard R W, Bourne A J 1991 Testicular regression syndrome — a pathological study of 77 cases. Histopathology 19: 269–272

Spires S E 1999 Testicular regression syndrome: histologic recognition among pathologists. American Journal of clinical Pathology 112: 547

Swain A, Lovell-Badge R 1997 A molecular approach to sex determination in mammals. Acta Paediatrica 86: 46–49

Tanaka Y, Sasaki Y, Tachibana K et al 1994a Gonadal mixed germ cell tumor combined with a large hemangiomatous lesion in a patient with turner's syndrome and 45,X/46,X, +mar karyotype. Archives of Pathology & Laboratory Medicine 118: 1135–1138

Tanaka Y, Sasaki Y, Tachibana K, Suwa S, Terashima K, Nakatani Y 1994b Testicular juvenile granulosa cell tumor in an infant with X/XY mosaicism clinically diagnosed as true hermaphroditism. American Journal of Surgical Pathology 18: 316–322

Tateno T, Sasagawa I, Ashida J, Nakada T 1999 Deletion of Y chromosome involving the DAZ (deleted in azoospermia) gene in XX males. Archives of Andrology 42: 179–183

Telvi L, Lebbar A, Del Pino O, Barbet J P, Chaussain J L 1999 45,X/46,XY mosaicism: report of 27 cases. Pediatrics 104: 304–308

Uehara S, Funato T, Yaegashi N et al 1999a SRY mutation and tumor formation on the gonads of XY pure gonadal dysgenesis patients. Cancer Genetics & Cytogenetics 113: 78–84

Uehara S, Tamura M, Nata M et al 1999b Complete androgen insensitivity in a 47,XXY patient with uniparental disomy for the X chromosome. American Journal of Medical Genetics 86: 107–111

van Niekerk W A, Retief A E 1981 The gonads of human true hermaphrodites. Human Genetics 58: 117–122

Vanderbijl A E, Fleuren G J, Kenter G G, Dejong D 1994 Unique combination of an ovarian gonadoblastoma, dysgerminoma, and mucinous cystadenoma in a patient with turners syndrome — a cytogenetic and molecular analysis. International Journal of Gynecological Pathology 13: 267–272

Vanslooten A J, Rechner S F, Dodds W G 1992 Recurrent maternal virilization during pregnancy caused by benign androgen-producing ovarian lesions. American Journal of Obstetrics and Gynecology 167: 1342–1343

Vauthier-Brouzes D, Vanna Lim-You K, Sebagh E, Lefebvre G, Darbois Y 1997 Krukenberg tumor during pregnancy with maternal and fetal virilization: a difficult diagnosis. A case report. Journal de Gynecologie, Obstetrique et Biologie et la Reproduction (Paris) 26: 831–833

Veitia R, Ion A, Barbaux S et al 1997 Mutations and sequence variants in the testis-determining region of the Y chromosome in individuals with a 46,XY female phenotype. Human Genetics 99: 648–652

Vilain E, McCabe E R B 1998 Mammalian sex determination: From gonads to brain. Molecular Genetics & Metabolism 65: 74–84

Viner R M, Teoh Y, Williams D M, Patterson M N, Hughes I A 1997 Androgen insensitivity syndrome: a survey of diagnostic procedures and management in the UK. Archives of Diseases of Children 77: 305–309

Vlasak I, Plochl E, Kronberger G et al 1999 Screening of patients with Turner syndrome for 'hidden' Y-mosaicism. Klinische Padiatrica 211: 30–34

Winters J L, Chapman P H, Powell D E, Banks E R, Allen W R, Wood D P 1996 Female pseudohermaphroditism due to congenital adrenal hyperplasia complicated by adenocarcinoma of the prostate and clear cell carcinoma of the endometrium. American Journal of Clinical Pathology 106: 660–664

Zhu Y S, Katz M O, Imperato-McGinley J 1998 Natural potent androgens: lessons from human genetic models. Baillière's Clinical Endocrinology and Metabolism 12: 83–113

37

Development and anatomy of the placenta

B. Huppertz   M. Castellucci   P. Kaufmann

Early development of the human placenta   1233
Prelacunar stage   1233
Lacunar stage   1234
Early villous stages   1235

Basic villous structure and villous components   1236
Villous trophoblast   1236
Turnover and apoptosis of villous trophoblast   1239
Villous stroma   1242
Immunohistochemical markers for villous components   1245

Villous trees   1246
Structure of villous types   1246
Development of the villous trees   1249
Angioarchitecture of the villous trees   1249
Intervillous space and placentone architecture   1251
Three-dimensional interpretation of villous cross-sectional
    features   1253

Non-villous parts of the placenta   1253
Chorionic plate, umbilical cord, and membranes   1253
Basal plate and uteroplacental vessels   1257
Placental septa   1259
Cell columns and cell islands   1259
Extravillous trophoblast   1260
Fibrinoid   1261

Appendix: Brief description of developmental stages   1261

EARLY DEVELOPMENT OF THE HUMAN PLACENTA

PRELACUNAR STAGE

The development of the placenta begins as soon as the blastocyst implants. The implanting blastocyst, composed of 107–256 cells (Hertig 1960), is a flattened vesicle. Most of the cells make up the outer wall (trophoblast), surrounding the blastocystic cavity (Fig. 37.1a). Apposed to its inner surface is a small group of cells that form the embryoblast.

The embryonic, or implantation, pole of the blastocyst is attached to the endometrium first (Fig. 37.1a, cf. also Fig. 37.12). The usual implantation site is the upper part of the posterior wall of the uterine body, near to the mid-sagittal plane (Fig. 37.14a); for additional details see Boyd & Hamilton (1970) and Denker & Aplin (1990).

During attachment, and following invasion of the endometrial epithelium, the trophoblastic cells of the implanting embryonic pole of the blastocyst proliferate to form a double-layered trophoblast (Heuser & Streeter 1941). The outer of the two layers, directly facing the maternal tissue, is transformed into a syncytiotrophoblast by fusion of neighbouring trophoblast cells. The remaining cellular components of the blastocyst wall, which have not yet achieved contact with maternal tissues, remain discrete and are called cytotrophoblast (Fig. 37.1a,b). Throughout the following days, and with progressive invasion, additional parts of the blastocyst surface come into close contact with maternal tissues. This is followed by trophoblastic proliferation with subsequent fusion. The syncytiotrophoblastic mass increases by expanding over the surface of the implanting blastocyst as implantation progresses (Fig. 37.1b). At the implantation pole, it is not a smooth-surfaced mass but rather is covered with branching, finger-like extensions which deeply invade the endometrium. This first stage, lasting from day 7–8 post-conception, has been defined as the prelacunar period by Wislocki & Streeter (1938).

The syncytiotrophoblast has no generative potency. The cytotrophoblast acts as stem cells which guarantee growth of the trophoblast by continuous proliferation, with subsequent fusion to form the syncytiotrophoblast. The latter is a continuous acellular system, not interrupted by intercellular spaces and not composed of individual syncytial units. Terms such as 'syncytial cells' or 'syncytiotrophoblasts' are inappropriate.

LACUNAR STAGE

At day 8 post-conception, small vacuoles appear in the enlarging syncytiotrophoblastic mass at the implantation pole. The vacuoles quickly enlarge and become confluent to form a system of so-called lacunae (Fig. 37.1b–d). The separating lamellae, or pillars, of syncytiotrophoblast are called the trabeculae. Their appearance marks the begin-

ning of the lacunar or trabecular stage of placentation which lasts from day 8–13 post-conception. Lacuna formation starts at the implantation pole. With advancing implantation and expansion of the syncytiotrophoblastic mass the process extends all over the blastocyst within a few days.

At day 12 post-conception the blastocyst is so deeply implanted that the uterine epithelium closes over the implantation site (cf. Fig. 37.1c). At this time, the outer surface of the blastocyst is completely transformed into syncytiotrophoblast. At its inner surface, it is covered by a locally incomplete layer of cytotrophoblast. Since trophoblastic proliferation and syncytial fusion have started at the implantation pole, the trophoblastic wall is considerably thicker at this point, as compared to the anti-implantation pole (Figs 37.1c, 37.10, day 13 and 18). The thicker trophoblast of the implantation pole is later

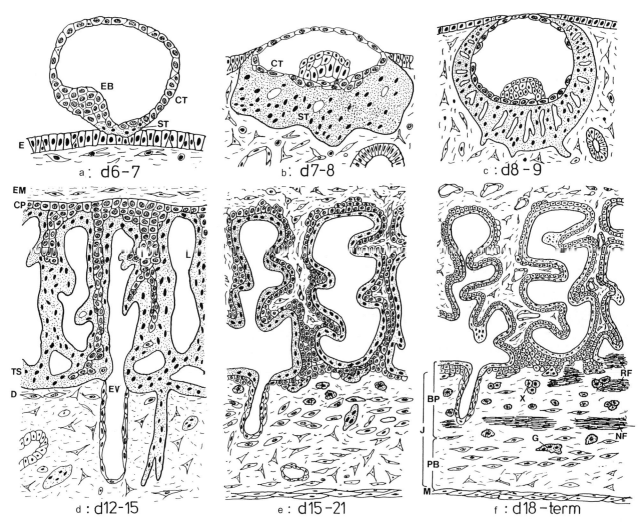

Fig. 37.1 Typical stages of early placental development: **a** and **b** prelacunar stages; **c** early lacunar stage; **d** transition from late lacunar to primary villous stage; **e** secondary villous stage; **f** tertiary villous stage. EB = embryoblast; CT = cytotrophoblast; ST = syncytiotrophoblast; E = endometrial epithelium; EM = extraembryonic mesoderm; CP = primary chorionic plate; T = trabeculae and primary villi; L = maternal blood lacunae; TS = trophoblastic shell; EV = endometrial vessel; D = decidua; J = junctional zone; BP = basal plate; PB = placental bed; M = myometrium; RF = Rohr fibrinoid; NF = Nitabuch fibrinoid; X = extravillous trophoblast (x cells); G = trophoblastic giant cell. (Modified with permission from Kaufmann & Scheffen 1992.)

transformed into the placenta, whereas the opposing thinner trophoblastic circumference only initially attempts to establish the same structure; later, it shows regressive transformation into the smooth chorion, the 'membranes' (Fig. 37.12, day 40). All data of placental development given in the following sections refers to the situation at the implantation pole.

Lacuna formation subdivides the trophoblastic covering of the blastocyst into three layers (Fig. 37.1d):

a. the primary chorionic plate, facing the blastocystic cavity;
b. the lacunar system, together with the trabeculae;
c. the trophoblastic shell, facing the endometrium.

The primary chorionic plate is composed of a more or less continuous stratum of cytotrophoblast. Towards the lacunae, the cytotrophoblast is covered by syncytiotrophoblast (Fig. 37.1d). At day 14 post-conception, mesenchymal cells spread around the inner surface of the cytotrophoblast layer (Fig. 37.1d). There they transform into a loose network of branching cells, the extraembryonic mesenchyme. Luckett (1978) found evidence that these primitive connective tissue cells were derived from the embryonic disc rather than being of trophoblastic origin.

Below the primary chorionic plate is the lacunar system. The lacunae are separated from each other by septa or pillars of syncytiotrophoblast, the trabeculae (Fig. 37.1c,d). Originally, these are solely syncytiotrophoblastic in nature. Around day 12 post-conception, however, they are invaded by cytotrophoblast cells (Fig. 37.1d), which are derived from the primary chorionic plate. Within a few days, the cytotrophoblast spreads down the entire length of the trabeculae. Where the peripheral ends of the trabeculae join together, they form the outermost layer of the trophoblast, the trophoblastic shell (Hertig & Rock 1941; Boyd & Hamilton 1970). In the beginning, this is a purely syncytiotrophoblastic structure (Fig. 37.1d), but as soon as the cytotrophoblast reaches the shell via the trabeculae (about day 15 post-conception), the former achieves a more heterogeneous structure (Fig. 37.1e).

In the early stages of implantation, the erosion of the maternal tissues occurs under the lytic influence of the syncytial trophoblast. The existence of cytotrophoblast at the base of the shell changes this situation. The proliferative activity of the cytotrophoblast and its rapid migration into the depth of the endometrium appear to be responsible for the further invasion and, thus, for the further expansion of the implantation area (Boyd & Hamilton 1970; Pijnenborg et al 1981). In the course of this process, numerous syncytial elements can be observed far removed from the trophoblastic shell (Fig. 37.1f), partly in the depth of the uterine wall. These multinuclear giant cells are derived from invading cytotrophoblast which later fuse (Park 1971; Robertson & Warner 1974; Pijnenborg et al 1981).

The endometrial stroma undergoes remarkable changes throughout this process. The presence of eroding trophoblast, by being a mechanical irritant and by hormonal activity, causes the endometrial stromal cells to proliferate and to enlarge, thus giving rise to the decidual cells (Welsh & Enders 1985).

The invasive activities of the basal syncytiotrophoblast cause disintegration of the maternal endometrial vessel walls from day 12 post-conception onwards, starting with the superficial capillary loops. Blood cells, leaving the altered capillaries, are found inside the lacunae (Boyd & Hamilton 1970). At the same time, the disintegrating capillaries are surrounded by the basally expanding syncytiotrophoblast, which gradually replaces the capillary walls (as revealed by animal studies; Leiser & Beier 1988). Further invasion of the trophoblast, with progressive destruction of the capillary limbs down to their arteriolar beginnings and their venular endings, provides the anatomical basis for the final formation of separate arterial inlets into the lacunar system as well as venous outlets.

Morphological (Hustin et al 1988) and clinical studies in the human using Doppler, ultrasound and endoscopy (Schaaps & Hustin 1988) suggested that true maternal blood flow in the normal human placenta is only established after the 12th week of pregnancy. In the earlier stages, it was postulated, only maternal plasma perfuses the intervillous space while the entrance of erythrocytes is blocked by cytotrophoblast plugs within the spiral arterial lumina. These data were controversial since they are difficult to bring into harmony with many other morphological, physiological and clinical data (for review see Moll 1995; Carter 1997). Today, most placentologists agree that during the first trimester a moderate flow of intervillous blood must be present resulting in generally hypoxic conditions. Only from the second trimester onwards is intervillous circulation fully established (Benirschke & Kaufmann 2000).

EARLY VILLOUS STAGES

Shortly after the first appearance of maternal erythrocytes in the lacunae, around day 13 post-conception, blindly ending syncytial side branches form which protrude into the lacunae (Fig. 37.1d,e). With increasing length and diameter, these so-called primary villi are invaded by cytotrophoblast. Both processes mark the beginning of the villous stages of placentation. Further proliferative activities, with branching of the primary villi, initiate the development of villous trees, the stems of which are derived from the former trabeculae. Where the latter keep their contact with the trophoblastic shell, they are called anchoring villi (Fig. 37.1e,f). At the same time, the lacunar system is, by definition, transformed into the intervillous space.

Only two days later, mesenchymal cells derived from the extra-embryonic mesenchyme of the primary chorionic plate begin to invade the villi, thus transforming them into secondary villi (Fig. 37.1e). Within a few days, the mesenchyme expands peripherally to the villous tips and to near the base of the anchoring villi (Wislocki & Streeter 1938; Boyd & Hamilton 1970). It does not, however, reach the trophoblastic shell which, during these early stages of placentation, remains free of fetal connective tissue.

Beginning between days 18 and 20 post-conception, the first fetal capillaries can be observed in the mesenchyme (Fig. 37.1f). They are derived from haemangioblastic progenitor cells which locally differentiate from the mesenchyme (King 1987; Demir et al 1989). The same progenitor cells give rise to groups of haematopoietic stem cells which are always surrounded by the early endothelium and are thus positioned within the primitive capillaries. The appearance of capillary cross-sections in the villous stroma marks the development of the first tertiary villi. Until term, all fetally vascularised villi can be subsumed under this name; these form the vast majority of the villi. Henceforth, only transitory developmental stages of new villus formation (trophoblastic and villous sprouts) correspond to primary or secondary villi.

At about the same time as the fetal vascularisation of the villi starts, the fetally vascularised allantois reaches the chorionic plate (Fig. 37.12) and fuses with the villous vessels. A complete feto-placental circulation is established around the beginning of the 5th week post-conception, as soon as enough capillary segments are fused with each other to form a true capillary bed. Also during the following weeks, in confined areas of the placenta, intravascular haematopoiesis may be observed.

The expansion of the early villous trees takes place in the following way (Castellucci et al 1990b, 2000): at the surfaces of the larger villi, local cytotrophoblast proliferation, with subsequent syncytial fusion, causes the production of syncytial sprouts. These are structurally comparable to the early primary villi, and are composed solely of trophoblast. Most of the syncytial sprouts degenerate, probably due to inappropriate local conditions, and only some are invaded by villous mesenchyme. Formation of fetal vessels within the stroma, with subsequent growth in length and width, is characteristic of the transformation into new mesenchymal villi. Along their surfaces new sprouts are produced.

Fetal and maternal circulations come into close proximity with each other as soon as an intravillous, i.e. fetal circulation, is established. Both bloodstreams are always separated by the placental barrier (Fig. 37.2c,d) which is made up of the following layers:

1. a continuous, uninterrupted layer of syncytiotrophoblast covering the villous surface and thus lining the intervillous space
2. an initially (first trimester) complete, but later (second and third trimesters) discontinuous layer of cytotrophoblast (Langhans cells)

3. a trophoblastic basal membrane
4. connective tissue
5. fetal endothelium, which is only surrounded by an ultrastructurally evident basal membrane in the last trimester.

Throughout the following periods of development, the tertiary villi undergo a complex process of differentiation, which results in various villous types which differ from each other in terms of structure and function. This differentiation process is paralleled by qualitative and quantitative changes of the placental barrier (cf. Table 37.1): the syncytiotrophoblast is reduced in thickness from more than 20 μm to a mean of 3.5 μm. The cytotrophoblast diminishes and, at term, can be found in only 20% of the villous surface. The mean villous diameter decreases since the newly formed villous types are generally smaller than those preceding. Because of this latter process, the intravillous position of the fetal capillaries comes closer to the villous surface with advanced maturation. In many places, the capillary basal lamina may even fuse with that of the trophoblast, thus considerably reducing the barrier in terms of thickness and number of layers.

In summary, all these factors result in a reduction of the mean maternal–fetal diffusion distance from between 50 and 100 μm in the second month to between 4 and 5 μm at term (Table 37.1).

BASIC VILLOUS STRUCTURE AND VILLOUS COMPONENTS

VILLOUS TROPHOBLAST

The basic morphology of the placental villi can be seen from Figs 37.2, 37.3. The maternal blood in the intervillous space is directly in contact with the syncytiotrophoblast which is the superficial layer of the placental villi. It must be pointed out that the syncytiotrophoblast is a continuous, uninterrupted syncytial layer (Fig. 37.3) that extends over the surfaces of all villous trees and is thus completely lining the intervillous space. The few reports that point to the existence of lateral cell membranes, subdividing the syncytium into 'syncytial units', appear to have an artifactual rather than a real basis. However, with advancing pregnancy, focal degeneration of the syncytiotrophoblast may occur, predominantly at the surfaces of the chorionic plate and the trophoblastic shell, but also at the villous surfaces. These local interruptions of the syncytiotrophoblast are closed within a few days by fibrinoid material mostly resulting from blood clotting (fibrin-type fibrinoid; Frank et al 1994). Below the syncytiotrophoblast varying numbers of cytotrophoblast cells (Langhans cells) can be found. The two components of the trophoblast layer are separated from the centrally located villous stroma by a basement membrane (Fig. 37.3).

Table 37.1 Summary of mean data on placental development. All data refer to the end of the corresponding week or to the end of the corresponding month of pregnancy.

week post conception (p.c.)	week post menstruation (p.m.)	month post menstruation (p.m.)	crown–rump length (Kaufmann, 1981)	embryonic/fetal weight (Kaufmann, 1981)	placental weight (Kaufmann, 1981)	placental weight per fetal weight (Kaufmann, 1981)	mean length of umbilical cord (Winckel, 1893)	mean placental diameter (Boyd & Hamilton, 1970)	placental thickness postpartum (Boyd & Hamilton, 1970)	placental thickness, incl. uterine wall by ultrasound (Johannigmann et al, 1972)	villous volume per placenta (Knopp, 1960)	villous surface per placenta (Knopp, 1960)	mean trophoblastic thickness (Benirschke & Kaufmann, 2000)	volume of fetal vessel lumina per villous volume (Kaufmann, 1981)	percentage of villous surface covered by Langhans cells (Kaufmann, 1972)	mean maternofetal diffusion distance (Kaufmann & Scheffen, 1992)
			mm	g	g	g/g	mm	mm	mm	mm	g (%)	cm²	μm	%	%	μm
	1															
	2	1														
1	3															
2	4															
3	5		2.5													
4	6	2	5				5									
5	7		9										18.9	2.7		55.9
6	8		14	1.1	6	5.5					5 (83%)	830			85	
7	9		20	2									19.1	3.0		
8	10	3	26	5	14	2.8										
9	11		33	11									21.6	4.0		
10	12		40	17	26	1.5					18 (29%)	3020			80	
11	13		48	23			160	50								
12	14	4	56	30	42	1.4			10							
13	15		65	40												
14	16		75	60	65	1.1	180	75	12		28 (43%)	5440		6.0	80	40.2
15	17		88	90			220	75								
16	18	5	99	130	90	0.69							11.6	6.3		
17	19		112	180												
18	20		125	250	115	0.46	300	100	15	28	63 (55%)	14 800		6.6	60	22.4
19	21		137	320			330	100								
20	22	6	150	400	150	0.38										
21	23		163	480												
22	24		176	560	185	0.33	350	125	18	34	102 (55%)	28 100			55	21.6
23	25		188	650			370	125								
24	26	7	200	750	210	0.28										
25	27		213	870												
26	28		226	1000	250	0.25	400	150	20	33	135 (54%)	42 200	9.7	9.1	45	
27	29		236	1130			420	150								
28	30	8	250	1260	285	0.23										
29	31		263	1400												
30	32		276	1550	315	0.20	450	170	22	43	191 (61%)	72 200			35	20.6
31	33		289	1700			460	170								
32	34	9	302	1900	355	0.19										
33	35		315	2100												
34	36		328	2300	390	0.17	490	200	24	45	234 (50%)	101 000	5.2	21.3	25	11.7
35	37		341	2500			500	200								
36	38	10	354	2750	425	0.15										
37	39		367	3000												
38	40		380	3400	470	0.14	520	220	25	45	273 (58%)	125 000	4.1	28.4	23	4.8

The trophoblastic mantle of the villi is the principal site for placental transfer and secretory functions. Most of these take place in the syncytiotrophoblast, whereas the underlying Langhans cells (Fig. 37.3b) act as proliferating stem cells that contribute to syncytiotrophoblastic growth by syncytial fusion (Fig. 37.4). Not only does syncytial growth depend on continuous incorporation of fusing cytotrophoblastic cells, but the regeneration of

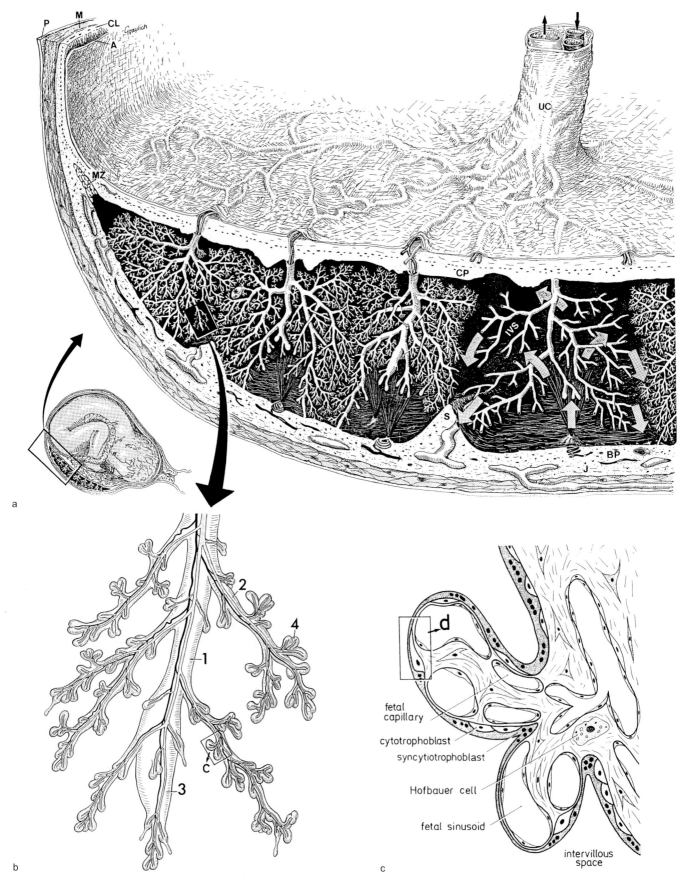

Fig. 37.2 Basic structure of the mature human placenta.

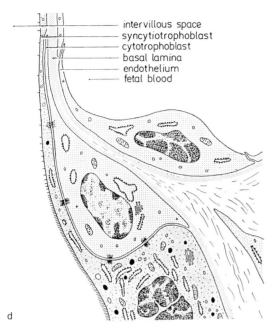

intervillous space
syncytiotrophoblast
cytotrophoblast
basal lamina
endothelium
fetal blood

d

Fig. 37.2 Basic structure of the mature human placenta.
a The maternal blood flow leaving the endometrial spiral arteries is directed into loose centres of the villous trees, so-called placentone centres. UC = umbilical cord; A = amnion; CL = chorion laeve; M = myometrium; P = perimetrium; MZ = marginal zone between placenta and fetal membranes, with obliterated intervillous space and ghost villi; CP = chorionic plate; IVS = intervillous space; S = placental septa; * = cell island, connected to a villous tree; BP = basal plate; J = junctional zone.
b Peripheral ramifications of a mature villous tree, consisting of a stem villus (1) which continues in a bulbous immature intermediate villus (3); the slender side branches are the mature intermediate villi (2); its surface is densely covered with grape-like terminal villi (4).
c Simplified lightmicroscopic diagram of two terminal villi, branching off a mature intermediate villus (right).
d Simplified electronmicroscopic diagram of the placental barrier, demonstrating its typical layers.
(a Reproduced with permission from Kaufmann & Scheffen 1992; **b–d** modified with permission after Benirschke & Kaufman 2000.)

degenerating syncytial organelles and enzyme systems does so as well (Pierce & Midgley 1963; Kaufmann et al 1983). Thus, the villous cytotrophoblast (Langhans cells) act as stem cells, proliferating, differentiating, and subsequently fusing with the syncytium (Fig. 37.4). Proliferation of the cytotrophoblast is regulated by the oxygen supply (Fox 1970), as in many other cell populations.

Corresponding to its functional pluripotency, the syncytiotrophoblast is structurally composed of mosaic-like patches (Fig. 37.3a) with varying ultrastructural and enzyme patterns:

1. The epithelial plates, or vasculo-syncytial membranes, offer a minimal maternofetal diffusion distance of 1–2 μm; these are the main sites of diffusional transfer of gases, water and the carrier transfer of glucose.
2. The thicker syncytial segments, with prevailing rough or smooth endoplasmic reticulum, are specialised areas for the secretion of proteo-hormones and placental proteins, metabolism of steroid hormones and maternofetal protein transfer.
3. The so-called syncytial knots and sprouts are very heterogeneous structures, characterised by accumulations of nuclei protruding into the intervillous space. Most of those found in histological sections are merely tangential sections of the villous surfaces (Fig. 37.10c) (Cantle et al 1987). The remaining true syncytial sprouts are direct evidence of trophoblastic proliferation as first steps of villus formation (Fig. 37.5). Syncytial knots are local aggregations of old, mostly apoptotic syncytial nuclei which have been accumulated within the syncytiotrophoblast by continuous incorporation of cytotrophoblast (Fig. 37.4f).

TURNOVER AND APOPTOSIS OF VILLOUS TROPHOBLAST

The villous syncytiotrophoblast has no generative potency. For its growth, repair and regeneration it depends on syncytial fusion of cytotrophoblast which represent the proliferating stem cells of the villous trophoblast layer (Richart 1961; Benirschke & Kaufmann 2000). Moreover, it has been shown that syncyntial fusion is used as a mechanism to transfer RNA from the trophoblastic stem cells into the syncytium, the latter showing downregulation of RNA synthesis (transcription) (Kaufmann et al 1983; Huppertz et al 1999a; for review see, Benirschke & Kaufmann 2000). In order to fulfil the syncytial needs for RNA-transfer, considerably more trophoblast cells fuse syncytially than are needed for syncytial growth. Aged excess nuclei are accumulated within the syncytiotrophoblast and are shed into the maternal circulation within 3 to 4 weeks after syncytial fusion (Huppertz et al 1998; Huppertz & Kaufmann 1999). These data lead to the suggestion that proliferation, differentiation, and syncytial fusion of villous cytotrophoblast are tightly regulated events, as is the 'aging' of syncytiotrophoblast with extrusion of excess nuclei.

Recently, evidence has been provided that the cascade of apoptosis is involved in this regulation. The data available show that the apoptosis cascade starts at the cellular stage of trophoblast, initiating subsequent syncytial fusion (Huppertz et al 1998, 1999a). Figure 37.6 demonstrates the apoptotic events found in villous trophoblast as related to turnover of villous trophoblast.

The presence of the tumour necrosis factor-receptor 1 (TNF-R1) on the cytotrophoblast (Yui et al 1996; Huppertz et al 1998) and of TNFα in cytotrophoblast (Lea et al 1997) and in fetal villous macrophages (Hofbauer cells) (Steinborn et al 1998) make it very tempting to speculate about a rôle of the TNFα/TNF-R1 system for induction of apoptosis in villous trophoblast. One of the very early events during apoptosis is the switch of phosphatidylserine from the inner to the outer leaflet of

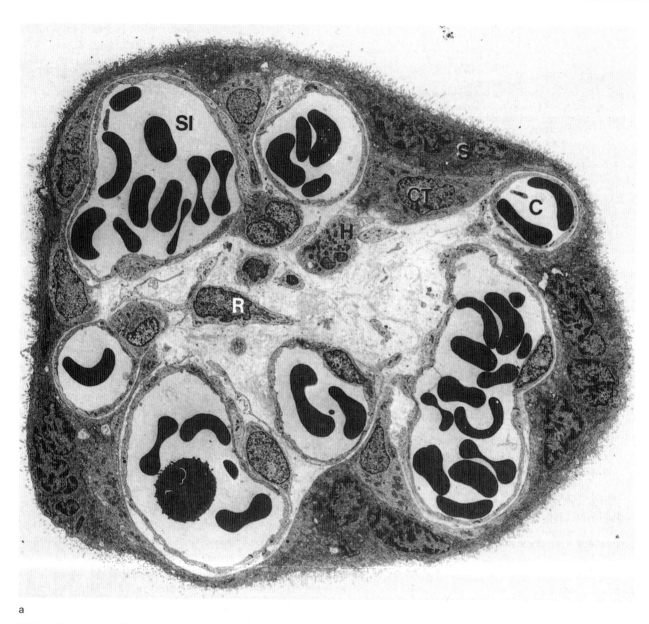

a

Fig. 37.3 a Ultrastructural features of a typical, well-fixed terminal villus. It illustrates the high degree of fetal capillarisation with narrow capillaries (C) and dilated sinusoids (SI). The sparse connective tissue is composed of fixed connective tissue cells (R) and macrophages (H), enmeshed in loosely arranged connective tissue fibres. The stromal core is surrounded by the outer syncytiotrophoblast (S) which is composed of mosaic-like patches which vary in structure and thickness. Below the syncytiotrophoblast a few Langhans cells (villous cytotrophoblast) (CT) can be seen.

the plasma membrane. This event, also known to be a prerequisite for syncytial fusion, has been shown to take place at least in some of the cytotrophoblast cells, maybe restricted to higher differentiated cells (Huppertz et al 1998). The switch of phosphatidylserine in some of the trophoblast cells makes it very likely that syncytial fusion in the villous trophoblast depends upon commencement of the apoptosis cascade in the cellular stage of trophoblast (Huppertz & Kaufmann 1999).

At the present time it is not known what controls syncytial fusion: whether it is only the stage of apoptosis of the cytotrophoblast or of both cyto- and syncytiotrophoblast. Ultrastructural findings have shown that matu-

ration of cytotrophoblast to highly differentiated cells as well as subsequent fusion, only takes place beneath syncytiotrophoblast that is largely void of ribosomes (Benirschke & Kaufmann 2000). Mi et al (2000) have shown that the retroviral fusogenic protein HerrW-env ('syncytin') is involved. As its receptor RDR, a neutral amino acid transporter was identified (for review see Pötgen et al 2002).

High levels of apoptosis inhibitors, such as Bcl-2 and Mcl-1, in cytotrophoblast as well as in areas of the syncytiotrophoblast (e.g. Sakuragi et al 1994; Huppertz et al 1998) lead to the assumption that syncytial fusion is also a mechanism to 'transplant' large numbers of these

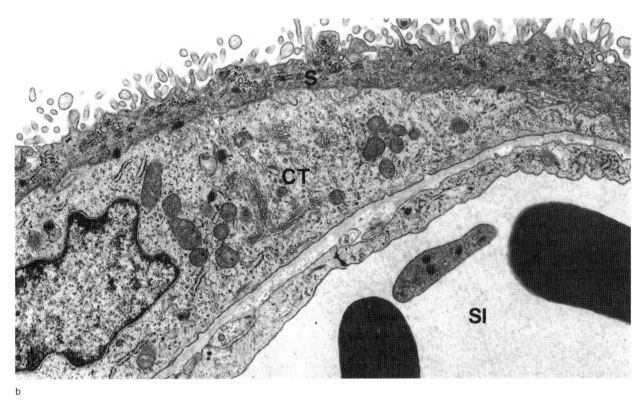

b

Fig. 37.3 b Higher magnification of a Langhans cell (CT) of the villus shown in **a.** Most of the Langhans cells belong to this undifferentiated type of proliferating or resting stem cell. (Reproduced with permission from Schiebler & Kaufmann 1981.)

proteins into the syncytiotrophoblast. In the cytotrophoblast the expression of these mitochondrial proteins enables the stem cells to make use of early apoptosis mechanisms for initiation of syncytial fusion without the need to irreversibly enter the execution stages of the apoptosis cascade. In the syncytiotrophoblast these inhibitory proteins provide the machinery to reversibly block the progression of the apoptosis cascade for a specific time interval. The time lapse between syncytial fusion and apoptotic extrusion of a particular nucleus has been calculated to be about two to three weeks (Huppertz et al 1998; Huppertz & Kaufmann 1999) showing that the blockage by transferred and/or de novo transcribed inhibitors must be highly effective.

The cytotrophoblast only displays the very early stages of apoptosis while the late and final stages of apoptosis are restricted to the syncytiotrophoblast. Typical characteristics of late apoptotic nuclei (condensed chromatin, annular localisation of chromatin and TUNEL positivity) are restricted to rather inconspicuous areas of the syncytiotrophoblast. These comprise degenerative syncytium mostly adjacent to fibrin-type fibrinoid (Yasuda et al 1995; Nelson 1996) and syncytial knots (Smith et al 1997; Huppertz et al 1998, 1999a,b; Mayhew at el 1999).

Apoptotic nuclei are aggregated as syncytial knots and are pinched off into the maternal circulation. The extruded nuclei had been postulated as 'aging nuclei' long

before, even though not discussed in terms of apoptosis (Martin & Spicer 1973; Jones & Fox 1977; Cantle et al 1987; Benirschke & Kaufmann 2000). The further fate of the syncytial knots remains open. They have been reported to impact in lung capillaries where they may undergo further breakdown and finally phagocytosis.

The findings and data listed above explain why the vast majority of trophoblast cells incorporated into the syncytiotrophoblast by syncytial fusion are not required for syncytial growth but rather are part of the apoptotic turnover of villous trophoblast. Relating proliferative activity to incidence of apoptosis in villous trophoblast, Huppertz et al (1998) concluded that throughout the third trimester only about 10% of the cytotrophoblast included by fusion is needed for growth of the villous surface, about 85% are shed again by apoptosis as syncytial knots into the maternal circulation. This may amount to up to 3 g trophoblast per day delivered into the maternal circulation.

It is well known that apoptosis requires a functional energy-producing system (Cotter et al 1990). Accordingly, this process takes place only in normoxic or slightly hypoxic pregnancies. Under severely hypoxic condition, the apoptosis cascade is interrupted and results in a secondary necrosis of syncytiotrophoblast (Huppertz et al 1999c). This necrotic material composed of syncytial knots and smaller syncytial fragments is also shed into the maternal blood.

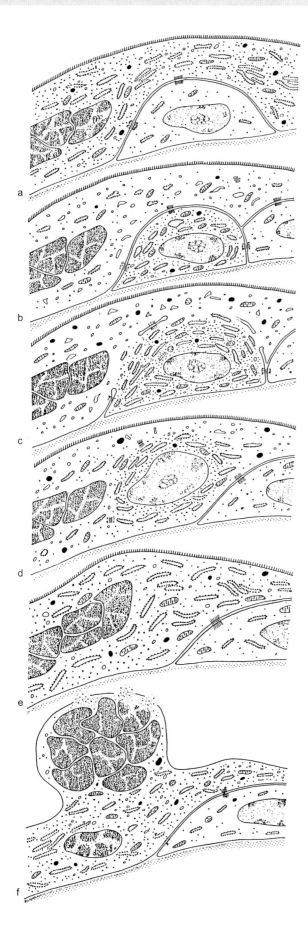

VILLOUS STROMA

The villous stromal core consists of fixed connective tissue cells, connective tissue fibres, macrophages (Hofbauer cells), occasional mast cells and fetal vessels.

The endothelium of the villous vessels (Fig. 37.3b) acts as a filter, limiting macromolecular transfer across the vessel wall to a certain molecular size (probably below 20 000 Dalton). The cells that surround the endothelium, i.e. the pericytes and smooth muscle cells, are thought to be active in vaso-regulation (Nikolov & Schiebler 1973). Since nerves have never been observed in the placenta, vaso-regulation must be accomplished by humoral means and/or by local mechanisms.

The connective tissue cells of the vessel adventitia shade into the components of the surrounding villous stroma, without any sharp demarcation line. We can differentiate between fixed stromal cells and Hofbauer cells. The former are responsible for the production of the extracellular matrix of the villous core. They show different morphological aspects related to the stromal architecture of the different villous types (see below).

The Hofbauer cells are fetal macrophages present throughout pregnancy in the human placenta (Figs 37.7c, and 37.8). The surface morphology of these cells is characterised by lamellipodia, blebs, and microplicae. Moreover they have numerous, large intracytoplasmic vacuoles in the first half of pregnancy. As gestation progresses these vacuoles decrease in number and size, and intracytoplasmic granules, probably lysosomes, become more apparent (Enders & King 1970; Castellucci et al 1980; Castellucci & Kaufmann 2000, review Vince & Johnson 1996). The vacuoles and the large lamellipodia have been considered to be involved in the reduction of the quantity of fetal serum proteins in the stroma of the villus. This view is in agreement with the fact that the placenta lacks a lymphatic system to return proteins from the interstitial space to the blood vascular system (Enders & King 1970; Castellucci et al 1984).

Fig. 37.4 Cytotrophoblastic contribution to growth and regeneration of syncytiotrophoblast. Below areas of syncytiotrophoblast which undergo loss of ribosomes (degranulation of the rough endoplasmic reticulum), Langhans cells start differentiation by developing a large number of organelles **a**, **b**. After disintegration of the separating cell membranes **c**, these organelles are transferred into the syncytiotrophoblast and thus regenerate the latter **d**. As soon as these organelles age again, this process starts anew. In this way increasing numbers of trophoblastic nuclei are accumulated in the syncytiotrophoblast **e**. The oldest are clustered as syncytial knots, thereafter protruded as 'syncytial sprouts' and finally extruded into the intervillous space **f**. (Reproduced with permission from Kaufmann 1983.)

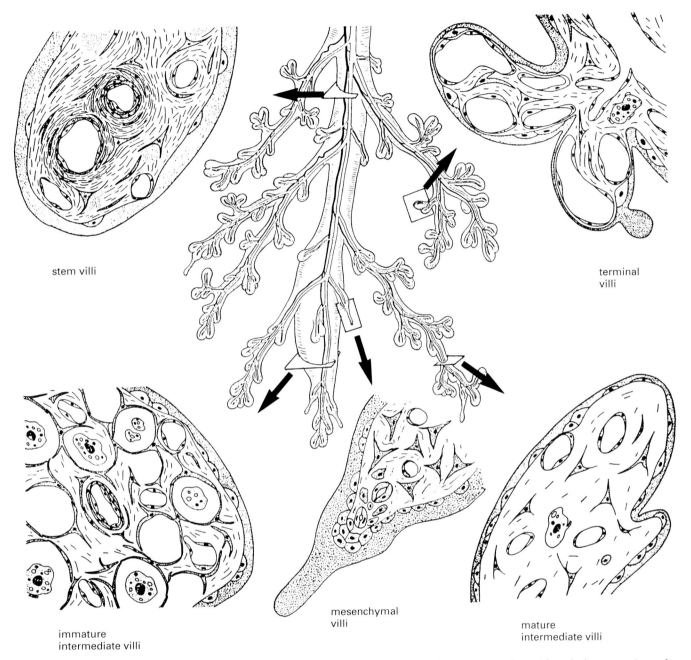

stem villi

terminal
villi

immature
intermediate villi

mesenchymal
villi

mature
intermediate villi

Fig. 37.5 Simplified representation of the peripheral branches of a mature placental villous tree, together with typical cross-sections of the five villous types. For further details see text. (Modified with permission after Kaufmann & Scheffen 1992.)

Concerning the immunological aspects of these cells, it has been demonstrated that they possess Fc receptors for IgG (Moskalewski et al 1975; Kameda et al 1991; Sedmak et al 1991), express CR3 (CD11) and are capable of immune and non-immune phagocytosis (Goldstein et al 1988; Zaccheo et al 1989). Hofbauer cells can express class I and II MHC determinants and, concerning the latter, first-trimester Hofbauer cells are rarely DR- and DP-positive; DQ antigens are not expressed (Bulmer & Johnson 1984; Goldstein et al 1988). Class II MHC antigens are acquired by increasing numbers of placental macrophages from the second

trimester onwards (Castellucci et al 1990a; Castellucci & Kaufmann 2000). Several CD (cluster of differentiation) antigens are expressed by the Hofbauer cells as, for example, CD4 and CD14 (Goldstein et al 1988; Zaccheo et al 1989). Immunohistochemical application of antibodies against macrophage specific antigens has indicated that more macrophages are present in the placental villi than is evident from histological and electron-microscopical studies. Hofbauer cells produce IL1 (Flynn et al 1982), which has diverse biological functions within and without the immune response (Platanias & Vogelzang 1990; Dinarello 1991). IL1 may regulate the remodelling

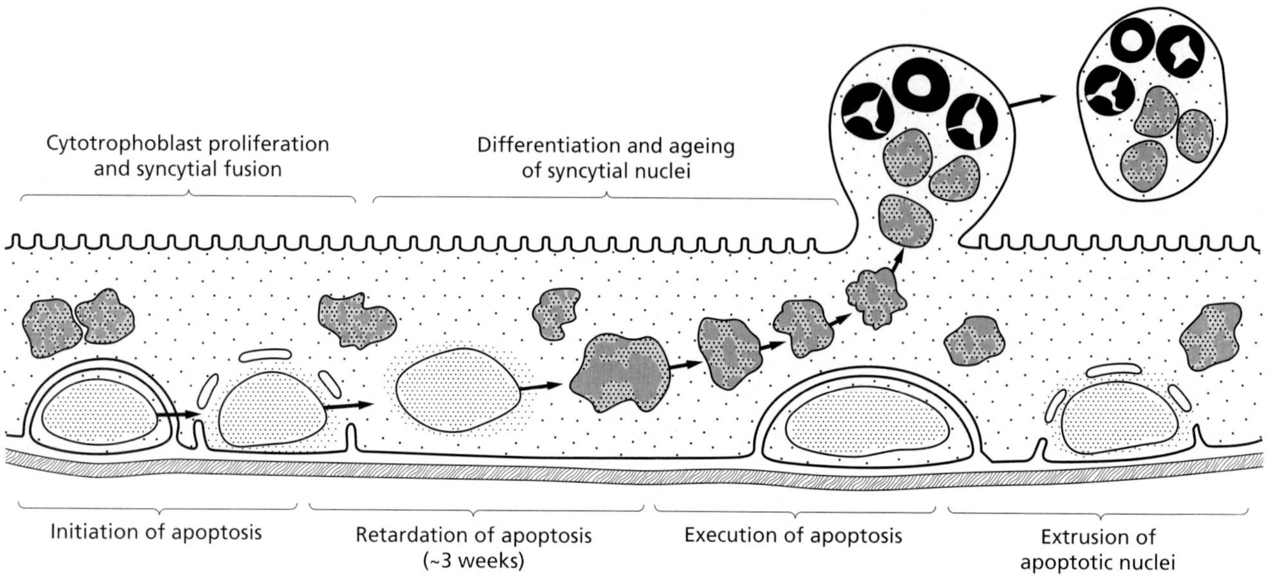

Fig. 37.6 The role of apoptosis for the turnover of villous trophoblast. Apoptosis of villous trophoblast is initiated already in the cytotrophoblast where it is involved in the fusion process. After syncytial fusion, the cascade is retarded and only after about 3 weeks the execution stages of the apoptosis cascade lead to the extrusion of old and apoptotic nuclei into the maternal circulation.

of the core of the placental villi by influencing the behaviour of villous fibroblasts (Glover et al 1987; Thornton et al 1990; Castellucci & Kaufmann 2000). Moreover, Hofbauer cells, it has been suggested, influence angiogenesis and vasculogenesis in the human placenta (Castellucci et al 1980; King 1987; Demir et al 1989).

IMMUNOHISTOCHEMICAL MARKERS FOR VILLOUS COMPONENTS

Several antibodies are available that may be used as easily applicable markers for the various villous components:

- trophoblast: anti-cytokeratin (Beham et al 1988; Daya & Sabet 1991)
- syncytiotrophoblast: anti-hPL (Beck et al 1986; Gosseye & Fox 1984); anti-βhCG (Kurman et al 1984a,b); anti-transferrin receptor (Yeh et al 1987; Bierings et al 1988); the monoclonal NDOG1 (Sunderland et al 1981)

- stromal cells: anti-vimentin (Khong et al 1986; Beham et al 1988)
- fibroblasts: anti-desmin (Beham et al 1988)
- smooth muscle cells, including myofibroblasts: anti-gamma-smooth muscle actin (Kohnen et al 1996); this antibody is also a useful marker for stem villi and their immature precursors which are the only villous types equipped with fully differentiated myofibroblast and smooth muscle cells
- macrophages (Hofbauer cells): anti-CD-14/anti-leu-M3 (Zaccheo et al 1989); anti-CD68 (Reister et al 1999)
- endothelium: anti-CD34/Qbend/10 (Kadyrov et al 1998); anti-von Willebrand factor (Jaffe 1987)
- fibrin-type fibrinoid (blood clot product): anti-fibrin (β-peptide) (Hui et al 1983; Frank et al 1994)
- matrix-type fibrinoid (fibrin-like extracellular matrix secreted by trophoblast): anti-oncofetal fibronectins/BC-1 or FDC-6 or blood group antigen precursor 'i' (Frank et al 1995)

Fig. 37.7 Semithin plastic sections of human placental villi. **a** This survey picture demonstrates the structural and staining variability of villous cross sections. s = stem villus; m = mature intermediate villus; t = terminal villus; * = tangential sections of villous trophoblastic surfaces; p = perivillous fibrin (fibrin-type ibrinoid); v = villous fibrinoid necrosis (mostly fibrin-type fibrinoid). (Reproduced with permission from Benirschke & Kaufmann 2000.) **b** Cross-section of a large stem villus, surrounded by smaller stem villi (s) and terminal villi (t). Note that the adventitia of the artery (above) and of the vein (below) continue directly into the surrounding villous stroma. Superficially, numerous smaller cross-sections of the paravascular capillary net of the stem villi are seen. (Reproduced with permission from Leiser et al 1985.) **c** Section of an immature intermediate villus from the 22nd week of pregnancy with its typical reticular stroma. The rounded, vacuolated macrophages (Hofbauer cells) are located in stromal channels which are devoid of collagen fibres and appear as empty holes (cf. Fig. 37.7). In faintly stained paraffin sections, such features can be misinterpreted as villous oedema. (Reproduced with permission from Kaufmann 1981). **d** Cross-section of the typical poorly vascularised mature intermediate villus. Note the peripheral position of the narrow capillaries and the loose connective tissue. (Reproduced with permission from Benirschke & Kaufmann 2000.) **e** Longitudinal section of a richly vascularised terminal villus. The capillaries are locally dilated making the so-called sinusoids. The latter protrude the trophoblastic surface forming epithelial plates. (Reproduced with permission from Kaufmann et al 1979.)

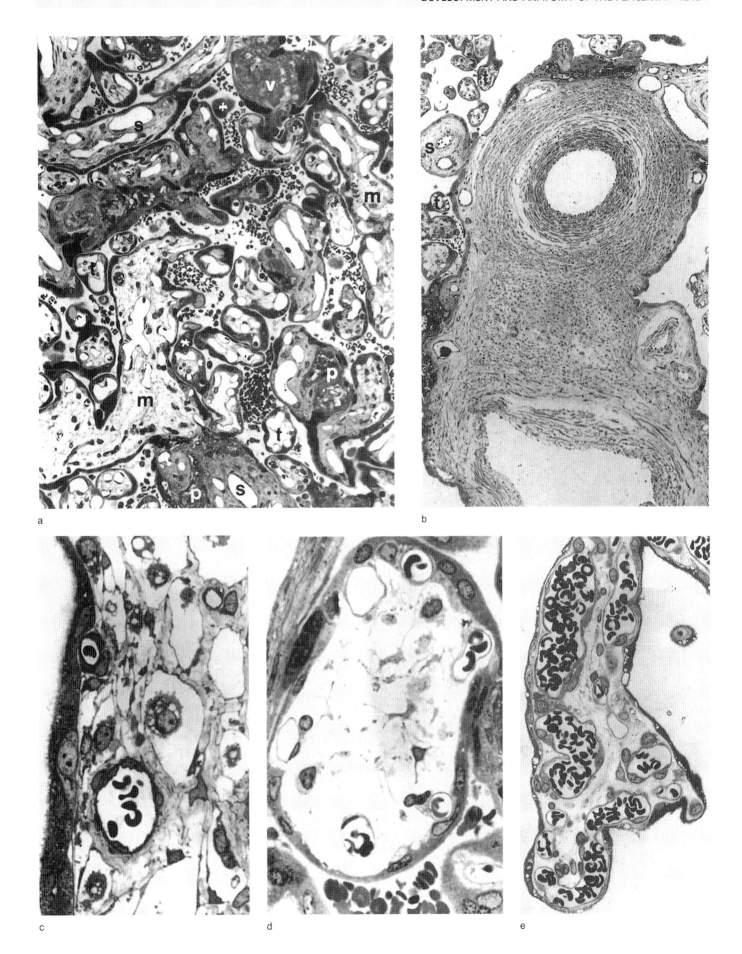

a

b

c

d

e

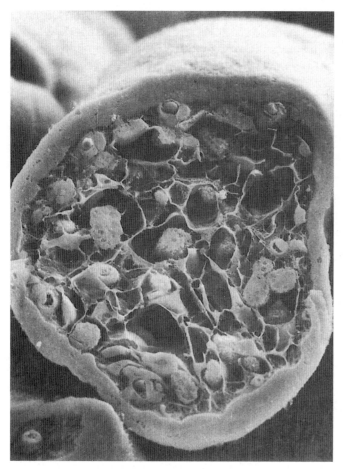

Fig. 37.8 Scanning electronmicrograph of a freeze-cracked immature intermediate villus demonstrating the three-dimensional view of reticular stroma with fixed connective tissue cells surrounding the stromal channels in which the macrophages can be found. (Reproduced with permission from Castellucci & Kaufmann 1982.)

VILLOUS TREES

STRUCTURE OF VILLOUS TYPES

The ramifications of the villous trees can be subdivided into segments which differ mainly in their calibre, stromal structure, vessel structure, and position within the villous tree (Figs 37.5, 37.7a). Five villous types have been described (Kaufmann et al 1979; Sen et al 1979; Castellucci & Kaufmann 1982; Kaufmann 1982; Castellucci et al 1984, 1990b; Burton 1987). Some can be further subdivided. As will be discussed, all villous types derive from single precursors, the mesenchymal villi, which correspond to the so-called tertiary villi of the early stages of placentation.

The following villous types can be histologically identified:

1. Stem villi (Figs 37.5, 37.7b) are characterised by a compact fibrous stroma, arteries and veins or arterioles, and by venules with a lightmicroscopically identifiable media and/or adventitia. Fetal capillaries are poorly developed and make up the so-called paravascular net (Arts 1961; Leiser et al 1985) which is underlying the trophoblast. The stem villi comprise the following structures:

a. the main stem (truncus chorii) (Fig. 37.13) of a villous tree which connects the latter with the chorionic plate (diameter 1000–3000 μm)

b. about four generations of short, thick branches (rami chorii) which are usually derived from the truncus already in the vicinity of the chorionic plate

c. up to 20 further generations of asymmetric dichotomous branchings (ramuli chorii) which are more slender branches (diameter ranging from 80–300 μm), extending into the periphery of the villous trees

d. a special group of stem villi is represented by the anchoring villi. These are ramuli chorii which connect to the basal plate by a cell column. The latter acts as the growth zone for this ramulus as well as for the basal plate.

The functional role of the stem villi is to support the mechanical stability of the villous tree and to provide the peripheral villi with fetal blood. About one-third of the total villous volume of the mature placenta is made up of this villous type.

2. Mature intermediate villi (Figs 37.5, 37.7d, 37.10b) are peripheral ramifications of villous stems, arranged in bundles of long, slender, multiply branching villi, their calibre at term ranging from 80 to about 120 μm. Most of their vessels are fetal capillaries, in between which are some small arterioles and venules. The vessels are embedded in a very loose connective tissue, with scanty fibres and cells, and occupy more than half of the villous volume. To their surfaces at least 95% of all terminal villi are connected (Fig. 37.10b,d). This demonstrates that these are the main sites of growth and differentiation of the terminal villi. As concluded from the increased degree of fetal vascularisation, their share in materno-fetal exchange cannot be ignored. Highly active enzyme patterns indicate their metabolic and endocrine activities. About 25% of the villous branches are of this type. The first typical mature intermediate villi are formed in the 25th week post-menstruation.

3. Terminal villi (Figs 37.3a, 37.5, 37.7e, 37.10b) are the final, grape-like ramifications of the intermediate villi, characterised by their high degree of capillarisation (>50% of the stromal volume) and the presence of highly dilated sinusoids, showing mean capillary diameters of about 14 μm and maximum values of more than 40 μm (Kaufmann et al 1985). Moreover, they are characterised by the presence of epithelial plates (Amstutz 1960) or vasculo-syncytial membranes. These are thinned anuclear syncytiotrophoblastic lamellae which are directly apposed to the sinusoidally dilated segments of the fetal capillaries (Fig. 37.3a).

One or a small group of terminal villi are connected to the intermediate villi by a narrow neck region (diameter about 40 μm), characterised by thin trophoblast surrounding a scant stromal core, most of which is occupied by two to four narrow capillaries. The extremely high degree of fetal vascularisation in the terminal villi and neck region, and the minimal materno-fetal diffusion distance of less than 4 μm, make this villous type the most appropriate for diffusional exchange. The terminal villous volume amounts to 30–40% of the villous tree. Terminal villi develop shortly after the first mature intermediate villi, roughly around the 27th week post-menstruation (Table 37.2).

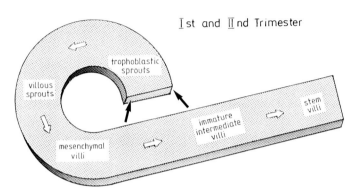

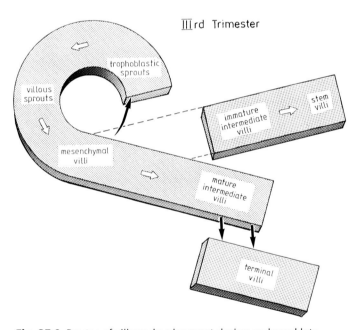

Fig. 37.9 Routes of villous development during early and late pregnancy. White arrows indicate the transformation of one villous type into another, whereas black arrows symbolise the formation of new villi along the surfaces of others. Throughout the first and second trimesters, trophoblastic sprouts are produced along the surfaces of mesenchymal and immature intermediate villi. They are transformed into mesenchymal villi and then differentiate into immature intermediate villi before they are transformed into stem villi. Throughout the third trimester, the mesenchymal villi become transformed into mature intermediate villi, which later produce terminal villi along their surfaces. The remaining immature intermediate villi continue to differentiate into stem villi. Thus their number steeply decreases towards term. Only in the centres of the villous trees may the villous developmental mode of the first and the second trimester persist until term. Because of this, the base for the formation of new sprouts is reduced and the growth capacity of the villous trees gradually slows. (Reproduced with permission from Castellucci et al 1990b.)

4. Immature intermediate villi (Figs 37.5, 37.7c, 37.8) are peripheral continuations of stem villi. They prevail in immature placentas and normally persist, in small groups, in the centres of the villous trees (placentones). They represent the immature forerunners of stem villi. By lightmicroscopy their typical structural feature is the presence of a voluminous reticularly structured connective tissue that is rich in Hofbauer cells and poor in fibres. As can be seen by electronmicroscopy, sail-like processes of the fixed stromal cells form a system of collagen-free intercommunicating channels oriented in parallel to the major axis of the villi (Castellucci & Kaufmann 1982). The Hofbauer cells lie mostly inside the channels. Functionally, the rôle of immature intermediate villi in the materno-fetal exchange at maturity should be negligible. Their main functions probably are, firstly, to act as precursors of the stem villi, into which they are continuously transformed, and secondly to produce villous sprouts.

Immature intermediate villi may cause diagnostic problems, since their reticular stromal core has only a weak affinity for conventional stains due to the lack of collagen. The resulting histological picture is that of a seemingly oedematous villus which has accumulated much interstitial fluid (cf. Fig. 37.16c,d). We believe that many villi referred to as 'oedematous villi' in the literature are in fact normal, immature intermediate villi. They can be very numerous in several pathological conditions in which villous development and differentiation is impaired, as in, for example, most cases of materno-fetal rhesus incompatibility (Pilz et al 1980; Kaufmann et al 1987).

5. Mesenchymal villi (Figs 37.5, 37.16d). These are the first tertiary villi. They prevail in the early stages of pregnancy, where they are the forerunners of immature intermediate villi. In the mature placenta, the mesenchymal villi are inconspicuous. They are transient stages of villous development, derived from villous sprouts. They differentiate either via immature intermediate villi into stem villi (first to second trimester), or directly into mature intermediate villi (third trimester). Structurally, the mesenchymal villi can be identified by their slender shape, by numerous Langhans cells, poorly developed fetal capillaries, and a connective tissue that consists mostly of large, poorly branched cells, surrounded by scanty bundles of connective tissue fibres. Immunohistochemically, they can be identified by the presence of tenascin (Castellucci et al 1991) and hyaluronic acid (Castellucci et al 2000) which are strongly expressed throughout the villous stroma.

DEVELOPMENT OF THE VILLOUS TREES

The five villous types described above represent different stages of development and differentiation of the villous trees (Fig. 37.9) (Castellucci et al 1990b). The process starts with trophoblastic sprouts which are produced by trophoblastic proliferation along the surfaces of mes-

Table 37.2 Summary of the structural and developmental characteristics of the five villous types from the 4th to the 40th week post-menstruation

Weeks post menstruation	Stem villi	Immature intermediate villi	Mesenchymal villi	Mature intermediate villi	Terminal villi
4			Only mesenchymal villi (120–250 μm) and trophoblastic sprouts (30–60 μm) are present. Large mesenchymal villi (>200 μm) may show diffuse and moderate stromal fibrosis.		
5					
6					
7		Within the mesenchymal villi, the first stromal channels appear.			
8		Numerous immature intermediate villi (100–200 μm) with reticular stroma; calibre of the largest vessels is 20–30 μm.	Numerous short mesenchymal villi (60–100 μm), partly continuous with slim trophoblastic sprouts, branching from the surfaces of immature intermediate villi.		
9					
10					
11		Increasing amount and size of immature intermediate villi (100–400 μm); calibre of stem vessels increased up to 100 μm; vessel walls with 2 to 3 concentric layers of cells.			
12					
13					
14		Lightmicroscopically apparent bundles of collagen fibres arranged around vessel walls.			
15					
16			The amount of mesenchymal villi and of trophoblastic sprouts is slowly decreasing.		
17	About 50% of all villi with calibres >150 μm show fusion of the fibrosed adventitial sheaths around the primitive arteries with those of the veins. This is the first step towards formation of the fibrosed stromal core of stem villi.				
18					
19	First true stem villi appear. Smaller ones (150–300 μm) show centrally fibrosed core with arterial and venous adventitia being fused. Those >300 μm show a largely fibrosed core.	Immature intermediate villi are still the dominating villous type. Those with calibres from 100–150 μm show no stromal fibrosis. The larger ones show fibrosis of the walls of larger vessels.			
20					
21			The number of mesenchymal villi with poorly fibrosed and poorly vascularized stroma, rich in cells, considerably increases. They grow in length and in width (calibres 80–150 μ) and show a continuous transition into mature intermediate villi.		
22					
23					
24	Calibre >300 μm: completely fibrosed stroma; calibre <300 μm: superficial layer of reticular stroma below the trophoblast.	Number and size of immature intermediate villi is decreasing.			
25			Typical mesenchymal villi are rare and mostly located near to immature intermediate villi.		
26					
27				Coiling of capillaries causes outpocketings of mature intermediate villi.	Local spot-like groups of first typical terminal villi appear; they show calibres of about 60 μm, about half of their stromal volume being occupied by capillary lumina. superficial rim of reticular
28				Mature intermediate villi with dense stroma, rich in stromal cells and poor in fibres, with calibres ranging from 100–150 μm are the dominating villous type.	
29	Calibre >200 μm: completely fibrosed stroma; calibre <200 μm: incomplete stroma.				
30					
31					
32		Still few evenly distributed immature intermediate villi can be found; the stroma is only partly reticular in nature.			Increasing amount of evenly distributed terminal villi with sinusoidally dilated capillaries and few epithelial plates.
33					

Table 37.2 (contd.)

	Stem villi	Immature intermediate villi	Mesenchymal villi	Mature intermediate villi	Terminal villi
Weeks post menstruation: 34 35 36 37 38 39 40	Usually, all stem villi are devoid of reticular stroma; however, below the trophoblast there still is a less densely fibrosed rim, rich in fibroblasts. All stem villi (except a few around the central cavity) are completely fibrosed. The trophoblast of the larger ones often is replaced by fibrinoid.	The few remaining immature intermediate villi are no longer evenly dispersed but rather concentrated as small groups in the centres of the villous trees lining the central cavities. The extremely loose reticular stroma shows only a few typical stromal channels.	Mesenchymal villi are histologically inconspicuous; the few identifiable ones are usually located around the central cavities.	The relative amount of mature intermediate villi is decreasing to about 25% of total villous volume. The calibre is reduced to 80–120 μm.	Terminal villi are the dominating villous type; they amount to about 40% of total villous volume.

enchymal and immature intermediate villi. Mesenchymal invasion into the trophoblastic sprouts leads to the formation of villous sprouts. As soon as capillaries are formed these villi are called mesenchymal villi. Until the 7th week post-menstruation, mesenchymal villi may progress directly to primitive stem villi. However, from the 8th week post-menstruation onwards, mesenchymal villi differentiate into immature intermediate villi, which produce ample new sprouts before they are transformed into stem villi (Fig. 37.9). From this date onwards, this is the only route for the formation of stem villi. As long as these processes are active, the placenta is rapidly growing though not differentiating.

This situation changes considerably during the third trimester, in which placental growth slows and villous differentiation starts. The mesenchymal villi no longer transform into immature intermediate villi but rather into mature intermediate ones which later produce terminal villi along their surfaces (Fig. 37.9). The remaining immature intermediate villi differentiate into stem villi. As a consequence, the number of immature intermediate villi steeply decreases towards term. Because of this fact, the base for the formation of new sprouts is also reduced, and the growth capacity of the villous trees gradually slows. Only in the centres of the villous trees (placentone centres) do some mesenchymal villi persist and continue to produce immature intermediate villi. It follows that at term these two villous types can only be found around the central cavity where they are responsible for the typical loose and apparently immature structure of the placentone centres (Fig. 37.2a) (cf. section on intervillous space and placentone architecture). There they serve as persistent growth zones of the villous trees (Schuhmann 1981).

The above described events at the beginning of the last trimester are the most important steps for understanding villous development. At this time, the transformation of newly formed mesenchymal villi into immature intermediate villi switches to a transformation of the former into mature intermediate villi (Fig. 37.9, Table 37.2). If this switch takes place early in gestation, the placenta differentiates prematurely but stops growing too soon, due to the deficit of immature intermediate and mesenchymal villi. By contrast, if the switch is delayed, the placenta is characterised by persisting immaturity and striking growth since immature, quickly growing villi prevail.

ANGIOARCHITECTURE OF THE VILLOUS TREES

Large fetal arteries and veins are restricted to the main stem villi (Fig. 37.7b), whereas arterioles and venules are mainly located in the smaller stem villi, as well as in mature and immature intermediate villi (Kaufmann et al 1985; Leiser et al 1985). All of the above larger fetal vessels are accompanied by a system of long, slender capillaries, the so-called paravascular net (Arts 1961). In the mature, intermediate villi, the arterioles and venules turn into long coiled terminal capillary loops. In areas of maximum coiling, the capillaries stretch the surface of the mature intermediate villi, producing bulges, the terminal villi. This mechanism takes place in the course of the last trimester. As soon as the longitudinal growth of the capillaries exceeds that of the mature intermediate villi, the capillaries coil and cause the protrusion of the terminal villi. This process is accentuated under hypoxic conditions when capillary growth is stimulated (Bacon et al 1984), resulting in a higher number of multiply branched terminal villi (Tenny-Parker changes) (cf. Fig. 37.10c,d) (Jackson et al 1987; Kaufmann et al 1987, 1988).

Particularly within the terminal villi, the capillaries may dilate considerably, thus forming sinusoids (Figs 37.3a,

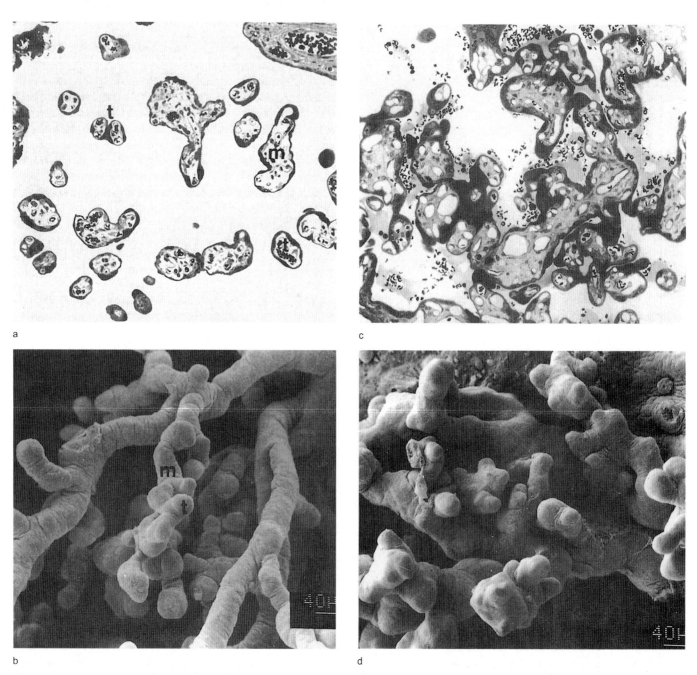

a

c

b

d

Fig. 37.10 Comparison of cross-sectional features with the three-dimensional shape of the villi. **a** and **b** Normal mature placenta. Sectioning of slender mature intermediate villi (m) covered with grape-like terminal villi (t) like those in the scanning electronmicrograph **b** results in numerous roundish to oval villous sections **a** and only a few trophoblastic flat sections, so-called sprouts and bridges. **c** and **d** Severe pre-eclampsia near term. Multiply indented, fist-like terminal villi branching off irregularly shaped mature intermediate villi like those in the scanning electronmicrograph **d** increase the chance of flat sectioning across trophoblastic surfaces. The resulting picture **c** is that of a seemingly net-like system with numerous trophoblastic 'sprouts' and 'bridges'. (Reproduced with permission from Kaufmann et al 1987.)

37.7e). One capillary loop may supply several terminal villi 'in series', dilating and narrowing several times for each single terminal villus. The main function of the sinusoids is probably to reduce blood flow resistance and, thus, to guarantee an even blood supply to the long terminal capillary loops (mean 4000 μm) and the shorter paravascular capillaries (1000 μm) (Kaufmann et al 1985). There is no convincing proof for the earlier view that the sinusoids are dilated, specialised venous parts of the capillary loops, which were thought to increase the maternofetal exchange rate by reducing the blood flow velocity.

Normal oxygen supply during pregnancy leads to a balanced growth and maturation of vessels and villi resulting in mature intermediate villi with capillary loops bulging into the terminal villi (Fig. 37.11). Under reduced oxygen concentrations (e.g. maternal anaemia, pregnancy at high altitude) the mature intermediate villi show increased branching angiogenesis, resulting in an increased number of highly branched terminal villi

(Fig. 37.11). In contrast, under elevated oxygen levels (e.g. intrauterine growth restriction with absent or reversed enddiastolic blood flow in the umbilical arteries) the mature intermediate villi remain largely unbranched ending in a single terminal villus (Fig. 37.11). This is a result of predominance of non-branching angiogenesis (Kingdom & Kaufmann 1997; Todros et al 1999).

INTERVILLOUS SPACE AND PLACENTONE ARCHITECTURE

The human placenta is of the haemochorial, villous type. After leaving the spiral arteries, the maternal blood circulates through the diffuse intervillous space and flows directly around the villi (Fig. 37.2a). Most anatomical investigations of the intervillous space have been made on delivered placentas which are no longer exposed to the in vivo effect of maternal blood pressure distending the intervillous space. Therefore, the usual appearance of the

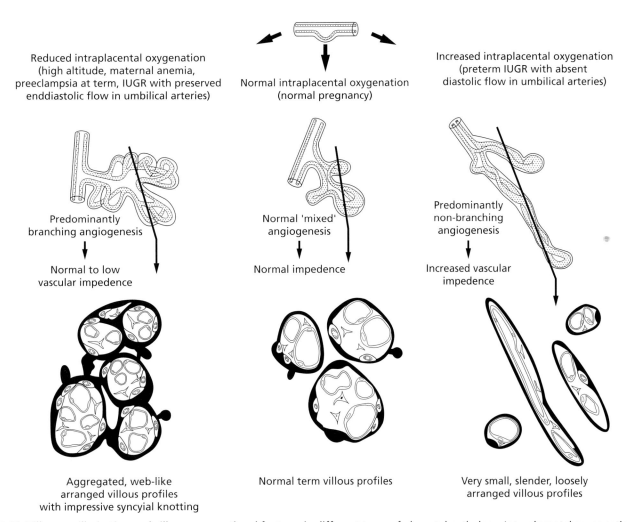

Fig. 37.11 Villous capillarisation and villous cross-sectional features in different types of placental pathology. Intraplacental oxygenation is critical for capillary development: Hypoxia causes branching angiogenesis (left). Abnormally good oxygenation induces non-branching angiogenesis (right). Normal placental oxygenation results in a mixture of both (central pathway). The differences in vascular geometry are reflected by obvious differences in villous cross-sectional features.

intervillous space of the delivered placenta is that of a system of extremely narrow clefts. Calculations based on intervillous blood volume and villous surface make it likely that the mean width ranges between 16 and 32 μm (Benirschke & Kaufmann 2000).

Wigglesworth (1967) studied corrosion casts of fetal vessels and suggested that most villous trees are arranged as hollow-centered bud-like structures. When he injected the spiral arteries, he found that the injection mass collected in the loose centres of the villous trees. This is in agreement with Schuhmann's description of the 50–100 maternal arterial inlets as being located near the centres of the villous trees (Schuhmann & Wehler 1971; Schuhmann 1981). The 50–200 maternal venous outlets per placenta are thought to be arranged around the periphery of the villous trees. Thus, each feto-maternal circulatory unit is composed of one villous tree with a corresponding, centrifugally perfused, part of the intervillous space (Fig. 37.2a). This unit was called a 'placentone' by Schuhmann & Wehler (1971). Most placentologists agree that, under in vivo conditions, the majority of the 40–60 placentones are in contact with each other and that they overlap more or less broadly, since structural borderlines, such as real placental septa, are absent (Becker & Jipp 1963). It is our experience that the peripheral placentones are more clearly separated from each other and thus exhibit typical structural differences between their central and their peripheral zones. In the thicker, more central regions of the placenta, most villous trees overlap. This causes less distinct differences between maternal inflow and outflow areas of the placentone.

According to Schuhmann & Wehler (1971), the centres of typical placentones exhibit loosely arranged villi, mostly of the immature intermediate type, and provide a large intervillous space for the maternal arterial inflow. Schuhmann (1981) suggested that these central cavities are pressure-dependent in vivo structures which rapidly collapse after delivery. Sonographic findings support this view. According to Moll (1981) the central cavity guarantees fast and homogeneous distribution of blood into the surrounding mantle of smaller, more densely packed villi of mature intermediate and terminal type, without much loss of pressure (Fig. 37.2a).

The perilobular zone of a placentone is that loosely arranged area of mature intermediate and terminal villi which separates neighbouring villous trees and which, subchorially, is connected to the subchorial lake. This is the venous outflow area.

The radioangiographic studies of Ramsey et al (1963) in the rhesus monkey, and of Borell et al (1958) in human placentas, are consistent with the placentone concept. Physiological studies concerning the intervillous circulation (Moll 1981; Schmid-Schönbein 1988) indicate that the actual filling velocities of the central cavities amount only to a few centimeters per second. After passage of the central cavity, a subsequent rather slow centrifugal spreading of the blood towards the subchorial and peripheral zone is observed. Wallenburg et al (1973) ligated single spiral arteries in rhesus monkeys and obtained obliteration of the intervillous space and degeneration of the corresponding villous tree. This experiment demonstrates that each villous tree depends on its own spiral artery. Even though the intervillous space is a widely open, freely communicating system, villous arrangement and pressure gradients are co-ordinated in such a way that blood perfusion depends strictly on the original flow arrangement. Reversal of the direction seems to be impossible.

If one accepts these considerations, the zones of highest pO_2 in the intervillous space are in the placentone's centres where the immature intermediate villi, together with their sprouting mesenchymal side branches, are concentrated. ^{3}H-thymidine incorporation is twice as high in the placentone centre as in the periphery (Geier et al 1975). This is in seeming contrast to experimental and histological findings which suggested that low oxygen concentration serves as a stimulus for trophoblastic proliferation and villous sprouting (Alvarez 1967; Alvarez et al 1970; Fox 1970). The most likely explanation for this discrepancy is that oxygen delivery to the centrally located, large villi in the central cavity and its vicinity is reduced, due to high blood flow velocity and long diffusion distances. The surrounding densely packed mantle of the placentone, although located nearer the venous pole, probably has the much higher oxygen delivery since blood flow velocity is reduced in the slender intervillous clefts and diffusion distances are short. This results in high mean pO_2 values at the villous surfaces and supports effective materno-fetal oxygen transfer. At the same time, it inhibits villous proliferation and stimulates villous differentiation.

Whereas the centre of the placentone acts as a proliferative zone which guarantees placental growth until term, the periphery is the functionally fully active exchange and secretory area. This has also been demonstrated histochemically and biochemically by the higher activity of enzymes such as alkaline phosphatase (Schuhmann et al 1976), and by the higher conversion rate of steroid hormones (Lehmann et al 1973) in the placentones' periphery.

In most placentas, the immature placentone centres are present until term, at least in the more peripheral areas of the organ. Due to their size and distribution they are rarely present in routine histological sections. Only in cases of preterm maturation of the placenta (hypermaturity, maturitas praecox) do we regularly find mature placentone centres. Thus, such a placenta has lost its capacity to grow since only the immature intermediate villi and their immediate mesenchymal branches are able to sprout and act as growth zones.

For the histopathologist, the heterogeneity of the villous tree causes considerable problems. Since the average diameter of a placentone is two to four centimetres, histological sections will often not cover a representative part of the placentone and may not include both the immature growth zones and the highly differentiated mature tissue. Prevalence of one or the other tissue may influence the diagnosis. This danger is even greater when one considers that neighbouring villous trees may show varying degrees of maturation. This is of particular importance when performing morphometric evaluations of the placenta. Burton (1987) remarked: '. . . strict attention must be paid to the sampling regime if meaningful results are to be obtained. Sadly this has not always been taken into consideration in the past, and so many of the published claims must be qualified accordingly'. This problem is greater still when one uses small tissue samples — for example, those obtained from the placenta at Caesarean section (Schweikhart & Kaufmann 1977) or by chorionic biopsy.

THREE-DIMENSIONAL INTERPRETATION OF VILLOUS CROSS-SECTIONAL FEATURES

Placental histopathology is based on the lightmicroscopy of paraffin sections. Thus, the normal and pathological features of the placenta are usually described in terms of the two dimensions apparent in the lightmicroscope. The studies by Küstermann (1981), using reconstructions of serial paraffin sections, and by Burton (1986a,b, 1987), working with plastic serial sections, as well as those by Cantle et al (1987) and Kaufmann et al (1987), comparing lightmicroscopy of villous sections with scanning electromicroscopy of comparable and identical material, revealed that the two-dimensional impression does not always reflect the real three-dimensional structure.

This is particularly true for the so-called syncytial knots (aggregations of apoptotic syncytial nuclei), syncytial sprouts (mushroom-shaped syncytial protrusions with aggregated nuclei due to villous sprouting), and syncytial bridges (syncytiotrophoblastic connections between neighbouring villi), most of which prove to be only tangential sections of the villous surface. Their true interpretation is of importance for placental pathology since the histological appearance of syncytial sprouts, for example, is often accepted as a diagnostic indicator of placental ischaemia (Alvarez et al 1964, 1969, 1970; Schuhmann & Geier 1972). Burton (1986a) and Cantle et al (1987) have shown that most of the above mentioned structures were flat sections but that also occasional true sprouts, knots and bridges were present. At the same time, it became apparent (Kaufmann et al 1987) that the diagnostic value of the so-called sprouts, even though mainly trophoblastic flat sections, was still useful. These are significant 'sectional artifacts' which point to a characteristic deformation of the terminal villi (Tenny-Parker changes). It became evident from Cantle's material (1987) that branching, twisting, and coiling of villi (e.g. as a result of hypoxia) enhances the chance of tangential sectioning of

trophoblastic surface (Fig. 37.10a–d). Since this deformation is usually caused by ischaemia the above conclusions drawn by Alvarez et al (1969, 1970) are generally correct. The diagnostic value of the two-dimensional finding of 'syncytial sprouts' still remains.

Although most knots, sprouts and bridges in the mature placenta must be considered sectional artifacts, there is a certain proportion of true syncytial protrusions. These trophoblastic specialisations may serve as first steps of villous sprouting (sprouts), i.e. formation of new villi (Fig. 37.5) (Boyd & Hamilton 1970; Cantle et al 1987; Castellucci et al 1990b), as a mechanism of extrusion of old syncytial nuclei (knots) (Fig. 37.4f) (Martin & Spicer 1973; Jones & Fox 1977), or as simple mechanical aids to establish junctions between neighbouring villi (bridges) (Cantle et al 1987). Generally, in the young placenta, the majority of sprouts are true trophoblastic outgrowths. In paraffin sections of the mature placenta, the vast majority of these structures are artifacts due to thick sectioning and villous deformation (Fig. 37.10a–d).

The question of how to interpret 'knots', 'sprouts', and 'bridges' relates to the more relevant question of how to interpret villous shapes and branching patterns three-dimensionally. Burton (1986a) showed that three factors increase the chance of tangential sectioning of villi. These are branching, curving, and superficial notching. Long, slender, stretched villi (e.g. derived from a slightly immature placenta of about 32–36 weeks menstrual age) have an extremely low incidence of tangential sectioning. Thicker, bulbous villi, as in the early stages of pregnancy (Fig. 37.16a–d), gestational diabetes mellitus, persisting immaturity at term, and rhesus incompatibility, may show some more tangential sections due to the irregular surfaces of the bulbous immature intermediate villi. However, these cases also show an increased incidence of real trophoblastic sprouting as the first step of formation of new villi. The normal mature placenta, which has numerous short terminal villi branching from the surfaces of the mature intermediate villi (Fig. 37.10a,b), has a slightly higher incidence. The hypoxic, hypercapillarised placenta (e.g. pre-eclampsia) is characterised by multiply branched, fist-like terminal villi (Fig. 37.10d); it shows such a degree of flat sectioning that the two-dimensional picture may achieve a net-like appearance (Fig. 37.10c), in which most terminal villi are seemingly connected to each other by syncytial 'bridges'.

NON-VILLOUS PARTS OF THE PLACENTA

CHORIONIC PLATE, UMBILICAL CORD, AND MEMBRANES

The development of the chorionic plate, the umbilical cord and the membranes is closely related to that of the amnion. Throughout the last days of the 2nd week post-conception, the blastocystic cavity is being filled by a loose meshwork of mesoderm cells, the so-called extra-embryonic mesoblast, which surrounds the embryoblast (Fig. 37.12, day 13). The embryoblast is composed of two vesicles, the amnionic vesicle and the primary yolk sac.

Where both vesicles are in contact with each other, they form the double-layered embryonic disc. During the course of the following days, the extra-embryonic meso-derm cells are rearranged in such a way that they only

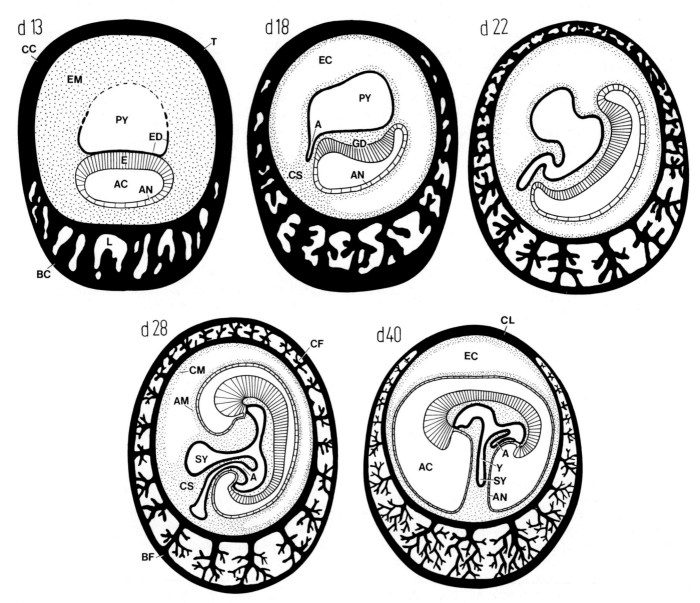

Fig. 37.12 Highly simplified, not true to scale, drawing of the development of the umbilical cord and amnion. Day 13 post-conception: the embryonic disc consists of two epithelial layers — the ectoderm (E), which is contiguous with the amnionic epithelium (AN) and surrounds the amnionic cavity (AC), and the entoderm (ED), which partially surrounds the primary yolk sac cavity (PY). Both vesicles are surrounded by the extra-embryonic mesoderm (EM) and by the trophoblast (black) which shows some lacunar spaces (L). BC = basal chorion; CC = capsular chorion; T = trophoblast. Day 18 post-conception: at this stage at the presumptive caudal end of the germinal disk (GD), the allantoic invagination (A) has occurred. In the extra-embryonic mesoderm, the exocoelom (EC) has cavitated. A mesenchymal bridge has developed that will ultimately form the umbilical cord, the 'connecting stalk' (CS). Day 22 and day 28 post-conception: the embryo has begun to rotate and fold. The primary yolk sac is being subdivided into the intra-embryonic intestinal tract and the secondary (extra-embryonic) yolk sac (SY). Secondary yolk sac and allantois extrude from the future embryonic intestinal tract into the connecting stalk. The amnionic cavity amnionic mesoderm (AM) and chorionic mesoderm (CM) largely surround the embryo because of its folding and rotation. Villous formation has occurred at the entire periphery of the chorionic vesicle, forming the so-called chorion frondosum (CF). BF = basal chorion frondosum. Day 40 post-conception: the embryo has now fully rotated and folded. It is completely surrounded by the amnionic cavity. The umbilical cord has developed from the connecting stalk, as it has become covered by amnionic membrane. The exocoelom has become largely compressed by the expansion of the amnionic cavity. At the abembryonic pole of the chorionic vesicle, the recently formed placental villi gradually atrophy, thus forming the chorion laeve (CL). Only that portion which retains villous tissue, that which has the insertion of the umbilical cord, develops into the placental disc. Y = omphalo-mesenteric duct. (Modified with permission after Benirschke & Kaufmann 2000.)

line the inner surface of the primary chorionic plate and the surfaces of the two embryonic vesicles (Fig. 37.12, day 18). Between both mesoderm layers the exocoelom cavity forms. It largely separates the embryo, together with its mesodermal cover, from the chorionic mesoderm. The exocoelom is only bridged by the mesoderm in one place, which lies basal to the amnionic vesicle. This mesenchymal connection is referred to as the connecting stalk: this is the early forerunner of the umbilical cord and fixes the early embryo to the membranes.

During the same period (around day 18 post-conception), a duct-like extension of the yolk sac, originating from the presumptive caudal region of the embryo, extends into the connecting stalk: this is the allantois, the primitive extra-embryonic urinary bladder.

The three subsequent weeks are characterised by three developmental processes (Fig. 37.12):

a. The embryo rotates in such a way that the yolk sac vesicle, originally facing the region opposite the implantation site, is turned towards the implantation pole.
b. The amnionic vesicle enlarges considerably, extending around the embryo.
c. The originally flat embryonic disc is bent in the anterior–posterior direction, and rolled up in the lateral direction. It thus 'herniates' into the amnionic vesicle. The bending fetus subdivides the yolk sac into an intra-embryonic duct (the gut) and into an extra-embryonic part (the omphalo-enteric or omphalo-mesenteric duct), which is peripherally dilated to form the extra-embryonic yolk sac vesicle.

Both the allantois and the extra-embryonic yolk sac extend into the mesenchyme of the connecting stalk (Fig. 37.12, day 28). Fluid accumulation within the amnionic cavity causes its expansion, so that it slowly compresses the exocoelom. Between days 28 and 40 post-conception, the expanding amnionic cavity has surrounded the embryo to the extent that the connecting stalk, together with the allantois and the yolk sac, are compressed to a slender cord, which is surrounded by amnionic epithelium (Fig. 37.12, day 40): they thus form the umbilical cord. The cord lengthens as the embryo 'prolapses' backwards into the amnionic sac (Hertig 1962).

By the 3rd week post-conception, the extra-embryonic yolk sac, the omphalo-mesenteric duct which connects with the embryonic gut, and the allantois become supplied with fetal vessels. All mammals use either allantoic or yolk sac vessels for the vascularisation of the placenta. The human allantoic vessels — two allantoic arteries originating from the internal iliac arteries, and one allantoic vein which enters into the hepatic vein — invade the placenta and become connected to the villous vessels. The allantoic participation in placental vascularisation gave rise to the name 'chorio-allantoic' placenta. The allantoic epithelium gradually disappears. Fusion of the allantoic

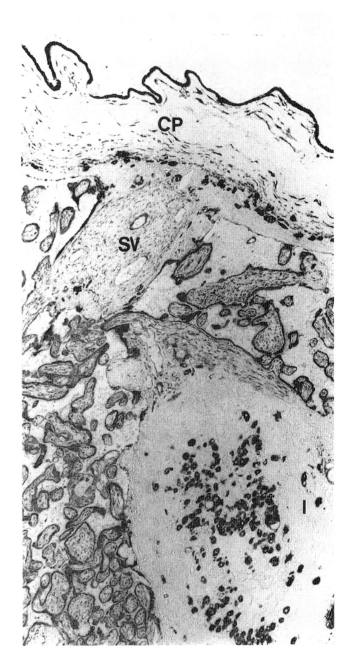

Fig. 37.13 Cryostat survey section at the 40th week post-menstruation, showing the chorionic plate (CP) which is covered with the folded amnion, an off-branching stem villus (SV), numerous peripheral villous branches and a cell island (I). Because of the histochemical reaction for malate dehydrogenase, the amnionic epithelium and the large extravillous trophoblast cells within the chorionic plate and within the cell island show intense staining, whereas villous trophoblast and connective tissue cells are weaker stained; the fibrinoid (matrix-type fibrinoid) of the cell island (I), embedding and surrounding the extravillous trophoblast cells, remains unstained. (Reproduced with permission from Schiebler & Kaufmann 1981.)

vessels with the intravillous vessel system establishes a complete feto-placental circulation in the course of the 5th week post-conception.

During the same process of expansion that leads to the formation of the cord, the amnionic mesenchyme locally touches and finally fuses with the chorionic mesoderm, thus occluding the exocoelomic cavity. This process starts in the surroundings of the cord insertion at the chorionic plate and persists until the middle of pregnancy, when the amnionic cavity completely occupies the exocoelom, so that amnionic and chorionic mesenchyme fuse everywhere (Figs 37.12, day 40; 37.14a,b). Only cleft-like remnants of the exocoelom may be detectable in the later stages of pregnancy. As distinct from the cord, where the amnion firmly fuses with the underlying connective tissue, fusion of the amnion with chorionic plate or membranes is never perfect, but rather amnion and chorion can always easily slide against each other. Histologically they seem to be separated by a system of slender, fluid-filled clefts, the intermediate, or spongy, layer of the chorionic plate and of the membranes (Figs 37.13 and 37.15a).

At day 14 post-conception, the primary chorionic plate consists of three layers: extra-embryonic mesenchyme, cytotrophoblast, and syncytiotrophoblast (Fig. 37.1f). They separate the intervillous space from the blastocystic cavity. Trophoblastic proliferation with subsequent degeneration and fibrinoid transformation, together with fibrin deposition from the intervillous space (Langhans fibrinoid), cause continuous growth of the primary chorionic plate. Around the 5th week of pregnancy, allantoic blood vessels reach the primary chorionic plate via the connective stalk (Benirschke 1965). Where stem villi branch off from the chorionic plate, branches of the allantoic vessels protrude into the stroma and fuse with the intravillous capillary system.

As soon as the amnionic sac has expanded to such a degree that the amnionic mesenchyme comes into close contact with the mesenchymal surface of the chorionic plate (8th–10th week post-conception), the definitive chorionic plate is formed (Fig. 37.12, day 40; Fig. 37.15a). For further details regarding the mature chorionic plate, see Weser & Kaufmann (1978) and Wiese (1975).

As already mentioned earlier, all villous developmental steps described above are valid only for the implantation pole, i.e. that part of the blastocystic circumference which was attached to the endometrium and which implanted first. The other parts of the blastocystic circumference, implanted a few days later, undergo a corresponding, although delayed development (Fig. 37.12, day 28). These areas are called the capsular chorion frondosum. Here, the first regressive changes can be observed, even during the process of villous vasculogenesis in the early part

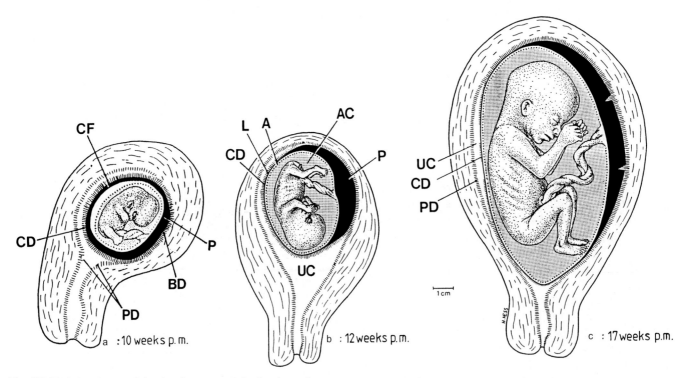

Fig. 37.14 Later stages of the development of the fetal membranes. **a** Up to 10 weeks post-menstruation, the embryo is surrounded by the chorion frondosum (CF); its later specialisation into chorion laeve and the placenta is indicated by a slight local increase in thickness (P) only. The chorion frondosum is covered by the capsular decidua (CD) which is continuous with basal decidua (BD) at the placental site, and with the parietal decidua (PD) which lines the uterine cavity. The amnion (dotted line) is not fused in most places with the chorion frondosum. **b** Two weeks later (12th week post-menstruation), the original chorion frondosum has differentiated into the thick placenta (P) and the thinner fetal membranes that surround the amnionic cavity (AC). At this stage, the membranes are composed of inner amnion (A), intermediate chorion laeve (L), and outer capsular decidua (CD). Because of the embryo's small size, the uterine cavity (UC) is largely open. **c** From 17 weeks on, the membranes come into close contact with the uterine wall. The remainder of the capsular decidua (CD) fuse with the parietal decidua (PD) and largely close the uterine cavity (UC). From then on, the chorion laeve contacts the parietal decidua. (Modified with permission after Kaufmann 1981.)

of the 4th week. The newly formed villi degenerate, and the surrounding intervillous space is obliterated. Finally, the chorionic plate, the obliterated intervillous space, villous remnants, and the basal plate fuse, forming a multilayered compact lamella, the smooth chorion or chorion laeve (Fig. 37.12, day 40). The first patches of the smooth chorion appear opposite to the implantation pole at the so-called anti-implantation pole. From there, they spread over about 70% of the surface of the chorionic sac until the 4th lunar month, when this process comes to a halt.

With complete implantation, the decidua closes again over the blastocyst, bulging into the uterine lumen, and is called the capsular decidua (Fig. 37.14a). With increasing diameter of the chorionic sac, the capsular decidua locally comes into contact with the parietal decidua of the opposing uterine wall and between the 15th and 20th week post-conception the two decidual layers fuse with each other, thus obstructing the uterine cavity (Fig. 37.14d). From this point onwards, the smooth chorion has contact over almost its entire surface with the decidual surface of the uterine wall, and may function as a paraplacental exchange organ. Due to the lack of fetal vascularisation of both the smooth chorion and the amnion, all paraplacental exchange between fetal membranes and fetus has to pass the amnionic fluid.

The structure of the fetal membranes at term was defined by Bourne (1962). Apart from the amnion's involvement in the production and resorption of the amnionic fluid, there are findings which suggest that it is metabolically active; Mühlhauser et al (1994) found that the amnionic epithelium contains abundant carbonic anhydrase, an enzyme involved in removal of CO_2 and in pH regulation.

BASAL PLATE AND UTEROPLACENTAL VESSELS

The trophoblastic shell is formed as the base of the lacunar system at day 8 post-conception (Fig. 37.1c,d). In the beginning, it is a purely syncytiotrophoblastic layer. From day 13 post-conception onwards, cytotrophoblast reaches

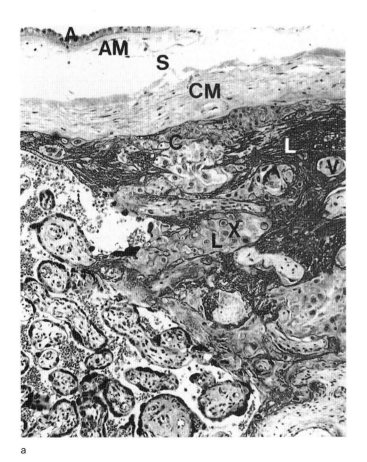

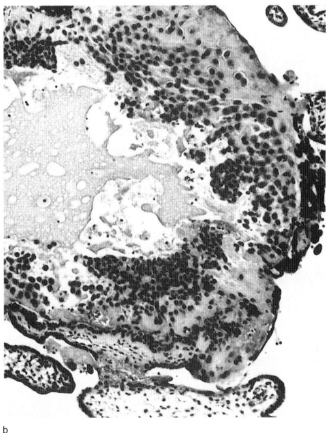

a   b

Fig. 37.15 Paraffin sections of non-villous parts of the placenta. **a** The chorionic plate at the 40th week post-menstruation; the typical layering of the mature chorionic plate with amnionic epithelium (A), amnionic mesenchyme (AM), spongy layer (S), chorionic mesenchyme (CM), chorionic cytotrophoblast (C), and Langhans fibrinoid (L) is evident. Clusters of trophoblast cells (X) and residues of buried villi (V) are typically incorporated in the Langhans fibrinoid. Note the histologically different appearance of the light, glossy fibrinoid (matrix-type fibrinoid) surrounding the trophoblast cells as compared to the darker, reticular fibrinoid (fibrin-type fibrinoid, derived from blood clot) in between. (Reproduced with permission from Benirschke & Kaufmann 2000.) **b** A cell island at the 19th week post-menstruation. It is composed of matrix-type fibrinoid and clusters of extravillous trophoblast cells. In the centre a central cavity, a so-called cyst, can be observed. Such cavities have to be considered a result of degeneration with subsequent liquefaction. (Reproduced with permission from Kaufmann 1981.)

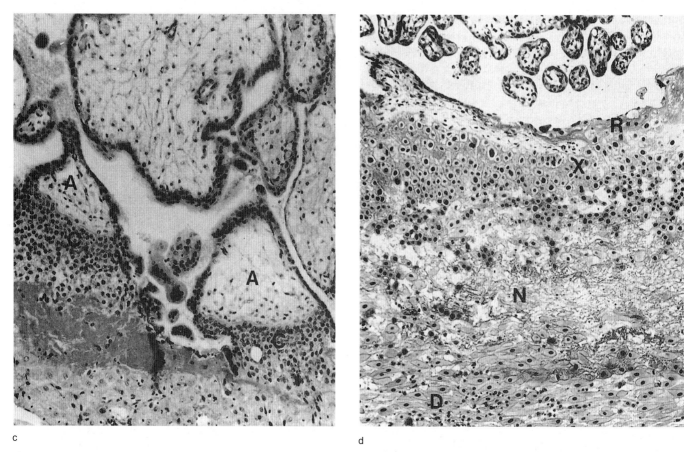

c

d

Fig. 37.15 c Cell columns at the 15th week post-menstruation. In early stages of pregnancy the anchoring villi (A) are connected to the basal plate (below) by broad or slender feet consisting of cytotrophoblast, the so-called cell columns. These are proliferative zones for the villous trophoblast as well as for the trophoblast of the basal plate. × 110. (Reproduced with permission from Benirschke & Kaufmann 2000.) **d** The basal plate at the 23rd week post-menstruation. The typical layering of the basal plate is evident. Facing the intervillous space it is covered by an interrupted layer of Rohr's fibrinoid (R), followed by a nearly complete layer of cytotrophoblast (X). The latter is largely separated from the decidua cells (D) by a loose layer of Nitabuch's fibrinoid (N). The heterogeneous staining patterns of both fibrinoid layers point to their mixed composition of matrix-type and of fibrintype fibrinoids. (Reproduced with permission from Benirschke & Kaufmann 2000.)

the shell, penetrates it (Fig. 37.1e), and intermingles with neighbouring cells of the endometrium; many of the latter have meanwhile transformed into decidual cells. As soon as invading trophoblast cells come into close contact with each other they may fuse to form the syncytial giant cells of the junctional zone. Where they are separated from each other, they undergo differentiation into so-called extravillous trophoblast (Fig. 37.1f).

The entire materno-fetal 'battlefield' stretches from the intervillous space down to the myometrium and is described as the junctional zone (Fig. 37.1f). The superficial part of this, which adheres to the placenta after placental separation, is the basal plate (Fig. 37.15d). It consists of the remainders of the original trophoblastic shell, together with the attached trophoblastic and endometrial cells, and much fibrinoid material (Hein 1971; Kaufmann & Stark 1971; Stark & Kaufmann 1971). Those parts of the junctional zone that remain in the uterus after delivery are called the placental bed. This consists mainly of endometrial tissue, with intermingled trophoblastic cells (Robertson & Warner 1974).

Following erosion of the first endometrial capillaries at day 12 post-conception, larger endometrial arteries (spiral arteries) and veins also become eroded and thus connected with the intervillous space. There is general agreement that the number of corresponding maternal vessels that supply the placenta, although originally high, is reduced considerably towards term by obliteration (Boyd & Hamilton 1970). The final number of spiral arteries for the term placenta is below 100, that for venous openings 50–200.

As early as in the second month of pregnancy, the walls of the spiral arteries and veins show regressive changes which are accompanied by infiltration of vessel walls and vessel lumina by trophoblast cells. Endothelial necrosis is followed by focal and, later, general degeneration or dedifferentiation of the muscle cells of the media. In some places, all endothelial and muscular elements may degenerate, thus transforming the vessels into flaccid tubes, constructed of amorphous extracellular material infiltrated by trophoblast cells (Brosens et al 1967; de Wolf et al 1973). This process is accompanied by dilatation of the lumina, in particular those near the intervillous space. Rounded trophoblast cells, so-called intra-arterial trophoblast, invade the arterial lumina and in some places may completely obstruct the arterial lumina whilst in others they replace the degenerate endothelium to form a new vascular lining. Uteroplacental veins undergo similar changes, though to a much lesser degree: they always remain free of intravascular trophoblast.

Even though they appear degenerative in nature, these pregnancy changes in the uteroplacental vessels are described as 'physiological processes' (Brosens 1988), necessary for normal implantation. Complete absence of, or reduced, physiological vessel alterations is regularly combined with fetal growth restriction and may be complicated by hypertensive pregnancy (Brosens 1988; Sheppard & Bonnar 1988).

PLACENTAL SEPTA

Placental septa are bizarre-shaped conglomerations of fibrinoid, intermingled with groups of trophoblastic and/or decidual cells, connected to the basal plate. They are not vascularised. They are columnar, or sail-like, structures rather than real septa (Becker & Jipp 1963), dividing the

intervillous space into separately maternally perfused chambers (Fig. 37.2a). They are interpreted as dislocations of basal plate tissue into the intervillous space, caused by lateral movement and folding of the uterine wall and basal plate over each other (Benirschke & Kaufmann 2000).

CELL COLUMNS AND CELL ISLANDS

Cell columns are the trophoblastic connections of larger stem villi, the so-called anchoring villi, to the basal plate. These are segments of the villous tree that persist in the primary villus stage, since mesenchymal invasion during formation of secondary villi does not reach the most basal segments of the anchoring villi (Fig. 37.1f, 37.15c). Because of continuing cytotrophoblastic proliferation, the cell columns serve as segments of longitudinal growth of the anchoring villi. From their bases, cytotrophoblast invades the basal plate (Fig. 37.15c), thus also contributing to the growth of the latter. The cell columns represent the growth zones of extravillous trophoblast found in basal plate, placental bed and placental septa. Fibrinoid deposition at the surface of the cell columns slowly

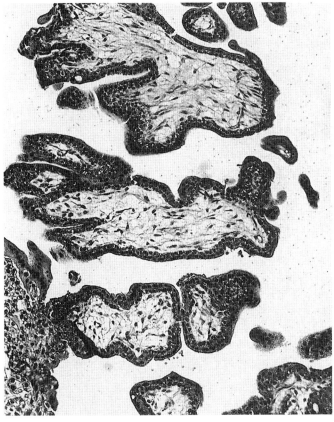

a

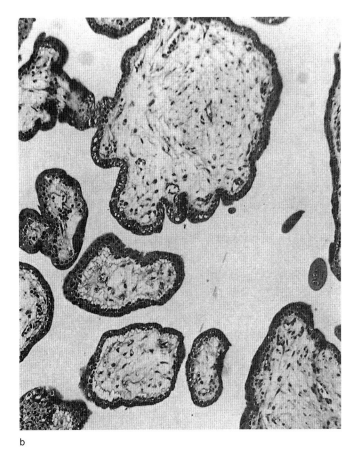

b

Fig. 37.16 a Paraffin section of placental villi of the 6th week post-menstruation. Note the thick trophoblastic covering consisting of complete layers of cytotrophoblast and syncytiotrophoblast. Fetal capillaries are poorly developed or, in some places, still lacking. In the lower left corner, an early step in the formation of a cell island can be seen, attached to the villous surface. **b** Paraffin section of placental villi of the 8th week post-menstruation. All villi are vascularised. As one can see from the diffuse stromal structure, the villi still belong to the mesenchymal type.

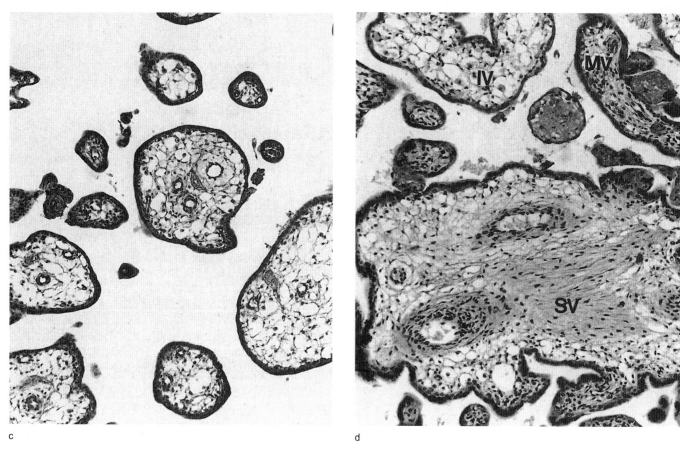

c

d

Fig. 37.16 c Paraffin section of placental villi of the 12 week post-menstruation. The larger villi have achieved the reticular stroma of typical immature, intermediate villi. The smaller villi are mesenchymal in structure. The first small fetal arteries and veins can be seen. **d** Paraffin section of placental villi of the 15th week post-menstruation. The larger immature intermediate villi exhibit the first signs of central stromal fibrosis, originating from the larger fetal vessels, thus establishing the first stem villi (SV). Several typical immature intermediate villi (IV), as well as mesenchymal villi (MV) can be seen. As this is typical for mesenchymal villi of the second and third trimester, they are associated with degenerating villi being more or less transformed into fibrinoid. (Reproduced with permission from Benirschke & Kaufmann 2000.)

'buries' them into the basal plate. As soon as they are completely incorporated into the latter, the cytotrophoblastic proliferation slows down. Following partial degeneration of the cells and complete disintegration of their structure, cell columns largely disappear in the course of the last trimester and can only rarely be observed in the term placenta.

Cell islands obviously are largely comparable structures. They, too, are formed from villous tips which have not been opened up by connective tissue and fetal vessels during the transition from primary, via secondary, to tertiary villi (Fig. 37.16a). The only difference is that these villous tips were not connected to the basal plate as anchoring villi. Also the cytotrophoblast of the cell islands proliferates and, afterwards, becomes largely embedded into fibrinoid which surrounds the clusters and strings of extravillous cytotrophoblast (Fig. 37.13). Sometimes central degeneration and liquefaction causes the development of fluid-filled cysts inside the cell islands.

EXTRAVILLOUS TROPHOBLAST

The vast majority of cellular and syncytial trophoblast from the implanted blastocyst is consumed in the development of the placental villi. The remaining trophoblast, which is not used for villus formation, the extravillous trophoblast, is the basic material for the development of all other parts of the placenta. These are the chorion laeve, the marginal zone, the chorionic plate, the basal plate including the cell columns, the septa and the cell islands.

The nomenclature of the extravillous trophoblast

Because some doubt originally existed regarding its derivation, the first name employed was 'X cells'. The trophoblastic nature of these cells was, however, finally proved by Y-specific fluorescence studies in placentas of male infants (Faller & Ferenci 1973; Khudr et al 1973).

Since the cells are obviously heterogeneous in structure, many authors proposed new designations: extravillous trophoblast, extravillous cytotrophoblast, non-villous trophoblast, intermediate trophoblast, specialised trophoblast, interstitial trophoblast, intravascular trophoblast, intra-arterial trophoblast, trophoblastic giant cells, trophocytes, spongiotrophoblast-like cells, placental site giant cells, etc. Regrettably, each of these terms has a slightly different definition. We, therefore, use the term 'extravillous trophoblast' as the most general heading for all types of trophoblast occurring outside the villi. When syncytial elements can be excluded, the name 'extravillous cytotrophoblast' may be more appropriate.

One may speculate that all these forms of extravillous cytotrophoblast merely represent different stages of differentiation from a proliferating stem cell, via highly differentiated, metabolically active forms towards cellular degeneration (Kaufmann & Stark 1971; Okudaira et al 1971). The extravillous trophoblast in the various placental locations may differ in some characteristics (e.g. antigens, morphology, proliferation, behaviour) due to the different micro-environments. There are immunohistochemical findings (Gosseye & Fox 1984; Kurman et al 1984a,b; Beck et al 1986) which make it very likely that the extravillous cytotrophoblast is composed of several parallel lines of cell differentiation.

We propose the following nomenclature for the extravillous trophoblast in the junctional zone:

a. extravillous syncytiotrophoblast (multinucleated giant cells — most probably newly fused syncytial elements only in the depth of the placental bed)
b. extravillous cytotrophoblast (this term probably being largely identical with what has been called 'intermediate trophoblast' by Kurman et al 1984a); this again is composed of two different entities:
   i. the endovascular trophoblast, lining the spiral artery lumina and partly occluding these, and infiltrating the medias of spiral arteries and partly even uteroplacental veins,
   ii. the interstitial trophoblast, comprising all those extravillous trophoblast cells that are not located inside vessel lumina and vessel walls, showing various degrees of differentiation from proliferation to degeneration, being more or less in contact with fibrinoid; also this subgroup may not be homogeneous in nature.

In the pathological literature (Benirschke & Kaufmann 2000) a population of cells is referred to as 'placental site giant cells' or 'placental site cells', located at the materno-fetal interface: these are, in fact, cells of the interstitial extravillous trophoblast. They have a basophilic cytoplasm and penetrate deeply into the decidua. Pathologists are often faced with the need to establish beyond doubt that an intrauterine pregnancy has been present and such cells allow them to distinguish clearly a placental site.

One of the crucial problems in histopathology is the discrimination between extravillous cytotrophoblast and decidua. Reliable markers for decidual cells, as opposed to trophoblastic cells, are anti-prolactin (Rosenberg et al 1980) and anti-vimentin (Beham et al 1988). Extravillous trophoblast can be identified by binding anti-cytokeratins (Beham et al 1988; Daya & Sabet 1991) and anti-hPL (Gosseye & Fox 1984; Kurman et al 1984a,b; Beck et al 1986).

FIBRINOID

Fibrinoid material is present in both normal and pathological placentas at all stages of development. Fibrinoid deposition is a regular feature at all those locations where syncytiotrophoblast, as the usual lining of the intervillous space, has disappeared as a result of degenerative changes. Another important location is in the immediate materno-fetal 'battlefield' of the junctional zone, the deeper part of the basal plate (Nitabuch's fibrinoid) (Fig. 37.15d).

Immunohistochemical studies (Frank et al 1994; Lang et al 1994) have shown that placental fibrinoid is heterogeneous in nature, two different types being distinguished. Fibrin-type fibrinoid shows intense reaction with anti-fibrin antibodies but does not contain extravillous trophoblast cells or extracellular matrix molecules. It is found particularly in perivillous fibrin and in the Rohr stria of the basal plate. Matrix-type fibrinoid is largely devoid of fibrin but contains numerous extracellular matrix molecules such as laminin, collagen IV and oncofetal fibronectin. These molecules embed clusters of extravillous trophoblast which are involved in the production of this material. Matrix-type fibrinoid is found within degenerating villi, cell islands, septa and the basal plate. Locally, both types may mix with each other.

Several functional roles have been proposed for the two forms of placental fibrinoid, these including a contribution to the mechanical stability of the placenta, a substitute for the degenerating syncytiotrophoblast at the villous surface, shaping of the intervillous space, an immunological barrier and growth promotion for trophoblast.

APPENDIX: BRIEF DESCRIPTION OF DEVELOPMENTAL STAGES

It is the intention of this synopsis to present only information on developmental stages that is directly applicable to the pathological and histological examination of human material. For this purpose, data from various sources has been pooled. Information concerning the embryo and fetus will only be given as far as it is of importance for the definition of the stage. Some of the quantitative data are summarised in Table 37.1. Qualitative data concerning villous development is outlined in Table 37.2. The data are based on the following publications (in parentheses): embryonic staging post-conception (p.c.) (Carnegie staging — O'Rahilly, 1973); crown–rump length, embryonic and fetal weight, mean diameter of the chorionic sac, placental diameter and thickness, placental weight (Boyd & Hamilton 1970; O'Rahilly 1973; Kaufmann 1981); placental and uterine thickness in vivo (Johannigmann et al 1972); length of umbilical cord (Winckel 1893); structural and quantitative data concerning villous development (Benirschke & Kaufmann 2000).

Day 1 post-conception, Stage 1: one fertilised cell; diameter 0.1 mm.

Day 2 post-conception, Stage 2a: from 2 to 4 cells; diameter 0.1–0.2 mm.

Day 3 post-conception, Stage 2b: from 4 to ± 16 cells; diameter 0.1–0.2 mm.

Day 4 post-conception, Stage 3: from 16 to ± 64 cells; diameter about 0.2 mm; free blastocyst.

Day 5 to early day 6 post-conception, Stage 4: from about 128 to ± 256 cells; diameter 0.2–0.3 mm; blastocyst attached to the endometrium.

Late day 6 to early day 8 post-conception, Stage 5a: implantation, prelacunar stage of the trophoblast; the flattened blastocyst measures about 0.3×0.3×0.15 mm. The blastocyst is partially implanted. The embryonic disc measures about 0.1 mm in diameter.

Late day 8 to day 9 post-conception, Stage 5b, early lacunar or trabecular stage: diameter of chorionic sac 0.5×0.5×0.3 mm; embryonic disc about 0.1 mm. The syncytiotrophoblast at the implantation pole exhibits vacuoles as forerunners of the lacunar system.

Day 10 to day 12 post-conception, Stage 5c, late lacunar or trabecular stage: diameter of chorionic sac 0.9×0.9×0.6 mm. Around day 11, implantation is complete; the defect in the endometrial epithelium becomes closed by a blood coagulum, and covered by epithelium on day 12. The syncytiotrophoblastic vacuoles fuse to form the lacunar system. First contact of lacunar system with eroded endometrial capillaries. At the implantation site, the endometrial thickness is 5 mm; first signs of decidualisation.

Day 13 post-conception, Stage 6, early primary villous stage (first free primary villi): the nearly round chorionic sac has a diameter of 1.2–1.5 mm; length of embryonic disc is 0.2 mm.

With expansion of the lacunar system, the syncytiotrophoblast becomes reduced to radially oriented trophoblastic trabeculae, the forerunners of the stem villi. After invasion of cytotrophoblast into the trabeculae, free trophoblastic outgrowths into the lacunae, so-called free primary villi, are formed. The trabeculae are now called 'villous stems'. By definition, from this date onwards, the lacunae are transformed into the intervillous space. Cytotrophoblast from the former trabeculae penetrates the trophoblastic shell and invades the endometrium.

Day 14 post-conception, Stage 6, late primary villous stage: diameter of chorionic sac 1.6–2.1 mm; length of embry-

onic disc 0.2–0.4 mm. First appearance of primitive streak and of yolk sac. Placenta cf. day 13.

Day 15 to 16 post-conception, Stage 7, early secondary villous stage: diameter of chorionic sac about 5 mm; length of embryonic disc <0.9 mm. Appearance of notochordal process and primitive node (Hensen). Starting at the implantation pole and continuing to the anti-implantation pole, extra-embryonic mesenchyme from the chorionic cavity invades the villi, transforming them into secondary villi. The bases of the villous stems, connecting the latter with the trophoblastic shell, remain free of mesenchyme and thus persist in the primary villous stage (forerunners of the cell columns).

Day 17 to 18 post-conception, Stage 8, late secondary villous stage: diameter of chorionic sac <8 mm; length of embryonic disc <1.3 mm. On the embryonic disc, the notochordal and neurenteric canals, and the primitive pit can be discerned. For the structure of the placenta cf. days 15, 16.

Day 19 to 21 post-conception, Stage 9, early tertiary villous stage: diameter of chorionic sac <12 mm; length of embryonic disc = crown–rump length of the embryo 1.5–2.5 mm; 1–3 somites. Neural folds appear; first heart contractions.

In the villous mesenchyme fetal capillaries develop (tertiary villi). The villous diameters are largely homogeneous, presenting two differently sized groups of villi. The larger villi and their branches exhibit diameters of 120–250 μm. Histologically, the stroma of both is mesenchymal in nature. Along their surfaces, one finds numerous small (30–60 μm) sprouts.

Day 22 to 23 post-conception, Stage 10: diameter of chorionic sac <15 mm; crown–rump length 2–3.5 mm; 4–12 somites. Neural folds start to fuse, two visceral arches. Placenta cf. days 19 to 21.

Day 23 to 26 post-conception, Stage 11: diameter of the chorionic sac <18 mm; crown–rump length 2.5–4.5 mm; 13–20 somites. Closure of the rostral neuropore; optic vesicles identifiable.

The length of villi connecting chorionic plate with trophoblastic shell varies from 1 mm (anti-implantation pole) to 2 mm (implantation pole). The central two-thirds are supplied with mesenchyme and capillaries, the peripheral one-third remain in the primary villous stage (cell columns). Most villi contain loose mesenchyme, together with centrally positioned fetal capillaries (mesenchymal villi) (Fig. 37.16a). Peripherally, they continue into massive trophoblastic sprouts. The larger villi (>200 μm) show moderate net-like fibrosis. The villous trophoblastic surface is composed of the outer syncytiotrophoblast and complete inner layer of cytotrophoblast. The chorionic plate, consisting of fetal mesenchyme, cytotrophoblast and syncytiotrophoblast, still lacks fibrinoid. The trophoblastic shell is transformed into the basal plate by intense mixing of decidual and trophoblastic cells. Tissue necrosis in the contact zone of both cell populations causes the appearance of the first loci of Nitabuch fibrinoid.

Day 26 to 29 post-conception, Stage 12: diameter of chorionic sac <21 mm; crown–rump length 3–5 mm; 21–29 somites. Closure of the caudal neuropore; three visceral arches; upper limb buds appear. Placenta cf. days 23 to 26.
Day 29 to 42 post-conception, Stages 13 to 16: diameter of chorionic sac from 21–33 mm; crown–rump length 4–12 mm. Thirty and more somites; four limb buds and otic vesicle, first appearance of lens pit and optic cup, thereafter closure of lens vesicle; clear evidence of cerebral vesicles; hand plates; retinal pigment visible; foot plates.

Thickness of the chorion at the implantation pole about 6 mm, at the anti-implantation pole about 3 mm. The uterine lumen is still open, parietal and capsular decidua are not yet in contact. The largest villi reach diameters <400 μm. The overwhelming share of the villous stroma is still mesenchymal in nature (Fig. 37.16b). The villous cytotrophoblastic layer is incomplete. Near the end of this period, the majority of mesenchymal villi show increased numbers of macrophages, as well as appearance of the first stromal channels. These are the first signs of reticular transformation of their stroma towards immature intermediate villi. In the course of the 7th week post-conception the newly formed medium-sized villi (150–250 μm) more or less completely show reticular stroma of immature intermediate villi. Peripheral portions of villous side branches, persisting in the primary villous stage, may increase in size by continuous cell proliferation with subsequent fibrinoid degeneration; they establish the first cell islands.

3rd month post-menstruation 9th–12th week post-menstruation, days 43–70 post-conception; Stages 17 to 23: diameter of chorionic sac from 38–63 mm; crown–rump length from 10–31 mm. Finger rays, toe rays, nipples and eyelids appear; upper limbs bent at the elbow region; first signs of finger separation. The embryonic weight increases throughout the 3rd month from 2 to 17 g.

The chorionic sac is covered by villi over its entire surface, and there is, as yet, no subdivision into smooth chorion and placenta. However, around the anti-implantation pole, increased degenerative changes in the villi and considerable fibrinoid deposition initiate formation of the chorion laeve. Parietal and capsular decidua may locally come into contact, but they remain still unfused. The early, moderately fibrosed mesenchymal villi (cf. days 23–26) near the chorionic plate meanwhile have achieved a diameter of up to 500 μm. The majority of villi measuring between 100 and 400 μm establish the typical reticular appearance of immature intermediate villi (Fig. 37.16c,d). Small-sized villi with diameters below 100 μm show mesenchymal stroma. Trophoblastic and villous sprouts are numerous. In the 8th week post-conception stem vessels are formed (luminal diameters 20–30 μm) with vessel walls consisting of two to three

layers of cells. They do not show surrounding adventitial fibrosis. Until the 12th week post-conception (Fig. 37.16c) some of these vessels show an increase in luminal width up to 100 μm; however, there is no change in their wall structure. Fibrinoid deposition at the intervillous surface of the chorionic plate is still an exception. The amnionic cavity has extended to such a degree that the amnionic mesoderm in many places comes into contact with the connective tissue layer of the chorionic plate.

4th month post-menstruation, 13th–16th week post-menstruation, 11th–14th week post-conception: The maximum diameter of the chorionic sac increases throughout this period from 68 mm to 80–90 mm. The crown–rump length grows from 45 to 80 mm.

The continuous degeneration of placental villi at the anti-implantation pole, which is free of villi from the middle of the 4th months onwards, as well as the villous proliferation at the implantation pole, initiate the differentiation of the chorionic sac into smooth chorion and placenta. The first real placental septa become visible. The cell columns become more deeply incorporated into the basal plate by fibrinoid deposition in their surroundings. The chorionic plate is in close contact with the amnion over its entire surface, giving it the definitive shape and layering.

Among the villi the immature intermediate ones with diameters of 100 to about 300 μm dominate (Fig. 37.16d). Their larger, centrally positioned fetal vessels show concentric adventitial fibrosis. Until the end of this month, this fibrosis increases to such an extent that in about half of the cases arterial and venous adventitia fuse, thus forming a fibrous central villous core (first real stem villi). The remaining parts of the stroma remain reticular in structure. In this stage, the first real stem villi can be easily distinguished from the much larger fibrosed original mesenchymal villi near the chorionic plate, which show only moderate fibrosis in a net-like pattern, extending all over the villous core. Mesenchymal villi (60–100 μm in diameter) and sprouts are numerous but, because of their size, they occupy only a minority of the total villous volume. Perivillous fibrinoid deposition becomes a usual finding on the villous surfaces.

5th month post-menstruation, 17th–20th week post-menstruation, 15th–18th week post-conception: The crown–rump length increases from 80 to 130 mm. The placenta is clearly separated from the smooth chorion.

The structure of the stem villi is nearly the same as in the previous month; however, their number is considerably increased. In the 18th week post-conception, the majority of the large-calibre villi, those exceeding 300 μm, are more or less completely fibrosed. Those ranging from 150–300 μm show central stromal fibrosis surrounding artery and vein, and a broad superficial layer of reticular stroma (Fig. 37.17a). Most villi have diameters between 100 and 150 μm and are still immature

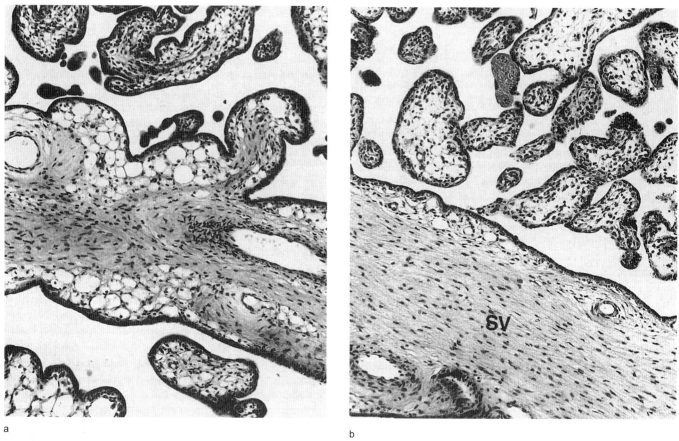

a

b

Fig. 37.17 a Paraffin section of placental villi of the 18th week post-menstruation. The picture is comparable to that of the preceding stage. Formation of stem villi with stromal fibrosis is a little more expressed. **b** Paraffin section of placental villi of the 21st week post-menstruation. The stroma of the stem villi (SV) is largely fibrous. Only a thin superficial rim of reticular connective tissue hints at their derivation from immature intermediate villi.

intermediate in character without, or with only sparse, adventitial fibrosis around the central vessels. Continuous development of fetal capillaries causes the reduction of mean maternal–fetal diffusion distance. Septa and cell islands, which originally consisted mainly of accumulations of cells, now grow considerably by apposition of fibrinoid. In their centres, cysts sometimes form.

6th month post-menstruation, 21st–24th week post-menstruation, 19th–22nd week post-conception: The fetus grows from 130 to 180 mm crown–rump length.

The histological features change considerably: the majority of immature intermediate villi become transformed into stem villi. Those exceeding 300 µm in calibre are more or less completely fibrosed, those ranging from 100–300 µm still have a discontinuous thin superficial layer of reticular stroma (Fig. 37.17b) The majority of stem villi measure around 200 µm in thickness, some achieve diameters of more than 1000 µm. Size and number of immature intermediate villi is slowly decreasing. Unlike all earlier stages, the originally stub-like mesenchymal villi expand in diameter (80–150 µm) and in length, achieving nearly filiform shapes. Their stroma is characterised by an increasing number of cells. These

events mark their initial transformation into mature intermediate villi rather than immature intermediate villi. In this stage, in routine paraffin sections it is impossible to distinguish between mesenchymal and newly formed mature intermediate villi (Fig. 37.17c).

7th month post-menstruation, 26th–28th week post-menstruation, 23rd–26th week post-conception: As compared to the 6th month, there are only quantitative changes. The crown–rump length increases from 180 to 230 mm.

The distribution of structure and calibre of the villi is similar to what was seen during the 6th month. The number of immature intermediate villi with reticular stroma decreases in favour of stem villi and mature intermediate villi. The latter represent the dominating villous type, being identifiable by their calibre (100–150 µm), their mostly elongated sectional shape and their highly numerical density of stromal cells. In locally restricted areas, obviously in the periphery of the villous trees, the first small groups of grape-like, highly capillarised terminal villi (calibre 60–80 µm) appear. Cell columns are surrounded by increasing amounts of fibrinoid and become deeply invaginated into the basal plate. The syncytiotrophoblastic covering of the chorionic plate becomes replaced by an initially

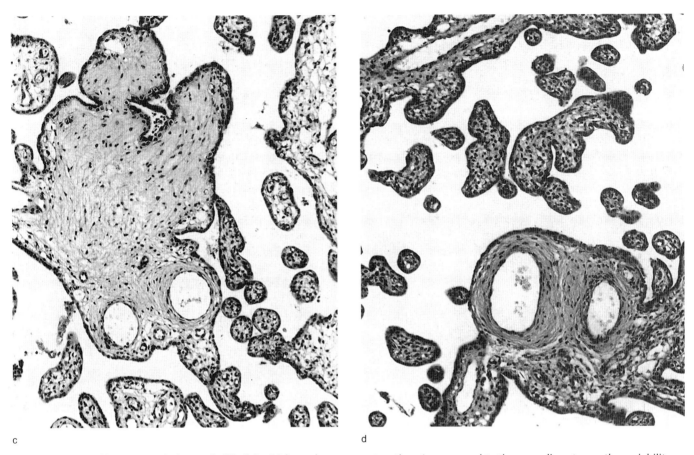

c

d

Fig. 37.17 c Paraffin section of placental villi of the 24th week post-menstruation. As compared to the preceding stages, the variability in villous shapes and diameters is sharply increasing. The population of small slender villi, originally referred to as mesenchymal villi, has achieved structural characteristics of mature intermediate villi. **d** Paraffin section of placental villi of the 29th week post-menstruation. In this period, the mature intermediate villi and the stem villi are the prevailing villous types. (Reproduced with permission from Benirschke & Kaufmann 2000.)

thin layer of fibrinoid which, throughout the following weeks, grows in thickness and forms the Langhans stria.

8th month post-menstruation, 29th–32nd week post-menstruation, 27th–30th week post-conception: crown–rump length 230 to 280 mm.

Steeply increasing numbers of mature intermediate villi and of terminal villi, which both exhibit calibres from 40–150 μm, are the reason for considerably increased numbers of villi per section (Fig. 37.17d). Besides a majority of villi of small calibre there are mainly stem villi of large calibre. Stem villi exceeding 20 μm in diameter are more or less completely fibrosed. Smaller ones still exhibit a discontinuous superficial reticular rim. The few still existing immature intermediate villi are rather evenly dispersed. As a result of beginning sinusoidal dilatation of the fetal capillaries in the newly formed terminal villi, the amount of vasculo-syncytial membranes (epithelial plates) is increased, and the mean trophoblastic thickness as well as the mean materno-fetal diffusion distance are considerably reduced.

9th month post-menstruation, 33rd–36th week post-menstruation, 31st–34th week post-conception: crown–rump length 280 to 330 mm.

Histologically, the developmental processes described for the preceding month become even more prominent: the mean maternal–fetal diffusion distance and the mean trophoblastic thickness are further reduced. Cytotrophoblast is present only at 25% of the villous surfaces and difficult to identify in paraffin sections, due to the slender form and light staining of the cells. The largest stem villi reach 500–1500 μm in diameter. The originally reticular superficial zone of the stroma shows an increased number of fibroblasts for a few weeks, as compared to the more central highly fibrous parts of the stem villi (Fig. 37.18a). This difference usually is no longer observed at term. Larger parts of the syncytiotrophoblast of the stem villi are replaced by fibrinoid. The vast majority of villi are mature intermediate and terminal villi (Fig. 37.18b). The mature intermediate ones still have large diameters of 100–150 mm. A few evenly distributed immature intermediate villi, with calibres of 100–200 μm, can regularly be found in nearly all villous trees, indicating still active placental growth.

10th month post-menstruation, 37th–40th week post-menstruation, 35th–38th week post-conception: the mean crown–rump length is raised from 330 mm to its final

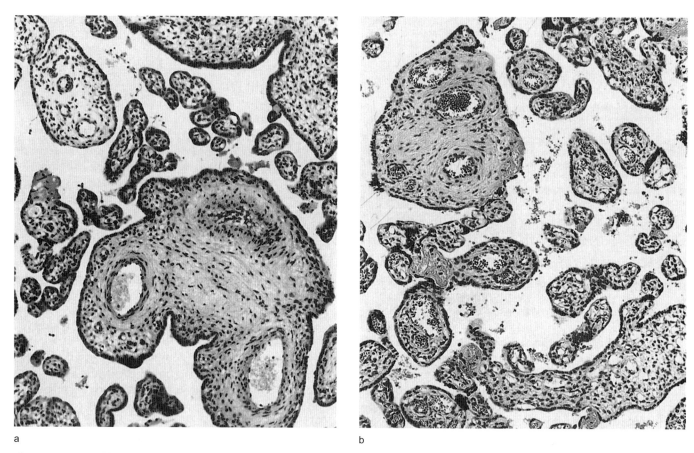

a

b

Fig. 37.18 a Paraffin section of placental villi of the 33rd week post-menstruation. The number of immature intermediate villi is decreasing. The majority of villi are stem villi and mature intermediate villi; the latter are intermingled with the first few terminal villi which, because of their similar diameters, are difficult to differentiate from mature intermediate villi in paraffin sections. The stem villi are still not fully fibrosed but rather show a thin superficial stromal layer which has few fibres and is rich in connective tissue cells.
b Paraffin section of placental villi of the 35th week post-menstruation. The distribution of villous types is largely comparable to that demonstrated for the preceding stage.

value of 380 mm. The mean placental weight increases from 400 to 470 g. There are considerable individual variations. Early clamping of the cord following delivery of the baby may even increase placental weight by as much as 100 g.

The permutation of villous types differs from the foregoing stage in several aspects. There are considerably increased numbers of terminal villi (about 40% of the total villous volume of the placenta) (Fig. 37.18c,d) and a higher degree of capillarisation of the latter. This is mainly due to the fact that many of the capillary cross-sections are dilated sinusoidally to maximum values of 40 μm. In well-preserved, early-fixed placentas, which did not suffer from fetal vessel collapse, the terminal fetal villous capillary lumina amount to 40% or more of the villous volume. About 20% of the villi are stem villi. In the fully mature placenta, the fibrous stroma reaches the trophoblastic or fibrinoid surface of the stem villi everywhere; a superficial reticular rim, or a superficial accumulation of fibroblasts, as in the 9th month, should be absent at term (Fig. 37.18c,d). This has to be interpreted as a sign of persisting immaturity. The syncytiotro-

phoblastic mantle of the larger stem villi is degenerate in most places, and very often it is replaced by fibrinoid (Fig. 37.18d). About 30–40% of the villous volume is made up of mature intermediate villi which, histologically, can be differentiated from the terminal villi by their slender, elongated and usually winding and branching shape, by the reduced degree of fetal capillarisation, by the absence of larger fetal vessels with lightmicroscopically identifiable media and adventitia, and by the high proportion of connective tissue cells. Their diameter has reached its definitive value of 80–120 μm. In normal mature placentas, the few persisting immature intermediate villi should be concentrated in the centre of the villous trees rather than being evenly distributed. The latter situation always indicates persisting immaturity of the placenta. If the central cavities of the placentones are not collapsed the immature intermediate villi delineate the remains of the latter. The cell bodies of the still existing villous cytotrophoblast are so thin at times that they may be difficult to identify; thus many investigators tend to underestimate their quantity, or even deny their existence. The amount of perivillous fibrinoid is extremely variable.

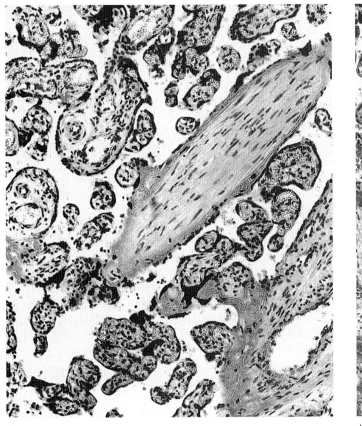

c

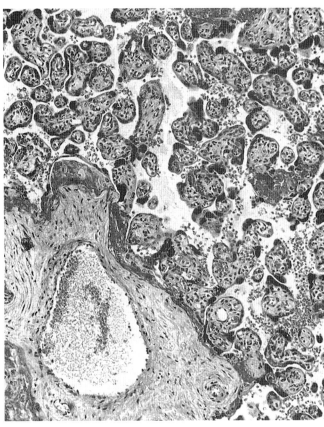

d

Fig. 37.18 c Paraffin section of placental villi of the 38th week post-menstruation. Dominating villous types are mature intermediate villi and terminal villi, both of small calibre. In between, several stem villi of varying calibre can be seen. As is typical for near-term placentas, the trophoblastic cover of the stem villi is partly replaced by fibrinoid. The stromal core is completely fibrosed. Reticular stroma or cellular connective tissue (which, as a typical sign of immaturity, was visible below the trophoblast in earlier stages throughout the last few weeks) is absent. **d** Paraffin section of placental villi of the 40th week post-menstruation. The calibre distribution is not very different from that of the 38th week. Despite this, some remarkable changes exist: the fibrinoid deposits around the larger stem villi (mostly fibrin-type fibrinoid) are considerably increased; also, because of the irregular shapes of terminal villi at term, numerous flat sections of villous surfaces can be seen. In this figure, these appear as dark spots of seemingly accumulated nuclei. (Reproduced with permission from Benirschke & Kaufmann 2000.)

In normal placentas we have never observed complete absence.

Additional quantitative results concerning placental development and composition of the term placenta are given in Tables 37.1 and 37.2. When examining these tables and comparing the results from different authors, it is important to note that placental morphometry is heavily influenced by the mode of sampling and by the preparation of the material. Because of the high degree of maternal and fetal vascularisation, the placenta reacts immediately to changes in intravascular pressure. Thus, the mode of birth, the time elapsing from cessation of maternal and fetal blood flows to tissue fixation and the nature of cord clamping directly influence the volumetric relations of villi and intervillous space. Normally, immersion fixation of the entire placenta or of small pieces should be sufficient. The more advanced methods, such as perfusion fixation (Burton et al 1987) or puncture biopsy of the still maternally perfused placenta during Caesarean section (Voigt et al 1978; Sen et al 1979), are

very time-consuming. When studying immersion-fixed material, however, one should keep in mind that this material differs quantitatively and qualitatively from the in vivo conditions.

For further details we refer to the following publications: placental growth development in relation to birth weight (Bouw et al 1978); relationship of placental weight to body size at 7 years of age, and to abnormalities in children (Naeye 1987); fetal and placental weights in relation to maternal weight (Auinger & Bauer 1974); ultrasonographic measurements of volumetric growth of the placenta (Bleker et al 1977); weight development of placenta and membranes in early pregnancy (Abramovich 1969); ratio of gestational sac volume to crown–rump length in early pregnancy (Goldstein et al 1986); villous surface area and villous volume densities in various placental regions and along different levels of the chorial basal axis (Teasdale 1978; Boyd et al 1980; Cabezon et al 1985; Bacon et al 1986); local variations of villous surface, fetal vascularisation, and amount of vasculo-syncytial membranes in the placentone (maternal–fetal circulatory unit) (Schuhmann et al 1986); total villous surface in relation to fetal weight, in normal and various pathological cases (Clavero-Nunez & Botella-Llusia 1963); morphometric data affecting placental oxygen diffusion (Mayhew et al 1984, 1986); computer measurement of the mass of syncytiotrophoblast (Boyd et al 1983); ultrastructural morphometric analysis of the villous syncytiotrophoblast (Sala et al 1983); microvillous surface enlargement of the villous surface (Teasdale & Jean-Jacques 1985); comparison of villous structure following immersion and perfusion fixation (Burton et al 1987).

REFERENCES

Abramovich D R 1969 The weight of placenta and membranes in early pregnancy. Journal of Obstetrics and Gynaecology of the British Commonwealth 76: 523–526

Alvarez H 1967 Syncytial proliferation in normal and toxemic pregnancies. Obstetrics and Gynecology 29: 637–643

Alvarez H, De Bejar R, Aladjem S 1964 La placenta human: aspectos morfologicos y fisio-patologicos. 4th Uruguayan Congress for Obstetrics and Gynecology 1: 190–261

Alvarez H, Morel R L, Benedetti W L, Scavarelli M 1969 Trophoblast hyperplasia and maternal arterial pressure at term. American Journal of Obstetrics and Gynecology 105: 1015–1021

Alvarez H, Benedetti W L, Morel R L, Scavarelli M 1970 Trophoblast development gradient and its relationship to placental hemodynamics. American Journal of Obstetrics and Gynecology 106: 416–420

Amstutz E 1960 Beobachtungen über die Reifung der Chorionzotten in der menschlichen Placenta mit besonderer Berücksichtigung der Epithelplatten. Acta Anatomica 42: 122–130

Arts N F T 1961 Investigations on the vascular system of the placenta. Part I. General introduction and the fetal vascular system. American Journal of Obstetrics and Gynecology 82: 147–158

Auinger W, Bauer P 1974 Zum Zusammenhang zwischen Kindsgewicht, Placentagewicht, Muttergewicht und Muttergrösse. Archiv für Gynäkologie 217: 69–83

Bacon B J, Gilbert R D, Kaufmann P et al 1984 Placental anatomy and diffusing capacity in guinea pigs following long-term maternal hypoxia. Placenta 5: 475–488

Bacon B J, Gilbert R D, Longo L D 1986 Regional anatomy of the term human placenta. Placenta 7: 233–241

Beck T, Schweikhart G, Stolz E 1986 Immunohistochemical location of HPL, SP1 and β-HCG in normal placentas of varying gestational age. Archives of Gynecology 239: 63–74

Becker V, Jipp P 1963 Über die Trophoblastschale der menschlichen Plazenta. Geburtshilfe und Frauenheikunde 23: 466–474

Beham A, Denk H, Desoye G 1988 The distribution of intermediate filament proteins, actin and desmoplakins in human placental tissue as revealed by polyclonal and monoclonal antibodies. Placenta 9: 479–492

Benirschke K 1965 In: Wynn R M (ed) Fetal homeostasis. Academic Press, New York, p 328

Benirschke K, Kaufmann P 2000 Pathology of the human placenta, 4th edn. Springer, New York.

Bierings M B, Adriaansen H J, Van Dijk J P 1988 The appearance of transferrin receptors on cultured human cytotrophoblast and in vitro formed syncytiotrophoblast. Placenta 9: 387–396

Bleker O P, Kloosterman G J, Breur W, Mieras D J 1977 The volumetric growth of the human placenta: a longitudinal ultrasonic study. American Journal of Obstetrics and Gynecology 127: 657–661

Borell U, Fernström I, Westman A 1958 Eine arteriographische Studie des Plazentarkreislaufs. Geburtshilfe und Frauenheilkunde 18: 1–9

Bourne G L 1962 The human amnion and chorion. Lloyd-Luke, London

Bouw G M, Stolte L A M, Baak J P A, Oort J 1978 Quantitative morphology of the placenta. 3. The growth of the placenta and its relationship to birth weight. European Journal of Obstetrics, Gynecology and Reproductive Biology 8: 73–76

Boyd J D, Hamilton W J 1970 The human placenta. Heffer & Sons, Cambridge

Boyd P A, Brown R A, Stewart W J 1980 Quantitative structural differences within the normal term human placenta: a pilot study. Placenta 1: 337–344

Boyd P A, Brown R A, Coghill G R, Slidders W, Stewart W J 1983 Measurement of the mass of syncytiotrophoblast in a range of human placentae using an image analysing computer. Placenta 4: 255–262

Brosens I 1988 The utero-placental vessels at term — the distribution and extent of physiological changes. Trophoblast Research 3: 61–68

Brosens I, Robertson W B, Dixon H G 1967 The physiological response of the vessels of the placental bed to normal pregnancy. Journal of Pathology and Bacteriology 93: 569–579

Bulmer J N, Johnson P M 1984 Macrophage populations in the human placenta and amniochorion. Clinical and Experimental Immunology 57: 393–403

Burton G J 1986a Intervillous connections in the mature human placenta: instances of syncytial fusion or section artifacts? Journal of Anatomy 145: 13–23

Burton G J 1986b Scanning electron microscopy of intervillous connections in the mature human placenta. Journal of Anatomy 147: 245–254

Burton G J 1987 The fine structure of the human placental villus as revealed by scanning electron microscopy. Scanning Microscopy 1: 1811–1828

Burton G J, Ingram S C, Palmer M E 1987 The influence of mode of fixation on morphometrical data derived from terminal villi in the human placenta at term: a comparison of immersion and perfusion fixation. Placenta 8: 37–51

Cabezon C, De La Fuente F, Jurado M, Lopez G 1985 Histometry of the placental structures involved in the respiratory interchange. Acta Obstetricia et Gynecologica Scandinavica 64: 411–416

Cantle S J, Kaufmann P, Luckhardt M, Schweikhart G 1987 Interpretation of syncytial sprouts and bridges in the human placenta. Placenta 8: 221–234

Carter A M 1997 When is the maternal placental circulation established in man? Placenta 18: 83–87

Castellucci M, Kaufmann P 1982 A three-dimensional study of the normal human placental villous core: II. Stromal architecture. Placenta 3: 269–285

Castellucci M, Kaufmann P 2000 Hofbauer cells. In: Benirschke K, Kaufmann P (eds) Pathology of the human placenta, 4th edn. Springer, New York, pp 82–88

Castellucci M, Zaccheo D, Pescetto G 1980 A three-dimensional study of the normal human placental villous core. I. The Hofbauer cells. Cell and Tissue Research 210: 235–247

Castellucci M, Schweikhart G, Kaufmann P, Zaccheo D 1984 The stromal architecture of immature intermediate villus of the human placenta: functional and clinical implications. Gynecological and Obstetrical Investigation 18: 95–99

Castellucci M, Mühlhauser J, Zaccheo D 1990a The Hofbauer cell: the macrophage of the human placenta. In: Andreani D, Bompiani G, Di Mario U, Faulk W P, Galluzzo A (eds) Immunobiology of normal and diabetic pregnancy. John Wiley & Sons, Chichester, pp 135–144

Castellucci M, Scheper M, Scheffen I, Celona A, Kaufmann P 1990b The development of the human placental villous tree. Anatomy and Embryology 181: 117–128

Castellucci M, Classen-Linke I, Mühlhauser J, Kaufmann P, Zardi L, Chiquet-Ehrismann R 1991 The human placenta: a model for tenascin expression. Histochemistry 95: 449–458

Castellucci M, Kosanke G, Verdenelli F, Huppertz B, Kaufmann P 2000 Villous sprouting: fundamental mechanisms of human placental development. Human Reproduction Update, 6: 485–494

Clavero-Nunez J A, Botella-Llusia J 1963 Ergebnisse von Messungen der Gesamtoberfläche normaler und krankhafter Placenten. Archiv für Gynäkologie 198: 56–60

Cotter T G, Lennon S V, Glynn J G, Martin S J 1990 Cell death via apoptosis and its relationship to growth, development and differentiation of both tumour and normal cells. Anticancer Research 10: 1153–1159

Daya D, Sabet L 1991 The use of cytokeratin as a sensitive and reliable marker for trophoblastic tissue. American Journal of Clinical Pathology 95: 137–141

Demir R, Kaufm0ann P, Castellucci M, Erbengi T, Kotowski A 1989 Fetal vasculogenesis and angiogenesis in human placental villi. Acta Anatomica 136: 190–203

Denker H-W, Aplin J D (eds) 1990 Trophoblast invasion and endometrial receptivity: novel aspects of the cell biology of embryo implantation. Trophoblast Research IV Kluwer Academic, Boston, MA

de Wolf F, de Wolf-Peeters C, Brosens I 1973 Ultrastructure of the spiral arteries in the human placental bed at the end of normal pregnancy. American Journal of Obstetrics and Gynecology 117: 833–848

Dinarello C A 1991 Interleukin-1 and interleukin-1 antagonism. Blood 77: 1627–1652

Enders A C, King B F 1970 The cytology of Hofbauer cells. Anatomical Record 167: 231–252

Faller T H, Ferenci P 1973 Der Aufbau der Placenta-Septen. Untersuchungen mir Hilfe der Quinacrinfluorescenzfärbung des Y-Chromatins. Zeitschrift für Anatomie und Entwicklungsgeschichte 142: 207–217

Flynn A, Finke J H, Hilfiker M L 1982 Placental mononuclear phagocytes as a source of interleukin-1. Science 218: 475–477

Fox H 1970 Effect of hypoxia on trophoblast in organ culture. American Journal of Obstetrics and Gynecology 107: 1058–1064

Frank H G, Malekzadeh F, Kertschanska S, Crescimanno C, Castellucci M, Lang I, Desoye G, Kaufmann P 1994 Immunohistochemistry of two different types of placental fibrinoid. Acta Anatomica 150: 55–68

Frank H G, Huppertz B, Kertschanska S, Blanchard D, Roelcke D, Kaufmann P 1995 Anti-adhesive glycosylation of fibronectin-like molecules in human placental matrix-type fibrinoid. Histochemistry and Cell Biology 104: 317–329

Geier G, Schuhmann R, Kraus H 1975 Regional unterschiedliche Zellproliferation innerhalb der Plazentone reifer menschlicher Plazenten: autoradiographische Untersuchungen. Archiv für Gynakologie 21: 31–37

Glover D M, Brownstein D, Burchette S, Larsen A, Wilson C B 1987 Expression of HLA class II antigens and secretion of interleukin-1 by monocytes and macrophages from adults and neonates. Immunology 61: 195–201

Goldstein J, Braverman M, Salafia C, Buckley P 1988 The phenotype of human placental macrophages and its variation with gestational age. American Journal of Pathology 133: 648–659

Goldstein S R, Subramanyam B R, Snyder J R 1986 Ratio of gestational sac volume to crown–rump length in early pregnancy. Human Pathology 31: 320–321

Gosseye S, Fox H 1984 An immunohistological comparison of the secretory capacity of villous and extravillous trophoblast in the human placenta. Placenta 5: 329–348

Hein K 1971 Licht- und elektronenmikroskopische Untersuchungen an der Basalplatte der reifen menschlichen Plazenta. Zeitschrift für Zellforschung 122: 323–349

Hertig A T 1960 La nidation des oeufs humains fecondes normaux et anormaux. In: Ferin J, Gaudefroy M (eds) Les fonctions de nidation uterine et leurs troubles. Masson, Paris, pp 169–213

Hertig A T 1962 The placenta: some new knowledge about an old organ. Obstetrics and Gynecology 20: 859–866

Hertig A T, Rock J 1941 Two human ova of the previllous stage having an ovulation age of about eleven and twelve days respectively. Contributions to Embryology, Carnegie Institution of Washington 29: 127–156

Heuser C H, Streeter G L 1941 Development of the macaque embryo. Contributions to Embryology, Carnegie Institution of Washington 29: 15–55

Hui K Y, Haber E, Matsueda G R 1983 Monoclonal antibodies to a synthetic fibrin-like peptide bind to human fibrin but not fibrinogen. Science 222: 1129–1132

Huppertz B, Kaufmann P 1999 The apoptosis cascade in human villous trophoblast. A review. Trophoblast Research 13: 215–242

Huppertz B, Frank H G, Kingdom J C P, Reister F, Kaufmann P 1998 Villous cytotrophoblast regulation of the syncytial apoptotic cascade in the human placenta. Histochemistry and Cell Biology 110: 495–508

Huppertz B, Frank H G, Reister F, Kingdom J, Korr H, Kaufmann P 1999a Apoptosis cascade progresses during turnover of human trophoblast: analysis of villous cytotrophoblast and syncytial fragments in-vitro. Laboratory Investigation 79: 1687–1702

Huppertz B, Frank H G, Kaufmann P 1999b The apoptosis cascade — morphological and immunohistochemical methods for its visualization. Anatomy and Embryology 200: 1–18

Huppertz B, Kingdom J, Caniggia I, Kaufmann P 1999c Oxygen modulates the balance between apoptosis and necrosis in human villous trophoblast. Placenta 20: A32

Hustin J, Schaaps J P, Lambotte R 1988 Anatomical studies of the utero-placental vascularization in the first trimester of pregnancy. Trophoblast Research 3: 49–60

Jackson M R, Mayhew T M, Haas J D 1987 Morphometric studies on villi in human term placentae and the effects of altitude, ethnic grouping and sex of newborn. Placenta 8: 487–495

Jaffe E A 1987 Cell biology of endothelial cells. Human Pathology 18: 234–239

Johannigmann J, Zahn V, Thieme V 1972 Einführung in die Ultraschalluntersuchung mit dem Vidoson. Elektromedica 2: 1–11

Jones C J P, Fox H 1977 Syncytial knots and intervillous bridges in the human placenta: an ultrastructural study. Journal of Anatomy 124: 275–286

Kadyrov M, Kosanke G, Kingdom J, Kaufmann P 1998 Increased fetoplacental angiogenesis during first trimester in anaemic women. Lancet 352: 1747–1749

Kameda T, Koyama M, Matzuzaki N, Taniguchi T, Saji F, Tanizawa O 1991 Localization of three subtypes of Fc P receptors in human placenta by immunohistochemical analysis. Placenta 12: 15–26

Kaufmann P 1972 Untersuchungen über die Langhanszellen in der menschlichen Placenta. Zeitschrift fur Zellforschung 128: 283–302

Kaufmann P 1981 Entwicklung der Plazenta. In: Becker V, Schiebler Th H, Kubli F (eds) Die Plazenta des Menschen. Thieme, Stuttgart

Kaufmann P 1982 Development and differentiation of the human placental villous tree. Bibliotheca Anatomica 22: 29–39

Kaufmann P 1983 Vergleichend-anatomische und funktionelle Aspekte des Placenta-Baues. Funktionelle Biologie und Medizin 2: 71–79

Kaufmann P, Scheffen I 1992 Placental development. In: Polln R, Fox W (eds) Neonatal and fetal medicine — physiology and pathophysiology. Saunders, Orlando

Kaufmann P, Stark J 1971 Die Basalplatte der reifen menschlichen Placenta. I. Semidünnschnitt-Histologie. Zeitschrift für Anatomie und Entwicklungsgeschichte 135: 1–19

Kaufmann P, Sen D K, Schweikhart G 1979 Classification of human placental villi. I Histology and scanning electron microscopy. Cell and Tissue Research 200: 409–423

Kaufmann P, Nagi W, Fuhrmann B 1983 Die funktionelle Bedeutung der Langhanszellen der menschlichen Plazenta. Verhandlungen der Anatomischen Gesellschaft 77: 435–436

Kaufmann P, Bruns U, Leiser R, Luckhardt M, Winterhager E 1985 The fetal vascularization of term human placental villi. II Intermediate and terminal villi. Anatomy and Embryology 173: 203–214

Kaufmann P, Luckhardt M, Schweikhart G, Cantle S J 1987 Cross sectional features and three-dimensional structure of human placental villi. Placenta 8: 235–247

Kaufmann P, Luckhardt M, Leiser R 1988 Three-dimensional representation of the fetal vessel system in the human placenta. Trophoblast Research 3: 113–137

Khong T Y, Lane E B, Robertson W B 1986 An immunocytochemical study of fetal cells at the maternal-placental interface using monoclonal antibodies to keratins, vimentin and desmin. Cell and Tissue Research 246: 189–195

Khudr G, Soma H, Benirschke K 1973 Trophoblastic origin of the X-cell and the placental giant cell. American Journal of Obstetrics and Gynecology 115: 530–533

King B F 1987 Ultrastructural differentiation of stromal and vascular components in early macaque placental villi. American Journal of Anatomy 178: 30–44

Kingdom J C P, Kaufmann P 1997 Oxygen and placental villous development: origins of fetal hypoxia. Placenta 18: 613–621

Knopp J 1960 Das Wachstum der Chorionzotten vom 2. bis 10. Monat. Zeitschrift für Anatomie und Entwicklungsgeschichte 122: 42–59

Kohnen G, Kertschanska S, Demir R, Kaufmann P 1996 Placental villous stroma as a model system for myofibroblast differentiation. Histochemistry and Cell Biology 105: 415–429

Kurman R J, Main C S, Chen H-C 1984a Intermediate trophoblast: a distinctive form of trophoblast with specific morphological, biochemical and functional features. Placenta 5: 349–370

Kurman R J, Young R H, Norris H J, Main C S, Lawrence W D, Scully R E 1984b Immunocytochemical localization of placental lactogen and chorionic gonadotropin in the normal placenta and trophoblastic tumors, with emphasis on intermediate trophoblast and the placental site trophoblastic tumor. International Journal of Gynecological Pathology 3: 101–121

Küstermann W 1981 Über 'Proliferationsknoten' und 'Syncytialknoten' der menschlichen Placenta. Anatomischer Anzeiger 150: 144–157

Lang I, Hartmann M, Blaschitz A et al 1994 Differential lectin binding to the fibrinoid of human full term placenta: correlation with a fibrin antibody and the PAF-Halmi method. Acta Anatomica 150: 170–177

Lea R G, Tulppala M, Critchley H O 1997 Deficient syncytiotrophoblast tumour necrosis factor-alpha characterises failing first trimester pregnancies in a subgroup of recurrent miscarriage patients. Human Reproduction 12: 1313–1320

Lehmann W D, Schuhmann R, Kraus H 1973 Regionally different steroid biosynthesis within materno-fetal circulation units (placentones) of mature human placentas. Journal of Perinatal Medicine 1: 198–204

Leiser R, Beier H M 1988 Morphological studies of lacunar formation in the early rabbit placenta. Trophoblast Research 3: 97–110

Leiser R, Luckhardt M, Kaufmann P, Winterhager E, Bruns U 1985 The fetal vascularisation of term human placental villi. I. Peripheral stem villi. Anatomy and Embryology 173: 71–80

Luckett W P 1978 Origin and differentiation of the yolk sac and extraembryonic mesoderm in presomite human and rhesus monkey embryos. American Journal of Anatomy 152: 59–97

Martin B J, Spicer S S 1973 Ultrastructural features of cellular maturation and aging in human trophoblast. Journal of Ultrastructure Research 43: 133–149

Mayhew T M, Joy C F, Haas J D 1984 Structure-function correlation in the human placenta: the morphometric diffusing capacity for oxygen at full term. Journal of Anatomy 139: 691–708

Mayhew T M, Jackson M R, Haas J D 1986 Microscopical morphology of the human placenta and its effects on oxygen diffusion: a morphometric model. Placenta 7: 121–131

Mayhew T M, Leach L, McGee R, Ismail W W, Myklebust R, Lammiman M J 1999 Proliferation, differentiation and apoptosis in villous trophoblast at 13–41 weeks of gestation (including observations on annulate lamellae and nuclear pore complexes). Placenta 20: 407–422

Mi S, Lee X, Li X, Veldman G M, Finnerty H, Racie L, LaVallie E, Tang X Y, Edouard P, Howes S, Keith J C, McCoy J M 2000 Syncytin is a captive retroviral envelope protein involved in human placental morphogenesis. Nature 403: 785–789

Moll W 1981 Physiologie der maternen plazentaren Durchblutung. In: Becker V, Schiebler Th H, Kubli F (eds) Die Plazenta des Menschen. Thieme, Stuttgart, pp 172–194

Moll W 1995 Absence of intervillous blood flow in the first trimester of human pregnancy. Placenta 16: 333–334

Moskalewski S, Ptak W, Czarnik Z 1975 Demonstration of cells with IgG receptor in human placenta. Biology of the Neonate 26: 268–273

Mühlhauser J, Crescimanno C, Rajaniemi H, Parkkila S, Milovanov A P, Castellucci M, Kaufmann P 1994 Immunohistochemistry of carbonic anhydrase in human placenta and fetal membranes. Histochem 101: 91–98

Naeye R L 1987 Do placental weights have clinical significance? Human Pathology 18: 387–391

Nelson D M 1996 Apoptotic changes occur in syncytiotrophoblast of human placental villi where fibrin type fibrinoid is deposited at discontinuities in the villous trophoblast. Placenta 17: 387–391

Nikolov S D, Schiebler T H 1973 Über das fetale Gefäßsystem der reifen menschlichen Placenta. Zeitschrift for Zellforschung 139: 333–350

Okudaira Y, Hashimoto T, Hamanaka N, Yoshinare S 1971 Electron microscopic study on the trophoblastic cell column of human placenta. Journal of Electron Microscopy 20: 93–106

O'Rahilly R 1973 Developmental stages in human embryos. Part A, Publication 631. Carnegie Institute of Washington, Washington

Park W W 1971 Choriocarcinoma: a study of its pathology. Heinemann, London, pp 13–27

Pierce G B, Midgley A R 1963 The origin and function of human syncytiotrophoblastic giant cells. American Journal of Pathology 43: 153–173

Pijnenborg R, Robertson W B, Brosens I, Dixon G 1981 Trophoblast invasion and the establishment of haemochorial placentation in man and laboratory animals. Placenta 2: 71–92

Pilz I, Schweikhart G, Kaufmann P 1980 Zur Abgrenzung normaler, artefizieller und pathologischer Strukturen in reifen menschlichen Plazentazotten. III. Morphometrische Untersuchungen bei Rh-Inkompatibilität. Archives of Gynecology and Obstetrics 229: 137–154

Platanias L C, Vogelzang N J 1990 Interleukin-1: biology, pathophysiology, and clinical prospects. American Journal of Medicine 89: 621–629

Pötgens A J G, Schmitz U, Bose P, Versmold A, Kaufmann P, Frank H G 2002 Mechanisms of syncytial fusion: a review. Placenta 23, Suppl A: 107–113

Ramsey E M, Corner G W Jr, Donner M W 1963 Serial and cineradioangiographic visualization of maternal circulation in the primate (hemochorial) placenta. American Journal of Obstetrics and Gynecology 86: 213–225

Reister F, Frank H G, Heyl W et al 1999 The distribution of macrophages in spiral arteries of the placental bed in pre-eclampsia differs from that in healthy patients. Placenta 20: 229–233

Richart R 1961 Studies of placental morphogenesis. I. Radioautographic studies of human placenta utilizing tritiated thymidine. Proceedings of the Society for Experimental Biology and Medicine 106: 829–831

Robertson W B, Warner B 1974 The ultrastructure of the human placental bed. Journal of Pathology 112: 203–211

Rosenberg S M, Maslar I A, Riddick D H 1980 Decidual production of prolactin in late gestation: further evidence for a decidual source of amniotic fluid prolactin. American Journal of Obstetrics and Gynecology 138: 681–685

Sakuragi N, Matsuo H, Coukos G et al 1994 Differentiation-dependent expression of the Bcl-2 proto-oncogene in the human trophoblast lineage. Journal of the Society for Gynecological Investigation 1: 164–172

Sala A M, Valeri V, Matheus M 1983 Stereological analysis of syncytiotrophoblast from human mature placenta. Archives of Anatomy and Microscopy 72: 99–106

Schaaps J P, Hustin J 1988 In vivo aspect of the maternal-trophoblastic border during the first trimester of gestation. Trophoblast Research 3: 3–48

Schiebler T H, Kaufmann P 1981 Reife Plazenta. In: Becker V, Schiebler T H, Kubli F (eds) Die Plazenta des Menschen. Georg Thieme, Stuttgart, pp 51–100

Schmid-Schönbein H 1988 Conceptional proposition for a specific microcirculatory problem: Maternal blood flow in hemochorial multivillous placentae as percolation of a 'porous medium'. Trophoblast Research 3: 17–38

Schuhmann R 1981 Plazenton: Begriff, Entstehung, funktionelle Anatomie. In: Becker V, Schiebler T H, Kubli H (eds) Die Plazenta des Menschen. Thieme Verlag, Stuttgart, pp 199–207

Schuhmann R, Geier G 1972 Histomorphologische Placentabefunde bei EPG-Gestose. Archiv für Gynäkologie 213: 31–47

Schuhmann R, Wehler V 1971 Histologische Unterschiede an Plazentazotten innerhalb der materno-fetalen Strömungseinheit. Ein Beitrag zur funktionellen Morphologie der Plazenta. Archiv für Gynäkologie 210: 425–439

Schuhmann R, Kraus H, Borst R, Geier G 1976 Regional unterschiedliche Enzymaktivität innerhalb der Placentone reifer menschlicher Placenten. Histochemische und biochemische Untersuchungen. Archiv für Gynäkologie 220: 209–226

Schuhmann R, Stoz F, Maier M 1986 Histometrische Untersuchungen an Plazentonen menschlicher Plazenten. Zeitschrift für Geburtshilfe und Perinatologie 190: 196–203

Schweikhart G, Kaufmann P 1977 Zur Abgrenzung normaler, artefizieller und pathologischer Strukturen in reifen menschlichen Plazentazotten. I Ultrastruktur des Syncytiotrophoblasten. Archiv für Gynäkologie 222: 213–230

Sedmak D D, Davis D H, Singh U, van de Winkel J G J, Anderson C L 1991 Expression of IgG Fc receptor antigens in placenta and on endothelial cells in humans: an immunohistochemical study. American Journal of Pathology 138: 175–181

Sen D K, Kaufmann P, Schweikhart G 1979 Classification of human placental villi. II. Morphometry. Cell and Tissue Research 200: 425–434

Sheppard B L, Bonnar J 1988 The maternal blood supply to the placenta in pregnancy complicated by intrauterine fetal growth retardation. Trophoblast Research 3: 69–82

Smith S C, Baker P N, Symonds E M 1997 Placental apoptosis in normal human pregnancy. American Journal of Obstetrics and Gynecology 177: 57–65

Stark J, Kaufmann P 1971 Die Basalplatte der reifen menschlichen Placenta. II. Gefrierschnitthistochemie. Zeitschrift für Anatomie und Entwicklungsgeschichte 135: 185–201

Steinborn A, von Gall C, Hildenbrand R, Stutte H J, Kaufmann M 1998 Identification of placental cytokine-producing cells in term and preterm labor. Obstetrics and Gynecology 91: 329–335

Sunderland C A, Redman C W G, Stirrat G M 1981 Monoclonal antibodies to human syncytiotrophoblast. Immunology 43: 541–546

Teasdale F 1978 Functional significance of the zonal morphologic differences in the normal human placenta. American Journal of Obstetrics and Gynecology 130: 773–778

Teasdale F, Jean-Jacques G 1985 Morphometric evaluation of the microvillous surface enlargement factor in the human placenta from mid-gestation to term. Placenta 6: 375–381

Thornton S C, Por S B, Walsh B J, Penny R, Breit S N 1990 Interaction of immune and connective tissue cells: I. The effect of lymphokines and monokines on fibroblast growth. Journal of Leukocyte Biology 47: 312–320

Todros T, Sciarrone A, Piccoli E, Guiot C, Kaufmann P, Kingdom J 1999 Umbilical Doppler waveforms and placental villous angiogenesis in pregnancies complicated by fetal growth restriction. Obstetrics and Gynecology 93: 499–503

Vince G S, Johnson P M 1996 Immunobiology of human uteroplacental macrophages — friend and foe? Placenta 17: 191–199

Voigt S, Kaufmann P, Schweikhart G 1978 Zur Abgrenzung normaler, artefizieller und pathologischer Strukturen in reifen menschlichen Plazentazotten. II. Morphometrische Untersuchungen zum Einfluss des Fixationsmodus. Archiv für Gynäkologie 226: 347–362

Wallenburg H C S, Hutchinson D L, Schuler H M, Stolte L A M, Janssens J 1973 The pathogenesis of placental infarction. II. An experimental study in the rhesus monkey placenta. American Journal of Obstetrics and Gynecology 116: 841–846

Welsh A O, Enders A E 1985 Light and electron microscopic examination of the mature decidual cells of the rat with emphasis on the antimesometrial decidua and its degeneration. American Journal of Anatomy 172: 1–29

Weser H, Kaufmann P 1978 Lichtmikroskopische und histochemische Untersuchungen an der Chorionplatte der reifen menschlichen Placenta. Archiv für Gynäkologie 225: 15–30

Wiese K-H 1975 Licht-und elektronenmikroskopische Untersuchungen an der Chorionplatte der reifen menschlichen Placenta. Archiv für Gynäkologie 218: 243–259

Wigglesworth J S 1967 Vascular organization of the human placenta. Nature 216: 1120–1121

Winckel F K L W 1893 Lehrbuch der Geburtshilfe, 2. Aufl. Veit, Leipzig

Wislocki G B, Streeter G L 1938 On the placentation of the macaque (Macaca mulatta) from the time of implantation until the formation of the definitive placenta. Contributions to Embryology of the Carnegie Institute 27: 1–66

Yasuda M, Umemura S, Osamura Y R, Kenjo T, Tsutsumi Y 1995 Apoptotic cells in the human endometrium and placental villi: pitfalls in applying the TUNEL method. Archives of Histology and Cytology 58: 185–190

Yeh C-J G, Hsi B L, Samson M et al 1987 Monoclonal antibodies (GB 16, GB 18, GB 19, GB 22) raised against human placental microvilli recognise the transferrin receptor. Placenta 8: 627–638

Yui J, Hemmings D, Garcia Lloret M I, Guilbert L J 1996 Expression of the human p55 and p75 tumor necrosis factor receptors in primary villous trophoblasts and their role in cytotoxic signal transduction. Biology of Reproduction 55: 400–409

Zaccheo D, Pistoia V, Castellucci M, Martinoli C 1989 Isolation and characterization of Hofbauer cells from human placental villi. Archives of Gynecology and Obstetrics 246: 189–200

38

General pathology of the placenta, umbilical cord and fetal membranes

H. Fox

Pathology of the placenta   1273
Macroscopic abnormalities of the placenta   1273
Histological abnormalities of the placenta   1285

Pathology of the umbilical cord   1293
Developmental abnormalities   1293
Mechanical lesions   1297
Vascular lesions   1298
Ulceration and necrosis   1299
Inflammation   1300
Cysts   1300
Tumours   1301

Pathology of the membranes   1301
Squamous metaplasia   1301
Amnion nodosum   1302
Meconium staining   1303
Inflammation of the membranes   1303
Premature rupture of the membranes   1306
Extramembranous pregnancy   1306
Extra-amniotic pregnancy   1307
Amniotic bands and strings   1307

Clinicopathological value of pathological examination of the
    placenta, cord and membranes   1308
Pre-eclampsia   1309
Intrauterine fetal growth retardation   1310
Preterm delivery   1311
Intrauterine fetal death   1312
Maternal infections   1314

PATHOLOGY OF THE PLACENTA

Placental abnormalities have to be assessed in functional terms and no lesion, however pathologically impressive it may appear, can be considered as significant if it cannot be shown to impair fetal oxygenation, development or growth. It is readily accepted, however, that the pathologist committed to this attitude is faced with a grave disadvantage when examining the delivered placenta for many, probably most, of the complications of pregnancy traditionally attributed to 'placental insufficiency' are a result, not of intrinsic changes within the placenta, but of abnormalities in maternal uteroplacental blood flow. These in turn appear to be largely due to inadequate conversion, by extravillous trophoblast, of the spiral arteries into uteroplacental vessels (see Chapter 39). The pathologist must therefore examine the placenta in the light of the frustrating knowledge that the most important pathological processes affecting the organ are present in vessels which are not usually available for study. It should be noted that this chapter is largely concerned with the pathology of the third-trimester placenta: changes encountered in placentas from pregnancies terminating during the early stages are discussed in Chapter 41. Certain specialised aspects of placental pathology are considered in Chapters 40, 42 and 48.

MACROSCOPIC ABNORMALITIES OF THE PLACENTA

These can be usefully, though obviously arbitrarily and somewhat artificially, grouped into four categories:

1. Developmental abnormalities
2. Lesions which reduce the mass of functioning villi
3. Haematomas and thrombi
4. Miscellaneous abnormalities which are devoid of functional significance.

Developmental abnormalities

Placenta extrachorialis

This is the commonest developmental anomaly of the placenta, being found in about 25% of all placentas (Fox 1997a). In this abnormality the chorionic plate, from which the villi arise, is smaller than the basal plate and hence the transition from villous to membranous chorion takes place not at the edge of the placenta but at some distance within the circumference of the fetal surface of the placenta, thus leaving a ridge of villous tissue projecting beyond the limits of the chorionic plate (Fig. 38.1). If the transition from villous to membranous chorion is marked by a flat ring of membranes the placenta is classed as 'circummarginate' (Fig. 38.2) whilst if this ring is plicated with a raised, often rolled, edge the placenta is

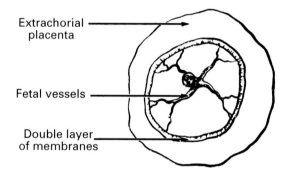

Fig. 38.1 Diagrammatic representation of an extrachorial placenta as viewed from the fetal aspect. (From Fox 1997a. Reproduced by permission of W B Saunders.)

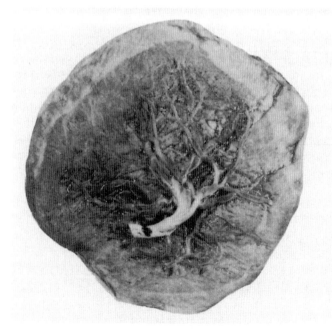

Fig. 38.2 A circummarginate placenta viewed from the fetal aspect. (From Fox 1997a. Reproduced by permission of W B Saunders.)

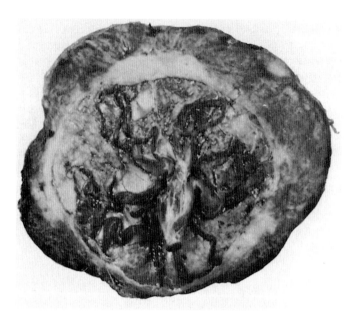

Fig. 38.3 A circumvallate placenta viewed from the fetal aspect. (From Fox 1997a. Reproduced by permission of W B Saunders.)

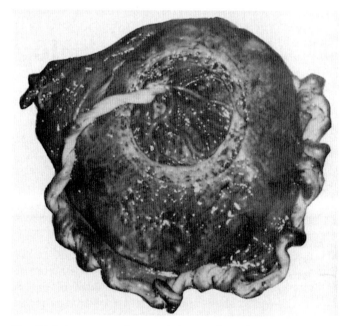

Fig. 38.4 An extreme degree of circumvallate placentation: viewed from the fetal aspect.

of the 'circumvallate' type (Figs 38.3, 38.4). Either of these two anomalies may be either complete or partial (Fig. 38.5) whilst a placenta may be circummarginate in one area and circumvallate in another.

The pathogenesis of placenta extrachorialis is unknown but suggested theories include poor development of the chorion frondosum, low intra-amniotic pressure, unduly shallow implantation of the ovum, marginal haemorrhage during early pregnancy and genetic factors: none of these hypotheses carries much conviction and a more persuasive view is that extrachorial placentation is

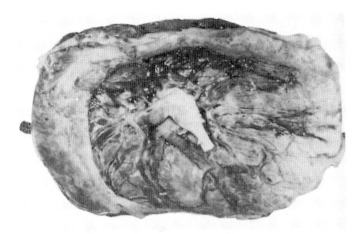

Fig. 38.5 A partially circumvallate placenta viewed from the fetal aspect. On the left side the placenta is vallate but on the right side it is normal. (From Fox 1997a. Reproduced by permission of W B Saunders.)

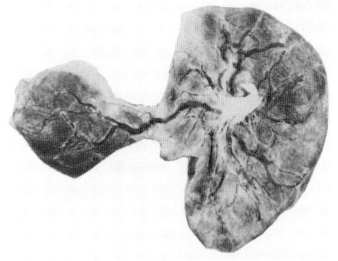

Fig. 38.6 A placenta with an accessory lobe which is joined to the main placental mass by a bridge of membranes. The cord is inserted into the main placenta and a vessel is running intramembranously to the lobe.

a consequence of excessively deep implantation of the blastocyst.

Opinion has been sharply divided about the clinical significance of extrachorial placentation, some maintaining that it is simply an anatomical variant of no clinical importance and others claiming that it is causally related to a high incidence of miscarriage, antepartum bleeding, premature labour and perinatal death. Some of this confusion has been due to the inclusion of both circummarginate and circumvallate placentas under the single heading of placenta extrachorialis for it is now clear that the circummarginate form is totally devoid of clinical significance. By contrast the circumvallate placenta, whether partial or complete, is associated with an increased incidence of low birth weight (Fox 1997a) though it should be noted that the affected infants are, to use a paradoxical phase, 'heavy' small babies, a point emphasised by the fact that circumvallate placentation is not associated with any excess of perinatal mortality. It is not currently known whether the increased incidence of low birth weight associated with circumvallate placentas is because this is, possibly because of distortion or constriction of the intervillous space, an inadequate form of placentation or whether both the abnormal placental form and the fetal growth defect are mutually dependent upon a common causal factor.

It has been claimed that circumvallate placentas are associated with an increased incidence of congenital malformations (Lademacher et al 1981) whilst Kaplan (1993b) has maintained that circumvallate placentation is associated with prematurity: there have been no subsequent data to support either of these contentions.

Placenta membranacea

In this anomaly all, or most, of the membranes are covered on their outer aspect by placental villi.

Exceptionally there may be focal thickening to form a placental disc (Hurley & Beischer 1987; Wilkins et al 1991) but more commonly the gestational sac is diffusely covered by villous tissue. This condition, which is extremely rare occurring in between 1 in 20 000 and 1 in 40 000 pregnancies (Greenberg et al 1991), has been variously attributed to pre-existing endometritis, poor development of the decidual blood supply, endometrial hyperplasia, unduly deep blastocyst implantation and a faulty trophoblastic anlage (Fox 1997a). Irrespective of pathogenesis, this anomaly is of grave import for the fetus: a placenta membranacea must of necessity also be a placenta praevia and in virtually every case recurrent antepartum bleeding, often from quite an early stage of pregnancy, is associated with either miscarriage or premature onset of labour. The outlook for fetal survival is particularly poor for not only is the fetus at risk from early delivery but it is also usually markedly underweight for the length of the gestational period, suggesting that this is an inefficient mode of placentation. In about one-third of cases a placenta membranacea is also a placenta increta (Greenberg et al 1991).

Accessory lobe

Adjacent to the main placenta may be found one or more accessory lobes of variable size (Fig. 38.6). The accessory lobe may be linked to the main placental mass by a narrow isthmus of chorionic tissue but it is not infrequently entirely separate and connected only by the membranes. The vascular supply to the lobe is usually from a vessel which runs an intramembranous course as a branch from an artery on the fetal surface of the placenta. Accessory lobes are found in about 30% of pregnancies and are usually devoid of clinical significance: occasionally, however, the lobe is retained in utero after delivery of the main placenta, this leading to subinvolution and postpartum bleeding, whilst very rarely trauma to the vessels running intramembranously to the lobe results in serious fetal haemorrhage (Hata et al 1988).

An accessory lobe has been variously attributed to unduly superficial implantation of the blastocyst with subsequent development on both anterior and posterior walls of the uterus, to implantation into the lateral or apical sulcus or to partial failure of the normal process of villous atrophy in the chorion laeve.

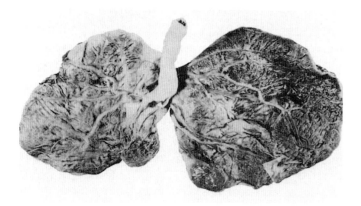

Fig. 38.7 A bilobate placenta with the cord inserted between the two placental lobes.

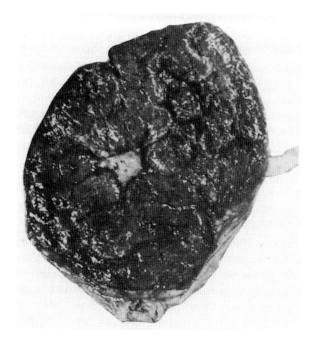

Fig. 38.8 A fenestrate placenta viewed from the maternal aspect. There is a focal deficiency of villous tissue in the centre of the placenta but the chorionic plate is complete.

Bilobate placenta

This consists of two approximately equal lobes which may be connected by a bridge of chorionic tissue or which may be quite discrete from each other (Fig. 38.7). The umbilical cord is usually inserted between the two lobes, sometimes into a connecting bridge but often velamentously. This anomaly occurs in approximately one in 350 pregnancies and its only clinical association is with an unusually high incidence of first-trimester bleeding (Fox 1997a). The pathogenesis of this anomaly is believed to be superficial implantation of the fertilised ovum with subsequent attachment of the placenta to both anterior and posterior uterine walls.

Fenestrate placenta

This is an exceptionally rare abnormality of unknown pathogenesis in which the central portion of a discoidal placenta is missing (Fig. 38.8): sometimes there is an actual hole in the centre of the placenta but more commonly the deficit is of villous tissue only. The only clinical significance of this abnormality is that it may be mistakenly thought that the missing portion is still retained in the uterus and the mother thus subjected to an unnecessary uterine exploration.

Lesions reducing mass of functional villi

Perivillous fibrin deposition

Some degree of fibrin deposition around villi occurs in almost all placentas but in a proportion is sufficiently extensive to be macroscopically visible either as a firm white plaque, often but not invariably in the marginal angle (Fig. 38.9), or as an area of irregular, whitish

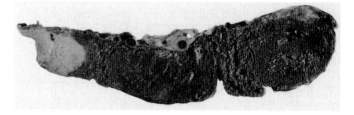

Fig. 38.9 A peripherally situated plaque of perivillous fibrin which fills in the lateral angle of the placenta.

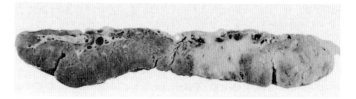

Fig. 38.10 A centrally situated focus of perivillous fibrin which is irregular in outline and rather poorly delineated.

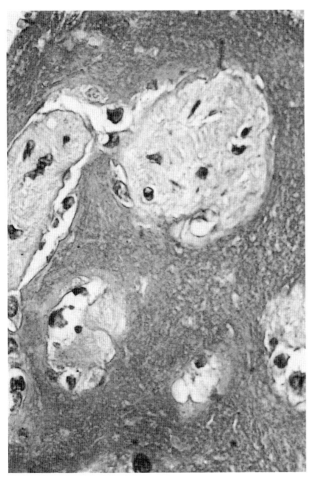

Fig. 38.11 Villi entrapped in a plaque of perivillous fibrin. The villi are fibrotic, avascular and have lost their trophoblastic covering.

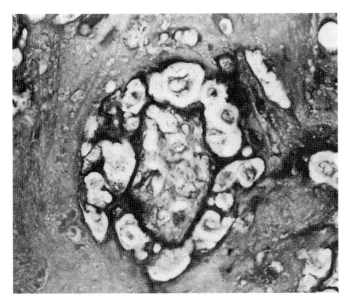

Fig. 38.12 Proliferation of cytotrophoblastic cells to form a mantle around a villus embedded in a plaque of fibrin.

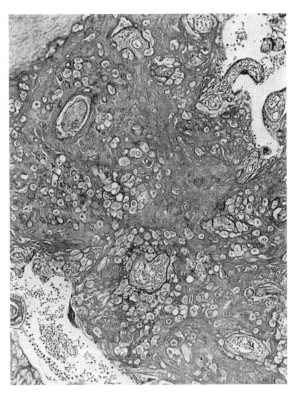

Fig. 38.13 A plaque of perivillous fibrin in which there has been marked proliferation of the villous cytotrophoblastic cells, many of which have become detached from their parent villi and have spread out into the enveloping fibrin. (From Fox 1997a. Reproduced by permission of W B Saunders.)

mottling (Fig. 38.10). Histologically these lesions are seen to consist of widely separated villi entrapped in fibrin which fills in and obliterates the intervillous space (Fig. 38.11). The syncytiotrophoblast of the entrapped villi degenerates and disappears but the villous cytotrophoblast persists and may proliferate not only to form a cellular mantle around individual villi (Fig. 38.12) but also to spread out into the surrounding fibrin (Fig. 38.13). The stroma of the included villi becomes markedly fibrotic whilst their fetal vessels undergo sclerosis and eventual obliteration. Lesions of this type occur in about 25% of placentas from uncomplicated term pregnancies and this incidence is not increased in prolonged pregnancy or in pre-eclampsia, indeed it is often unusually low in placentas from the latter group (Fox 1997a).

The entrapped villi are not, in any sense of the word, infarcted but are nevertheless of no functional value to the fetus in so far as they are clearly excluded from playing any rôle in materno-fetal transfer mechanisms. However, macroscopically visible perivillous fibrin plaques, despite clearly reducing the mass of functional villous tissue, are, in the author's experience, devoid of any clinical significance, this applying not only to small lesions but also to those in which as many as 25–30% of the villi are entrapped in fibrin (Fox 1997a): it is only fair to add that some have claimed that perivillous fibrin of this degree is associated with preterm labour and fetal growth retardation (Redline & Patterson 1994; Salafia et al 1995). The clinical banality of this lesion is explicable in terms of its pathogenesis. The fibrin surrounding the villi is formed from maternal blood in the intervillous space. As the villous syncytiotrophoblast is in direct contact with the maternal blood, and can thus be regarded as playing an endothelial-like rôle, it was in the past thought that thrombosis occurred as a result of syncytial 'degeneration': indeed, this view is still held by some (Salafia & Pijnenborg 1999; Benirschke & Kaufmann 2000) who argue that syncytial damage will result in the exposure of the maternal blood to the villous trophoblastic basement membrane which, with its content of collagens, laminin and fibrinectins, activates the coagulation system in the maternal blood. Electronmicroscopy has, however, clearly shown that the initial stage in the development of a perivillous fibrin plaque is an adherence of platelets to healthy villous syncytiotrophoblast (Moe & Jorgensen 1968) and there can be little doubt that fibrin deposition occurs as a result of turbulence, eddy currents and stasis of maternal blood within the intervillous space. The greater, therefore, the maternal blood flow through the closed irregular intervillous space the greater is the possibility of turbulence, stasis and fibrin deposition and it thus follows that perivillous fibrin plaques tend to form particularly in placentas with an excellent maternal blood supply, this accounting for the low incidence of these plaques in placentas from pre-eclamptic women and the very low incidence of fetal hypoxic complications associated with the presence of this placental lesion (Fox 1997a).

The outstanding significance of perivillous fibrin plaques is that they bear eloquent witness to the fact that the placenta can withstand the loss of up to 30% of its functioning villous population without any evidence of physiological embarrassment. Very occasionally, however, there is a truly massive perivillous deposition of fibrin, with 80–90% of the villous parenchyma being incorporated into fibrinous masses (Fig. 38.14): the placenta can clearly not withstand a loss of villous tissue of this magnitude and, very exceptionally, fetal death can ensue from perivillous fibrin deposition of this degree. This condition of very extensive perivillous fibrin deposition blends, almost imperceptibly, with that of maternal floor infarction (see below).

Maternal floor infarction

This term is applied to an excess deposition of fibrin on the basal plate. This lesion is not an infarct and a better term would be 'massive basal plate fibrin deposition'.

On gross examination the maternal surface of a placenta showing this abnormality appears greyish-yellow and has a somewhat gyriform appearance. In the sliced placenta the basal plate is seen to be markedly thickened by firm white material which can diminish considerably the height of the intervillous space (Fig 38.15). Histologically, there is simply excess fibrin deposited on the basal plate: as the fibrin increases in amount basally situated villi will become entrapped in the enlarging fibrinous mass and then undergo the same changes as do those enmeshed in a plaque of perivillous fibrin deposition. In many cases there is also extensive perivillous fibrin deposition at sites away from the basal plate.

Maternal floor infarction is very uncommon and is of unknown pathogenesis. In the past it was thought that the lesion developed after fetal death but sufficient cases of maternal floor infarction associated with a live born infant have now been described (Clewell & Manchester 1983; Katz et al 1987; Andres et al 1990; Mandsager et al 1994) for this view to be no longer tenable. Nevertheless, the lesion is associated with a high incidence of fetal

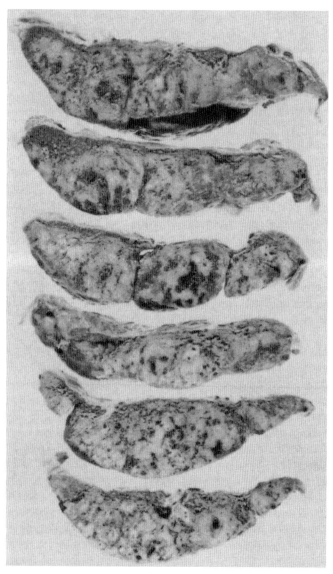

Fig. 38.14 An extreme example of perivillous fibrin deposition: approximately 90% of the villous parenchyma is incorporated into fibrinous plaques.

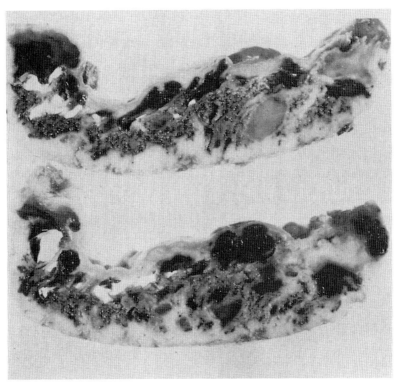

Fig. 38.15 A placenta showing marked basal deposition of fibrin, this being an example of maternal floor infarction. (From Fox 1997a. Reproduced by permission of W B Saunders.)

death and intrauterine growth retardation (Naeye 1985a; Nickel 1988; Andres et al 1990) possibly because the fibrin interferes with the perfusion of the intervillous space by maternal blood (Gersell 1993).

Maternal floor infarction tends to recur in successive pregnancies and may be associated with elevated alpha-fetoprotein levels.

Infarction

A fresh placental infarct is well demarcated, dark red and moderately firm (Fig. 38.16). As the infarct ages it becomes progressively harder and its colour changes successively to brown, yellow and white, an old infarct thus appearing as a hard white plaque with a smooth, or slightly granular, amorphous cut surface (Fig. 38.17). Histologically the early infarct is characterised by aggregation of the villi in the affected area with marked narrowing, often obliteration, of the intervillous space (Fig. 38.18): the villous fetal vessels are dilated and congested whilst the syncytial nuclei show early necrotic changes, such as pyknosis or karyorrhexis (Fig. 38.19). As the infarct ages the syncytial nuclei eventually disappear and there is a progressive coagulative necrosis of the villi: the fetal erythrocytes trapped in the vessels of the infarcted villi undergo haemolysis and the endothelium of these vessels degenerates (Fig. 38.20). The old infarct simply consists therefore of crowded 'ghost villi' showing,

it should be noted, no fibrosis or cytotrophoblastic proliferation (Fig. 38.21). There is no evidence of circulation of maternal blood through the narrowed intervillous space within the infarct though what little is left of this space often contains fibrin which is probably derived from plasma which has leaked out from the necrotic fetal villous vessels: there is commonly deposition of fibrin, derived from maternal blood, around the periphery of the infarct and non-infarcted villi are frequently entrapped within this peripheral fibrinous shell. There may be a polymorphonuclear leucocytic infiltration of the infarcted area but such a cellular infiltrate is often either scanty or entirely absent.

Small areas of infarction, involving less than 5% of the villous parenchyma, are common, occurring in 25% of placentas from uncomplicated pregnancies, and are of no clinical importance (Fox 1997a). It is widely agreed, however, that extensive placental infarction, involving more than 10% of the villous parenchyma, is associated with a high incidence of fetal hypoxia, growth retardation and intrauterine death (Naeye 1977; Fox 1997a; Lewis & Benirschke 1999). At first sight it appears obvious that these fetal complications are a direct result of loss of viable villous tissue and, indeed, it has been these apparent ill-effects of placental infarction which have led many to the belief that the placenta is normally at the full stretch of its physiological capacity and has little or no functional reserve. This is an apparently logical corollary

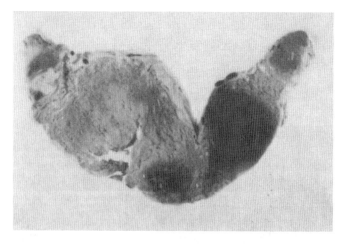

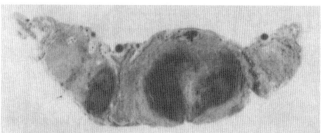

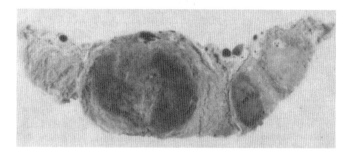

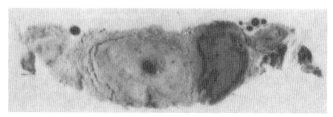

Fig. 38.16 Multiple fresh infarcts in a placenta. The infarcted areas are dark red, firm and well delineated.

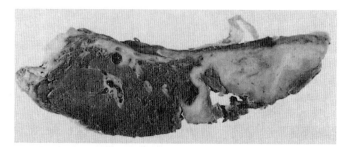

Fig. 38.17 An old placental infarct. This is seen as a white, amorphous plaque. (From Fox 1997a. Reproduced by permission of W B Saunders.)

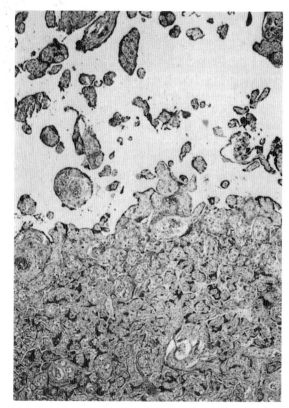

Fig. 38.18 Low-power view of a fresh placental infarct (below). The villi are aggregated and the intervillous space obliterated. (From Fox 1997a. Reproduced by permission of W B Saunders.)

of the assumption that the placenta can not withstand the loss of 10% of its functioning tissue without dire consequences for the continuing growth and viability of the fetus: this is, however, too simplistic a view for, as already discussed, a similar, or even greater, loss of villi due to their entrapment in fibrin is of no importance. This is an apparent paradox unless it is borne in mind that the villi are oxygenated from the maternal blood and that although many maternal vessels open into the intervillous space there is little or no mixing of arterial streams, the individual vessels being, in functional terms, end arteries; an infarct is therefore due to a localised obstruction to

the maternal uteroplacental circulation either by a retroplacental haematoma or by a thrombus. If the comparatively uncommon infarcts due to retroplacental haematomas are excluded it is clear that extensive infarction is due to widespread thrombotic occlusion of maternal uteroplacental vessels: this is not an event which would be expected to occur in a healthy vascular tree and it is therefore no coincidence that extensive placental infarction is usually only seen in placentas from preeclamptic women for it is in these that a vascular abnormality, in the form of acute atherosis (Robertson 1976, 1981; Khong 1991), is found which predisposes to thrombosis. Far more importantly, however, there is in this condition, whether thrombosis is superadded or not,

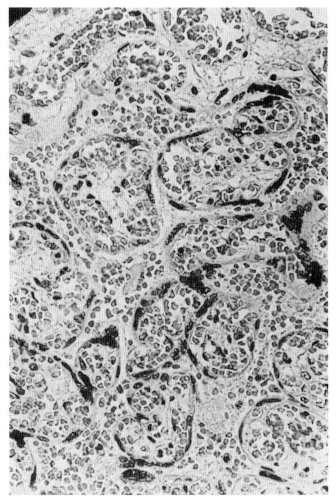

Fig. 38.19 Higher-power view of a fresh placental infarct. The villous vessels are congested and the intervillous space is markedly narrowed.

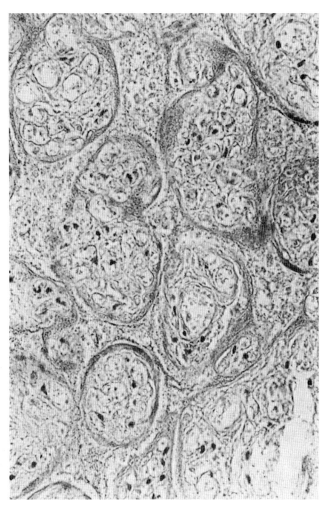

Fig. 38.20 Villi in an infarct which is somewhat older than that shown in Fig. 38.19. Villous congestion is less obvious and many of the erythrocytes in the fetal vessels have undergone haemolysis. The villous syncytiotrophoblast is almost entirely necrotic.

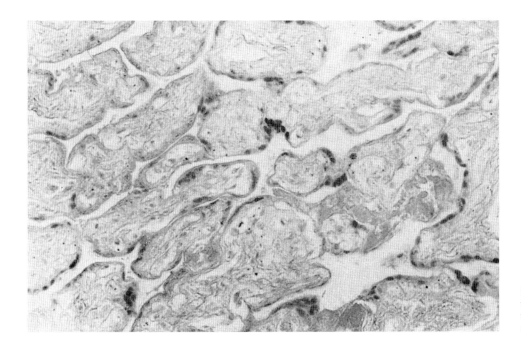

Fig. 38.21 Villi in an old infarct. The villi have a 'ghost-like' appearance whilst the villous trophoblast is almost entirely lost.

a severely restricted maternal blood flow to the placenta as a result of inadequate transformation of the spiral arteries into uteroplacental vessels (Robertson et al 1975; Robertson 1976, 1981). Thus extensive infarction occurs only against a background of a markedly abnormal maternal vasculature and a restricted maternal blood flow to the placenta and it is these factors, rather than the loss of villi due to infarction, which are the real cause of the fetal complications. The true significance of extensive placental infarction is therefore that it is the visible hallmark of a severely compromised circulation to the placenta. It is true that the situation is further worsened in such cases by infarction being superimposed on a placenta, the functional reserve of which may have been already dissipated by uteroplacental ischaemia, but the infarction per se is not the cause of the fetal complications and would be of no consequence if it occurred in a placenta with an adequate maternal blood supply.

Fetal artery thrombosis

This lesion is seen macroscopically as a roughly triangular area of pallor within the placental substance, the base of the triangle abutting onto the basal plate (Fig. 38.22): there is no alteration in parenchymal texture or consistency. Histological examination reveals a sharply localised area of avascular villi (Fig. 38.23) which contrast starkly with their immediately adjacent fully vascularised neighbours (Fig. 38.24): the stroma of these villi becomes fibrotic and the fetal vessels undergo an obliterative sclerosis though their trophoblast remains intact and viable. An organising, or organised, thrombosis is seen occluding a fetal stem artery at the apex of the lesion.

The cause of fetal artery thromboses is usually unknown but it has been suggested that they are indicative of a hypercoagulable state in the fetus and may be associated with a maternal coagulopathy, such as that found in association with anticardiolipin antibodies or protein C deficiency (Kraus 1993; Rayne & Kraus 1993; Redline & Pappin 1995). Fetal artery thrombosis is a rel-

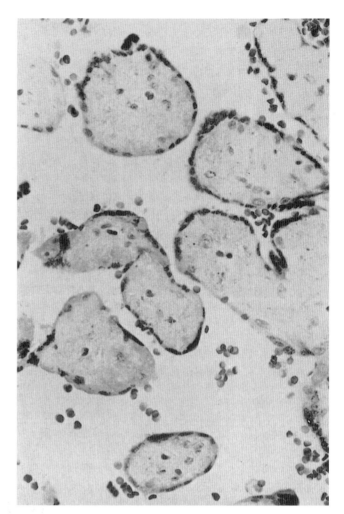

Fig. 38.23 Avascular villi resulting from a fetal artery thrombosis. (From Fox 1997a. Reproduced by permission of W B Saunders.)

atively common condition, found in about 4% of placentas from live births, and is usually clinically unimportant. The banal nature of this abnormality is still further evidence of the functional reserve capacity of the placenta, for even lesions in which 20–30% of the villi are rendered avascular are not associated with any effect on fetal wellbeing, despite the obvious fact that the avascular villi are effectively excluded from playing any rôle in materno-fetal transfer activity. Very occasionally, it is true, placentas are encountered in which multiple occlusions of fetal vessels, again occurring for no discernible cause, result in 50%, or more, of the villi being rendered avascular (Fox 1997a): under such circumstances fetal death can, and does, occur, for the placenta can not withstand a deletion of villous tissue of this magnitude.

Primary defect in placental growth

It is widely assumed that a below normal villous mass may result in inadequate growth of the placenta, that the physiological capacity of the placenta is related to its

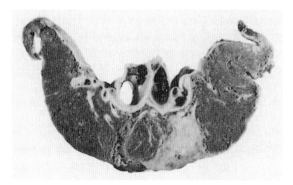

Fig. 38.22 A localised area of pallor in a placenta, due to a fetal artery thrombosis. (From Fox 1997a. Reproduced by permission of W B Saunders.)

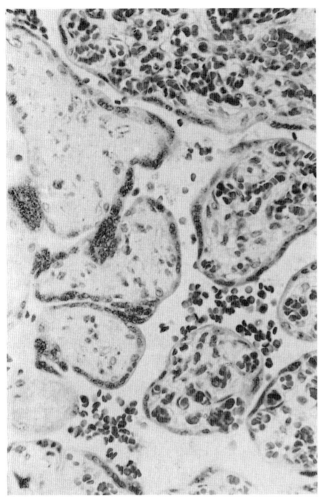

Fig. 38.24 Avascular villi consequent on thrombosis of a fetal stem artery (left) contrast with their immediately adjacent fully vascularised neighbours (right). (From Fox 1997a. Reproduced by permission of W B Saunders.)

weight and that the functional deficiencies of a small placenta will restrict fetal growth: in other words, a small placenta will result in an abnormally small fetus. However, a knowledge of placental weight is, in itself, of

little or no value, especially when taking into account the extreme difficulty of obtaining an accurate assessment of placental mass and the grossly inaccurate and misleading nature of the values obtained by weighing the placenta in the delivery room or in the laboratory (Fox 1997a). Placental:fetal weight ratios are clearly more meaningful but, although there have been a number of reviews of the significance of this ratio it would not be an undue over-simplification to draw the conclusion that these studies suggest only that small babies have small placentas and large babies have large placentas. It then becomes almost a matter of faith whether one believes that the baby is small because the placenta is small or that the placenta is small because the baby is small.

Certain facts suggest, however, that placental mass is unlikely to be a limiting factor for fetal growth. Thus if fetal weight were narrowly limited by placental mass this would imply that the term placenta does not have any functional reserve capacity. Simple pathological studies of such trivial lesions as perivillous fibrin deposition and fetal artery thrombosis indicate that this is most unlikely to be true whilst experimental studies, involving either surgical reduction of placental mass (Cefalo et al 1977; Robinson et al 1979) or artificially increased fetal oxygen consumption (Lorijn & Longo 1980), have confirmed the striking functional reserve of the placenta. Furthermore, the placenta has a normally unrealised potential for further incremental growth, a fact indicated by the unduly large placentas found in conditions such as pregnancy at high altitude, severe maternal anaemia and maternal heart failure (Clavero-Nunez 1963; Beischer et al 1970; Kruger & Arias-Stella 1970; Agboola 1975; Godfrey et al 1991).

The combination of a considerable reserve capacity and of a potential for further growth makes it unlikely that placental mass limits fetal weight, the placenta, in fact, usually being small because the baby is small. Under these circumstances the placenta, although small, has probably reached a size sufficient either to meet the nutritional and gaseous needs of the small fetus or one which

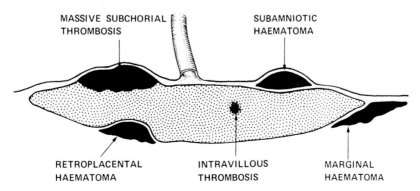

Fig. 38.25 Diagram of the sites of the various haematomas and thrombi that can occur in and around the placenta. (From Fox 1978. Reproduced by permission of W B Saunders.)

is fully capable of transferring to the fetus the limited supply of maternal oxygen and nutrients. A knowledge of placental weight is therefore of very little value in attempting to elucidate the cause of diminished fetal growth.

Haematomas and thrombi (Fig. 38.25)

Retroplacental haematoma

This is a haematoma which lies between, and separates, the basal plate of the placenta and the uterine wall: it is apparent on the maternal aspect of the placenta and bulges up towards the fetal surface with compression and often, though not invariably, infarction of the overlying villous tissue. An old haematoma is firmly adherent to the placenta and although a fresh one may become detached during delivery it leaves a characteristic crater-like depression in the maternal surface: it should be noted that adherent clot is always easily separated from the placenta and does not indent the surface.

Retroplacental haematomas have been variously attributed to rupture of a maternal uteroplacental artery or obstruction of the placental venous outflow; placental bed biopsies have suggested that, in some cases, the bleeding may originate from vascular malformations in the placental bed (Dommisse & Tiltman 1992). They are found in approximately 5% of all placentas, though their incidence is increased three-fold in those from pre-eclamptic women (Fox 1997a); there is no consistent relationship between the presence of a retroplacental haematoma and a clinical history of abruptio placentae.

The haematoma separates the overlying villi from the maternal blood vessels, but many haematomas are small,

detected only on pathological examination and of no clinical significance. It is, however, not surprising that large lesions, in which 40% or more of the villous population is acutely deprived of its blood supply, are associated with a high incidence of fetal hypoxia and death.

Subamniotic haematoma

This occurs on the fetal surface of the placenta as a plum-coloured tumefaction which lifts the amnion off from the chorion. Most are fresh and result from tearing of surface chorionic veins by excessive cord traction during delivery. Old haematomas, which are often accompanied by thrombosis of chorionic veins, tend to be associated with a low birth weight (DeSa 1971); though the nature of this relationship is far from clear.

Marginal haematoma

This is seen as a crescentic lesion at one edge of the placenta: the haematoma is usually also adherent to the maternal surface of the immediately adjacent membranes. It is usually thought that haematomas of this type occur in cases where the placenta is partially implanted in the lower uterine segment but with its lateral margin being some distance from the internal os, i.e. a lateral placenta praevia: marginal bleeding is therefore thought to result from rupture of venous channels at the lower placental margin during the process of obliteration of the lower uterine segment. Harris (1988) has disputed this view but did not provide any convincing alternative explanation. This lesion may be associated with maternal antepartum bleeding but is usually thought to be of no other clinical importance (Fox 1997a); Harris (1988) has maintained

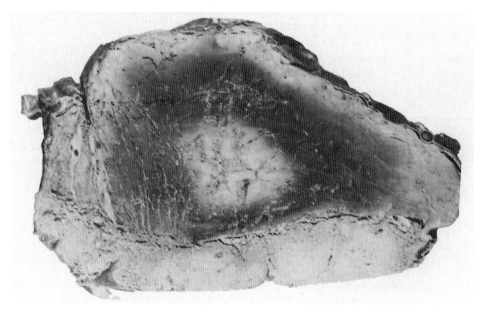

Fig. 38.26 A massive subchorial haematoma. The chorionic plate (above) has been completely stripped off from the villous tissue (below) by a massive accumulation of thrombus.

that marginal haematomas are associated with preterm labour but this claim awaits confirmation.

Massive subchorial thrombosis

This lesion, also known as a Breus' mole, is a thrombus, measuring more than 1 cm in thickness, which separates the chorionic plate from the underlying villous tissue (Fig. 38.26). The thrombus is often lobulated or bulbous and may distort the fetal surface of the placenta by forming bulging protuberances into the amniotic cavity. The thrombus probably originates from maternal blood and it has been speculated that it results from extensive obliteration of the venous channels draining the intervillous space. Massive subchorial thrombi are usually found in placentas from miscarriages but Shanklin & Scott (1975) described seven examples associated with the delivery, usually prematurely, of a liveborn child: their clinical significance is not known.

Not all subchorial thrombi are massive and although small lesions of this type have attracted little attention it is probable that they are more common than is usually realised: such lesions are, however, probably of no clinical significance (Pearlstone & Baxi 1993).

Intervillous thrombosis

This is a villus-free nodular thrombus within the intervillous space (Fig. 38.27). The thrombi usually lie approximately midway between the maternal and fetal surfaces of the placenta, measure between 1 cm and 2 cm in diameter and are soft and dark red when fresh, such early lesions also being known as Kline's haemorrhages: as the thrombi age they become gradually converted into hard, white, laminated plaques.

Thrombi of this type are found in up to 40% of all placentas (Fox 1997a), contain an admixture of fetal and maternal blood (Kaplan et al 1982) and mark a site of fetal bleeding into the intervillous space. Fetal haemorrhage is almost certainly a consequence of rupture of a villus at a site of syncytial attenuation and it is probable that thrombosis occurs because of release of a thromboplastic substance from the site of villous syncytial damage

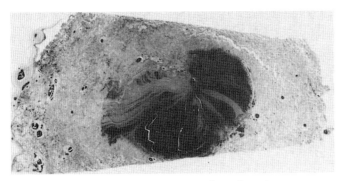

Fig. 38.27 A fresh, red laminated intervillous thrombus.

(Batcup et al 1983). Large intervillous thrombi may be associated with elevated maternal serum alpha-fetoprotein levels (Salafia et al 1988; Jauniaux et al 1990).

Miscellaneous macroscopic abnormalities

These include subchorionic fibrin plaques, septal cysts and grossly visible calcification, all of which are devoid of functional significance. It is probably worth stressing that placental calcification, often regarded as evidence of either placental senescence or 'degeneration', is of no pathological or clinical importance. Calcification is not more common, or extreme, in placentas from prolonged or abnormal pregnancies than it is in placentas from uncomplicated term pregnancies and is not associated with any fetal complications (Fox 1997a). The cause of the calcification is unknown though in biochemical terms the calcification is of the metastatic type, i.e. occurs in a calcium-saturated environement (Poggi et al 2001). Calcification occurs most commonly in first pregnancies and its incidence is related directly to low maternal age, high maternal socioeconomic status and delivery during the summer months. Placental calcification appears to occur earlier in pregnancy in cigarette smokers (Brown et al 1988).

HISTOLOGICAL ABNORMALITIES OF THE PLACENTA

Villous abnormalities

It is preferable to classify villous abnormalities, as far as possible, on a functional, rather than a purely morphological, basis. These may be grouped into:

1. Abnormalities of villous maturation
2. Changes secondary to a reduced maternal uteroplacental blood flow
3. Changes secondary to a reduced fetal villous blood flow
4. Abnormalities of unknown pathogenesis
5. Inflammatory lesions.

Abnormalities of villous maturation

During the nine months of a normal gestation there is, as discussed in Chapter 37, a progressive maturation and evolution of the villous tree. Most of the villi present in the first trimester are stem villi whilst intermediate-type villi dominate during the second trimester: from about the 30th week of gestation terminal villi (Fig. 38.28) begin to bud off from the intermediate villi and these form the bulk of the villous population in the term placenta. Histologically this changing pattern is reflected in a progressive change from large villi with small, centrally placed, fetal vessels to small villi with sinusoidally dilated

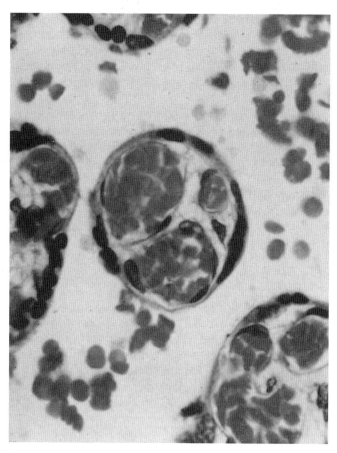

Fig. 38.28 A typical terminal villus. It is small and sinusoidally dilated vessels occupy most of its cross-sectional area. (From Fox 1997a. Reproduced by permission of W B Saunders.)

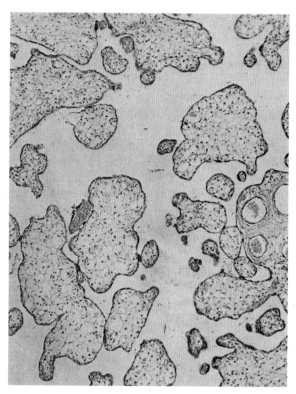

Fig. 38.29 Villi in a placenta from an uncomplicated pregnancy terminating spontaneously at the 36th week of gestation. There is, for this stage of pregnancy, a marked deficiency of terminal villi, most of the villi being of the intermediate type. (From Fox 1997a. Reproduced by permission of W B Saunders.)

fetal capillaries which lie in an immediately subtrophoblastic position. The net result of these villous changes is a marked increase in the surface area of the trophoblast which is in contact with the maternal blood in the intervillous space, an approximation to each other of the maternal and fetal circulatory systems, an increased concentration gradient between maternal and fetal blood and a crowding of flow lines, the small terminal villi being the form of villous structure which is optimally adapted for materno-fetal transfer. It is thus clear that villous tree maturation is essential for fully effective functioning of the placenta and the corollary of this is that a failure of the villous tree to undergo full maturation, with a resulting dominance of mature intermediate villi and a paucity of terminal villi at term, will result in a decreased functional efficiency of the placenta. It is therefore not surprising that a deficiency of the terminal villi (Fig. 38.29) in a late third trimester placenta (a phenomenon usually simply classed as 'villous immaturity') is associated with a high incidence of fetal growth retardation (Fox 1997a), though it should be remarked that most small for gestational age infants have fully mature placentas. Villous immaturity should only be diagnosed if there is a generalised immaturity of the villous tree for in all term placentas a few intermediate villi are always to be found scattered

amongst an otherwise fully mature villous population, usually in the centre of a lobule: these are an indication of continuing placental growth with the formation of fresh villi. It should be noted that it is very difficult to assess minor degrees of villous immaturity: there is considerable interobserver variation in making such an assessment (Khong et al 1995) and statements that gestational age of the placenta can be determined within +/− two weeks (Redline 1999) should be regarded with considerable scepticism.

The reverse of the coin, accelerated villous maturation, is also sometimes encountered, preterm infants having a fully mature placenta: this is seen particularly in pregnancies complicated by pre-eclampsia and may be a compensatory mechanism to counter the effects of a diminished maternal blood flow.

It should be noted here that the histological features which characterise maturation of the villous tree have been widely misinterpreted as ageing changes and accelerated villous maturation has been considered to represent premature ageing. A critical review of the evidence for placental ageing reveals, however, little or no indication that the placenta undergoes a true ageing process and indicates that the mature placenta is far from being senescent in either morphological or functional terms (Fox 1997b).

Changes secondary to a reduced maternal uteroplacental blood flow

Villi in placentas subjected to a reduced maternal utero-placental blood flow, e.g. in severe maternal pre-eclampsia, show a consistent and characteristic pattern of abnormalities which is identical to that noted in villous tissue grown in vitro under conditions of low oxygen tension (Fox 1970; MacLennon et al 1972; Amalados & Burton 1985; Burton et al 1989). There is an undue prominence and number of villous cytotrophoblastic cells (Fig. 38.30), together with irregular thickening of the trophoblastic basement membrane: although the syncytiotrophoblast usually appears remarkably normal on light microscopy, small focal areas of syncytial necrosis are seen on ultrastructural examination (Jones & Fox 1980).

The cytotrophoblastic cells are the trophoblastic stem cells for, even during rapid periods of trophoblastic growth, it is only in these cells that DNA synthesis and mitotic activity occurs, the syncytiotrophoblast appearing

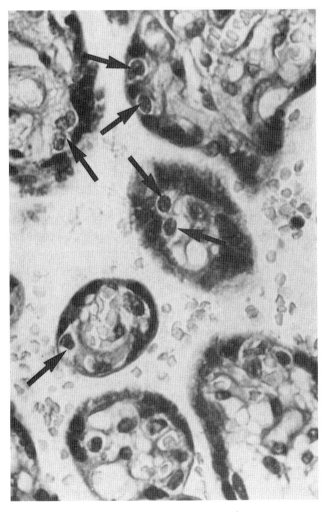

Fig. 38.30 Villi in a placenta from a woman with severe pre-eclampsia. Many prominent cytotrophoblastic cells (arrowed) are seen.

to be formed by a breaking down of the limiting membrane of the cytotrophoblastic cells. The electronmicroscope has also allowed for the recognition that some villous cytotrophoblastic cells have a cytoplasmic complexity lying somewhere between that of the simple, rather primitive, resting cytotrophoblastic cell, with its paucity of cytoplasmic organelles, and that of the organelle-rich syncytiotrophoblast: such cells are regarded as being in the process of conversion into syncytiotrophoblast. The cytotrophoblastic stem cells can therefore be considered as forming a germinative zone though one which is, in the later stages of pregnancy, largely quiescent, the cytotrophoblastic cells becoming progressively less prominent as gestation proceeds and appearing to diminish in number; there is, in reality, an increase in their number as pregnancy progresses, their apparent sparcity being a reflection of their wider dispersal in an increased volume of trophoblast (Simpson et al 1992). The normal inactivity of the villous cytotrophoblastic cells at term indicates that there is little need for the formation of fresh trophoblast at this time.

If, however, the necessity of forming new syncytiotrophoblast arises, as is the case when this tissue suffers ischaemic damage as a result of a reduced maternal blood flow, the germinative zone will be reactivated and the cytotrophoblastic cells proliferate in an attempt to repair and replace injured syncytial tissue: thus the cytotrophoblastic cells become more numerous and unusually prominent whilst mitotic figures are seen with modest frequency, all features suggesting a resurgence of activity. That there is a true proliferation of these cells has been confirmed by Arnholdt et al (1991) using a monoclonal antibody to Ki-67. At the electronoptical level many of the proliferating cells are seen to be of the type with an increased cytoplasic complexity, this indicating rapid and continuing conversion into syncytiotrophoblast, and freshly formed syncytial tissue can sometimes be recognised. This repair process is a highly successful one for it often requires prolonged search to detect residual focal areas of syncytial damage at the ultrastructural level (Jones & Fox 1980).

The trophoblastic basement membrane thickening which is seen in the villi of placentas subjected to ischaemia is probably an incidental by-product of the cytotrophoblastic cell hyperplasia for basement membrane protein is almost certainly secreted, in part at least, by these cells and an unusual degree of proliferative activity on their part would therefore be accompanied by an excessive production of basement membrane material: this is a situation akin to that found in diabetic microangiopathy, in which thickening of the capillary basement membrane is secondary to an increased turnover of endothelial cells (Vracko & Benditt 1970).

The essential response of the placenta to ischaemia is therefore a reparative one, with gross trophoblastic damage being efficiently repaired.

Changes secondary to a reduced fetal blood flow

These are seen in their purest form in the localised group of villi which, whilst fully oxygenated from the maternal blood, have been deprived of their fetal circulation by thrombosis of a fetal stem artery: such villi invariably show stromal fibrosis and an excess formation of syncytial knots and it is of interest to note that identical changes occur in the monkey placenta after ligation of a fetal stem artery (Myers & Fujikura 1968). These changes, stromal fibrosis and excess syncytial knot formation, are seen in generalised form whenever there is an overall reduction of fetal perfusion of the placenta as occurs, for example, in some cases of prolonged pregnancy, and are invariably found as a post-mortem change (Fig. 38.31) in placentas from fetuses which have been dead in utero for several days or weeks before delivery (Genest 1992; Fox 1997a). Why these particular changes should result from an impairment of fetal blood flow through the placenta is

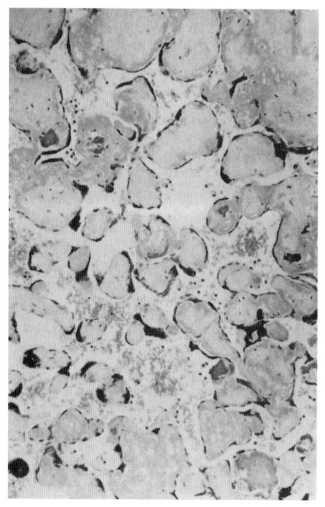

Fig. 38.31 Villi in placenta from a case of longstanding fetal intrauterine death. The villi show stromal fibrosis and a marked excess of syncytial knots. (From Fox 1997a. Reproduced by permission of W B Saunders.)

unknown but the placental villi do not in any way depend upon the fetal blood supply for either their oxygenation or supply of nutrients and hence there is no good reason why a reduced fetal perfusion should affect the functional activity of the placenta: it is therefore not surprising that neither stromal fibrosis nor excess syncytial knot formation can, in themselves, be correlated with any evidence of adverse effects, during life, on the fetus (Fox 1997a).

It should be noted that true syncytial knots have to be differentiated from syncytial sprouts which form drumstick-shaped protrusions from the villous surface and contain large nuclei; these represent the early stages of villous growth and branching and are seen on immature villi (Benirschke & Kaufmann 2000). Tangential flat cutting of the surface syncytiotrophoblast can also give an appearance which can be misinterpreted as true syncytial knots (Burton 1986; Cantle et al 1987; Kaufmann et al 1987) but the synctial nuclei in these apparent 'knots' cases are fully normal. True syncytial knots are focal clumps of aggregated syncytial nuclei with condensed nuclear chromatin which protrude into the intervillous space from the villous surface: it is now clear that these are aged syncytial nuclei which have undergone apoptosis (Jones & Fox 1977; Huppertz et al 1998; Huppertz & Kaufmann 1999). Syncytial knots are not, as is often thought to be the case, a manifestation of any degenerative change in the trophoblast: their progressive increase in the placenta as gestation progresses is a time-related phenomenon but is not a true ageing change. Excessive syncytial knotting is often attributed to uteroplacental ischaemia (Altshuler 1993; Kaplan 1993b; Kliman et al 1995) but there is no firm evidence for this view and many pertinent arguments against it (Fox 1997a).

Abnormalities of unknown pathogenesis

Prominent amongst these is fibrinoid necrosis of placental villi. The first stage in the evolution of this lesion is the appearance of a small nodule of homogeneous, acidophilic, PAS-positive material at one point in the villous trophoblast. This nodule progressively enlarges as fresh fibrinoid material is laid down on its deep aspect so as to form a mass which gradually bulges into, and compresses, the villous stroma, this process continuing until the whole villus is converted into a fibrinoid nodule (Fig. 38.32). The syncytiotrophoblast of the affected villus is normal in the early stages of evolution of this lesion but eventually atrophies and is largely lost, though even at a late stage a few remnants of this tissue remain around the periphery of the fibrinoid material. This particular villous abnormality remains as something of an enigma: there is clear evidence that the fibrinoid material appears first in a cytotrophoblastic cell and is not due to deposition within the villus of fibrin derived from the maternal blood in the intervillous space (Wilkin 1965; Fox 1997a) but how and why it develops is far from clear. The lesion has often

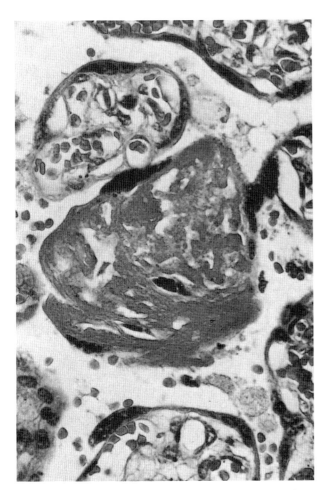

Fig. 38.32 A villus which has undergone complete fibrinoid necrosis.

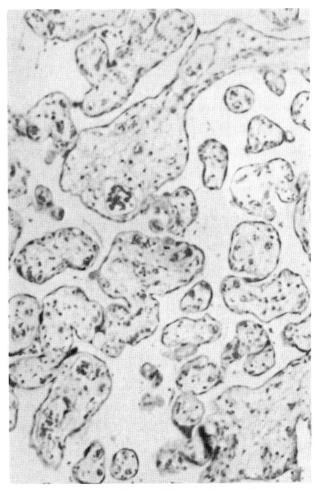

Fig. 38.33 Oedematous villi in a full-term placenta from a diabetic woman. (From Fox 1997a. Reproduced by permission of W B Saunders.)

been attributed to an immunological reaction within villous tissue, a view which currently receives little support but has not yet been totally excluded. A pathologist noting an excess of villi showing this change in a placenta is not currently in a position to draw any conclusions from this observation.

Villous oedema (Fig. 38.33) is usually of unknown origin: most accounts of placental pathology indicate that this abnormality is easy to recognise but, in practice, its distinction from villous immaturity is difficult and there is no doubt that normal intermediate villi are often wrongly classed as oedematous (Kaufmann et al 1987; Benirschke & Kaufmann 2000). Nevertheless, villous oedema does occur, though it can probably only be recognised when of quite marked degree; under such circumstances the presence of villous oedema correlates well with an increased placental water content (Barker et al 1994).

It is clearly tempting to attribute villous oedema to a functional inadequacy of the villous fetal circulation but no firm evidence exists to support this view. It is usually considered that villous oedema is of no functional importance but Naeye et al (1983) considered villous oedema

to be indicative of fetal hypoxia, a view that Sen-Schwarz et al (1989) could not confirm.

In some placentas there is an obvious excess of fetal vessels within the terminal villi (Fig. 38.34), a condition described as chorangiosis by Altshuler (1984). For recognition of this entity Altshuler suggested that there should be at least 10 different light microscopic fields in 10 different placental areas with 10 villi that have 10 capillary lumens in each villus. He correlated this villous abnormality with a poor neonatal outcome and suggested that it represented a response to chronic fetal hypoxia (Altshuler 1993), a view supported by Benirschke & Kaufmann (2000). There have, however, been no reported prospective studies of this villous abnormality and Burton et al (1996) and Espinoza et al (2001) have shown that the villous vascular response to hypoxic stress is dilatation, rather than proliferation, of the villous capillaries. It should also be noted that chorangiosis is usually focal rather than diffuse and it is difficult to see how chronic fetal oxygen lack could result in a patchy villous hypervascularisation. Chorangiosis should certainly be noted but its significance remains uncertain.

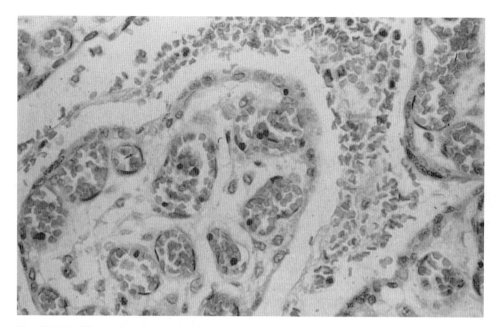

Fig. 38.34 Villi showing chorangiosis.

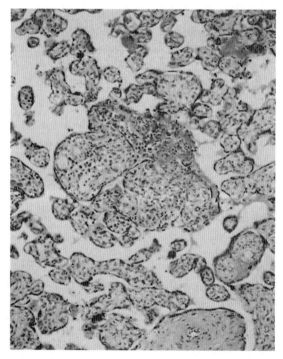

Fig. 38.35 Mild focal villitis showing a small group of villi with an inflammatory cell infiltrate.

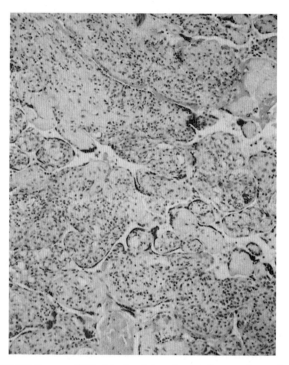

Fig. 38.36 Severe villitis. Much of the placental parenchyma is involved in the chronic inflammatory process with scarred villi in areas where inflammation has subsided.

Inflammatory lesions

A villitis is an inflammatory lesion of the villous substance which is due to infections reaching the placenta from the maternal blood. The villitis may be focal, with lesions present in random isolated villi (Fig. 38.35), or diffuse, with extensive involvement of contiguous villi in many areas of the placenta (Fig. 38.36): the focal form is the more common and very few villi may be involved, to the extent that lesions may be missed unless the placenta is extensively sampled.

A villitis may be characterised only by an inflammatory cell infiltrate but there can also be tissue necrosis: reparative changes may be seen and villous fibrosis and shrinkage may be found as an end result of the inflammatory process. Villitides may be further subdivided in terms of both the topography of the inflammatory lesions and the

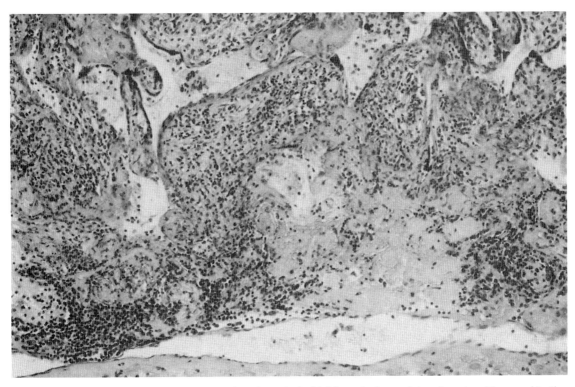

Fig. 38.37 Basal or parabasal villitis. Chronic lymphocytic deciduitis at the base of the placenta with spread to the adjacent placental villi.

type of inflammatory cells found in the villi (Russell 1980). Thus a villitis may be basal, the inflamed villi being predominantly those adjacent to the basal plate (Fig. 38.37), or non-basal, the inflamed villi being randomly distributed with no obvious relationship to the basal plate.

A villitis is usually chronic and characterised by a mixed villous infiltrate of lymphocytes, plasma cells and histiocytic cells, though in a minority of cases the infiltrate is either purely lymphocytic or wholly histiocytic. A pure lymphocytic villitis is commonly basal in type and associated with little tissue destruction, while a histiocytic villitis is invariably randomly distributed and frequently associated with trophoblastic necrosis and villous destruction. The lesions of villitis may be very scattered but all except a tiny minority of cases will be detected if four sections of placental tissue are examined.

Some infections, such as syphylis, toxoplasmosis, rubella, listeriosis or cytomegalovirus infection, produce specific, or at least characteristic, histological features which are detailed in a later section. Nevertheless, in the vast majority of cases of villitis (98%) there are no specific histological features and no infective organism can be identified. The incidence of villitis of unknown aetiology in large unselected series of third trimester placentas in Western countries ranges from 6 to 14% (Altshuler & Russell 1975; Russell 1979, 1980; Knox & Fox 1984) but the incidence of villitis is influenced by ethnic, environmental and socioeconomic factors and varies in different populations.

Furthermore, although some cases of villitis of unknown origin are very extensive and easily recognised it is not uncommon for only 2–4% of the villous population to show an inflammatory infiltrate and lesions as scanty as these can, as already mentioned, easily be missed on routine histological examination. It can also be very difficult to recognise a villitis and Khong et al (1993) found that even amongst experienced pathologists there is a significant degree of interobserver variation in diagnosing villitis.

Because so many cases of villitis are of unknown aetiology the view that villitis is a pathognomonic hallmark of infection has been challenged by the suggestion that this lesion is the morphological expression of an immunological reaction within villous tissue: it has been argued that infection is one, but by no means the sole, cause of such an immune lesion, other possibilities being a maternal graft rejection or a graft-versus-host reaction (Labarrere et al 1990; Redline 1995, 1999). It is, however, quite possible that in many cases an immune reaction is superimposed on, or is provoked by, an initial infectious insult (Gersell 1993) and in our present state of knowledge it would still be prudent to regard a villitis of anything more than a trivial degree as being indicative of an infection.

There is an undoubted association between villitis of unknown aetiology and an increased incidence of intrauterine fetal growth retardation (Altshuler & Russell 1975; Labarrere et al 1982; Knox & Fox 1984; Althabe & Labarrere 1985; Salafia et al 1992a,b; Redline &

Patterson 1994; Redline 1999) though it must be stressed that in prospective studies the vast majority of neonates whose placentas show a villitis are of normal weight. A villitis of unknown aetiology can recur in successive pregnancies and this recurrent form of villitis tends to be unusually extensive and shows a particularly strong association with fetal growth retardation (Russell et al 1980; Redline & Abramowsky 1985; Labarrere & Althabe 1987).

The nature of the link between villitis of unknown aetiology and diminished fetal growth is far from being clear. Benirschke & Kaufmann (2000) consider that the restriction of fetal growth is related to the elimination of a considerable amount of placental parenchyma from nutrient transfer. This may be true in occasional rare cases but is clearly not true in the vast majority of cases of villitis in which the inflammatory damage wreaked upon the placenta is far too limited in extent to dissipate the functional reserve of the organ. Hence some other cause must be sought. If, and it is admittedly quite a large 'if', a chronic villitis is commonly due to an unrecognised viral infection then it is perfectly possible that the virus passes through the inadequate barrier of the placenta to infect the fetus and restrict it's growth, the inhibitory effect of viruses on fetal DNA synthesis being well established (Fox 1993, 1994, 2001). It is true that neonates whose placentas show evidence of a villitis do not usually have any clinical evidence of an infection but the infection may have been relatively transitory and the growth restriction temporary.

Abnormalities of the fetal stem arteries

Fibromuscular sclerosis

This is characterised by a marked hyperplasia of the fibrous and muscular tissue of the media with a proliferation of intimal fibrous tissue which grows into, and eventually obliterates, the vascular lumen (Fig. 38.38). Fibromuscular sclerosis is seen in localised form in stem arteries supplying areas of villous infarction and in stem arteries distal to an occluding thrombus whilst a generalised fibromuscular sclerosis of the fetal stem arteries is found only in placentas from stillbirths, being absent from placentas of fresh stillbirths but becoming increasingly more prominent as the time interval between fetal demise and delivery increases (Genest 1992; Fox 1997a). These observations point inescapably to the conclusion that fibromuscular sclerosis is a reactive change consequent upon a cessation of fetal blood flow through the affected vessels.

Obliterative endarteritis

This term is applied to an abnormality of the fetal stem arteries of the placenta which is characterised by apparent

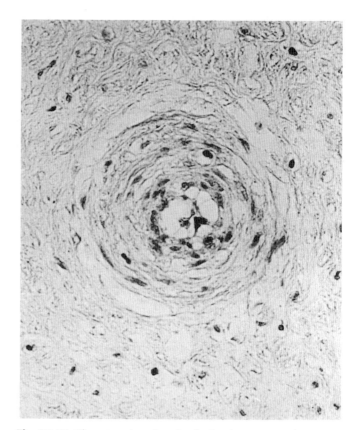

Fig. 38.38 Fibromuscular sclerosis of a fetal stem artery in a placenta from a case of intrauterine fetal death.

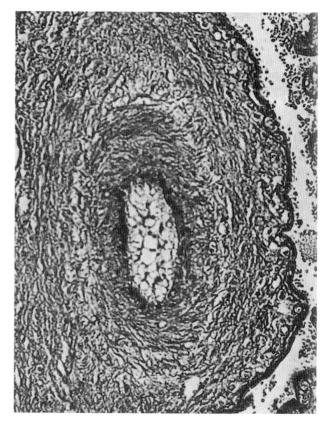

Fig. 38.39 Obliterative endarteritis in a fetal stem artery. (From Fox 1997a. Reproduced by permission of W B Saunders.)

swelling and proliferation of clear endothelial cells with narrowing, sometimes to an extreme degree, of the vascular lumen (Fig. 38.39). Ultrastructural studies of stem arteries showing this change have revealed, however, that the apparent swelling and proliferation of the endothelial cells is due to their partial displacement into the vascular lumen by herniations of medial smooth muscle cell cytoplasm into the intima: the clarity of the apparently swollen endothelial cells is a fixation artifact (van der Veen et al 1982). An obliterative endarteritis appears therefore not to be a pathological lesion in the true sense of the word for the smooth muscle herniation is almost certainly a reflection of, and due to, vasoconstriction. If vasoconstriction is prolonged it can lead to widespread sclerosis of small vessels in the distal part of the villous tree (Giles et al 1985; McCowan et al 1988; Fok et al 1990), a change associated with an increased resistance in the placental vascular bed (Trudinger et al 1985b; Bracero et al 1989; Zacutti et al 1992; Hitschold et al 1993).

Constriction of the fetal stem arteries is usually an indirect response to diminished maternal uteroplacental blood flow (Stock et al 1980) and is part of an attempt by the deprived fetus to divert blood to the cerebral and coronary circulations.

PATHOLOGY OF THE UMBILICAL CORD

Today the umbilical cord, in the past strangely neglected, is now seen to be vitally important though possibly the pendulum has swung too far the other way with a tendency to overstress the clinical significance of even relatively minor abnormalities of the cord. These is no doubt that cord lesions can, and do, cause fetal hypoxia and even demise but claims that such lesions are responsible for approximately 1 in 6 perinatal deaths (Wessell et al 1992) seem somewhat exaggerated. The pathologist has to evaluate cord lesions very critically before concluding that they are functionally significant and a cause, rather than a result, of fetal death or damage.

DEVELOPMENTAL ABNORMALITIES

Abnormal length of the cord

The factors controlling cord length are still not fully understood but there is some evidence that cord length is related to the degree of fetal mobility, and hence to the tensile force placed upon the cord, particularly during the early stages of pregnancy.

The average length of the normal umbilical cord is between 54 and 61 cm (Fox 1997a) whilst it is thought that a cord length of 32 cm or less should be regarded as abnormally short. Most infants with an unduly short cord pass through delivery unscathed and although there have been claims that a significant proportion develop either intrauterine distress or neonatal asphyxia, presumed to be because of excessive traction on the cord during descent of the fetus and occlusion of the cord vessels, this has never actually been demonstrated to be the case and, indeed, umbilical blood pH and base deficit values are the same for neonates with short cords as they are for those with cords of normal length (Berg & Rayburn 1995).

Quite apart from the complications that can occur during labour, Naeye (1985b) has shown that there is a correlation between an unduly short cord and an increased frequency of subsequent childhood mental and motor impairment: he considered, probably quite correctly, that the short cord was the result rather than the cause of the psychomotor abnormalities, these being associated with diminished fetal movement and hence with less stretching stress to the cord.

An abnormally long cord is thought to predispose to knotting, torsion and prolapse but it is rather difficult to define the limit that should be exceeded for the cord to be considered as unduly long: Berg & Rayburn (1995) defined an unusually long cord as being more than 80 cm whilst Heifetz (1999) regarded a length of 60 cm or more as excessive.

Vestigial remnants

Remnants of the allantoic or omphalomesenteric ducts may be apparent on microscopic examination of the cord. Allantoic remnants were present in 14.5% of the 1000 cords examined by Jauniaux et al (1989). They are usually seen between the two umbilical arteries and appear either as a solid cord or as a duct: in the latter case the lumen is lined by flattened epithelium and only very occasionally is transitional epithelium found.

Remains of the omphalomesenteric duct (Fig. 38.40), found in 1.4% of cords by Jauniaux et al (1989), are situated at the margin of the cord, are lined by a cuboidal or columnar epithelium, and may contain a little mucus. Very occasionally the omphalomesenteric duct remnants

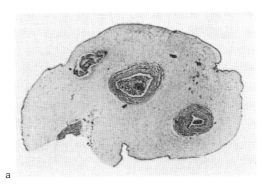

a

Fig. 38.40a Low-power view of umbilical cord containing a persistent remnant of the omphalomesenteric duct: this is seen above and to the left and is situated towards the margin of the cord. (From Fox 1997a. Reproduced by permission of W B Saunders.)

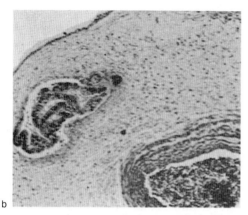

Fig. 38.40b Detail of Fig 38.40a showing a remnant of the omphalomesenteric duct above and to the left. (From Fox 1997a. Reproduced by permission of W B Saunders.)

show differentiation into gastrointestinal-type structures (Fig 38.41) with well-formed gastric or intestinal-type epithelium within, or on the surface of, the cord; the gastrointestinal epithelium may appear as a nodule or polyp and in one such case the presence of gastric-type mucosa appeared to be a causal factor in ulceration of an umbilical vein with massive fetal haemorrhage (Blanc & Allan 1961).

Single umbilical artery

The incidence of a single umbilical artery in prospective studies of white term infants is about 1%, though this figure is significantly higher in black infants and in twins (Heifetz 1984, 1999; Benirschke & Kaufmann 2000). If, however, naked-eye examination of the fresh cord is relied upon as the sole means of diagnosis a misleadingly low incidence will be obtained; a higher, and more accurate, yield of this abnormality is found if the cord is subjected to histological examination.

One further point of technique should be emphasised. The two umbilical arteries may fuse at their lower end into a single trunk which subsequently divides into two rami. If the cord is sectioned too closely to the chorionic plate (i.e. at a distance of less than 3 cm from the placental surface) this normal variation may be wrongly interpreted, and therefore a diagnosis of single umbilical artery should always be confirmed by a second section taken at a higher level.

A single umbilical artery is accompanied very often by fetal malformation, the reported frequency of this association varying considerably but being, in most studies, between 25 and 50% (Fox 1997a). Malformations do not, despite occasional claims to the contrary, show a bias towards any particular organ or system; they are frequently multiple and often lethal. The malformations may not be apparent at birth for Leung & Robson (1989) and Bourke et al (1993) have shown that there is a high incidence of clinically silent renal anomalies in infants with a single umbilical artery. Infants with a single umbilical artery often have a low birth weight and a high perinatal mortality even in the absence of malformations (Bryan & Kohler 1974; Heifetz 1984).

There has been considerable debate as to whether a single umbilical artery is due to a primary aplasia or to a secondary atrophy of the missing vessel; in fact it is almost certain that both of these mechanisms can be invoked, for, whilst in some cases there is an absolute absence of a second artery in the cord, in others there is

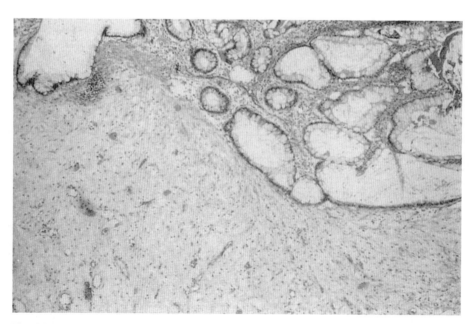

Fig. 38.41 Large intestinal-like epithelium in the umbilical cord which was derived from a persistent remnant of the omphalomesenteric duct. (From Fox 1997a. Reproduced by permission of W B Saunders.)

evidence of a previously present vessel, sometimes seen histologically as a small, shrivelled and involuted artery with an obliterated lumen but occasionally only recognisable by the presence of remnants of the muscular or elastic wall.

Supernumary umbilical vessels

The significance of an increased number of umbilical vessels has attracted little attention and no firm association with congenital malformation has been established. Most apparent examples of supernumerary cord vessels are, in reality, examples of excessive looping or branching of the umbilical arteries. Gupta et al (1993) found more than three vascular profiles on cross-section in 40 (6%) of 644 cords from which samples at fetal end, midportion and placental end were examined; the extra vascular profiles were seen most commonly in sections taken from the central portion of the cord and longitudinal dissection of the vessels showed that the appearances were due to branching rather than to looping or the presence of true supernumary vessels. In this study an increased number of vascular profiles was found more commonly in cords from stillbirths than in those from live births and there was a clear association between this anomaly and a history of maternal cigarette smoking.

Eccentric and marginal insertion (Fig. 38.42)

Eccentric insertion of the cord can hardly be classed as an anomaly, for it is found more commonly than is a central insertion. Marginal insertion (the so-called 'battledore placenta') is less common than an eccentrically placed cord but appears to be devoid of clinical significance (Fox 1997a).

Velamentous insertion

A velamentously inserted cord is inserted, not into the placenta, but into the membranes (Fig. 38.42), and hence the unprotected umbilical vessels run for some distance between the amnion and chorion before passing on to the placental surface. Velamentous insertion is found in about 1% of singleton placentas but is significantly more common in multiple pregnancies (Benirschke & Kaufmann 2000). Other proposed associations, such as fetal malformation and low birth weight, are more open to debate.

Neither the aetiology nor the pathogenesis of velamentous insertion is fully understood but Benirschke & Kaufmann (2000) favour the concept of 'trophotropism', arguing that the cord is originally normally inserted but becomes stranded in the membranes by a process, during placental expansion, of central atrophy and unidirectional lateral growth of the chorion frondosum.

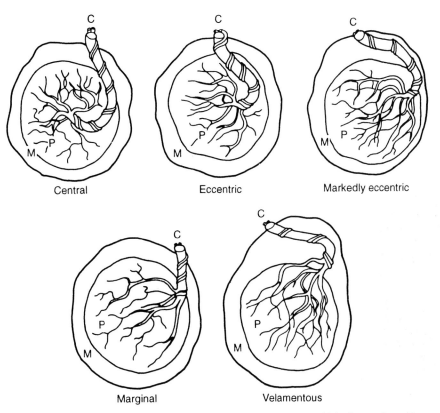

Fig. 38.42 Diagrammatic representation of the various sites at which the cord may be inserted. C, cord; P, placenta; M, membranes (From Fox 1997a. Reproduced by permission of W B Saunders.)

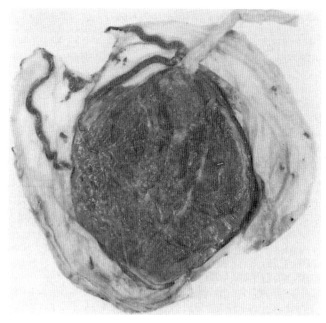

Fig. 38.43 An example of velamentous cord insertion in which a fetal vessel running through the membranes has been torn (above and to the left) during delivery. (From Fox 1997a. Reproduced by permission of W B Saunders.)

Velamentous insertion of the cord is of serious import for the fetus because of the risk of damage to the exposed and unprotected fetal vessels during labour and delivery (Fig. 38.43). This danger is, of course, most prominent when the intramembranous vessels run across the internal os; serious or fatal fetal bleeding from tearing of such a vessel (which produces the clinical picture of 'vasa praevia') is associated with a very high fetal mortality rate. Although the bleeding is usually from fetal vessels in the region of the internal os, it is well established that haemorrhage can also occur from velamentous vessels if the upper uterine segment for the vessels in the chorion laeve are firmly bound down by perivascular collagen, an anatomical arrangement which makes them particularly susceptible to damage during uterine contractions. It should not be thought, however, that the vessels of a velamentously inserted cord are only susceptible to damage during labour, for there have been a number of well-authenticated reports of bleeding from such vessels during the antepartum period (Fox 1997a).

Despite the obvious and dangerous possibility of bleeding from velamentous vessels the vast majority of infants whose cords are velamentously inserted pass through labour and delivery without haemorrhage, it being estimated that this complication occurs in only 2% of such cases (Quek & Tan 1972). The fetus is, however, at still further risk, for its life may be endangered by compression of the velamentous vessels against the wall of the pelvis during delivery; fetal distress under such circumstances is common and fetal demise by no means rare (Cordero et al 1993).

Interposito velamentosa

This is a very rare anomaly in which the cord appears to be inserted velamentously into the chorion laeve but the cord substance surrounds the fetal vessels until they reach the placenta; its pathogenesis is unknown.

Insertion funiculi furcata (furcate insertion)

In this condition the site of cord insertion is normal, but, prior to insertion, the vessels lose their protective covering of Wharton's jelly and branch before reaching the placental surface; the exposed vessels are liable to damage with resultant fetal haemorrhage.

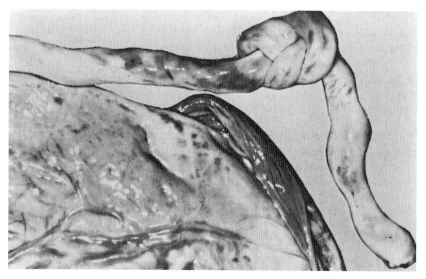

Fig. 38.44 A knot in an umbilical cord. (From Fox 1997a. Reproduced by permission of W B Saunders.)

MECHANICAL LESIONS

Knots

True knots can be formed in the umbilical cord (Fig. 38.44) and these are to be distinguished from 'false knots', which are either local dilatations of umbilical vessels or focal accumulations of Wharton's jelly. True knots are found in about 0.5% of all deliveries (McLennan et al 1988; Heifetz 1999). The incidence is notably high in monoamniotic twins and it is thought that a long cord, an excess of amniotic fluid and over-vigorous fetal movements all predispose to knot formation.

The functional significance of cord knotting is disputed but it seems likely that a tight knot can obstruct the fetal circulation through the cord and lead to fetal hypoxia. In assessing the significance of a tight knot, it should, however, be borne in mind that a previously loose knot may be suddenly tightened as the infant descends during delivery: recently formed knots of this type can be distinguished from longstanding knots on the following grounds:

1. In an old knot there is marked and permanent grooving of the cord at the site of the knot.
2. At the site of a longstanding knot there is a loss of Wharton's jelly and a constriction of the umbilical vessels.
3. When an old knot is undone there is persistent curling of the cord at the site of the knot.

A knot formed during early labour will not usually show these features, but may nevertheless be responsible for intrapartum death, fetal distress or neonatal asphyxia; examination of such a knot will, however, show oedema, congestion or thrombosis, and in the absence of these changes it would not be justifiable to attribute any functional significance to a knot. Failure to look carefully for such changes and lack of histological examination may be factors in some of those studies in which true knots have not been of any clinical importance and not associated with fetal hypoxia (McLennan et al 1988).

Rupture

A rupture of the cord may be partial or complete. The term 'incomplete rupture' is usually taken to mean tearing of, or damage to, an umbilical vessel and thus represents one mechanism of cord haematoma formation (see section on vascular lesions); the extravasated blood is often confined to the cord but sometimes it ruptures into the amniotic sac; such cases should be classed as 'rupture of an umbilical vessel' rather than as rupture of the cord, as should be also those cases in which rupture of velamentous vessels results in separation of the abnormally inserted cord from the placenta.

Complete rupture of the cord is extremely rare for the cord has considerable tensile strength and can withstand a severe degree of stretching, partly because of its high content of elastic tissue and partly because of the tortuous course which its vessels pursue. This being the case, it is not surprising that most ruptures of the cord complicate precipitate delivery, especially from the upright or squatting posture, and occur immediately after the birth of the child though, exceptionally, cord rupture may occur either during the early stages of labour or even before labour begins for which no cause can be determined (Lurie et al 1990).

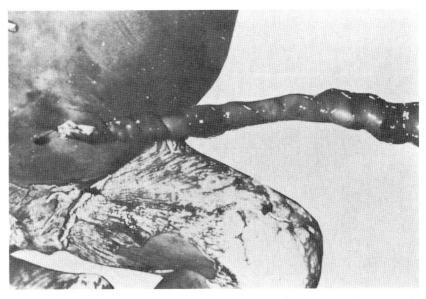

Fig. 38.45 A tightly twisted cord in a macerated stillbirth. The torsion has occurred at the characteristic site, at the fetal end of the cord. (From Fox 1997a. Reproduced by permission of W B Saunders.)

The effects of cord rupture can obviously be catastrophic but some infants do survive rupture of the cord during the late stages of labour and delivery.

Torsion

The cord is normally twisted in so far as its vessels run a spiral course, but pathological torsion is usually readily distinguishable from the normal spiralling. The torsion may affect the whole cord, but is more commonly localised, and whilst a single lesion is usually found, there may occasionally be multiple twists. The characteristic site of torsion is at the fetal end of the cord (Fig. 38.45), but examples of torsion at the placental end have been recorded.

The incidence of this complication is unknown but it is certainly rare, A tight cord torsion will clearly obstruct the umbilical vessels and can cause fetal death. It has been argued that cord torsion is a post-mortem event and there is no doubt that excessive twisting of the cord may occur after fetal death. An ante-mortem torsion can, however, be distinguished from post-mortem twisting by demonstrating that it remains permanently after separation of the fetus and placenta and by histological examination, which will show congestion, oedema and, possibly, thrombosis at the site of torsion, all features absent from post-mortem twisting of the cord.

Stricture

A stricture of the cord is rare and is often, though by no means invariably, complicated by torsion. The stricture is usually well defined, short, single and at the fetal end of the cord (Fig. 38.46) and is characterised by a focal, and often extreme, deficiency of Wharton's jelly, this being accompanied, sometimes, by well-marked fibrosis. The lack of Wharton's jelly has been attributed to a focal congenital lack, but Benirschke (1994) thought that the loss of Wharton's jelly was secondary to a torsion whilst Heifetz (1999) considered that loss of Wharton's jelly at the fetal end of the cord is virtually physiological. Although commonly present in stillbirths a stricture does not appear to be a post-mortem phenomenon related to maceration for occasional babies with a cord stricture have been born alive; in the stillbirths the evidence suggests strongly that cord stricture played a role, possibly a very important one, in fetal demise in such cases.

VASCULAR LESIONS

Haematoma

Haematomas of the cord may be iatrogenic, complicating amniocentesis, umbilical blood sampling or intrauterine intravascular blood transfusion.

Spontaneous haematomas of the cord are found in 1–2% of deliveries (Heifetz 1999) but their pathogenesis awaits clarification and their clinical significance remains uncertain. The picture has been unduly confused by the tendency of some authors to limit their attention to those 80% of cord haematomas which are of the 'simple' variety, i.e. which are entirely intrafunicular; the findings in such studies will clearly contrast with those of workers who have also included within their remit the 20% of haematomas which rupture through the covering sheath into the amniotic cavity. Furthermore, the distinction between a ruptured haematoma and bleeding from a torn cord has not always been clearly drawn.

The simple haematomas, which consist of an extravasation of blood into Wharton's jelly, are usually single and occur most commonly towards, or at, the fetal end of the cord; they present as a rounded or sausage-shaped turgid

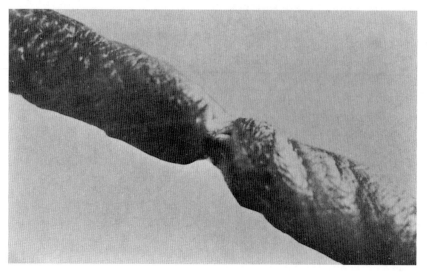

Fig. 38.46 A sharply localised stricture in a cord from a stillborn infant. (From Fox 1997a. Reproduced by permission of W B Saunders.)

tumefaction which is usually reddish-purple or 'aubergine' coloured. The haematomas vary considerably in size, and range from a diameter of just over 1 cm to a swelling 'the thickness of a child's arm'; they can be from 4 to 40 cm in length.

The aetiology of cord haematomas is usually obscure and amongst the suggested aetiological factors have been torsion, traction of an unduly short cord, trauma during delivery, non-specific inflammation of the cord, prolapse of the cord, a deficiency of Wharton's jelly, and a haemorrhagic diathesis in the infant. Benirschke (1994) considered excessive cord length and prolapse to be the most important aetiological factors.

The perinatal mortality rate in infants whose cord contains a haematoma has been reported, incorrectly in the view of Heifetz (1999), as being in the region of 40 to 50%, but it is far from clear, in many cases, whether the haematoma is responsible for fetal demise or whether both the haematoma and fetal death are mutually dependent upon some common causal factor. In our present state of knowledge it would be unwise to attribute fetal death to a cord haematoma until all other possible causes of demise have been excluded.

Thrombosis of umbilical vessels

This is rare, being found in 1 in 1290 unselected deliveries by Heifetz (1988). A majority of cord thrombi appear to accompany, and are probably a complication of, cord compression, torsion, stricture, or haematoma whilst most of the remainder occur in association with obstetrical complications or fetal abnormalities. In the few remaining cases the pathogenesis of the thrombosis is obscure.

The thrombi are usually (85%) in the umbilical vein, these occurring in isolation in about two-thirds of cases and being associated with thrombi in one or both arteries in about 20% of cases: only in a small proportion (11–15%) does an arterial thrombus occur alone. There is a theoretical risk, which is occasionally realised, of embolic spread from a cord thrombus to placental or fetal vessels (Heifetz 1988; Cook et al 1995).

A very high incidence of fetal death is found in association with an umbilical vessel thrombosis, but in most such cases it appears probable that fetal demise has been due principally to the condition of which the thrombotic episode is a complication, rather than to the thrombosis itself. There is no doubt that an infant can survive an umbilical vessel thrombosis, and this lesion is, in itself, likely to serve as a primary cause of fetal death in only a small minority of cases.

ULCERATION AND NECROSIS

Bendon et al (1991) described three cases of linear ulceration of the umbilical cord associated with congenital intestinal atresia and Khong et al (1994) subsequently described a further example of this combination of lesions. The similarity of all these cases suggests that this association of cord and intestinal abnormalities is more than coincidental and represents a true syndrome. In three of the four cases there was severe haemorrhage from the ulcerated cord.

Meconium induced necrosis

Altshuler and his colleagues (Altshuler & Hyde 1989; Altshuler et al 1992) delineated a characteristic lesion of the umbilical arteries that appears to be induced by meconium and their description of this entity has been fully confirmed by Benirschke (1994). The lesion is always associated with prolonged passage of meconium

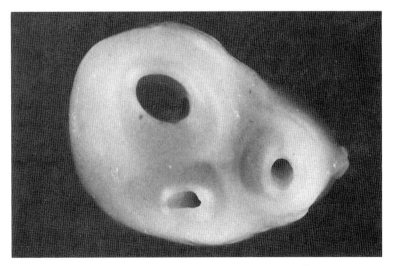

Fig. 38.47 Necrotising funisitis: macroscopic appearances of a cross-section of the umbilical cord. (Courtesy of Dr V J Baldwin, Vancouver, and from Fox 1997a. Reproduced by permission of W B Saunders.)

and consists of segmental necrosis of the arterial wall, the vein usually not being involved: the necrotic segment of the artery always faces towards the cord surface and there are numerous meconium-laden macrophages within the Wharton's jelly. In long-standing cases there may be an accumulation of polymorphonuclear leucocytes within the necrotic segment of the vessel wall and in some instances there is also linear ulceration of the cord surface.

INFLAMMATION

Acute funisitis, inflammation of Wharton's jelly, is a late feature of the amniotic fluid infection syndrome and is discussed later.

A specific form of funisitis is necrotising funisitis. This term was introduced by Navarro & Blanc (1974) to describe a form of chronic inflammation of the umbilical cord which is also sometimes classed as 'sclerosing funisitis' or 'constrictive sclerosis of the cord'. The cord may appear somewhat rigid and taut ('cooked macaroni' appearance) and on cross-section there are visible yellow–white or chalky bands surrounding thickened vessel walls (Fig. 38.47), an appearance likened to that seen in an Ouchterlony diffusion plate. Histologically there are concentric perivascular bands of necrotic Wharton's jelly containing acute and chronic inflammatory cells in various stages of degeneration (Fig. 38.48); calcification may occur in the necrotic areas. There is nearly always an associated chorioamnionitis.

Claims that this form of funisitis is a specific feature of, and is confined to, syphilis (Fojaco et al 1989;

Knowles & Frost 1989) have not been confirmed, others finding that this lesion can be found in a wide range of infections (Craver & Baldwin 1992; Jacques & Qureshi 1992): there is, however, no doubt that it is a common finding in congenital syphilis, being present in about one-third of cases (Schwartz et al 1995). Heifetz and Bauman (1994) considered that whilst no single pathogen causes necrotising funisitis there is, nevertheless, a strong association with latent Herpes simplex infection of the endometrium.

It would appear that necrotising funisitis is a non-specific lesion which results from long-standing chronic inflammation at a site from which inflammatory debris can not be removed. Clinically there is an association between necrotising funisitis and a high incidence of premature rupture of the membranes, preterm labour, intrauterine growth retardation and intrauterine fetal death; the basis for these associations is not known.

CYSTS

Umbilical cord cysts are of several varieties:

1. *Derived from vestigial remnants*. A cyst, usually situated near the fetal end of the cord, may develop from remnants of either the allantois or the omphalomesenteric duct. Those of allantoic origin are lined by a cuboidal or flattened epithelium, which may, however, show a transitional epithelial pattern in some areas, whilst those arising from omphalomesenteric duct remnants are usually lined by an epithelium of gastric or intestinal type, can have

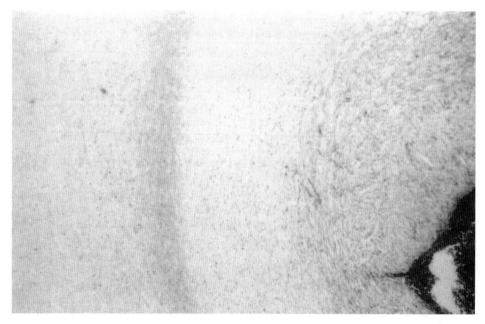

Fig. 38.48 Necrotising funisitis. Concentric bands of necrosis are seen in the wall of the cord. (Courtesy of Dr V J Baldwin, Vancouver, and from Fox 1997a. Reproduced by permission of W B Saunders.)

smooth muscle and nerve ganglia in their wall and are often surrounded by many small vessels which can appear almost angiomatoid. Cysts of this type are commonly small and of no clinical importance, but they may sometimes reach the size of a hen's egg.

2. *Derived from amniotic inclusions.* These are uncommon; they are usually small, and are lined by amniotic-type epithelium.

3. *Formed by degeneration of Wharton's jelly.* These are not true cysts but are cavitations which result from a mucoid degeneration of Wharton's jelly; they lack an epithelial lining and contain clear mucoid material. Pseudocysts of this type have been described in cases of fetal trisomy 18 (Jauniaux et al 1988a) but whether this is a real, or even a frequent, association remains to be determined.

TUMOURS

Haemangiomas

Cord haemangiomas are rare (Fox 1997a), present as rounded or ovoid swellings in the cord and those described have usually ranged from 3 to 17 cm in diameter: they are very variable in colour and consistency. In some cases attention may be drawn to the haemangioma by the presence of a cord haematoma, this presumably being due to local leakage from the neoplasm. Histologically, the neoplasms have the appearances of either a capillary or cavernous haemangioma, but the microscopic features have often been somewhat distorted by the loose, rather myxoid, stroma in which the tumour is set.

In some cases the haemangioma has clearly been supplied by one umbilical artery, in others it has apparently been connected with both an umbilical vein and an umbilical artery, and in yet others the tumour has been quite separate from the major vessels and appears to have arisen from capillaries in Wharton's jelly. It would appear highly probable that the haemangioma is a hamartoma rather than a true neoplasm and that it arises as a malformation of the primitive angiogenic mesenchyme of the developing cord.

Cord hemangiomas can be associated with an elevated maternal alpha-fetoprotein level; the elevation may be only slight but very high levels are sometimes attained (Barson et al 1980; Resta et al 1988; Yavner & Redline 1989; Bruhwiler et al 1994).

The cord haemangioma can thus be considered as very similar in origin and nature to the more common placental haemangioma, but whereas a whole range of complications have been recorded for the placental haemangioma the clinical significance of cord haemangiomas is less well defined. An association with polyhydramnios, fetal disseminated intravascular coagulation or fetal hydrops has been described but such complications are inconsistent and of debatable pathogenesis.

Teratoma

Very few teratomas of the cord have been recorded (Fox 1997a). Some pathologists have a conceptual difficulty in accepting that a teratoma can occur in the cord and consider that all such apparent cases are a fetus acardius but it is doubtful if an acardiac twin could be entirely intrafunicular and there are no theoretical or practical reasons why a teratoma should not occur in the cord. Teratomas are derived from germ cells: these originally arise in the dorsal wall of the yolk sac, later migrate into the primitive gut wall, and then continue out through the root of the mesentery eventually to reach the genital folds. Not all germ cells complete this rather complicated journey and some may go astray to extragonadal sites, where they may eventually give rise to a teratoma. During the first few months of pregnancy there is an evagination of primitive gut into the umbilical cord, and it is possible that primordial germ cells may migrate out through the wall of this evaginated gut into the connective tissue of the cord, where they may then give rise to a teratoma.

PATHOLOGY OF THE MEMBRANES

SQUAMOUS METAPLASIA

Squamous metaplasia is seen on the fetal surface of the amnion and umbilical cord, though in the latter site it would better be termed squamous hyperplasia. Any number of lesions may be present and they tend to be aggregated most strikingly around the site of cord insertion. The foci of squamous metaplasia are grey or white,

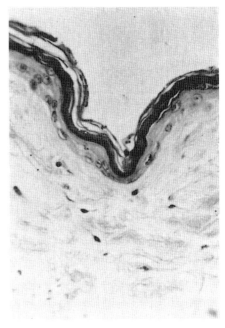

Fig. 38.49 Squamous metaplasia of the amnion. (From Fox 1997a. Reproduced by permission of W B Saunders.)

range in size up to a few millimetres in diameter, are slightly elevated, are rough and granular to the touch, and can only be separated from the amnion with difficulty; occasionally the foci may coalesce to form large, smooth plaques measuring several centimetres across. Histologically (Fig. 38.49) the foci consist of stratified squamous epithelial cells, the number of layers varying from six to 20. There is usually a sharp transition at the edge of the lesion from columnar to squamous epithelium.

Squamous metaplasia is common and of no clinical or pathological significance.

AMNION NODOSUM

This condition, in which the fetal surface of the amnion is studded with multiple small nodules, is associated with oligohydramnios and thus particularly likely to be found in cases of fetal renal agenesis, congenital obstruction of the fetal urinary tract or extramembranous pregnancy. There are, however, well-documented examples of amnion nodosum occurring in the membranes of healthy infants. Although the condition is usually seen in term pregnancies, it has been noted in first-trimester miscarriages.

On naked-eye inspection, amnion nodosum is seen as small, slightly elevated plaques or nodules on the fetal surface of the amnion (Fig. 38.50); these occur with greatest frequency on that part of the amnion directly overlying the placenta, particularly around the site of insertion of the cord, but they do also develop on the extraplacental amnion and on that covering the umbilical cord. The nodules measure 1 to 5 mm across, are usually round, often geometrically so, but may be ovoid: they are shiny, greyish-yellow and may be easily detached from the amnion to leave a ragged saucer-like depression. The nodules not infrequently coalesce to form irregular plaques, and if one of these is picked off it is found to be soft, waxy and rather granular to the touch.

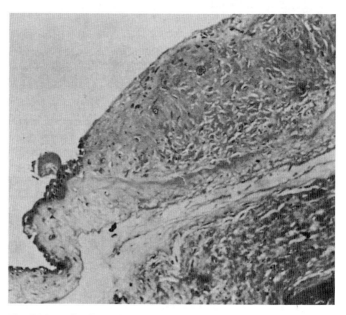

Fig. 38.51 Histological appearances of a nodule of amnion nodosum (above and to the right). Cellular fragments are embedded in amorphous eosinophilic material. (From Fox 1997a. Reproduced by permission of W B Saunders.)

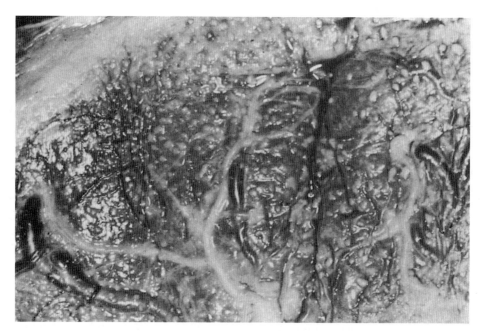

Fig. 38.50 Macroscopic appearances of amnion nodosum in the amnion covering the fetal surface of the placenta. The tiny nodules are seen most clearly above and to the right. (From Fox 1997a. Reproduced by permission of W B Saunders.)

On light microscopy (Fig. 38.51) the nodules, which are deposits of vernix caseosa, consist largely of amorphous or granular eosinophilic material which is sometimes arranged in broad fibrillar bands; embedded in this are cells, cell fragments and, occasionally, fragments of hair. The amorphous material is PAS and Alcian Blue positive, but stains negatively for keratin, amyloid and fibrin. The amnion may grow over the superficial surface of the nodule in an attempt to 'epithelialise' it.

The only pathological or clinical significance of amnion nodosum is that it is an excellent, though not entirely absolute, hallmark of oligohydramnios, and its presence should alert one to the possibility of a congenital abnormality in the newborn infant.

MECONIUM STAINING

Meconium staining of the membranes is found in nearly 20% of placentas (Nathan et al 1994; Benirschke & Kaufmann 2000) but occurs most commonly in placentas from pregnancies prolonged beyond the 42nd week of gestation (Usher et al 1988; Steer et al 1989). Meconium staining has traditionally been regarded as evidence of intrauterine fetal hypoxia and distress but in recent years it has been shown that there is no clear-cut correlation between meconium passage and either the clinical status of the neonate or laboratory measures of fetal hyoxia and acidosis (Houlihan & Knuppel 1994; Fox 1997a). The vast majority of fetuses with meconium staining of the membranes have not been subjected to a hypoxic insult and meconium passage is now thought to be a result of normal fetal gut maturation and motilin secretion (Lewis & Gilbert-Barness 1999). Any increase in perinatal mortality associated with heavy meconium passage is due principally to an increased incidence of the meconium aspiration syndrome.

If meconium has been in contact with the amnion for several hours degenerative changes, such as vacuolation, piling up of cells and, later, necrosis may be seen on histological examination of the stained membranes. Meconium-laden macrophages may be seen, first in the amnion and then later in the chorion. It may be necessary to distinguish between meconium and haemosiderin in amniotic macrophages, a distinction easily accomplished with a Prussian blue stain.

INFLAMMATION OF THE MEMBRANES

Chorioamnionitis is the term applied to those infections of the placenta and membranes which are due to an entry of organisms into the amniotic sac from the maternal birth canal. In this form of infection the brunt of the inflammatory process is borne by the membranes rather than by the placental tissue. It is currently thought that inflammation of the membranes is virtually always due to infection and that a chorioamnionitis is indicative of infection of the amniotic fluid; nevertheless infection of the amniotic fluid, as assessed by positive cultures, is not necessarily associated with histological evidence of chorioamnionitis and histologically proven chorioamnionitis occurs far more commonly than does clinically evident intra-amniotic infection.

In most cases of chorioamnionitis the placenta and membranes appear macroscopically normal. In the relatively uncommon cases of severe and well-established bacterial infection the membranes may be friable, oedematous, opaque, slimy and foul-smelling, whilst in infections of moderate severity there will be a variable degree of loss of the normal translucency of the membranes, which may have a slightly granular appearance. In the rare examples of chorioamnionitis due to *Candida albicans* the membranes, and particularly the umbilical cord, may be studded with tiny yellow–white nodules or plaques which are usually of pin-point size.

Chorioamnionitis is, with rare exceptions, an acute inflammatory lesion and characteristically the first histological evidence of an ascending infection is a polymorphonuclear leucocytic infiltration of the extraplacental membranes (Fig. 38.52). The infiltrate appears first, and is subsequently most marked, at the lower pole of the amniotic sac. This is followed by an accumulation of polymorphonuclear leucocytes in the intervillous space immediately below the chorionic plate, which forms the roof of this space (Fig. 38.53); these cells are often enmeshed in fibrin, not because there is a fibrinous exudate but because the cells have infiltrated, and become embedded in, a pre-existing layer of subchorionic fibrin. This aggregation of leucocytes is known as a 'subchorial intervillositis'; inflammatory cells are rarely seen elsewhere in the intervillous space, whilst a villitis is rarely, with the possible exception of listeriosis, a feature of an ascending

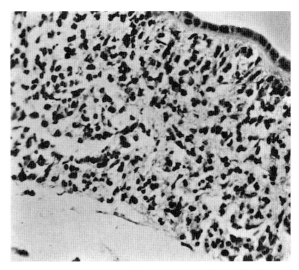

Fig. 38.52 Chorioamnionitis due to an ascending infection. There is a polymorphonuclear leucocytic infiltration of the extraplacental membranes. These cells are of maternal origin. (From Fox 1997a. Reproduced by permission of W B Saunders.)

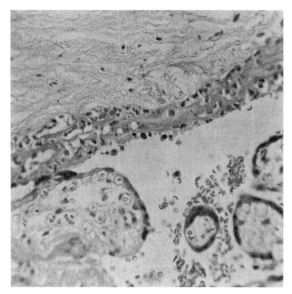

Fig. 38.53 An accumulation of maternal polymorphonuclear leucocytes in the roof of the intervillous space ('intervillositis'): the leucocytes are infiltrating the subchorionic fibrin. (From Fox 1997a. Reproduced by permission of W B Saunders.)

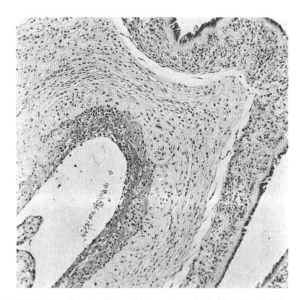

Fig. 38.54 A polymorphonuclear leucocytic infiltration of the chorionic plate of a placenta involved in an asending infection: a subchorial intervillositis is also present and this is a later stage in the evolution of the inflammatory process than that which is shown in Fig. 38.53. Most, if not all, of these leucocytes are, however, still of maternal origin. (From Fox 1997a. Reproduced by permission of W. B. Saunders.)

infection. The inflammatory cells in the roof of the intervillous space later extend upwards into the chorionic plate (Fig. 38.54) and at this stage the inflammatory cellular response is purely maternal in origin, the leucocytes in the extraplacental membranes coming from maternal decidual vessels and those in the chorionic plate being derived from maternal blood in the intervillous space. Later, however, fetal leucocytes begin to migrate out from fetal vessels in the chorionic plate (Fig. 38.55), first from

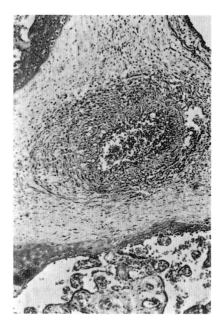

Fig. 38.55 A vasculitis in a fetal vessel which is situated in the chorionic plate of a placenta involved in an ascending infection. (From Fox 1997a. Reproduced by permission of W B Saunders.)

the veins and then later from the arteries, and subsequently an angiitis of the umbilical vessels is seen (Fig. 38.56) with eventual migration of fetal leucocytes into Wharton's jelly.

It is characteristic of ascending infections that the cellular migration from the fetal vessels is not concentric but is orientated towards the uterine cavity; furthermore, the vasculitis is limited to vessels in the chorionic plate and does not extend along their branches that run into the placental parenchyma. Similarly, any umbilical angiitis is

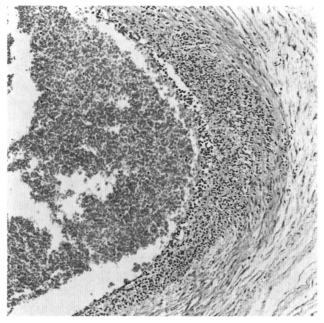

Fig. 38.56 An umbilical angiitis found in association with a chorioamnionitis. (From Fox 1997a. Reproduced by permission of W B Saunders.)

confined to the vessels of the cord and stops short at the anterior abdominal wall of the fetus. The funiculitis is often very patchy and may be limited to an area of the cord that lay near to the cervical os, whilst occasionally an isolated funiculitis, unassociated with a chorioamnionitis, is seen; nearly always when this occurs there has been a prolapse of the cord.

Chorioamnionitis commonly has a polymicrobial aetiology and the organisms frequently isolated from inflamed membranes include enterococci, coagulase-positive staphylococci, anaerobic streptococci and *Escherichia coli*, all organisms normally found inhabiting the lower female genital tract during pregnancy. Group B haemolytic streptococci, which intermittently colonise the genital tract, cause more perinatal morbidity and mortality than any other bacteria (Katz 1993) and are an important cause of chorioamnionitis (Beecroft et al 1976; Vigorita & Parmley 1979; Novak & Platt 1985; Yancey et al 1994); nevertheless there is a rather poor correlation between neonatal streptococcal infection and the presence of a chorioamnionitis, the organisms appearing to have the ability to pass rapidly through the membranes whilst only inducing a minimal inflammatory response.

In recent years there has been an increasing tendency to implicate *Chlamydia trachomatis*, Ureaplasma and the mycoplasmas as important factors in chorioamnionitis (Embree et al 1980; Gibbs et al 1982; Kundsin et al 1984; Dong et al 1987; Quinn et al 1987; Hillier et al 1988; Jacob-Cormier et al 1989; Donders et al 1991; Eschenbach 1993; Smith & Taylor-Robinson 1993) though it has to be admitted that the aetiological significance of these organisms, particularly that of *Chlamydia*, has been challenged (Romero et al 1989a; Ismail et al 1992).

The role played by *Gardnerella vaginalis* in the aetiology of chorioamnionitis is a complex one. This organism, by itself, does not appear to be pathogenic when present in the amniotic fluid (Gibbs et al 1987) but the combination of *G. vaginalis* together with those other organisms implicated in bacterial vaginosis, namely *M. hominis* and anaerobes, does appear to be quite an important cause of inflammation of the membranes (Silver et al 1989; Gibbs 1992).

Mycotic chorioamnionitis is uncommon and is nearly always due to *Candida albicans* (Schwartz & Reef 1990) whilst the only virus which has been identified as a possible cause of chorioamnionitis is *Herpes simplex*.

The long held belief that the intact membranes offer a virtually impregnable bar to the spread of bacteria has suffered considerable recent attrition and it is now clear that, especially in preterm pregnancies, amniotic sac infection and chorioamnionitis can occur in the presence of intact membranes (Guvenc et al 1989; Romero et al 1989c; Armer & Duff 1991). It still remains true, however, that at term the fluid within an intact amniotic sac is usually sterile.

Many cases of chorioamnionitis develop without any predisposing factor but there is a significant relationship between prolonged rupture of the membranes and a high incidence of chorioamnionitis (Fox & Langley 1971) whilst prolonged labour is also a risk factor (Soper et al 1989). The incidence of amniotic infection rises with an increasing number of vaginal examinations during labour (Newton et al 1989; Soper et al 1989).

There is now overwhelming evidence that an association exists between chorioamnionitis and preterm delivery, particularly when this occurs before the 35th week of gestation (Perkins et al 1987; Hillier et al 1988, 1991; Romero et al 1989a,b,c; Gibbs et al 1992; Hyde & Altshuler 1999; Taylor 2000). The exact nature of this association is, however, not always clear for whilst it is almost certain that chorioamnionitis can both precipitate preterm labour and induce premature rupture of the membranes (Naeye & Peters 1980; Romero et al 1993) it is also possible that premature rupture of the membranes, due to non-infective factors, may be complicated by chorioamnionitis. Despite these uncertainties it is clear that chorioamnionitis is common in cases of early preterm labour, the incidence in various studies ranging from 19 to 74% (Chellam & Rushton 1985; Guzick & Winn 1985; Hillier et al 1988; Mueller-Heubach et al 1990; van der Elst et al 1991).

It has been suggested that bacterial infection of the membranes may lead to their premature rupture because of the release of elastases and collagenases from the neutrophil polymorphonuclear leucocytes infiltrating the membranes (Naeye 1991). Bacteria, by themselves, also diminish the tensile strength, elasticity and 'work to rupture' of the membranes by the release of proteolytic enzymes (McGregor et al 1987) but the combination of some, but not all, bacteria and neutrophil polymorphonuclear leucocytes causes more damage to the membranes than either bacteria or acute inflammatory cells alone (Schoonmaker et al 1989). The relationship between chorioamnionitis and premature onset of labour is more complex. Prostaglandins are thought to play a vital rôle in stimulating parturition and there is considerable evidence that infection is associated with a greatly increased production of prostaglandins by the amnion (Lopez-Bernal et al 1987, 1989; Romero et al 1987; van der Elst et al 1991). Cytokines play a predominant role, not only in stimulating the excess prostaglandin synthesis found in chorioamnionitis but also in evoking labour (Mitchell et al 1993). The cytokines, produced by activated macrophages in response to infection, which have been particularly implicated in this respect, are interleukin-1, interleukin-2, tumour necrosis factor, granulocyte colony stimulating factor, interleukin-8 and interleukin-6; high levels of these cytokines are found in the amniotic fluid in cases of chorioamnionitis (Romero et al 1989a,b, 1990, 1992a,b; Hillier et al 1993), they can stimulate prostaglandin synthesis by the amnion and decidua

(Romero et al 1989d; Mitchell et al 1993), inhibit progesterone synthesis (Ohno et al 1994) and, under experimental conditions, directly elicit uterine contractility (Gibbs et al 1992).

A particular risk presented to the fetus by chorioamnionitis is clearly that of spread of infection to the fetus from the inflamed membranes. The fetus may inhale infected amniotic fluid and develop a 'congenital' pneumonia, whilst entry of the fluid into the upper respiratory tract can cause meningitis. The fetal skin or eyes can be infected by direct contact with organisms in the fluid, which is probably the aetiological mechanism in a proportion of cases of neonatal pyogenic dermatitis or ophthalmia. Swallowing of the fluid may be responsible for some cases of neonatal gastritis, enteritis or peritonitis. All these complications occur infrequently in chorioamnionitis; on the other hand they rarely occur in its absence.

Other possible risks posed to the fetus by amniotic fluid infection are considerably more nebulous. It has been suggested that the cytokines which are activated by amniotic fluid infection may cause fetal brain damage (Yoon et al 1997) but, as Edwards & Duggan (2000) have remarked, the data to support a rôle for intrauterine infection in human cerebral damage are largely circumstantial and, to some degree, inconsistent. It has also been suggested that umbilical cord inflammation may cause constriction of the umbilical vessels and fetal hypoxia (Hyde & Altshuler 1999): this view is currently speculative but merits further study.

Chorioamnionitis may be associated with maternal pyrexia and tachycardia; there is also an unduly high incidence of postpartum pelvic sepsis, uterine tenderness and maternal leucocytosis. The most serious risk presented to the mother by an amniotic infection is, however, the fortunately uncommon complication of endotoxic shock, this being confined to infections due to Gram-negative organisms.

PREMATURE RUPTURE OF THE MEMBRANES

The term 'premature rupture of the membranes' is used here in its conventional obstetrical sense, i.e. rupture of the membranes during the later months of pregnancy but before the 37th week of gestation with subsequent onset of premature labour and delivery. The membranes may, of course, rupture at a much earlier stage of gestation and this can result in miscarriage, extramembranous pregnancy or extra-amniotic pregnancy, subjects which are considered separately.

Premature rupture of the membranes is an important cause of preterm delivery; it is estimated that in approximately one-third of such deliveries the membrane rupture is the initial event, occurring prior to, and presumably being responsible for, the early onset of labour (Lockwood 1994). It has been variously proposed that

under such circumstances there may be an inherent weakness, a mechanical deficiency or a degenerative change. There is now no doubt that infection, in the form of a chorioamnionitis, is an important factor in the aetiology of premature rupture, accounting for up to 55% of cases (Romero et al 1988), and this relationship is discussed above. Nevertheless, premature membrane rupture can occur in the complete absence of any clinical or pathological evidence of infection and it is in these cases that the possibility of a mechanical defect in the membranes has been raised (Polzin & Brady 1991): a deficiency of collagen III has often been canvassed in this respect but nevertheless there is no consistent evidence of any decreased mechanical strength in prematurely ruptured membranes (Bell 2000).

Whether there is or is not a subtle change in membrane collagen content or metabolism is not, of course, a matter of great moment for the pathologist looking at conventionally stained sections of ruptured membranes. No consistent histological abnormality in prematurely ruptured membranes has been described and most such membranes appear normal.

EXTRAMEMBRANOUS PREGNANCY

In this condition, gestation continues after rupture of both amnion and chorion during early or mid-pregnancy so that the fetus develops, either partly or fully, outside the membranes. In most cases the membranes have ruptured between the 11th and 23rd week of pregnancy, and delivery has occurred between the 27th and 35th weeks, with there being, in the intervening period, a continuous or intermittent loss of liquor. A very high proportion of the infants have died during the neonatal period, either from prematurity alone or from this combined with infection.

The placenta from an extramembranous pregnancy is invariably circumvallate, whilst the membranous sac is unduly small and clearly of too limited a capacity to have contained the fetus; characteristically, the sac wall is rather firm and usually has, at the margins of the rupture site, a thick, rolled edge (Fig. 38.57), though this is not invariably the case (Perlman et al 1980). Nodules of amnion nodosum may be present and there may be extensive deposition of haemosiderin in the membranes (Benirschke & Kaufmann 2000).

EXTRA-AMNIOTIC PREGNANCY

In this form of gestation, rupture of the amnion occurs in early pregnancy but the fetus continues to survive in the intact chorion. This appears, at first sight, to be an extremely infrequent phenomenon but the frequency of this form of gestation has probably been underestimated, for amniotic band formation, now widely though not universally held to be a complication of early amniotic rupture and often used as a surrogate for this diagnosis, is much less uncommon.

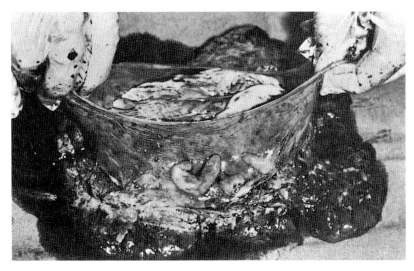

Fig. 38.57 Placenta and membranes from an extramembranous pregnancy. The placenta is circumvallate, whilst the membranes are short and thick with a rolled edge. The membranous sac was too small to have contained the fetus. (From Fox 1997a. Reproduced by permission of W BSaunders.)

Following amniotic rupture there is no external loss of liquor, though there may be oligohydramnios, and the pregnancy, though probably often failing, may well proceed to term; the placenta is of normal form and the infant may be completely normal. The diagnosis can be made by recognising that the amnion is represented only by a small apron-like 'cuff' or 'collar' around the insertion of the cord (Fig. 38.58) or by noting the presence of amniotic strings. Amnion nodosum may be present in some cases (Yang et al 1984).

The aetiology of amniotic rupture in the early months of gestation is a matter of conjecture. Some cases of amniotic band syndrome appear to have followed diagnostic amniocentesis or chorionic villus sampling in early pregnancy but in the vast majority of cases no aetiological factor can be identified.

AMNIOTIC BANDS AND STRINGS

A wide, but characteristic, range of fetal abnormalities (including constriction rings, intrauterine amputations,

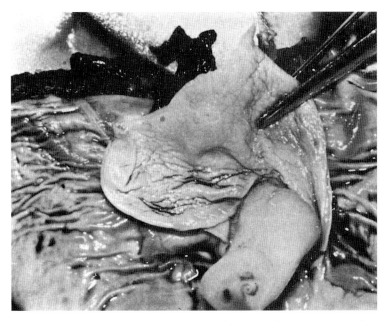

Fig. 38.58 An extra-amniotic pregnancy. The amnion is represented only by a small shrunken, but grossly thickened, remnant which forms a 'collar' around the insertion of the cord. (From Fox 1997a. Reproduced by permission of W B Saunders.)

syndactyly, fusion defects of the cranium and face, and club-feet) are often found in association with amniotic bands, strings and adhesions.

Torpin (1968) proposed that amniotic bands and strings were a consequence of amniotic rupture during early pregnancy. He showed that following this event the amnion tends to become partially or totally detached from the chorion and may then fragment, shred, and shrink down to form a collar around the insertion of the cord, or roll up to form a rope-like structure, the distal end of which may be free or still attached to the chorion. Following amniotic detachment, the mesoblastic tissue on the maternal surface of the separated amnion and that on the fetal surface of the denuded chorion tends to be drawn out into thin fibrous strings. The stage is then set for the possible entanglement of fetal limbs or digits within these bands or strings, with the subsequent development of constriction rings which, in extreme cases, lead to intrauterine amputations. Furthermore, the raw chorion rapidly absorbs liquor, and in the resulting oligohydramniotic state, which is probably responsible for the development of club-feet, the fetus may rub against the rough chorion and sustain abrasions to which the mesoblastic strings may become attached, there producing fusion deformities, particularly of the head and face. Finally, the fetus may actually swallow a mesoblastic string, and this will result eventually in an adhesion between membranes and face, with a further risk of fusion deformities at this site.

The bands can also cause syndactyly, by encircling the developing digits, or abdominal constriction rings (Imber et al 1974), and can, even more alarmingly, encircle the neck and cause intrauterine decapitation (Ehrhardt 1956;

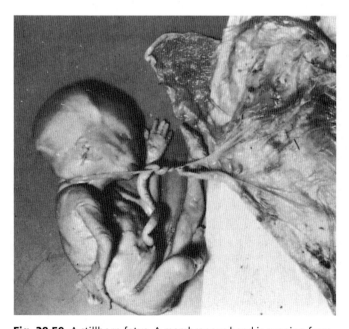

Fig. 38.59 A stillborn fetus. A membranous band is running from the placenta to the fetal occipital region and is constricting the umbilical cord. (From Fox 1997a. Reproduced by permission of W B Saunders.)

Swinburne 1967). Even if the fetus escapes malformation by amniotic bands or strings, it still faces a threat to its continued existence, for a band may encircle the umbilical cord and constrict it (Fig. 38.59), often sufficiently to cause fetal compromise and, not uncommonly, death (Reles et al 1991; Pommerenke & Sadenwasser 1992; Kanayama et al 1995).

If called upon to examine a placenta from a child with presumed amniotic band deformities, the pathologist would be well advised to immerse the organ in water, a technique which allows for the delicate amniotic strings to be more easily seen and recognised; subsequent histological examination will show that the amnion is absent from the placental surface.

CLINICOPATHOLOGICAL VALUE OF PATHOLOGICAL EXAMINATION OF THE PLACENTA, CORD AND MEMBRANES

There is considerable confusion in the minds of both pathologists and obstetricians as to which placentas should be subjected, in routine hospital practice, to pathological examination and about the information that may be derived from such studies. Some consider that all placentas should be examined by a pathologist (Salafia & Vintzileos 1990), an opinion with which Benirschke & Kaufmann (2000) agree. In most countries today there are, however, obvious logistic and financial reasons why this is not possible and, indeed, no truly viable scientific reasons have been given for advocating such a Herculean task. The College of American Pathologists (Langston et al 1997) has recommended a more selective approach as, more recently, have Lewis & Benirschke (1999) and Porter (2000). Whilst these selective lists of indications for placental examination are probably valid in specialised centres with a specific interest in placental studies they also are too all-encompassing for routine practice. Thus, for example, maternal diabetes mellitus is usually given as an indication for placental examination and it is true that examination of placentas from diabetic women commonly shows a characteristic, but non-specific, pattern of changes (Fox 1997a). What information does this give, however, to the obstetrician? The obstetrician knows that the patient is diabetic and has tried to control blood sugar levels as tightly as possible throughout pregnancy. The results of a placental examination add nothing to the obstetrician's knowledge of the present pregnancy and will not influence the management of future pregnancies. Under these circumstances routine pathological examination of the diabetic's placenta would appear to be a waste of time and money. It could be said that exactly the same considerations apply to the examination of placentas from women with pre-eclampsia or eclampsia but in these conditions the obstetrician frequently wishes to know how much damage, if any, the placenta has suffered and whether the condition has been complicated by retroplacental bleeding. Maternal drug or alcohol abuse are also often considered as indications for examination of the placenta: the results of studies of placentas from such cases are of considerable interest to both research placentologists and toxicologists but, again, add nothing to the obstetrician's understanding of the present pregnancy and are not predictive for future pregnancies.

With this attitude in mind a realistic view of the indications for placental examination in routine practice would be:

Preterm delivery before the 36th week of gestation
Maternal infection
Maternal pre-eclampsia or eclampsia
Fetal intrauterine growth retardation
Fetal or neonatal hypoxia
Fetal or neonatal death
Fetal hydrops
Suspected fetal metabolic disorder
Multiple pregnancy
Maternal malignant disease

The most important of these from the view of routine practice are maternal pre-eclampsia, fetal intrauterine growth retardation, preterm delivery, fetal intrauterine death and maternal infection and these topics will be briefly considered here. The placental findings in respect to fetal hydrops, fetal metabolic disorders, neonatal hypoxia and neonatal death are covered in texts of placental and perinatal pathology (Keeling 1993; Fox 1997a; Benirschke & Kaufmann 2000) whilst the placenta in multiple pregnancy is discussed in Chapter 48 and involvement of the placenta in maternal malignant disease is considered in Chapter 42.

PRE-ECLAMPSIA

Placentas from pre-eclamptic women tend, on average, to be smaller than those from uncomplicated pregnancies but the decrease is only slight and a proportion of such placentas are unusually large: the placental:fetal weight ratio is generally increased. There is no excess of extrachorial placentation and the incidence of placental infarction ranges from about 33% in cases of mild pre-eclampsia to approximately 60% in patients with the severe form of the disease: extensive infarction (involving more than 10% of the parenchyma) is found in about 30% of placentas from cases of severe pre-eclampsia but is not a feature of the milder forms of this disease (Fox 1997a). It will be appreciated that most placentas from pre-eclamptic women therefore either show no infarction or are only infarcted to an extent too limited to be of functional significance. Retroplacental haematomas are found unduly frequently, occurring in about 12–15% of cases, but there is no excess of any other gross lesion.

Histologically, the villi are usually of normal maturity for the length of the gestational period though some appear to show accelerated maturation. The only consistent abnormalities are hyperplasia of the villous cytotrophoblastic cells (Fig. 38.60) and thickening of the villous trophoblastic basement membrane. The villi are often normally vascularised but in a significant proportion of placentas they are hypovascular with small, non-dilated and relatively inconspicuous vessels: this change is associ-

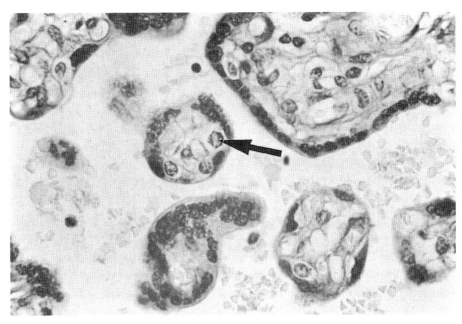

Fig. 38.60 Villi in a placenta from a woman with pre-eclampsia. The syncytiotrophoblast shows no obvious damage but the cytotrophoblastic cells (one of which is arrowed) are unduly numerous and prominent.

ated with, and parallels in severity the degree of, an obliterative arteritis of the fetal stem arteries (Las Heras et al 1983, 1985), a lesion that is found to a greater or lesser extent in about a third of placentas from pre-eclamptic patients. The hypovascular villi, but not those which are adequately perfused from the fetal side, have an abundance of syncytial knots and show increased stromal fibrosis.

If decidua is found attached to the basal plate of the placenta it may be possible to discern that some of the spiral vessels have not undergone physiological change, even in their intradecidual segments (Khong et al 1986) and atherosis characterised by a fibrinoid necrosis of the arterial wall together with an intramural accumulation of lipid-laden marophages and a perivascular lymphocytic cuffing: it should be noted that these changes in the decidual vessels, whilst characteristic of pre-eclampsia, are not specific to that condition (Khong 1991; Khong & Robertson 1992).

At the ultrastructural level the cytotrophoblastic hyperplasia and the basement membrane thickening are confirmed whilst the villous syncytiotrophoblast shows patchy focal necrosis, loss and distortion of microvilli on the free surface, diminished pinocytotic activity, a reduced number of secretory droplets and dilatation of the rough endoplasmic reticulum (Jones & Fox 1980).

The changes seen in the placenta of the pre-eclamptic woman therefore exemplify those, previously described, which are associated with a reduced maternal uteroplacental blood flow and all the abnormalities in the trophoblast are explicable on this basis. That maternal uteroplacental blood flow is decreased in pre-eclampsia is well established (Campbell et al 1983, 1986; McParland & Pearce 1988; Steel et al 1988; Bewley et al 1991; Mires et al 1998) and the pathological basis for this, which is an inadequate transformation by extravillous intravascular trophoblast of the spiral arteries into uteroplacental vessels, has been clearly defined in recent years (see Chapter 39) and there is in pre-eclampsia a clear correlation between inadequate development of the uteroplacental vessels, as noted in placental bed biopsies, and an abnormal uterine flow velocity waveform in Doppler studies (Oloffson et al 1993; Lin et al 1995). All the changes seen in placentas from pre-eclamptic patients can reasonably be attributed to this reduction in maternal blood flow and no other pathogenetic factor need be invoked. Cytotrophoblastic proliferation is a direct response to trophoblastic ischaemia but the excess of syncytial knots and villous stromal fibrosis is an indirect consequence in so far as it results from diminished fetal villous perfusion as a result of the oblitertative endarteritis of the fetal stem vessels, this change being a morphologic surrogate for vasoconstriction. This vasoconstriction leads to a significant increase in placental vascular resistance (Trudinger et al 1985b) and almost certainly represents a fetal haemodynamic response to the uteroplacental

ischaemia for it has been clearly shown in experimental studies that restriction of maternal blood flow and/or reduced oxygenation of placental tissue results in a marked decrease in fetal blood flow through the placenta, presumably as a result of vasoconstriction (Stock et al 1980; Howard et al 1987; Clapp 1994). This diminished placental perfusion in response to uteroplacental ischaemia results in a preferential diversion of blood to the vitally important cerebral and cardiac circulations.

The functional consequences of the ischaemic damage to the placenta are, however, hard to assess. The reduced syncytial pinocytotic activity is indicative of a decreased transfer capacity whilst the paucity of secretory droplets attests to impaired synthetic activity. Whether, however, these functional changes reflect true syncytial damage or are simply a consequence of a diminished oxygen supply is debatable. It is nevertheless clear that any damaging effects of pre-eclampsia on the placenta are limited by the extremely efficient repair process which the trophoblast mounts against ischaemic attack and it is highly probable that the ill effects of pre-eclampsia on fetal growth, oxygenation and viability are due, not to placental damage, but to an inadequate maternal supply of oxygen and nutrients (Fox 1988).

The maternal ill effects are thought, by contrast, to be due to the release into the circulation of some substance from the ischaemic placenta which causes maternal endothelial cell dysfunction (Roberts et al 1989; Redman 1991). It has been suggested that in pre-eclampsia an excess of cellular, subcellular and molecular debris is shed from the syncytium as a result of both oxidative stress-induced apoptosis and necrosis and that this is capable in some, but not all, women of activating an inflammatory response of which endothelial cell dysfunction is one aspect (Baker 2000; Redman & Sargent 2000).

INTRAUTERINE FETAL GROWTH RETARDATION

There are many well-established causes of intrauterine fetal growth retardation, such as pre-eclampsia, fetal infection, congenital fetal malformation, fetal chromosomal abnormality, maternal cigarette smoking, etc., but after elimination of these there remains a residue of cases for which there is no obvious maternal or fetal cause: it is the placenta of such infants which is considered here, whilst recognising, of course, that even these instances of 'idiopathic' intrauterine growth retardation are almost certainly a heterogeneous group in aetiological terms.

Placentas from cases of idiopathic intrauterine growth retardation are small but placento-fetal weight ratios are usually normal. They usually show no excess of macroscopic abnormalities (Fox 1994, 1997a, 2000) though an increased incidence of infarcts, albeit usually small ones, has been noted in some studies (Salafia et al 1992b). Maternal floor infarction, very extensive perivillous fibrin deposition, widespread thrombosis of fetal arteries and unusually large, or multiple, placental haemangiomas may all be associated with diminished fetal growth but such lesions are found in only a small minority of placentas from growth retarded infants.

Histological examination of placentas from small for gestational age infants reveals no constant or diagnostic pathological picture (Fox 1997a, 2000). Many, probably about 25%, are histologically normal in all respects and the vast majority are normally mature for the length of the gestational period though a few show a delay in villous maturation. Villitis of unknown aetiology is seen with undue frequency in placentas from small for gestational age infants: the reported proportion of such placentas in which this lesion has been found has been very variable but averages in the region of 30%. The remainder commonly show evidence of having been subjected to ischaemia or, most commonly, an admixture of both ischaemic and diminished fetal perfusion patterns, i.e. their appearances are very similar to those found in pre-eclamptic patients. That there is, in many cases of idiopathic intrauterine growth retardation, a diminished maternal blood flow to the placenta is now well established, both by the use of older techniques (Lunell et al 1979) and by Doppler studies of the uteroplacental circulation (Trudinger et al 1985a,b; McCowan et al 1988; Bewley et al 1991; Iwata et al 1993). The pathological basis for a diminished maternal blood supply to the placenta in many cases of intrauterine fetal growth retardation is now reasonably well established for inadequate conversion of spiral arteries into uteroplacental vessels, in a manner identical to that seen in pre-eclampsia, is found, though less consistently, in cases of normotensive idiopathic intrauterine fetal growth retardation (Sheppard & Bonnar 1976; Robertson 1981; Khong et al 1986; Khong & Robertson 1992) and this defect in placentation is specifically associated with abnormal uterine flow velocity waveforms (Lin et al 1995). There must be strong grounds for presuming that the resultant restriction of maternal blood flow is a crucially important factor in the failure of fetal growth, for in experimental studies artificially induced limitation of placental blood flow will result in an unduly small fetus (Robinson & Owens 1993; Clapp 1994). Acute atherosis is also often present in the maternal vessels in cases of idiopathic fetal growth retardation (Althabe et al 1985; Khong 1991).

Histological examination of placentas from small for gestational age infants also often shows, as in pre-eclampsia, evidence of diminished fetal perfusion of the villous vessels, e.g. small or sclerosed fetal vessels, stromal fibrosis, an increased number of syncytial knots. It is therefore not surprising that Doppler studies have shown that there is, in many placentas from growth retarded fetuses, an increased resistance in the fetal placental vascular bed and a diminished fetal placental blood flow (Trudinger et al 1985 a,b; Gudmunsson & Marsal 1988; Bracero et al 1989; Gill et al 1993; Hitschold et al 1993). There

has been some dispute amongst those performing Doppler studies as to the morphological basis for the increased resistance in the placental fetal vasculature of growth retarded fetuses. Some have thought that there is obliteration of stem vessels (Giles et al 1985; Bracero et al 1989; Fok et al 1990), whilst others consider that there is a reduction in the vascularity of the terminal villi (Hitschold et al 1993; Macara et al 1995, 1996). There has also been some disagreement between those who consider that the reduced fetal perfusion is a response to uteroplacental ischaemia (Giles et al 1985) and others who invoke a developmental arrest of placental angiogenesis (Bracero et al 1989; Jackson et al 1995; Kreczy et al 1995).

A characteristic feature of many placentas from small for gestational age fetuses is, however, an 'endarteritis obliterans' in the large stem arteries (van der Veen & Fox 1983). This lesion is, as previously discussed, the hallmark of a prolonged vasoconstriction. This occurs as a response to uteroplacental ischaemia and is part of an attempt by the deprived fetus to divert blood to the cerebral and coronary circulations. This haemodynamic view of the basis for an increased fetal vascular resistance in the placenta of low birth weight infants is conceptually more appealing than the alternative concept of arrested angiogenesis for it is difficult both to reconcile this latter view with the proven inadequate placentation in many such cases and to suggest an aetiological factor for arrested vascular development; furthermore the concept of a fixed vascular deficiency accords ill with the observation that in many, though not all, cases of fetal growth retardation maternal hyperoxygenation decreases fetal intraplacental vascular resistance (Bilardo et al 1991; de Rochembeau et al 1992).

This view of the major importance of a restricted maternal uteroplacental flow with consequent placental and fetal hypoxia in intrauterine fetal growth retardation has recently been challenged, especially for those cases in which Doppler studies show absent end diastolic flow velocity (Krebs et al 1996; Macara et al 1996; Kingdom et al 1997; Kingdom & Kaufmann 1997; Kingdom 1998; Kohnen & Kingdom 2000). Whilst accepting the evidence, derived from fetal umbilical venous blood studies, that there is fetal hypoxia in such cases (Nicolaides et al 1988) it has nevertheless been maintained that there is no placental hypoxia, this claim being based on the finding of an unusually high oxygen content in uteroplacental venous blood in cases of intrauterine fetal growth retardation (Pardi et al 1992). This apparent discrepancy between 'placental hyperoxia' and fetal hypoxia has led to the view that under such circumstances there may be a primary defect in placental nutrient and gas transfer, a defect due to inhibition of the angiogenic drive to form terminal villi by the high oxygen levels in the intervillous space. This interesting and original hypothesis suffers from two major defects, both of which have been pointed out by Burton (1997). Firstly, the theory is heavily dependent upon a single study which demonstrated that the oxygen content and saturation of the uterine venous blood was higher in cases of intrauterine growth retardation than in normal controls. Secondly, the theory invokes a circular argument: abnormal villous development reduces fetal uptake of oxygen with resultant placental hyperoxia which causes abnormal villous development.

Clearly, no consensus has been reached as yet about the rôle of the placenta in intrauterine fetal growth retardation. The most that a pathologist can do in the majority of cases is to describe the findings whilst refraining from drawing clear-cut conclusions about cause and effect. The pathologist should also accept that the introduction of molecular and cytogenetic techniques may reveal abnormalities of the placenta that are associated with fetal growth retardation but which are not discernible by microscopy, confined placental mosaicism (Kalousek et al 1991; Kalousek 1994; Kalousek & Langlois 1994) being a classical example.

PRETERM DELIVERY

Between 5 and 10% of babies are delivered prematurely but deliveries before the 32nd week of gestation account for only about 1.5% of births and deliveries under 28 weeks account for only 0.2–0.6% of births; it is however

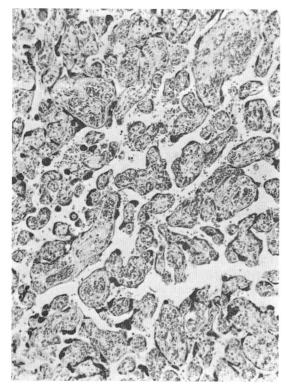

Fig. 38.61 Histological appearances of the villi in a placenta from a pregnancy terminating spontaneously at the 35th week of gestation. The villi are morphologically fully mature in all respects. This is an example of 'maturitas praecox placentae'.

in this last group that prematurity poses its greatest threat for two-thirds of deaths in preterm infants occur in infants born at less than 28 weeks of gestation (Walkinshaw 1995). In a considerable proportion of cases early delivery is related to an obvious obstetrical complication such as twin pregnancy, abruptio placentae, cervical incompetence, placenta praevia or severe pre-eclampsia; in a high proportion of the remainder premature labour is a consequence of, and is secondary to, either chorioamnionitis or idiopathic premature rupture of the membranes: chorioamnionitis, with or without membrane rupture, is the most important precipitating factor of very early preterm delivery, certainly before the 28th week of gestation and, though to a slightly lesser extent, before the 32nd week of gestation. True idiopathic primary premature onset of labour in women with intact, non-inflamed membranes is a relatively uncommon event, Lettieri et al (1993) being unable to find a potential aetiological factor in only 4% of preterm births.

The prematurely delivered placenta is usually smaller and lighter than a term placenta but is otherwise generally unremarkable on naked-eye examination. There is no excess of extrachorial placentation or of abnormal insertion of the cord whilst infarcts, perivillous fibrin deposition and calcification are distinctly uncommon.

On histological examination the fetal stem arteries rarely show any abnormality and the villi are, in most instances, of apparently normal maturity for the length of the gestational period. It is almost invariably the case, however, that a proportion of prematurely delivered placentas depart from this pattern and have a villous morphology which is that of the fully mature term organ (Fig. 38.61): this proportion is about 10% in most series (Fox 1997a). In some such cases the estimate of the length of the gestational period may have been faulty but fully mature placentas are sometimes encountered from women who are undoubtedly only 30 to 32 weeks pregnant and who give birth to babies whose weight and length were fully compatible with a pregnancy of this duration. These are then true examples of 'maturitas praecox placentae' and as such are a manifestation of an asynchrony between the rates of placental and fetal maturation. Naeye (1987, 1989, 1992) has argued that premature placental maturation in preterm deliveries is an adaptive response to a reduced maternal uteroplacental blood flow whilst Arias et al (1993) maintained that some cases of preterm delivery were associated with a maternal vasculopathy. This view has been strengthened by claims that in some cases of otherwise idiopathic premature onset of labour, particularly those in which the fetus had a very low birth weight or was hypoxic, there are maternal vascular abnormalities which are qualitatively, though not quantitatively, identical to those found in pre-eclampsia (Salafia et al 1991, 1995, 2000; Salafia & Mill 1996; Salafia & Pijnenborg 1999). This concept has won some support from Doppler studies (Strigini et al 1995) and is certainly a feasible one for it is becoming increasingly clear that the spectrum of obstetrical disorders which may result from abnormal placentation is very wide.

INTRAUTERINE FETAL DEATH

There is some debate as to where the line should be drawn between a miscarriage and a stillbirth but it would be generally agreed that an intrauterine fetal death after the 22nd week of gestation is a stillbirth.

It is a time-honoured cliche that examination of the placenta is an integral component of an autopsy on a still-born infant. The extent to which placental examination helps in elucidating the cause of intrauterine demise is, however, still a matter of dispute. Hovatta et al (1983) studied 243 stillbirths and considered that just over 50% of these were due to placental factors and that nearly 12% resulted from cord complications. Included, however, as instances of 'placental failure' were, inter alia, pre-eclampsia, twin births, preterm labour and uterine anomalies, conditions for which terminology indicating a functional failure of the placenta seems quite inappropriate: further, death was attributed in just over 25% of cases to abruptio placentae or large placental infarcts without adequate consideration of the many live infants whose placentas show such lesions. Rayburn et al (1985) claimed that they were able to establish the cause of fetal death in 88 of 89 stillbirths examined: placental histological abnormalities were the sole abnormal findings in 11% of these cases and these consisted of a poorly defined entity of 'vascular insufficiency'. Volker (1992) considers that 50% of still-births are directly due to placental causes and lists delayed villous maturation, 'endarteritis obliterans' of the placental stem vessels and placental infarction as causes of a 'chronic placental insufficiency' which leads to fetal demise, a viewpoint which ignores the fact that such abnormalities can be found in many placentas from live births. It seems often to be the case that pathologists seize on any abnormality, no matter how functionally unimportant, which is present in the placenta and attribute fetal death to this, thus effectively disguising the true cause of death or, perhaps even more importantly, concealing our ignorance, in many cases, of the factors which have led to the adverse pregnancy outcome. Any claim that a particular placental lesion has been the direct cause of fetal demise must be stringently evaluated, a procedure which tends to reduce dramatically the proportion of such deaths due to placental causes. Macroscopic examination of the placenta of a stillbirth is clearly of some value though it would be over-optimistic to expect such an examination to yield a causal factor for fetal death in anything more than a small minority of cases. It is true that, on occasion, inspection of the placenta may reveal an obvious presumptive cause for fetal demise, e.g. ruptured vasa praevia, massive infarction, a very large retroplacental haematoma, a huge haemangioma, very extensive fetal artery thrombosis or well-marked placental floor infarc-

tion, but such findings are very much the exception rather than the rule. It is of particular importance not to overstress the significance of gross lesions and to bear in mind that even quite extensive infarction or perivillous fibrin deposition is compatible with continuing fetal viability. Examination of the umbilical cord is just as important as placental examination and may yield important, sometimes critical, clues as to the cause of death.

Those undertaking histological examination of the placenta from a stillborn fetus must take into account the time interval that has elapsed between fetal demise and delivery. After fetal death in utero the placenta remains fully viable, is still a living, functioning organ, and can, indeed invariably does, undergo a series of morphological changes. These changes, which are now well documented, show a consistent pattern and are progressive (Wilkin 1965; Emmrich 1966a,b, 1992; Davies & Glasser 1967; Fox 1968; Theuring 1968; Hustin and Gaspard 1977). There is a considerable increase in the number of villous syncytial knots though the syncytiotrophoblast of the villi usually appears otherwise normal; the villous cytotrophoblastic cells become more numerous and prominent, whilst the trophoblastic basement membrane undergoes a gradual thickening. The villous stroma becomes increasingly dense and fibrotic, and the villous fetal vessels undergo a progressive sclerosis which leads eventually to their obliteration. The fetal stem vessels show striking changes, with their lumens becoming greatly narrowed, and eventually obliterated, by a process of fibromuscular sclerosis.

Genest (1992) has re-examined the placental changes that occur after fetal death in an attempt to relate them with a greater degree of precision to the duration of intrauterine retention of the dead fetus. His findings were very similar to those described above but, in addition, he noted villous intravascular karyorrhexis, probably of leucocytic nuclei, as the earliest post-mortem change. Genest showed that three histological features can be used to determine the approximate time interval between death and delivery, these being villous intravascular karyorrhexis, changes in the villous stem arteries and villous fibrosis. Thus if none of these changes is present the fetus has been dead for less than 6 hours whilst if karyorrhexis is the only change noted the time interval is between 6 and 48 hours: the presence of this change together with stem vessel abnormalities and fibrosis of 50%, or less, of the villi indicates that fetal demise had occurred between 2 and 14 days before delivery whilst changes more marked than these indicate a retention period of over 14 days.

The pathogenesis of these post-mortem changes in villous morphology is reasonably clear. The death of the fetus is, of course, followed by a complete cessation of the fetal circulation through the placenta, and this will lead to fibromuscular sclerosis of the fetal stem arteries, obliteration of the villous capillaries, villous stromal fibrosis, and a proliferation of villous syncytial knots. The trophoblastic basement membrane thickening and the cytotrophoblastic hyperplasia are, on the other hand, a response to a reduced maternal blood flow to the placenta; it is known that maternal uteroplacental blood flow decreases notably after fetal death (Browne & Veall 1953), though the decrease is not of a degree such as to impair the continuing viability of the trophoblast. The teleological advantages of this reduction in uteroplacental blood flow are obvious, but the mechanism by which it is produced is obscure; one possibility is that it is a consequence of the loss of the fetal circulation through the villi, for ten Berge (1955) has described a villous 'pulse' which may help the circulation of maternal blood through the intervillous space, and a loss of this could lead to the stagnation of blood in the intervillous space, a rise in intervillous space pressure and a consequent decrease in uteroplacental blood flow; this is, of course, a somewhat simplistic (though not necessarily incorrect) view for there must be many feto-maternal 'messages' which are interrupted by fetal death.

These post-mortem alterations in the placenta of the dead fetus are of no importance in themselves but do have two unfortunate consequences. The first is that they may be wrongly considered to have been present at the time of, and to have contributed to, fetal demise; the second is that histological examination of these placentas may be of limited value. Examination of a placenta from a stillbirth dead in utero for less than 48 hours is just as valid and worthwhile as is examination of a placenta from a live born infant; if the retention period is longer than this, however, the ability to detect villous changes due to alterations in either uteroplacental or fetoplacental blood flow progressively diminishes whilst histological examination of the placental tissue from a fetus dead in utero for more than 14 days is largely a worthless procedure in this respect. Histological study of the villous tissue of a macerated fetus may yield limited information, such as detecting the presence of a severe or widespread villitis, but is very often unrewarding.

MATERNAL INFECTIONS

As discussed earlier maternal infection involving the placenta usually results in a villitis. Most cases of villitis are of unknown, or at least unrecognised, aetiology but some systemic maternal infections produce a reasonably characteristic, and sometimes diagnostic, pattern of placental lesions.

Syphilis

The infected placenta is typically large and pale (Malan et al 1990) and usually, though far from invariably, presents a triad of histological appearances, none of which is spe-cific but which when taken together are are highly suggestive of syphilitic infection (Russell & Altschuler 1974; Horn et al 1992; Qureshi et al 1993; Samson et al 1994). Firstly, there are changes which are secondary to infective haemolytic anaemia in the fetus, namely, villous immaturity and the presence of nucleated erythrocytes in the fetal vessels. Secondly, there is an endarteritis and perivascultis of the villous stem vessels and, thirdly, there is a focal proliferative villitis which varies from lymphocytic to granulomatous but in which many plasma cells are characteristically present (Fig. 38.62); the number of Hofbauer cells tends to be increased.

The spirochaetes may be identified in the placental tissues with a Warthin–Starry stain or by immunofluorescence (Schwartz et al 1994) but demonstration of spirochaetal DNA with the polymerase chain reaction is probably now the technique of choice (Genest et al 1996).

Listeriosis

This organism may reach the placenta by either the ascending or the haematogenous route; indeed in most cases it is not possible to determine which of these routes has been involved for there are usually both lesions in the villous parenchyma and a chorioamnionitis (Lallemand

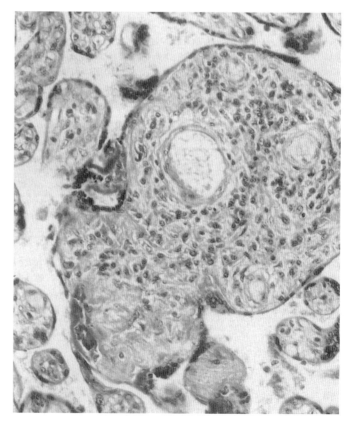

Fig. 38.62 Congenital syphilis. There is a focal villitis showing an almost pure plasma cell infiltrate with only occasional lymphocytes.

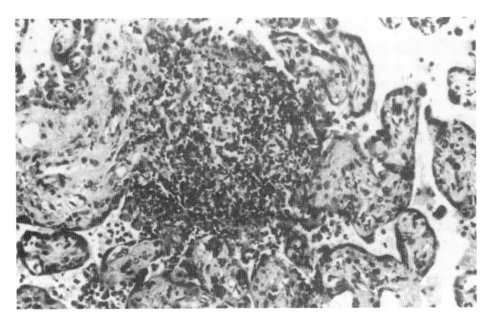

Fig. 38.63 A microabscess in a case of placental listeriosis; this consists of necrotic debris and polymorphonuclear leucocytes.

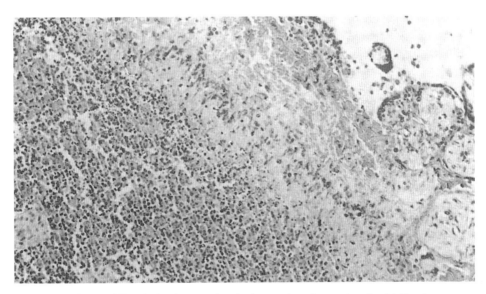

Fig. 38.64 Placental listeriosis. The margin of a large microabscess showing histiocytes palisaded around polymorphonuclear leucocytes.

et al 1992; Gersell 1993). Infected placentas may be somewhat bulky but most are of normal size. There are usually seen within the parenchyma or on the placental surface minute or small scattered whitish-yellow lesions which, histologically, are microabscesses consisting of foci of necrosis in which many polymorphonuclear leucocytes and organisms are present (Fig. 38.63); at the margin of the larger of these foci (Fig. 38.64) there is often a rim of palisaded histiocytic cells; much larger macroabscesses may also be present (Topalovski et al 1993). Villi can be caught up and enmeshed in intervillous fibrin and inflammatory debris, whilst large masses of necrotic villi may be present, these often appearing to be contiguous with an inflamed and necrotic septum. In addition to these gross lesions, a focal villitis may also be present, in which, characteristically, localised collections of polymorphonuclear leucocytes are seen between the trophoblast and the villous stroma.

Rubella

The findings in rubella infection of the placenta have been described by, inter alia, Garcia et al (1985); Kaplan (1990, 1993a,b); Horn & Becker (1992) and Horn et al (1993). In the acute stage of the infection there is a focal necrotising villitis (Fig. 38.65) and a necrotising endarteritis of the fetal villous vessels. The villitis is very variable: some involved villi show only focal necrosis of the trophoblast, whilst in others the trophoblast is totally necrotic with perivillous deposition of fibrin and poly-morphs; small groups of villi are sometimes agglutinated by fibrin. The villous stroma can be hypercellular or oede-matous and often contains prominent Hofbauer cells, in the cytoplasm of which eosinophilic granules may be seen. The villous fetal vessels show, very characteristically, endothelial necrosis, whilst fragmented erythrocytes may be present in their lumina; there is sometimes also a well-marked perivasculitis. Eosinophilic inclusion bodies may be seen in the endothelial cells or, less frequently, in the villous trophoblast.

In placentas obtained after the acute stage of the disease has passed there may be only scattered, avascular, shrunken fibrotic villi (Fig. 38.66), but in some both active and healed lesions are present simultaneously, which suggests continuing and progressive villous damage.

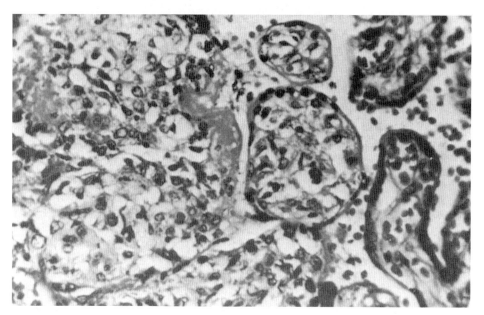

Fig. 38.65 Placenta from a woman with rubella. There is a focal necrotising villitis involving the villi in the left of the field.

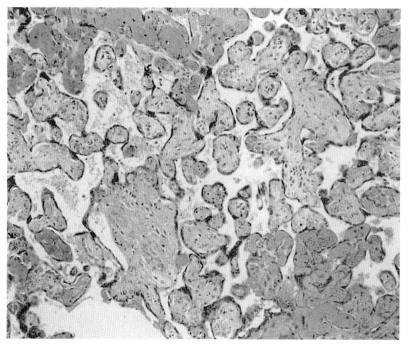

Fig. 38.66 Placenta from a women with rubella. Villous inflammation has subsided leaving scarred avasular villi.

A not inconsiderable proportion of placentas from which rubella virus is isolated do not show any inflammatory lesions or morphological abnormality.

Parvovirus B 19 infection

Parvovirus B 19 infection is an important cause of fetal hydrops and death (Abdel-Fattah & Soothil 2001). Placentas infected by this virus tend to be large and may be oedematous; histologically, the placental infection is characterised by the presence, within the fetal vessels, of a markedly increased number of nucleated red blood cells, some of which contain intranuclear inclusions consisting of a central clear or eosinophilic area with peripheral chromatin condensation (Kaplan 1993a,b,c); the diagnostic nuclear inclusions are not always found in the placenta, being present in only two of five placentas from fatal cases of fetal parvovirus infection studied by Rogers et al (1993). Patchy villous immaturity and oedema is common and although Kaplan (1993a) maintained that a villitis is not seen in this infection Morey et al (1992) noted that a vasculitis, affecting villous capillaries and occasionally stem arteries, is a common finding and is associated with a perivascular round cell inflammatory infiltrate.

Cytomegalovirus infection

The placental changes induced by this virus have been documented quite extensively (Altshuler & McAdams 1971; Benirschke et al 1974; Mostoufi-Zadeh et al 1984; Garcia et al 1989). Grossly, the infected placenta is often unremarkable but is sometimes bulky and oedematous, whilst histologically there is characteristically a low-grade focal or diffuse lymphoplasmacytic villitis. The villi show, however, a spectrum of histological changes, ranging from, in the early stages, a focal necrotising and proliferative villitis, sometimes with granulomatous features (Kaplan 1993a), to, in the later stages, atrophy and fibrosis. The brunt of the inflammatory damage is borne by the villous stroma rather than by the trophoblast, and whilst there is usually an infiltration of lymphocytes into the stroma it is not uncommon to also find plasma cells, these often being most numerous in the immediately perivascular areas; the lymphocytes appear to be all T cells whilst the plasma cells may be IgM- or IgG-secreting (Schwartz et al 1992). An increased number of Hofbauer cells may be present. Focal or generalised villous oedema is sometimes seen, and thrombosis of fetal vessels may occur. Deposition of haemosiderin pigment in the villi is often a particularly striking feature. Cytomegalovirus inclusion bodies can often be found in the infected placenta (Fig. 38.67) though they are usually few in number and are sometimes only detected after a prolonged search; they are usually seen in the endothelial cells of the fetal vessels but may occasionally be located in the stromal cells or in the trophoblast.

In many cases of documented intrauterine fetal cytomegalovirus infection the placenta appears normal on histological examination (Muhlemann et al 1994) and it is known that cytomegalovirus can be isolated from such placentas (Davis et al 1971; Hayes & Gibas 1971); furthermore, a villitis which is evoked by cytomegalovirus infection may show no specific features and can masquerade as a villitis of unknown aetiology. It is in cases such as these that immunoflourescence (Garcia et al 1989) immunocytochemistry (Muhlemann et al 1994; Sinzger et al 1993), in situ hybridisation (Sachdev et al 1990) and the polymerase chain reaction (Nakamura et al 1994) have proven to be of great value in demonstrating the presence of the virus in placental tissue.

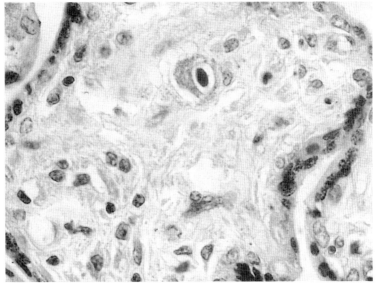

Fig. 38.67 Cytomegalovirus infection of the placenta. A typical cytomegalic cell with an intra-nuclear inclusion is seen in a villus.

Human immunodeficiency virus infection

Vertical materno-fetal transmission of human immunodeficiency virus occurs, in different settings, in between 14 and 48% of pregnancies in seropositive mothers and in at least some of these cases the transmission occurs before the onset of labour, presumably by a transplacental route (McIntyre 2001). The virus has been identified within placental tissue by electronmicroscopy (Jauniaux et al 1988b), immunocytochemistry (Mattern et al 1992; Backe et al 1994), in situ hybridisation (Backe et al 1992; Anderson et al 1994), polymerase chain reaction and in situ polymerase chain reaction (Zevallos et al 1994) and has been detected most frequently in the Hofbauer cells and less commonly in the trophoblast and fetal endothelial cells.

Placentas from women who are seropositive for human immunodeficiency virus usually appear macroscopically normal though in a few studies the placentas have been unduly heavy (Caretti et al 1988; Jauniaux et al 1988b). Chorioamnionitis is unusually common (Jauniaux et al 1988b; Chandwani et al 1991, 1992) but this is almost certainly because of a secondary opportunistic infection. Histologically there has been a widespread consensus that a villitis is not seen and that no specific abnormalities are present (Jauniaux et al 1988; Chandwani et al 1991, 1992; Schwartz et al 1992; Backe et al 1994).

Toxoplasmosis

Placentas infected by *Toxoplasma gondii* are often macroscopically normal, but a proportion are large, bulky and pale. Histologically there is a low-grade smouldering chronic villitis which may involve single villi or groups of villi (Fig. 38.68); these show a mononuclear cell infiltration (predominantly lymphocytic but sometimes with a sprinkling of plasma cells), fibrosis, an excessive number of Hofbauer cells and, sometimes, necrosis (Elliot 1970; Garcia et al 1983). Occasionally a granulomatous type of lesion may be seen in the villi (Elliott 1970; Popek 1992), whilst the fetal vessels often show an endarteritis. The intervillous space may contain nodular masses of histiocytes. Encysted and free forms of *Toxoplasma* may be seen, usually the former, and commonly in the chorionic plate or amnion rather than in the villi; the cysts are morphologically characteristic but can, if necessary, be specifically identified by a fluorescent antibody technique (Foulon 1990). The polymerase chain reaction is of considerable value for the recognition of toxoplasmosis if the diagnostic cysts are not present (Savva & Holliman 1990). In the hydropic form of placental toxoplasmosis the villi are oedematous, hypercellular and contain many Hofbauer cells: the resemblance to the placenta of severe materno-fetal rhesus incompatibility may be further accentuated by the presence, because of fetal anaemia, of numerous nucleated red blood cells in the fetal vessels. The focal chronic villitis and the presence of encysted forms of the parasite allow for the differentiation of this form of placentitis from the placental changes of rhesus incompatibility.

Placentas have been described which contained numerous encysted forms of *Toxoplasma* but which did not show any morphological abnormality or evidence of inflammation (Werner et al 1963).

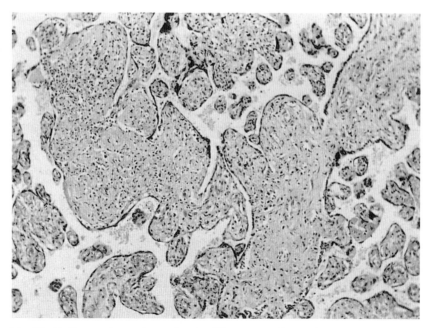

Fig. 38.68 Placental toxoplasmosis. The villi are somewhat oedematous and there is a mononuclear cell villous inflammatory infiltrate.

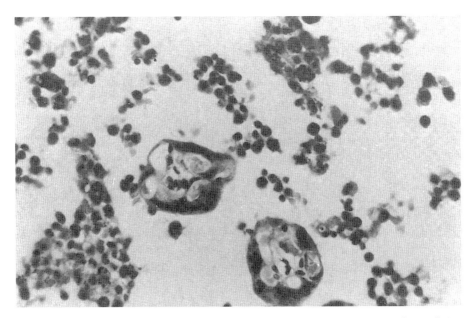

Fig. 38.69 Placental malaria. There are large aggregates of maternal mononuclear cells in the intervillous space.

Malaria

Malaria in pregnancy is consistently associated with a significant reduction in birth weight ((Shulman et al 2001) and malarial infection of the placenta is common in areas in which this disease is endemic. On histological examination (Galbraith et al 1980; Yamada et al 1989; Bulmer et al 1993a,b; Ordi et al 1998; Ismail et al 2000) parasites can often be seen in maternal red blood cells in the intervillous space and a variable amount of dark brown, coarse, granular malarial pigment is present. Much of the pigment appears within maternal monocytes in the intervillous space but it is sometimes apparent within villous Hofbauer cells: in some cases free pigment is present within the villous syncytiotrophoblast and this is associated with focal syncytial necrosis. The pigment-bearing monocytes can form large aggregates within the intervillous space (Fig. 38.69) and these, together with parasitised erythrocytes, may be bound by intervillous fibrin to form an inflammatory-like mass. Within the villous tissue there may be some thickening of the trophoblastic basement membrane, an undue prominence of the villous

cytotrophoblastic cells and an excess number of villi showing a variable degree of fibrinoid necrosis. It is noteworthy that parasitised maternal erythrocytes appear to be sequestrated in the intervillous space possibly because certain strains of the parasite have an ability to adhere to chondroitin sulphate A on the surface of the syncytiotrophoblast (Fried & Duffy 1996) and such strains are frequently found infecting pregnant women (Maubert et al 1997); a further factor contributing to the accumulation of mononuclear cells in the intervillous space is that these cells conspicuously express intercellular adhesion molecule 1 (Sugiyama et al 2001). It seems quite possible that the accumulation, sometimes massive, of mononuclear cells in the intervillous space could impair maternal blood flow to the placenta and thus inhibit fetal growth: in support of this view there does appear to be a correlation between the presence of these cells in large numbers and low birth weight (Ordi et al 1998; Rogerson & Beeson 1999) and there is some evidence, derived from Doppler studies, that materno-fetal blood flow is reduced in active cases of malaria (Arbeille et al 1998; Shulman et al 2001).

REFERENCES

Abdel-Fattah S A, Soothill P W 2001 Parvovirus B19 infection in pregnancy. In: MacLean A B, Regan L, Carrington D (eds) Infection and pregnancy. RCOG Press, London, pp 271–282

Agboola A 1975 Placental changes in patients with a low haematocrit. British Journal of Obstetrics and Gynaecology 82: 225–227

Althabe O, Labarrere C 1985 Chronic villitis of unknown aetiology and intrauterine growth retarded infants of normal and low ponderal index. Placenta 6: 265–276

Althabe O, Labarrere C, Telenta M 1985 Maternal vascular lesions in placentae of small-for-gestational age infants. Placenta 6: 369–373

Altshuler G 1984 Chorangiosis: an important placental sign of neonatal morbidity and mortality. Archives of Pathology and Laboratory Medicine 108: 71–74

Altshuler G 1993 A conceptual approach to placental pathology and pregnancy outcome. Seminars in Diagnostic Pathology 10: 204–221

Altshuler G, Hyde S 1989 Meconium-induced vasoconstricton: a potential cause of cerebral and other fetal hypoperfusion and of poor pregnancy outcome. Journal of Childhood Neurology 4: 137–142

Altshuler G, McAdams A J 1971 Cytomegalic inclusion disease of a nineteen-week fetus: case report including a study of the placenta. American Journal of Obstetrics and Gynecology 111: 295–298

Altshuler G Russell P 1975 The human placental villitides: a review of chronic intrauterine infection. Current Topics in Pathology 60: 64–112

Altshuler G, Arizawa M, Molnar-Nadasty G 1992 Meconium-induced umbilical cord necrosis and ulceration: a potential link between the placenta and poor pregnancy outcome. Obstetrics and Gynecology 79: 760–766

Alvarez H, Sala M A, Benedetti W L 1972 Intervillous space reduction in the edematous placenta. American Journal of Obstetrics and Gynecology 112: 819–820

Amalados A S, Burton G J 1985 Organ culture of human placental villi in hypoxic and hyperoxic conditions: a morphometric study. Journal of Developmental Pathology 7: 113–118

Anderson V M, Zevallos E, Gu J 1994 The HIV-exposed placenta: morphologic observations and interpretation. Trophoblast Research 8: 47–65

Andres R L, Kuyper W, Resnik R, Piacquadio R M, Benirschke K 1990 The association of maternal floor infarction of the placenta with adverse perinatal outcome. American Journal of Obstetrics and Gynecology 163: 935–938

Arbeille P, Carles G, Bousquet F, Body G, Lansac J 1998 Fetal cerebral and umbilical artery blood flow changes during pregnancy complicated by malaria. Journal of Ultrasound Medicine 17: 223–229

Arias F, Rodriquez L, Rayne S C, Kraus F T 1993 Maternal placental vasculopathy and infection: two distinct subgroups among patients with preterm labor and preterm ruptured membranes. American Journal of Obstetrics and Gynecology 168: 585–591

Armer T L, Duff P 1991 Intraamniotic infection with intact membranes and preterm labor. Obstetrical and Gynecological Survey 46: 598–593

Arnholdt H, Meisel F, Fandrey K, Lohrs U 1991 Proliferation of villous trophoblast of the human placenta in normal and abnormal pregnancies. Virchows Archiv B Cellular Pathology 60: 365–372

Backe E, Jiminez E, Unger M, Schafer A, Jauniaux E, Vogel M 1992 Demonstration of HIV-1 infected cells in human placenta by *in situ* hybridization and immunostaining. Journal of Clinical Pathology 45: 871–874

Backe E, Jiminez E, Unger M et al 1994 Vertical human immunodeficiency virus transmission: a study of placental pathology in relation to maternal risk factors. American Journal of Perinatology 11: 326–330

Baker P N 2000 The maternal effects of abnormal placentation. In: Kindom J C P, Jauniaux E R M, O'Brien P M S (eds) The placenta: basic science and clinical practice. RCOG Press, London, pp 97–108

Barker G, Boyd R D H, D'Souza S W et al 1994 Placental water content and distribution. Placenta 15: 47–56

Barson A J, Donnai P, Ferguson A, Donnai D, Reed A P 1980 Haemangioma of the cord: further cause of raised alphafetoprotein. British Medical Journal 281: 1252

Batcup G, Tovey L A D, Longster G 1983 Feto-maternal blood group incompatibility studies in placental intervillous thrombosis. Placenta 4: 449–453

Beecroft D M C, Farmer K, Mason G H, Morris M C, Stewart J H 1976 Perinatal infection by group B-haemolyic streptococci. British Journal of Obstetrics and Gynaecology 83: 960–966

Beischer N A, Sivasamboo R, Vohra S, Silpisornkosal S, Reid S 1970 Placental hypertrophy in severe pregnancy anaemia. Journal of Obstetrics and Gynaecology of the British Commonwealth 77: 398–409

Bell S C 2000 Mechanisms underlying premature rupture of the fetal membranes. In: Kingdom J C P, Jauniaux E R M, O'Brien P M S (eds) The placenta: basic science and clinical practice. RCOG Press, London, pp 187–203

Bendon R W, Tyson R W, Baldwin V J et al 1991 Umbilical cord ulceration and intestinal atresia: a new association? American Journal of Obstetrics and Gynecology 164: 582–586

Benirschke K 1994 Obstetrically important lesions of the umbilical cord. Journal of Reproductive Medicine 39: 262–272

Benirschke K, Kaufmann P 2000 Pathology of the human placenta, 4th edn. Springer-Verlag, New York

Benirschke K, Mendoza G R, Bazeley P L 1974 Placental and fetal manifestations of cytomegalovirus infection. Virchows Archiv Abteilung B Zell Pathologie 16: 121–139

Berg T G, Rayburn W E 1995 Umbilical cord length and acid-base balance at delivery. Journal of Reproductive Medicine 40: 9–12

Bewley S, Cooper D, Campbell S 1991 Doppler investigation of uteroplacental blood flow resistance in the second trimester: a screening study for pre-eclampsia and intrauterine growth retardation. British Journal of Obstetrics and Gynaecology 98: 871–879

Bilardo C M, Snijders R N, Campbell S, Nicolaides K 1991 Doppler study of the fetal circulation during long-term maternal hyper-oxygenation for severe early onset intrauterine growth retardation. Ultrasound in Obstetrics and Gynecology 1: 250–257

Blanc W A, Allan G W 1961 Intrafunicular ulceration of persistent omphalomesenteric duct with intra-amniotic hemorrhage and fetal death. American Journal of Obstetrics and Gynecology 82: 1392–1396

Bourke W G, Clarke T A, Mathews T G, O'Halpin D, Donoghue V B 1993 Isolated single umbilical artery — the case for routine renal screening. Archives of Disease in Childhood 68: 600–601

Bracero L A, Beneck D, Kirshenbaum N et al 1989 Doppler velocimetry and placental disease. American Journal of Obstetrics and Gynecology 161: 388–393

Brown H L, Miller J M, Khawli D, Gabert H A 1988 Premature placental calcification in maternal cigarette smokers. Obstetrics and Gynecology 71: 914–917

Browne J C Mc C, Veall N 1953 The maternal placental blood flow in normotensive and hypertensive women. Journal of Obstetrics and Gynaecology of the British Empire 60: 141–147

Bruhwiler H, Rabner M, Luscher K P 1994 Pranatale Diagnose eines Nabelschnur-Hamangioms bei Alphafetoprotein. Ultraschall in der Medizin 15: 140–142

Bryan E M, Kohler H G 1974 The missing umbilical artery. I. Prospective study based on a maternity hospital. Archives of Disease in Childhood 50: 714–718

Bulmer J N, Rasheed F N, Francis N, Morrison L, Greenwood B M 1993a Placental malaria. I. Pathological classification. Histopathology 22: 211–218

Bulmer J N, Rasheed F N, Morrison L, Francis N, Greenwood B M 1993b Placental malaria. II. A semi-quantitative investigation of the pathological features. Histopathology 22: 219–225

Burton G J 1986 Intervillous connections in the mature human placenta: instances of syncytial fusion or section artefacts? Journal of Anatomy 145: 13–23

Burton G J 1997 Invited commentary on 'oxygen and placental villous development: origins of fetal hypoxia'. Placenta 18: 625–626

Burton G J, Mayhew T M, Robertson L A 1989 Stereological re-examination of the effects of varying oxygen tensions on human placental villi maintained in organ culture for up to 12 h. Placenta 10: 263–273

Burton G J, Reshetnikova O S, Milaovanov A P, Teleshova O V 1996 Stereologic evaluation of vascular adaptions in human placental villi to differing forms of hypoxic stress. Placenta 17: 49–55

Campbell S, Griffin D R, Pearce J M et al 1983 New Doppler technique for assessing uteroplacental blood flow. Lancet 1: 675–677

Campbell S, Pearce J M, Hackett G et al 1986 Qualitative assessment of uteroplacental blood flow: early screening test for high-risk pregnancies. Obstetrics and Gynecology 68: 649–653

Cantle S J, Kaufmann P, Luckhardt M, Schweikhart G 1987 Interpretation of syncytial sprouts and bridges in the human placenta. Placenta 8: 221–234

Caretti N, Bertolin A, Dalla Pria S 1988 Placental alterations and fetal conditions in relation to the presence of anti-human immunodeficiency virus (HIV) in pregnant mothers. Panminerva Medica 30: 77–80

Cefalo R C, Simkovich K W, Abel F, Hellegers A E, Chez R A 1977 Effect of potential surface area reduction on fetal growth. American Journal of Obstetrics and Gynecology 129: 434–439

Chandwani S, Greco M A, Mittal K, Antoine C, Krasinski K, Borkowsky W 1991 Pathology of human immunodeficiency virus expression in placentas of seropositive women. Journal of Infectious Diseases 163: 1134–1138

Chandwani S, Greco M A, Krasinski K, Borkowsky W 1992 Pathology of the placenta in HIV-11 infection. Progress in AIDS Pathology 3: 65–81

Chatfield W R, Rogers T G H, Brownlee B E W, Rippon P E 1975 Placental scanning with computer-linked gamma camera to detect impaired placental blood flow and intrauterine growth retardation. British Medical Journal 2: 120–122

Chellam V G, Rushton D I 1985 Chorioamnionitis and funiculitis in the placentas of 200 births weighing less than 2.5 kg. British Journal of Obstetrics and Gynaecology 92: 808–814

Clapp J F 1994 Physiological adaptation to intrauterine growth retardation. In: Ward R H T, Smith S K, Donnai D (eds) Early fetal growth and development. RCOG Press, London, pp 275–281

Clavero-Nunez J A 1963 La placenta de las cardiacas. Revista Espanola de Obstetricia y Ginecologia 22: 129–134

Clewell W H, Manchester D K 1983 Recurrent maternal floor infarction: a preventable cause of fetal death. American Journal of Obstetrics and Gynecology 147: 346–347

Cook V, Weeks J, Brown J, Bendon R 1995 Umbilical artery obstruction and fetoplacental thromboembolism. Obstetrics and Gynecology 85: 870–872

Cordero D R, Helfgott A W, Landy H J et al 1993 A non-hemorrhagic manifestation of vasa previa: a clinicopathological case report. Obstetrics and Gynecology 82: 698–700

Craver R D, Baldwin V J 1992 Necrotizing funisitis. Obstetrics and Gynecology 79: 64–70

Davies J, Glasser S R 1967 Light and electron microscopic observations on a human placenta 2 weeks after fetal death. American Journal of Obstetrics and Gynecology 98: 1111–1124

Davis L E, Tweed G V, Steward J A et al 1971 Cytomegalovirus mononucleosis in a first trimester pregnant female with transmission to the fetus. Pediatrics 48: 200–206

de Rochembeau B, Poix D, Mellier G 1992 Maternal hyperoxygenation: a fetal blood flow velocity prognosis test in small-for-gestational-age fetuses. Ultrasound in Obstetrics and Gynecology 2: 279–282

deSa O J 1971 Rupture of foetal vessels on placental surface. Archives of Disease in Childhood 46: 495–501

De Wolf F, Carreras L O, Moerman P et al 1982 Decidual vasculopathy and extensive placental infarction in a patient with repeated thromboembolic accidents, recurrent fetal loss, and a lupus anticoagulant. American Journal of Obstetrics and Gynecology 142: 834–929

Dommisse J, Tiltman A J 1992 Placental bed biopsies in placental abruption. British Journal of Obstetrics and Gynaecology 99: 651–654

Donders C G G, Moerman P, de-Wet G H, Hooft P, Goubau P 1991 The association between Chlamydia cervicitis, chorioamnionitis and neonatal complications. Archives of Gynecology and Obstetrics 249: 79–85

Dong Y, St Clair P G, Ramzy I, Kagan-Hallets, Gibbs R S 1987 A morphologic and clinical study of placental inflammation at term. Obstetrics and Gynecology 70: 175–186

Edwards A D, Duggan P J 2000 Placental inflammation and brain injury in preterm infants. In: Kingdom J C P, Jauniaux E R M, O'Brien P M S (eds) The placenta: basic science and clinical practice. RCOG Press, London, pp 204–208

Elliot W G 1970 Placental toxoplasmosis. American Journal of Clinical Pathology 53: 413–417

Embree J E, Krause V W, Embil J A, Macdonald S 1980 Placental infection with mycoplasma hominis and Ureaplasma urealyticum: a clinical correlation. Obstetrics and Gynecology 56: 475–481

Emmrich P 1966a Untersuchungen au Placenten mazerierter Totgeburten im Hinblick auf die mogliche Ursache des intrauterinen Fruchttodes. Zeitschrift fur Geburtshilfe und Gynakologie 165: 185–194

Emmrich P 1966b Morphologie und Histochemie der Placenta bei intrauterinen Fruchttod mit Mazeration. Gyaecologia 162: 241–253

Emmrich P 1992 Pathologie der Plazenta. IX. Intrauteriner Fruchttod. Regression, Odem und Fibrosierung. Zentralblat fur Pathologie 138: 1–8

Erhardt L 1956 Seltene Spontanamputation durch Amnionstrang. Zentralblatt fur Gynakologie 78: 1509–1513

Eschenbach D A 1993 Ureaplasma urealyticum and premature bith. Clinical Infectious Diseases Supplement 1, S100–S106

Espinoza J, Sebira N J, McAuliffe F, Krampl E, Nicolaides K H 2001 Placental villus morphology in relation to maternal hypoxia at high altitude. Placenta 22: 606–608

Fojaco R M, Hensley G T, Moskowitz L 1989 Congenital syphilis and necrotizing funisitis. Journal of the American Medical Association 261: 1788–1790

Fok R Y, Pavlova Z, Benirschke K et al 1990 The correlation of arterial lesions with umbilical artery Doppler velocimetry in the placentae of small-for-dates pregnancies. Obstetrics and Gynecology 75: 578–583

Foulon W, Naessens A, de Catto L, Amy J-J 1990 Detection of congenital toxoplasmosis by chorionic villus sampling and early amniocentesis. American Journal of Obstetrics and Gynecology 163: 1511–1513

Fox H 1968 Morphological changes in the human placenta following fetal death. Journal of Obstetrics and Gynaecology of the British Commonwealth 75: 839–843

Fox H 1970 Effect of hypoxia on trophoblast in organ culture: a morphologic and autoradiographic study. American Journal of Obstetrics and Gynecology 107: 1058–1064

Fox H 1988 The placenta in pregnancy hypertension. In: Rubin P C (ed) Handbook of hypertension, vol 10, Hypertension in pregnancy. Elsevier, Amsterdam, pp 16–37

Fox H 1993 The placenta and infection. In: Redman C W G, Sargent I L, Starkey P M (eds) The human placenta. Blackwells, Oxford, pp 313–333

Fox H 1994 The placenta in intrauterine growth retardation. In: Ward R H T, Smith S K, Donnai D (eds) Early fetal growth and development. RCOG Press, London, pp 223–235

Fox H 1997a Pathology of the placenta, 2nd edn. W B Saunders, London

Fox H 1997b Aging of the placenta. Archives of Disease in Childhood 77: 165–170

Fox H 2000 Placental pathology. In: Kingdom J, Baker P (eds) Intrauterine growth restriction: aetiology and management. Springer-Verlag, London, pp 187–201

Fox H 2001 The effects of viruses on the placenta. In: Infection in pregnancy. RCOG Press, London, pp 195–206

Fox H, Jones C J P 1983 Pathology of trophoblast. In: Loke Y W, Whyte A (eds) Biology of trophoblast. Elsevier, Amsterdam, pp 137–185

Fox H, Langley F A 1971 Leucocytic infiltration of the placenta and umbilical cord: a clinicopathologic study. Obstetrics and Gynecology 37: 451–458

Fried M, Duffy P E 1996 Adherence of plasmodia falciparum to chondroitin sulphate A in the human placenta. Science 272: 1502–1504

Frusca T, Morassi L, Pecorelli S et al 1989 Histological features of uteroplacental vessels in normal and hypertensive patients in relation to birthweight. British Journal of Obstetrics and Gynaecology 96: 835–839

Galbraith R M, Fox H, Hsi B, Galbraith G M P, Bray R S, Faulk W P 1980 The human materno-fetal relationship in malaria. II. Histological, ultrastructural and immunopathological studies of the placenta. Transactions of the Royal Society of Tropical Medicine and Hygiene 74: 61–72

Garcia A G P 1982 Placental morphology of low-birth-weight infants born at term: gross and microscopic study of 50 cases. Contributions to Gynecology and Obstetrics 9: 100–112

Garcia A G P, Coutinho S G, Amendoeira M R, Assumpacao M R, Albano M 1983 Placental morphology of newborns at risk for congenital toxoplasmosis. Journal of Tropical Pediatrics 29: 95–103

Garcia A G P Marques R L S, Lobato Y Y, Fonseca M E F, Wigg M D 1985 Placental pathology in congenital rubella. Placenta 6: 281–295

Garcia A G P, Fonseca M E F, Marques R L S, Lobato Y Y 1989 Placental morphology in cytomegalovirus infection. Placenta: 10: 1–19

Genest D R 1992 Estimating the time of death in stillborn fetuses. II. Histologic evaluation of the placenta: a study of 71 stillborns. Obstetrics and Gynecology 80: 585–592

Genest D R, Choi-Hong S R, Tate J E et al 1996 Diagnosis of congenital syphilis from placental examination: comparison of histopathology, Steiner stain, and polymerase chain reaction for Treponoma pallidum DNA. Human Pathology 27: 366–373

Gersell D J 1993 Chronic viritis, chronic chorioamnionitis and maternal floor infarction. Seminars in Diagnostic Pathology 10: 251–266

Gibbs R S 1993 Chorioanionitis and bacterial vaginosis. American Journal of Obstetrics and Gynecology 169: 460–462

Gibbs R S, Blanco J D, St Clair P J, Castaneda Y S 1982 Quantitative bacteriology of amniotic fluid from women with intra-amniotic infection at term. Journal of Infectious Diseases 145: 1–8

Gibbs S R, Weiner M H, Walmer K, St Clair P 1987 Microbiologic and serologic studies of Gardnerella vaginalis in intra-amniotic infection. Obstetrics and Gynecology 70: 187–190

Gibbs S R, Romero R, Hillier S L, Eschenbach D A, Sweet R L 1992 A review of premature birth and and subclinical infection. American Journal of Obstetrics and Gynecology 166: 1515–1528

Giles W B, Trudinger B J, Baird P J 1985 Fetal umbilical flow velocity wavelengths and placental resistance: pathologic correlation. British Journal of Obstetrics and Gynaecology 92: 31–38

Gill R W, Warren P S, Garrett W J, Kossoff G, Stewart A 1993 Umbilical vein blood flow. In: Chervenak F A Isaacson G C, Campbell S (eds) Ultrasound in obstetrics and gynecology. Little Brown, Boston, pp 587–595

Godfrey K M, Redman C W, Barker D J, Osmond C 1991 The effect of maternal anaemia and iron deficiency on the ratio of fetal weight to placental weight. British Journal of Obstetrics and Gynaecology 98: 886–891

Greenberg J A, Sorem K A, Shifren J L, Riley L E 1991 Placenta membranacea with placenta increta: a case report and literature review. Obstetrics and Gynecology 78: 512–514

Gudmundsson S, Marsal K 1998 Umbilical and uteroplacental blood flow velocity waveforms in pregnancies with fetal growth retardation. European Journal of Obstetrics, Gynecology and Reproductive Biology 27: 187–196

Gupta I, Hillier V F, Edwards J M 1993 Vascular branching in the umbilical cord: an indication of maternal smoking habits and intrauterine distress. Placenta 14: 117–123

Guvenc M, Guvenc H, Cengiz L, Cengiz T, Uslu T 1989 Subclinical amnionitis in patients with intact membranes in preterm labour. Paediatrics and Perinatal Epidemiology 3: 367–374

Guzick D S, Winn K 1985 The association of chorioamnionitis with preterm delivery. Obstetrics and Gynecology 65: 11–16

Harris B A 1988 Peripheral placental seperation: a review. Obstetrical and Gynecological Survey 43: 577–581

Hata K, Hata T, Aoki T et al 1988 Succenturiate placenta diagnosed by ultrasound. Gynecological and Obstetrical Investigation 25: 273–276

Hayes K, Gibas H 1971 Placental cytomegalovirus infection without fetal involvement following primary infection in pregnancy. Journal of Pediatrics 79: 401–405

Heifetz S A 1984 Single umbilical artery: a statistical analysis of 237 autopsy cases and review of the literature. Perspectives in Pediatric Pathology 8: 345–378

Heifetz F A 1988 Thrombosis of the umbilical cord: analysis of 52 cases and literature review. Pediatric Pathology 8: 37–54

Heifetz S A 1999 Pathology of the umbilical cord. In: Lewis S L, Perrin E (eds) Pathology of the placenta, 2nd edn. Churchill Livingstone, New York, pp 107–135

Heifetz S A, Bauman M 1994 Necrotizing funisitis and herpes simplex infection of placental and decidual tissues: study of four cases. Human Pathology 25: 715–722

Hillier S L, Martius J, Krohn M A, Kiviat N B, Holmes K K, Eschenbach D A 1988 A case control study of of chorioamnionic-infection and histologic chorioamnionitis in pregnancy. New England Journal of Medicine 319: 972–978

Hillier S L, Krohn M A, Kiviat N B, Watts D H, Eschenbach D A 1991 Microbiologic causes and neonatal outcomes associated with chorioamnion infection. American Journal of Obstetrics and Gynecology 165: 955–961

Hillier S L, Witkin S S, Krohn M A, Kiviat N B, Eschenbach D A 1993 The relationship of amniotic fluid cytokines and preterm delivery, amniotic fluid infection, histologic chorioamnionitis, and chorioamnion infection. Obstetrics and Gynecoogy 81: 941–948

Hitschold T, Weiss E, Beck T et al 1993 Low target birth weight or growth retardation? Umbilical Doppler flow velocity waveforms and histometric analysis of fetoplacental vascular tree. American Journal of Obstetrics and Gynecology 168: 1260–1264

Horn L C, Becker V 1992 Morphologische Plazentabefunde bei klinisch-serologisch gesichterter und vermuteter Rotelninfektion in der zweiten Schwangerschaftshalfte. Zeitschrift fur Geburtshilfe und Perinatologie 196: 199–204

Horn L C Emmrich P, Krugmann J 1992 Plazentabefunde bei Lues connata. Pathologe 13: 146–151

Horn L C, Buttner W, Horn E 1993 Rotelnbedingte Plazentaveranderungen. Perinatale Medizin 5: 5–10

Houlihan C M, Knuppel R A 1994 Meconium-stained amniotic fluid: current controversies. Journal of Reproductive Medicine 39: 888–898

Hovatta O, Lipasti A, Rapola J, Karjalainen O 1983 Causes of stillbirth: a clinicopathological study of 243 patients. British Journal of Obstetrics and Gynaecology 90: 691–696

Howard R B, Hosokawa T, Maguire M H 1987 Hypoxia-induced fetoplacental vasoconstriction in perfused human placental cotyledons. American Journal of Obstetrics and Gynecology 157: 1261–1266

Huppertz B, Kaufmann P 1999 The apoptosis cascade in human villous trophoblast: a review. Trophoblast Research 13: 215–242

Huppertz B, Frank H G, Kingdom J C P, Reister F, Kaufmann 1998 Villous cytotrophoblast regulation of the syncytial apoptotic cascade in the human placenta. Histochemistry and Cell Biology 110: 495–508

Hurley V A, Beischer N A 1987 Placenta membranacea: case report. British Journal of Obstetrics and Gynaecology 94: 798–802

Hustin J, Gaspard U 1977 Comparison of hidstological changes seen in placental tissue cultures and in placentae obtained after fetal death. British Journal of Obstetrics and Gynecology 84: 210–215

Hyde S R, Altshuler G 1999 Infectious disorders of the placenta In: Lewis S H, Perrin E (eds) Pathology of the placenta, 2nd edn. Churchill Livingstone, New York, pp 317–342

Imber G, Guthrie R H, Goulian D 1974 Congenital band of the abdomen and the amniotic etiology of bands. American Journal of Surgery 127: 753–754

Ismail M A, Pridjian G, Hibbard J U, Harth G, Moawad A A 1992 Significance of positive cervical cultures for Chlamydia trachomatis in patients with preterm premature rupture of the membranes. American Journal of Perinatology 9: 368–370

Ismail M R, Ordi J, Menendez C et al 2000 Placental pathology in malaria: an histological, immunohistochemical and quantitative study. Human Pathology 31: 85–92

Iwata M, Matsuzaki N, Shimizu I, Nakayama M, Suehara N 1993 Prenatal detection of ischemic changes in the placenta of the growth-retarded fetus by Doppler flow velocimetry of the maternal uterine artery. Obstetrics and Gynecology 82: 494–499

Jackson M R, Walsh A J, Morrow R J, Mullen J B, Lye S J, Ritchie J W K 1995 Reduced placental villous tree elaboration in small-for-gestational-age newborn pregnancies: relationship with umbilical artery Doppler waveforms. American Journbal of Obstetrics and Gynecology 172: 518–525

Jacob-Cormier B, Petitjean J, Asselin D, Quibriac M, von Theobald F 1989 Ureaplasma urealyticum et chorioamniotite. Revue Francais de Gynecologie et d'Obstetrique 84: 25–28

Jacobson S L, Imhof R, Manning M et al 1990 The value of Doppler assessment of the uteroplacental circulation in predicting preeclampsia or intrauterine growth retardation. American Journal of Obstetrics and Gynecology 162: 110–114

Jacques S M, Qureshi F 1992 Necrotizing funisitis: a study of 45 cases. Human Pathology 23: 1278–1283

Jauniaux E, Donner C, Thomas C et al 1988a Umbilical cord pseudocyst in trisomy 18. Prenatal Diagnosis 8: 274–275

Jauniaux E, Nessmann C, Imbert M C, Meuris S, Puissant F, Hustin J 1988b Morphological aspects of the placenta in HIV pregnancies. Placenta 8: 633–642

Jauniaux E De Munter C, Vanesse M, Wilkin P, Hustin J 1989 Embryonic remnants of the umbilical cord: morphologic and clinical aspects. Human Pathology 20: 458–462

Jauniaux E, Gidd D, Moscoso G, Campbell S 1990 Ultrasonographic diagnosis of a large placental intervillous thrombosis associated with elevated maternal serum alpha-fetoprotein level. American Journal of Obstetrics and Gynecology 163: 1558–1560

Jones C J P, Fox H 1977 Syncytial knots and intervillous bridges in the human placenta: an ultrastructural study. Journal of Anatomy 124: 275–286

Jones C J P, Fox H 1980 An ultrastructural and ultrahistochemical study of the human placenta in maternal pre-eclampsia. Placenta 1: 61–76

Kalousek D K 1994 Current topic: confined placental mosaicism and intrauterine fetal development. Placenta 15: 219–230

Kalousek D K, Langlois S 1994 The effects of placental and somatic chromosomal mosaicism on fetal growth. In: Ward R H T, Smith S K, Donnai D (eds) Early fetal growth and development. RCOG Press, London, pp 245–256

Kalousek D K, Howard-Peebles P N, Olson P B et al 1991 Confirmation of CVS mosaicism in term placentae and high frequency of intrauterine growth retardation association with confined placental mosaicism. Pre-natal Diagnosis 11: 743–750

Kanayama M D, Gaffey T A, Ogburn P L 1995 Constriction of the umbilical cord by an amniotic band, with fetal compromise illustrated by reverse diastolic flow in the umbilical artery: a case report. Journal of Reproductive Medicine 40: 71–73

Kaplan C 1990 The placenta and viral infections. Clinical Obstetrics and Gynecology 33: 232–241

Kaplan C 1993a The placenta and viral infections. Seminars in Diagnostic Pathology 10: 232–250

Kaplan C 1993b Placental pathology for the nineties. Pathology Annual 28: 15–72

Kaplan C, Blanc W A, Elias J 1982 Identification of erythrocytes in intervillous thrombi: a study using inmunoperoxidase identification of hemoglobins. Human Pathology 13: 554–557

Katz V L 1993 Management of group B stretococcal disease in pregnancy. Clinical Obstetrics and Gynecology 36: 832–842

Katz V L, Bowes W A, Sierkh A E 1987 Maternal floor infarction of the placenta associated with elevated second trimester alpha-fetoprotein. American Journal of Perinatology 4: 225–228

Kaufmann P, Gentzen D M, Davidoff M 1977 Die Ultrastruktur von Langhanszellen in pathologischen menschlichen Plazenten. Archiv fur Gynakologie 222: 319–322

Kaufmann P, Luckhardt M, Schweikhart G, Cantle S J 1987 Cross sectional features and three dimensional structure of the human placental villi. Placenta 8: 235–247

Keeling J W 1993 Fetal and neonatal pathology, 2nd edn. Springer-Verlag, London

Khong T Y 1991 Acute atherosis in pregnancies complicated by hypertension, small-for-gestational-age infants, and diabetes mellitus. Archives of Pathology and Laboratory Medicine 115: 722–725

Khong T Y, Robertson W B 1992 Spiral artery disease. In: Coulam C B,

Faulk W P, McIntyre J A (eds) Immunological obstetrics. Norton, New York, pp 492–501

Khong T Y, De Wolf F, Robertson W B et al 1986 Inadequate maternal vascular response to placentation in pregnancies complicated by pre-eclampsia and by small-for-gestational-age infants. British Journal of Obstetrics and Gynaecology 93: 1049–1059

Khong T Y, Staples A, Moore L, Byard R W 1993 Observer reliability in assessing villitis of unknown aetiology. Journal of Clinical Pathology 46: 208–210

Khong T Y, Ford W D, Haan E A 1994 Umbilical cord ulceration in association with intestinal atresia in a child with deletion 13q and Hirschsprung's disease. Archives of Disease in Childhood 71: 212–213

Khong T Y, Staples A, Bendon R W et al 1995 Observer reliability in assessing placental maturity by histology. Journal of Clinical Pathology 48: 420–423

Kingdom J 1998 Current topic: placental pathology in obstetrics: adaptation or failure of the villous tree. Placenta 19: 347–351

Kingdom J C P, Kaufmann P 1997 Current topic: oxygen and placental villous development: origins of fetal hypoxia. Placenta 18: 613–621

Kingdom J C P, Macara L, Krebs C, Leiser R, Kaufmann P 1997 Pathological basis for abnormal umbilical artery doppler waveforms in pregnancies complicated by intrauterine growth retardation: a review. Trophoblastic Research 10: 291–309

Kliman H, Perrotta P L, Jones D C 1995 The efficacy of placental biopsy. American Journal of Obstetrics and Gynecology 173: 1084–1088

Knowles S, Frost T 1989 Umbilical cord sclerosis as an indicator of congenital syphilis. Journal of Clinical Pathology 42: 1157–1159

Knox W F, Fox H 1984 Villitis of unknown aetiology: its incidence and significance in placentae from a British population. Placenta 5: 395–402

Kohnen G, Kingdom J 2000 Villous development and the pathogenesis of IUGR. In: Kingdom J, Baker P (eds) Intrauterine growth restriction: aetiology and management. Springer, London, pp 131–147

Kovalovszki L, Villanyi E, Banko G 1990 Placental villous edema: a possible cause of antenatal hypoxia. Acta Paediatrica Hungarica 30: 209–215

Kraus F T 1993 Placental thrombi and related problems. Seminars in Diagnostic Pathology 10: 275–283

Krebs C, Macara L, Leiser R, Bowman A W, Greer I A, Kingdom J C P 1996 Intrauterine growth restriction with absent end-diastolic flow velocity in the umbilical artery is associated with maldevelopment of the terminal placental villous tree. American Journal of Obstetrics and Gynecology 175: 1534–1542

Kreczy A, Fusi L, Wigglesworth J S 1995 Correlation between umbilical artery flow and placental morphology. International Journal of Gynecological Pathology 14: 306–309

Kruger H, Arias-Stella J 1970 The placenta and the newborn infant at high altitudes. American Journal of Obstetrics and Gynecology 106: 586–591

Kundsin R B, Driscoll S G, Monson R R, Yeh C, Biano S A, Cochran W D 1984 Association of Ureaplasma urealyticum in the placenta with perinatal morbidity and mortality. New England Journal of Medicine 310: 941–945

Labarrere C A, Althabe O 1987 Chronic villitis of unknown aetiology in recurrent intrauterine fetal growth retardation. Placenta 8: 167–173

Labarrere C A, Althabe O, Telenta M 1982 Chronic villitis of unknown aetiology in placentae of idiopathic small for gestational age infants. Placenta 3: 309–318

Labarrere C A, McIntyre J A, Faulk W P 1990 Immunohistologic evidence that villitis in human normal term placentas is an immunologic lesion. American Journal of Obstetrics and Gynecology 162: 515–522

Lademacher D S, Vermeulen R C W, Harten J J, Arts N F T 1981 Circumvallate placenta and congenital malformation. Lancet i: 732

Lallemand A V, Gaillard D A, Paradis P H, Chippaux C G 1992 Fetal listeriosis during the second trimester of gestation. Pediatric Pathology 12: 665–671

Langston C, Kaplan C, MacPherson T et al 1997 Practice guide-lines for examination of the placenta. Developed by the placental pathology practice guideline development task force of the College of American Pathologists. Archives of Pathology and Laboratory Medicine 121: 449–476

Las Heras J, Haust M D, Harding P G 1983 Morphology of fetal placental stem arteries in hypertensive disorders ('toxaemia') of pregnancy. Applied Pathology 1: 301–309

Las Heras J, Baskerville J C, Harding P G, Haust M D 1985 Morphometric studies of fetal placental stem arteries in hypertensive disorders ('toxaemia') of pregnancy. Placenta 6: 217–227

Lemtis H, Hadrich G 1974 Uber die Gewichtsabname des Mutterkuchens nach der Geburt und die Bedeutung fur die Quotienten aus Plazenta und Kindsgewicht. Geburstshilfe und Frauenheilkunde 34: 618–622

Lettieri L, Vintzileos A M, Rodis J F, Albini S M, Salafia C M 1993 Does 'idiopathic' preterm labor resulting in preterm birth exist? American Journal of Obsytetrics and Gynecology 160: 1480–1485

Leung A K C, Robson W L M 1989 Single umbilical artery — a report of 159 cases. American Journal of Diseases of Children 143: 108–111

Lewis S H, Benirschke K 1999 Overview of placental pathology and justification for examination of the placenta. In: Lewis S H, Perrin E (eds) Pathology of the placenta, 2nd edn. Churchill Livingstone, New York, pp 1–26

Lewis S H, Gilbert-Barness E 1999 Placental membranes. In: Lewis S H, Perrin E (eds) Pathology of the placenta, 2nd edn. Churchill Livingstone, New York, pp 137–160

Lin S, Shimizu I, Suehara N, Nakayama M, Aono T 1995 Uterine artery Doppler velocimetry in relation to trophoblast migration into the myometrium of the placental bed. Obstetrics and Gynecology 85: 760–765

Lippert T H, Cloeren S F, Kidess E, Fridrich R 1980 Assessment of uteroplacental haemodynamics in pre-eclampsia. In: Bonnar J, MacGillivray I, Symonds E M (eds) Pregnancy hypertension. MTP Press, Lancaster, pp 267–270

Liu Q X 1990 Pathology of the placenta from small for gestational age infants. Chinese Journal of Obstetrics and Gynecology 25: 331–334

Lockwood C J 1994 Recent advances in elucidating the pathogenesis of preterm delivery, the detection of patients at risk, and preventative therapies. Current Opinion in Obstetrics and Gynecology 6: 7–18

Longo L D 1981 The interrelations of maternal–fetal transfer and placental blood flow. Placenta (suppl 2): 45–64

Lopez-Bernal A, Hansell D J, Canete Soler R, Keeling J W, Turnbull A C 1987 Prostaglandins, chorioamnionitis and preterm labour. British Journal of Obstetrics and Gynaecology 94: 1156–1158

Lopez-Bernal A, Hansell D J, Khong T Y, Keeling J W, Turnbull A C 1989 Prostaglandin E production by the fetal membranes in unexplained preterm labour and labour associated with chorioamnionitis. British Journal of Obstetrics and Gynaecology 96: 1133–1139

Lorijn R H W, Longo L D 1980 Clinical and physiologic implications of increased fetal oxygen consumption. American Journal of Obstetrics and Gynecology 136: 451–457

Lunell N O, Sarby B 1979 Utero-placental blood flow: methods of determination, clinical application and the effect of beta-mimetic agonists. In: Sutherland H W, Stowers J M (eds) Carbohydrate metabolism in pregnancy and the newborn 1978. Springer, Berlin, pp 86–101

Lunell N O, Sarby B, Lewander R, Nylund L 1979 Comparison of uteroplacental blood flow in normal and in intrauterine growth-retarded pregnancy. Gynecologic and Obstetric Investigation 10: 106–118

Lurie S, Fenakel K, Gorbacz S 1990 Antenatal maceration of the umbilical cord: a case report. European Journal of Obstetrics, Gynecology and Reproductive Biology 35: 279–281

McCormick J N, Faulk W P, Fox H, Fudenberg H H 1971 Immunohistological and elution studies of the human placenta. Journal of Experimental Medicine 91: 1–13

McCowan L M, Ritchie K, Mo L Y Bascom P A, Sherret H 1988 Uterine artery flow velocity waveforms in normal and growth-retarded pregnancies. American Journal of Obstetrics and Gynecology 158: 499–504

McFadyen I R, Price A B, Geirsson R T 1986 The relation of birth weight to histological appearances in vessels of the placental bed. British Journal of Obstetrics and Gynaecology 93: 47–51

McGregor J A, French J I, Lawellin D, Franco-Buff A, Smith C, Todd J K 1987 Bacterial protease-induced reduction of chorioamniotic membrane strength and elasticity. Obstetrics and Gynecology 69: 164–175

McIntyre J 2001 HIV and pregnancy. In: MacLean A B, Regan L, Carrington D (eds) Infection and pregnancy. RCOG Press, London, pp 253–264

MacLennon A H, Sharpe F, Shaw-Dunn J 1972 The ultrastructure of human trophoblast in spontaneous and induced hypoxia using a system of organ culture: a comparison with ultrastructural changes in pre-eclampsia and placental insufficiency. Journal of Obstetrics and Gynaecology of the British Commonwealth 79: 113–121

McLennan H, Price E, Urbanska M, Craig N, Fraser M 1988 Umbilical cord knots and encirclements. Australian and New Zealand Journal of Obstetrics and Gynaecology 28: 116–119

McParland P, Pearce J M 1988 Doppler blood flow in pregnancy. Placenta 9: 427–450

Macara L, Kingdom J C P, Kohnen G, Bowman A W, Greer I A, Kaufmann P 1995 Elaboration of stem villous vessels in growth restricted pregnancies with abnormal umbilical artery Doppler waveforms. British Journal of Obstetrics and Gynaecology 102: 578–583

Macara L, Kingdom J C P, Kaufmann P, Kohnen G, Hair J, More I A R 1996 Structural analysis of placental terminal villi from growth-restricted pregnancies with abnormal umbilical artery Doppler waveforms. Placenta 17: 37–48

Malan A F, Woods D L, van der Elst C W, Meyer M P 1990 Relative placental weight in congenital syphilis. Placenta 11: 3–6

Mandsager N T, Bendon R, Mostello D et al 1994 Maternal floor infarction of the placenta: prenatal diagnosis and clinical significance. Obstetrics and Gynecology 83: 750–754

Mattern C F T, Murray K, Jensen A 1992 Localization of human immunodeficiency virus core antigen in term human placentas. Pediatrics 89: 207–209

Maubert B, Guilbert I J, Deloron P 1997 Cytoadherence of *Plasmodium falciparum* to intercellular adhesion molecule 1 and chondroitin-4-sulfate expressed by the syncytiotrophoblast in the human placenta. Infection and Immunology 65: 1251–1257

Mires G J, Williams F L, Leslie J, Howie P W 1998 Assessment of uterine arterial notching as a screening test for adverse pregnancy outcome. American Journal of Obstetrics and Gynecology 179: 1317–1323

Mitchell M D, Trautman D S, Dudley D J 1993 Cytokine networking in the placenta. Placenta 14: 249–275

Moe N, Jorgensen I 1968 Fibrin deposits on the syncytium of the normal human placenta: evidence of their thrombogenic origin. Acta Pathologica et Microbiologica Scandinavica 72: 519–541

Molteni R A, Stanley J S S, Battaglia F C 1978 Relations of fetal and placental weight in human beings: fetal/placental weight ratios at various gestational ages and birthweight distributions. Journal of Reproductive Medicine 21: 327–332

Morey A L, Keeling J W, Porter H J, Fleming K A 1992 Clinical and histopathological features of parvovirus B19 infection in the human fetus. British Journal of Obstetrics and Gynaecology 99: 566–574

Mostoufi-Zadeh M, Driscoll S G, Biano S A, Kundsin R B 1984 Placental evidence of cytomegalovirus infection of the fetus and neonate. Archives of Pathology and Laboratory Medicine 108: 403–406

Mueller-Heubach E, Rubinstein D N, Schwartz S S 1990 Histologic chorioamnionitis and preterm delivery in different patient populations. Obstetrics and Gynecology 75: 622–626

Muhlemann K, Miller R A, Meday L, Menegus M A 1994 Characterization of cytomegalovirus infection by immunocytochemistry. Trophoblast Research 8: 215–222

Myers R A, Fujikura T 1968 Placental changes after experimental abruptio placentae and fetal vessel ligation of rhesus monkey placenta. American Journal of Obstetrics and Gynecology 100: 846–851

Naeye R L 1977 Placental infarction leading to fetal or neonatal death: a prospective study. Obstetrics and Gynecology 50: 583–588

Naeye R L 1985a Maternal floor infarction. Human Pathology 16: 823–828

Naeye R L 1985b Umbilical cord length: clinical significance. Journal of Pediatrics 107: 278–281

Naeye R L 1987 Functionally important disorders of the placenta, umbilical cord and fetal membranes. Human Pathology 17: 680–691

Naeye 1989 Pregnancy hypertension, placental evidences of low uteroplacental blood flow and spontaneous preterm delivery. Human Pathology 21: 441–444

Naeye R L 1991 Acute chorioamnionitis and the disorders that produce placental insufficiency. In: Kraus F T, Damjanov I, Kaufman N (eds) Pathology of reproductive failure. Williams & Wilkins, Baltimore, pp 286–307

Naeye R L 1992 Disorders of the placenta, fetus, and neonate: diagnosis and clinical significance. Mosby, St Louis

Naeye R L, Peters E C 1980 Causes and consequences of premature rupture of fetal membranes. Lancet i: 192–194

Naeye R L, Maisels J, Lorenz R P, Botti J J 1983 The clinical significance of placental villous edema. Pediatrics 71: 588–594

Nakamura Y, Sakuma S, Ohta Y, Kawano K, Hashimoto T 1994 Detection of the human cytomegalovirus gene in placental chronic villitis by polymerase chain reaction. Human Pathology 25: 815–818

Nathan L, Leveno K J, Carmody T J, Kelly M A, Sherman M I 1994 Meconium: a 1990's perspective. Obstetrics and Gynecology 83: 329–333

Navarro C, Blanc W A 1974 Subacute necrotizing funisitis: a variant of cord inflammation with a high rate of perinatal infection. Journal of Pediatrics 85: 689–697

Newton E R, Prihoda T J, Gibbs R S 1989 Logistic regression analysis of risk factors for intramniotic infection. Obstetrics and Gynecology 73: 571–575

Nickel R E 1988 Maternal floor infarction: an unusual cause of intrauterine growth retardation. American Journal of Diseases of Children 142: 1270–1271

Nicolaides K H, Bilardi C M, Soothill P W, Campbell S 1988 Absence of end-diastolic frequencies in the umbilical artery: a sign of fetal hypoxia and acidosis. British Medical Journal 297: 1026–1027

Novak R W, Platt M S 1985 Significance of placental findings in early-nset group B streptococcal neonatal sepsis. Clinical Pediatrics 24: 256–259

Nummi S 1972 Relative weight of the placenta and perinatal mortality: a retrospective clinical and statistical analysis. Acta Obstetricia et Gynecologica Scandinavica (suppl 17): 1–69

Ohno Y, Kasugi M, Kurauchi O, Mizutani S, Tomoda Y 1994 Effect of interleukin-2 on the production of progesterone and prostaglandin E2 in human fetal membranes and its consequence for preterm uterine contractions. European Journal of Endocrinology 130: 478–484

Olofsson P, Laurini R N, Marsal K 1993 A high uterine pulsatility index reflects a defective development of placental bed spiral arteries in pregnancies complicated by hypertension and fetal growth retardation. European Journal of Obstetrics, Gynecology and Reproductive Biology 49: 161–168

Ordi J, Ismail M R, Ventura P J et al 1998 Massive chronic intervillositis of the placenta associated with malarial infection. American Journal of Surgical Pathology 22: 1006–1011

O'Shaughnessy R W 1981 Uterine blood flow and fetal growth. In: van Assche F A, Robertson W B (eds) Fetal growth retardation. Churchill Livingstone, Edinburgh, pp 101–116

Pardi G, Cetin L, Marconi A M, et al 1992 Venous drainage of the human uterus: respiratory gas studies in normal and fetal growth retarded pregnancies. American Journal of Obstetrics and Gynecology 166: 699–706

Pearlstone M, Baxi L 1993 Subchorionic hematoma: a review. Obstetrical and Gynecological Survey 48: 65–68

Perkins R P, Zhou S M, Butler C, Skipper B J 1987 Histologic chorioamnionitis in pregnancies of various gestational ages: implications in preterm rupture of the membranes. Obstetrics and Gynecology 70: 856–860

Perlman M, Tennenbaum A, Menash M, Ornoy A 1980 Extramembranous pregnancy: maternal, placental, and perinatal implications. Obstetrics and Gynecology 55: 34s–37s

Poggi S H, Bostrom K I, Demer L L, Skinner H C, Koos B J 2001 Placental calcification: a metastatic process. Placenta 22: 591–596

Polzin W J, Brady K 1991 Mechanical factors in the etiology of premature rupture of the membranes. Clinical Obstetrics and Gynecology 34: 702–714

Pommerenke F, Sadenwasser W 1992 Nabelschnurkompression durch Amniostrang. Zentralblatt fur Gynakologie 114: 557–559

Popek E J 1992 Granulomatous villitis due to *Toxoplasma gondii*. Pediatric Pathology 12: 281–288

Porter H L 2000 The role of placental examination as a perinatal investigation. In: Kingdom J C P, Jauniaux E R M, O'Brien P M S (eds) The placenta: basic science and clinical practice. RCOG Press, London, pp 109–120

Quek S P, Tan K L 1972 Vasa praevia. Australian and New Zealand Journal of Obstetrics and Gynaecology 12: 206–209

Quinn P A, Butany J, Taylor J, Hannah W 1987 Chorioamnionitis and its association with pregnancy outcome and microbiol infection. American Journal of Obstetrics and Gynecology 156: 379–387

Qureshi F, Jacques S M, Reyes M P 1993 Placental histopathology in syphilis. Human Pathology 24: 779–784

Rayburn W, Sander C, Barr M Jr, Rygiel R 1985 The stillborn fetus: placental histologic examination in determining a cause. Obstetrics and Gynecology 65: 637–641

Rayne S C, Kraus F T 1993 Placental thrombi and other vascular lesions: classification, morphology, and clinical correlations. Pathology Research and Practice 189: 2–17

Redline R W 1995 Placental pathology: a neglected link between basic disease mechanisms and untoward pregnancy outcome. Current Opinion in Obstetrics and Gynecology 7: 10–15

Redline R W 1999 Disorders of the placental parenchyma. In: Lewis S H, Perrin E (eds) Pathology of the placenta, 2nd edn. Churchill Livingstone, New York, pp 161–184

Redline R W, Abramowsky C R 1985 Clinical and pathologic aspects of recurrent placental villitis. Human Pathology 16: 727–731

Redline R W, Pappin A 1995 Fetal thrombotic vasculopathy: the clinical significance of extensive avascular villi. Human Pathology 26: 80–85

Redline R W, Patterson P 1993 Villitis of unknown etiology is associated with major infiltration of fetal tissue by maternal inflammatory cells. American Journal of Pathology 143: 332–336

Redline R W, Patterson P 1994 Patterns of placental injury: correlations with gestational age, placental weight, and clinical diagnosis. Archives of Pathology and Laboratory Medicine 118: 698–701

Redman C W G 1991 Pre-eclampsia and the placenta. Placenta 12: 301–308

Redman C W G, Sargent I L 2000 Placental debris, oxidative stress and pre-eclampsia. Placenta 21: 597–602

Reles A, Friedmann W, Vogel M, Dudenhausen J W 1991 Intrauteriner Fruchttod nach Strangulation der Nabelschnur durch Amniobänder. Geburtshilfe und Frauenheilkunde 51: 1006–1008

Resta R G, Luthy D A, Mahoney B S 1988 Umbilical cord hemangioma associated with extremely high alphafetoprotein levels. Obstetrics and Gynecology 72: 488–491

Roberts J M, Taylor R N, Musci T J et al 1989 Pre-eclampsia: an endothelial cell disorder. American Journal of Obstetrics and Gynecology 161: 1200–1204

Robertson W B 1976 Utero-placental vasculature. Journal of Clinical Pathology 20: Supplement, Royal College of Pathologists 10: 9–17

Robertson W B 1981 Maternal blood supply in fetal growth retardation. In: van Assche F A, Robertson W B (eds) Fetal growth retardation. Churchill Livingstone, Edinburgh, pp 126–138

Robertson W B, Dixon H G 1969 Uteroplacental pathology. In: Klopper A, Diczfalusy E (eds) Fetus and placenta. Blackwell, Oxford

Robertson W B, Brosens I, Dixon H G 1975 Uteroplacental vascular pathology. European Journal of Obstetrics, Gynecology and Reproductive Biology 5: 47–65

Robinson J S, Owens J 1993 The placenta and intrauterine growth retardation. In: Redman C W G, Sargent H, Starkey P M (eds) The human placenta. Blackwell Scientific, Oxford, pp 558–578

Robinson J S, Kingston E J, Jones C T, Thornburn G D 1979 Studies on experimental growth retardation in sheep: the effect of removal of endometrial caruncles on fetal size and metabolism. Journal of Developmental Physiology 1: 379–398

Rogers B B, Mark Y, Oyer C E 1993 Diagnosis and incidence of fetal parvovirus infection in an autopsy series. I. Histology. Pediatric Pathology 13: 371–379

Rogerson S J, Beeson J G 1999 The placenta in malaria: mechanisms of infection, disease and fetal morbidity. Annals of Tropical Medicine and Parasitology 93: S35–S42

Rolschau J 1978 Circumvallate placenta and intrauterine growth retardation. Acta Obstetricia et Gynecologica Scandinavica (suppl) 72: 11–14

Romero R, Quintero R, Emamian M, Wan M, Hobbins J C, Mitchell M D 1987 Prostaglandin concentrations in amniotic fluid of women with intramniotic infection and preterm labor. American Journal of Obstetrics and Gynecology 157: 1461–1467

Romero R, Roslawsky T, Oyarzun E et al 1988 Infection and labor. II. Bacterial endotoxin in amniotic fluid and its relationship to the onset of preterm labor. American Journal of Obstetrics and Gynecology 158: 1044–1049

Romero R, Brody D T, Oyarzun E et al 1989a Infection and labor. III Interleukin-1: a signal for the onset of partuition. American Journal of Obstetrics and Gynecology 160: 1117–1123

Romero R, Manogue K R, Mitchell M D et al 1989b. Infection and labor. IV. Cachectin-tumor necrosis factor in the amniotic fluid of women with intraamniotic infection and preterm labor. American Journal of Obstetrics and Gynecology 161: 336–341

Romero R, Sirtori M, Oyarzun E et al 1989c Infection and labor. V. Prevelance, microbiology and clinical significance of intraamniotic infection in women with preterm labor and intact membranes. American Journal of Obstetrics and Gynecology 161: 817–824

Romero R, Durum S, Dinarello C A, Oyarzun E, Hobbins J C, Mitchell M D 1989d Interleukin-1 stimulates prostaglandin synthesis by human amnion. Prostaglandins 37: 13–22

Romero R, Avila C, Santhanam U, Sehgal P B 1990 Amniotic fluid interleukin-6 in preterm labor: association with infection. Journal of Clinical Investigation 65: 1392–1400

Romero R, Mazor M, Sepulveda W, Avila C, Copeland D, Wiliams J 1992a Tumor necrosis factor in preterm and term labor. American Journal of Obstetrics and Gynecology 166: 1576–1587

Romero R, Mazor M, Brandt F et al 1992b Interleukin-1 alpha and interleukin-1 beta in preterm and term human partuition. American Journal of Reproductive Immunology 27: 117–123

Romero R, Nores J, Mazor M et al 1993 Microbiol invasion of the amniotic cavity during term labor: prevalence and clinical significance. Journal of Reproductive Medicine 38: 543–548

Russell P 1979 Inflammatory lesions of the human placenta. II. Villitis of unknown etiology in perspective. American Journal of Diagnostic Gynecology and Obstetrics 1: 339–346

Russell P 1980 Inflammatory lesions of the human placenta. III. The histopathology of villitis of unknown aetiology. Placenta 1: 227–244

Russell P, Altshuler G 1974 The placental abnormalities of congenital syphilis. American Journal of Diseases of Children 128: 160–163

Russell P, Atkinson A, Krishnan I 1980 Recurrent reproductive failure due to severe placental villitis of unknown etiology. Journal of Reproductive Medicine. 24: 93–98

Sachdev R, Nuovo G R, Kaplan C, Greco M A 1990 In situ hybridization analysis for cytomegalovirus in chronic villitis. Pediatric Pathology 10: 909–917

Salafia C M, Mill J F 1996 The value of placental pathology in studies of spontaneous prematurity. Current Opinion in Obstetrics and Gynecology 8: 89–95

Salafia C M, Pijnenborg R 1999 Disorders of the decidua and maternal vasculature. In: Lewis S H, Perrin E (eds) Pathology of the placenta, 2nd edn. Churchill Livingstone, New York, pp 185–212

Salafia C M, Vintzileos A M 1990 Why all placentas should be examined by a pathologist in 1990. American Journal of Obstetrics and Gynecology 163: 1282–1293

Salafia C M, Silberman L, Herrera N E, Mahoney M J 1988 Placental pathology at term associated with elevated midtrimester maternal serum alpha-fetoprotein cocentration. American Journal of Obstetrics and Gynecology 158: 1064–1066

Salafia C M, Vogel C A, Vintzileos A M et al 1991 Placental pathologic findings in preterm birth. American Journal of Obstetrics and Gynecology 165: 934–938

Salafia C M, Vintzileos A M, Silberman L, Bantham K F, Vogel C A 1992a Placental pathology of idiopathic intrauterine growth retardation at term. American Journal of Perinatology 9: 179–184

Salafia C M, Vintzileos A M, Silberman L et al 1992b Placental pathology of idiopathic intrauterine growth retardation at term. American Journal of Perinatology 9: 179–184

Salafia C M, Ernst L, Pezzullo J P, Wolf W, Rosenkrantz T S, Vintzileos A M 1995 The very low birth weight infant: maternal complications leading to preterm birth, placental lesions, and intrauterine growth retardation. American Journal of Perinatology 12: 106–110

Salafia C M, Thorp J, Starzyk K A 2000 Placental pathology in spontaneous prematurity. In: Kingdom J C P, Jauniaux E R M, O'Brien P M S (eds) The placenta: basic science and clinical practice. RCOG Press, London, pp 168–186

Samson G R, Meyer M P, Blake D R B, Cohen M C, Mouton S C E 1994 Syphilitic placentitis: an immunopathy. Placenta 15: 67–77

Sandstedt B 1979 The placenta and low birth weight. Current Topics in Pathology 66: 1–55

Savva D, Holliman R E 1990 PCR to detect toxoplasma. Lancet 336: 1325

Schiebler T H, Kaufmann P 1981 Reife Placenta. In: Becker V, Schiebler T H, Kubli F (eds) Die Plazenta des Menschen. Thieme, Stuttgart, pp 51–100

Schoonmaker J N, Lawellin D W, Lunt B, McGregor J A 1989 Bacteria and inflammatory cells reduce chorioamniotic membranes integrity and tensile strength. Obstetrics and Gynecology 74: 590–596

Schulman H 1993 Uteroplacental flow velocity. In: Chervenak F A, Isaacson G C, Campbell S (eds) Ultrasound in obstetrics and gynecology. Little Brown, Boston, pp 569–577

Schwartz D A, Reef S 1990 Candida albicans placentitis and funisitis: early diagnosis of congenital candidemia by histopathologic examination of umbilical cord vessel. Pediatric Infectious Disease Journal 9: 661–665

Schwartz D A, Khan R, Stoll B 1992 Characterization of the fetal inflammatory response to cytomegalovirus placentitis. Archives of Pathology and Laboratory Medicine 116: 518–524

Schwartz D A, Zhang W, Larsen S Rice R J 1994 Placental pathology of congenital syphilis — immunohistochemical aspects. Trophoblast Research 8: 223–229

Schwartz D A, Larsen D A, Beck-Sague C, Fears M, Rice R J 1995 Pathology of the umbilical cord in congenital syphilis: analysis of 25 cases. Human Pathology 26: 781–784

Sen-Schwarz S, Ruchelli E, Brown D 1989 Villous oedema of the placenta: a clinicopathological study. Placenta 10: 297–307

Shanklin D R, Scott J S 1975 Massive subchorial thrombohaematoma (Breus' mole). British Journal of Obstetrics and Gynaecology 82: 476–487

Sheppard B L, Bonnar J 1976 The ultrastructure of the arterial supply of the human placenta in pregnancy complicated by fetal growth retardation. British Journal of Obstetrics and Gynaecology 83: 948–959

Sheppard B L, Bonnar J 1980a Uteroplacental arteries and hypertensive pregnancy. In: Bonnar J, MacGillivray I, Symonds E M (eds) Pregnancy hypertension. MTP Press, Lancaster, pp 213–219

Sheppard B L, Bonnar J 1980b Ultrastructural abnormalities of placental villi in placentae from pregnancies complicated by fetal growth retardation: their relationship to decidual spiral arterial lesions. Placenta 1: 145–156

Sheppard B L, Bonnar J 1981 An ultrastructural study of uteroplacental spiral arteries in hypertensive and normotensive pregnancy and fetal growth retardation. British Journal of Obstetrics and Gynaecology 88: 695–705

Shulman C, Dorman E, Brabin B 2001 Malaria in pregnancy. In: MacLean A B, Regan L, Carrington D (eds) Infection and pregnancy. RCOG Press, London, pp 124–136

Silver H M, Sperling R S, St Clair P J, Gibbs R S 1989 Evidence relating bacterial vaginosis to intraamniotic infection. American Journal of Obstetrics and Gynecology 161: 808–812

Simpson R A, Mayhew T M, Barnes P R 1992 From 13 weeks to term, the trophoblast of human placenta grows by the continuous recruitment of new proliferative units: a study of nuclear number using the dissector. Placenta 13: 501–512

Sinzger C, Muntefering H, Loning T, Stoss H, Plachter B, Jahn G 1993 Cell types infected in human cytomegalovirus placentitis identified by immunohistochemical double staining. Virchows Archiv A Pathological Anatomy and Histopathology 423: 249–256

Smith J R, Taylor-Robinson D 1993 Infection due to Chlamydia trachomatis in pregnancy and the newborn. Balliere's Clinics in Obstetrics and Gynaecology 7: 237–255

Soper D E, Mayhall C G, Dalton H P 1989 Risk factors for intraamniotic infection: a prospective epidemiological study. American Journal of Obstetrics and Gynecology 161: 562–566

Steel S A, Pearce J M, Chamberlain G V P 1988 Doppler ultrasound of the uteroplacental circulation as a screening test for severe preeclampsia with intrauterine growth retardation. European Journal of Obstetrics, Gynecology and Reproductive Biology 28: 279–287

Steer P J, Eigbe F, Lissauer T J, Beard R W 1989 Interrelationships among abnormal cardiotocograms in labor, meconium staining of the amniotic fluid, arterial cord blood pH, and Agpar scores. Obstetrics and Gynecology 74: 715–721

Stock M A, Anderson D F, Phernetton T M et al 1980 Vascular response of the fetal placenta to local occlusion of the maternal placental vasculature. Journal of Developmental Physiology 2: 339–346

Strigini F A L, Lancioni G, de Luca G et al 1995 Uterine artery velocimetry and spontaneous preterm delivery. Obstetrics and Gynecology 85: 374–377

Sugiyama T, Cuevas L E, Bailey W et al 2001 Expression of intercellular adhesion molecule 1 (ICAM-1) in *Plasmodium falciparum*-infected placenta. Placenta 22: 573–579

Swinburne L M 1967 Spontaneous intrauterine decapitation. Archives of Disease in Childhood 42: 636–641

Taylor D J 2000 The role of intrauterine infection in preterm birth. In: Kingdom J C P, Jauniaux E R M, O'Brien P M S (eds) The placenta: basic science and clinical practice. RCOG Press, London, p 161–168

Teasdale F 1982 Morphometric evaluation. Contributions to Gynecology and Obstetrics 9: 17–28

ten Berge B S 1955 Capillaraktion in der Placenta. Archiv fur Gynakologie 186: 253–256

Theuring F 1968 Fibrose Obliterationen an Deckplatten und Stammzottengefassen der Placenta nach intrauterinem Fruchttod. Archiv fur Gynakolgie 206: 237–251

Thomson A M, Billewicz W Z, Hytten F E 1969 The weight of the placenta in relation to birthweight. Journal of Obstetrics and Gynaecology of the British Commonwealth 76: 865–872

Topalovski M, Yang S S, Boonpasat Y 1993 Listeriosis of the placenta: clinicopathologic study of seven cases. American Journal of Obstetrics and Gynecology 169: 616–620

Torpin R 1968 Fetal malformation caused by amnion rupture during gestation. Charles C Thomas, Springfield, Illinois

Trudinger B J, Giles W B, Cook C M 1985a Uteroplacental blood flow velocity time waveforms in normal and complicated pregnancy. British Journal of Obstetrics and Gynaecology 92: 39–45

Trudinger B J, Giles W B, Cook C M et al 1985b Fetal umbilical flow velocity waveforms and placental resistance: clinical significance. British Journal of Obstetrics and Gynaecology 92: 23–30

Usher R H, Boyd M E, McLean F H, Kramer M S 1988 Assessment of fetal risk in postdate pregnancies. American Journal of Obstetrics and Gynecology 158: 259–264

van der Elst C W, Lopez-Bernal A, Sinclair-Smith C C 1991 The role of chorioamnionitis and prostaglandins in preterm labor. Obstetrics and Gynecology 77: 672–676

van der Veen F, Fox H 1983 The human placenta in idiopathic intrauterine growth retardation: a light and electron microscopic study. Placenta 4: 65–78

van der Veen F, Walker S, Fox H 1982 Endarteritis obliterans of the fetal stem arteries of the human placenta: an electron microscopic study. Placenta 3: 181–190

Vigorita V J, Parmley T H 1979 Intramembranous localization of bacteria in beta-hemolytic group B streptococcal chorioamnionitis. Obstetrics and Gynecology 53: 13S–15S

Volker U 1992 Gewichts- und Grossenvergleich von Plazenten und Feten bei intrauterinem Fruchttod. Perinatal Medizin 4: 8–16

Vracko R, Benditt E 1970 Capillary basal lamina thickening: its relationship to endothelial cell death and replacement. Journal of Cell Biology 47: 281–285

Walkinshaw S A 1995 Preterm labour and delivery of the preterm infant. In: Chamberlain G (ed) Turnbull's obstetrics, 2nd edn. Churchill Livingstone, Edinburgh, pp 609–632

Werner J, Schmidtke L, Thomasheck G 1963 *Toxoplasma* Infektion und Schwangerschaft, der histologische Nachweis des intrauteriner Infektionweges. Klinische Wochenschrift 41: 96–101

Wessell J, Gerhold W, Unger M, Lichtenegger W, Vogel M 1992 Nabelschnurkomplikationen als Ursache des intrauterinen Fruchttodes. Zeitschrifte for Geburtshilfe und Perinatologie 196: 173–176

Wigglesworth J S 1964 Experimental growth retardation in the foetal rat. Journal of Pathology and Bacteriology 88: 1–13

Wilkin P 1965 Pathologie du placenta. Masson, Paris

Wilkins B S, Batcup G, Vinall P S 1991 Partial placenta membranacea. British Journal of Obstetrics and Gynaecology 98: 675–679

Wilson D, Paalman R J 1967 Clinical significance of circumvallate placenta. Obstetrics and Gynecology 29: 774–778

Wingerd J, Christianson R E, Levitt W V, Schoen E J 1976 Placental ratio in white and black women: relation to smoking and anemia. American Journal of Obstetrics and Gynecology 124: 671–675

Yamada M, Steketee R, Abramowsky C et al 1989 *Plasmodium falciparum* associated placental pathology: a light and electron microscopic and immunohistologic study. American Journal of Tropical Medicine and Hygiene 41: 161–168

Yancey M K, Duff P, Clark P, Kurtzer T, Frentzen B H, Kublis P 1994 Peripartum infection associated with vaginal group B streptococcal colonization. Obstetrics and Gynecology 84: 816–819

Yang S S, Levine A J, Sanborn J R, Delp R A 1984 Amniotic rupture, extra-amniotic pregnancy, and vernix granulomata. American Journal of Surgical Pathology 8: 117–122

Yavner D L, Redline R W 1989 Angiomyxoma of the umbilical cord with massive cystic degeneration of Wharton's jelly. Archives of Pathology and Laboratory Medicine 113: 935–937

Yoon B H, Jun J K, Romero R et al 1997 Amniotic fluid inflammatory cytokines (interleukin-6, interleukin-1-beta, and tumor necrosis factor-alpha), neonatal brain white matter lesions, and cerebral palsy. American Journal of Obstetrics and Gynecology 177: 19–26

Zacutti A, Borruto F, Bottacci G et al 1992 Umbilical blood flow and placental pathology. Clinical and Experimental Obstetrics and Gynecology 19: 63–69

Zevallos E A, Anderson V M, Baird E Gu J 1994 Detection of HIV-1 sequences in placentas of HIV infected mothers by in situ polymerase chain reaction. Cell Vision 1: 116–121

39

Pathology of the pregnant uterus

J. Hustin   M. Wells

Introduction   1327

Normal uterine adaptations to pregnancy   1328
Endometrium   1328
Myometrium   1330
Blood vessels   1331

Early placentation   1332
Migratory trophoblast   1332
Development of the uteroplacental vasculature   1335

Placental bed pathology   1336
Hypertensive disorders of pregnancy   1336
Intrauterine fetal growth retardation   1344
Other systemic disorders   1344

Other defects of placentation   1345
Spontaneous miscarriage   1345
Trophoblastic disease   1346
Placenta creta   1347
Antepartum haemorrhage   1349
Postpartum haemorrhage   1353

INTRODUCTION

The female genital tract undergoes extensive physiological and structural adaptations to pregnancy. Because it has to contain and nurture the growing fetus, the uterus manifests such adaptations to a greater extent than other parts of the genital tract, but there is still much ignorance of the mechanisms involved. There is even less understanding of those defects in uterine adaptation to the pregnant state that may have a bearing on the aetiology and pathogenesis of many disorders of pregnancy. In the great majority of abnormal pregnancies, for obvious reasons, the uterus is not available for histopathological study so that deductions about the disorder in question must be made from the delivered fetal placenta and, in cases of perinatal death, from autopsy studies of the neonate. The uterus involutes postpartum and any pregnancy-associated defect on the maternal side of the placenta disappears in the process and may not recur in subsequent pregnancies. Important additional information has been gleaned from occasional pregnancy hysterectomy specimens, from the technique of placental bed biopsy (Dixon & Robertson 1958; Hustin et al 1983; Robertson et al 1986) and from autopsies in cases of maternal death (Rushton & Dawson 1982), that are fortunately now an uncommon occurrence. Regrettably, such deaths are usually the subject of a coroner's inquiry where the emphasis is more upon the cause of death and less upon the elucidation of the pathology of the condition leading to the fatality.

It is reasonable to assume that any serious anatomical or physiological abnormality, congenital or acquired, of the uterine tissues will be inimical to a pregnancy. It follows that aberrations in the normal symbiotic interaction between fetal and maternal tissues are likely to be crucial determinants of many disorders of pregnancy. Pre-eclampsia, fetal intrauterine growth retardation, spontaneous miscarriage, antepartum and postpartum haemorrhage are but a few examples in which feto-maternal interactions are probably defective. This chapter will therefore be devoted to a review of what is currently known and, perhaps more importantly, to what remains to be discovered about human placentation and its imperfections.

NORMAL UTERINE ADAPTATIONS TO PREGNANCY

ENDOMETRIUM

Conception probably occurs in most instances soon after release of the oocyte from the follicle at mid-cycle, that is on about day 15 or 16 of a normal 28-day cycle. The zygote then develops through the morula stage in the Fallopian tube and, if it survives the journey, reaches the cavity of the uterus a few days later to mature into a blastocyst prior to nidation in the primed endometrium on about day 21 of the cycle. By this time the endometrium, having been primed by oestrogen in the first half of the cycle, is at full glandular secretory activity but the stroma, at this stage, shows no evidence of predecidualisation. The maturation of the conceptus to a blastocyst and the secretory activity of the endometrium appear to require fairly precise synchronisation if nidation is to be successful.

However, with the application of new reproductive technologies, priming of the endometrium is achieved by different hormonal regimens: the resulting mucosal pattern usually differs markedly from the physiological state but a substantial number of implantations do occur (Deligdisch 1993). It is clear that the amount of progestagen administered is always less than that necessary to induce full decidualisation. It has been suggested that it is the status of the surface epithelium which is crucial for successful implantation (Hustin & Franchimont 1992). Certain properties of the apical pole of the cells, as expressed by the binding of lectins, play a very important rôle in the phenomenon of apposition.

There is evidence (Noyes 1972) that a predecidualised stroma is inhibitory to implantation and this may be a factor, amongst others, that could help to explain the high loss of early pregnancies, in the first two weeks following conception (Edmonds et al 1982).

It is remarkable that histopathologists are still unable to differentiate the features of a luteal phase endometrium where conception, but not nidation, has occurred from those of the more usual secretory endometrium of a non-conception cycle (Arronet et al 1973). In the latter circumstance the glands begin to undergo involutionary change on about day 23 whereas the stroma flourishes to produce a pronounced predecidual reaction by the time of menstruation. In the former circumstance two factors operate to produce subtle changes in the endometrium. If the conceptus is viable and has begun to produce hCG the corpus luteum is sustained instead of involuting, ensuring a rising level of plasma progesterone and a direct effect on the endometrium (Arias-Stella 1973). Most observers (Hertig 1964; Buxton & Olson 1969; Karow et al 1971) agree that the glands, instead of collapsing into the typical 'saw-tooth' appearance associated with secretory exhaustion (Fig. 39.1), continue to secrete with the epithelium becoming increasingly vacuolated and thrown into pseudopapillary folds, giving a hypersecretory impression

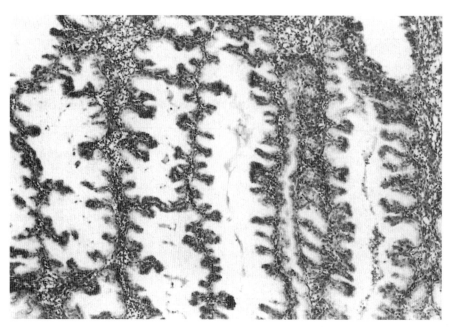

Fig. 39.1 Mid to late luteal phase endometrium with collapse of the glands due to resorption of interstitial oedema producing the characteristic 'saw-tooth' appearance.

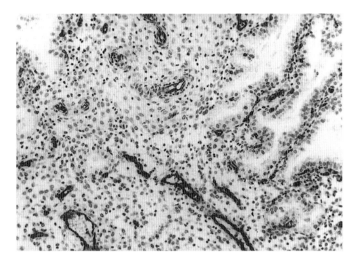

Fig. 39.2 Endometrium of early gestation glands are actively secreting and spiral arteries cuffed with predecidua underlined by endothelial immunostaining (anti-CD31 antibody with Avidin Biotin Complex and hematoxylin counterstain are outlined).

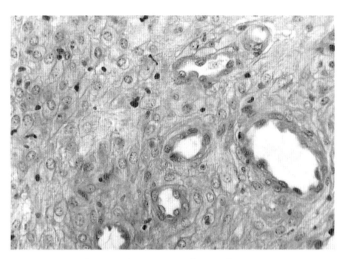

Fig. 39.3 Decidua vera in curettings from a first-trimester voluntary termination of pregnancy. The stroma has been converted to a sheet of plump glycogen-rich cells. The spiral artery is not modified.

(Fig. 39.2). The stroma is quite similar to that of late secretory phase (Fig. 39.3) with obvious decidualisation beginning around spiral arteries and under the surface epithelium. Complete decidualisation is however not evident before pregnancy is well established. The Arias-Stella phenomenon, with its nuclear pleomorphism added to the hyperplastic glandular changes, is present only during a limited period before a true decidua is complete (Fig. 39.4). It is more easily recognised in cases of ectopic pregnancy since the intrauterine compression due to the presence of the conceptus, which adds considerably to the decidualisation process, is lacking.

One cell type, prominent in late secretory endometrium and in the decidua of early pregnancy, the endometrial granulocyte or K cell (Kornchenzellen), is now recognised to be a large granular lymphocyte. It is of natural killer (NK) lineage and thus displays CD56 positivity (Bulmer 1994). It contains large phloxinophilic granules (Fig. 39.5) and is seen best in the decidua vera clustered around vessels and the slit-like glands of early pregnancy (Fig. 39.6). When degranulated these lymphocytes are difficult to distinguish from the other round cells seen at the site of placentation.

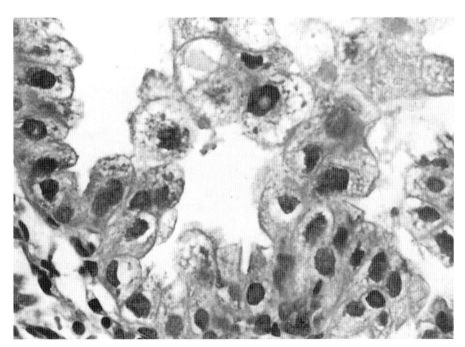

Fig. 39.4 Cytological detail of the Arias-Stella phenomenon: the glandular epithelial nuclei vary in size and are hyperchromatic with crenated nuclear membranes while the cytoplasm is vacuolated to a greater or lesser degree.

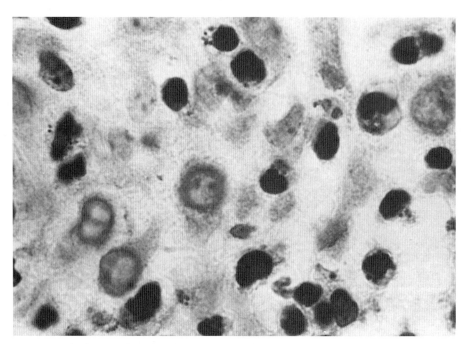

Fig. 39.5 The large, pale decidual cells contrast with the smaller, darkly staining endometrial granulocytes which contain spherical phloxinophilic granules. Phloxine tartrazine.

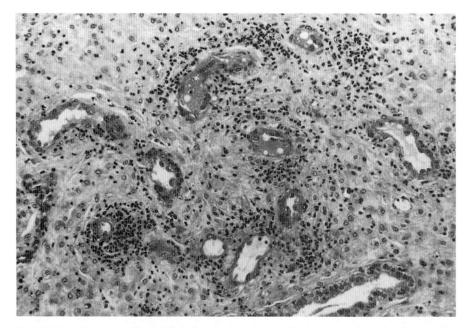

Fig. 39.6 Decidua vera (parietalis) of early pregnancy with concentration of endometrial granulocytes in the region of glands and spiral arteries.

MYOMETRIUM

It is self-evident that the uterus must enlarge pari passu with the growing conceptus but whether it does so by hypertrophy of existing smooth muscle or by hyperplasia is still debated. The answer is almost certainly that both processes are at work as mitoses are not difficult to find in the myometrium of the early pregnant uterus (Fig. 39.7). The relative contributions of the two mechanisms to increasing uterine bulk remain to be determined. It is clear that uterine smooth muscle cells enlarge very early in pregnancy. Their length can attain more than 200 μm for a width of around 15 μm. A significant addition to the weight and size of the uterus is made by increased collagen synthesis, the production of more of the complex ground substance and, no doubt, from increased fluid storage (Hytten & Leitch 1971). This increase explains why uterine muscle layers glide smoothly over each other.

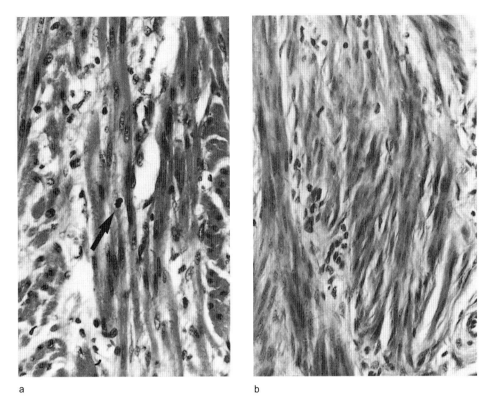

a

b

Fig. 39.7 Myometrium in the first trimester of pregnancy **a** showing hypertrophied smooth muscle, mitosis (arrow) and increase in intercellular constituents. Non-pregnant uterus **b** at same magnification for contrast.

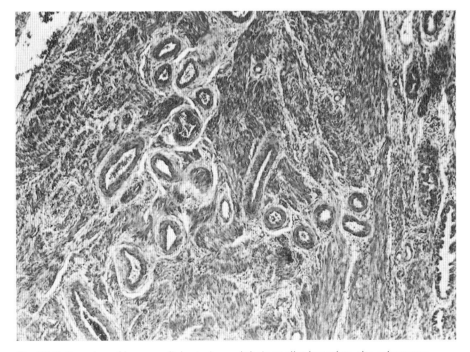

Fig. 39.8 Complex of larger radial arteries and their smaller branches, the subarcuate arteries, in the inner myometrium (endometrium, right).

BLOOD VESSELS

The major vessels of the uterus are involved also in the processes of hypertrophy and hyperplasia (Burchell et al 1978; Ramsey & Donner 1980). The uterine and ovarian arteries and their accompanying veins increase in length and calibre dramatically as the pregnant uterus enlarges, which is only to be expected as there is a ten-fold increase in blood supply to the pregnant uterus during the third trimester (Browne & Veall 1953). Similar accommodating changes have to take place in the arcuate system of blood vessels and its radial branches in the substance of the uterus. In the non-pregnant state, uterine arteries are markedly coiled. As a result, intimal cushions are formed which disappear as soon as the arteries become elongated to follow the growth of the pregnant uterus. The arcuate and radial arteries usually lose their internal elastic lamina; their media is reduced to a limited layer of muscle cells. These changes had been noticed as early as 1903 by Argaud. The latter arteries are the parent vessels of the spiral arteries supplying the endometrium of the non-pregnant uterus, some of which are destined to become the uteroplacental arteries of the pregnant uterus (Fig. 39.8).

Figure 39.9 gives a diagrammatic representation of the blood supply to the non-pregnant uterus as an aid to the understanding of human placentation and its disorders.

EARLY PLACENTATION

The development of the fetal placenta has been dealt with in Chapter 37, but because human placentation is haemochorial and, as such, requires a more intimate and complex reaction of fetal with maternal tissues, it is necessary to return to the subject to deal with the maternal aspect.

MIGRATORY TROPHOBLAST

A phenomenon common to all species with haemochorial placentation is the elaboration of migratory tropho-

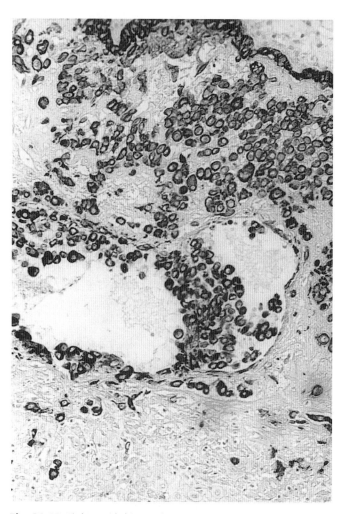

Fig. 39.10 Eight-week (six weeks post-conception) gestation: streamers of non-villous trophoblast from the trophoblast shell (top) infiltrating the basal decidua. A portion of an artery is also occupied by trophoblast (centre). Cytokeratin immunostaining.

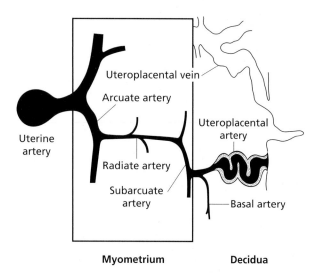

Fig. 39.9 Diagram of the blood supply to the non-pregnant uterus. During pregnancy the spiral arteries of the placental site or bed are converted to uteroplacental arteries by the action of migratory trophoblast. The small basal arteries are not involved and remain as nutritive vessels to the inner myometrium and basal decidua.

blast, the pattern of which varies in different species (Pijnenborg et al 1981a; Ramsey 1982). Invasion of uterine tissues occurs to a greater or lesser degree, depending on the species, but an essential feature is the opening up of maternal vessels by non-villous trophoblast. In the early stages of human placentation, the migratory trophoblast derives from the primary trophoblast which encircles the conceptus and which will later, i.e. after 2 or 3 weeks, differentiate as the trophoblastic shell (Boyd & Hamilton 1970). In the ensuing weeks, placental villi will form through expansion of the mesenchyme of the chorionic plate, within trophoblastic cells of the shell (Fig. 39.10). Simultaneously, streamers of such cells can be seen emanating from the outer part of the shell in the basal decidua, that is on the abembryonic side of the conceptus. By about six weeks post-conception, or eight weeks gestation by dating from the last menstrual period, the basal decidua is extensively overrun by migratory cytotrophoblast (Fig. 39.11), some

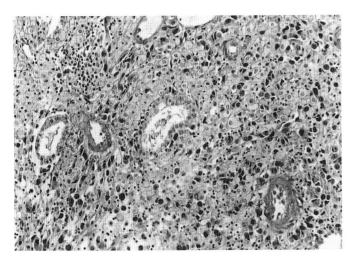

Fig. 39.11 First-trimester pregnancy: the basal decidua is extensively overrun by migratory interstitial cytotrophoblast, some of which has converted to syncytial placental bed giant cells.

of which, usually that nearer to the myometrium, is in the early stage of symplasmic fusion to form syncytiotrophoblast (Pijnenborg et al 1980), the characteristic placental bed (or site) giant cells. Extravillous trophoblast can be readily detected in routine histopathological practice by its immunohistochemical reactivity for cytokeratins (Wells & Bulmer 1988).

By about 10 weeks gestation the inner few millimetres of the myometrium of the placental bed are heavily colonised by this interstitial migratory cytotrophoblast (Fig. 39.12) but here the scene is altogether different with cytotrophoblast and smooth muscle coexisting in apparent harmony (Pijnenborg et al 1981b). The function of non-villous interstitial migratory trophoblast is not at all clear. There is evidence (Boyd & Hamilton 1970; Pijnenborg et al 1981b) that it is an important source of the hormones elaborated by trophoblast but even if this is so it still does not explain the functions of these cells. A good case has been made that one function is the 'priming' of the myometrial segments of the spiral arteries of the placental bed preparatory to their conversion to uteroplacental arteries (Pijnenborg et al 1983). There is a tendency for the interstitial migratory cytotrophoblast to concentrate around the myometrial blood vessels and this proximity is associated with the development of oedema and disruption of the normal architecture of the vessel wall (Fig. 39.13). There have been many recent studies of the possibility that extravillous trophoblast and various cells of the maternal compartment interact in the organisation of a materno-embryonic dialogue (Tabibzadeh & Bakaknia 1995; Aplin 1996). In particular, regulation of the interstitial penetration of the migratory trophoblast is evident. Production of numerous molecules which bind to their specific receptors on both sides is of considerable help for the development of the conceptus (Nawrocki et al 1997). The ultimate fate of migratory cytotrophoblast that reaches the myometrium is unknown although much of it is converted to placental bed giant cells (Robertson

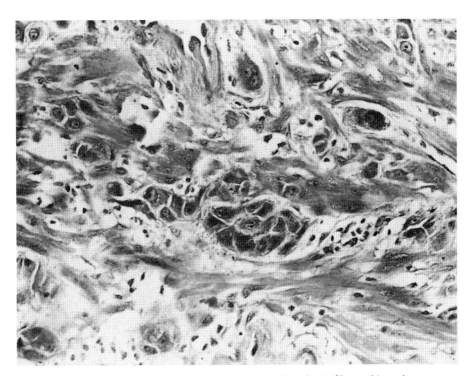

Fig. 39.12 Ten week gestation: migratory cytotrophoblast has infiltrated into the myometrium and clumps of cells are in the process of forming syncytial giant cells.

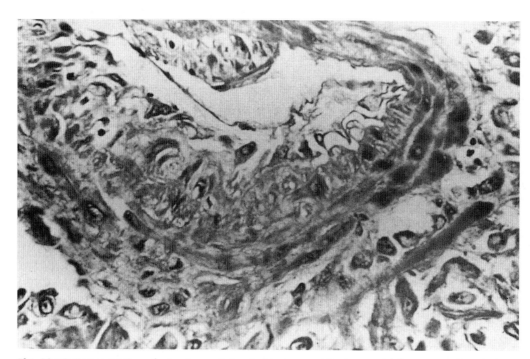

Fig. 39.13 Concentration of migratory cytotrophoblast around the myometrial segment of a spiral artery associated with oedema and disruption of the architecture of the vessel wall.

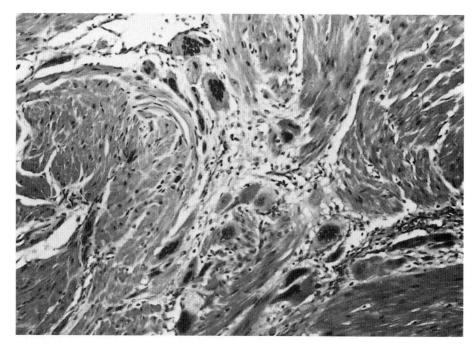

Fig. 39.14 Placental bed at term: residual, partially effete, syncytial giant cells in the myometrium.

& Warner 1974; Pijnenborg et al 1981b). These latter cells are almost certainly static end cells; only the uninuclear cytotrophoblast apparently has the property of mobility. It seems likely that an undetermined proportion of the original invasive trophoblast perishes in the myometrium or is simply dispersed by the expansion of the placental site. The placental bed giant cells can be regarded as the sur-vivors until term (Fig. 39.14) and it is doubtful that they have a rôle to play in the second half of pregnancy. Be that as it may, they usually disappear within about a week after parturition (Boyd & Hamilton 1970). In pregnancies in which physiological changes fail to occur in spiral arteries at the decidual–myometrial junction, there is normal migration of interstitial trophoblast into the

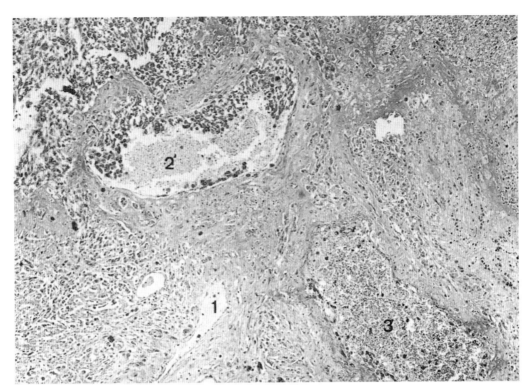

Fig. 39.15 First-trimester pregnancy: several cuts (1,2,3) through a tortuous, decidual spiral (uteroplacental) artery. In 1 the lumen is empty while in 2, the opening into the intervillous space, endovascular cytotrophoblast is entering the vessel from the surrounding shell.

uterine wall, but the prevalence of multinucleated giant cells at this junction is much increased before 36 weeks gestation. This may be an expression of disturbed migration of trophoblastic cells into the arterial wall (Gerretsen et al 1983).

DEVELOPMENT OF THE UTEROPLACENTAL VASCULATURE

One subset of non-villous trophoblast, if indeed it is a distinctive variety, does have an observable function, the attack upon and opening up of the maternal vessels. In the early weeks of gestation sheets of cytotrophoblast proliferating from the original cytotrophoblastic shell (Harris & Ramsey 1966), and later from the tips of villi (Pijnenborg et al 1980), can be seen penetrating the walls of decidual spiral arteries and forming plugs of such cells in the lumens (Fig. 39.15). These plugs are loose and often intermingled with detached endothelial cells. They migrate in a retrograde fashion. It is, however, uncertain whether they are truly incorporated in the vessel wall. In fact, extravillous interstitial trophoblast cells usually concentrate around and possibly within uteroplacental arteries. The interaction between the mural trophoblast and the tissues native to the vessel wall is accompanied by extensive fibrinoid deposition (Fig. 39.16), a mixture of maternal fibrin and microfibrillary material elaborated by the trophoblast (De Wolf et al 1973). The net effect is the

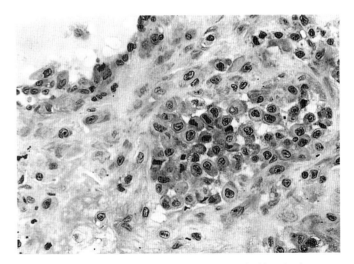

Fig. 39.16 Decidual spiral artery with cytotrophoblast in the lumen and within its wall, the latter phenomenon accompanied by fibrinoid deposition. Plentiful cyto and syncytial interstitial non-villous trophoblast and endometrial granulocytes can be seen in the surrounding decidua.

ultimate conversion of the decidual segments of the spiral arteries of the placental bed to distended sinusoidal vessels lacking musculoelastic tissue so that they become virtually passive fibrinoid tubes (Fig. 39.17). It was to this mode of conversion of the small spiral arteries to large capacity uteroplacental arteries that Brosens et al (1967) gave the name 'physiological changes'.

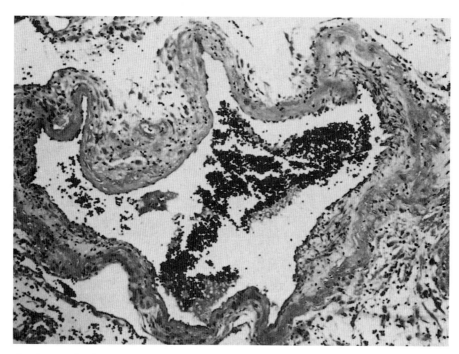

Fig. 39.17 Third-trimester pregnancy: at this stage the decidual segment of the uteroplacental artery has evolved into a distended, sinusoidal vessel, the wall of which is composed largely of fibrinoid and fibrous tissue with little musculo-elastic tissue remaining.

In many species there are separate waves of endovascular trophoblast migration (Pijnenborg et al 1981a) and this feature has been found also in human pregnancy (Robertson et al 1975; Pijnenborg et al 1983. It is, however, unclear how a second wave of migration could exist against a truly established blood flow in the uteroplacental arteries. The physiological vascular changes of the decidual segments of the spiral arteries are essentially completed by about the tenth week of gestation as is the definitive form of the fetal placenta. Subsequent growth of the placental site would then appear to occur simply by expansion commensurate with growth of the feto-placental unit (Gruenwald 1972). However, two recent papers have demonstrated the presence of endothelial cells in the lining of the basal plate; these are explained by the peripheral extension of the placenta incorporating peripheral veins (Craven et al 2000; Nanaev et al 2000). Clearly, Fig. 39.18 depicts a continuous endothelial lining beneath the periphery of an early (6 weeks) placenta. This evolution could be a link between the early deciduochorial and late haemochorial placenta. However, the process is not yet complete because it is doubtful if the uteroplacental vasculature elaborated for the first trimester could satisfy the increasing demands made upon it in the second and third trimesters. At about 14–16 weeks gestation, the remnants of the trophoblastic shell are freed in the uteroplacental arteries and probably migrate to the myometrial segments of vessels (second wave of endovascular migration) (Fig. 39.18) which, it will be recalled, have already been altered in their morphology

(Fig. 39.19), presumably because of their close association with migratory interstitial cytotrophoblast. An interaction indentical to that which took place in the decidual arteries between the endovascular trophoblast and the vessel wall now ensues in the myometrial segments (De Wolf et al 1980a) with progressive distension of the vessel, probably going on well into the third trimester (Fig. 39.20) (Table 39.1). Although no detailed studies of the decidual or myometrial veins have been undertaken, a similar transformation of the decidual veins has been noted (Brosens et al 1967) but for some unknown reason the myometrial veins are left relatively undisturbed in their morphology although they increase enormously in calibre. A system has thus been elaborated of a low resistance, high conductance (Moll et al 1975) arterial supply to the intervillous space of the fetal placenta capable of delivering something in excess of half a litre of blood per minute during the third trimester. Figure 39.21 gives a diagrammatic representation of the fully developed blood supply to the placenta.

PLACENTAL BED PATHOLOGY

HYPERTENSIVE DISORDERS OF PREGNANCY

During a normal pregnancy there is a tendency for the blood pressure to fall slightly until mid-gestation then to rise gradually to the pre-pregnancy level or somewhat higher in the last few weeks and during labour (Hytten & Leitch 1971). Particularly in primipara (Chesley 1980),

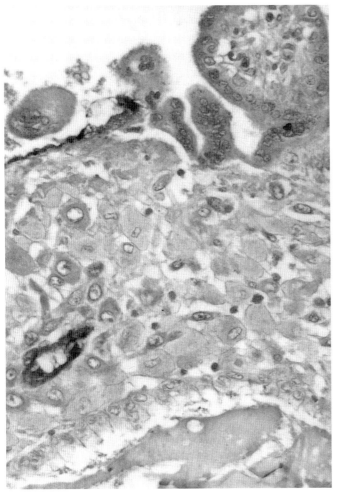

Fig. 39.18 Endothelial cells are clearly delineated in a small basal artery and within the lining of the basal plate facing the intervillous space. (Immunostain for CD31 with hematoxylin counterstain.)

1. a hypoxic state at the materno-embryonic interface is a prerequisite for the development of the illness;
2. the function of extravillous trophoblast is defective and physiological changes of maternal vessels are deficient;
3. endothelial cells, especially the maternal ones, are altered and produce vasoconstrictive molecules;
4. there is a production of oxygen free radicals and lipid peroxides which are quite toxic for endothelial cells. A recent study has shown that invasive cytotrophoblast from pre-eclamptic women shows increased expression of xanthine oxidase which is implicated in the generation of superoxide anion radicals and hydrogen peroxide (Many et al 2000);
5. vascular endothelial growth factor (VEGF) of placental origin is produced in increased amounts and can induce endothelial dysfunction (Dekker & Sibai 1998; Roberts 1998; Zhou et al 1998; Hayman et al 1999).

The pathology of pre-eclampsia is now better defined, at least in its morphological aspects, providing a more logical approach to the determination of aetiological factors. In the first place it seems likely that the stage is set during the second trimester for the clinical manifestations of the disorder in the third trimester. Consistently in cases of pre-eclampsia, whether arising de novo or superimposed upon essential hypertension or renal disease, the second wave of endovascular trophoblast migration into the myometrial segments of the spiral (uteroplacental) arteries does not occur (Brosens et al 1972) so that these arterial segments remain unaffected by the adaptive physiological vascular changes (Fig. 39.22, cf. Fig. 39.20) throughout the whole course of pregnancy. In addition, complete absence of physiological changes throughout the entire length of both decidual and myometrial segments of some spiral arteries has been demonstrated in a study of basal plates of placentas (Khong et al 1986). Partial and incomplete physiological changes restricted to less than 50% of the circumference of vessels have been noted in a study of placental bed spiral arteries in hypertensive pregnancies (Pijnenborg et al 1991), suggesting that the inhibition of trophoblastic invasion is by no means a uniform process or an 'all or none' phenomenon. These findings all point to a defect in the normal interaction between migratory trophoblast and maternal uterine tissues, which could be due to increased resistance on the part of maternal tissue or to decreased aggressiveness of the trophoblast or to a combination of both. Whatever the mechanism may be, the consequence during the late second trimester and for the whole of the third is a compromised blood supply to the intervillous space (Fig. 39.23). Previously, it was puzzling why the rise in blood pressure and the onset of proteinuria should be delayed by up to 10 weeks or more, since the second wave of endovascular trophoblast migration normally gets under way by the 16th week of gestation at the latest. However, the timing and

the disorder now known as pre-eclampsia (the terms 'toxaemia of pregnancy' and 'pre-eclamptic toxaemia' should be abandoned as there is no evidence of a toxin in the disorder) may appear in the third trimester and is characterised by a rapidly rising blood pressure, proteinuria and, in severe cases, generalised oedema. Diagnosis and definitions present difficulties when the clinical manifestations are mild or variable, but the classification of Davey & MacGillivray (1988), which groups patients with hypertension and/or proteinuria in pregnancy into clearly defined categories, is useful. Failing intervention by the clinician the disorder may be complicated by epileptiform fits, overt eclampsia, before, during, or after labour and death may result from cerebral haemorrhage, renal or liver failure and other complications. Women who have essential hypertension or renal disease have a greater than average risk of developing superimposed pre-eclampsia.

The aetiology of the disorder is not completely understood but there is evidence that:

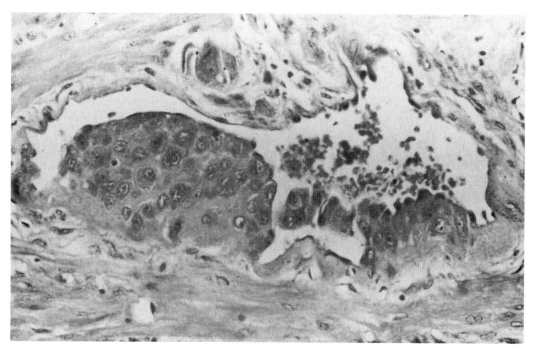

Fig. 39.19 Sixteen weeks gestation: myometrial spiral artery, already altered in morphology (see Fig. 39.13) to resemble a vein, containing an intimal collection of cytotrophoblast from the second endovascular migration. Note that endothelial cells cover the trophoblast.

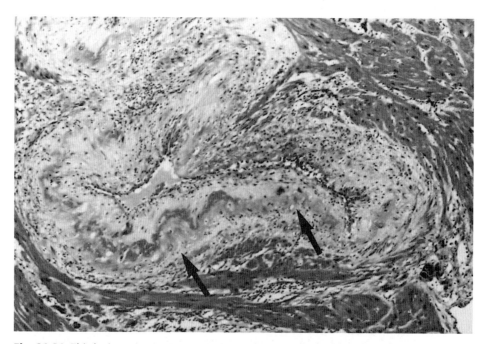

Fig. 39.20 Third-trimester pregnancy: myometrial spiral artery with fully developed physiological changes. The uteroplacental artery, which is artifactually collapsed, has a wall composed largely of fibrinoid with incorporated trophoblast (arrows) and fibrous tissue, there being little residual musculo-elastic tissue.

extent of trophoblastic invasion may be more variable than is usually assumed. In normal pregnancy, about 32% of spiral arteries have undergone physiological changes by 16–18 weeks (Pijnenborg et al 1983), but almost all of the 100–150 arteries show physiological changes by term. This suggests that trophoblastic invasion of the myome-

trial segments, and the development of physiological changes in the spiral arteries, continues throughout pregnancy and is not restricted to the first two trimesters (Pijnenborg et al 1991).

Nevertheless, Khong et al (1986) consider there to have been sufficient investigations of the placental bed at

Table 39.1 Physiological changes of intra-uterine arteries

I. Myometrial radiate arteries
- Loss of internal elastic lamina
- Decrease of the thickness of the media

II. Uteroplacental arteries
- Loss of elastic fibers and smooth muscle cells
- Decrease of the content of extracellular matrix
- Incorporation of extravillous trophoblast
- Widening of the lumen
- Important tortuosity

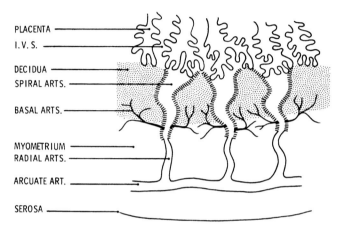

PLACENTA
I.V.S.
DECIDUA
SPIRAL ARTS.
BASAL ARTS.
MYOMETRIUM
RADIAL ARTS.
ARCUATE ART.
SEROSA

Fig. 39.21 Diagram of the uteroplacental blood supply during the third trimester. The venous drainage, which in general parallels the arterial supply, is not shown. Note that the basal arteries (black) are not involved with physiological vascular changes.

or near term in normal pregnancies and enough of normal preterm pregnancies to confirm that intraluminal/endovascular trophoblast is a rare finding in the third trimester of normal pregnancy (Brosens et al 1967). Therefore the presence of luminal endovascular trophoblast in uteroplacental arteries in the third trimester in abnormal pregnancies complicated by pre-eclampsia and/or babies with a birth weight less than the tenth centile for gestational age, is taken as evidence of defective interaction between fetal and maternal tissues (Khong et al 1986).

When the clinical manifestations of pre-eclampsia do appear, pathological lesions are inflicted upon the uteroplacental arteries and their branches and upon small arteries in the decidua vera remote from the placental bed. The archetypal lesion, acute atherosis (Fig. 39.24), was first described by Hertig (1945), elaborated upon by Zeek & Assali (1950), and has been the subject of many studies since (Dixon & Robertson 1958; Brosens 1964; Maqueo et al 1964; Robertson et al 1967, 1975, 1976; Sheppard & Bonnar 1976, 1980; Gerretsen et al 1981; Hustin et al 1983) with more recent reviews by Labarrere (1988) and Khong (1991). The arteriopathy is characterised by a fibrinoid-type necrosis of the whole vessel wall in small decidual arteries with the distinctive feature of an accumulation of lipophages in the damaged wall and an inconstant infiltrate of round cells in the vicinity. Ultrastructural studies (De Wolf et al 1975; Sheppard & Bonnar 1976; Shanklin & Sibai 1989) have

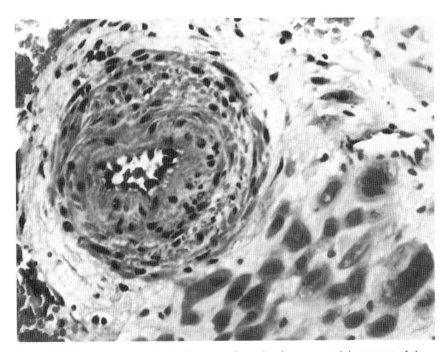

Fig. 39.22 Pregnancy complicated by pre-eclampsia: the myometrial segment of the spiral artery, having *not* been colonised by the second wave of endovascular trophoblast migration, shows no physiological changes (cf. Fig. 39.19) despite the presence of abundant interstitial trophoblast, including giant cells, near the vessel.

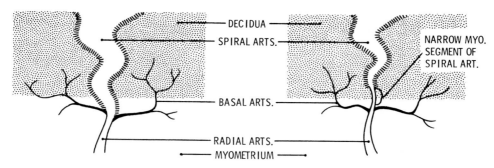

Fig. 39.23 Extent of physiological changes in the uteroplacental arteries in normal and pre-eclamptic pregnancies. In the latter the failure of the second wave of endovascular trophoblast migration leaves the myometrial segments of the spiral arteries as constricted high-resistance vessels from the second trimester until term.

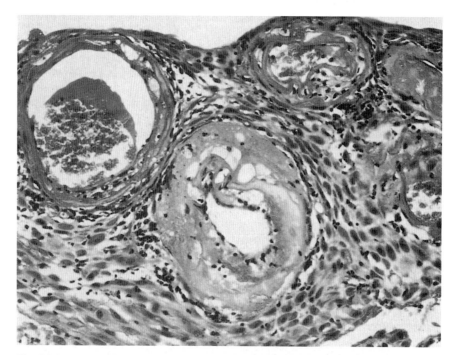

Fig. 39.24 Acute atherosis in the decidua vera of a pregnancy complicated by pre-eclampsia. The spiral arteries show extensive fibrinoid necrosis with intramural lipophages and a mild perivascular mononuclear infiltrate.

shown that the lipid-bearing cells are of two types: damaged myointimal cells and macrophages phagocytosing cell debris, so that there is some analogy with the development of atheroma to justify the name given to this idiosyncratic vasculopathy of pre-eclampsia. The pathogenesis of the lesion is unresolved with altered haemodynamic influences and inappropriate immunological feto-maternal reactions or a combination of both as the current chief contenders (Robertson et al 1967; Kitzmiller & Benirschke 1973). Immunohistochemical studies often reveal extensive deposition of IgM and C3 in decidual arteries with acute atherosis in pre-eclampsia (Hustin et al 1983) and these deposits have also been found in similar vessels in pregnant patients with autoim-

mune diseases (Labarrere et al 1986) and in atherosis-like lesions from rejected renal and cardiac homograft transplants (Porter 1974; Palmer et al 1985) and after hepatic transplantation (Demetris et al 1985). Acute atherosis is restricted to the pregnant uterus, however, and its topography is of interest in that it is seen best and in its pure form in the small arteries in the decidua vera or parietalis remote from any trophoblast, the nearest being the thin rim of chorion of the membranes. Similarly, in the placental bed, it affects small basal arteries which do not communicate with the intervillous space and also the decidual and myometrial segments of the uteroplacental spiral arteries that have *not* undergone physiological changes (Fig. 39.25) and therefore contain no trophoblast

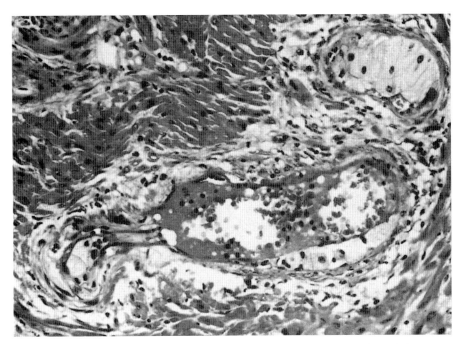

Fig. 39.25 Pre-eclampsia: myometrial spiral artery, unaffected by physiological changes, showing advanced acute atherosis.

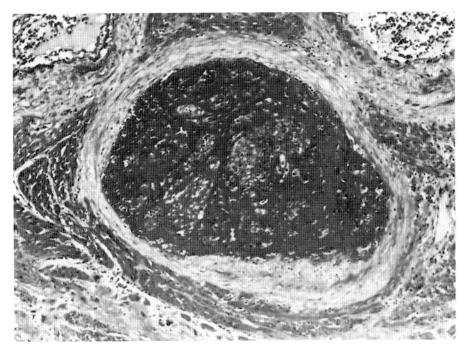

Fig. 39.26 Placental bed biopsy from a case of severe pre-eclampsia showing occlusive thrombosis of a uteroplacental artery.

in their walls. It is therefore difficult to accept that some form of immunological reaction between trophoblast and the maternal vessel wall is involved. If such a reaction were humoral, with the formation of immune complexes, it could be anticipated that acute atherosis would be found in pre-eclamptic women at sites other than the uterus and such lesions have never been reported

although necrotising arterial lesions occur in the liver, brain and other organs in fatal cases of eclampsia (Govan 1976). The higher incidence and severity of chronic villitis of unknown aetiology in placentas from pre-eclamptic cases has led to the suggestion that this may represent a feto-maternal immunological reaction (Labarrere & Althabe 1985, 1986). Whatever the pathogenesis of the

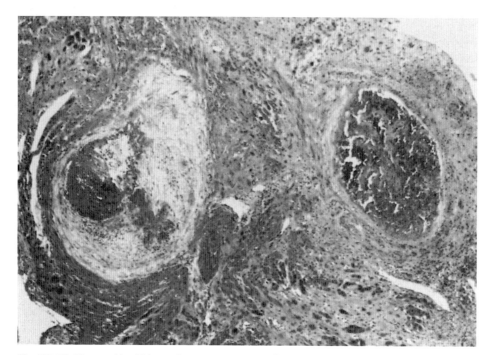

Fig. 39.27 Placental bed biopsy from a severe case of pre-eclampsia with placental abruption: recent upon organising thrombosis of a uteroplacental artery with decidual necrosis (right).

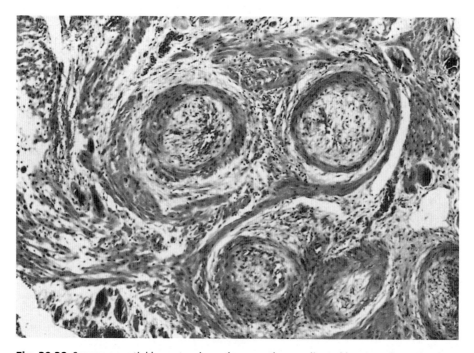

Fig. 39.28 Severe essential hypertension subsequently complicated by pre-eclampsia: the myometrial segments of the spiral (uteroplacental) arteries show marked hyperplastic arteriosclerosis but no trophoblast-induced physiological changes. The myometrium contains placental bed giant cells.

vasculopathies of pre-eclampsia may be, there can be little doubt that they offer the best explanation for occlusive thrombosis (Fig. 39.26) with resultant placental infarction (Brosens & Renaer 1972), decidual necrosis, placental abruption and antepartum haemorrhage (Fig. 39.27),

all of which are relatively common complications of the hypertensive disorders of pregnancy.

Recently, it has been demonstrated that an excess of macrophages in and around uteroplacental arteries showing reduced trophoblast invasion in pre-eclampsia may be responsible for inducing apoptosis in extravillous trophoblast and thereby limiting trophoblastic invasion of those spiral arteries (Reister et al 2001).

When pre-eclampsia is superimposed upon pre-existing essential hypertension or renal disease the resultant pathology is more complex. Women with essential hypertension who complete their pregnancies without developing pre-eclampsia usually deliver babies of normal or even above normal weight (MacGillivray 1975). In these circumstances it will be found that the maternal vascular response to placentation is perfectly adequate with the development of physiological changes in the uteroplacental arteries right down to the terminations of the parent radial arteries. In other cases of chronic hypertension, and where pre-eclampsia does complicate the pregnancy, the physiological changes will be found to be restricted to the decidual segments of the uteroplacental arteries but, presumably because of the effect of the hypertension on the high-resistance myometrial segments which are unchanged by the action of endovascular trophoblast, these segments show remarkable hyperplastic changes with apparent luminal stenosis (Fig. 39.28). Since such vascular pathology is not usually seen outside the uterus in hypertensive women of this age group, this exaggerated response to hypertension in the uteroplacental vasculature is probably related to the special haemodynamic requirements of the pregnant uterus (Table 39.2). However, there is a suggestion that, in arteries with partial physiological changes in hypertensive pregnancies, subintimal proliferation may represent an overreaction to physiological trophoblastic invasion (Pijnenborg et al

Table 39.2 Intra-uterine arteries and pre-eclampsia

I.	**Myometrial radiate arteries**
	• 'Normal' thickness of the media
	• Persistence of the internal elastic lamina
	• Myofibroblastic subintimal proliferation
II.	**Uteroplacental arteries**
	• Presence of a more or less preserved media
	• Reduction in mural trophoblastic incorporation
	• Acute atherosis (segmental)
	• Endothelial cell lesions
	• Thromboses

1991). We have not encountered internal cushion formation in the absence of an internal elastic lamina. Endothelial vacuolation in uteroplacental arteries is also common in cases of chronic hypertension (Pijnenborg et al 1991) and is probably the visible expression of endothelial dysfunction. It must be remembered that the placental floor is covered at term with tens of thousands of maternal endothelial cells. Therefore this part of the intervillous space must be considered an important extension of the maternal vascular space. Any endothelial alteration will of course have rapid and obvious manifestations (Hustin & Jauniaux 2000).

The deleterious effects of pre-eclampsia upon the hyperplastic vessels make bad matters worse as acute atherosis is now superimposed upon arteriosclerosis (Fig. 39.29). It is scarcely surprising that a pregnant woman with essential hypertension who subsequently develops pre-eclampsia carries a much higher than average risk of perinatal morbidity and mortality for her

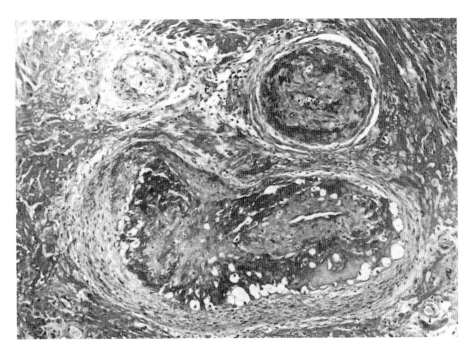

Fig. 39.29 Essential hypertension with superimposed pre-eclampsia: the hyperplastic myometrial spiral arteries are further damaged by acute atherosis with numerous foam cells in the fibrinoid necrosis.

baby. A similar sequence of events may occur in women with overt or latent renal disease during pregnancy and, in fact, a woman who has recurrent pre-eclampsia in sequential pregnancies should be investigated for the possibility of latent renal disease or other predisposing disorders (Chesley 1980).

INTRAUTERINE FETAL GROWTH RETARDATION

In most, but not in all, cases of pregnancy hypertension with proteinuria the neonate is in the lower centiles for birth weight, even allowing for the higher incidence of premature delivery. The inadequate uteroplacental blood supply and associated vascular and placental lesions provide an acceptable explanation for this outcome but what about those cases of intrauterine growth retardation (IUGR) where there is no hypertension or other cause, such as maternal cigarette smoking, to incriminate? It has been claimed (Sheppard & Bonnar 1976, 1980) that severe intrauterine growth retardation is always associated with atherotic lesions of the uteroplacental arteries and resultant placental damage irrespective of the level of the blood pressure and that an inadequate physiological vascular response to placentation is inconstant in intrauterine growth retardation and in pre-eclampsia. Others disagree (Brosens et al 1977; Gerretsen et al 1981), maintaining that acute atherosis, defined as a necrotising arteriopathy affecting vessels *not* showing trophoblast-induced physiological changes, is virtually pathognomonic of pre-eclampsia and that restriction of the physiological changes to the decidual vessels is consistent in pre-eclampsia but inconstant and variable in idiopathic intrauterine growth retardation.

It has been shown that in those cases with intrauterine growth retardation without pre-ecelampsia, the myo-

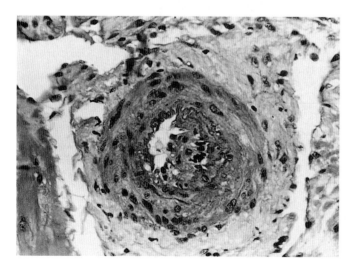

Fig. 39.30 Placental bed biopsy from a case of intrauterine growth retardation *not* due to hypertensive disorders. Note the eccentric intimal cushion, the presence of an internal elastic lamina and of a thick layer of smooth muscle cells. Orcein + H & E.

metrial radiate arteries may exhibit an almost normal non-gravid structure, i.e. with a normal media and a prominent internal elastic lamina (Hustin et al 1983). Moreover, subintimal myofibroblastic cushions may be prominent with new formation of elastic tissue (Fig. 39.30).

The aetiology of intrauterine growth retardation is complex and whilst, logically, an insufficient blood flow to the placenta is the first abnormality to suspect, quite clearly many other factors may play a rôle including infections and genetic abnormalities. Moreover, a significant proportion of intrauterine growth retardation cases are associated with placental findings which point to problems in the organisation and efficiency of the feto-placental circulation.

A small fetus is usually attached to a small placenta and it could be argued that the placenta is small commensurate with the fetus (Gruenwald 1975; Fox 1976) rather than that the fetus is small because of a damaged and inadequate placenta. In a majority of cases of intrauterine growth retardation the small fetus cannot be explained by so-called 'placental insufficiency' for which there is little morphological or other evidence (Fox 1976, 1981, 2000). Intrauterine growth retardation probably starts early in gestation although it is usually only detected clinically in the third trimester and it is also false to argue that the small feto-placental unit is the result of acute lesions occurring late in the third trimester (Robertson et al 1981).

OTHER SYSTEMIC DISORDERS

Diabetes mellitus

Diabetes mellitus complicating pregnancy brings its own special problems. Despite better control of glucose metabolism there is still a higher than average incidence of complications during pregnancy, of perinatal morbidity and mortality and of congenital malformations in babies born to diabetic mothers. Not unnaturally, because of the well-known deleterious effect of diabetes on large and small blood vessels, attention has been focused on the placenta (Fox 1979, 1997) and, in particular, upon the uteroplacental vasculature (Driscoll 1965). The results of many studies, however, have been equivocal because of the failure by the authors to distinguish vasculopathies attributable to other complications of diabetic pregnancies, such as hypertensive disorders, from those due to the diabetes per se (Robertson 1979). A study (Kitzmiller et al 1981), carefully avoiding these pitfalls, recorded acute vasculopathies (extensive atherosis and fibrinoid deposits) in the decidua of 30% of pregnant diabetic women who did not have established hypertension or pre-eclampsia and similar vasculopathies in 50% of diabetic women with hypertension. Deposits of IgM and C3 were detected in arteries with atherosis. Hustin et al (1983) could not confirm these findings.

Systemic lupus erythematosus

On becoming pregnant a woman with systemic lupus erythematosus (SLE) may experience a worsening of her condition and have miscarriage, stillbirth or deliver a baby with intrauterine growth retardation (Jungers et al 1982). Hypertension with proteinuria due to lupus nephritis produces a syndrome akin to pre-eclampsia and acute atherosis may be found in the decidua (Abramowsky et al 1980). Labarrere et al (1986) have also found this lesion in the basal and parietal decidua of patients with SLE, associated with an absence of physiological changes in the basal plate. Massive deposits of IgM and a smaller amount of C3 and C1q were also present in these acute atherotic lesions. Similar findings were also noted in cases of scleroderma and idiopathic thrombocytopenic purpura. In some women with SLE and in others without the stigmata of SLE a plasma factor, somewhat paradoxically called lupus anticoagulant, may be present (Carreras et al 1981; Vermulen et al 1981; Branch et al 1985). This factor and another antibody, i.e. anticardiolipin, are associated with various pathological conditions of pregnancy encompassing pre-eclampsia, fetal loss, thromboses, autoimmune thrombocytopenia and placental infarction. Several mechanisms have been postulated to explain the syndrome: they include — inhibition of vascular-prostacyclin production (by blockade of the release of arachidonic acid from endothelial cells (Rustin et al 1988) — interference with thrombomodulin (Cariou et al 1988), tissue plasminogen activity (Francis et al 1988), protein S (Moreb & Kitchens 1989) or antithrombin III (Cosgriff & Martin 1981).

The complete antiphospholipid syndrome is thus linked to maternal vascular problems either through endothelial dysfunction or platelet activation. The first site to be involved is of course the uterus: most cases of second or early third trimester fetal deaths, with significant placental ischaemic lesions show arterial thromboses with or without acute atherosis in the basal plate. They are significantly associated with autoimmune problems. It has been recently demonstrated that a significant subset of patients with recurrent miscarriages have elevated levels of antibodies against endothelial cells (Roussev et al 1998).

OTHER DEFECTS OF PLACENTATION

It is self-evident that the complex interactions between fetal and maternal tissues essential for the establishment and maintenance of haemochorial placentation will be defective on occasions but we know remarkably little, as is obvious from the situation in pre-eclampsia, about the mechanisms and even of the morphological background of many such mishaps. Perhaps the most compelling aspect of human placentation requiring elucidation relates to the promotional and controlling factors regulating trophoblast migration, which appears to be an essential prerequisite of haemochorial placentation. Many papers have been published in recent years discussing the regulation of trophoblast penetration in the decidua and into the inner portion of the myometrium. It has been demonstrated, for example, that extravillous trophoblast possesses several membrane molecules which can bind to proteins of the extracellular matrix (Nawrocki et al 1997) and thereby undertake progressive invasion of the decidua. Intravascular trophoblastic cells are, for a while, attached to the trophoblastic shell; they form loose plugs in the vessel lumen. When the growth of the conceptus has stretched the trophoblast shell to the limits of rupture, the plugs are freed in the uteroplacental artery and isolated trophoblastic cells detach and stick to the endothelial layer. A significant blood flow has been initiated by this time. It is clear that early pathological events in pregnancy are linked to these phenomena which occur during the early weeks when the placenta is still deciduochorial and when the embryo must rely on the extraplacental adnexa (extra-embryonic coelom and secondary yolk sac) for transfer functions. Later on, the initiation of a timely blood flow in the intervillous space is critical.

SPONTANEOUS MISCARRIAGE

Although the pathology of early pregnancy loss or miscarriage is dealt with fully elsewhere, new insights into its pathogenesis suggest that defective placentation is highly relevant. In particular it has become evident that the presence of intravascular trophoblast plugs is critical. Fox & Wells (1998), have emphasised the harmful consequences of inadequate placentation, which could lead to premature entry of maternal blood into the intervillous space.

It has been suggested that, in quite a number of aneuploid pregnancies, abnormalities of heart activity and umbilical blood flow can be detected (Jauniaux et al 1996). In most of these cases, trophoblast development, especially extravillous, is impaired. It has been demonstrated that in a substantial number of miscarriages, there is an almost complete absence of intravascular trophoblast plugs (Fig. 39.31). Physiological changes of uteroplacental arteries are frequently lacking and the trophoblast shell is markedly hypoplastic or absent (Hustin et al 1990). All these findings point to an untimely initiation of significant maternal blood flow in the intervillous space. This uncontrolled flow is associated with an increase in the pressure within the intervillous space which in turn induces collapse of villous capillaries and eventually arrest of the embryoplacental circulation (Fig. 39.31).

A secondary event is abruptio: the excessive maternal flow pours through the remnants of the trophoblastic shell and dissects the maternal decidua which in its turn undergoes necrosis (Hustin & Jauniaux 2000) (Fig. 39.32).

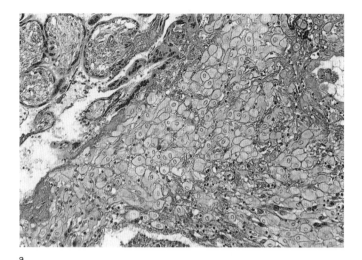

a

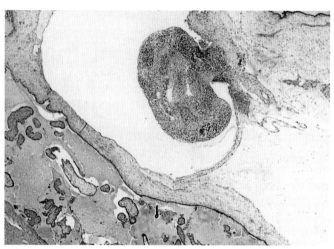

Fig. 39.32 Spontaneous expulsion of first trimester pregnancy. The amniotic cavity contains a stunted embryo. The placenta is markedly hypoplastic and the intervillous space is filled with fresh blood.

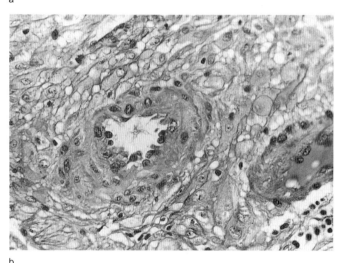

b

Fig. 39.31 Curettage specimen of first-trimester miscarriage
a The placental bed is almost devoid of interstitial trophoblast.
b This spiral artery does not contain intravascular trophoblast. Physiological changes are practically absent.

TROPHOBLASTIC DISEASE

Once again, although this subject is dealt with at length in Chapter 40 it may well have a bearing on placentation and its regulatory mechanisms. In the typical example of complete molar pregnancy there is failure to form an embryo but placental development, albeit abnormal, continues and excessive villous trophoblast proliferation is a common feature. Interestingly, except in the very rare case of placental site trophoblastic tumour, the extravillous trophoblast accompanying hydatidiform moles does not display the usual infiltrative pattern. Instead, one encounters a more or less straight superficial lining of trophoblast covering a layer of necrotic tissue.

In some cases where hysterectomy has been performed with hydatidiform mole in situ, we have been impressed by the absence of true physiological changes in the decidual spiral arteries. A recent study has confirmed the lack of physiological change in these vessels in cases of com-

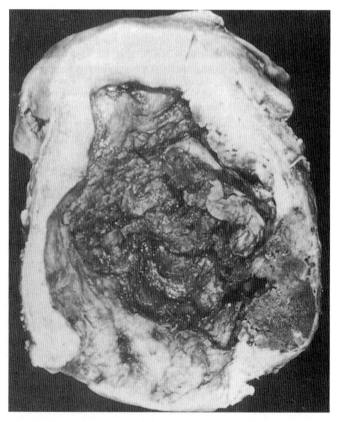

Fig. 39.33 Hysterectomy specimen from a case of placenta increta: penetration by placental villi deep into the lower segment myometrium has almost reached the serosa.

plete hydatidiform mole, though placentation appeared to occur normally in partial moles (Sebire et al 2001). Persistent trophoblastic disease with, as the term implies, survival and continued growth of trophoblast beyond its normal life span following a miscarriage or term pregnancy, is yet another example of failure of control of this inherently aggressive fetal tissue. At the worst extreme is the fortunately rare development of choriocarcinoma. Wells & Bulmer (1988) have summarised the results of immunohistological studies which, overall, are similar to those described in normal pregnancy.

PLACENTA CRETA

This condition is subdivided into placenta accreta where there is undue adhesion to the placental bed, increta where anchoring villi penetrate deeply into the myometrium (Fig. 39.33) and percreta where villi infiltrate right through the wall of the uterus. This undue adhesiveness or invasiveness may be total, more commonly partial or focal, and the depth of penetration may vary in different areas of the placental bed. The aetiology and pathogenesis of the condition are still debated but analysis of series of cases (Benirschke & Driscoll 1967; Fox 1972, 1978) provides information about its incidence, associations and natural history.

Fox (1972, 1997) has made a thorough survey of the aetiology of placenta creta, from a very large (622 cases) series. The most important predisposing factors are placenta praevia, previous uterine curettage and previous Caesarean section, all three accounting for 25 to 35% percent of cases. Also significant are previous manual removal of the placenta, cornual implantation, previous uterine sepsis and uterine fibroids (Khong & Robertson 1987), whereas previous uterine surgery and uterine malformation are of only marginal significance. Caesarean section is an important predisposing factor (Clark et al 1985).

The increasing use of endometrial resection by laser or electrosurgery is usually performed in women who do not wish to conceive. Nevertheless, pregnancy and the problem of placenta creta can occur just as it did previously following endometrial cauterisation (Wood & Rogers 1993).

The popular explanation for the development of placenta creta is a focal or diffuse deficiency of decidua permitting the anchoring villi and the fibrinoid basal plate to attach directly to the underlying myometrium and, in more severe cases, to penetrate deeply into the myometrium. Examination of sections (Fig. 39.34) through the adherent areas reveals an absence or paucity of decidua but with an excess of the cytotrophoblast that is a normal feature of the basal plate in late pregnancy (Fig. 39.35). Decidua has been regarded as a barrier to prevent undue invasiveness of trophoblast (Kirby & Cowell 1968; Finn & Porter 1975). The depth of trophoblast penetration in the decidua is linked to the presence of adhesion molecules which bind to extracellular matrix components (Damsky et al 1992; Aplin 1996). The relationship is complex and varies qualitatively according to the depth of trophoblast (i.e. trophoblast shell level, superficial or deep decidua). Fox (1997) has discussed the point in detail and largely favours, just like Benirschke & Kaufmann (1995), the concept of deficient or absent decidua. Other workers have claimed that a pericellular coating of glycoproteinous fibrinoid protects trophoblastic cells from immune attack (Kirby et al 1964; Currie & Bagshawe 1967). Both postulates have been questioned on morphological and other grounds (Wynn 1972; Robertson & Warner 1974; Pijnenborg et al 1981a)

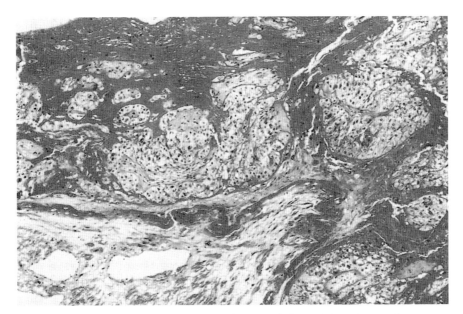

Fig. 39.34 Placenta accreta: the fibrinoid of the basal plate, without intervening decidua, abuts directly on the myometrium. The cytotrophoblast, a normal feature of the basal plate, is unusually prominent and hypertrophic.

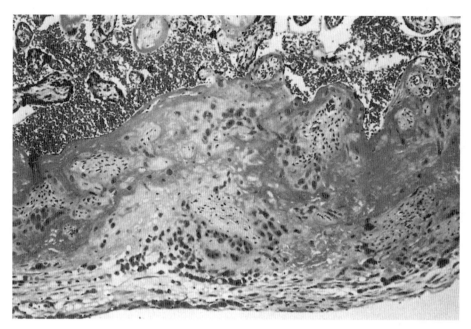

Fig. 39.35 Basal plate of a normal placenta showing fibrinoid, non-villous cytotrophoblast and adherent basal decidua.

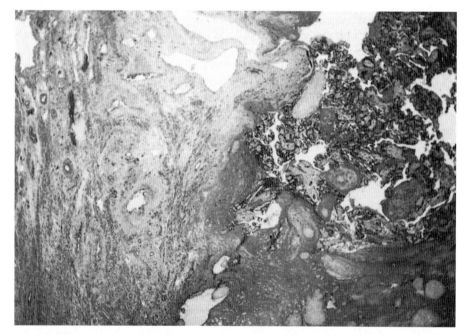

Fig. 39.36 Placenta praevia creta: the placenta (right) is deeply embedded in the lower uterine segment (left) in close proximity to large distended blood vessels.

and any barrier effect must at best be temporary as cytotrophoblast clearly sweeps through the decidua early in pregnancy to reach the myometrium. The example of ectopic pregnancy where implantation can and does occur without a constituted decidua is probably the best and most frequently encountered example of placenta creta. In utero, the decidua appears to constitute a temporary restraining, rather than an obstructive, tissue. A likely explanation of the pathogenesis of placenta accreta

is that nidation is achieved and the early stage of placentation is effected in a normal part of the endometrium but, as the placental site extends and enlarges, in areas of the placental bed such as those near scars or in the lower segment, isthmus or upper cervical canal of the uterus where decidualisation is less than adequate, the invasive non-villous trophoblast overwhelms the poorly decidualised mucosa to achieve deep penetration (Robertson et al 1985). This would account for the fact that placenta creta is usually only partial and, in cases of placenta praevia, restricted to that part of the placenta embedded in the lower segment, isthmus and cervical canal (Fig. 39.36).

Placenta creta is rare in primiparae; its incidence increases with age and parity; this may reflect the number of 'injuries' that a uterus must sustain during the reproductive years. It may also be that the regulation of trophoblast penetration varies with time and increases with the number of gestations. This idea would be in keeping also with the not infrequent history in cases of placenta creta of the necessity for manual removal of the placenta in the previous pregnancy. The deep penetration of anchoring villi in placenta creta is accompanied by an extension of endovascular trophoblast migration with physiological vascular changes in larger calibre arteries such as the radials (Fig. 39.37) accounting for the torrential haemorrhage that may accompany attempted removal of the placenta in cases of placenta praevia with creta.

Khong & Robertson (1987) have confirmed the presence of an unusual uteroplacental vasculature in which physiological changes were present much more deeply than normally, in large arteries of the radial/arcuate system deep in the myometrium, while there were some superficial spiral arteries and some arteries deeper in the placental bed in closer proximity to abundant trophoblast, without physiological changes. They also found that there was no apparent diminution of decidua parietalis or, in cases of focal accreta, of adjacent basalis. The extravillous trophoblast was mainly uninuclear or binuclear, with a paucity of placental bed syncytial giant cells, in contrast to the findings in late normal placentation. There was an apparent proliferation of interstitial trophoblast at the junction of placenta with myometrium, but the density of interstitial trophoblast deeper in the myometrium was lower than in normal placentation. These findings suggest that there is defective interaction between maternal tissues, particularly decidua, and migratory trophoblast in the early stages of placentation, resulting in undue adherence of the placenta or penetration into the uterus coupled with the development of an abnormal uteroplacental circulation.

This hypothesis is supported by the albeit rare presentation of placenta creta before 20 weeks gestation: only about 10 such cases have been reported (Harden et al 1990) and the incidental finding of direct attachment of villi to the uterine musculature at the implantation site of an unsuspected 2.5 cm embryo in a uterus from a 'grand multipara' removed during the course of a prolapse repair (Begneaud et al 1965).

Immunohistologically, the phenotype of extravillous trophoblast populations is identical to that seen in normal placental tissue (Earl et al 1987).

ANTEPARTUM HAEMORRHAGE

The pathology of uterine bleeding during the second half of pregnancy, apart from that associated with late miscarriage, premature labour, placenta praevia and/or creta, and blood dyscrasias, is something of a mystery.

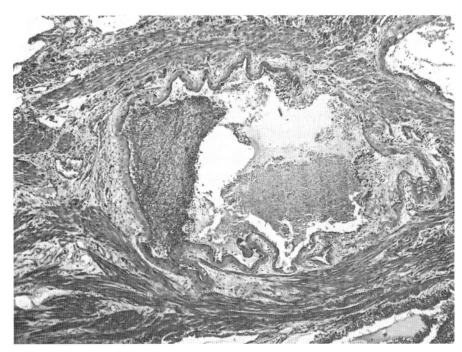

Fig. 39.37 Placenta accreta: physiological vascular changes in a radial artery deep in the myometrium.

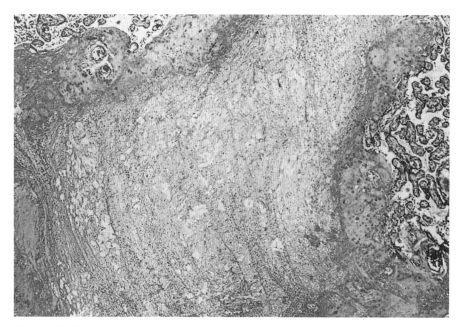

Fig. 39.38 Placenta from a normal pregnancy with a small retroplacental haematoma of some age in the basal decidua.

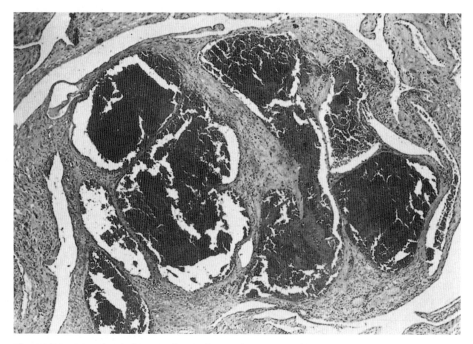

Fig. 39.39 Antepartum haemorrhage ultimately requiring hysterectomy, related to abnormal vascular configuration.

Clinically, antepartum haemorrhage (APH) presents as revealed or concealed 'accidental haemorrhage' of varying degrees of severity from the trivial to the potentially life-threatening for the fetus and mother. Pathologically, it is associated with placental abruption, retroplacental bleeding and haematoma formation. That the condition is, to a minor degree, relatively common is evidenced by the not infrequent finding of small retroplacental haematomas (Fig. 39.38) of various ages on the maternal surface of delivered placentas where the pregnancies and deliveries

have been perfectly normal. Manifestly the bleeding is maternal and comes from the uteroplacental circulation but the precise cause of the bleeding is unknown (Fox 1997), although it is presumed by most to be triggered off by decidual necrosis with involvement of uteroplacental arteries; only a minority consider the bleeding to come from ruptured veins.

Ignorance of the pathogenesis of the various lesions of the basal decidua and basal plate is due to the fact that all pathological studies and deductions so far have had to be made on the delivered fetal placenta. An extensive review of the placentas from 21 784 deliveries by Gruenwald et al (1968) produced valuable clinicopathological correlations of what they termed clinical 'abruption' and pathological 'separation', the former obviously detected by the obstetricians and the latter only by the pathologists. They could shed no light on the actual pathogenesis of the retroplacental pathology. A similar state of affairs emerges from a later review (Gorodeski et al 1982). It is remarkable that serious vascular complications occur but rarely in the uteroplacental circulation during its establishment and evolution considering that Virchow's classical triad for thrombogenesis — damage to the vessel wall, changes in haemodynamics and alteration in the constituents of the blood — all occur during placentation. No doubt adjustments to systemic haemostatic mechanisms afford some protection against vascular complications but, as previously suggested, trophoblast must be equipped to prevent thrombosis in the vessels it colonises. In fact, trophoblast which enters the uteroplacental arteries changes its membrane expression and presents with intercellular adhesion proteins characteristic of endothelial cells. Moreover, new proteins are also expressed which allow interaction between trophoblast and endothelial cells (Zhou et al 1997). It can safely be assumed however that, as in all biological processes, there are occasional failures. This is certainly the case in the hypertensive disorders of pregnancy where decidual necrosis, placental abruption and haemorrhage are common, as already illustrated, but here the vascular lesions are a consequence, inter alia, of the raised blood pressure and, in general, they occur in vessels that have not been altered by trophoblast invasion. Furthermore, antepartum haemorrhage generally coexists with placental infarction only when a large retroplacental haematoma is formed, the latter most likely the immediate cause of the former. It would therefore seem likely that mechanisms other than thromboses in the uteroplacental vasculature will have to be found to explain antepartum haemorrhage in otherwise normal pregnancies, which constitute the largest proportion of this category of pregnancy complications.

In the very occasional hysterectomy specimen available from normotensive pregnancies complicated by severe antepartum haemorrhage, abnormal vascular configurations akin to arteriovenous malformations have been detected (Fig. 39.39). This finding, however, can be taken only as a hint that not every uteroplacental artery of the 120 or so transformed spiral arteries in normal pregnancy (Brosens & Dixon 1966) results in an architecturally perfect, or even adequate, vessel following the complicated interactions between trophoblast and the vessel wall in the first and second trimesters of pregnancy.

In a relatively recent study of placental bed biopsy specimens in placenta abruption, however, Dommisse & Tiltman (1992) found vascular malformations in four out of 12 biopsies, three of which were from normotensive

pregnancies. These lesions appeared to be somewhat different in structure to those previously detected. Although varying in size, each was a markedly dilated, complex vessel which, for the most part, resembled a vein with recent, non-occlusive thrombus in the lumen and a thin wall which contained no elastic lamina, trophoblast or fibrin. Elsewhere, however, the wall was thickened and showed sub-intimal fibrosis with fibrin and trophoblast deep to the thickening, and numerous smaller channels at the periphery. Near two of these malformations there was marked intramyometrial haemorrhage and, in one, this appeared to arise from the abnormal vessel. These lesions may represent arteriovenous communications and the sub-intimal fibrosis may indicate attempts at 'arterialisation' of veins subjected to arterial pressures; haemorrhages from such vessels may well be under sufficient

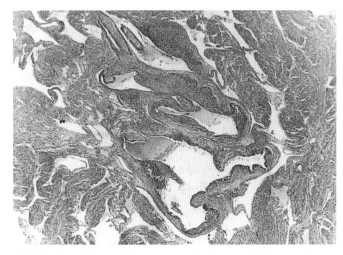

Fig. 39.40 Peripartum hysterectomy for intractable haemorrhage. The implantation site at the myometrial level had the appearance of a sponge filled with blood. It was composed of enormously distended lakes suggesting a vascular malformation.

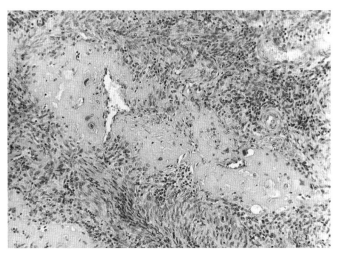

Fig. 39.41 Placental bed about one week postpartum with early involution of uteroplacental arteries. Note some residual trophoblast in the vessel wall.

pressure to track between muscle fibres. In seven of the 12 biopsies, there was absence of physiological transformation of uteroplacental arteries, but four of these were from hypertensive patients.

It must be remembered that arteriovenous shunts probably do exist in the pregnant uterus. Their existence has been postulated by Hustin & Jauniaux (1997) in the general scheme of uteroplacental vascularisation in early pregnancy. During the first weeks, the amount of maternal blood which effectively enters the intervillous space is extremely limited and very slowly percolates through the slits of the trophoblastic shell. Functional arteriovenous communications would significantly limit the flow of maternal blood in the uteroplacental arteries: most probably, these shunts cease to function in the second trimester when blood flow in the intervillous space is fully established. There may, however, be exceptions: we have, for example, encountered a patient with a twin pregnancy in a bicornuate uterus. Delivery by Caesarean section was followed by torrential life-threatening haemorrhage which necessitated hysterectomy. The left uterine cornu which hosted the implantation site was completely filled with numerous blood lakes giving the uterine wall a completely spongy appearance (Fig. 39.40).

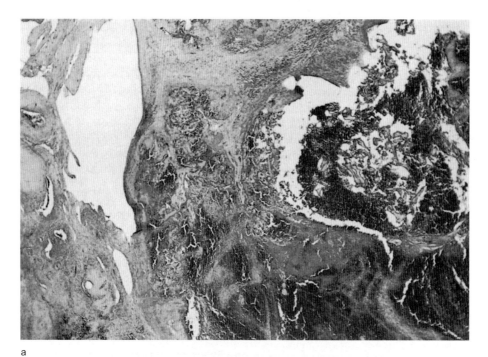

a

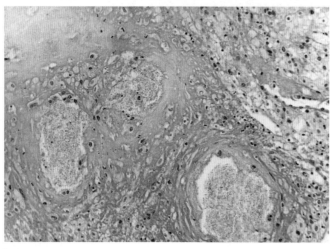

b

Fig. 39.42 Curettage specimen from a case of postpartum haemorrhage (PPH):
a A 'placental polyp' including retained villi admixed with haemorrhagic fibrinoid and partial involution of uteroplacental vessels (left). **b** Necrotic foci involving a uteroplacental artery.

POSTPARTUM HAEMORRHAGE

After delivery of the newborn and its placenta there is a rapid contraction of the parturient uterus accompanied by an equally rapid adjustment of haemostatic mechanisms (Bonnar et al 1969) to promote closure and thrombosis in the sheared decidual segments of the uteroplacental arteries and veins (Fig. 39.41). Failure of either or both processes may lead to serious primary postpartum bleeding. A commoner mishap occurring at various intervals after labour is secondary postpartum haemorrhage. It is often assumed that this form of haemorrhage is due to 'retained products of conception', implying retention of portions of the fetal placenta, but only in a minority of cases is a so-called placental polyp revealed on curettage (Fig. 39.42). In some, postpartum infection undoubtedly plays a rôle but, in the majority, curetted material yields neither placental villi nor evidence that infection is a major factor. The usual finding is of organising hyaline and decidualised tissue, perhaps containing effete nonvillous trophoblast, but the most significant feature is the presence of distended and partially hyalinised portions of the uteroplacental vessels containing organising thrombi of various ages, much of it very recent (Fig. 39.43), indicating partial failure or delay in the involution of the placental bed (Ober & Grady 1961; Robertson 1976; Khong & Khong 1993).

Involution of the pregnant uterus to the non-pregnant state is an ill-understood subject. It is remarkable that by the time of the first menstrual period following parturition the myometrial and endometrial segments of the spiral arteries, that were altered almost beyond recognition to become uteroplacental arteries, have reverted to the original morphology of small arteries in the uterus, or elsewhere in the body for that matter.

No systemic study has documented the disappearance of extravillous trophoblast from the placental bed following normal delivery, but it is generally considered that trophoblast persists for only 7–10 days postpartum. In a study of 22 cases of subinvolution, Andrew et al (1989) demonstrated the presence of extravillous trophoblast in a perivascular location and this was seen in larger amounts and more frequently around subinvoluted vessels than around involuted vessels in the same specimen. Trophoblast was not seen in control tissues which contained no subinvoluted vessels. Normally involuted vessels showed intimal proliferation with regeneration of the internal elastic lamina and hyalinisation of the medial tissue. Normal uteroplacental arteries showed replacement of endothelium by endovascular trophoblast in the first two trimesters, but they had generally re-endothelialised in the third trimester. The subinvoluted vessels possessed *no* endothelial lining and this may account for the presence of thrombi within these vessels. Persistence of endovascular trophoblast was seen in two of the cases of subinvolution. In a subsequent study these same workers showed that complement component and immunoglobulin deposition can be demonstrated in the walls of normally involuted vessels, but are absent in subinvoluted vessels (Andrew et al 1993). These findings suggest yet another abnormal materno-fetal relationship in vessels of the placental bed, possibly with an immunological dimension, this time in the postpartum period, manifesting itself as subinvolution.

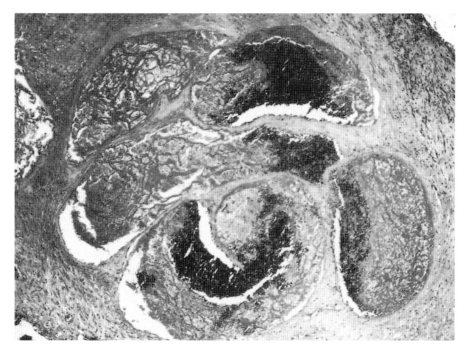

Fig. 39.43 Secondary postpartum haemorrhage: subinvolution of a leash of uteroplacental vessels which contain recent thrombi of various ages.

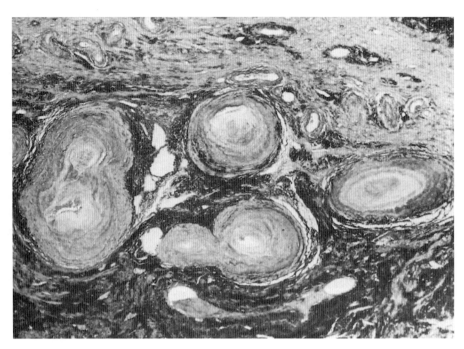

Fig. 39.44 Non-pregnant uterus from a 'grand multipara': the arcuate and radial arteries show laminated medial and intimal thickenings and there is much elastica-like material around the vessels. Orcein-van Gieson.

It would appear that it is interference with this process of vascular involution and reconstitution which is the commonest cause of secondary postpartum haemorrhage. The larger blood vessels of the uterus, that is the radials and arcuates, hardly ever involute completely so that it is usually easy to distinguish the histology of the parous from the nulliparous myometrium by the legacies of pregnancies left in the blood vessels. When the residua of pregnancies are excessive, the characteristic vascular features of intimal hyperplasia and medial lamination of hyalinised material (Fig. 39.44) form part of the bulky uterus of so-called subinvolution. Whether or not these features account for the symptoms, such as menorrhagia, associated with a clinical diagnosis of subinvolution of the uterus in the older parous woman has not been established.

REFERENCES

Abramowsky C R, Vegas M E, Swinehart G, Gyves M T 1980 Decidual vasculopathy of the placenta in lupus erythematosus. New England Journal of Medicine 303: 668–672

Althabe D, Labarrere C, Telenta M 1985 Maternal vascular lesions in placentae of small-for-gestational-age infants. Placenta 6: 265–276

Andrew A C, Bulmer J N, Wells M, Morrison L, Buckley C H 1989 Subinvolution of the uteroplacental arteries in the human placental bed. Histopathology 15: 395–405

Andrew A, Bulmer J N, Morrison L, Wells M, Buckley C H 1993 Subinvolution of the uteroplacental arteries: an immunohistochemical study. International Journal of Gynecological Pathology 12: 28–33

Aplin J 1996 The cell biology of human implantation. Placenta 17: 269–276

Argaud R 1903 Recherches sur la structure des artères chez l'homme. MD Thesis Toulouse, pp 56–69

Arias-Stella J 1973 Gestational endometrium. In: Norris H J, Hertig A T, Abell M R (eds) The uterus. Williams & Wilkins, Baltimore, pp 185–212

Arronet G H, Berquist C A, Parekh M C, Latour J P A, Marshall K G 1973 Evaluation of endometrial biopsy in the cycle of conception. International Journal of Fertility 18: 220–225

Begneaud W, Dougherty C M, Mickal A 1965 Placenta accreta in early gestation; report of 2 cases. American Journal of Obstetrics and Gynecology 92: 267–268

Benirschke K, Kaufmann P 1995 Pathology of the human placenta, 3rd edn. Springer-Verlag, Heidelberg

Bonnar J, McNicol C P, Douglas A S 1969 Fibrinolytic enzyme system and pregnancy. British Medical Journal 3: 387–389

Boyd J D, Hamilton W J 1970 The human placenta. Heffer, Cambridge

Branch D W, Scott J R, Kochenour N K, Hershgold E 1985 Obstetric complications associated with the lupus anticoagulant. New England Journal of Medicine 313: 1322–1326

Brosens I 1964 A study of the spiral arteries of the decidua basalis in normotensive and hypertensive pregnancies. Journal of Obstetrics and Gynaecology of the British Commonwealth 71: 222–230

Brosens I, Dixon H G 1966 The anatomy of the maternal side of the placenta. Journal of Obstetrics and Gynaecology of the British Commonwealth 73: 357–363

Brosens I, Renaer M 1972 On the pathogenesis of placental infarcts in preeclampsia. Journal of Obstetrics and Gynaecology of the British Commonwealth 79: 794–799

Brosens I, Robertson W B, Dixon H G 1967 The physiological response of the vessels of the placental bed to normal pregnancy. Journal of Pathology and Bacteriology 93: 569–579

Brosens I, Robertson W B, Dixon H G 1972 The role of the spiral arteries in the pathogenesis of preeclampsia. In: Wynn R M (ed) Obstetrics and gynecology annual 1. Appleton-Century-Crofts, New York, pp 177–191

Brosens I, Dixon H G, Robertson W B 1977 Fetal growth retardation and the arteries of the placental bed. British Journal of Obstetrics and Gynaecology 84: 656–664

Browne J C M, Veal L N 1953 The maternal placental blood flow in normotensive and hypertensive women. Journal of Obstetrics and Gynaecology of the British Empire 60: 141–147

Bulmer J N 1994 Human endometrial lymphocytes in normal pregnancy and pregnancy loss. Annals of the New York Academy of Sciences 734: 185–192

Burchell R C, Creed F, Rasoulpour M, Whitcomb M 1978 Vascular anatomy of the human uterus and pregnancy wastage. British Journal of Obstetrics and Gynaecology 85: 698–706

Buxton C L, Olson L E 1969 Endometrial biopsy inadvertently taken during conception cycle. American Journal of Obstetrics and Gynecology 105: 702–706

Cariou R O, Tobelem G, Bellucci S et al 1988 Effect of lupic anticoagulant on antithrombogenic properties of endothelial cells, inhibition of thrombomodulin dependent protein C activation. Thrombosis and Haemostasis 40: 54–58

Carreras L O, Machin S J, Denman R et al 1981 Arterial thrombosis, intrauterine death and lupus anticoagulant: detection of immunoglobulin interfering with prostacyclin formation. Lancet 1: 244–246

Chesley L C 1980 Evolution of concepts of eclampsia. In: Bonnar J, MacGillivray I, Symonds E M (eds) Pregnancy hypertension. MTP Press, Lancaster, pp 1–11

Clark S L, Koonings P P, Phelan J P 1985 Placenta previa/accreta and prior caesarean section. Obstetrics and Gynecology 66: 89–92

Cosgriff T M, Martin B A 1981 Low functional and high antigenic antithrombin III level in patient with the lupus anticoagulant and recurrent thrombosis. Arthritis and Rheumatism 24: 94–96

Craven C M, Zhao L, Ward K 2000 Lateral placental growth occurs by trophoblast cell invasion of decidual veins. Placenta 21: 160–169

Currie G A, Bagshawe K D 1967 The masking of antigens on trophoblast and cancer cells. Lancet 1: 708–710

Damsky C H, Fitzgerald M L, Fisher S J 1992 Distribution patterns of extracellular matrix components and adhesion receptors are intricately modulated during first trimester cytotrophoblast differentiation along the invasive pathway in vivo. Journal of Clinical Investigation 89: 210–222

Davey D A, MacGillivray I 1988 The classification and definition of the hypertensive disorders of pregnancy. American Journal of Obstetrics and Gynecology 158: 892–898

Dekker G A, Sibai B M 1998 Etiology and pathogenesis of preeclampsia: current concepts. American Journal of Obstetrics and Gynecology 179: 1359–1375

Deligdisch L 1993 Effects of hormone therapy on the endometrium. Modern Pathology 6: 94–106

Demetris A J, Lasky S, Van Thiel D H et al 1985 Pathology of hepatic transplantation: a review of 62 adult allograft recipients immunosuppressed with a cyclosporin/steroid regimen. American Journal of Pathology 118: 151–161

De Wolf F, De Wolf-Peeters C, Brosens I 1973 Ultrastructure of the spiral arteries in the human placental bed at the end of normal pregnancy. American Journal of Obstetrics and Gynecology 117: 833–848

De Wolf F, Robertson W B, Brosens I 1975 The ultrastructure of acute atherosis in hypertensive pregnancy. American Journal of Obstetrics and Gynecology 123: 164–174

De Wolf F, De Wolf-Peeters C, Brosens I, Robertson W B 1980a The human placental bed: electron microscopic study of trophoblastic invasion of spiral arteries. American Journal of Obstetrics and Gynecology 137: 58–70

De Wolf F, Brosens I, Renaer M 1980b Fetal growth retardation and the maternal arterial supply of the human placenta in the absence of sustained hypertension. British Journal of Obstetrics and Gynaecology 87: 678–685

Dixon H G, Robertson W B 1958 A study of the vessels of the placental bed in normotensive and hypertensive women. Journal of Obstetrics and Gynaecology of the British Empire 65: 803–809

Dommisse J, Tiltman A J 1992 Placental bed biopsies in placental abruption. British Journal of Obstetrics and Gynaecology 99: 651–654

Driscoll S G 1965 The pathology of pregnancy complicated by diabetes mellitus. Medical Clinics of North America 49: 1053–1067

Earl U, Bulmer J N, Briones A 1987 Placenta accreta: an immunohistological study of trophoblast populations. Placenta 8: 273–282

Edmonds D K, Lindsay K S, Miller J F et al 1982 Early embryonic mortality in women. Fertility and Sterility 38: 447–453

Finn C A, Porter D G 1975 The uterus. Elek Science, London, pp 74–85

Fox H 1972 Placenta accreta, 1945–1969. Obstetrical and Gynecological Survey 27: 475–490

Fox H 1976 The histopathology of placental insufficiency. Journal of Clinical Pathology 29 suppl (Royal College of Pathologists) 10: 1–8

Fox H 1979 Placental changes in gestational diabetes. In: Sutherland H W, Stowers J M (eds) Carbohydrate metabolism in pregnancy and the newborn 1978. Springer-Verlag, Berlin, pp 102–113

Fox H 1981 Placental malfunction as a factor in intrauterine growth retardation. In: Van Assche A, Robertson W B (eds) Fetal growth retardation. Churchill Livingstone, Edinburgh, pp 117–125

Fox H 1997 Pathology of the placenta, 2nd ed. W B Saunders, London

Fox H 2000 Placental pathology. In: Kingdom J, Barer P (eds) Intrauterine growth restriction: aetiology and management. Springer, London, pp 187–201

Fox H, Wells M 1998 Pathology of the first trimester of pregnancy. In: Kurjak A (ed) Textbook of perinatal medicine. Parthenon, London pp 991–998

Francis R B, Mac Ghee W G, Feinstein D I 1988 Endothelial dependent fibrinolysis in subjects with the lupus anticoagulant and thrombosis. Thrombosis and Haemostasis 39: 412–414

Freeman R M 1991 Placenta accreta and myotonic dystrophy: two case reports. British Journal of Obstetrics and Gynaecology 98: 594–595

Frosca T, Morassi L, Pecorelli S, Grigolato P, Gastaldi A 1989 Histological features of uteroplacental vessels in normal and hypertensive patients in relation to birthweight. British Journal of Obstetrics and Gynaecology 96: 835–839

Gerretsen G, Huisjes H J, Elema J D 1981 Morphological changes of the spiral arteries in the placental bed in relation to preeclampsia and fetal growth retardation. British Journal of Obstetrics and Gynaecology 88: 876–881

Gerretsen G, Huisjes H J, Hardouk M J, Elema J D 1983 Trophoblast alterations in the placental bed in relation to physiological changes in spiral arteries. British Journal of Obstetrics and Gynaecology 90: 34–39

Gorodeski I G, Bahari C M, Schachter A, Neri A 1982 Abruption and premature separation of placenta previa. European Journal of Obstetrics, Gynecology and Reproductive Biology 13: 75–85

Govan A D T 1976 The histology of eclamptic lesions. Journal of Clinical Pathology 29 suppl (Royal College of Pathologists) 10: 63–69

Gruenwald P 1972 Expansion of placental site and maternal blood supply of primate placentas. Anatomical Record 173: 189–204

Gruenwald P 1975 The supply line of the fetus: definitions relating to fetal growth. In: Gruenwald P (ed) The placenta and its maternal supply line. MTP Press, Lancaster, pp 1–17

Gruenwald P, Levin H, Yousen H 1968 Abruption and premature separation of the placenta. American Journal of Obstetrics and Gynecology 102: 604–614

Harden M A, Walters M, Valente P T 1990 Postabortal hemorrhage due to placental increta: a case report. Obstetrics and Gynecology 75 (2): 523–526

Harris J W S, Ramsey E M 1966 The morphology of human uteroplacental vasculature. Contributions to embryology, no 260. Carnegie Institution of Washington Publication 625, 38: 43–58

Hayman R, Brockelsby J, Kenny L, Baker P 1999 Preeclampsia: the endothelium, circulating factor(s) and vascular endothelial growth factor. Journal of the Society for Gynecologic Investigation 6: 3–10

Hertig A T 1945 Vascular pathology in the hypertensive albuminuric toxemias of pregnancy. Clinics 4: 602–613

Hertig A T 1964 Gestational hyperplasia of endometrium. Laboratory Investigation 13: 1153–1157

Hustin J 1995 Vascular physiology and pathophysiology of early pregnancy. In: Bourne T H, Jauniaux E, Jurkovic D (eds) Transvaginal colour doppler. Springer-Verlag, Heidelberg, pp 47–56

Hustin J, Franchimont P 1992 The endometrium and implantation. In: Barnea E R, Hustin J, Jauniaux E (eds) The first twelve weeks of pregnancy. Springer-Verlag, Heidelberg, pp 26–44

Hustin J, Jauniaux E 1997 Mechanisms and pathology of miscarriage. In: Grndzinskas J G, O'Brien P M S (eds) Problems in early pregnancy: advances in diagnosis and management. RCOG Press, London, pp 19–30

Hustin J, Jauniaux E R M 2000 Histology of miscarriage: its relation to pathogenesis. In: Kingdom J C P, Jauniaux E R M, O'Brien P M S (eds) The placenta: basic science and clinical practice. RCOG Press, London, pp 121–132

Hustin J, Foidart J M, Lambotte R 1983 Maternal vascular lesions in pre-eclampsia and intra-uterine growth retardation: light microscopy and immunofluorescence. Placenta 4: 489–498

Hustin J, Jauniaux E, Schaaps J P 1990 Histological study of the materno-embryonic interface in spontaneous abortion. Placenta 11: 477–486

Hutton R A, Chow F P R, Craft I L, Dandona P 1980 Inhibitors of platelet aggregation in the fetoplacental unit and myometrium with particular reference to the ADP-degrading property of placenta. Placenta 1: 125–130

Hytten F E, Leitch I 1971 The physiology of human pregnancy, 2nd edn. Blackwell, Oxford

Jauniaux E, Gavriil P, Khun P, Kurdi P, Hyett J, Nicolaides K 1996 Fetal heart rate and umbilicoplacental doppler flow velocity waveforms in early pregnancies with a chromosomal abnormality and/or increased nuchal translucency thickness. Human Reproduction 11: 435–439

Jungers P, Dougados M, Pelissier C et al 1982 Lupus nephropathy and pregnancy: report of 104 cases in 36 patients. Archives of Internal Medicine 142: 771–776

Karow W G, Gentry W C, Skeels R F, Payne S A 1971 Endometrial biopsy in the luteal phase of the cycle of conception. Fertility and Sterility 22: 482–495

Khong T Y 1991 Acute atherosis in pregnancies complicated by hypertension, small-for-gestational-age infants and diabetes mellitus. Archives of Pathology and Laboratory Medicine 115: 722–725

Khong T Y, Khong T K 1993 Delayed post-partum hemorrhage: a morphologic study of causes and their relation to other pregnancy disorders. Obstetrics and Gynecology 82: 17–22

Khong T Y, Robertson W B 1987 Placenta creta and placenta praevia creta. Placenta 8: 399–409

Khong T Y, De Wolf F, Robertson W B, Brosens I 1986 Inadequate maternal vascular response to placentation in pregnancies complicated by pre-eclampsia and by small-for-gestational-age infants. British Journal of Obstetrics and Gynaecology 93: 1049–1059

Khong T Y, Liddell H S, Robertson W B 1987 Defective haemochorial placentation as a cause of miscarriage: a preliminary study. British Journal of Obstetrics and Gynaecology 94: 649–655

Kirby D R S, Cowell T P 1968 Trophoblast-host interactions. In: Fleischmajer P, Billingham R E (eds) Epithelial–mesenchymal interactions. Williams & Wilkins, Baltimore, pp 64–77

Kirby D R S, Billington W D, Bradbury S, Goldstein D J 1964 Antigen barrier of the mouse placenta. Nature London 204: 548–549

Kitzmiller J L, Benirschke K 1973 Immunofluorescent study of placental bed vessels in preeclampsia of pregnancy. American Journal of Obstetrics and Gynecology 115: 248–251

Kitzmiller J L, Watt N, Driscoll S G 1981 Decidual arteriopathy in hypertension and diabetes in pregnancy: immunofluorescent studies. American Journal of Obstetrics and Gynecology 141: 773–779

Labarrere C 1988 Review article: acute atherosis: a histopathological hallmark of immune aggression? Placenta 9: 95–108

Labarrere C, Althabe O 1985 Chronic villitis of unknown etiology and maternal arterial lesions in pre-eclamptic pregnancies. European Journal of Obstetrics, Gynecology and Reproductive Biology 20: 1–11

Labarrere C, Althabe O 1986 Chronic villitis of unknown etiology and decidual maternal vasculopathies in sustained chronic hypertension. European Journal of Obstetrics, Gynecology and Reproductive Biology 21: 27–32

Labarrere C A, Catoggio L J, Mullen E G, Althabe O H 1986 Placenta lesions in maternal auto-immune diseases. American Journal of Reproductive Immunology and Microbiology 12: 78–86

McFadyen I R, Price A B, Geirsson R T 1986 The relation of birthweight to histological appearances in vessels of the placental bed. British Journal of Obstetrics and Gynaecology 93: 476–481

MacGillivray I 1975 Clinical aspects of uteroplacental insufficiency. European Journal of Obstetrics, Gynecology and Reproductive Biology 5: 101–108

MacGillivray I 1983 Preeclampsia: the hypertensive disease of pregnancy. W B Saunders, London

Many A, Hubel C A, Fisher S J, Roberts J M, Zhou Y 2000 Invasive cytotrophoblasts manifest evidence of oxidative stress in preeclampsia. American Journal of Pathology 156: 321–331

Maqueo M, Azuela J C, De la Vega M D 1964 Placental pathology in eclampsia and preeclampsia. Obstetrics and Gynecology 24: 350–356

Moll W, Kunzel W, Herberger J 1975 Hemodynamic implications of hemochorial placentation. European Journal of Obstetrics, Gynecology and Reproductive Biology 5: 67–74

Moreb J, Kitchens C J 1989 Acquired functional protein S deficiency, cerebral venous thrombosis and coumarin skin necrosis in association with antiphospholipid syndrome: report of two cases. American Journal of Medicine 87: 207–210

Nanaev A K, Kosanke G, Kemp B, Frank H G, Huppertz B, Kaufmann P 2000 The human placenta is encircled by a ring of smooth muscle cells. Placenta 21: 122–125

Nawrocki B, Polette M, Maquoi E, Birembaut P 1997 Expression of matrix metalloproteinases and their inhibitors during human placental development. Trophoblast Research 10: 97–113

Noyes R W 1972 Disorders of gamete transport and implantation. In: Assali N S (ed) Pathophysiology of gestation, vol 1. Academic Press, New York, pp 64–143

Ober W B, Grady H G 1961 Subinvolution of the placental site. Bulletin of the New York Academy of Medicine 37: 713–730

Palmer D C, Tsar C C, Roodman S T et al 1985 Heart graft arteriosclerosis: an ominous finding on endomyocardial biopsy. Transplantation 39: 385–388

Pijnenborg R, Dixon G, Robertson W B, Brosens I 1980 Trophoblastic invasion of human decidua from 8 to 18 weeks of pregnancy. Placenta 1: 3–19

Pijnenborg R, Robertson W B, Brosens I, Dixon H G 1981a Trophoblast invasion and the establishment of haemochorial placentation in man and laboratory animals. Placenta 2: 71–92

Pijnenborg R, Bland J M, Robertson W B, Dixon H G, Brosens I 1981b The pattern of interstitial trophoblastic invasion of the myometrium in early human pregnancy. Placenta 2: 303–316

Pijnenborg R, Bland J M, Robertson W B, Brosens I 1983 Uteroplacental arterial changes related to interstitial trophoblast migration in early human pregnancy. Placenta 4: 397–414

Pijnenborg R, Anthony J, Davey D A et al 1991 Placental bed spiral arteries in the hypertensive disorders of pregnancy. British Journal of Obstetrics and Gynaecology 98: 648–655

Porter K A 1974 Renal transplantation. In: Heptinstall R M (ed) Pathology of the kidney. Little Brown, London, pp 977–1042

Ramsey E M 1982 The placenta: human and animal. Praeger, New York

Ramsey E M, Donner M W 1980 Placental vasculature and circulation. Thieme, Stuttgart

Reister F, Frank H G, Kingdom J C et al 2001 Macrophage-induced apoptosis limits endovascular trophoblast invasion in the uterine wall of preeclamptic women. Laboratory Investigation 81: 1143–1152

Roberts J M 1998 Endothelial dysfunction in preeclampsia. Seminars in Reproductive Endocrinology 16: 5–15

Robertson W B 1976 Uteroplacental vasculature. Journal of Clinical Pathology 29 suppl (Royal College of Pathologists) 10: 9–17

Robertson W B 1979 Utero-placental blood supply in maternal diabetes. In: Sutherland H W, Stowers J M (eds) Carbohydrate metabolism in pregnancy and the newborn. Springer-Verlag, Berlin, pp 63–75

Robertson W B, Warner B 1974 The ultrastructure of the human placental bed. Journal of Pathology 112: 203–211

Robertson W B, Brosens I, Dixon H G 1967 The pathological response of the vessels of the placental bed to hypertensive pregnancy. Journal of Pathology and Bacteriology 93: 581–592

Robertson W B, Brosens I, Dixon H G 1975 Uteroplacental vascular pathology. European Journal of Obstetrics, Gynecology and Reproductive Biology 5: 47–65

Robertson W B, Brosens I, Dixon H G 1976 Maternal uterine vascular lesions in the hypertensive complications of pregnancy. In: Lindheimer M D (ed) Hypertension in pregnancy. Wiley, New York, pp 115–127

Robertson W B, Brosens I, Dixon H G 1981 Maternal blood supply in fetal growth retardation. In: Van Assche A, Robertson W B (eds) Fetal growth retardation. Churchill Livingstone, Edinburgh, pp 126–138

Robertson W B, Brosens I, Landells W N 1985 Abnormal placentation. Obstetrics and Gynecology Annual 14: 411–426

Robertson W B, Khong T Y, Brosens I, De Wolf F, Sheppard B L, Bonnar J 1986 The placental bed biopsy: review from three European centres. American Journal of Obstetrics and Gynecology 155: 401–412

Roussev R G, Stern J J, Kaider B D, Thaler C J 1998 Anti-endothelial cell antibodies: another cause for pregnancy loss. American Journal of Reproductive Immunology 39: 89–95

Rushton D I, Dawson I M P 1982 The maternal autopsy. Journal of Clinical Pathology 35: 909–921

Rustin M H, Bull H A, Machin S J, Isenberg D A, Snaith M L, Dowd P M 1988 Effects of the lupus anticoagulant in patients with systemic lupus erythematosus on endothelial cell prostacyclin release and procoagulant activity. Journal of Investigative Dermatology 90: 744–748

Sebire N J, Rees H, Paradinas F et al 2001 Extra villus endovascular implantation site trophoblast invasion is abnormal in complete versus partial molar pregnancies. Placenta 22: 725–728

Shanklin D R, Sibai B M 1989 Ultrastructural aspects of preeclampsia: placental bed and uterine boundary vessels. American Journal of Obstetrics and Gynecology 161: 735–741

Sheppard B L, Bonnar J 1976 The ultrastructure of the arterial supply of the human placenta in pregnancy complicated by fetal growth retardation. British Journal of Obstetrics and Gynaecology 83: 948–959

Sheppard B L, Bonnar J 1980 Uteroplacental arteries and hypertensive pregnancy. In: Bonnar J, MacGillivray I, Symonds E M (eds) Pregnancy hypertension. MTP Press, Lancaster, pp 213–219

Tabibzadeh S, Bakaknia A 1995 The signals and molecular pathways involved in implantation, a symbiotic interaction between blastocyst and endometrium involving adhesion and tissue invasion. Human Reproduction 10: 1579–1602

Vermulen J, Carreras L O, Van Assche A 1981 Repeated abortion and intrauterine death in women with a lupus anticoagulant. In: Van Assche A, Robertson W B (eds) Fetal growth retardation. Churchill Livingstone, Edinburgh, pp 156–160

Wallenburg H C S 1981 Prostaglandins and the maternal placental circulation: review and perspectives. Biological Research in Pregnancy 2: 15–22

Wells M, Bulmer J N 1988 The human placental bed: histology, immunohistochemistry and pathology. Histopathology 13: 493–498

Wood C, Rogers P 1993 A pregnancy after planned partial endometrial resection. Australian and New Zealand Journal of Obstetrics and Gynaecology 33: 316–318

Wynn R M 1972 Cytotrophoblastic specialisations: an ultrastructural study of the human placenta. American Journal of Obstetrics and Gynecology 114: 339–355

Zeek P M, Assali N S 1950 Vascular changes in the decidua associated with eclamptogenic toxemia of pregnancy. American Journal of Clinical Pathology 20: 1099–1109

Zhou Y, Fisher S J, Janatpour M et al 1997 Human cytotrophoblasts adopt a vascular phenotype as they differentiate. A strategy for successful endovascular invasion? Journal of Clinical Investigation 99: 2139–2151

Zhou Y, Genbacev O, Damsky C H, Fisher S J 1998 Oxygen regulates human cytotrophoblast differentiation and invasion: implications for endovascular invasion in normal pregnancy and in preeclampsia. Journal of Reproductive Immunology 39: 197–213

40

Gestational trophoblastic diseases

F. J. Paradinas   C. W. Elston

Introduction, history and classification   1359

Hydatidiform moles   1361
Aetiology and pathogenesis of moles   1361
Relative incidence and clinical presentation of molar
  pregnancy   1367
The pathology of complete and partial hydatidiform
  moles   1370
Special investigations in the diagnosis of molar
  pregnancy   1381
Prognosis of complete and partial moles   1383

Invasive moles and persistent trophoblastic disease   1388
Pathogenesis of invasive moles   1388
Incidence and clinical presentation   1388
Pathology of invasive moles   1389
Prognosis of invasive mole   1391

Trophoblastic neoplasms   1392
Aetiology and pathogenesis of trophoblastic
  neoplasms   1394
Incidence and clinical presentation of trophoblastic
  neoplasms   1396
Pathology of choriocarcinoma   1398
Pathology of placental site trophoblastic tumour   1405
Pathology of epithelioid trophoblastic tumour   1409
Non-gestational carcinomas with trophoblastic
  metaplasia   1411

Biopsy and differential diagnosis of trophoblastic
  lesions   1412
Differential diagnosis of lesions containing chorionic
  villi   1413
Differential diagnosis of lesions not containing chorionic
  villi   1413

INTRODUCTION, HISTORY AND CLASSIFICATION

The lesions grouped together under this broad title represent a wide range of diseases, from a specific type of miscarriage, hydatidiform mole, to the malignant neoplasm, choriocarcinoma. This apparent paradox is explained by the similarities in therapeutic approach in both. Because of their secretion of an ideal tumour marker, human chorionic gonadotrophin (hCG), the treatment of gestational trophoblastic diseases can be accurately monitored, and this has proved invaluable in almost eliminating the previously high mortality. These diseases evoke further interest because of their unique status as naturally occurring allografts and their study could help us to understand the normal mechanisms of nidation and intrauterine fetal survival.

Gestational trophoblastic diseases comprise two separate groups: non-neoplastic conditions, which may behave in an aggressive way or predispose to a neoplasm, that is, hydatidiform moles, and trophoblastic neoplasms.

Hydatidiform moles are described in old Greek medical texts, when they were already regarded as abnormal pregnancies (Ober & Fass 1961), but our understanding of what causes these abnormal pregnancies has been elusive until recently. Colourful explanations include the story of Margaret Countess of Henneberg, who after recriminating a poor woman for having too many children, was herself subject to a curse and in 1276 was delivered of 365 small vesicles; these were interpreted as gestational sacs, which the attendants to her labour proceeded to baptise (Ober & Fass 1961). A plaque recording the event can still be seen in Loosdoinen church, now part of The Hague. Descriptions and illustrations of moles in renaissance medical literature are not rare (Östör 1996) and the explanations given for their occurrence are no less colourful (the result of a fright, frequent coitus, etc). Authors often fail to distinguish between hydatidiform or vesicular moles and the more solid 'carneous' moles caused by other forms of miscarriage but by the beginning of the 19th century the origin of hydatidiform moles from placental tissue became generally accepted (Östör 1996). The pathology of moles when their course was not interrupted or modified by early diagnosis and therapy can be found in the seminal studies of Hertig (Hertig & Sheldon 1947; Hertig 1950; Hertig & Mansell 1956), Park (Park & Lees 1950; Park 1971) and Brewer (1959, 1967).

A common denominator of hydatidiform moles is swelling of chorionic villi. The idea that this could be caused by some external influence on the developing conceptus dominated the medical literature of the first half of the 20th century, culminating with the ideas of Hertig (Hertig & Edmonds 1940). They classified specimens with hydropic swelling into three groups: type I (hydropic abortuses) in which the swelling was mild, an embryo was often found and the disease affected the conceptus early in the first trimester, type II (transitional moles) in which swelling was more intense but focal, an embryo or fetus was present and the disease manifested itself in the second trimester, and type III (true or classical moles) in which hydrops was generalised and intense, no embryo developed and the disease could progress into the third trimester. Implied in this classification was the idea that a single cause could affect the conceptus either in different degrees or at different times, resulting in different forms of a wide spectrum of disease. On the factual evidence then available, this theory was appealing, gained wide acceptance and stimulated the search for possible environmental causes of the disease. However, the most significant advance in understanding the pathogenesis of moles has come from the field of cytogenetics and shows that moles are genetically determined by chromosomal abnormalities. These occur at the time of fertilisation or earlier and result in the various molar types.

Ewing (1910) devised the term chorioadenoma destruens to denote the type of hydatidiform mole which retained its villous stroma and penetrated into the myometrium, occasionally extending into pelvic structures and rarely metastasising. It behaved as a locally malignant process and Ewing considered the lesion intermediate between a classical hydatidiform mole and choriocarcinoma. The more straightforward descriptive term 'invasive mole' is now preferred (Park 1971; Elston 1978; Hertz 1978). In the vast majority of cases, invasive moles are genetically and morphologically complete moles and the invasive potential of partial moles is probably extremely low. The reasons why some complete moles invade and others do not are still unknown.

The most important feature of moles, as stressed by Park (1971), is the excessive growth of their trophoblastic epithelium which makes them more prone to invade than a normal placenta (invasive moles) and more likely to develop into neoplasms. This seems to occur often in complete or classical moles but very rarely in transitional moles, now renamed partial moles (Vassilakos & Kajii

1976; Vassilakos et al 1977). The main interest of Hertig's third group (the much more common hydropic abortuses or type I), is in the differential diagnosis from the other two.

The realisation that certain neoplasms arose from trophoblast was first noted in Germany towards the end of the 19th century. The first description of choriocarcinoma was probably by Chiari in 1877. He stressed the origin from the placental bed, and the relationship with a previous gestation but failed to recognise that it arose from the trophoblast. Sänger (1889) produced a comprehensive classification of primary uterine neoplasms, but he incorrectly presumed that trophoblastic tumours were sarcomatous and arose from decidua.

The correct origin from trophoblast was finally deduced by Marchand (1894) after a classical clinicopathological study. He later established the fetal origin of the trophoblast, and introduced the term 'chorionepithelioma' (Marchand 1898). This interpretation was quickly accepted in continental Europe and the United States, but not in England due to the obstinacy of the Obstetrical Society of London (Ober & Fass 1961). It finally took a Scotsman to convince the learned members of the Society (Teacher 1903a,b) and the trophoblastic origin of choriocarcinoma has not been challenged seriously since then.

When Marchand (1895) correctly established the histogenesis of choriocarcinoma from the villous trophoblast, he recognised an uncommon variant, which he termed atypical choriocarcinoma. Ewing (1910) subsequently divided the latter entity into two forms, syncytial endometritis and syncytioma. Ewing recognised that the histological appearances in trophoblastic lesions were more important in relation to their degree of malignancy than previously thought. He devised a morphological classification under the broad term 'chorioma' with the following subdivisions:

1. Hydatid mole
2. Chorioadenoma destruens (invasive mole)
3. Choriocarcinoma
4a. Syncytial endometritis
4b. Syncytioma.

Ewing's classification has only required modification recently. It was devised at a time when histological material was available in nearly all cases. Today, most patients with persistence of trophoblastic proliferation following a hydatidiform mole are monitored by hCG assay and may receive chemotherapy without a firm tissue diagnosis of invasive mole of choriocarcinoma. The International Union Against Cancer (1967) used the unsatisfactory category 'uncertain' to denote such cases, but the more precise terminology 'persistent trophoblastic disease' is preferred (Elston 1976, 1978; Hertz 1978).

The lesion which Ewing termed syncytial endometritis is characterised by infiltration of decidua and adjacent myometrium by intermediate (non-villous or extravillous) trophoblast in the placental bed. His terminology is inappropriate, because it is not an inflammatory pathological process, but a rather florid form of the physiological permeation normally present in implantation sites. The preferred terminology is 'exaggerated placental site reaction' (Elston 1991; Silverberg & Kurman 1992) and the lesion is worth including in a classification of trophoblastic disease for two reasons: it defines the normal end of the spectrum and its presence in a curettage for postpartum or abortal bleeding may lead the unwary into a mistaken histological diagnosis of malignancy.

Placental site reactions, particularly myometrial, can persist long after the last known pregnancy. Some of these lesions were described as placental site nodules or plaques by Young et al (1988, 1990). In our view a clear distinction should be made between a decidual exaggerated placental site reaction in the placental bed of a very recent pregnancy and a myometrial placental site reaction which has persisted longer than usual, since the latter probably has a different biological explanation and certainly has different clinical implications.

The lesion which Ewing termed syncytioma proved much more difficult to characterise because of its relative rarity. The striking resemblance to the placental site trophoblast and the benign course without metastatic spread led a number of authorities to conclude that the process was not neoplastic (Ober et al 1971; Kurman et al 1976; Elston 1981). However, subsequent reports of fatal cases associated with metastasis clearly indicated a neoplastic process (Scully & Young 1981; Twiggs et al 1981; Eckstein et al 1982; Young & Scully 1984). It is now accepted that these lesions are tumours differentiating towards the intermediate trophoblast of the placental bed and the terminology proposed by Scully & Young (1981) 'placental site trophoblastic tumour' (PSTT), has been adopted by the International Society of Gynecological Pathologists (Young et al 1988; Silverberg & Kurman 1992).

In more recent years, the name epithelioid trophoblastic tumour (ETT) has been proposed for a tumour lacking the dimorphic pattern of choriocarcinoma but different morphologically from placental site tumour. The term would include tumours predominantly composed of mononuclear cells, a pattern often seen in choriocarcinoma metastases after chemotherapy (Mazur 1989; Jones et al 1993), and uterine tumours, also composed of mononuclear cells, in patients who may not have been treated and which may present long after the last known pregnancy (Mazur & Kurman 1994; Shih & Kurman 1998a). In our view, there is a danger of confusing under the term 'epithelioid' two forms of atypical choriocarcinoma which have different clinical presentation, different behaviour and different immunocytochemical profiles. The first has been previously described by us as predominantly cytotrophoblastic choriocarcinoma (Paradinas 1992, 1998b; Elston 1996) and the second, a very rare

tumour indeed, we have regarded as a placental site tumour of long evolution (Paradinas 1997, 1998b). We think that the two should be clearly separated, but agree that the term ETT is acceptable to describe rare uterine trophoblastic tumours with long evolution. However, it should be recognised that the names do not imply origin from a specific type of trophoblastic cell, but describe the predominant line of differentiation at a particular time and — as in other human neoplasms — this can change due to environmental or therapeutic influences. This probably explains the tumours of mixed morphology which are encountered occasionally (Paradinas 1992, 1998b; Fukunaga & Ushigome 1993a; Shih & Kurman 1998a). It is therefore suggested that a modern histopathological classification of trophoblastic disease should include the categories indicated below:

Hydatidiform moles
- complete
- partial
- invasive

Persistent trophoblastic disease
Choriocarcinoma
- dimorphic (classical)
- monomorphic (predominantly mononuclear)

Placental site trophoblastic tumour
Epithelioid trophoblastic tumour
Exaggerated placental site reaction
Persistent placental site reaction (placental site trophoblastic nodule)
Trophoblastic lesions, unclassified.

This classification is based on that proposed by the International Society of Gynecological Pathologists (Silverberg & Kurman 1992), but incorporates more recent developments.

HYDATIDIFORM MOLES

Complete and partial hydatidiform moles may be regarded as abnormal products of conception which are usually associated with either a 'blighted' ovum (Elston 1978; Fox 1989), or a malformed embryo/fetus. They are characterised by swelling of chorionic villi and excessive proliferation of trophoblast epithelium, which may result in myometrial invasion or give rise to a neoplasm. Invasive moles are moles which invade the myometrium and may metastasise: they will be discussed separately.

AETIOLOGY AND PATHOGENESIS OF MOLES

Genetic abnormalities in complete mole

The fact that hydatidiform moles result from genetically abnormal pregnancies is now firmly established. It was first noted that most classical (complete) moles were of female (XX) genetic sex. Early studies estimated genetic sex by the distribution of Barr bodies in the trophoblastic and stromal cells of the mole. Although the reported prevalence varied widely, there was general agreement that moles were predominantly of XX female genetic sex (Park 1957; Atkin 1965; Tominaga & Page 1966; Elston 1970). It has since been shown convincingly by determination of karyotype, that the great majority of complete hydatidiform moles are of 46,XX constitution (Kajii & Ohama 1977; Vassilakos et al 1977; Jacobs et al 1978a, 1980; Szulman & Surti 1978a, 1978b; Lawler et al 1979, 1982b). The application of chromosome marker studies, based on the technique of quinacrine staining (Q-banding) described by Caspersson et al (1971), which allows precise identification of each chromosome in the human karyotype, produced a more significant advance. Data derived from Q and C banding (Giemsa staining of centromeric regions) suggested that most complete moles are of androgenetic origin (Kajii & Ohama 1977; Wake et al 1978; Lawler et al 1979; Jacobs et al 1980; Lawler et al 1982b) with two paternal sets of chromosomes but no maternal contribution and, as a rule, maternal DNA can be found only in mitochondria (Wallace et al 1982). Analysis of results of karyotyping in over 400 complete moles have indicated that between 92 and 96% had a 46, XX karyotype, due to fertilisation of an egg with no effective maternal genome by a haploid (23,X) sperm which then duplicates without cytokinesis (Kajii & Ohama 1977; Jacobs et al 1980; Wake et al 1984; Lawler & Fisher 1986, 1987a; Surti 1987), that is, they are homozygous and androgenetic in origin. These conclusions have been supported by HLA studies (Yamashita et al 1979; Bateman et al 1997) and gene probing using restriction fragment length polymorphisms (RFLP) (Wallace et al 1982; Surti et al 1983; Fisher et al 1989; Ko et al 1991).

Some complete moles are heterozygous with a 46,XY karyotype. They arise from dispermy: fertilisation of the 'empty' ovum by two separate haploid sperms carrying 23,X and 23,Y chromosomes respectively (Wake et al 1978; Surti et al 1979; Ohama et al 1981; Pattillo et al 1981; Kajii et al 1984; Lawler & Fisher 1987a; Surti 1987). Heterozygous 46,XX complete moles have also been described (Lawler & Fisher 1987a). Although the reported incidences of dispermic heterozygous complete moles vary, recent studies have shown a higher prevalence of heterozygosity than had been reported previously (Fisher et al 1989; Kovacs et al 1991). In Kovacs' study, genetic 'fingerprinting' of 22 complete moles showed heterozygosity in 40% but in most other series this is about 20 to 25%. No cases of YY moles have been described and it is presumed that such a combination results in non-viable pregnancies.

The reasons for molar development when all DNA comes from the father are explained by the phenomenon of genetic imprinting. Some genes responsible for trophoblastic and fetal development are imprinted genes: that is, only the paternal or the maternal genes are active.

When only female genes are present, such as in mature ovarian teratomas (Parrington et al 1984), there is growth of fetal tissues but no significant trophoblastic development. When only male genes are active, such as in complete moles, there is exuberant trophoblastic growth but development of the inner cell mass is arrested very early (Barton et al 1984). The nature of imprinting in biochemical terms is not fully understood, although it is thought to involve methylation of side chains of DNA bases (Reik 1989; Mutter 1997). Again, the precise moment at which this occurs during maturation of germ cells is not known, nor is the exact location of the imprinted genes controlling trophoblast growth, although recent research points towards areas of chromosomes 7, 11 and 19 (Ariel et al 1994; Rachmilewitz et al 1995; Walsh et al 1995; Lustig et al 1997; Matsuda et al 1997; Wake et al 1998; Moglabey et al 1999). Complete moles are therefore due to an imbalance of paternal versus maternal imprinted genes which in most cases is due to fertilisation of an egg which loses all its maternal genome, but why and how this is lost is not known.

Some reported complete moles contain maternal contributions (Jacobs et al 1982a; Vejerslev et al 1991; Sunde et al 1993; Fisher et al 1997). It is possible that some early reports of these biparental complete moles included partial moles or non-molar conceptions mistaken for complete moles, but the findings have been substantiated by more recent research (Helwani et al 1999; Fisher et al 2000) and suggest that the pathogenesis of complete mole is more heterogeneous than previously suspected and that complete moles can occur rarely even if the maternal DNA is not lost. This is probably due to relaxation of imprinting, a mechanism which rarely causes imbalance between paternal and maternal imprinted genes in other human genetic disorders such as Beckwith–Wiedemann syndrome and Angleman's syndrome (Reik 1989; Ariel et al 1994; Ohlsson et al 1993). Clearly, half the chromosomes inherited by a woman are inherited from her father and a failure or relaxation of the normal imprinting mechanisms during maturation of the egg could result in excess of male imprinted genes. This would result in a mole with biparental karyotype and no chromosomal abnormality detectable with the techniques used so far. Support for this theory comes from the demonstration that there are alterations of some imprinted genes, such as H19 and IGF2 in trophoblastic diseases (Ariel et al 1994; Rachmilewitz et al 1995; Walsh et al 1995; Lustig et al 1997; Wake et al 1998; Ohlsson et al 1999). Relaxation of imprinting may be an important mechanism when several complete moles occur in the same patient — so called repetitive moles — and in patients with a family history of moles, since in these situations, complete moles are often biparental rather than androgenetic (Helwani et al 1999; Fisher et al 2000). Recent studies in two families have shown a defective maternal imprinted gene in chromosome 19 (Moglabey et al 1999).

If an imbalance between paternal and maternally imprinted genes is the main mechanism of molar development, there is — at least in theory — the possibility of this occurring as a result of uniparental disomies, trisomies and translocations. All these have been reported as a cause of imbalance of imprinted genes in other human genetic disorders, such as Beckwith–Wiedemann syndrome (Reik 1989), and there is no reason why these should not explain some moles, but it is unlikely, because areas of the genome controlling trophoblastic development may be on more than one chromosome and — so far — isolated reports of moles due to these chromosomal abnormalities remain unconfirmed.

A few cases of androgenetic complete mole showing triploidy and tetraploidy have been reported (Habibian & Surti 1987; Hemming et al 1987, 1988; Vejerslev et al 1987; Lage et al 1989, 1992; Lawler & Fisher 1991; Fukunaga et al 1995a, 1996b; Paradinas et al 1996). In the majority of karyotyped cases, there was an excess of paternal over maternal chromosomes, supporting the view that it is the ratio of paternally to maternally imprinted genetic material and not ploidy that is important in the evolution of molar gestations (Vejerslev et al 1987). These cases are nevertheless rare. More modern techniques (see page 1381–1383) have confirmed that the majority of complete moles are diploid but with higher aneuploid and hyperdiploid cell populations than previously suspected (Habibian & Surti 1987; Fisher et al 1987; Hemming et al 1987; Lage et al 1988, 1992; Sunde et al 1989; Koenig et al 1993; Van de Kaa et al 1993). This probably reflects the progressive genetic imbalance that accompanies the development of neoplasia in predisposing conditions such as moles and has been used in trying to predict prognosis (see page 1386).

Genetic abnormalities in partial mole

Early cytogenetic studies of partial moles were difficult to interpret because of a lack of consistency in the morphological classification, but several showed an association between hydropia and triploidy (Makino et al 1964; Schlegel et al 1966; Carr 1969). Vassilakos et al (1977) included in their category of partial hydatidiform mole some cases with no excess trophoblast and found a variety of chromosomal abnormalities, predominantly triploidy but also trisomies. Szulman & Surti (1978a,b) defined the syndrome of partial mole more precisely and included only those cases which exhibit definite circumferential trophoblastic excess. In their studies, the great majority of partial moles have had a triploid karyotype and this has been substantially confirmed by other groups (Jacobs et al 1982a, 1982b; Lawler et al 1982a; Surti 1987; Lawler & Fisher 1991) and also by using flow cytometry (Fisher et al 1987; Lage et al 1988; Jeffers et al 1995; Paradinas et al 1996), by image analysis of appropriately stained sections (Van de Kaa et al 1991, 1993;

Barclay et al 1993; Jeffers et al 1995) and by counting argyrophilic nucleolar organiser regions (Suresh et al 1990; Neudeck et al 1997; Watanabe et al 1998). Triploidy occurs in approximately 1% of conceptions that lead to clinically apparent pregnancies, and about 80% of triploid first trimester miscarriages appear to be partial moles (Szulman et al 1981a,b). Jacobs et al (1982b) have shown that if the additional haploid component is paternal (diandry) then a molar gestation ensues, and if it is maternal (digyny) the result is usually a non-molar gestation. Some digynic triploid pregnancies abort early in the first trimester but in others there is significant fetal development and the disease is only diagnosed in the second trimester. At this later stage, the proportion of digynic triploids is higher (McFadden et al 1993; Redline et al 1998). The diandric origin of triploid partial moles has been confirmed by cytogenetic studies, chromosomal heteromorphisms, (restriction fragment length polymorphisms and minisatellite polymorphisms) and HLA polymorphisms, in the same way as in complete mole (Couillon et al 1978; Szulman et al 1981a; Lawler et al 1982b; Vejerslev et al 1987; Lawler & Fisher 1991). Redline et al (1998) have reported some histological similarities between diandric and dyginic triploids and the latter have in some cases been diagnosed morphologically as partial moles (Jacobs et al 1982b; Repiska et al 1998), but there is no evidence that they have excessive trophoblast proliferation or increased risk of persistent trophoblastic disease. Although most partial moles are triploid, there are well-documented cases of tetraploid partial moles (Lage et al 1989) also explained by more than one paternal set of chromosomes in the presence of a maternal genome. Isolated cases of triploid mosaicism with partial hydrops of the placenta have been reported (Ikeda et al 1996) and may account for some previously reported hydropic placentas with a live birth, but these are rare.

Early studies determining ploidy by either flow cytometry or image analysis also report variable proportions of diploid partial moles (Teng & Ballon 1984; Fisher et al 1987; Hemming et al 1987; Lage et al 1988) which in one instance reached 83% (Davis et al 1987). In our experience (Paradinas 1994a, 1996, 1998; Paradinas et al 1996) most cases initially diagnosed as diploid partial moles are either non-molar miscarriages or complete moles evacuated at a young gestational age and erroneously classified as partial moles because hydrops is not yet generalised. This is also the experience of others (Gschwendtner et al 1998; Watanabe et al 1998; Zhang et al 1998; Bell et al 1999). Nevertheless, there is the theoretical possibility that an imbalance between paternal and maternal genetic material could occur due to uniparental disomy, trisomy, translocations or relaxation of imprinting as in complete mole although, to our knowledge, this has not yet been demonstrated.

Cases of trophoblastic hyperplasia in a significant number of trisomies have been reported (Van Oven et al 1989; Redline et al 1998) but a critical assessment of this problem is difficult without better definition of what constitutes hyperplasia in a conceptus and a clear differentiation between the common finding of abundant trophoblast from the trophoblastic shell and columns in early miscarriages and the abnormal distribution of excess trophoblast seen in moles. Nevertheless, even in experienced hands, correlation of partial mole with triploidy has never been 100% (Lawler & Fisher 1987a, 1991; Lage et al 1992; Paradinas et al 1996; Gschwendtner et al 1998). This probably reflects the similarities between some of the clinical and morphological features of partial mole and those of other chromosomal abnormalities which may cause hydropic miscarriages, such as monosomies (Byrne et al 1984), trisomies (Paradinas 1994a, 1996; Jauniaux et al 1998; Geisler et al 1999), digynic triploidy (Redline et al 1998) and placental mosaicism (Ikeda et al 1996).

For practical purposes, it can be said that the majority of partial moles are triploid and rarely tetraploid. Aneuploid populations in partial moles are also present but less frequently than in complete moles (Van de Kaa et al 1993).

Genetic abnormalities in non-molar hydropic miscarriages

Over 50% of miscarriages after 4 weeks gestation have abnormal karyotypes incompatible with life (Boué et al 1976; Honoré et al 1976; Szulman 1995; Jauniaux et al 1996) and hydropic change is common in them as well as in genetically normal conceptuses. Chromosomal abnormalities include trisomies, digynic triploids, tetraploids, monosomies, translocations and mosaics. Flow cytometry and image analysis are helpful in their differential diagnosis from partial mole (Fukunaga et al 1993a,b,c 1996b; Cheville et al 1995) since they will show diploidy in the majority of trisomies, monosomies and translocations, but cannot differentiate between digynic and diandric triploids. Most trisomies and digynic triploids miscarry significantly earlier than partial moles and no evidence that they have increased risk of persistand throphoblastic disease compared with a normal pregnancy has yet emerged.

In the second trimester, there is a condition in which large, often cystic placentas may be mistaken by ultrasound and on pathological examination for partial moles and the offspring may be affected by Beckwith–Wiedemann syndrome (Shapiro et al 1982; Takayama et al 1986). The condition has been described under various, often descriptive, names (Lage 1991; Moscoso et al 1991; Sander 1993; McCowan & Becroft 1994; Pridmore et al 1994). The term placental mesenchymal dysplasia (Jauniaux et al 1997) seems, however, appropriate because in some cases the baby is apparently normal. These placentas are usually diploid and with a normal karyotype but the possibility of subtle genetic abnormalities has not been investigated. We know that Beckwith–Wiedemann syndrome is due to an imbalance of imprinted genes: paternally active genes regulating insulin growth factor-2 (IGF2) located in chromosome 11 are overexpressed and there is underexpression of adjacent maternally imprinted genes responsible for some fetal development. The imbalance can be due to trisomies, translocations and uniparental disomies of chromosome 11, but also to relaxation of imprinting in probably about half the cases (Reik 1989; Ohlsson et al 1993; Polychronacos 1993; Mutter 1997). It is interesting that an imbalance of imprinted genes is also the mechanism underlying molar development and that there is evidence of abnormal expression of the same genes causing Beckwith–Wiedemann syndrome in hydatidiform moles and trophoblastic neoplasms (Mutter et al 1993a; Mutter 1997; Ohlsson et al 1999). Two cases with this placental abnormality seen by us and one previously reported (McCowan & Becroft 1994) were twin pregnancies with a complete mole, but in our cases the moles are androgenetic. Some reported cases of pseudo-partial mole, partial mole with a live birth, diploid partial mole and trisomic partial mole (Leroy et al 1976; Jauniaux et al 1998; Geisler et al 1999; Hsieh et al 1999; Lembet et al 2000) could in fact be examples of mesenchymal dysplasia.

There are also rare cases in which chromosomal abnormalities such as triploidy or polyploidy appear to affect only part of the placenta (Ikeda et al 1996; Benirschke et al 2000). These placental mosaics are rare but can also be diagnosed as partial moles. However, there is no evidence that focal development of hydrops in partial moles is due to different chromosomal constitution of hydropic and non-hydropic areas, although the cause of this focal hydrops is still unknown.

Risk factors which may influence molar development

It is firmly established that moles are genetically determined but there is still no scientifically proven explanation of how some ova lose their maternal nuclear DNA, why fertilisation by more than one sperm can occur, or what controls genetic imprinting. It is therefore still relevant to study risk factors, including genetic and environmental factors, which may influence the incidence of molar pregnancies.

ABO and HLA antigens may be of some importance in the development of persistent trophoblastic disease and choriocarcinoma after a mole (see prognosis of moles), but there is no strong evidence that any specific ABO or HLA antigen occurs more often in patients with moles than in the general population (Lawler et al 1971; Lawler 1978; Berkowitz et al 1981; Yamashita et al 1981). Souka et al (1993) have reported a higher incidence of HLA-A1 in patients with moles and Bassaw & Roopnarinesingh (1990) a higher incidence in group O; their studies are not controlled and involve small numbers of patients.

Clearly, further studies are needed. There are no studies of partial moles.

Maternal and paternal age

A complete mole may occur at any time during the childbearing period, but there is a markedly increased risk for women over the age of 40 and a significant increase, at the lower end of the reproductive range, particularly in teenagers (Smalbraak 1957; Yen & MacMahon 1968; Stone & Bagshawe 1976; Elston 1978; Hayashi et al 1982; Berkowitz et al 1985; Atrash et al 1986; Bagshawe et al 1986; Graham et al 1990; Paradinas et al 1996; Di Cintio et al 1997). The reasons for this are unknown, although it has been presumed that abnormal ova may be commoner in these age groups. Although an increase in complete moles has also been reported in women with older partners (Parazzini et al 1986), this has not been confirmed by other groups.

The more recent characterisation of partial mole means that there are no comparable data, but in most series partial moles occur with the same incidence at any maternal age (Jacobs et al 1978b, 1982a; Szulman & Surti 1982; Parazzini et al 1986; Paradinas et al 1996; Evans et al 1997). No associations of partial mole with paternal age have been found (Parazzini et al 1986). It is therefore possible that paternally derived triploidy occurs by chance in a proportion of fertilisations though a defective zona pellucida in the oocyte has been suggested as a possible reason for fertilisation by more than one sperm. Non-molar hydropic miscarriages are considerably commoner in older women (Roman & Stevenson 1983; Paradinas et al 1996). This has been known for some time and probably represents progressive damage of genetic material with age.

Previous personal or family history of molar pregnancies is a significant factor in complete moles (Franke et al 1983; Sand et al 1984; La Vecchia et al 1985). Bagshawe et al (1986) estimated that the risk after one mole increased to 1 in 56 and after two moles to 1 in 6.5. The reasons for this are probably varied. In some cases the patients are in the older age group and have had previous normal pregnancies and in others they are very young and eventually have normal pregnancies. In both situations, repetitive moles could be explained by whatever causes maternal DNA loss by the oocyte at both extremes of fertile life. The fact that the problem may occur with different partners (Tuncer et al 1999) certainly favours this. However, repetitive and familial moles may be biparental rather than androgenetic (see page 1362) when the tendency to develop moles could be related to relaxation of imprinting. Some patients with repetitive moles may have as many as 6 or 7 moles and never achieve a normal pregnancy (Fisher et al 2000). To date, very few families with a tendency to develop complete moles have been reported (Ambani et al 1980;

Parazzini et al 1984; Helwani et al 1999) and information on the underlying genetic defects responsible is still sketchy.

Some patients who have had more than one mole also have normal pregnancies (Rice et al 1989; Berkowitz et al 1998). Some moles may be complete, some partial and sometimes a mixture of both is seen. Partial moles are more common than complete moles and the chances of having more than one by chance are greater. There is a report of four partial moles and no normal pregnancies (Narayan et al 1991), but we have had the opportunity of reviewing the histology and analysing polymorphisms in molar tissue from that particular patient and found that in fact the moles are all diploid biparental early complete moles. The information available at present does not suggest a predisposition for several partial moles to occur in certain patients or in certain families, as is the case in complete moles.

There is also an association between history of repeated spontaneous miscarriages and molar pregnancy (Yen & MacMahon 1968; La Vecchia et al 1985; Messerli et al 1985; Parazzini et al 1986; Acaia et al 1988; Coulam et al 1991; Talati 1998) although none was found in some studies (Atrash et al 1986). In some patients referred to our unit with a mole, histological review of evacuated material from these, supposedly non-molar, previous miscarriages, has shown that they were also molar, usually complete moles miscarrying at an early stage. Failure to recognise clinically and pathologically early molar pregnancies probably accounts for some of these cases, particularly in patients with a tendency to develop biparental complete moles, but the reasons for the association may be multifactorial and merit further investigation. Increased numbers of pregnancies increase the chances of one of them being molar but, overall, parity does not appear to be a risk factor after correction for maternal age (Yen & MacMahon 1968; La Vecchia et al 1985).

Race, geographical distribution, nutrition and other socioeconomic factors

These have been reviewed by Elston (1981); Grimes (1984); Bracken (1987) and more recently by others (Parazzini et al 1991; Chung et al 1995; Di Cintio et al 1997). It was long suspected that trophoblastic diseases occur more frequently in the Far East and developing countries than in the Western Hemisphere and this was confirmed by a geographical study based on small samples from the United States and several Asian countries (Joint Project 1959). Initial estimates suggested that the difference in frequency amounted to some 10 to 20 times. This was based on comparison of such frequencies for hydatidiform mole as 1:125 for Taiwan (Wei & Ouyang 1963) and 1:200 for the Philippines (Acosta-Sison 1967a,b) with 1:2000 for the United States (Hertig & Sheldon 1947). Unfortunately, as pointed out by Hertz

Table 40.1 Estimated frequency of trophoblastic disease in relation to the number of gestations

Author	Year	Country	Frequency	
			Hydatidiform mole	**Choriocarcinoma**
Asia				
King	1956	Hong Kong	1:530 pregnancies	1:496 deliveries
Reddy & Rao	1969	India	1:463 pregnancies	
Poen & Diojopranoto	1965	Indonesia	1:85 pregnancies[a]	1:570 pregnancies[a]
			1:373 pregnancies[b]	1:1800 pregnancies[b]
			1:522 pregnancies	
Ishizuka	1976	Japan	1:760 pregnancies	1:8000 pregnancies
Llewellyn-Jones	1965	Malaysia	1:200 pregnancies	1:1382 pregnancies
Acosta-Sison	1967	Philippines	1:868 deliveries	
Tan et al	1982	Singapore	1:125 deliveries	1:8000 pregnancies
Wei & Ouyang	1963	Taiwan		
Africa				
Agboola	1979	Nigeria Uganda	1:379 deliveries	
Leighton	1973		1:971 deliveries	
Australasia				
Duff	1989	New Zealand	1:1497 pregnancies	
Olesnicky et al	1985	Australia	1:1357 deliveries	
Europe				
Bagshawe et al	1986	UK	1:650 pregnancies	
Franke et al	1983	Netherlands	1:1580 pregnancies	
Kolstad & Hognestad	1965	Norway	1:1300 deliveries	1:20 000 deliveries
Ringertz	1970	Sweden	1:1560 pregnancies	1:41 000 deliveries
Vejerslev et al	1984	Denmark	1:3158 pregnancies	
Womack & Elston	1985	UK	1:1400 deliveries	
Middle East				
Ghali	1969	Iraq	1:276 deliveries	
Graham et al	1990	United Arab Emirates	1:491 deliveries	
Matalon & Modan	1972	Israel	1:1300 pregnancies	
Latin America				
Aguero et al	1973	Venezuela	1:1088 pregnancies	
Marquez-Monter et al	1963	Mexico	1:220 pregnancies	
North America				
Hayashi et al	1982	USA	1:923 pregnancies	
Hertig & Sheldon	1947	USA	1:2000 deliveries	
Martin	1978	USA (Alaska)[c]	1:257 deliveries	
Yen & MacMahon	1968	USA	1:1450 deliveries	
Yuen & Cannon	1981	Canada	1:1205 pregnancies	

[a] Incidence in hospital serving 'low' socioeconomic population
[b] Incidence in hospital serving 'high' socioeconomic population
[c] Population of relatively recent East Asian descent

(1978), the WHO Scientific Group (1983) and Bracken (1987), much of the epidemiological data are of dubious value due to differences in methods of recording data and problems of diagnostic accuracy. Some studies have included both complete and partial hydatidiform moles whilst others, particularly those published more than two decades ago, recorded only complete moles. This is reflected in the wide range of frequencies reported throughout the world (Table 40.1); Bracken (1987) estimated that for hydatidiform mole this varied from 0.5 to 2.5:1000 pregnancies. For the reasons stated above it is still difficult to obtain accurate comparisons between 'high' and 'low' risk areas. Womack & Elston (1985), using the frequency of hydatidiform mole per live births only, compared figures from Nottingham, UK, with those from Aichi, Japan (Ishizuka 1976), and found a four-fold

increase in the latter. Closely similar results were obtained by Graham et al (1990) who used the Nottingham data as a comparison for the frequency in Abu Dhabi. Higher rates in the Middle East for complete moles have also been reported in Saudi Arabia (Felemban et al 1998). It is clear that complete hydatidiform mole, in particular, occurs more frequently in the 'high risk' areas of Asia, Africa, Latin America and the Middle East than in the 'low risk' areas of Australasia, Europe and North America. However, recent studies suggest considerably less variation than previously, perhaps explained by recent migrations of Asian populations to Australia, Europe and America and by a real decline in incidence in some Asian countries such as South Korea and Japan (Hando et al 1998; Kanazawa 1998; Kim et al 1998; Martin & Kim 1998). The reasons for this decline are probably complex, but there have been improvements in nutrition and a decrease in pregnancies at both extremes of fertile life (Martin & Kim 1998). Both of these could have contributed to the high incidences previously observed in these Asian countries (Editorial 1975).

Socioeconomic factors, and nutrition in particular, were suggested as important by the Joint Project (1959). This was not substantiated by others (Bracken 1987; Buckley 1987). Indeed, in some studies the risk seems to be greatest for women of higher social class (La Vecchia et al 1985; Messerli et al 1985). However, higher incidences in socially deprived communities continue to be reported (Guo et al 1994; Lira-Plascencia et al 1995; Gul et al 1997; Talati 1998). Several studies have suggested diets with a low protein intake as a possible risk factor (Marquez-Monter et al 1963; Acosta-Sison 1967b) but this does not explain the higher incidences in some communities with high protein intake, such as Alaskans (Martin 1978). Nevertheless, more recent and better controlled studies also suggest a possible link of higher incidences of complete mole with a poor diet (Berkowitz et al 1985; Parazzini et al 1988; Ha et al 1996).

Reports on ethnic differences have also been conflicting, partly because of the difficulty in carrying out truly multiracial studies. No association with ethnic group was found by the Joint Project (1959) but in Hawaii McCorriston (1968) found a higher incidence of trophoblastic disease in Orientals compared with Europeans of the same socioeconomic class and native Hawaiians of a lower status. Jacobs et al (1982a) estimated that the incidence of complete moles in Hawaiians of Filipino origin was five times that of Caucasians. In Malaysia no ethnic difference was found in Kuala Lumpur in an initial study (Llewellyn-Jones 1965) but a higher incidence in Chinese was reported by Sivanesaratnam (1998). In Singapore Teoh et al (1971) reported a higher incidence in Indians and Eurasians but this was not confirmed by Lee et al (1981), and more recently Chong & Koh (1999) found a higher incidence in Singaporean Indians and Malays. In the United States, Yen & MacMahon (1968) found a higher incidence of moles in blacks than in whites, but this was not confirmed by Hayashi et al (1982). Martin (1978), however, showed that the risk is increased in Alaskan natives compared with Caucasian Americans. In the Middle East, Graham et al (1990) found that the increased risk of complete mole was greater in Gulf Arabs than in other ethnic groups.

In conclusion it can be said that complete mole is more common in the Far East, Middle East, Southern and Central America, but that the recent decrease in incidence in developing countries in these areas suggests that social and dietary habits are probably as important or more important than racial differences. There is no comparable information regarding partial moles.

Other environmental factors

Information on other environmental factors is limited. Cigarette smoking has only been investigated in a small number of studies and the data are conflicting and inconclusive: some reports suggesting an association (La Vecchia et al 1985; Parazzini et al 1985) and others none (Yen & MacMahon 1968; Berkowitz et al 1985; Messerli et al 1985). Bracken (1987) has reviewed studies on exposure to herbicides, especially in South East Asia, and concluded that case selection bias renders the data unreliable, and more specifically Ha et al (1996) did not find any association between moles and exposure to agent orange during the Vietnam war. Previous use of oral contraceptives has been found to be unrelated to risk of hydatidiform mole (Berkowitz et al 1985; La Vecchia et al 1985; Messerli et al 1985) but it may have an influence in subsequent development of persistent trophoblastic disease (Bagshawe & Lawler 1982; WHO 1983; Bagshawe et al 1986; Palmer et al 1999). De Ruyck (1951) claimed to have isolated a virus from both hydatidiform mole and choriocarcinoma, but this has never been confirmed by other workers, nor has any other infective agent been incriminated. Radiation to the abdomen has been suggested as an aetiological factor in triploidy (Uchida & Freeman 1985) but it has not been corroborated by further studies.

RELATIVE INCIDENCE AND CLINICAL PRESENTATION OF MOLAR PREGNANCIES

The incidence of complete mole and its geographical variation has already been discussed (see aetiology and pathogenesis). In Europe and North America it is of the order of 0.5 to 1.5 per 1000 births and in high-risk areas about 1.5 to 5 per 1000 births (see Table 40.1).

The incidence of partial mole throughout the world is not yet known, but paternally derived triploidy, the genetic abnormality which appears to cause most partial moles, is considerably more common than androgenesis, the cause of most complete moles (Szulman et al 1981a; Jacobs et al 1982a; Szulman & Surti 1982; Paradinas 1998a). Jacobs et al (1982a) in a histological review of 1602 miscarriages from about 28 000 pregnancies in Hawaii, found 88 partial and 40 complete moles. Partial moles were 3.2 per 1000 births and complete moles 1.5 per 1000 births. If we assume that all paternally derived triploids are partial moles and assess the frequency of paternally derived triploidy in failed pregnancies, we can reach a rough estimate of what the real frequency of partial mole could be. Approximately 10% of pregnancies end in spontaneous miscarriages and in most surveys (Boué et al 1976; Honoré et al 1976; Brajenovic-Milic et al 1998) about half of these are found to be due to genetic abnormalities. Triploidy is found in about 15 to 28% of chromosomally abnormal first trimester miscarriages and over two-thirds of these triploids appear to be paternally derived (Jacobs et al 1982b). We should therefore expect at least 5 partial moles per 1000 births. This is only a little higher than the incidence reported in Hawaii (3.2 per 1000) but considerably higher than the proportions of partial moles to complete moles reported in many other series. In early reports these vary enormously from 3% to 35% of all moles (Berkowitz et al 1979, 1986c; Czernobilsky et al 1982; Womack & Elston 1985; Bagshawe et al 1986, 1990). In a relatively recent study (Lawler & Fisher 1991) 25% of all moles were partial and Fukunaga et al (1995b) found 1.7 per 1000 births complete and 2 per 1000 partial moles in a Tokyo hospital. In a histological review of 670 unselected cases referred to the London Registry in 12 months in 1986–87, only 28% of histologically proven moles were partial but this had increased to 47% in 1994 (Paradinas 1998a) and to 52% in 1998. The Registry covers an area with about 500 000 births per year and the mole numbers registered in 1994 represent 0.7 per 1000 births for complete moles and 0.6 per 1000 births for partial moles. In 1998, the numbers of registered complete moles remain at a similar level, but partial moles have increased to 0.8 per 1000 births; however, if the incidence of partial mole is similar throughout the world, partial moles appear still to be grossly underdiagnosed. Underdiagnosis is not confined to Britain, and authors in other countries stress the fact that the use of ploidy analysis and more strict histological criteria enabled them to reclassify as partial moles specimens previously regarded as non-molar (Fukunaga et al 1993c, 1995a; Gschwendtner et al 1998; Bell et al 1999). Partial moles miscarrying early may be unsuspected and not sent for histological examination, or specimens sent are either inadequate for diagnosis or inadequately sampled by histopathologists. In Sweden, Lindholm & Flam (1999) found that 70% of partial moles and 16% of complete moles in their practice were clinically and radiologically unsuspected and would have been missed if histological examination had not been performed.

Clinical presentation

Like other forms of miscarriage, moles can present as inevitable or missed miscarriages in the first trimester of pregnancy. However, unlike other miscarriages, in which early death of the embryo is usually followed by arrest of trophoblastic growth, in moles the latter may continue proliferating. In the case of partial mole, the fetus may not die until the second trimester and the disease may not be diagnosed clinically as an abnormal pregnancy until much later. Technical improvements and extensive use of vaginal ultrasound in the management of pregnancy has resulted in earlier evacuation of complete and partial moles (Paradinas 1994a, 1996; Paradinas & Fisher 1995; Fox 1997; Mosher et al 1998; Coukos 1999), so that in developed countries, early moles are now a majority. The

clinical and pathological features of moles evacuated late and early can be very different. It is therefore necessary to describe and to compare not only the differences between complete and partial moles, but also the clinical and pathological features of moles evacuated early and late.

Second trimester complete moles usually show all the characteristic clinical and ultrasound symptoms and signs well known to obstetricians (Lurain 1987), that is: vaginal bleeding, anaemia, hyperemesis, toxaemia, clinical or subclinical hyperthyroidism, uterus larger than dates, ovarian theca-lutein cysts and a classical snow storm appearance on ultrasound. Vaginal, vulval, pelvic or pulmonary metastases occurred if the mole was invasive in about 10% of patients evacuated late (Kohorn 1984; Bagshawe et al 1986; Berkowitz & Goldstein 1988, 1997a). Pulmonary complications due to trophoblast embolisation or to other reasons (cardiovascular complications of toxaemia, thyroid storm, pulmonary oedema due to fluid replacement) used to occur in about 27% of complete moles of at least 16 weeks gestation (Twiggs et al 1979). In addition, hCG values in retained complete moles at this stage are significantly higher than expected for a non-molar pregnancy and high hCG in a patient with the clinical features described is usually due to a complete mole in about 90% of cases (Romero et al 1985). In developing countries, a significant proportion of complete moles still present as described above (Lira-Plascencia et al 1995).

First trimester complete moles often present with vaginal bleeding as threatened or inevitable miscarriages between the 6th and 12th week of gestation. Even at this stage, uterine size may be larger than dates in about 28% of cases (Berkowitz & Goldstein 1997a) but this means that in the majority it is not. In their series of 74 early complete moles, hyperemesis was present in only 8%, anaemia in 5% and toxaemia in 1%. There were no patients with hyperthyroidism or respiratory complications and hyperthyroidism is nowadays rare (Hershman 1999). Theca-lutein cysts are rare and ultrasound may not be diagnostic of a mole (Lindholm & Flam 1999), although it usually shows no evidence of an embryo. We have nevertheless seen two patients in whom ultrasound scan showed a 1 cm embryo and who were later delivered of a complete mole (Paradinas et al 1997). Others have also detected the presence of a gestational sac by ultrasound (Zaki & Bahar 1996). This could be explained by a twin non-molar pregnancy or by embryonic development in some complete moles (see page 1374). The level of hCG varies markedly from case to case. Serum values in excess of 1×10^6 IU/l are not uncommon in patients with a complete mole before evacuation, but hCG may be normal or low due to early losses of molar tissue before hCG determination. This and the very high hCG levels seen sometimes in early normal pregnancy and in twin pregnancies makes hCG levels less useful in diagnosis than they are in monitoring patients. AFP determinations, helpful in diagnosis of partial moles, are seldom performed in complete moles. Transient and early AFP elevations have been noted in some, but in most cases this is due to the coexistence of a twin non-molar pregnancy and are explained by fetal development of the non-molar twin (Jauniaux et al 1999). In summary, the early clinical and radiological features of complete moles are often similar to those of a miscarriage due to other causes and the proportion of moles diagnosed only when the evacuated specimen is examined by the pathologist has increased (Paradinas 1998a; Lindholm & Flam 1999).

Second trimester partial moles are more difficult to recognise clinically but usually easy to diagnose by ultrasound (Mittal et al 1998; Jauniaux 1999). At this stage, toxaemia is not uncommon (Rijhsinghani et al 1997) and hCG values are often elevated. The uterus may be enlarged due to a large cystic placenta but this is not as marked as in complete mole and the uterus may be normal or smaller in size for dates due to oligohydramnios and fetal growth restriction. There are characteristic congenital abnormalities in more than 80% of fetuses (Doshi et al 1983; McFadden et al 1993) and AFP may be high if there are neural tube defects. Theca-lutein cysts and hyperthyroidism are considerably less common than in complete moles (Ludwig et al 1998). Nowadays the pregnancy seldom progresses beyond this stage and most triploid fetuses die in utero or the pregnancy is terminated, but in the past, rare cases have progressed to term, the baby dying in the first few weeks of extrauterine life. Some of these rare triploids with a live birth may not be complete triploids but triploid mosaics (Doshi et al 1983) and both digynic and diandric triploids are regarded as non-viable pregnancies.

First trimester partial moles are even more difficult to separate clinically and radiologically from non-molar miscarriages. Not uncommonly the fetus dies about the 8th or 10th week but is retained (missed miscarriage); then the uterus may be smaller than dates, with a collapsed gestational sac in which the fetus may or not be discernible and the pregnancy is not usually diagnosed as molar before evacuation. In a series of 81 cases including partial moles of all gestational ages (Berkowitz et al 1986c) excessive uterine size was observed in only 4% and hyperemesis, toxaemia, hyperthyroidism or respiratory complications were not found. Others (Naumoff et al 1981; Czernobilsky et al 1982; Szulman & Surti 1982), report similar experience and the numbers of correct preoperative diagnoses in most of these series was about 10%. It has been suggested that if the products of conception are not examined histologically, some 70 to 90% of partial moles will be missed (Berkowitz & Goldstein 1997a; Lindholm & Flam 1999). Because of the low incidence of complications after partial mole (page 1387) this does not have serious consequences for the majority of patients, and may give a false sense of security to both gynaecologist and pathologist dealing with diagnosis and management of partial moles, but in a large referral centre we see, about once a year, persistent trophoblastic disease or choriocarcinoma after an unrecognised partial mole.

The rare condition of mesenchymal dysplasia (see page 1364) can mimic the clinical and ultrasound appearances of a second trimester partial mole (Reid et al 1983; Hillstrom et al 1995; Jauniaux & Nicolaides 1997). These large placentas can produce abnormally high levels of hCG; as in partial mole maternal AFP can be also high and there may be toxaemia. In some cases, there is a stillbirth or the pregnancy is terminated if there are associated fetal abnormalities, but in others, the pregnancy may end in a normal live birth. Chorionic villus sampling usually shows a normal diploid karyotype and may be helpful in differential diagnosis from partial mole.

Twin molar pregnancies are not uncommon; usually a complete mole with a non-molar twin of which there are numerous reports (Jones & Lauersen 1975; Suzuki et al 1980; Fisher et al 1982; Vejerslev et al 1986; Deaton et al 1989; Miller et al 1993). Rarely, complete moles also occur in a triplet pregnancy (Azuma et al 1992; Amr et al 2000) and these have become more frequent recently due to multiple egg implantations in IVF programmes (Shozu et al 1998). A significant proportion of these pregnancies end in first trimester miscarriages (Paradinas et al 1997) but some may progress to the second trimester, when the combination of a fetus and a cystic placenta may result in the mistaken diagnosis of partial mole. In some cases this has led to termination of pregnancy but experience has shown that the presence of a complete mole may not result in stillbirth and present advice is that the pregnancy is continued until there is a chance of a viable birth (Fishman et al 1998; Matsui et al 2000) although frequently labour has to be induced or Caesarean section performed because of the dangers to the mother due to toxaemia. The association between complete moles and twin mesenchymal dysplasia has already been mentioned and its genetic implications deserve further study.

Twin pregnancies of a partial mole with a non-molar pregnancy are more difficult to detect but we have seen a few examples. Cases of twin partial mole with complete mole and twin partial moles have also been reported (Dalrymple et al 1995; Frates & Feinberg 2000). The main lesson to be learned from twin molar pregnancies is that allowing the pregnancy to continue until the normal pregnancy is viable, does not increase the risk of eventually needing chemotherapy, but overall they appear to have a higher incidence of persistent trophoblastic disease than complete mole alone.

Ectopic tubal complete and partial moles have been described. Because tubal pregnancies abort very early, diagnosis is often difficult and many of the single case reports published may not be genuine. This was the opinion of Ober & Maier (1982) who found only 4 acceptable cases amongst 22 reported in the literature and Burton et al (2001) could only substantiate 3 out of

25 cases registered in Sheffield as true molar pregnancies. Most cases reported are 'hydatidiform moles', presumably complete moles, but a few partial moles in which triploidy has been confirmed are on record (Montgomery et al 1993). Ectopic moles are too few to know if they present a higher risk than intrauterine moles but the available evidence to date suggests that they do not.

THE PATHOLOGY OF COMPLETE AND PARTIAL HYDATIDIFORM MOLES

Macroscopic appearances

The gross appearances of a fully developed complete hydatidiform mole in the second and third trimester are very characteristic. The 'bunch of grapes' appearance from which the name is derived (Figs 40.1, 40.2) is due to the conversion of chorionic villi into strings and clusters of vesicles which vary in diameter from approximately 1 to 30 mm. The molar placenta is increased in weight, often in excess of 2000 g. It is rare for a gesta-

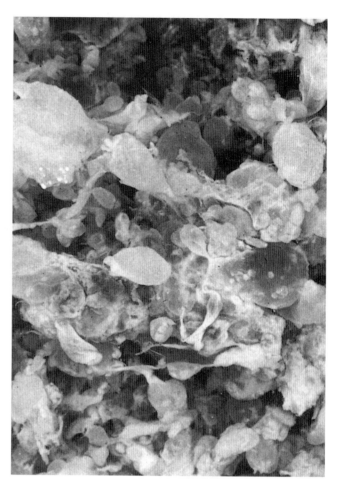

Fig. 40.2 Close-up view of another complete mole to show the variation in size of vesicles.

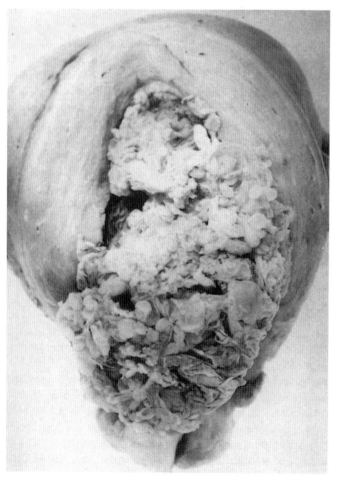

Fig. 40.1 An opened uterus containing a complete hydatidiform mole within the endometrial cavity. (From Fox H 1997 *Pathology of the placenta*, Saunders, Philadelphia. Reproduced by permission of Professor Fox and W B Saunders.)

tional sac or fetal tissues to be identified at this stage and if they are present, they are usually due to a separate twin pregnancy (page 1369).

Due to greater clinical awareness and the use of ultrasonography, an increasing number of patients with complete mole have the uterus evacuated at an earlier stage, often in the first trimester. In the London Mole Registry, gestational age at evacuation was on average 17 weeks in the decade of the 1960s (Elston 1970) but only 12 weeks in the 1980s (Paradinas 1994a; Paradinas et al 1996) and a survey of the first 100 histologically confirmed complete moles registered in the year 2000 shows an average of 9.4 weeks. A similar trend has been reported in other centres in developed countries (Keep et al 1996; Berkowitz & Goldstein 1997a; Fox 1997; Mosher et al 1998). In these cases the classical gross appearances described above are not fully developed and only occasional vesicles may be seen, leading to an erroneous assumption that this focal hydrops represents a partial rather than a complete mole (Paradinas 1994a). Evacuation, or spontaneous miscarriage, at around 6 to 8 weeks gestation may not show any vesicles and the correct diagnosis may be unsuspected until the products are examined histologically.

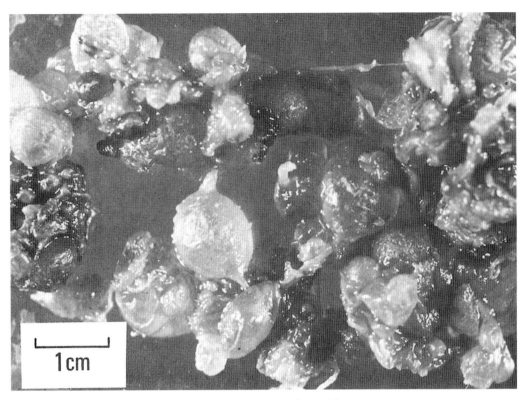

Fig. 40.3 A partial hydatidiform mole, showing scanty molar vesicles.

The gross appearances of partial moles are also variable depending on the time of evacuation. Hydropic change, even when moles are fully developed in the second trimester, is characteristically focal rather than generalised (hence the term partial mole, Fig. 40.3). Hydrops is usually less intense than in a complete mole, but vesicles can reach 20 mm in diameter. A recognisable fetus, or fetal parts, are frequently found. More often than not the fetus is malformed, this being a contributory cause of miscarriage or stillbirth. Fetal abnormalities associated with triploidy are varied (Doshi et al 1983; Tayson & Kalousek 1992) and better described in second trimester fetuses. At this stage, pathological diagnosis is usually confirmatory of the condition already suspected clinically. However, a proportion of triploids (in our experience a majority) miscarry or are diagnosed as abnormal pregnancies earlier in the first trimester. Like complete moles, the average gestational age at evacuation is getting shorter (15.4 weeks in 1990 but only 12.1 weeks in a survey of the first 160 histologically confirmed cases registered in the year 2000). In these early specimens the placental tissue is never as bulky as in a complete mole and, in general, is less often accompanied by haemorrhagic material. Vesicles may be few or absent and the obstetrician may not suspect molar pregnancy either before or after evacuation. In this situation, the specimen may not be sent for histology, or only a small sample is sent to confirm intrauterine pregnancy. Not infrequently most of the conceptus is sent for karyotype analysis and the pathologist receives only decidua. Poor sampling of specimens from spontaneous miscarriages in the laboratory is less common but also occurs. All these factors help to explain the low reported incidences of partial moles.

First trimester non-molar miscarriages may become hydropic but vesicles do not usually reach more than 3 mm in size and a suspicion of molar pregnancy seldom arises from naked-eye examination. However, they present considerable problems in the microscopic differential diagnosis. It is more difficult to separate partial moles from rare instances of mesenchymal dysplasia (see page 1372), since hydrops of some terminal villi closely mimics partial mole (Fig. 40.4) but most of the cysts are to be found in stem villi and examination of the fetal aspect of the placenta can show prominent aneurysmatic vessels (Sander 1994) not usually seen in partial moles.

Microscopic appearances of complete mole

There are three features which should be carefully analysed in miscarriages and molar specimens: 1 – the amount, distribution and appearance of the trophoblastic epithelium, 2 – the presence of hydropic change and stromal appearances of non-hydropic villi and 3 – the presence or absence of embryonic inner cell mass derivatives.

As stressed by Park (1971), excessive amounts, abnormal distribution and pleomorphism of trophoblast are the hallmark of complete moles. These abnormalities can be defined as more than the normal two layers of

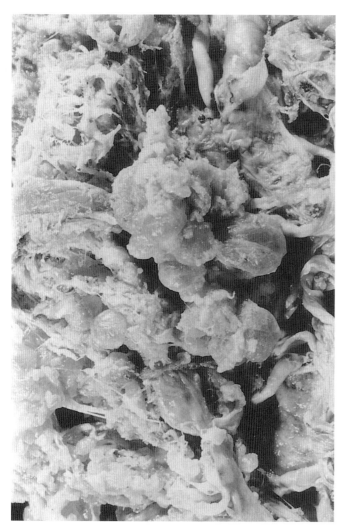

Fig. 40.4 Placental mesenchymal dysplasia showing focal hydropic change. It was diagnosed as partial mole clinically and by ultrasound and Caesarean section performed at 26 weeks. The fetus was normal and died soon after birth. The placenta weighed 1400 g. Both placenta and fetus had 46,XX karyotype.

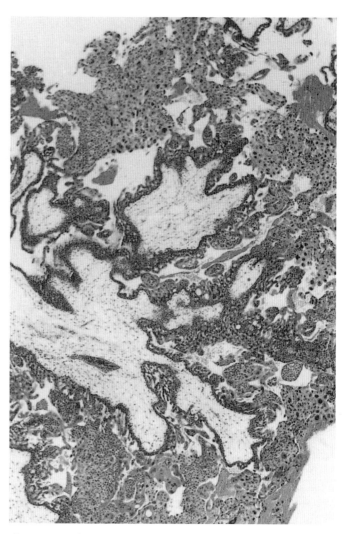

Fig. 40.5 Androgenetic complete hydatidiform mole evacuated at 7 weeks gestation. There is little hydropic change but small sprouts on the surface give villi a polypoid appearance.

trophoblastic cells (cyto- and syncytiotrophoblast) proliferating at various points on the surface of villi (multifocal) or completely surrounding them (circumferential). This is well-illustrated in Figs 40.5 (a first trimester complete mole) and 40.6 (a second trimester complete mole). However, it is important to understand that trophoblast is not firmly attached to villi and that cell clusters unrelated to villi are often found. Indeed, villous trophoblast excess in abnormal distribution is usually found only on a small proportion of molar villi, but it is naïve to think that these are the only areas where trophoblast is proliferating excessively. The presence or absence of trophoblast excess on slides can be influenced by numerous factors, such as previous losses before evacuation, method of evacuation (prostaglandin, suction or curettage), whether evacuation has been complete or not, degree of myometrial invasion of a mole, adequacy of sampling in the theatre and in the laboratory etc.

Excess multifocal or circumferential trophoblast is already present in very early first trimester complete moles of about 6–7 weeks gestation (Fig. 40.5) and in general it is easier to detect at this stage than in later gestations but care should be taken not to interpret as excess trophoblast the abundant trophoblast present in early normal placentation and in early miscarriages (See Fig. 40.18).

A great deal has been written about inclusions or pseudoinclusions of the trophoblast layer into underlying stroma in partial moles, but invaginations and pseudoinclusions in complete moles are also common. They can be cystic or solid but are irregular or oval in shape and different from the round inclusions of partial moles (compare Figs 40.7, 40.13). Finding inclusions in a mole does not necessarily mean that it is partial.

Pleomorphic trophoblast is characteristically present in moles, particularly complete moles (Fig. 40.8). It

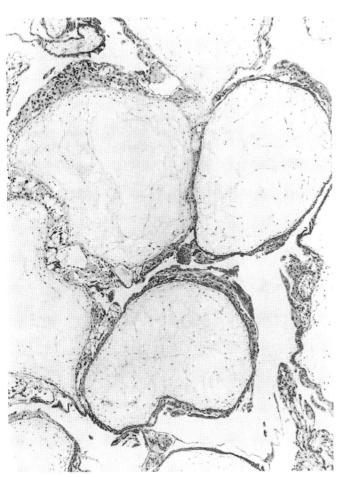

Fig. 40.6 Second trimester complete hydatidiform mole exhibiting villous hydropia with central liquefaction and absent stromal blood vessels. There is a slight degree of trophoblastic hyperplasia.

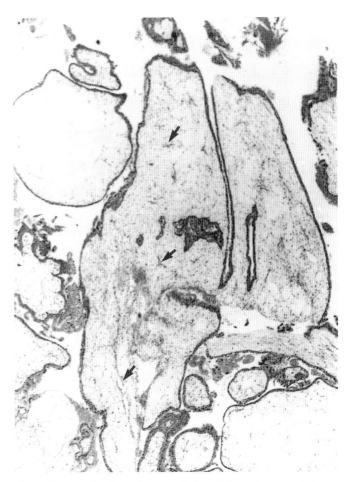

Fig. 40.7 Invagination of the trophoblastic layer in a complete mole often results in irregular pseudoinclusions. Practically all complete moles of less than 12 weeks gestation contain vessels (arrows) but in most cases these are never functional, probably due to early arrest in the development of the inner cell mass.

represents aneuploid cell populations (Van de Kaa et al 1991, 1993; Montes et al 1996) and is a feature important in molar diagnosis, although the amounts in a particular specimen can vary from abundant to none due to sampling error. In addition, it is difficult for the general histopathologist, reporting only a few molar cases per year, to acquire the experience necessary to assess the significance of trophoblastic atypia in miscarriage specimens, since some is usually present in normal pregnancies, particularly in retained, degenerate material. However, finding it may be helpful if no excess is found on the villous surface, such as in the specimen shown in Fig. 40.9, which corresponds to an androgenetic complete mole evacuated at 14 weeks gestation and which shows attenuated rather than excessive trophoblast.

The second important diagnostic feature of complete moles is hydropic change, but this is only generalised (complete) and intense in the second trimester. The chorionic villi become distended by the accumulation of stromal fluid, resulting in either mild oedema or central liquefaction, so called cisterns (Fig. 40.6). The enlarged

villi are generally rounded, but collapsed villi may have an irregular shape. In older moles there is absence or paucity of fetal stromal blood vessels and Elston (1970) found them in only 12% of cases of 17 weeks average gestational age. Collagen in the stroma of villi is usually scant and hydropic villi may appear as empty sacs. Some villi may be completely necrotic, but even if the entire mole is necrotic, complete, rather than partial, mole can be suspected by the prominent and generalised hydrops and the lack of significant stromal fibrosis.

In younger first trimester complete moles (now a majority in developed countries), hydrops may be microscopical and only present in a few villi, but villi are generally larger than normal and have abnormal shapes (Figs 40.5, 40.7) described as branching or polypoid (Szulman & Surti 1978a,b; Kajii et al 1984; Paradinas 1994a; Keep et al 1996; Paradinas et al 1996; Lage & Sheikh 1997) and have been compared to the formation of secondary villi in the development of the normal placenta (Kajii et al 1984). Occasionally, tangential sections of polypoid villi result in a characteristic lobulated appearance (Fig. 40.10).

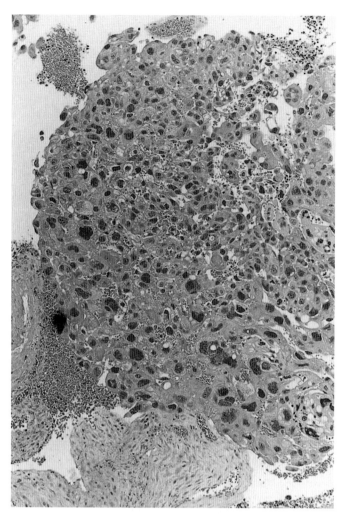

Fig. 40.8 Marked pleomorphism of trophoblast in complete mole. This usually represents aneuploidy but usually behaves in a benign fashion if molar villous stroma is also present. It can be mistaken for choriocarcinoma if the sample is unrepresentative.

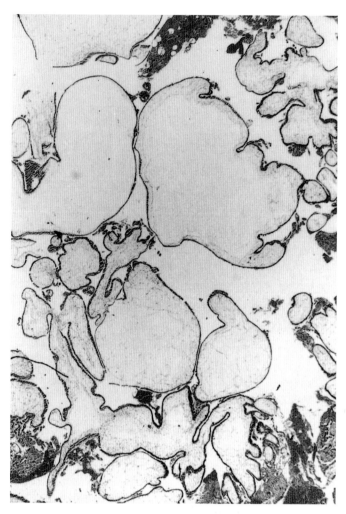

Fig. 40.9 Androgenetic complete mole showing attenuated rather than excessive trophoblast on the villous surface. This is not an uncommon event and more extensive sampling showed hyperplastic trophoblast on some villi and clusters of pleomorphic trophoblast.

In early complete moles there are numerous vessels (Fig. 40.7) and large amounts of acid muco-polysaccharides (Suster & Robinson 1992) which give it an immature appearance (Kajii et al 1984; Paradinas 1994a; Qiao et al 1997). Stromal cells tend to have spindle shapes and stromal mitoses may be seen. Except in rare instances (see below), vessels are usually collapsed and devoid of fetal red cells, but they may also show open lumina and are occasionally malformed (Paradinas et al 1996). Early complete moles have little collagen or reticulin and this may only be demonstrated around vessels. Fibrosis does not increase with molar age in distinction from partial moles. Stromal nuclear debris in villi of complete moles (Fig. 40.11) in the absence of necrosis or degeneration of their trophoblast surface epithelium is very common (Szulman & Surti 1978a,b) and has been confirmed by us (Paradinas 1994a; Paradinas et al 1996). This is presumed to be due to apoptosis of stromal cells and should be differentiated from cell debris in the wall

and lumina of vessels, which occurs in all forms of miscarriage after embryonic demise, reflecting the progressive loss of vessels. The cause of this apoptosis is, so far, unknown but its presence can be very helpful in diagnosis when other features, such as excess trophoblast or hydrops are absent in scanty or unrepresentative material. However, it should not be interpreted as molar in isolation, or when the trophoblast surface epithelium is itself necrotic. A significant proportion of complete moles miscarry spontaneously in early gestation and a failure to recognise the changes described above as molar could explain the high rates of persistent trophoblastic disease after presumed non-molar miscarriages reported by early workers (Hertig & Mansell 1956).

The third important diagnostic feature in the diagnosis of complete moles is that amnion, yolk sac, nucleated red cells or other embryonic tissues are not usually found, although this statement must now be qualified. Complete moles were originally thought to be anembryonic

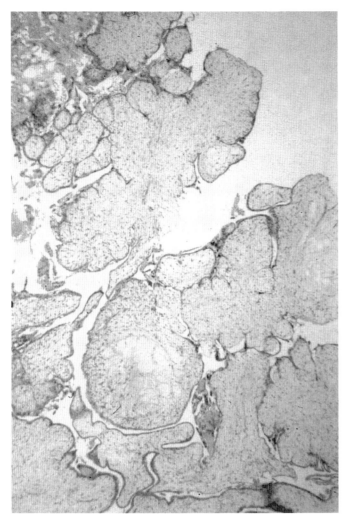

Fig. 40.10 Tangential section of irregular villi from a complete mole may result in a characteristic lobulated appearance.

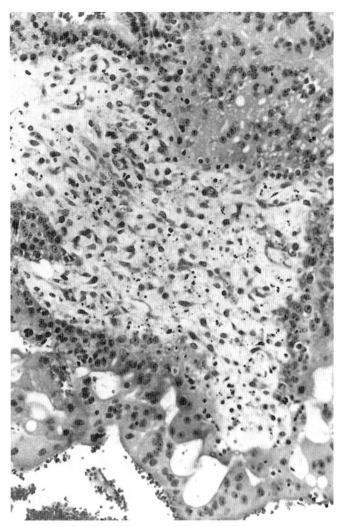

Fig. 40.11 Nuclear debris in the stroma of a complete mole. This is very often present in some villi in first trimester complete moles and is useful in diagnosis.

pregnancies (Hertig & Mansell 1956) and the finding of embryonic structures with a mole was taken as an indication of either a twin non-molar gestation with a complete mole, or of the mole being partial. However, nucleated red cells in molar vessels or amniotic or yolk sac epithelium are found rarely in diploid complete moles (Jacobs 1982a; Paradinas 1994a, 1997; Paradinas et al 1996, 1997; Fisher et al 1997; Van de Kaa 1997a; Zaragoza et al 1997; Sheikh & Lage 1998). In some cases, these are biparental (Jacobs 1982a; Sunde et al 1993; Fisher et al 1997), but in others they are androgenetic (Fisher et al 1997; Weaver et al 2000). Molar sex and red cell sex are similar (Van de Kaa et al 1997a) and DNA minisatellite polymorphisms in amnion and mole are identical (Weaver et al 2000). It is therefore probable that the absence of maternally imprinted genes results in early arrest of embryonic development rather than its absence. This is in accordance with experiments by Surani et al (1984a,b) in mice, where fertilisation of empty eggs resulted in exuberant trophoblastic proliferation but also showed inner cell mass development in some cases. It also explains better the presence of stroma and vessels in complete moles, since in normal placenta these are derived from extraembryonic mesoderm.

It must be stressed that the amounts of amniotic epithelium or yolk sac found with a complete mole are usually microscopical and that nucleated red cells are only rarely found in first trimester complete moles and almost never in second trimester. We have searched for them in many complete moles of 6 to 8 weeks gestational age and they are absent in most, suggesting that in most cases development of the inner cell mass stops before the 4th week of gestation, when haemopoiesis begins in extraembryonic yolk sac. From the practical point of view, this means that finding amnion, nucleated red cells in molar villi or embryonic tissue in moles evacuated early is not enough reason to classify a mole as partial, since it can be a complete mole with or without a twin pregnancy, with a much higher incidence of complications than a partial mole.

In most cases, histological diagnosis of a complete hydatidiform mole is relatively straightforward if the pathologist receives the total amount of tissue evacuated, as is usually the case when modern disposal vacuum suction systems are used: if a small specimen only is sent to the laboratory, or there is inadequate sampling, the diagnosis of molar pregnancy can be missed. In our experience, and that of others, diagnostic uncertainties decrease with increasing amounts of placental tissue available for study and if the morphology of young complete moles described above is taken into consideration.

Microscopical appearance of partial moles

Assessment of trophoblastic appearances in a putative partial mole is usually more difficult than in a complete mole, since even extensive sampling may only show excess trophoblast around occasional villi, and as many as 5 or even 10 blocks containing villi may be necessary before it is detected (Szulman & Surti 1978b; Lage

1990). In our experience, no more than 7% of partial moles show extensive or intense trophoblast excess (Fig. 40.12) and the excess on individual villi is more often multifocal than circumferential. Unlike the excess trophoblast of complete moles, where both cyto- and syncytiotrophoblast are obvious, most of the trophoblast in partial moles is syncytium and mononuclear cytotrophoblast is less conspicuous. Syncytial cells may be separated by empty spaces and are often referred to as 'vacuolated' (Fig. 40.12). As in complete moles, the main differential diagnosis is with the abundant trophoblastic shell and columns present in early miscarriages, but polar trophoblast may be present rarely in partial moles evacuated very early. As pointed out by Howat et al (1993), it is the abnormal distribution of trophoblast that is readily apparent in partial moles. Its excess is much more difficult to evaluate morphologically.

There are sharp indentations on the surface of villi in partial moles which can result in inclusions similar to

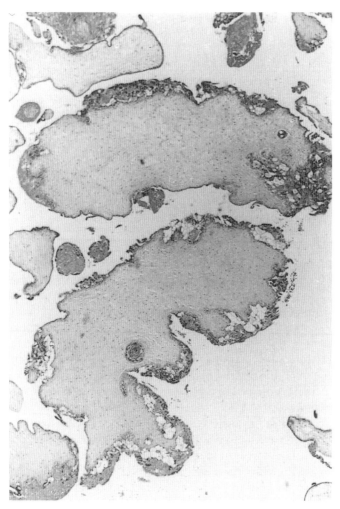

Fig. 40.12 Partial mole showing scalloped irregular villi and abundant syncytiotrophoblast on the surface. This trophoblastic excess is seldom as intense as in this case and is more often localised to a few villi.

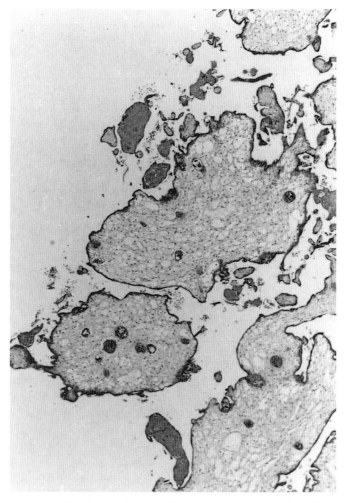

Fig. 40.13 Small, round trophoblastic inclusions may be found in partial mole. When numerous, such as in this case, they represent trophoblast excess growing inwards into the stroma. Scanty similar inclusions can be found in other chromosomal abnormalities causing miscarriage.

those seen in complete moles, but also inclusions which are characteristically round, either solid or cystic and occasionally calcified. If excess trophoblast around villi grows mainly outwards, inclusions are few and if it grows inwards inclusions can be numerous (Fig. 40.13). Unfortunately, although round inclusions are very characteristic of partial mole, they are not pathognomonic and can be seen in small numbers in digynic triploids, some trisomies, monosomies and translocations, particularly when associated with the irregular villi occasionally seen in these conditions (Byrne et al 1984; Paradinas et al 1994; Redline et al 1998).

In an ideal world, a diagnosis of partial mole should only be entertained if definite trophoblast excess is seen somewhere in the specimen (Szulman 1987; Lage 1990; Elston 1991; Conran et al 1993; Howat et al 1993) but, even more often than with complete moles, samples from partial moles are frequently inadequate and unrepresentative. We have seen a significant number of patients with persistent trophoblastic disease and choriocarcinoma after triploid partial moles, where no excess trophoblast

was found and the diagnosis initially missed (Bagshawe et al 1990; Paradinas 1994; Paradinas 1998a; Seckl et al 2000). This was due either to poor sampling or to unfamiliarity with subtle histological changes which should at least suggest the possibility of partial mole and which are described below.

In partial moles evacuated in the second trimester there is hydropic change and some vesicles can be 20 or 30 mm in diameter, but hydrops is focal (partial) and mirrors the gross appearances. Cisterns present in some villi (Fig. 40.14) alternate with non-hydropic villi. Some of the latter, particularly when the fetus survives well into the second trimester, may have a relatively normal structure, but others have abnormal shapes, abnormal vascularity or excessive trophoblast. Therefore, abnormalities in partial mole affect the whole placenta and not just those villi that become hydropic (Paradinas 1997). In both hydropic and non-hydropic villi blood vessels containing fetal red cells may be preserved (Fig. 40.15), depending on the age of the gestation and the interval between embryonic or fetal death and evacuation. In

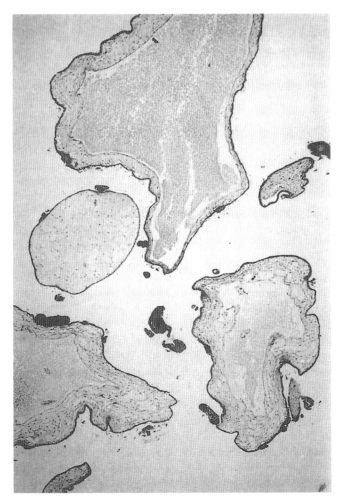

Fig. 40.14 Partial hydatidiform mole. Note the irregular 'scalloped' outline, cisternal formation and scanty circumferential collections of trophoblast.

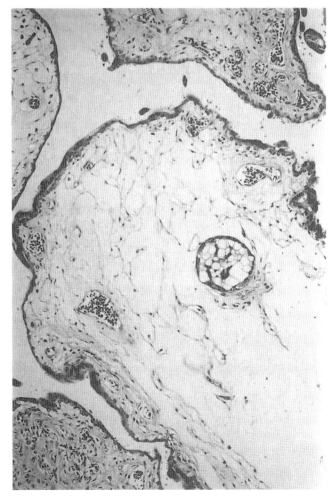

Fig. 40.15 Villus from a partial mole. A trophoblastic inclusion is present and blood vessels containing red cells are also seen. (Reprinted with permission from Elston 1989.)

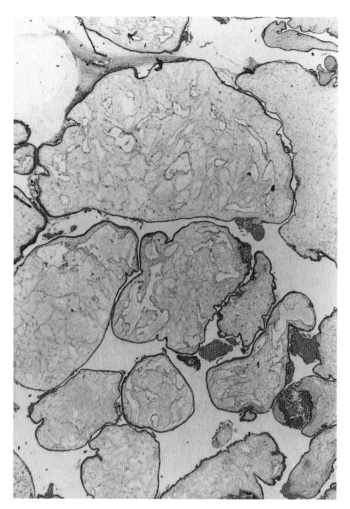

Fig. 40.16 Angiomatoid vascular malformations in partial mole. These are commoner in the second trimester, involve only a few villi and are usually empty of blood after fetal demise.

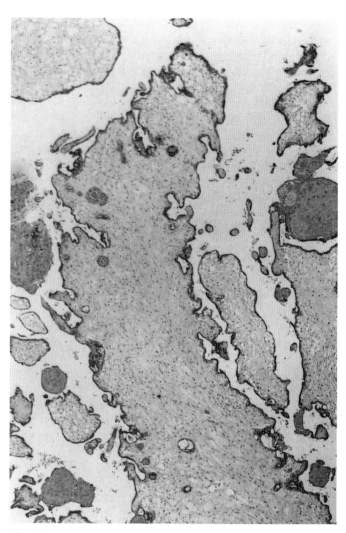

Fig. 40.17 Scalloped villi from a partial mole. There are numerous small but angulated invaginations. These may be absent in some partial moles and involve only occasional villi in others.

partial moles evacuated late, characteristic angiomatoid malformations often occur (Fig. 40.16). These were interpreted as branching cisterns by Szulman & Surti (1978a,b) and were noted but thought unrelated to molar pregnancy by Park (1971). Their vessels are usually empty of fetal blood, suggesting development just before fetal demise (Paradinas 1994a, 1997). Abnormal angiectatic vessels are rare in complete moles and non-molar miscarriages but in our study (Paradinas et al 1996) they were seen in 28% of partial moles and have been well described by others (Klausen & Larsen 1994; Lage & Sheikh 1997). In partial moles retained for long periods the stroma may be avascular and this progressive avascularity is accompanied by fibrosis (Fukunaga 2000). Presence of significant amounts of collagen in villous stroma is therefore more suggestive of partial than complete mole. Nuclear debris is only seen within and around disintegrating vessels. Very characteristic of partial mole is the presence of irregular villi with a dentate outline (Fig. 40.17) often described as scalloped or Norwegian fjord type. In contrast to the irregular villi of early com-

plete mole, the invaginations are sharply angulated rather than polypoid (compare Fig. 40.17 with Fig. 40.5). The numbers of such villi in a partial mole may vary from few to a majority and may not be seen if the sample is small. Hydropic villi are less likely to show irregular outlines, but the fact that hydrops affects only some villi means that non-hydropic irregular villi are often seen in second trimester specimens.

As in complete mole, the average gestational age at evacuation of partial moles is getting shorter and in partial moles of 8 to 12 weeks hydrops may be very mild, cisterns absent or small and fibrosis not yet developed (Fukunaga 2000). At this stage, vessels are usually numerous and reticulin more abundant than in complete moles, forming a web which extends amongst vessels and stromal cells, the latter often being stellate in shape. Villi may have irregular scalloped outlines but invaginations are less marked and round inclusions less numerous than later on. At this stage, and depending on the amount available for study, the differentiation between early partial mole and some non-molar miscarriages can be very difficult or even impossible on morphological grounds alone. Miscarriages due to other chromosomal abnormalities such as monosomy XO (Byrne et al 1984); trisomies (Van Oven et al 1989; Van Lijnschoten et al 1993; Genest et al 1995; Paradinas 1997) and digynic triploidy (Redline et al 1998) can also have villi with irregular outlines and only the presence of trophoblast excess and cisterns appears to have significant predictive value in the diagnosis of triploidy. However, these two features may be difficult to assess in partial moles, since occasional small cisterns (usually smaller than 3 mm) may be present in non-molar miscarriages and trophoblast in them can be very abundant and easily misinterpreted as excessive. In doubtful cases, patients are followed up with hCG measurements until this is normal, which in non-molar specimens is usually within 8 weeks and follow-up is then discontinued. The number of cases in which diagnosis is doubtful is, however, increasing due to poor sampling and to earlier evacuation.

With the rare exceptions described earlier (see page 1375) the finding of fetal or embryonic derivatives in a mole is a strong indication that it may be partial, but has little value in the differential diagnosis of partial mole versus hydropic miscarriage. In our series of over 150 triploid partial moles (Paradinas et al 1996), they were present in over 50% of specimens of all gestational ages. Obviously, they are found more frequently in second trimester partial moles, in those extensively sampled and in those with a short interval between fetal death and evacuation. Fetal red cells may persist in fetal vessels long after fetal death (Szulman 1995). They are commoner in partial moles than in first trimester non-molar miscarriages, since the embryo tends to survive longer.

Microscopical appearances of non-molar miscarriages

The two main reasons for confusion between moles and non-molar miscarriages are unfamiliarity with the abundant trophoblast normally present in early gestation and with the fact that hydrops can occur in some non-molar specimens. Trophoblast in early miscarriage is polar or intervillous in distribution (Fig. 40.18), representing the trophoblastic columns that anchor the conceptus to maternal tissues and are the source of the trophoblastic cells infiltrating the placental bed. In non-molar early implantation sites, the conceptus has a small gestational sac from which sprouting secondary villi develop, and is encased in a circumferential trophoblast shell (Fig. 40.19). Amnion and embryo are often lost and this structure can be interpreted as a hydropic villus from an early complete mole. However, in early gestational sacs, more than two layers of trophoblast are only present at the tips of the secondary villi and there is no significant

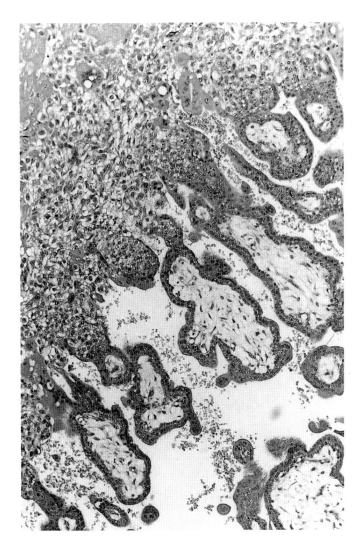

Fig. 40.18 First trimester spontaneous miscarriage, with apparent proliferation of cytotrophoblast at poles of villi. This is normal and commonly seen in early miscarriage. Trophoblast is less pleomorphic than in moles.

trophoblast cellular pleomorphism (Fig. 40.18). Additionally, one should always suspect an early gestational sac and not a branching villus from a complete mole if only one such structure has been obtained at curettage, a most unusual event in complete moles if the specimen sent to the laboratory is abundant and has been adequately sampled. Unfortunately, this is not always so and when in doubt, a clinicopathological discussion or hCG determination may help to reach the correct interpretation, since in early non-molar miscarriages hCG after evacuation will quickly return to normal. Early non-molar miscarriages are nevertheless often mistaken for moles because some small terminal villi embedded in the trophoblastic shell may appear, on tangential sections, completely surrounded by several layers of trophoblast. Because of this, finding more than two layers of trophoblast around small non-hydropic villi in early gestation is not as significant as finding them around larger hydropic villi later in pregnancy. Trisomies and other

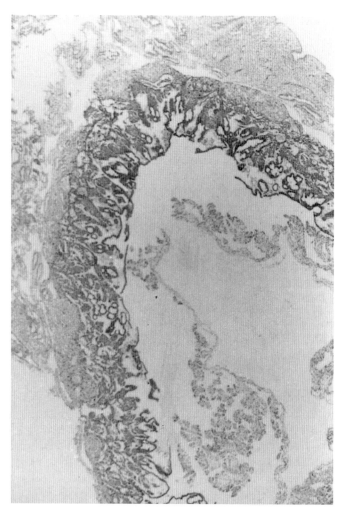

Fig. 40.19 Chorion from an early gestation. Secondary villi are regular and radiate from a central cavity. Amnion has detached from chorion and is folded within the cavity.

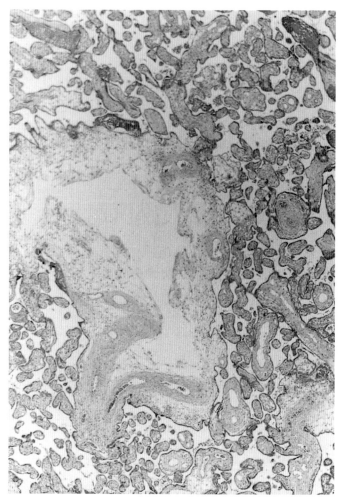

Fig. 40.20 Hydrops of stem villi with cistern formation in mesenchymal dysplasia. Thick muscular vessels are separated by abundant oedema fluid.

non-molar miscarriages often contain single cell trophoblastic inclusions which have been regarded as useful in diagnosis but they can be seen in partial and complete moles (Szulman & Surti 1978b; Paradinas et al 1996) and are not helpful in difficult cases. Between 12 and 18% of specimens sent to us each year with a diagnosis of molar pregnancy are easily recognisable non-molar miscarriages interpreted as moles. Hydropic change in non-molar miscarriages is usually mild, and when present, more generalised than in partial mole, but cisterns are seldom present and hydropic villi larger than 3 mm very rare. There is one exception to this: mesenchymal dysplasia (page 1372). The latter are large placentas and although some terminal villi may be hydropic, most of the cisterns are found in stem villi containing large muscular vessels (Fig. 40.20). Quite often there are foci of chorangiosis (Fig. 40.21) composed of small regular capillaries localised to a few neighbouring villi and very different to the branching angiectatic vessels seen in partial moles. In some cases, there is a stillbirth of a malformed fetus with omphalocele and other congenital malformations but in others, there is a live birth, with or without growth retardation, or with features of Beckwith–Wiedemann syndrome. None of the 15 cases seen by us showed excess trophoblast and no patient with this condition has developed persistent trophoblastic disease (Paradinas et al 2001).

In conclusion, diagnosis of molar pregnancy and molar type can improve with a knowledge of gestational age, extensive sampling of placental material, awareness of the appearances and distribution of trophoblast in early gestation and awareness of the appearances of moles in early gestation. Some of these are easily achieved, but extensive sampling of miscarriages can be time-consuming and expensive in terms of pathologists' time. We find that as the time before evacuation of abnormal pregnancies shortens, the numbers of specimens in which a diagnosis of partial mole is uncertain increases and we agree with others (Benirschke 1989) that more extensive use of flow cytometry or image analysis could be very helpful in refining the morphological diagnosis of molar pregnancy and in selecting patients likely to benefit from follow-up.

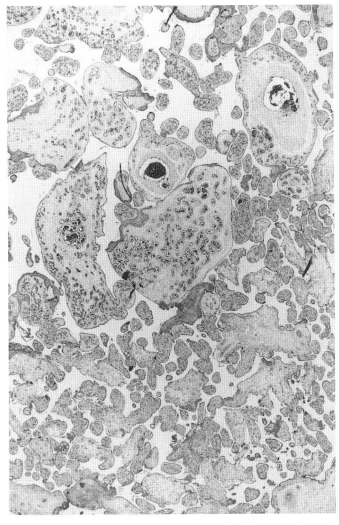

Fig. 40.21 Chorangiosis involving occasional villi in mesenchymal dysplasia.

SPECIAL INVESTIGATIONS IN THE DIAGNOSIS OF MOLAR PREGNANCY

In ideal circumstances the diagnosis of hydatidiform mole would be made on the basis of clinical features combined with histological and genetic data, but this is not a practical proposition for the vast majority of cases, especially as fresh tissue is required for cytogenetic analysis. For this reason, several other techniques have been investigated to evaluate their usefulness in the diagnosis of moles and their differential diagnosis from hydropic products of conception.

Histochemistry and immunocytochemistry

Stains for collagen, reticulin, basement membranes, mucosubstances, calcium and ribonucleic acids can be used to emphasise some of the features described earlier in the stroma of molar and non-molar villi but with a little experience these features are readily appreciated in ordinary H & E stained sections. The same can be said for immunocytochemistry to demonstrate vessels in the stroma of a complete mole (Paradinas 1994b; Qiao et al

1997) or placental hormones in the trophoblastic epithelium. Brescia et al (1987) and Losch & Kainz (1996) found that demonstration of hCG, hPL, PLAP and cytokeratins was of some use in differentiating both types of mole but the minor variations reported appear to reflect the gestational age of the specimen rather than molar type. Other workers (Fukunaga et al 1993a; Martinazzi et al 1996) regard immunocytochemistry for placental hormones as of little use and this is also our experience. The presence of oestrogen and progesterone receptors in moles has been investigated immunocytochemically by Cheung et al (1995) and that of inhibin by Minami et al (1993), McCluggage et al (1998) and Shih & Kurman (1999). This work may be important in understanding the biology of trophoblastic lesions but to date it has proved of little use in the diagnosis and differential diagnosis of moles.

Immunohistochemistry for the gene product of $p57^{kip2}$, a maternally expressed imprinted gene, has recently been shown to be of value in the distinction between partial (p57-positive and complete (p57-negative) moles (Chilosi et al 1998; Genest et al 2002).

Markers of cell proliferation have been extensively studied. Proliferating cell nuclear antigen (PCNA) is a 36 kD nuclear protein which is an auxiliary protein of DNA polymerase delta and is present in proliferating cells (Mathews et al 1984; Bravo et al 1987). The monoclonal antibody PC 10 recognises nuclear PCNA in routinely fixed paraffin-embedded tissues and has been used to study cell proliferation in a variety of tissues (Hall et al 1990; Hall & Woods 1990). Cheung et al (1993a) have examined the expression of PC 10 in choriocarcinoma, complete and partial mole and spontaneous miscarriages. They found much higher counts in choriocarcinoma than in the other three entities, but no difference between the moles and the miscarriages. Similarly, Suresh et al (1993) have shown no differences in PC 10 expression between spontaneous miscarriage and partial mole; these studies do not compare pregnancies of similar gestational age and this is likely to influence the results, but in practice it means that they are of little value in differentiation between both types of mole and between moles and non-molar miscarriages. Immunocytochemistry and/or in situ hybridisation have also been used to demonstrate other proliferation markers, oncogenes and cell products known to be overexpressed in neoplasia and preneoplastic conditions. These studies are less relevant to molar diagnosis than to the development of persistent trophoblastic disease and choriocarcinoma and will be discussed later.

Ultrastructural studies

Ultrastructural studies have contributed little to either diagnosis of moles or to our understanding of molar pathology. Wynn & Davies (1964b) examined a single mole and concluded that in general the trophoblast resembled that of the normal placenta. An intermediate trophoblastic cell was prominent, with a spectrum of

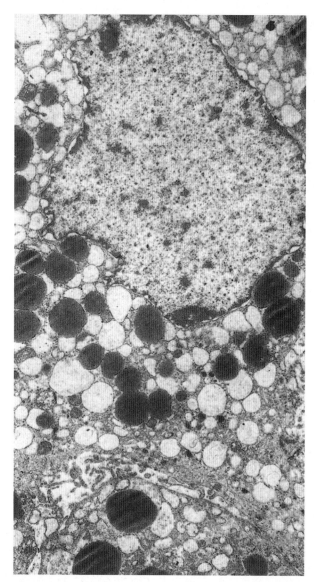

Fig. 40.22 Electronmicrograph of syncytiotrophoblast from a complete mole. There is abundant dilated endoplasmic reticulum with numerous lipid droplets.

transition from typical cytotrophoblast to mature secretory syncytiotrophoblast. They considered that the hydropic change in hydatidiform mole was dependent on the functional activity of the overlying trophoblast, ceasing if the trophoblast became atrophic or degenerate. Most other studies have confirmed the similarity of molar cytotrophoblastic cells to the normal (Gonzalez-Angulo et al 1966; Okudaira & Strauss 1967; Fox & Kharkongor 1971; Sen et al 1973). The appearances of molar syncytiotrophoblast appear to be more variable and abnormal (Ockleford & Clode 1983). Prominent and irregular surface microvilli are frequently seen and lipid droplets are increased (Fig. 40.22) with an expanded dilated endoplasmic reticulum (Gonzalez-Angulo et al 1966; Fox & Kharkongor 1971; Sen et al 1973). Ockleford & Clode (1983), using scanning electronmicroscopy, have found

abnormal microvillous structures, which they refer to as 'microgibbosities'. Mitochondrial appearances have been remarkably variable: small with irregular cristae (Larsen 1973), normal (Sen et al 1973), and enlarged (Fox & Kharkongor 1971). The presence of intermediate trophoblastic cells was noted by Gonzalez-Angulo et al and by Sen et al but not by Fox & Kharkongor.

There has been little speculation on the significance of these ultrastructural findings; Fox & Kharkongor (1971) concluded that the appearances seen by them were more akin to trophoblastic hyperplasia than neoplasia, whilst Ockleford & Clode (1983) suggested that the microgibbous elongated microvilli were consistent with a dysplastic epithelium. The ultrastructure of invasive mole has been studied by Wynn & Harris (1967) and Okudaira & Strauss (1967). Apart from evidence of more active trophoblast, the appearances are similar to those seen in a complete hydatidiform mole.

Ploidy analysis

A problem of cytogenetic analysis is that fresh tissue is required. Furthermore, selection bias may occur, since only a few cells are examined and can only be carried out on cells that can be induced to grow; cells that do not grow, and those with a long cell cycle, will be missed. Flow cytometry and image analysis permit the evaluation of the DNA content of many cells in all stages of the cycle, including interphase. A considerable further advantage has been conferred by the development of techniques for extracting DNA from formalin-fixed tissues (Hedley et al 1983) thus obviating the need for fresh specimens.

Routine histological material is therefore available for analysis and large numbers of cells from many specimens can be assessed in a short time. Several studies have confirmed the diploid status of the great majority of complete moles and the presence of triploidy in most partial moles (Fisher et al 1987; Hemming et al 1987; Lage et al 1988, 1991; Koenig et al 1993). This technique is therefore a useful alternative to cytogenetics, particularly in the distinction of partial from complete mole (Bagshawe et al 1990) and partial moles from non-molar miscarriages. However, there are exceptions (digynic triploids which are not molar, rare triploid androgenetic complete moles, tetraploid complete and partial moles) and ploidy can only be used in conjunction with morphology. The method has also been used to detect aneuploid and polyploid cell populations which may reflect genetic instability associated with development of neoplasia and cell proliferation.

Information similar to that obtained by flow cytometry can be obtained by image analysis. This was initially done by assessing the number of copies of one or several chromosomes using fluorochromes which stain specifically heterochromatic regions in interphase nuclei (Tommerup & Vejerslev 1985). It can be done either in sections (correcting results for the fact that a proportion of nuclei in sections will be incomplete depending on section thickness) or in smears of cell suspensions which can be also prepared from paraffin-embedded tissue. More recently, this has been superseded by assessing the DNA content of individual cells with an image analyser, preferably in smears from cell suspensions. The method gives results comparable to flow cytometry and uses less expensive equipment but is more time consuming (Jeffers et al 1995).

Some information about ploidy can be obtained from the study of silver-stained nucleolar organiser region-associated proteins (AgNORs). These tend to be more numerous in the nuclei of malignant than benign tumours or hyperplastic conditions (Crocker & Skilbeck 1987; Smith & Crocker 1988; Suarez et al 1989), where they may reflect aneuploidy and cell proliferation. In moles, Suresh et al (1990) found that AgNOR counts could not be correlated with proliferative activity and concluded that they were more likely to be a reflection of ploidy status. This has been confirmed by Watanabe et al (1998) and it appears that AgNOR counts do not provide useful information about proliferative activity of moles but are of some use in detecting triploids.

Interphase cytogenetics

Chromosomal aberrations at the cellular level can be demonstrated by in situ hybridisation (ISH) using chromosome specific probes, so-called 'interphase cytogenetics'. Van de Kaa and colleagues (1991) used this technique to study paraffin sections from a small number of hydatidiform moles. By using probes for the centromeric region of chromosomes 1 and X and the Q arm of Y they demonstrated that it is a useful technique which enables chromosome ploidy analysis and molar sex to be established, with preservation of histological appearances. They have now applied the technique to a larger series of cases of hydatidiform mole, complete and partial, and compared the results with cases of hydropic miscarriage (Van de Kaa et al 1993). In combination with DNA cytometry they have found DNA polyploidy in complete moles with a high GO/G1 exceeding rate, significantly different from hydropic miscarriages, and concluded that these techniques are useful in distinguishing those two entities. However, no significant differences were found between triploid partial moles and hydropic miscarriages. The finding that a high proportion of complete moles in this series exhibited aneuploidy and polyploidy rather than diploidy has been confirmed in other studies using image analysis (Williams et al 1995) and flow cytometry (Lage et al 1992; Fukunaga et al 1993b; Bewtra et al 1997). This does not invalidate the facts ascertained by chromosomal analysis that most complete moles are diploid and most partial moles triploid, but shows that the trophoblast from moles, particularly complete moles, has heterogeneous cell populations which were not detected when only a few cells from a mole were karyo-typed. The relationship of aneuploidy to molar prognosis is discussed later. Van de Kaa et al (1997a) also demonstrated by this method that the sex of nucleated red cells in vessels of complete moles was identical to that of the moles, suggesting some degree of embryonic development in complete mole, an event previously regarded as impossible.

DNA polymorphisms

The most significant advances in our understanding of molar pregnancies in recent years have come from the study of variable number tandem repeat sequences of DNA. The number of times that pairs of amino acids are repeated in specific areas of the genome is constant in each individual, but highly polymorphic. They are relatively short and withstand fixation and paraffin processing. The polymerase chain reaction (PCR) is used to amplify the amounts of DNA obtained and specific primers to identify each tandem repeat (Jeffreys et al 1988). This is the method used in forensic investigations and applied to moles can detect the sex of the mole by detecting Y chromosome specific sequences (Witt & Erickson 1989), the androgenetic nature of complete moles (Fisher et al 1989; Azuma et al 1991; Fukuyama et al 1991; Lane et al 1993) and the origin of moles and tumours from specific pregnancies (Fisher et al 1992a,b; Fisher & Newlands 1993). In recent years, it has also been used to investigate the possible embryonic development in complete moles (Fisher et al 1997; Weaver et al 2000) and the characterisation of biparental complete moles (Helwani et al 1999; Fisher et al 2000). Facilities for such specialised techniques as flow cytometry, ISH and PCR are, of course, not available in most routine laboratories, but in cases of diagnostic difficulty arrangements should be made for paraffin blocks to be sent to expert centres for analysis.

In conclusion, the great majority of cases of hydatidiform mole will continue to be diagnosed on morphological grounds alone, but, increasingly, newer molecular biological techniques will be necessary to evaluate difficult or borderline cases. Those techniques which can be applied to formalin-fixed paraffin-embedded material clearly have the greater potential in routine practice, and in this respect flow cytometry, interphase cytogenetics using in situ hybridisation and the study of DNA polymorphisms show the most promise. Understanding the mechanisms of imprinting and the various forms of molar development in pregnancies with apparently normal chromosomal constitution are future goals probably in the realm of DNA biochemistry.

PROGNOSIS OF COMPLETE AND PARTIAL MOLES

The careful follow-up of patients with hydatidiform mole has undoubtedly contributed to the dramatic reduction in mortality from choriocarcinoma, but paradoxically there is an unnecessary anxiety concerning the overall prognosis of molar gestations. It must be stressed that the majority of patients with hydatidiform mole have no sequelae, and in modern clinical practice persistent trophoblastic disease ensues in no more than 10% of patients for all molar types (Curry et al 1975; Womack & Elston 1985; Bagshawe et al 1986; Lurain & Sciarra 1991). There would be a significant benefit in reduction of unnecessary follow-up if the small group of patients who will develop persistent trophoblastic disease could be identified at the time of the original diagnosis. Since persistent trophoblastic disease is common after complete mole and rare after partial mole, accurate diagnosis of mole type is the best and simplest way of achieving this. However, updated morphological criteria valid to differentiate between both types of mole at an earlier stage of development are not yet widely used and accurate diagnosis of molar type is therefore poor (Paradinas 1998a). It is also relevant to ask if within each molar type one could identify patients likely to develop persistent trophoblastic disease (that is, invasive mole or choriocarcinoma), by looking at clinical, histopathological, genetic and other biological characteristics of the growing trophoblast which may indicate a higher propensity to invasion or to neoplastic transformation. These are reviewed separately for both types of mole.

Complete moles

The risk of persistent trophoblastic disease has been variously estimated to be as little as 8% for all mole types (Bagshawe et al 1986) and as high as 20–29% for complete moles (Ishizuka 1976; Kohorn 1982; Womack & Elston 1985). As commented by Berkowitz & Goldstein (1997b) and Paradinas (1998a) these differences reflect differences in criteria to diagnose molar pregnancy and differences in criteria to diagnose persistent trophoblastic disease. The lowest rates reported are from units with regional hCG follow-up systems, where moles are registered after a diagnosis made elsewhere (Fasoli et al 1982; Franke et al 1983; Bagshawe et al 1986). These are likely to include higher proportions of uncomplicated molar pregnancies and higher proportions of misdiagnosed non-molar miscarriages (Paradinas 1998a). The highest rates come from units specialised in the treatment of trophoblastic tumours and likely to see a higher proportion of patients with complications. A survey of over 2000 patients seen in five USA specialised centres shows an average incidence of 20% with persistent trophoblastic disease (Berkowitz & Goldstein 1997b). Estimates at Charing Cross Hospital for 1998 show 15% patients with persistent trophoblastic disease after a histologically confirmed diagnosis of complete mole. Many factors which could influence persistence of the disease have been studied. Some relate to the method of evacuation, some

to the environment in which the mole grows, that is the patient, and some to the biological characteristics of the mole itself.

Adequate evacuation

In most patients adequate evacuation is curative and vacuum aspiration is recommended as the initial method to avoid the dangers of perforation. Prostaglandin and oxytocin-induction may have a higher incidence of persistent disease (Bagshawe at al 1986), although the possibility that this is due to their use in more advanced pregnancies has been suggested (Flam et al 1991). Vacuum aspiration followed by curettage is commonly practised and a second curettage is sometimes necessary if the initial evacuation has not succeeded. However, repeated curettage increases the dangers and does not reduce the incidence of patients who will need chemotherapy (Bagshawe et al 1986). In recent years, earlier chemotherapy has reduced the incidence of metastases but earlier evacuation has not reduced the need for chemotherapy (Paradinas et al 1996; Berkowitz et al 1997b) suggesting that some complete moles may be invasive from the onset and therefore difficult to eradicate by evacuation alone.

Influence of the maternal environment

The patient's age, as well as hormones and immunological factors have been suggested as important. In some series (Stone & Bagshawe 1979; Ayhan et al 1996) chemotherapy was more frequent in older patients and those who had had previous moles. In Charing Cross, the use of contraceptive hormones during follow-up is not recommended, at least until hCG is normal, since patients receiving them had a higher incidence of persistent disease (Stone et al 1976) possibly due to reactivation of residual trophoblast populations. Even the hormonal changes of new pregnancies can reactivate molar trophoblast and choriocarcinomas genetically related to complete moles evacuated many years before have been described (Fisher et al 1995). This increased risk has been confirmed in a large multicentre study in the United States (Palmer et al 1999) but is not considered by them serious enough to restrict the use of oral contraceptives.

There has been considerable research on the immunogenicity of trophoblastic tissue, and in particular on antigenic differences between patients and their partners, using both the HLA and ABO systems (Berkowitz et al 1986a,b; Lawler & Fisher 1987a). Circulating immune complexes including paternal HLA antigens have been identified in the serum of women following evacuation of complete moles (Lahey et al 1984; Lawler & Fisher 1987b). The majority of patients who require chemotherapy for postmolar trophoblastic disease have antibodies to paternal HLA antigens and it appears that hydatidiform mole may be more immunogenic than a normal conceptus (Bagshawe et al 1971; Lawler & Fisher 1987c). This may be related to the androgenetic origin of most complete moles which expose the maternal immune system to a double dose of paternal antigen. Class I HLA antigens were first demonstrated in the stroma of chorionic villi (Faulk & Temple 1976; Sunderland et al 1981, Fisher & Lawler 1984b) but were not readily demonstrable in trophoblastic epithelium, although non-polymorphic class I determinants were identified in non-villous trophoblast and in proliferating trophoblast of complete moles (Sunderland et al 1985). HLA antigens have been difficult to localise by immunofluorescence (Sasagawa et al 1988), suggesting blocking antibodies. Higher incidences of HLA-DR-6 have been reported in association with persistent disease as well as a higher incidence of shared loci between patient and partner (Sbracia et al 1996) but these studies are preliminary and require confirmation. The expression of HLA-G on trophoblast surface and susceptibility of these cells to the effects of lymphocytes is receiving some attention (Zdravkovic et al 1999; Kilburn et al 2000) but these studies are of no practical value in assessing prognosis. Initial studies reported higher incidences of choriocarcinoma after term pregnancy and molar pregnancy in patients with ABO groups incompatible with those of their partners, but no differences have been found after molar pregnancies in subsequent research involving larger numbers of patients (Fisher et al 1993).

There have been attempts to assess immunological reactions by quantifying the cellular reaction around choriocarcinoma and moles (Elston 1969; Mogensen & Olsen 1973) and improved prognosis reported when this is intense. More recent studies (Wongweragiat et al 1999) show qualitative differences between the cellular reaction of moles and that of non-molar placentas, moles showing greater numbers of CD4 T-lymphocytes. Lymphocyte and macrophage function studies show depressed T-cell reactions in persistent disease and this could be related to production of cytokines and other factors by abnormal trophoblast (Guilbert et al 1993; Kamada et al 1993; Shaarawy et al 1996). Not enough is known about the physiological and pathological mechanisms of placentation to assess the usefulness of these studies in prognosis of moles.

Genetic type of complete mole

It has been suggested that heterozygous complete moles have a greater disposition to persistent trophoblastic disease than homozygous complete moles (Sasaki et al 1982; Wake et al 1984, 1987). Heterozygosity has been demonstrated in four cases of invasive mole (Wake et al 1984) and three cases of postmolar choriocarcinoma (Wake et al 1981; Sasaki et al 1982; Fisher & Lawler 1984a). However, in a relatively large series Lawler & Fisher (1991) found no difference in the requirement for

chemotherapy between patients with homozygous and heterozygous complete moles, and Mutter et al (1993b), using PCR on paraffin-embedded tissue, have shown that there is no increase in risk of metastasis for Y-chromosome positive compared with Y-chromosome negative moles. Only a few cases of biparental complete moles have been identified. We have seen two patients with repetitive biparental complete moles and one of them has required chemotherapy. The risk could be similar to that of other forms of complete mole.

Clinical prognostic indicators

It would appear logical that patients who present with vaginal metastases at the time of diagnosis (a reflection of invasive potential) should have a worse prognosis, but early studies (Elston 1970) showed that they did not. Patients with large uterus for dates, with high hCG levels (which to some extent reflect trophoblastic activity), and with hyperthyroidism, toxaemia or ovarian lutein cysts (which reflect thyroid and ovarian stimulation by hCG) have been said to have higher incidences of persistent trophoblastic disease (Curry et al 1975; Morrow et al 1977; Murad et al 1990). However, only patients with high pre-evacuation levels of hCG had higher incidences of chemotherapy in several studies (Deligdisch et al 1978; Ayhan et al 1996; Balaram et al 1999). Mungan et al (1996) found no predictive value in any of the clinical features mentioned above. It is interesting that early evacuation of moles has resulted in a remarkable decrease in the incidence of metastases, toxaemia and other complications of complete molar pregnancy but has not reduced the incidence of moles that need chemotherapy (Paradinas et al 1996; Berkowitz & Goldstein 1997b). Some clinical features, such as high pre-evacuation hCG levels, may have some predictive value in moles diagnosed in the second trimester, as is still the case in some countries, but they are of less practical use in early complete moles.

Histological grading systems

Before the introduction of accurate methods for the measurement of hCG, it was advocated that the morphological appearances of the trophoblast of complete moles could be used to predict which patients were likely to develop choriocarcinoma (Hertig & Sheldon 1947; Hertig & Mansell 1956). Hertig and colleagues proposed a grading system, initially with six categories and subsequently with three, and claimed that there is an increasing risk of malignancy with increasing trophoblastic 'hyperplasia' and atypia. Although some studies have supported these findings (Schiffer et al 1960; Douglas 1962; Deligdisch et al 1978; Sugimori et al 1980) most have not (Hunt et al 1953; Smalbraak 1957, 1959; Logan & Motyloff 1958; Tow & Yung 1967; Elston & Bagshawe

1972a; Genest et al 1991; Montes et al 1996). Elston & Bagshawe examined a series of hydatidiform moles, which, because of the referral nature of their unit, had a higher than average rate of subsequent choriocarcinoma (21% compared with 2%). They found no comparable excess of grade 3 moles, nor was there any increase in the number of choriocarcinomas derived from the grade 3 moles which did occur. They concluded that there is no value in attempting to predict potential malignant behaviour from the histological appearances of a hydatidiform mole and this view became generally accepted, although Hertig's teaching still has its adherents (Driscoll 1977; Deligdisch et al 1978; Balaram et al 1999). Genest et al (1991), from the New England Trophoblastic Disease Centre, have confirmed Elston & Bagshawe's work, and it is to be hoped that histological grading of hydatidiform mole will finally be abandoned as uninformative.

Hyperdiploidy and aneuploidy

Malignant neoplasms tend to have high proportions of aneuploid and hyperdiploid cells and this is also true of trophoblastic disease. Trophoblast from complete moles has been shown to have higher proportions of aneuploid cells than normal trophoblast and to be more vulnerable to chromosomal breakage (Habibian & Surti 1987). This genetic instability could lead to oncogene activation and could therefore be a measure of a tendency to develop invasion or neoplasia. Hemming et al (1988) investigated the value of flow cytometry in this respect. Although they found that cases which developed persistent trophoblastic disease had high hyperdiploid fractions, the values fell within the range for all diploid hydatidiform moles. The authors concluded that flow cytometry cannot be used to predict the possible behaviour of hydatidiform mole in an individual patient. Measurement of aneuploid fractions by flow cytometry also has difficulties of interpretation, since some diploid cells in the sample can be maternal, rather than molar and their variable numbers in different samples can affect results (Wersto et al 1991). Image cytometry of cell suspensions or in sections also has limitations, but to date no author has found significantly greater aneuploidy in patients who develop persistent trophoblastic disease (Fukunaga et al 1995a; Jeffers et al 1995; Sunde et al 1996; Van de Kaa et al 1996) and it appears that it has limited predictive value, although there is agreement that it is greater in neoplasms than in moles and greater in moles than in non-molar miscarriages.

Proliferative activity

The markers of cell proliferation PCNA and Ki-67 have been extensively studied (Cheung et al 1993a, 1994; Jeffers et al 1994, 1996; Schammel & Bocklage 1996; Ostrzega et al 1998). In general, proliferative activity is greater in complete moles than in partial moles or non-molar abor-

tions but it does not predict which complete moles will require chemotherapy.

AgNOR counts

It is uncertain if AgNORs reflect cell ploidy, cell proliferation or a combination of the two (Suresh et al 1990) and in many ways, their limitations are those of flow cytometry. Statistically significant differences in AgNOR counts between complete moles which do and do not need chemotherapy have been reported (Yang 1993); this has not yet been confirmed by any other group although, like ploidy, their usefulness in correct classification of mole types is emphasised in recent publications (Neudeck et al 1997; Watanabe et al 1998).

Oncogenes and growth factors

Some oncogenes and proto-oncogenes are more widely expressed in cells from complete moles than in normal placentas (Goustin et al 1985; Cheung et al 1993b; Lee 1995; Cheville et al 1996a,b; Fulop et al 1998; Halperin et al 2000). Their products, in particular growth factors, have been extensively studied and most have been found overexpressed in choriocarcinoma cells and in moles, particularly complete and invasive moles (Holmgrem et al 1993; Mutter et al 1993a; John et al 1997; Molykutty et al 1999). These studies help to understand autocrine and paracrine regulation of trophoblast growth and patterns of deregulation in tumours, but some reports are conflicting; for instance, Cameron et al (1994) found only 1 of 20 patients with persistent trophoblastic disease and *C-erbB-2* expression whereas Bauer et al (1997) found *C-erbB-2* mainly in invasive moles and choriocarcinomas and together with ploidy studies, suggested a rôle in predicting outcome. Another mechanism thought to play a rôle in eluding the programmed senescence of cells and development of neoplasia is increased telomerase activity, but this is also present in actively proliferating normal trophoblast (Kyo et al 1997). Increased telomerase activity has been reported in complete moles, particularly those developing persistent trophoblastic disease (Bae & Kim 1999; Cheung et al 1999; Nishi et al 1999; Sukcharoen et al 1999). At present these studies are time consuming and results difficult to evaluate. They have not yet contributed significantly to the differential diagnosis or prognostic assessment of moles. The same can be said of expression of apoptotic markers (Mochizuki et al 1998; Wong et al 1999; Halperin et al 2000; Chiu et al 2001) which may merely reflect regulation of trophoblastic proliferation.

Conclusions

It must be concluded that at present there is no alternative to careful hCG follow-up for all patients with complete hydatidiform mole. In the United Kingdom this is done by registration of patients with hydatidiform mole and accurate radioimmunoassay in specialised laboratories (Bagshawe et al 1986; Newlands et al 1992, 1997). When the hCG level returns to normal patients are advised not to start another pregnancy until the hCG level has been normal for at least six months. If the hCG level is still elevated beyond eight weeks from the date of evacuation follow-up is continued for two years. This caution is highlighted by a report from Elmer et al (1993). They cited the case of a patient who required chemotherapy for persistent trophoblastic disease after hCG levels had returned to normal within 25 weeks of the evacuation of a complete hydatidiform mole and remained normal for over a year before rising again. The main criteria for treatment are a raised serum hCG (>20 000 IU/l) more than 4 weeks after evacuation, rising hCG values, prolonged uterine haemorrhage and radiological evidence of metastatic lesions (Newlands et al 1992). Following a complete mole, about 15% of patients require chemotherapy (Newlands 1997), and the mortality is extremely low at 0.2% (Bagshawe et al 1986).

Partial moles

The case for adequate follow-up for patients with complete hydatidiform moles is clearly established, but until comparatively recently, much less has been known about the behaviour of partial moles. Some groups suggested that follow-up was not required (Vassilakos & Kajii 1976; Lawler et al 1982a) and the absence of persistent trophoblastic disease in early series appeared to support this view (Szulman & Surti 1982; Lawler & Fisher 1987a; Lawler & Fisher 1991). However, the total number of cases studied was too small to reach a definite conclusion and a number of case reports have demonstrated that persistent trophoblastic disease does develop after partial hydatidiform mole. Cases with histopathological confirmation include metastatic disease after partial mole (Elston 1976), invasive mole (Szulman et al 1978, 1981b; Gaber et al 1986) and choriocarcinoma (Looi & Sivanesaratnam 1981; Bagshawe et al 1990; Gardner & Lage 1992). Genetic proof of origin of choriocarcinoma from previous partial moles has been shown in three cases (Seckl et al 2000). Several series of patients who required chemotherapy for persistent trophoblastic disease after the evacuation of partial moles have now been reported, from New England, USA (Berkowitz et al 1986a; Berkowitz et al 1988; Berkowitz & Goldstein 1988; Rice et al 1990), Charing Cross Hospital, UK (Bagshawe et al 1990) and Aichi Prefecture, Japan (Goto et al 1993), although they provide greatly differing estimates of the risk: 5.5% (New England), 2.8% (Aichi) and 0.5% (Charing Cross). This reflects differences in referral patterns and criteria for post-evacuation chemotherapy but also differences in morphological criteria to diagnose partial mole (Paradinas 1994, 1998a). For instance,

several partial moles which required chemotherapy in one series (Lage et al 1991) were diploid and may have been reclassified as complete moles if updated criteria had been used. Until the features of early complete moles are more widely recognised by pathologists, many are being called partial moles. This confusion probably explains occasional reports of 83% of diploid partial moles with 20% needing chemotherapy (Davis et al 1987). It is also uncertain if cases of reported metastases after partial mole (Jones et al 1980; Szepesi et al 1988; Goto et al 1993; Chen et al 1994; Menczer et al 1999) are real partial moles, complete moles or choriocarcinomas complicating moles. More recent studies report lower incidences of persistent trophoblastic disease after partial mole, with Sunde et al (1996) estimating an incidence between 0 and 2.7% and Zalel & Dgani (1997) an incidence of 2.9%. In our experience there is no doubt that hCG takes longer to return to normal in patients with partial mole than after non-molar miscarriages. Chemotherapy after partial mole is needed about once a year but this is exceedingly rare after a histologically proven non-molar miscarriage (Paradinas et al 1996).

We therefore feel that partial moles need follow-up. The fact that many initial diagnoses of partial mole are wrong (they are in fact early complete moles), makes this a greater need. Since follow-up is recommended for a minimum of 6 months during which time contraception should be practised (Bagshawe et al 1986; Gal & Friedman 1987; Newlands et al 1992) it is not a procedure to be undertaken lightly and accurate patient selection is vital. Shorter follow-up for partial mole is desirable (Szulman 1987), but, at present, follow-up cannot be relaxed until the diagnosis has been supported by genetic studies, ploidy studies or by histological examination in a specialised centre.

There are no studies of prognostic factors in partial mole comparable to those of complete mole. Only 35 patients with histologically confirmed partial moles who needed chemotherapy after molar evacuation have been registered at Charing Cross in 28 years. As a group, they do not have more abundant multifocal or circumferential trophoblast than those from patients who did not need chemotherapy. Indeed in some cases, there was no excess trophoblast in inadequate samples, but patients later developed choriocarcinoma. The very mild excess and very focal distribution of trophoblast in partial moles means that sampling error is common. Proliferative activity is also much less intense than in complete moles when measured with proliferation markers such as PCNA and Ki-67. Unless moles and spontaneous non-molar miscarriages of similar gestational age are compared, increased proliferation may not be apparent (Suresh et al 1993; Jeffers et al 1994; Cheville et al 1996b). We have compared partial moles which needed chemotherapy with partial moles which did not, matched for gestational age and patient's age (Halls & Paradinas 2001). The Ki-67 index was higher in the treated group but only reached statistical significance when counts were restricted to cytotrophoblast forming villous and intervillous clusters. These studies are time consuming, subject to sampling error and unlikely to be of use in the follow-up of partial moles. Like complete moles, partial moles do express oncogenes and their products but less frequently and with less intensity (Cheville et al 1996a; Fulop et al 1998; Halperin et al 2000) and like proliferative activity, it is more difficult to detect differences between them and non-molar miscarriages or normal first trimester placentas.

INVASIVE MOLES AND PERSISTENT TROPHOBLASTIC DISEASE

In most instances, hydatidiform moles are cured by adequate evacuation achieved by suction, curettage or a combination of the two. This suggests that, as in a normal pregnancy, molar tissue is located mainly in endometrium and decidua. However, in some cases it invades myometrium and vessels and can metastasise, although, unlike choriocarcinoma, is still forming villous stroma. Park (1967) proposed that abnormal trophoblast which forms villous stroma has only a locally malignant potential, whilst that which does not form villous stroma has a 'metastasising' malignant potential, but this is not supported by cases of trophoblastic disease in which metastatic nodules have been shown to contain villi (Delfs 1957; Ring 1972; Kohorn et al 1978). Tow (1966), based on his experience in treating trophoblastic disease in Singapore, suggested that invasive mole be renamed 'villous choriocarcinoma' and that classical choriocarcinoma be called 'avillous choriocarcinoma'. He argued that the villous form was merely an early stage of avillous choriocarcinoma and that, in his practice at least, both lesions received the same treatment. These ideas received some support on theoretical grounds from Brewer (1967) and the classification continued in Singapore for some time (Ratnam & Chew 1976). The available evidence, however, indicates that invasive mole only rarely progresses to true choriocarcinoma (Chun & Braga 1967; Park 1971), and that the presence of molar villi is a marker of an inherently less aggressive trophoblastic proliferation. Tow's proposal was not incorporated into the classification recommended by the International Union Against Cancer (1967), nor has it been supported elsewhere (Bagshawe 1969; Park 1971; Elston 1978; WHO Scientific Group 1983; Silverberg & Kurman 1992; Mazur & Kurman 1994). Since the prognosis of invasive mole is very different from that of choriocarcinoma and the presence of molar villous stroma is a clear distinguishing feature, there are excellent practical reasons for keeping the two lesions separate. This distinction has been accepted by most authorities (Hertig & Mansell 1956; Ober et al 1971; Park 1971; Elston 1991; Silverberg & Kurman 1992).

Dehner (1980) has commented that invasive mole has ceased to be an important clinicopathological entity, because hysterectomy is rarely performed now in trophoblastic disease and invasion is difficult to assess in curettings. However, in most instances in which persistent trophoblastic disease develops, this is due to the presence of myometrial lesions detectable by ultrasound or CT scan and likely to be invasive moles. This is usually confirmed in the few cases in which hysterectomy is performed electively or when the disease proves to be chemoresistant. Therefore, although pathological diagnosis will be made less frequently, there are strong practical reasons for retaining invasive mole as a separate diagnostic category.

PATHOGENESIS OF INVASIVE MOLES

We do not know why some complete moles readily invade myometrium and others do not. It seems logical to postulate that the longer the mole remains in utero, the higher the chances of invasion should be, but earlier evacuation in recent years has not reduced the incidence of persistent trophoblastic disease likely to be due to myometrial invasion, although it has reduced the incidence of molar metastases (Paradinas et al 1996; Mosher et al 1998). It seems likely that some moles have from the onset a higher invasive tendency than others due to deregulation of the normal mechanisms controlling invasion at the implantation site. Knowledge of these mechanisms is at present sketchy (see prognosis of molar pregnancies) and no consistent chromosomal or genetic abnormality has yet been described in specific association with invasive moles. The factors that influence trophoblastic invasion and regulate it in normal and molar placentas, such as collagenases, adhesion molecules and plasminogen activator amongst others, are being extensively studied (Fernandez et al 1992; Goshen et al 1996; Crescimanno et al 1999; Floridon et al 1999) but there are still no clues as to the reasons for the differences in invasive tendency of moles.

INCIDENCE AND CLINICAL PRESENTATION

In the days when hysterectomy was common in the management of molar pregnancies, invasive moles occurred in about 16% of molar pregnancies (Hertig & Mansell 1956). Most of these were probably invasive complete moles, since few partial moles were recognised at that time. Very similar figures (10% to 20%) are reported in recent years for the incidence of persistent trophoblastic disease after complete mole. Documented partial moles in hysterectomy specimens are a rarity (Szulman et al 1981b; Gaber et al 1986) and the incidence of persistent gestational trophoblastic disease after partial mole likely to be due to an invasive mole is in our experience of the order of 0.5% (Bagshawe et al 1990). Higher incidences have been reported by others (see prognosis of partial mole) but recent publications (Matsui et al 1996; Zalel & Dgani 1997) using updated criteria for molar diagnosis, report incidences close to those seen by us at Charing Cross.

In most cases the clinical presentation is that of a complete mole which remains unresolved after adequate evacuation. Rarely, vaginal metastases are present initially but the clinical picture is otherwise that of a complete mole. Hysterectomy specimens with invasive moles seen by us in recent years fall into three categories: elective hysterectomy before or after a trial of chemotherapy for a mole, hysterectomy for vaginal bleeding in perimenopausal women on HRT in whom the diagnosis was unsuspected and hysterectomies in women of any age presenting with uterine perforation and haemoperitoneum.

PATHOLOGY OF INVASIVE MOLES

The macroscopical appearances are variable and dependent on the extent of invasion. There may be little abnormality in the uterine cavity except for the presence of haemorrhage and vesicles at the implantation site. A haemorrhagic cavity of variable size may be present, with obvious penetration into the myometrium (Fig. 40.23). Less commonly the molar tissue extends so deeply that the uterus is perforated, or there is extension into adjacent structures such as the broad ligament. In some cases the original hydatidiform mole is still present within the uterine cavity.

Microscopically the main diagnostic feature is the presence within the myometrium of molar villi showing trophoblastic proliferation. The villi may vary considerably in size and occasionally are inconspicuous. It is therefore important that in any uterus containing a proliferative trophoblastic lesion a careful search should be made for molar villi in order to avoid an erroneous diagnosis of choriocarcinoma. The amount of trophoblast is also variable, and although there is usually at least a moderate increase, in some cases little trophoblastic overgrowth is seen. In the majority of cases a florid placental site reaction will persist, and this should not be mistaken for choriocarcinomatous invasion.

Fig. 40.23 Invasive mole of the increta type. Molar villi penetrate into the myometrium at the fundus. (Reproduced by kind permission of Professor D Hourihan.)

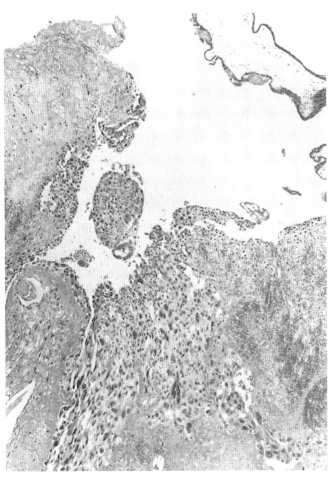

Fig. 40.24 Invasive mole of the accreta type. This field shows the molar implantation site with a villus above and trophoblast attached to decidua below.

Hertig (1950) drew an analogy between the degree of invasion of an invasive mole and placenta accreta, increta and percreta. It is probable that in all hydatidiform moles there is at least a technical breach of the decidua and therefore minimal invasion, and the sooner a hysterectomy is performed after evacuation of a mole the more likely it is that evidence of local invasion will be found (Gore & Hertig 1967). In the accreta type of invasive mole, seen most frequently when the original hydatidiform mole is still contained in the uterus at hysterectomy, or where the mole was aborted shortly before hysterectomy, molar villi are attached directly to superficial myometrium without intervening decidua (Figs 40.24, 40.25). There is no deep invasion of the myometrium, although small trophoblastic emboli may be found (Fig. 40.26). The majority of cases fall into the increta category. Hydropic villi extend deeply into the myometrium, but the serosa remains intact. Most of the invasion takes place through dilated venous channels (Fig. 40.27) and direct myometrial muscle invasion is limited. Foci of haemorrhage may occur but are usually confined to the molar tissue rather than myometrium. In a minority of cases molar villi penetrate through the full thickness of the uterine wall (percreta type). This results in

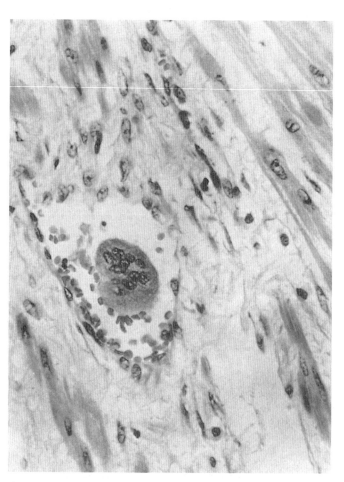

Fig. 40.26 A blood vessel deep in the myometrium contains a small trophoblastic embolus. Same case as Figs 40.24 and 40.25.

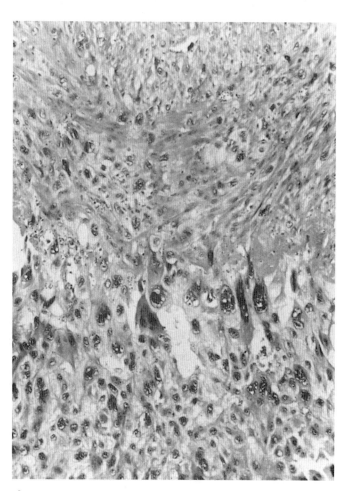

Fig. 40.25 Same case as Fig. 40.24. Proliferating trophoblast above is attached to myometrium below.

uterine perforation or extension into the adjacent parametrium.

Vascular invasion can also result in the development of metastases. For most tumours the development of metastases is one of the main criteria for the diagnosis of malignancy. Because trophoblastic disease covers a wide spectrum of processes which includes both neoplastic and non-neoplastic conditions, such a simplistic view is inappropriate. Trophoblastic cells have been detected in the peripheral blood of pregnant women (Couone et al 1984; Mueller et al 1990) and deportation of benign trophoblastic fragments has also been described in normal pregnancy (Attwood & Park 1961) and in eclampsia (Schmorl 1893; Veit 1901; Bardawil & Toy 1959). Metastatic lesions are also well recognised in molar pregnancies, but it is extremely important to appreciate that their development does not necessarily mean that choriocarcinoma has supervened; indeed they more usually indicate simply that the mole is invasive.

Before the advent of early evacuation and early chemotherapy, the reported frequency of metastases in hydatidiform mole varied widely, with a range from 24% (Greene 1959) to 40% (Wilson et al 1961). In a selected

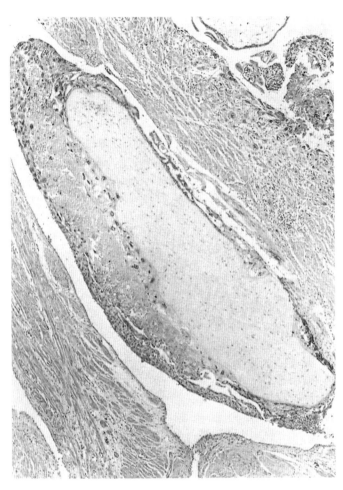

Fig. 40.27 Invasive mole of the increta type. A molar villus lies within a dilated venous sinus deep in the myometrium.

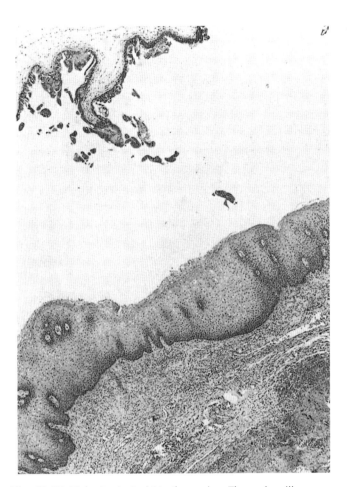

Fig. 40.28 Molar 'metastasis' to the vagina. The molar villus was obtained at biopsy of a haemorrhagic vaginal nodule, part of which is visible at the bottom right.

series of patients in the United Kingdom, Elston (1970) found a frequency of 36% which agrees closely with the figure of 35% obtained by Tow (1966) from a review of the literature. Such figures are clearly an overestimate of the true frequency, due to selection of patients who have developed complications, and it must be re-emphasised that persistent trophoblastic disease with metastatic lesions only occurred in approximately 10% of patients with complete hydatidiform mole (Womack & Elston 1985; Bagshawe et al 1986) and in most instances this included radiological metastases rather than just those confirmed histologically. Nowadays, early diagnosis and early chemotherapy has reduced this dramatically and no more than 1% of patients admitted to our institution with persistent trophoblastic disease after a complete mole have metastases. This is also the experience of the New England Trophoblastic Disease Unit (Berkowitz & Goldstein 1997b) where an incidence of metastases of 4% for all types of gestational trophoblastic disease (including choriocarcinomas) is quoted.

In most cases metastatic lesions occur in the lungs. Their detection is usually based on clinical assessment and radiological evidence, without histological confirma-

tion. There are, however, a number of reports in which lung lesions contained molar villi or benign deported trophoblastic fragments (Delfs 1957; Jacobson & Enzer 1959; Reed et al 1959; Wilson et al 1961; Ring 1972; Johnson et al 1979). Vaginal metastases (Figs 40.28 to 40.30) which contain molar villi or benign trophoblast have also been recorded (Haines 1955; Bardawil et al 1957; Dinh-De & Minh 1961; Hsu et al 1962; Thiele & de Alvarez 1962; Elston 1976) and rarer metastatic sites include brain (Ishizuka 1967), spinal cord (Hsu et al 1962) and paraspinal connective tissue (Delfs 1957). Such metastatic lesions are almost always benign in nature and usually regress after evacuation of the mole. Death attributed to histologically proven metastases has only rarely been reported (Hsu et al 1962; Ishizuka 1967). Malignancy can only be assumed to have developed when metastases have been confirmed histologically and have the appearances of choriocarcinoma.

PROGNOSIS OF INVASIVE MOLE

Most published figures concerning the mortality of invasive mole have been from the era before chemotherapy

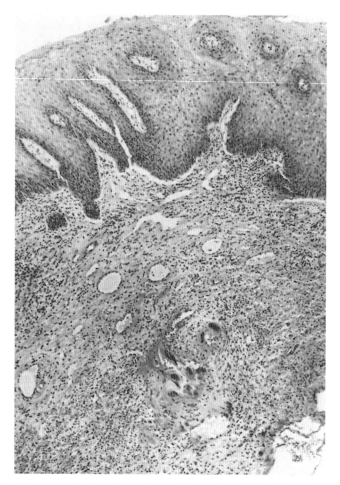

Fig. 40.29 Benign trophoblastic deportation in a patient with a hydatidiform mole. This is a vaginal nodule showing part of a haemorrhagic cavity in which syncytial giant cells are seen. (Reprinted with permission from Elston 1989.)

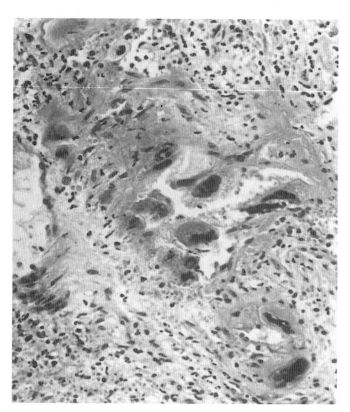

Fig. 40.30 Higher magnification of nodule shown in Fig. 40.29 There are scanty syncytiotrophoblastic cells but no chorionic villi. (Reprinted with permission from Elston, 1989.)

became available. The highest recorded mortality is 20% in the Far East (Prawirohardjo et al 1957), whilst a figure of 14% was obtained by Greene (1959) in a selected series in the United States. Ober (1965) reviewed the world literature and found nine deaths in 145 cases (6%), which is closely similar to Ishizuka's (1967) figures for Japan of an 8% mortality. Since the introduction of chemotherapy a pathological diagnosis of invasive mole is made less frequently than before, with a decline in the use of hysterectomy, and most cases will be included within the broad classification of persistent trophoblastic disease. Accurate statistics are not readily available, but no deaths from histologically confirmed invasive mole occurred in the Charing Cross series (Elston 1978), and this now seems to be the general experience (Du Beshter et al 1987). Most deaths in the past were attributable to local catastrophic events such as haemorrhage or uterine perforation rather than to the development of malignant trophoblastic disease. It is clear that the mortality from invasive mole is now very low, emphasising the limited aggressiveness of the lesion.

TROPHOBLASTIC NEOPLASMS

To have a proper understanding of the histogenesis of trophoblastic tumours it is important to outline the morphological and physiological features of normal trophoblast. During placentation the outer cell layer of the blastocyst proliferates to form the trophoblastic cell mass. After about seven days the trophoblast differentiates into two layers: the inner layer is composed of large mononuclear cells with clear cytoplasm, the cytotrophoblast, and the outer layer is made up of a multinucleated syncytium, the syncytiotrophoblast. It is well established that the syncytiotrophoblast is derived from the cytotrophoblast by cell fusion, but does not divide further. A third type of trophoblastic cell, which is also derived from the cytotrophoblast, has now been recognised. These cells are mononuclear but exhibit amphophilic cytoplasm like syncytiotrophoblast. Since they share morphological characteristics with cyto- and syncytiotrophoblast they have been designated intermediate trophoblast (Kurman et al 1984). During implantation, intermediate trophoblast migrates from the cytotrophoblastic cell columns at the anchoring tips of villi to infiltrate widely in the placental bed (Pijnenborg et al 1981). It is these cells which also invade and partially replace the endothelium of the decidual portion of spiral arteries (Kurman et al 1984), a facet

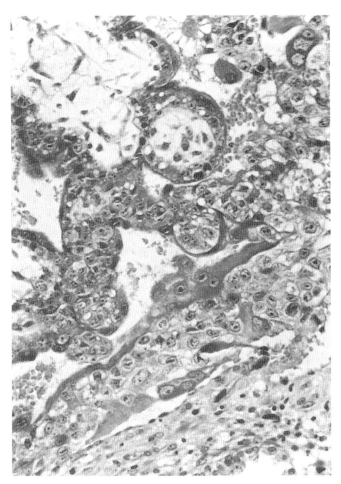

Fig. 40.31 Implanting 15-day blastocyst. The villous stroma is above and the decidua below. In the centre cores of mononuclear cytotrophoblast are surrounded by multinucleated syncytiotrophoblast which forms the margins of the intervillous space containing maternal red cells.

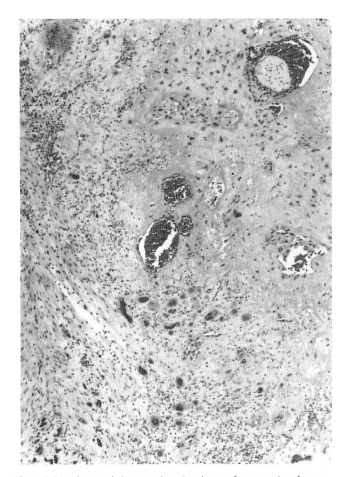

Fig. 40.32 Placental site reaction. Products of conception from a spontaneous abortion. A villus at the top right is embedded in decidua. Extravillous trophoblastic cells are seen at the bottom left.

of implantation essential for subsequent fetal development. Thus the villous trophoblast comes to be composed predominantly of cytotrophoblast and syncytiotrophoblast (Fig. 40.31) with a small component of intermediate trophoblast, and the extravillous trophoblast is composed mainly of intermediate trophoblast with a minor amount of syncytiotrophoblast (Figs 40.32, 40.33). Another recently described cell type is vacuolated trophoblast (Yeh et al 1989), mainly present in the chorion in late pregnancy.

A range of protein hormones, steroid hormones and enzymes is secreted by the placenta. The majority are confined to the syncytiotrophoblast but the localisation of two, hCG and human placental lactogen (hPL), has led to a more complete characterisation of the various types of trophoblast (Heyderman et al 1981; Kurman et al 1984). Cytotrophoblast does not contain hCG or hPL. Syncytiotrophoblast contains hCG in large amounts in the first trimester, decreasing as pregnancy proceeds, and only small amounts of hPL at any stage. Intermediate tro-

phoblast, in contrast, contains moderate amounts of hPL throughout (Fig. 40.34), with only focal amounts of hCG. Vacuolated trophoblast expresses some hPL but placental alkaline phosphatase (PLAP) is more often found (Yeh et al 1989). Inhibin is also produced by most forms of trophoblast but is less specific.

Trophoblastic tumours show differentiation towards villous trophoblast (choriocarcinoma), intermediate trophoblast (placental site tumour) and vacuolated trophoblast (epithelioid trophoblastic tumour). There are, however, tumours with mixtures of various cell types and tumours which change morphology in time or after therapy (Paradinas 1998b) and we should not regard these tumour types as mutually exclusive or to imply that they arise from specific types of trophoblast.

Trophoblastic differentiation can occur in germ cell tumours and by metaplasia in other forms of cancer but by definition, gestational trophoblastic neoplasms are the result of a pregnancy. As with molar pregnancies, both the maternal environment and genetic abnormalities may be relevant to their development.

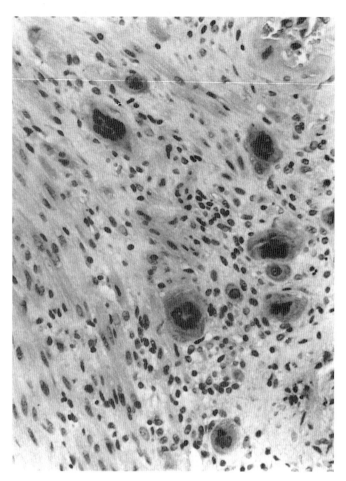

Fig. 40.33 Higher magnification of the field shown in Fig. 40.32, to show intermediate trophoblastic cells infiltrating between muscle bundles.

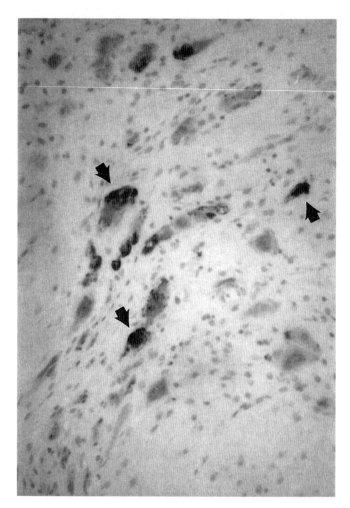

Fig. 40.34 Localisation of hPL in intermediate trophoblast of placental site (arrowheads). Same case as Figs 40.25 and 40.26. Immunoperoxidase–hPL.

AETIOLOGY AND PATHOGENESIS OF TROPHOBLASTIC NEOPLASMS

Influence of the maternal environment

In some series, choriocarcinoma patients have been older than in series of pregnant patients as a whole and with a greater incidence of miscarriages (WHO 1983). Like moles, choriocarcinoma occurs more often in the Orient but no associations with particular ethnic groups have been reported. Epidemiological studies are difficult because of the rarity of the condition and even more difficult nowadays because tissue diagnosis is often not available.

Choriocarcinoma is derived from a fetal tissue proliferating in the maternal host and occupies a unique status as a neoplastic allograft. The remarkable success of cytotoxic therapy in gestational trophoblastic disease, particularly in comparison with the far less favourable results in trophoblastic tumours of germ cell origin, points strongly to a genetic disparity between the patient and the tumour. This is supported by morphological studies which show that a lymphoplasmacytoid cell infiltrate, similar to that

seen in cellular allograft rejection, is present in approximately 90% of choriocarcinomas (Elston 1969). The intensity of the infiltrate is related to prognosis, and survival is better in patients with a marked reaction (Elston 1969; Elston & Bagshawe 1973; Elston 1976). Similar findings have been reported by Park (1971), Mogensen & Olsen (1973) and Ito et al (1981), who advocate a reporting system which includes both intensity of cellular reaction and vascular permeation by tumour cells. Junaid et al (1976) found a cellular reaction in less than half their cases in Nigeria, with no correlation with prognosis. This may be due to the late presentation of many of their patients, since prognosis deteriorates markedly the longer the interval between the antecedent gestation and the start of treatment (Bagshawe 1976). Confirmation that the lymphoplasmacytoid infiltrates are the morphological expression of tumour rejection is as yet incomplete, and much of the evidence is conflicting. Although Bagshawe (1969) has demonstrated that patients with gestational choriocarcinoma may develop tolerance to skin grafts from their husbands, results of immunotherapy have been inconclusive (Hertz 1978; Goldstein & Berkowitz 1982). Lymphoid infiltrates surrounding moles and choriocarcinoma differ significantly from those in normal pregnancy (Wongweragiat et al 1999) and products from choriocarcinoma cell lines and from patients with choriocarcinoma can cause immunosuppression (Guilbert et al 1993; Shaarawy et al 1996; Mor et al 1998; Kilic et al 1999).

Several studies indicate that HLA class I antigens are also expressed in gestational choriocarcinoma (Tursz et al 1981; Berkowitz et al 1986a,b). Circulating immune complexes containing paternal antigens have been detected in the sera of patients with choriocarcinoma (Shaw et al 1979; Lahey et al 1984) and immunohistological studies have identified HLA class I antigen in malignant trophoblastic cells, including the BeWo cell line (Trowsdale et al 1980; Anderson & Berkowitz 1985; Berkowitz et al 1986a,b). Of particular interest in recent years has been the detection of HLA-G on the surface of trophoblast and its modulation of maternal immune responses (Yang et al 1995; Dorling et al 2000). Theoretically HLA compatibility may influence the progression of gestational trophoblastic neoplasia. If the patient and her partner are histocompatible the trophoblastic tumour that bears paternal antigens might not be immunogenic in the maternal host. Some groups have claimed that histocompatibility is more common with metastatic trophoblastic disease (Mogensen & Kissmeyer-Nielsen 1968, 1971; Tomoda et al 1976) but this has not been confirmed by others (Rudoph & Thomas 1970; Lawler et al 1971; Lewis & Terasaki 1971; Mittal et al 1975; Berkowitz et al 1981; Yamashita et al 1981). Lawler (1978) concluded that the HLA system does not exert a strong influence on the chances of a woman developing a trophoblastic tumour.

An increased frequency of blood group A has been reported in women with choriocarcinoma (Llewellyn-Jones 1965; Dawood et al 1971). Bagshawe et al (1971) reported an increased incidence of trophoblastic tumours in patients with a different ABO group than their husbands, particularly in choriocarcinoma after term pregnancies. Initial studies (Bagshawe 1976; Lawler & Fisher 1987b) appeared to support this and it was incorporated as a risk factor in the WHO and Charing Cross scoring systems (Bagshawe 1973; WHO 1983; Smith et al 1993). These studies have not been supported by more recent research by the same group (Fisher et al 1993): it is now possible to ascertain the ABO group of molar tissue without the presence of red cells and a study of 48 patients who needed chemotherapy has shown equal numbers of compatible and incompatible cases. Assessment of ABO compatibility is now of little practical importance due to the more successful regimes available for the treatment of gestational trophoblastic tumours and is no longer included in the scoring system at Charing Cross (Newlands 1997).

Genetic abnormalities in the trophoblast

The comparative rarity of choriocarcinoma has limited the opportunities for detailed cytogenetic analysis, and no consistent pattern of abnormality has emerged. Observations made in cells growing in tissue culture or in nude mice may not be relevant to the situation in vivo, since cells often undergo further mutations. Aneuploidy is common (Galton et al 1963; Makino et al 1963) and many studies have shown grossly abnormal karyotypes with a wide range of ploidies and a number of chromosomal rearrangements (Wake et al 1981; Sasaki et al 1982; Sheppard et al 1985; Lawler & Fisher 1986; Rodriguez et al 1995). In a study by Davis & Foster (1984), using quinacrine staining on histological sections, 14 of 19 choriocarcinomas were found to be Y-body positive, but other studies have not found higher incidences of persistent trophoblastic disease after XY moles (Fisher & Lawler 1984a), nor is choriocarcinoma more frequent after term pregnancies with a male liveborn (Schoen et al 1954).

Most of the oncogenes and growth factors found in moles (page 1386) are more easily demonstrable in choriocarcinomas. Expression of four oncogenes c-*fms*, c-*fos*, c-*myc* and c-*ras* has been identified by in situ hybridisation in BeWo and JaR cell lines (Muller et al 1983; Bartocci et al 1986; Rettenmier et al 1986; Sarkar et al 1986; Pollard et al 1987). The c-*fms* proto-oncogene product is related to the receptor for colony stimulating factor 1 (CSF-1) (Sheer et al 1985) and c-*fms* expression has been identified in the syncytiotrophoblast of hydatidiform moles (Yokoyama et al 1988; Cheung et al 1993b). Increasing use of molecular genetic techniques has resulted in increasing numbers of mitogenes and gene products which have been found to be altered in choriocarcinoma (Huch et al 1998; Vegh et al 1999; Xu et al 1999) but there is no consistent abnormality, suggesting that there may be many different pathways in the development of trophoblastic neoplasms. Ahmed et al (2000) have shown by comparative genomic hybridisation that there is amplification of 7q21-q31 and loss of 8p12-p21 in choriocarcinoma, but not in moles. These or similar studies of genetic differences between trophoblast from moles and that from choriocarcinoma could help to define trophoblastic neoplasia better and differentiate it from the more controlled growth disturbance of moles. An approach to the study of these genetic abnormalities is the creation of cell hybrids by introducing normal chromosomes into immortalised choriocarcinoma cell lines (Matsuda et al 1997) and assessing the effect of the new genetic material in modulating trophoblastic growth. The results suggest the existence of one or more tumour suppressor genes in chromosome 7 but further studies are needed to see if this is a constant abnormality in choriocarcinomas and to define the abnormality further.

Genetic studies in placental site trophoblastic tumour are few. Cytogenetic and ploidy studies have shown less aneuploidy than in choricarcinoma and a majority of tumours are reported to be diploid on flow cytometry (Eckstein et al 1985; Lathrop et al 1988; Fukunaga & Ushigome 1993a,b). It is, however, clear from histological examination than some tumours are very pleomorphic and some cases have been aneuploid and near triploid or tetraploid (Kashimura et al 1990; Remadi et al 1997). Oncogenes, tumour suppressor genes and their products have been described (Muller-Hocker et al 1997) and proliferation markers have been used to differentiate tumours from benign placental site reactions (Ichikawa et al 1998; Shih & Kurman 1998b; Shih et al 1999).

Environmental factors in the development of trophoblastic neoplasms

The possibility of a link between choriocarcinoma and oncogenic viruses has been suggested in the past (De Ruyck 1951; Nastac et al 1980). These studies have little relevance today, but the possibility of viruses altering the proliferative and invasive properties of trophoblast is nevertheless possible and has been demonstrated in trophoblast tissue cultures with SV40 (Aboagye-Mathiesen et al 1996; Khoo et al 1998) and the retrovirus ERV-3 (Lin et al 1999). The relevance of this to human disease is yet to be investigated.

There is remarkably little information on the possible effects of chemicals on the aetiology of human trophoblastic tumours. The effects that contraceptive hormones and hormonal changes from new pregnancies may have in activating residual 'dormant' trophoblast has already been mentioned. An association between high ethanol consumption and mortality from choriocarcinoma has been suggested (Guo et al 1994).

One factor which has limited research into the aetiology of trophoblastic disease is the relative lack of a suitable experimental model. The spontaneous development of choriocarcinoma in animals is exceedingly rare, the first convincing account being in a rhesus monkey (Lindsey et al 1969). The experimental induction of choriocarcinoma has also proved difficult. For example, the uterine tumour induced in pregnant rats by dimethylbenzanthracene (Stein-Werblowksy 1960) and originally classified as choriocarcinoma has since been designated as sarcomatous (Bagshawe 1969). Other experiments have met with limited success; for example, one animal out of a batch of pregnant armadillos given oral thalidomide developed metastatic choriocarcinoma (Marin-Padilla & Benirschke 1963), and a tumour resembling choriocarcinoma was produced in two out of 15 pregnant rabbits after electrocoagulative destruction of the lateral thalamic nucleus (Kushima et al 1967). However, in Japan several groups have been able to produce histologically confirmed malignant trophoblast by reverting to the use of dimethylbenzathracene in pregnant rats, with evidence of hormonal activity in some cases (Shintani et al

1966; Miyamoto et al 1972; Komuro 1976; Tanaka 1976). Because of the difficulties referred to above, other workers have preferred to develop techniques involving the heterologous transplantation of human choriocarcinoma cell lines (Hertz 1967; Pattillo & Gey 1968; Lewis et al 1969; Grummer et al 1999) and basic insights into the endocrinology, ultrastructure and immunology of trophoblastic neoplasia have been obtained (Hertz 1978).

Little is known about environmental factors in placental site or epithelioid trophoblastic tumours. Some could arise from choriocarcinomas as chemoresistant cell populations (Paradinas 1998b) but these tumours are rare and no epidemiological information is available.

INCIDENCE AND CLINICAL PRESENTATION OF TROPHOBLASTIC NEOPLASMS

It is now known that implantation is unsuccessful in many fertilisation events which are not clinically apparent (Miller et al 1980) and the possibility of trophoblastic tumours occurring 'ab initio' (Acosta-Sison 1959) is no longer fanciful. It is generally assumed that the directly preceding pregnancy is that causing the tumour and in most instances this is probably the case, but recent studies of genetic polymorphisms have shown that trophoblast from previous pregnancies, particularly previous molar pregnancies, can be the origin of a choriocarcinoma occurring after a term pregnancy (Fisher et al 1992a; Suzuki et al 1993; Arima et al 1994; Fisher et al 1995). This may explain anecdotal cases of choriocarcinoma occurring many years after the last known pregnancy and after a new normal pregnancy in patients who have had a mole, or a previous miscarriage in which the products of conception have not been examined.

Persistent trophoblastic disease occurs in about 15 to 20% of patients with a complete hydatidiform mole (Womack & Elston 1985; Berkowitz & Goldstein 1997b; Newlands 1997), but the majority of these are probably invasive moles and Hertig & Mansell (1956) estimated that the incidence of choriocarcinoma after a mole was only about 2.5%. This is, however, considerably higher than after a term pregnancy (1 in 100 000). The most accurate estimates of the nature of the preceding gestation are derived from the era before cytotoxic therapy for gestational trophoblastic disease became fully established; from published data choriocarcinoma is preceded by hydatidiform mole in approximately 50% of cases in the Western Hemisphere, but in the Far East this association appears to be stronger (Table 40.2). In the period 1960 to 1970 complete mole was the preceding gestation in at least 50% of cases of choriocarcinoma registered at Charing Cross (Elston 1978), but only 26% of histologically confirmed cases in 1990–2000 were preceded by a mole. The incidence of choriocarcinoma after a term pregnancy has not increased in absolute terms, although they are now 52% of those registered. Similar trends have

Table 40.2 Percentage of each type of antecedent gestation in choriocarcinoma

Author	Antecedent gestation Hydatidiform mole		Miscarriage	Term delivery	Tubal pregnancy
Novak & Seah (1954)	USA	39	38	23	2
Hertig & Mansell (1956)	USA	50	25	22.5	2.5
Elston (1970)	UK	49	28	20.5	2.5
Acosta-Sison (1967)[a]	Philippines	60	23	11	0
Ratnam & Chew (1976)	Singapore	78.3	7.5	11.3	2.9

[a] Six cases ab initio

been reported in Asia in recent years (Hando et al 1998; Kim et al 1998) and have been attributed to improvements in follow-up and management of molar pregnancies. We still see significant numbers (22%) after miscarriages or stillbirths in which products of conception have not been examined and this includes therapeutic terminations. Some of these could be unrecognised molar pregnancies, possibly early moles, which could also explain the high incidences reported by Hertig & Mansell (1956) after miscarriages (1 in 15 000). No pregnancy is devoid of risk but we have seen remarkably few cases in which the preceding pregnancy is a histologically documented non-molar miscarriage.

Very rarely, gestational choriocarcinoma is not the result of a pregnancy but due to organ transplantation from a woman harbouring the disease into immunosuppressed recipients (Knoop et al 1994; Doutrelepont et al 1995). Unexpected death of a woman of child-bearing age from intracerebral haemorrhage can be due to haemorrhage within unsuspected choriocarcinoma and this should be kept in mind.

Overall, gestational choriocarcinoma occurs in approximately 1:20 000 to 1:40 000 pregnancies in the Western Hemisphere; higher figures are quoted for Third World countries but the accuracy of some studies is dubious (Table 40.1, p. 1366). It may present at any age during the reproductive period. Elston (1970) found a range from 17 to 56 years with an average age of 27 years; there was a mean gravidity of 2 with a range of 1 to 9.

There is little information on the epidemiology and frequency of placental site trophoblastic tumour. The age range and parity of the patients appear similar to those of

patients with choriocarcinoma. It can occur after a molar pregnancy or a term pregnancy and this has been confirmed genetically (Fisher et al 1992b; Bower et al 1996), but preceding molar pregnancies are less common than in choriocarcinoma. At Charing Cross, 1351 patients were treated for gestational trophoblastic disease in 20 years (Bower et al 1996); during those years choriocarcinoma was proved histologically in 175 patients and placental site tumour in 19. The lack of tissue diagnosis in most treated cases means that the figures may not be accurate but indicate that placental site tumour is considerably rarer than choriocarcinoma. Nearly 100 cases were collected from the literature by Chang et al (1999) and more have been reported since. Presentation is often more insidious and tumour growth slower than in choriocarcinoma and tumours have been diagnosed in perimenopausal or postmenopausal women (McLellan et al 1991).

Epithelioid trophoblastic tumours are even rarer and only 7 examples have been found in the Charing Cross files since histology was regularly reviewed from 1970 onwards. However, excluded from this figure are numerous monomorphic metastatic tumours removed after chemotherapy for choriocarcinoma.

The commonest presenting symptom of choriocarcinoma is vaginal haemorrhage, often severe and prolonged, and this usually occurs within a few weeks or months of the related preceding gestation (Magrath et al 1971). Frequently (27% in Magrath et al series), patients will present with a distant metastasis, occasionally many years after the pregnancy of origin (Magrath et al 1971; Suzuki et al 1999). The commonest site of metastases is

Table 40.3 Distribution of distant metastases in choriocarcinoma

Study		Percentage involvement						No of cases
		Lung	Brain	Liver	Kidney	Intestines	Lymph node	
Park & Lees	(1950)	60	17	16	13	9	6	263
Hou & Pang	(1956)	96	90	50	43	21	0	25
Piston	(1970)	80	40	20	20	15	0	27
Oher et al	(1971)	100	61	60	47	40	15	44
Junaid et al	(1974)	94	33	39	26	17	5	100
Mazur et al	(1982)	97	50	50	33	23	23	30

the lung, patients presenting with cough, pleuritic pain or haemoptysis. Rarely this may be as multiple pulmonary emboli or pulmonary hypertension due to intravascular tumour growth in the pulmonary arteries (Bagshawe & Brooks 1959; Seckl et al 1991). Neurological presentations are less common but sometimes, intracerebral haemorrhage or cerebral pseudoaneurysms in a woman of child-bearing age are the initial events (Magrath et al 1971; Dana et al 1996; Kalafut et al 1998). Metastases to other sites are less common (see Table 40.3) but have been reported in the liver, pancreas, gastrointestinal tract, kidney, spleen, thyroid, nasal cavity, bone and choroid amongst others (Devasia et al 1994; Erdogan et al 1994; Challis et al 1996; Flam & Kock 1996). Haemorrhages, including haemoperitoneum secondary to organ rupture, pain or other symptoms referred to these sites in a young woman should raise suspicion of choriocarcinoma.

As with hydatidiform moles, hyperthyroidism can occur and cases of virilisation (Rajatanavin et al 1995) have been described, perhaps related to hCG overstimulation of ovarian theca cells. Other hormones sometimes elevated in patients with choriocarcinoma are prolactin (Ranta et al 1981) and parathormone (Deftos et al 1994).

In those cases in which choriocarcinoma follows an apparently normal pregnancy it is assumed that the tumour arose in the 'normal' placenta; direct evidence for this occurrence is available in case reports reviewed by Christopherson et al (1992) and Lage & Roberts (1993). It is unusual for choriocarcinoma to present during pregnancy but rare cases are described and the literature has been reviewed recently by Jacques et al (1998) and Steigrad et al (1999). It should be remembered that the tumour can metastasise to the baby as well as the mother (Buckell & Owen 1954) and that symptoms in the baby may be noticed before they are apparent in the mother (Andreitchouk et al 1996; Kishkurno et al 1997), so that hCG follow-up should include both mother and child.

Placental site tumour also presents mainly with uterine symptoms but haemorrhages are rarer and amenorrhoea commoner than in choriocarcinoma. Eight of 20 cases reviewed by us (Dessau et al 1990; Bower et al 1996) were found in hysterectomy specimens after failed chemotherapy for persistent trophoblastic disease. In one of these, typical choriocarcinoma was present in endometrial curettings prior to chemotherapy showing that placental site tumour is not necessarily a separate entity from the onset. One patient presented with uterine perforation and two small lung metastases and had no chemotherapy prior to hysterectomy. The uterus contained typical placental site tumour and the lung metastases, removed at the same time, showed choriocarcinoma. Hyperprolactinaemia is common and one of our patients was initially misdiagnosed as having a pituitary adenoma. In about 10% of cases reported, the patient had a nephrotic syndrome, apparently due to chronic intravascular coagulation with fibrin deposition in glomeruli (Park 1975; Eckstein et al 1982; Young & Scully 1984; Young et al

1985). The nephrotic syndrome resolves after hysterectomy (Eckstein et al 1982; Young & Scully 1984). Only one patient presented with brain metastases in our series. Virilisation has also been reported (Nagelberg & Rosen 1985).

Epithelioid trophoblastic tumours may also present with disturbances of menstruation. Patients may be perimenopausal and diagnosis is often delayed. The preceding pregnancy may be a term pregnancy or a molar pregnancy occurring many years before. We have seen 10 and 14 year intervals and an 18 years interval has been reported (Shih & Kurman 1998a). It is rare for this tumour to present with metastases if post-chemotherapy cases are excluded.

The literature on the rare occurrence of gestational choriocarcinoma in the Fallopian tube was reviewed comprehensively by Ober & Maier (1982) and the numerous single case reports published since add little to our knowledge of the condition. It usually presents with the signs and symptoms of an ectopic pregnancy or an ovarian tumour (Muto et al 1991) and has been reported in association with tubal adenocarcinoma (Tagaki et al 1985). Only rare cases of ovarian choriocarcinoma have been confirmed genetically as gestational rather than germ cell in origin (Lorigan et al 1996). One case of placental site tumour confined to the tube has been reported (Su et al 1999) and a second one has been recently seen by us.

PATHOLOGY OF CHORIOCARCINOMA

Macroscopic appearances

The gross appearances of choriocarcinoma are remarkably similar from case to case. Typically there is a well-circumscribed nodular lesion, 0.5 cm up to 5 cm in diameter, with a dominantly haemorrhagic structure. The coloration depends largely on the age of the nodule; in recent lesions there is a consistent red colour throughout, but in older lesions the central part gradually takes on a more yellow–brown appearance due to organisation of the haemorrhagic and necrotic tumour tissue. In the uterus the primary nodules may be single or multiple, and may project into the endometrial cavity or extend deeply into the myometrium (Fig. 40.35). Local metastatic nodules may be present in the cervix or vagina. At distant metastatic sites the same haemorrhagic nodular pattern is usually seen (Fig. 40.36), but in the lungs in rare cases, as noted previously, the malignant trophoblast may be entirely intravascular, causing occlusion of pulmonary arteries by thromboembolus (Fig. 40.37).

Microscopical appearances

In the typical primary nodule the malignant trophoblast is located at the periphery and little is found in the centre. This occurs to a much greater extent in choriocarcinoma

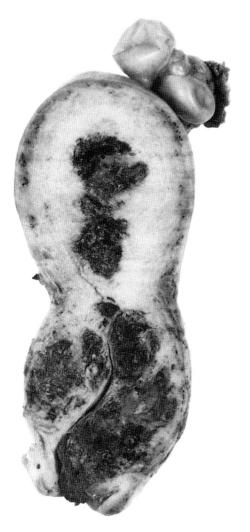

Fig. 40.35 Sagittal section of uterus to show dark haemorrhagic nodules of choriocarcinoma in the body, and similar deposits in the cervix. (From Fox H 1997 *Pathology of the placenta*, W B Saunders, Philadelphia. Reproduced by permission of Professor H Fox and W B Saunders).

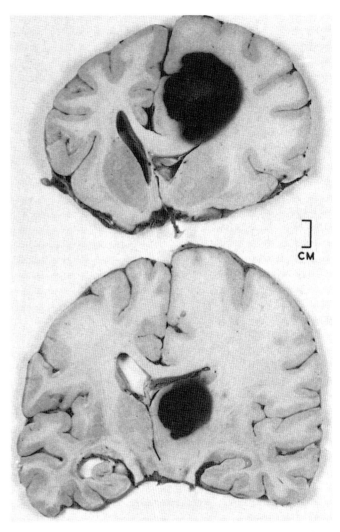

Fig. 40.36 Metastatic choriocarcinoma in brain. The coronal slices show two separate haemorrhagic nodules.

than in other solid tumours, because, uniquely, it lacks intrinsic tumour vasculature. The malignant trophoblast relies for cell nutrition on its permeation of the host blood vessels and such vessels are only present at the peripheral tumour–host interface. In this respect choriocarcinoma behaves in exactly the same way as the normal trophoblast of human placenta. The analogy can be taken further in considering the detailed microscopical structure. Choriocarcinoma has a very characteristic bilaminar pattern which recapitulates the appearances of the trophoblast of the early implanting blastocyst (Fig. 40.38). Central cores of mononuclear cytotrophoblastic cells are surrounded by rims of multinucleated syncytiotrophoblastic cells (Figs 40.38–40.40). The syncytiotrophoblast is usually arranged around maternal blood spaces which resemble the intervillous space of normal placentation (Fig. 40.38), but occasionally cytotrophoblast and syncytiotrophoblast are present as separate

sheets of tumour tissue (Figs 40.41, 40.42). It is rare for a tumour to be composed entirely of one cell type but one element may sometimes be greatly in excess of the other and metastases after chemotherapy may have little syncytium. The nuclei of the cytotrophoblastic cells are large and vesicular with prominent nucleoli which are often multiple. The cytoplasm is generally clear but occasionally focally granular. The syncytial nuclei may also appear vesicular with prominent nucleoli, but are smaller than cytotrophoblastic nuclei. The syncytial cytoplasm is deeply eosinophilic and frequently appears as a lacy network. Mitoses are confined to the cytotrophoblast and are more numerous than in other trophoblastic tumours but there is no correlation between the degree of mitotic activity and prognosis. A variable infiltrate of lymphoplasmacytoid cells may be present in close association with malignant trophoblast. This may be intense, and the severity correlates with prognosis (Elston & Bagshawe 1973).

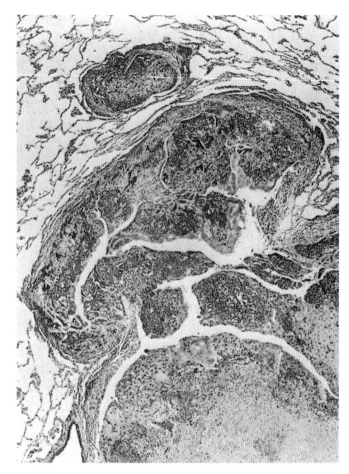

Fig. 40.37 Metastatic choriocarcinoma in lung. The tumour is located entirely within branches of the pulmonary artery. The patient presented with pulmonary hypertension.

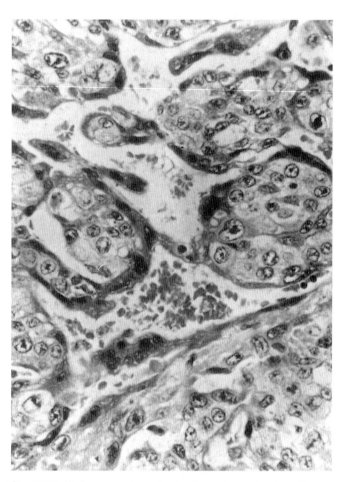

Fig. 40.39 High-power view of a choriocarcinoma to show the typical bilaminar structure. Note the maternal red cells in pseudointervillous spaces.

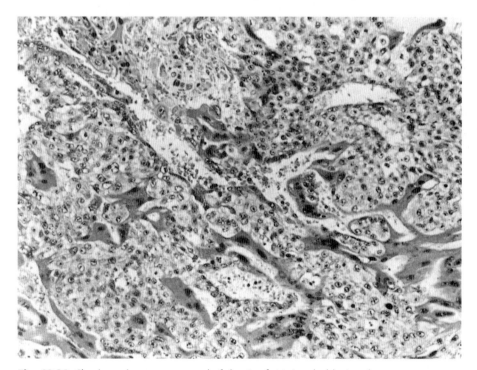

Fig. 40.38 Choriocarcinoma, composed of sheets of cytotrophoblast and syncytiotrophoblast.

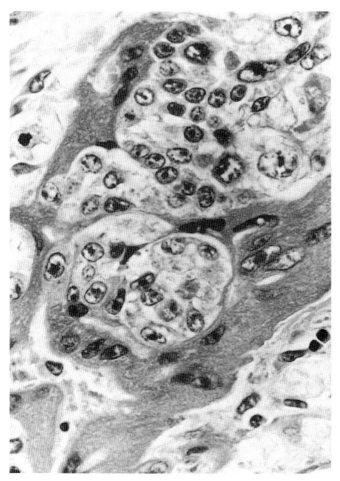

Fig. 40.40 Another choriocarcinoma, showing central cores of cytotrophoblast surrounded by syncytiotrophoblast. Note the prominent nucleoli, particularly in the cytotrophoblast.

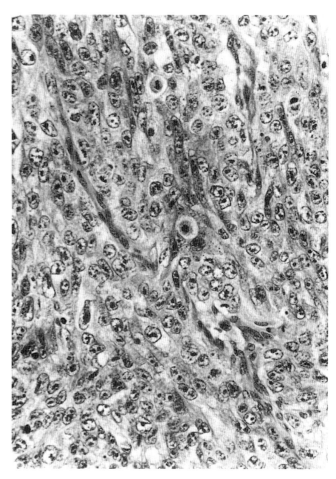

Fig. 40.41 Choriocarcinoma in which there is a predominance of cytotrophoblast.

Although extensive myometrial invasion is a prominent feature of typical choriocarcinoma, it is unusual to find muscle destruction or necrosis, and, where malignant trophoblast is in contact with myometrium, preservation of the latter is excellent. This is mainly because invasion rarely takes place directly into muscle but rather via the venous sinuses, which become markedly dilated.

As noted previously, choriocarcinoma lacks an intrinsic stromal vasculature and there is, therefore, always some permeation of the venous sinuses at the periphery of the tumour (Fig. 40.43). This is the first step in the progression of myometrial invasion towards the uterine venous plexus (Fig. 40.44). Tumour cells can also proliferate within the vessels and embolise along the venous sinuses until they impact and occlude the lumen (Fig. 40.45). The tumour nodule thus formed erodes the endothelium of the vessels and expands into the adjacent myometrium (Fig. 40.46). In this way it is possible for uterine perforation to occur, although the great bulk of the tumour in the myometrium is intravascular.

Choriocarcinoma is distinguished from invasive mole by the absence of true chorionic villi. Occasional non-molar cases have been described in which residual chorionic villi have been identified within the tumour or in adjacent myometrium (Novak & Seah 1954; Elston 1978; Ober & Maier 1982). In such cases the villi do not exhibit molar change and are either degenerate or appear normal microscopically (Fig. 40.47). There is no reason why the vestiges of the placental tissue from which the tumour has arisen should not persist, and, indeed, it is surprising that it does not happen more often, but the occurrence is exceedingly rare. Of even greater rarity is the finding of very early choriocarcinomatous change within an otherwise normal placenta (MacRae 1951; Driscoll 1963; Brewer & Mazur 1981; Tsukamoto et al 1981; Fox & Laurini 1988; Hallam et al 1990; Christopherson et al 1992; Lage & Roberts 1993). The placental primary is often very small and may only be found after a careful and extensive search. Microscopically intraplacental choriocarcinoma arises from the cytotrophoblast of apparently normal chorionic villi which do not show hydropic change. The characteristic bilaminar structure is seen as a mantle investing the villi, but true invasion of villous stroma is rare (Fox & Laurini 1988; Lage & Roberts 1993). Metastases, when they occur, also have the typical bilaminar structure, without

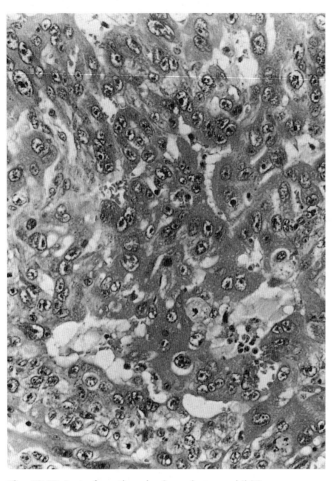

Fig. 40.42 Part of another choriocarcinoma exhibiting a predominantly syncytiotrophoblastic structure.

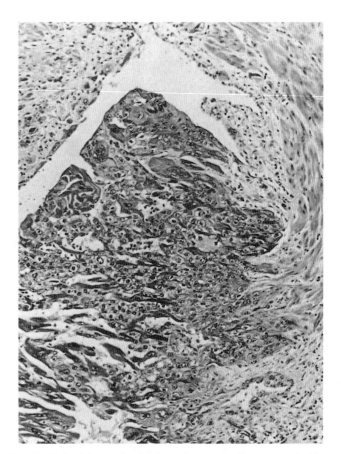

Fig. 40.43 Periphery of a choriocarcinoma. Malignant trophoblast is seen invading into a dilated venous sinus.

the presence of formed villi. Such findings suggest that in the majority of cases of choriocarcinoma which follow a normal pregnancy the tumour arises in situ from villous trophoblast rather than in retained or persistent trophoblast following the gestation. There are, however, cases in which the pregnancy merely reactivates dormant trophoblast from a mole evacuated years before (Fisher et al 1995). In rare instances, prolonged follow-up of both mother and child after placental choriocarcinoma has shown no metastases (Barghorn et al 1998; Jacques et al 1998).

Unusual cases have recently been reported in which an intraplacental chorangioma was associated with a proliferation of trophoblast resembling choriocarcinoma (Jauniaux et al 1988; Trask et al 1994; Aonahata et al 1998). This is likely to be a chance association.

Fox & Laurini (1988) speculated on the possible existence of in situ molar choriocarcinoma, which at that time had not been described. There is no doubt that the trophoblast of a mole and even that of a first trimester non-molar miscarriage could become neoplastic, but unlike in a third trimester placenta neoplasia is much more difficult to detect in a background of highly proliferative trophoblast in the first trimester and even more so in molar

trophoblast, which is already very pleomorphic and aneuploid. Carcinoma in situ in a partial mole (Heifetz & Czaja 1992), and in early non-molar placenta (Fukunaga et al 1996a) has been described but the findings should be interpreted with caution. The patients did not require chemotherapy and similar florid proliferating trophoblast to that described by Heifetz & Czaja is present in moles in which there is no subsequent persistent trophoblastic disease (Elston & Bagshawe 1972a).

Microscopical appearances in metastases

Little variation in microscopical pattern is seen between tumours at primary and metastatic sites when removed together and the same bilaminar structure is preserved in the metastases. In our experience (Paradinas 1992, 1998b) metastases removed after chemotherapy are more often composed predominantly of mononuclear cells regardless of the initial histology, reflecting perhaps chemoresistant cell clones. This has also been reported by others (Duncan & Mazur 1989; Mazur 1989; Jones et al 1993) and the tumours interpreted as epithelioid trophoblastic tumours (Shih & Kurman 1998a) but unlike epithelioid tumours, they are mitotically very active, show central haemorrhagic necrosis, predominantly intravascular invasion at the periphery and abundant hCG. They

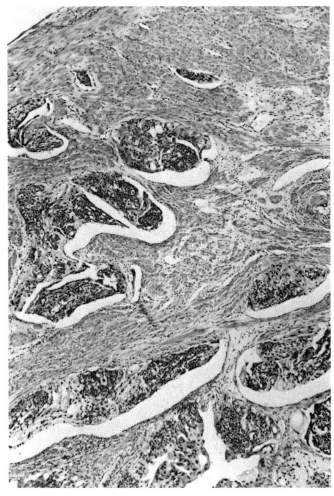

Fig. 40.44 Choriocarcinoma with extensive vascular invasion. The main tumour mass is at the bottom right and embolic tumour is present in dilated venous sinuses out to the serosa at the top left; intervening myometrium is intact. (From Fox H 1997 *Pathology of the placenta*. W B Saunders, Philadelphia. Reproduced by permission of Professor H Fox and W B Saunders).

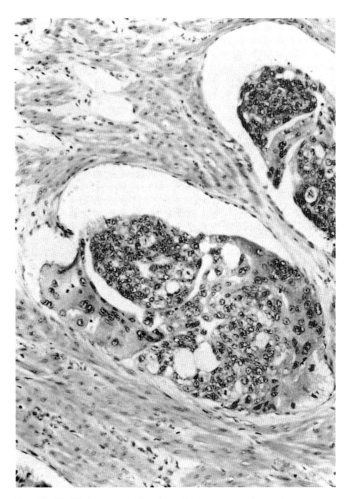

Fig. 40.45 Higher magnification of the tumour shown in Fig. 40.44. A tumour embolus has impacted in a venous sinus and is attached to the vessel wall, replacing the endothelium. (From Fox H 1997 *Pathology of the placenta*. W B Saunders, Philadelphia. Reproduced by permission of Professor H Fox and W B Saunders)

have been referred to as predominantly cytotrophoblastic choriocarcinomas in previous publications (Paradinas 1992, 1998b; Elston 1996) but unlike cytotrophoblast, many of the mononuclear cells have dense cytoplasm and are hormonally active. It would be more precise to regard them as monomorphic choriocarcinomas. In longstanding metastases and in patients successfully treated with cytotoxic therapy the tumour nodule may be almost completely necrotic with little or no surviving tumour tissue.

It is difficult to obtain an accurate estimate for the frequency of metastases in choriocarcinoma due to the wide variation in published figures (Table 40.3). Some studies are based entirely on autopsy records, whilst others include clinical data without histological confirmation. The series reported by Hou & Pang (1956); Elston (1970); Ober et al (1971); Junaid et al (1974) and Mazur et al (1982) are all composed of personal or collective autopsy cases. Those reported by Elston and Mazur et al are probably the most representative of the modern chemotherapy era, and

confirm that the lungs, brain and liver are the most frequent metastatic sites. They are in keeping with clinical estimates obtained by Hunter et al (1990).

Ultrastructure of choriocarcinoma

In the small number of studies reported, the general appearances have resembled those of normal early placental trophoblast, although nuclei are slightly larger with infolded nuclear membranes. The cytotrophoblastic mitochondria tend to be enlarged and prominent, and the endoplasmic reticulum of the syncytiotrophoblast is slightly increased (Wakitani 1962; Knoth et al 1969; Larsen 1973). Phagocytic activity, not normally present in trophoblast, has been observed in the syncytiotrophoblast of choriocarcinoma (Knoth et al 1969; Larsen 1973). Infererra et al (1967) found both intermediate and undifferentiated trophoblastic cells in addition to relatively normal cytotrophoblast and syncytiotrophoblast.

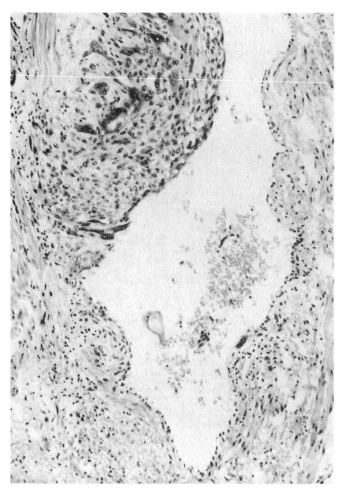

Fig. 40.46 Choriocarcinoma within a venous sinus. Part of the vessel wall is replaced by tumour which is invading into the adjacent myometrium. (From Fox H 1997 *Pathology of the placenta*. W B Saunders, Philadelphia. Reproduced by permission of Professor H Fox and W B Saunders)

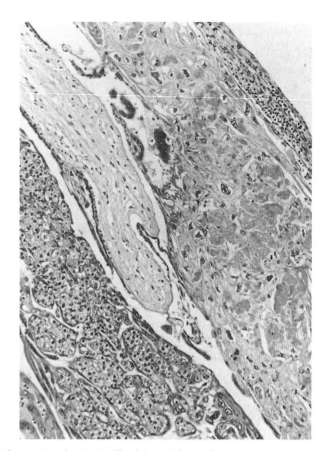

Fig. 40.47 Chorionic villus lying within a choriocarcinoma. The neoplastic trophoblast does not arise from the villus, nor is the latter invasive.

Because of the scarcity of suitable material from patients with choriocarcinoma, studies have also been carried out on cell lines of transplanted human choriocarcinoma in experimental animals (Wynn & Davies 1964a; Larsen et al 1967; Knoth et al 1969). Essentially similar appearances to those described above were found. In addition Larsen et al (1967), studying choriocarcinoma transplanted to the hamster liver, noted desmosomes connecting tumour cells to liver cells and compared the invasiveness of choriocarcinoma with that of the normal fertilised ovum. The differences between choriocarcinoma, atypical choriocarcinoma and placental site tumour have been discussed by Duncan & Mazur (1989) but in general, electronmicroscopy contributes little to either diagnosis (mixtures of trophoblastic cell types are usually found) or to our understanding of the biology of choriocarcinoma.

Immunocytochemistry of choriocarcinoma

In contrast, immunocytochemistry for placental hormones, markers of cell proliferation and other cell pro-

ducts has a rôle in the differential diagnosis of choriocarcinoma from other gestational trophoblastic tumours. In choriocarcinomas hCG is positive in a significant number of cells, particularly in syncytiotrophoblast, but even in predominantly monomorphic tumours hCG is the hormone found in the highest number of cells. Fewer cells stain for hPL and it is rare to find PLAP. Choriocarcinoma cells are consistently positive for cytokeratins, including low molecular weight cytokeratins and occasional cells may be positive for epithelial membrane antigen (EMA) and CEA. Ki-67 is positive in numerous cells (Shih & Kurman 1998b) and this correlates with a high mitotic rate (60 or more mitoses per 10 high-power fields are not unusual). Frequently, material obtained at curettage or in needle biopsies is very necrotic and remaining viable cells may not show the typical bilaminar structure typical of choriocarcinoma. Finding cells which are predominantly hCG positive and with a high Ki-67 index favours choriocarcinoma. Unfortunately, germ cell tumours and non-gestational carcinomas can have trophoblastic differentiation (see below) and produce placental hormones, particularly hCG. Positivity for placental hormones is therefore no absolute proof that the tumour is a gestational choriocarcinoma.

Genetic polymorphisms

The same techniques applied in forensic investigations to determine identity can be used to determine origin of choriocarcinomas from specific pregnancies and to determine if the tumour is gestational (Fisher et al 1992a,b, 1995; Suzuki et al 1993; Arima et al 1994). These can be performed on archival material and carried out in a few days. They are becoming very useful, not only in understanding the biology of trophoblastic tumours, but also in helping to define prognosis and influencing therapeutic decisions.

Prognosis of choriocarcinoma

Prior to the establishment of the Mathieu Memorial Chorioepithelioma Registry in the United States in 1946 (Brewer 1959) anecdotal evidence suggested that choriocarcinoma was highly malignant and always fatal. This over-gloomy view was dispelled by the first statistical report from the Registry, as Novak & Seah (1954) found a minimum two-year survival of 15% in the 74 patients on whom data was available. Treatment in all cases was hysterectomy, with pelvic irradiation in one. In a later report from the Registry based on 147 cases, a similar figure for five-year survival was obtained (Brewer et al 1961).

The dramatic improvement in survival due to the use of cytotoxic therapy began as a result of observations made by Hertz and co-workers that folic acid was essential for the growth of the female genital tract and embryonic development (Hertz 1978). Thiersch (1952) also found that it was possible to induce abortion in women treated with small doses of the folic acid antagonist 4-aminopteroyl-glutamic acid. These facts led to the treatment of the first patient with choriocarcinoma by methotrexate, and in 1956 Li et al reported complete remission in two patients with choriocarcinoma and one with invasive mole. By 1961 Hertz et al were able to present the results of 5 years experience with chemotherapy in 63 patients, 44 of whom had choriocarcinoma. They estimated that in comparison with previous results from the literature prolonged survival had been raised from 6 to 48%. As more experience was gained results improved and it was possible to obtain sustained remission in over 80% of patients if treatment was initiated early in the course of the disease.

Sustained remission rates of nearly 90% for metastatic trophoblastic disease and virtually 100% for localised disease have now been achieved, and it is clear that the best results are obtained in patients in whom treatment is monitored in an expert centre (Berkowitz & Goldstein 1988; Jones 1990; Lurain & Sciarra 1991; Newlands et al 1992, 1997). At Charing Cross Hospital, London, a prognostic scoring system is used to stratify patients so that they receive appropriate therapy (Newlands et al 1997).

This is based on a number of factors, including the type of antecedent gestation, interval from pregnancy to diagnosis, hCG level at diagnosis and number of metastases. Patients are divided into low, medium and high risk categories. Even in the high risk category overall survival is 87%. The poorest prognosis occurs in those patients with choriocarcinoma after a term pregnancy, when therapy is delayed and in patients previously given inappropriate chemotherapy in non-specialised centres.

PATHOLOGY OF PLACENTAL SITE TROPHOBLASTIC TUMOUR

Macroscopic appearances

The gross appearances are much more variable than in choriocarcinoma. There may be a localised nodule, which in some cases projects into the endometrial cavity, but more often there is an ill-defined mass in the myometrium. The lesion is usually tan to yellow in colour, without striking haemorrhage, and foci of necrosis may

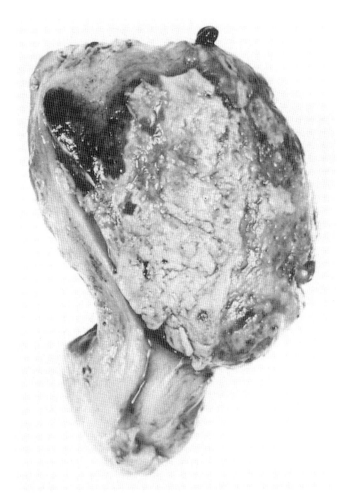

Fig. 40.48 Hysterectomy specimen with a placental site trophoblastic tumour. There is extensive necrosis but only a little haemorrhage.

be present (Fig. 40.48). The degree of invasion is variable; in some cases only superficial involvement of the myometrium occurs whilst in others there may be penetration through to the serosa.

Microscopical appearances

The pattern of infiltration by the trophoblastic cells recapitulates the appearances seen at the normal placental bed (Figs 40.49, 40.50). There is a diffuse infiltrate of mononuclear and multinucleated trophoblastic cells arranged in cords, islands and sheets between myometrial bundles. In contrast with the bilaminar pattern of choriocarcinoma the infiltrate is rather monotonous and resembles the intermediate trophoblast. The majority of cells are mononuclear (Fig. 40.51) with clear or eosinophilic cytoplasm but multinucleated forms having amphophilic cytoplasm are also present. Where cords of cells infiltrate amongst myometrial bundles they may have a spindle cell appearance. A major point of distinction from choriocarcinoma is the preservation of intact venous sinuses or capillaries within the tumour mass (Fig. 40.52), but areas of increased vascularity are rare. Infiltration of vessel walls

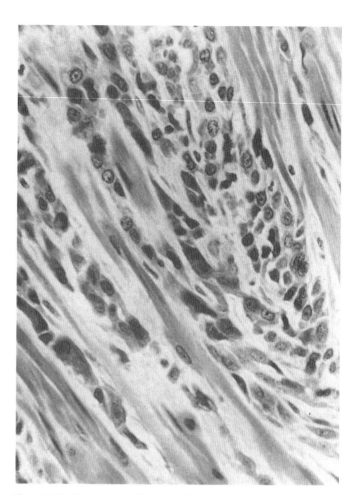

Fig. 40.50 Higher magnification of Fig. 40.49 showing mononuclear and multinucleated intermediate trophoblastic cells, with preservation of muscle bundles.

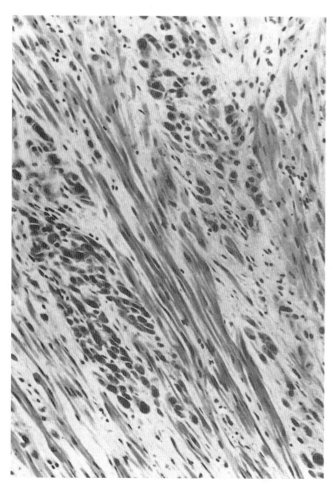

Fig. 40.49 Placental site trophoblastic tumour. Cords and sheets of intermediate trophoblastic cells infiltrate between muscle bundles.

may be seen but intravascular proliferation is less obvious. Islands of tumour necrosis may be present, usually in areas of poor vascularity. Mitoses can usually be identified, but counts are variable and rarely high; usually between 1 and 10 mitoses per 10 high-power fields. A major difference between placental site tumour and exaggerated or persistent placental site reactions is that tumours show confluent growth and large sheets of cells, whereas non-neoplastic infiltrates consist of isolated cells or clusters of only a few cells. In hysterectomy specimens the distinction is usually clear but small biopsies may not be representative and small clusters at the periphery of the mass may show features indistinguishable from those of a placental site reaction (Collins et al 1990).

Placental site tumour has less tendency to vascular invasion and remains localised to the uterus for longer, so that FIGO stages are more relevant than they are for choriocarcinoma. Tumours can extend to the parametrium, ovaries, bladder and rectum and may metastasise to regional lymph nodes (a very unusual event in choriocarcinoma). Distant metastases are common in the lung, but are rare in other sites, although we have seen them in brain and pancreas and a patient presenting with

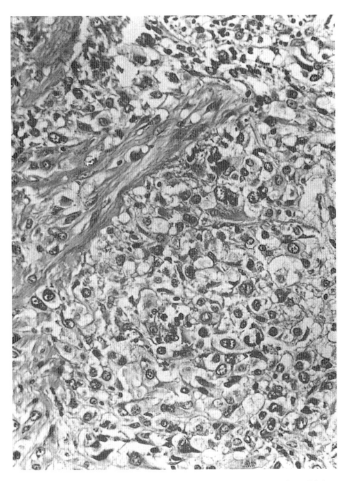

Fig. 40.51 Another placental site trophoblastic tumour in which the cells are predominantly mononuclear.

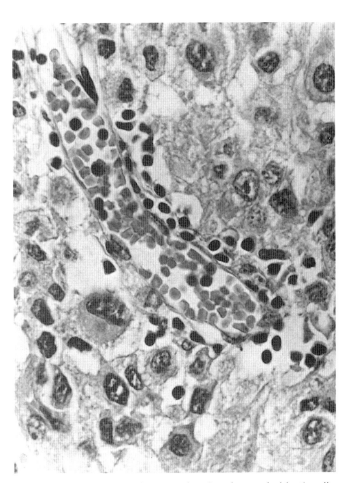

Fig. 40.52 Same case as Fig. 40.51 showing the trophoblastic cells infiltrating around a preserved myometrial capillary.

scalp metastases has been reported (Yuen et al 1998). Ectopic tumours can occur: we have seen a hybrid placental site/epithelioid trophoblastic tumour located in a tubo-ovarian mass. Cervical (Horn et al 1997) and tubal (Su et al 1999) placental site tumours have also been recorded.

Ultrastructure of placental site tumour

There are several reports (Blackwell & Papadimitrou 1979; Gloor & Hurlimann 1981; Berger et al 1984; Duncan & Mazur 1989; Motoyama et al 1994). They stress the fact that the main cell has similarities with normal intermediate trophoblast from the placental bed and also that other cells resembling cyto- and syncytiotrophoblast are often seen, reinforcing the relationship between different forms of trophoblastic neoplasia. They do not help significantly in diagnosis.

Immunocytochemistry of placental site tumour

This reveals an entirely different pattern to that seen in choriocarcinoma. Abundant amounts of hPL are seen in a diffuse pattern (Fig. 40.53) whilst hCG is present only focally (Fig. 40.54). As a rule, PLAP is only present in

occasional cells. This pattern is usually present also in the metastases when they occur but we have noted reversal of immunostaining pattern in some metastases, which showed more hCG than hPL positive cells and were more haemorrhagic. This has also been observed by others in aggressive cases (Zhang & Kraus 1986) and may reflect a change in biological behaviour, tumours becoming more like monomorphic choriocarcinomas. Recent studies of proliferation markers such as Ki-67 are more accurate than mitotic counts and show that mitotic indexes are much higher than in placental site reactions but lower than in choriocarcinomas (Ichikawa et al 1998; Shih & Kurman 1998b). Placental site tumours may express other placental hormones, such as SP1, pregnancy-associated major basic protein (pBSM) (Rhoton-Vlasak et al 1998) and inhibin (Minami et al 1993; McCluggage 1998; Pelkey et al 1999) but neither their demonstration in tissues nor in serum appear to have advantages over the use of hCG, hPL and PLAP (Badonnel et al 1994).

Genetic polymorphisms

As with choriocarcinoma, these can pinpoint the pregnancy of origin of the tumour (Fisher et al 1992b; Bower

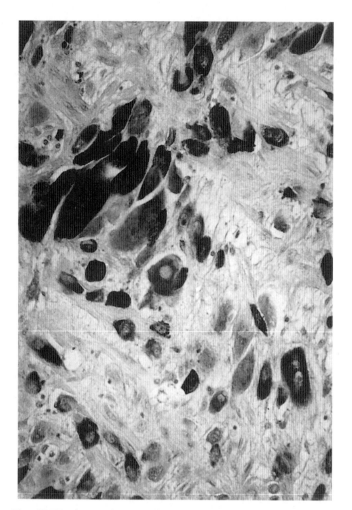

Fig. 40.53 Placental site trophoblastic tumour. The majority of cells show diffuse staining for hPL. Immunoperoxidase–hPL.

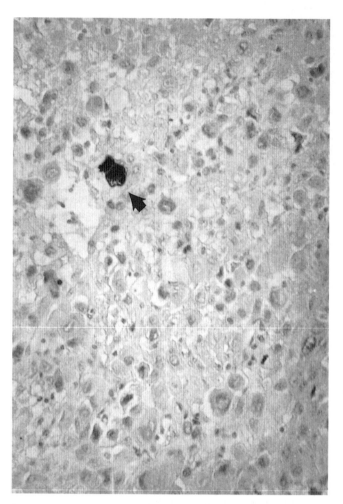

Fig. 40.54 Same case as Fig. 40.53. Immunostaining reveals hCG in only one cell in this field (arrowhead). Immunoperoxidase–hCG.

et al 1996) and have shown that complete mole is the pregnancy origin more often than thought previously.

Prognosis of placental site tumour

Until comparatively recently it appeared that placental site trophoblastic tumour was a relatively benign and frequently self-limiting process; in 1981 Elston found only one death in 19 cases from the literature, and that was due to postoperative complications. Subsequently several fatal cases were reported (Scully & Young 1981; Twiggs et al 1981; Eckstein et al 1982; Gloor et al 1983) and Young et al (1988) in a further review found seven deaths out of 38 fully documented cases in whom follow-up data of over one year's duration or to death was available. They were aware of a further 48 cases seen in consultation, four of whom were considered to have malignant tumours. Young et al (1988) therefore estimated that between 10 and 15% of patients with placental site trophoblastic tumour have a malignant outcome, with an overall mortality of up to 10%. A review of 19 cases managed at Charing Cross (Bower et al 1996) showed a 20% mortal-

ity, but it did not include patients treated initially by hysterectomy in the referring hospital and never seen at Charing Cross. In a recent review of 88 cases from the literature, Chang et al (1999) recorded a 30% mortality for stages FIGO III and IV at presentation. The tumour stage on presentation and the length of the interval between the preceding pregnancy and diagnosis (Bower et al 1996) seem to be significant prognostic variables.

The histological features of placental site trophoblastic tumour cannot be used with confidence to predict prognosis and malignant cases have been described in which the original appearances suggested exaggerated placental site reaction (Collins et al 1990; Orrell & Sanders 1991). It has been proposed that estimation of the number of mitoses may be a helpful prognostic factor (Scully & Young 1981; Mazur & Kurman 1987; Lathrop et al 1988; Young et al 1988), since most fatal cases which have been reported have had counts of 5 or more per high-power field. Leaving aside the inherent inaccuracy of expressing counts per 'high-power field' without stating the field area (Ellis & Whitehead 1981), fatal cases with low mitotic counts have occurred (Gloor et al 1983; Young et al

1985). Conversely, a patient with a very high count (11 per 10 high-power fields) seen by us, refused hysterectomy, the tumour apparently regressed and she has had two normal pregnancies since (Bower et al 1996). It should be noted that a curettage specimen from a placental site trophoblastic tumour may not be representative of the whole tumour and counts may appear falsely high or low. In a study of 23 patients with PSTT in 1994 (Paradinas 1994b), we found a statistically significant difference between good and bad prognostic groups when counts were performed in hysterectomy specimens, but not in curettings. It is therefore necessary to conduct full follow-up in all patients (Finkler et al 1988; Dessau et al 1990; Bower et al 1996) and this has to be long term, because metastases can occur many years after initial treatment. In marked contrast with choriocarcinoma the treatment of choice is surgical rather than cytotoxic therapy (Newlands et al 1997). In some cases curettage alone seems to have been curative (Ober et al 1971; Kurman et al 1976) and this indicates that the tumour may regress even if excision is incomplete. For the majority of patients, however, hysterectomy is indicated (Finkler et al 1988; Lathrop et al 1988; Dessau et al 1990; Newlands et al 1997) and this has the added advantage that the extent of local involvement can be assessed properly from full histopathological examination of the specimen. Hoffman et al (1993) have also advocated pelvic node dissection for staging purposes, but we have not yet found tumour in lymph nodes which were not obviously involved either clinically or by imaging techniques. Ovarian involvement is usually macroscopically apparent if present and Berkowitz et al (1990) have pleaded for a conservative approach if the ovaries are apparently normal. Cytotoxic therapy has been used in some cases (Twiggs et al 1981; Finkler et al 1988; Lathrop et al 1988; Dessau et al 1990) but the results have been disappointing and only occasionally has long-term remission been achieved (Dessau et al 1990; Hoffman et al 1993; Bower et al 1996; Chang et al 1999).

PATHOLOGY OF EPITHELIOID TROPHOBLASTIC TUMOUR

Although biologically inaccurate (all trophoblastic tumours are epithelial), the above name was first used by Mazur (1989) for a form of choriocarcinoma predominantly composed of mononuclear cells surrounding vessels and present in lung metastases from two patients after multiple courses of chemotherapy. The cells were different from intermediate trophoblast on light and electron microscopy and contained only a little hCG and hPL. There was extensive necrosis but haemorrhage was only mild. No PLAP immunocytochemistry was done.

In our experience, and that of others (Jones et al 1993), a majority of metastases from choriocarcinoma removed after chemotherapy are predominantly mononuclear and

composed of highly atypical trophoblast (Paradinas 1997, 1998b). In spite of the paucity of syncytium, hCG is still present in most and is the marker found in highest cell numbers. Vascular invasion is common at the periphery and haemorrhagic necrosis in the middle. Therefore, they still have the macroscopical appearances and biological behaviour of choriocarcinomas, although they are chemorresistant. This tumour pattern is occasionally seen before chemotherapy and has been previously classified by us as predominantly cytotrophoblastic choriocarcinoma (Paradinas 1992, 1997, 1998b; Elston 1996) and as atypical choriocarcinoma by others (Wang 1990). However, the tumour described by Mazur (Mazur 1989; Mazur & Kurman 1994) differs from the above description in that viable tumour cells at the periphery show mainly interstitial infiltration and there is little haemorrhage.

Shih & Kurman (1998a, 2001) have described 14 patients with epithelioid trophoblastic tumours and defined their clinical, histological and immuno-

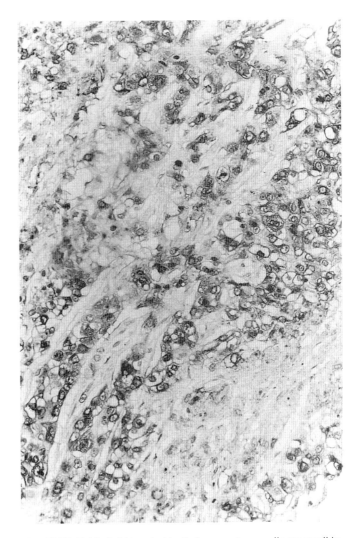

Fig. 40.55 Epithelioid trophoblastic tumour. Some cells are small in size and regular, others show vacuolated cytoplasm.

cytochemical profiles better. In 12 patients the diagnosis was made on hysterectomy or curettage specimens and only 2 presented as metastases. The interval between the preceding pregnancy and diagnosis was long (up to 18 years); in 8 cases it was a term delivery, in 2 it was a mole, in 2 a miscarriage and in 2 unknown. Characteristically, tumours had a nodular, expansive pattern of growth and were composed of a mixture of mononuclear cells with either eosinophilic or clear (often vacuolated) cytoplasm (Fig. 40.55). Necrosis and hyaline fibrillar material surrounded groups of cells, which often survived only near vessels (Figs 40.56, 40.57). Dystrophic calcification was common in areas of necrosis (Fig. 40.57). The mitotic rate was low (in the range of 0 to 10 mitoses per 10 high-power fields) and the Ki-67 index averaged 18%. Interestingly, five tumours also had mixtures of choriocarcinoma, placental site tumour or both. Immunocytochemistry was consistently positive for cytokeratins and EMA but hCG and hPL were only found focally and PLAP was also focal, although present in most tumours.

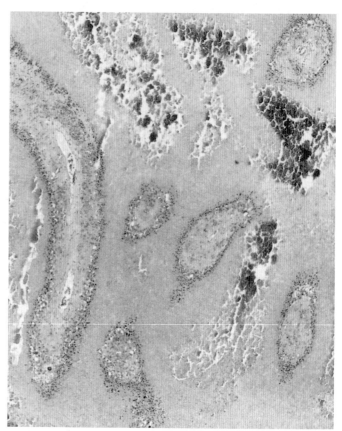

Fig. 40.57 Low magnification of epithelioid trophoblastic tumour showing extensive necrosis and dystrophic calcification. Viable cells survive around vessels only.

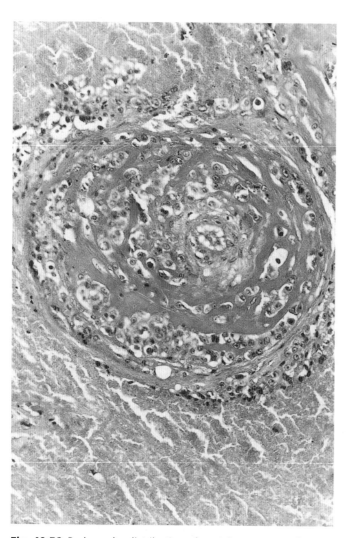

Fig. 40.56 Perivascular distribution of surviving tumour cells is characteristically found in epithelioid trophoblastic tumours.

Inhibin was consistently positive, as were other non-specific markers of trophoblast.

Seven out of 56 specimens, received in consultation at Charing Cross and diagnosed as placental site tumours had microscopical features similar to those described above. Three were from perimenopausal patients who presented with stage III tumours; two of them are now dead of disease and one is alive after thoracotomy, which showed metastases of similar histological pattern. Two are from patients with stage I tumours apparently cured by hysterectomy. The last two tumours are interesting: in one there are areas with the appearance of monomorphic choriocarcinoma, high Ki-67 index and many hCG-positive cells; this patient is lost to follow-up; in the other, the tumour was tubo-ovarian and had foci of typical placental site tumour with abundant hPL expression; she is alive but follow-up is short. Some hCG and hPL were present in most tumours but PLAP was present in all, although only in 3 was it expressed in numerous cells (Fig. 40.58).

We have previously regarded this tumour as a variant of placental site tumour of long standing (Paradinas 1997, 1998b) and in all our cases the preceding pregnancy was many years before (14 in one case). Shih & Kurman (1998) suggest that this is a different tumour type derived not from villous or implantation site

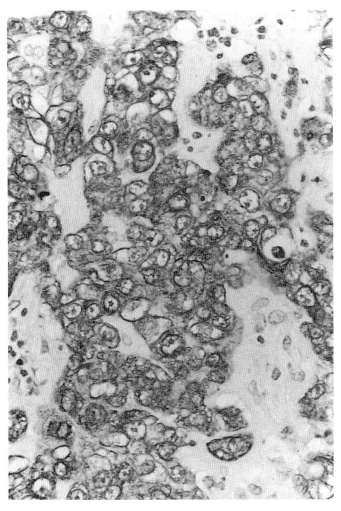

Fig. 40.58 Most cells were positive for PLAP in this epithelioid trophoblastic tumour. PLAP is only found rarely in choriocarcinomas and placental site tumours. Immunoperoxidase-PLAP.

trophoblast but from trophoblast from the chorion laeve (Yeh et al 1989). This is an interesting suggestion but the fact that mixtures of tumour types are often found speaks against it. Trophoblast, and particularly its stem cells (cytotrophoblast), has all the genetic information to differentiate in various directions and this could be altered in time by therapeutic intervention or by changes in the environment in which the tumour grows. We nevertheless agree that this is a very distinctive tumour type in which many cells resemble vacuolated and non-vacuolated trophoblast normally present in the chorion of third trimester placentas and deserves further study.

From the practical point of view, the rationale of separating the epithelioid variant from other trophoblastic tumours is less obvious. Firstly, it is a very rare tumour and its behaviour, form of infiltration and metastatic potential are very similar to those of placental site tumour (Paradinas 1997; Shih & Kurman 1998). Secondly, mixed tumours are common. Thirdly, there is the danger that more aggressive examples of predominantly mononuclear

choriocarcinoma may be misdiagnosed as epithelioid trophoblastic tumour. The latter are rapidly growing tumours, often intravascular, frequently haemorrhagic and produce mainly hCG; but some tumours with these features have already been reported as epithelioid (Hamazaki et al 1999). Fourthly, there is the danger of misdiagnosing as epithelioid trophoblastic tumours non-gestational carcinomas with hCG production. We have received in consultation with such a diagnosis material from several patients, including one with lung and intraplacental metastases; the tumour proved to be non-gestational on genetic studies but the fact that the diagnosis was entertained at all shows that the clinical and pathological features of this rare tumour are not yet well known. Diagnosis should be confirmed in specialised centres.

NON-GESTATIONAL CARCINOMAS WITH TROPHOBLASTIC METAPLASIA

Most histopathologists are familiar with the fact that germ cell tumours and some anaplastic carcinomas can have morphological trophoblastic differentiation or produce hCG. The problem cannot be reviewed in detail here but the fact that immunocytochemistry for placental hormones is readily available means that many more patients are being referred to specialist centres with the diagnosis of possible choriocarcinoma. The distinction is important, because in disseminated gestational choriocarcinoma chemotherapy is almost always curative, whereas disseminated anaplastic carcinomas are almost always lethal and remissions short-lived. It is our experience that a clear morphological differentiation in small biopsies is often impossible, but DNA analysis with PCR amplification detects polymorphisms foreign to the patient in gestational tumours and is invaluable in reaching therapeutic decisions (Fisher et al 1992a).

Morphological differentiation can be very close to that of gestational choriocarcinoma and when typical cyto- and syncytiotrophoblast are present, the tumour tends to invade vessels and is haemorrhagic. More often, the pathologist receives a very anaplastic tumour with occasional uncharacteristic giant cells and in which some mononuclear or multinucleated cells are positive for hCG. Serum hCG values are relatively low for the bulk of the tumour and seldom higher than 1000 IU/l. Immunocytochemistry is unhelpful, since epithelial markers such as cytokeratins, EMA and CEA can be present in trophoblastic tumours. In large biopsies or resected tumours the distinction may be easier. The two most useful criteria are the presence of differentiation towards other structures (usually glandular or squamous) and the presence of intrinsic vasculature in non-gestational tumours (Paradinas 1997, 1998b).

The range of neoplasms in which trophoblastic differentiation has been reported and a primary trophoblastic tumour must be considered is very wide (see Dehner 1980 for an early review) and includes intracranial and liver neonatal tumours (Watanabe et al 1987; Kim et al 1993) in which the possibility of metastases from maternal choriocarcinoma has to be excluded, tumours in women of reproductive age and even tumours in postmenopausal patients, since we know trophoblast can lie dormant and be reactivated long after a pregnancy. The commonest reported sites of non-gestational choriocarcinomas with hCG production are the lung (Dehner 1980; Pushchak & Farhi 1987; Kuida et al 1988; Attanoos et al 1998; Ikura et al 2000), gastrointestinal tract including liver and pancreas (Ishikawa et al 1986; Matthews et al 1986; Nakanuma et al 1986; Östör et al 1993; Imai et al 1994; Wasan et al 1994), urinary tract including prostate (Rodenburg et al 1985, Shah et al 1986; Kuida et al 1988; Nishimura et al 1995; Sheaff et al 1996), breast (Kuida et al 1988; Green 1990; Murata et al 1999) and other sites (Maeyama et al 1985). A few sarcomas with hCG production have been recorded (Kalra et al 1984; Meredith et al 1985) but this is rare. Occasionally tumours also produce alpha-fetoprotein (AFP) (Östör et al 1993) which would be unusual in a gestational neoplasm. In most reported cases no genetic studies have been done, but these are often a part of the diagnostic work-up in recent reports and may help to assess the real magnitude of the problem.

Of particular interest is the differential diagnosis of gestational choriocarcinoma from trophoblastic differentiation in non-gestational gynaecological cancer. This is rare but it can occur in endometrial carcinomas (Civantos & Rywlin 1972; Pesce et al 1991; Hoffman et al 1995; Kalir et al 1995; Black et al 1998; Tunc et al 1998), squamous or anaplastic cervical and vaginal carcinomas (Ohara et al 1993; Morimura et al 1996; Duru et al 1998; Hameed et al 1999) and mixed Müllerian tumours (Khuu et al 2000). Tumours may be diagnosed initially as gestational but they usually fail to respond to chemotherapy and the correct diagnosis is only established when the features described above are found in surgically resected specimens or when no paternal DNA is found in them. Their differential diagnosis from placental site tumour, epithelioid trophoblastic tumour and placental site nodules (see below), particularly those located in the cervix, can be very difficult in small biopsies.

BIOPSY AND DIFFERENTIAL DIAGNOSIS OF TROPHOBLASTIC LESIONS

In the general field of tumour pathology it has become increasingly important that a tissue diagnosis of malignancy is established before potentially dangerous treatment, such as radiotherapy or cytotoxic therapy, is embarked upon. Paradoxically, this maxim is no longer true for the one solid tumour in which it is possible to obtain a high level of lasting cures, choriocarcinoma. This is largely due to the secretion by trophoblastic cells of hCG,

which has proved to be an ideal tumour marker. The development of the radioimmunoassay method for the measurement of gonadotrophin excretion in the urine (Bagshawe 1969) and the beta subunit of hCG in the serum (Kardana & Bagshawe 1976) means that initial tumour load and response to therapy can now be assessed with great accuracy (Newlands et al 1992; Newlands 1997). These are undeniable facts, but hydatidiform moles and tumours often produce abnormal forms of hCG and fragments of hCG which are not detected by kits prepared to diagnose normal pregnancy (Cole 1997) and there are pitfalls in the performance and interpretation of tests which result in false negative and false positive results (Cole 1997, 1998). Also, placental site and epithelioid trophoblastic tumours produce little hCG and so far, other hormones present in them (hPL and PLAP), have not been found useful to monitor treatment, because the amounts in serum do not reflect tumour bulk as closely as hCG in choriocarcinoma. The ectopic production of placental hormones, particularly hCG and hCG fragments by many non-gestational anaplastic carcinomas complicates the picture. Therefore, the histopathologist still plays a fundamental role in the management of trophoblastic lesions, although many patients with postmolar trophoblastic disease are treated without a definite histological diagnosis ever being established.

Although most patients with trophoblastic disease are eventually treated in special centres, the initial diagnosis is usually made in the referring hospital. Patients most frequently present with menstrual irregularity or frank uterine haemorrhage, and histological examination of endometrial curettings is still the most widely used diagnostic procedure in this situation. Indeed, curettings containing chorionic villi or fragments of trophoblast are one of the commonest diagnostic problems in routine gynaecological histopathology. Whilst most specimens are straightforward retained products of conception, in a minority the trophoblast may appear abnormal and the possibility of trophoblastic disease has to be considered. Such biopsies may prove difficult to interpret, and there is unfortunately a tendency amongst pathologists to overdiagnose malignancy.

Elston & Bagshawe (1972b) carried out a detailed investigation into the reliability of the histological diagnosis of trophoblastic disease from uterine curettings. They stressed the importance of the clinical, and in particular, obstetric history, and defined three histological groups: trophoblast associated with villous structures, simple or suspicious trophoblast and trophoblast diagnostic of choriocarcinoma. In a subsequent review Elston (1981) suggested that for practical purposes the interpretation of trophoblastic curettings could be considered in two broad groups, depending on the presence or absence of chorionic villi. Since the establishment of placental site and epitheliod trophoblastic tumours as neoplastic processes, it has also become necessary to include lesions derived from the extravillous trophoblast in the differential diagnosis of non-villous trophoblastic curettings.

DIFFERENTIAL DIAGNOSIS OF LESIONS CONTAINING CHORIONIC VILLI

The majority of specimens containing chorionic villi are derived from spontaneous miscarriages or induced terminations. In our experience many gynaecologists send these to the laboratory (if at all) only for confirmation that they are intrauterine products of conception. Many pathologists are happy to confirm this if they see a few chorionic villi in just one section and go no further because correlation between morphological features and karyotypic abnormalities is poor (Fox 1993; Van Lijneshoten et al 1993). However, many clinically unsuspected complete and partial moles are now received with no other information than 'products of conception'. Correct diagnosis of these moles is less of a problem if the pathologist is familiar with the appearances of a normal conceptus in the first trimester or with the mild hydropic change and loss of vessels present in most non-molar miscarriages retained for some days after embryonic death (see page 1379). However, review of specimens from patients registered for hCG follow-up at Charing Cross in the last 30 years has convinced us that some pathologists are not (Paradinas et al 1991; Paradinas 1998a). Between 12% and 18% patients initially registered for follow-up each year do not have a mole and in most, the distinction from molar pregnancy is easy.

Genuine diagnostic difficulty does occur when there are irregular villi, round trophoblastic inclusions or focal hydropic change (Rushton 1981) and it has been shown that pathologists are poor at recognising correlations between villous morphology and karyotypic abnormalities (Van Lijnschoten et al 1993). Consistency and reproducibility of diagnosis of moles is poor when old histological criteria are used to distinguish between hydropic miscarriage and partial hydatidiform mole and partial mole and complete mole (Javey et al 1979; Messerli et al 1987; Conran et al 1993; Howat et al 1993; Koenig et al 1993). The last three groups concluded that the histological criteria were either not being applied correctly or they were lacking in practical use. Our experience indicates that this is because histological criteria defined for moles evacuated in the second trimester are no longer valid for first trimester disease. However, good agreement is achieved when data concerning DNA content is included in the analysis (Conran et al 1993; Fukunaga et al 1995a) and if updated criteria are used (Paradinas et al 1996; Gschwendtner et al 1998).

Excessive trophoblast in abnormal distribution is still the best criterion to diagnose moles. If this is absent but hydropic change greater than 3 mm and cisterns are present, the possibility of a mole must still be seriously considered and the pathologist should search for trophoblast excess by examining more tissue. A complete mole can be suspected if the chorionic villi are large, polypoid and have nuclear debris; a partial mole can be suspected if there are branching angiomatoid vessels in the stroma of dentate villi or frequent round inclusions. Complete moles evacuated in the first trimester have vessels and hydrops is mild and focal in them. They should not be called partial on this account. A knowledge of gestational age at the time of evacuation is therefore very useful in the histological assessment.

The need for adequate sampling of placental tissue in spontaneous miscarriages cannot be overemphasised, but extensive sampling is time consuming and likely to overload already busy laboratories. Thus, the use of flow cytometry for the diagnosis of triploidy, perhaps done centrally, could be very helpful. If placental material is scanty it may not be adequate to diagnose or exclude a mole and this should be stated in the report. The aim should be to identify the excessive and abnormal distribution of trophoblast characteristic of moles but this may not be possible in the available material and a short hCG follow-up is advisable in doubtful cases.

Curettings taken in the investigation of haemorrhage after delivery or after a molar evacuation may also reveal villous placental tissue, which is often degenerate and inflamed. The introduction of hCG assay in the management and follow-up of patients with hydatidiform mole has reduced the need for uterine curettage (Newlands et al 1992) but if curettage is performed within 48 hours of molar evacuation hydropic molar villi are nearly always present and this finding has no particular diagnostic or prognostic significance. During follow-up it may be appropriate to carry out further curettage. It is of great importance that these specimens are interpreted with caution by the histopathologist. If they contain obvious molar villi a diagnosis of choriocarcinoma cannot, by definition, be made. The correct terminology is persistent mole or postmolar trophoblastic disease, and therapeutic decisions will be based more on hCG levels and radiographic findings than the histological appearances. Nevertheless, the presence of molar villi is an indication that the patient is more likely to have an invasive mole than choriocarcinoma and only a small proportion of these patients will require cytotoxic therapy. It follows that with any trophoblastic proliferation a careful search must be made for formed villi; all available material should be blocked and multiple sections examined if necessary. The majority of postmolar curettages will be carried out within the first three months of follow-up, but molar villi may persist in the uterus for many months if the mole is still growing (Elston & Bagshawe 1972b).

DIFFERENTIAL DIAGNOSIS OF LESIONS NOT CONTAINING CHORIONIC VILLI

Interpretation of curettings containing trophoblast without chorionic villi depends to a large extent on the nature of the preceding gestation. If this was a hydatidiform mole then the same cautious approach as that employed with villous curettings is indicated. A diagnosis of persistent trophoblastic disease is applied and careful follow-up continued. A minority of patients will subsequently require cytotoxic therapy. If the preceding gestation was a normal pregnancy and three or more months have elapsed since delivery, then the presence of pleomorphic trophoblast in abundance is an almost certain indication that the patient has developed choriocarcinoma or placental site trophoblastic tumour. Immediate full investigation should be implemented, and virtually every patient in this group will require further therapy.

After a miscarriage, trophoblastic fragments may be encountered together with a decidual placental site reaction. The presence of villous and decidual placental site trophoblast together is likely to be from a recent pregnancy. If the material from the miscarriage was not sent for histology, the possibility that this could have been molar should always be considered. There may be small collections of monomorphous, usually syncytial, trophoblastic cells set within necrotic debris (Fig. 40.59). Considerable nuclear abnormality may be present and care must be taken not to ascribe these atypical features to neoplastic change; they probably indicate hypoxia due to the growth pattern of trophoblast lacking an intrinsic vasculature. If larger sheets of trophoblast are seen with a

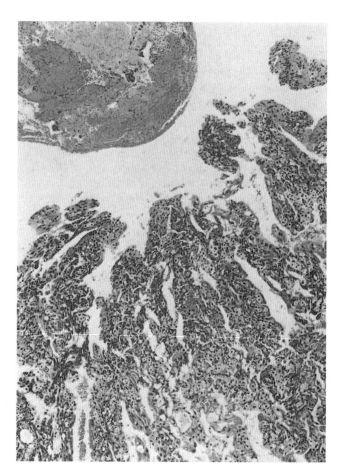

Fig. 40.60 Suspicious trophoblast. The large sheet of trophoblastic tissue on the right has a recognisable bilaminar structure, but no invasion was present.

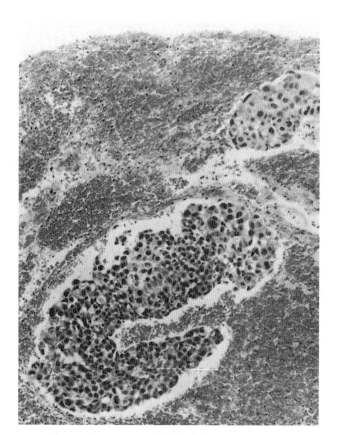

Fig. 40.59 Simple trophoblast in an endometrial curetting. Small fragments of trophoblast with pyknotic nuclei are seen; no clear distinction into cyto- or syncytiotrophoblast is evident.

bilaminar arrangement of cyto- and syncytiotrophoblast reminiscent of choriocarcinoma (Figs 40.60, 40.61) but without evidence of invasion, the appearances are labelled as suspicious trophoblast. Only when bilaminar trophoblast is very pleomorphic, very abundant or exhibits unequivocal myometrial invasion can the appearances be considered diagnostic of choriocarcinoma (Fig. 40.62). This is even more likely if there is a long time interval (months) since the previous miscarriage.

In many curettages performed for 'missed' miscarriage or 'retained products' the only finding is haemorrhagic and necrotic decidua in which residual placental site reaction may be visible (see Figs 40.32, 40.33). Even though chorionic villi are not present, it may be helpful to the clinicians to report the presence of the placental site reaction, thus indicating that a gestation has taken place. In doubtful cases the presence of extravillous trophoblast can be confirmed very easily using immunostaining for low molecular weight cytokeratin, which distinguishes trophoblast from decidua (Sasagawa et al 1986) or by demonstrating placental hormones in them. Similar appearances may also be found in postpartum curettings. In some cases the placental site trophoblast may be particularly florid, placing the appearances in the category of

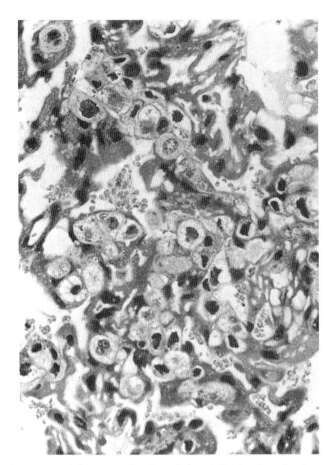

Fig. 40.61 Higher magnification of Fig. 40.59, showing clearly separate cytotrophoblast and syncytiotrophoblast.

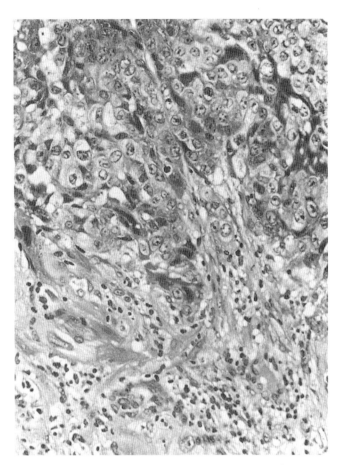

Fig. 40.62 Biopsy diagnostic of choriocarcinoma. Typical bilaminar trophoblast invades myometrium.

exaggerated placental site reaction. The differential diagnosis of placental site trophoblastic tumour should be considered in these circumstances and the distinction between the two may on occasion be difficult, especially if the tissue sample is small (Young et al 1988; Orrell & Sanders 1991). Proximity to the preceding gestation, limited degree of decidual and myometrial infiltration and scanty mitoses favour a diagnosis of placental site reaction and we have never seen a placental site tumour less than five months after the preceding pregnancy. Shih & Kurman (1998b) have reported a high Ki-67 index in placental site tumour but not in exaggerated placental site of a recent pregnancy. There was no significant overlap between the results from the two groups and if confirmed, this should be a useful test. In a small number of cases it is impossible to make a definite diagnosis and careful follow-up is advisable. In placental site tumours hCG tends to remain elevated, whereas in placental site reactions it tends to become normal.

A slightly different problem is the differential diagnosis between placental site tumour, epithelioid trophoblastic tumour and placental site nodules (Young et al 1988, 1990). The latter are usually of small size and circumscribed (Fig. 40.63). They show extensive hyalinisation, a degenerative appearance and paucity of mitoses

(Fig. 40.64). There is a mixture of cells with eosinophilic and with clear vacuolated cytoplasm and Mallory bodies may be found in them (Tsang et al 1993). hCG is only infrequently found in them but epithelial markers such as cytokeratins and EMA are consistently present and scattered cells may contain hPL and PLAP. In fact the morphological and immunocytochemical profile of placental site nodule is very similar to that of epithelioid trophoblastic tumour (Shih et al 1999), possibly because in both the trophoblast has been there for a long time and shows regressing features. The Ki-67 index in placental site nodule has been reported as ranging from 3 to 10% (Shih et al 1999; Shih & Kurman 2001), higher than in exaggerated placental site reaction but lower than in neoplasms. There are now many reported cases of this condition (Lee & Chan 1990; Silva et al 1993; Huettner et al 1994; Shitabata & Rutgers 1994; Buettner et al 1996; Santos et al 1999) including examples in the cervix (Buettner et al 1996; Kase 1996; Van Dorpe & Moerman 1996) and Fallopian tube (Nayar et al 1996; Campello et al 1998). They can be mistaken for cervical squamous cell carcinoma and the differential diagnosis from epithelioid and placental site tumour may be impossible in small biopsies, which should always be interpreted in the light of serological and radiological information. We do

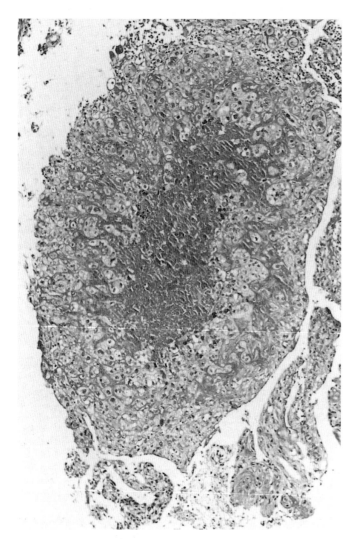

Fig. 40.63 Myometrial placental site nodule showing central necrosis and pericellular hyalinisation.

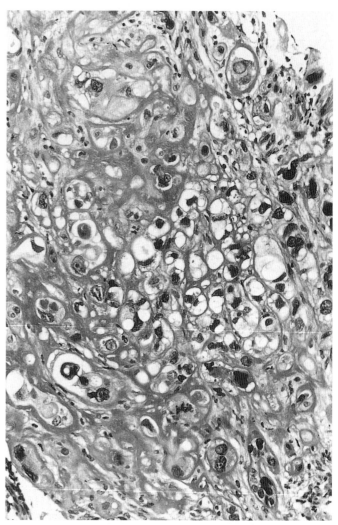

Fig. 40.64 Higher magnification of placental site nodule showing a mixture of vacuolated and non-vacuolated cells similar to those seen in epithelioid trophoblastic tumour.

not know how long these nodules can remain in the myometrium but have seen them at least a year after the last known pregnancy. They should always be treated with caution if the interval between the last pregnancy and diagnosis is long (months or years rather than weeks). We have recently seen a case that illustrates this very well: the patient was delivered of a twin molar pregnancy (normal male baby and complete mole), had placental site nodules in two curettages done one and three months after delivery, but hCG was still marginally elevated and she had chemotherapy after which hCG and uterine ultrasound became normal; she became pregnant in the third year of follow-up, but she had a spontaneous miscarriage of a conceptus with Turner's syndrome. Her hCG failed to return to normal after evacuation and a 1 cm myometrial lesion was seen on ultrasound. Hysterectomy showed typical choriocarcinoma

genetically related to the mole and to placental site nodules 3 years before. This illustrates both the potential of trophoblast to differentiate in various directions and the reactivation of dormant trophoblast by a new pregnancy.

Differentiation of choriocarcinoma from placental site trophoblastic tumour should not be difficult on morphological grounds because of the contrast between the bilaminar structure of the former and the largely monomorphous appearance of the latter. Immunostaining for hCG and hPL should be used to resolve doubtful cases. It is important to make the distinction between the two lesions if at all possible. As pointed out previously, if the features point towards choriocarcinoma cytotoxic therapy is indicated, but if placental site trophoblastic tumour is suspected the treatment of choice is surgery.

REFERENCES

Aboagye-Mathiesen G, Zdravkovic M, Toth F D, Graham C H, Lala P K, Ebbesen P 1996 Altered expression of the tumor suppressor/oncoprotein p53 in SV40 Tag-transformed human placental trophoblast and malignant trophoblast cell lines. Early Pregnancy 2: 102–112

Acaia B, Parazzini F, La Vecchia C et al 1988 Increased frequency of complete hydatidiform mole in women with repeated abortion. Gynecologic Oncology 31: 310–314

Acosta-Sison H 1959 Ab initio choriocarcinoma. Two unusual cases. Obstetrics and Gynecology 13: 350–354

Acosta-Sison H 1967a Trophoblastic or chorionic tumors as observed in the Philippines. In: Holland J F, Hreshchyshyn M M (eds) Choriocarcinoma: transactions of a conference of the International Union against Cancer. Springer-Verlag, Berlin, pp 35–36

Acosta-Sison H 1967b Observation which may indicate the etiology of hydatidiform mole and explain its high incidence in the Philippines and Asiatic countries. Philippine Journal of Surgery 14: 209–297

Agboola A 1979 Trophoblastic neoplasia in an African urban population. Journal of the National Medical Association 71: 935–937

Aguero O, Kizer S, Pinedo G 1973 Hydatidiform mole in Concepcion Palacios Maternity Hospital. American Journal of Obstetrics and Gynecology 116: 1117–1120

Ahmed M N, Kim K, Haddad B, Berchuck A, Qumsiyeh M B 2000 Comparative genomic hybridization studies in hydatidiform moles and choriocarcinoma: amplification of 7q21-q31 and loss of 8p12-p21 in choriocarcinoma. Cancer Genetics and Cytogenetics 116: 10–15

Ambani L M, Vaidya R A, Rao C S, Daftary S D, Motashaw N D 1980 Familial occurrence of trophoblastic disease: report of recurrent molar pregnancies in sisters in three families. Clinical Genetics 18: 27–29

Amr M F, Fisher R A, Foskett M A, Paradinas F J 2000 Triplet pregnancy with hydatidiform mole. International Journal of Gynecological Cancer 10: 76–81

Anderson D J, Berkowitz R S 1985 Gamma-interferon enhances expression of Class I MHC antigens in the weakly HLA-positive human choriocarcinoma cell line BeWo but does not induce MHC expression in the HLA-negative choriocarcinoma cell line Jar. Journal of Immunology 135: 2498–2501

Andreitchouk A E, Takahashi O, Kodama H et al 1996 Choriocarcinoma in infant and mother: a case report. Journal of Obstetrics and Gynaecology Research 22: 585–588

Aonahata M, Masuzawa Y, Tsutsui Y 1998 A case of intraplacental choriocarcinoma associated with placental hemangioma. Pathology International 48: 897–901

Ariel I, Lustig O, Oyer C E et al 1994 Relaxation of imprinting in trophoblastic disease. Gynecologic Oncology 53: 212–219

Arima T, Imamura T, Amada S, Tsuneyoshi M, Wake N 1994 Genetic origin of malignant trophoblastic neoplasms. Cancer Genetics and Cytogenetics 73: 95–102

Atkin N B 1965 In: Park W W (ed) The early conceptus, normal and abnormal. Livingstone, London, pp 130–134

Atrash H K, Hogue C J R, Grimes D A 1986 Epidemiology of hydatidiform mole during early gestation. American Journal of Obstetrics and Gynecology 154: 906–909

Attanoos R L, Papagiannis A, Suttinont P, Goddard H, Papotti M, Gibbs A R 1998 Pulmonary giant cell carcinoma: pathological entity or morphological phenotype? Histopathology 32: 225–231

Attwood H D, Park W W 1961 Embolism to the lungs by trophoblast. Journal of Obstetrics and Gynaecology of the British Commonwealth 68: 611–617

Ayhan A, Tuncer Z S, Halilzade H, Kucukali T 1996 Predictors of persistent disease in women with complete hydatidiform mole. Journal of Reproductive Medicine 41: 591–594

Azuma C, Saji F, Tokugawa Y et al 1991 Application of gene amplification by polymerase chain reaction to genetic analysis of molar mitochondrial DNA: the detection of anuclear empty ovum as the cause of complete mole. Gynecologic Oncology 40: 29–33

Azuma C, Saji F, Takemura M et al 1992 Triplet pregnancy involving complete hydatidiform mole and two fetuses: genetic analysis by deoxyribonucleic acid fingerprint. American Journal of Obstetrics and Gynecology 166: 664–667

Badonnel Y, Barbe F, Legagneur H, Poncelet E, Schweitzer M 1994 Inhibin as a marker for hydatidiform mole: a comparative study with the determinations of intact human chorionic gonadotrophin and its free beta-subunit. Clinical Endocrinology 41: 155–162

Bae S N, Kim S J 1999 Telomerase activity in complete hydatidiform mole. American Journal of Obstetrics and Gynecology 180: 328–333

Bagshawe K D 1969 The clinical biology of the trophoblast and its tumours. Arnold, London

Bagshawe K D 1973 Recent observations related to chemotherapy and immunology of gestational choriocarcinoma. Advances in Cancer Research 18: 231–263

Bagshawe K D 1976 Risk and prognostic factors in trophoblastic neoplasia. Cancer 38: 1373–1385

Bagshawe K D, Brooks W D W 1959 Subacute pulmonary hypertension due to chorionepithelioma. Lancet 1: 653–658

Bagshawe K D, Lawler S D 1982 Unmasking moles. British Journal of Obstetrics and Gynaecology 89: 255–257

Bagshawe K D, Rawlings G, Pike M, Lawler S D 1971 ABO blood groups in trophoblastic neoplasia. Lancet i: 553–557

Bagshawe K D, Dent J, Webb J 1986 Hydatidiform mole in England and Wales 1973–83. Lancet 2: 673–677

Bagshawe K D, Lawler S D, Paradinas F J, Dent J, Brown P, Boxer G M 1990 Gestational trophoblastic tumours following initial diagnosis of partial hydatidiform mole. Lancet 335: 1074–1076

Balaram P, John M, Rajalekshmy T N, Mathew A, Enose S, Gangadharan V P 1999 A multivariate analysis of prognostic indicators in complete hydatidiform moles (CHM). European Journal of Obstetrics, Gynecology and Reproductive Biology 87: 69–75

Barclay I D, Dabbagh L, Babiak J, Poppema S 1993 DNA analysis (ploidy) of molar pregnancies with image analysis on paraffin tissue sections. American Journal of Clinical Pathology 100: 451–455

Bardawil W A, Toy B L 1959 The natural history of choriocarcinoma; problems of immunity and spontaneous regression. Annals of the New York Academy of Sciences 60: 197–251

Bardawil W A, Hertig A T, Velardo J T 1957 Regression of trophoblast. 1 Hydatidiform mole: a case of unusual features; possible metastasis and regression; review of literature. Obstetrics and Gynecology 10: 614–625

Barghorn A, Bannwart F, Stallmach T 1998 Incidental choriocarcinoma confined to a near-term placenta. Virchows Archiv 433: 89–91

Bartocci A, Pollard J W, Stanley E R 1986 Regulation of colony-stimulating factor-1 during pregnancy. Journal of Experimental Medicine 164: 956–961

Barton S C, Surani M A H, Norris M L 1984 Role of paternal and maternal genomes in mouse development. Nature 311: 374–376

Bassaw B, Roopnarinesingh S 1990 The epidemiology and management of patients with hydatidiform mole. West Indian Medical Journal 39: 43–46

Bateman A C, Hemmatpour S K, Theaker J M, Howell W M 1997 Genetic analysis of hydatidiform moles in paraffin-embedded tissue using rapid, polymerase chain reaction-based HLA class II typing. Journal of Clinical Pathology 50: 288–293

Bauer M, Horn L C, Kowalzik J, Mair W, Czerwenka K 1997 C-erbB-2 amplification and expression in gestational trophoblastic disease correlates with DNA content and karyotype. General and Diagnostic Pathology 143: 185–190

Bell K A, Van Deerlin V, Addya K, Clevenger C V, Van Deerlin P G, Leonard D G 1999 Molecular genetic testing from paraffin-embedded tissue distinguishes nonmolar hydropic abortion from hydatidiform mole. Molecular Diagnosis 4: 11–19

Benirschke K 1989 Flow cytometry for all mole-like abortion specimens. Human Pathology 20: 403–404

Benirschke K, Spinosa J C, McGinniss M J, Marchevsky A, Sanchez J 2000 Partial molar transformation of the placenta of presumably monozygotic twins. Pediatric and Developmental Pathology 3: 95–100

Berger G, Verbaere J, Feroldi J 1984 Placental site trophoblastic tumor of the uterus: an ultrastructural and immunohistochemical study. Ultrastructural Pathology 6: 319–329

Berkowitz B J, Jones J G, Merkatz I R, Runowicz C O 1990 Ovarian conservation in placental site trophoblastic tumor. Gynecologic Oncology 37: 239–243

Berkowitz R S, Goldstein D P 1988 Diagnosis and management of the primary hydatidiform mole. Obstetrics and Gynecology Clinics of North America 15: 491–502

Berkowitz R S, Goldstein D P 1997a Presentation and management of molar pregnancy. In: Hancock B W, Newlands E S, Berkowitz R S (eds) Gestational trophoblastic disease. Chapman & Hall Medical, London, pp 127–142

Berkowitz R S, Goldstein D P 1997b Presentation and management of persistent trophoblastic disease and gestational trophoblastic tumours in the USA. In: Hancock B W, Newlands E S, Berkowitz R S (eds) Gestational trophoblastic disease. Chapman & Hall Medical, London, pp 157–172

Berkowitz R S, Goldstein D P, Bernstein M 1979 Natural history of partial hydatidiform moles. Lancet i: 719

Berkowitz R S, Hornig-Rohan J, Martin-Alosco S et al 1981 HL-A antigen frequency distribution in patients with gestational choriocarcinoma and their husbands. Placenta (suppl 3): 263–267

Berkowitz R S, Cramer D W, Bernstein M R, Cassells S, Driscoll S G, Goldstein D P 1985 Risk factors for complete molar pregnancy from a case-control study. American Journal of Obstetrics and Gynecology 152: 1016–1020

Berkowitz R S, Umpierre S A, Taylor-Emery S, Goldstein D P, Anderson D J 1986a Immunobiology of complete molar pregnancy and gestational trophoblastic tumor. Cancer and Metastasis Reviews 5: 109–123

Berkowitz R S, Umpierre S A, Johnson P M, McIntyre J A, Anderson D J 1986b Expression of trophoblast-leukocyte common antigens and placental-type alkaline phosphatase in complete molar pregnancy. American Journal of Obstetrics and Gynecology 155: 443–446

Berkowitz R S, Goldstein D P, Bernstein M R 1986c Natural history of partial molar pregnancy. Obstetrics and Gynecology 66: 677–681

Berkowitz R S, Goldstein D P, Bernstein M R 1988 Partial molar pregnancy: a separate entity. Contemporary Obstetrics and Gynecology 31: 99–102

Berkowitz R S, Im S S, Bernstein M R, Goldstein D P 1998 Gestational trophoblastic disease. Subsequent pregnancy outcome, including repeat molar pregnancy. Journal of Reproductive Medicine 43: 81–86

Bewtra C, Frankforter S, Marcus J N 1997 Clinicopathologic differences between diploid and tetraploid complete hydatidiform moles. International Journal of Gynecological Pathology 16: 239–244

Black K, Sykes P, Ostor A G 1998 Trophoblastic differentiation in an endometrial carcinoma. Australian and New Zealand Journal of Obstetrics and Gynaecology 38: 472–473

Blackwell J B, Papadimitriou J M 1979 Trophoblastic pseudotumour of the uterus. Case report and ultrastructure. Cancer 43: 1734–1741

Boué J, Phillipe E, Giroud E, Boué A 1976 Phenotypic expression of lethal chromosomal abnormalities in human abortuses. Teratology 14: 3–13

Bower M, Paradinas F J, Fisher R A et al 1996 Placental site trophoblastic tumor: molecular analysis and clinical experience. Clinical Cancer Research 2: 897–902

Bracken M B 1987 Incidence and aetiology of hydatidiform mole: an epidemiological review. British Journal of Obstetrics and Gynaecology 94: 1123–1135

Brajenovic-Milic B, Petrovic O, Krasevic M, Ristic S, Kapovic M 1998 Chromosomal anomalies in abnormal human pregnancies. Fetal Diagnosis and Therapy 13: 187–191

Bravo R, Frank R, Blundell P A, MacDonald-Bravo H 1987 Cyclin/PCNA is the auxiliary protein of DNA delta. Nature 326: 515–517

Brescia R J, Kurman R J, Main C S, Surti U, Szulman A E 1987 Immunocytochemical localization of chorionic gonadotropin, placental lactogen, and placental alkaline phosphatase in the diagnosis of complete and partial hydatidiform moles. International Journal of Gynecological Pathology 6: 213–229

Brewer J I 1959 The Albert F Mathieu Chorionepithelioma Registry. Annals of the New York Academy of Sciences 80: 140–142

Brewer J I 1967 Light microscopy of gestational trophoblastic disease. In: Lund C W, Choate J W (eds) Transcript of 4th Rochester Trophoblast Conference. Rochester, New York, pp 6–24

Brewer J I, Mazur M T 1981 Gestational choriocarcinoma: its origin in the placenta during seemingly normal pregnancy. American Journal of Surgical Pathology 5: 267–277

Brewer J I, Rhinehart J I, Dunbar R W 1961 Choriocarcinoma: a report of the 5 or more years survival from the Albert Mathieu Chorionepithelioma Registry. American Journal of Obstetrics and Gynecology 81: 574–583

Buckell E W C, Owen T K 1954 Chorionepithelioma in mother and infant. Journal of Pathology and Bacteriology 61: 329–330

Buckley J 1987 Epidemiology of gestational trophoblastic diseases. In: Szulman A E, Buchsbaum H J (eds) Gestational trophoblastic disease. Springer-Verlag, New York, pp 8–26

Buettner R, Schleicher P, Schleicher B, Ruschoff J, Hofstadter F 1996 Benign placental trophoblast nodule. Case report with overview of proliferative diseases of the intermediate stage trophoblast. Geburtshilfe und Frauenheilkund 56: 257–261

Burton J L, Corps E A, Gillespie A M et al 2001 Over-diagnosis of hydatidiform mole in early tubal ectopic pregnancy. Histopathology 38: 409–417

Byrne J, Blanc W A, Warburton D, Wigger J 1984 The significance of cystic hygroma in fetuses. Human Pathology 15: 61–67

Cameron B, Gown A M, Tarnimi H K 1994 Expression of c-erb-B 2 oncogene product in persistent gestational trophoblastic disease. American Journal of Obstetrics and Gynecology 170: 1616–1621

Campello T R, Fittipaldi H, O'Valle F, Carvia R E, Nogales F F 1998 Extrauterine (tubal) placental site nodule. Histopathology 32: 562–565

Carr D H 1969 Cytogenetics and the pathology of hydatidiform degeneration. Obstetrics and Gynecology 33: 333–342

Caspersson T, Lomakka G, Lech L 1971 The 24 fluorescence patterns of human metaphase chromosomes distinguishing characters and variability. Hereditas 67: 89–102

Challis D E, Rew K J, Steigrad S J 1996 Choriocarcinoma complicated by splenic rupture: an unusual presentation. Journal of Obstetrics and Gynaecology Research 22: 395–400

Chang Y L, Chang T C, Hsueh S et al 1999 Prognostic factors and treatment for placental site trophoblastic tumor — report of 3 cases and analysis of 88 cases. Gynecologic Oncology 73: 216–222

Chen R J, Huang S C, Chow S N, Hsieh C Y, Hsu H C 1994 Persistent gestational trophoblastic tumour with partial hydatidiform mole as the antecedent pregnancy. British Journal of Obstetrics and Gynaecology 101: 330–334

Cheung A N, Ngan H Y, Chen W Z, Loke S L, Collins R J 1993a The significance of proliferating cell nuclear antigen in human trophoblastic disease: an immunohistochemical study. Histopathology 22: 565–568

Cheung A N Y, Srivastava G, Pittaluga S, Mam T K, Collins R J 1993b Expression of C-myc and C-fms oncogenes in trophoblastic cells in hydatidiform mole and normal human placenta. Journal of Clinical Pathology 46: 204–207

Cheung A N, Ngan H Y, Collins R J, Wong Y L 1994 Assessment of cell proliferation in hydatidiform mole using monoclonal antibody MIB1 to Ki-67 antigen. Journal of Clinical Pathology 47: 601–604

Cheung A N, Ngan H Y, Ng W F, Khoo U S 1995 The expression of cathepsin D, oestrogen receptor and progestogen receptor in hydatidiform mole. An immunohistochemical study. Histopathology 27: 341–347

Cheung A N, Zhang D K, Liu Y, Ngan H Y, Shen D H, Tsao S W 1999 Telomerase activity in gestational trophoblastic disease. Journal of Clinical Pathology 52: 588–592

Cheville J C, Greiner T, Robinson R A, Benda J A 1995 Ploidy analysis by flow cytometry and fluorescence in situ hybridization in hydropic placentas and gestational trophoblastic disease. Human Pathology 26: 753–757

Cheville J C, Robinson R, Benda J A 1996a p53 expression in placentas with hydropic change and hydatidiform moles. Modern Pathology 9: 392–396

Cheville J C, Robinson R, Benda J A 1996b Evaluation of Ki-67 (MIB-1) in placentas with hydropic change and partial and complete hydatidiform mole. Pediatric Pathology and Laboratory Medicine 16: 41–50

Chiari H 1877 Über drei Fälle von primären Carcinom im Fundus and Corpus des Uterus. Medizinische Jährbücher 7: 364–368

Chilosi M, Piazzola E, Lestani M et al 1998 Differential expression of p57^{kip2}, a maternally imprinted cdk inhibitor, in normal human placenta and gestational trophoblastic disease. Laboratory Investigation 78: 269–276

Chiu P M, Ngan Y S, Khoo Y S, Cheung A N Y 2001 Apoptotic activity in gestational trophoblastic disease correlates with clinical outcome: assessment by the caspase related M30 CytoDeath antibody. Histopathology 38: 243–249

Chong C Y, Koh C F 1999 Hydatidiform mole in Kandang Kerbau Hospital — a 5-year review. Singapore Medical Journal 40: 265–270

Christopherson W A, Kanbour A, Szulman A E 1992 Choriocarcinoma in a term placenta with maternal metastases. Gynecologic Oncology 46: 239–245

Chun D, Braga C A 1967 Choriocarcinoma in Hong Kong. In: Wood C, Walters W A W (eds) Proceedings of the 5th World Congress of Gynaecology and Obstetrics. Butterworth, New South Wales, pp 398–405

Chung T K H, Cheung T H, Lam S K, Chang A M Z 1995 Epidemiology and aetiology of trophoblastic disease. Current Obstetrics and Gynaecology 5: 2–5

Civantos F, Rywlin A M 1972 Carcinomas with trophoblastic differentiation and secretion of chorionic gonadotrophins. Cancer 29: 789–798

Cole L A 1997 Human chorionic gonadotropin assay. In: Hancock B W, Newlands E S, Berkowitz R S (eds) Gestational trophoblastic disease. Chapman & Hall Medical, London, pp 143–172

Cole L A 1998 Phantom hCG and phantom choriocarcinoma. Gynecologic Oncology 71: 325–329

Collins R J, Ngan H Y S, Wong L C 1990 Placental site trophoblastic tumor: with features between an exaggerated placental site reaction and a placental site trophoblastic tumor. International Journal of Gynecological Pathology 9: 170–177

Conran R M, Hitchcock C L, Popek E J et al 1993 Diagnostic considerations in molar gestations. Human Pathology 24: 41–48

Couillon P, Hors J, Boué A 1978 Identification of the origin of triploidy by HLA markers. Human Genetics 41: 35–44

Coukos G, Makrigiannakis A, Chung J, Randall T C, Rubin S C, Benjamin I 1999 Complete hydatidiform mole. A disease with a changing profile. Journal of Reproductive Medicine 44: 698–704

Coulam C B, Wagenknetch D, McIntrye J A, Faulk W P, Annegers J F 1991 Occurrence of other reproductive failures among women with recurrent spontaneous abortion. American Journal of Reproductive Immunology 25: 96–98

Couone A W, Multon D, Johnson P M, Adolfini M 1984 Trophoblast cells in peripheral blood from pregnant women. Lancet ii: 841–843

Crescimanno C, Marzioni D, Paradinas F J et al 1999 Expression pattern alterations of syndecans and glypican-1 in normal and pathological trophoblast. Journal of Pathology 189: 600–608

Crocker J, Skilbeck N 1987 Nucleolar organiser region associated proteins in cutaneous melanocytic lesions: a quantitative study. Journal of Clinical Pathology 40: 885–889

Curry S L, Hammond C B, Tyrey L, Creasman W T, Parker R T 1975 Hydatidiform mole: diagnosis, management and long term follow-up of 347 patients. Obstetrics and Gynecology 45: 1–3

Czernobilsky B, Barash A, Lancet M 1982 Partial moles: a clinicopathological study of 25 cases. Obstetrics and Gynecology 59: 75–77

Dalrymple C, Russell P, Murray J 1995 Coexistent complete and partial hydatidiform moles in a twin pregnancy. Journal of Obstetrics and Gynaecology 21: 325–330

Dana A, Saldanha G J, Doshi R, Rustin G J 1996 Metastatic cerebral choriocarcinoma coexistent with a viable pregnancy. Gynecologic Oncology 61: 147–149

Davis J P, Foster K J 1984 Sex assignment in gestational trophoblastic neoplasia. American Journal of Obstetrics and Gynecology 148: 722–725

Davis J, Kerrigan D P, Way D L, Weiner S A 1987 Partial hydatidiform moles: deoxyribonucleic acid content and course. American Journal of Obstetrics and Gynecology 157: 969–973

Dawood M Y, Teoh E S, Ratnam S S 1971 ABO blood group in trophoblastic neoplasia. American Journal of Obstetrics and Gynecology 78: 918–923

Deaton J L, Hoffman J S, Saal H, Allred C, Koulos J P 1989 Molar pregnancy coexisting with a normal fetus: a case report. Gynecologic Oncology 32: 394–397

Deftos L J, Burton D W, Brandt D W, Pinar H, Rubin L P 1994 Neoplastic hormone-producing cells of the placenta produce and secrete parathyroid hormone-related protein. Studies by immunohistology, immunoassay, and polymerase chain reaction. Laboratory Investigation 71: 847–852

Dehner L P 1980 Gestational and nongestational trophoblastic neoplasia. A historic and pathobiologic survey. American Journal of Surgical Pathology 4: 43–58

Delfs E 1957 Quantitative chorionic gonadotrophin: prognostic value in hydatidiform mole and chorionepithelioma. Obstetrics and Gynecology 9: 1–24

Deligdisch L, Driscoll S G, Goldstein D P 1978 Gestational trophoblastic neoplasms: morphologic correlations of therapeutic response. American Journal of Obstetrics and Gynecology 130: 801–806

De Ruyck R 1951 Mise en évidence du virus choriotrope dans quatre case de môle hydatidiforme, et dans un cas de métastase pulmonaire de chorio-épithéliome. Bulletin de L'Assocation Francaise pour l'Etude du Cancer 38: 252–268

Dessau R, Rustin G J S, Dent J, Paradinas F J, Bagshawe K D 1990 Surgery and chemotherapy in the management of placental site tumor. Gynecologic Oncology 39: 56–59

Devasia A, Nath V, Abraham B, Gopalkrishnan G, Nair S 1994 Hematuria, renal mass and amenorrhea: indicators of a rare diagnosis. Journal of Urology 151: 409–410

Di Cintio E, Parazzini F, Rosa C, Chatenoud L, Benzi G 1997 The epidemiology of gestational trophoblastic disease. General Diagnostic Pathology 143: 103–108

Dinh-De T, Minh H N 1961 Hydatidiform mole with recurrent vaginal metastasis. American Journal of Obstetrics and Gynecology 82: 660–663

Dorling A, Monk N J, Lechler R I 2000 HLA-G inhibits the transendothelial migration of human NK cells. European Journal of Immunology 30: 586–593

Doshi N, Surti U, Szulman A E 1983 Morphologic anomalies in triploid liveborn fetuses. Human Pathology 14: 716–723

Douglas G W 1962 Malignant change in trophoblastic tumors. American Journal of Obstetrics and Gynecology 84: 884–894

Doutrelepont J M, Mat O, Abramowicz D et al 1995 Inadvertent transfer of choriocarcinoma with renal transplantation: characteristics of the donor-recipient pairs. Transplantation Proceedings 27: 1789–1790

Driscoll S G 1963 Choriocarcinoma: an 'incidental finding' within a term placenta. Obstetrics and Gynecology 21: 96–101

Driscoll S G 1977 Gestational trophoblastic neoplasms: morphologic considerations. Human Pathology 8: 529–539

Du Beshter B, Berkowitz R S, Goldstein D P, Cramer D W, Bernstein M R 1987 Metastatic gestational trophoblastic disease: experience at the New England Trophoblastic Disease Centre, 1965–1985. Obstetrics and Gynecology 69: 390–395

Duff G B 1989 Gestational trophoblastic disease in New Zealand, 1980–1986. Australian and New Zealand Journal of Obstetrics and Gynaecology 29: 139–142

Duncan D A, Mazur M T 1989 Trophoblastic tumors: ultrastructural comparison of choriocarcinoma and placental-site trophoblastic tumor. Human Pathology 20: 370–381

Duru N K, Dilek S, Yenen M C, Atay V, Dede M, Tokac G 1998 Bulky vaginal choriocarcinoma unrelated to pregnancy in the reproductive period. European Journal of Gynaecologic Oncology 19: 85–86

Eckstein R P, Paradinas F J, Bagshawe K D 1982 Placental site trophoblastic tumour (trophoblastic pseudotumour): a study of four cases requiring hysterectomy including one fatal case. Histopathology 6: 221–226

Eckstein R P, Russell P, Friedlander M M, Tattersall M H N, Bradfield A 1985 Metastasizing placental site tumor: a case study. Human Pathology 16: 632–636

Editorial 1975 Epidemiological aspects of choriocarcinoma. British Medical Journal ii: 606–607

Ellis P S J, Whitehead R 1981 Mitosis counting — a need for reappraisal. Human Pathology 12: 3–4

Elmer D B, Granai C O, Ball H G, Curry S L 1993 Persistence of gestational trophoblastic disease for longer than 1 year following evacuation of hydatidiform mole. Obstetrics and Gynecology 81: 888–890

Elston C W 1969 Cellular reaction to choriocarcinoma. Journal of Pathology 97: 261–268

Elston C W 1970 A histopathological study of trophoblastic tumours: with special reference to the cellular reaction to choriocarcinoma. MD Thesis, University of London

Elston C W 1976 The histopathology of trophoblastic tumours. Journal of Clinical Pathology 29 (suppl 10): 111–131

Elston C W 1978 Trophoblastic tumours of the placenta. In: Fox H (ed) Pathology of the placenta. W B Saunders, London, pp 368–425

Elston C W 1981 Gestational tumours of trophoblast. In: Anthony P P, MacSween R N M (eds) Recent advances in histopathology. Churchill Livingstone, Edinburgh, pp 149–161

Elston C W 1989 Trophoblastic disease: A review with emphasis on recent advances and problems in differential diagnosis. In: Damjanov I, Cohen A H, Mills S E, Young R H (eds) Progress in reproductive and urinary tract pathology. Field and Wood, New York, pp 31–71

Elston C W 1991 Trophoblastic disease: a review with emphasis on recent advances and problems in differential diagnosis. In: Damjanov I, Cohen A H, Mills S E, Young R H (eds) Progress in reproductive and urinary tract pathology. Field & Wood, New York, pp 31–72

Elston C W 1995 Gestational trophoblastic disease. In: Fox H and Wells M (eds) Haynes & Taylor: gynaecological pathology. Churchill Livingstone, Edinburgh, pp 1597–1639

Elston C W, Bagshawe K D 1972a The value of histological grading in the management of hydatidiform mole. Journal of Obstetrics and Gynaecology of the British Commonwealth 79: 717–724

Elston C W, Bagshawe K D 1972b The diagnosis of trophoblastic tumours from uterine curettings. Journal of Clinical Pathology 25: 111–118

Elston C W, Bagshawe K D 1973 Cellular reaction in trophoblastic tumours. British Journal of Cancer 28: 245–256

Erdogan G, Cesur V, Unal M, Ortac F, Balci M K 1994 Choriocarcinoma metastasis in the thyroid gland. Thyroid 4: 301–303

Evans A C, Soper J T, Hammond C B 1997 Clinical manifestations of molar pregnancies and gestational trophoblastic tumours. In: Hancock B W, Newlands E S, Berkowitz R S eds. Gestational trophoblastic disease. Chapman & Hall Medical, London, pp 109–125

Ewing J 1910 Chorioma: a clinical and pathological study. Surgery, Gynecology and Obstetrics 10: 366–392

Fasoli M, Ratti E, Franceschi S et al 1982 Management of gestational trophoblastic disease: results of a cooperative study. Obstetrics and Gynecology 60: 205–209

Faulk W P, Temple A 1976 Distribution of B2 microglobulin and HLA in chorionic villi of human placentae. Nature 262: 799–802

Felemban A A, Bakri Y N, Alkharif H A, Altuwaijri S M, Shalhoub J, Berkowitz R S 1998 Complete molar pregnancy. Clinical trends at King Fahad Hospital, Riyadh, Kingdom of Saudi Arabia. Journal of Reproductive Medicine 43: 11–13

Fernandez P L, Merino M J, Nogales F F et al 1992 Immunohistochemical profile of basement membrane proteins and 72 kilodalton type IV collagenase in the implantation placental site. An integrated view. Laboratory Investigation 66: 572–579

Finkler N J, Berkowitz R S, Driscoll S G, Goldstein D P, Bernstein M R 1988 Clinical experience with placental site trophoblastic tumors at the New England Trophoblastic Disease Centre. Obstetrics and Gynecology 71: 854–857

Fisher R A, Lawler S D 1984a Heterozygous complete hydatidiform moles: do they have a worse prognosis than homozygous complete moles? Lancet ii: 51

Fisher R A, Lawler S D 1984b The expression of major histocompatibility antigens in the chorionic villi of molar placentae. Placenta 5: 237–242

Fisher R A, Newlands E S 1993 Rapid diagnosis and classification of hydatidiform moles with polymerase chain reaction. American Journal of Obstetrics and Gynecology 168: 563–569

Fisher R A, Sheppard D M, Lawler S D 1982 Twin pregnancy with complete hydatidiform mole (46,XX) and fetus (46,XY): genetic origin proved by analysis of chromosome polymorphisms. British Medical Journal 284: 1218–1220

Fisher R A, Lawler S D, Ormerod M G, Imrie P R, Povey S 1987 Flow cytometry used to distinguish between complete and partial hydatidiform moles. Placenta 8: 249–256

Fisher R A, Povey S, Jeffreys A J et al 1989 Frequency of heterozygous complete hydatidiform moles, estimated by locus-specific minisatellite and Y chromosome-specific probes. Human Genetics 82: 259–263

Fisher R A, Newlands E S, Jeffreys A J et al 1992a Gestational and nongestational trophoblastic tumors distinguished by DNA analysis. Cancer 69: 839–845

Fisher R A, Paradinas F J, Newlands E S, Boxer G M 1992b Genetic evidence that placental site trophoblastic tumours can originate from a hydatidiform mole or a normal conceptus. British Journal of Cancer 65: 355–358

Fisher R A, Johnson P H, Povey S, Hopkinson D A, Lawler S D 1993 ABO genotyping of complete hydatidiform moles. Disease Markers 11: 179–185

Fisher R A, Soteriou B A, Meredith L, Paradinas F J, Newlands E S 1995 Previous hydatidiform mole identified as the causative pregnancy of choriocarcinoma following birth of normal twins. International Journal of Gynecological Cancer 5: 64–70

Fisher R A, Paradinas F J, Soteriou B A, Foskett M, Newlands E S 1997 Diploid hydatidiform moles with fetal red cells in molar villi. 2-Genetics. Journal of Pathology 181: 189–195

Fisher R A, Khatoon R, Paradinas F J, Roberts A P, Newlands E S 2000 Repetitive complete hydatidiform mole can be biparental in origin and either male or female. Human Reproduction 15: 594–598

Fishman D A, Padilla L A, Keh P, Cohen L, Frederiksen M, Lurain J R 1998 Management of twin pregnancies consisting of a complete hydatidiform mole and normal fetus. Obstetrics and Gynecology 91: 546–550

Flam F, Kock E 1996 Metastatic choroidal choriocarcinoma. Acta Obstetricia et Gynecologica Scandinavica 75: 688–689

Flam F, Lundstrom V, Pettersson F 1991 Medical induction prior to surgical evacuation of hydatidiform mole: is there a greater risk of persistent trophoblastic disease? European Journal of Obstetrics, Gynaecology and Reproductive Biology 42: 57–60

Floridon C, Nielsen O, Holund B et al 1999 Localization and significance of urokinase plasminogen activator and its receptor in placental tissue from intrauterine, ectopic and molar pregnancies. Placenta 20: 711–721

Fox H 1989 Editorial: hydatidiform moles. Virchows Archives A, Pathological Anatomy 415: 387–389

Fox H 1993 Commentary: histological classification of tissue from spontaneous abortions: a valueless exercise? Histopathology 22: 599–600

Fox H 1997 Differential diagnosis of hydatidiform moles. General and Diagnostic Pathology 143: 117–125

Fox H, Kharkongor N F 1971 Ultrastructure of molar trophoblast. Journal of Obstetrics and Gynaecology of the British Commonwealth 78: 652–659

Fox H, Laurini R N 1988 Intraplacental choriocarcinoma: a report of two cases. Journal of Clinical Pathology 41: 1085–1088

Franke H R, Risse E K J, Kenemans P, Vooijs G P, Stolke J G 1983 Epidemiologic features of hydatidiform mole in the Netherlands. Obstetrics and Gynecology 62: 613–616

Frates M C, Feinberg B B 2000 Early prenatal sonographic diagnosis of twin triploid gestation presenting with fetal hydrops and theca-lutein ovarian cysts. Journal of Clinical Ultrasound 28: 137–141

Fukunaga M 1994 Histopathologic study of partial hydatidiform moles and DNA triploid placentas. Pathology International 44: 528–534

Fukunaga M 2000 Early partial hydatidiform mole prevalence, histopathology, DNA ploidy, and persistence rate. Virchows Archiv 437: 180–184

Fukunaga M, Ushigome S 1993a Malignant trophoblastic tumors: immunohistochemical and flow cytometric comparison of choriocarcinoma and placental site trophoblastic tumors. Human Pathology 24: 1098–1106

Fukunaga M, Ushigome S 1993b Metastasizing placental site trophoblastic tumor. An immunohistochemical and flow cytometric study of two cases. American Journal of Surgical Pathology 17: 1003–1010

Fukunaga M, Ushigome S, Fukunaga M 1993a Spontaneous abortions and DNA ploidy. An application of flow cytometric DNA analysis in detection of non-diploidy in early abortions. Modern Pathology 6: 619–624

Fukunaga M, Ushigome S, Fukunaga M, Sugishita M 1993b Application of flow cytometry in diagnosis of hydatidiform moles. Modern Pathology 6: 353–359

Fukunaga M, Miyazawa Y, Sugishita M, Ushigome S 1993c Immunohistochemistry of molar and non-molar placentas with special reference to their differential diagnosis. Acta Pathologica Japonica 43: 683–689

Fukunaga M, Endo Y, Ushigome S 1995a Flow cytometric and clinicopathological study of 197 hydatidiform moles with special reference to the significance of cytometric aneuploidy and literature review. Cytometry 22: 135–138

Fukunaga M, Ushigome S, Endo Y 1995b Incidence of hydatidiform mole in a Tokyo hospital: a 5 year (1989 to 1993) prospective morphological and flow cytometric study. Human Pathology 26: 758–764

Fukunaga M, Nomura K, Ushigome S 1996a Choriocarcinoma in situ at a first trimester. Report of two cases indicating an origin of trophoblast of a stem villus. Virchows Archiv 429: 185–188

Fukunaga M, Endo Y, Ushigome S 1996b Clinicopathologic study of tetraploid hydropic villous tissues. Archives of Pathology and Laboratory Medicine 120: 569–572

Fukuyama R, Takata M, Kudoh J et al 1991 DNA diagnosis of hydatidiform mole using the polymerase chain reaction. Human Genetics 87: 216–218

Fulop V, Mok S C, Genest D R, Szigetvari I, Cseh I, Berkowitz R S 1998 c-myc, c-erbB-2, c-fms and bcl-2 oncoproteins. Expression in normal placenta, partial and complete mole, and choriocarcinoma. Journal of Reproductive Medicine 43: 101–110

Gaber L W, Redline R W, Mostoufi-Zadeh M, Driscoll S G 1986 Invasive partial mole. American Journal of Clinical Pathology 85: 722–724

Gal D, Friedman M 1987 Follow up and contraception. In: Szulman A E, Buchsbaum H J (eds) Gestational trophoblastic disease. Springer-Verlag, New York, pp 179–185

Galton M, Goldman P B, Holt S F 1963 Karyotypic and morphologic characterisation of a serially transplanted human choriocarcinoma. Journal of the National Cancer Institute 31: 1019–1035

Gardner H A R, Lage J L 1992 Choriocarcinoma following a partial mole: a case report. Human Pathology 23: 468–471

Geisler J P, Mernitz C S, Hiett A K, Geisler H E, Cudahy T J 1999 Trisomy 21 fetus co-existent with a partial molar pregnancy: case report. Clinical and Experimental Obstetrics and Gynecology 26: 149–150

Genest D R, Laborde O, Berkowitz R S, Goldstein D P, Bernstein M R, Lage J 1991 A clinicopathologic study of 153 cases of complete hydatidiform mole (1980–1990): histologic grade lacks prognostic significance. Obstetrics and Gynecology 78: 402–409

Genest D R, Roberts D, Boyd T, Bieber F R 1995 Fetoplacental histology as a predictor of karyotype: a controlled study of spontaneous first trimester abortions. Human Pathology 26: 201–209

Genest D R, Dorfman D M, Castrillon D H 2002 Ploidy and imprinting in hydatidiform moles. Complementary use of flow cytometry and immunohistochemistry of the imprinted gene product p57kip2 to assist molar classification. Journal of Reproductive Medicine 47: 342–346

Ghali F H 1969 Incidence of trophoblastic neoplasia in Iraq. American Journal of Obstetrics and Gynecology 105: 992–993

Gloor E, Hurlimann J 1981 Trophoblastic pseudotumor of the uterus. Clinicopathologic report with immunohistochemical and ultrastructural studies. American Journal of Surgical Pathology 5: 5–13

Gloor E, Ribolzi J, Dialdas J, Barrelet L, Hurlimann J 1983 Placental site trophoblastic tumors (trophoblastic pseudotumor) of the uterus with metastases and fatal outcome. American Journal of Surgical Pathology 7: 483–486

Goldstein D P, Berkowitz R S 1982 Gestational trophoblastic neoplasms: clinical principles of diagnosis and management. W B Saunders, Philadelphia

Gonzalez-Angulo A, Marquez-Monter H, Zavala B J, Yabur E, Salazar H 1966 Electron microscopic observations in hydatidiform mole. Obstetrics and Gynecology 27: 455–467

Gore H, Hertig A T 1967 Problems in the histologic interpretation of the trophoblast. Clinical Obstetrics and Gynecology 10: 269–289

Goshen R, Ariel I, Shuster S et al 1996 Hyaluronan, CD44 and its variant exons in human trophoblast invasion and placental angiogenesis. Molecular Human Reproduction 2: 685–691

Goto S, Yamada A, Ishizuka T, Tomoda Y 1993 Development of postmolar trophoblastic disease after partial molar pregnancy. Gynecologic Oncology 48: 165–170

Goustin A S, Betsholtz C, Pfeifer-Ohlsson S et al 1985 Coexpression of the sis and myc proto-oncogenes in developing human placenta suggests autocrine control of trophoblast growth. Cell 41: 301–312

Graham I H, Fajardo A M, Richards R L 1990 Epidemiological study of complete and partial hydatidiform mole in Abu Dhabi: influence of maternal age and ethnic group. Journal of Clinical Pathology 43: 661–664

Green 1990 Mucoid carcinoma of the breast with choriocarcinoma in its metastases. Histopathology 16: 504–506

Greene R R 1959 Chorioadenoma destruens. Annals of the New York Academy of Sciences 80: 143–151

Grimes D A 1984 Epidemiology of gestational trophoblastic disease. American Journal of Obstetrics and Gynecology 150: 309–318

Grummer R, Donner A, Winterhager E 1999 Characteristic growth of human choriocarcinoma xenografts in nude mice. Placenta 20: 547–553

Gschwendtner A, Neher A, Kreczy A, Muller-Holzner E, Volgger B, Mairinger T 1998 DNA ploidy determination of early molar pregnancies by image analysis: comparison to histologic classification. Archives of Pathology and Laboratory Medicine 122: 1000–1004

Guilbert L, Robertson S A, Wegmann T G 1993 The trophoblast as an integral component of a macrophage-cytokine network. Immunology and Cell Biology 71: 49–57

Gul T, Yilmazturk A, Erden A C 1997 A review of trophoblastic diseases at the medical school of Dicle University. European Journal of Obstetrics, Gynecology and Reproductive Biology 74: 37–40

Guo W D, Chow W H, Li J Y, Chen J S, Blot W J 1994 Correlations of choriocarcinoma mortality with alcohol drinking and reproductive factors in China. European Journal of Cancer Prevention 3: 223–226

Ha M C, Cordier S, Bard D et al 1996 Agent orange and the risk of gestational trophoblastic disease in Vietnam. Archives of Environmental Health 51: 368–374

Habibian R, Surti U 1987 Cytogenetics of trophoblasts from complete hydatidiform moles. Cancer Genetics and Cytogenetics 29: 271–287

Haines M 1955 Hydatidiform mole and vaginal nodules. Journal of Obstetrics and Gynaecology of the British Empire 62: 6–11

Hall P A, Woods A L 1990 Immunohistochemical markers of cell proliferation: achievements, problems and prospects. Cell and Tissue Kinetics 23: 531–549

Hall P A, Levison D A, Woods A L et al 1990 Proliferating cell nuclear antigen (PCNA) immunolocalisation in paraffin sections: an index of cell proliferation with evidence of deregulated expression in some neoplasms. Journal of Pathology 162: 285–294

Halls J, Paradinal F J 2000 (unpublished observations)

Hallam L A, MacLaren K M, El-Jabbour J N, Helm C W, Smart G E 1990 Intraplacental choriocarcinoma: a case report. Placenta 11: 247–251

Halperin R, Peller S, Sandbank J, Bukovsky I, Schneider D 2000 Expression of the p53 gene and apoptosis in gestational trophoblastic disease. Placenta 21: 58–62

Hamazaki S, Nakamoto S, Okino T et al 1999 Epithelioid trophoblastic tumor: morphological and immunohistochemical study of three lung lesions. Human Pathology 30: 1321–1327

Hameed A, Miller D S, Muller C Y, Coleman R L, Albores-Saavedra J 1999 Frequent expression of β-human chorionic gonadotropin (β-hCG) in squamous cell carcinoma of the cervix. International Journal of Gynecological Pathology 18: 381–386

Hando T, Ohno M, Kurose T 1998 Recent aspects of gestational trophoblastic disease in Japan. International Journal of Gynaecology and Obstetrics 60(suppl 1): S71–S76

Hayashi K, Bracken M B, Freeman D H, Hellenbrand K 1982 Hydatidiform mole in the United States (1970–1977): a statistical and theoretical analysis. American Journal of Epidemiology 115: 67–77

Hedley D W, Friedlander M L, Taylor I W, Rugg C A, Musgrove E A 1983 Method for analysis of cellular DNA content of paraffin embedded pathological material using flow cytometry. Journal of Histochemistry and Cytochemistry 31: 1333–1335

Heifetz S A, Czaja J 1992 In situ choriocarcinoma arising in partial hydatidiform mole: implications for the risk of persistent trophoblastic disease. Pediatric Pathology 12: 601–611

Helwani M N, Seoud M, Zahed L, Zaatari G, Khalil A, Slim R 1999 A familial case of recurrent hydatidiform molar pregnancies with biparental genomic contribution. Human Genetics 105: 112–115

Hemming J D, Quirke P, Womack C et al 1987 Diagnosis of molar pregnancy and persistent trophoblastic disease by flow cytometry. Journal of Clinical Pathology 40: 615–620

Hemming J D, Quirke P, Womack C et al 1988 Flow cytometry in persistent trophoblastic disease. Placenta 9: 615–621

Hershman J M 1999 Human chorionic gonadotropin and the thyroid: hyperemesis gravidarum and trophoblastic tumors. Thyroid 9: 653–657

Hertig A T 1950 Hydatidiform mole and chorionepithelioma. In: Meigs J B, Sturgis S H (eds) Progress in gynecology, vol 2. Grune & Stratton, New York, pp 372–394

Hertig A T, Edmonds H W 1940 Genesis of hydatidiform mole. Archives of Pathology 30: 260–291

Hertig A T, Mansell H 1956 Tumors of the female sex organs. Part 1. Hydatidiform mole and choriocarcinoma. In: Atlas of tumour pathology, section 9, fascicle 33. Armed Forces Institute of Pathology, Washington DC

Hertig A T, Sheldon W H 1947 Hydatidiform mole: a pathologicoclinical correlation of 200 cases. American Journal of Obstetrics and Gynecology 53: 1–36

Hertz R 1967 Serial passage of choriocarcinoma of women in the hamster cheek pouch. In: Holland J F, Hreshchyshyn M M (eds) Choriocarcinoma: transactions of a conference of the International Union against Cancer. Springer-Verlag, Berlin, pp 26–28

Hertz R 1978 Choriocarcinoma and related gestational trophoblastic tumors in women. Raven Press, New York

Hertz R, Lewis J L Jr, Lipsett M B 1961 Five years experience with the chemotherapy of metastatic choriocarcinoma and related trophoblastic tumors in women. American Journal of Obstetrics and Gynecology 82: 631–640

Heyderman E, Gibbons A R, Rosen S W 1981 Immunoperoxidase localisation of human placental lactogen: a marker for the placental origin of the giant cells in 'syncytial endometritis' of pregnancy. Journal of Clinical Pathology 34: 303–307

Hillstrom M M, Brown D L, Wilkins-Haug L, Genest D R 1995 Sonographic appearance of placental villous hydrops associated with Beckwith-Wiedemann syndrome. Journal of Ultrasound Medicine 14: 61–64

Hoffman J S, Silverman A D, Gelber J, Cartun R 1993 Placental site trophoblastic tumor: a report of radiologic, surgical and pathologic methods of evaluating the extent of disease. Gynecologic Oncology 50: 110–114

Hoffman K, Nekhlyudov L, Deligdisch L 1995 Endometrial carcinoma in elderly women. Gynecologic Oncology 58: 198–201

Holmgren L, Flam F, Larsson E, Ohlsson R 1993 Successive activation of the platelet-derived growth factor beta receptor and platelet-derived growth factor B genes correlates with the genesis of human choriocarcinoma. Cancer Research 53: 2927–2931

Honoré L H, Dill F J, Poland B J 1976 Placental morphology in spontaneous human abortuses with normal and abnormal karyotypes. Teratology 14: 151–166

Horn L C, Goretzlehner U, Dirnhofer S 1997 Placental site trophoblastic tumor (PSTT) initially misdiagnosed as cervical carcinoma. Pathology Research and Practice 193: 225–230

Hou P C, Pang S C 1956 Chorionepithelioma: an analytical study of 28 necropsied cases with special reference to the possibility of spontaneous regression. Journal of Pathology and Bacteriology 72: 95–104

Howat A J, Beck S, Fox H et al 1993 Can histopathologists reliably diagnose molar pregnancy? Journal of Clinical Pathology 46: 599–602

Hsieh C C, Hsieh T T, Hsueh C, Kuo D M, Lo L M, Hung T H 1999 Delivery of a severely anaemic fetus after partial molar pregnancy: clinical and ultrasonographic findings. Human Reproduction 14: 1122–1126

Hsu C T, Huang I C, Chen T Y 1962 Metastases in benign hydatidiform mole and chorioadenoma destruens. American Journal of Obstetrics and Gynecology 84: 1414–1424

Huch G, Hohn H P, Denker H W 1998 Identification of differentially expressed genes in human trophoblast cells by differential-display RT-PCR. Placenta 19: 557–567

Huettner P C, Gersell D J 1994 Placental site nodule: a clinicopathologic study of 38 cases. International Journal of Gynecological Pathology 13: 191–198

Hunt W, Dockerty M B, Randall L M 1953 Hydatidiform mole: clinico-pathological study involving 'grading' as a measure of possible malignant change. Obstetrics and Gynecology 1: 593–609

Hunter V, Raymond E, Christensen C et al 1990 Efficacy of the metastatic survey in the staging of gestational trophoblastic disease. Cancer 65: 1647–1650

Ichikawa N, Zhai Y L, Shiozawa T et al 1998 Immunohistochemical analysis of cell cycle regulatory gene products in normal trophoblast and placental site trophoblastic tumor. International Journal of Gynecological Pathology 17: 235–240

Ikeda Y, Jinno Y, Masuzaki H, Niikawa N, Ishimaru T 1996 A partial hydatidiform mole with 2N/3N mosaicism identified by molecular analysis. Journal of Assisted Reproduction and Genetics 13: 739–744

Ikura Y, Inoue T, Tsukuda H, Yamamoto T, Ueda M, Kobayashi Y 2000 Primary choriocarcinoma and human chorionic gonadotrophin-producing giant cell carcinoma of the lung: are they independent entities? Histopathology 2000 36: 17–25

Imai Y, Kawabe T, Takahashi M et al 1994 A case of primary gastric choriocarcinoma and a review of the Japanese literature. Journal of Gastroenterology 29: 642–646

Infererra C, Pullé C, Rigano A, Palmara D 1967 Aspetti ultrastrutturali e citochimici del coriocarcinoma uterino. Archivo di Ostetricia e Ginecologia 72: 707–744

International Union Against Cancer 1967 In: Holland J F, Hreshchyshyn M M (eds) Choriocarcinoma: transactions of a conference of the International Union Against Cancer. Appendix 1. Springer-Verlag, Berlin, pp 116–118

Ishikawa H, Tsutsumi H, Ikoma M, Yoshida H, Murayama N, Watanabe M 1986 Undifferentiated carcinoma of the pancreas with choriocarcinomatous features producing human chorionic gonadotropin. Gan No Rinsho. 32: 1041–1045

Ishizuka N 1967 Chemotherapy of chorionic tumors. In: Holland J F, Hreshchyshyn M M (eds) Choriocarcinoma: transactions of a conference of the International Union against Cancer. Springer-Verlag, Berlin, pp 116–118

Ishizuka N 1976 Studies of trophoblastic neoplasia. Gann 18: 203–216

Ito H, Sekine T, Komuro N et al 1981 Histologic stromal reaction of the host with gestational choriocarcinoma and its relation to clinical stage, classification and prognosis. American Journal of Obstetrics and Gynecology 140: 781–786

Jacobs P A, Hassold T J, Matsuyama A M, Newlands I M 1978a Chromosome constitution of gestational trophoblastic disease. Lancet ii, p 49

Jacobs P A, Angell R R, Buchanan I M, Hassold T J, Matsuyama A M, Manuel B 1978b The origin of human triploids. Annals of Human Genetics 42: 49–52

Jacobs P A, Wilson C M, Sprenkle J A, Rosenshein N B, Migeon B R 1980 Mechanism of origin of complete hydatidiform moles. Nature 286: 714–716

Jacobs P A, Hunt P A, Matsuura J S, Wilson C C, Szulman A E 1982a Complete and partial hydatidiform mole in Hawaii: cytogenetics, morphology and epidemiology. British Journal of Obstetrics and Gynaecology 89: 258–266

Jacobs P A, Szulman A E, Funkhouser J, Matsuura J S, Wilson C C 1982b Human triploidy: relationship between parental origin of the additional haploid complement and development of partial hydatidiform mole. Annals of Human Genetics 46: 223–231

Jacobson F J, Enzer N 1959 Hydatidiform mole with 'benign' metastasis to lung. American Journal of Obstetrics and Gynecology 78: 868–875

Jacques S M, Qureshi F, Doss B J, Munkarah A 1998 Intraplacental choriocarcinoma associated with viable pregnancy: pathologic features and implications for the mother and infant. Pediatric and Developmental Pathology 1: 380–387

Jauniaux E 1999 Partial moles: from postnatal to prenatal diagnosis. Placenta 20: 379–388

Jauniaux E, Nicolaides K H 1997 Early ultrasound diagnosis and follow-up of molar pregnancies. Ultrasound in Obstetrics and Gynecology 9: 17–21

Jauniaux E, Zucker M, Meuris S et al 1988 Chorangiocarcinoma: an unusual tumour of the placenta: the missing link? Placenta 9: 607–613

Jauniaux E, Kadri R, Hustin J 1996 Partial mole and triploidy: screening patients with first trimester spontaneous abortion. Obstetrics and Gynecology 88: 616–619

Jauniaux E, Nicolaides K H, Hustin J 1997 Perinatal features associated with placental mesenchymal dysplasia. Placenta 18: 701–706

Jauniaux E, Halder A, Partington C 1998 A case of partial mole associated with trisomy 13. Ultrasound in Obstetrics and Gynecology 11: 62–64

Jauniaux E, Bersinger N A, Gulbis B, Meuris S 1999 The contribution of maternal serum markers in the early prenatal diagnosis of molar pregnancies. Human Reproduction 1999 14: 842–846

Javey H, Borazjani G, Behmard S, Langley F A 1979 Discrepancies in the histological diagnosis of hydatidiform mole. British Journal of Obstetrics and Gynaecology 86: 480–483

Jeffers M D, Greehan D, Gillan G E 1994 Comparison of villous trophoblast proliferation rate in hydatidiform mole and non-molar abortion by assessment of proliferating cell nuclear antigen expression. Placenta 15: 551–556

Jeffers M D, Michie B A, Oakes S J, Gillan J E 1995 Comparison of ploidy analysis by flow cytometry and image analysis in hydatidiform mole and non-molar abortion. Histopathology 27: 415–421

Jeffers M D, Richmond J A, Smith R 1996 Trophoblast proliferation rate does not predict progression to persistent gestational trophoblastic disease in complete hydatidiform mole. International Journal of Gynecological Pathology 15: 34–38

Jeffreys A J, Wilson V, Neumann R, Keyte J 1988 Amplification of human minisatellites by the polymerase chain reaction: towards DNA fingerprinting of single cells. Nucleic Acids Research 16: 10953–10971

John M, Rajalekshmy T N, Nair M B et al 1997 Expression of epidermal growth factor in gestational trophoblastic disease (GTD). Journal of Experimental and Clinical Cancer Research 16: 129–134

Johnson T R, Comstock C H, Anderson D G 1979 Benign gestational trophoblastic disease metastatic to pleura: unusual cause of hemothorax. Obstetrics and Gynecology 53: 509–511

Joint Project for Study of Choriocarcinoma and Hydatidiform Mole in Asia 1959 Geographic variation in the occurrence of hydatidiform mole and choriocarcinoma. Annals of the New York Academy of Sciences 80: 178–195

Jones I S, Buntine D, Vesey E J 1980 Ectopic vaginal trophoblast in association with a partial mole. Australian and New Zealand Journal of Obstetrics and Gynaecology. 20: 242–244

Jones W B 1990 Gestational trophoblastic disease: what have we learned in the past decade? American Journal of Obstetrics and Gynecology 162: 1286–1295

Jones W B, Lauersen N H 1975 Hydatidiform mole with coexistent fetus. American Journal of Obstetrics and Gynecology 122: 267–272

Jones W B, Romain K, Erlandson R A, Burt M E 1993 Thoracotomy in the management of gestational choriocarcinoma: a clinicopathologic study. Cancer 72: 2175–2181

Junaid T A, Hendrickse H P de V, Oladiran B, Edington G M, Williams A O 1974 Choriocarcinoma in Ibadan, Nigeria. Journal of the National Cancer Institute 53: 1597–1599

Junaid T A, Hendrickse H P de V, Oladiran B, Edington G M, Williams A O 1976 Choriocarcinoma in Ibadan: clinicopathological studies. Human Pathology 7: 215–222

Kajii T, Ohama K 1977 Androgenic origin of hydatidiform mole. Nature 268: 633–634

Kajii T, Kurashigo H, Ohama K, Uchino F L 1984 XY and XX complete moles: clinical and morphological correlations. American Journal of Obstetrics and Gynecology 150: 57–64

Kalafut M, Vinuela F, Saver J L, Martin N, Vespa P, Verity M A 1998 Multiple cerebral pseudoaneurysms and hemorrhages: the expanding spectrum of metastatic cerebral choriocarcinoma. Journal of Neuroimaging 8: 44–47

Kalir T, Seijo L, Deligdisch L, Cohen C 1995 Endometrial adenocarcinoma with choriocarcinomatous differentiation in an elderly virginal woman. International Journal of Gynecological Pathology 14: 266–269

Kalra J K, Mir R, Kahn L B, Wessely Z, Shah A B 1984 Osteogenic sarcoma producing human chorionic gonadotrophin. Case report with immunohistochemical studies. Cancer 53: 2125–2128

Kamada M, Ino H, Naka O et al 1993 Immunosuppressive 30-kDa protein in urine of pregnant women and patients with trophoblastic diseases. European Journal of Obstetrics, Gynecology and Reproductive Biology 50: 219–225

Kanazawa K 1998 Trophoblastic disease: twenty years experience at Niigata University. International Journal of Gynecology and Obstetrics 60(suppl 1): S97–S103

Kardana A, Bagshawe K D 1976 A rapid, sensitive and specific radioimmunoassay for human chorionic gonadotrophin. Journal of Immunological Methods 9: 297–305

Kase H, Kodama S, Yahata T, Aoki Y, Tanaka K 1996 Case report: an exaggerated placental site with a cervical pregnancy. Journal of Obstetrics and Gynaecological Research 22: 379–383

Kashimura M, Kashimura Y, Oikawa K, Sakamoto C, Matsuura Y, Nakamura S 1990 Placental site trophoblastic tumor: immunohistochemical and nuclear DNA study. Gynecologic Oncology 38: 262–367

Keep D, Zaragoza M V, Hassold T, Redline R W 1996 Very early complete hydatidiform mole. Human Pathology 27: 708–713

Khoo N K, Bechberger I F, Shepherd T et al 1998 SV 40 Tag transformation of the normal invasive trophoblast results in a premalignant phenotype. I Mechanisms responsible for hyperinvasiveness and resistance to anti-invasive action of TGFbeta. International Journal of Cancer 77: 429–439

Khuu H M, Crisco C P, Kilgore L, Rodgers W H, Conner M G 2000 Carcinosarcoma of the uterus associated with a nongestational choriocarcinoma. South Medical Journal 93: 226–228

Kilburn B A, Wang J, Duniec-Dmuchkowski Z M, Leach R E, Romero R, Armant D R 2000 Extracellular matrix composition and hypoxia regulate the expression of HLA-G and integrins in a human trophoblast cell line. Biology of Reproduction 62: 739–747

Kilic M, Flossmann E, Flossmann O et al 1999 Jeg-3 human choriocarcinoma-induced immunosuppression: downregulation of interleukin-2, interleukin-2 receptor alpha-chain, and its Jak/Stat signaling pathway. American Journal of Reproductive Immunology 41: 61–69

Kim S J, Bae S N, Kim J H et al 1998 Epidemiology and time trends of gestational trophoblastic disease in Korea. International Journal of Gynaecology and Obstetrics 60(suppl 1): S33–S38

Kim S N, Chi J G, Kim Y W et al 1993 Neonatal choriocarcinoma of liver. Pediatric Pathology 13: 723–730

King G 1956 Hydatidiform mole and chorion epithelioma. The problem of the borderline case. Proceedings of the Royal Society of Medicine 49: 381–390

Kishkurno S, Ishida A, Takahashi Y et al 1997 A case of neonatal choriocarcinoma. American Journal of Perinatology 14: 79–82

Klausen S, Larsen L G 1994 Partial moles with maze-like vascular anomaly. APMIS 102: 638–640

Knoop C, Jacobovitz D, Antoine M, de Francquen P, Yernault J C, Estenne M 1994 Donor transmitted tumors in lung allograft recipients: report on two cases. Transplantation 57: 1679–1680

Knoth M, Hesseldahl H, Larsen J F 1969 Ultrastructure of human choriocarcinoma. Acta Obstetricia et Gynecologica Scandinavica 48: 100–118

Ko T M, Hsieh C Y, Ho H N, Hsieh F J, Lee T Y 1991 Restriction fragment length polymorphism analysis to study the genetic origin of complete hydatidiform mole. American Journal of Obstetrics and Gynecology 164: 901–906

Koenig C, Demopoulos R I, Vamvakos E C et al 1993 Flow cytometric DNA ploidy and quantitative histopathology in partial moles. International Journal of Gynecological Pathology 12: 235–240

Kohorn E I 1982 Hydatidiform mole and gestational trophoblastic disease in Southern Connecticut. Obstetrics and Gynecology 59: 78–84

Kohorn E I 1984 Molar pregnancy: presentation and diagnosis. Clinical Obstetrics and Gynecology 27: 181–191

Kohorn E I, McGinn R C, Gee B L, Goldstein D P, Osathanondh R 1978 Pulmonary embolisation of trophoblastic tissue in molar pregnancy. Obstetrics and Gynecology 51: 155–205

Kolstad P, Hognestad J 1965 Trophoblastic tumours in Norway. Acta Obstetricia et Gynecologica Scandinavica 44: 80–88

Komuro N 1976 Experimental induction of chorionepithelioma in pregnant rats. Acta Obstetrica et Gynaecologica Japonica 23: 32–42

Kovacs B W, Shahbahrami B, Tast D E, Curtin J P 1991 Molecular genetic analysis of complete hydatidiform moles. Cancer Genetics and Cytogenetics 54: 143–152

Kuida C A, Braunstein G D, Shintaku P, Said J W 1988 Human chorionic gonadotropin expression in lung, breast and renal carcinomas. Archives of Pathology and Laboratory Medicine 112: 282–285

Kurman R J, Scully R E, Norris H J 1976 Trophoblastic pseudotumor of the uterus: an exaggerated form of 'syncytial endometritis' simulating a malignant tumor. Cancer 38: 1214–1226

Kurman R J, Young R H, Norris H J, Lawrence W D, Scully R E 1984 Immunocytochemical localisation of placental lactogen and chorionic gonadotrophin in the normal placenta and trophoblastic tumors with emphasis on intermediate trophoblast and the placental site trophoblastic tumor. International Journal of Gynecological Pathology 3: 101–121

Kushima K, Noda K, Makita M 1967 Experimental production of chorionic tumour in rabbits. Tohuku Journal of Experimental Medicine 91: 209–214

Kyo S, Takakura M, Tanaka M et al 1997 Expression of telomerase activity in human chorion. Biochemical and Biophysical Research Communications 241: 498–503

Lage J M 1990 Diagnostic dilemmas in gynecologic and obstetric pathology. Seminars in Diagnostic Pathology 7: 146–155

Lage J M 1991 Placentomegaly with massive hydrops of placental stem villi, diploid DNA content, and fetal omphaloceles: possible association with Beckwith-Wiedemann syndrome. Human Pathology 22: 591–597

Lage J M, Roberts D J 1993 Choriocarcinoma in a term placenta: pathologic diagnosis of tumor in an asymptomatic patient with metastatic disease. International Journal of Gynecological Pathology 12: 80–85

Lage J M, Sheikh S S 1997 Genetic aspects of gestational trophoblastic diseases: a general overview with emphasis on new approaches in determining genetic composition. General Diagnostic Pathology 143: 109–115

Lage J M, Driscoll S G, Yavner D L et al 1988 Hydatidiform moles: application of flow cytometry in diagnosis. American Journal of Clinical Pathology 89: 596–600

Lage J M, Weinberg D S, Yavner D L, Bieber F R 1989 The biology of tetraploid hydatidiform moles: histopathology, cytogenetics and flow cytometry. Human Pathology 20: 419–425

Lage J M, Berkowitz R S, Rice L W, Goldstein D P, Bernstein M R, Weinberg D S 1991 Flow cytometric analysis of DNA content in partial hydatidiform moles with persistent gestational trophoblastic tumor. Obstetrics and Gynecology 77: 111–115

Lage J M, Mark S D, Roberts D J, Goldstein D P, Bernstein M R, Berkowith R S 1992 A flow cytometric study of 137 fresh hydropic placentas: correlation between types of hydatidiform moles and nuclear DNA ploidy. Obstetrics and Gynecology 79: 403–410

Lahey S J, Steele G, Rodrick M L et al 1984 Characterisation of antigenic components from circulating immune complexes in patients with gestational trophoblastic neoplasia. Cancer 53: 1316–1321

Lane S A, Taylor G R, Ozols B, Quirke P 1993 Diagnosis of complete molar pregnancy by microsatellites in archival material. Journal of Clinical Pathology 46: 346–348

Larsen J F 1973 Ultrastructure of the abnormal human trophoblast. Acta Anatomica Supplement 1: 47–74

Larsen J F, Ehrmann R L, Bierring F 1967 Electron microscopy of human choriocarcinoma transplanted into hamster liver. American Journal of Obstetrics and Gynecology 99: 1109–1124

Lathrop J C, Lauchlan S, Nayak R, Ambler M 1988 Clinical characteristics of placental site trophoblastic tumor (PSTT). Gynecologic Oncology 31: 32–42

La Vecchia C, Franceschi S, Parazzini F et al 1985 Risk factors for gestational trophoblastic disease in Italy. American Journal of Epidemiology 121: 457–464

Lawler S D 1978 HLA and trophoblastic tumours. British Medical Bulletin 34: 305–308

Lawler S D, Fisher R A 1986 Genetic aspects of gestational trophoblastic tumors. In: Ichinoe K (ed) Trophoblastic diseases. Ikagu-Shoin, Tokyo, pp 23–33

Lawler S D, Fisher R A 1987a Genetic studies in hydatidiform mole with clinical correlations. Placenta 8: 77–88

Lawler S D, Fisher R A 1987b Immunological aspects. In: Szulman A E, Buchsbaum H J (eds) Gestational trophoblastic disease. Springer-Verlag, New York, pp 77–87

Lawler S D, Fisher R A 1987c Immunogenicity of hydatidiform mole. Placenta 8: 195–199

Lawler S D, Fisher R A 1991 A prospective genetic study of complete and partial hydatidiform moles. American Journal of Obstetrics and Gynecology 164: 1270–1277

Lawler S D, Klouda P T, Bagshawe K D 1971 The HL-A system in trophoblastic neoplasia. Lancet ii: 834–837

Lawler S D, Pickthall V J, Fisher R A et al 1979 Genetic studies of complete and partial hydatidiform moles. Lancet ii: 580

Lawler S D, Fisher R A, Pickthall V J, Povey S, Evans M W 1982a Genetic studies on hydatidiform moles. I — The origin of partial moles. Cancer Genetics and Cytogenetics 5: 309–320

Lawler S D, Povey S, Fisher R A, Pickthall V J 1982b Genetic studies on hydatidiform moles. II — The origin of complete moles. Annals of Human Genetics 46: 209–222

Lee K C, Chan J K 1990 Placental site nodule. Histopathology 16: 193–199

Lee Y S 1995 p53 expression in gestational trophoblastic disease. International Journal of Gynecological Pathology 14: 119–124

Lee Y S, Cheah E, Szulman A E 1981 The pattern of hydatidiform moles in Singapore. Australian and New Zealand Journal of Obstetrics and Gynaecology 21: 230–233

Leighton P C 1973 Trophoblastic disease in Uganda. American Journal of Obstetrics and Gynecology 117: 341–344

Lembet A, Zorlu C G, Yalcin H R, Seckin B, Ekici E 2000 Partial hydatidiform mole with diploid karyotype in a live fetus. International Journal of Gynaecology and Obstetrics 69: 149–152

Leroy J P, Goude H, Cozic A, Philippe E 1976 Placenta pseudo-molaire avec enfant normal. Journal de Gynecologie, Obstetrice et Biologie de Reproduction 5: 743–748

Lewis J L Jr, Terasaki P T 1971 HL-A leukocyte antigen studies in women with gestational trophoblastic neoplasms. American Journal of Obstetrics and Gynecology 111: 547–554

Lewis J L Jr, Davis C R, Ross G T 1969 Hormonal, immunologic and chemotherapeutic studies of transplantable human choriocarcinoma. American Journal of Obstetrics and Gynecology 104: 472–478

Li M C, Hertz R, Spencer D B 1956 Effect of methotrexate therapy upon choriocarcinoma and chorioadenoma. Proceedings of the Society of Experimental Biology and Medicine 93: 361–366

Lin L, Xu B, Rote N S 1999 Expression of endogenous retrovirus ERV-3 induces differentiation in BeWo, a choriocarcinoma model of human placental trophoblast. Placenta 20: 109–118

Lindholm H, Flam F 1999 The diagnosis of molar pregnancy by sonography and gross morphology. Acta Obstetricia et Gynecologica Scandinavica 78: 6–9

Lindsey J R, Wharton C R, Woodruff J D, Baker J H 1969 Intrauterine choriocarcinoma in a rhesus monkey. Pathologica Veterinaria 6: 378–384

Lira-Plascencia J, Tenorio-Gonzalez F, Gomezpedroso-Rea J, Novoa-Vargas A, Aranda-Flores C, Ibarguengoitia-Ochoa F 1995 [Gestational trophoblastic disease. A 6-year experience at the Instituto Nacional de Perinatologia]. Ginecologia y Obstetricia de Mexico 63: 478–482

Llewellyn-Jones D 1965 Trophoblastic tumours: geographical variations in incidence and possible aetiological factors. Journal of Obstetrics and Gynaecology of the British Commonwealth 72: 242–248

Logan B J, Motyloff L 1958 Hydatidiform mole: a clinical and pathological study of 72 cases, with reference to their malignant tendencies. American Journal of Obstetrics and Gynecology 75: 1134–1148

Looi L M, Sivanesaratnam V 1981 Malignant evolution with fatal outcome in a patient with partial hydatidiform mole. Australian and New Zealand Journal of Obstetrics and Gynaecology 21: 51–52

Lorigan P C, Grierson A J, Goepel J R, Coleman R E, Goyns M H 1996 Gestational choriocarcinoma of the ovary diagnosed by analysis of tumor DNA. Cancer 104: 27–30

Losch A, Kainz C 1996 Immunohistochemistry in the diagnosis of the gestational trophoblastic disease. Acta Obstetricia et Gynecologica Scandinavica 75: 753–756

Ludwig M, Gembruch U, Bauer O, Diedrich K 1998 Ovarian hyperstimulation syndrome (OHSS) in a spontaneous pregnancy with fetal and placental triploidy: information about the general pathophysiology of OHSS. Human Reproduction 13: 2082–2087

Lurain J R 1987 Natural history. In: Szulman A E, Buchsbaum H J (eds) Gestational trophoblastic disease. Springer-Verlag, New York, pp 69–76

Lurain J R, Sciarra J J 1991 Study and treatment of gestational trophoblastic disease at the John I Brewer Trophoblastic Disease Center, 1962–1990. European Journal of Gynaecological Oncology 12: 425–428

Lustig O, Schulze E, Komitowski D et al 1997 The expression of the imprinted genes H19 and IGF-2 in choriocarcinoma cell lines. Is H19 a tumour suppressor gene? Oncogene 15: 169–177

McCluggage W G, Ashe P, McBride H, Maxwell P, Sloan J M 1998 Localization of the cellular expression of inhibin in trophoblastic tissue. Histopathology 32: 252–256

McCorriston C C 1968 Racial incidence of hydatidiform mole: a study in a contained polyracial community. American Journal of Obstetrics and Gynecology 101: 377–381

McCowan L M, Becroft D M 1994 Beckwith-Wiedemann syndrome, placental abnormalities and gestational proteinuric hypertension. Obstetrics and Gynecology 83: 813–817

McFadden D E, Kwong L C, Yam I Y, Langlois S 1993 Parental origin of triploidy in human fetuses: evidence for genomic imprinting. Human Genetics 92: 465–469

McLellan R, Buscema J, Currie J L, Woodruff J D 1991 Placental site trophoblastic tumor in a postmenopausal woman. American Journal of Clinical Pathology 95: 670–675

MacRae D J 1951 Chorionepithelioma occurring during pregnancy. Journal of Obstetrics and Gynaecology of the British Empire 58: 373–380

Maeyama M, Furuki Y, Munemura M, Tanaka N, Iwamasa T 1985 In vivo and in vitro studies on the production of placental proteins (human chorionic gonadotropin, human placental lactogen, and pregnancy-specific beta 1-glycoprotein) in an adrenal choriocarcinoma. Obstetrics and Gynecology 65: 593–596

Magrath I T, Golding P R, Bagshawe K D 1971 Medical presentations of choriocarcinoma. British Medical Journal 2: 633–637

Makino S, Sasaki M S, Fukuschima T 1963 Preliminary notes on the chromosomes of human chorionic lesions. Proceedings of the Japanese Academy 39: 54–58

Makino S, Sasaki M S, Fukuschima T 1964 Triploid chromosome constitution in human chorionic lesions. Lancet ii: 1273–1275

Marchand F 1894 Verhandlung ärztlicher Verein zu Marburg. Klinische Wochenschrift Berlin 31: 813–814

Marchand F 1895 Über die sogenannten 'decidualen, Geschwülste Anschluss an normale Geburt, Abort, Blasenmole, und Extrauterinschwangerschaft. Monatsschrift für Geburtshilfe und Gynäkologie 1: 419–428 and 513–562

Marchand F 1898 Über das maligne Chorion-Epitheliom, nebst Mittheilung von 2 neuen Fallen. Zeitschrift für Geburtshilfe und Gynakologie 39: 173–258

Marin-Padilla M, Benirschke K 1963 Thalidomide-induced alterations in the blastocyst and placenta of the armadillo, dasypus novemcintus mexicanus, including a choriocarcinoma. American Journal of Pathology 43: 999–1016

Marquez-Monter H, de la Vega G A, Robles M, Bolio-Cicero A 1963 Epidemiology and pathology of hydatidiform mole in the General Hospital of Mexico: study of 104 cases. American Journal of Obstetrics and Gynecology 85: 856–864

Martin B H, Kim J H 1998 Changing face of gestational trophoblastic tumour. International Journal of Gynaecology and Obstetrics 60 (suppl 1): S111–S120

Martin P M 1978 High frequency of hydatidiform mole in native Alaskans. International Journal of Gynaecology and Obstetrics 15: 395–396

Martinazzi S, Zampieri A, Todeschin P et al 1996 Correlazione tra aspetti istologici e quadri citogenetici nei tessuti placentari da aborto precoce.

L'immunoistochimica ha un ruolo? [Correlation of the histological and cytogenetic pictures in placental tissue from early abortion. Does immunohistochemistry have a role?]. Pathologica 88: 275–285

Matalon M, Modan B 1972 Epidemiologic aspects of hydatidiform mole in Israel. American Journal of Obstetrics and Gynecology 112: 107–112

Mathews M B, Berstein R M, Franza B R Jr, Garrels J I 1984 Identity of the proliferating cell nuclear antigen and cyclin. Nature 303: 374–376

Matsuda T, Sasaki M, Kato H et al 1997 Human chromosome 7 carries a putative tumor suppressor gene(s) involved in choriocarcinoma. Oncogene 15: 2773–2781

Matsui H, Izuka Y, Sekiya S, Takamizawa H 1996 System for registering gestational trophoblastic disease in Chiba prefecture in the past 20 years. Nippon Sanka Fujinka Gakkai Zasshi 40: 199–205

Matsui H, Sekiya S, Hando T, Wake N, Tomoda Y 2000 Hydatidiform mole coexistent with a twin live fetus: a national collaborative study in Japan. Human Reproduction 15: 608–611

Matthews T H, Heaton G E, Christopherson W M 1986 Primary duodenal choriocarcinoma. Archives of Pathology and Laboratory Medicine 110: 550–552

Mazur M T 1989 Metastatic gestational choriocarcinoma. Unusual pathologic variant following therapy. Cancer 63: 1370–1377

Mazur M T, Kurman R J 1987 Choriocarcinoma and placental site trophoblastic tumor. In: Szulman A E, Buchsbaum J H (eds) Gestational trophoblastic disease. Springer-Verlag, New York, pp 45–68

Mazur M T, Kurman R J 1994 Gestational trophoblastic disease and related lesions. In: Kurman R J (ed) Blaustein's pathology of the female genital tract. New York, Springer-Verlag, pp 1049–1093

Mazur M T, Lurain J R, Brewer J J 1982 Fatal gestational choriocarcinoma: clinicopathological study of patients treated at a trophoblastic disease center. Cancer 50: 1833–1846

Menczer J, Girtler O, Zajdel L, Glezerman M 1999 Metastatic trophoblastic disease following partial hydatidiform mole: case report and literature review. Gynecologic Oncology 74: 304–307

Meredith R F, Wagman L D, Piper J A, Mills A S, Neifeld J P 1986 Beta-chain human chorionic gonadotropin-producing leiomyosarcoma of the small intestine. Cancer 58: 131–135

Messerli M L, Lilienfeld A M, Parmley T, Woodruff J D, Rosenshein N B 1985 Risk factors for gestational trophoblastic neoplasia. American Journal of Obstetrics and Gynecology 153: 294–300

Messerli M L, Parmley T, Woodruff J D et al 1987 Inter- and intra-pathologist variability in the diagnosis of gestational trophoblastic neoplasia. Obstetrics and Gynecology 69: 622–626

Miller D, Jackson R, Ehlen T, McMurtrie E 1993 Complete hydatidiform mole coexistent with a twin live fetus: clinical course of four cases with complete cytogenetic analysis. Gynecologic Oncology 50: 119–123

Miller J F, Williamson E, Glue J, Gordon Y B, Grudzinska G, Sykes A 1980 Fetal loss after implantation. a Prospective Study. Lancet ii: 554–556

Minami S, Yamoto M, Nakano R 1993 Immunohistochemcial localization of inhibin-activin subunits in hydatidiform mole and invasive mole. Obstetrics and Gynecology 82: 414–418

Mittal K K, Kachru R B, Brewer J I 1975 The HL-A and ABO antigens in trophoblastic disease. Tissue Antigens 6: 57–69

Mittal T K, Vujanic G M, Morrissey B M, Jones A 1998 Triploidy: antenatal sonographic features with post-mortem correlation. Prenatal Diagnosis 18: 1253–1262

Miyamoto M, Nilsuwarn N, Angsubhakorn S 1972 The morphology of experimental chorionic tumours in rats. Acta Pathologica Japonica 22: 343–352

Mochizuki M, Maruo T, Matsuo H, Samoto T, Ishihara N 1998 Biology of human trophoblast. International Journal of Gynaecology and Obstetrics 60(suppl 1): S21–S28

Mogensen B, Kissmeyer-Nielsen F 1968 Histocompatibility antigens of the HL-A locus in generalised gestational choriocarcinoma. Lancet i: 721–725

Mogensen B, Kissmeyer-Nielsen F 1971 Current data on HL-A and ABO typing in gestational choriocarcinoma and invasive mole. Transplantation Proceedings 3: 1267–1269

Mogensen B, Olsen S 1973 Cellular reaction to gestational choriocarcinoma and invasive mole. Acta Pathologica et Microbiologica Scandinavica Section A 81: 453–456

Moglabey Y B, Kircheisen R, Seoud M, El Mogharbel N, Van den Veyver I, Slim R 1999 Genetic mapping of a maternal locus responsible for familial hydatidiform moles. Human Molecular Genetics 8: 667–671

Molykutty J, Schultz G, Rajalekshmy T N, Enose S, Nair M K, Balaram P 1999 Immunolocalization and quantitation of transforming growth factor alpha in hydatidiform mole. Tumori 85: 183–187

Montes M, Roberts D, Berkowitz R S, Genest D R 1996 Prevalence and significance of implantation site trophoblastic atypia in hydatidiform moles and spontaneous abortions. American Journal of Clinical Pathology 105: 411–416

Montgomery E A, Roberts E F, Conran R M, Hitchcock C L 1993 Triploid abortus presenting as an ectopic pregnancy. Archives of Pathology and Laboratory Medicine 117: 652–653

Mor G, Gutierrez L S, Eliza M, Kahyaoglu F, Arici A 1998 Fas-fas ligand system-induced apoptosis in human placenta and gestational trophoblastic disease. American Journal of Reproductive Immunology 40: 89–94

Morimura Y, Yazawa M, Hoshi K et al 1996 Uterine cervical clear-cell adenocarcinoma with a choriocarcinomatous component: a case report. Journal of Obstetrics and Gynaecology Research 22: 437–441

Morrow C P, Kletzky O A, Disaia P J, Townsend D E, Mishell D R, Nakamura R M 1977 Clinical and laboratory correlates of molar pregnancy and trophoblastic disease. American Journal of Obstetrics and Gynecology 128: 424–430

Moscoso G, Jauniaux E, Hustin J 1991 Placental vascular anomaly with diffuse mesenchymal stem villous hyperplasia. A new clinico-pathological entity? Pathology Research and Practice 187: 324–328

Mosher R, Goldstein D P, Berkowitz R, Bernstein M, Genest D R 1998 Complete hydatidiform mole. Comparison of clinicopathologic features, current and past. Journal of Reproductive Medicine 43: 21–27

Motoyama T, Ohta T, Ajioka Y, Watanabe H 1994 Neoplastic and non-neoplastic intermediate trophoblasts: an immunohistochemical and ultrastructural study. Pathology International 44: 57–65

Mueller U W, Hawes C S, Wright A E et al 1990 Isolation of fetal trophoblast cells from peripheral blood of pregnant women. Lancet 336: 197–200

Muller R, Tremblay J M, Adamson E D, Verman I M 1983 Tissue and cell type-specific expression of two human c-onc genes. Nature 304: 454–456

Muller-Hocker J, Obernitz N, Johannes A, Lohrs U 1997 P53 gene product and EGF-receptor are highly expressed in placental site trophoblastic tumor. Human Pathology 28: 1302–1306

Mungan T, Kuscu E, Dabakoglu T, Senoz S, Ugur M, Cobanoglu O 1996 Hydatidiform mole: clinical analysis of 310 patients. International Journal of Gynaecology and Obstetrics 52: 233–236

Murad T M, Longley J V, Lurain J R, Brewer J I 1990 Hydatidiform mole: clinicopathologic associations with the development of postevacuation trophoblastic disease. International Journal of Gynaecology and Obstetrics 32: 359–367

Murata T, Ihara S, Nakayama T et al 1999 Breast cancer with choriocarcinomatous features: A case report with cytopathologic details. Pathology International 49: 816–819

Muto M G, Lage J M, Berkowitz R S, Goldstein D P, Bernstein M R 1991 Gestational trophoblastic disease of the fallopian tube. Journal of Reproductive Medicine 36: 57–60

Mutter G L 1997 Role of imprinting in abnormal human development. Mutation Research 396: 141–147

Mutter G L, Stewart C L, Chaponot M L, Pomponio R J 1993a Oppositely imprinted genes H19 and insulin-like growth factor 2 are coexpressed in human androgenetic trophoblast. American Journal of Human Genetics 53: 1096–1102

Mutter G L, Pomponio R J, Berkowitz R S, Genest D R 1993b Sex chromosome composition of complete hydatidiform moles: relationship to metastasis. American Journal of Obstetrics and Gynecology 168: 1547–1551

Nagelberg S, Rosen S W 1985 Clinical and laboratory investigation of a virilized woman with placental-site trophoblastic tumour. Obstetrics and Gynecology 65: 527–534

Nakanuma Y, Unoura M, Noto H, Ohta G 1986 Human chorionic gonadotropin in primary liver carcinoma in adults. An immunohistochemical study. Virchows Archiv A 409: 365–373

Narayan H, Mansour P, McDougall W W 1991 Recurrent consecutive partial molar pregnancy. Gynecologic Oncology 46: 122–127

Nastac E, Athanasiu P, Predescu E et al 1980 Experimental investigations in hamsters and rabbits with DNA extracted from human uterine tumors. Virologie 31: 37–39

Naumoff P, Szulman A E, Weinstein B, Mazer J, Surti U 1981 Ultrasonography of partial hydatidiform mole. Radiology 140: 467–470

Nayar R, Snell J, Silverberg S G, Lage J M 1996 Placental site nodule occurring in a fallopian tube. Human Pathology 27: 1243–1245

Neudeck H, Unger M, Hufnagl P et al 1997 Villous cytotrophoblast proliferating potential in complete and partial hydatidiform mole: diagnostic value of silver-stained nucleolar organizer region (AgNOR)-associated proteins. General Diagnostic Pathology 143: 179–184

Newlands E S, Fisher R A, Searle F 1992 The immune system in disease: gestational trophoblastic tumours. Balliere's Clinical Obstetrics and Gynaecology 6: 519–538

Newlands E S 1997 Presentation and management of persistent gestational trophoblastic disease and gestational trophoblastic tumours in the UK. In: Hancock B W, Newlands E S, Berkowitz R S (eds) Gestational trophoblastic disease. Chapman & Hall Medical, London, pp 143–172

Nishi H, Ohyashiki K, Fujito A et al 1999 Expression of telomerase subunits and localization of telomerase activation in hydatidiform mole. Placenta 20: 317–323

Nishimura R, Koizumi T, Morisue K et al 1995 Expression and secretion of the beta subunit of human chorionic gonadotropin by bladder carcinoma in vivo and in vitro. Cancer Research 55: 1479–1484

Novak E, Seah C S 1954 Choriocarcinoma of the uterus: study of 74 cases from the Mathieu Memorial Chorionepithelioma Registry. American Journal of Obstetrics and Gynecology 67: 933–957

Ober W B 1965 Clinical and pathological aspects of abnormal trophoblast: discussion. In: Park W W (ed) The early conceptus, normal and abnormal. Livingstone, London, pp 141–144

Ober W B, Fass R O 1961 The early history of choriocarcinoma. Journal of the History of Medicine and Allied Sciences 16: 49–73

Ober W B, Maier R C 1982 Gestational choriocarcinoma of the Fallopian tube. Diagnostic Gynecology and Obstetrics 3: 213–231

Ober W B, Edgcomb J R, Price E B Jr 1971 The pathology of choriocarcinoma. Annals of the New York Academy of Sciences 172: 299–426

Ockleford C D, Clode A 1983 Microgibbosities in hydatidiform mole. Journal of Pathology 141: 181–189

Ohama K, Kajii T, Okamoto E et al 1981 Dispermic origin of XY hydatidiform moles. Nature 292: 551–552

Ohara A, Yamada S, Suzuki N et al 1993 A case of hCG producing cervical carcinoma of the uterus. Nippon Sanka Fujinka Gakkai Zasshi 45: 1333–1336

Ohlsson R, Nystrom A, Pfeifer-Ohlsson S et al 1993 IGF2 is parentally imprinted during human embryogenesis and in the Beckwith–Wiedemann syndrome. Nature Genetics 4: 94–97

Ohlsson R, Flam F, Fisher R et al 1999 Random monoallelic expression of the imprinted IGF2 and H19 genes in the absence of discriminative parental marks. Development, Genes and Evolution 209: 113–119

Okudaira Y, Strauss L 1967 Ultrastructure of molar trophoblast: observations on hydatidiform mole and chorioadenoma destruens. Obstetrics and Gynecology 30: 172–187

Olesnicky G, Long A R, Quinn M A et al 1985 Hydatidiform mole in Victoria: aetiology and natural history. Australian and New Zealand Journal of Obstetrics and Gynaecology 21: 1–6

Orrell J M, Sanders D S A 1991 A particularly aggressive placental site trophoblastic tumour. Histopathology 18: 559–561

Östör A 1996 God's first cancer and man's first cure: milestones in gestational trophoblastic disease. In: Fecher & Rosen (eds) ASCP reviews in Pathology. Anatomical Pathology, part 3, pp 165–178

Östör A G, McNaughton W M, Fortune D W, Rischin D, Hillcoat B L, Riley C B 1993 Rectal adenocarcinoma with germ cell elements treated with chemotherapy. Pathology 25: 243–246

Ostrzega N, Phillipson J, Liu P 1998 Proliferative activity in placentas with hydropic change and hydatidiform mole as detected by Ki-67 and proliferating cell nuclear antigen immunostaining. American Journal of Clinical Pathology 110: 776–781

Palmer J R, Driscoll S G, Rosenberg L et al 1999 Oral contraceptive use and risk of gestational trophoblastic tumors. Journal of the National Cancer Institute 91: 635–640

Paradinas F J 1992 Pathology and classification of trophoblastic tumours. In: Coppleson M, Monaghan J M, Tattersall M N H (eds) Gynecologic oncology. Churchill Livingstone, Edinburgh, pp 1013–1026

Paradinas F J 1994a The histological diagnosis of hydatidiform mole. Current Diagnostic Pathology 1: 24–31

Paradinas 1994b Value of histopathology in the diagnosis and prognosis of placental site trophoblastic tumour (PSTT). Proceedings of the VII World Congress on Gestational Trophoblastic Diseases, Hong Kong, p 49 (Abstract)

Paradinas F J 1997 Pathology of gestational trophoblastic disease. In: Hancock B W, Newlands E S, Berkowitz R S (eds) Gestational trophoblastic disease. Chapman & Hall Medical, London, pp 43–75

Paradinas F J 1998a The diagnosis and prognosis of molar pregnancy: the experience of the National Referral Centre in London. International Journal of Gynaecology and Obstetrics 60(suppl 1): S57–S64

Paradinas F J 1998b The differential diagnosis of choriocarcinoma and placental site tumour. Current Diagnostic Pathology 5: 93–101

Paradinas F J, Fisher R A 1995 Pathology and molecular genetics of trophoblastic disease. Current Obstetrics and Gynaecology 5: 6–12

Paradinas F J, Browne P, Dent J, Boxer G, Bagshawe K D 1991 Problems in the histological diagnosis of hydatidiform mole: a survey from the UK. Journal of Pathology 163: 168A

Paradinas F J, Browne P, Fisher R A, Foskett M, Bagshawe K D, Newlands E 1996 A clinical, histopathological and flow cytometric study of 149 complete moles, 146 partial moles and 107 non-molar hydropic abortions. Histopathology 28: 101–109

Paradinas F J, Fisher R A, Browne P, Newlands E S 1997 Diploid hydatidiform moles with fetal red blood cells in molar villi. I Pathology, incidence and prognosis. Journal of Pathology 181: 183–188

Paradinas F J, Sebire N J, Fisher R A et al 2001 Pseudopartial moles; placental stem vessel hydrops and the association with Beckwith–Wiedemann syndrome and complete moles. Histopathology 39: 447–454

Parazzini F, La Vecchia C, Franceschi S, Mangili G 1984 Familial trophoblastic disease: case report. American Journal of Obstetrics and Gynecology 149: 382–383

Parazzini F, La Vecchia C, Pampallona S, Franceschi S 1985 Reproductive patterns and the risk of gestational trophoblastic disease. American Journal of Obstetrics and Gynecology 152: 866

Parazzini F, La Vecchia C, Pampallona S 1986 Parental age and risk of complete and partial hydatidiform mole. British Journal of Obstetrics and Gynaecology 93: 582–585

Parazzini F, La Vecchia C, Caminiti C, Negri E, Cecchetti G, Fasoli M 1988 Dietary factors and risk of trophoblastic disease. American Journal of Obstetrics and Gynecology 158: 93–99

Parazzini F, Mangili G, La Vecchia C, Negri E, Bocciolone L, Fasoli M 1991 Risk factors for gestational trophoblastic disease: a separate analysis of complete and partial hydatidiform moles. Obstetrics and Gynecology 78: 1039–1045

Park W W 1957 The occurrence of sex chromatin in chorionepitheliomas and hydatidiform moles. Journal of Pathology and Bacteriology 74: 197–206

Park W W 1967 The pathology of trophoblastic tumors. In: Holland J F, Hreshchyshyn M M (eds) Choriocarcinoma: transactions of a conference of the International Union against Cancer. Springer-Verlag, Berlin, pp 3–8

Park W W 1971 Choriocarcinoma: a study of its pathology. Heinemann, London

Park W W 1975 Possible functions of nonvillous trophoblast. European Journal of Obstetrics, Gynecology and Reproductive Biology 5: 35–46

Park W W, Lees J C 1950 Choriocarcinoma. A general review, with analysis of 516 cases. Archives of Pathology 49: 73–104 and 205–241

Parrington J M, West L F, Povey S 1984 The origin of ovarian teratomas. Journal of Medical Genetics 21: 4–12

Pattillo R A, Gey G O 1968 The establishment of a cell line of human hormone synthesising trophoblastic cells in vitro. Cancer Research 28: 1231–1236

Pattillo R A, Sasaki S, Katayama K P, Roesler M, Mattingly R F 1981 Genesis of 46 XY hydatidiform mole. American Journal of Obstetrics and Gynecology 141: 104–105

Pelkey T J, Frierson H F Jr, Mills S E, Stoler M H 1999 Detection of the alpha-subunit of inhibin in trophoblastic neoplasia. Human Pathology 30: 26–31

Pesce C, Merino M J, Chambers J T, Nogales F 1991 Endometrial carcinoma with trophoblastic differentiation: an aggressive form of uterine cancer. Cancer 68: 1799–1802

Pijnenborg R, Bland J M, Robertson W B, Dixon G, Brosens I 1981 The pattern of interstitial trophoblastic invasion of the myometrium in early human pregnancy. Placenta 2: 303–316

Poen H T, Djojopranoto M 1965 The possible etiologic factors of hydatidiform mole and choriocarcinoma: preliminary report. American Journal of Obstetrics and Gynecology 92: 510–513

Pollard J W, Bartocci A, Arceci R, Orlofsky A, Ladner M B, Stanley E R 1987 Apparent role of the macrophage growth factor CSF-1, in placental development. Nature 330: 484–486

Polychronakos C 1993 Parental imprinting of the genes for IGF-II and its receptor. Advances in Experimental Medicine and Biology 343: 189–203

Prawirohardjo S, Martiono K S, Sutomo T 1957 Hydatidiform mole and choriocarcinoma in Indonesia. First Asiatic Congress of Obstetrics and Gynecology, Tokyo, pp 112–129

Pridmore B R, Khong T Y, Wells W A 1994 Ultrasound placental cysts associated with massive placental stem villous hydrops, diploid DNA content, and exomphalos. American Journal of Perinatology 11: 14–18

Pushchak M J, Farhi D C 1987 Primary choriocarcinoma of the lung. Archives of Pathology and Laboratory Medicine 111: 477–479

Qiao S, Nagasaka T, Nakashima N 1997 Numerous vessels detected by CD34 in the villous stroma of complete hydatidiform moles. International Journal of Gynecological Pathology 16: 233–238

Rachmilewitz J, Elkin M, Rosensaft J et al 1995 H19 expression and tumorigenicity of choriocarcinoma derived cell lines. Oncogene 11: 863–870

Rajatanavin R, Chuahirun S, Chailurkit L, Srisupundit S, Tungtrakul S 1995 Virilization associated with choriocarcinoma. Journal of Endocrinological Investigation 18: 653–655

Ranta T, Wahlstrom T, Rutanen E M, Stenman U H, Seppala M 1981 Serum prolactin levels and immunohistochemical localization of prolactin in trophoblastic disease. Acta Pathologica et Microbiologica Scandinavica. Sect. A, 89: 235–239

Ratnam S S, Chew S C 1976 The natural history of gestational trophoblastic disease. In: First Inter-Congress of the Asian Federation of Obstetrics and Gynaecology, pp 1–7

Reddy D, Rao N 1969 Trophoblastic tumours. I. Hydatidiform mole. Indian Journal of Medical Science 23: 527–537

Redline R W, Hassold T, Zaragoza M V 1998 Prevalence of the partial molar phenotype in triploidy of maternal and paternal origin. Human Pathology 29: 505–511

Reed S, Coe J I, Bergquist K 1959 Invasive hydatidiform mole metastatic to the lungs: report of a case. Obstetrics and Gynecology 13: 749–753

Reid M H, McGahan J P, Oi R 1983 Sonographic evaluation of hydatidiform mole and its look-alikes. American Journal of Roentgenology 140: 307–311

Reik W 1989 Genomic imprinting and genetic disorders in man. Human Genetic Disease Reviews 5: 331–337

Remadi S, Lifschitz Mercer B, Ben Hur H, Dgani R, Czernobilsky B 1997 Metastasizing placental site trophoblastic tumor: immunohistochemical and DNA analysis. 2 case reports and a review of the literature. Archives of Gynecology and Obstetrics 259: 97–103

Repiska V, Vojtassak J, Korbel M et al 1998 Molekularno geneticka diagnostika parcialnej moly hydatidozy. Ceska Gynekologie 63: 189–192

Rettenmier G W, Sacca R, Furman W L et al 1986 Expression of the human c-fms proto-oncogene product (colony-stimulating factor-1 receptor) on peripheral blood mononuclear cells and choriocarcinoma cell lines. Journal of Clinical Investigation 77: 1740–1743

Rhoton-Vlasak A, Wagner J M, Rutgers J L et al 1998 Placental site trophoblastic tumor: human placental lactogen and pregnancy-associated major basic protein as immunohistologic markers. Human Pathology 29: 280–288

Rice L W, Lage J M, Berkowitz R S, Goldstein D P, Bernstein M R 1989 Repetitive complete and partial hydatidiform mole. Obstetrics and Gynecology 74: 217–219

Rice L W, Berkowitz R S, Lage J M, Goldstein D P, Bernstein M R 1990 Persistent gestational trophoblastic tumor after partial hydatidiform mole. Gynecologic Oncology 36: 358–362

Rijhsinghani A, Yankowitz J, Strauss R A, Kuller J A, Patil S, Williamson S 1997 Risk of preeclampsia in second-trimester triploid pregnancies. Obstetrics and Gynecology 90: 884–888

Ring A M 1972 The concept of benign metastasizing hydatidiform moles. American Journal of Clinical Pathology 58: 111–117

Ringertz N 1970 Hydatidiform mole, invasive mole and choriocarcinoma in Sweden, 1958–1965. Acta Obstetricia et Gynecologica Scandinavica 49: 195–203

Rodenburg G J, Nieuwenhuyzen-Kruseman A G, de Maaker H A, Fleuren G J, van Oosterom A T 1985 Immunohistochemical localization and chromatographic characterization of human chorionic gonadotropin in a bladder carcinoma. Archives of Pathology and Laboratory Medicine 109: 1046–1048

Rodriguez E, Melamed J, Reuter V, Chaganti R S 1995 Chromosomal abnormalities in choriocarcinomas of the female. Cancer Genetics and Cytogenetics 80: 9–12

Roman E, Stevenson A C 1983 Spontaneous abortion In: Baron S L,

Thomson A M (eds) Obstetrical Epidemiology. Academic Press, London, pp 61

Romero R, Horgan G, Kohorn E I et al 1985 New criteria for the diagnosis of gestational trophoblastic disease. Obstetrics and Gynecology 66: 553–558

Rudolph R H, Thomas E D 1970 Histocompatibility studies in patients with trophoblastic tumors. American Journal of Obstetrics and Gynecology 108: 1126–1129

Rushton D I 1981 Examination of products of conception from previable human pregnancies. Journal of Clinical Pathology 34: 819–835

Sand P K, Lurain J R, Brewer J I 1984 Repeat gestational trophoblastic disease. Obstetrics and Gynecology 63: 140–144

Sander C M 1993 Angiomatous malformation of placental chorionic stem vessels and pseudo-partial molar placentas: report of five cases. Pediatric Pathology 13: 621–633

Sänger M 1889 Zwei aussergewöhnliche Falle von Abortus. Zentralblatt für Gynäkologie 13: 132–134

Santos L D, Fernando S S, Yong J L, Killingsworth M C, Wu X J, Kennerson A R 1999 Placental site nodules and plaques: a clinicopathological and immunohistochemical study of 25 cases with ultrastructural findings. Pathology 31: 328–336

Sarkar S, Kacinski B M, Kohorn E I et al 1986 Demonstration of myc and ras oncogene expression by hybridisation in situ in hydatidiform mole and in the Be Wo choriocarcinoma cell line. American Journal of Obstetrics and Gynecology 154: 390–393

Sasagawa M, Watanabe S, Ohmomo Y et al 1986 Reactivity of two monoclonal antibodies (Troma I and CAM 5.2) on human tissue sections: analysis of their usefulness as a histological trophoblast marker in normal pregnancy and trophoblastic disease. International Journal of Gynecological Pathology 5: 345–356

Sasagawa M, Sasaki T, Yasuda M et al 1988 [HLA-DP and HLA-DQ antigen expression on trophoblasts of normal human pregnancy and trophoblastic diseases]. Nippon Sanka Fujinka Gakkai Zasshi 40: 1525–1530

Sasaki M, Katayama P K, Roesler M et al 1982 Cytogenetic analysis of choriocarcinoma cell lines. Acta Obstetrica et Gynecologica Japonica 36: 2253–2256

Sbracia M, Scarpellini F, Mastrone M, Grasso J A 1996 HLA antigen sharing in Italian couples in which women were affected by gestational trophoblastic tumors. American Journal of Reproductive Immunology 35: 252–255

Schammel D P, Bocklage T 1996 p53 PCNA, and Ki-67 in hydropic molar and nonmolar placentas: an immunohistochemical study. International Journal of Gynecological Pathology 15: 158–166

Schiffer M A, Pomerance W, Mackles A 1960 Hydatidiform mole in relation to malignant disease of the trophoblast. American Journal of Obstetrics and Gynecology 90: 516–531

Schlegel R J, Nen R, Leao J C et al 1966 Arborising amniotic polyps in triploid conceptuses: a diagnostic anatomic lesion? American Journal of Obstetrics and Gynecology 96: 357–361

Schmorl G 1893 Pathologisch-anatomische Untersuchungen über Puerperal-eklampsie. Vogel, Leipzig

Schoen I, Konwaler B E, Novak E 1954 The sex incidence of the fetus or child in maternal choriocarcinoma. Journal of Pathology and Bacteriology 67: 1134–1138

Scully R E, Young R H 1981 Trophoblastic pseudotumor: a reappraisal. American Journal of Surgical Pathology 5: 75–76

Seckl M J, Rustin G J S, Newlands E S, Gwyther S J, Bomanji J 1991 Pulmonary embolism, pulmonary hypertension and choriocarcinoma. Lancet 338: 1313–1315

Seckl M J, Fisher R A, Salerno G et al 2000 Choriocarcinoma and partial hydatidiform moles. Lancet 356: 36–39

Sen D K, Sinnatharay T A, Lau K A 1973 The ultrastructure of molar trophoblast. Australian and New Zealand Journal of Obstetrics and Gynaecology 13: 35–39

Shaarawy M, Darwish N A, Abdel-Aziz O 1996 Serum interleukin-2 and soluble interleukin-2 receptor in gestational trophoblastic diseases. Journal of the Society for Gynecolgic Investigation 3: 39–46

Shah V M, Newman J, Crocker J et al 1986 Ectopic beta-human chorionic gonadotropin production by bladder urothelial neoplasia. Archives of Pathology and Laboratory Medicine 110: 107–111

Shapiro L R, Duncan P A, Davidian M M, Singer N 1982 The placenta in familial Beckwith-Wiedemann syndrome. Birth Defects 18: 203–206

Shaw A R E, Dasgupta M K, Kovithavongs T et al 1979 Humoral and cellular immunity to paternal antigen in trophoblastic neoplasia. International Journal of Cancer 24: 586–593

Sheaff M T, Martin J M, Badenoch D F, Baithun S I 1996 β-hCG as a prognostic marker in adenocarcinoma of the prostate. Journal of Clinical Pathology 49: 329–332

Sheer C J, Rettenmier C W, Sacca R, Roussel M F, Look A T, Stanley E R 1985 The c-fms proto-oncogene product is related to the receptor for the mononuclear phagocyte growth factor, CSF-1. Cell 41: 665–676

Sheikh S S, Lage J M 1998 Diagnosis of early complete hydatidiform mole (ECM): a study of 35 cases. Modern Pathology 11: 114A

Sheppard D M, Fisher R A, Lawler S D 1985 Karyotypic analysis and chromosomal polymorphisms in four choriocarcinoma cell lines. Cancer Genetics and Cytogenetics 16: 251–258

Shih I M and Kurman R J 1998a Epithelioid trophoblastic tumour. A neoplasm distinct from choriocarcinoma and placental site trophoblastic tumour simulating carcinoma. American Journal of Surgical Pathology 22: 1393–1403

Shih I M, Kurman R J 1998b Ki-67 labeling index in the differential diagnosis of exaggerated placental site, placental site trophoblastic tumor, and choriocarcinoma: a double immunohistochemical staining technique using Ki-67 and Mel-CAM antibodies. Human Pathology 29: 27–33

Shih I M, Kurman R J 1999 Immunohistochemical localization of inhibin-alpha in the placenta and gestational trophoblastic lesions. International Journal of Gynecological Pathology 18: 144–150

Shih I M, Kurman R J 2001 The pathology of intermediate trophoblastic tumors and tumor-like lesions. International Journal of Gynecological Pathology 20: 31–47

Shih I M, Seidman J D, Kurman R J 1999 Placental site nodule and characterization of distinctive types of intermediate trophoblast. Human Pathology 30: 687–694

Shintani S, Glass L E, Page E W 1966 Studies of induced malignant tumors of placental and uterine origin in the rat. 1. Survival of placental tissue following fetectomy. 2. Induced tumors and their pathogenesis with special reference to choriocarcinoma. 3. Identification of experimentally induced choriocarcinoma by detection of placental hormone. American Journal of Obstetrics and Gynecology 95: 542–563

Shitabata P K, Rutgers J L 1994 The placental site nodule: an immunohistochemical study. Human Pathology 25: 1295–1301

Shozu M, Akimoto K, Kasai T, Inoue M, Michikura Y 1998 Hydatidiform moles associated with multiple gestations after assisted reproduction: diagnosis by analysis of DNA fingerprint. Molecular Human Reproduction 4: 877–880

Silva E G, Tornos C, Lage J, Ordonez N G, Morris M, Kavanagh J 1993 Multiple nodules of intermediate trophoblast following hydatidiform moles. International Journal of Gynecological Pathology 12: 324–332

Silverberg S G, Kurman R J 1992 Tumors of the uterine corpus and gestational trophoblastic disease. Atlas of tumor pathology, third series, fascicle 3. Armed Forces Institute of Pathology, Washington DC

Sivanesaratnam V 1998 The management of gestational trophoblastic disease in developing countries such as Malaysia. International Journal of Gynaecology and Obstetrics 60(suppl 1): S105–S109

Smalbraak J 1957 Trophoblastic growths: a clinical, hormonal and histopathologic study of hydatidiform mole and choriocarcinoma. Elsevier, Amsterdam

Smalbraak J 1959 Problems in the classification of hydatidiform moles. Annals of the New York Academy of Sciences 80: 105–120

Smith D B, Newlands E S, Bagshawe K D 1993 Correlation between clinical staging (FIGO) and prognostic groups with gestational trophoblastic disease. British Journal of Obstetrics and Gynaecology 100: 157–160

Smith R, Crocker J 1988 Evaluation of nucleolar organiser region-associated proteins in breast malignancy. Histopathology 12: 113–125

Souka A R, Kholeif A, Zaki S, Rocca M, Ghanem I 1993 Human leukocyte antigen in hydatidiform mole. International Journal of Gynaecology and Obstetrics 41: 257–260

Steigrad S J, Cheung A P, Osborn R A 1999 Choriocarcinoma co-existent with an intact pregnancy: case report and review of the literature. Journal of Obstetrics and Gynaecology Research 25: 197–203

Stein-Werblowsky R 1960 Induction of chorionepitheliomatous tumour in the rat. Nature 186: 980

Stone M, Bagshawe K D 1976 Hydatidiform mole: two entities. Lancet i: 535–536

Stone M, Bagshawe K D 1979 An analysis of the influence of maternal age, gestational age, contraceptive method and the mode of primary treatment of patients with hydatidiform moles on the incidence of subsequent chemotherapy. British Journal of Obsterics and Gynaecology 86: 782–792

Stone M, Dent J, Kardana A, Bagshawe K D 1976 Relationship of oral contraception to development of trophoblastic tumour after evacuation of a hydatidiform mole. British Journal of Obstetrics and Gynaecology 83: 913–916

Su Y N, Cheng W F, Chen C A et al 1999 Pregnancy with primary tubal placental site trophoblastic tumor. A case report and literature review. Gynecologic Oncology 73: 322–325

Suarez V, Newman J, Hiley C, Crocker J, Collins M 1989 The value of AgNOR numbers in neoplasms and non-neoplastic epithelium of the stomach. Histopathology 14: 61–66

Sugimori H, Kashiuara Y, Tsukamoto N, Taki I 1980 Histological grading of hydatidiform mole. Acta Obstetrica et Gynaecologica Japonica 32: 1951–1956

Sukcharoen N, Mutirangura A, Limpongsanurak S 1999 Telomerase activity in complete hydatidiform mole. Journal of Reproductive Medicine 44: 465–470

Sunde L, Vejerslev L O, Larsen J K et al 1989 Genetically different cell subpopulations in hydatidiform moles. A study of three cases by RFLP, flow cytometric, cytogenetic, HLA and morphological analyses. Cancer Genetics and Cytogenetics 37: 179–192

Sunde L, Vejerslev L O, Jensen M P, Pedersen S, Hertz J M, Bolund L 1993 Genetic analysis of repeated, biparental, diploid, hydatidiform moles. Cancer Genetics and Cytogenetics 66: 16–22

Sunde L, Mogensen B, Olsen S, Nielsen V, Christensen I J, Bolund L 1996 Flow cytometric DNA analyses of 105 fresh hydatidiform moles, with correlations to prognosis. Analytic Cellular Pathology 12: 99–114

Sunderland C A, Redman C W, Stirrat G M 1981 HLA A, B, C antigens are expressed on nonvillous trophoblast of the early human placenta. Journal of Immunology 127: 2614–2615

Sunderland C A, Redman C W G, Stirrat G M 1985 Characterisation and localisation of HLA antigens on hydatidiform mole. American Journal of Obstetrics and Gynecology 151: 130–135

Surani M A H, Barton S C, Norris M L 1984a Nuclear transplantation in the mouse: heritable differences between parental genomes after activation of the embryonic genome. Cell 45: 127–136

Surani M A H, Barton S C, Norris M L 1984b Development of reconstituted mouse eggs suggests imprinting of the genome during gametogenesis. Nature 308: 548–550

Suresh U R, Chawner L, Buckley C H, Fox H 1990 Do AgNOR counts reflect cellular ploidy or cellular proliferation? A study of trophoblastic tissue. Journal of Pathology 160: 213–215

Suresh U R, Hale R J, Fox H, Buckley C H 1993 Use of proliferation cell nuclear antigen immunoreactivity for distinguishing hydropic abortions from partial hydatidiform moles. Journal of Clinical Pathology 46: 48–50

Surti U 1987 Genetic concepts and techniques. In: Szulman A E, Buchsbaum H J (eds) Gestational trophoblastic disease. Springer-Verlag, New York, pp 111–121

Surti U, Szulman A E, O'Brien S 1979 Complete (classic) hydatidiform mole with 46 XY karyotype of paternal origin. Human Genetics 51: 153–155

Surti U, Leppert K, White R 1983 Analysis of hydatidiform moles by RFLPs and chromosome heteromorphisms. American Journal of Human Genetics 35: 72A

Suster S, Robinson M J 1992 Placental intravillous accumulation of sulphated mucosubstances: a reevaluation of so-called hydropic degeneration of the villi. Annals of Clinical and Laboratory Science 22: 175–181

Suzuki M, Matsunobu A, Wakita K, Nishijima M, Osanai K 1980 Hydatidiform mole with a surviving coexisting fetus. Obstetrics and Gynecology 56: 384–388

Suzuki T, Goto S, Nawa A, Kurauchi O, Saito M, Tomoda Y 1993 Identification of the pregnancy responsible for gestational trophoblastic disease by DNA analysis. Obstetrics and Gynecology 82: 629–634

Suzuki T, Kitami A, Hori G, Notake Y, Mitsuya T, Sagawa F 1999 Metastatic lung choriocarcinoma resected nine years after hydatidiform mole. Scandinavian Cardiovascular Journal 33: 180–182

Szepesi J, Szigetvari I, Toth A, Hadju K, Laszlo J 1988 Partial mole with lung metastases and multiple abnormalities of the fetus. Zentralblatt fur Gynakologie 110: 246–249

Szulman A E 1987 Partial hydatidiform mole. In: Szulman A E, Buchsbaum H J (eds) Gestational trophoblastic disease. Springer-Verlag, New York, pp 37–44

Szulman A E 1995 Embryonic death: pathology and forensic implications. In: Oimmick J E, Singer O B (eds) Forensic aspects in pediatric pathology. Perspectives in pediatric pathology. Basel, Karger 119: 43–58

Szulman A E, Surti U 1978a The syndromes of hydatidiform mole. I — Cytogenetic and morphologic correlations. American Journal of Obstetrics and Gynecology 131: 665–671

Szulman A E, Surti U 1978b The syndromes of hydatidiform mole. II — Morphologic evolution of the complete and partial mole. American Journal of Obstetrics and Gynecology 132: 20–27

Szulman A E, Surti U 1982 The clinicopathologic profile of the partial hydatidiform mole. Obstetrics and Gynecology 59: 597–602

Szulman A E, Surti U, Berman M 1978 Patient with partial mole requiring chemotherapy. Lancet ii: 1099

Szulman A E, Philippe E, Boué J G, Boué A 1981a Human triploidy: association with partial hydatidiform moles and nonmolar conceptuses. Human Pathology 12: 1016–1021

Szulman A E, Ma H K, Wong E, Hsu C 1981b Residual trophoblastic disease in association with partial hydatidiform mole (retrospective study in Hong Kong). Obstetrics and Gynecology 57: 392–394

Takagi M, Sato Y, Cho R, Koh K, Nagayama T 1985 Choriocarcinoma coexisting with adenocarcinoma in the pars interstitialis of the oviduct: a case report. Asia-Oceania Journal of Obstetrics and Gynaecology 11: 255–260

Takayama M, Soma H, Yaguchi S et al 1986 Abnormally large placenta associated with Beckwith–Wiedemann syndrome. Gynecologic and Obstetric Investigation. 22: 165–168

Talati N J 1998 The pattern of benign gestational trophoblastic disease in Karachi. Journal of the Pakistan Medical Association 48: 296–300

Tan K C, Karim S M, Ratnam S S 1982 Hydatidiform mole in Singapore. Annals of Academic Medicine of Singapore 11: 545–548

Tanaka T 1976 Studies on histogenesis of experimentally induced chorioepithelioma in rats. Acta Obstetrica et Gynecologica Japonica 23: 43–54

Tayson R W, Kalousek D K 1992 Chromosomal abnormalities in stillbirth and neonatal death. In: Dimmick J E, Kalousek D K (eds) Developmental pathology of the embryo and fetus. Lippincott, Philadelphia, pp 83–110

Teacher J H 1903a On chorionepithelioma (the so-called deciduoma malignum) and the occurrence of chorionepitheliomatous and hydatidiform mole-like structures in tumours of the testis. Transactions of the Obstetrical Society of London 45: 256–302

Teacher J H 1903b On chorionepithelioma and the occurrences of chorionepitheliomatous and hydatidiform mole-like structures in teratoma. Journal of Obstetrics and Gynaecology of the British Empire 4: 1–64 and 145–199

Teng N N H, Ballon S C 1984 Partial hydatidiform mole with diploid karyotype: report of three cases. American Journal of Obstetrics and Gynecology 150: 961–964

Teoh E S, Dawood M Y, Ratnam S S 1971 Epidemiology of hydatidiform mole in Singapore. American Journal of Obstetrics and Gynecology 110: 415–420

Thiele R A, de Alvarez R R 1962 Metastasizing benign trophoblastic tumors. American Journal of Obstetrics and Gynecology 84: 1395–1406

Thiersch J B 1952 Therapeutic abortions with a folic acid antagonist, 4-aminopteroylglutamic acid (4 amino PGA) administered by the oral route. American Journal of Obstetrics and Gynecology 63: 1298–1304

Tominaga T, Page E W 1966 Sex chromatin of trophoblastic tumors. American Journal of Obstetrics and Gynecology 96: 305–309

Tommerup N, Vejerslev L O 1985 Identification of triploidy by DA/DAPI staining of trophoblastic interphase nuclei. Placenta 6: 363–367

Tomoda Y, Fuma M, Saiki N, Ishizuka N, Akaza T 1976 Immunologic studies in patients with trophoblastic neoplasia. American Journal of Obstetrics and Gynecology 126: 661–667

Tow W S H 1966 The classification of malignant growths of the chorion. Journal of Obstetrics and Gynaecology of the British Commonwealth 73: 1000–1001

Tow W S H, Yung R H 1967 The value of histological grading in prognostication of hydatidiform mole. Journal of Obstetrics and Gynaecology of the British Commonwealth 74: 292–293

Trask C, Lage J M, Roberts D J 1994 A second case of 'chorangiocarcinoma' presenting in a term asymptomatic twin pregnancy: choriocarcinoma in situ with associated villous vascular proliferation. International Journal of Gynecological Pathology 13: 87–91

Trowsdale J, Travers P, Bodmer W F, Patillo R 1980 Expression of HL-A, -B, and -C and B2-microglobulin antigens in choriocarcinoma cell lines. Journal of Experimental Medicine 152: 11S–17S

Tsang W Y, Chum N P, Tang S K, Tse C C, Chan J K 1993 Mallory's bodies in placental site nodule. Archives of Pathology and Laboratory Medicine 117: 547–550

Tsukamoto N, Kashimura Y, Sano M, Saito T, Kanda S, Taki I 1981 Choriocarcinoma occurring within the normal placenta with breast metastasis. Gynecologic Oncology 11: 348–363

Tunc M, Simsek T, Trak B, Uner M 1998 Endometrial adenocarcinoma with choriocarcinomatous differentiation: a case report. European Journal of Gynaecological Oncology 19: 489–491

Tuncer Z S, Bernstein M R, Wang J, Goldstein D P, Berkowitz R S 1999 Repetitive hydatidiform mole with different male partners. Gynecologic Oncology 75: 224–226

Tursz T, Lipinski M, Guillard M et al 1981 Characterisation of antibodies reacting with husband's lymphocytes in sera from patients with trophoblastic malignancies. Tissue Antigens 17: 376–385

Twiggs L B, Morrow C P, Schlaerth J B 1979 Acute pulmonary complications of molar pregnancy. American Journal of Obstetrics and Gynecology 135: 189–194

Twiggs L B, Okagaki T, Phillips G L, Stroemer J R, Adcock L L 1981 Trophoblastic pseudotumor — evidence of malignant disease potential. Gynecologic Oncology 12: 238–248

Uchida I A, Freeman V P C 1985 Triploidy and chromosomes. American Journal of Obstetrics and Gynecology 151: 65–69

Van de Kaa C A, Nelson K A M, Ramaekers F C S, Vooijs P G, Hopman A H N 1991 DNA Interphase cytogenetics of routinely processed hydatidiform moles and hydropic abortions. Journal of Pathology 165: 281–287

Van de Kaa C A, Hanselaar A G J, Hopman A H N et al 1993 DNA cytometric and interphase cytogenetic analyses of paraffin-embedded hydatidiform moles and hydropic abortions. Journal of Pathology 170: 229–238

Van de Kaa C A, Schijf C P, de Wilde P C et al 1996 Persistent gestational trophoblastic disease: DNA image cytometry and interphase cytogenetics have limited predictive value. Modern Pathology 9: 1007–1014

Van de Kaa C A, Poddighe P J, Nillesen W N, Smeets J M, Robben C M, Vooijs P G 1997a Early embryonal tissues do not exclude a diagnosis of complete hydatidiform mole. In: Van de Kaa C A (eds) DNA analysis of hydatidiform mole, MD thesis Catholic University, Nijmegen, pp 79–94

Van de Kaa C A, Schijf C P, de Wilde P C, Hanselaar A G, Vooijs P G 1997b The role of deoxyribonucleic acid image cytometric and interphase cytogenetic analyses in the differential diagnosis, prognosis and clinical follow up of hydatidiform moles. A report from the Central Molar Registration in the Netherlands. American Journal of Obstetrics and Gynecology 177: 1219–1229

Van Dorpe I, Moerman P H 1996 Placental site nodule of the uterine cervix. Histopathology 29: 379–382

Van Lijnschoten G, Arends J W, Leffers P et al 1993 The value of histomorphological features of chorionic villi in early spontaneous abortion for the prediction of karyotype. Histopathology 22: 557–563

Van Oven M W, Schoots C J F, Oosterhuis J W, Keij J F, Dam-Meiring A, Huisjes H J 1989 The use of DNA flow cytometry in the diagnosis of triploidy in human abortions. Human Pathology 20: 238–242

Vassilakos P, Kajii T 1976 Hydatidiform mole; two entities. Lancet i: 259

Vassilakos P, Riotton G, Kajii T 1977 Hydatidiform mole: two entities: a morphologic and cytogenetic study with some clinical considerations. American Journal of Obstetrics and Gynecology 127: 167–170

Vegh G L, Fulop V, Liu Y et al 1999 Differential gene expression pattern between normal human trophoblast and choriocarcinoma cell lines: downregulation of heat shock protein-27 in choriocarcinoma in vitro and in vivo. Gynecological Oncology 75: 391–396

Veit J 1901 Über deportation von Chorionzotten. Zeitschrift für Geburtshilfe und Gynäkologie 44: 466–504

Vejerslev L O, Mogensen B, Olsen S 1984 Hydatidiform mole: preliminary results from the current Danish investigation. Second World Congress on Trophoblastic Neoplasms, Singapore, p 1 (abstract)

Vejerslev L O, Dueholm M, Nielsen F H 1986 Hydatidiform mole: cytogenetic marker analysis in twin gestation: report of two cases. American Journal of Obstetrics and Gynecology 155: 614–617

Vejerslev L O, Fisher R A, Surti U, Wake N 1987 Hydatidiform mole: cytogenetically unusual cases and their implications for the present classification. American Journal of Obstetrics and Gynecology 157: 180–184

Vejerslev L O, Sunde L, Hansen B F, Larsen J K, Christensen I J, Larsen G 1991 Hydatidiform mole and fetus with normal karyotype: support of a separate entity. Obstetrics and Gynecology 77: 868–874

Wake N, Takagi N, Sasaki M 1978 Androgenesis as a cause of hydatidiform mole. Journal of the National Cancer Institute 60: 51–53

Wake N, Chapman V, Matski S, Sandberg A A 1981 Chromosomes and cellular origin of choriocarcinoma. Cancer Research 41: 3137–3143

Wake N, Seki T, Fujita H et al 1984 Malignant potential of homozygous and heterozygous complete moles. Cancer Research 44: 1226–1230

Wake N, Fujino T, Hoshi S 1987 The propensity to malignancy of dispermic heterozygous moles. Placenta 8: 319–326

Wake N, Arima T, Matsuda T 1998 Involvement of IGF2 and H19 imprinting in choriocarcinoma development. International Journal of Gynaecology and Obstetrics 60(suppl 1): S1–S8

Wakitani T 1962 Electron microscopic observations on the chorionic villi of the normal human placenta and chorioepithelioma malignum. Mie Medical Journal 12: 43–64

Wallace D C, Surti U, Adams C W, Szulman A E 1982 Complete moles have paternal chromosomes but maternal mitochondrial DNA. Human Genetics 61: 145–147

Walsh C, Miller S J, Flam F, Fisher R A, Ohlsson R 1995 Paternally derived H19 is differentially expressed in malignant and nonmalignant trophoblast. Cancer Research 55: 1111–1116

Wang Y E 1990 Atypical choriocarcinoma. Analysis of 3 cases. Chung Hua Fu Chan Ko Tsa Chih 25: 355–357

Wasan H S, Schofield J B, Krausz T, Sikora K, Waxman J 1994 Combined choriocarcinoma and yolk sac tumor arising in Barrett's esophagus. Cancer. 73: 514–517

Watanabe I, Yamaguchi M, Kasai M 1987 Histologic characteristics of gonadotropin-producing hepatoblastoma: a survey of seven cases from Japan. Journal of Pediatric Surgery 22: 406–411

Watanabe M, Ghazizadeh M, Konishi H, Araki T 1998 Interphase cytogenetic and AgNOR analyses of hydatidiform moles. Journal of Clinical Pathology 51: 438–443

Weaver D, Fisher R A, Newlands E S, Paradinas F J 2000 Amniotic tissue in complete hydatidiform moles can be androgenetic. Journal of Pathology 191: 67–70

Wei P Y, Ouyang P C 1963 Trophoblastic diseases in Taiwan: a review of 157 cases in a 10 year period. American Journal of Obstetrics and Gynecology 85: 844–849

Wersto R P, Liblit R A L, Koss L G 1991 Flow cytometric DNA analysis of human solid tumors: a review of the interpretation of DNA histograms. Human Pathology 22: 1085–1098

WHO Scientific Group 1983 Gestational trophoblastic disease. WHO Technical Report Series 692. WHO, Geneva

Williams R A, Charlton I G, Howat A J 1995 Image analysis DNA densitometry measurements on complete and partial hydatidiform mole and nonmolar products of conception. International Journal of Gynecological Pathology 14: 300–305

Wilson R B, Hunter J S, Dockerty M B 1961 Chorioadenoma destruens. American Journal of Obstetrics and Gynecology 81: 546–559

Witt M, Erickson R P 1989 A rapid method for detection of Y-chromosomal DNA from dried blood specimens by the polymerase chain reaction. Human Genetics 82: 271–274

Womack C, Elston C W 1985 Hydatidiform mole in Nottingham: a 12-year retrospective epidemiological and morphological study. Placenta 6: 95–105

Wong S Y, Ngan H Y, Chan C C, Cheung A N 1999 Apoptosis in gestational trophoblastic disease is correlated with clinical outcome and Bcl-2 expression but not Bax expression. Modern Pathology 12: 1025–1033

Wongweragiat S, Searle R F, Bulmer J N 1999 Decidual T lymphocyte activation in hydatidiform mole. Journal of Clinical Pathology 52: 888–894

Wynn R M, Davies J 1964a Ultrastructure of transplanted choriocarcinoma and its endocrine implications. American Journal of Obstetrics and Gynecology 88: 618–634

Wynn R M, Davies J 1964b Ultrastructure of hydatidiform mole: correlative electron microscopic and functional aspects. American Journal of Obstetrics and Gynecology 90: 293–307

Wynn R M, Harris J A 1967 Ultrastructure of trophoblast and endometrium in invasive mole (chorioadenoma destruens). American Journal of Obstetrics and Gynecology 99: 1125–1135

Xu B, Lin L, Rote N S 1999 Identification of a stress-induced protein during human trophoblast differentiation by differential display analysis. Biology of Reproduction 61: 681–686

Yamashita K, Wake N, Araki T, Ichinoe K, Makoto K 1979 Human lymphocyte antigen expression in hydatidiform mole: androgenesis following fertilization by a haploid sperm. American Journal of Obstetrics and Gynecology 135: 597–600

Yamashita K, Ishikawa M, Shimizu T, Kuroda M 1981 HLA antigens in husband-wife pairs with trophoblastic tumor. Gynecologic Oncology 12: 68–74

Yang B L 1993 AgNOR of gestational trophoblastic tumors and its clinical significance. Chung Hua Fu Chan Ko Tsa Chih 28: 408–410

Yang Y, Geraghty D E, Hunt J S 1995 Cytokine regulation of HLA-G expression in human trophoblast cell lines. Journal of Reproductive Immunology 29: 179–195

Yeh I T, O'Connor D M, Kurman R J 1989 Vacuolated cytotrophoblast: a subpopulation of trophoblast in the chorion laeve. Placenta 10: 429–438

Yen S, MacMahon B 1968 Epidemiologic features of trophoblastic disease. American Journal of Obstetrics and Gynecology 101: 126–132

Yokoyama S, Niimi S, Tsuroaka M 1988 The expression of c-myc, c-fms, c-sis oncogenes in the trophoblast of normal pregnancy and trophoblastic disease. Acta Obstetrica et Gynaecologica Japonica 40: 1867–1874

Young R H, Scully R E 1984 Placental site trophoblastic tumor: current status. Clinical Obstetrics and Gynecology 27: 248–258

Young R H, Scully R E, McCluskey R T 1985 A distinctive glomerular lesion complicating placental site trophoblastic tumor: report of two cases. Human Pathology 16: 35–42

Young R H, Kurman R J, Scully R E 1988 Proliferations and tumors of the placental site. Seminars in Diagnostic Pathology 5: 223–237

Young R H, Kurman R J, Scully R E 1990 Placental site nodules and plaques: a clinicopathological analysis of 20 cases. American Journal of Surgical Pathology 14: 1001–1009

Yuen B H, Cannon W 1981 Molar pregnancy in British Columbia: estimated incidence and post evacuation regression patterns of the beta subunit of human chronic gonadotrophin. American Journal of Obstetrics and Gynecology 139: 316–319

Yuen Y F, Lewis E J, Larson J T, Wilke M S, Rest E B, Zachary C B 1998 Scalp metastases mimicking alopecia areata. First case report of placental site trophoblastic tumor presenting as cutaneous metastasis. Dermatologic Surgery 24: 587–591

Zaki Z M, Bahar A M 1996 Ultrasound appearance of a developing mole. International Journal of Gynaecology and Obstetrics 55: 67–70

Zalel Y, Dgani R 1997 Gestational trophoblastic disease following the evacuation of partial hydatidiform mole: a review of 66 cases. European Journal of Obstetrics, Gynecology and Reproductive Biology 71: 67–71

Zaragoza M V, Keep D, Genest D R, Hassold T, Redline R W 1997 Early complete hydatidiform moles contain inner cell mass derivatives. American Journal of Medical Genetics 70: 273–277

Zdravkovic M, Aboagye-Mathiesen G, Guimond M J, Hager H, Ebbesen P, Lala P K 1999 Susceptibility of MHC class I expressing extravillous trophoblast cell lines to killing by natural killer cells. Placenta 20: 431–440

Zhang J, Kraus F T 1986 Placental site trophoblastic tumor (PSTT): immunocytochemical correlations. Laboratory Investigation 54: 73A

Zhang X, Zhang L, Zhou X 1998 The relationship between the pathological classifications and molecular genetics of hydatidiform moles. Chung Hua Fu Chan Ko Tsa Chih 33: 163–164

41

The pathology of miscarriage

H Fox   L Regan

Definition of miscarriage   1431

Incidence   1432

Aetiological factors   1432
Infections   1432
Physical factors   1432
Endocrinological abnormalities   1433
Psychological factors   1433
Immunological factors   1433
Thrombophilias   1434
Congenital abnormalities of the fetus   1435
Genetic abnormalities   1435

Pathogenesis of miscarriage   1435

Pathology   1436
General anatomico-pathological classification of material
  from miscarriages   1436
Macroscopic abnormalities of the cord and placenta   1437
Histological abnormalities in the placenta   1438

DEFINITION OF MISCARRIAGE

There has in the past been much pedantic quibbling as to the definition of a spontaneous miscarriage but for practical purposes any pregnancy that terminates before the fetus is viable is a miscarriage. The most widely used definition is that employed by the World Health Organization (1977) which defines a miscarriage as 'expulsion of an embryo or fetus weighing 500 gram or less'; using this definition pregnancies that terminate in a spontaneous miscarriage will always do so before the 22nd week of gestation. It will be noted that this definition evades the issue as to whether a liverborn infant weighing less than 500 g should be considered as a miscarriage and whilst including some cases of partial hydatidiform mole excludes complete moles. In reality, of course, most miscarriages occur during the first trimester or in the early second trimester and thus pose no difficulties of recognition or definition. By convention a miscarriage is classed as early if it occurs before the 13th week of pregnancy and as late if pregnancy loss occurs at or after the 13th week of gestation.

Because spontaneous miscarriage is so common, and because most miscarriages are followed by a perfectly normal subsequent pregnancy, early pregnancy loss only becomes a real clinical problem in women who recurrently, or 'habitually', miscarry. There are, however, differing views as what exactly constitutes 'recurrent' miscarriage for it is certainly possible for a woman to have two consecutive miscarriages simply by pure chance; the odds against miscarriage occurring in three successive pregnancies simply by chance are, however, very high and therefore a woman who miscarries in three successive pregnancies can be regarded as suffering recurrent pregnancy loss (Berry et al 1995), although in fact this will occur in 0.3% of women as a result of bad luck alone (Hatasaka 1994). The distinction between sporadic and recurrent miscarriages is important for it is certain that the aetiological factors differ considerably for the two forms of miscarriage: thus, for instance, fetal chromosomal abnormalities are a major aetiological factor for sporadic miscarriages but not for recurrent miscarriage. Unfortunately, the pathologist examining material from a miscarriage is only rarely informed as to whether the miscarriage is sporadic or recurrent whilst even the obstetrician will not know if a woman suffering her first miscarriage is having a sporadic miscarriage or the first of what is later seen to be a sequence of recurrent miscarriages. To complicate the matter still further it is quite possible for a sporadic miscarriage, due possibly to a fetal chromosomal abnormality, to interrupt a series of recurrent miscarriages due to a quite different factor.

INCIDENCE

It is widely agreed that about 15% of recognised pregnancies spontaneously miscarry (Alberman 1988; Daya 1994; Hatasaka 1994; Berry et al 1995; Regan 1997); there is no doubt, however, that a significant proportion of conceptuses are lost without the woman being aware that she is, or has been, pregnant. Roberts & Lowe (1975), with the aid of an ingenious mathematical formula, calculated that 78% of conceptuses in women aged 20 to 29 in England and Wales miscarry whilst Edmonds et al (1982), using highly sensitive beta-hCG assays, found that the rate of clinically undetectable early pregnancy loss was as high as two thirds of all conceptions. Later studies have yielded more conservative estimates, suggesting that 18–22% of conceptions fail to survive as a clinically recognisable pregnancy (Sweeney et al 1988; Wilcox et al 1988). Most of these early pregnancy failures occur prior to, or very soon after, implantation and possible causes of pregnancy loss at this stage include a failure of gene activation, a chromosomal abnormality or errors of cytokinesis and karyokinesis (Chard 1991).

AETIOLOGICAL FACTORS

Any attempt to categorise the factors responsible for spontaneous miscarriage must, in our present state of knowledge, be both riddled with lacunae of ignorance and, at least partially, based on hypotheses or unproven assumptions. Amongst the suggested aetiological factors are the following.

INFECTIONS

Any infection in early pregnancy that is accompanied by a severe maternal systemic disturbance, e.g. lobar pneumonia, can cause miscarriage without there being any direct involvement of the placenta or fetus (Kline et al 1985). A number of organisms appear, however, to have a specifically abortifacient effect although often producing few or no systemic symptoms in the mother; the organisms which have been particularly stigmatised in this respect include rubella virus, *Treponoma pallidum,*

Listeria monocytogenes, cytomegalovirus, Toxoplasma gondii, Campylobacter sp. and, possibly, *Herpes simplex* virus and Coxsackie virus (Charles & Larsen 1990). The mechanism of pregnancy loss in such infections is obscure but it is probable that fetal infection is an important factor and that the pregnancy does not fail because of any presumed placental dysfunction caused by inflammatory damage. *Chlamydia trachomatis,* and *Mycoplasma hominis* have not, despite some claims to the contrary (Stray-Pederson et al 1978; Quinn et al 1987; Witkin & Ledger 1992), been clearly linked to miscarriage (Charles & Larsen 1990; Rae et al 1994; Summers 1994; Feist et al 1999; Regan & Jivraj 2001) but a high incidence of positive cultures for *Ureaplasma urealyticum* has been obtained from placentas of spontaneous miscarriages (Fox 1997). Bacterial vaginosis, which is not strictly an infection but a change in vaginal flora with reduced lactobacilli, is associated with an increased risk of late miscarriage (Kurki et al 1992; Llahi-Camp et al 1996), though the nature of this relationship is unknown.

The actual quantitative contribution of infections to sporadic human miscarriage is not known with any degree of certainty but is probably low (Summers 1994; Simpson et al 1996) whilst infection appears to play little or no role in recurrent miscarriage (Plouffe et al 1992; Regan & Jivraj 2001).

PHYSICAL FACTORS

Claims that uterine leiomyomas, especially those in a submucous site, are associated with a high incidence of early pregnancy loss and that myomectomy results in a much improved reproductive performance (Buttram & Reiter 1981; Garcia & Tureck 1984) are difficult to evaluate for they are based on uncontrolled studies: the most that can be said is that leiomyomas may be a very infrequent cause of miscarriage (Treffers 1990).

It has been widely conceded that uterine malformations are a cause of early pregnancy loss and that they may be an important factor in cases of recurrent miscarriage (Bennett 1987). The foundations for this belief are, however, not as firm as is generally thought to be the case. Treffers (1990) reviewed critically the then available evidence for a causal relationship between uterine malformations and miscarriage and came to the iconoclastic but scientifically impeccable conclusion that the statistical basis for such a belief was weak and largely explicable in terms of selective reporting. Nevertheless, reports continue to appear claiming a very high incidence of miscarriage, often recurrent, both generally for women with uterine anomalies (Ludmir et al 1990; Stein & March 1990; Golan et al 1992; Makino et al 1992; Acien 1996) and specifically in unicornuate uteri (Donderwinkel et al 1992; Moutos et al 1992; Goldberg & Falcone 1999) and septate uteri (Manchesi et al 1989; Michalas 1991). It is difficult to draw any firm conclusions from these conflicting views but, on balance, it does appear that the incidence of miscarriage is increased in women with uterine malformations, though probably not dramatically. The association with early pregnancy loss appears to be strongest for septate uteri (Patton 1994; Grimbiz et al 1998; Homer et al 2000) and it is of interest that this only appears to be true if the placenta is actually implanted on the septum (Fedele et al 1989).

Cervical incompetence is widely believed to be a well-documented cause of second-trimester miscarriage but in fact there is no agreement about the criteria for the diagnosis of this abnormality, no agreement about its incidence and no agreement about the value of cervical cerclage (Treffers 1990; Quinn 1993).

External trauma to the uterus occupies a much lower place in the aetiological hierarchy of miscarriage than that which would be afforded to it by the general public (Baker 1982; Sorensen et al 1986)

ENDOCRINOLOGICAL ABNORMALITIES

Luteal phase defect, also known as corpus luteum deficiency, has been thought to be an important factor in the pathogenesis of early pregnancy loss and this concept served as the basis for the administration of progesterone to prevent spontaneous miscarriage. It is certainly true that adequate progesterone levels are necessary to sustain an early pregnancy and also true that progesterone levels are often low in patients who miscarry (Li et al 2000) but there is considerable doubt about the value, in terms of prevention of miscarriage, of progestational therapy (Goldstein et al 1989; Stirrat 1990; Simpson 1992; Coulam & Stern 1994; Dawood 1994): further, serum progesterone levels are not reliably predictive of pregnancy outcome (Ogasawasa et al 1997). It is indeed probable that low progesterone levels in early pregnancy are a reflection of a pregnancy that has already failed because the trophoblast cannot produce sufficient progesterone rather than an aetiological factor in pregnancy loss (Regan 1997).

There is a high incidence of polycystic ovaries amongst women who recurrently miscarry (Sagle et al 1988; Balen et al 1993a; Clifford et al 1994) and it has been thought that the hypersecretion of luteinizing hormone (LH), which is a feature of this disorder, could be an important factor in recurrent miscarriage (Regan et al 1990; Balen et al 1993b; Watson et al 1993). However, a prospective randomised placebo-controlled study concluded that pre-pregnancy pituitary suppression of endogenous LH does not improve the live birth rate of women with recurrent miscarriage and polycystic ovary syndrome who hypersecrete LH (Clifford et al 1996). Furthermore, in a recent very large study it was shown that whilst indeed polycystic ovaries were unduly common in women with recurrent miscarriage the miscarriage rate was no higher in those with polycystic ovaries than was that in women with

normal ovaries: further, elevated LH levels were not associated with an increased miscarriage rate (Rai et al 2000).

There is no increased risk of spontaneous miscarriage in women with well-controlled diabetes mellitus (Mills et al 1988) but there is an excess incidence of early pregnancy loss in diabetic women with inadequate glucose control (Hanson et al 1990; Miodovnick et al 1990; Simpson 1992; Clifford & Regan 1994).

The presence of thyroid autoantibodies has been noted in women who suffer recurrent miscarriage (Stagnaro-Green et al 1990; Pratt et al 1993; Abramson & Stagnaro-Green 2001; Matalon et al 2001). The patients in whom such antibodies are found are clinically euthyroid and clinically diagnosable hypo- or hyperthyroidism are not currently considered as risk factors for spontaneous miscarriage (Huisjes 1990; Coulam & Stern 1994). Hence, it is generally thought that the anti-thyroid antibodies are an epiphenomenal manifestation of a generalised autoimmune abnormality rather than being related to specific thyroid dysfunction (Gleicher et al 1993; Silver & Branch 1994; Regan 1997) and two prospective studies have shown that pregnancy outcome is unaffected by the presence of these antibodies (Muller et al 1999; Rushworth et al 2000). Nevertheless, it has been claimed that thyroid replacement therapy increases the incidence of live births in women with thyroid autoantibodies who recurrently miscarry (Vaquero et al 2000) and this does raise the possibility of a very mild thyroid dysfunction or an impaired thyroid adaptation to pregnancy.

PSYCHOLOGICAL FACTORS

Evidence has been adduced that psychogenic factors may be of aetiological importance in a small proportion of first-trimester miscarriages (Michel-Wolfromm 1967; Silverman 1970; Hertz 1973). This evidence is, however, anecdotal, uncontrolled and based upon the study of women who had already suffered repeated pregnancy failures, no information being available about the prior personality or psychological status of women who subsequently suffer recurrent miscarriages (Huisjes 1990; Keye 1994). It is, of course, not surprising that women who have suffered repeated miscarriages develop stress-related symptoms, anxiety states or depression (Hopper 1997; Engelhard et al 2001; Geller et al 2001).

IMMUNOLOGICAL FACTORS

The concept of miscarriage being due, in some instances, to an alloimmune-mediated graft rejection process is seductively attractive; indeed, many have succumbed to the temptation and have supported this view on purely conjectural grounds. There is, in fact, no convincing evidence that cytotoxic antibodies, serum blocking factors or HLA-sharing influence pregnancy outcome and no direct scientific evidence that alloimmune factors play any role in early pregnancy loss (Stirrat 1990, 1992; Silver & Branch 1994; Berry et al 1995).

The role played by autoimmune mechanisms has been explored at length and has centred, in recent years, on antiphospholipid antibodies. It had long been recognised that women suffering from systemic lupus erythematosus have a high incidence of spontaneous miscarriage and it later became apparent that pregnancy loss in this disease is related to the presence of antiphospholipid antibodies (lupus anticoagulant and anticardiolipin antibody) which, it is now recognised, are not confined to patients with lupus but can also occur in women who are otherwise apparently well. There is no relationship between sporadic miscarriage and the presence of antiphospholipid antibodies (Infante-Rivard et al 1991), this contrasting with the apparently clear-cut association of these antibodies with recurrent early pregnancy loss (Triplett 1992; Silver & Branch 1994; Rai et al 1995a,b; Rai & Regan 1998; Vinatier et al 2001). There have, however, been wide differences in the reported incidence of these antibodies in both women with uncomplicated pregnancies and in patients suffering repeated miscarriages; this probably reflects both patient selection bias and variations in laboratory testing but not everybody has been fully convinced that there is a real correlation between antiphospholipid antibodies and early, as opposed to late, fetal loss (Petri et al 1987; Simpson 1992; Melk et al 1995). Even allowing for a causal role of antiphospholipid antibodies in recurrent miscarriage the mechanism by which they cause fetal loss is disputed for the finding of a decidual vasculopathy, thrombotic lesions and extensive placental infarction in some studies (De Wolf et al 1982; Hanley et al 1988; Out et al 1991; Erlendsson et al 1993; Levy et al 1998) has not been confirmed in all (Branch 1994; Silver & Branch 1994; Arnout et al 1995; Sebire et al 2002): experimental studies have suggested that antiphospholipid antibodies may, in fact, have a direct embryotoxic effect (Sthoeger et al 1993).

Evidence that antinuclear antibodies are associated with recurrent pregnancy loss is, at best, flimsy (Branch 1994).

THROMBOPHILIAS

Antiphospholipid antibodies (discussed above) have been thought to predispose to thrombosis and in recent years other thrombophilic conditions, such as deficiencies of the naturally occurring inhibitors of coagulation — antithrombin III, protein S and protein C, have been explored as potential causes of early and late pregnancy loss (Preston et al 1996; Sanson et al 1996; Brenner 2000; Ward 2000), it being claimed that up to 55% of recurrent miscarriages are caused by procoagulant disorders (Bick 2000). It is widely assumed that these thrombophilic disorders lead to thrombotic placental lesions

which, in turn, lead to fetal loss (Arias et al 1998; Ward 2000): evidence to support this claim is, however, scanty (Khong & Hague 1999; Mousa & Alfirevic 2000).

It has been estimated that the overall prevalance of activated protein C resistance in patients with recurrent miscarriage is 14% (Cohen et al 1997) and Rai et al (1996) noted that such resistance was associated with late but not early miscarriage. Activated protein C resistance is commonly inherited as an autosomal dominant trait and is due to a point mutation in the factor V gene. The mutated factor V, known as factor V Leiden, is resistant to proteolytic inactivation by activated protein C, this resulting in increased thrombin generation. In some studies no relationship has been found between factor V Leiden mutation and recurrent miscarriage (Dizon-Townson et al 1997; Metz et al 1997; Kutteh et al 1999) but in others this mutation has been associated with a high incidence of recurrent pregnancy loss (Grandone et al 1997; Hatzis et al 1999; Meinardi et al 1999; Souza et al 1999; Bare et al 2000), either principally in the second trimester (Rai et al 1996) or in both first and second trimesters (Younis et al 2000). A factor V Leiden mutation in the fetus may be of either maternal or paternal origin and fetal factor V Leiden mutation appears to be associated with an increased risk of miscarriage even if there is no maternal mutation (Ward 2000). Activated protein C resistance may be acquired as well as inherited and Clark et al (2001) failed to find any relationship between acquired activated protein C resistance and fetal loss. However, in the largest published study of 1000 recurrent miscarriage sufferers screened for both inherited and acquired forms of activated protein C resistance Rai et al (2001) showed that the prevalence of acquired activated protein C resistance was significantly higher in women with a history of both early and late miscarriage than that found in a normal parous control group although the Factor V Leiden allele frequency was identical in both groups.

Hyperhomocysteinaemia is a marker of a potential for thrombosis. Congenital hyperhomocysteinaemia may be due to a genetic deficiency of the enzyme cystothionine-beta-synthase which converts homocysteine into cytothionine: increasingly, however, a genetic thermolabile variant (C677T) of the enzyme methylenetetrahydrifolate reductase (MTHFR) is thought to be of greater quantitative importance as a cause of congenital hyperhomocysteinaemia. Acquired hyperhomocysteinaemia is usually due to a folate deficiency. Wouters et al (1993) found a high incidence of hyperhomocysteinaemia in women suffering recurrent miscarriages, a finding confirmed in most subsequent studies (Nelen et al 1997; Ray & Laskin 1999; Aubard et al 2000; Nelen et al 2000a; Raziel et al 2001) but not in all (Kutteh et al 1999; Foka et al 2000). The nature of the association between hyperhomocysteinaemia and recurrent miscarriage is uncertain but high homocysteine levels cause endothelial dysfunction

(Chambers et al 1998) and it is suggested that placentas from women with hyperhomocysteinaemia show evidence of endothelial damage and impairment of nitric oxide mediated vasodilatation (Khong & Hague 1999), together with defective chorionic villous vascularisation (Nelen et al 1998, 2000b).

A further thrombophilic syndrome is due to a mutation in the prothrombin gene which results in the variant 20210A prothrombin. So far, this mutation has been linked to recurrent pregnancy loss in two studies (Souza et al 1999; Foka et al 2000) but no association was found in three others (Brenner et al 1999; Kutteh et al 1999; Pickering et al 2001).

Thrombophilic disorders are of rapidly increasing importance in the study of recurrent miscarriage. However, the simple presence of a single genetic prothrombotic factor is a poor predictor of future pregnancy complications. Thus, in a recent prospective pregnancy outcome study it was found that women with a factor V Leiden gene mutation were at increased risk of miscarriage than were women with a normal factor V genotype; nevertheless a significant proportion of women with factor V Leiden mutation had a fully successful pregnancy (Rai et al 2002). Because haemostasis is a highly complex function it is probable that functional coagulation studies may be required to identify those women at risk of miscarriage.

CONGENITAL ABNORMALITIES OF THE FETUS

This term is used here to denote anatomical abnormalities in karyotypically normal embryos; it is, however, difficult to disentangle these two variables for whilst, for instance, cleft lip and palate is found three times as commonly in embryos from miscarriages than in liveborn infants these abnormalities are not uncommon in chromosomal abnormalities. Despite this caveat it is clear that the incidence of anatomical malformations in spontaneous miscarriages is unduly high; thus, for example the incidence of isolated neural tube defects, which are not usually associated with an abnormal karyotype, is very much higher in spontaneously miscarried fetuses than in either live newborns or in therapeutically aborted fetuses (Fantel et al 1980; Byrne & Warburton 1986; McFadden & Kalousek 1989).

GENETIC ABNORMALITIES

There is little doubt that chromosomal abnormalities are the single most important factor in spontaneous sporadic miscarriage, for at least 50% of early spontaneous miscarriages are cytogenetically abnormal (Boué et al 1975; Lauritsen 1976; Hassold et al 1980; Warburton et al 1980; Simpson & Bombard 1987; Creasy 1988; Davison & Burn 1990; Eiben et al 1990; Ohno et al 1991; Cowchock et al 1993; Kalousek et al 1993; Goddijn &

Leschot 2000). There has been fairly general agreement that autosomal trisomy, 45 XO monosomy, triploidy, and tetraploidy account respectively for about 45 to 55, 20 to 30, 15 to 20, and 5% of abnormal karyotypes in spontaneous miscarriages (Creasy 1988; Davison & Burn 1990; Simpson 1992; Byrne & Ward 1994). Trisomies involving every chromosome have been described in spontaneous miscarriages with the exceptions of number 1 and the Y chromosome: between a third and a half of such trisomies involve chromosome 16 whilst chromosomes 2, 7, 13, 14, 15, 21 and 22 each account for between 5 and 10% of trisomic pregnancy losses. It is of interest that not only does the incidence of miscarriage vary considerably amongst the differing various types of chromosomal abnormality but that each particular karyotypic abnormality is associated with a specific and consistent incidence of pregnancy loss; thus, for instance, 98% of monosomy XO embryos are lost and, whilst virtually all cases of trisomy 16 miscarry, this is only true for 70 per cent of those with trisomies 17–18 or 21–22 (Fox 1997).

Most cytogenetic abnormalities associated with miscarriage arise de novo but a small number of abnormal karyotypes result from parental abnormalities, these accounting for about 4–6% of recurrent miscarriages (Simpson et al 1981; de Braekeleer & Dao 1990; Regan 1997; Fryns & van Buggenhout 1998; Goddijn & Leschot 2000). The parental abnormalities encountered most commonly in recurrent miscarriages are balanced reciprocal translocations with Robertsonian translocations being less frequent (Stray-Pederson & Stray-Pederson 1984; de Braekeleer & Dao 1990; Clifford et al 1994).

A particular form of chromosomal abnormality, confined placental mosaicism, appears to be associated with an increased risk of spontaneous miscarriage (Kalousek et al 1992; Wang et al 1993) but this is a double edged weapon for, as discussed below, confined placental mosaicism may also actually prevent pregnancy loss.

It is probable that consideration only of cytogenetic abnormalities underestimates the genetic contribution to spontaneous miscarriage; the application of DNA technology will almost certainly reveal a range of genetic deletions and rearrangements that are not detectable by standard cytogenetic techniques. It has, indeed, been suggested that molecular research will reveal that early pregnancy loss is, with few exceptions, related entirely to genetic causes (Byrne & Ward 1994) though this is, perhaps, the view of enthusiasts for a particular approach.

PATHOGENESIS OF MISCARRIAGE

A mere listing of possible aetiological factors in miscarriage gives no indication as to why and how early pregnancy loss actually occurs. To say that a conceptus has miscarried *because* of a neural tube defect or a 45 XO monosomy is an easy but over-facile explanation for, quite obviously, many fetuses with similar abnormalities do not miscarry but attain viability. Furthermore, we have very little knowledge as to how a chromososomal abnormality is recognised and of the mechanisms by which such an abnormality results in miscarriage.

Some light has, however, been shed on the pathogenesis of spontaneous miscarriage in recent years for it is becoming increasingly clear that placental factors are of considerable importance. Thus there is strong evidence that a confined placental mosaicism may prevent miscarriage of an aneuploid fetus: whilst the vast majority of cases of fetal trisomy 13 or 18 miscarry, those with an associated confined placental mosaicism, in which a proportion of the cytotrophoblastic cells have a normal diploid chromosomal complement, survive (Kalousek et al 1989; Kalousek 1993, 1994). This suggests that placental or trophoblastic function, rather than maternal recognition of a trisomic fetus, determines survival in trisomic conceptuses.

Khong et al (1987) and Michel et al (1990) suggested that there is, in many cases of early pregnancy loss, inadequate placentation with a failure of extravillous trophoblast to adequately invade the spiral arteries of the placental bed. This was confirmed by Hustin et al (1990) who found absent or reduced physiological change in the placental bed spiral arteries in over 60% of early spontaneous miscarriages: Hustin & Jauniaux (1992) have suggested that inadequate trophoblastic migration and invasion may be secondary to a fetal chromosomal abnormality or a severe fetal abnormality in which there is failure of trophoblastic growth and migration. In a recent study, however, a failure of endovascular trophoblastic invasion was found in placentas from cases of early pregnancy loss associated with the presence of antiphospholipid antibodies but was not a feature of placentas from miscarriages associated with fetal aneuploidy (Sebire et al 2002).

If inadequate placentation is a common feature in many spontaneous miscarriages why should it result in pregnancy failure at this early stage? One view has been that the miscarriage is due to uteroplacental ischaemia as a result of inadequate conversion of spiral arteries into uteroplacental vessels (Rushton 1988). It is, however, extremely unlikely that ischaemia could be held responsible for fetal demise at a stage of pregnancy when there is little or no true perfusion of the intervillous space by maternal blood (Hustin & Schaaps 1987; Exalto 1995) and, indeed, Doppler studies have not shown any abnormality of the uteroplacental circulation in patients who miscarry (Alcazar & Ruiz-Perez 2000). The alternative view, championed by Hustin and his colleagues (Hustin et al 1990, 1996; Hustin & Jauniaux 1992, 1997, 2000; Jauniaux et al 1994), and one that has much to commend it, is that miscarriage is due to premature entry of maternal blood into the intervillous space. They argue that the migrating extravillous trophoblast normally forms intravascular cellular plugs in the placental bed vessels

which restrict free passage of maternal blood into the intervillous space: if these plugs are not adequately formed maternal blood will enter the intervillous space prematurely and disrupt the trophoblastic shell with resultant miscarriage. A less mechanistic view is that an unduly early free maternal blood flow into the intervillous space subjects the placenta, which at this stage is normally hypoxic, to an episode of oxidative stress which may result in placental damage and pregnancy failure (Jauniaux et al 2000).

PATHOLOGY

GENERAL ANATOMICO-PATHOLOGICAL CLASSIFICATION OF MATERIAL FROM MISCARRIAGES

The pathologist will find that the tissue presented for the study of a miscarriage ranges from a complete placenta and fetus to a few scanty curettings. It is therefore necessary to adopt an overall anatomical classification of miscarriage material; several such classifications have been proposed (Mall & Meyer 1921; Geneva Conference 1966; Hertig 1968; Laurini 1990) but the one suggested by Fujikura et al (1966) is, with slight modifications, probably the most useful in practice. Miscarriage material is grouped as follows:

I. Incomplete specimen
   a. Villi only
   b. Villi and decidua
   c. Decidua and trophoblastic cells
II. Ruptured empty sac
   a. With cord stump
   b. Without cord stump
III. Intact empty sac
IV. Fetus present
   a. With chorionic sac
      i. Normal non-macerated fetus
      ii. Normal macerated fetus
      iii. Grossly disorganised fetus
      iv. Focal abnormality of fetus
   b. Without chorionic sac
      i. Normal non-macerated fetus
      ii. Normal macerated fetus
      iii. Grossly disorganised fetus
      iv. Focal abnormality of fetus.

In this classification the term 'focal abnormality' refers to a defect such as spina bifida, whilst the expression 'grossly disorganised' is applied to those fetuses which are so ill-formed that they can only be classed as 'nodular' or 'cylindrical'. Most of the other terms used in this classification are self-explanatory, though it should be noted that 'intact empty sac' is used instead of 'blighted ovum', this latter expression being open to widely differing interpretations and being, in itself, meaningless. The term 'anembryonic pregnancy' is also synonymous with 'intact empty sac' and is, when applied to conventional miscarriages, quite a useful terminology: unfortunately this description has also been applied, misleadingly, to complete hydatidiform moles. These latter are not included in this classification though they are simply an unusual form of miscarriage: this omission is deliberate, for a mole is a distinctive entity which falls outside the general group of run-of-the-mill miscarriages and merits the separate attention which it is afforded in Chapter 40.

Although the above classification has many merits the reality of the situation is that most miscarriage material reaching the pathologist either consists only of decidua and placental tissue or is decidual tissue which contains a placental site reaction; fetal tissues may or may not be present but it is uncommon to receive an intact fetus or a complete sac. The embryo is, therefore, not considered further in this account and those requiring information on this aspect of the pathology of early pregnancy failure are referred to specialist texts on embryonic and fetal pathology (Kalousek et al 1990).

MACROSCOPIC ABNORMALITIES OF THE CORD AND PLACENTA

Abnormalities of the cord

Javert and Barton (1952) and Javert (1957) have, with considerable justification, maintained that abnormalities of the umbilical cord have been largely ignored in studies of spontaneous miscarriage claiming that lesions or abnormalities of the cord are a major aetiological factor in early pregnancy loss. As Fox (1997) has pointed out, however, analysis of Javerts 1000 cases of miscarriage shows that in only 3% was a significant lesion of the cord, such as torsion, stricture or true knots, present.

A single umbilical artery is found more frequently in spontaneous miscarriages than in full-term live births, this anomaly being present in about 2.5% of miscarried conceptuses (Thomas 1962). In view of the known association between this abnormality and chromosomal disorders (Saller et al 1990; Khong & George 1992) this is a not unexpected finding, and there are certainly no grounds for assuming that the lack of one umbilical vessel is a cause of early pregnancy loss.

Hathout (1964) and Monie (1965) have maintained that there is an association between miscarriage and velamentous or marginal insertion of the cord, but this has been specifically denied by Philippe et al (1968) and this interesting point remains to be settled.

Abnormalities of the placenta

It is rather unusual to have the opportunity to examine complete placentas from spontaneous miscarriages and,

in general terms, macroscopic examination of such placentas commonly reveals little, if anything, that is helpful in elucidating the possible cause of the pregnancy failure. It is usually very difficult to say if placentas from first trimester miscarriages are of normal shape or not, but Scott (1960) convincingly refuted earlier claims (Hobbs & Rollins 1934) of an excess of extrachorial placentation in miscarriage material.

Gaither & Sampson (1968) have suggested that perivillous fibrin deposition is an important feature of placentas from miscarriages whilst Salafia et al (1993) have noted a relatively high incidence of placental infarcts in first trimester miscarriages. Bret et al (1967) and Fox (1997) thought, however, that gross lesions, such as infarcts, intervillous thrombi and perivillous fibrin plaques, are uncommonly seen in tissue from early pregnancy failures and occur no more frequently in placentas from spontaneous miscarriages than in placentas from induced therapeutic abortions of the same gestational age. Philippe et al (1968) found a high incidence of retroplacental haematomas in miscarriage material, but there must be considerable doubt as to whether the formation of such haematomas is a primary or a secondary change. Marginal placental haematomas have been noted in ultrasonic studies of miscarriages (Mantoni 1985) but these have received little pathological attention in first trimester placentas.

Some authors have commented on the relatively frequent occurrence of a massive subchorial thrombosis (Breus's mole) in placentas from spontaneous miscarriages (Levy 1956; Dydowicz & Pisarki 1967; Abaci & Aterman 1968; Bret & Grepinet 1968; Philippe et al 1968). This lesion (figs 41.1, 41.2) is not confined to placentas from miscarriages as it is also sometimes found in placentas from liveborn infants (Shanklin & Scott 1975): it may play a rôle in some cases of early pregnancy loss but this remains to be determined.

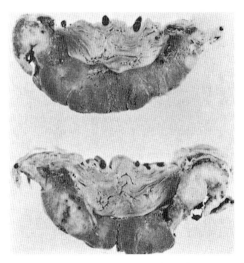

Fig. 41.1 A massive laminated subchorial thrombus in an otherwise normal placenta from a chromosomally normal miscarriage.

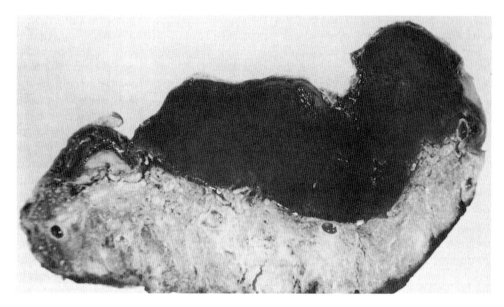

Fig. 41.2 A massive subchorial thrombus in a placenta from a triploid miscarriage. The placenta shows focal microcystic change.

A very small number of placentas from spontaneous miscarriages show maternal floor infarction (Rushton 1988): there is no convincing evidence that this lesion is linked to maternal thrombophilia (Mousa & Alfirevic 2000).

HISTOLOGICAL ABNORMALITIES IN THE PLACENTA

About 40% of placentas from spontaneous miscarriages have villi that are fully normal for the length of the gestational period (fig. 41.3), whilst a further 20 to 30% show only the changes that occur after fetal death, i.e.

sclerosis and obliteration of fetal vessels and stromal fibrosis (fig. 41.4). In between 20 and 40% of placentas from miscarried fetuses the villi show, either focally or diffusely, hydropic change, i.e. they appear swollen and oedematous, either hypovascular or, much more commonly, avascular and have an attenuated trophoblastic mantle (figs 41.5, 41.6). Hydropic change, sometimes wrongly and misleadingly classed as 'hydatidiform degeneration' of the villi, is not associated with the formation of central cisterns and is not apparent macroscopically as visible vesicles. It is worth noting that although hydropic change is usually considered to be due to villous oedema (Genest 1994), a recent study has suggested that the villous swelling is due to an

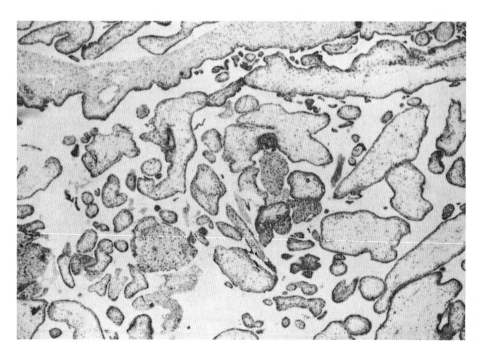

Fig. 41.3 Normal histological appearances of the placental villi in a placenta miscarried at the sixth week of gestation.

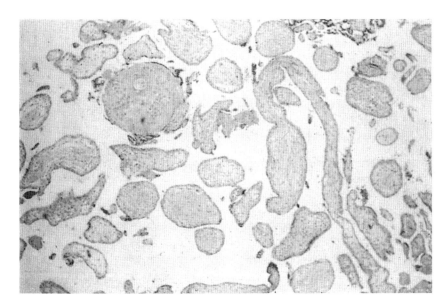

Fig. 41.4 Placental tissue from a spontaneous miscarriage. The villi show only the changes that occur after fetal death.

accumulation, within the villous stroma, of sulphated mucosubstances (Suster & Robinson 1992), a finding that requires confirmation. An unusual finding is a massive chronic intervillositis occurring repetitively in placentas of women who suffer recurrent miscarriages (Doss et al 1995; Boyd & Redline 2000): the cause of this intervillositis is obscure but the vast majority of the infiltrating cells are CD45Rb and CD68 positive.

In addition to these general findings there have been many claims that it is possible to correlate villous morphology in cases of early pregnancy failure either with specific chromosomal abnormalities or, less ambitiously, with an abnormal, as opposed to a normal, karyotype (Bret & Grepinet 1968; Philippe & Boué 1969, 1970; Carr 1971a,b; Cohen 1972; Philippe 1973, 1986; Honoré et al 1976; Geisler & Kleinebrecht 1978; Gocke et al 1982, 1985; Canki et al 1988; Muntefering et al 1988; Rockelein et al 1989; Horn et al 1991). Those making

these claims have stressed the diagnostic value of such features as vesicular change in the villi, irregular villous contours, the presence of trophoblastic pseudoinclusions, trophoblastic hyperplasia, the finding of abnormal stromal cells and, in the case of XO monosomy, villous fibrosis and hypoplasia.

It will be appreciated that many of these studies antedate the delineation of the partial hydatidiform mole and the recognition that this is the pathological hallmark of a diandrous fetal triploidy. Removal from many of these series of cases clearly seen to be, in retrospect, partial moles dilutes considerably the significance of their findings. Further, some of these analyses have failed to take into account the changes that occur in the placental villi after fetal death.

Recent studies have cast considerable doubt on the ability of pathologists to identify villous changes that are characteristic of fetal karyotypic abnormalities with, as

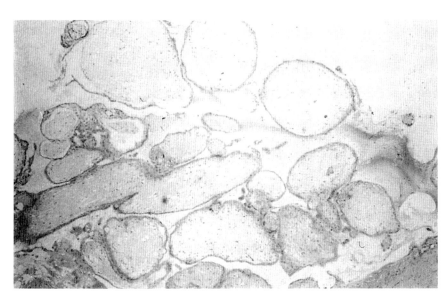

Fig. 41.5 Hydropic change in the villi of a placenta from a miscarried fetus.

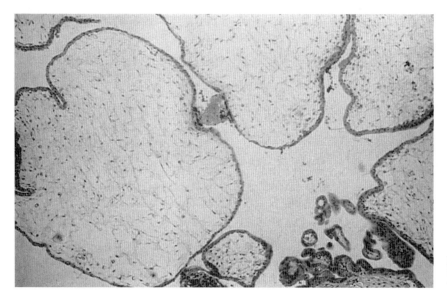

Fig. 41.6 Higher-power view of hydropic villi in a placenta of a miscarriage: there is no trophoblastic hyperplasia.

ever, the exception of diandrous triploidy. firstly, it has been shown that the inter-observer variation in the detection of histological features thought to be associated with fetal karyotypic abnormalities is very considerable (van Lijnschoten et al 1993a). Secondly, prospective studies have demonstrated, with some considerable clarity, that villous histology is an insensitive and inaccurate indicator of fetal chromosomal abnormalities (Novak et al 1988; Minguillon et al 1989; Rehder et al 1989; Hustin & Jauniaux 1992; van Lijnschoten et al 1993b; Fukunaga et al 1995;.Genest et al 1995) a finding that has also been our experience (figs 41.7, 41.8). Morphometric analysis of villous tissue has proved equally unrewarding in this respect (van Lijnschoten et al 1993b), though it is only fair to say that this conclusion has been disputed by

Rockelein and his colleagues who believe that karyotypic abnormalities can be identified by morphometry and scanning electronmicroscopy of placental villi (Rockelein et al 1990a,b). It is certainly possible that karyotypic abnormalities alter villous growth in a rather subtle fashion, too subtle, however, to be detected on light microscopy but neither morphometry or scanning electron microscopy is likely to have great appeal or value for histopathologists who have to deal with an abundance of tissue from early pregnancy failures. Studies of the trophoblastic apoptotic index have also failed to show any difference between placentas from chromosomally abnormal miscarriages and those from pregnancy failures in which the karyotype was normal (Halperin et al 2000; Qumsiyeh et al 2000), though in one of these studies

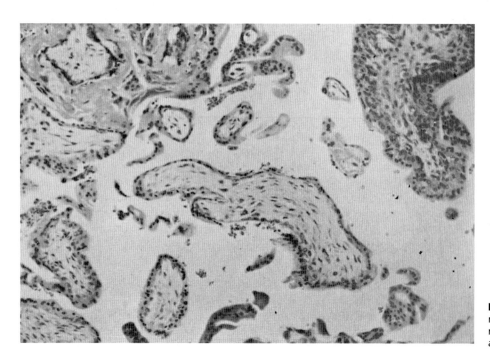

Fig. 41.7 Villi in a placenta from an XO miscarriage: the appearances cannot be readily distinguished from those seen in a placenta showing post-mortem change.

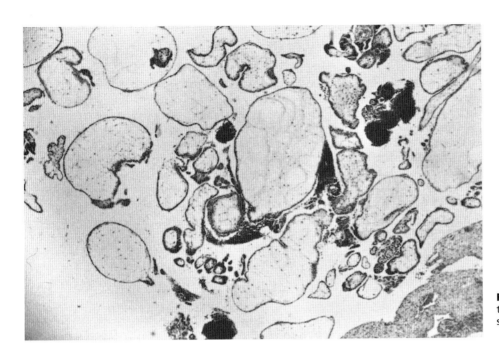

Fig. 41.8 Villi in a placenta from a trisomic miscarriage: the appearances are simply those of a hydropic miscarriage.

there was increased apoptosis of stromal cells in the villi of the cytogenetically abnormal placentas (Qumsiyeh et al 2000).

It appears therefore that an accurate histological classification of placental villous morphology in spontaneous miscarriages, in terms of normal and abnormal karyotypes, is not attainable. Is there then anything that can be gleaned from the histology of placentas from miscarriages that gives any indication as to the cause of the pregnancy failure or affords any hint as to the prognosis of future pregnancies?

Rushton (1981, 1984, 1988) has codified the villous patterns seen in placental tissue from spontaneous miscarriages and has produced a morphological classification which, after excluding partial moles, may be paraphrased along the following lines:

Group 1. A considerable proportion of the villi show hydropic change.
Group 2. Some villi are hydropic but most show postmortem change with stromal fibrosis.
Group 3. The villi show no evidence of hydropic or postmortem change and are of normal appearance for the length of the gestational period.

Rushton has emphasised that each of these groups is, in terms of the aetiology of the miscarriage, heterogeneous and that the appearances reflect more the stage of gestation at which the pregnancy failed than any specific factor. Nevertheless, it would be reasonable to assume that placentas from Group 1 are either from anembryonic pregnancies or from cases of very early fetal death; under such circumstances the factor leading to pregnancy failure is more likely to be intrinsic to the fetus than to lie in the maternal environment and therefore a

fetal karyotypic abnormality is statistically the most likely cause. In Group 2 cases it is certain that, as in Group 1 cases, fetal death preceded the miscarriage, the fetus having been dead for some time before the pregnancy terminated. It is therefore probable, though not certain, that in this group also, the primary factor leading to pregnancy failure was fetal rather than maternal. finally, in Group 3 cases, which are usually from miscarriages occurring later in gestation than the other two groups, the normal appearance of the placental tissue indicates that the fetus was either alive at the time of the miscarriage or had died only very shortly before the pregnancy terminated. It appears reasonable to postulate that in this group the pregnancy failed because of a fault in the maternal environment rather than because of any fetal abnormality.

The reasoning behind Rushton's approach is impeccable but how useful is this classification in practice? Any morphological classification of miscarriage material is probably only of real value in recurrent miscarriages and it is probable that most cases of repetitive pregnancy failure are due to maternal rather than fetal factors. A valid morphological classification of miscarriage material should therefore tend to identify those apparently sporadic cases of spontaneous miscarriage which are likely to recur and should reveal a different pattern in sporadic and repetitive pregnancy failures. Houwert-de Jong and his colleagues (Houwert-de Jong 1989; Houwert-de Jong et al 1990) have used Rushton's classification to examine placental material from both sporadic and recurrent miscarriages: they found that the pattern of placental changes was identical in these two groups and that, furthermore, they could not correlate the histopathological findings with the outcome of subsequent pregnancies. This does imply that current approaches to placental histological abnormalities in miscarriage material are unlikely to be of any great value in the study and management of cases of recurrent miscarriage.

In realistic terms, therefore, what is the value of histological examination of tissue from spontaneous miscarriages?

firstly, of course, to confirm that the patient has actually been pregnant, an aim achieved by the finding either of fetal tissue, villous tissue or of a placental site reaction in decidual tissue.

Secondly, to confirm that the pregnancy has been intrauterine, the only proof of which is the detection of a placental site reaction in decidual tissue; the mere presence of placental villi in uterine curettings is not proof of an intrauterine gestation for these may be from a tubal pregnancy which has miscarried and prolapsed into the uterus. Detection of a placental site reaction is usually a straightforward task but in debatable cases staining for cytokeratins or human placental lactogen is of considerable help in identifying trophoblastic tissue (Khong et al 1994).

Thirdly, to exclude gestational trophoblastic disease. It is in most cases relatively easy to exclude a complete hydatidiform mole though with complete moles increasingly being diagnosed by ultrasound at an early stage in their morphological evolution this diagnosis is becoming somewhat more difficult (Paradinas 1994). In theory the distinction between a hydropic miscarriage and a partial hydatidiform mole is straightforward but in practice there is very considerable inter- and intra-observer error in making this differential diagnosis (Howat et al 1993). It is often suggested that the distinction between these two forms of miscarriage rests upon the finding of villous trophoblastic hyperplasia in a partial mole but not in a hydropic abortus. This is a wrong approach for, in fact, there is often no real trophoblastic hyperplasia in a partial hydatidiform mole and the differential diagnosis rests upon the evidence of an abnormal pattern of trophoblastic growth in a partial mole, circumferential or multifocal trophoblastic growth being a feature of partial moles but never present in a non-molar pregnancy. In truly doubtful

cases flow or image cytometry may be of considerable diagnostic value in distinguishing triploid partial moles from diploid hydropic abortions (van Oven et al 1989; Fukunaga et al 1993; Lage & Popek 1993; Topalovski et al 1995; Kaspar et al 1998) though it must be borne in mind that some hydropic non-molar miscarriages will also be triploidies (Szulman 1995): it has been thought that these non-molar triploidies are usually digynic but recent studies have shown that many are in fact diandrous (Zaragoza et al 2000).

Fourthly, it may occasionally be necessary for medicolegal purposes to attempt to estimate the time of embryonic or fetal death. If the villi are hydropic and avascular and do not contain any erythrocytes it is reasonable to assume that embryonic death occurred before the fifth week of gestation, i.e. before vascularisation of the villi. After this stage the ratio of nucleated to non-nucleated red cells in the fetal vessels may be of value as a chronological marker (Salafia et al 1988; Szulman 1991). Initially, the red cells are of yolk sac origin and are nucleated but these are progressively replaced by non-nucleated red cells of fetal hepatic origin; thus the ratio of nucleated to non-nucleated red cells is 9:1 at the 7th week of gestation and changes gradually to 1:9 at the 9th week of pregnancy, all the cells being non-nucleated by the 10th gestational week. After embryonic or fetal death the fetal red cells may persist in the collapsed villous vessels for several weeks and their nucleation status can provide a clue to the approximate date of fetal death.

These comments about the histological findings in spontaneous miscarriage refer principally to pregnancy failure in the first trimester or early second trimester. In the later stages of the second trimester cases of miscarriage merge almost imperceptibly into cases that could almost be classed as very early premature onset of labour. In these cases chorioamnionitis becomes a relatively common and important finding (Gaillard et al 1993).

A final point is that in 'iatrogenic spontaneous miscarriages', i.e. those following chorionic villus sampling, the placental tissue is usually fully normal for the length of the gestational period (McCormack et al 1991).

REFERENCES

Abaci F, Aterman K 1968 Changes of the placenta and embryo in early spontaneous abortion. American Journal of Obstetrics and Gynecology 102: 252–263

Abramson J, Stagnaro-Green A 2001 Thyroid antibodies and fetal loss: an evolving story. Thyroid 11: 57–63

Acien P 1996 Uterine anomalies and recurrent miscarriage. Obstetrics and Gynecology Clinics of North America 49: 944–955

Alberman E 1988 The epidemiology of repeated abortion. In: Beard R W, Sharp F (eds) Early pregnancy loss: mechanisms and treatment. Springer-Verlag, London, pp 9–17

Alberman E, Elliott M, Creasy M, Dhadial R 1975 Previous reproductive history in mothers presenting with spontaneous abortion. British Journal of Obstetrics and Gynaecology 82: 366–373

Alcazar J L, Ruiz-Perez M L 2000 Uteroplacental circulation in patients with first-trimester threatened abortion. Fertility and Sterility 73: 130–135

Arias F, Romero R, Joist H, Kraus F T 1998 Thrombophilia: a mechanism of disease in women with adverse pregnancy outcome and thrombotic

lesions in the placenta. Journal of Maternal Fetal Medicine 7: 277–286

Arnout J, Spitz, Van Assche A, Vermylen J 1995 The antiphospholipid syndrome in pregnancy. Hypertension in Pregnancy 14: 147–178

Aubard Y, Dorodes Y, Cantaloube M 2000 Hyperhomocysteinemia and pregnancy—a review of our present understanding and therapeutic implications. European Journal of Obstetrics, Gynecology and Reproductive Biology 93: 157–165

Baker D P 1982 Trauma in the pregnant patient. Surgical Clinics of North America 62: 275–289

Balen A H, Tan S L, MacDougall J, Jacobs H S 1993a Miscarriage rates following in-vitro fertilisation are increased in women with polycystic ovaries and reduced by pituitary desensitization with buserelin. Human Reproduction 8: 959–964

Balen A H, Tan S L, Jacobs H S 1993b Hypersecretion of luteinizing hormone: a significant cause of infertility and miscarriage. British Journal of Obstetrics and Gynaecology 100: 1082–1089

Bare S N, Poka R, Balogh I, Ajzner E 2000 Factor V Leiden as a risk factor for miscarriage and reduced fertility. Australian and New Zealand Journal of Obstetrics and Gynaecology 40: 186–190

Bennett M J 1987 Congenital abnomalities of the fundus. In: Bennett M J, Edmonds D K (eds) Spontaneous and recurrent abortion. Williams & Wilkins, Baltimore, pp 109–129

Berry C W, Brambati B, Eskes T K A B et al 1995 The Euro-team early pregnancy (ETEP) protocol for recurrent miscarriage. Human Reproduction 10: 1516–1520

Bick R L 2000 Recurrent miscarriage syndrome due to blood coagulation protein/platelet defects: prevalence, treatment and outcome results. DRW Metroplex Recurrent Miscarriage Syndrome Cooperative Group. Clinical and Applied Thrombosis and Hemostasis 6: 115–125

Boué J, Boué A, Lazar P 1975 Retrospective and prospective epidemiological studies of 1500 karyotyped spontaneous human abortions. Teratology 12: 11–26

Boyd T K, Redline R W 2000 Chronic histiocytic intervillositis: a placental lesion associated with recurrent reproductive loss. Human Pathology 31: 1389–1396

Branch D W 1994 Thoughts on the mechanism of pregnancy loss associated with the antiphospholipid syndrome. Lupus 3: 275–280

Brenner B 2000 Inherited thrombophilia and fetal loss. Current Opinion in Hematology 7: 290–295

Brenner B, Sarig G, Weiner Z, Younis J, Blumenfeld Z, Lanir N 1999 Thrombophilic polymorphisms are common in women with fetal loss without apparent cause. Thrombosis and Haemostasis 82: 6–9

Bret J, Grepinet J 1968 Etude comparative des éléments anatomo-cliniques dans une série d'avortements chromosomiques, dans une série témoin au cours de la mole de Breus. Gynécologie et Obstétrique 67: 313–328

Bret J, Lancret P, Bourel M 1967 Enquete anatomopathologique 'standard' sur le placenta dans 425 cas d'avortements. Revue Francaise de Gynécologie et d'Obstétrique 62: 409–412

Buttram V C, Reiter R C 1981 Uterine leiomyomata: etiology, symptomatology, and management. Fertility and Sterility 32: 40–46

Byrne J, Warburton D 1986 Neural tube defects in spontaneous abortion. American Journal of Medical Genetics 25: 327–333

Byrne L B J, Ward K 1994 Genetic factors in recurrent abortion. Clinical Obstetrics and Gynecology 37: 691–704

Canki N, Warburton D, Byrne J 1988 Morphological characteristics of monosomy X in spontaneous abortions. Annales de Genetique 31: 4–13

Carr D H 1971a Chromosomes and abortion. In: Harris H, Hirschorn K (eds) Advances in human genetics, vol 2. Plenum Press, New York, pp 201–257

Carr D H 1971b The abortus. In: Abramson H (ed) Symposium on the functional physiopathology of the fetus and neonate. C. V. Mosby, St Louis, pp 94–109

Chambers J C, McGregor A, Jean-Marie J, Kooner J S 1998 Acute hyperhomocysteinaemia and endothelial dysfunction. Lancet 351: 36–37

Chard T 1991 Frequency of implantation and early pregnancy loss in natural cycles. Balliere's Clinical Obstetrics and Gynaecology 5: 179–189

Charles D, Larsen B 1990 Spontaneous abortion as a result of infection. In: Huisjes H J, Lind T (eds) Early pregnancy failure. Churchill Livingstone, Edinburgh, pp 161–176

Clark P, Sattar N, Walker I D, Greer I A 2001 The Glasgow Outcome, APCR and lipid (GOAL) Pregnancy Study: significance of pregnancy associated activated protein C resistance. Thrombosis and Haemostasis 85: 30–35

Clifford K A, Regan L 1994 Recurrent pregnancy loss. In: Studd J (ed) Progress in obstetrics & gynaecology, vol 11. Churchill Livingstone, Edinburgh, pp 97–110

Clifford K A, Rai R, Watson H, Regan L 1994 An informative protocol for the investigation of recurrent miscarriage: preliminary experience of 500 consecutive cases. Human Reproduction 9: 1328–1332

Clifford K A, Rai R, Watson H, Franks S, Regan L 1996 Does suppressing luteinising hormone secretion reduce the miscarriage rate? Results of a randomised controlled trial. British Medical Journal 312: 1508–1511

Cohen H, Atoyebi W, Pickering W, Regan L 1997 Factor V Leiden and acquired activated protein C resistance in women with recurrent miscarriage. British Journal of Haematology 97: 300–301

Cohen J 1972 Intéret de l'examen du placenta dans les avortements spontanés du premier trimestre. Revue Francaise de Gynécologie et d'Obstétrique 67: 123–126

Coulam C B, Stern J J 1994 Endocrine factors associated with recurrent spontaneous abortion. Clinical Obstetrics and Gynecology 37: 730–744

Cowchock F S, Gibas S, Jackson L G 1993 Chromosome errors as a cause of spontaneous abortion: the relative importance of maternal age and obstetric history. Fertility and Sterility 59: 1011–1014

Creasy R (1988) The cytogenetics of spontaneous abortion in humans. In: Beard R W, Sharp F (eds) Early pregnancy loss: mechanisms and treatment. Springer-Verlag, London, pp 293–304

Davison E V, Burn J 1990 Genetic causes of early pregnancy loss. In: Huisjes H J, Lind T (eds) Early pregnancy failure. Churchill Livingstone, Edinburgh, pp 55–78

Dawood M Y 1994 Corpus luteal insufficiency. Current Opinion in Obstetrics and Gynecology 6: 121–127

Daya S 1994 Issues in the etiology of recurrent spontaneous abortion. Current Opinion in Obstetrics and Gynecology 6: 153–159

de Braekeleer M, Dao T N 1990 Cytogenetic studies in couples experiencing repeated pregnancy losses. Human Reproduction 5: 519–528

De Wolf F, Carreras I O, Moerman P, Vermylen J, van Assche A, Renaer M 1982 Decidual vasculopathy and extensive placental infarction in a patient with repeated thromboembolic accidents, recurrent fetal loss and a lupus anticoagulant. American Journal of Obstetrics and Gynecology 142: 829–834

Dizon-Townson D S, Kinney S, Branch D W, Ward K 1997 The factor V Leiden mutation is not a common cause of recurrent miscarriage. Journal of Reproductive Immunology 34: 217–223

Donderwinkel P F, Dorr J P, Willemsen W N 1992 The unicornuate uterus: clinical implications. European Journal of Obstetrics, Gynecology and Reproductive Biology 47: 135–139

Doss B J, Greene M F, Hill J, Heffner L J, Bieber F R, Genest D R 1995 Massive chronic intervillositis associated with recurrent abortions. Human Pathology 26: 1245–1251

Dydowicz M, Pisarki T 1967 Estimation and classification of morphological changes in chorions on spontaneous abortions. Bulletin Societe des Amis des Science et des Lettres de Poznan 16: 143–158

Edmonds D K, Lindsay K S, Miller J F, Williamson R, Woods P J 1982 Early embryonic mortality in women. Fertility and Sterility 38: 447–453

Eiben B, Bartels I, Bahr-Porsch S et al 1990 Cytogenetic analysis of 750 spontaneous abortions with the direct-preparation method of chorionic villi and its implications for studying genetic causes of pregnancy wastage. American Journal of Human Genetics 47: 656–663

Engelhard I M, van den Hout M A, Arntz A 2001 Posttraumatic stress disorder after pregnancy loss. General Hospital Psychiatry 23: 62–66

Erlendsson K, Steinsson K, Johansson J H, Geirsson R T 1993 Relation of antiphospholipid antibody and placental bed inflammatory vascular changes to the outcome of pregnancy in successive pregnancies of two women with systemic lupus erythematosus. Journal of Rheumatism 20: 1779–1785

Exalto N 1995 Early human nutrition. European Journal of Obstetric, Gynecology and Reproductive Biology 61: 3–6

Fantel A G, Shepard T H, Vadheim-Roth C, Stephens T D, Coleman C 1980 Embryonic and fetal phenotypes: prevalence and other associated factors in a large study of spontaneous abortion. In: Porter I H, Hook E B (eds) Human embryonic and fetal death. Academic Press, New York, pp 71–87

Fedele L, Dorta M, Brioschi D et al 1989 Pregnancies in septate uteri: outcome in relation to site of uterine implantation as determined by sonography. American Journal of Roentgenology 152: 781–784

Feist A, Sydler T, Gebbers J J, Popischil A, Guscetti F 1999 No association of Chlamydia with abortion. Journal of the Royal Society of Medicine 92: 237–238

Foka Z J, Lambropoulos A F, Saravelos H et al 2000 Factor V leipen and prothrombic G20210A mutations, but not methylenetrahydrofolate reductase C677T, are associated with recurrent miscarriages. Human Reproduction 15:458–462

Fox H 1997 Pathology of the placenta, 2nd edition. Saunders, London

Fryns J P, van Buggenhout G 1998 Structural chromosomal rearrangements in couples with recurrent fetal wastage. European Journal of Obstetrics, Gynecology and Reproductive Biology 81: 171–176

Fujikura J, Froehlich L A, Driscoll S G 1966 A simplified anatomic classification of abortions. American Journal of Obstetrics and Gynecology 95: 902–905

Fukunaga M, Ushigome S, Fukunaga M 1993 Spontaneous abortions and DNA ploidy: an application of flow cytometric DNA analysis in detection of non-diploidy in early abortions. Modern Pathology 6:619–624

Fukunaga M, Onda T, Endo Y, Ushigome S 1995 Is there a correlation between histology and karotype in early spontaneous abortion? International Journal of Surgical Pathology 2: 295–300

Gaillard D A, Paradis P, Lallemand A V et al 1993 Spontaneous abortions during the second trimester of gestation. Archives of Pathology and Laboratory Medicine 117: 1022–1026

Gaither D B, Sampson C C 1968 Intervillous fibrin deposition associated with spontaneous abortion: analysis of 100 cases. Journal of the National Medical Association 60: 497–499

Garcia C R, Tureck R W 1984 Submucosal leiomyomas and infertility. Fertility and Sterility 42: 16–19

Geisler K, Kleinebrecht J 1978 Cytogenetic and histologic analysis of spontaneous abortion. Human Genetics 45: 239–251

Geller P A, Klier C M, Neugebauer R 2001 Anxiety disorders following miscarriage. Journal of Clinical Psychiatry 62: 432–438

Genest D R 1994 The pathology of early pregnancy wastage. Advances in Pathology and Laboratory Medicine 7: 281–312

Genest D R, Roberts D, Boyd D, Bieber F R 1995 Fetoplacental pathology as a predictor of karyotype: a controlled study of spontaneous first trimester abortions. Human Pathology 26: 201–209

Geneva Conference 1966 Standardisation of procedures for chromosome studies in abortions. Cytogenetics 5: 361–393

Gleicher N, Pratt D, Dudkiewicz A 1993 What do we really know about autoantibody abnormalities and reproductive failure: a critical review. Autoimmunity 16: 115–140

Gocke H, Muradow I, Cremer H 1982 Morphologische und zytogenetische Befunde bei Fruhaborten. Verhandlungen der Deutschen Gesellschichte fur Pathologe 66: 141–146

Gocke H, Schwanitz G, Muradow I, Zerres K 1985 Pathomorphologie und Genetik in der Fruhschwangerschaft. Pathologe 6: 249–259

Gooddijn M, Leschot N J 2000 Genetic aspects of miscarriage. Balliere's Best Practice and Research in Clinical Obstetrics and Gynaecology 14: 855–865

Golan A, Langer R, Neuman M et al 1992 Obstetric outcome in women with congenital uterine malformations. Journal of Reproductive Medicine, 37, 233–236

Goldberg J M, Falcone T 1999 Müllerian anomalies: reproduction, diagnosis and treatment. In: Gidwani G, Falcone T (eds) Congenital malformations of the female genital tract: diagnosis and management. Lipincott, Williams & Wilkins, Philadelphia, pp 177–204

Goldstein P, Berrier J, Rosen S, Sacks H S, Chalmers T C 1989 A meta-analysis of randomized controlled trials of progestational agents in pregnancy. British Journal of Obstetrics and Gynaecology 96: 365–374

Grandone E, Margaglione D, Colaizzo D, D'Addedda M 1997 Factor V Leiden is associated with repeated and recurrent unexplained fetal loss. Thrombosis and Haemostasis 77L 822–824

Grimbiz G, Camus M, Clasen K, Tournaye H, De Muncke L, Devroey P 1998 Hysteroscopic septum resection in patients with recurrent abortion or infertility. Human Reproduction 13: 1188–1193

Halperin R, Peller S, Rotschild M, Bukovsky I, Schneider D 2000 Placental apoptosis in normal and abnormal pregnancies. Gynecologic and Obstetric Investigation 50: 84–87

Hanley J G, Gladman D D, Rose T H, Laskin C A, Urowitz M B 1988 Lupus pregnancy: a prospective study of placental changes. Arthritis and Rheumatism 31: 356–366

Hanson U, Perrson B, Thunell S 1990 Relationship between haemoglobin AIC in early type (insulin dependant) diabetic pregnancy and the occurrence of spontaneous abortion and fetal malformation in Sweden. Diabetologia 33: 100–104

Hassold T J, Chen N, Funkhouser J et al 1980 A cytogenetic study of 1000 spontaneous abortions. Annals of Human Genetics 44: 151–178

Hatasaka H H 1994 Recurrent miscarriage: epidemiologic factors, definitions, and incidence. Clinical Obstetrics and Gynecology 37: 625–634

Hathout H 1964 The vascular pattern and mode of insertion of the umbilical cord in abortion material. Journal of Obstetrics and Gynaecology of the British Commonwealth 71: 963–964

Hatzis T, Cardamakis E, Drivalas E et al 1999 Increased resistance to activated protein C and factor V Leiden in recurrent abortions: review of other hypercoagulability factors. European Journal of Contraception and Reproductive Health Care 4: 135–144

Hertig A T 1968 Human trophoblast. Thomas, Springfield, Illinois

Hertz D G 1973 Rejection of motherhood: a psychosomatic appraisal of habitual abortion. Psychosomatics 14: 241–244

Hobbs J E Rollins P R 1934 Fetal death from placenta circumvallata. American Journal of Obstetrics and Gynecology 28: 78–83

Homer H A, Li T Cooke S D 2000 The septate uterus: a review of management and reproductive outcome. Fertility and Sterility 73: 1–14

Honoré L H, Dill F J, Poland B J 1976 Placental morphology in spontaneous human abortuses with normal and abnormal karyotypes. Teratology 14: 151–166

Hopper E 1997 Psychological consequences of early pregnancy loss. In: Grudzinskas J G, O'Brien P M S (eds) Problems in early pregnancy: advances in diagnosis and management. RCOG Press, London, pp 296–308

Horn L C, Rosenkranz M, Bilek K 1991 Wertigkeit der Plazentahistologie fur die Erkennung genetisch bedingter Aborte. Zeitschrift fur Geburtshilfe und Perinatologie 195: 47–53

Houwert-de-Jong M H 1989 Habitual abortion; views and fact finding. Thesis, University of Utrecht

Houwert-de-Jong M H, Bruinse H W, Eskes T K A B et al 1990 Early recurrent miscarriage: histology of conception products. British Journal of Obstetrics and Gynaecology 97: 533–535

Howat A J, Beck S, Fox H et al 1993 Can histopathologists reliably diagnose molar pregnancy? Journal of Clinical Pathology 46: 599–602

Huisjes H J 1990 Maternal disease and early pregnancy loss. In: Huisjes H J, Lind T (eds) Early pregnancy failure. Churchill Livingstone, Edinburgh, pp 148–153

Hustin J, Jauniaux E R M 1992 Morphology and mechanisms of abortion. In: Barnea E R, Hustin J, Jauniaux E R M (eds) The first twelve weeks of gestation. Springer-Verlag, Berlin, pp 280–296

Hustin J, Jauniaux E R M 1997 Mechanisms and pathology of miscarriage. In: Grudzinskas J G, O'Brien P M S (eds) Problems in early pregnancy: advances in diagnosis and management. RCOG Press, London, pp 19–30

Hustin J, Jauniaux E R M 2000 Histology of miscarriage: its relation to pathogenesis. In: Kingdom J C P, Jauniaux E R M, O'Brien P M S (eds) The placenta: basic science and clinical practice. RCOG Press, London, 121–132

Hustin J, Schaaps J P 1987 Echographic and anatomic studies of the maternotrophoblastic border during the first trimester of pregnancy. American Journal of Obstetrics and Gynecology 157: 162–168

Hustin J, Jauniaux E, Schaaps J P 1990 Histological study of the materno-embryonic interface in spontaneous abortion. Placenta 11: 477–486

Hustin J, Kadri R, Jauniaux E 1996 Spontaneous and habitual abortion: a pathologist's point of view. Early Pregnancy 2: 85–95

Infante-Rivard C, David M, Gauthier R, Rivard G E 1991 Lupus anticoagulants, anticardiolipin antibodies, and fetal loss: a case control study. New England Journal of Medicine 325: 1063–1066

Jauniaux E R M, Zaidi J, Jurcovic D, Campbell S Hustin J 1994 Comparison of colour Doppler features and pathological findings in complicated early pregnancy. Human Reproduction 9: 2432–2437

Jauniaux E R M, Watson E L, Hempstock J, Bao Y P, Skepper J N, Burton G J 2000 Onset of maternal arterial blood flow and placental oxidative stress: a possible factor in human early pregnancy failure. American Journal of Pathology 157: 2111–2122

Javert C T 1957 Spontaneous and habitual abortion. McGraw-Hill, New York

Javert C T, Barton B 1952 Congenital and acquired lesions of the umbilical cord and spontaneous abortion. American Journal of Obstetrics and Gynecology 63: 1065–1077

Kalousek D K 1993 The effect of confined placental mosaicism on development of the human aneuploid conceptus. Birth Defects: Original Article Series 29: 39–51

Kalousek D K 1994 Current topic: confined placental mosaicism and intrauterine fetal development. Placenta 15: 219–230

Kalousek D K, Barrett I, McGillivray B C 1989 Placental mosaicism and intrauterine survival of trisomies 13 and 18. American Journal of Human Genetics 44: 338–343

Kalousek D K, fitch N, Paradice B A 1990 Pathology of the human embryo and previable fetus: an atlas. Springer-Verlag, New York

Kalousek D K, Barrett I J, Gartner A B 1992 Spontaneous abortion and confined chromosomal mosaicism. Human Genetics 88: 642–646

Kalousek D K, Pantzar T, Tsai M, Paradice B 1993 Early spontaneous abortion: morphologic and karotypic findings in 3,912 cases. Birth Defects 29: 53–61

Kaspar H G, Kraemer B B, Kraus F T 1998 DNA ploidy by image cytometry and karotype in spontaneous abortions. Human Pathology 29: 1013–1016

Keye W 1994 Psychologic relationships. Clinical Obstetrics and Gynecology 37: 671–680

Khong T Y, George K 1992 Chromosomal abnormalities associated with a single umbilical artery. Prenatal Diagnosis 12: 965–968

Khong T Y, Hague W M 1999 The placenta in maternal hyperhomocysteinaemia. British Journal of Obstetrics and Gynaecology 106: 272–278

Khong T Y, Liddell H S, Robertson W B 1987 Defective haemochorial placentation as a cause of miscarriage: a preliminary study. British Journal of Obstetrics and Gynaecology 94: 649–655

Khong T Y, Stewart C J, Mott C, Chambers H M, Staples A J 1994 The usefulness of human placental lactogen and keratin immunohistoochemistry in the assessment of tissue from purported intrauterine pregnancies. American Journal of Clinical Pathology 102: 72–75

Kline J, Stein Z, Susser W D 1985 Fever during pregnancy and spontaneous abortion. American Journal of Epidemiology 121: 832–842

Kurki T, Sivonen A, Renkonen O, Savia E, Ylikorkala O 1992 Bacterial vaginosis in early pregnancy and pregnancy outcome. Obstetrics and Gynecology 80: 173–177

Kutteh E H, Park V M, Deitcher S R 1999 Hypercoagulable state mutation analysis in white patients with early first-trimester recurrent pregnancy loss. Fertility and Sterility 71: 1048–1053

Lage J M, Popek E J 1993 The role of DNA flow cytometry in evaluation of partial and complete hydatidiform moles and hydropic abortions. Seminars in Diagnostic Pathology 10: 267–274

Laurini R N 1990 Abortion from a morphological viewpoint. In: Huisjes H J, Lind T (eds) Early pregnancy failure. Churchill Livingstone, Edinburgh, pp 79–113

Lauritsen J G 1976 Aetiology of spontaneous abortion: a cytogenetic and epidemiological study of 288 abortuses. Acta Obstetricia et Gynecologica Scandinavica Supplement 52: pp 1–29

Levy H 1956 Mola de Breus — revisao des conceitos patogeneticos a proposito de nove casos proprios. Gazeta Medica Portuguesa 9: 341–363

Levy R A Avvad E, Oliveira J, Porto L C 1998 Placental pathology in antiphospholipid syndrome. Lupus 7, Supplement 2: S81–S85

Li T C, Spuijbroek M D, Tuckerman E, Anstie B, Loxley M, Laird S 2000 Endocrinological and endometrial factors in recurrent miscarriage. British Journal of Obstetrics and Gynaecology 107: 1471–1479

Llhai-Camp J M, Rai R, Ison C, Regan L, Taylor-Robinson D 1996 Association of bacterial vaginosis with a history of second trimester miscarriage. Human Reproduction 11: 1578–1588

Ludmir J, Samuels P, Brooks S, Mennuti M T 1990 Pregnancy outcome of patients with uncorrected uterine anomalies managed in a high-risk obstetric setting. Obstetrics and Gynecology. 75: 906–910

McCormack M J, Mackenzie W E, Rushton D I, Newton J R 1991 Clinical and pathological factors in spontaneous abortion following chorionic villus sampling. Prenatal Diagnosis 11: 841–846

McFadden D E, Kalousek D 1989 Survey of neural tube defects in spontaneously aborted embryos. American Journal of Medical Genetics 32: 356–358

Makino T, Umeuchi M, Nakada K et al 1992 Incidence of congenital uterine anomalies in repeated reproductive wastage and prognosis for pregnancy after metroplaty. International Journal of Fertility 37: 167–170

Mall F P, Meyer A W 1921 Studies on abortuses: a survey of pathologic ova in the Carnegie embryological collection. Contributions to Embryology, Carnegie Institution of Washington 12: 1–364

Manchesi I, Manchesi F, Parlato F et al 1989 Reproductive performance in women with uterus didelphys. Acta Europaea Fertilitas 20: 121–124

Mantoni M 1985 Ultrasound signs in threatened abortion and their prognostic significance. Obstetrics and Gynecology 65: 471–475

Matalon S T, Blank M, Ornoy A, Shoenfeld Y 2001 The association between anti-thyroid antibodies and pregnancy loss. American Journal of Obstetrics and Gynecology 45: 72–77

Meinardi J R, Middeldorp S, de Kam P J et al 1999 Increased risk for fetal loss in carriers of the factor V Leiden mutation. Annals of Internal Medicine 130: 736–739

Melk A, Mueller-Eckhardt G, Polten B, Lattermann A, Heine O, Hoffmann O 1995 Diagnostic and prognostic significance of anticardiolipin antibodies in patients with recurrent spontaneous abortions. American Journal of Reproductive Immunology 33: 228–233

Metz J, Kloss M, O'Malley C J et al 1997 Prevalence of factor V Leiden is not increased in women with recurrent miscarriage. Clinical Applied Thrombosis and Hemostasis 3: 137–140

Michalas S P 1991 Outcome of pregnancy in women with uterine malformation: evaluation of 62 cases. International Journal of Gynaecology and Obstetrics 35: 557–559

Michel M Z, Khong T Y, Clark D A, Beard R W 1990 A morphological and immunological study of human placental bed biopsies in miscarriage. British Journal of Obstetrics and Gynaecology 97: 984–988

Michel-Wolfromm H 1967 Le facteur psychique dans l'avortement spontanés. Revue Francaise de Gynécologie et d'Obstétrique 62: 533–536

Mills J L, Simpson J L, Driscoll S G et al 1988 Incidence of spontaneous abortion among normal women and insulin-dependent diabetic women whose pregnancies were identified within 21 days of conception. New England Journal of Medicine 319: 1617–1623

Minguillon C, Eiben B, Bahr-Porsch S, Vogel M, Hansmann H 1989 The predictive value of chorionic villus histology for identifying chromosomally normal and abnormal spontaneous abortions. Human Genetics 82: 373–376

Miodovnik M, Mimoni F, Siddiqi T, Khoury J Berk M A 1990 Spontaneous abortions in repeat diabetic pregnancies: a relationship with glycemic control. Obstetrics and Gynecology 75: 75–78

Monie I W 1965 Velamentous insertion of the cord in early pregnancy. American Journal of Obstetrics and Gynecology 93: 276–281

Mousa H A, Alfirevic Z 2000 Do placental lesions reflect thrombophilia state in women with adverse pregnancy outcome? Human Reproduction 15: 1830–1833

Moutos D H, Damewood M D, Schlaff W D, Rock J A 1992 A comparison of the reproductive outcome between women with a unicornuate uterus and women with a didelphic uterus. Fertility and Sterility 58: 88–93

Muller A F, Verhoeff A, Mantel M J, Berghout A 1999 Thyroid autoimmunity and abortion: a prospective study in women undergoing in vitro fertilization. Fertility and Sterility 71: 30–34

Muntefering R, Dallenbach-Hellweg G, Ratscheck M 1989 Pathologische-anatomische Befunde bei der gestorten Fruhschwangerschaft. Gynakologie 21: 262–272

Nelen W L D, Steegers E A P, Eskes T K A, Blom H J 1997 Genetic risk factor for unexplained recurrent early pregnancy loss. Lancet 350: 861

Nelen W L D, Bulten J, Blom H J, Steegers E A P, Hanselaar A G J, Eskes T K A 1998 Association between chorionic villous vascularization and homocysteine concentration in women with unexplained recurrent pregnancy loss? Netherland Journal of Medicine 52: 57

Nelen W L D, Blom H J, Steegers E A P, den Heijer M, Eskes T K A B 2000a Hyperhomocysteinemia and recurrent early pregnancy loss: a meta analysis. Fertility and Sterility 74: 1196–1199

Nelen W L D, Bulten J, Steegers E A P, Blom H J, Hanselaar A G J, Eskes T K A B 2000b Maternal homocysteine and chorionic vascularization in recurrent early pregnancy loss. Human Reproduction 15: 954–960

Novak R W, Agamonalis D, Dasu S et al 1988 Histological analysis of placental tissue in first trimeter abortions. Pediatric Pathology 8: 477–482

Ogasawasa M, Kajiura S, Katano K, Aoyama T, Aoki K 1997 Are serum progesterone levels predictive of recurrent miscarriage in future pregnancies? Fertility and Sterility 68: 806–809

Ohno M, Meada T, Matsunobu A 1991 A cytogenetic study of spontaneous abortions with direct analysis of chorionic villi. Obstetrics and Gynecology 77: 394–398

Out H J, Kooijman C D, Bruinse H W, Derksen R H 1991 Histopathological findings in placentas from patients with intrauterine death and antiphospholipid antibodies. European Journal of Obstetrics, Gynecology and Reproductive Biology 41: 179–185

Paradinas F J 1994 The histological diagnosis of hydatidiform moles. Current Diagnostic Pathology 1: 24–31

Patton P E 1994 Anatomic uterine defects. Clinical Obstetrics and Gynecology 37: 705–721

Petri M, Golbus M, Anderson R, Whiting-O'Keefe Q, Corash L, Hellmann D 1987 Antinuclear antibody, lupus anticoagulant, and anticardiolipin antibody in women with idiopathic habitual abortion. Arthritis and Rheumatism 30: 601–606

Philippe E 1973 Morphologie et morphometrie des placentas d'aberration chromosomique lethale. Reue Francaise de Gynecologie et d'Obstetrique 68: 645–653

Philippe E 1986 Pathologie foeto-placentaire. Masson, Paris

Philippe E, Boué J G 1969 Le placenta des aberations chromosomiques fétales. Annales d'Anatomie Pathologique 14: 249–266

Philippe E, Boué J G 1970 Placenta et aberrations chromosomiques au cours des avortements spontanés. Presse Médicale 78: 641–646

Philippe E, Ritter J, Dehalleux J M, Renaud R, Gandar R 1968 De la pathologie des avortements spontanés. Gynécologie et Obstétrique 67: 97–118

Pickering W, Marriott K, Regan L 2001 G20210A prothrombin gene mutation: prevalence in a recurrent miscarriage population. Clinical and Applied Thrombosis and Hemostasis 7: 25–28

Plouffe L, White E W, Tho S P et al 1992 Etiologic factors of recurrent abortion and subsequent reproductive performance of couples: have we made any progress in the past 10 years? American Journal of Obstetrics and Gynecology 167: 313–321

Pratt D, Novotny M, Kaberlein G, Dudkiewicz A, Gleicher N 1993 Antithyroid antibodies and the association with non-organ specific antibodies in recurrent pregnancy loss. American Journal of Obstetrics and Gynecology 168: 837–841

Preston F E, Rosendaal F R, Walker I D, Briet F, Berntorp E 1996 Increased fetal loss in women with heritable thrombophilia. Lancet 348: 913–916

Quinn M 1993 final report of the Medical Research Council/Royal College of Obstetricians and Gynaecologists multicentre randomised trial of cervical cerclage. British Journal of Obstetrics and Gynaecology 100: 1154–1155

Quinn P A, Petric M, Barkin M et al 1987 Prevalence of antibody to Chlamydia trachomatis in spontaneous abortion and infertility. American Journal of Obstetrics and Gynecology 156: 291–296

Qumsiyeh M B, Kim K R, Ahmed M N, Bradford W 2000 Cytogenetics and mechanisms of spontaneous abortions: increased apoptosis and decreased cell proliferation in chromosomally abnormal villi. Cytogenetics and Cell Genetics 88: 230–235

Rae R, Smith I W, Liston W A, Kilpatrick D C 1994 Chlamydial serologic studies and recurrent spontaneous abortion. American Journal of Obstetrics and Gynecology 170: 782–785

Rai R S, Regan L 1998 Antiphospholipid syndrome and pregnancy loss. Hospital Medicine 59: 637–639

Rai R S, Clifford K, Cohen H, Regan L 1995a High prospective fetal loss rate in untreated pregnancies of women with recurrent miscarriage and antiphospholipid antibodies. Human Reproduction 10: 3301–3304

Rai R S, Regan L, Clifford K et al 1995b Antiphospholipid antibodies and beta2-glcoprotein-I in 500 women with recurrent miscarriage: results of a comprehensive screening approach. Human Reproduction 10: 2001–2005

Rai R S, Regan L, Hadley E, Dave M, Cohen H 1996 Second-trimester pregnancy loss is associated with activated protein C resistance. British Journal of Haematology 92: 489–490

Rai R S, Backos M, Rushworth F, Regan L 2000 Polycystic ovaries and recurrent miscarriage — a reappraisal. Human Reproduction 15: 612–615

Rai R S, Shlebak A, Cohen H et al 2001 Factor V Leiden and acquired protein C resistance among 1000 women with recurrent miscarriage. Human Reproduction 16: 961–965

Rai R S, Backos M, Elgaddal S, Shlebak A, Regan L 2002 Factor V Leiden and recurrent miscarriage — a prospective outcome of untreated pregnancies. Human Reproduction 17: 101–104

Ray J G, Laskin C A 1999 Folic acid and homocystine metabolic defects and the risk of placental abruption, pre-eclampsia and spontaneous pregnancy loss: a systematic review. Placenta 20: 519–529

Raziel A, Kornberg Y, Friedler S, Schachter M, Sela B A, Ron-El R 2001 Hypercoagulable thrombophilic defects and hyperhomocysteinemia in patients with recurrent pregnancy loss. American Journal of Reproductive Immunology 45: 65–71

Regan L 1997 Sporadic and recurrent miscarriage. In: Grudzinskas J G, O'Brien P M S (eds) Problems in early pregnancy: advances in diagnosis and management. RCOG Press, London, pp 31–52

Regan L, Jivraj S 2001 Infection and pregnancy loss. In: MacLean A, Regan L, Carrington D (eds) Infection and pregnancy. RCOG Press, London, pp 291–304

Regan L, Owen E J, Jacobs H S 1990 Hypersecretion of luteinising hormone, infertility, and miscarriage. Lancet 336: 1141–1144

Rehder H, Coerdt W, Egger R, Klink F, Schwinger E 1989 Is there a correlation between morphological and cytogenetic findings in placental tissue from early missed abortions? Human Genetics 82: 377–385

Roberts C J, Lowe C R 1975 Where have all the conceptions gone? Lancet i: 498–499

Rockelein G, Schroder J, Ulmer R 1989 Korrelation von Karyotype und Plazentamorphologie beim Fruhabort. Pathologe 10: 306–314

Rockelein G, Ulmer R, Schroder J 1990a Karyotype and placental structure of first trimester spontaneous abortions; a morphometrical study. European Journal of Obstetrics, Gynecology and Reproductive Biology 38: 25–32

Rockelein G, Ulmer R, Schwille R 1990b Surface and branching of placental villi in early abortion: relationship to karyotype: scanning electron microscopic study. Virchows Archiv A. Pathological Anatomy and Histopathology 417: 151–158

Rushton D I 1981 Examination of products of conception from previable human pregnancies. Journal of Clinical Pathology 34: 819–835

Rushton D I 1984 The classification and mechanisms of spontaneous abortion. Perspectives in Pediatric Pathology 8: 269–287

Rushton D I 1988 Placental pathology in spontaneous miscarriage. In: Beard R W, Sharp F (eds) Early pregnancy loss: mechanisms and treatment. Springer-Verlag, London, pp 149–157

Rushworth F H, Backos M, Rai R, Chilcott I, Baxter N, Regan L 2000 Prospective pregnancy outcome in untreated recurrent miscarriers with thyroid autoantibodies. Human Reproduction 15: 1637–1639

Sagle M, Bishop K, Ridley N et al 1988 Recurrent early miscarriage and polycystic ovaries. British Medical Journal 297: 1027–1028

Salafia C M, Weigl C A, Foy G J 1988 Correlation of placental erythrocyte morphology with gestational age. Pediatric Pathology 8: 495–502

Salafia C, Maier D, Vogel C, Burns J, Silberman L 1993 Placental and decidual histology in spontaneous abortion: detailed description and correlations with chromosome number. Obstetrics and Gynecology 82: 295–303

Saller D N, Keene C L, Sun C-C J, Schwartz S 1990 The association of single umbilical artery with cytogenetically abnormal pregnancies. American Journal of Obstetrics and Gynecology 163: 922–925

Sanson B, Freidrich P W, Simioni P et al 1996 The risk of abortion and stillbirth in antithrombin-, protein C-, and protein S-deficient women. Thrombosis and Haemostasis 75: 387–388

Scott J S 1960 Placenta extrachorialis (placenta marginata and placenta circumvallata): a factor in antepartum haemorrhage. Journal of Obstetrics and Gynaecology of the British Empire 67: 904–918

Sebire N J, Fox H, Backos M, Rai R, Paterson C, Regan L 2002 Defective endovascular trophoblast invasion in primary antiphospholipid antibody syndrome-associated early pregnancy failure. Human Reproduction 17: 1067–1071

Shanklin D R, Scott J S 1975 Massive subchorial thrombohaematoma (Breus' mole). British Journal of Obstetrics and Gynaecology 82: 476–487

Silver R M, Branch D W 1994 Recurrent miscarriage: autoimmune considerations. Clinical Obstetrics and Gynecology 37: 745–760

Silverman M 1970 Psychological aspects of habitual abortion. Psychiatric Communications 13: 35–40

Simpson J L 1992 The aetiology of pregnancy failure. In: Stabile E, Grudzinskas G, Chard T (eds) Spontaneous abortion: diagnosis and treatment. Springer-Verlag, London, pp 21–47

Simpson J L, Bombard A T 1987 Chromosomal abnormalities in spontaneous abortions: frequency, pathology and genetic counselling. In: Edmonds K, Bennet M J (eds) Spontaneous abortion. Blackwell, London, pp 51–76

Simpson J L, Elias S, Martin A O 1981 Parental chromosomal rearrangements associated with repetitive spontaneous abortions. Fertility and Sterility 36: 584–590

Simpson J L, Gray R H, Queenan J T et al 1996 Further evidence that infection is an infrequent cause of first trimester spontaneous abortion. Human Reproduction 11: 2058–2060

Sorensen V J, Bivins B A, Obeid F N, Horst H M 1986 Trauma in pregnancy. Henry Ford Hospital Medical Journal 34: 101–104

Souza S S, Ferriani R A, Pontes A G, Zago M A, Franco R F 1999 Factor V leiden and factor II G20210A mutations in patients with recurrent abortion. Human Reproduction 14: 2448–2450

Stagnaro-Green A, Roman S H, Cobin R H, El-Harazy E, Alvarez-Marfany M, Davies T F 1990 Detection of at-risk pregnancy by means of highly sensitive assays for thyroid autoantibodies. Journal of the American Medical Association 264: 1422–1425

Sthoeger Z M, Mozes E, Tartakovsky B 1993 Anti-cardiolipin antibodies induce pregnancy failure by impairing embryonic implantation. Proceedings of the National Academy of Sciences USA 90: 6464–6467

Stein A L, March C M 1990 Pregnancy outcome in women with müllerian anomalies. Journal of Reproductive Medicine 35: 411–414

Stirrat G M 1990 Recurrent miscarriage. II Clinical associations, causes and management. Lancet 336: 728–733

Stirrat G M 1992 Recurrent spontaneous abortion. In: Coulam C B, Faulk W P, McIntyre J A (eds) Immunological obstetrics. Norton, New York, pp 357–376

Stray-Pederson B, Eng J, Reikvam T M 1978 Uterine T-mycoplasma colonization in reproductive failure. American Journal of Obstetrics and Gynecology 130: 307–311

Stray-Pederson B, Stray-Pederson S 1984 Etiologic factors and subsequent reproductive performance in 195 couples with a prior history of habitual abortion. American Journal of Obstetrics and Gynecology 148: 140–146

Summers P R 1994 Microbiology relevant to recurrent miscarriage. Clinical Obstetrics and Gynecology 37: 722–729

Suster S, Robinson M J 1992 Placental intravillous accumulation of sulphated mucosubstances: a reevaluation of so-called hydropic degeneration of the villi. Annals of Clinical and Laboratory Science 22: 175–181

Sweeney A M, Meyer M R, Aarons J H et al 1988 Evaluation of methods for the prospective identification of early fetal losses in environemental epidemiology studies. American Journal of Epidemiology: 127: 843–849

Szulman A E 1991 Examination of the early conceptus. Archives of Pathology and Laboratory Medicine 115: 696–700

Szulman A E 1995 Embryonic death: pathology and forensic implications. Perspectives in Pediatric Pathology 19: 43–58

Thomas J 1962 Die Entwicklung von Fetus und Placenta bei Nabelgefssanomalien. Archiv für Gynakologie 198: 216–223

Topalovski M, Hankin R C, Michael C et al 1995 Ploidy analysis of products of conception by image and flow cytometry with cytogenetic correlation. American Journal of Clinical Pathology 103: 409–414

Treffers P E 1990 Uterine causes of early pregnancy failure — a critical evaluation. In: Huisjes H J, Lind T (eds) Early pregnancy failure. Churchill Livingstone, Edinburgh, pp 114–147

Triplett D A 1992 Obstetrical complications associated with antiphospholipid antibodies. In: Coulam C B, Faulk W P, McIntyre J A (eds) Immunological obstetrics. Norton, New York, pp 377–403

van Lijnschoten G, Arends J W, De la Fuente A A, Schouten H J A, Geraedts J P M 1993a Intra- and inter-observer variation in the interpretation of histological features suggesting chromosomal abnormality in early abortion specimens. Histopathology 22: 25–29

van Lijnschoten G, Arends J W, Leffers P et al 1993b The value of histomorphological features of chorionic villi in early spontaneous abortion for the prediction of karotype. Histopathology 22: 557–563

van Oven M W, Schoots C J, Osterhuis J W et al 1989 The use of DNA flow cytometry in the diagnosis of triploidy in human abortions. Human Pathology 20: 238–242

Vaquero E, Lazzarin N, De Carolis C, Valensise H, Moretti C, Ramanini C 2000 Mild thyroid abnormalities and recurrent spontaneous abortion: diagnosis and therapeutical approach. American Journal of Reproductive Immunology 43: 204–208

Vinatier D, Dufour P, Cosson M, Houpeau J L 2001 Antiphospholipid syndrome and recurrent miscarriages. European Journal of Obstetrics, Gynecology and Reproductive Biology 96: 37–50

Wang B B T, Rubin C H, Williams J 1993 Mosaicism in chorionic villus sampling: an analysis of incidence and chromosomes involved in 2612 consecutive cases. Prenatal Diagnosis 13: 179–190

Warburton D, Stein Z, Kline J, Susser M 1980 Chromosome abnormalities in spontaneous abortions: data from the New York City study. In: Porter I H, Hook E B (eds) Human embryonic and fetal death. Academic Press, New York, pp 261–287

Ward K 2000 Inherited thrombophilias and placental thrombosis. In: Kingdom J C P, Jauniaux E R M, O'Brien P M S (eds) The placenta: basic science and clinical practice. RCOG Press, London, pp 133–143

Watson H, Kiddy D S, Hamilton-Fairley D et al 1993 Hypersecretion of luteinizing hormone and ovarian steroids in women with recurrent early miscarriage. Human Reproduction 8: 829–833

Wilcox A J, Weinberg C R, O'Connor J F et al 1988 Incidence of early loss of pregnancy. New England Journal of Medicine 319: 189–194

Witkin S S, Ledger W J 1992 Antibodies to *Chlamydia trachomatis* in sera of women with recurrent spontaneous abortions. American Journal of Obstetrics and Gynecology 167: 135–139

World Health Organization 1977 Recommended definitions, terminology and format for statistical tables related to the perinatal period. Acta Obstetricia et Gynecologica Scandinavica 56: 247–253

Wouters M G, Boers G H, Blom H J et al 1993 Hyperhomocysteinemia: a risk factor in women with unexplained recurrent early pregnancy loss. Fertility and Sterility 60: 820–825

Younis J S, Brenner B, Ohel G, Tal J, Lanir N, Ben-Ami M 2000 Activated protein C resistance and factor V Leiden mutation can be associated with first- as well as second-trimester recurrent pregnancy loss. American Journal of Reproductive Immunology 43: 31–35

Zaragoza M V, Surti U, Redline R W, Millie E, Chakravarti A, Hassold T J 2000 Parental origin and phenotype of triploidy in spontaneous abortions: predominance of diandry and association with the partial hydatidiform mole. American Journal of Human Genetics 66: 1807–1820

42

Non-trophoblastic tumours of the placenta

H. Fox

Introduction   1449

Primary non-trophoblastic tumours of the placenta   1449
Haemangioma   1449
Teratoma   1454
Hepatocellular adenoma   1455
Leiomyoma   1455

Placental metastases from maternal neoplasms   1455

Placental metastases from fetal neoplasms   1457

INTRODUCTION

Non-trophoblastic tumours of the placenta fall into three groups:

1. Tumours arising within the placenta
2. Metastatic deposits from a maternal neoplasm
3. Metastases from a fetal neoplasm.

PRIMARY NON-TROPHOBLASTIC TUMOURS OF THE PLACENTA

The only primary non-trophoblastic tumours of the placenta which have been convincingly described are the relatively common haemangioma, the extremely rare teratoma and the even rarer hepatocellular adenoma. Even these arouse some doubt as to their nosological status for the haemangioma is probably a hamartomatous malformation rather than a true neoplasm, whilst many believe that all apparent teratomas of the placenta are, in reality, examples of fetus acardius amorphus.

HAEMANGIOMA

Haemangiomas, also known as 'chorangiomas' or 'chorioangiomas', are relatively common and occur in approximately 1% of all placentas (Fox 1997). Placental haemangiomas are usually single but occasionally multiple, the apparent record being the 25 discrete tumours, each with its own pedicle, in the placenta described by Fisher (1940). Rarely, a placenta may be diffusely infiltrated by haemangiomatous tissue (Jaffe et al 1985; Angelone et al 1989), a condition known as chorangiomatosis.

Most placental haemangiomas are not visible on the external surface of the placenta: they are small and within the placental substance and hence are unlikely to be noticed unless the placenta is systematically sliced. These small intraplacental tumours are usually round and well demarcated from the surrounding normal villous tissue, often appearing encapsulated: their cut surface is smooth and firm and may be yellow, brown, tan, red or white. They often bear a superficial resemblance to an intervillous thrombus from which, however, they can be distinguished by their lack of lamination. Large haemangiomas, i.e. measuring more than 5 cm in diameter (Fig. 42.1), are rare and usually readily apparent on naked-eye examination of the intact placenta; they are seen most commonly as bulging protuberances on the fetal surface but a minority occur on the maternal aspect where they may appear to replace the whole, or part, of a lobe. Occasionally a haemangioma is situated entirely within the membranes and is attached to the placenta only by a vascular pedicle. These large haemangiomas usually have a purplish-red, glistening, encapsulated, smooth or bosselated outer surface which is sometimes deeply grooved by bands of fibrous tissue; they may be round, ovoid or reniform and on section appear highly vascular.

Histologically, most placental haemangiomas have a microscopic appearance similar to that seen in haemangiomas elsewhere in the body, with numerous blood vessels set in a loose, scanty, fibrous stroma (Fig. 42.2); the vessels are usually small and of capillary size but may be markedly dilated to give a cavernous appearance. Sometimes, however, there is a predominance of the stromal component (Fig. 42.3) with only a few ill-formed vessels set in abundant loose, immature, cellular mesenchymal tissue. Degenerative changes, such as necrosis, calcification, myxoid change, hyalinisation or even fat accumulation (Reddy et al 1969), may complicate and confuse the histological picture. This variation in histological pattern is often used as a basis for classifying

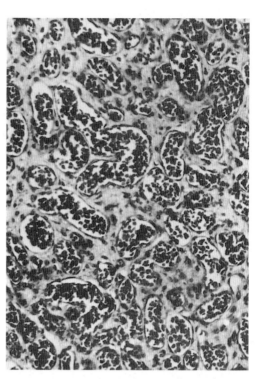

Fig. 42.2 Histological appearances of a placental haemangioma which is showing a typical 'angiomatous' pattern. (From H Fox 1997 *Pathology of the placenta* by courtesy of W B Saunders.)

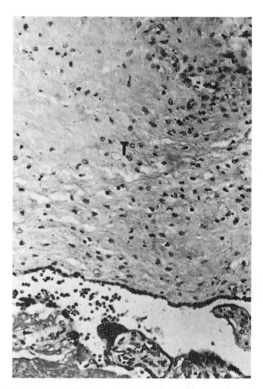

Fig. 42.3 A placental haemangioma (above) which shows a 'cellular' pattern and is formed largely of loose, mesenchymal tissue. Elsewhere there was a transition to a more typical 'angiomatous' pattern (see Fig. 42.4). (From H Fox 1997 *Pathology of the placenta* by courtesy of W B Saunders.)

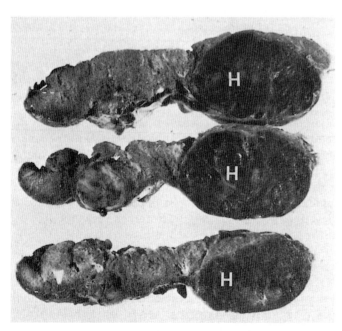

Fig. 42.1 A large haemangioma (H) in a placenta. (From *Pathology of the placenta* by courtesy of the Editor, Dr E V D K Perrin.)

placental haemangiomas into 'angiomatous', 'cellular' and 'degenerate' types (Marchetti 1939). This histological classification is useful for descriptive purposes but is basically a false subdivision for the cellular type is simply a less mature and less differentiated form of the angiomatous variety. Furthermore many haemangiomas show a variable picture, being cellular in some areas and angiomatous in others, often with a gradual transition between the two histological patterns (Fig. 42.4). Most haemangiomas do, however, show a predominantly angiomatous appearance and thus present little in the way of diagnostic difficulty, though those rare tumours which have a cellular pattern throughout have occasionally been misdiagnosed as fibromas, myxomas or leiomyomas.

Mitotic figures are occasionally seen in placental haemangiomas and very rarely these are fairly numerous and associated with some degree of endothelial or stromal cell atypia. Such findings have sometimes led to a diagnosis of sarcoma (Ahrens 1953) but no placental haemangioma has ever behaved in a malignant fashion: it has nevertheless been suggested that such tumours be regarded as 'atypical' haemangiomas (Majlessi et al 1983; Mesia et al 1999) and this is probably a prudent form of terminology.

In most instances a haemangioma has a distinct capsule of either fibrous tissue or attenuated syncytiotrophoblast (Fig. 42.5) but occasionally there is only a pseudocapsule of compressed villous tissue. Two very unusual, and conceptually challenging, placental tumours

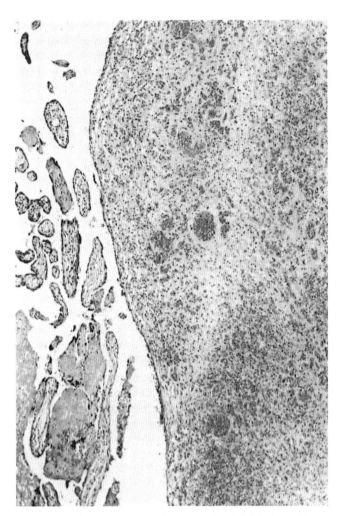

Fig. 42.5 A placental haemangioma (on the right) is limited by a distinct capsule of attenuated syncytiotrophoblast. (From *Pathology of the placenta* by courtesy of the Editor, Dr E V D K Perrin.)

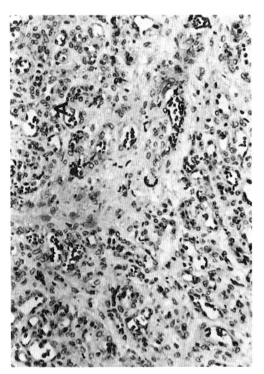

Fig. 42.4 Another area of the placental haemangioma shown in Fig. 42.3: here there is a transition from a 'cellular' to an 'angiomatous' pattern. (From H Fox 1997 *Pathology of the placenta* by courtesy of W B Saunders.)

have been described by Jauniaux et al (1988) and Trask et al (1994). Both of these were typical haemangiomas but with a surrounding mantle of atypical proliferating trophoblast which closely resembled choriocarcinomatous tissue. These neoplasms were classed as 'chorangiocarcinomas' but Khong (2000) has claimed that capsular trophoblastic proliferation with nuclear atypia is quite a common phenomenon in placental haemangiomas and considered that such tumours should simply be classed as 'haemangiomas with trophoblastic proliferation': certainly there has been no evidence of persistent trophoblatic disease in any of these cases.

Chorangiomatosis, in which multiple nodules of angiomatous tissue are scattered throughout the placental substance (Fig. 42.6), should be distinguished from 'chorangiosis', a condition in which a significant proportion of the villi contain an excess of fetal vessels (Altshuler 1984). In a number of reports in the literature chorangiosis has been incorrectly used as a synonym for chorangiomatosis whilst it has often been mooted that chorangiosis forms

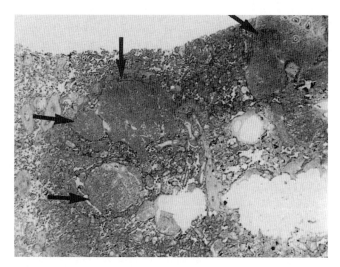

Fig. 42.6 Multiple nodules of haemangiomatous tissue (arrowed) in the substance of a placenta. (From H Fox 1997 *Pathology of the placenta* by courtesy of W B Saunders.)

a link between normal villi and a haemangioma (Benirschke 1999). The concept of chorangiosis, which is defined as 10 or more villi in 10 fields, viewed under a × 10 objective, containing 10 or more fetal vessels has been subjected to criticism but nevertheless appears to be valid: there is, however, no evidence that chorangiosis is a transitional phase in the development, or a forme fruste, of chorangiomatosis.

Associated changes

Placentas containing a haemangioma are usually otherwise normal but a small proportion are unduly heavy, sometimes weighing, after removal of the tumour, over 1000 g (Sen 1970; Potashnik et al 1973). The cause of this placentomegaly is obscure but occasional placentas containing a haemangioma are notably oedematous.

A unique example of a coexistent haemangioma and a hydatidiform mole has been reported (Vermelin et al 1957), a combination which is rather curious in view of the avascularity of a mole. Two placentas have been described in which there was a coexistence of a haemangioma and the findings characteristic of placental mesenchymal dysplasia (Chen et al 1997). One placental haemangioma has been associated with bilateral ovarian theca-lutein cysts (King et al 1991), a somewhat surprising finding because there is no evidence that placental haemangiomas secrete hCG.

Nature and origin

The angiomatous nature of these tumours has been fully confirmed by electronmicroscopic and immunohistochemical studies (Kim et al 1971; Cash & Powell 1980) but it is still a matter of dispute as to whether they are true neoplasms or hamartomas. The occasional presence

of mitotic figures and the frequent evidence of disproportionate growth between the haemangioma and the rest of the placenta have persuaded some that they are true neoplasms but it is probably a majority opinion that haemangiomas are hamartomas which arise as a malformation of the primitive angioblastic tissue of the placenta, i.e. the chorionic mesenchyme. The appearances of the cellular type of placental haemangioma mimic closely those seen in a primary villous stem during the stage of angiogenesis and it is indeed probable that haemangiomas arise as a result of distorted angiogenesis within a single primary villous stem, a view fully supported by an immunohistochemical study of their cytoskeletal profile (Lifschitz-Mercer et al 1989). This hypothesis implies that haemangiomas arise during the early stages of placental development and it has therefore to be admitted that haemangiomas have never been observed in placentas from first-trimester miscarriages or terminations, being apparently confined to second- and third-trimester placentas. Chorangiomas occur with unusual frequency in pregnancies at high altitude (Reshetnikova et al 1996; Benirschke 1999) and this may indicate that reduced oxygen levels have some effect on vascular growth factors.

Clinical effects

Most placental haemangiomas are of no clinical importance but those measuring more than 5 cm in diameter may be associated with a variety of complications which can affect the mother, the developing fetus or the neonate. It has been claimed that some haemangiomas of smaller size may be clinically important (Mucitelli et al 1990) but this remains to be confirmed by further studies.

Complications during pregnancy

A high proportion of large haemangiomas are accompanied by polyhydramnios, the reported incidence of this association ranging from 16–33% (Fox 1997). The development of polyhydramnios is clearly related to the size of the haemangioma for there have been no convincing reports of polyhydramnios complicating haemangiomas measuring less than 5 cm in diameter. The excess of fluid is independent of associated fetal abnormalities and is of obscure cause but it is not due to compression of the umbilical veins or to transudation from vessels on the fetal surface of the haemangioma (Fox 1997). McInroy & Kelsey (1954) put forward the ingenious view that the polyhydramnios was a result of an increased excretion of fetal urine, the stimulus for this being the return to the fetus of waste products in blood which had bypassed the placenta by circulating through the functionally inactive haemangioma. Wallenburg (1971) has raised the possibility that the excess of amniotic fluid is due to a fluid imbalance consequent upon fetal congestive cardiac failure, this is turn being secondary to the haemangioma acting as a peripheral arteriovenous shunt. Which, if any, of these theories is correct is a matter for conjecture but it is worth pointing out that a few haemangiomas have been accompanied by oligohydramnios (Engel et al 1981), the cause of this being even more cryptic.

Antepartum bleeding may occasionally complicate a placental haemangioma, either as a result of retroplacental haemorrhage from a tumour on the maternal aspect of the placenta or as a consequence of rupture of the vascular pedicle of a pedunculated tumour, a catastrophe that may lead to fetal exsanguination. It has been suggested that there may be an association between placental haemangioma and abruptio placentae which is independent of bleeding from the tumour and is due to increased stress being brought to bear on the uteroplacental vasculature by altered haemodynamics in the intervillous space (Kohler et al 1976), but this remains to be proven. There have also been recurrent claims for an association between placental haemangioma and an increased incidence of pre-eclampsia but the evidence for this is unconvincing.

It is often thought that placental haemangiomas predispose to premature onset of labour and, indeed, in many series almost a third of pregnancies have terminated prematurely; nearly always, however, this is due to labour being precipitated by polyhydramnios, and pregnancies not complicated by an excess of liquor usually proceed to term (Wallenburg 1971; Fox 1997).

It should be noted that placental haemangiomas, especially those large enough to be of possible clinical significance, can now be readily diagnosed by ultrasound (Spirt et al 1980; O'Malley et al 1981; Liang et al 1982; Scharl & Shlensker 1987), even as early as the 19th week of gestation (Nahmanovici et al 1982); furthermore, a placental haemangioma may be associated with elevated levels of alpha-fetoprotein either only in the maternal blood (Mann et al 1983; Kapoor et al 1989; Franca-Martins et al 1990; Thomas & Blakemore 1990) or in both maternal blood and amniotic fluid (Schnitger et al 1980). Elevation of alpha-fetoprotein levels is, however, by no means a constant finding and is indeed present in only a minority of cases (Khong & George 1994).

Complications during labour

There have been exceptional instances in which a very large placental haemangioma has obstructed vaginal delivery whilst on rare occasions the tumour may become detached from the placenta during labour and either passed separately per vaginam or retained in utero after expulsion of the placenta with subsequent subinvolution and postpartum bleeding.

Complications affecting the fetus and neonate

The overall mortality in cases of placental haemangioma is only minimally increased (Fox 1997) and this slight excess of deaths is confined to those rare cases in which there is either a very large tumour or multiple tumours in the placenta. Intrauterine fetal distress and death can occur in such cases and have been generally ascribed to hypoxia consequent upon fetal blood passing through the physiological dead space of the tumour and thus being returned to the fetus in an oxygen-depleted state (Ito et al 1994). Fetal death can be due, however, to cardiac failure as a consequence of the haemangioma acting as a peripheral arteriovenous shunt (Knoth et al 1976) or to compression of the cord by an unusually bulky tumour (Rodan & Bean 1983).

The liveborn infant whose placenta contains a haemangioma is usually normal though a few, again those with large or multiple tumours, are small for gestational age (King & Lourien 1978), this growth deficit being also attributed to bypassing of the functional placental tissue by fetal blood which is shunted through the tumour and returned to the fetus in a nutrient-poor state.

There is some dispute as to whether placental haemangiomas are associated with an excess of fetal malformations (Glaser et al 1988). There does certainly appear to be a rather high incidence of skin angiomas in infants whose placenta contained a haemangioma (Froehlich et al 1971; Leblanc & Carrier 1979) but whilst in some studies there has not been an increased incidence of any other form of malformation in others there was a remarkably high incidence of congenital abnormalities (15%), albeit all of a rather trivial nature (Froehlich et al 1971). Examples have been reported of placental haemangiomas occurring, probably coincidentally, in association with the Beckwith–Wiedemann (Drut et al 1992) and the Wolf–Hirschhorn (Verloes et al 1991; Ulrich et al 1999) syndromes.

The newborn infant whose placenta contains a large mass of haemangiomatous tissue is subject to a number of complications, usually of a transitory nature, which are thought to be a direct consequence of the placental tumour (Fox 1997). Prominent amongst these is transient cardiomegaly (Tonkin et al 1980; Eldar-Geva et al 1988; Nuttinen et al 1988; Ito et al 1994) which is probably due to the increased cardiac output required for shunting blood through the haemangioma which can, in haemodynamic terms, be considered as a peripheral arteriovenous shunt. Neonatal oedema is uncommon and in some cases is a manifestation of cardiac failure (Eldar-Geva et al 1988; Imakita et al 1988; Nuttinen et al 1988; Koivu & Nuttinen 1990): in others, however, it is a consequence of neonatal hypoalbuminaemia (Sweet & Robertson 1973), a deficiency which may be due either to transudation of protein from the vessels of the tumour or to chronic feto-maternal bleeding (Vettenranta et al 1987). Large haemangiomata may be associated with neonatal anaemia and Du et al (1968) suggested that this is a result of sequestration of blood within the haemangioma but the anaemia can also be due to a massive feto-maternal haemorrhage (Sims et al 1976; Stiller & Skafish 1986; Santamaria et al 1987) or to a microangiopathic haemolytic anaemia following injury inflicted on fetal red cells as they traverse the labyrinthine vascular channels of the tumour (Bauer et al 1978). The infrequently encountered neonatal thrombocytopenia has been attributed to platelet injury within the tumour vessels (Du et al 1968) but can also be a manifestation of disseminated intravascular coagulation triggered off by a thromboplastic substance released from the haemangioma (Jones et al 1972; Jaffe et al 1985): neonatal thrombocytopenia due to a placental haemangioma has led to fatal intracranial haemorrhage (Lopez-Herce Cid et al 1983).

Recurrence

Very little is known about the possibility of recurrence of placental haemangiomas in successive pregnancies but Ludighausen & Sahiri (1983) have described a case in which multiple large haemangiomas were present in the placenta of a woman's first and third pregnancies, both of which resulted in intrauterine fetal death; her second pregnancy was uncomplicated by placental haemangiomas and resulted in a live child. Chan & Leung (1988) have reported a not dissimilar patient who, in successive pregnancies, had a placenta containing multiple haemangiomas, these being associated in both gestations with intrauterine fetal death.

TERATOMA

Placental teratomas are rare: up to 1994 only 17 examples had been reported (Fox 1997) and only a few subsequent cases have since been described (Jaswal et al 1995; Wang et al 1995; Koumantakis et al 1996; Shimojo et al 1996; Elagoz et al 1998; Meinhard et al 1999; Gillet et al 2001). These tumours always lie between the amnion and chorion, usually on the fetal surface of the placenta but sometimes within the membranes at the placental margin (Fig. 42.7): they are smooth, round or oval and their diameter ranges from 2.5 to 7.5 cm. The tumour has no umbilical cord and receives its blood supply from a branch of the fetal artery on the surface of the placenta. All reported placental teratomas have been solid throughout and have contained a melange of squamous epithelium, skin appendages, gastrointestinal epithelium, fat, muscle, thyroid tissue, neural tissue and mesenchyme: these tissues have always been mature and no example of an immature teratoma of the placenta has been described.

Not everyone agrees, however, that placental teratomas exist and some argue that all such apparent tumours are examples of fetus acardius amorphus (Smith & Pounder 1982). It has been suggested that a distinction can be drawn between these two conditions (Fox & Butler-Manuel 1964) on the following grounds:

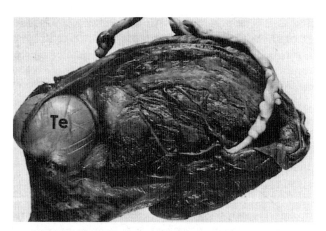

Fig. 42.7 A placental teratoma (Te) which is situated in the membranes adjacent to the main placental mass. The teratoma did not have an umbilical cord, showed no evidence of axial organisation and contained skin, neural tissue, fat, cartilage and bone. (From H Fox *Pathology of the placenta* 1997 by courtesy of W B Saunders.)

1. A fetus acardius amorphus has a separate umbilical cord which is attached either to the placenta of its twin or to a separate placenta: such a cord may be poorly developed or rudimentary. By contrast a teratoma does not have a cord and is vascularised by a branch of a fetal artery on the placental surface.
2. It is usual to regard a fetus acardius amorphus as being totally disorganised but in fact a complete failure of organisation is very unusual and in most cases central skeletal development is apparent with partial or complete formation of a vertebral column. This degree of organisation is not seen in a teratoma, in which any bone present is usually totally disorganised.

These distinguishing criteria have, however, been criticised by Stephens et al (1989), who claimed, in particular, that lack of an umbilical cord does not help in the distinction between a teratoma and a fetus amorphus. These authors do allow that the extent of skeletal development is a more valid criterion but nevertheless come to the conceptually nihilistic conclusion that distinction of a placental teratoma from a fetus amorphus is meaningless.

At first sight it seems difficult to explain the histogenesis of placental teratomas but it is possible that they are derived from germ cells which migrate out from the evagination of primitive gut which is always present in the umbilical cord during the early stages of embryogenesis. Such germ cells could be arrested in the connective tissue of the cord and could give rise to a teratoma of the cord. If, however, they continue their migration they will pass into the loose connective tissue between the amnion and the fetal surface of the placenta and could then continue into the extraplacental membranes between amnion and chorion. All the placental teratomas which have been described have developed along the line of this proposed route of aberrant migration of germ cells.

Placental teratomas are of no clinical significance except for their ability to produce a puzzling image on radiological or ultrasonic examination (Fox & Butler-Manuel 1964; Williams & Williams 1994).

HEPATOCELLULAR ADENOMA

A few placental tumours of this type have been described (Chen et al 1986; Khalifa et al 1998; Vesoulis & Agamanolis 1998; Dargent et al 2000). The lesion described by Chen et al (1986) measured 7 cm in diameter but the remainder have had a diameter of 1 cm or less: the tumours appear as rounded tan or dark red nodules either in the placental parenchyma or in a sub-chorionic site. Histologically, these tumours were formed of lobulated cords and nests of polygonal cells resembling fetal liver: the cells branched in a semi-trabecular fashion with intervening endothelium-lined spaces. Portal tracts, bile ducts, central veins and bile pigment were absent but extramedullary haematopoiesis was seen. It is probable that these tumours, if they are indeed tumours, arise from displaced yolk sac elements and they do not appear to have any clinical significance.

LEIOMYOMA

Two intraplacental smooth muscle tumours have been described (Tapia et al 1985; Ernst et al 2001). It is highly probable that these were, in reality, myometrial or endometrial leiomyomas that had become incidentally incorporated into the placenta and, indeed, in the case described by Ernst et al it was clearly shown by genetic studies that the neoplasm was of maternal rather than fetal origin.

PLACENTAL METASTASES FROM MATERNAL NEOPLASMS

Malignant disease in a pregnant woman, although uncommon, is by no means rare: nevertheless, there have been fewer than 60 reports of metastasis of a solid, non-lymphomatous maternal neoplasm to the placenta (Fox 1997), this possibly bearing greater witness to the infrequency of pathological examination of the placenta than to the rarity of placental involvement in disseminated maternal malignant disease. By far the commonest maternal neoplasm to involve the placenta is malignant melanoma which accounts for approximately half of the reported cases of placental metastatic disease. This predominance of malignant melanoma is not, however, surprising for tumour spread to the placenta occurs only by the bloodstream and only in patients with widely disseminated neoplastic disease: these criteria are exactly met by many cases of malignant melanoma, a neoplasm which, further, is not uncommon in relatively young women of reproductive age. Next in frequency to malignant melanoma are carcinomas of the breast and bronchus, this being probably a reflection not only of the high incidence of these neoplasms but also of their tendency to spread by the bloodstream at an early stage. There have been remarkably few instances of gastrointestinal neoplasms which have metastasised to the placenta whilst there has been only one report of cervical carcinoma involving the placenta (Cailliez et al 1980); this latter deficiency is particularly striking in view of the fact that cervical neoplasms are amongst the commonest tumours to complicate pregnancy but one which is probably explicable by the tendency of cervical carcinomas to spread principally by the lymphatic, rather than the vascular, route. There have been two instances of placental metastases from a medulloblastoma (Pollack et al 1993b; Brossard et al 1994) and one from a primitive neuroectodermal tumour (Sakurai et al 1998). The only well-documented maternal sarcomas which have metastasised to the placenta have been a vaginal angiosarcoma (Frick et al 1997), a Ewing's sarcoma of bone (Greenberg et al 1982), an orbital rhabdomyosarcoma (O'Day et al 1994) and an angiosarcoma of the breast (Sedgely et al 1985). Two cases of endometrial stromal sarcoma involving the placenta have been described (Katsanis et al 1998) but these were examples of direct spread of the uterine tumour to the decidua rather than real metastases.

Placentas involved by a malignant melanoma are often, though not invariably, macroscopically abnormal: tumour deposits may be visible as black or brown nodules of varying size within the placental substance though the deposits may appear white, and can be mistaken for infarcts, if the melanoma is of the amelanotic variety. Not uncommonly the placenta is generally rather firm and has a brown or grey tinge. Histologically, malignant melanoma cells are seen as clumps or sheets within the intervillous space (Fig. 42.8): central necrosis is not uncommon in large masses of tumour cells and it should be noted that, to the unwary eye, the neoplastic cells may be mistaken for proliferating cytotrophoblast (Fig. 42.9). Invasion of the villi by melanoma cells is an inconstant finding, the villi often being enveloped by tumour cells without any obvious tissue invasion (Fig. 42.10): nevertheless, infiltration of the villous stroma, and sometimes the fetal villous vessels, has been noted in approximately half of the reported cases. The villous Hofbauer cells often contain abundant melanin pigment, this occurring independently of the villous invasion by malignant cells and being responsible for the generalised discoloration of the placenta.

Placentas containing metastatic deposits of non-melanotic neoplasms often appear normal to the naked eye, visible tumour deposits being present in only about a third of cases; the tumour nodules may be of pin-head size only but can attain a diameter of 2 cm. Histologically, sheets of neoplastic cells are seen in the intervillous space (Fig. 42.11); villous or fetal vascular invasion is uncommon.

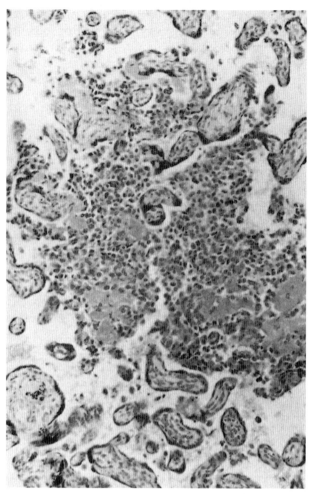

Fig. 42.8 Sheet-like masses of metastatic malignant melanoma cells in the intervillous space. (From *Pathology of the placenta* by courtesy of the Editor, Dr E V D K Perrin. Sections kindly supplied by Dr P Russell, Sydney.)

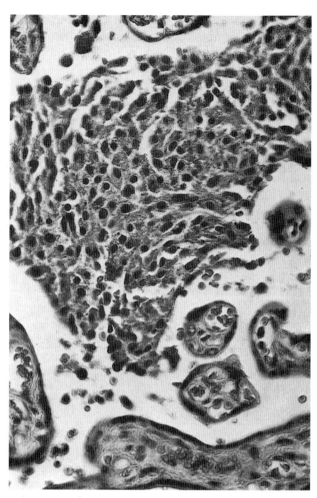

Fig. 42.9 A higher-power view of a placental metastasis from a cutaneous malignant melanoma. The malignant cells are forming sheets within the intervillous space. (From H Fox 1997 *Pathology of the placenta* by courtesy of W B Saunders.)

The presence of malignant cells within the intervillous space is usually classed as a placental 'metastasis' but it should be noted that the tumour cells are still within the maternal vascular system and are often not obviously invading placental tissue: this has led some to decry the use of the term 'metastasis' in this context and to regard the presence of intervillous tumour cells as simply a sequestration effect. Nevertheless, the large sheets of malignant cells found in the intervillous space in many instances do suggest that tumour growth is occurring in this intravascular site and that the cells must have a point of contact with placental structures. The reasons for the common failure of neoplastic cells in the intervillous space to invade villous tissue are, however, far from clear. Possibly the trophoblast simply acts as a physical or mechanical barrier though it has often been suggested that the fetal tissue of the placenta rejects the antigenically alien maternal tumour cells by an immunological reaction; proponents of this latter view have, however, not usually remarked on the lack of immunocompetent cells in the villi which are resisting attack.

Whatever the true nature of the placental 'barrier' may be, it is clearly not always inviolate for, as already noted, it is breached in a proportion of cases with resulting malignant infiltration of the villous stroma and, occasionally, of the fetal villous vessels. Indeed malignant cells can pass over into the fetus though, despite some claims to the contrary, there have been only three fully documented and definite cases of transplacental spread of a maternal neoplasm to the fetus, both being malignant melanomas. The child described both by Weber et al (1930) and by Holland (1949) died at 8 months of age whilst the infant reported by Brodsky et al (1963) died after 48 days of life; widespread deposits of malignant melanoma were present in both children and it is of particular interest that in both cases malignant cells had been seen in the fetal vessels of the placenta. In a recently reported case hepatic and pulmonary metastases developed in a five-month-old child whose mother had a bronchial carcinoma (Tolar et al 2002). It cannot be assumed, however, that the mere presence of tumour cells within fetal vessels is absolute proof of spread to the

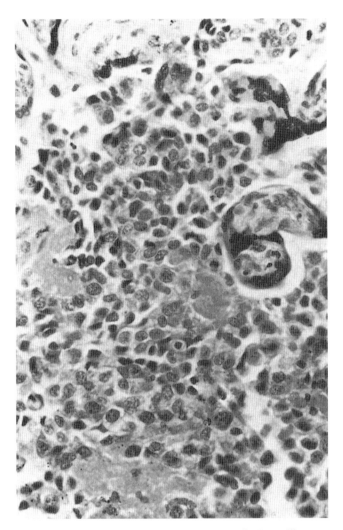

Fig. 42.10 Metastatic malignant melanoma in the intervillous space. The neoplastic cells surround, but do not invade, a villus. (Courtesy of Dr P Russell, Sydney.)

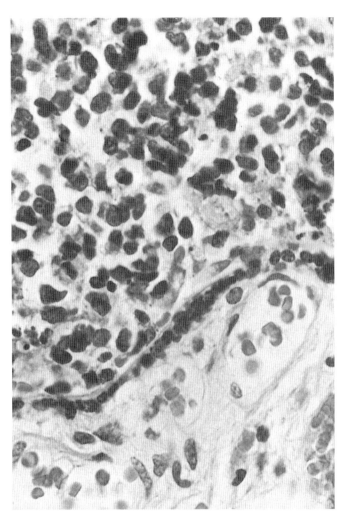

Fig. 42.11 A metastatic deposit of Ewing's sarcoma in the intervillous space adjacent to an intact villus. (From Greenberg et al 1982. Courtesy of Dr P Greenberg and W B Saunders.)

fetus for in a number of cases in which this phenomenon has been noted there has been no subsequent evidence of neoplastic disease in the infant.

There have been five well-documented reports of placental involvement by maternal malignant lymphoma (Kurtin et al 1992; Pollack et al 1993a; Tsujimura et al 1993; Meguerian-Bedoyan et al 1997; Nishi et al 2000) all these being non-Hodgkins lymphomas, and there have been a few scattered reports of spread of leukaemic cells to the placenta in women suffering from acute or subacute leukaemia during pregnancy (Bierman et al 1956; Rigby et al 1964; Nummi et al 1973; Honoré & Brown 1990), the leukaemic cells being confined to the intervillous space (Fig. 42.12) where they have usually appeared as groups, sheets or clumps. There must, however, be some scepticism about the validity of the term 'placental involvement' in cases of leukaemia: clearly, if the mother has an extremely high peripheral white count many leukaemic cells will be seen in the maternal blood in the intervillous space and such a finding alone does not mean

that the placenta is 'involved' in the malignant process: such an involvement should only be considered if large clumps or sheets of leukaemic cells are seen.

No instance of villous involvement by leukaemic cells has ever been reported. Some light has possibly been shed on this phenomenon by a study of a placenta from a woman with acute lymphoblastic leukaemia in which phagocytosis and destruction of tumour cells within the villous trophoblast was clearly demonstrable on electron-microscopic examination (Wang et al 1983). Whether this remarkable finding is confined to leukaemic cells or is typical of a more generalised trophoblastic response to neoplastic cells awaits further elucidation.

PLACENTAL METASTASES FROM FETAL NEOPLASMS

Dissemination of a malignant fetal neoplasm to the placenta is extremely uncommon though it is probable that

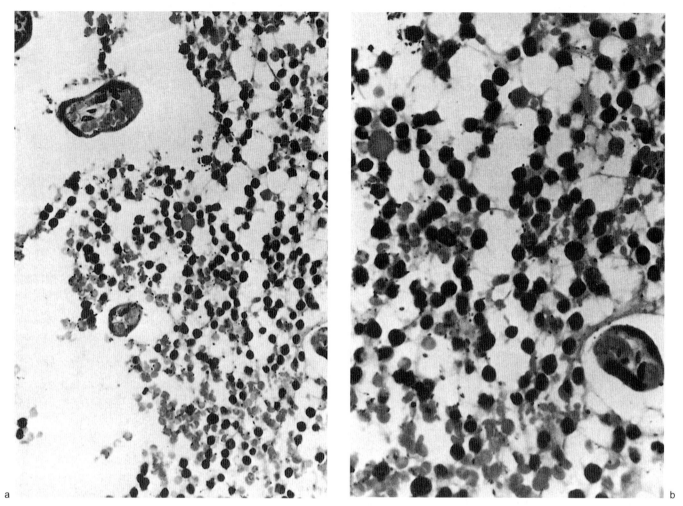

a   b

Fig. 42.12 a Leukaemic cells in the intervillous space of a placenta from a woman suffering from acute leukaemia. **b** Higher-power view of part of the field shown in a. (Courtesy of Professor D Jenkins, Cork.)

the apparent rarity of this phenomenon has been accentuated by the fact that most congenital tumours are not clinically apparent at birth and by the infrequency with which placentas are submitted to routine histological examination.

The fetal neoplasm which has attracted most attention has been the neuroblastoma and there have been approximately a dozen well-documented reports of placental involvement by such a tumour (Strauss & Driscoll 1964; Anders et al 1970; Hustin & Chef 1972; Jurkovic et al 1973; Johnson & Halbert 1974; Perkins et al 1980; Stovring 1980; van der Slikke & Balk 1980; Smith et al 1981; Mutz & Sterling 1991; Lynn et al 1997; Ohyhama et al 1999). The descriptions given of the gross and microscopic features of the placentas in these cases have been strikingly uniform for all were bulky, pale, oedematous and heavy (commonly weighing over 1000 g) and all bore a close resemblance to the hydropic placenta of severe erythroblastosis fetalis. Tumour deposits were not macroscopically visible in any case and the detection of neoplastic involvement was dependent upon histological examination. Microscopy revealed plugging of the fetal stem and villous vessels (Figs 42.13, 42.14) by clumps and nests of

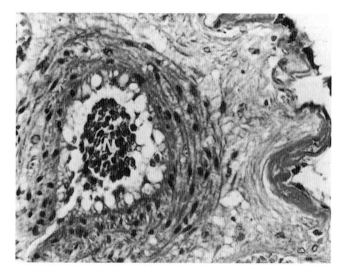

Fig. 42.13 A fetal stem artery in a placenta from a fetus with a widely metastasising thoracic neuroblastoma. The arterial lumen is plugged by a clump of neuroblastomatous cells. (Photograph kindly supplied by Dr I Jurkovic, Czechoslovakia, and reprinted from H Fox 1997 *Pathology of the placenta* by courtesy of W B Saunders.)

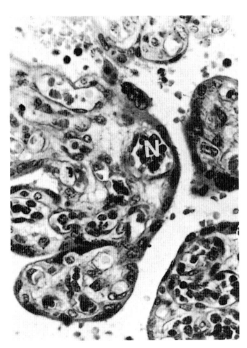

Fig. 42.14 Villi from the placenta illustrated in Fig. 42.13. Many of the fetal villous vessels contain groups of neuroblastoma cells. (Photograph kindly supplied by Dr I Jurkovic, Czechoslovakia, and reprinted from H Fox 1997 *Pathology of the placenta* by courtesy of W B Saunders.)

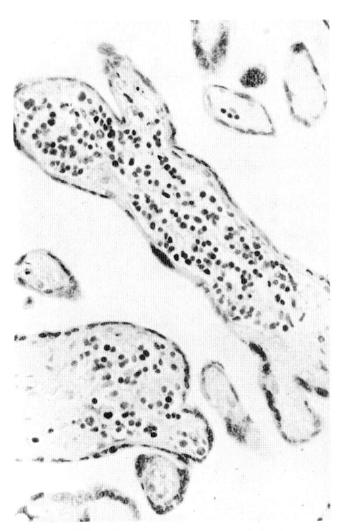

Fig. 42.15 Villi in a placenta containing metastatic fetal neuroblastoma. The neoplastic cells have broken out from the fetal vessels and are infiltrating the villous stroma. (Section kindly supplied by Dr D Haust, London, Ontario, and reprinted from *Pathology of the placenta* by courtesy of the Editor, Dr E V D K Perrin.)

neuroblastomatous cells, the extent of fetal vascular invasion being, however, very variable. In some placentas the tumour cells were widely disseminated throughout the fetal vasculature and were, in one case, seen in every villus (Strauss & Driscoll 1964); more commonly, neoplastic cells were seen within the fetal vessels in at least one villus per low power field. In only one case (Fig. 42.15) have neuroblastomatous cells extended out from the fetal vessels to invade the villous stroma (Perkins et al 1980).

The villi in the involved placentas are usually large, immature and oedematous with, sometimes, a proliferation of villous stromal mesenchymal cells; these villous abnormalities are present both in villi vascularised by tumour-containing vessels and in villi free of neoplastic cells.

It is not clear whether the failure, in most cases, of the neuroblastomatous cells to penetrate into the villous stroma is due to mechanical or immunological factors. Strauss & Driscoll (1964) thought that an immunological defence mechanism of some type was involved, basing this view on the resemblance of these placentas to those seen in severe materno-fetal rhesus incompatibility and on their finding, in one case, of nuclear debris in the perivascular villous stroma. The validity or otherwise of this concept is currently an imponderable but the placental abnormalities are certainly not due solely to the presence of neoplastic cells, for identical villous abnormalities have been observed in a placenta from a baby with congenital neuroblastoma which had not spread to involve the placenta (Birner 1961). This observation

lends credence to the view that placental oedema and bulkiness is due simply to mechanical obstruction of placental venous return by a large fetal intra-abdominal mass.

There have been two instances of a fetal hepatoblastoma metastasising to the placenta (Robinson & Rolande 1985; Doss et al 1998) and one report of placental metastases from a congenital primitive epithelial liver tumour (Ohyama et al 2000). Fetal malignant melanoma, arising in a giant melanocytic naevus, has also metastasised to the placenta (Schneiderman et al 1987): the placenta in the latter case was extremely bulky and malignant melanoma cells were present both within the fetal villous vessels and within the stroma of the villi. Nests, or aggregates, of intravillous naevus cells have also been described in placentas from fetuses with benign giant skin naevi (Holaday & Castrow 1968; Werner 1972; Demian et al 1974; Sotelo-Avila et al

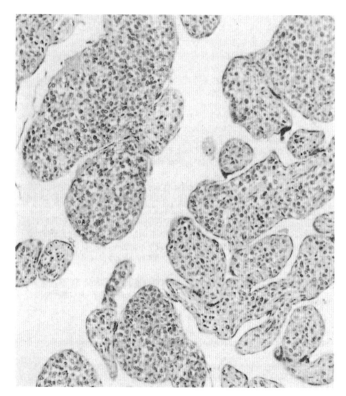

Fig. 42.16 Placental villi from a case of fetal leukaemia. Villous vessels and stroma contain numerous leukaemic cells. (From *Pathology of the placenta* by courtesy of the Editor, Dr E V D K Perrin.)

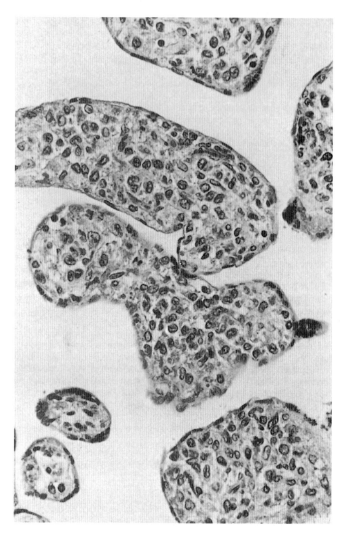

Fig. 42.17 Higher-power view of placenta shown in Fig. 42.16. Leukaemic cells are present in both vessels and stroma of the villi. (From *Pathology of the placenta* by courtesy of the Editor, Dr E V D K Perrin.)

1988; Jauniaux et al 1993; Antaya et al 1995; Ball et al 1998) and have usually been described as 'metastases': it is, however, more probable that the naevus cell aggregates represent aberrant migration of neural crest elements in early gestation.

A few examples of placental involvement in fetal leukaemia have been reported (Las Heras et al 1980; Gray et al 1986). In these cases leukaemic cells have been present in the fetal villous vessels and usually, though not invariably, in the villous stroma (Figs 42.16, 42.17). Placentas involved in fetal leukaemia are usually unduly bulky and oedematous.

A single case of a fetal lymphoma involving the placenta, and indeed apparently confined to the placenta, has been described (Fritsch et al 1999). There was an infiltrate of the villi by a monoclonal population of B cells which was proven genetically to be of fetal origin.

REFERENCES

Ahrens C A 1953 Vier Falle von Plazentatumoren. Zeitschrift fur allgemeinen Pathologie und pathologische Anatomie 90: 144

Altshuler G 1984 Chorangiosis: an important placental sign of neonatal morbidity and mortality. Archives of Pathology and Laboratory Medicine 108: 71–74

Anders D, Frick R, Kindermann G 1970 Metastasierendes Neuroblastom des Feten mit Aussaat in die Plazenta. Geburtshilfe und Frauenheilkunde 30: 969–975

Angelone A, Caruso A, Berghella A, Sindici G, Bianchi O 1989 Sur un caso di emangioma diffuso della placenta. Minerva Ginecologica 41: 625–628

Antaya R J, Keller R A, Wilkerson J A 1995 Placental nevus cells associated with giant congenital pigmented nevi. Pediatric Dermatology 12: 260–262

Ball R A, Genest D, Sander M, Schmidt B, Barnhill R L 1998 Congenital melanocytic nevi with placental infiltration by melanocytes: a benign condition that mimics metastatic melanoma. Archives of Dermatology 134: 711–714

Bauer C R, Fojaco R M, Bancalari E, Fernandez-Rocha L 1978 Microangiopathic hemolytic anemia and thrombocytopenia in a neonate associated with a large placental chorioangioma. Pediatrics 62: 574–577

Benirschke K 1999 Recent trends in chorangiomas, especially those of multiple and recurrent choriangiomas. Pediatric and Developmental Pathology 2: 264–269

Bierman H R, Aggeler P M, Thelander H, Kely K H, Cordes L 1956 Leukemia and pregnancy: a problem in transmission in man. Journal of the American Medical Association 161: 220–223

Birner W F 1961 Neuroblastoma as a cause of antenatal death. American Journal of Obstetrics and Gynecology 82: 1388–1391

Brodsky I, Baron M, Kahn S B, Lewis G Jr, Teillem M 1965 Metastatic malignant melanoma from mother to fetus. Cancer 18: 1048–1050

Brossard J, Abish S, Bernstein M L et al 1994 Maternal malignancy involving the products of conception: a report of malignant melanoma and medulloblastoma. American Journal of Pediatric Medicine and Oncology 16: 380–383

Cailliez D, Moirot M H, Fessaro C, Hemet J, Philippe E 1980 Localization placentaire d'un carcinome du col uterin. Journal de Gynecologie, Obstetrique et Biologie de la Reproduction 9: 461–463

Cash J, Powell D 1980 Placental chorangioma. American Journal of Surgical Pathology 4: 87–92

Chan K W, Leung C Y 1988 Recurrent multiple chorioangiomas and intrauterine death. Pathology 20: 77–78

Chen C P, Chern S R, Wang T Y, Huang Z D, Huang M C, Chuang C Y 1997 Pregnancy with concomitant chorangioma and placental vascular malformation with mesenchymal hyperplasia. Human Reproduction 12: 2553–2556

Chen K T, Ma C K, Kassel S H 1986 Hepatocellular adenoma of the placenta. American Journal of Surgical Pathology 10: 436–440

Dargent J L, Verdebout J M, Barlow P, Thomas D, Hoorens A, Goossens A 2000 Hepatocellular adenoma of the placenta: report of a case associated with maternal bicornuate uterus and fetal renal dysplasia. Histopathology 37: 287–288

Demian S D E, Donnelly W H, Frias J L, Monif C R G 1974 Placental lesions in congenital giant pigmented nevi. American Journal of Clinical Pathology 61: 438–442

Doss B J, Vicari J, Jacques S M, Qureshi F 1998 Placental involvement in congenital hepatoblastoma. Pediatric and Developmental Pathology 1: 538–542

Drut R, Drut R M, Toulouse J C 1992 Hepatic hemangioendotheliomas, placental chorioangiomas and dysmorphic kidneys in Beckwith-Wiedemann syndrome. Pediatric Pathology 12: 197–203

Du J, Ko C, Lauchlan S C 1968 Multiple choriangiomata of the placenta associated with fetal anemia. Canadian Medical Association Journal 99: 862–864

Elagoz S, Aker H, Cetin A 1998 Placental teratoma: a case report. European Journal of Obstetrics, Gynecology and Reproductive Biology 80: 263–265

Eldar-Geva T, Hochner-Ceinikier D, Ariel I, Ron M, Yagel S 1988 Fetal high-output cardiac failure and acute hydramnios caused by large placental chorioangioma: a case report. British Journal of Obstetrics and Gynaecology 95: 1200–1203

Engel K, Hahn T, Kayschnia R 1981 Sonographische Diagnose eines Plazentatumors mir hochgradiger Mangelentwicklung, Aysbiloug einer Anhydramnie und nachfollen dem Fruction. Geburtshilfe und Frauenheilkunde 41: 570–573

Ernst L M, Hui P, Parkash V 2001 Intraplacental smooth muscle tumor: a case report. International Journal of Gynecological Pathology 20: 284–288

Fisher J F 1940 Chorioangioma of the placenta. American Journal of Obstetrics and Gynecology 40: 493–498

Fox H 1997 Pathology of the placenta. W B Saunders, London

Fox H, Butler-Manuel R 1964 A teratoma of the placenta. Journal of Pathology and Bacteriology 88: 137–140

Franca-Martins A M, Graubard Z, Holloway G A, Van der Merwe F J 1990 Placental haemangioma associated with acute fetal anaemia in labour. Acta Medica Portugesa 3: 187–189

Frick R, Rummell H H, Heberling D, Schmidt W D 1997 Placenta-Metastasen mutterlicher Neoplasien: Angioblastische Sarkom der Vagina mit Placentarer Aussatt. Geburtshilfe und Frauenheilkunde 37: 216–220

Fritsch M, Jaffe E S, Griffin C, Camacho J, Raffeld M, Kingma D W 1999 Lymphoproliferative disorder of fetal origin presenting as oligohydramnios. American Journal of Surgical Pathology 23: 595–601

Froehlich L, Fujikura T, Fisher P 1971 Choriangiomas and their clinical implications. Obstetrics and Gynecology 37: 51–59

Gillet N, Hustin J, Magritte J P, Givron O, Longueville E 2001 Placental teratoma: a differential diagnosis with fetal acardia. Journal de Gynecologie, Obstetrique et Biologie de la Reproduction 30: 789–792

Glaser G, Junemann A, Tunte W et al 1988 Plazentares Chorangiom und kindliche Fehlbildungen. Geburtshilfe und Frauenheilkunde 48: 450–452

Gray E S, Balch N J, Kohler H, Thompson W D, Simpson J G 1986 Congenital leukaemia: an unusual cause of stillbirth. Archives of Disease in Childhood 61: 1001–1006

Greenberg P, Collins J D, Voet R L, Jariwala L 1982 Ewing's sarcoma metastatic to placenta. Placenta 3: 191–197

Holaday W J, Castrow F F 1968 Placental metastasis from fetal giant pigmented nevus. Archives of Dermatology 98: 486–488

Holland E 1949 A case of transplacental metastasis of malignant melanoma of mother to foetus. Journal of Obstetrics and Gynaecology of the British Empire 56: 529–536

Honoré L H, Brown L B 1990 Intervillous placental metastasis with maternal myeloid leukemia. Archives of Pathology and Laboratory Medicine 114: 450

Hustin J, Chef R 1972 Nephroblastome diffuse bilaterale: reflexions sur un nouveau cas. Journal de Gynecologie, Obstetrique et Biologie de la Reproduction 1: 373–384

Imakita M, Yutani C, Ishibashi-Ueda H, Murakami M, Chiba Y 1988 A case of hydrops fetalis due to placental chorangioma. Acta Pathologica Japonica 38: 941–945

Ito M, Kumamoto T, Yamamoto H et al 1994 A case report of placental hemangioma resulting in severe fetal distress. Acta Pediatrica Japonica 36: 207–211

Jaffe R, Seigal A, Rat J et al 1985 Placental chorioangiomatosis: a high risk pregnancy. Postgraduate Medical Journal 64: 453–455

Jaswal T S, Sen R, Singh S, Punia R P, Singh H, Sen J 1995 Teratoma of the placenta. Journal of the Indian Medical Association 93: 342–345

Jauniaux E, Zucker M, Meuris S et al 1988 Chorangiocarcinoma: an unusual tumour of the placenta: the missing link? Placenta 9: 607–613

Jauniaux E, deMeeus M-C, Verellen G, Lachapele J M, Hustin J 1993 Giant congenital melanocytic nevus with placental involvement: long term follow up of a case and review of the literature. Pediatric Pathology 13: 717–721

Johnson A T, Halbert D 1974 Congenital neuroblastoma presenting as hydrops fetalis. North Carolina Medical Journal 35: 289–291

Jones C E M, Rivers R P A, Taghizadeh A 1972 Disseminated intravascular coagulation and fetal hydrops in a newborn infant in association with a chorangioma of placenta. Pediatrics 50: 901–907

Jurkovic I, Fric I, Boor A 1973 Placenta pri neuroblastome. Ceskoslovenska Pediatrie 28: 443–445

Kandom-Moyo J, Jajeri H, Winisdoerffer C, Philippe E, Beauvais P, Dreyfus J 1972 Souffrance foetal et chorio-angiome: etude du rhythme cardiaque foetal: a propos de 2 cas. Journal de Gynecologie, Obstetrique et Biologie de la Reproduction 1: 575–579

Kapoor R, Gupta A K, Sing S, Sood A, Saha M M 1989 Antenatal sonographic diagnosis of chorioangioma of the placenta. Australasian Radiology 33: 288–289

Katsanis W A, O'Connor D M, Gibb R K, Bendon R W 1998 Endometrial stromal sarcoma involving the placenta. Annals of Diagnostic Pathology 2: 301–305

Khalifa M A, Gersell D J, Hansen C H, Lage J M 1998 Hepatic (hepatocellular) adenoma of the placenta: a study of four cases. International Journal of Gynecological Pathology 17: 241–244

Khong T Y 2000 Chorangioma with trophoblastic proliferation. Virchows Archiv 436: 167–171

Khong T Y, George K 1994 Maternal serum alphafetoprotein levels in chorangiomas. American Journal of Perinatology 11: 245–248

Kim C G, Benirschke K, Connolly K S 1971 Chorangioma of the placenta: chromosomal and electron microscopic studies. Obstetrics and Gynecology 37: 372–376

King C R, Lourien E 1978 Chorioangioma of the placenta and intrauterine growth failure. Journal of Pediatrics 93: 1027–1028

King P A, Lopes A, Tang M H, Lam S K, Ma H K 1991 Theca-lutein ovarian cysts associated with placental chorioangioma: case report. British Journal of Obstetrics and Gynaecology 98: 322–323

Knoth M, Rygaard J, Hesseldahl H 1976 Chorangioma with hydramnios and intrauterine fetal death. Acta Obstetricia et Gynecologica Scandinavica 55: 279–281

Kohler H G, Iqbal N, Jenkins D M 1976 Chorionic haemangiomata and abruptio placentae. British Journal of Obstetrics and Gynaecology 83: 667–670

Koivu M K, Nutinen E N 1990 Large placental chorioangioma as a cause of congestive heart failure in newborn infants. Pediatric Cardiology 11: 221–224

Koumantakis E, Makrigiannakis A, Froudarakis G, Datseris G, Matalliotakis J 1996 Teratoma of the placenta: a case report. Clinical and Experimental Obstetrics and Gynecology 23: 268–271

Kurtin P J, Gaffrey T A, Habermann T M 1992 Peripheral T-cell lymphoma involving the placenta. Cancer 70: 2963–2968

Las Heras J, Leal G, Haust M D 1986 Congenital leukemia with placental involvement: report of a case with ultrastructural study. Cancer 58: 2278–2281

Leblanc A, Carrier C 1979 Chorio-angiome placentaire, angiomes cutanes et cholestase neonatale. Archives Francaises de Pediatrie 36: 484–486

Liang S T, Wood J S K, Wong V C W 1982 Chorioangioma of the placenta: an ultrasonic study. British Journal of Obstetrics and Gynaecology 89: 480–482

Lifschitz-Mercer B, Fogel M, Kushnir I, Czernobilsky B 1989 Chorangioma: a cytoskeletal profile. International Journal of Gynecological Pathology 8: 349–356

Lopez-Herce Cid J, Escriba Polo R, Escudero Loy R 1983 Corioangioma placentario y hemorraghia intracraneal neonatal. Anales Espanoles de Pediatria 19: 405–406

Ludighausen M V, Sahiri I 1983 Chorangiome der Plazenten als Ursache wiederhalter Totgeburten. Geburtshilfe und Frauenheilkunde 43: 233–235

Lynn A A, Parry S I, Morgan M A, Mennuti M T 1997 Disseminated congenital neuroblastoma involving the placenta. Archives of Pathology and Laboratory Medicine 121: 741–744

McInroy R A, Kelsey H A 1954 Chorio-angioma (haemangioma of placenta) associated with acute hydramnios. Journal of Pathology and Bacteriology 68: 519–523

Majlessi H F, Wagner K M, Brooks J 1983 Atypical cellular chorangioma of the placenta. International Journal of Gynecological Pathology 1: 403–408

Mann L, Alroomf L, McNay M, Ferguson-Smith M A 1983 Placental haemangioma: case report. British Journal of Obstetrics and Gynaecology 90: 983–984

Marchetti A A 1939 Consideration of certain types of benign tumors of the placenta. Surgery, Gynecology and Obstetrics 68: 733–743

Meguerian-Bedoyan Z, Lamant L, Hopfner C, Pulford K, Chittal S, Delsol G 1997 Anaplastic large cell lymphoma of maternal origin involving the placenta: case report and literature review. American Journal of Surgical Pathology 21: 1236–1241

Meinhard K, Dimitrov S, Nicolov A, Dimitrova V, Vassilev N 1999 Placental teratoma: a case report. Pathology Research and Practice 195: 649–651

Mesia A F, Mo P, Ylagan L R (1999) Atypical cellular chorangioma. Archives of Pathology and Laboratory Medicine 123: 536–538

Mucitelli D R, Charles E Z, Kraus F T 1990 Chorioangiomas of intermediate size and intrauterine growth retardation. Pathology Research and Practice 186: 455–458

Mutz I D, Sterling R 1991 Konnatales Neuroblastom und Plazentametastasen. Monatsschrift fur Kinderheilkunde 139: 154–156

Nahmanovici C, Pancrazi J, Philippe E 1982 Chorioangiome placentaire: diagnostie echographique a la 19° semaine. Journal de Gynecologie, Obstetrique et Biologie de la Reproduction 11: 593–597

Nishi Y, Suzuki S, Otsubo Y et al 2000 B-cell-type malignant lymphoma with placental involvement. Journal of Obstetrical and Gynecological Research 26: 39–43

Nummi S, Koivisto M, Hakosalo J 1973 Acute leukaemia in pregnancy with placental involvement. Annales Chirurgiae et Gynaecologiae Fenniae 62: 394–398

Nuttinen E N, Puistola A, Herva R, Joivisto M 1988 Two cases of large placental chorioangioma with fetal and neonatal complications. European Journal of Obstetrics, Gynaecology and Reproductive Biology 29: 315–320

O'Day M P, Nielsen P, Al-Bolomi I, Wilkins I A 1994 Orbital rhabdomyosarcoma metastatic to the placenta. American Journal of Obstetrics and Gynecology 171: 1382–1383

Ohyama M, Kobayashi S, Aida N, Toyoda Y, Ijiri R, Tanaka Y 1999 Congenital neuroblastoma diagnosed by placental examination. Medical Pediatric Oncology 33: 430–431

Ohyama M, Ijiri R, Tanaka Y et al 2000 Congenital primitive epithelial tumor of the liver showing focal rhabdoid features, placental involvement, and clinical features mimicking multifocal hemangioma or stage 4S neuroblastoma. Human Pathology 31: 259–263

O'Malley B P, Toi A, deSa D J, Williams G L 1981 Ultrasound appearances of placental chorioangioma. Radiology 138: 159–160

Perkins D G, Kopp C M, Haust M D 1980 Placental infiltration in congenital neuroblastoma: a case study with ultrastructure. Histopathology 4: 383–389

Pollack R N, Sklarin N T, Rao S, Divon M Y 1993a Metastatic placental lymphoma associated with maternal human immunodeficiency virus infection. Obstetrics and Gynecology 81: 856–857

Pollack R N, Pollack M, Rochon L 1993b Pregnancy complicated by medulloblastoma with metastases in the placenta. Obstetrics and Gynecology 81: 858–859

Potashnik. G, Ben Adereth N, Leventhal H 1973 Chorioangioma of the placenta: clinical and pathological implications. Israel Journal of Medical Sciences 9: 904–908

Reddy C R R, Rao A V N, Sulochana G 1969 Haemangiolipoma of placenta. Journal of Obstetrics and Gynaecology of India 19: 653–655

Reshetnikova O S, Burton G J, Milovanov A P 1996 Increased incidence of placental chorioangioma in high-altitude pregnancies: hypovaric hypoxia as a possible etiological factor. American Journal of Obstetrics and Gynecology 174: 557–561

Rigby P G, Hanson T A, Smith R S 1964 Passage of leukemic cells across the placenta. New England Journal of Medicine 271: 124–127

Robinson H B Jr, Rolande R P 1985 Fetal hepatoblastoma with placental metastases. Pediatric Pathology 4: 163–167

Rodan B A, Bean W J 1983 Chorioangioma of the placenta causing intrauterine fetal demise. Journal of Ultrasound Medicine 2: 95–97

Sakurai H, Mitsuhashi N, Ibuki Y, Joshita T, Fukusato T, Nibe H 1998 Placental metastasis from maternal primitive neuroectodermal tumor. American Journal of Clinical Oncology 21: 39–41

Santamaria M, Benirschke K, Carpenter P M, Baldwin V J, Pritchard J A 1987 Transplacental hemorrhage associated with placental neoplasms. Pediatric Pathology 7: 601–615

Scharl A, Schlensker K H 1987 Chorioangiome – sonographische Diagnose und klinische Bedeutung. Zeitschrift fur Perinatologie 191: 250–253

Schneiderman H, Wa A Y, Campbell W A et al 1987 Congenital melanoma with multiple prenatal metastases. Cancer 60: 1371–1377

Schnitger A, Lieogren S, Radberg C, Johansson S G O, Kjessler B 1980 Raised maternal serum and amniotic fluid alpha-fetoprotein levels associated with a placental haemangioma. British Journal of Obstetrics and Gynaecology 87: 824–826

Sedgely M G, Östör A G, Fortune D W 1985 Angiosarcoma of the breast metastatic to breast and ovary. Australian and New Zealand Journal of Obstetrics and Gynaecology 25: 299–302

Sen D K 1970 Placental hypertrophy associated with chorioangioma. American Journal of Obstetrics and Gynecology 107: 652–654

Shimojo H, Itoh N, Shigematsu H, Yamazaki T 1996 Mature teratoma of the placenta. Pathology International 46: 372–375

Sims D G, Barron S L, Wadhera V, Ellis H A 1976 Massive chronic feto-maternal bleeding associated with placental chorio-angiomas. Acta Paediatrica Scandinavica 65: 271–273

Smith C R, Chan H S L, de Sa D J 1981 Placental involvement in congenital neuroblastoma. Journal of Clinical Pathology 34: 785–789

Smith L A, Pounder D J 1982 A teratoma-like lesion of the placenta: a case report. Pathology 14: 85–87

Sotelo-Avila C, Graham M, Hanby D E, Rudolph A J 1988 Nevus cell aggregates in the placenta: a histochemical and electron microscopic study. American Journal of Clinical Pathology 89: 395–400

Spirt B, Gordon L, Cohen W, Yambao T 1980 Antenatal diagnosis of chorioangioma of the placenta. American Journal of Roentgenology 13: 1273–1275

Stephens T D, Spall R, Urter A G, Martin R 1989 Fetus amorphus or placental teratoma? Teratology 40: 1–10

Stephenson H E Jr, Terry C W, Lukens J N et al 1971 Immunologic factors in human melanoma 'metastatic' to products of gestation (with exchange transfusion of infant to mother). Surgery 69: 515–522

Stiller A C, Skafish P R 1986 Placental chorioangioma: a rare cause of feto-maternal transfusion with maternal hemorrhage and fetal distress. Obstetrics and Gynecology 67: 296–298

Stovring S 1980 Kongenit neuroblastom med metastaser til placenta. Ugeskrift for Laeger 142: 2977–2978

Strauss L, Driscoll S G 1964 Congenital neuroblastoma involving the placenta: reports of two cases. Pediatrics 34: 23–31

Sweet L, Robertson N R C 1973 Hydrops fetalis with chorioangioma of the placenta. Journal of Pediatrics 82: 91–94

Tapia R H, White V A, Ruffolo E H 1985 Leiomyoma of the placenta. Southern Medical Journal 78: 863–864

Thomas R L, Blakemore K J 1990 Chorioangioma: a new inclusion in the prospective and retrospective evaluation of elevated maternal serum alpha-fetoprotein levels. Prenatal Diagnosis 10: 691–696

Tolar J, Coad J E, Neglia J P 2002 Transplacental transfers of small cell carcinoma of the lung. New England Journal of Medicine 346: 1501–1502

Tonkin I L, Setzer E S, Ermocilla R 1980 Placental chorangioma: a rare cause of congestive heart failure and hydrops fetalis in the newborn. American Journal of Roentgenology 134: 181–183

Trask C, Lage J M, Roberts D J 1994 A second case of 'chorangiocarcinoma' presenting in a term pregnancy: choriocarcinoma in situ with associated villous vascular proliferation. International Journal of Gynecological Pathology 13: 87–91

Tsujimura T, Matsumoto K, Aozasa K 1993 Placental involvment by maternal non-Hodgkin's lymphoma. Archives of Pathology and Laboratory Medicine 117: 325–327

Ulrich B, Heidenreich W, Borgmann U 1999 Das Chorangiom der Plazenta. Zeitschrift fur Geburtshilfe und Neonatologie 203: 173–175

van der Slikke J W, Balk A G 1980 Hydramnios with hydrops fetalis and disseminated fetal neuroblastoma. Obstetrics and Gynecology 55: 250–253

Verloes A, Schaaps J P, Herens C et al 1991 Prenatal diagnosis of cystic hygroma and chorioangioma in the Wolf-Hirschhorn syndrome. Prenatal Diagnosis 11: 129–132

Vermelin H, Braye M, Collectte C I 1957 Association de chorioangiome placentaire et de degenerescence molaire. Bulletin de la Federation des Societes de Gynecologie et d'Obstetrique de Langue Francaise 9: 225

Vesoulis Z, Agamanolis D 1998 Benign hepatocellular tumor of the placenta. American Journal of Surgical Pathology 22: 355–359

Vettenranta K, Heikinheimo M, Sipponen P, Rapola J, Ruth V 1987 Placental hemangioma: a cause of neonatal hypovolemia. Duodecima 103: 1095–1097

Wallenburg H C S 1971 Chorioangioma of the placenta: thirteen new cases and a review of the literature from 1939 to 1970 with special reference to clinical complications. Obstetrical and Gynecological Survey 26: 411–425

Wang L, Du X, Li M 1995 Placental teratoma: case report and review of the literature. Pathology Research and Practice 191: 1267–1270

Wang T, Harman W, Hartge R 1983 Structural aspects of a placenta from a case of maternal acute lymphatic leukaemia. Placenta 4: 185–196

Weber F P, Schwartz K, Hellenschied R 1930 Spontaneous inoculation of melanotic sarcoma from mother to foetus. British Medical Journal 1: 537–539

Werner C 1972 Melaninablagerungen in der Plazenta bei neurokutaner Melanophakomatose des Feten. Geburtshilfe und Frauenheilkunde 32: 891–894

Williams V L, Williams R A 1994 Placental teratoma: prenatal ultrasonographic diagnosis. Journal of Ultrasound in Medicine 13: 587–589

43

Pathology of the liver and gallbladder in pregnancy

S. G. Hübscher

Introduction   1465

Liver function during normal pregnancy   1465
Biochemical changes   1466
Clinical manifestations   1466
Morphological changes   1466

Liver diseases peculiar to pregnancy   1467
Intrahepatic cholestasis of pregnancy   1467
Acute fatty liver of pregnancy   1469
The liver in toxaemia of pregnancy   1474
The HELLP syndrome   1475
Spontaneous rupture of the liver   1476
Miscellaneous group   1477

Liver diseases developing concurrently with pregnancy   1478
Acute viral hepatitis   1478
Herpes simplex hepatitis   1479
Other infectious diseases   1479
Drug-induced hepatic injury   1479
Hepatic neoplasms and tumour-like conditions   1480
Other thrombotic microangiopathies occurring during pregnancy   1480
Budd–Chiari syndrome   1481
Spontaneous rupture of the splenic artery   1481
Spontaneous rupture of the biliary tract   1481
Primary biliary cirrhosis and fetal microchimerism   1481

Pregnancy in pre-existing liver disease   1482
Chronic viral hepatitis   1482
Autoimmune hepatitis   1483
Cirrhosis and portal hypertension   1483
Metabolic liver diseases   1483
Miscellaneous group   1484
Pregnancy and liver transplantation   1484

Bile composition, gallbladder function and cholelithiasis   1484

INTRODUCTION

Liver disease is uncommon in pregnancy and can be divided into three main categories: liver diseases which are peculiar to pregnancy, liver disease developing concurrently with pregnancy, and established liver diseases complicated by pregnancy. This chapter will focus mainly on liver diseases which are peculiar to pregnancy. A number of other conditions, which are not unique to pregnancy, but in which there are particular pregnancy related problems will also be discussed. A detailed discussion of all liver diseases which may be seen in the pregnant woman is beyond the scope of this chapter. For those conditions which have essentially the same manifestations in pregnant women as those seen in non-pregnant individuals, the reader is referred to standard texts dealing with liver pathology. A brief review of changes in gallbladder function and gallbladder disease in pregnancy is included at the end of the chapter.

LIVER FUNCTION DURING NORMAL PREGNANCY

Some of the physiological changes which occur in the pregnant woman to support fetal growth and development have an impact on liver function. The serum levels of oestrogen and progesterone increase throughout pregnancy and these hormones have effects on hepatic metabolic, synthetic and excretory functions (Kern et al 1978; van Thiel & Gavaler 1987; Bacq et al 1996). Total blood volume and cardiac output are increased by some 50%: total hepatic blood flow, however, remains unchanged (Munnell & Taylor 1947) such that in the third trimester there is a relative decrease of 25–30% in the proportion of the cardiac output which passes through the liver (Robson et al 1990). Consequently drugs that are cleared by the liver in a blood-flow dependent manner have a reduced clearance rate in pregnancy (Rustgi et al 1993). The increase in plasma volume causes haemodilution, which results in a decrease in serum protein levels.

BIOCHEMICAL CHANGES

Standard biochemical liver function tests that show changes in the course of pregnancy are summarised in Table 43.1 (Haemmerli 1966; Seymour & Chadwick 1979; Krejs & Haemmerli 1982; Krejs 1983; Bacq et al 1996; Wolf 1996; Girling et al 1997).

Serum levels of alanine transaminase (ALT) and aspartate transminase (AST) tend to rise during pregnancy. Significantly higher levels of ALT and AST have been found in late pregnancy compared with early pregnancy and/or normal controls (Elliott & O'Kell 1971; Cerutti et al 1976; Knopp et al 1985; Salgo & Pal 1989). However in the study of Girling et al (1997) AST and ALT levels were lower in uncomplicated pregnancy (including late pregnancy) than the non-pregnant reference range. Overall, ALT and AST levels still remain within the normal range and an increase in serum transaminases therefore warrants further investigation (Bacq et al 1996).

The serum alkaline phosphatase (AP) shows a progressive increase and in the third trimester the levels are two to four times normal. The increase is largely due to placental alkaline phosphatase which constitutes 50% of the serum content at term; the bone iso-enzyme is also increased (Adeniyi & Olatunbosun 1984; Valenzuela et al 1987; Rodin et al 1989). However, the hepatic iso-enzyme also shows an increase in the last trimester, a change which suggests that pregnancy normally exerts a cholestatic effect. The serum levels of alkaline phosphatase may remain elevated for four to six weeks postpartum (Krejs 1983).

Serum bilirubin levels tend to fall during pregnancy (Knopp et al 1985; Jarnfelt-Samisoe et al 1986; Bacq et al 1996; Girling et al 1997). This may be due to haemodilution resulting in lower concentrations of serum proteins including albumin, which is the protein that transports bilirubin.

Total serum protein concentration falls by 10 g/l in the first half of pregnancy and remains fairly constant thereafter. The reduction is due to haemodilution and mainly affects the albumin level with a small decrease in immunoglobulin levels. The albumin level is reduced by 35% at term. In contrast, fibrinogen levels are significantly increased from mid-term; α and β globulins, caeruloplasmin, transferrin and a number of other carrier proteins are slightly increased in the third trimester. These serum protein changes may persist for six to 12 weeks after delivery (Krejs 1983).

Bromsulphthalein (BSP) excretion tests (Combes et al 1963) show an increased uptake from the plasma and increased storage in the liver in the last trimester, with reduced active secretion into bile such that the maximal secretory rate (Tm) is reduced by 25%.

There is a slight increase in the level of bile acids during pregnancy (Fulton et al 1983; Jarnfelt-Samisoe et al 1986; Carter 1991) and a reduction in the enterohepatic circulation of bile acids.

Serum levels of gamma glutamyl transpeptidase (GGT) tend to decrease in late pregnancy (Bacq et al 1996; Girling et al 1997). This may reflect hormone-induced impairment of hepatic synthesis of GGT. A similar phenomenon has also been observed in women taking oral contraceptives and in cholestasis of pregnancy (Combes et al 1977; Jacquemin et al 1988).

Serum lipids of all classes increase through to term. The greatest changes affect triglycerides and cholesterol, which increase by 300% and 60%, respectively, while phospholipids increase by 5% (Svanborg & Vikrot 1965).

CLINICAL MANIFESTATIONS

Although biochemical changes are well documented, in the great majority of cases these are not associated with any obvious clinical problems. (McNair & Jaynes 1960; Hytten & Leitch 1971; Seymour & Chadwick 1979). Spider naevi and palmar erythema, stigmata of chronic liver disease, may appear in late pregnancy but disappear soon after parturition. Liver size remains normal.

MORPHOLOGICAL CHANGES

Histological and ultrastructural studies have shown a number of mild non-specific changes. (Ingerslev & Teilum 1945; Antia et al 1958; Gonzalez-Angulo et al 1970; Perez et al 1971). Histological changes include variation in liver cell size, increased numbers of binucleate cells, a light lymphocytic infiltrate in portal tracts, variable changes in glycogen and fat content and Kupffer cell enlargement. Electron microscopic examination has revealed an increase in smooth and rough endoplasmic reticulum, increased numbers of peroxisomes and giant

Table 43.1 Liver function tests in normal pregnancy

Remain within normal range		
Serum transaminases		
Serum 5–nucleotidase		
Prothrombin time		

Increase		
Serum alkaline phosphatase	x	2–4
Serum fibrinogen		50%
Serum cholesterol	x	1.5–2
Serum triglycerides	x	3–5
Serum bile acids		slight

Decrease		
Serum bilirubin		slight, variable
Serum albumin		35%
Serum gamma glutamyl transpeptidase		slight
Bromusulphthalein dye secretion		25%

mitochondria with crystalline inclusions. These changes may represent an adaptive response related to hormonal changes in pregnancy.

LIVER DISEASES PECULIAR TO PREGNANCY

INTRAHEPATIC CHOLESTASIS OF PREGNANCY

First described by Ahlfeld in 1883 (Ikonen 1964), the classical accounts of intrahepatic cholestasis of pregnancy (ICP) are those of Svanborg (1954) and Thorling (1955) from Sweden. More recently the subject has been reviewed by others (Reyes et al 1976, 1978; Reyes 1982, 1992; Reyes & Simon 1993; Reyes 1997; Davidson et al 1998; Fagan et al 1999; Lammert et al 2000). Other terms which have been used to describe the syndrome include hepatitis of pregnancy, jaundice of late pregnancy, recurrent jaundice of pregnancy, cholestatic jaundice of pregnancy, *pruritus gravidarum* and *icterus gravidarum*.

Incidence and risk factors

In most countries intrahepatic cholestasis is a rare complication of pregnancy, with a prevalence rate in the region of 1 in 1000 pregnancies (Haemmerli 1966; Reyes 1982; Reyes 1992; Bacq et al 1997; Lammert et al 2000). A higher prevalence rate (1–1.5%) has been observed in Scandinavian countries. Higher prevalence rates still have been reported (10–20%) in Chile and Bolivia (Reyes 1982, 1992), where members of the ethnic Indian population are at particular risk of developing ICP. There is a very low incidence in Oriental countries and among Negro populations. The prevalence of the syndrome has also shown changes with time (Reyes 1992). A seasonal variation in incidence was reported in Finland with a higher incidence in winter (Laatikainen & Ikonen 1975).

Other possible risk factors for ICP include twin or multiple pregnancies, progesterone therapy to prevent premature delivery (Bacq et al 1997), and hepatitis C infection (Locatelli et al 1999).

Clinical features

The typical clinical presentation is that of pruritus developing in the third trimester of pregnancy (*pruritus gravidarum*). In up to a third of cases pruritus develops during the second or, rarely, the first trimester (Lammert et al 2000). The pruritus varies in intensity, is worse at night and can be severe and incapacitating. Only about 10–25% of cases become clinically jaundiced (*icterus gravidarum*) and these are considered to be more severe examples of the spectrum of ICP. Icterus without pruritus is rare. The pruritus and jaundice persist until term and then quickly resolve in the great majority of cases, usually within 24–48 hours of delivery. In some cases pruritus and/or jaundice persist for up to 4 weeks. There have been a

small number of patients in whom a chronic cholestatic syndrome appears to have developed as a complication of ICP (Olsson et al 1993). However, rapid resolution of changes related to ICP postpartum is such a characteristic feature that persistence of pruritus or biochemical abnormalities for more than three months should raise the suspicion of some other cholestatic liver disorder, such as primary biliary cirrhosis.

The development of ICP in one pregnancy is associated with a 45–70% risk of recurrent ICP in subsequent pregnancies (Lammert et al 2000). However, there is considerable individual variability. Some patients have recurrent cholestasis in each pregnancy, others have one or more asymptomatic pregnancies before the first cholestatic episode, and still others have pruritus and/or cholestasis in an unpredictable sequence and with variation in time of onset and severity in consecutive pregnancies (Furhoff 1974; Reyes 1982).

Vanjak et al (1991) reported a single case in which there was an association between intrahepatic cholestasis of pregnancy and acute fatty liver of pregnancy (Vanjak et al 1991). Coexistence of these two disorders has also been reported from Chile (Reyes et al 1994) but the association was considered to be fortuitous.

Biochemical changes

Liver function tests show a cholestatic pattern. The most sensitive indicator is a rise in serum bile acid levels, which may increase up to 100-fold normal. There is a proportionately greater increase in cholic acid, compared with chenodeoxycholic and deoxycholic acid, (Laatikainen & Ikonen 1977; Laatikainen et al 1978). Hyperbilirubinaemia not usually exceeding 100 μmol/l is only detected in 10–20% of cases and fluctuates from week to week. Alkaline phosphatase and gamma GT levels are also increased above those seen in normal pregnancy.

Other biochemical changes which are seen in ICP include a 2–10-fold elevation in the serum levels of transaminases, a 2–3-fold increase in serum 5-nucleotidase and varying elevations in serum lipids including cholesterol, triglycerides and phospholipids (Johnson 1975; Johnson et al 1975b).

Histological features

In the presence of typical clinical and biochemical changes, liver biopsy is not required. The histological changes which occur in ICP are not specific and resemble those seen in other forms of 'pure' intrahepatic cholestasis. There is a mild, often inconspicuous, bilirubinostasis with perivenular hepatocellular and canalicular bile retention. This may be focal in the liver, suggesting a heterogeneous acinar response to the factor(s) causing ICP. Mild reactive Kupffer cell hyperplasia is also evident. There is minimal or no liver cell necrosis and the portal tracts are normal. In cases associated with chronic cholestatic features, varying degrees of periportal fibrosis have been described, rarely progressing to a biliary-type cirrhosis (Olsson et al 1993; Leevy et al 1997).

Ultrastructural studies have also shown non-specific changes comprising liver cell swelling and loss of canalicular microvilli, features common to bile retention from any cause (Haemmerli 1966; Adlercreutz et al 1967; Kater & Mistilis 1967).

Pathogenetic mechanisms

The precise mechanisms of cholestasis in ICP are not clear. However, the evidence available points to a combination of genetic, hormonal and environmental factors. (Schorr-Lesnick et al 1991; Reyes 1992; Reyes & Simon 1993; Wolf 1996; Lammert et al 2000).

The striking variation in the incidence of ICP according to geographical and ethnic differences suggests that genetic predisposition may be important. Familial aggregation of cases (Reyes et al 1978; Reyes 1982) and retrospective studies showing familial aggregation of intrahepatic cholestasis of pregnancy and contraceptive steroid induced cholestasis (Dalen & Westerholm 1974) further support this concept. Until recently no specific genetic or phenotypic markers had been identified (Reyes 1982). However, the discovery of mutations in genes encoding biliary transport proteins has shed further light on the genetic basis of a number of familial intrahepatic cholestatic syndromes. These include progressive familial intrahepatic cholestasis (PFIC) and benign recurrent intrahepatic cholestasis (BRIC) (Oude Elferink & van Berge Henegouwen 1998; Jacquemin & Hadchouel 1999; Luketic & Shiffman 1999; Kullak-Ublick et al 2000; Jacquemin et al 2001). A higher incidence of ICP has been observed in the mothers of patients with PFIC or BRIC, suggesting that heterozygote mutations of hepatobiliary transport proteins may predispose to ICP (Clayton et al 1969; De Pagter et al 1976; Whitington et al 1994). A mutation in the multidrug resistance gene 3 (*MDR3*), which encodes for the canalicular phosphatidylcholine translocase enzyme, has been identified in six members of a family with a history of ICP and PFIC (Jacquemin et al 1999). A heterozygous missense mutation in the *MDR3* gene has also been described in a single patient with ICP in whom there was no family history of PFIC (Dixon et al 2000). However, specific defects in hepatobiliary transport proteins have not been identified in the great majority of cases of ICP.

Hormonal factors related to oestrogens and progesterones have also been implicated in the pathogenesis of ICP. The disease presents in the last trimester, when hormone levels are highest, and resolves rapidly after delivery, when the levels of hormones return to normal. Twin pregnancies, in which rises in hormone levels are more pronounced, are associated with a higher incidence of ICP (Gonzales et al 1989). Factors which may promote the cholestatic effects of sex hormones include genetically determined variations in individual susceptibility (see below), increased levels (endogenously produced or exogenously administered) and defects in their metabolism and excretion. Women with intrahepatic cholestasis of pregnancy have a tendency to develop pruritus and abnormal liver function tests following oestrogen administration (Kreek et al 1967a,b; Kreek & Sleisenger 1970; Reyes et al 1981; Kreek 1987). A history of 'pill-induced' cholestasis is commonly found in patients with intrahepatic cholestasis of pregnancy (Dalen & Westerholm 1974; Kreek 1987). These observations suggest an increased sensitivity to steroid hormones, which is independent of pregnancy itself (Vore 1987). The mechanism of action of oestrogens and progesterones in producing cholestasis is not fully understood (Reyes & Simon 1993). Postulated effects include diminished uptake of bile acids at the basolateral membrane of hepatocytes due to inhibition of basolateral bile acid transporter proteins, decreased fluidity of the sinusoidal membrane with a resultant change in lipid composition, increased permeability of tight junctions and inhibition of canalicular bile acid export proteins resulting in decreased bile flow (Lammert et al 2000). However, a number of these changes may also occur as secondary effects of cholestasis itself and their importance in the pathogenesis of ICP is therefore uncertain. Sulphation of bile acids is important in attenuating their cholestatic potential, and the elevation in oestrogens, which occurs in pregnancy, has been associated with impairment in sulphation capacity (Davies et al 1994).

Exogenous factors that may contribute to the development of ICP include environmental factors, which may account for the decline in prevalence rates of ICP in Chile during recent years and for the seasonal variation that has been noted in certain countries. Some studies have linked ICP to low serum selenium levels (Kauppila et al 1987; Humberto et al 2000).

Fetal effects

ICP is associated with increased risks of premature delivery, which occurs in 19–60% of pregnancies, fetal distress complicating 22–33% of deliveries and stillbirths, which occur in 1–2% of ICP pregnancies (Shaw et al 1982; Laatikainen & Tulenheimo 1984; Berg et al 1986; Fisk & Storey 1988; Rioseco et al 1994; Alsulyman et al 1996; Bacq et al 1997; Lammert et al 2000). Perinatal mortality rates in the region of 10–20% have been observed in some studies of ICP (Fisk & Storey 1988; Rioseco et al 1994; Bacq et al 1997). However, with improvements in obstetric management, perinatal mortality rates have greatly improved and approach those seen in normal pregnancies (Rioseco et al 1994; Bacq et al 1997).

The pathogenesis of fetal complications of ICP is uncertain. Increased bile acid levels have been found in amniotic fluid and cord plasma suggesting increased flux of bile acids from mother to fetus (Lammert et al 2000). High maternal serum bile acid levels have been found in cases of sudden fetal death (Bacq et al 1997) and high fetal bile acid levels in cases of fetal distress (Laatikainen 1975). High levels of bile acids may result in a reduction in placental flow. They are also associated with increased meconium passage, which may cause umbilical vein obstruction and reduction in umbilical blood flow (Lammert et al 2000).

Maternal outcome

ICP causes considerable morbidity, mainly related to severe pruritus. Steatorrhoea, occurring as a consequence of reduced bile secretion, may have an adverse impact on maternal nutrition (Johnson et al 1975a; Reyes et al 1987). There is also an increased risk of postpartum haemorrhage, probably related to vitamin K deficiency. However the prognosis is otherwise good with no evidence of any long-term effects on hepatic function in the great majority of cases (Furhoff & Hellstrom 1974). There is an increased frequency of gallstones, particularly cholesterol stones, the overall prevalence being twice or more that found in a similar normal population (Thorling 1955; Furhoff 1974; Furhoff & Hellstrom 1974; Glasinovic et al 1989). The effects of normal pregnancy on gallbladder function are discussed elsewhere in this chapter. However, it is noteworthy that the fasting volume of the gallbladder may show an even greater increase in pregnancy complicated by intrahepatic cholestasis (Ylostalo et al 1981). ICP is associated with reduction in gallbladder motility which may predispose to cholesterol stone formation (Lammert et al 2000). In addition, some of the biliary transport protein gene mutations which have been identified in cases of ICP have also been implicated in the pathogenesis of cholesterol gallstone disease (Lammert 2001).

ACUTE FATTY LIVER OF PREGNANCY

The distinctive pathological features of acute fatty liver of pregnancy (AFLP) were first described by Sheehan (1940), who recognised and differentiated obstetric acute yellow atrophy of the liver from acute yellow atrophy complicating viral and toxic hepatitis.

Incidence and risk factors

The prevalence is approximately 1 in 5–15 000 pregnancies. A higher incidence has been reported in first pregnancies, multiple gestations and in male births (Rolfes & Ishak 1985; Davidson 1998). Although occasional cases of recurrent AFLP have been described (Barton et al

1990; Schoeman et al 1991; MacLean et al 1994; Reyes et al 1994; Visconti et al 1995), there is no clear evidence of a genetic predisposition.

Clinical features

These are reviewed in a large series of papers (Ober & Le Compte 1955; Moore 1956; Breen et al 1970; Davies et al 1980; Varner & Rinderknechts 1980; Burroughs et al 1982; Hague et al 1983; Pockros et al 1984; Rolfes & Ishak 1985; Riely 1987; Schorr-Lesnick et al 1991a; Mabie 1992; Reyes et al 1994; Bacq 1998; Castro et al 1999). Patients typically present in the last trimester of pregnancy, the majority after the 35th week. Occasional cases present during the second trimester (Buytaert et al 1996; Monga & Kratz 1999; Suzuki et al 2001) and rare cases postpartum. Following a prodromal illness of three to seven days with general malaise, there is nausea and severe vomiting associated with upper abdominal pain and tenderness. Polydipsia with or without polyuria is a frequent feature, which in some cases has been attributed to transient diabetes insipidus (Kennedy et al 1994). Jaundice then develops and is usually followed by rapid progression to fulminant liver failure. Many cases have hypertension, proteinuria and oedema, features characteristic of pre-eclampsia. The relationship between AFLP and toxaemia of pregnancy is discussed further below.

Laboratory investigations

There is usually haematological evidence of disseminated intravascular coagulation with increased prothrombin- and partial thromboplastin times (Liebman et al 1983; Pockros et al 1984; Riely 1987) and decreased antithrombin III levels (Castro et al 1996a). This disturbance of coagulation accounts for many of the fatal complications of the disease and may worsen after delivery (Pockros et al 1984). Other haematological abnormalities which are frequently seen in AFLP include a marked neutrophil leucocytosis, circulating normoblasts and giant platelets.

Radiological techniques including ultrasonography (Campillo et al 1986), computed tomography (CT) (Mabie et al 1989) and magnetic resonance imaging (MRI) are potentially useful non-invasive methods of confirming fatty infiltration in the liver. However, these imaging techniques have limited value in diagnosing fatty change in AFLP (Castro et al 1996b; Castro et al 1999).

Biochemical changes include a modest elevation in serum bilirubin levels, usually less than 150 μmol/l, with peak levels occurring postpartum, alkaline phosphatase levels slightly greater than those present in normal pregnancy and variably raised aminotransferases, usually between 100–500 U/l. Hypoglycaemia is often severe and may contribute to early coma. There is marked elevation in serum ammonia but, in contrast to fulminant viral or drug-induced hepatitis, there is a generalised fall in serum amino acids although glutamine, alanine and lysine levels may be raised (Burroughs et al 1982). Hyperuricaemia regularly occurs in the early stages and may, in part, be due to reduced renal clearance. Serum amylase and lipase levels may also be elevated due to the presence of an associated pancreatitis.

Histological features

The most characteristic histological abnormality in acute fatty liver of pregnancy is the presence of severe microvesicular steatosis, principally involving hepatocytes in acinar zones 2 and 3, but in severe cases extending to an almost panacinar distribution (Burroughs et al 1982). These features are shown in Figs 43.1–43.3. A pattern of mid-zonal necrosis was noted in one case by Joske and his colleagues (1968). Because fatty change is present in a microvesicular form, it may produce an appearance resembling the hepatocyte ballooning which is seen in other conditions such as toxic liver injury or acute viral

hepatitis. As the degree of fat accumulation may not be readily appreciated in paraffin-embedded sections, in cases where a diagnosis of AFLP is suspected clinically a portion of the biopsy should be retained for lipid staining of frozen sections (Fig. 43.2). Canalicular and hepatocellular bilirubinostasis are also present, sometimes to a marked degree. There is Kupffer cell hyperplasia and aggregates of ceroid-laden macrophages are conspicuous. There is usually only a very mild inflammatory cell reaction (Fig. 43.3) characterised by a mononuclear cell infiltrate in the parenchyma and portal tracts, sometimes with a few eosinophils and occasional plasma cells. Extramedullary haemopoiesis is often present. Intrasinusoidal fibrin deposits have also been noted and may occasionally be associated with small haemorrhages (Burroughs et al 1982).

Although liver cell death is not a conspicuous feature in haematoxylin and eosin stained tissue sections, collapse of the reticulin framework is often seen indicating significant liver cell loss presumably as a consequence of lytic

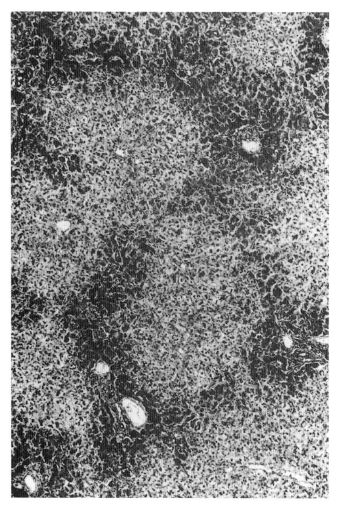

Fig. 43.1 Acute fatty liver of pregnancy: the darker staining periportal areas (zone 1 of the acinus) contrast with the paler fat-containing areas surrounding the hepatic veins and involving zones 2 and 3 of the acinus. Masson trichrome.

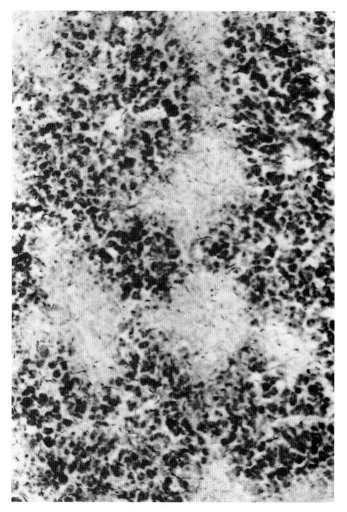

Fig. 43.2 Acute fatty liver of pregnancy: the distribution and the extent of lipid deposition is better appreciated on an oil Red-O stained frozen section.

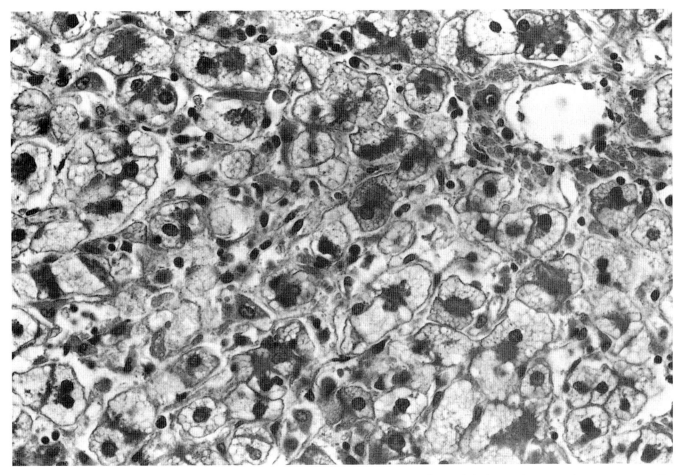

Fig. 43.3 Acute fatty liver of pregnancy: the liver cells in the perivenular area are swollen and their cytoplasm contains numerous small fat vesicles which surround the nucleus. There is a very light mononuclear cell infiltrate and some Kupffer cell hyperplasia. Masson trichrome.

necrosis (Fig. 43.4) (Burroughs et al 1982; Malatjalian & Badley 1983). At autopsy the liver is usually small and this reduction in liver weight in the presence of fat accumulation does indicate substantial liver cell loss.

Biopsies in survivors have demonstrated progressive disappearance of the fat from the periportal to the perivenular zone (Duma et al 1965), usually within a few days of parturition.

Ultrastructural studies (Weber et al 1979; Burroughs et al 1982) have shown that the fat is not membrane bound: there is dilatation of the rough endoplasmic reticulum and some cells show cytoplasmic degeneration with autophagic vacuoles (Figs 43.5, 43.6). The mitochondria show considerable variation in size, with many of giant and elongated appearance, and contain crystalline inclusions of varying sizes and shapes (Ockner et al 1990; Reyes et al 1994). A honeycomb appearance of the smooth endoplasmic reticulum has also been reported (Duma et al 1965).

With increasing awareness of the clinical features and other laboratory findings in AFLP, liver biopsy is now rarely required to confirm the diagnosis (Minakami et al 1988; Castro et al 1999). In the study of Castro et al (1999), only one of 28 cases considered to have typical features of AFLP was confirmed histologically. In the absence of histological confirmation, Castro and her colleagues suggest that the term 'reversible peripartum liver failure' be used instead (Castro et al 1999). However, liver biopsy may still be required in occasional cases where there are atypical features (particularly if there is an alternative diagnosis for which immediate delivery is not indicated therapeutically, e.g. acute viral hepatitis) or where the condition fails to resolve postpartum.

Maternal and fetal complications

Very high maternal and fetal mortality rates, in the order of 75–85%, have been noted in some earlier studies of AFLP (Hatfield et al 1972; Varner & Rinderknechts 1980). However, more recently there has been a substantial reduction in maternal and fetal mortality. In a combined series of 85 cases reported by Reyes et al (1994), Usta et al (1994), Pereira et al (1997) and Castro et al (1999) there were no maternal deaths. Fetal mortality was also less than 10% in three of these studies (Usta et al 1994; Pereira et al 1997; Castro et al 1999). Factors

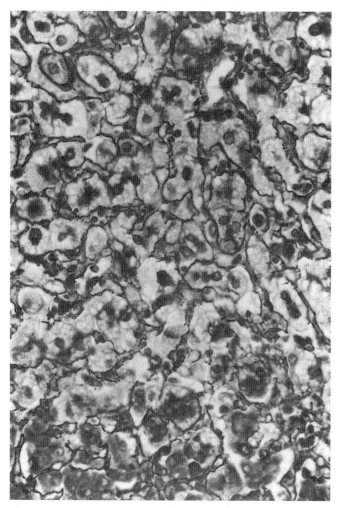

Fig. 43.4 Acute fatty liver of pregnancy: perivenular condensation of the reticulin framework as shown here indicates that there has been earlier hepatocytolysis. Gordon & Sweet's reticulin.

which may have contributed to the improved outcome of AFLP include: an increased awareness of the condition resulting in earlier diagnosis, improvements in supportive therapy for the complications of AFLP and prompt delivery by Caesarean section. In addition, it is now recognised that the illness may vary considerably in severity and that milder, non-fatal forms of the disease also occur (Bernuau et al 1982; Ebert et al 1984; Hou et al 1984; Pockros et al 1984; Riely 1984; Tsuki et al 1984; Schapiro & Thorp 1996). Liver transplantation has been carried out in two cases (Ockner et al 1990; Amon et al 1993). Because of the potentially reversible nature of the liver injury, AFLP may be a suitable indication for auxiliary liver transplantation (Franco et al 2000).

Maternal death is usually due to extrahepatic manifestations such as massive gastrointestinal haemorrhage, usually from the oesophagus and/or stomach, disseminated intravascular coagulation or renal failure. Fatty infiltration of renal tubular epithelium has been reported (Slater & Hague 1984). Pancreatitis may occur, sometimes with peripancreatic bleeding (Riely 1987). In mothers who recover there is no evidence of any residual chronic liver disease and subsequent uncomplicated pregnancy is well documented (Duma et al 1965; Breen et al 1972; Mackenna et al 1977; Davies et al 1980; Jenkins & Darling 1980; Burroughs et al 1982; Riely 1984).

Fetal death is due to stillbirth or prematurity. Mild fatty change has been noted in the livers of stillborn infants (Haemmerli 1966). Surviving infants have no abnormalities.

Pathogenetic mechanisms

The aetiology of acute fatty liver of pregnancy is uncertain. Studies in mice have shown that pregnancy, or repeated administration of female sex hormones, impairs the ultrastructure and function of liver mitochondria (Grimbert et al 1993; Grimbert et al 1995). However, these changes are insufficient alone to result in microvesicular fat deposition and an additional triggering factor is therefore required. Several studies have suggested that defects in the mitochondrial beta-oxidation pathway of fatty acid metabolism may be important in this respect (Treem et al 1994; Treem et al 1996; Tyni et al 1998; Ibdah et al 1999; Strauss et al 1999; Ibdah et al 2000). Similar mechanisms have also been implicated in the pathogenesis of other liver diseases characterised by microvesicular steatosis, such as Reye's syndrome (Fromenty & Pessayre 1997; Burt et al 1998). The combination of a heterozygous state for long-chain 3-hydroxyacyl-coenzyme A dehydrogenase (LCHAD) in the mother and a homozygous state for the same enzyme in the fetus appears to be associated with a particularly high risk of pregnancy complications, including AFLP. The higher incidence of AFLP which has been noted in multiple pregnancies may relate to further stressing of the fatty acid oxidation capacity of the susceptible woman.

Although the bulk of evidence points to LCHAD deficiency as being important in the pathogenesis of AFLP, there has been a single cases in which AFLP has been associated with short-chain acyl-coenzyme A dehydrogenase deficiency (Matern et al 2001).

Studies on the nature of the fat accumulation in acute fatty liver of pregnancy have shown that it is mainly composed of triglycerides, with smaller amounts of free fatty acids also present (Fromenty & Pessayre 1997). A similar lipid composition has also been observed in other conditions associated with microvesicular steatosis, such as Reye's syndrome (Fromenty & Pessayre 1995).

Acute fatty liver of pregnancy often occurs in patients with signs of toxaemia of pregnancy leading to the suggestion that it is part of the spectrum of pre-eclampsia (Riely 1987; Sibai et al 1994; Pereira et al 1997). In addition the fatty acid oxidation defects, which have been implicated in the pathogenesis of AFLP, have also been associated with other pregnancy-related complications

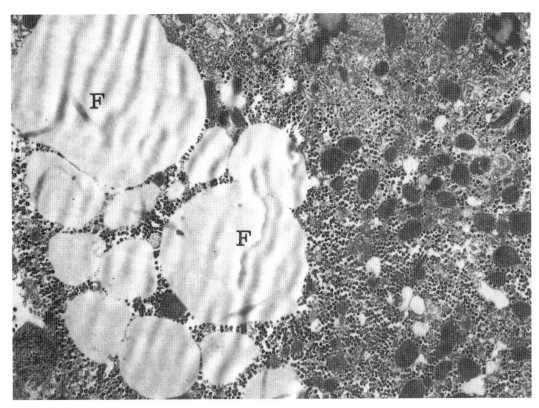

Fig. 43.5 Acute fatty liver of pregnancy: electronmicrograph showing non-membrane bound fat vacuoles (F) containing slightly osmophilic material. (Reprinted with permission from Burroughs et al 1982.)

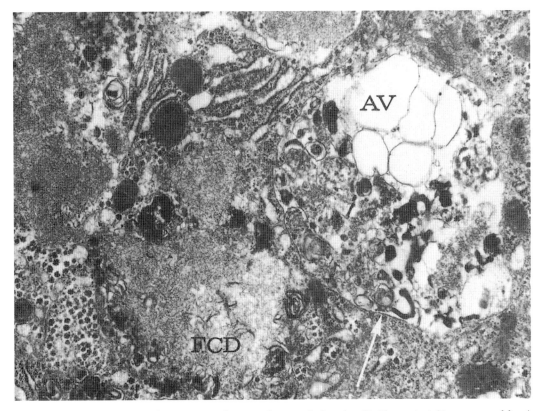

Fig. 43.6 Acute fatty liver of pregnancy: electronmicrograph showing fibrillar material in an area of focal cytoplasmic degeneration (FCD) and a single-membrane-bound autophagic vacuole (AV). (Reprinted with permission from Burroughs et al 1982.)

including pre-eclampsia and the HELLP syndrome (Tyni et al 1998; Strauss et al 1999). Histological studies have demonstrated that less severe degrees of microvesicular steatosis are frequently present in liver biopsies obtained from patients with pre-eclampsia, (Minakami et al 1988; Barton et al 1992; Dani et al 1996) although in many cases fat is not evident in routine haematoxylin and eosin stained sections. These observations suggest that pre-eclampsia, the HELLP syndrome and AFLP are part of a spectrum of pregnancy-induced microvesicular fatty disease in the liver, with AFLP being the most severe form. The presence of overlapping clinical and haemato-logical features would also support this hypothesis (Pereira et al 1997). However, it is worth noting that microvesicular steatosis can also be detected frequently in autopsy specimens obtained from people with no history of liver disease and the significance of this lesion as an isolated finding is therefore uncertain (Fraser et al 1995). Furthermore, other authors have concluded that the clini-cal, histological and other laboratory findings in most cases of AFLP and toxaemia are sufficiently different to enable a clear distinction to be made (Rolfes & Ishak 1986a,b; Vigil-De Gracia 2001).

THE LIVER IN TOXAEMIA OF PREGNANCY

Toxaemia of pregnancy is characterised by hypertension, proteinuria and oedema. It is more common in primi-paras than in multiparas. Pre-eclampsia is usually defined on the basis of new onset hypertension and albuminuria developing after 20 weeks of pregnancy (Higgins & de Swiet 2001), most cases presenting in the last trimester. Although oedema is now omitted from the definition of pre-eclampsia, it remains an important clinical manifesta-tion of the condition. In more severe cases there are central nervous system complications characterised by convulsions and eventual coma (eclampsia). Many of the serious complications of eclampsia are related to dissemi-nated intravascular coagulation (DIC). The pathogenesis of toxaemia of pregnancy is discussed elsewhere in this book. Only the pathological effects of toxaemia on the liver will be considered here.

Minor degrees of hepatic dysfunction are commonly present in toxaemia. Upper abdominal pain related to liver enlargement and tenderness is a common symptom (Barron 1992). Jaundice is usually mild with serum bilirubin levels of less than 100 μmol/l. Occasional cases present with severe jaundice (Killam et al 1975; Long et al 1977). Elevations in the serum levels of alkaline phosphatase are frequently present, usually to a mild degree. In the study of Girling et al (1997), 34% of patients had abnormal liver function tests (LFTs) com-pared to the normal reference range. The prevalence of elevated LFTs rose to 54% when the reference range was amended to take account of normal pregnancy related changes.

In pre-eclampsia, minor non-specific histological changes have been noted in the liver including hepatocel-lular pleomorphism and reactive Kupffer cell hyperplasia (Antia et al 1958). The distinctive liver lesion which characterises more severe and fatal cases of toxaemia of pregnancy comprises periportal intrasinusoidal fibrin deposition associated with irregular areas of liver cell necrosis and intraparenchymal haemorrhage (Figs 43.7, 43.8). Inflammatory changes are usually minimal or absent. The hepatic arteries and arterioles in the immedi-ately adjacent portal tracts show plasmatic vasculosis with seepage of fibrin into their walls (Fig. 43.8). Most of these changes can be attributed to endothelial damage (Lyall & Greer 1996) and other effects of DIC. Vasospasm and/or vasodilation of hepatic arterioles may also be involved (Sheehan & Lynch 1973; Rolfes & Ishak 1986a,b). Immunohistochemical studies carried out by Arias & Marcilla-Jimenez (1976) showed that sinusoidal deposits of fibrin (or fibrinogen) were present in all of 12 liver biopsies obtained from pre-eclamptic women.

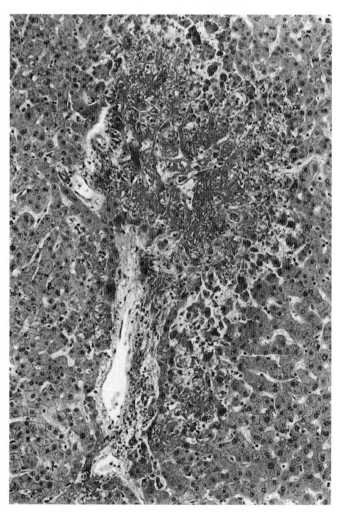

Fig. 43.7 Toxaemia of pregnancy: an irregular flame-shaped area of necrosis with fibrin deposition involving part of the periportal area. MSB.

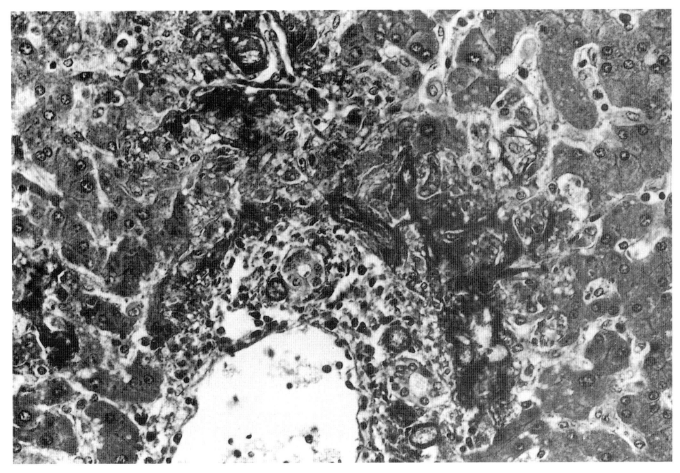

Fig. 43.8 Toxaemia of pregnancy: intrasinusoidal fibrin deposition and related liver cell necrosis is present in the periportal area; note also the dark staining of the peribiliary arterioles due to plasmatic vasculosis with escape of fibrin into their walls. Masson trichrome.

Ten of the 12 biopsies showed only mild histological changes. The two other biopsies contained small foci of necrosis, in which there were larger nodular aggregates of fibrin and, to a lesser extent, IgG, IgM and C3. Similar changes have also been observed in the glomerular lesions occurring in toxaemia of pregnancy (Vassalli et al 1963).

THE HELLP SYNDROME

Weinstein (1982) described 29 cases of severe pre-eclampsia/eclampsia complicated by haemolysis (H), elevated liver enzymes (EL) and a low platelet (LP) count. Although in this initial description, it was suggested that the HELLP syndrome constituted a distinct entity, which was separate from severe pre-eclampsia, it is now generally accepted that the HELPP syndrome is a variant of severe pre-eclampsia (Curtin & Weinstein 1999; Haddad et al 2000b). The criteria used to define the HELLP syndrome are: (i) haemolysis (characteristic peripheral blood smear, in which burr cells, schistocytes and spherocytes are present and serum lactate dehydrogenase >600 U/L or serum bilirubin >1.2 mg/dL); (ii) elevated liver enzymes

(serum aspartate aminotransferase level >70 U/l) and (iii) low platelet count (less than 100 000/mm³) (Sibai 1990; Barton & Sibai 1992; Haddad et al 2000b).

It is estimated that the HELLP syndrome occurs in 2–12% of cases of toxaemia of pregnancy and 0.2–0.8% of all pregnancies (Jones 1998; Rath et al 2000). As with pre-eclampsia, the HELLP syndrome typically presents during the third trimester. A small proportion of cases present during the second trimester (Haddad et al 2000b) and occasional cases a few hours to six days postpartum, (Barton & Sibai 1992; Risseeuw et al 1999). It occurs predominantly in multiparous women over 25 years old. Patients present with nausea or vomiting, epigastric or right upper quadrant pain, and headache. There may be oedema and the diastolic blood pressure is usually greater than 100 mmHg. Maternal complications include cerebral haemorrhage, eclampsia, disseminated intravascular coagulopathy, adult respiratory distress syndrome, placental abruption, acute renal failure and hepatic haemorrhage/rupture (Portis et al 1997; Isler et al 1999; Haddad et al 2000a). Maternal mortality rates as high as 24% have been reported (Portis et al 1997), but appear to be declining. In one recent study of 183 women with the

HELLP syndrome, the maternal mortality was only 1% (Haddad et al 2000a). There is an increased risk of obstetric complications in subsequent pregancies including recurrence of the HELLP syndrome (Sibai et al 1986; Sullivan et al 1994; Sibai et al 1995). The incidence of intrauterine growth retardation and prematurity is also increased, and infants of affected mothers may have thrombocytopenia with DIC. The severity of neonatal complications correlate with the severity of maternal disease, and the overall perinatal mortality rate ranges from 10–60% (Sibai et al 1995; Wolf 1996; Portis et al 1997).

Liver biopsies frequently show features of a non-specific reactive hepatitis with a mild portal tract chronic inflammatory cell infiltrate. In some cases there is focal parenchymal necrosis and haemorrhage with fibrin deposition. These changes typically have a periportal distribution, similar to that described in eclampsia (Schorr-Lesnick 1991). Fatty change, usually microvesicular, and neutrophilic infiltration may also be seen (Barton & Sibai 1992; Halim et al 1996). Intrahepatic haemorrhage, subcapsular haematomas, extracapsular perihepatic haematomas and hepatic infarction have all been reported as complications of pre-eclampsia and HELLP syndrome (Barton & Sibai 1992; Chan & Gerscovich 1999; Zissin 1999). In some cases these haemorrhagic manifestations may be associated with rupture of the liver (Barton & Sibai 1992; Sheikh et al 1999), discussed further below. A small number of cases have undergone liver transplantation for hepatic complications of the HELLP syndrome (Strate et al 2000). A poor correlation has been observed between the severity of the histological changes and the other laboratory findings in the HELLP syndrome (Barton et al 1992).

The presence of antiphospholipid antibodies has been associated with an earlier presentation of the HELLP syndrome and with more extensive ischaemic damage (Alsulyman et al 1996; Amant et al 1997). Other prothrombotic factors, which have been implicated in the pathogenisis of HELLP syndrome, include mutations in coagulation factor V (Brenner et al 1996; Bozzo et al 2001), although evidence for this is controversial (Livingston et al 2001). Other factors which have also been implicated in the pathogenesis of hepatocyte necrosis in the HELLP syndrome are vasospasm of the hepatic arterial blood supply, cytokines, including TNF-alpha, and neutrophil-mediated mechanisms (Sibai 1990; Halim et al 1996).

SPONTANEOUS RUPTURE OF THE LIVER

This rare complication of pregnancy has been estimated to occur in approximately 1 in 45 000 live births (Sherbahn 1996). It occurs most commonly in association with toxaemia in the last trimester of pregnancy but in a minority of cases there is no associated hypertension

Neerhof et al 1989; (Smith et al 1991; Matsuda et al 1997; Schwartz & Lien 1997). Some cases develop immediately postpartum. It more commonly affects multiparous women and tends to occur at an older age than typical pre-eclampsia (Ralston & Schwaitzberg 1998). Other pregnancy related conditions which may predispose to rupture of the liver are AFLP (Minuk et al 1987) and the HELLP syndrome (Barton & Sibai 1992). A small number of cases have been associated with pre-existing liver lesions including haemangioma (Yen 1964), amoebic abscess (Yen 1964), liver cell adenoma (Hibbard 1976; Kent et al 1978) and liver cell carcinoma (Roddie 1957; Bis & Waxman 1976).

There is usually a history of trauma, often minor. The clinical presentation is acute with profound shock, sometimes out of proportion to the amount of blood which is found in the peritoneal cavity (Golan & White 1979). In some cases, upper abdominal pain, hepatic tenderness, nausea and vomiting have been present for some days. In a patient with toxaemia, clinical awareness of the risk of rupture may allow an early diagnosis to be made ultrasonically or by CT scanning, and may improve the prognosis (Sommer et al 1979; Greca et al 1984; Smith et al 1991). The management of cases is surgical and requires emergency laparotomy with hepatic artery ligation, hepatic artery embolisation or lobectomy (Loevinger et al 1985; Terasaki et al 1990). The maternal mortality rate is high (up to 75% — Bis & Waxman 1976; Cozzi & Morris 1996) with a correspondingly high fetal loss (Severino et al 1970; Bis & Waxman 1976; Golan & White 1979). Early recognition and prompt surgical treatment of liver rupture have improved the outcome in some cases (Ralston & Schwaitzberg 1998), but high maternal and fetal mortality rates still persist (Sheikh et al 1999).

Spontaneous rupture predominantly involves the right lobe (Severino et al 1970; Bis & Waxman 1976; Hibbard 1976; Golan & White 1979). The rupture is thought to occur from subcapsular haematomas, which may be found without peritoneal haemorrhage and which may be continuous with haemorrhage within the liver substance (Lavery & Bowes 1971; Sheehan & Lynch 1973). In a case described by MacSween (1995) focal sharply circumscribed intrahepatic haemorrhages were present together with larger areas of subcapsular haemorrhage (Fig. 43.9). The areas of haemorrhage contained periportal foci showing appearances closely resembling those described in toxaemia of pregnancy (Fig. 43.10) Arteriography has demonstrated pseudoaneurysms associated with areas of subcapsular haemorrhage in some cases of pregnancy — associated intrahepatic haemorrhage and rupture (Wagner et al 1985; Greenstein et al 1994).

The aetiology of the condition is uncertain. The increased vascular reactivity and disseminated intravascular coagulation which occur in toxaemia of pregnancy could predispose to focal parenchymal haemorrhage, which, in some cases, becomes confluent, giving rise to

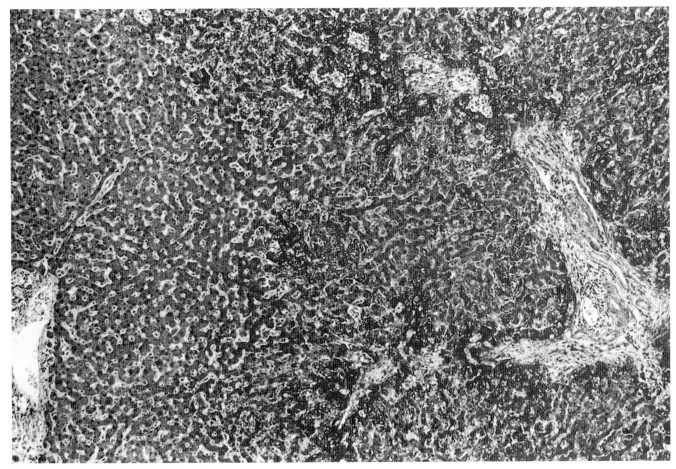

Fig. 43.9 Spontaneous rupture of the liver at 27 weeks' gestation in a patient with mild toxaemia: there is a fairly sharp delineation between normal liver (left) and the area showing haemorrhage and extensive sinusoidal fibrin deposition. MSB.

intrahepatic and subcapsular haematomas (Chesley 1966; Sheehan & Lynch, 1973; Sheikh et al 1999). Abdominal trauma may then be the precipitating factor leading to rupture of the liver capsule.

MISCELLANEOUS GROUP

Hyperemesis gravidarum

This poorly understood condition, which typically occurs in the first trimester of pregnancy, may be associated with dysfunction in a variety of organs, notably the liver and thyroid gland (Abell & Riely 1992). It occurs in 0.2 to 1.6% of pregnancies. It has been estimated that liver involvement occurs in up to 50% of patients with hyperemesis gravidarum, but in the majority of cases this represents mild subclinical disease. In a minority of patients who do develop jaundice, this is usually mild (Wallstedt et al 1990; Abell & Riely 1992). Biochemical changes include a slight increase in aminotransferases, generally less than four times the upper limit of normal (Morali & Braverman 1990). Wallstedt et al (1990) found elevated levels of transaminases in 6 of 12 patients, with some having levels

higher than 800 U/l. Elevations in bilirubin levels are present less commonly (Wallstedt et al 1990; Riely 1994). Histological examination of the liver in a small number of cases has shown mild non-specific changes, including cholestasis, hepatocyte ballooning and/or vacuolisation and focal hepatocyte dropout (Sheehan 1940; Adams et al 1968; Richards et al 1970; Wallstedt et al 1990; Wolf 1996).

Liver pregnancy

This is very rare but in eight of a series of 236 extrauterine pregnancies placental attachment to the liver was recorded (Cornell & Lash 1933). More recently, single case reports have been published (Murley 1956; Meare et al 1965; Kirby 1969; Hietala et al 1983; Mitchell & Teare 1984a; Shukla et al 1985; Veress & Wallmander 1987; Borlum & Blom 1988; Harris et al 1989; De Almeida Barbosa et al 1991; Delabrousse et al 1999). Most cases present in early pregnancy with acute abdominal symptoms resembling those occurring in other forms of ruptured ectopic pregnancy. Occasional pregnancies have gone to term (Meare et al 1965; Shukla et al 1985) and in one of these a live infant was born (Shukla et al 1985).

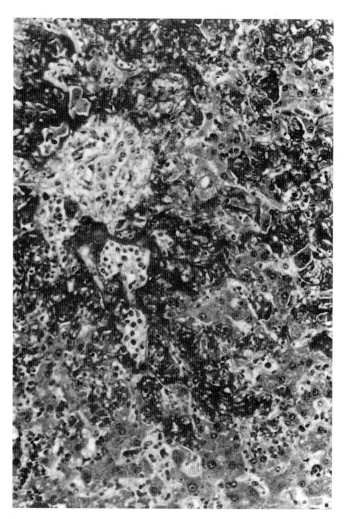

Fig. 43.10 From the same patient as Fig. 43.9. There is periportal haemorrhage, liver cell necrosis and fibrin deposition. There is a mild acute inflammatory cell reaction. MSB.

LIVER DISEASES DEVELOPING CONCURRENTLY WITH PREGNANCY

ACUTE VIRAL HEPATITIS

Viral hepatitis is the commonest cause of jaundice in pregnancy (Haemmerli 1966; Mishra & Seef 1992; Dinsmoor 1997; Hunt & Sharara 1999). Although all of the main types of hepatitis virus can theoretically present as acute infections during pregnancy, in practice most cases can be attributed to hepatitis E or B (Jaiswal et al 2001). In the great majority of cases, the clinical and pathological features of acute viral hepatitis occurring in pregnancy are the same as seen in the non-pregnant individual, and the reader is referred to other standard texts which describe these features in detail. For an overview of viral hepatitis in pregnancy the reader is referred to Mishra & Seef (1992); Rustgi et al (1993); Simms & Duff (1993); Dinsmoor (1997); Duff (1998); Magriples (1998). Only those issues which

specifically relate to viral infection in pregnancy will be considered here.

Most cases of hepatitis B infection and the great majority of cases of hepatitis C infection which occur in pregnancy are ones where infection was acquired prior to pregnancy. The effects of pregnancy on chronic viral hepatitis and vice versa will be discussed later, together with fetal complications, including the transmission of viral infection.

Hepatitis A

There are some reports of prematurity and stillbirths when hepatitis A infection occurs in the last trimester but there is no evidence that it causes congenital defects (Meadow 1968; Waterson 1979). Transmitted hepatitis A has been reported as a rare cause of neonatal hepatitis (Schwer & Moosa 1978; Tong et al 1981; Williams & Ede 1981; Mishra & Seef 1992; Tanaka et al 1995; Fagan et al 1999).

Hepatitis B

Infection in the third trimester has been associated with an increased risk of prematurity, sometimes with an increased fetal mortality (Steven 1981). There is no increase in congenital malformations.

Hepatitis E

Hepatitis E virus (HEV) is an important cause of acute viral hepatitis in developing countries and, in a small proportion of cases, results in acute liver failure (Mast & Krawcynzski 1996; Kar et al 1997; Coursaget et al 1998; Acharya et al 2000; Jaiswal et al 2001). HEV has also been implicated as a rare cause of fulminant hepatic failure in non-endemic areas such as the UK (Sallie et al 1994). Chronic infection is not seen (Aggarwal & Krawcynski 2000). A higher incidence and more severe course of presumed HEV infection have been observed in pregnant women, with mortality rates reaching as high as 25% (Melnick 1957; Wong et al 1980; Khuroo et al 1981; Hla-Myint et al 1985; Tsega et al 1992; Aggarwal & Krawcynski 2000). In the study of Khuroo et al (1981) fulminant hepatitis occurred exclusively in the third trimester. Distinction between fulminant HEV infection and acute fatty liver of pregnancy (AFLP), which also presents during the third trimester, cannot be made on the basis of clinical and biochemical features and demonstration of anti-HEV antibodies is required to confirm a diagnosis of acute HEV infection (Hamid et al 1996). Disseminated intravascular coagulation, which is a characteristic finding in AFLP, has also been reported as a feature of HEV infection (Krawczynski 1993). Histological features of HEV infection resemble those seen in other types of acute viral hepatitis. In some cases there are prominent cholestatic features, which may mimic changes seen in biliary obstruction (Aggarwal & Krawcynski 2000). In cases presenting with fulminant hepatitis, there is extensive hepatocyte destruction resulting in submassive or massive hepatic necrosis.

The reasons for the variations in HEV infection in pregnancy in developing countries are not clear. Defects in maternal nutrition and immunosuppresive effects of pregnancy have been postulated as possible mechanisms.

Vertical transmission of HEV infection from mother to infant has been reported to occur in a small number of cases (Khuroo et al 1995), the effects ranging from mild anicteric hepatitis to severe hepatitis associated with massive hepatic necrosis resulting in death.

HERPES SIMPLEX HEPATITIS

This is a rare but serious complication of pregnancy. Herpes simplex virus (HSV) hepatitis in adults usually presents as part of a disseminated systemic infection occurring as a complication of immunosuppression, and this has been postulated as the mechanism for pregnancy as a risk factor. Most cases present with fever and severe hepatic dysfunction in the last trimester of pregnancy. Occasional cases have occurred during the second or, rarely, the first trimester (Young et al 1996). The mucocutaneous lesions, which characterise herpes simplex infection, are frequently absent and, because of the low index of suspicion, the diagnosis is frequently overlooked (Jacques & Qureshi 1992; Kang & Graves 1999). The majority of cases are due to HSV-2 infection, and primary infection during the latter part of pregnancy appears to constitute the greatest risk (Mudido et al 1993). The clinical, biochemical and other laboratory findings lack diagnostic specificity and liver biopsy is regarded as the most reliable technique for establishing a diagnosis of HSV hepatitis (Kaufman et al 1997). The characteristic histological features include scattered areas of coagulative hepatocyte necrosis surrounded by a zone of congestion. Inflammation is generally mild or absent. At the periphery of necrotic areas hepatocytes containing nuclear inclusions may be seen. Immunohistochemistry is useful to confirm the presence of HSV antigens in hepatocyte inclusions. Rarely, there may be massive hepatic necrosis without obvious viral inclusions (Jacques & Qureshi 1992). Hepatic involvement is a severe manifestation of systemic HSV infection and high maternal and fetal mortality rates have been reported. Early diagnosis and treatment with antiviral therapy in the form of acyclovir improves the outcome for both the mother and infant (Klein et al 1991; Johnson & Saldana 1994; Young et al 1996; Kang & Graves 1999). Neonatal herpes hepatitis, usually due to transmission of the virus from the genital herpes in the mother is well recognised (Overall 1994).

OTHER INFECTIOUS DISEASES

Amoebic abscess

This is caused by the protozoan organism *Entamoeba histolytica*, which is endemic in many parts of the developing world. Several cases of hepatic amoebiasis in pregnancy have been reported in endemic areas (de Silva 1970; Navaraine 1972; Wagner et al 1975; Cowan & Houlton 1978; Katzeff & Moore 1984; Mitchell & Teare 1984b; Mabina et al 1998; Patial et al 1998; Gangwal et al 2000; Read et al 2001). It is possible that an increased susceptibility to amoebiasis in the pregnant woman is related to impaired immune responsiveness (Abioye et al 1972). Complications of hepatic amoebiasis in pregnancy include preterm labour and intraperitoneal rupture.

Miscellaneous

Other infectious diseases which have presented with hepatic complications during pregnancy include pyogenic abscess (Kopernick et al 1988), echinococcal cysts (Kain & Keystone 1988; Crow et al 1990; Golaszewski et al 1995; van Vliet et al 1995), in some cases requiring surgical intervention, leptospirosis (Burroughs 1991) and malaria (Arya & Prasad 1988).

DRUG-INDUCED HEPATIC INJURY

The spectrum of complications associated with drug toxicity in the pregnant woman is similar to that seen in nonpregnant individuals. For a detailed description of drug-induced liver injury, the reader is referred to appropriate standard texts. Because of increasing awareness of the possible direct effects or teratogenic effects on the fetus considerable care is exercised in the administration of most drugs during pregnancy.

The toxic effects of certain drugs may be exacerbated by pregnancy. The best known example is tetracycline, for which there is a strong association between high-dose therapy, pregnancy and liver toxicity (Kunelis et al 1965). Histologically, tetracycline toxicity is characterised by microvesicular steatosis. In less severe cases fatty change is confined to peripheral acinar regions, but in other cases it has a panacinar distribution (Farrell 1994). These changes closely resemble those seen in acute fatty liver of pregnancy (AFLP) and have been associated with severe, often fatal, disease affecting the liver and other organs. The hepatotoxic effects of tetracyclines are thought to relate to two main mechanisms: inhibition of mitochondrial beta oxidation of lipids and decreased egress of triglycerides from the liver (Fromenty & Pessayre 1997). The first of these two pathways has also been implicated in the pathogenesis of AFLP, as discussed earlier. Hormonal changes related to pregnancy also impair function of liver mitochondria (Grimbert et al 1993; Grimbert et al 1995), which may account for pregnancy as a contributory factor. Because the dose-dependent nature of tetracycline toxicity is now well recognised, serious hepatic complications are no longer seen (Fromenty & Pessayre 1997). There is some evidence to suggest that the toxic effects of drugs associated with cholestatic reactions (e.g. chlorpromazine) may be exacerbated if they develop during pregnancy. There have been a small number of patients in whom chlorpromazine therapy during pregnancy has been complicated by a chronic cholestatic syndrome associated with bile duct loss and biliary cirrhosis (Moradpour 1994; Chlumska et al 2001). However, a similar pattern of liver injury has also been reported as a rare complication of chlorpromazine therapy in non-pregnant individuals (Degott et al 1992) and definite evidence for pregnancy as a risk factor for chlorpromazine toxicity is lacking (Ishak & Irey 1972).

HEPATIC NEOPLASMS AND TUMOUR-LIKE CONDITIONS

Liver masses presenting in pregnancy are rare. The majority are benign lesions. In some parts of the world infectious agents are the commonest cause for hepatic masses presenting in pregnancy.

Benign intrahepatic lesions which have been observed during pregnancy include liver cell adenoma, focal nodular hyperplasia, haemangioma, angiomyolipoma and inflammatory pseudotumour (Kent et al 1978; Knowles et al 1978; Gong et al 1988; Livneh et al 1988; Imagawa et al 1994; Maze et al 1999; Mathieu et al 2000). Hormonal factors are known to be important in the aetiology of liver cell adenomas and hormonal changes occurring during pregnancy may result in increased growth and vascularity of these tumours. Rupture and hemorrhage from adenomas may occur during pregnancy and in the puerperium (Hayes et al 1977; Kent et al 1977; Rooks et al 1979). Hepatic haemangiomas are usually incidental findings but there have been two reports in which these lesions were associated with high-output cardiac failure during pregnancy (Gong et al 1988; Livneh et al 1988).

There have been a few reports describing liver cell adenoma occurring as a primary placental lesion (Chen et al 1986; Khalifa et al 1998; Vesoulis & Agamanolis 1998; Dargent et al 2000). The histogenesis of this lesion is uncertain. A monodermal teratoma, possibly related to displaced yolk sac elements, or heterotopia of liver tissue in the placenta are two main possibilities that have been postulated.

Primary hepatocellular carcinoma (HCC) is a common neoplasm, but presentation during pregnancy is very uncommon. In a review of the published literature, Lau et al could only identify 23 reported cases, to which they added five of their own (Lau et al 1995). The male preponderance of HCC, its occurrence at a late age in women and the decreased fertility associated with cirrhosis (an important risk factor in the pathogenesis of HCC) may all be factors contributing to the rarity of HCC in pregnancy. It should be noted that serum alpha-fetoprotein (AFP) levels are normally elevated in late pregnancy, with still greater increases occurring in the event of intrauterine fetal death (Adinolfi et al 1975), and the diagnostic value of AFP as a tumour marker for HCC is thus reduced in the pregnant woman. However, levels above 200 ng/100 ml are still considered to be diagnostic of primary liver cell carcinoma. Human chorionic gonadotrophins may also be demonstrated in 14% of patients with hepatocellular carcinoma (Braunstein et al 1973). Pregnancy appears to have an adverse impact on the outcome of HCC, with the median survival time being shorter than in non-pregnant women (Lau et al 1995). In occasional cases rupture of the liver has complicated liver cell carcinoma (Roddie 1957; Purtilo et al 1975). Although the fibrolamellar variant of HCC typically occurs in young adults without antecedent liver disease, there have only been two reports of this neoplasm presenting during pregnancy (Kroll et al 1991; Gemer et al 1994).

Cholangiocarcinoma occurs very rarely in pregnancy (Purtilo et al 1975; Devoe et al 1983; Nakamoto & vanSonnenberg 1985). There has been one case in which intrahepatic cholangiocarcinoma presented with features mimicking those of the HELLP syndrome (Balderston et al 1998).

The liver is a rare site for metastatic choriocarcinoma (Barnard et al 1986; Alveyn & Loehry 1988; Erb & Gibler 1989).

OTHER THROMBOTIC MICROANGIOPATHIES OCCURRING DURING PREGNANCY

The term thrombotic microangiopathy (TMA) has been used to describe a range of conditions characterised by occlusion of small blood vessels by platelet rich thrombi (McCrae & Cines 1997). Endothelial cell injury and platelet activation are thought to be important pathogenetic mechanisms. Pregnancy is associated with a variety of changes that enhance blood coagulation, which also predispose to the development of TMA.

Examples of TMA unique to pregnancy are preeclampsia, the HELLP syndrome and acute fatty liver of pregnancy. These three conditions have already been discussed. Pregnancy is also recognised as a risk factor for haemolytic uraemic syndrome (HUS) and thrombotic thrombocytopenic purpura (TTP) (Ezra et al 1996; McCrae & Cines 1997; Esplin & Branch 1999). In addition to problems related to thrombocytopenia, the microangiopathy which occurs in HUS and TTP results in changes involving the kidneys and central nervous system, respectively. Hepatic damage is rarely seen.

Although the clinicopathological features of HUS and TTP are usually fairly distinctive, areas of overlap exist between these two conditions and other pregnancy associated thrombotic microangiopathies (Sibai et al 1994; Uslu et al 1994; Hsu et al 1995; Kaiser & Distler 1996; Kahra et al 1998; Kemp et al 1999) and it has been suggested that these various diseases may be part of a spectrum of 'thrombotic microangiopathy of pregnancy' (Kemp et al 1999).

BUDD–CHIARI SYNDROME

It is of historical interest that in Chiari's first patient the clinical picture developed following childbirth (Chiari 1899). Other cases of the Budd–Chiari syndrome occurring in association with pregnancy have been reviewed by Rosenthal et al (1972); Tiliacos et al (1978); Khuroo & Datta (1980); Artigas et al (1982). The aetiology is not clear, although it has been postulated that it is due to a hypercoagulable state in pregnancy, possibly related to the effects of oestrogens. This might also explain the reported association of the Budd–Chiari syndrome with the use of contraceptive steroids. Other prothrombotic factors which have been implicated in the pathogenesis of pregnancy-related Budd–Chiari syndrome include factor V Leiden mutation (Fickert et al 1996; Deltenre et al 2001), pre-eclampsia (Gordon et al 1991) and thrombotic thrombocytopenic purpura (Hsu et al 1995). Pregnancy appears to be a particularly important risk factor for the Budd–Chiari syndrome in the Indian subcontinent (Dilawari et al 1994; Singh et al 2000).

The syndrome usually develops in the late stages of pregnancy or postpartum. Typically there is thrombosis of the major hepatic veins without involvement of the inferior vena cava. In some cases there is an acute fulminant presentation, with rapidly progressive liver failure (Dilawari et al 1994; Valentine et al 1995). The prognosis is usually poor; in Khuroo & Datta's series of 16 patients (1980) eight died within one year despite portacaval shunting. However, Vons et al (1984) reported three uneventful pregnancies in two women with this syndrome. Occasional cases have been treated by liver transplantation (Jamieson et al 1991; Valentine et al 1995; Salha et al 1996; Schilling et al 2000).

Histological changes in the liver are common to the syndrome irrespective of its aetiology. They comprise severe sinusoidal congestion associated with atrophy and necrosis of liver cells in peripheral acinar regions. In the chronic stages, there is replacement fibrosis and periportal nodular regeneration. In some cases a true cirrhosis supervenes. Features of venous outflow obstruction are often inconspicuous at this stage and distinction from other causes of cirrhosis may be difficult. Large regeneration nodules are sometimes seen in the chronic stages of Budd–Chiari syndrome and may be difficult to distinguish from neoplastic nodules (Tanaka & Wanless 1998). Liver nodules resembling focal nodular hyperplasia have been described in one woman who underwent liver transplantation for chronic Budd–Chiari syndrome,

occurring as a complication of pregnancy 7 years earlier (Schilling et al 2000).

Veno-occlusive disease, associated with pyrrolizidine alkaloids ingested in Jamaican bush tea, has been reported in one infant, presumably due to placental transfer (Roulet et al 1988).

SPONTANEOUS RUPTURE OF THE SPLENIC ARTERY

Although this is a rare event, more than 100 cases of spontaneous rupture of the splenic artery in pregnancy have now been reported (O'Grady et al 1977; Angelakis et al 1993). The haemodynamic and endocrine changes that occur in pregnancy have been implicated in causing arterial alterations, which predispose to the formation of new aneurysms and weakening of pre-existing aneurysms (Barrett et al 1982). Multiparity and the presence of portal hypertension appear to increase the risk of aneurysm formation and rupture (Barrett & Caldwell 1981; de Vries et al 1982; Holdsworth & Gunn 1992; Caillouette & Merchant 1993; Hillemanns et al 1996). Other sites in which pregnancy-associated aneurysms occur include the aorta, cerebral, renal, coronary and ovarian arteries. More than 50% of ruptured arterial aneurysms in women under the age of 40 are pregnancy related (Barrett et al 1982) and up to 50% of ruptured splenic artery aneurysms occur in pregnancy (Holdsworth & Gunn 1992). Most cases present during the third trimester, labour or the puerperium (Macfarlane & Thorbjarnarson 1966; O'Grady et al 1977). The mortality rate is disproportionately high at 75% in pregnant women, compared with 25% in non-pregnant individuals (Caillouette & Merchant 1993). Fetal mortality rates in excess of 90% have been reported (Holdsworth & Gunn 1992; Caillouette & Merchant 1993).

SPONTANEOUS RUPTURE OF THE BILIARY TRACT

Spontaneous rupture of the bile duct or cystic duct has been reported as a rare complication of pregnancy (Lemay et al 1980; Hendrickx et al 1981; Piotrowski et al 1990). In common with the cases seen in non-pregnant patients, bile duct rupture in pregnancy has been associated with cholelithiasis. Choledochal cysts may first come to clinical notice during pregnancy, local kinking of the cyst presumably interfering with bile flow and resulting in cholangitis (Hopkins et al 1990). There are two case reports of rupture of a choledochal cyst in pregnancy (Friend 1958; Saunders & Jackson 1969).

PRIMARY BILIARY CIRRHOSIS AND FETAL MICROCHIMERISM

Primary biliary cirrhosis (PBC) is a disease which predominantly affects women of child bearing age. Although primary biliary cirrhosis presenting during pregnancy is not well described it has been suggested that fetal microchimerism occurring during pregnancy may be an initiating factor for the subsequent development of PBC (Jones 2000; Tanaka et al 2000). Pregnancy is associated with two-way trafficking of cells from mother to fetus and vice versa. Fetal cells entering the maternal circulation are predominantly CD34+ haematological precursor cells, which appear to have the potential to persist for many years (Bianchi et al 1996). CD34 is also expressed in cells of the embryonic ductal plate, from which intrahepatic bile ducts eventually develop (Blakolmer et al 1995; Lemmer et al 1998). There is also evidence to suggest that haemopoietic stem cells of bone marrow origin can migrate to the liver in the adult, where they can differentiate into hepatocytes or biliary epithelial cells (Theise et al 2000; Sell 2001). There is thus the potential for fetal cells to trigger immune reactions cross-reacting with biliary epithelial cells. A number of studies have attempted to investigate this intriguing possibility further by using molecular techniques to look for DNA sequences derived from the Y chromosome in peripheral blood and/or liver tissue from PBC patients who had delivered a male child prior to onset of the illness (Rubbia-Brandt et al 1999; Tanaka et al 1999; Corpechot et al 2000; Fanning et al 2000). One of these studies found that Y chromosome DNA was more commonly present in the liver of PBC patients with male children than a control group of non-PBC patients with a similar pregnancy history (Fanning et al 2000). However, a similar association was not observed in the other three studies and the significance of fetal microchimerism as a potential trigger for primary biliary cirrhosis or other autoimmune liver diseases is uncertain (Jones 2000; Tanaka et al 2000).

PREGNANCY IN PRE-EXISTING LIVER DISEASE

Chronic liver disease is associated with an increased incidence of infertility. In cases when pregnancy does occur an increased risk of maternal and fetal complications has been observed. The risks of suffering fertility problems and obstetric complications appear to be related to the severity of chronic liver disease, most problems being seen in women who have developed an established cirrhosis particularly when related to alcohol abuse. The topic has been extensively reviewed by Varma (1987) and Lee (1992).

CHRONIC VIRAL HEPATITIS

Hepatitis B

Pregnancy does not appear to have any impact on liver damage related to chronic hepatitis B virus (HBV) infection.

The most important consequence of maternal HBV infection is vertical transmission to the neonate. The main risk factor for vertical transmission is the level of maternal viral replication. In women who are HBsAg and HBeAg positive, the risk of neonatal infection is 80–90%. By contrast, only 10–15% of children born to mothers who are HBsAg positive and HBeAg negative become infected (Berger et al 1998; Michielsen & Van Damme 1999). Measurement of serum viral DNA levels may be helpful in the latter group to determine the risk of vertical transmission. Acute infection in the last trimester has also been associated with a high risk of vertical transmission (Cossart 1977; Isenberg 1977). The precise mode of transmission from mother to baby is uncertain, but it is most likely to be related to exposure to infected maternal blood and amniotic fluid at the time of delivery. Breast milk also contains viral antigens, but there is no definite evidence for transmission of HBV infection via this route.

More than 90% of those who become infected as neonates develop a chronic carriers state and develop chronic hepatitis (Thomas et al 1988; Mulligan & Stiehm 1994; Michielsen & Van Damme 1999). This contrasts with infection acquired in adulthood, where the risk of developing chronic infection is substantially lower — less than 10%. The precise mechanisms involved in the induction of tolerance to the virus in the neonate are unclear. It is possible that maternal antibodies to HBV antigens cross the placenta and block recognition of virus-infected cells by cytotoxic T cells. It has also been postulated that HBeAg, which is one of the targets for a cellular immune response against HBV, crosses the placenta and induces tolerance (Thomas et al 1988). Immaturity of the neonatal immune system may also result in failure to eradicate the virus from infected hepatocytes (Mulligan & Stiehm 1994). A small proportion of neonates infected with HBV present with an acute hepatitis with rare cases of fulminant hepatitis. Vaccination of newborn infants born to HBV infected mothers has greatly reduced the risk of developing chronic HBV infection in this group of children and universal vaccination of neonates has been advocated as a mechanism for achieving global eradication of hepatitis B (MacIntyre 2001).

Hepatitis C

During pregnancy HCV infected women frequently experience a fall in serum transaminase levels, which then rise again following delivery (Conte et al 2000; Latt et al 2000). There is a concomitant rise in HCV-RNA levels during pregnancy, which return to baseline levels after delivery (Wejstal et al 1998). These observations suggest that immune mechanisms controlling viral replication are impaired during pregnancy. Histological changes have not been documented and the long-term impact of transient changes in viral replication during pregnancy is unknown.

HCV infection is not associated with an increased risk of obstetric complications during pregnancy (Floreani et al 1996; Jabeen et al 2000). However, approximately 1–5% of HCV-positive pregnancies result in transmission of HCV to the infant (Conte et al 2000; Yeung et al 2001). Maternal risk factors for mother-to-infant transmission include co-infection with HIV and high levels of viraemia (Hunt et al 1997; Zanetti et al 1999; Yeung et al 2001). It is not clear if viral transmission occurs in utero or as a perinatal infection complicating delivery (Conte et al 2000). Spontaneous clearance of maternally acquired HCV infection has been described in 17% of cases reviewed by Yeung et al (2001).

Hepatitis D

Transmission of HDV from mother to infant is extremely rare and can only occur with simultaneous transmission of HBV (Zanetti et al 1982).

Hepatitis G

Hepatitis G virus (HGV) is a parenterally transmitted RNA virus which is frequently acquired in association with HCV infection. Although HGV is hepatotropic, there is no clear evidence that it has a pathogenetic role in causing liver disease. Studies of pregnant women have shown high prevalence rates of HGV infection, between 10 and 60%, in HCV-positive and HIV-positive individuals (Hino et al 1998; Palomba et al 1999; Westjal et al 1999), but this does not appear to have any effect on liver disease. High rates of vertical transmission (between 40 and 80%) have been observed (Inaba et al 1997; Lin et al 1998; Palomba et al 1999; Westjal et al 1999) but these have not been associated with any clinical evidence of hepatitis in infected infants.

AUTOIMMUNE HEPATITIS

Problems relating to reduced fertility and fetal complications of pregnancy occurring in women with autoimmune hepatitis have been reviewed by Steven et al (1979). There are conflicting data regarding the effects of pregnancy on autoimmune hepatitis. Beneficial effects, related to pregnancy-associated immunosuppression (Colle & Hautekeete 1999) and flares in disease activity (Heneghan et al 2001) have both been reported.

CIRRHOSIS AND PORTAL HYPERTENSION

Pregnancy in patients with cirrhosis is uncommon (Aggarwal et al 1999). Cirrhosis is associated with amenorrhoea and sub-fertility but the reasons for this are not clear.

Maternal complications of pregnancy occurring in cirrhosis include gastrointestinal haemorrhage and hepatocellular failure (Whelton & Sherlock 1968; Cheng 1977; Pajor & Lehoczhy 1994; Russell & Craigo 1998). However, whilst it is generally accepted that pregnancy aggravates liver disease in cirrhotic patients, the extent to which hepatic complications exceed those occurring in non-pregnant women with cirrhosis is not clear. In some women with primary biliary cirrhosis jaundice and/or worsening of cholestatic biochemistry have developed during the third trimester (Whelton & Sherlock 1968; Nir et al 1989). Rapidly progressive liver disease, necessitating listing for liver transplantation within a year of presentation, has been observed in one woman who was diagnosed with primary biliary cirrhosis during the third trimester of pregnancy (Rabinovitz et al 1995). Pregnancy does not appear to have an adverse effect on liver disease in primary sclerosing cholangitis (Janczewska et al 1996). An increased risk of postpartum haemorrhage has also been reported in cirrhotic women (Cheng 1977).

Fetal complications of pregnancy associated with cirrhosis include spontaneous miscarriage, intrauterine growth retardation and preterm delivery, all of which contribute to increased fetal morbidity and mortality (Whelton & Sherlock 1968; Pajor & Lehoczhy 1994; Russell & Craigo 1998; Aggarwal et al 1999).

An increased risk of variceal bleeding has also been observed in pregnant women with non-cirrhotic portal hypertension, with associated fetal complications of spontaneous miscarriage, prematurity, small for gestational age babies and perinatal death (Cheng 1977; Aggarwal et al 2001).

METABOLIC LIVER DISEASES

Wilson's disease

Secondary amenorrhoea, reduced fertility and an increased incidence of spontaneous miscarriage occur in women with Wilson's disease (Sternlieb 2000; Tarnacka et al 2000). These problems partly represent non-specific consequences of chronic liver disease, as already discussed above. In addition, there is some evidence that free copper circulating in serum may have a direct effect in impairing ovarian follicular function (Kaushansky et al 1987). In a review of published and unpublished reports from various sources, Sternlieb identified a total of 153 infants born to 111 women with Wilson's disease (Sternlieb 2000). In women with well-controlled disease, maternal and fetal outcome is good. Interruption of therapy has been associated with haemolytic episodes and fulminant hepatic failure (Shimono et al 1991). There is no evidence that the drugs used to treat Wilson's disease have any teratogenic effects (Sternlieb 2000).

Hereditary hepatic porphyria

The effects of pregnancy on various disturbances of porphyrin metabolism have been reviewed by Brodie and his colleagues (1976, 1977). The perinatal mortality is increased to 8% in the acute intermittent form and to 15% in hereditary coproporphyria. Pregnancy may exacerbate the cutaneous lesions of porphyria cutanea tarda (Loret de Mola et al 1996), but the impact on hepatic manifestations of this condition is uncertain. While frequent attacks of porphyria have been observed during pregnancy and in the puerperium there is no clear evidence that these result in increased maternal mortality (Brodie 1976, 1977).

MISCELLANEOUS GROUP

Hyperbilirubinaemia syndromes

Unconjugated bilirubin may cross the placenta. Cotton et al (1981) reported kernicterus in one infant delivered by Caesarean section in a case of fulminant liver failure due to cirrhosis.

Dubin–Johnson syndrome

This rare familial condition is characterised by chronic intermittent jaundice and conjugated hyperbilirubinaemia, which may first come to clinical notice when the patient is using oral contraceptives or during pregnancy, especially in the third trimester (Arias 1961; Cohen et al 1972; Dizoglio & Cardillo 1973). Although pregnancy may exacerbate the condition, progressive liver disease does not occur and the prognosis remains very good. Miscarriage rates are said to be increased (Krejs 1983).

Other familial syndromes

Gilbert's syndrome is probably not affected by pregnancy (Krejs 1983). In Rotor's syndrome, similar to the Dubin–Johnson syndrome but without hepatic accumulation of pigment (Wolpert et al 1977), jaundice has been reported to improve following pregnancy (Haverback & Wirtschafter 1960).

Polycystic liver disease

There has been a single case report of adult polycystic disease presenting during pregnancy (Kesby 1998).

PREGNANCY AND LIVER TRANSPLANTATION

Liver transplantation has been carried out successfully during pregnancy on a small number of occasions. The indications for liver transplantation in this setting have included liver diseases unrelated to pregnancy, such as fulminant hepatitis B infection (Fair et al 1990; Laifer et al 1990) and decompensated cirrhosis due to autoimmune hepatitis (Laifer et al 1997), and pregnancy-related conditions, including acute fatty liver of pregnancy (Ockner et al 1990; Amon et al 1993) and the HELLP syndrome (Strate et al 2000).

Following liver transplantation for whatever cause normal menses return within a few weeks or months in most women (Cundy et al 1990), although some still experience persisting menstrual abnormalities (Mass et al 1996). The first documented pregnancy in a liver allograft recipient was in 1978 and numerous successful pregnancies have been reported since then (Burroughs et al 1991; Armenti et al 2000).

In most cases pregnancy does not appear to have a major impact on liver allograft function. An increased incidence of rejection has been observed when conception occurs within 6 months of transplantation (Casele & Laifer 1998), but otherwise pregnancy does not appear to predispose to graft rejection. Worsening of graft function due to presumed recurrence of hepatitis C infection has also been reported during pregnancy, in occasional cases resulting in rapidly progressive graft failure (Armenti et al 2000).

A higher incidence of obstetric complications, mainly hypertension and pre-eclampsia, has been observed in liver allograft recipients, with associated fetal complications of intrauterine growth retardation and premature delivery (Radomski et al 1995; Casele & Laifer 1998). Hypertension and renal dysfunction, occurring as side effects of immunsuppressive drug therapy, are commonly present in liver allograft recipients and may predispose to or exacerbate changes related to toxaemia. With increased experience in the management of pregnancy following liver transplantation, the overall risk of maternal and fetal complications is low (Jain et al 1998).

Cytomegalovirus (CMV) is an important cause of opportunistic infection in liver allograft recipients. Although pregnancy does not appear to have a major impact on cytomegalovirus disease in the mother, cytomegalovirus infection is the leading cause of neonatal mortality in some post-liver transplant pregnancy series (Armenti et al 2000). Neonatal mortality has been ascribed to prematurity, low birthweight and overwhelming sepsis although it is not clear how these relate to maternal cytomegalovirus infection.

Immunosuppressive regimes are often modified during pregnancy because of potentially harmful effects on the fetus. According to guidelines issued by the United States Food and Drug Administration Agency azathioprine can cause fetal harm and should not be used in pregnant women. However, there is no clear evidence that any of the immunosuppressive agents used routinely in liver transplantation have proven teratogenic effects in humans.

BILE COMPOSITION, GALLBLADDER FUNCTION AND CHOLELITHIASIS

Pregnancy is a well-recognised risk factor for the development of cholesterol gallstones, the risk increasing according to the number of pregnancies (Scragg et al 1984; Everson 1993; Tsimoyiannis et al 1994; Beckingham

2001). Gallstones are found in 6–8% of nulliparous women and in 18–20% of women with two or more pregnancies (Gilat & Konikoff 2000). As discussed earlier, intrahepatic cholestasis of pregnancy is associated with a further increase in the risk of developing gallstones.

There are a number of ways in which pregnancy may be implicated in the pathogenesis of gallstones. Firstly, the hormonal changes that occur during pregnancy result in an increased cholesterol saturation index of bile, making it more lithogenic. These changes are most marked in the second and third trimester (Kern et al 1981; Everson et al 1991; Valdivieso et al 1993). A similar mechanism has been proposed for the development of gallstones in users of contraceptive steroids. Secondly, there is an increase in the size and change in the composition of the bile acid pool, with a reduction in the ratio between chenodeoxycholic acid (CDCA) and cholic acid (CA) (Kern et al 1981; Kern et al 1982). These changes also occur in the later two-thirds of pregnancy and have been described in association with the use of contraceptive steroids (Bennion et al 1976; Kern et al 1982), suggesting that hormonal factors may again be important. Enterohepatic cycling of the bile acid pool is also reduced in pregnancy, partly as a result of slowing in the intestinal transit time, but also due to changes in gallbladder function. Thirdly, pregnancy is associated with an increase in fasting gallbladder volume and with incomplete emptying of the gallbladder (Braverman et al 1980; Cohen 1980; Everson et al 1982; Kapicioglu et al 2000). These changes predispose to the development of biliary stasis and sludge formation. It is not clear if changes in gallbladder function in pregnancy are also hormonally induced, and there are conflicting data regarding the effects of contraceptive steroids on gall bladder volume and function in non-pregnant women (Braverman et al 1980; Everson et al 1982). However, oestrogen and progesterone receptors are present in the human gallbladder (Singletary et al 1986) and it is possible that they may play a rôle in regulating its contractility (Daignault et al 1988; Hould et al 1988). As discussed earlier intrahepatic cholestasis of pregnancy is also associated with an increase in volume and reduction in motility of the gallbladder.

Ultrasonographic studies have shown that biliary sludge and/or gallstones commonly develop during pregnancy (Maringhini et al 1993; Valdivieso et al 1993; Van Bodegraven et al 1998; Gilat & Konikoff 2000). The incidence of biliary sludge formation is approximately 25% (Maringhini et al 1993) and gallstone neoformation occurs in 3–10% of cases (Valdivieso et al 1993; Gilat & Konikoff 2000). The biliary sludge which forms during pregnancy is usually asymptomatic and disappears a few months postpartum in most cases (Maringhini et al 1993). Many of the small stones which develop during pregnancy also disappear postpartum, presumably due to reversal of the pregnancy-related lithogenic factors.

Although symptomatic gall bladder disease is considered to be an uncommon problem in pregnant women (Seymour & Chadwick 1979), it represents the commonest non-gynaecological indication for surgery during pregnancy (Sungler et al 2000). Cholecysectomy has generally been avoided, because of an increased risk of fetal complications, including fetal loss (Ghumman et al 1997). However, improvements in peri-operative monitoring of mother and fetus and advances in surgical technique, including laparoscopic cholecystectomy, have improved fetal outcome and cholecystectomy can now be regarded as a safe technique at any stage during pregnancy (Cosenza et al 1999; Sungler et al 2000). Biliary obstruction by gallstones was considered to be the cause of jaundice in 27 of 450 cases in Haemmerli's series (1966), but has been rarely observed in other studies.

Acknowledgements

The author is indebted to Professor R N M MacSween, who wrote this chapter for the previous edition of Haines & Taylor, from which many of the illustrations and references have been used with kind permission. Thanks are also due to Miss T E Claridge, who has helped with typing the manuscript.

REFERENCES

Abell T L, Riely C A 1992 Hyperemesis gravidarum. Gastroenterology Clinics of North America 21: 835–849

Abioye A A, Lewis E A, McFarlane H 1972 Clinical evaluation of serum immunoglobulin in amoebiasis. Immunology 23: 937–946

Acharya S K, Panda S K, Saxena A, Gupta S D 2000 Acute hepatic failure in India: a perspective from the East. Journal of Gastroenterology and Hepatology. 15: 473–479

Adams R H, Gordon J, Combes B 1968 Hyperemesis gravidarum. I. Evidence of hepatic dysfunction. Obstetrics and Gynecology 31: 659–664

Adeniyi F A, Olatunbosun D A 1984 Origins and significance of the increased plasma alkaline phosphatase during normal pregnancy and pre-eclampsia. British Journal of Obstetrics and Gynaecology 91: 857–862

Adinolfi A, Adinolfi M, Lessoff M H 1975 Alpha-feto-protein during development and in disease. Journal of Medical Genetics 12: 138–151

Adlercreutz H, Svanborg A, Anberg A 1967 Recurrent jaundice in pregnancy. II. A study of the estrogens and their conjugation in late pregnancy. American Journal of Medicine 42: 341–347

Aggarwal R, Krawczynski K 2000 Hepatitis E: an overview and recent advances in clinical and laboratory research. Journal of Gastroenterology and Hepatology 15: 9–20

Aggarwal N, Sawnhey H, Suril V, Vasishta K, Jha M, Dhiman R K 1999 Pregnancy and cirrhosis of the liver. Australian and New Zealand Journal of Obstetrics and Gynaecology 39: 503–506

Aggarwal N, Sawhney H, Vasishta K, Dhiman R K, Chawla Y 2001 Non-cirrhotic portal hypertension in pregnancy. International Journal of Gynaecology and Obstetrics 72: 1–7

Alsulyman O M, Castro M A, Zuckerman E, McGehee W, Goodwin T M 1996 Preeclampsia and liver infarction in early pregnancy associated with the antiphospholipid syndrome. Obstetrics and Gynecology 88: 644–646

Alveyn C G, Loehry C A 1988 Hepatic metastases due to choriocarcinoma. Postgraduate Medical Journal 64: 941–942

Amant F, Spitz B, Arnout J, Van Assche F A 1997 Hepatic necrosis and haemorrhage in pregnant patients with antiphospholipid antibodies. Lupus 6: 552–555

Amon E, Allen S R, Petrie R H et al 1993 Acute fatty liver of pregnancy associated with preeclampsia; management of hepatic failure with postpartum liver transplantation. American Journal of Perinatology 8: 278–279

Angelakis E J, Bair W E, Barone J E, Lincer R M 1993 Splenic artery aneurysm rupture during pregnancy. Obstetrical and Gynecological Survey 48: 145–148

Antia F P, Bharadwaj T P, Watsa M C, Master J 1958 Liver in normal pregnancy, pre-eclampsia and eclampsia. Lancet 2: 776–778

Arias F, Marchilla-Jimenez R 1976 Hepatic fibrinogen deposits in preeclampsia: immunofluorescent evidence. New England Journal of Medicine 295: 578–582

Arias I M 1961 Studies of chronic familial non-haemolytic jaundice with conjugated bilirubin in the serum with and without an unidentified pigment in the liver cells. American Journal of Medicine 31: 510–518

Armenti V T, Herrine S K, Radomski J S, Moritz M J 2000 Pregnancy after liver transplantation. Liver Transplantation 6: 671–685

Artigas J M G, Estabanez J S, Faure M R A 1982 Pregnancy and the Budd–Chiari syndrome. Digestive Diseases and Sciences 27: 89–90

Arya T V, Prasad R N 1988 Malarial hepatitis. Journal of the Association of Physicians of India 36: 294–295

Bacq Y 1998 Acute fatty liver of pregnancy. Seminars in Perinatology 22: 134–140

Bacq Y, Zarka O, Brechot J F et al 1996 Liver function tests in normal pregnancy: a prospective study of 103 pregnant women and 103 matched controls. Hepatology 23: 1030–1034

Bacq Y, Sapey T, Brechot M C, Pierre F, Fignon A, Dubois F 1997 Intrahepatic cholestasis of pregnancy: a French prospective study. Hepatology 26: 358–364

Balderston K D, Tewari K, Azizi F, Yu J K 1998 Intrahepatic cholangiocarcinoma masquerading as the HELLP syndrome (hemolysis, elevated liver enzymes, and low platelet count) in pregnancy: case report. American Journal of Obstetrics and Gynecology. 179: 823–824

Barnard D E, Woodward K T, Yancy S G, Weed J C Jr, Hammond C B 1986 Hepatic metastases of choriocarcinoma: a report of 15 patients. Gynecologic Oncology 25: 73–83

Barrett J M, Caldwell B H 1981 Association of portal hypertension and ruptured splenic artery aneurysm in pregnancy. Obstetrics and Gynecology 57: 255–257

Barrett J M, Van Hooydonk J E, Boehm F H 1982 Pregnancy-related rupture of arterial aneurysms. Obstetrical and Gynecological Survey 37: 557–566

Barron W M 1992 The syndrome of pre-eclampsia. Gastroenterology Clinics of North America 21: 851–872

Barton J R, Sibai B M 1992 Care of the pregnancy complicated by HELLP syndrome. Gastroenterology Clinics of North America 21: 937–950

Barton J R, Sibai B M, Mabie W C et al 1990 Recurrent acute fatty liver of pregnancy. American Journal of Obstetrics and Gynecology 163: 534–538

Barton J R, Riely C A, Adamec T A, Shanklin D R, Khoury A D, Sibai B 1992 Hepatic histopathologic condition does not correlate with laboratory abnormalities in HELLP syndrome (hemoloysis, elevated liver enzyme and low platelet count). Americal Journal of Obstetrics and Gynecology 167: 1538–1543

Beckingham I J 2001 ABC of diseases of liver, pancreas, and biliary system. Gallstone disease. British Medical Journal 322: 91–94

Bennion L J, Ginsberg R L, Garnick M B, Bennett P 1976 Effects of oral contraceptives on the gallbladder bile of normal women. New England Journal of Medicine 294: 189–192

Berg B, Helm G, Petersohn L, Tryding N 1986 Cholestasis of pregnancy. Clinical and laboratory studies. Acta Obstetricia et Gynecologica Scandanavia; 65: 107–113

Berger A, Doerr H W, Weber B 1998 Human immunodeficiency virus and hepatitis B virus infection in pregnancy: diagnostic potential of viral genome detection. Intervirology; 41: 201–207

Bernuau J, Degott C, Nouel O, Rueff B, Benhamou J P 1982 Non-fatal acute fatty liver of pregnancy. Gut 24: 340–344

Bianchi D, Williams J M, Sullivan L M, Hanson F W, Klinger K W, Shuber A P 1996 PCR quantitation of fetal cells in maternal blood in normal aneuploid pregnancies. American Journal of Human Genetics 61: 822–829

Bis K A, Waxman B 1976 Rupture of the liver associated with pregnancy: a review of the literature and report of two cases. Obstetrical and Gynecological Survey 31: 763–773

Blakolmer K, Jaskiewicz K, Dunsford H A, Robson S C 1995 Hematopoietic stem cell markers are expressed by ductal plate and bile duct cells in developing human liver. Hepatology 21: 1510–1516

Borlum K G, Blom R 1988 Primary hepatic pregnancy. International Journal of Gynaecology and Obstetrics 27: 427–429

Bozzo M, Carpani G, Leo L et al 2001 HELLP syndrome and factor V Leiden. European Journal of Obstetrics, Gynecology and Reproductive Biology 95: 55–58

Braunstein G D, Vogel C L, Vaitukaitis J L, Ross G T 1973 Ectopic production of human chorionic gonadotrophin in Ugandan patients with hepatocellular carcinoma. Cancer 32: 223–226

Braverman D Z, Johnson M L, Kern F Jr 1980 Effects of pregnancy and contraceptive steroids on gallbladder function. New England Journal of Medicine 302: 362–364

Braverman D Z, Herbet D, Goldstein R et al 1988 Postpartum restoration of pregnancy-induced cholecystoparesis and prolonged intestinal transit time. Journal of Clinical Gastroenterology 10: 642–646

Breen K J, Perkins K W, Mistilis S P, Shearman R 1970 Idiopathic acute fatty liver of pregnancy. Gut 11: 822–825

Breen K J, Perkins K W, Schenker S, Dunkerley R C, Moore H C 1972 Uncomplicated subsequent pregnancy after idiopathic fatty liver of pregnancy. Obstetrics and Gynecology 40: 813–815

Brenner B, Lanir N, Thaler I 1996 HELLP syndrome associated with factor V R506Q mutation. British Journal of Haematology. 92: 999–1001

Brodie M J, Beattie A D, Moore M R, Goldberg A 1976 Pregnancy and hereditary hepatic porphyria. In: Doss M (ed) Porphyrins in human diseases. Karger, Basel, pp 251–254

Brodie M J, Moore M R, Thompson G G, Goldberg A, Low R A L 1977 Pregnancy and the acute porphyrias. British Journal of Obstetrics and Gynaecology 84: 726–731

Burroughs A K 1991 Liver disease and pregnancy. In: McIntyre N, Benhamou J P, Bircher J, Rizzetto M, Rodes J (eds) Oxford textbook of clinical hepatology, vol 2. Oxford University Press, Oxford, pp 1319–1332

Burroughs A K, Seong N H, Dojcinov D M et al 1982 Idiopathic acute fatty liver of pregnancy in 12 patients. Quarterly Journal of Medicine 205: 481–497

Burt A D, Mutton A, Day C P 1998 Diagnosis and interpretation of steatosis and steatohepatitis. Seminars in Diagnostic Pathology 15: 246–258

Buytaert I M, Elewaut G P, Van Kets H E 1996 Early occurrence of acute fatty liver in pregnancy. American Journal of Gastroenterology 91: 603–604

Caillouette J C, Merchant E B 1993 Ruptured splenic artery aneurysm in pregnancy. Twelfth reported case with maternal and fetal survival. American Journal of Obstetrics and Gynecology 168: 1810–1811

Campillo B, Bernau J, Witz M-O et al 1986 Ultrasonography in acute fatty liver of pregnancy. Annals of Internal Medicine 105: 383–384

Carter J 1991 Serum bile acids in normal pregnancy. British Journal of Obstetrics and Gynecology 98: 540–543

Casele H L, Laifer S A 1998 Pregnancy after liver transplantation. Seminars in Perinatology 22: 149–155

Castro M A, Goodwin T M, Shaw K J, Ouzounian J G, McGehee W G 1996a Disseminated intravascular coagulation and antithrombin III depression in acute fatty liver of pregnancy. American Journal of Obstetrics and Gynecology 174: 211–216

Castro M A, Ouzounian J G, Colletti P M, Shaw K J, Stein S M, Goodwin T M 1996b Radiological studies in acute fatty liver of pregnancy. A review of the literature and 19 new cases. Journal of Reproductive Medicine 41: 839–843

Castro M A, Fassett M J, Reynolds T B, Shaw K J, Goodwin T M 1999 Reversible peripartum liver failure: a new perspective on the diagnosis, treatment, and cause of acute fatty liver of pregnancy, based on 28 consecutive cases. American Journal of Obstetrics and Gynecology 181: 389–395

Cerutti R, Ferrari S, Grella P, Castelli G P, Rizzotti P 1976 Behaviour of serum enzymes in pregnancy. Clinical Experimental Obstetrics and Gynecology 9: 22–24

Chan A D, Gerscovich E O 1999 Imaging of subcapsular hepatic and renal hematomas in pregnancy complicated by preeclampsia and the HELLP syndrome. Journal of Clinical Ultrasound 27: 35–40

Chen K T, Ma C K, Kassel S H 1986 Hepatocellular adenoma of the placenta. American Journal of Surgical Pathology 10: 436–440

Cheng Y-S 1977 Pregnancy in liver cirrhosis and/or portal hypertension. American Journal of Obstetrics and Gynecology 128: 812–822

Chesley L C 1966 Vascular reactivity in normal and toxemic pregnancy. Clinical Obstetrics and Gynecology 9: 871–881

Chiari H 1899 Uber die selbstandige Phlebitis obliterans der Hauptstamme der Venae hepaticae als Todesursache. Beitrage zur pathologischen Anatomie und zur allgemeinen Pathologie 26: 1–18

Chlumska A, Curik R, Boudova L et al 2001 Chlorpromazine-induced cholestatic liver disease with ductopenia. Cesk Patol 37: 118–122

Clayton R J, Iber F L, Ruebner B H, McKusick V A 1969 Byler disease. Fatal familial intrahepatic cholestasis in an Amish kindred. American Journal of Diseases in Childhood 117: 112–124

Cohen L, Lewis C, Arias I M 1972 Pregnancy, oral contraceptives and chronic familial jaundice with predominantly conjugated hyperbilirubinemia (Dubin–Johnson syndrome). Gastroenterology 62: 1182–1190

Cohen S 1980 The sluggish gallbladder of pregnancy. New England Journal of Medicine 302: 397–398

Colle I, Hautekeete M 1999 Remission of autoimmune hepatitis during pregnancy: a report of two cases. Liver 19: 55–57

Combes B, Shore G M, Cunningham F G, Walker F B, Shorey J W, Ware A 1977 Serum gamma-glutamyl transpeptidase activity in viral hepatitis: suppression in pregnancy and by birth control pills. Gastroenterology 72: 271–274

Combes E, Shibata H, Adams R, Mitchell B D, Tramell V 1963 Alteration in sulfabromophthalein sodium removal mechanisms from blood during normal pregnancy. Journal of Clinical Investigation 42: 1431–1436

Conte D, Fraquelli M, Prati D, Colucci A, Minola E 2000 Prevalence and clinical course of chronic hepatitis C virus (HCV) infection and rate of HCV vertical transmission in a cohort of 15,250 pregnant women. Hepatology 31: 751–755

Cornell E L, Lash A F 1933 Abdominal pregnancy. International Abstracts of Surgery 8: 98–104

Corpechot C, Barbu V, Chazouilleres O, Poupon R 2000 Fetal michrochimerism in primary biliary cirrhosis. Journal of Hepatology 33: 696–700

Cosenza C A, Saffari B, Jabbour N et al 1999 Surgical management of biliary gallstone disease during pregnancy. American Journal of Surgery 178: 545–548

Cossart Y E 1977 The outcome of hepatitis B virus infection in pregnancy. Postgraduate Medical Journal 53: 610–613

Cotton D B, Brock B J, Schifrin B S 1981 Cirrhosis and fetal hyperbilirubinemia. Obstetrics and Gynecology 57: 25s–27s

Coursaget P, Buisson Y, N'Gawara M N, Van Cuyck-Gandre H, Roue R 1998 Role of hepatitis E virus in sporadic cases of acute and fulminant hepatitis in an endemic area (Chad). American Journal of Tropical Medicine and Hygiene 58: 330–334

Cowan D B, Houlton C C 1978 Rupture of an amoebic liver abscess in pregnancy: a case report. South African Medical Journal 53: 460–461

Cozzi P J, Morris D L 1996 Two cases of spontaneous liver rupture and literature review. Hepatic Pancreatic and Biliary Surgery 9: 257–260

Crow J P, Larry M, Vento E G et al 1990 Echinococcal disease of the liver in pregnancy. Hepatic Pancreatic and Biliary Surgery 2: 115–151

Cundy T F, O'Grady J G, Williams R 1990 Recovery of menstruation and pregnancy after liver transplantation. Gut 31: 337–338

Curtin W M, Weinstein L V 1999 A review of HELLP syndrome. Journal of Perinatology 19: 138–143

Daignault P G, Fazekas A G, Rosenthall L et al 1988 Relationship between gallbladder contraction and progesterone receptors in patients with gallstones. American Journal of Surgery 155: 147–151

Dalen E, Westerholm B 1974 Occurrence of hepatic impairment in women jaundiced by oral contraceptives and in their mothers and sisters. Acta Medica Scandinavica 195: 459–463

Dani R, Mendes G S, Medeiros J D, Peret F J, Nunes A 1996 Study of the liver changes occurring in preeclampsia and their possible pathogenetic connection with acute fatty liver of pregnancy. American Journal of Gastroenterology 91: 292–294

Dargent J L, Verdebout J M, Barlow P, Thomas D, Hoorens A, Goossens A 2000 Hepatocellular adenoma of the placenta: report of a case associated with maternal bicornuate uterus and fetal renal dysplasia. Histopathology 37: 287–289

Davidson K M 1998 Intrahepatic cholestasis of pregnancy. Seminars in Perinatology 22: 104–111

Davidson K M, Simpson L L, Knox T A, D'Alton M E 1998 Acute fatty liver of pregnancy in triplet gestation. Obstetrics and Gynecology 91: 806–808

Davies M H, Wilkinson S P, Hanid M A et al 1980 Acute liver disease with encephalopathy and renal failure in late pregnancy and the early puerperium: a study of fourteen patients. British Journal of Obstetrics and Gynaecology 87: 1105–1114

Davies M H, Ngong J M, Yucesoy M et al 1994 The adverse influence of pregnancy upon sulphation: a clue to the pathogenesis of intrahepatic cholestasis of pregnancy? Journal of Hepatology 21: 1127–1134

De Almeida Barbosa A Jr, Rodriguez de Freitas L A, Andrade Mota M 1991 Primary pregnancy in the liver: a case report. Pathology Research and Practice 187: 329–331

Degott C, Feldmann G, Larrey D et al 1992 Drug-induced prolonged cholestasis in adults: a histological semiquantitative study demonstrating progressive ductopenia. Hepatology 15: 244–251

Delabrousse E, Site O, Le Mouel A, Riethmuller D, Kastler B 1999 Intrahepatic pregnancy: sonography and CT findings. American Journal of Roentgenology 173: 1377–1378

Deltenre P, Denninger M H, Hillaire S 2001 Factor V Leiden related Budd–Chiari syndrome. Gut 48: 264–268

De Pagter A G, van Berge Henegouwen G P, ten Bokkel Huinink J A, Brandt K H 1976 Familial benign recurrent intrahepatic cholestasis. Interrelation with intrahepatic cholestasis of pregnancy and from oral contraceptives? Gastroenterology 71: 202–207

de Silva K 1970 Intraperitoneal rupture of an amoebic liver abscess in a pregnant woman at term. Ceylon Medical Journal 15: 51–53

Devoe L D, Moossa A R, Levin B 1983 Pregnancy complicated by extrahepatic biliary tract carcinoma. A case report. Journal of Reproductive Medicine 28: 153–155

De Vries J E, Schattenkerk M E, Malt R A 1982 Complications of splenic artery aneurysm other than intraperitoneal rupture. Surgery 91: 200–204

Dilawari J B, Bambery P, Chawla Y et al 1994 Hepatic outflow obstruction (Budd–Chiari syndrome). Experience with 177 patients and a review of the literature. Medicine (Baltimore) 73: 21–36

Dinsmoor M J 1997 Hepatitis in the obstetric patient. Infectious Disease Clinics of North America 11: 77–91

Dixon P H, Weerasekera N, Linton K J et al 2000 Heterozygous MDR3 missense mutation associated with intrahepatic cholestasis of pregnancy: evidence for a defect in protein trafficking. Human Molecular Genetics 9: 1209–1217

Dizoglio J A, Cardillo E 1973 The Dubin–Johnson syndrome and pregnancy. Obstetrics and Gynecology 42: 560–563

Duff P 1998 Hepatitis in pregnancy. Seminars in Perinatology 22: 277–283

Duma R J, Dowling E A, Alexander H J, Sibrons D, Dempsey H 1965 Acute fatty liver of pregnancy: report of surviving patient studied with serial liver biopsies. Annals of Internal Medicine 63: 851–858

Ebert E C, Sun E A, Wright S H et al 1984 Does early diagnosis and delivery in acute fatty liver of pregnancy lead to improvement in maternal and infant survival? Digestive Diseases and Science 29: 453–455

Elliott J R, O'Kell R T 1971 Normal clinical chemistry values for pregnant women at term. Clinical Chemistry 17: 156–157

Erb R E, Gibler W B 1989 Massive hemoperitoneum following rupture of hepatic metastases from unsuspected choriocarcinoma. American Journal of Emergency Medicine 7: 196–198

Esplin M S, Branch D W 1999 Diagnosis and management of thrombotic microangiopathies during pregnancy. Clinical Obstetrics and Gynecology 42: 360–367

Everson G T 1993 Pregnancy and gallstones. Hepatology 17: 159–161

Everson G T, McKinley C, Lawson M, Johnson M, Kern F Jr 1982 Gallbladder function in the human female: effect of the ovulatory cycle, pregnancy, and contraceptive steroids. Gastroenterology 82: 711–719

Everson G T, McKinley C, Kern F Jr 1991 Mechanisms of gallstone formation in women: effects of exogenous estrogen (premarin) and dietary cholesterol on hepatic lipid metabolism. Journal of Clinical Investigation 87: 237–246

Ezra Y, Rose M, Eldor A 1996 Therapy and prevention of thrombotic thrombocytopenic purpura during pregnancy: a clinical study of 16 pregnancies. American Journal of Hematology 51: 1–6

Fagan E A 1999 Intrahepatic cholestasis of pregnancy. Clinics in Liver Disease 3: 603–632

Fagan E A, Hadzic N, Saxena R, Mieli-Vergani G 1999 Symptomatic neonatal hepatitis A disease from a virus variant acquired in utero. Pediatric Infectious Diseases Journal 18: 389–391

Fair J, Klein A G, Feng T, Merritt W T, Burdick J F 1990 Intrapartum orthotopic liver transplantation with successful outcome of pregnancy. Transplantation 50: 534–535

Fanning P A, Jonsson J R, Clouston A D et al 2000 Detection of male DNA in the liver of female patients with primary biliary cirrhosis. Journal of Hepatology 33: 690–695

Farrell G C 1994 Drug-induced liver disease. Churchill Livingstone, Edinburgh, pp 226–229

Ferris T F, Herdson P B, Dunnill M S, Lee M R 1969 Toxemia of pregnancy in sheep: a clinical, physiological and pathological study. Journal of Clinical Investigation 48: 1643–1655

Fickert P, Ramschak H, Kenner L et al 1996 Acute Budd–Chiari syndrome with fulminant hepatic failure in a pregnant woman with factor V Leiden mutation. Gastroenterology 111: 1670–1673

Fisk N M, Storey G N 1988 Fetal outcome in obstetric cholestasis. British Journal of Obstetrics and Gynaecology 95: 1137–1143

Floreani A, Paternoster D, Zappala F et al 1996 Hepatitis C virus infection in pregnancy. British Journal of Obstetrics and Gynaecology 103: 325–329

Franco J, Newcomer J, Adams M, Saeian K 2000 Auxiliary liver transplant in acute fatty liver of pregnancy. Obstetrics and Gynecology 95: 1042

Fraser J L, Antonioli D A, Chopra S, Wang H H 1995 Prevalence and nonspecificity of microvesicular fatty change in the liver. Modern Pathology 8: 65–70

Friend W D 1958 Rupture of choledochal cyst during confinement. British Journal of Surgery 46: 155

Fromenty B, Pessayre D 1995 Inhibition of mitochondrial β-oxidation as a mechanism of hepatotoxicity. Pharmacology and Therapeutics 67: 101–154

Fromenty B, Pessayre D 1997 Impaired mitochondrial function in microvesicular steatosis. Effects of drugs, ethanol, hormones and cytokines. Journal of Hepatology 26: 43–53

Fulton I C, Douglas J G, Hutchon D J R, Beckett G J 1983 Is normal pregnancy cholestatic? Clinica Chimica Acta 130: 171–176

Furhoff A K 1974 Itching in pregnancy: a 15 year follow up study. Acta Medica Scandinavica 196: 403–410

Furhoff A K, Hellstrom K 1974 Jaundice in pregnancy: a follow up study of the series of women originally reported by L Thorling. II. Present health of the women. Acta Medica Scandinavica 196: 181–189

Gangwal P, Gupta M D, Agarwal A et al 2000 Amoebic liver abscess in pregnancy. Tropical Gastroenterology 21: 29–30

Gemer O, Segal S, Zohav E 1994 Pregnancy in a patient with fibrolamellar hepatocellular carcinoma. Archives of Gynecology and Obstetrics 255: 211–212

Ghumman E, Barry M, Grace P A 1997 Management of gallstones in pregnancy. British Journal of Surgery 84: 1646–1650

Gilat T, Konikoff F 2000 Pregnancy and the biliary tract. Canadian Journal of Gastroenterology 4 Suppl D: 55D–59D

Girling J C, Dow E, Smith J H 1997 Liver function tests in pre-eclampsia: importance of comparison with a reference range derived for normal pregnancy. British Journal of Obstetrics and Gynaecology 104: 246–250

Glasinovic J C, Mage R M, Ferreiro O et al 1989 Cholelithiasis in a Chilean female population: prevalence and associated risk factors. Gastroenterology 96: A 601

Golan A, White R G 1979 Spontaneous rupture of the liver associated with pregnancy: a report of 5 cases. South African Medical Journal 56: 133–136

Golaszewski T, Susani M, Golaszewski S, Sliutz G, Bischof G, Auer H 1995 A large hydatid cyst of the liver in pregnancy. Archives of Gynecology and Obstetrics 256: 43–47

Gong B, Baken L A, Julian T M et al 1988 High output heart failure due to hepatic arteriovenous fistula during pregnancy: a case report. Obstetrics and Gynecology 72: 440–442

Gonzales M C, Reyes H, Arrese M et al 1989 Intrahepatic cholestasis of pregnancy in twin pregnancies. Journal of Hepatology 9: 84–90

Gonzales-Angulo A, Aznar-Ramos R, Marquez-Monter H et al 1970 The ultrastructure of liver cells in women under steroid therapy. I. Normal pregnancy and trophoblastic growth. Acta Endocrinologica 65: 193–206

Gordon S C, Polson D J, Shirkhoda A 1991 Budd–Chiari syndrome complicating pre-eclampsia: diagnosis by magnetic resonance imaging. Journal of Clinical Gastroenterology 13: 460–462

Greca F H, Coelho J C U, Filho O D B, Wallbach A 1984 Ultrasonographic diagnosis of spontaneous rupture of the liver in pregnancy. Journal of Clinical Ultrasound 12: 515–516

Greenstein D, Henderson J M, Boyer T D 1994 Liver hemorrhage: recurrent episodes during pregnancy complicated by preeclampsia. Gastroenterology 106: 1668–1671

Grimbert S, Fromenty B, Fisch C et al 1993 Decreased mitochondrial oxidation of fatty acids in pregnant mice: possible relevance to development of acute fatty liver of pregnancy. Hepatology 17: 628–637

Grimbert S, Fisch C, Deschamps D et al 1995 Effects of female sex hormones on liver mitochondria in non-pregnant female mice: possible

role in acute fatty liver of pregnancy. American Journal of Physiology 268: G107–G115

Haddad B, Barton J R, Livingston J C, Chahine R, Sibai B M 2000a Risk factors for adverse maternal outcomes among women with HELLP (hemolysis, elevated liver enzymes, and low platelet count) syndrome. American Journal of Obstetrics and Gynecology 183: 444–448

Haddad B, Barton J R, Livingston J C, Chahine R, Sibai B M 2000b HELLP (hemolysis, elevated liver enzymes, and low platelet count) syndrome versus severe preeclampsia: onset at < or =28.0 weeks' gestation. American Journal of Obstetrics and Gynecology 183: 1475–1479

Haemmerli U P 1966 Jaundice during pregnancy with special reference on recurrent jaundice during pregnancy and its differential diagnosis. Acta Medica Scandinavica (suppl) 444: 1–111

Hague W M, Fenton D W, Duncan S L B, Slater D N 1983 Acute fatty liver of pregnancy: a review of the literature and six further cases. Journal of the Royal Society of Medicine 76: 752–761

Halim A, Kanayama N, El Maradny E et al 1996 Immunohistological study in cases of HELLP syndrome (hemolysis, elevated liver enzymes and low platelets) and acute fatty liver of pregnancy. Gynecological and Obstetric Investigations 41: 106–112

Hamid S S, Jafri S M, Khan H, Shah H, Abbas Z, Fields H J 1996 Fulminant hepatic failure in pregnant women: acute fatty liver or acute viral hepatitis? Journal of Hepatology 25: 20–27

Harris G J, Al-Jurf A S, Yuh W T, Abu-Yousef M M 1989 Intrahepatic pregnancy. A unique opportunity for evaluation with sonography, computed tomography, and magnetic resonance imaging. Journal of the American Medical Association 261: 902–904

Hatfield A K, Stein J H, Greenberger N J, Abernethy R W, Ferris T F 1972 Idiopathic acute fatty liver of pregnancy: death from extrahepatic manifestations. American Journal of Digestive Disease 17: 167–178

Haverback B J, Wirtschafter S K 1960 Familial nonhemolytic jaundice with normal liver histology and conjugated bilirubin. New England Journal of Medicine 262: 113–117

Hayes D, Lamki H, Hunter I W E 1977 Hepatic cell adenoma presenting with intraperitoneal haemorrhage in the puerperium. British Medical Journal 12: 1394

Hendrickx L, Van Hee R H, Hubens A 1981 Spontaneous rupture of the cystic duct during pregnancy. Netherlands Journal of Surgery 33: 247–249

Heneghan M A, Norris S M, O'Grady J G, Harrison P M, McFarlane J G 2001 Management and outcome of pregnancy in autoimmune hepatitis. Gut 48: 97–102

Hibbard L T 1976 Spontaneous rupture of the liver in pregnancy: a report of eight cases. American Journal of Obstetrics and Gynecology 126: 324–328

Hietala S-O, Anderson M, Emdin S O 1983 Ectopic pregnancy in the liver: report of a case and angiographic findings. Acta Chirurgica Scandinavica 149: 633–635

Higgins J R, de Swiet M 2001 Blood-pressure measurement and classification in pregnancy. Lancet 357: 131–135

Hillemanns P, Knitza R, Muller-Hocker J 1996 Rupture of splenic artery aneurysm in a pregnant patient with portal hypertension. American Journal of Obstetrics and Gynecology 174: 1665–1666

Hino K, Moriya T, Ohno N et al 1998 Mother-to-infant transmission occurs more frequently with GB virus C than hepatitis C virus. Archives of Virology 143: 65–72

Hla-Myint, Myint-Myint Soe, Tun-Khin et al 1985 A clinical and epidemiological study of an epidemic of non-A non-B hepatitis in Rangoon. American Journal of Tropical Medicine and Hygiene 34: 1183–1189

Holdsworth R J, Gunn A 1992 Ruptured splenic artery aneurysm in pregnancy. A review. British Journal of Obstetrics and Gynaecology 99: 595–597

Hopkins N F, Benjamin I S, Thompson M H et al 1990 Complications of choledochal cysts. Annals of the Royal College of Surgeons of England 74: 229–235

Hou S H, Levin S, Ahola S et al 1984 Acute fatty liver of pregnancy: survival with early Cesarean section. Digestive Diseases and Science 29: 449–452

Hould F S, Fried G M, Fazekas A G et al 1988 Progesterone receptors regulate gallbladder motility. Journal of Surgical Research 45: 505–512

Hsu H W, Belfort M A, Vernino S, Moake J L, Moise K J Jr 1995 Postpartum thrombotic thrombocytopenic purpura complicated by Budd–Chiari syndrome. Obstetrics and Gynecology 85: 839–843

Humberto R, Baez M E, Gonzalez M C et al 2000 Selenium, zinc and copper plasma levels in intrahepatic cholestasis of pregnancy, in normal pregnancies and in healthy individuals in Chile. Journal of Hepatology 32: 542–549

Hunt C M, Sharara A I 1999 Liver disease in pregnancy. American Family Physician. 59: 829–836

Hunt C M, Carson K L, Sharara A I 1997 Hepatitis C in pregnancy. Obstetrics and Gynecology 89: 883–890

Hytten F E, Leitch I 1971 The physiology of human pregnancy, 2nd edn. Blackwell Scientific Publications, Oxford

Ibdah J A, Bennet M J, Rinaldo P et al 1999 A fetal fatty-acid oxidation disorder as a cause of liver disease in pregnant women. New England Journal of Medicine 340: 1723–1731

Ibdah J A, Yang Z, Bennett M J 2000 Liver disease in pregnancy and fetal fatty acid oxidation defects. Molecular Genetics and Metabolism 71: 182–189

Ikonen E 1964 Jaundice in late pregnancy. Acta Obstetricia et Gynecologica Scandinavica 43: suppl 5

Imagawa D K, Lien J M, Dugan M C, Tompkins R K 1994 Angiomyolipoma of the liver presenting in pregnancy. American Journal of Surgery 60: 824–826

Inaba N, Okajima Y, Kang X S, Ishikawa K, Fukasawa I 1997 Maternal–infant transmission of hepatitis G virus. American Journal of Obstetrics and Gynecology 117: 1537–1538

Ingerslev M, Teilum G 1945 Biopsy studies on the liver in pregnancy. II. Liver biopsy on normal pregnant women. Acta Obstetricia et Gynecologica Scandinavica 25: 352–360

Ishak K G, Irey N 1972 Hepatic injury associated with the phenothiazines. Clinicopathologic and follow-up study of 36 patients. Archives of Pathology 93: 283–304

Isenberg J N 1977 The infant and hepatitis B virus infection. Advances in Paediatrics 24: 445–498

Isler C M, Rinehart B K, Terrone D A, Martin R W, Magann E F, Martin J N Jr 1999 Maternal mortality associated with HELLP (hemolysis, elevated liver enzymes, and low platelets) syndrome. American Journal of Obstetrics and Gynecology 181: 924–928

Jabeen T, Cannon B, Hogan J et al 2000 Pregnancy and pregnancy outcome in hepatitis C type 1b. Quarterly Journal of Medicine 93: 597–601

Jacquemin E, Hadchouel M 1999 Genetic basis of progressive familial intrahepatic cholestasis. Journal of Hepatology 31: 377–381

Jacquemin E, Hadchouel M, Congard B, Laugier J 1988 Cholestase gravidique et activité serique normale de la gamma glutamyl transpeptidase (Letter). Gastroenterology Clinical Biology 12: 768–769

Jacquemin E, Cresteil D, Manouvrier S, Boute O, Hadchouel M 1999 Heterozygous non-sense mutation of the MDR3 gene in familial intrahepatic cholestasis of pregnancy. Lancet 353: 210–211

Jacquemin E, De Vree J M, Cresteil D et al 2001 The wide spectrum of multidrug resistance 3 deficiency: from neonatal cholestasis to cirrhosis of adulthood. Gastroenterology 120: 1448–1458

Jacques S M, Qureshi F 1992 Herpes simplex virus hepatitis in pregnancy: a clinicopathologic study of three cases. Human Pathology 23: 183–187

Jain A, Venkataramanan R, Fung J J et al 1997 Pregnancy after liver transplantation under tacrolimus. Transplantation 64: 559–565

Jaiswal S P, Jain A K, Naik G, Soni N, Chitnis D S 2001 Viral hepatitis during pregnancy. International Journal of Gynaecology and Obstetrics 72: 103–108

Jamieson N V, Williams R, Calne R Y 1991 Liver transplantation for Budd–Chiari syndrome, 1976–1990. Annales de Chirugie 45: 362–365

Janczewska I, Olsson R, Hultcrantz R, Broome U 1996 Pregnancy in patients with primary sclerosing cholangitis. Liver 16: 326–330

Jarnfelt-Samsioe A, Eriksson B, Waldenstrom J, Samsioe G 1986 Serum bile acids, gamma-glutamyltransferase and routine liver tests in emetic and nonemetic pregnancies. Gynecological and Obstetric Investigation 21: 169–176

Jenkins W F, Darling M R 1980 Idiopathic acute fatty liver of pregnancy: subsequent uncomplicated pregnancy. Journal of Obstetrics and Gynaecology 1: 100–101

Johnson L G, Saldana L R 1994 Herpes simplex virus hepatitis in pregnancy. A case report. Journal of Reproductive Medicine 39: 544–546

Johnson P 1975 Studies on cholestasis of pregnancy. IV. Serum lipids and lipoprotein in relation to duration of symptoms and severity of the disease and fatty acid composition of lecithin in relation to duration of symptoms. Acta Obstetricia et Gynecologica Scandinavica 54: 307–313

Johnson P, Samsioe G, Gustafson A 1975a Studies in cholestasis of pregnancy. I. Clinical aspects and liver function tests. Acta Obstetricia et Gynecologica Scandinavica 54: 77–84

Johnson P, Samsioe G, Gustafson A 1975b Studies on cholestasis of pregnancy. II. Serum lipids and lipoproteins. Acta Obstetricia et Gynecologica Scandinavica 54: 105–111

Jones D E J 2000 Fetal microchimerism: an aetiological factor in primary biliary cirrhosis? Journal of Hepatology 33: 834–837

Jones S L 1998 HELLP! A cry for laboratory assistance: a comprehensive review of the HELLP syndrome highlighting the role of the laboratory. Haematopathology and Molecular Haematology. 11: 147–171

Joske R A, McCully D J, Mastaglia F L 1968 Acute fatty liver of pregnancy. Gut 9: 489–493

Kahra K, Draganov B, Sund S, Hovig T 1998 Postpartum renal failure: a complex case with probable coexistence of hemolysis, elevated liver enzymes, low platelet count, and hemolytic uremic syndrome. Obstetrics and Gynecology 92: 698–700

Kain K C, Keystone J S 1988 Recurrent hydatid disease during pregnancy. American Journal of Obstetrics and Gynecology 159: 1216–1219

Kaiser C, Distler W 1996 Thrombotic thrombocytopenic purpura and HELLP (hemolysis, elevated liver enzymes and low platelets) syndrome: differential diagnostic problems. American Journal of Obstetrics and Gynecology 175: 506–507

Kang A H, Graves C R 1999 Herpes simplex hepatitis in pregnancy: a case report and review of the literature. Obstetrical and Gynecological Survey 54: 463–468

Kapicioglu S, Gurbuz S, Danalioglu A, Senturk O, Uslu M 2000 Measurement of gallbladder volume with ultrasonography in pregnant women. Canadian Journal of Gastroenterology 175: 403–405

Kar P, Budhiraja S, Narang A, Chakravarthy A 1997 Etiology of sporadic acute and fulminant non-A, non-B viral hepatitis in north India. Indian Journal of Gastroenterology. 16: 43–45

Kater R H M, Mistilis S B 1967 Obstetric cholestasis and pruritis of pregnancy. Medical Journal of Australia 54: 638–640

Katzeff T C, Moore P J 1984 Ruptured amoebic liver abscess in pregnancy: a case report. Central African Journal of Medicine 30: 257–258

Kaufman B, Gandhi S A, Louie E, Rizzi R, Illei P 1997 Herpes simplex virus hepatitis: case report and review. Clinics in Infectious Diseases 24: 334–338

Kauppila A, Korpela H, Makila U-M, Yrjanheikki E 1987 Low selenium concentration and glutathione peroxidase activity in intrahepatic cholestasis of pregnancy. British Medical Journal 294: 150–152

Kaushanksy A, Frydman M, Kaufman H, Homburg R 1987 Endocrine studies on the ovulatory disturbances in Wilson's disease. Fertility and Sterility 47: 270–273

Kemp W L, Barnard J J, Prahlow J A 1999 Death due to thrombotic thrombocytopenic purpura in pregnancy: case report with review of thrombotic microangiopathies of pregnancy. American Journal of Forensic Medicine and Pathology 20: 189–198

Kennedy S, Hall P M, Seymour A E, Hague W M 1994 Transient diabetes insipidus and acute fatty liver of pregnancy. British Journal of Obstetrics and Gynaecology 101: 387–391

Kent D R, Nissen E D, Nisen S E, Chambers C 1977 Maternal death resulting from rupture of liver adenoma associated with oral contraceptives. Obstetrics and Gynecology (suppl) 50: 5s–6s

Kent D R, Nissen S E, Ziehm D J 1978 Effect of pregnancy on liver tumor associated with oral contraceptives. Obstetrics and Gynecology 55: 148–151

Kern F Jr, Erfling W, Simon F R, Dahl R, Mallory A, Starzl T E 1978 Effect of estrogen on the liver. Gastroenterology 75: 512–522

Kern F Jr, Everson G T, De Mark B et al 1981 Biliary lipids, bile acids, and gallbladder function in the human female: effects of pregnancy and the ovulatory cycle. Journal of Clinical Investigation 68: 1229–1242

Kern F Jr, Everson G T, De Mark B et al 1982 Biliary lipids, bile acids, and gallbladder function in the human female: effects of contraceptive steroids. Journal of Laboratory and Clinical Medicine 99: 798–805

Kesby G J 1998 Pregnancy complicated by symptomatic adult polycystic liver disease. American Journal of Obstetrics and Gynecology. 179: 266–267

Khalifa M A, Gersell D J, Hansen C H, Lage J M 1998 Hepatic (hepatocellular) adenoma of the placenta: a study of four cases. International Journal of Gynecological Pathology 17: 241–244

Khuroo M S, Datta D V 1980 Budd–Chiari syndrome following pregnancy: report of 16 cases with roentgenologic, hemodynamic and histologic studies of the hepatic outflow tract. American Journal of Medicine 68: 113–121

Khuroo M S, Teli M R, Skidmore S, Sofi M A, Khuroo M I 1981 Incidence and severity of viral hepatitis in pregnancy. American Journal of Medicine 70: 252–255

Khuroo M S, Kamili S, Jameel S 1995 Vertical transmission of hepatitis E virus. Lancet 345: 1025–1026

Killam A P, Dillard S H, Patton R C, Pedersen P R 1975 Pregnancy-induced hypertension complicated by acute liver disease and disseminated intravascular coagulation. American Journal of Obstetrics and Gynecology 123: 823–828

Kirby N G 1969 Primary hepatic pregnancy. British Medical Journal 1: 296

Klein N A, Mabie W C, Shaver D C et al 1991 Herpes simplex virus hepatitis in pregnancy. Two patients successfully treated with acyclovir. Gastroenterology 100: 239–244

Knopp R H, Bergelin R O, Wahl P W, Walden C E, Chapman M B 1985 Clinical chemistry alterations in pregnancy and oral contraceptive use. Obstetrics and Gynecology 66: 682–690

Knowles D M, Casarella W J, Johnson P M, Wolff M 1978 The clinical, radiologic and pathologic characterisation of benign hepatic neoplasms: alleged associations with oral contraceptives. Medicine 57: 223–237

Kopernik G, Mazor M, Leiberman J R et al 1988 Pyogenic liver abscess in pregnancy. Israeli Journal of Medical Science 24: 245–246

Krawczynski K 1993 Hepatitis E. Hepatology 17: 932–941

Kreek M J 1987 Female sex steroids and cholestasis. Seminars in Liver Disease 7: 8–23

Kreek M J, Sleisenger H E 1970 Estrogen induced cholestasis due to endogenous and exogenous hormones. Scandinavian Journal of Gastroenterology (suppl) 7: 122–131

Kreek M J, Sleisenger M H, Jeffries G H 1967a Recurrent cholestatic jaundice of pregnancy with demonstrated estrogen sensitivity. American Journal of Medicine 43: 795–798

Kreek M J, Wester E, Sleisenger M H et al 1967b Idiopathic cholestasis of pregnancy: the response to challenge with the synthetic estrogen, ethinyl estradiol. New England Journal of Medicine 277: 1391–1395

Krejs G J 1983 Jaundice during pregnancy. Seminars in Liver Disease 3: 73–82

Krejs G J, Haemmerli U P 1982 Jaundice during pregnancy. In: Schiff L, Schiff E R (eds) Diseases of the liver, 5th edn. Lippincott, Philadelphia, pp 1561–1580

Kroll D, Mazor M, Zirkin H, Schulman H, Glezerman M 1991 Fibrolamellar carcinoma of the liver in pregnancy. A case report. Journal of Reproductive Medicine 36: 823–827

Kullak-Ublick G A, Beuers U, Paumgartner G 2000 Hepatobiliary transport. Journal of Hepatology 32: 3–18

Kunelis C T, Peters J L, Edmondson H A 1965 Fatty liver of pregnancy and its relationship to tetracycline therapy. American Journal of Medicine 38: 359–377

Laatikainen T 1975 Fetal bile acid levels in pregnancies complicated by maternal intrahepatic cholestasis. American Journal of Obstetrics and Gynecology 122: 852–856

Laatikainen T, Ikonen E 1975 Fetal prognosis in obstetric hepatosis. Annales Chirurgiae et Gynaecologiae Fenniae 64: 155–164

Laatikainen T, Ikonen E 1977 Serum bile acids in cholestasis of pregnancy. Obstetrics and Gynecology 50: 313–318

Laatikainen T, Tulenheimo A 1984 Maternal serum bile acid levels and fetal distress in cholestasis of pregnancy. International Journal of Gynaecology and Obstetrics 22: 91–94

Laatikainen T, Lehtonen P, Hesso A 1978 Biliary bile acids in uncomplicated pregnancy and in cholestasis of pregnancy. Clinica Chimica Acta 85: 145–150

Laifer S A, Darby M J, Scantlebury V P et al 1990 Pregnancy and liver transplantation. Obstetrics and Gynecology 76: 1083

Laifer S A, Abu-Elmagd K, Fung J J 1997 Hepatic transplantation during pregnancy and the puerperium. Journal of Maternal and Fetal Medicine. 6: 40–44

Lammert F, Marschal H-U, Glantz A, Matern S 2000 Intrahepatic cholestasis of pregnancy: molecular pathogenesis, diagnosis and management. Journal of Hepatology 33: 1012–1021

Lammert F, Carey M C, Paigen B 2001 Chromosomal organization of candidate genes involved in cholesterol gallstone formation: a murine gallstone map. Gastroenterology 120: 221–238

Latt N C, Spencer J D, Beeby P J et al 2000 Hepatitis C in injecting drug-using women during and after pregnancy. Journal of Gastroenterology and Hepatology 15: 175–181

Lau W Y, Leung W T, Ho S et al 1995 Hepatocellular carcinoma during pregnancy and its comparison with other pregnancy-associated malignancies. Cancer 75: 2669–2676

Lavery D W, Bowes R M 1971 Subcapsular haematoma of the liver in pregnancy: report of four cases. South African Medical Journal 45: 603–605

Lee W M 1992 Pregnancy in patients with chronic liver disease. Gastroenterology Clinics of North America 21: 889–903

Leevy C B, Koneru B, Klein K M 1997 Recurrent familial prolonged intrahepatic cholestasis of pregnancy associated with chronic liver disease. Gastroenterology. 113: 966–972

Lemay M, Granger L, Verschelden G et al 1980 Spontaneous rupture of the common bile duct during pregnancy. Canadian Medical Association Journal 122: 14–15

Lemmer E R, Shepard E G, Blakolmer K, Kirsch R E, Robson S C 1998 Isolation from human fetal liver of cells co-expressing CD34 haematopoietic stem cell and CAM 5.2 pancytokeratin markers. Journal of Hepatology 29: 450–454

Liebman H A, McGeehee W G, Patak M J, Fienstein D I 1983 Severe depression of antithrombin III associated with disseminated intravascular coagulation in women with fatty liver of pregnancy. Annals of Internal Medicine 98: 330–333

Lin H H, Kao J H, Yeh K Y et al 1998 Mother to infant transmission of GB virus C/hepatitis G virus: the role of high-titered maternal viremia and mode of delivery. Journal of Infectious Diseases 177: 1202–1206

Livingston J C, Barton J R, Park V et al 2001 Maternal and fetal inherited thrombophilias are not related to the development of severe preeclampsia. American Journal of Obstetrics and Gynecology 185: 153–157

Livneh A, Langevitz P, Morag B 1988 Functionally reversible hepatic arteriovenous fistulas during pregnancy in patients with hereditary hemorrhagic telangiectasia. Southern Medical Journal 81: 1047–1049

Locatelli A, Roncaglia N, Arreghini A, Bellini P, Bergani P, Ghidini A 1999 Hepatitis C virus infection is associated with a higher incidence of cholestasis of pregnancy. British Journal of Obstetrics and Gynaecology 106: 498–500

Loevinger E H, Vujic I, Lee W M, Anderson M C 1985 Hepatic rupture associated with pregnancy: treatment with transcatheter embolotherapy. Obstetrics and Gynecology 65: 281–284

Long R G, Scheuer P J, Sherlock S 1977 Pre-eclampsia presenting with deep jaundice. Journal of Clinical Pathology 30: 212–215

Loret de Mola J R E, Muise K L, Duchon M A 1996 Porphyria cutanea tarda and pregnancy. Obstetrical and Gynecological Survey 51: 493–497

Luketic V A, Shiffman M L 1999 Benign recurrent intrahepatic cholestasis. Clinics in Liver Disease 3: 509–528

Lyall F, Greer I A 1996 The vascular endothelium in normal pregnancy and pre-eclampsia. Reviews in Reproduction 1: 107–116

Mabie W C 1992 Acute fatty liver of pregnancy. Gastroenterology Clinics of North America 21: 951–960

Mabie W C, Dacus J V, Sibai B M et al 1989 Computed tomography in acute fatty liver of pregnancy. American Journal of Obstetrics and Gynecology 158: 142–145

Mabina M H, Moodley J, Pitsoe S B, Monokoane S 1998 Amoebic liver abscess in pregnancy: report of two cases. East African Medical Journal 75: 57–60

McCrae K R, Cines D B 1997 Thrombotic microangiopathy during pregnancy. Seminars in Haematology 34: 148–158

Macfarlane J, Thorbjarnarson B 1966 Rupture of splenic artery aneurysm during pregnancy. American Journal of Obstetrics and Gynecology 95: 1025–1037

MacIntyre C R 2001 Hepatitis B vaccine: risks and benefits of universal neonatal vaccination. Journal of Paediatrics and Child Health 37: 215–217

Mackenna J, Pupkin M, Crenshaw L, MacLeod M, Parker R 1977 Acute fatty metamorphosis of liver. American Journal of Obstetrics and Gynecology 127: 400–404

MacLean M A, Cameron A D, Cumming G P, Murphy K, Mills P, Hillan K J 1994 Recurrence of acute fatty liver of pregnancy. British Journal of Obstetrics and Gynaecology 101: 453–454

McNair R D, Jaynes R V 1960 Alterations in liver function during normal pregnancy. American Journal of Obstetrics and Gynecology 80: 500–507

MacSween R N M 1995 Pathology of the liver and gallbladder in pregnancy: Fox H (ed) Haines & Taylor, 4th edn, Churchill Livingstone, Edinburgh, pp 1735–1758

Magriples U 1998 Hepatitis in pregnancy. Seminars in Perinatology 22: 112–117

Malatjalian D A, Badley B W D 1983 Acute fatty liver of pregnancy: light and electron microscopic studies. Gastroenterology 84: 1384 (abstract)

Maringhini A, Ciambra M, Baccelliere P, Raimondo M, Pagliaro L 1988 Sludge, stones and pregnancy. Gastroenterology 95: 1160–1161

Mass K, Quint E H, Punch M R, Merion R M 1996 Gynecological and reproductive function after liver transplantation. Transplantation 62: 476–479

Mast E E, Krawczynski K 1996 Hepatitis E: an overview. Annual Reviews in Medicine. 47: 257–266

Matern D, Hart P, Murtha A P et al 2001 Acute fatty liver of pregnancy associated with short-chain acyl-coenzyme A dehydrogenase deficiency. Journal of Pediatrics 138: 585–588

Mathieu D, Kobeiter H, Maison P et al 2000 Oral contraceptive use and focal nodular hyperplasia of the liver. Gastroenterology. 118: 560–564

Matsuda Y, Maeda T, Hatae M 1997 Spontaneous rupture of the liver in an uncomplicated pregnancy. Journal of Obstetric and Gynaecological Research. 23: 449–452

Maze G L, Lee M, Schenker S 1999 Inflammatory pseudotumor of the liver and pregnancy. American Journal of Gastroenterology 94: 529–530

Meadow S R 1968 Infectious hepatitis and stillbirth. British Medical Journal 1: 426

Meare Y, Elena J B, Raolison S 1965 Un cas de grossesse à inplantation hepatique avec enfant vivant. Semaine des Hospitaux de Paris 41: 1430–1433

Melnick J L 1957 A waterborne urban epidemic of hepatitis. In: Hartman F W, Lo Grippo G A, Mateer J G, Barron J (eds) Hepatitis frontiers. Little Brown, Boston, pp 211–225

Michielsen P P, Van Damme P 1999 Viral hepatitis and pregnancy. Acta Gastroenterolica Belgica 62: 21–29

Minakami H, Oka N, Sato T et al 1988 Preeclampsia: a microvesicular fat disease of the liver? American Journal of Obstetrics and Gynecology 159: 1043–1047

Minuk G Y, Lui R C, Kelly J K 1987 Rupture of the liver associated with acute fatty liver of pregnancy. American Journal of Gastroenterology 82: 457–460

Mishra L, Seef L B 1992 Viral hepatitis, A through E complicating pregnancy. Gastroenterology Clinics of North America 21: 883–887

Mitchell R W, Teare A J 1984a Primary hepatic pregnancy: a case report and review. South African Medical Journal 65: 200–202

Mitchell R W, Teare A J 1984b Amoebic liver abscess in pregnancy: case report. British Journal of Obstetrics and Gynaecology 91: 393–395

Monga M, Katz A R 1999 Acute fatty liver in the second trimester. Obstetrics and Gynecology 93: 811–813

Moore H C 1956 Acute fatty liver of pregnancy. British Journal of Obstetrics and Gynaecology 63: 189–198

Moradpour D, Altorfer J, Flury R et al 1994 Chlorpromazine-induced vanishing bile duct syndrome leading to biliary cirrhosis. Hepatology 20: 1437–1441

Morali G A, Braverman D Z 1990 Abnormal liver enzymes and ketonuria in hyperemesis gravidarum. A retrospective review of 80 patients. Journal of Clinical Gastroenterology 12: 303–305

Mudido P, Marshall G S, Howell R S, Schmid D S, Steger S, Adams G 1993 Disseminated herpes simplex virus infection during pregnancy. A case report. Journal of Reproductive Medicine 38: 964–968

Mulligan M J, Stiehm E R 1994 Neonatal hepatitis B infection: clinical and immunologic considerations. Journal of Perinatology 14: 2–9

Munnell E W, Taylor H C 1947 Liver blood flow in pregnancy — hepatic vein catheterisation. Journal of Clinical Investigation 26: 952–956

Murley A H G 1956 Liver pregnancies. Lancet i: 994–995

Nakamoto S K, vanSonnenberg E 1985 Cholangiocarcinoma in pregnancy: the contributions of ultrasound-guided interventional techniques. Journal of Ultrasound Medicine 4: 557–559

Navaraine R A 1972 Postpartum intraperitoneal rupture of an amoebic liver abscess. Ceylon Medical Journal 17: 160–163

Neerhof M G, Zelman W, Sullivan T 1989 Hepatic rupture in pregnancy: a review. Obstetrical and Gynecological Survey 44: 407–409

Nir A, Sorokin Y, Abramovici H et al 1989 Pregnancy and primary biliary cirrhosis. International Journal of Gynaecology and Obstetrics 28: 279–282

Ober W B, Le Compte P M 1955 Acute fatty metamorphosis of the liver associated with pregnancy: a distinctive lesion. American Journal of Medicine 19: 743–758

Ockner S A, Brunt E M, Cohn S M et al 1990 Fulminant hepatic failure caused by acute fatty liver of pregnancy treated by orthotopic liver transplantation. Hepatology 11: 59–64

O'Grady J, Day E, Toole A, Paust J C 1977 Splenic artery aneurysm rupture in pregnancy: a review and case report. Obstetrics and Gynecology 50: 627–630

Olsson R, Tysk C, Aldenborg F, Holm B 1993 Prolonged postpartum course of intrahepatic cholestasis of pregnancy. Gastroenterology 105: 267–271

Oude Elferink R P, van Berge Henegouwen G P 1998 Cracking the genetic code for benign recurrent and progressive familial intrahepatic cholestasis. Journal of Hepatology 29: 317–320

Overall J C Jr 1994 Herpes simplex virus infection of the fetus and newborn. Pediatric Annual 23: 131–136

Pajor A, Lehoczky D 1994 Pregnancy in liver cirrhosis. Assessment of maternal and fetal risks in eleven patients and review of the management. Gynecological and Obstetric Investigation 38: 45–50

Palomba E, Bairo A, Tovo P A 1999 High rate of maternal-infant transmission of hepatitis G virus in HIV-1 and hepatitis C virus infected women. Acta Paediatrica 88: 1392–1395

Patial R K, Kapoor D, Gupta H, Patial S 1998 Amoebic liver abscess in pregnancy. Journal of the Association of Physicians of India 46: 570

Pereira S P, O'Donohue J, Wendon J, Williams R 1997 Maternal and perinatal outcome in severe pregnancy-related liver disease. Hepatology 26: 1258–1262

Perez V, Gorodisch S, Casavilla F, Maruffo C 1971 Ultrastructure of human liver at the end of normal pregnancy. American Journal of Obstetrics and Gynecology 110: 428–430

Piotrowski J J, Van Stiegmann G, Liechty R D 1990 Spontaneous bile duct rupture in pregnancy. Hepatic, Pancreatic and Biliary Surgery 2: 205–209

Pockros P J, Peters R L, Reynolds T B 1984 Idiopathic fatty liver of pregnancy: findings of ten cases. Medicine 63: 1–11

Portis R, Jacobs M A, Skerman J H, Skerman E B 1997 HELLP syndrome (hemolysis, elevated liver enzymes, and low platelets) pathophysiology and anesthetic considerations. AANA Journal 65: 37–47

Purtilo D T, Clark J V, Williams R 1975 Primary hepatic malignancy in pregnant women. American Journal of Obstetrics and Gynecology 121: 41–44

Rabinovitz M, Appasamy R, Finkelstein S 1995 Primary biliary cirrhosis diagnosed during pregnancy. Does it have a different outcome? Digestive Disease and Science 40: 571–574

Radomski J S, Moritz M J, Munoz S J, Cater J R, Jarrell B E, Armenti V T 1995 National Transplantation Pregnancy Registry: analysis of pregnancy outcomes in female liver transplant recipients. Liver Transplantation and Surgery 1: 281–284

Ralston S J, Schwaitzberg S D 1998 Liver hematoma and rupture in pregnancy. Seminars in Perinatology 22: 141–148

Rath W, Faridi A, Dudenhausen J W 2000 HELLP syndrome. Journal of Perinatal Medicine 28: 249–60

Read K M, Kennedy-Andrews S, Gordon D L 2001 Amoebic liver abscess in pregnancy. Australian and New Zealand Journal of Obstetrics and Gynaecology 41: 236–237

Reyes H 1982 The enigma of intrahepatic cholestasis of pregnancy: lessons from Chile. Hepatology 1: 87–96

Reyes H 1992 The spectrum of liver and gastrointestinal disease seen in cholestasis of pregnancy. Gastroenterology Clinics of North America 21: 905–921

Reyes H 1997 Review: intrahepatic cholestasis. A puzzling disorder of pregnancy. Journal of Gastroenterology and Hepatology 12: 211–216

Reyes H, Simon F R 1993 Intrahepatic cholestasis of pregnancy: an estrogen related disease. Seminars in Liver Disease 13: 289–301

Reyes H, Ribalta J, Gonzalez-Cerou M 1976 Idiopathic cholestasis of pregnancy in a large kindred. Gut 17: 709–713

Reyes H, Gonzalez M C, Ribalta J et al 1978 Prevalence of intrahepatic cholestasis of pregnancy in Chile. Annals of Internal Medicine 88: 487–493

Reyes H, Ribalta J, Gonzalez M C, Segovia N, Oberhauser O 1981 Sulfobromophthalein clearance tests before and after ethinyl estradiol administration in women and men with familial history of intrahepatic cholestasis of pregnancy. Gastroenterology 81: 226–331

Reyes H, Rodrigan M E, Gonzalez M C 1987 Steatorrhoea in patients with intrahepatic cholestasis of pregnancy. Gastroenterology 93: 584–590

Reyes H, Sandovat L, Wainstein A et al 1994 Acute fatty liver of pregnancy: a clinical study of 12 episodes in 11 patients. Gut 35: 101–106

Richards R L, Willocks J, Dow T G B 1970 Jaundice in pregnancy. Scottish Medical Journal 15: 52–57

Riely C A 1984 Acute fatty liver of pregnancy (editorial). Digestive Diseases and Science 29: 456–457

Riely C A 1987 Acute fatty liver of pregnancy. Seminars in Liver Disease 7: 47–54

Riely C A 1994 Hepatic disease in pregnancy. American Journal of Medicine 96:(Suppl 1A) 18S–22S

Rioseco A J, Ivankovic M B, Manzur A et al 1994 Intrahepatic cholestasis of pregnancy: a retrospective case-control study of perinatal outcome. American Journal of Obstetrics and Gynecology 170: 890–895

Risseeuw J J, de Vries J E, van Eyck J, Arabin B 1999 Liver rupture postpartum associated with preeclampsia and HELLP syndrome. Journal of Maternal and Fetal Medicine. 8: 32–35

Robson S C, Mutch E, Boys R J, Woodhouse K W 1990 Apparent liver blood flow during pregnancy: a serial study using indocyanine green clearance. British Journal of Obstetrics and Gynaecology 97: 720–724

Roddie T W 1957 Haemorrhage from primary carcinoma of the liver complicating pregnancy. British Medical Journal 1: 31–39

Rodin A, Duncan A, Quartero H W P et al 1989 Serum concentrations of alkaline phosphatase isoenzymes and osteocalcin in normal pregnancy. Journal of Clinical Endocrinology and Metabolism 68: 1123–1127

Rolfes D B, Ishak K G 1985 Acute fatty liver of pregnancy: a clinicopathologic study of 35 cases. Hepatology 5: 1149–1158

Rolfes D B, Ishak K G 1986a Liver disease in toxemia of pregnancy. American Journal of Gastroenterology 81: 1138–1144

Rolfes D B, Ishak K G 1986b Liver disease in pregnancy. Histopathology 10: 555–570

Rooks J B, Ory H W, Ishak K G et al 1979 Epidemiology of hepatocellular adenoma: the role of oral contraceptive use. Journal of the American Medical Association 242: 644–648

Rosenthal T, Shani M, Deutsch V, Samra H 1972 The Budd–Chiari syndrome after pregnancy: report of two cases and a review of the literature. American Journal of Obstetrics and Gynecology 113: 789–792

Roulet M, Laurini R, Rivier L et al 1988 Hepatic veno-occlusive disease in newborn infant of a woman drinking herbal tea. Journal of Pediatrics 112: 433–436

Rubbia-Brandt L, Philippeaux M M, Chavez S, Mentha G, Borisch B, Hadengue A 1999 FISH for Y chromosome in women with primary biliary cirrhosis: lack of evidence for leucocyte microchimerism. Hepatology 30: 821–822

Russell M A, Craigo S D 1998 Cirrhosis and portal hypertension in pregnancy. Seminars in Perinatology 22: 156–165

Rustgi V K, Fagiuoli S, Van Thiel D H 1993 The liver in pregnancy. In: Rustgi V K, Van Thiel D H (eds) The liver in systemic disease. Raven Press, New York, pp 267–283

Salgo L, Pal A 1989 Variation in some enzymes in amniotic fluid and maternal serum during pregnancy. Enzyme 41: 101–107

Salha O, Campbell D J, Pollard S 1996 Budd–Chiari syndrome in pregnancy treated by caesarean section and liver transplant. British Journal of Obstetrics and Gynaecology 103: 1254–1256

Sallie R, Silva A E, Purdy M et al 1994 Hepatitis C and E in non-A non-B fulminant hepatic failure: polymerase chain reaction and serological study. Journal of Hepatology 20: 580–588

Saunders P, Jackson B T 1969 Rupture of choledochus cyst in pregnancy. British Medical Journal 3: 573–574

Schapiro L, Thorp J M Jr 1996 Diagnosis of early acute fatty liver of pregnancy. Journal of Maternal and Fetal Medicine 5: 314–316

Schilling M K, Zimmermann A, Redaelli C et al 2000 Liver nodules resembling focal nodular hyperplasia after hepatic venous thrombosis. Journal of Hepatology 33: 673–676

Schoeman M N, Batey R G, Wilcken B 1991 Recurrent acute fatty liver of pregnancy associated with a fatty-acid oxidation defect in the offspring. Gastroenterology 100: 544–548

Schorr-Lesnick B, Lebovics E, Dworkin B, Rosenthal W S 1991 Liver disease unique to pregnancy. American Journal of Gastroenterology 86: 659–670

Schwartz M L, Lien J M 1997 Spontaneous liver hematoma in pregnancy not clearly associated with preeclampsia: a case presentation and literature review. American Journal of Obstetrics and Gynecology 176: 1328–1332

Schwer M, Moosa A 1978 The effects of hepatitis A and B in pregnancy on mother and fetus. South African Medical Journal 54: 1092–1095

Scragg R K R, McMichael A J, Seamark R F 1984 Oral contraceptives, pregnancy and endogenous oestrogen in gall stone disease — a case-control study. British Medical Journal 288: 1795–1799

Sell S 2001 Heterogeneity and plasticity of hepatocyte lineage cells. Hepatology 33: 738–750

Severino L J, Freedman W L, Makeshkumar A P 1970 Spontaneous subcapsular hematoma of liver during pregnancy. New York State Journal of Medicine 70: 2818–2821

Seymour C A, Chadwick V S 1979 Liver and gastrointestinal function in pregnancy. Postgraduate Medical Journal 55: 343–352

Shaw D, Frohlich J, Wittmann B A, Willms M 1982 A prospective study of 18 patients with cholestasis of pregnancy. American Journal of Obstetrics and Gynecology 142: 621–625

Sheehan H L 1940 The pathology of acute yellow atrophy and delayed chloroform poisoning. Journal of Obstetrics and Gynaecology of the British Empire 47: 49–62

Sheehan H L, Lynch J B 1973 Pathology of toxaemia of pregnancy. Churchill Livingstone, Edinburgh

Sheikh R A, Yasmeen S, Pauly M P, Riegler J L 1999 Spontaneous intrahepatic hemorrhage and hepatic rupture in the HELLP syndrome: four cases and a review. Journal of Clinical Gastroenterology 28: 323–328

Sherbahn R 1996 Spontaneous ruptured subcapsular liver hematoma associated with pregnancy. A case report. Journal of Reproductive Medicine 41: 125–128

Shimono N, Ishibashi H, Ikematsu H et al 1990 Fulminant hepatic failure during perinatal period in a pregnant woman with Wilson's disease. Hepatogastroenterology 37 (suppl 2): 122

Shimono N, Ishibashi H, Ikematsu H et al 1991 Fulminant hepatic failure during perinatal period in a pregnant woman with Wilson's disease. Gastroenterologica Japonica 26: 69–73

Shukla V K, Pandey S, Pandey L K, Roy S K, Vaidya M P 1985 Primary hepatic pregnancy. Postgraduate Medical Journal 61: 831–832

Sibai B M 1990 The HELLP syndrome (hemolysis, elevated liver enzyme levels, and low platelets): much ado about nothing? American Journal of Obstetrics and Gynecology 162: 311–316

Sibai B M, Taslimi M M, El-Nazer A et al 1986 Maternal-perinatal outcome associated with the syndrome of hemolysis, elevated liver enzymes, and low platelets in severe preeclampsia-eclampsia. American Journal of Obstetrics and Gynecology 155: 501–509

Sibai B M, Kustermann L, Velasco J 1994 Current understanding of severe preeclampsia, pregnancy-associated hemolytic uremic syndrome, thrombotic thrombocytopenic pupura, hemolysis, elevated liver enzymes and low platelet syndrome, and postpartum acute renal failure: different clinical syndromes or just different names? Current Opinions in Nephrology and Hypertension 3: 436–445

Sibai B M, Ramadan M K, Chari R S, Friedman S A 1995 Pregnancies complicated by HELLP syndrome (hemolysis, elevated liver enzymes, and low platelets): subsequent pregnancy outcome and long-term prognosis. American Journal of Obstetrics and Gynecology 172: 125–129

Simms J, Duff P 1993 Viral hepatitis in pregnancy. Seminars in Perinatology 17: 384–393

Singh V, Sinha S K, Nain C K et al 2000 Budd–Chiari syndrome: our experience of 71 patients. Journal of Gastroenterology and Hepatology. 15: 550–554

Singletary B K, Van Thiel D H, Eagon P K 1986 Estrogen and progesterone receptors in human gallbladder. Hepatology 6: 574–578

Slater D N, Hague W M 1984 Renal morphological changes in idiopathic acute fatty liver of pregnancy. Histopathology 8: 567–581

Smith L G, Moise K J, Dildy G A, Carpenter R J 1991 Spontaneous rupture of liver during pregnancy: current therapy. Obstetrics and Gynecology 77: 171–175

Sommer D G, Greenway G D, Bookstein J J, Orloff M P 1979 Hepatic rupture with toxemia of pregnancy: angiographic diagnosis. American Journal of Radiology 132: 455–456

Sternlieb I 2000 Wilson's disease and pregnancy. Hepatology 31: 531–532

Steven M M 1981 Pregnancy and liver disease. Gut 22: 592–614

Steven M M, Buckley J D, Mackay I R 1979 Pregnancy in chronic active hepatitis. Quarterly Journal of Medicine 48: 519–531

Strate T, Broering D C, Bloechle C et al 2000 Orthotopic liver transplantation for complicated HELLP syndrome. Case report and review of the literature. Archives in Gynecology and Obstetrics 264: 108–111

Strauss A W, Bennett M J, Rinaldo P et al 1999 Inherited long-chain 3-hydroxyacyl-CoA dehydrogenase deficiency and a fetal-maternal interaction cause maternal liver disease and other pregnancy complications. Seminars in Perinatology 23: 100–112

Sullivan C A, Magann E F, Perry K G Jr, Roberts W E, Blake P G, Martin J N Jr 1994 The recurrence risk of the syndrome of hemolysis, elevated liver enzymes, and low platelets (HELLP) in subsequent gestations. American Journal of Obstetrics and Gynecology 171: 940–943

Sungler P, Heinerman P M, Steiner H et al 2000 Laparoscopic cholecystectomy and interventional endoscopy for gallstone complications during pregnancy. Surgical Endoscopy 14: 267–271

Suzuki S, Watanabe S, Araki T 2001 Acute fatty liver of pregnancy at 23 weeks of gestation. British Journal of Obstetrics and Gynaecology 108: 223–224

Svanborg A 1954 A study of recurrent jaundice in pregnancy. Acta Obstetricia et Gynecologica Scandinavica 33: 434–444

Svanborg A, Vikrot O 1965 Plasma lipid fractions, including individual phospholipids at various stages of pregnancy. Acta Medica Scandinavica 178: 615–630

Tanaka A, Lindor K, Gish R et al 1999 Fetal microchimerism alone does not contribute to the induction of primary biliary cirrhosis. Hepatology 30: 833–888

Tanaka A, Lindor K, Ansari A et al 2000 Fetal microchimerisms in the mother: immunologic implications. Liver Transplantation 6: 138–143

Tanaka I, Shima M, Kubota Y et al 1995 Vertical transmission of hepatitis A virus. Lancet 345: 397

Tanaka M, Wanless I R 1998 Pathology of the liver in Budd–Chiari syndrome: portal vein thrombosis and the histogenesis of veno-centric cirrhosis, veno-portal cirrhosis, and large regenerative nodules. Hepatology 27: 488–496

Tarnacka B, Rodo M, Cichy S, Czlonkowska A 2000 Procreation ability in Wilson's disease. Acta Neurologica Scandinavia 101: 395–398

Terasaki K K, Quinn M F, Lundell C J, Finck E J, Pentecost M J 1990 Spontaneous hepatic hemorrhage in pre-eclampsia: treatment with hepatic arterial embolization. Radiology 174: 1039–1041

Theise N D, Nimmakayalu M, Gardner R et al 2000 Liver from bone marrow in humans. Hepatology 32: 11–16

Thomas H C, Jacyna M, Waters J, Main J 1988 Virus–host interaction in chronic hepatitis B virus infection. Seminars in Liver Disease 8: 342–349

Thorling L 1955 Jaundice in pregnancy: a clinical study. Acta Medica Scandinavica (suppl) 151: 302

Tiliacos M, Tsantoulas D, Tsoulias A et al 1978 The Budd–Chiari syndrome in pregnancy. Postgraduate Medical Journal 54: 686–691

Tong M J, Thursby M, Takela J et al 1981 Studies on the maternal–infant transmissions of the viruses which cause acute hepatitis. Gastroenterology 80: 999–1004

Treem W R, Rinaldo P, Hale D E et al 1994 Acute fatty liver of pregnancy and long-chain 3-hydroxyacyl-coenzyme A dehydrogenase deficiency. Hepatology 19: 339–345

Treem W R, Shoup M E, Hale D E et al 1996 Acute fatty liver of pregnancy, hemolysis, elevated liver enzymes, and low platelets syndrome, and long chain 3-hydroxyacyl-coenzyme A dehydrogenase deficiency. American Journal of Gastroenterology 91: 2293–2300

Tsega E, Hansson B G, Krawczynski E, Nordenfeld E 1992 Acute sporadic viral hepatitis in Ethiopia: causes, risk factors and effects on pregnancy. Clinical and Infectious Diseases 14: 961–965

Tsimoyiannis E C, Antoniou N C, Txaboulas C, Papanikolaou N 1994 Cholelithiasis during pregnancy and lactation. Prospective study. European Journal of Surgery 160: 627–631

Tsuki Y, Sakamoto S, Fujimoto Y et al 1984 Two cases of idiopathic acute fatty liver of pregnancy with a milder clinical course. Acta Hepatologica Japonica 25: 666–673

Tyni T, Ekholm E, Pihko H 1998 Pregnancy complications are frequent in long-chain 3-hydroxyacyl-coenzyme A dehydrogenase deficiency. American Journal of Obstetrics and Gynecology 178: 603–608

Uslu M, Guzelmeric K, Asut I 1994 Familial thrombotic thrombocytopenic purpura imitating HELLP syndrome (hemylosis, elevated liver enzymes, and low platelets) in two sisters during pregnancy. American Journal of Obstetrics and Gynecology 170: 699–700

Usta I M, Barton J R, Amon E A, Gonzalez A, Sibai B M 1994 Acute fatty liver of pregnancy: an experience in the diagnosis and management of fourteen cases. American Journal of Obstetrics and Gynecology 171: 1342–1347

Valdivieso V, Covarrubias C, Siegel F, Cruz F 1993 Pregnancy and cholelithiasis: pathogenesis and natural course of gallstones diagnosed in early puerperium. Hepatology 17: 1–4

Valentine J M, Parkin G, Pollard S G, Bellamy M C 1995 Combined orthotopic liver transplantation and caesarean section for the Budd–Chiari syndrome. British Journal of Anaesthesia 75: 105–108

Valenzuela G J, Munson L A, Tarbaux N M, Farley J R 1987 Time-dependent changes in bone, placental, intestinal and hepatic alkaline phosphatase activities in serum during human pregnancy. Clinical Chemistry 33: 1801–1806

Van Bodegraven A A, Bohmer C J, Manoliu R A et al 1998 Gallbladder contents and fasting gallbladder volumes during and after pregnancy. Scandinavian Journal of Gastroenterology 33: 993–997

Vanjak D, Moreau R, Roche-Sicot J, Soulier A, Sicot C 1991 Intrahepatic cholestasis of pregnancy and acute fatty liver of pregnancy. Gastroenterology 100: 1123–1125

Van Thiel D H, Gavaler J S 1987 Pregnancy associated sex steroids and their effects on the liver. Seminars in Liver Disease 7: 1–7

van Vliet W, Scheele F, Sibinga-Mulder L, Dekker G A 1995 Echinococcosis of the liver during pregnancy. International Journal of Gynaecology and Obstetrics 49: 323–324

Varma R 1987 Course and prognosis of pregnancy in women with liver disease. Seminars in Liver Disease 7: 59–66

Varner M, Rinderknechts N 1980 Acute fatty metamorphosis of pregnancy: a maternal mortality and literature review. Journal of Reproductive Medicine 24: 177–180

Vassalli P, Morris R H, McCluskey R T 1963 The pathogenic role of fibrin deposition in the glomerular lesions of toxemia of pregnancy. Journal of Experimental Medicine 118: 467–477

Veress B, Wallmander T 1987 Primary hepatic pregnancy. Acta Obstetricia et Gynecologica Scandinavica 66: 563–564

Vesoulis Z, Agamanolis D 1998 Benign hepatocellular tumor of the placenta. American Journal of Surgical Pathology 22: 355–359

Vigil-De Gracia P 2001 Acute fatty liver and HELLP syndrome: two distinct pregnancy disorders. International Journal of Gynaecology and Obstetrics 73: 215–220

Visconti M, Manes G, Giannattasio F, Uomo G 1995 Recurrence of acute fatty liver of pregnancy. Journal of Clinical Gastroenterology 21: 243–245

Vons C, Smadja C, Franco D et al 1984 Successful pregnancy after Budd–Chiari syndrome. Lancet i: 975

Vore M 1987 Estrogen cholestasis: membranes, metabolites or receptors. Gastroenterology 93: 643–649

Wagner V P, Smale L E, Lischke J H 1975 Amebic abscess of the liver and spleen in pregnancy and the puerperium. Obstetrics and Gynecology 45: 562–565

Wagner W H, Lundell C G, Donovan A J 1985 Percutaneous angiographic embolization for hepatic arterial hemorrhage. Archives of Surgery 120: 1241–1249

Wallstedt A, Riely C A, Shaver D et al 1990 Prevalence and characteristics of liver dysfunction in hyperemesis gravidarum. Clinical Research 38: 970–976

Waterson A P 1979 Virus infections (other than rubella) during pregnancy. British Medical Journal 2: 564–566

Weber F L, Snodgrass P J, Powell D E et al 1979 Abnormalities of hepatic mitochondrial urea-cycle enzyme activities and hepatic ultrastructure in acute fatty liver of pregnancy. Journal of Laboratory and Clinical Medicine 94: 27–41

Weinstein L 1982 Syndrome of hemolysis, elevated liver enzymes, and low platelet count: a severe consequence of hypertension in pregnancy. American Journal of Obstetrics and Gynecology 142: 159–167

Weinstein L 1985 Preeclampsia/eclampsia with hemolysis, elevated liver enzymes, and thrombocytopenia. Obstetrics and Gynecology 66: 657–660

Wejstal R, Widell A, Norkrans G 1998 HCV-RNA levels increase during pregnancy in women with chronic hepatitis C. Scandinavian Journal of Infectious Diseases 30: 111–113

Wejstal R, Manson A S, Widell A, Norkrans G 1999 Perinatal transmission of hepatitis G virus (GB virus type C) and hepatitis C virus infections — a comparison. Clinics in Infectious Disease 28: 816–821

Whelton M J, Sherlock S 1968 Pregnancy in patients with hepatic cirrhosis: management and outcome. Lancet 2: 995–999

Whitington P F, Freese D K, Alonso E M, Schwarzenberg S J, Sharp H L 1994 Clinical and biochemical findings in progressive familial intrahepatic cholestasis. Journal of Pediatric Gastroenterology and Nutrition 18: 134–141

Williams R, Ede R J 1981 Hepatitis in pregnancy (editorial). British Medical Journal 283: 1074–1075

Wojcicka-Jagodzinska J, Kuczyriska-Sicinska J, Czaykowski K, Smolarczyk R 1989 Carbohydrate metabolism in the course of intrahepatic cholestasis of pregnancy. American Journal of Obstetrics and Gynecology 161: 959–964

Wolf J L 1996 Liver disease in pregnancy. Medical Clinics of North America 80: 1167–1187

Wolpert E, Pascasio F M, Wolkoff A W, Arias I M 1977 Abnormal sulphobromophthalein metabolism in Rotor's syndrome and obligate heterozygotes. New England Journal of Medicine 296: 1099–1101

Wong D C, Purcell R H, Sreenivasan M A, Prasad S R, Pavri K M 1980 Epidemic and endemic hepatitis in India: evidence for a non A, non B hepatitis virus aetiology. Lancet ii: 876–879

Yen S C 1964 Spontaneous rupture of liver during pregnancy. Obstetrics and Gynecology 23: 783–787

Yeung L T, King S M, Roberts E A 2001 Mother-to-infant transmission of hepatitis C virus. Hepatology 34: 223–229

Ylostalo P, Kirkinen P H, Heikkinen J et al 1981 Gallbladder volume in cholestasis of pregnancy. New England Journal of Medicine 304: 359

Young E J, Chafizadeh E, Oliveira V L, Genta R M 1996 Disseminated herpes virus infection during pregnancy. Clinics in Infectious Disease 22: 51–58

Zanetti A R, Ferroni P, Magliano E M et al 1982 Perinatal transmission of the hepatitis B virus and of the HBV associated delta agent from mothers to offspring in northern Italy. Journal of Medical Virology 9: 139–148

Zanetti A R, Tanzi E, Newell M L 1999 Mother-to-infant transmission of hepatitis C virus. Journal of Hepatology 31 Suppl 1: 96–100

Zimmerman H J, Ishak K G 1982 Valproate-induced hepatic injury: analysis of 23 fatal cases. Hepatology 2: 591–597

Zissin R, Yaffe D, Fejgin M, Olsfanger D, Shapiro-Feinberg M 1999 Hepatic infarction in preeclampsia as part of the HELLP syndrome: CT appearance. Abdominal Imaging 24: 594–596

44

Pathology of the kidney in pregnancy

D. R. Turner

Introduction   1495

Infection   1495
Acute pyelonephritis   1495
Chronic pyelonephritis   1497
Interstitial nephritis   1499
Renal tuberculosis   1499

Acute renal failure in pregnancy   1500
Acute tubular necrosis   1500
Bilateral renal cortical necrosis   1501
Acute renal failure in pregnancy septicaemia   1503
Pre-eclampsia   1503
Abruptio placentae   1503
Prolonged intrauterine death and amniotic fluid
   embolism   1503
Acute fatty liver of pregnancy   1503
HELLP syndrome   1503
Idiopathic postpartum acute renal failure   1503

Pre-eclampsia and hypertension   1505
Pathogenesis of pre-eclampsia   1506
Renal changes in pre-eclampsia   1506

Renal diseases coexisting with pregnancy   1511
Glomerular diseases which may coexist with
   pregnancy   1512
Non-glomerular renal diseases coexisting with
   pregnancy   1519

INTRODUCTION

Before considering renal disease in pregnancy it is important to appreciate that even in normal pregnancy there are major alterations in the results of tests of renal function which complicate the assessment of renal disease. Thus the glomerular filtration rate normally increases by up to 50% (Sims & Krantz 1958) and the effective renal plasma flow increases correspondingly, particularly during the second trimester, returning to normal values at the time of delivery. In consequence, serum creatinine and urea levels fall during the second trimester and return to normal at term. Other parameters which change in pregnancy are glycosuria and proteinuria which tend to increase. Therefore tests of renal function in pregnancy must be viewed against this background since a 'normal' value obtained in a pregnant woman may in fact represent impaired renal function.

When a patient is found to have evidence of renal disease in pregnancy it may prove to be a chronic process which preceded the pregnancy or a recent development which has either been precipitated by some aspect of the pregnancy itself or has occurred coincidentally. In any of these cases it is necessary to consider the effect of the disease on the pregnancy as well as the effect of pregnancy on the progression of the disease. The problems which need to be covered can be conveniently included under the following headings: infections, causes of acute renal failure in pregnancy and the puerperium, pre-eclampsia, hypertension and renal diseases coexisting with pregnancy.

INFECTION

ACUTE PYELONEPHRITIS

Acute pyelonephritis is an important and serious complication of pregnancy which usually develops in women with asymptomatic bacteriuria (Eschenbach 1976). Clinically these patients develop loin pain and fever, and are obviously ill with symptoms of coexisting lower urinary tract infection. Most patients are treated with antibiotics and recover, so histological examination is not relevant, but where material has become available the classical pathology of acute pyelonephritis is observed. The kidney is enlarged and acutely inflamed. The surface may show areas containing yellowish 'spots' (Fig. 44.1) which on cut surfaces are seen to overlie yellowish streaks extending out from the medulla into the cortex. The renal pelvis is also acutely inflamed as are the ureters and bladder. Histological examination of the renal parenchyma confirms the patchy involvement of the organ with groups of renal tubules filled with neutrophil polymorphs spilling over into the surrounding renal interstitium which is correspondingly distended by the cellular infiltrate and oedema (Fig. 44.2). It should be noted that in addition to the neutrophil polymorphs the cellular infiltrate contains numerous macrophages, lymphocytes and plasma cells, the proportions varying according to the time scale of the infection.

If the acute inflammation progresses unchecked then destruction of the renal parenchyma can occur causing extensive loss of tubular epithelial cells, invasion of glomeruli, abscess formation, septicaemia and even necrosis of renal papillae. However, the most usual result is resolution of infection assisted by antibiotic therapy.

As mentioned above, the majority of patients who are likely to develop acute pyelonephritis during pregnancy can be identified at their first antenatal visit as having 'asymptomatic bacteriuria'. This has been defined by Whalley (1967) as 'a condition consisting of an absence of symptoms at a time when the patient has true bacteriuria (as opposed to simple contamination)'.

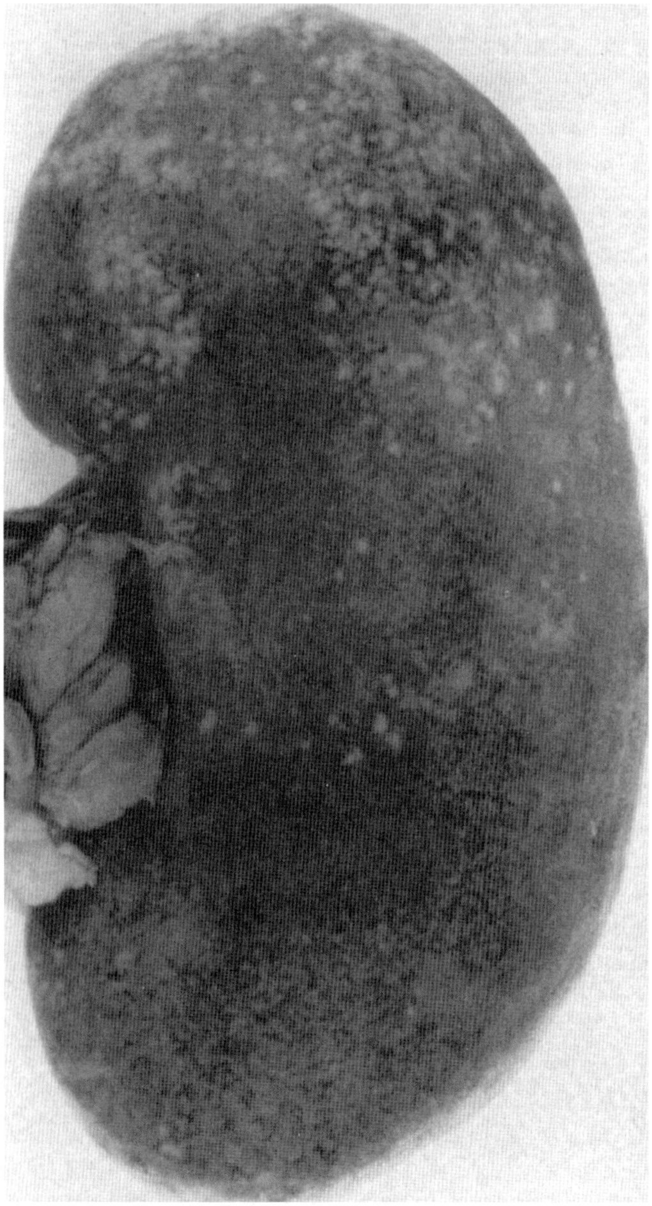

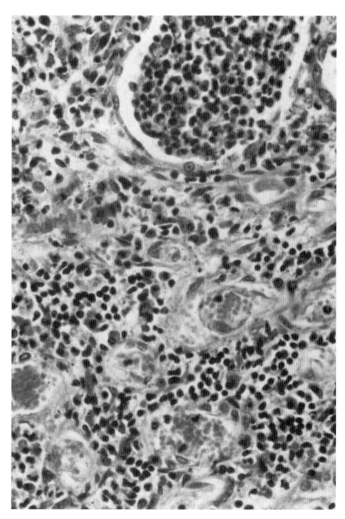

Fig. 44.1 Macroscopic appearance of severe acute pyelonephritis with almost confluent yellow 'spots' on the capsular surface of the kidney.

Fig. 44.2 Severe acute pyelonephritis with neutrophils distending a tubule top right and inflammatory cells within the interstitial tissues.

Normal urine is sterile and with symptomatic infection of the urinary tract one would expect to find a pathogenic organism such as *Escherichia coli* present with a bacterial colony count in excess of 10^5 organisms/ml in the vast majority of cases. Accidental contamination of the urine by nonpathogenic organisms during collection of the specimen usually gives a colony count of less than 10^4 organisms/ml.

Assuming a clean specimen of urine has been collected, a colony count of 10^5 organisms/ml in a patient without symptoms is highly likely to represent bacteriuria. Colony counts of between 10^4 and 10^5 are equivocal and should be confirmed in a repeat test. Obviously the precision of the urine collection is important in these assessments and needs to be performed in a uniform manner so that comparisons between groups of patients can be meaningful. The clean catch method with cleansing of the hands and periurethral area with antiseptic soap followed by spreading of the labia prior to voiding urine is probably the most practical technique. There is an 80% reliability with one test and a 95% reliability when repeated.

The prevalence of bacteriuria in pregnancy is quoted at between 2 and 10% in different studies with the figures being consistently higher in the lower social classes. Whether this relates to the greater use of antibiotics by the upper social classes or lack of hygiene in the lower social classes is not established.

What is clearly established is that antibiotics given to those pregnant women with bacteriuria will largely prevent them from developing acute pyelonephritis (Lindheimer & Katz 1977a). Only about one-third of cases of bacteriuria will proceed to clinical infection if left untreated which suggests that the bacteriuric patients are not a homogeneous group. Indeed, it seems that those with upper urinary tract involvement are more likely to proceed to clinical infection than those with lower tract involvement. A number of methods have been examined for their suitability in distinguishing between these two categories. Fairley (1970) described the use of ureteral catheterisation to identify asymptomatic infection involving the upper urinary tract. The maximal urinary concentrating ability is impaired in some 14–40% of pregnancy bacteriurics and this impairment is restored by eradicating the bacteria (Norden & Tuttle 1965). Similar circumstantial evidence can be cited in relation to serum antibody levels which tend to be elevated in about a third of bacteriurics (Reeves & Brumfitt 1968). The fluorescent antibody test (Thomas et al 1974) is capable of demonstrating the presence of a coating of immunoglobulin on the surface coat of bacteria when infection of the upper urinary tract is present. However, there is dispute about the interpretation of this test. So far there is no perfect system for identifying with certainty all cases with infection of the upper urinary tract and it is therefore prudent to treat all bacteriurias. Indeed even the test system for bacteriuria is not perfect and a small percentage of patients with subclinical urinary tract infection will not be identified and treated. This probably explains why some cases of acute pyelonephritis in pregnancy have no preceding history of bacteriuria.

The bacteriuria which is seen in early pregnancy is almost certainly an extension of the asymptomatic bacteriuria seen in schoolgirls (1.2% of population) with some enhancement following the onset of regular sexual intercourse, rather than representing something special to pregnancy.

When a patient has had one or more attacks of acute pyelonephritis in pregnancy it is recommended that the urinary tract should be examined postpartum for abnormalities. This is best delayed for several weeks (12 or so) to give time for the changes of pregnancy to regress. Only occasionally do such examinations demonstrate scarring of the kidneys. In those cases the scarring is generally taken to represent damage due to reflux nephropathy acquired in childhood and not the result of recent infection. Other structural abnormalities such as aberrant collecting systems, calculi and neurogenic bladders are also relatively uncommon findings in women who have had acute pyelonephritis in pregnancy. The predisposition of the urinary tract to infection during pregnancy was originally blamed solely on obstruction of the ureters by pressure on the pelvic brim by the enlarging uterus. However, it is now appreciated that inhibition of peristalsis of the smooth muscle in the wall of the ureter by progesterone is also an important factor in causing dilatation of the ureters and urinary stasis, which thereby predisposes to bacterial infection. Although *E. coli* accounts for 80% of urinary tract infections in pregnancy, other organisms such as Klebsiella, enterobacter, proteus species and enterococci may be responsible. The *E. coli* which are associated with acute pyelonephritis seem to represent a non-random set of closely related isolates and some of these strains may be characteristic of pregnancy patients only (Hart et al 1996).

It appeared clearly established that patients with symptomatic pyelonephritis in pregnancy have approximately twice the expected rate of premature deliveries (Lancet leading article, 1985). However Fan et al (1987) found no threat to pregnancy in patients successfully treated with antibiotics. They did point out the danger of failing to control infection due to bacterial resistance to antibiotics. Conflicting results have been obtained for the relationship between bacteriuria in pregnancy and prematurity, presumably because the bacteriurias represent a non-homogeneous group. As mentioned above this non-homogeneity is increased by treatment with antibiotics and subsequent relapse of a proportion of cases.

CHRONIC PYELONEPHRITIS

Chronic pyelonephritis represents a chronic inflammatory destruction of renal parenchyma which may be related to

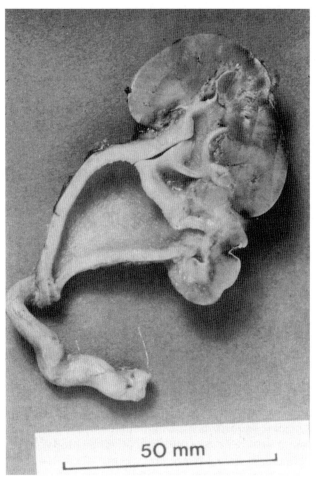

Fig. 44.3 Macroscopic appearance of segmental scarring in a kidney from a young child with reflux and secondary infection.

a variety of causes including obstruction in the renal tract and vesico-ureteric reflux. The pattern of scarring is often of a segmental nature with a predilection for the upper and lower poles of the kidney. The calyces of the renal pelvis may be dilated and pulled outwards in relation to the scarred areas (Fig. 44.3). The evidence of chronic inflammation is usually seen best in the renal parenchyma adjacent to the renal pelves where aggregates of lymphocytes and plasma cells are found. Even germinal centres may develop in this site. Elsewhere in the renal parenchyma chronic inflammatory cells may also be present in a patchy distribution. In the early stages destruction of renal tubules is evident in scarred areas with a tendency to crowding of residual glomeruli. The residual atrophic tubules contain protein casts which stain intensely with eosin giving an appearance similar to that seen in thyroid follicles (Fig. 44.4). As the scarring progresses the glomeruli develop sclerotic changes, which may be either segmental or involve whole glomeruli, followed by their disappearance. Thus gradually both tubules and glomeruli disappear from the scarred areas leaving the blood vessels as a dominant feature, the latter having become more prominent as a result of thickening of their walls and crowding due to loss of intervening parenchyma.

Where obstruction is a major factor in the genesis of chronic pyelonephritis the effect of pressure atrophy contributes to the loss of renal parenchyma, which may become generally thinned as a consequence in addition to segmental scarring.

In non-obstructive pyelonephritis the causative factors include vesico-ureteric reflux in infancy together with abnormal structure of some renal papillae (Ransley &

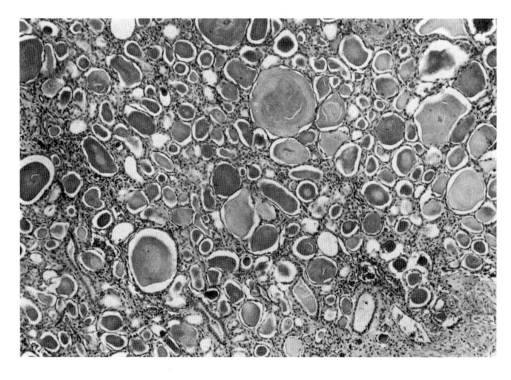

Fig. 44.4 End-stage picture of atrophic tubules in chronic pyelonephritis with intensely staining eosinophilic casts within the renal tubules.

Risdon 1978) which permit the ingress of urine into the corresponding collecting ducts (so-called intrarenal reflux). However the situation is complicated by the fact that vesico-ureteric reflux and obstruction may coexist and furthermore vesico-ureteric reflux tends to disappear with time so the basic cause of renal scarring may well not be demonstrable by the time a woman in the reproductive phase of life is found to have scarred kidneys.

For the woman who begins pregnancy with chronic pyelonephritis, however acquired, there is a higher chance of both asymptomatic and symptomatic bacteriuria as compared with control groups. The overall prognosis for pregnancy is determined more by the presence or absence of hypertension and by the adequacy of residual renal function. The prognosis is usually favourable in the absence of hypertension, assuming that renal function is adequate, while the presence of hypertension and renal insufficiency are associated with a poor prognosis (Lindheimer & Katz 1977b). Indeed Kincaid-Smith (1983) reported rapid deterioration of renal function in four patients with reflux nephropathy who started pregnancy with impaired renal function. Jungers et al (1996) confirmed these findings and Kincaid-Smith (1983) also showed that increased proteinuria is the best indicator of progression of reflux nephropathy.

INTERSTITIAL NEPHRITIS

A variety of different disease processes have been included with chronic pyelonephritis under the general term interstitial nephritis. These include analgesic nephropathy, Balkan nephropathy, drug-induced interstitial nephritis, sarcoidosis and metabolic disturbances such as hyperuricaemia,

oxalosis and nephrocalcinosis. No detailed studies of the inter-relationship of these disorders with pregnancy seem to be available. The general impression, however, is gained that provided renal function is not seriously impaired at the start of pregnancy the prognosis is good.

RENAL TUBERCULOSIS

The diagnosis of renal tuberculosis is usually heralded by the finding of symptoms of dysuria, frequency and haematuria accompanied by sterile pyuria. Acid-fast bacilli may be identified in a smear of centrifuged urine or a positive culture may be required to establish the diagnosis. It is considered safe for pyelography to be carried out after the 20th week of pregnancy to establish the extent of the disease.

Renal involvement in tuberculosis is never primary and always results from blood-borne spread (although the primary site of infection may have healed). Furthermore it cannot be assumed to be limited to one site; the whole of the renal tract must be regarded as being potentially involved.

The disease begins with the development of tuberculoid granulomas within the renal interstitium. The granulomas are composed of Langerhans' type giant cells and epithelioid macrophages. The acid-fast bacilli may be very difficult to identify both in terms of their size and relative scarcity in histological sections. As the granulomas enlarge they undergo necrosis centrally and coalesce to form a larger necrotic mass surrounded by a palisade of macrophages and giant cells (Fig. 44.5). Ultimately this mass may encroach upon one of the calyces and can then discharge its cheese-like contents into the urinary system

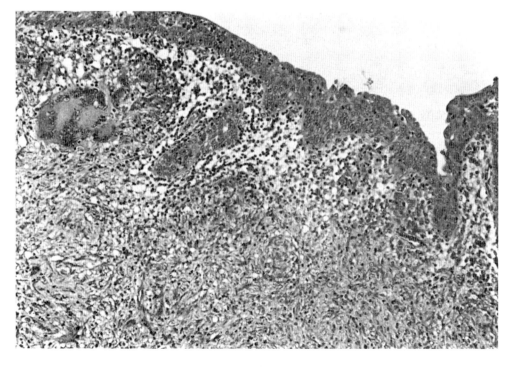

Fig. 44.5 Numerous granulomas and giant cells beneath the calyceal epithelium in a case of renal tuberculosis.

leaving a cavity within the renal parenchyma. Such cavities remain as a permanent marker of renal destruction and indeed have a predisposition to dystrophic calcification which fortuitously makes them more readily visible by X-rays. Involvement of the urinary tract may lead to progressive chronic inflammation of the ureters and bladder. However, modern anti-tuberculous chemotherapy usually cuts short the disease process before it has become extensive.

There is general agreement that pregnancy does not significantly affect the course and prognosis of patients with tuberculosis apart, perhaps, from the possibility of more frequent relapses in the puerperium (Sulavick 1975). Indeed, provided the patient has adequate renal function and a normal blood pressure at the start, renal tuberculosis is not a contraindication to a successful pregnancy (Felding 1968).

ACUTE RENAL FAILURE IN PREGNANCY

This can be defined as the sudden development of renal insufficiency from any cause in a pregnant patient previously thought to have normal kidneys. A marked rise in blood urea nitrogen and serum creatinine levels are found together with a decrease in urine output to less than 400 ml/day in the majority of cases, although a non-oliguric form of acute renal failure with impaired function but normal urine volume is also recognized. Causative factors include events which may occur at any time and are not therefore specific to pregnancy (1a below) and others which are particular complications of pregnancy (1b below).

1a. *Causative factors not limited to pregnancy which may lead to acute renal failure*
   Septicaemic shock
   Hypovolaemic shock due to haemorrhage or
      dehydration
   Intravascular haemolysis
   Administration of nephrotoxic agents
   Urinary tract obstruction
   Fulminant glomerulonephritis
   Myoglobinuria
1b. *Special complications of pregnancy which may lead to acute renal failure*
   Septic abortion
   Acute pyelonephritis
   Eclampsia
   Hyperemesis gravidarum
   Acute fatty liver in pregnancy
   HELLP syndrome
   Abruptio placentae ⎫ Particularly
   Prolonged intrauterine death ⎪ prone to
   Amniotic fluid embolism ⎬ progress to
   Uterine haemorrhage ⎪ bilateral renal
   Postpartum idiopathic acute ⎭ cortical necrosis
      renal failure

Studies using angiography and isotope methods indicate that there is usually a demonstrable vasoconstriction and/or reduction of vascular supply to the renal cortex in cases of acute renal failure (Hollenberg et al 1970). The corollary of this is a reduction in renal blood flow to less than half its normal value and almost total cessation of glomerular filtration. If this condition is of short duration, due either to a relatively transient problem or due to rapid and effective therapeutic measures, the functional disturbance is entirely reversible. This readily reversible type of acute renal failure is described as prerenal failure, and one would not expect to find any significant morphological abnormality within the renal tissue.

According to some authors (Stratta et al 1996) acute renal failure has become an increasingly rare event in pregnancy as a result of improved health care. However, this will clearly depend on the quality and extent of healthcare systems available and numerous studies from countries with less well developed systems show that acute renal failure is still an important and potentially dangerous condition (Chugh et al 1994).

ACUTE TUBULAR NECROSIS

The longer the period in which renal cortical blood flow is severely restricted, the greater the chance that tissue necrosis will occur. The most vulnerable cells in terms of metabolic activity are the proximal tubular epithelial cells, closely followed by the distal tubular epithelial cells. The first morphological evidence of cell damage occurs in the thick ascending loop of Henle (Brezis et al 1984). Cytoplasmic swelling and vacuolation may be seen first in a focal distribution, subsequently becoming confluent, as the ischaemic period increases (Fig. 44.6). Nuclear degeneration and loss are the markers of cell death (Fig. 44.7). Fortunately the regenerative capacity of the tubular epithelial cells is considerable, such that, provided the devastation is not complete, a sufficient number of cells will survive with the capacity to reconstitute the tubular epithelium. If a renal biopsy is performed in the early regenerative stage, the tubular epithelial cells may be seen to be much flatter than normal and lack many of their normal features of differentiation (Fig. 44.8). Occasional mitotic figures are an encouraging sign that regeneration is progressing. In many cases necrosis is not identified at any stage but by electronmicroscopy a loss of differentiation can be identified; microvilli and basolateral infoldings disappear, together with a marked reduction in mitochondria.

The patient will require to be supported during the period of functional failure of her kidneys by peritoneal dialysis or haemodialysis according to what local facilities are available. Mortality is less than for acute renal failure in non-obstetric patients (Grünfeld et al 1980; Turney et al 1990).

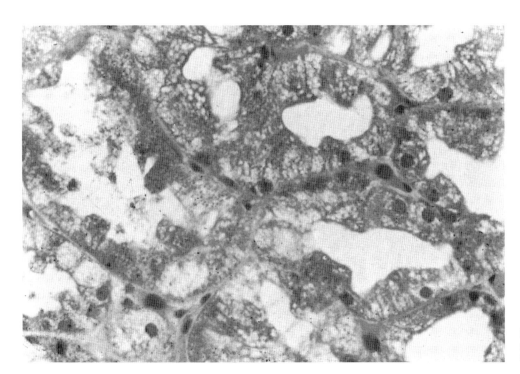

Fig. 44.6 Tubular necrosis with cytoplasmic swelling and vacuolation.

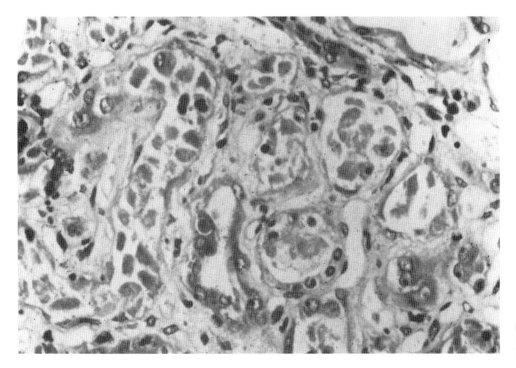

Fig. 44.7 Tubular necrosis with nuclear loss and shedding of cells into the lumen.

BILATERAL RENAL CORTICAL NECROSIS

When renal ischaemia is particularly severe and prolonged the degree of necrosis is correspondingly severe, and affects all the constituent structures of the renal cortex where vascular spasm exerts its major effect (Fig. 44.9). Much weight has been placed on the finding of intravascular thrombi involving glomeruli and arterial vessels. However, the relative infrequency of these lesions in many cases suggests that they could not solely account for the extent or distribution of the necrosis which occurs. Although cortical necrosis is seen in both pregnant and non-pregnant states there is a marked predisposition for it to be associated with obstetric complications (Kleinknecht et al 1973). This suggests that there are some facets of pregnancy which aggravate renal cortical ischaemia when it occurs. In normal pregnancy the levels of fibrinogen, factor VII, factor VIII and factor X are all

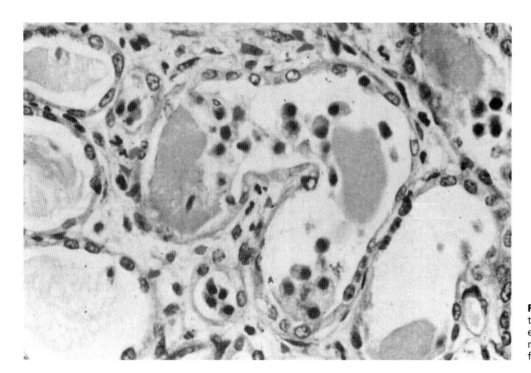

Fig. 44.8 The reparative stage of tubular necrosis with the epithelial cells represented by a relatively undifferentiated flattened layer of cells.

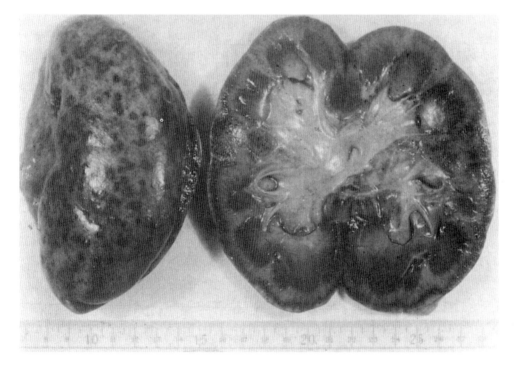

Fig. 44.9 Bilateral renal cortical necrosis with pallor of the cortical tissue due to infarction of all its tissue components. (Provided by Professor R Risdon.)

increased and fibrinolysis is reduced (Bonnar 1976) so that it is tempting to assume that intravascular thrombi could develop more readily than in the non-pregnant state. However, therapeutic attempts to prevent or reverse the assumed intravascular coagulation with heparin and fibrinolytic agents have proved remarkably ineffective in preventing cortical necrosis. Although it is often possible to demonstrate evidence of defibrination in patients with obstetric complications this does not seem to be consis-

tently greater in those cases which proceed to cortical necrosis. Furthermore, when intravascular thrombi are identified in renal cortical necrosis they tend to be identified in the terminal stages rather than in early biopsies, suggesting that they are more likely to represent an additional feature rather than the primary event.

It would seem therefore that Sheehan's original hypothesis (Sheehan & Moore 1952) that the usual primary event in renal cortical necrosis is severe and prolonged vascular spasm is still supported by the available evidence. He regarded the intravascular thrombi as evidence of a terminal relaxation of vascular spasm leading to blood flow through necrotic vessels and glomeruli and consequent thrombosis of these vessels. It would perhaps be naïve to assume that all examples of cortical necrosis were explicable by a single pathogenetic mechanism. The prognosis for renal cortical necrosis is obviously poor and often leads to death, haemodialysis or renal transplantation (Grünfeld et al 1980). It should be noted that some cases of patchy involvement of the renal cortex have been known to recover a useful degree of renal function (Heptinstall 1992). There is therefore a danger that a renal biopsy may provide a falsely gloomy picture if only a small piece of totally necrotic material is obtained.

ACUTE RENAL FAILURE IN PREGNANCY SEPTICAEMIA

Following the change in social attitudes which permitted the legalisation of abortion the incidence of septic abortion has fallen considerably. It remains, however, an important cause of acute renal failure in early pregnancy with a peak incidence around 16 weeks gestation. Septicaemia may also occur in pregnancy as a complication of acute pyelonephritis and puerperal sepsis. The marked hypotensive effect of overwhelming infection causes renal ischaemia, and intravascular coagulation may be superimposed. This latter process may be triggered by endotoxins in the circulation or by intravascular haemolysis due to clostridial infection (Emmanuel & Lindheimer 1976).

Parallels are inevitably drawn between the occasional development of renal cortical necrosis as a consequence of pregnancy septicaemia and the generalised Shwartzman reaction, which can be triggered by giving a single dose of endotoxin in pregnant animals. Certainly endotoxin has the capacity to induce intravascular coagulation. In practice, however, pregnancy septicaemia does not usually progress to renal cortical necrosis.

PRE-ECLAMPSIA

Acute renal failure may develop within the setting of severe pre-eclampsia. Here it is postulated that renal cortical ischaemia is caused by the severe swelling of the glomerular capillary endothelium to the extent that the capillary lumens are obliterated causing post-glomerular ischaemia. A minority of such cases progress to cortical necrosis. There is some evidence that the older multiparous patients are more liable to have such a fatal outcome, possibly due to undetected hypertension or renal vascular disease (Grünfeld et al 1980). Intravascular haemolysis has also been postulated as being responsible in part for the renal cortical ischaemia in eclampsia but the mechanism for this is uncertain.

ABRUPTIO PLACENTAE

There is a particularly high incidence of renal cortical necrosis developing in patients with acute renal failure due to abruptio placentae. The estimated blood loss is usually less than would be expected from the degree of renal ischaemia produced, suggesting that hypovolaemia is only part of the problem. The defibrination syndrome is usually also present (Kleiner & Greston 1976).

PROLONGED INTRAUTERINE DEATH AND AMNIOTIC FLUID EMBOLISM

The defibrination syndrome is often encountered in association with prolonged intrauterine death and amniotic fluid embolism. These complications of pregnancy are then particularly prone to lead to acute renal failure and renal cortical necrosis.

ACUTE FATTY LIVER OF PREGNANCY

This rare complication of pregnancy, which is primarily a problem from the hepatological aspects, has been linked with tetracycline usage by some authors (Kunelis et al 1965). Acute renal failure is a frequent complication but the morphological changes seen in the kidneys are usually unimpressive apart from fatty vacuolation of the tubular epithelial cells. The liver failure is the main clinical problem. In some cases where renal failure has developed, thrombi have been seen in the microvasculature of the renal cortex (Morrin et al 1967) but this development has not been shown convincingly to be a prime cause of the renal failure. Slater & Hague (1984) have described sub-endothelial electron-dense deposits and mesangial cell interposition in four cases of acute fatty liver of pregnancy with renal involvement. The precise mechanism responsible for these effects is unclear.

HELLP SYNDROME

This is an association of haemolysis, elevated liver enzymes and low platelets which may occur in pregnancy and lead to acute renal failure. Its relationship with pre-eclampsia, haemolytic uraemic syndrome and postpartum acute renal failure is discussed by Sibai et al (1994).

IDIOPATHIC POSTPARTUM ACUTE RENAL FAILURE

This syndrome was first described by Scheer & Jones (1967), Wagoner et al (1968) and Robson et al (1968) and is relatively rare yet often fatal when it does occur. Microangiopathic haemolytic anaemia is often present and accelerated hypertension frequently develops. The pregnancy has usually been uneventful until shortly after parturition when a typical case will present with a flu-like

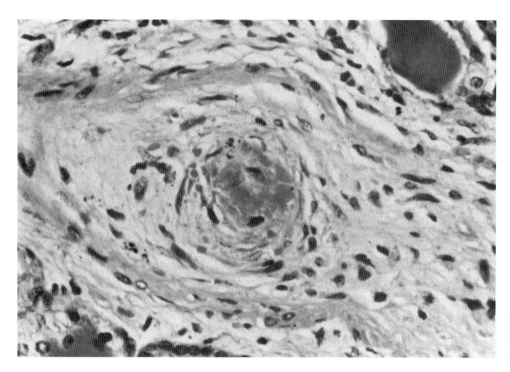

Fig. 44.10 Florid intimal proliferation in a small artery with occlusion of the lumen by fibrin in postpartum acute renal failure.

illness reminiscent of the prodromal phase of the haemolytic uraemic syndrome. The histological changes seen in the kidney are very similar to those seen in scleroderma with renal involvement. There is marked cellular proliferation and accumulation of mucopolysaccharide ground substance in the subintimal zone of arterial vessels (Fig. 44.10). Fibrinoid necrosis is seen particularly in the walls of arterioles (Fig. 44.11). The glomeruli may show ischaemic changes as a consequence of the vascular occlusion or segmental necrosis with crescent formation

may occur. Fibrin is usually demonstrable, using immunohistochemical techniques, in the walls of arterioles and small arteries and in parts of some glomeruli. In glomeruli which are showing neither ischaemic collapse nor necrosis the capillary walls are initially thickened by a pale material in the subendothelial zone which may contain fibrin tactoids. Subsequently, mesangial cell interposition may occur and cause a reduplication of the glomerular capillary basement membranes. These features suggest that the coagulation mechanism is involved and,

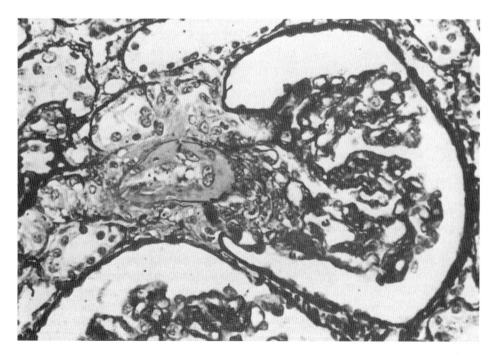

Fig. 44.11 Fibrinoid necrosis of the wall of an afferent arteriole and ischaemic collapse of the glomerular tuft in postpartum acute renal failure.

indeed, although many patients die, recovery has been reported after anticoagulant therapy (Donadio & Holley 1974).

There is a striking similarity between postpartum acute renal failure and the development of haemolytic uraemic syndrome in women taking oral contraceptives. This latter complication of oestrogen consumption was described by Tobon (1972). However, women who develop either one of these conditions do not show any increased susceptibility to the other. Yet women who develop the haemolytic uraemic syndrome after using the contraceptive pill have a greater chance of developing acute rejection following renal transplantation.

PRE-ECLAMPSIA AND HYPERTENSION

The term toxaemia of pregnancy has been used in an ill-defined way to describe the occurrence of hypertension, proteinuria and oedema in pregnancy. This syndrome has encompassed not only patients with pre-eclampsia/eclampsia but also patients with essential hypertension and hypertension secondary to other causes such as chronic renal disease. Since pre-eclampsia may be superimposed upon pre-existing hypertension or latent hypertension careful analysis is necessary to appreciate what is happening in an individual case (Lindheimer & Katz 1977c).

Pre-eclampsia/eclampsia is a condition peculiar to pregnancy with characteristic morphological changes in glomeruli which can be revealed by renal biopsy. Indeed, without biopsy pre-eclampsia is difficult to diagnose, and physicians are very reluctant to carry out biopsies in pregnancy although Packham and Fairley (1987) have shown a very low complication rate. The severity of the glomerular lesions tends to roughly parallel the degree of proteinuria found clinically (Sheehan 1980). Pre-eclampsia is uncommon before 20 weeks' gestation, unless associated with a hydatidiform mole or multiple pregnancy, and does not usually develop before 30 weeks' gestation. It is about seven times more frequent in first as compared with subsequent pregnancies. Other predisposing factors are essential hypertension, diabetes, fetal hydrops and extremes of reproductive age. The dramatic resolution of the syndrome following delivery tends to implicate the feto-placental unit in its aetiology although its marked association with first pregnancies has not been adequately explained.

In practice one does not normally have the assistance of the renal biopsy appearances in making the diagnosis of pre-eclampsia and therefore one is relying upon the interpretation of blood pressure readings and the assessment of proteinuria and oedema. Before analysing further the significance of various combinations of hypertension, oedema and proteinuria it is important to appreciate that accurate assessment of each of these three parameters can be difficult, particularly in deciding between the upper limits of normality and the first indication of pathological change. This area of uncertainty has no doubt contributed significantly to the confusion which surrounds the subject of pre-eclampsia.

The measurement of blood pressure is normally achieved by an indirect, non-invasive technique which is recognised as providing an estimation rather than an accurate reading. This makes the establishment of a normal value difficult, particularly when other factors such as age, smoking habits, family size, occupation, anxiety and discomfort are all known to be able to affect individual blood pressure readings. Furthermore, pregnancy itself induces a relative fall in blood pressure estimations to an average of about 70 mmHg diastolic by the 16th week of gestation with a subsequent rise to an average of about 80 mmHg by the 36th week of gestation. Clinically the figure of 140/90 has been regarded as abnormal but perinatal mortality figures (Friedman 1976) suggest that there is a sudden increase in mortality at blood pressure levels in excess of 125/75 throughout the period of observation in pregnancy.

Some degree of dependent oedema is almost universal in pregnancy and therefore pitting oedema in the legs cannot be assumed to be due to pre-eclampsia. Oedema of the hands and face is much more likely to have a significant pathological basis.

The assessment of proteinuria may be roughly performed by a dipstick method or more accurately estimated as grams per 24 h specimen or grams per litre. It is usual practice to ignore small degrees of proteinuria (i.e. less than 300 mg/24 h). A false high reading for proteinuria may occur as a result of contamination of the urine by vaginal discharge or bleeding and could theoretically be due to orthostatic proteinuria, violent exercise or exposure to severe cold. With these caveats a level of proteinuria in excess of 300 mg/24 h is usually taken to be indicative of either pre-eclampsia or possibly some other glomerular disorder.

In practice, however, the clinical diagnosis of pre-eclampsia has often been made on the sole criterion of an elevated blood pressure in late pregnancy and early puerperium which falls to normal levels within 10 days of delivery. This syndrome is sometimes termed gestational hypertension and may prove to be due to either pre-eclampsia, latent essential hypertension revealed by pregnancy, or hypertension, either essential or of renal origin, that has abated during the middle trimester of pregnancy. Consequently the diagnosis of pre-eclampsia is insecure in the absence of further evidence such as significant proteinuria (i.e. > 300 mg/24 h) or renal biopsy, the latter rarely being available.

It has been pointed out by Sheehan (1980) that the classical morphological findings of pre-eclampsia are almost never seen in the absence of proteinuria, lending support to the value of proteinuria as a clinical sign of pre-eclampsia.

Since many of the follow-up studies of patients with pre-eclampsia are confused by the inclusion of cases of gestational hypertension, the conclusions with regard to the long-term consequences must be drawn with care (Chesley 1980). Certainly such studies appear to show an increase in chronic hypertensive vascular disease in patients with 'pre-eclampsia'. However, when one begins to separate off the cases with gestational hypertension alone the incidence of development of chronic hypertensive disease falls correspondingly. Gestational hypertension tends to be much more common in heavy, obese females and increases sharply with age, which is also true of essential hypertension. Conversely the perinatal mortality is not increased in women with gestational hypertension nor are the infants small for gestational age as occurs with pre-eclampsia. Thus gestational hypertension appears to represent latent essential hypertension unmasked by pregnancy. Indeed, women with normotensive pregnancies have a much reduced chance of developing chronic hypertensive vascular disease than might be expected by comparison with matched unselected females. Thus pregnancy appears to be a useful screening test for chronic hypertension.

Although moderate proteinuria is a cardinal feature of pre-eclampsia, occasionally massive proteinuria with a full nephrotic syndrome may develop, as described in a series of patients by Roy First et al (1978).

PATHOGENESIS OF PRE-ECLAMPSIA

Innumerable theories have been propounded on the pathogenesis of pre-eclampsia, ranging from hormonal effects and the renin–angiotensin system through dietary excesses and deficiencies to more recent ideas carried along on the various cascade systems of haemostasis, kinins and prostaglandins (MacGillivray 1981). However, none of these theories provides an explanation for the well-established high incidence of pre-eclampsia in first pregnancies. Even a miscarriage appears to provide protection against the development of pre-eclampsia in a subsequent pregnancy.

Logic would seem to dictate that a system with the capacity to modify its functions with time, such as the specific immune system, must be involved. Indeed, it is generally accepted that a degree of immune tolerance is required in normal pregnancy to prevent rejection of the fetus and placenta. If immune tolerance were incompletely developed at the time of a first pregnancy then damage to the placental tissue would be expected and this could induce those changes we recognise as pre-eclampsia.

The fact that pre-eclampsia has a familial tendency (Chesley 1980; Cooper et al 1993) and also a racial predilection suggests that there may be a genetic abnormality which could be responsible for some women exhibiting impaired tolerance to the feto-placental unit, and thus being susceptible to the development of pre-eclampsia. Some caution needs to be observed in accepting that pre-eclampsia has a genetic basis since the clinical diagnosis of pre-eclampsia may include cases of essential hypertension which does have an inheritable basis.

The observation that twin pregnancies are particularly prone to induce pre-eclampsia, regardless of whether they are mono- or dizygotic, suggests that the phenomenon involves suppression or adaptation of a mechanism (i.e. tolerance) rather than an increased materno-fetal incompatibility (Campbell et al 1977). This idea is supported by the increased incidence of pre-eclampsia in association with other conditions where an enlarged placental mass develops: namely hydatidiform mole, triploidy, erythroblastosis fetalis and diabetes.

There seems to be no doubt that intravascular coagulation can be identified in many cases of pre-eclampsia, although this may well prove to be the consequence rather than the cause of pre-eclampsia. Many studies show that fibrin degradation products are elevated and when maternal tissues are available for examination some degree of intravascular thrombosis can be identified, particularly in severe disease. Certainly the changes seen in renal glomeruli (see below) are entirely consistent with a chronic low-grade fibrin deposition. Whether the final mechanisms which result in the pre-eclampsia syndrome depend on stimulation of the kinin system, a deficiency in prostacyclin production (Lewis 1982) or the renin–angiotensin system is not established although all these systems are under scrutiny. Experimentally, placental ischaemia in the rabbit can induce a syndrome resembling eclampsia (Abitbol et al 1976). Currently, the most logical explanation for pre-eclampsia would seem to be that the relatively underdeveloped uterine vasculature releases thromboplastins and/or other substances which induce vascular spasm affecting the renal glomeruli in particular. Occasional relaxation of spasm may then allow coagulation to occur around damaged endothelial cells. It is of interest that Clark et al (1992) have shown that endothelin levels are elevated in pre-eclampsia and may contribute to renal vasoconstriction. It is also of interest that women with a history of pre-eclampsia are relatively hypovolaemic and tend to have lower effective renal plasma flow and higher renal vascular resistance than control subjects and this is irrespective of their blood pressure (van Beek et al 1998).

RENAL CHANGES IN PRE-ECLAMPSIA

The descriptive label of glomerular capillary endotheliosis was proposed by Spargo et al (1959) and is broadly agreed to be the most characteristic lesion of pre-eclampsia. It describes an enlargement of the glomerular tuft (Fig. 44.12) due mainly to an increase in endothelial cell cytoplasm (Fig. 44.13). There is little overall increase in cellularity although there is a moderate widening of the mesangial areas. The endothelial cell cytoplasm shows a remarkable degree of swelling and vacuolation which

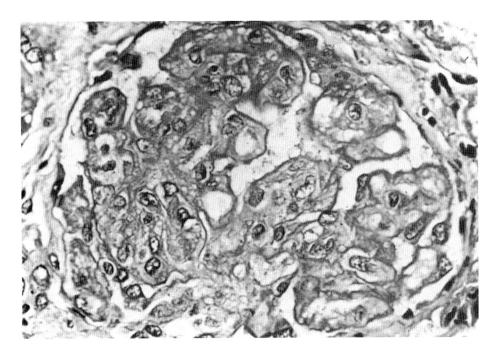

Fig. 44.12 Glomerular capillary endotheliosis due to swelling of endothelial cells in pre-eclampsia. The capillary lumens are largely obliterated.

encroaches considerably on the lumens of glomerular capillaries. Certainly the impression is that the endothelial cells have been damaged by vascular spasm or some agent or toxin, resulting in a markedly increased water content together with a variable degree of fatty change. The glomerular capillaries in pre-eclampsia usually appear bloodless in histological sections. However, this cannot be true in vivo or urine would not be produced at all. The most probable explanation of this observation is that as the intravascular pressure falls the blood in glomerular capillaries is expelled by the reflux of filtrate back from the urinary space and proximal tubule, and by the contraction of the glomerular tuft itself. The fatty change affecting the endothelial cells is variable both in degree and in the type of lipid present (Fig. 44.14). Neutral fat, phospholipid and cholesterol esters may be identified.

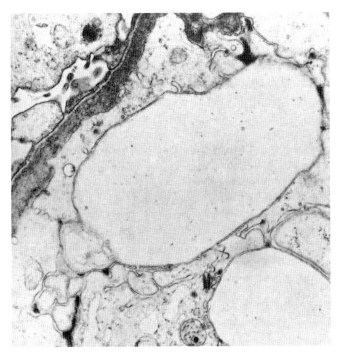

Fig. 44.13 Electronmicrograph showing swollen pale endothelial cell cytoplasm limited (top left) by a relatively normal glomerular capillary basement membrane in pre-eclampsia.

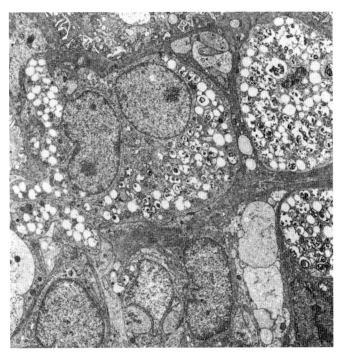

Fig. 44.14 Electronmicrograph showing swollen and vacuolated endothelial cells with numerous myelin bodies (residual bodies) from a case of pre-eclampsia.

The mesangial cells, although not increased in number, show a marked expansion of their cytoplasmic processes, some of which also show fatty change. It is the cytoplasmic increase which explains the widening of mesangial areas described above, and may be associated with an increased production of mesangial matrix material. In the more advanced cases of pre-eclampsia the mesangial cell processes may begin to grow round the capillary loops in the subendothelial region (Figs 44.15–44.17). This phenomenon is known as mesangial cell interposition and may lead to the laying down of a basement membrane-like material of mesangial matrix type in the subsendothelial space of the glomerular capillary wall (Fig. 44.18). The effect of this is to produce a double-contour effect in part or all of the glomerular capillary loop when stained with methanamine silver (Fig. 44.19).

The subendothelial space is expanded initially by a pale amorphous substance (Fig. 44.20) which gives a positive reaction with antisera to fibrinogen and has been referred to as fibrinoid (Kincaid-Smith 1991). Only occasionally are fibrin tactoids identified by electronmicroscopy, however. The subendothelial space may also contain occasional electron-dense deposits similar to those seen in immune complex disease. Immunofluorescent studies have given variable results but the general trend is for IgM and fibrin to be consistently identified (Tribe et al 1979) while other immunoglobulins and complement components are infrequent or unimpressive (Fig. 44.21). Foidart et al (1983) have shown that the material deposited in the subendothelial zone of the capillary loops consists of structural basement membrane components as well as plasma-derived proteins, and suggest that this may be mediated by prostaglandin secretion.

Despite the remarkable changes occurring in the endothelial cells and subendothelial space, the original glomerular basement membrane remains surprisingly intact in morphological terms although it is presumably sufficiently altered in biochemical terms to permit significant proteinuria.

The epithelial cells are altered to the extent that they may contain large hyaline cytoplasmic droplets and villous proliferation of the cytoplasmic membrane. However, the most significant feature is the relative normality of the epithelial foot processes despite proteinuria which may be of severe proportions (Fig. 44.18). This strongly suggests that the concept that proteinuria is solely due to foot process loss, as has been proposed in minimal change nephropathy and other glomerular disorders, is incorrect. Indeed Lafayette (1998) has shown that

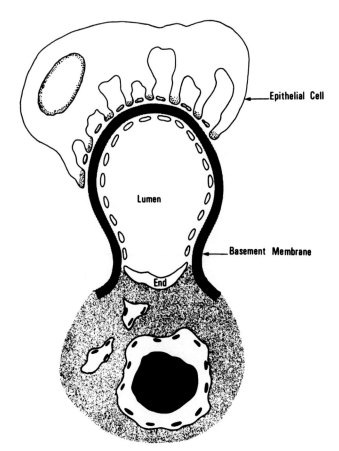

Fig. 44.15 Diagram of normal glomerular capillary loop with a mesangial or stalk cell at the base surrounded by mesangial matrix material. End = endothelial cell cytoplasm.

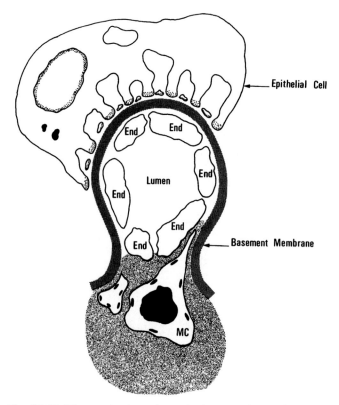

Fig. 44.16 Diagram to show the early changes of pre-eclampsia with endothelial cytoplasmic swelling and early mesangial cell interposition. End = endothelial cell cytoplasm; MC = mesangial cell.

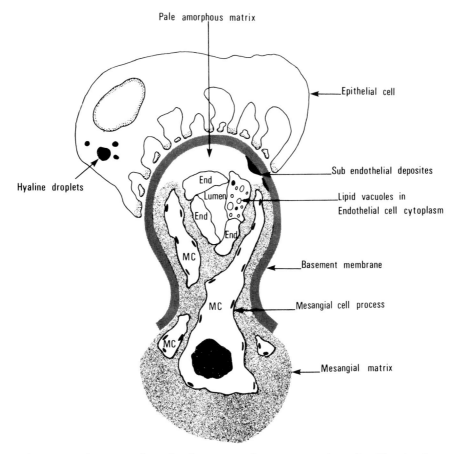

Fig. 44.17 Diagram to show the changes seen in severe pre-eclampsia with extensive mesangial cell interposition leading to reduplication of the glomerular capillary basement membrane. End = endothelial cell cytoplasm; MC = mesangial cell.

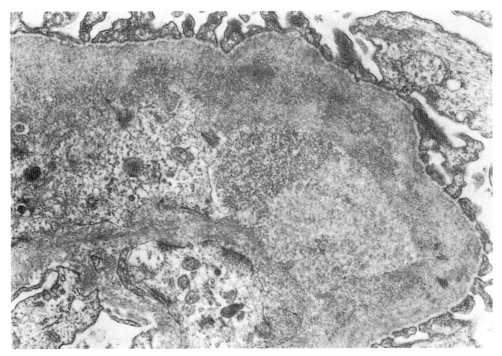

Fig. 44.18 Electronmicrograph showing normal foot processes at top and reduplicated glomerular capillary basement membrane adjacent to the residual capillary lumen (at bottom left) in pre-eclampsia.

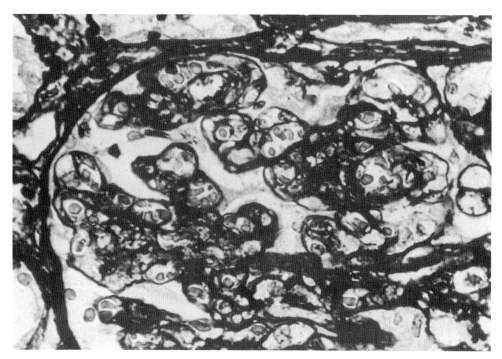

Fig. 44.19 Glomerulus with many capillary loops showing reduplication in pre-eclampsia.

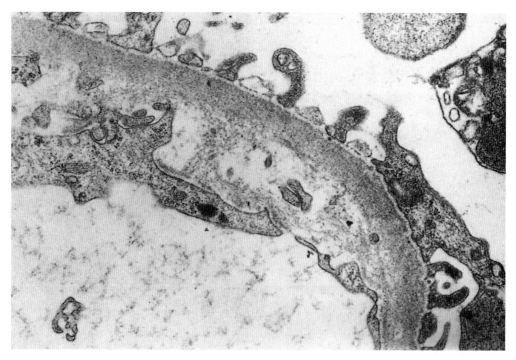

Fig. 44.20 Electronmicrograph with widening and pallor of the subendothelial zone of a glomerular capillary loop in pre-eclampsia.

the impaired glomerular filtration rate seen in pre-eclampsia correlates most accurately with the reduction of endothelial fenestral density and size and to the accumulation of fibrinoid deposits beneath the endothelium.

In up to 50% of cases of pre-eclampsia Seymour et al (1976) found adhesions between the glomerular tuft and the glomerular capsule. These were most likely to be identified at the site of origin of the proximal convoluted tubule from Bowman's capsule. In contrast to the other glomerular abnormalities seen in pre-eclampsia which resolve rapidly after parturition, the tuft adhesions have been shown to persist for many months or years as a

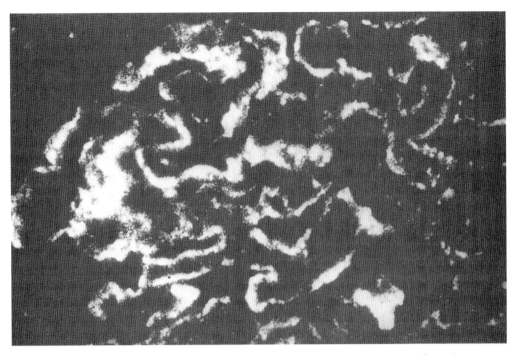

Fig. 44.21 Immunofluorescence photograph of glomerular IgM deposition in pre-eclampsia. (Provided by the late Dr C Tribe.)

permanent record of the episode of 'glomerular capillary endotheliosis' (Heaton & Turner 1985).

A variety of vascular changes have been described in the kidneys of patients with eclampsia (Sheehan 1980), including thickening of the media of arterioles, prominence of the juxtaglomerular apparatus, presence of 'elastic beads' in arterioles and fat in the walls of arterioles. However, none of these features is specific to pre-eclampsia and all may be seen in benign nephrosclerosis associated with hypertension.

The tubules are relatively unaffected by pre-eclampsia, showing only occasional non-specific features such as hyaline droplets and fatty change in occasional tubules. Even in eclampsia the tubular changes are relatively unimpressive being limited to some flattening of the epithelium of proximal tubules. Fully developed ischaemic necrosis of tubules is rare in eclampsia.

RENAL DISEASES COEXISTING WITH PREGNANCY

Some patients will enter pregnancy with pre-existing renal disease which may either be known or unsuspected. Alternatively the patients may acquire some form of renal disease coincidentally during the course of pregnancy. In either case if nephron loss has occurred it is likely to be masked, as far as conventional tests of renal function are concerned, by the considerable functional reserve which the healthy kidney possesses. Indeed, even when 75% of the renal mass has been destroyed the serum creatinine levels may be only slightly elevated.

In normal pregnancy the glomerular filtration rate rises by some 35%. Although few studies have been attempted on patients with renal disease in pregnancy, it would appear that a similar increase occurs in patients with mild to moderate renal impairment. Increases in creatinine clearance and reductions in serum creatinine have been noted in pregnancy by Bear (1976b) and Whalley et al (1975).

Bear (1976a) recommended that moderate or severe degrees of renal functional impairment should generally be regarded as a contraindication to pregnancy. However, a large study by Jones & Hayslett (1996) has shown that fetal survival has improved remarkably in recent years. This is important since 60% of infants born to women with a serum creatinine of >124 μm/litre are premature and these babies are also small for gestational age. The not so good news for the mother is that the risk of renal disease worsening in pregnancy rises sharply with moderate and severe degrees of renal impairment (from any cause) at the start of pregnancy, and this is further aggravated by the presence of hypertension. Hou (1999) has shown that for patients on dialysis the chance of a surviving infant is only 50%. He also showed that renal transplant patients have a risk of loss of renal function similar to controls so long as renal function is well preserved. While fertility is markedly depressed in women on dialysis, return of fertility is the rule in transplant patients although exposure to the risks of transplantation, cytotoxic drugs and infection pose a risk to both mother and child.

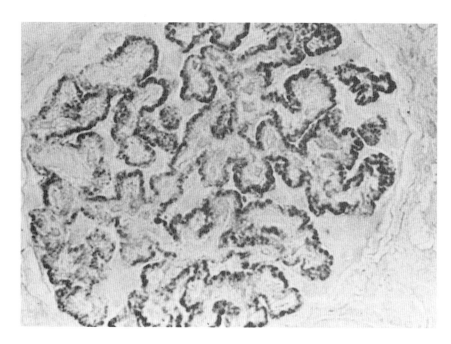

Fig. 44.22 Peripheral granular deposition of IgM in a glomerulus from a patient with membraneous glomerulonephritis. Immunoperoxidase technique.

GLOMERULAR DISEASES WHICH MAY COEXIST WITH PREGNANCY

The most obvious presenting symptom of glomerular disease is proteinuria which, if severe, may be associated with a full nephrotic syndrome (proteinuria in excess of 3.5 g/100 ml, oedema, albuminuria and hypercholesterolaemia). Obviously the difficulty here is to differentiate between pre-eclampsia and other types of glomerular disorder and this may only be possible if a renal biopsy is performed. Hill et al (1988) have shown a high correlation between pre-existing renal pathology and the endotheliosis lesions of pre-eclampsia, suggesting that pre-existing renal pathology increases the chances of developing pre-eclampsia in pregnancy. Ihle et al (1987) have pointed out that early onset 'pre-eclampsia' (before 37 weeks) contains a high proportion (>60%) of patients with renal disease.

Membranous glomerulonephritis

This form of chronic glomerular disease characterised by uniform thickening of glomerular capillary basement membranes is due to the accumulation of immunoglobulins and complement components (Figs 44.22, 44.23). These substances pass from the capillary lumen through the capillary

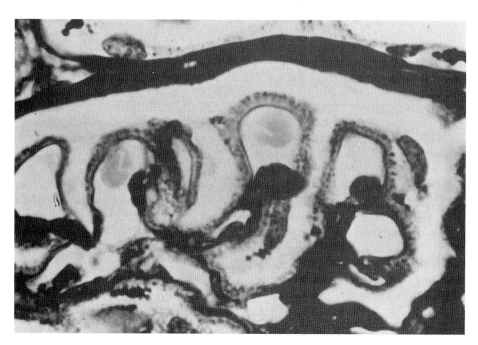

Fig. 44.23 Membranous glomerulonephritis showing thickening of glomerular capillary walls by spiky projections of the basement membrane interposed between immune deposits.

wall and complex with each other to form 'in situ' aggregates of electron-dense material beneath the foot processes of the epithelial cells. In only a few cases can antigens be identified in these electron-dense 'deposits'. The prognosis is difficult to determine in an individual case since 75% progress to chronic renal failure over a period of 5–10 years while 25% remit spontaneously during that time. Although steroids have been suggested as a therapeutic agent, the evidence for their value is insubstantial. In progressive cases the glomeruli become increasingly sclerosed resulting in extensive loss of nephrons.

When patients with membranous nephropathy enter pregnancy with normal renal function the prognosis for a successful outcome is good in some series although proteinuria may be increased during pregnancy (Katz et al 1980). Packham et al (1989a) showed increased fetal loss in their series and in some instances worsening of maternal renal function.

Minimal change glomerulonephropathy

Minimal change glomerulonephropathy may develop during the course of pregnancy and be characterised by heavy proteinuria and glomeruli which appear normal by light microscopy (Fig. 44.24). Electron microscopy demonstrates loss of the foot processes of the epithelial cells. The aetiology of this condition is unknown although it has sometimes been associated with a type 1 hypersensitivity reaction. The likely mechanism is a circulating factor which destroys or obliterates the glomerular polyanionic components thereby allowing polyanionic substances like serum albumin to pass freely into the urinary space.

Treatment with steroids is usually successful in this condition which has no tendency to progress to renal failure. There is, however, a tendency for proteinuria to be increased during pregnancy and for the infants to be small for gestational age (Katz et al 1980).

Primary focal and segmental sclerosis and hyalinosis

It has already been mentioned above that segmental sclerosing lesions may develop as a complication of pre-eclampsia. However, some patients enter pregnancy with what, for want of a better term, is called focal and segmental sclerosis and hyalinosis. Classically, this insidious condition presents with persistent proteinuria which fails to respond to steroid therapy. There may also be microscopic haematuria or even a full nephrotic syndrome. The segmental lesions tend to be progressive, leading eventually to hypertension and chronic renal failure. Packham et al (1988a) have shown that when these patients become pregnant both fetal loss and maternal complications are significantly increased.

Mesangiocapillary glomerulonephritis

Mesangiocapillary glomerulonephritis usually presents in adolescence or early adult life. It is always associated with a nephrotic syndrome and there may be some evidence of haematuria during acute exacerbations. The prognosis is

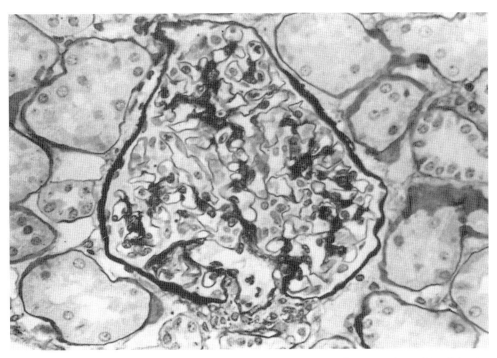

Fig. 44.24 A glomerulus which appears normal by light microscopy from a patient with minimal change disease.

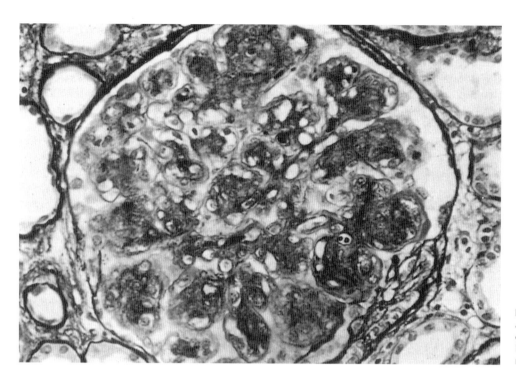

Fig. 44.25 A glomerulus from a patient with mesangiocapillary glomerulonephritis showing a lobular pattern due to marked mesangial cell proliferation.

uniformly poor with universal progression to chronic renal failure over a period of 5–10 years. Light microscopy shows that there are major abnormalities both in the capillary walls and in the mesangial regions of all glomeruli (Fig. 44.25). There is a tendency for the serum C3 levels to be low in this condition and a fraction called C3 nephritic factor may also be identified in the serum. In the most usual type of mesangiocapillary glomerulonephritis (type I) there are large subendothelial and

mesangial deposits of C3 (Fig. 44.26) which seem to stimulate mesangial cell proliferation and subsequent interpositional growth around capillary walls. The capillary lumens become progressively occluded and finally this leads to glomerular sclerosis and nephron loss. There exists a less common type of mesangiocapillary glomerulonephritis called linear-dense deposit disease (type II) in which C3 is deposited within proximal tubular basement membranes, Bowman's capsular basement membranes

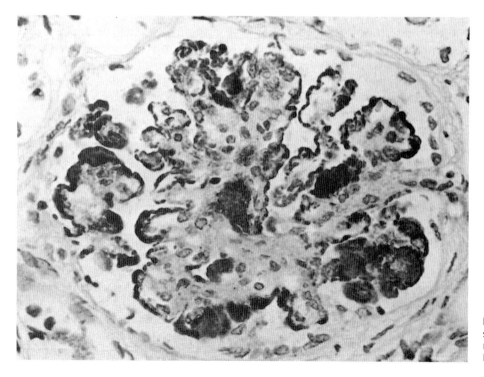

Fig. 44.26 A glomerulus stained to show C3 deposition in a patient with mesangiocapillary glomerulonephritis. Immunoperoxidase technique.

and the glomerular capillary basement membrane. Despite these differences in the morphological aspects the presentation, clinical features and prognosis are very similar to type I mesangiocapillary disease.

Cameron et al (1983) have shown that in patients with type I MCGN, 20 pregnancies resulted in eight live births, five spontaneous miscarriages and seven induced miscarriages. In five patients with type II MCGN there were nine pregnancies which resulted in five live births and four induced miscarriages. Those women who became pregnant and whose pregnancies were allowed to continue were those who still had good renal function and were without hypertension. No deterioration in their renal function was demonstrated during pregnancy. However, if pregnancy had been continued in those patients with hypertension and compromised renal function, it is probable that a decline in renal function would have been seen, as has been described for other forms of glomerulonephritis (Packham et al 1989b).

Lupus nephritis

The term lupus nephritis includes a spectrum of glomerular changes from mild mesangial proliferation through increasing degrees of segmental proliferation and necrosis (Fig. 44.27) to a severe diffuse proliferative glomerulonephritis with extensive cellular crescent formation. In addition a greater or lesser degree of membranous pattern of glomerulonephritis may also be superimposed. In contrast to the types of glomerular disorders previously described, where the degree of glomerular abnormality is fairly uniform in a given case, lupus nephritis is characterised by considerable variation of involvement between the glomeruli, such that some may appear only mildly abnormal with a small amount of mesangial proliferation, whilst their neighbours may show severe necrotising lesions with cellular crescent formation. As a consequence of the variety of immunological reactions which occur in systemic lupus a wide range of immunoglobulins and complement components are deposited within the glomeruli and may be identified using immunocytochemical techniques. They are also demonstrable as electron-dense deposits by electronmicroscopy and may occupy subepithelial, subendothelial or mesangial positions within the glomeruli. Similar but less obvious deposits may also be present along the tubular basement membranes associated with an interstitial nephritis. Although it is possible to suggest a diagnosis of lupus nephritis from the variable glomerular involvement and variety of immune reactants present in deposits at multiple sites the definitive diagnosis depends on satisfying the criteria of the American Rheumatology Society (Cohen et al 1971). Since systemic lupus occurs primarily in women during the child-bearing years, the chances of lupus nephritis coexisting with pregnancy must be considered both in patients with pre-existing disease who wish to have children and in pregnancy when systemic lupus may be first diagnosed.

According to an extensive survey by Hayslett & Lynn (1980) the onset of systemic lupus erythematosus during pregnancy causes significant maternal morbidity and fetal loss in the order of 37%. In contrast, patients with known systemic lupus who have been in clinical remission for six months prior to conception have a favourable prognosis for a normal pregnancy and live birth. When the disease has been active during the six months prior to conception

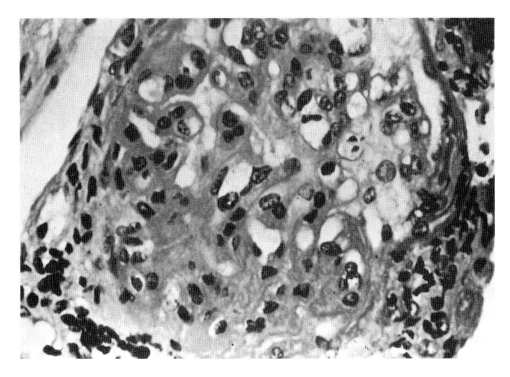

Fig. 44.27 A glomerulus from a patient with lupus nephritis showing cellular proliferation and sclerosis, particularly at the bottom left corner.

the possibility of further exacerbations is likely and the chances of a successful outcome are reduced by about 25%. Overall it appears that steroids are valuable in the suppression of active disease and do not induce developmental abnormalities in the fetus. Buyon (1990) suggests that by monitoring the levels of autoantibodies in the mother the damage to the fetus can be minimised. Bobrie et al (1987) provide a comprehensive review of pregnancy in patients with systemic lupus. Julkunen (1998) makes the point that patients with lupus nephritis need particularly careful management in pregnancy to achieve a successful outcome.

Mesangial IgA disease

This is a relatively benign form of glomerular disease which is common in childhood and usually associated with haematuria precipitated by upper respiratory tract infections. Some cases do not present until early adult life and are then more likely to be associated with proteinuria and the development of hypertension. Light microscopy shows mesangial proliferation within the glomerular tufts associated with mesangial deposits of IgA and C3 (Fig. 44.28). In a few glomeruli there may also be segmental proliferation with or without sclerosis. Kincaid-Smith et al (1980) have shown a very high incidence of segmental lesions in mesangial IgA disease following pregnancy and suggest that at least some of these lesions have been acquired as a consequence of pregnancy. They point out that intravascular coagulation

is a well-recognised feature of pregnancy and acute thrombotic lesions within a glomerular capillary could explain the development of a segmental sclerosis of the tuft. They also showed that hypertension prior to pregnancy was a poor prognostic feature for fetal survival in their series. Packham et al (1988b) showed that maternal renal function declined in pregnancy in 26% of cases of a series of 116 pregnancies associated with IgA disease.

Scleroderma

Fortunately scleroderma with renal involvement is an uncommon association with pregnancy but the few reports which do exist demonstrate a disastrous outcome, with maternal death in most cases. As has already been mentioned, the renal vascular lesions of idiopathic post-partum acute renal failure are very similar to those of renal scleroderma with subintimal fibrosis of an extreme degree in arterial walls and fibrinoid necrosis of arterioles (Figs 44.29, 44.30).

Acute post-infectious glomerulonephritis

The incidence of acute post-infectious glomerulonephritis has fallen to a very low level in recent years and seems to be particularly low in pregnancy, with even some of those cases suspected clinically proving to be acute exacerbations of more chronic forms of glomerulonephritis when renal biopsy is performed (Bear 1976b).

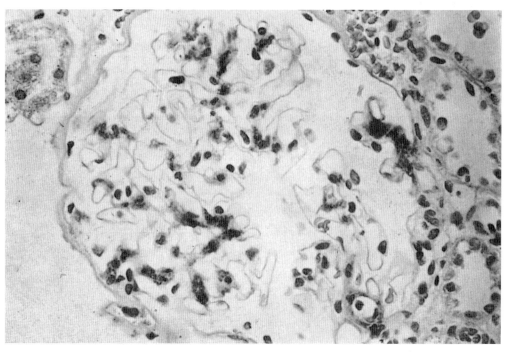

Fig. 44.28 A glomerulus with dark granular staining in the mesangial regions representing IgA deposits. Immunoperoxidase technique.

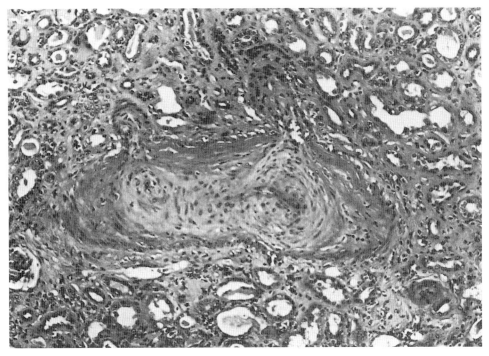

Fig. 44.29 Severe intimal proliferation in the wall of a small renal artery from a patient with scleroderma.

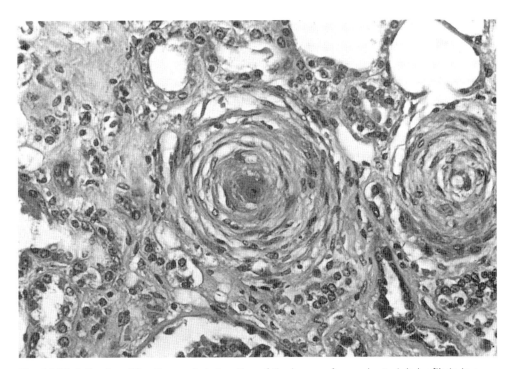

Fig. 44.30 Intimal proliferation and obstruction of the lumen of a renal arteriole by fibrin in a patient with scleroderma.

Diabetic glomerulopathy

Diabetic glomerulopathy is an important complication of juvenile diabetes and the average time for it to occur is 17 years after the onset of the disease. Therefore, some diabetic females will have developed the typical changes of diabetic glomerulopathy by the time they become pregnant. It certainly seems to be true that both pre-eclampsia and leg oedema are more frequent in diabetic women but there are conflicting views as to

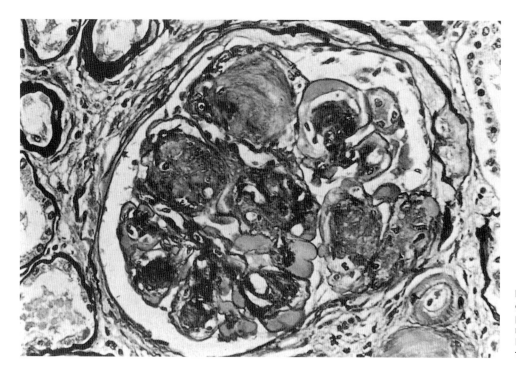

Fig. 44.31 Diabetic glomerulosclerosis with marked proliferation of the mesangial matrix leading to Kimmelstiel–Wilson nodule formation.

whether or not pregnancy has an adverse effect on diabetic glomerulopathy. Certainly, in patients who are only mildly affected, pregnancy appears to be well tolerated (Kitzmiller et al 1981).

In diabetic glomerulopathy there is an excess production of the mucopolysaccharide type of material of which both the glomerular capillary walls and mesangial matrix are formed. The result of this over-production is a uniform thickening of the glomerular basement membranes (so-called diffuse glomerulosclerosis) and an increase in mesangial matrix material (so-called nodular glomerulosclerosis). Usually both patterns coexist and occasional mesangial nodules may assume a considerable size, when they correspond to the description 'Kimmelstiel–Wilson nodules' (Fig. 44.31). Hyaline deposits due to the insudation of plasma proteins are usually particularly prominent in the walls of afferent arterioles in diabetic kidneys and this phenomenon is also seen in hypertensive vascular disease (Fig. 44.32). However, the presence of hyaline

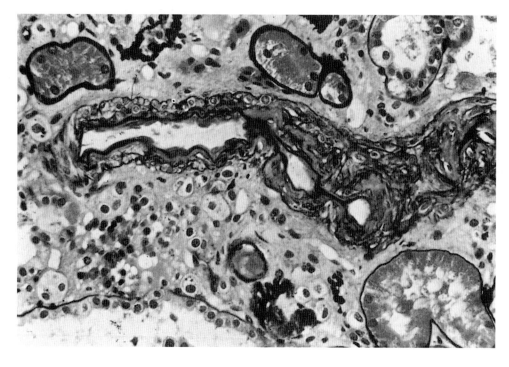

Fig. 44.32 A renal arteriole with irregular thickening of its wall on the right-hand side due to the insudation of hyaline material.

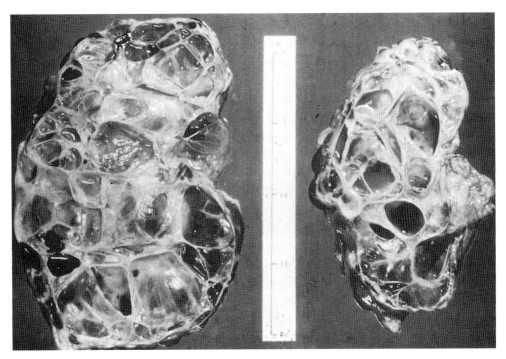

Fig. 44.33 Adult-type renal polycystic disease with extensive replacement of renal parenchyma by cysts of variable size.

deposits in the walls of efferent arterioles is diagnostic of diabetic nephropathy. Degenerative changes may also be seen in larger vessels but these do not differ in character from those which result from hypertensive disease. It is now fortunately rare for a patient with diabetes to present with uncontrolled hyperglycaemia. In such a case extensive vacuolation of the renal tubular epithelial cells due to intracytoplasmic glycogen accumulation is described. Both Purdy et al (1996) and Biesenback et al (1999) have shown that pregnancy in type 1 diabetic patients can cause a deterioration in renal function if it is significantly impaired pre-conceptually.

NON-GLOMERULAR RENAL DISEASES COEXISTING WITH PREGNANCY

Adult polycystic renal disease

Adult polycystic renal disease is almost always bilateral and may be discovered during the course of pregnancy. It is an autosomal dominant condition with massive enlargement of the kidneys by cysts of variable size into which haemorrhage may occur. The normal renal parenchyma is progressively destroyed leading eventually to chronic renal failure (Fig. 44.33). Provided the patient does not have hypertension and has reasonably normal renal function by conventional testing the pregnancy will normally proceed satisfactorily to term (Chapman et al 1994). The presence, however, of two massively enlarged kidneys as well as the enlarged uterus within the abdomen may result in difficulty with respiration.

Pelvic ectopic kidney

The presence of a congenital ectopic kidney within the pelvic cavity may cause difficulty with a normal vaginal delivery and a Caesarean section may therefore be required. It should also be noted that a pelvic ectopic kidney may represent a solitary kidney.

Renal tubular acidosis

This metabolic disorder has been shown to predispose to hypertension in pregnancy (Rowe et al 1999).

Urolithiasis

Urolithiasis is the commonest cause of severe abdominal pain in pregnancy and most of the stones which do occur contain calcium. There does seem to be an increased tendency for urinary tract infection to supervene in such cases (Coe et al 1978).

REFERENCES

Abitbol M M, Gallo G R, Pirani C L et al 1976 Production of experimental toxemia in the pregnant rabbit. American Journal of Obstetrics and Gynecology 124: 460

Bear R 1976a Pregnancy and lupus nephritis. Obstetrics and Gynecology 47: 715–719

Bear R A 1976b Pregnancy in patients with renal disease. Obstetrics and Gynecology 48: 13–18

Biesenbach G, Grafinger P, Stoger H, Zazgornik J 1999 How pregnancy influences renal function in nephropathic type 1 diabetic women depends on their pre-conceptual creatinine clearance. Journal of Nephrology 12: 41–46

Bobrie G, Liote F, Houillier P et al 1987 Pregnancy in lupus nephritis and related disorders. American Journal of Kidney Diseases 9: 339–343

Bonnar J 1976 Coagulation disorders. Journal of Clinical Pathology 29(suppl) 10: 35–41

Brezis M, Rosen S, Silva P, Epstein F H 1984 Renal ischaemia: a new perspective. Kidney International 26: 375–383

Buyon J P 1990 Systemic lupus erythematosus and the maternal-fetal dyad. Baillière's Clinical Rheumatology 4: 85–103

Cameron J S, Turner D R, Heaton J et al 1983 Idiopathic mesangiocapillary glomerulonephritis: comparison of Type I and II in children and adults and long term prognosis. American Journal of Medicine 74: 175–192

Campbell D M, MacGillivary I, Thompson B 1977 Twin zygosity and pre-eclampsia. Lancet ii: 97

Chapman A, Johnson A, Gabow P 1994 Pregnancy outcome and its relationship to progression of renal failure in autosomal dominant polycystic kidney disease. Journal of the American Society of Nephrology 5: 1178–1185

Chesley L C 1980 Hypertension in pregnancy: definition, familial factor and remote prognosis. Kidney International 18: 234–240

Chugh K, Jha V, Sachuja V, Joshu K 1994 Acute renal cortical necrosis — a study of 113 patients. Renal Failure 16: 37–47

Clark B A, Halvorson L, Sachs B, Epstein F H 1992 Plasma endothelin levels in pre-eclampsia, elevation and correlation with uric acid levels and renal impairment. American Journal of Obstetrics and Gynecology 166: 962–968

Coe F C, Parks J H, Lindheimer M D 1978 Nephrolithiasis during pregnancy. New England Journal of Medicine 298: 324–326

Cohen A S, Reynolds W E, Franklin E C 1971 Preliminary criteria for the classification of systemic lupus erythematosus. Bulletin of Rheumatological Diseases 21: 643–648

Cooper D W, Brennecke S P, Wilton A N 1993 Genetics of preeclampsia. Hypertension in Pregnancy 12: 1–23

Donadio J V, Holley K E 1974 Post-partum acute renal failure: recovery after heparin therapy. American Journal of Obstetrics and Gynecology 118: 510–519

Emmanuel D S, Lindheimer M D 1976 Recovery after prolonged anuria following septic abortion. Obstetrics and Gynecology 47: 36s–39s

Eschenbach D A 1976 Urinary tract infections. In: Russell Ramon de Alvarez (ed) The kidney in pregnancy. Wiley, New York, p 75

Fairley K F 1970 The routine determination of the site of infection in the investigation of patients with urinary tract infection. In: Kincaid-Smith P, Fairley K F (eds) Renal infection and renal scarring. Mercedes, Melbourne, p 107

Fan Y D, Pastorek J G, Miller J M Jr, Mulvey 1987 Acute pyelonephritis in pregnancy. American Journal of Perinatology 4: 324–326

Felding C F 1968 Pregnancy following renal diseases. Clinical Obstetrics and Gynecology 11: 579–592

Foidart J M, Nochy D, Nasgens B et al 1983 Accumulation of several basement membrane proteins in glomeruli of patients with pre-eclampsia and other hypertensive syndromes of pregnancy. Possible role of renal prostaglandins. Laboratory Investigation 49: 250–259

Friedman E A 1976 Effect of blood pressure on perinatal mortality. In: Friedman E A (ed) Blood pressure edema and proteinuria in pregnancy. A R Liss, New York

Grünfeld J P, Goneval D, Bournèrais F 1980 Acute renal failure in pregnancy. Kidney International 18: 179

Hart A, Pham T, Nowicki S et al 1996 Gestational pyelonephritis-associated Escherichia coli isolates represent a non-random, closely related population. American Journal of Obstetrics and Gynecology 174: 983–989

Hayslett J P, Lynn R I 1980 Effect of pregnancy in patients with lupus nephropathy. Kidney International 18: 207–220

Heaton J M, Turner D R 1985 Persistent renal damage following pre-eclampsia: a renal biopsy study of 13 patients. Journal of Pathology 147: 121–126

Heptinstall R H 1992 Pathology of the kidney, 4th edn. Little Brown, Boston, p 1289

Hill P A, Zimmerman M, Fairley K F, Kincaid-Smith P, Ryan G B 1988 Pre-eclampsia: a clinico-pathological study of 23 cases. Clinical and Experimental Hypertension, Part B — Hypertension in Pregnancy 7: 343–358

Hollenberg H K, Adams D F, Oken D E et al 1970 Acute renal failure due to nephrotoxins: renal hemodynamic and angiographic studies in man. New England Journal of Medicine 282: 1329–1336

Hou S 1999 Pregnancy in chronic renal insufficiency. American Journal of Kidney Diseases 33: 235–252

Ihle B, Long P and Oats J 1987 Early onset pre-eclampsia recognition of underlying renal disease. British Medical Journal 294: 65

Jones D, Hayslett J 1996 Outcome of Pregnancy in women with moderate or severe renal insufficiency. New England Journal of Medicine 335: 226–323

Julkunen H 1998 Renal lupus in pregnancy. Scandinavian Journal of Rheumatology Supplement 107: 80–83

Jungers P, Houllier P, Chauveau D et al 1996 Pregnancy in women with reflux nephropathy. Kidney International 50: 593–599

Katz A I, Davison J M, Hayslett J P, Singson E, Lindheimer M D 1980 Pregnancy in women with renal disease. Kidney International 18: 192–206

Kincaid-Smith P 1983 Reflux nephropathy. British Medical Journal 286: 2002–2003

Kincaid-Smith P 1991 The renal lesion of pre-eclampsia revisited. American Journal of Kidney Disease 17: 144–148

Kincaid-Smith P, Fairley K F 1987 Renal disease in pregnancy. Three controversial areas: mesangial IgA nephropathy, focal segmental sclerosis and reflux nephropathy. American Journal of Kidney Diseases 9: 328–333

Kincaid-Smith P S, Whitworth J A, Fairley K F 1980 Mesangial IgA nephropathy in pregnancy. Clinical and Experimental Hypertension 2: 821–838

Kitzmiller J L, Brown E R, Phillippe M et al 1981 Diabetic nephropathy and perinatal outcome. American Journal of Obstetrics and Gynecology 141: 741–751

Kleiner G J, Greston W M 1976 Current concepts of defibrination in the pregnant woman. Journal of Reproductive Medicine 17: 309–317

Kleinknecht D, Grünfeld J P, Gomes P C 1973 Diagnostic procedures and long-term prognosis in bilateral renal cortical necrosis. Kidney International 4: 390–400

Kunelis C T, Peters J L, Edmondson H A 1965 Fatty liver of pregnancy and its relationship to tetracycline therapy. American Journal of Medicine 38: 359–377

Lafayette R, Druzin M, Sibley R et al 1998 Nature of glomerular dysfunction in pre-eclampsia. Kidney International 54: 1240–1249

Leading Article 1985 Urinary tract infection during pregnancy. Lancet ii: 190

Lewis P 1982 The role of prostacyclin in pre-eclampsia. British Journal of Hospital Medicine 28: 393–395

Lindheimer M D, Katz A I 1977a Kidney function and disease in pregnancy. Lea & Febiger, Philadelphia, p 114

Lindheimer M D, Katz A I 1977b Kidney function and disease in pregnancy. Lea & Febiger, Philadelphia, p 168

Lindheimer M D, Katz A I 1977c Kidney function and disease in pregnancy. Lea & Febiger, Philadelphia, p 193

MacGillivray I 1981 Raised blood pressure in pregnancy: aetiology of pre-eclampsia. British Journal of Hospital Medicine 26: 110–119

Morrin P A F, Handa S P, Valberg L S 1967 Acute renal failure in association with fatty liver of pregnancy. Recovery after fourteen days of complete anuria. American Journal of Medicine 42: 844–851

Norden C W, Tuttle E P 1965 Impairment of urinary concentrating ability in pregnant women with asymptomatic bacteriuria. In: Kass E H (ed) Progress in pyelonephritis. Davis, Philadelphia, p 73

Packham D K, Fairley K F 1987 Renal biopsy indications and complications in pregnancy. British Journal of Obstetrics and Gynaecology 94: 935–939

Packham D K, North R A, Fairley K F, Hale B U, Whitworth J A, Kincaid-Smith P 1988a Pregnancy in women with primary focal and segmental hyalinosis and sclerosis. Clinical Nephrology 29: 185–192

Packham D K, North R A, Fairley K F, Whitworth J A, Kincaid-Smith P 1988b IgA glomerulonephritis in pregnancy. Clinical Nephrology 30: 15–21

Packham D K, North R A, Fairley K F, Whitworth J A, Kincaid-Smith P 1989a Membranous glomerulonephritis and pregnancy. Clinical Nephrology 28: 56–64

Packham D K, North R, Fairley et al 1989b Primary glomerulonephritis and pregnancy. Quarterly Journal of Medicine 71: 537–553

Purdy L, Hantsch C, Molitch M et al 1996 Effect of pregnancy on renal function in patients with moderate to severe diabetic renal insufficiency. Diabetes Care 19: 1067–1074

Ransley P G, Risdon R A 1978 Reflux and renal scarring. British Journal of Radiology 51 (suppl 14): 1–35

Reeves D S, Brumfitt W 1968 Localisation of urinary tract infection. In: O'Grady F, Brumfitt W (eds) Urinary tract infection. Oxford University Press, London, p 53

Robson J A, Martin A M, Ruckley V et al 1968 Irreversible postpartum renal failure: a new syndrome. Quarterly Journal of Medicine 37: 423–455

Rowe T, Magee K, Cunningham F 1999 Pregnancy and renal tubular acidosis. 16: 189–191

Roy First M, Ooi B S, Jao V, Pollak V E 1978 Pre-eclampsia with the nephrotic syndrome. Kidney International 13: 166–177

Scheer R L, Jones D B 1967 Malignant nephrosclerosis in women postpartum. Journal of the American Medical Association 201: 600–604

Seymour E Q, Petrucco O M, Clarkson A R et al 1976 Morphological and immunological evidence of coagulopathy in renal complications of pregnancy. In: Lindheimer M D, Katz A I, Zuspan F P (eds) Hypertension in pregnancy. Wiley, New York, p 139

Sheehan H L 1980 Renal morphology in pre-eclampsia. Kidney International 18: 241–252

Sheehan H L, Moore H C 1952 Renal cortical necrosis and the kidney of concealed accidental haemorrhage. Blackwell, Oxford

Sibai B, Kustermann L, Velaser J 1994 Current understanding of severe pre-eclampsia, pregnancy associated haemolytic uraemic syndrome, thrombotic thrombocytopaenic purpura, haemolysis, elevated liver enzymes and low platelet sydrome and post partum acute renal failure: different syndromes or just different names? Current Opinion in Nephrology & Hypertension 3: 436–445

Sims E A H, Krantz K E 1958 Serial studies of renal function during pregnancy and the puerperium in normal women. Journal of Clinical Investigation 37: 1764–1774

Slater D N, Hague W M 1984 Renal morphological changes in idiopathic acute fatty liver of pregnancy. Histopathology 8: 567–581

Spargo B, McCartney C P, Winemiller R 1959 Glomerular capillary endotheliosis in toxemia of pregnancy. Archives of Pathology 68: 593–599

Stratta P, Besso L, Canavese C, Segoloni G P 1996 Is pregnancy related acute renal failure a disappearing entity? Renal Failure 18: 575–584

Sulavik S B 1975 Pulmonary disease. In: Burrow G B, Ferris T F (eds) Medical complications during pregnancy. Saunders, Philadelphia, p 549

Thomas V, Shelkov A, Forland M 1974 Antibody-coated bacteria in urine and site of urinary tract infection. New England Journal of Medicine 290: 588–590

Tobon H 1972 Malignant hypertension, uremia and hemolytic anemia in a patient on oral contraceptives. Obstetrics and Gynecology 40: 681–685

Tribe C R, Smart G E, Davies D R, Mackenzie J C 1979 A renal biopsy study in toxaemia of pregnancy. Journal of Clinical Pathology 32: 681–692

Turney J H, Marshall D H, Brownjohn A M, Ellis C M, Parsons F M 1990 The evolution of acute renal failure 1956–1988. Quarterly Journal of Medicine 74: 83–104

van Beek E, Ekhart T, Schiffers et al 1998 Persistent abnormalities in plasma volume and renal haemodynamics in patients with a history of pre-eclampsia. American Journal of Obstetrics and Gynecology 179: 690–696

Wagoner R D, Holley K E, Johson W J 1968 Accelerated nephrosclerosis and post-partum acute renal failure in normotensive patients. Annals of Internal Medicine 69: 237–248

Whalley P 1967 Bacteriuria of pregnancy. American Journal of Obstetrics and Gynecology 97: 723–738

Whalley P J, Cunningham F G, Martin F G 1975 Transient renal dysfunction associated with acute pyelonephritis of pregnancy. Obstetrics and Gynecology 46: 174–177

45

Pathology of the nervous system in pregnancy

H. Reid

Introduction 1523

Chorea gravidarum 1524

Vascular disorders 1524
Encephalopathy of pre-eclampsia and eclampsia of
  pregnancy 1524
Cerebral venous thrombosis 1525
Benign intracranial hypertension 1527
Arterial obstruction 1527
Intracerebral haemorrhage 1528
Vascular malformations 1529

Migraine 1530

Wernicke's encephalopathy 1531

Central pontine myelinolysis 1531

Trauma 1532

Infections 1532

Acquired immunodeficiency syndrome (AIDS) 1532

Epilepsy 1533

Multiple sclerosis 1534

Neoplasms 1535

Pituitary 1535

Cranial and peripheral nerve lesions 1536

Myasthenia gravis 1536

Muscles 1536

INTRODUCTION

There are few, if any, diseases of the nervous system that are uniquely related to pregnancy, but there are a number that seem to be initiated or brought to light at this time, and others, previously known to be present, where management of the disease may have to be varied during the duration of pregnancy. In cases of maternal death it is important to examine the brain (Dawson 1988). If the case history is suggestive of any disease of the spinal cord, peripheral nerves or muscle these should also be examined, the spinal cord should be removed and appropriate samples of peripheral nerve and muscle taken.

By far the most common disease of the central nervous system (CNS) is the abnormality of mood which a majority of women suffer as postpartum depression and which is perhaps due to a relative inhibition of prolactin release. It is often associated with a delay in lactation and may be cured by small doses of chlorpromazine which stimulate prolactin release. Ten per cent of women need much more prolonged treatment, having perhaps an underlying depressive diathesis.

Pregnancy certainly precipitates a puerperal psychosis in one out of every 250 women but almost all have a previous history of delusional states and in many the condition recurs outside pregnancy. Its incidence is probably much the same now as when reported by Bates (1848) early in the 19th century. Both steroid and polypeptide hormone systems have important regulatory actions on neurone function in the brain. The needs of pregnancy require, of course, quite a different action by these substances on other tissues of the body and often the hormones are present in unusually large amounts. Minor changes in permeability of the blood–brain barrier, which appear to be quite common in pregnancy, will allow leakage into the brain of uncontrolled quantities of these hormonal modulators of neurone transmission. It is, therefore, not surprising that mental disorder may appear at this time.

CHOREA GRAVIDARUM

A disease which is now rare in this country, but which may still remain a problem in countries where rheumatic fever is common, is chorea gravidarum. This condition is essentially a recrudescence of the Sydenham's chorea associated with active rheumatic disease and is also found in women who have damaged basal ganglia as a result of hypoxic encephalopathy and in women with the antiphospholipid syndrome (Cervera et al 1997).

Chorea presents as an acute or subacute development of involuntary jerking movements of the face and extremities associated with hypotonia of the limbs and hyperreflexia. Most initial episodes occur during first pregnancies (80%), with up to a fifth of the women experiencing recurrences in subsequent pregnancies (Schipper 1988). Symptoms become less after 1–2 months of onset and rarely persist beyond the puerperium.

Chorea has also been reported as appearing in some women two or three months after starting hormonal contraceptive pills, this appearing to be independent of the type and dose of oral contraceptive ingested (Schipper 1988), although the oestrogen component may be important in the development of the movement disorder (Barber et al 1976).

Oestrogen may induce chorea in susceptible persons by enhancing dopaminergic neurotransmitters in the striatum (van Hartesveldt & Joyce 1986): dopamine agonists exacerbate pre-existing chorea and induce involuntary movements in asymptomatic non-pregnant patients with a history of rheumatic fever. Therefore, when chorea does develop during pregnancy, it is not necessary to assume that pregnancy has provoked an exacerbation of rheumatic disease: it has simply revealed an underlying weakness of basal ganglia function. As it is a self-limiting condition usually no therapy is required.

VASCULAR DISORDERS

The dangers of the encephalopathy associated with pre-eclampsia and eclampsia are well known: these and intracranial haemorrhage (Dorfman 1990; Simolke et al 1991) remain as important causes of maternal death (Department of Health 1998).

However, there are other vascular lesions which have been reported in pregnancy and although each condition individually accounts for a few cases only, taken together this is an important group as these other vascular lesions do cause a certain amount of morbidity and mortality.

The other vascular lesions that occur in, or are associated with, pregnancy are thromboembolism, atherosclerosis, migraine, coagulopathy, vasculitis and cerebral vasospasm (Weibers 1985; Geraghty et al 1991; Simolke et al 1991). Pregnancy has been said to increase the risk of stroke by about 3–13 times. In a study from Glasgow (Jennett & Cross 1967) of 65 female subjects aged 15–45 years with ischaemic stroke, 35% were pregnant or puerperal at the time of the stroke: an increase of 3–4 times the prevalence rate in non-pregnant women. In a more recent study (Leys et al 1997) the incidence of ischaemic stroke was the same in pregnancy and puerperium as in non-pregnant women of child bearing age, being 3.8 to 5 in 100 000 pregnancies. With the more widespread use of improved neuroradiological techniques other cerebro-vascular entities are being diagnosed; a rare one leading to haemorrhagic stroke is postpartum cerebral angiopathy (Ursell et al 1998). The clinical presentation includes headaches, focal neurological deficits and seizures which occur shortly after delivery. Angiography shows multiple narrowing of the intracranial cerebral arteries. The neurological signs are reversible although they can be worsened by giving toxic therapies for vasculitis and sympathomimetic agents.

ENCEPHALOPATHY OF PRE-ECLAMPSIA AND ECLAMPSIA OF PREGNANCY

Pre-eclampsia is characterised by a rapidly rising blood pressure, proteinuria and, in severe cases, generalised oedema; eclampsia is diagnosed when epileptiform fits supervene. Fully developed eclampsia is rare, but it is still one of the commonest causes of death related to pregnancy in the British Isles (Department of Health 1998) and one of the major causes of death related to pregnancy in the Western world. Eclampsia is an acute process and can be treated if the high blood pressure is lowered, in which case it is known as reversible posterior leukoencephalopathy syndrome (Mabie 1999).

Eclampsia occurs in around 1 per 2000 deliveries (Douglas & Redman 1992). As well as the mortality rate associated with pre-eclampsia and eclampsia there can also be severe morbidity due to cerebral haemorrhages, cortical blindness, renal failure, disseminated intravascular coagulation, pulmonary oedema and psychosis. Another syndrome may be associated with pre-eclampsia and eclampsia; that is the haemolysis, elevated liver enzymes and low platelet syndrome (HELLP) (Zunker et al 1995).

Although pre-eclampsia/eclampsia is a condition specifically linked with pregnancy (Kenny & Baker 1999), it shows much the same pathological changes in the brain as are to be found with the similar neurological picture that may accompany any rapidly developing or episodic hypertension, for example, with an amine-secreting phaeochromocytoma or a phase of primary or secondary malignant hypertension (Benedetti & Quilligan 1980; Zunker et al 1995; Hinchey et al 1996).

Pathologically the CNS changes occurring in eclampsia have been well described. Sheehan & Lynch (1973) found five major groups of cerebrovascular phenomena in eclampsia; these were:

1. petechial haemorrhages in patches in the cerebral cortex

2. multiple small areas of ischaemic softening, scattered throughout the brain, usually non-haemorrhagic
3. small areas of haemorrhage in subcortical white matter, usually localised to the upper part of the hemispheres
4. a single large haemorrhage in the white matter
5. haemorrhage in the basal ganglia or pons, often with rupture into the ventricles.

Not all of these lesions are present in every case that comes to post-mortem; for instance, intracerebral haemorrhage has been found only in 10–60% of fatal cases (Beck & Menezes 1981).

In a further small study only one out of seven cases had a large haemorrhage within the brain (Richards et al 1988). These workers reported a neuropathological study of seven patients who died, five with eclampsia and two with pre-eclampsia. They found that hypoxic-ischaemic damage and fibrinoid necrosis of the walls of small vessels were the most important neuropathological lesions. However, as oedema was not demonstrated histologically or on CT scan in pre-eclampsia they thought it unlikely that oedema formation was responsible for the prodromal signs and symptoms of eclampsia. They also thought it unlikely that oedema triggers the occurrence of seizures. The authors suggested that both the vasculopathy and hypoxic-ischaemic damage are involved in the pathogenesis of the oedema formation, which is present radiologically in eclampsia (Digre et al 1993). The vasculopathy is acute vessel wall damage with plasmatic vasculosis and fibrinoid necrosis. In only one case were there fibrin thrombi occluding damaged vessels. Three of the cases had perivascular microhaemorrhages similar to those shown in Fig. 45.1.

These lesions are also seen in hypertensive encephalopathy of different aetiology in which there is a breakdown of the blood–brain barrier, which can be due to a focal impairment of cerebral autoregulation (Manfredi et al 1997). The blood–brain barrier is constituted by the endothelial cells of cerebral capillaries, which have different characteristics to most endothelial cells elsewhere in the body. They have tight junctions between them and there are few pinocytotic vesicles within the endothelial cytoplasm and little if any pinocytotic transport through their cytoplasm. They are cells with a very high metabolic activity as indicated by the presence of an unusually large number of mitochondria in their cytoplasm; these are probably important in a number of processes whereby the endothelial cells control solute fluxes across the capillary wall (Miller & Ironside 1997). These features of the endothelial cells function as the blood–brain barrier. In an animal model of acute hypertension there are cerebral endothelial plasma membrane alterations which may lead to increased cerebrovascular permeability to proteins (Nag 1986). The basement membrane outside these endothelial cells has an important filtering function and beyond this again there is a

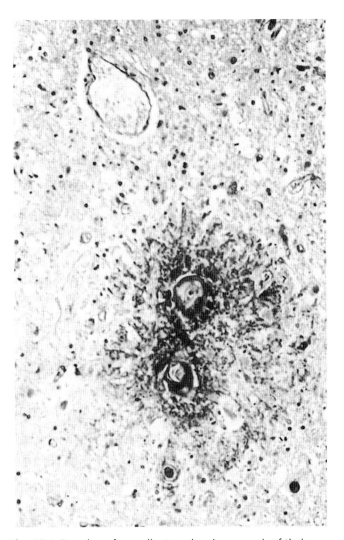

Fig. 45.1 Branches of a small artery showing necrosis of their walls and escape of fibrin into surrounding brain.

sheath of cytoplasmic foot processes of astrocytes which have a further selective function in the two-way tissue transport system; the brain is almost unique in having no lymphatic drainage and any resulting accumulation of extracellular solutes and fluid may be disturbing to the nutrition and function of nerve cells.

CEREBRAL VENOUS THROMBOSIS

It is difficult to ascertain the true incidence of this condition as it occurs in the puerperium 1–4 weeks after childbirth and only occasional cases have been reported during pregnancy (Cantu & Barinagarrementeria 1993). Srinivasan (1988) found that cerebral venous thrombosis had a frequency of 4–5 per 100 obstetric admissions in his centre in India, which suggests a much greater frequency than in Western countries where the incidence is 10 to 20 per 100 000 deliveries.

In Western countries, where antibiotics are more readily available, it is now unusual for there to be a septic cause of cerebral venous thrombosis. A major factor is more likely to be a hypercoagulable state from various abnormalities of the blood, such as an increase in platelets, factors VII and IX, and fibrinogen or decreased fibrinolysis predisposed to by dehydration, anaemia, cyanotic heart disease, polycythaemia vera, leukaemia or sickle cell disease. Other rarer causes are remote effects of carcinoma, Behçet's and Cogan's syndromes, cryofibrinogenaemias or the oral contraceptive pill (Srinivasan 1988).

In puerperal venous thrombosis there are reports of increased plasma fibrinogen with high erythrocyte sedimentation rate, decreased fibrinolytic activity, increased platelet adhesive index and increased levels of beta-lipoproteins and triglycerides with normal cholesterol values (Srinivasan 1984). Congenital disorders known to cause thrombophilia include deficiencies of antithrombin III, protein C, protein S and certain types of dysfibrinogenaemia as well as homocystenuria (Schutta et al 1991). Schutta and colleagues have also suggested that a deficiency of plasminogen might predispose to thrombosis by slowing the rate of fibrinolysis; this has been found in some patients with thrombosis. Another condition which has been associated with deep venous thrombosis and, in some cases cerebral venous thrombosis, is the primary antiphospholipid syndrome associated with an antiphospholipid antibody of IgG type 2 and 4 (Harris 1992). This syndrome is also associated with repeated fetal loss. These patients seem to have a systemic autoimmune disorder that overlaps with systemic lupus erythematosus (SLE). Some patients do have SLE but others only have the antiphospholipid antibodies and the venous thrombi (Asherson et al 1989; Brey et al 1990; Brey & Coull 1992) associated sometimes with cerebral ischaemic damage (Montalban et al 1991).

The anatomy of the superior sagittal sinus may also have a rôle to play in the formation of thrombi within it; the lumen has an inverted triangular shape and the arachnoid granulations project into the upper lateral angles and the cortical cerebral veins drain into its inferior angle. The lumen also contains fibrous trabeculae which favour thrombosis. If the upper half of the superior sagittal sinus is blocked, preventing the cerebrospinal fluid clearing function of the granulations, intracranial pressure increases without focal deficits, a condition known as pseudotumour cerebri. If the draining veins are blocked as well, focal seizures and neurological defects occur.

In venous stasis collateral drainage opens up and if the thrombosis is slight and slow in forming there is less damage as the venous blood is drained through the collateral branches.

The condition often presents clinically with headaches and, only in severe cases, with an epileptic fit which is soon followed by drowsiness, vomiting and hemiplegia (Chopra & Banerjee 1989; Donaldson & Lee 1994). The weakness and sensory disturbances can be unilateral or bilateral and involve the legs rather selectively. Confusion and psychotic symptoms may predominate and therefore puerperal psychosis needs to be excluded as do co-existing peripheral thrombosis, meningitis, postpartum eclampsia and space-occupying lesions. The radiological investigation of choice is magnetic resonance imaging (MRI) but if this is not available a CT scan should be followed by angiographic studies. CSF examination is rarely of diagnostic use and in many cases of venous sinus thrombosis, there is oedema of the brain. Obtaining CSF by lumbar puncture, therefore, is inadvisable for it may cause the death of the patient through brain movement and cerebellar coning.

It is the superior sagittal sinus and its draining veins which are commonly involved in the puerperium. However, occasional cases of thrombosis of the vein of Galen and its tributaries and associated straight sinus have been reported (Banerjee et al 1979). Bitemporal lobe infarction with occlusion of the veins of Labbe and the lateral sinuses is rare (Chopra & Banerjee 1989).

Pathology of superior sagittal sinus thrombosis

The brain is swollen and there is usually thrombosis of the cerebral veins as well as the superior sagittal sinus. In the latter the thrombus present in the sinus is usually older than that in the draining cerebral veins. There may be some degree of lateral brain shift and tentorial herniation or even cerebellar coning if the oedema is extensive. The cerebral veins that are thrombosed can be unilaterally or bilaterally involved, but more often they are involved unilaterally (Gettlefinger & Kokman 1977). There is discoloration of the cerebral gyri adjacent to the veins which are thrombosed; the brain surface is mottled and grey. Subarachnoid haemorrhage can be seen, within which are the cord-like rigid thrombosed veins. In these cases, on sectioning the brain, there is haemorrhagic infarction in the areas drained by the thrombosed veins (Fig. 45.2). As the patients die shortly after the onset of symptoms the infarcts are recent. Often the haemorrhagic infarcts have a central haematoma with softening of the surrounding brain with punctate haemorrhages. In those without a central haematoma there is softening of the brain with punctate haemorrhages.

Microscopically, in the early stages oedema is only seen with perineuronal and perioligodendrocytic haloes in the grey and white matter, respectively; degeneration of the neurones in the affected area is also seen. In the slightly older lesions there is haemorrhagic necrosis. Thrombosis is present in veins of all sizes and there are multiple satellite foci of ring or ball haemorrhages. Some of the venous walls show necrosis and there is polymorphonuclear leucocyte diapedesis. The affected neurones are shrunken and deeply staining (eosinophilic on H & E staining). Polymorphonuclear leucocytes and macrophages are present in small numbers; however if there are many polymorphonuclear leucocytes a septic cause should be suspected. Reactive astrocytes and haemosiderin

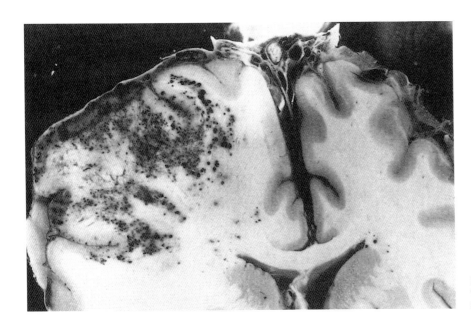

Fig. 45.2 Haemorrhagic infarction of one frontal lobe with thrombosis of surface veins and superior longitudinal sinus.

deposition are not usually evident. If there is a longer survival before the patient succumbs, the brain shows cavitation, focal cortical atrophy and organised thrombi.

Pathology of thrombosis in other venous sinuses

In the less common thrombosis of the straight sinus and vein of Galen there are bilateral haemorrhagic infarcts of the thalami, basal ganglia and corpus callosum (Banerjee et al 1979) or bilateral ischaemic necrosis with subcortical oedema (Milandre et al 1990).

Microscopically the older thrombi are in the smaller branches of the terminal veins with newer thrombus formation in the great vein of Galen and torcular. There is diapedesis of polymorphonuclear leucocytes, necrosis of parenchyma and confluent haemorrhages around the thrombosed vessels.

Outcome of venous thrombosis

In one study the mortality rate was 9% (Cantu & Barinagarrementeria 1993). The outlook is usually good in the survivors, many recovering without significant neurological deficit (Weibers 1985; Preter et al 1996). The prognosis is better than that in arterial stroke (Chopra & Banerjee 1989). However, the mortality rate in cases where there is deep cerebral venous sinus thrombosis, rather than in the superficial sagittal sinus, is worse — nine fatalities out of 15 cases in one series (Milandre et al 1990).

BENIGN INTRACRANIAL HYPERTENSION

Minor non-fatal venous and sinus obstructions may be the basis for the condition known as benign intracranial

hypertension or pseudotumour cerebri, which sometimes presents in pregnancy but also occurs in women of fertile age at other times of raised oestrogen levels (Caroscio & Pellmar 1979). The clinical presentation is one of raised intracranial pressure, without focal neurological signs, which usually subsides at the end of the pregnancy. Papilloedema, although transient, may cause a permanent loss of central vision. Occasionally the patient may show little clinical evidence of raised pressure but may have enlarged ventricles on CT scan and suffer a moderate degree of dementia. The condition is treatable by surgical procedures to provide alternative CSF drainage.

This condition is not, of course, confined to pregnancy and is seen as a sequel to head injury and to middle ear infections with related thrombosis of the lateral sinus and may be referred to as otitic hydrocephalus. Two mechanisms seem to be at work in pregnancy — the one already described above being a reduction of CSF absorption into partially occluded and thickened venous sinuses, the other being swelling of the brain due to hormonally related fluid imbalance (Powell 1972; Sussman et al 1998).

ARTERIAL OBSTRUCTION

It was thought in the past that cerebrovascular accidents due to arterial causes were more common among pregnant women, especially during the second or third trimester, than in non-pregnant women of similar age. This is probably not so today; Weibers & Whisnant (1985) could only find one case of cerebral infarction in 26 099 live births during 1955–1979 in Rochester, USA.

Although specific arterial diseases such as giant cell arteritis and Moyamoya arteritis have been described as a cause, they are rare (Karasawa et al 1980). Fibromuscular dysplasia has also been described (Ezra et al 1989).

Rheumatic heart disease with atrial and valvular lesions remains in some parts of the world as a fairly common source of emboli. Such emboli often lodge in quite peripheral cerebral arteries producing small strokes and often only minor residual disability. It must be remembered that the cerebral arterial tree has enormous anastomotic potential, both extracranially and on the brain surface. Thus, if an occlusion is confined to the common or internal carotid artery, there is often no neurological disability in this age group because of the good state of other collateral vessels. However, if the thrombus arises in or extends to the middle cerebral artery, thus losing the benefit of the cross-circulation from the circle of Willis, then hemiplegia, and sometimes death, is the outcome.

In these cases the infarct is usually found in the parietal and temporal lobes in the area supplied by the middle cerebral artery. It is usually an area of softening, with surrounding oedema; brain shift may also be present. The infarct shows varying degrees of liquefactive necrosis depending on how long the patient survived after the vessel was occluded. The infarct is usually pale and rarely haemorrhagic.

INTRACEREBRAL HAEMORRHAGE

The normal pathological mechanisms for the production of cerebrovascular disorders are not common in women of fertile age. Major intracerebral haemorrhage associated with essential hypertension is rare in this age group. Other factors associated with non-traumatic intracerebral bleeding in pregnancy are haematological disorders such as disseminated intravascular coagulation, often in association with placental abruption, leukaemia, thrombocytopenia, or carcinoma (Barno & Freeman 1976). Anticoagulant therapy (Hirsh et al 1972) is an obvious problem; however, illicit drugs can cause intracerebral haemorrhages (Sloan 1993).

Rupture of berry aneurysms and haemorrhage from vascular malformations, although not common, are important because they can be accurately diagnosed and treated (Weibers 1988).

Berry aneurysm of the circle of Willis

Subarachnoid haemorrhage from rupture of an aneurysm of the circle of Willis is an unduly frequent event during the gestational period and occurs in about one in 3000 pregnancies, 4% actually occurring during labour. Robinson et al (1972) thought they ruptured mainly after 26 weeks of gestation; however Dias & Sekhar (1990) thought they ruptured throughout gestation but that there was an increased incidence of rupture with advancing gestational age, but not during labour (Mas & Lamy 1998). There seems to be some special hormonal relationship here for there is an increase in the incidence of

rupture of other aneurysms during gestation (see Chapter 47). It may be relevant that, of the vascular deaths reported in a large British survey of women taking hormonal contraceptive pills, one of the significant increases was in subarachnoid haemorrhage from a cerebral aneurysm (Beral & Kay 1977). Similar findings were reported from the Framingham study (Sacco et al 1984).

Although these aneurysms, occurring at the junctional points of the circle of Willis (Fig. 45.3), are often referred to as congenital aneurysms, only a few are ever found in childhood; indeed the commonest age for presentation is 50–60 years. Seventy per cent of normal people have the congenital defect in the vessel wall at the branching of the vessels of the circle which has long been considered to be the basis for the disease. It seems, therefore, that other factors must be of major importance in those cases that produce an aneurysm which ruptures and, indeed, there is a type III collagen defect in at least some of these patients (Pope et al 1980). An innate difficulty with the healing of minor faults in the connective tissue of blood vessels together with the hormonally related changes in general collagenous tissues must combine in pregnancy to predispose to the rupture of aneurysms.

Dias & Sekhar (1990), in their review of 154 women in pregnancy and the puerperium who had intracranial

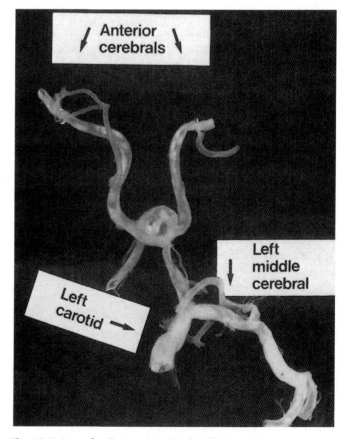

Fig. 45.3 Part of a dissected circle of Willis showing an aneurysmal sac arising at the junction of the left anterior cerebral and anterior communicating arteries.

haemorrhage from aneurysms and arteriovenous malformations, found 77% due to aneurysms and 23% due to arteriovenous malformations. The average maternal age for ruptured aneurysms was 29.4 years, slightly older than that for arteriovenous malformations (26.7 years). Of all the aneurysms causing the first intracerebral haemorrhage, 23% were diagnosed in the nulliparous group and the mean parity was two.

The sites of the aneurysms are similar to those reported in the non-gravid population: internal carotid artery (37%), posterior communicating artery (23%), anterior communicating/anterior cerebral artery (23%), middle cerebral artery (23%) and vertebrobasilar system (10%).

Pathology

In those dying suddenly from ruptured aneurysms there is marked subarachnoid haemorrhage, particularly over the area of the aneurysm, and there may be no other neuropathological findings. The aneurysm should be looked for at the time of the post-mortem, by dissecting off the haematoma in the subarachnoid space and identifying the aneurysm on the circle of Willis. Also the presence of other aneurysms should be excluded; in 17% of all aneurysmal cases more than one aneurysm is present. If an aneurysm is not found the vessels may be injected with water to see if there is a perforation where an aneurysm has been, and this is best done at the time of post-mortem examination. The aneurysms are usually 1 cm or less in diameter; occasionally aneurysms as large as 2 cm are found.

In those women with a longer survival after onset of symptoms there can be large intracerebral and intraventricular haemorrhages with evidence of brain shift. In other cases there may be evidence of brain shift and subarachnoid haemorrhage but with no further haemorrhage in other sites; the problem then may be due to arterial spasm leading to infarction of the brain with surrounding oedema. Oxyhaemoglobin is probably the principal pathological agent in causing vasospasm (Macdonald & Weir 1991).

In the Dias & Sekhar (1990) series the overall maternal mortality was 35% for aneurysms; these authors advocated surgical management of aneurysms in the pregnant woman which, they suggested, would also benefit the fetus. They pointed out, however, that the physiological changes of pregnancy need to be taken into account in the neurosurgical management of the patient, necessitating obstetrical and neonatological advice along with close monitoring.

VASCULAR MALFORMATIONS

These include arteriovenous malformations in which there are increased vessels per unit area with arterialised veins and thick-walled arteries and vascular hamartomas or angiomas. Not all arteriovenous malformations are associated with haemorrhages, some present with epilepsy and may never lead to intracerebral haemorrhage. Out of the various series of intracerebral haemorrhage in pregnant women 21–48% of cases are due to arteriovenous malformations (Dias & Sekhar 1990). Most arteriovenous malformations are present in the parietal region with fewer found in the occipital lobes followed by the frontal and temporal lobes (Dias & Sekhar 1990). Haemorrhage from an arteriovenous malformation tends to occur at a younger age than that due to a ruptured berry aneurysm. The haemorrhage can be subarachnoid, intracerebral or intraventricular. More commonly it is intracerebral with overlying subarachnoid haemorrhage; on careful examination of the brain enlarged surface veins may be seen. The abnormal vessels of the arteriovenous malformation can be obvious in the larger malformations (Fig. 45.4); smaller ones may only be seen on histological examination.

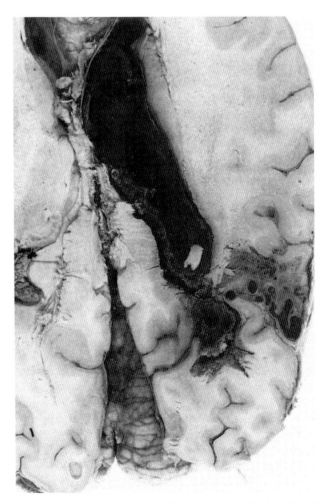

Fig. 45.4 Arteriovenous shunt malformation (so-called angioma) extending from the arachnoid surface of the occipital lobe to the wall of the ventricle. A large blood clot occupies the lateral ventricle.

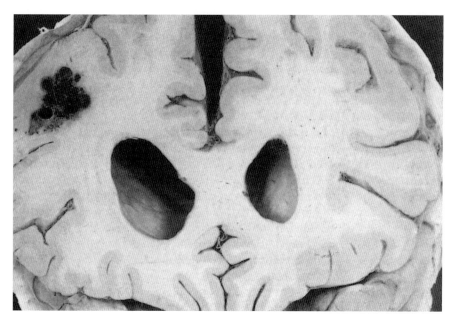

Fig. 45.5 Thin-walled venous angioma beneath cerebral cortex having no major arterial connection. There is some atrophy of white matter with dilatation of the lateral ventricle.

Haemorrhage from arteriovenous malformations in pregnancy may carry a higher risk than in the non-gravid population and may not benefit from surgical treatment (Dias & Sekhar 1990). In another survey (Horton et al 1990) of a group of 451 women who received proton beam therapy for their arteriovenous malformation there were 540 pregnancies resulting in 438 live births and 102 miscarriages, with 17 pregnancies complicated by a cerebral haemorrhage. They did not find that pregnancy significantly increased the rate of first cerebral haemorrhage from an arteriovenous malformation. Haemorrhage from an arteriovenous malformation occurs during gestation and not usually in the puerperium.

The other lesions which are a known cause of migrainous or epileptic attacks are capillary or venous angiomas (Fig. 45.5) but they have a low blood flow and never bleed significantly, though they can be associated with epilepsy (Awada et al 1997).

The argument is put forward by some that certain of the circulating steroids in pregnancy tend to cause relaxation of smooth muscle; certainly elastic tissues are more extendable. This may be the explanation for the first appearance, commonly in pregnancy, of an arteriovenous lesion of the spinal cord, loosely called an angioma, but resembling more a venous varix (Arseni & Simionescu 1959) (Fig. 45.6). This condition, once established with circulatory stasis and ischaemia, may persist after pregnancy as a varying degree of dysfunction of the lower spinal cord segments.

MIGRAINE

For most women who suffer from migraine, pregnancy brings temporary relief (Aube 1999); in a few it appears

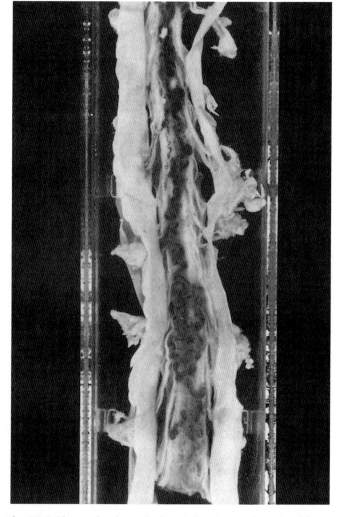

Fig. 45.6 Thoracolumbar spinal cord showing a subarachnoid venous varix.

for the first time and for about one in five it worsens. Hemiplegic migraine has been reported in pregnancy (Mandel 1988). It is thought to be due to an abnormal response of vessels, in that they dilate to 5-hydroxytryptamine (Pearce 1991). However, there are cases where the headache appears to be related to known aneurysms or arteriovenous malformations of the brain and where the attacks are more frequent and severe at certain points in the menstrual cycle. One would expect such a minority of cases to worsen during pregnancy even if subarachnoid haemorrhage does not occur. Obviously ergotamine therapy is contraindicated at this time.

WERNICKE'S ENCEPHALOPATHY

Women who develop hyperemesis gravidarum must be considered to be in danger of acute deficiency of B vitamins, especially thiamine. If this is not provided by, say, 50 mg intramuscularly at intervals, then there is a great danger of the abrupt onset of Wernicke's encephalopathy. This disease is not, of course, peculiar to pregnancy for it occurs in other cases of persistent vomiting such as pyloric stenosis or alcoholism. In Wernicke's encephalopathy transketolase activity is low; this is a thiamine-dependent enzyme in the pentose phosphate pathway. The most reliable test for thiamine deficiency is the thiamine pyrophosphate effect, where there is an increase in activity of transketolase when thiamine pyrophosphate is added to a preparation of the patient's red cells (Bergin & Harvey 1992). There is evidence that those patients who develop Wernicke's encephalopathy have a form of transketolase that binds thiamine less avidly than that of controls (Blass & Gibson 1977). Several other cases of Wernicke's

encephalopathy associated with hyperemesis gravidarum have been reported more recently (Guardian et al 1999).

The lesions are most obvious in the corpora mamillaria and adjacent parts of the wall of the third ventricle, the floor of the fourth ventricle and the midbrain. There appears to be a local breakdown of the adhesion between capillary and arteriolar endothelial cells and a loss of the blood–brain barrier to an extent where seepage of plasma and even small haemorrhages occur; there is also loss of neurones (Fig. 45.7).

Wernicke's encephalopathy clinically is recognised as nystagmus on upper gaze and gait ataxia; however the clinical signs related to damage to brain stem nuclei with, for example, extraocular palsies, may also be apparent. Damage to mamillary bodies will lead to confusion and, if treatment is not given early and urgently, a persistent loss of recent memory leading to Korsakoff's psychosis occurs. Other evidence of B vitamin deficiency may be seen with the hyperaesthesia and calf tenderness of polyneuropathy or the dyspnoea, palpitations and cardiac failure of beri beri.

CENTRAL PONTINE MYELINOLYSIS

Another rare complication of hyperemesis gravidarum is central pontine myelinolysis (Castillo et al 1989). This seems to follow a rapid correction of severe hyponatraemia. Bergin & Harvey (1992) reported a case of hyperemesis gravidarum where there was both central pontine myelinolysis and Wernicke's encephalopathy. Pathologically, there is extensive demyelination in the pons and other areas of white matter; there is no inflammatory cell infiltrate and little gliosis. The condition can lead to coma and death.

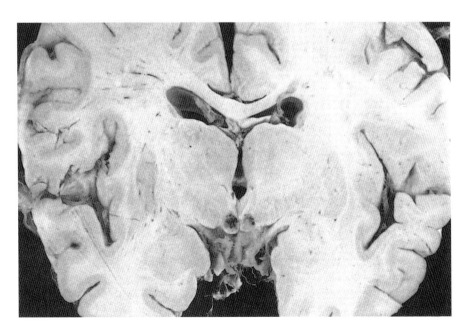

Fig. 45.7 Coronal slice through the brain at the level of the mamillary bodies. These show the characteristic focal petechial haemorrhagic lesions of Wernicke's encephalopathy.

TRAUMA

The commonest cause of death in young adults is trauma, and this can, unfortunately, happen to pregnant women; abdominal injuries are more likely than severe head injuries (Shah et al 1998) but the head may be injured alone or with other parts of the body. Head injuries in pregnant women are no different from head injuries generally; they can be minor, moderate or severe and the outcome depends upon their severity. In injuries from falls, the head hitting a hard surface, fractured skulls can occur and the development of an intracranial haematoma; with a fracture of the temporal bone the middle meningeal artery is torn and blood accumulates between the skull and the dura, an extradural haematoma, compressing the underlying cerebrum leading to ischaemic brain damage and brain shift. Loss of consciousness may not occur immediately after the fall but only after several hours, known as the lucid interval. Blunt head injuries from road traffic accidents can produce scalp lacerations, fractured skulls, acute subdural haematomas, traumatic subarachnoid haemorrhage, cerebral contusions and diffuse axonal injury. The latter is due to rotational shear damage to axons and is the underlying cause of coma and neurological damage; in this process axons are torn and, after 24 hours survival, axon bulb formation is seen microscopically. It is associated with petechial haemorrhages in an asymmetrical pattern in the corpus callosum and dorso-lateral areas of the upper brain stem. The brain in fatal cases can show evidence of oedema and brain shift; also in a substantial number of cases there is hypoxic/anoxic brain damage due to a hypoxic/anoxic episode at the time of the injury or shortly afterwards before adequate ventilation was commenced. This hypoxia/anoxia worsens the prognosis as it exacerbates the brain damage caused by the injury.

In one study the fetal outcome related mainly to direct fetal injury and to maternal haemodynamic insult (Drost et al 1990); four fetuses were lost and one neonate died because of the injuries received. There was only one maternal death in this series out of 318 cases.

INFECTIONS

Infections of the central nervous system do not seem as important in Western countries as in the developing world where tuberculosis is common and tuberculous meningitis still occurs in pregnancy. Bacterial leptomeningitis could occur but there are no factors in pregnancy to increase its incidence in Western countries.

A bacterial infection, listeriosis, is associated with repeated miscarriages and is a rare cause of infection of the CNS in the mother. *Listeria monocytogenes* is a Gram-positive rod and infection is often transmitted to adults by contaminated food, e.g. coleslaw, unpasteurised milk, raw milk and products made from unpasterurised milk, poultry, shellfish and processed meats. It is transmitted to the fetus by blood-borne spread or passage through the birth canal. Low rates of carriage are present in the general population; however, the relationship between carriage and the disease is not clear (Lamont & Postlethwaite 1986; Wenger & Broome 1991). When it has occurred in adults a variety of lesions have been found in the CNS; mortality may be up to 30% (Nieman & Lorber 1980). There may be meningitis, cerebritis or, more rarely, abscess formation; very occasionally there can be miliary granulomas in the meninges, but this is more common in infants. Listeria may produce suppuration of the brain substance in the absence of meningeal involvement.

At post-mortem in adults with listerial meningitis the brain shows thickened meninges which contain both polymorphs and macrophages in varying numbers. There have also been reports of infection localised to the brain stem (Kennard et al 1979). Multiple small abscesses in the pons and medulla have been reported (Howard et al 1981) and in such cases the brain stem is swollen and softened. The abscesses in the brain stem contain polymorphs and Gram-positive bacilli, found intra- and extracellularly. Fibrinoid material in concentric layers in small vessels with perivascular cuffing has also been described.

ACQUIRED IMMUNODEFICIENCY SYNDROME (AIDS)

There is an increasing incidence of positivity to human immunodeficiency virus (HIV) and this can be present in pregnancy, with infected infants being born. Brains from such cases should be handled as set out in the recommendations (Advisory Committee for Dangerous Pathogens 1990) for full precautions against infection by dangerous pathogens. The virus infects cells that carry CD4 antigen on their surface part of which acts as a receptor for entry of HIV into these cells. T lymphocytes of CD4 type (helper T cells) have the greatest CD4 surface antigen and therefore are easily infected by HIV; the virus can also infect B lymphocytes, monocytes and macrophages. The pathology of HIV infection can be divided into pre-AIDS and AIDS (acquired immunodeficiency syndrome). In pre-AIDS there is a latent period of relative well-being, which is of variable length, a few months to years, during which episodes of self-limiting Guillain–Barré-like acute or relapsing demyelinating peripheral neuropathy, mononeuritis multiplex or cranial neuropathies occur. In pre-AIDS, particularly in those who are drug misusers, there is a low-grade meningoencephalitis with increased numbers of mononuclear cells in the pia arachnoid and underlying brain tissue.

In the terminal stages of clinical AIDS there is progressive disease of the CNS in which, clinically, there is a varying combination of apathy, progressive behavioural or mental deterioration, ataxia, tremor and other involuntary movements (Price et al 1988). The mental deterioration is similar to that seen in subcortical dementia. The pathological changes of encephalopathy, in the absence of opportunistic infections or lymphoma, are of a relatively normal brain macroscopically but variable microscopic changes; these may be widespread but require adequate sampling of the brain. The changes can be non-specific and are found in the central white matter and the deep grey matter with the cerebral cortex being relatively spared (Gray et al 1988). These non-specific findings are diffuse or focal macrophage and microglial cell infiltration and reactive astrocytosis, which can be seen in cerebral and cerebellar white matter. The microglial cell infiltrates may be found in well-defined nodules in the grey or white matter. Perivascular cuffing by a few lymphocytes may be present as well. Prominent vacuolation of white matter is found in some cases, and most show pallor of the myelin. In some, but not all, cases, 25–69% in different reported series, there are multinucleated giant cells in the perivascular spaces, particularly in the cerebral white matter, basal ganglia and thalamus. These giant cells are thought to be derived from blood-derived monocytes and usually have 2–10 nuclei: HIV can be isolated from them (Esiri & Kennedy 1997).

In those cases with focal neurological symptoms there can also be opportunistic infection or even lymphoma in the brain. The commonest opportunistic infections are cytomegalovirus, cryptococcosis and toxoplasmosis. Other viral infections reported in AIDS brains are the JC virus which causes progressive multifocal leucoencephalopathy, Herpes simplex and varicella-zoster.

The lymphoma can be primary or systemic and occasional cases of metastatic Kaposi's sarcoma have been reported. Subarachnoid and intracerebral haemorrhage have also been reported as a result of thrombocytopenia, which is due to an autoimmune mechanism in AIDS. Cerebral infarction also occurs.

EPILEPSY

True, non-eclamptic, epilepsy is a fairly common disease with a prevalence of about one in 200 of the general population: the annual incidence in the third and fourth decades, the fertile years, is about one in 2000. As epilepsy is not uncommon, some women who already have epilepsy will become pregnant and some will have their onset of epilepsy during pregnancy. General information regarding the course of epilepsy during pregnancy and the type of epilepsy give no clear pointers on which to base predictions for the course of epileptic attacks during a single pregnancy (Gjerde et al 1988; Holmes 1988). There is no definite evidence that pregnancy worsens epilepsy. Bardy (1987) reported a series of cases where there was an increased frequency of seizures in 32% of

cases, a decrease in 14% and no change in 23%, with 31% being seizure free during 24 months. Knight & Rhind (1975) reported that 5% of women are improved in that they have fewer attacks during pregnancy. Rarely has there been reported a true gestational epilepsy recurring only in successive pregnancies (Teare 1980).

This variable picture is what might be expected when the many and various possible causes of such seizures are considered. There does not appear to be any prognostic help to be derived from the patient's age or previous history of precipitating factors.

The increases reported are mostly in the first trimester and are thought to be due in part to fluid retention, some women showing a considerable weight gain before the increase in the number of fits, and in part to poor drug control (Dimsdale 1959). For various reasons, including an increase of hydroxylating enzyme activity in the liver and vomiting, the dose of phenytoin required to control a known tendency to epilepsy needs to be increased during pregnancy and reduced in the puerperium (Swainman 1980; Leppik & Rask 1988). Factors such as maternal sleep deprivation, stress and inadequate anticonvulsant levels could be of greater importance than hormonal epileptogenesis.

Unfortunately, the maternal and fetal demand for folate increases at the same time as a larger dose of phenytoin is reducing (as a side effect) the absorption rate of folic acid from the gut (Dahlke & Mertens-Roesler 1967). Furthermore, increase of microsomal enzyme activity in liver cells may cause a more rapid folate metabolism and thus exaggerate a relative absorption deficiency (Bayliss et al 1971). It is, perhaps, this effect on folate that makes the problem of drug teratogenicity of great importance in the control of epilepsy during pregnancy. There is quite a lot of evidence that in cases where the mother is treated with anti-epileptic drugs there is an especially large increase in the occurrence of cleft palate and in congenital heart disease (in both conditions about 3 times the expected number) (Olafson et al 1998). These defects are probably multifactorial though some may be due to low blood folate levels (Dansky et al 1987). It is, however, quite clear that epileptic fits themselves will damage the fetus through the associated severe anoxia. The balance of risk in each case probably depends on the likely frequency of attacks. What is known is that if the pregnancies are carefully monitored throughout there is a good outcome for mother and fetus in most cases (Patterson 1989; Yerby 1996). Pregnancy can be a time when epilepsy first occurs and is not related to eclampsia; in these instances the gravid patient requires a complete examination to exclude an identifiable and treatable cause for the epilepsy. A patient with an astrocytoma had her first fits towards the end of pregnancy at the age of 31 years. Her attacks were of three types: (a) grand mal; (b) momentary unconsciousness with running eyes and nose; (c) ataxia with falling to the ground but no loss of consciousness. She continued to have these attacks for 18 years until her death because of a large astrocytoma in one temporal lobe and the basal ganglia. The tumour had shown very little other evidence of its presence by way of noticeable neurological deficits until a few months before death (Fig. 45.8).

Fatalities due to epilepsy in pregnancy are rare. The brain in patients dying acutely in status epilepticus may show oedema and brain shift but little else. In some cases there is no microscopic change but in others hippocampal sclerosis is seen, where the pyramidal neurones in Sommer's sector are lost with replacement gliosis and shrinkage of the hippocampus. This can be unilateral or bilateral. Neuronal loss may be seen in the cortex and Purkinje cell loss from the cerebellum. The brain should also be examined for the presence of neoplasms and evidence of old trauma with thinning of the cortical ribbon in areas of old contusions, particularly in the inferior aspects of the frontal and temporal lobes; these can also show yellow discoloration from the breakdown products of haemosiderin.

MULTIPLE SCLEROSIS

Multiple sclerosis is the most common disabling neurological disease of young people in the West, with a prevalence of up to one in 2000, varying greatly in different parts of the world with a gradual increase towards higher latitudes. Many women of fertile age will wish to be advised on whether the course of their disease will be affected by pregnancy. Statistically there is about two and a half times as great a relapse rate for such women but most relapses appear in the three months after delivery

(Birk et al 1988; Confavreux et al 1998). In one series (Birk et al 1988) only 10% had worsening of their symptoms during pregnancy: these authors also concluded that multiple sclerosis had no adverse effect on pregnancy, labour or delivery.

In pregnant women with multiple sclerosis there are protective soluble factors that cause the disease to be less active in pregnancy and this may be the underlying reason for the reduction in the onset of multiple sclerosis in pregnancy (Birk et al 1988): these protective factors are pregnancy-associated plasma protein and alpha-2-pregnancy-associated glycoprotein; fetal alpha-fetoprotein may also play some part in reducing the number of relapses of multiple sclerosis in pregnancy.

The pathology of multiple sclerosis varies depending on the length of time it has been present. In the established case the classic plaques of multiple sclerosis are seen throughout the CNS. Many are sited periventricularly around the lateral ventricles and are visible as well-defined grey lesions; sometimes they are seen at the surface of the pons and within the optic nerves. Microscopically, there is loss of myelin and oligodendrocytes with gliosis; axons are reduced in number, subsequent to the loss of the myelin sheaths around the axons. At the margins of the plaque there is not such a sharp line between myelinated and non-myelinated axons and in some lesions increased numbers of oligodendrocytes and lymphocytes are found here as well. When there is disease activity, macrophages and reactive astrocytes may also be found at the edges of plaques.

In the earlier stages of multiple sclerosis the lesions are pink or yellow, soft and associated more with sites around small veins. Microscopically, there is marked hypercellularity with macrophages and reactive astrocytes; myelin

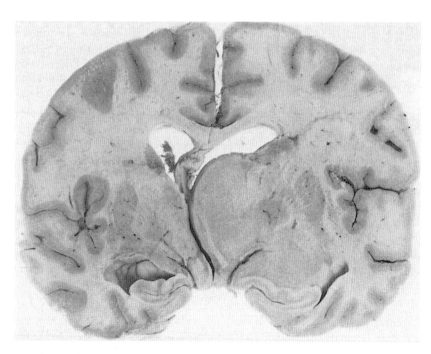

Fig. 45.8 Diffuse glioma infiltrating and expanding the basal ganglia and part of the temporal lobe on one side.

sheaths in these hypercellular areas show disintegration. Axons and nerve cells are preserved.

The aetiology is unknown, but is thought to be related to a hypersensitivity reaction to viral-damaged brain tissue after unidentified viruses have penetrated the blood–brain barrier. The macrophage infiltration in the earlier stages is thought to be important and there is damage to the myelin first with subsequent death of its associated oligodendrocyte. As some oligodendrocytes are known to proliferate at the edges of plaques remyelination does occur.

It is easier to correlate the plaques in the optic nerves and tracts as well as those in the brain stem and spinal cord to the clinical symptoms but much more difficult to correlate those in the rest of the cerebrum. Nerve conduction is slowed in demyelinated axons running through plaques, but such nerve processes, clothed only by astrocytes, may be very vulnerable to the disorders of the blood–brain barrier that have already been discussed. It may, therefore, be that clinical relapses in pregnancy are not necessarily evidence of the development of new lesions.

NEOPLASMS

Another situation in which it is difficult to assess the part that pregnancy plays in initiating or worsening the prognosis is intracranial neoplasia (Isla et al 1997; Tewari et al 2000). The commonest primary brain tumour in adults is the astrocytoma; this is a group of neoplasms arising from the astrocytic cells in the CNS which in the World Health Organization classification of brain tumors (Kleihues & Cavenee 2000) includes: pilocytic astrocytomas (commoner in children) WHO grade 1, fibrillary astrocytoma grade 2, anaplastic astrocytoma grade 3 and glioblastoma grade 4. In women, during the fertile period, the commonest primary brain tumours occur in the cerebral hemispheres and are usually the fibrillary astrocytomas; oligodendrogliomas can also occur but are infrequent. Glioblastoma is rarer in this age group — the peak incidence is 55–60 years and on average the survival after histological diagnosis is 9 months whereas fibrillary astrocytomas have on average a 48-month survival. Also fibrillary astrocytomas invariably undergo a rapid growth phase later on, as demonstrated in the previous case history. The potential doubling time for glioblastoma is around 11–12 days (Hoshino et al 1979) but as it is much slower in fibrillary astrocytomas these tumours when presenting in pregnancy have probably been present before conception; this is not necessarily so in the more rapidly growing glioblastoma. As well as the primary brain tumours, tumours arising from the meninges, meningiomas, the cranial nerves, usually the vestibular portion of the eighth cranial nerve, and the anterior pituitary gland can occur in the fertile years.

As it is such a dramatic event when occurring in pregnancy there have been many case reports describing intracranial neoplasms diagnosed in pregnancy, suggesting that pregnancy is associated with the growth of intracranial neoplasms. However, in one epidemiological study in Germany (Haas et al 1986) there were reduced numbers of primary brain tumours and meningiomas in observed to expected ratios that were statistically significant. Others agree that there is no higher incidence of primary brain tumours in pregnancy (Roelvink et al 1987; Simon 1988). Haas and co-workers (1986) did find an increase, though not statistically significant, in the number of intracranial schwannomas in their series.

It is known and well recognised that intracranial meningiomas and schwannomas can show accelerated growth during pregnancy (Michelsen & New 1968). The growth of meningiomas may be related to the presence of progesterone receptors on the tumour cells (Tilzer et al 1982); however more recently oestrogen receptors have also been found (Carroll et al 1999).

Haas and co-workers (1986) thought that the reduced incidence of astrocytomas in pregnancy could be due to the fact that women developing such a tumour may, because of disturbed hypothalamic function, have less chance of pregnancy due to reduced fertility, disturbances of ovulation, conception and implantation: these authors also suggested that even when pregnancy did start, abnormal embryonic development with early loss would affect their epidemiological figures.

Choriocarcinomas related to pregnancy have a high propensity for brain metastases, but this occurs in the postpartum period (Gurwitt et al 1975; Ishizuka et al 1983). In such cases intracranial metastases may result in death and they may need surgical extirpation as well as chemotherapy and radiotherapy. Primary intracranial choriocarcinoma has also been recorded in women; by 1982, 61 such cases had been reported (Furukawa et al 1986).

PITUITARY

As well as the brain suffering from ischaemia during pregnancy there can also be ischaemia of the pituitary gland, particularly after postpartum haemorrhage, and this can lead to Sheehan's syndrome (Sheehan & Davis 1982) with panhypopituitarism. With the ischaemia there is necrosis of the anterior pituitary gland which shrinks to produce an empty sella on radiological examination. In the empty sella syndrome the diaphragma sella is depressed and the suprasellar space is enlarged. Usually a rim of pituitary tissue is found in the fossa. There has also been a report of spontaneous resolution of Cushing's syndrome after pregnancy as a fortuitous result of pituitary necrosis (Aron et al 1990). Lymphocytic adenohypophysitis may present with a pituitary mass and mimic a pituitary adenoma (Saiwai et al 1998).

CRANIAL AND PERIPHERAL NERVE LESIONS

The changes in tissue fluid content which characterise pregnancy have their effect also on the peripheral nervous system, which includes the cranial as well as the peripheral nerves. This is apparent in patients who have type I neurofibromatosis. This autosomal dominantly inherited condition with variable penetrance shows the abnormal gene on chromosome 17q12 (Seizinger et al 1987). Neurofibromas are tumours but it is still not widely accepted that they are true neoplasms. They are oedematous and collagenous lesions of nerve sheath with increased numbers of axons and dystrophy of Schwann cells.

Further gelatinous enlargement by the accumulation of extracellular fluid makes the abnormal dermal nerve plexuses in neurofibromatosis more obvious in pregnancy but these subside later and there is no evidence of any permanent change (Swapp & Main 1973).

Various entrapment neuropathies are reported to occur more commonly in pregnancy (Massey & Cefalo 1979). Bell's palsy is thought to be due to a swollen facial nerve negotiating the long bony facial canal and occurs over three times more often than expected (about 45/100 000 births), mostly in the last few weeks of pregnancy (Hilsinger et al 1975).

Meralgia paraesthetica is due to bruising of the lateral cutaneous nerve of the thigh as it passes through the deep fascia. The carpal tunnel syndrome with tingling, numbness and pain in the median nerve distribution of hand and fingers may be a problem in as many as 20% of pregnant women (Gould & Wissinger 1978) in that it often disturbs sleep and provokes the unwise use of analgesic and hypnotic drugs. There are many women whose first attack of sciatica occurs in pregnancy, often during labour, when ligamentous laxity allows rupture of the intervertebral disc.

As well as the above single entrapment neuropathies there are cases of autoimmune neuropathy (acute inflammatory demyelinating polyneuropathy or Guillain–Barré syndrome), which does not appear to be altered in its frequency or severity in pregnancy (McCombe et al 1987). It causes a rapid onset of weakness and areflexia with few sensory symptoms. Cerebrospinal fluid shows an increase in protein with no increase in cells. About 60% of cases follow acute and infectious illness. The nerves show myelin stripping by macrophages and considerable perivascular lymphocytic cuffing in the epineurium. It is treated by supportive measures: however, as respiratory failure and cardiac arrhythmias occur, all patients need adequate and careful monitoring. Most get better; only occasionally is plasmapheresis required as it is thought to be caused by a humoral factor (Harrison et al 1984).

There is a chronic inflammatory demyelinating polyradiculoneuropathy which is known to occur during pregnancy, and the relapse rate is significantly increased in parous women; the relapses tend to occur during the third trimester and postpartum (McCombe et al 1987). It can recur in following pregnancies (Jones & Berry 1981). In this condition there is paraesthesia, weakness, hyporeflexia or areflexia and sensory impairment. The pathological changes in the nerves are similar to those seen in Guillain–Barré syndrome, without, however, such a high degree of inflammatory cell infiltrate in the nerves.

Trigeminal neuropathy can occur, although only occasionally, in pregnancy (Massey 1988). However, isolated mental nerve neuropathy even during pregnancy should always cause serious concern because of the association of numb chin with malignancy (Massey et al 1981).

MYASTHENIA GRAVIS

Myasthenia gravis is a disease which most commonly presents in women of child-bearing age and the strains of pregnancy may produce the first evidence of the condition. There is no reason to believe that the incidence of this disease is any higher in pregnancy, but it appears to be the case that deterioration may occur in about 45% of cases, particularly during the postpartum period. Conversely, around a third of patients undergo a remission of their symptoms during pregnancy (Batocchi et al 1999). A weakness and easy fatiguability of proximal muscles and difficulty with respiration are obvious disadvantages during labour which should, therefore, be shortened by a low forceps delivery (Scott 1976). Approximately 4% of pregnant women with myasthenia gravis die, usually as a result of entering either a myasthenic, or, less commonly, a cholinergic crisis (Plauche 1979).

The pathological basis of this disease lies not in the nervous system but in the acetylcholine receptor protein on the surface of muscle fibres with which motor axons relate. These receptors are damaged or rendered ineffective because of the production of autoantibodies to this protein. This abnormal antibody production may be reduced following removal of the enlarged thymus or thymoma which is found in 70% of sufferers.

Apart from the obstetrical management of these patients a significant problem exists for the 12–20% of children born to such women who show transient neonatal myasthenia gravis (Plauche 1979) due to the transplacental passage of anti-acetylcholine receptor antibodies.

MUSCLES

Polymyositis is an autoimmune disease which may have a subacute or chronic course of muscle weakness, predominantly proximal and usually symmetrical. In the florid forms there can be tenderness and pain of the affected muscles with swelling. The serum creatine kinase is raised and muscle biopsy shows mononuclear (lymphocytic) infiltration of muscle fibres with degeneration and regeneration, but these areas can be patchy and therefore not present in the muscle tissue sampled.

In pregnancy, polymyositis does occur, but it is rare and should be treated cautiously with steroids (Parry & Heiman-Patterson 1988).

REFERENCES

Advisory Committee for Dangerous Pathogens 1990 HIV: the causative agent of AIDS and related conditions. 2nd revised guidelines. Department of Health, London

Aron D C, Schnall A M, Sheeler L R 1990 Spontaneous resolution of Cushing's syndrome after pregnancy. American Journal of Obstetrics and Gynecology 162: 472–474

Arseni C, Simionescu M D 1959 Vertebral haemangiomata. Acta Psychiatrica et Neurologica Scandinavica 34: 1

Asherson R A, Khamastha M A, Ordi-Ros J et al 1989 The 'primary' antiphospholipid syndrome: major clinical and serological features. Medicine 68: 366–374

Aube M 1999 Migraine in pregnancy. Neurology 53 (4 Supplement 1): S26–S28

Awada A, Watson T, Obeid T 1997 Cavernous angioma presenting as pregnancy related seizures. Epilepsia 38: 844–846

Banerjee A K, Gulati D R, Chhuttani P N 1979 Primary internal cerebral vein thrombosis in a young adult. Neurology India 27: 135–139

Barber P, Arnold A, Evans G 1976 Recurrent hormone-dependent chorea: effects of estrogens and progesterone. Clinical Endocrinology 5: 23–29

Bardy A H 1987 Incidence of seizures during pregnancy, labor and puerperium in epileptic women: a prospective study. Acta Neurologica Scandinavica 75: 356–360

Barno A, Freeman D W 1976 Maternal deaths due to spontaneous subarachnoid hemorrhage. American Journal of Obstetrics and Gynecology 125: 384–392

Bates J 1848 Remarks on the statistics, pathology and treatment of puerperal insanity. London Medical Gazette 42: 990–992

Batocchi A P, Majolini L, Evoli A, Lino M M, Minisci C, Tonali P 1999 Course and treatment of myasthenia gravis during pregnancy. Neurology 52: 447–452

Bayliss E M, Crowley J M, Preece J M 1971 Influence of folic acid on blood phenytoin levels. Lancet i: 62–63

Beck D W, Menezes A H 1981 Intracerebral hemorrhage in a patient with eclampsia. Journal of the American Medical Association 246: 1442–1443

Benedetti T J, Quilligan E J 1980 Cerebral edema in severe pregnancy induced hypertension. American Journal of Obstetrics and Gynecology 137: 860–862

Beral V, Kay C R 1977 Mortality among oral contraceptive users. Lancet ii: 727–731

Bergin P S, Harvey P 1992 Wernicke's encephalopathy and central pontine myelinolysis associated with hyperemesis gravidarum. British Medical Journal 305: 517–518

Birk K, Smeltzer S C, Rudick R 1988 Pregnancy and multiple sclerosis. Seminars in Neurology 8: 205–213

Blass J, Gibson G 1977 Abnormality of a thiamine-requiring enzyme in patients with Wernicke-Korshoff syndrome. New England Journal of Medicine 297: 1367–1370

Brey R L, Coull B M 1992 Antiphospholipid antibodies: origin, specificity and mechanisms of action. Stroke 23 (suppl 1): 115–118

Brey R L, Hart R G, Sherman C G, Tegeler C H 1990 Antiphospholipid antibodies and cerebral ischaemia in young people. Neurology 40: 1190–1196

Cantu C, Barinagarrementeria F 1993 Cerebral venous thrombosis associated with pregnancy and puerperium. Review of 67 cases. Stroke 24: 1880–1884

Caroscio J T, Pellmar M 1978 Pseudotumor cerebri: occurrence during the third trimester of pregnancy. Mount Sinai Journal of Medicine (New York) 45: 539–541

Carroll R S, Zhang J, Black P M 1999 Expression of estrogen receptors alpha and beta in human meningiomas. Journal of Neurooncology 42: 109–116

Castillo R A, Ray R A, Vaghmai F 1989 Central pontine myelinolysis and pregnancy. Obstetrics and Gynecology. 73: 459–461

Cervera R, Asherson R A, Font J et al 1997 Chorea in the antiphospholipid syndrome. Clinical, radiologic, and immunologic characteristics of 50 patients from our clinics and the recent literature. Medicine (Baltimore) 76: 203–212

Chopra J S, Banerjee A K 1989 Primary intracranial sinovenous occlusions in youth and pregnancy. In: Toole J F (ed) Handbook of clinical neurology, vol 54 (revised series of vol 10). Vascular diseases, part II. Elsevier, New York, pp 425–452

Confavreux C, Hutchinson M, Hours M M, Cortinovis-Tourniaire P, Moreau T 1998 Rate of pregnancy-related relapse in multiple sclerosis. Pregnancy in Multiple Sclerosis Group. New England Journal of Medicine 339: 285–291

Dahlke M B, Mertens-Roesler E 1967 Malabsorption of folic acid due to diphenylhydantoin. Blood 30: 341–351

Dansky L V, Andermann E, Rosenblatt D, Sherwin A L, Andermann F 1987 Anticonvulsants, folate levels and pregnancy outcome: a prospective study. Annals of Neurology 21: 176–182

Dawson I 1988 The confidential enquiry into maternal deaths: its role and importance for pathologists. Journal of Clinical Pathology 41: 820–825

Department of Health 1998 Report on confidential enquiries into maternal deaths in England and Wales 1994–96. Her Majesty's Stationery Office, London

Dias M S, Sekhar L N 1990 Intracranial hemorrhage from aneurysms and arteriovenous malformations during pregnancy and the puerperium. Neurosurgery 27: 855–866

Digre K B, Varner M W, Osborn A G, Crawford S 1993 Cranial magnetic resonance imaging in severe preeclampsia vs eclampsia. Archives of Neurology 50: 399–406

Dimsdale H 1959 The epileptic in relation to pregnancy. British Medical Journal 2: 1147–1150

Donaldson J O, Lee N S 1994 Arterial and venous stroke associated with pregnancy. Neurology Clinics 12: 583–599

Dorfman S F 1990 Maternal mortality in New York city, 1981–1983. Obstetrics and Gynecology 76: 317–323

Douglas K A, Redman C W G 1992 Eclampsia in the United Kingdom: the 'BEST' way forward. British Journal of Obstetrics and Gynaecology 99: 355–356

Drost T F, Rosemurgy A S, Sherman H F, Scott L H, Williams J K 1990 Major trauma in pregnant women: maternal/fetal outcome. Journal of Trauma 30: 574–578

Esiri M M, Kennedy P G E 1997 Viral diseases. In: Graham D I, Lantos P L (eds) Greenfield's Neuropathology, 6th edn. Edward Arnold, London, vol 2, pp 19–21

Ezra Y, Kidron D, Beyth Y 1989 Fibromuscular dysplasia of the carotid arteries complicating pregnancy. Obstetrics and Gynecology 73: 840–843

Furukawa F, Haebara H, Hamashima Y 1986 Primary intracranial choriocarcinoma arising from the pituitary fossa. Report of an autopsy case with literature review. Acta Pathologica Japonica 36: 773–781

Geraghty J J, Hoch D B, Robert M E, Vinters H V 1991 Fatal puerperal cerebral vasospasm and stroke in a young woman. Neurology 41: 1145–1147

Gettlefinger D M, Kokman E 1977 Superior sagittal sinus thrombosis. Archives of Neurology (Chicago) 32: 2–4

Gjerde I O, Strandjord R E, Ulstein M 1988 The course of epilepsy during pregnancy: a study of 78 cases. Acta Neurologica Scandinavica 78: 198–205

Gould J S, Wissinger H A 1978 Carpal tunnel syndrome in pregnancy. Southern Medical Journal 71: 144–145

Gray F, Gheradi R, Scaravilli F 1988 The neuropathology of the acquired immune deficiency syndrome, AIDS; a review. Brain 111: 245–266

Guardian G, Voros E, Jardanhazy T, Ungurean A, Vecsei L 1999 Wernicke's encephalopathy induced by hyperemesis gravidarum. Acta Neurologica Scandanavia 99: 196–198

Gurwitt L J, Long J M, Clark R E 1975 Cerebral metastatic choriocarcinoma: a postpartum cause of 'stroke'. Obstetrics and Gynecology 45: 583–588

Haas J F, Janisch W, Staneczek W 1986 Newly diagnosed primary intracranial neoplasms in pregnant women: a population-based assessment. Journal of Neurology, Neurosurgery and Psychiatry 49: 874–880

Harris E N 1992 Serological detection of antiphospholipid antibodies. Stroke 23 (suppl 1): 13–16

Harrison B M, Hansen L A, Pollard J D, McLeod J G 1984 Demyelination induced by serum from patients with Guillain-Barre syndrome. Annals of Neurology 15: 163–170

Hilsinger R L, Adour K K, Doty H E 1975 Idiopathic facial paralysis, pregnancy and the menstrual cycle. Annals of Otology, Rhinology and Laryngology 84: 433–442

Hinchey J, Chaves C, Appignani B, et al 1996 A reversible posterior leukoencephalopathy syndrome. New England Journal of Medicine 334(8): 494–500

Hirsh J, Cade J F, Gallus A S 1972 Anticoagulants in pregnancy: a review of indications and complications (Editorial). American Heart Journal 83: 301–305

Holmes G L 1988 Effects of menstruation and pregnancy on epilepsy. Seminars in Neurology 8: 234–239

Horton J C, Chambers W A, Lyons S L, Adams R D, Kjellberg R N 1990 Pregnancy and the risk of hemorrhage from cerebral arteriovenous malformations. Neurosurgery 26: 867–872

Hoshino T, Wilson C B, Muraoka I 1979 The strathmokimetic (mitostatic) effect of vincristine and vinblastine on human gliomas. Acta Neuropathologica 47: 21–25

Howard A J, Kennard C, Eykyn S, Higgs I 1981 Listerial infections of the CNS in the previous healthy adult. Infection 9: 1067–1072

Ishizuka T, Tomoda Y, Kaseki S, Goto S, Hara T, Kobayashi T 1983 Intracranial metastasis of choriocarcinoma: a clinicopathologic study. Cancer 52: 1896–1903

Isla A, Alvarez F, Gonzalez A, Garcia-Grande A, Perez-Alvarez M, Garcia-Blazquez M 1997 Brain tumor and pregnancy. Obsterics Gynecology 89: 19–23

Jennett W B, Cross J N 1967 Influence of pregnancy and oral contraception on the incidence of strokes in women of childbearing age. Lancet i: 1019–1023

Jones M W, Berry K 1981 Chronic relapsing polyneuritis associated with pregnancy. Annals of Neurology 9: 413

Karasawa J, Kikuchi H, Furuse S 1980 Subependymal hematoma in Moyamoya disease. Surgical Neurology 13: 118–120

Kennard C, Howard A J, Scholtz C, Swash M 1979 Infection of the brain stem by L. monocytogenes. Journal of Neurology, Neurosurgery and Psychiatry 42: 931–933

Kenny L, Baker P N 1999 Maternal pathophysiology in pre-eclampsia. Bailliere's Best Practice Research Clinical Obstetrics 59–75

Kleihues P, Cavenee W K (eds) 2000 Pathology and genetics of tumours of the nervous system. WHO classification of tumours. IARC Press, Lyon, France

Knight A H, Rhind E G 1975 Epilepsy and pregnancy: a study of 153 cases in 59 patients. Epilepsia 16: 99–110

Lamont R J, Postlethwaite R 1986 Carriage of Listeria monocytogenes and related species in pregnant and non-pregnant women in Aberdeen, Scotland. Journal of Infection 13: 187–193

Leppik I E, Rask C A 1988 Pharmacokinetics of antiepileptic drugs during pregnancy. Seminars in Neurology 8: 240–246

Leys D, Lamy C, Lucas C et al 1997 Arterial ischemic strokes associated with pregnancy and puerperium. Acta Neurologica Belgium 97: 5–16

Mabie W C 1999 Management of acute severe hypertension and encephalopathy. Clinical Obstetrics and Gynaecology 42(3): 519–531

McCombe P A, McManis P G, Frith J A, Pollard J D, McLeod J G 1987 Chronic inflammatory demyelinating polyradiculoneuropathy associated with pregnancy. Annals of Neurology 21: 102–104

Macdonald R L, Weir B K A 1991 A review of hemoglobin and the pathogenesis of cerebral vasospasm. Stroke 22: 971–982

Mandel S 1988 Hemiplegic migraine in pregnancy. Headache 28: 414–416

Manfredi M, Beltramello A, Bongiovanni L G, Polo A, Pistoia L, Rizzulo N 1997 Eclamptic encephalopathy: imaging and pathogenetic considerations. Acta Neurologica Scandinavica 96: 277–282

Mas J L, Lamy C 1998 Stroke in pregnancy and the puerperium. Journal of Neurology 245: 305–313

Massey E W 1988 Mononeuropathies in pregnancy. Seminars in Neurology 8: 193–196

Massey E W, Cefalo R C 1979 Neuropathies of pregnancy. Obstetrical and Gynecological Survey 34: 489–492

Massey E W, Moore J, Schold C 1981 Mental neuropathy from systemic cancer. Neurology 31: 1277–1281

Michelsen J J, New P F J 1968 Brain tumour and pregnancy. Journal of Neurology, Neurosurgery and Psychiatry 32: 305–307

Milandre L, Pellissier J F, Vincentelli F, Khalil R 1990 Deep cerebral venous system thrombosis in adults. European Neurology 30: 93–97

Miller J D, Ironside J W 1997 Raised intracranial pressure, oedima and hydrocephalus. In: Graham D I, Lantos P L (eds) Greenfield's neuropathology, 6th edn. Arnold, London, vol 1, pp 161–164

Montalban J, Codina A, Ordi J, Vilardell M, Khamashta M A, Hughes G R V 1991 Antiphospholipid antibodies in cerebral ischaemia. Stroke 22: 750–753

Nag S 1986 Cerebral endothelial plasma membrane alteration in acute hypertension. Acta Neuropathologica 70: 38–43

Nieman R E, Lorber B 1980 Listeriosis in adults: a changing pattern: report of eight cases and review of the literature, 1968–1978. Review of Infectious Diseases 2: 207–227

Olafsson E, Halligrimsson J T, Hauser W A, Ludvigsson P, Gudmundsson G 1998 Pregnancies of women with epilepsy: a population-based study in Iceland. Epilepsia 39: 887–892

Parry G J, Heiman-Patterson T D 1988 Pregnancy and autoimmune neuromuscular disease. Seminars in Neurology 8: 197–204

Patterson R M 1989 Seizure disorders in pregnancy. Medical Clinics of North America 73: 661–665

Pearce J M S 1991 Sumaptriptan in migraine. British Medical Journal 303: 1491

Plauche W C 1979 Myasthenia gravis in pregnancy: an update. American Journal of Obstetrics and Gynecology 135: 691–695

Pope F M, Nicholls A C, Narsisi P, Bartlett J, Neil-Dwyer G, Dhoshi B 1980 Some patients with cerebral aneurysms are deficient in Type III collagen. Lancet i: 973–975

Powell J L 1972 Pseudotumor cerebri and pregnancy. Obstetrics and Gynecology 40: 713–718

Preter M, Tzourio C, Ameri A, Bousser M G 1996 Long term prognosis in cerebral venous thrombosis. Follow-up of 77 patients. Stroke 27: 243–246

Price R W, Brew B, Sidtis J, Rosenblum M, Scheck A C, Cleary P 1988 The brain in AIDS: central nervous system HIV-1 infection and AIDS dementia complex. Science 239: 586–591

Richards A, Graham D, Bullock R 1988 Clinicopathological study of neurological complications due to hypertensive disorders of pregnancy. Journal of Neurology, Neurosurgery and Psychiatry 51: 416–421

Robinson J L, Hall C J, Sedzimar C M 1972 Sub-arachnoid haemorrhage in pregnancy. Journal of Neurosurgery 36: 27–33

Roelvink N C A, Kamphorst W, van Alphen H A M, Rao B R 1987 Pregnancy-related primary brain and spinal tumors. Archives of Neurology 44: 209–215

Sacco R, Wolf P, Bharucha N 1984 Subarachnoid and intracerebral hemorrhage: natural history, prognosis and precursive factors in the Framingham Study. Neurology 34: 847–854

Saiwai S, Inoue Y, Ishihara T et al 1998 Lymphocytic adenohypophysitis: skull radiographs and MRI. Neuroradiology 40: 114–120

Schipper H M 1988 Sex hormones in stroke, chorea and anticonvulsant therapy. Seminars in Neurology 8: 181–186

Schutta H S, Williams E C, Baranski B G, Sutula T P 1991 Cerebral venous thrombosis with plasminogen deficiency. Stroke 22: 401–405

Scott J S 1976 Immunology of human reproduction. Academic Press, London, pp 229–288

Seizinger B R, Rouleau G A, Ozelius L J et al 1987 Genetic linkage of von Recklinghausen neurofibromatosis to the nerve growth factor receptor gene. Cell 49: 589–594

Shah K H, Simons R K, Holbrook T, Fortlage D, Winchell R J, Hoyt D B 1998 Trauma in pregnancy: maternal and fetal outcomes. Journal of Trauma 45: 83–86

Sheehan H L, Davis J C 1982 Post-partum hypopituitarism. Charles C Thomas, Springfield, Illinois

Sheehan H L, Lynch J B 1973 Pathology of toxaemia of pregnancy. Williams & Wilkins, Baltimore, pp 524–584

Simolke G A, Cox S M, Cunningham F G 1991 Cerebrovascular accidents complicating pregnancy and the puerperium. Obstetrics and Gynecology 78: 37–42

Simon R H 1988 Brain tumors in pregnancy. Seminars in Neurology 8: 214–221

Sloan M A 1993 Cerebrovascular disorders associated with licit and illicit drugs. In: Fisher M, Bogousslavsky J (eds), Current review of cerebrovascular disease, 1st edn. Current Medicine, Philadelphia 48–62

Srinivasan K 1984 Ischemic cerebrovascular disease in the young, two common causes in India. Stroke 15: 733–735

Srinivasan K 1988 Puerperal cerebral venous and arterial thrombosis. Seminars in Neurology 8: 222–225

Sussman J D, Sarkies N Pickard J D 1998 Benign intracranial hypertension. Pseudotumour cerebri: idiopathic intracranial hypertension. Advances in Technology in Standard Neurosurgery 24: 261–305

Swainman K F 1980 Antiepileptic drugs, the developing nervous system and the pregnant woman with epilepsy. Journal of the American Medical Association 244: 1477

Swapp G H, Main R A 1973 Neurofibromatosis in pregnancy. British Journal of Dermatology 80: 431–435

Teare A J 1980 True gestational epilepsy. South African Medical Journal 57: 546–547

Tewari K S, Cappuccini F, Asrat T et al 2000 Obstetric emergencies precipitated by malignant brain tumors. American Journal of Obstetrics and Gynecology 182: 1215–1221

Tilzer L L, Plapp F V, Evans J P, Stone D, Alward K 1982 Steroid receptor proteins in human meningiomas. Cancer 49: 633–636

Ursell M R, Marras C L, Farb R, Rowed D W, Black S E, Perry J R 1998 Recurrent intracranial heamorrhage due to postpartum cerebral angiopathy: implications for management. Stroke 29:1995–1998

Van Hartesveldt C, Joyce J 1986 Effects of estrogen on the basal ganglia. Neuroscience Biobehaviour Review 10: 1–14

Weibers D O 1985 Ischemic cerebrovascular complications of pregnancy. Archives of Neurology 42: 1106–1113

Weibers D O, 1988 Subarachnoid hemorrhage in pregnancy. Seminars in Neurology 8: 226–229

Weibers D O, Whisnant J P 1985 The incidence of stroke among pregnant women in Rochester, Minn, 1955 through 1979. Journal of the American Medical Association 254: 3055–3057

Wenger J D, Broome C V 1991 Bacterial meningitis: epidemiology. In: Lambert H P (ed) Infections of the central nervous system. Handbook of infectious diseases. Editors Kass E H, Weller T H, Woolff S M, Tyrrell D A p 27

Yerby M S 1996 Contraception, pregnancy and lactation in women with epilepsy. Bailliere's Clinical Neurology 5: 887–908

Zunker P, Ley-Pozo J, Louwen F, Schuierer G, Holzgreve W, Ringelstein E B 1995 Cerebral hemodynamics in pre-eclampsia/eclampsia syndrome. Ultrasound Obstetrics Gynecology 6: 411–415

46

Pathology of the cardiovascular system in pregnancy

E. G. J. Olsen   H. Fox

Introduction   1541

The effect of pregnancy on the normal heart   1542
Heart size   1542
Haemodynamic changes   1543
Changes in the blood coagulation system   1543

Effect of pregnancy on previously present cardiac disease   1543
Congenital and developmental heart disease   1543
Acquired cardiovascular disease   1547

Cardiovascular disease arising during pregnancy or the puerperium   1550
Myocardial infarction   1550
Arterial aneurysms   1550

INTRODUCTION

With the continuing excellence of antenatal care in the developed countries, patients with known cardiac disease are so carefully supervised during pregnancy, labour and

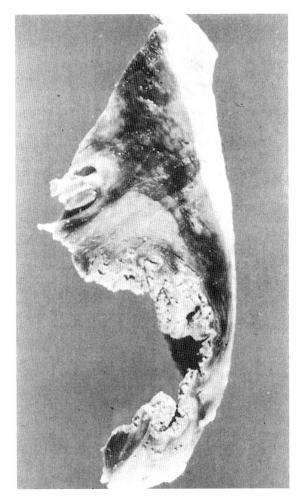

Fig. 46.1 An abscess in the left ventricular wall is illustrated which was due to staphylococcal septicaemia and myocarditis following delivery. (From Olsen, The Pathology of the Heart, 1980a, Macmillan, reproduced with permission of Palgrave.)

the puerperium that maternal deaths directly attributable to cardiac disorder rarely occur nowadays. Conversely, if pre-existing cardiac abnormalities are severe, either conception does not occur or termination of pregnancy is advised. It is therefore not surprising that material for the pathological study of the heart in pregnancy is now scarce.

This was not, however, the case in the past and one only has to refer to older texts of pathology to learn that, prior to the practice of antiseptic surgery, puerperal sepsis occurred in one in six women who were admitted to maternity hospitals, many of whom died as a result of bacterial septicaemia. The heart was not uncommonly involved in such a septicaemia with a resulting endocarditis or myocarditis. An example of this is shown in Fig. 46.1, which shows a staphylococcal abscess in the walls of the left ventricle (Fig. 46.2). Such cases are happily now extremely rare.

This chapter will describe the involvement of the heart during pregnancy and puerperium. The pathologist clearly needs to know the effects of pregnancy on the normal heart and may well be required to give an opinion not only as to whether pregnancy has contributed to the death of a cardiac patient but also as to whether cardiac disease has played a rôle in an obstetric death. The discussion will therefore be under three principal headings:

1. The effect of pregnancy on the normal heart
2. The effect of pregnancy on previously present cardiac disease
3. Cardiovascular disease arising during pregnancy or the puerperium.

Inevitably the effects of pregnancy on the heart are closely linked with physiological and clinical manifestations and these will therefore also be included in the various sections whenever appropriate.

THE EFFECT OF PREGNANCY ON THE NORMAL HEART

HEART SIZE

Heart weight can be related either to body weight or to height. Zeek (1942) constructed a table of normal values according to height (Table 46.1) and these figures provide an approximate guide to normal heart weights. Because, however, epicardial fat is commonly not removed when weighing the heart and because variable lengths of the great vessels are often included in the heart weight, values of 30 grams above or below the weights stated in the table are acceptable as being within the normal range. For more accurate assessment of heart weight, particularly in cases of mild hypertrophy, separate recordings of ventricular and septal weights, after removal of the atria, atrioventricular rings, valves, epicardial fat and coronary arteries, are essential. The free walls of the right and left

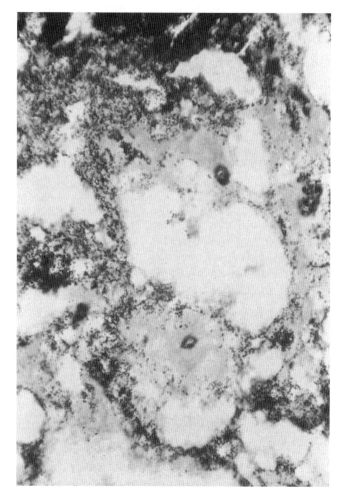

Fig. 46.2 Photomicrograph of the abscess illustrated in Fig. 46.1. The large number of staphylococci are clearly seen. Gram stain.

Table 46.1 Heart weight in relationship to height (From Zeek 1942)

Height	Heart weight (in grams)
150 cm	215–275
152 cm	221–281
155 cm	224–284
160 cm	233–293
165 cm	242–302
170 cm	251–311
175 cm	260–320
180 cm	269–329
183 cm	274–344
185 cm	277–337
191 cm	286–346

Table 46.2 Normal wall thickness in the heart

Atrial walls 2–2.5 mm thick
Right ventricle (at the conus) 2–3 mm thick
Left ventricle 12–15 mm thick

ventricles and the septum are separately weighed and the ratio is calculated (Fulton et al 1952).

Wall measurements are also helpful in the assessment of normal hearts (Table 46.2) but become unreliable if hypertrophy is accompanied by dilatation.

The haemodynamic changes of pregnancy (vide infra) have no lasting effect on the myocardium.

HAEMODYNAMIC CHANGES

Circulatory changes begin in the first trimester of pregnancy and these physiological adaptions become clearly manifest by mid-gestation. The blood volume expands by 30–40%, this increase commencing in the first trimester and reaching a sustained plateau at the 30th week of gestation (Elkayam & Gleicher 1998). Cardiac output also increases by up to 40% above that found in normal non-pregnant women, reaching a peak at mid-gestation and declining slightly during the last eight weeks of pregnancy (Hennessy et al 1996). Initially the increased cardiac output is achieved by an increased stroke volume but heart rate increases progressively throughout pregnancy, to reach a peak of 95 at term, and stroke volume gradually returns to normal levels (Ueland & Metcalfe 1975).

During labour and delivery there is a further increase in cardiac output with each contraction: there is also a transient rise in arterial blood pressure with each contraction and this is associated with a reflex bradycardia. Immediately following a vaginal delivery cardiac output increases by as much as 60% over pre-delivery levels, falling gradually to non-pregnant levels over the next two weeks.

These haemodynamic changes place no undue stress on the patient with a normal heart but may lead to cardiac decompensation if the functional capacity of the heart is impaired by pre-existing disease.

CHANGES IN THE BLOOD COAGULATION SYSTEM

Platelet adhesiveness does not alter during pregnancy or labour but increases slightly after delivery, this alteration persisting for about 72 hours (Shaper 1968). Fibrinolytic activity is depressed during pregnancy but assumes normal levels at delivery, this change occurring even before the umbilical cord is clamped (Shaper et al 1965; Shaper 1966). An initial rise above normal levels occurs for about 30 minutes with a subsequent return to sustained normal levels.

EFFECT OF PREGNANCY ON PREVIOUSLY PRESENT CARDIAC DISEASE

It is difficult to assess the true incidence of pre-existing heart disease complicating pregnancy as reports in the literature are often either studies of single cases or of large series emanating from specialised referral centres. Despite these limitations it is generally thought that about 1% of pregnant women will be suffering from some form of acquired or congenital heart lesion (Ehrenfeld et al 1964). Ueland (1978) has pointed out that over the last few decades there has been a decrease in the incidence of heart disease in pregnancy: thus during the years 1940–1950 the incidence was between 2.3 and 3.3% whilst between 1960 and 1970 this incidence had fallen to between 0.57 and 1.5%.

CONGENITAL AND DEVELOPMENTAL HEART DISEASE

Changes, over the past few decades, in the management of patients with congenital heart disease have led to increasing numbers of adult survivors reaching childbearing age (Perloff 1994; Warnes & Elkayam 1998; Schmaltz et al 1999). Early studies showed that many women with congenital heart lesions could sustain multiple pregnancies without untoward incident (Wooley et al 1961; Naeye et al 1967) whilst in later series there has been, for patients with New York Heart Association functional class I–II, a maternal mortality rate of 0.4% and no marked excess of fetal loss (Presbitero et al 1995; Sawhney et al 1998; Warnes & Elkayam 1998; Schmaltz et al 1999) there being only a few conditions, such as Marfan's syndrome with dilated aortic root, severe aortic stenosis and severe systemic ventricular dysfunction, which put the pregnant patient at increased risk of death (Colman et al 2000).

Coarctation of the aorta

This is defined as a significant narrowing of some part of the aorta, most commonly in the region of the ductus arteriosus. The classification of Edwards (1960) is recommended for precise anatomical categorisation. The coarctation may be string-like, flask-shaped or resemble an hour glass (Cleland et al 1956) and histologically there is thickening of the aortic media at the site of coarctation which may be associated with fibroelastic intimal thickening. The aortic media proximal to the coarctation shows an increase in elastic fibres whilst distal to the constriction there is a marked decrease in the medial content of such fibres.

It is generally held that pregnancy increases the risk of complications in patients with a coarctation, these complications including an exacerbation of systemic hypertension, heart failure, aortic rupture, cerebral haemorrhage and a small, but real, danger of aortic dissection (Pitkin et al 1990; Perloff 1994). In older studies there was a maternal mortality rate of about 10% (Benham 1949; Pritchard 1953; Goodwin 1958; Deal & Wooley 1973) with most deaths occurring before labour and delivery. This high death rate led to suggestions that either the coarctation should be corrected during pregnancy or the patient delivered by Caesarean section (Rosenthal 1955). With modern management, however, pregnancy is usually safe for the mother with an uncomplicated coarctation (Zeira & Zohar 1993; Warnes & Elkayam 1998) and most can be delivered vaginally. Surgical correction of a coarctation during pregnancy is only necessary if major complications occur but balloon angioplasty is contraindicated because of the risk of aortic dissection.

Patients with surgically corrected coarctations generally have fully normal pregnancies (Mortensen & Ellsworth 1965; Saidi et al 1998).

Left to right shunts

Left to right shunting occurs through an atrial septal defect, a ventricular septal defect or a patent ductus arteriosus, these being collectively the commonest congenital anomalies of the heart encountered in gravid women. As, during pregnancy, there is normally no significant alteration in the degree of shunting, the gravid state is well tolerated in patients with uncomplicated left to right shunts and there is no excess of maternal mortality (McAnulty et al 1982; Clarke 1991; Hess & Hess 1992; Zuber et al 1999). If, however, the shunt becomes reversed during pregnancy the patient is placed at serious risk of congestive cardiac failure and death. Shunt reversal tends usually to occur in the immediately postpartum period and is due to a sudden rise in pulmonary pressure. It has been suggested that this is due to haemodynamic changes in the pulmonary circulation but Naeye et al (1967) found extensive thrombosis of the pulmonary vessels in autopsies on four fatal cases of postpartum shunt reversal.

Right to left shunts

Eisenmenger's syndrome

This term applies to the development of high pulmonary vascular resistance in a patient with a previous left to right shunt, this occurring when pulmonary hypertension complicates a patent ductus arteriosus, ventricular septal defect or atrial septal defect. This association poses an extremely serious threat to a pregnant woman. Jones & Howitt (1965) reported a maternal mortality rate of 27.33% in women with this syndrome whilst in a later review of 70 pregnancies in 44 women with Eisenmenger's syndrome there was a maternal death rate of 52% (Gleicher et al 1979): the mortality was higher in those patients with a ventricular septal defect (60%) than in those with either an atrial septal defect or a patent ductus arteriosus (44% and 41.7%, respectively). Maarek-Charbit & Corone (1986) reviewed 42 pregnancies in women with Eisenmenger's syndrome and noted a 36% maternal mortality. Even in series reported during the last decade the maternal mortality has been between 27 and 39% (Antoine et al 1991; Corone et al 1992; Avila

et al 1995; Daliento et al 1998; Vongpatanasin et al 1998). Death occurs most commonly at, or soon after, delivery and is due to increased right to left shunting, either because of a fall in systemic pressure subsequent to blood loss or because of a rise in pulmonary pressure as a result either of haemodynamic changes or pulmonary embolism. Termination of pregnancy should be advised for all pregnant women with Eisenmenger's syndrome (Warnes & Elkayam 1998).

Fallot's tetralogy

This condition is defined as a ventricular septal defect with obstruction of the right ventricular outflow and a right to left shunt at rest or on effort. Four characteristic anatomical changes are seen in combination: a large ventricular septal defect, obstruction of pulmonary blood flow (which can occur at the infundibulum, at the pulmonary valve or above the pulmonary valve), overriding of the ventricular septal defect by the aorta and right ventricular hypertrophy.

This is the most common form of cyanotic congenital heart disease and when associated with pregnancy carries a high risk of cardiac failure or sudden death, the maternal mortality rate being between 4 and 12% (Mendelson 1951; Meyer et al 1964; Jones & Howitt 1965; Ueland 1978; Presbitero et al 1994). Currently, however, unoperated patients are seldom encountered during pregnancy and it is clear that surgical correction of Fallot's tetralogy allows for a fully normal pregnancy. Singh et al (1982) reported 40 uneventful pregnancies in 27 women with a corrected tetralogy, there being no cardiac complications or maternal deaths.

Aortic stenosis

Isolated stenosis of the aortic valve is almost always congenital and accounts for just over 1% of all congenital heart disease. Several forms, such as 'dome-shaped deformity' or 'unicommissural dome stenosis' have been described (Olsen 1980a) whilst stenosis may also occur in cases of bicuspid aortic valves. This condition is rare in pregnancy but Arias & Pineda (1978) reported one example and reviewed 38 pregnancies in previously described cases. These patients were particularly prone to cardiac failure and death during pregnancy and had a maternal mortality rate of 17.4%, demise occurring particularly during labour and delivery. Later, Easterling et al (1988) reviewed 5 cases of aortic stenosis during pregnancy: there were no maternal or fetal deaths. More recently, Lao et al (1993a) reviewed 25 pregnancies in 13 patients with congenital aortic stenosis: all the patients survived but clinical deterioration occurred in 8 of the pregnancies. There is no advantage to pregnancy termination in women with aortic stenosis for this procedure is also associated with a high mortality rate (Ramin et al

1989). If clinical deterioration does occur surgical valve replacement (Ben-Ami et al 1990) or balloon valvuloplasty (McIvor 1991; Banning et al 1993; Lao et al 1993b) can be safely undertaken.

Isolated pulmonary stenosis

Pregnant women with this congenital valvular abnormality run a high risk of congestive cardiac failure: death is, however, uncommon and Knapp & Arditi (1968) reviewed 75 cases of pulmonary stenosis in pregnant women in whom there were no deaths. Patients previously treated by surgery or balloon valvuloplasty have trouble-free pregnancies (Pitkin et al 1990).

Tricuspid atresia

Tricuspid atresia is characterised by an absent tricuspid valve orifice, hypoplasia of the right ventricle and an obligatory atrial septal defect. Presbitero et al (1994) reported 26 pregnancies in 10 women with tricuspid atresia: there were no maternal deaths though live births occurred in only 31% of cases, the incidence of fetal complications being directly related to the level of oxygen saturation in the maternal blood. For patients with marked right atrial enlargement there is a risk of atrial arrhythmia, thrombus formation and paradoxical embolism.

Ebstein's anomaly

This abnormality is characterised by varying degrees of displacement of the posterior and septal leaflets of the tricuspid valve into the right ventricle and is accompanied by right ventricular and atrial changes: in 50% of cases there is an associated atrial septal defect. Donnelly et al (1991) reported 36 pregnancies in 12 women with Ebstein's anomaly: there were no pregnancy-related deaths but there was an increased risk of preterm labour and dysmaturity to infants born of cyanotic mothers. Connolly & Warnes (1994) reported 111 pregnancies in 44 patients with this lesion. There were no serious maternal complications but there was an increased risk of fetal loss and prematurity.

Transposition of the great vessels

In transposition of the great vessels the aorta arises from the morphological right ventricle and the pulmonary artery from the morphological left ventricle. There are thus two parallel and separate circulations between which there is a communication via an atrial or ventricular septal defect. Patients who have had a surgical correction of transposition of the great vessels are now attaining childbearing age and a significant number of pregnancies in such women have now been reported (Lynch-Salamon et al 1993; Clarkson et al 1994; Lao et al 1994; Megerian et al 1994; Rousseil et al 1995; Connolly et al 1999;

Genoni et al 1999; Therrien et al 1999). These reports indicate that pregnancy is quite well tolerated in patients with good functional capacity: no maternal deaths have been reported but some patients have suffered a decline in right ventricular function and because of this occasional pregnancies have had to be terminated. There is a quite high incidence of fetal loss.

Developmental abnormalities

A number of conditions are rather arbitrarily designated as 'developmental' rather than 'congenital'.

Mitral valve prolapse

This is an entity common in otherwise normal women of childbearing age, its incidence in this group being variously estimated at between 4 and 28% (Markiewicz et al 1976; Procacci et al 1976; Boudoulas & Wooley 1988). Most individuals are asymptomatic but a minority suffer chest pain, arrhythmias, palpitations or effort intolerance (Alpert et al 1991; Alpert 1993). Rupture of chordae tendinae, congestive cardiac failure, infective endocarditis, cerebral embolism or sudden death may occur (Olsen 1980a; Kolibash 1988; Marks et al 1989; Alpert 1993). Clinically, there is typically a mid-systolic click followed by a late systolic murmur (Barlow et al 1968) whilst morphologically there is a mucoid change of the valve leaflets, affecting predominantly the posterior leaflet of the mitral valve which is enlarged, sometimes considerably so. The pathogenesis of this abnormality is obscure but suggested aetiological factors include an inborn excessive prominence of the zona spongiosa (Olsen & Al-Rufaie 1980), a biochemical abnormality (Davies et al 1981) and an anatomical abnormality of the chordae tendinae (Becker & DeWit 1979). Rayburn and his colleagues (Rayburn & Fontana 1981; Rayburn et al 1987; Rayburn 1998) studied 96 pregnancies in women with a mitral valve prolapse and found no cardiac complications, no increased risk of obstetrical complications and no maternal deaths. Further reports on pregnancies in 122 patients with mitral valve prolapse (Shapiro et al 1985; Tang et al 1985; Jana et al 1993; Chia et al 1994) have confirmed both the lack of any effect of pregnancy on the heart lesion and lack of any influence on pregnancy of the valvular disorder. Complications such as thromboembolism (Bergh et al 1988) or transient ischaemic attacks (Artal et al 1988) can occur during pregnancy but these are no more frequent in gravid patients than they are in non-pregnant women (Rayburn 1998). Bacterial endocarditis may occur as a complication of labour and these patients require antibiotic prophylaxis.

Marfan's syndrome

This is a hereditary disorder of the connective tissue characterised, in a high proportion of cases, by aneurysmal dilatation of the root of the aorta and/or the ascending part of the aorta, aortic valve insufficiency and thinning of the aortic wall: dissection of the ascending aorta is the major cause of morbidity and death (Chen 1998). The disorder is due to mutations in the fibrillin-1 gene which is located on chromosome 15q21 (Dietz et al 1991; Kainulainen et al 1992) with resulting abnormal patterns of synthesis, secretion and matrix deposition of the fibrillin protein which is a major building block in the formation of elastic tissue (Milewcz et al 1991; Aoyama et al 1995). This disorder also commonly affects the valve leaflets which are often thin, translucent and show a bluish tinge. Twenty-five per cent of patients have clinically detectable aortic regurgitation and if aortic insufficiency has been present for some time there is secondary valve thickening and, often, severe hypertrophy and dilatation of the left ventricle. Histologically, two features are seen in the aortic wall, the formation of medial mucoid pools and fragmentation of the medial elastic tissue (Fig. 46.3a, b): rarely, the mucoid pools attain cystic size (Keene et al 1971; Olsen 1975a). In the valve leaflets the zona spongiosa is particularly prominent whilst if there has been long-standing aortic regurgitation the aortic valve will be thickened by a superimposition of fibroelastic tissue. It should be noted that these pathological changes are sometimes found in patients with no other stigmata of Marfan's syndrome, the term 'Marfan forme fruste' being applied to such cases (Olsen 1975a,b).

Complications of Marfan's syndrome include aortic dissection and rupture and there is a general belief that

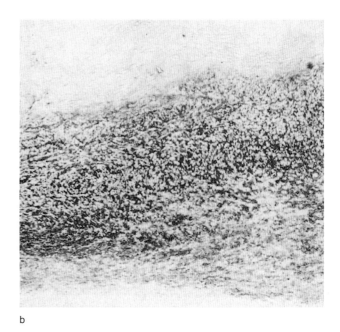

b

Fig. 46.3b From the same tissue as that in Fig. 46.3a, showing areas of acidic mucopolysaccharides. Alcian Blue.

the incidence of these complications is increased during pregnancy, a maternal mortality of 50% being quoted for gravid women with this disorder (Ueland 1978). Pyeritz (1981) reviewed all the 32 cases of previously reported Marfan's syndrome and confirmed this high mortality rate, 16 of the patients having died; he reported, however, a personal series of 105 pregnancies in women with Marfan's syndrome in which there was only one maternal death, this being in a woman who was in congestive cardiac failure before pregnancy supervened. Pyeritz concluded that whilst pregnancy in a woman with aortic root dilatation or aortic regurgitation was highly dangerous, those women without aortic root dilatation or aortic regurgitation usually did well in pregnancy and were not at increased risk of death. In a later prospective study of 45 pregnancies in 21 women with Marfan's syndrome Pyeritz and his colleagues (Rossiter et al 1995) showed that patients without major cardiac involvement tolerated pregnancy well and that pregnancy did not seem to aggravate aortic root dilatation. Although, therefore, the risk of aortic dissection and heart failure during pregnancy appears to be largely confined to those patients with pre-existing aortic root dilatation there have been reports of successful pregnancies in patients with quite well-marked root dilatation (Gordon & Johnson 1995; Mayet et al 1998). Furthermore, successful surgery for aortic valve and ascending aorta replacement has been carried out during pregnancy (Smith et al 1989) as has surgery for aortic dissection (Elkayam et al 1998b).

Vaginal delivery is well tolerated in women with Marfan's syndrome who have no aortic dilatation (Rossiter et al 1995) whilst those with aortic abnormalities should be delivered by Caesarean section (Elkayam

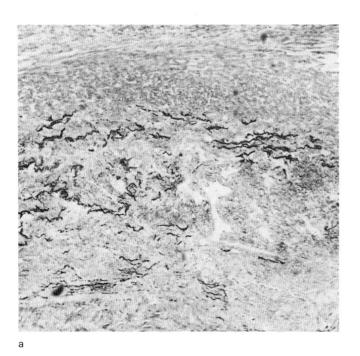

a

Fig. 46.3a The wall of the aorta in Marfan's disease. Extensive fragmentation of the medial elastic components is seen in all areas and is not confined to the region of mucoid pools. Miller's elastic van Gieson.

et al 1998b). Following either mode of delivery there is a high risk of postpartum haemorrhage (Pyeritz 1981; Irons & Pollard 1993), presumably because of abnormalities in the uterine vasculature.

Congenital heart block

Patients with this condition complicating pregnancy usually survive pregnancy with no untoward incident, though some will need temporary pacing (Eddy & Frankenfeld 1977; Dalvi et al 1992).

ACQUIRED CARDIOVASCULAR DISEASE

Rheumatic heart disease

In the past the ratio of rheumatic to congenital heart disease in pregnancy was 20:1; in recent years, however, the incidence of rheumatic heart disease declined to the extent that this ratio was only 3:1 (Ueland 1978). Today this ratio is probably approaching unity (Shime et al 1987).

The pathology of this disease, with its typical triad of valve thickening and commissural fusion together with chordal shortening and thickening, is well known, though predominantly commissural (Fig. 46.4) or largely chordal forms are less well recognised. Histologically, the valve leaflets are thickened by fibroelastic tissue and there is a chronic inflammatory cell infiltration of variable intensity: an increased valvular vascularity, characterised particu-

larly by the presence of thick-walled capillaries (Fig. 46.5), is a notable feature and is the only reliable criterion for distinguishing rheumatic from congenital valve disease.

In 75% of cases in which rheumatic heart disease complicates pregnancy the sole, or predominant, lesion is mitral stenosis. Women with this condition are at risk of developing pulmonary oedema, congestive heart failure, atrial fibrillation, acute circulatory failure and pulmonary thromboembolism, though the incidence of such complications has declined in recent years (Szekely et al 1973). The overall mortality rate for women with uncorrected mitral stenosis is now well under 1% (O'Driscoll et al 1962; Ueland 1978) though patients with either atrial fibrillation or pulmonary oedema have a mortality rate in the range of 17–20% (Ueland 1984). In theory, the woman with mitral stenosis is at most risk towards the end of the second trimester and during the immediately postpartum period. The latter of these assumptions appears to be correct for nearly half of the obstetric deaths due to mitral stenosis occur during the puerperium, almost invariably because of acute pulmonary oedema. Of those patients dying during pregnancy relatively few die at the end of the second trimester, nearly 75% succumbing after the 32nd week of gestation. Most patients can be successfully managed through pregnancy by careful medical care but some will require surgical treatment because of worsening symptoms and decreasing function. The surgical technique of choice is percutaneous balloon valvuloplasty with shielding of the fetus to

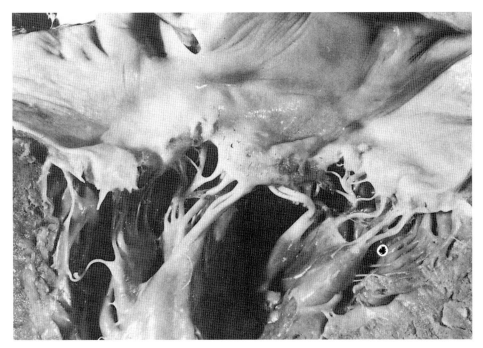

Fig. 46.4 Mitral valve stenosis in rheumatic heart disease. Valve involvement in this example is mainly commissural. The valve leaflets and some chordae are thickened but the latter are not shortened. A thrombus on the anterior leaflet can be seen.

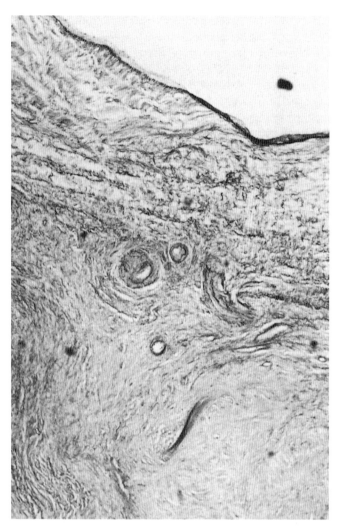

Fig. 46.5 Photomicrograph of the mitral valve showing increased vascularity. The capillary-sized vessels are invested with a thick muscular coat. From a patient with rheumatic heart disease who underwent valve replacement following successful pregnancy. Miller's elastic van Gieson.

limit radiation dosage: this procedure is well tolerated during pregnancy and usually results in considerable functional improvement (Esteves et al 1991; Lung et al 1994; Onderoglu et al 1995; Gupta et al 1998; Desai et al 2000; de Andrade et al 2001; Fawzy et al 2001). In occasional cases closed mitral valvotomy is a suitable alternative (Vosloo & Reichart 1987) whilst very occasionally a mitral valve replacement has been undertaken (Yaryura et al 1996). Patients with aortic stenosis of rheumatic origin are thought to be at considerable risk during pregnancy: any sudden drop in cardiac output, due to hypovolaemia, may lead to sudden death and a maternal mortality rate in the region of 17% has been noted (Arias & Pineda 1978). Women with mitral regurgitation, aortic regurgitation or with tricuspid valve disease usually tolerate pregnancy well (McAnulty et al 1982; Clarke 1991).

Infective endocarditis

This condition, which may be acute or subacute, usually develops in pregnancy as a complication of congenital or rheumatic valvular heart disease: it also complicates mitral valve prolapse or a prosthetic valve and can occur as a result of intravenous drug abuse. It is, however, rather uncommon in pregnancy and Payne et al (1982) were only able to find reports of 21 cases prior to that date; approximately 50 further cases have since been described (MacMahon et al 1987; Cox & Leveno 1989; Zamprogno et al 1990; Felice et al 1995; Garini et al 1995; Caraballo 1997; Kangavari et al 2000).

Pregnancy-related bacteraemia may occur following pregnancy termination, vaginal delivery or Caesarean section and although streptococcal infection is the most common cause of endocarditis in pregnancy, many of the organisms that have caused this infection have also been cultured from the normal vagina and postpartum uterus (Ebrahami et al 1998). The course of the disease, its management and its pathology are the same in the pregnant woman as in non-pregnant patients and until relatively recently there was an overall maternal mortality rate of 20–25% (Cox & Leveno 1989), most commonly due to heart failure: surgical intervention, especially valve replacement, has, however, had a dramatic impact on mortality in patients in whom medical treatment fails (Westaby et al 1992; Ebrahami et al 1998).

Prosthetic heart valves

The success attained in treating both acquired and congenital heart disease by artificial valve replacement has resulted in an increasing number of women with valve prostheses becoming pregnant. Accumulated experience of such cases has shown that most patients who are asymptomatic or only mildly symptomatic have a haemodynamic reserve that is fully adequate for a safe pregnancy (Pavankumar et al 1988; Sareli et al 1989; Uetsuka et al 1990; Ayhan et al 1991; Badduke et al 1991; Born et al 1992; Sbarouni & Oakley 1993; Caruso et al 1994; Hanania et al 1994; Lee et al 1994; Thomas et al 1994; Salazar et al 1996; Sadler et al 2000). However, decreased functional capacity and heart failure occur in a significant proportion of patients (Elkayam & Kahn 1998) and cases of acute pulmonary oedema in previously haemodynamically stable women have been recorded (Sareli et al 1989; Sbarouni & Oakley 1993; Salazar et al 1996).

A real danger is presented to pregnant women with a mechanical prosthetic valve by the increased risk of thromboembolism whilst gravid; thromboembolic events occur in about 10–15% of such patients and in two-thirds of these cases there is thrombosis of the valve which may be fatal (Elkayam & Khan 1998). This makes it necessary for patients with a mechanical valve, but not those with bioprosthetic or homograft valves, to receive anticoagulants during pregnancy (McColgin et al 1989; Clarke 1991). Anticoagulants reduce considerably the risk to the mother but do, unfortunately, pose some risks to the fetus. Coumarin derivatives, if taken early in pregnancy, are teratogenic and associated with a high incidence of miscarriage (Sareli et al 1989; Born et al 1992; Lecuru et al 1993; Wong et al 1993; Sadler et al 2000) whilst heparin, though not teratogenic, is less effective in preventing valve thrombosis (Salazar et al 1996; Abildgaard et al 1999). The arguments about the optimal anticoagulant regimen in pregnant women are therefore complex and outside the scope of this volume.

The use of anticoagulants in pregnancy may, of course, be complicated by severe vaginal bleeding during delivery and the puerperium and intracranial haemorrhage has also been reported (Bagga et al 2001).

Conditions of unknown aetiology

Hypertrophic cardiomyopathy

This condition, also known as idiopathic hypertrophic subaortic stenosis, belongs to the group of heart muscle diseases of unknown cause. It is recognised macroscopically by asymmetric, often severe, hypertrophy of the interventricular septum and is characterised histologically by severe hypertrophy and disarray of the myocardial fibres. The myocardial nuclei are often of a bizarre shape and frequently surrounded by a clear glycogen-containing zone. Ultrastructurally, there is extensive disarray of myocardial fibrils with many abnormal inter- and intrafibrillar connections (Olsen 1980b).

Pregnancy is potentially dangerous in this condition but Oakley et al (1979) have analysed a series of 54 pregnancies in 23 patients in which there were no maternal or fetal deaths, a result only achieved by careful management during the gestational period. A number of further cases of hypertrophic cardiomyopathy in pregnant women have since been reported (Boccio et al 1986; Minnich et al 1987; Tessler et al 1990; Van Kasteren et al 1991; Pelliccia et al 1992; Bascou et al 1993; Garcia Leon et al 1993; Coven et al 1994; Kazimudden et al 1998; Piacenza et al 1998; Wilansky et al 1998; Deiml et al 2000; Mokaddem et al 2000) and these have confirmed that these patients are at risk of haemodynamic and clinical deterioration, ventricular fibrillation, pulmonary oedema and, on rare occasions, sudden death. Patients with moderate or severe heart symptoms should be advised against becoming pregnant (Elkayam & Dave 1998).

Takayasu's disease

This condition affects particularly women aged between 15 and 40 and predominantly involves the aorta and its main branches. The walls of the affected arteries are thicker than normal despite aneurysmal dilatation. Histologically, intimal thickening is uniform and severe, consisting of loosely arranged connective tissue which is rich in acidic mucopolysaccharides but devoid of elastic tissue. There is destruction and fibrous replacement of the media with almost total loss of medial elastic tissue. The adventitia is often thickened to an extreme degree, anchoring the affected vessels to neighbouring structures (Olsen 1980a).

Ishikawa & Matsuura (1982) and Jonge et al (1983) supplemented an earlier review by Hauth et al (1977) of Takayasu's disease complicating pregnancy. Ishikawa & Matsuura, working in Japan, described a personally studied series of 33 pregnancies in 27 patients and reviewed reports of 50 pregnancies in 46 patients. Since then there have been a number of reports and reviews of this topic amongst the more recent of which are those of Rao et al (1992), Bassa et al (1995), Bloechle et al (1995), Elkayam & Hameed (1998b) and Sharma et al (2000). In general, the course of the disease does not appear to be influenced by pregnancy, some patients improving and others worsening during the gestational period. There is, however, a tendency for some patients to have an unusually marked elevation of blood pressure during labour and immediately after delivery and this has led to occasional cases of heart failure (Winn et al 1988) and cerebral haemorrhage (Ishikawa & Matsuura 1982).

Primary pulmonary hypertension

Primary pulmonary hypertension is an uncommon disease characterised by a mean pulmonary artery pressure of more than 25 mmHg at rest in the absence of left sided valvular disease, myocardial disease, congenital heart disease or respiratory, connective tissue or chronic thromboembolic disease (Rubin 1997). Despite a plethora of aetiological hypotheses the disease is of unknown origin. The haemodynamic changes of pregnancy throw a severe stress on the heart in this condition and a maternal mortality rate in the region of 50% was noted by McAnulty et al in 1981; Weiss et al (1998) reviewed all cases of primary pulmonary hypertension in pregnant women reported between 1978 and 1996 and found a maternal mortality rate of 30%. In cases reported since 1996 (O'Hare et al 1998; Takeuchi et al 1998; De Backer et al 1999; Easterling et al 1999; Low & Grange 1999; Robinson et al 1999; Badalian et al 2000; Olofsson et al 2001; Penning et al 2001; Stewart et al 2001) the maternal mortality appears to have fallen somewhat, to about 20%, and this may reflect the better medical results obtained with newer pulmonary vasodilator drugs.

Worsening of the clinical status is common during pregnancy and death may occur, usually in the immediately postpartum period, because of sudden cardiovascular collapse or progressive right ventricular failure.

Neither the duration of symptoms before pregnancy nor the severity of the pulmonary hypertension are predictors of the risk of death (Elkayam et al 1998a).

CARDIOVASCULAR DISEASE ARISING DURING PREGNANCY OR THE PUERPERIUM

MYOCARDIAL INFARCTION

During pregnancy total serum cholesterol values rise and the distribution between alpha and beta lipoproteins assumes a pattern similar to that found in men with ischaemic heart disease (Oliver & Boyd 1955). Furthermore, there is an increased risk of thrombosis during pregnancy as a result of marked alterations in the coagulation and fibrinolytic systems (Fletcher et al 1979). Despite these changes myocardial infarction is rare during pregnancy: only 26 cases had been reported by 1960 (Watson et al 1960), this figure rising to 30 by 1967 (Fletcher et al 1967) to 39 by 1970 and to 70 by 1985 (Hankins et al 1985): currently, nearly 150 cases have been reported (Roth & Elkayam 1998; Kulka et al 2001). Despite the fact that total plasma lipids reach a peak during the latter part of pregnancy, myocardial infarction is almost equally divided between the first and second half of pregnancy.

Reviews of reported cases of myocardial infarction during pregnancy (Badui & Enciso 1996; Roth & Elkayam 1996, 1998) have shown that when coronary artery morphology has been studied, coronary artery atherosclerosis with or without superimposed thrombosis was present in about 40% of cases and coronary thrombosis without evidence of atherosclerotic disease in around 20%: the coronary arteries have been normal in approximately 30% of cases whilst 15% of cases have been due to coronary artery dissection. This latter vascular catastrophe is particularly associated with pregnancy in the elderly multiparous woman and usually occurs in the immediately postpartum period (Shaver et al 1978; Barrett et al 1982; Coulson et al 1995; Samuels et al 1998; Koul et al 2001). Whatever the cause the infarction is usually anterior and commonly transmural (Nolan & Hankins 1989). Myocardial infarction may easily be missed during pregnancy, chest pain being misdiagnosed as abdominal in origin and electrocardiographic changes being difficult to interpret because of elevation of the diaphragm. Nevertheless, the prognosis is generally good with an overall mortality of 20% (Badui & Enciso 1996; Roth & Elkayam 1998): this overall death rate conceals the fact, however, that myocardial infarction in late pregnancy and during the early postpartum period has a mortality rate of 45% (Nolan & Hankins 1989). There is no reason to believe that the sequential healing process in the damaged myocardium differs in any way from that in the general non-pregnant population. There is, however, remarkably little information available about the risks of pregnancy in women who have suffered a previous myocardial infarction: it does appear, however, that there is no excess of deaths in such cases (Frenkel et al 1991).

ARTERIAL ANEURYSMS

There is a particular tendency for the pregnant woman to suffer rupture of an arterial aneurysm. This propensity has been attributed partly to the haemodynamic changes which characterise the gravid state and partly to hormone-induced changes, such as intimal hyperplasia and altered organisation of the media, in the arteries during pregnancy (Barrett et al 1982). Some doubt has, however, been expressed as to whether pregnancy per se is a true risk factor for aneurysm formation, it being suggested that complicating hypertension may be of greater importance (Wooley & Sparks 1992).

In the past it was thought that 50% of women aged less than 40 years who develop a dissecting aortic aneurysm are pregnant at the time this catastrophe occurs (Mandel et al 1954): in a more recent review, however, of 1235 patients with acute aortic dissection recorded in the literature no association was found with pregnancy (Oskoui & Lindsay 1994). This matter remains subjudice for nearly 200 cases of pregnancy-associated aortic dissection have been reported (Elkayam & Hameed 1998a). Advancing maternal age appears to be a significant risk factor during pregnancy but multiparity is not (Konishi et al 1980): dissection occurs most commonly during the third trimester (49% of cases), the first two days of the puerperium (19% of cases) or labour (13%). Only 19% of aortic dissections occur during the first two trimesters (Konishi et al 1980). The dissection is usually in the ascending aorta and has, in the past, been associated with a mortality rate in excess of 90%. There are, however, grounds for believing that the current aggressive surgical approach to a dissecting aortic aneurysm has much improved this gloomy prognosis (Barrett et al 1982).

More than 100 examples of rupture of a splenic artery aneurysm during pregnancy have been described (O'Grady et al 1977; Holdsworth & Gunn 1992; Angelakis et al 1993) and up to 50% of ruptured splenic artery aneurysms occur in pregnancy, predominantly during the first trimester (Vassalotti & Schaller 1967; Barrett et al 1982; Trastek et al 1985; Holdsworth & Gunn 1992). Nevertheless, a recent review of splenic artery aneurysms was unable to show any relationship with pregnancy (Dave et al 2000). The maternal mortality from rupture in pregnancy is about 70% and the fetal mortality is as high as 95% (Trastek et al 1985; Holdsworth & Gunn 1992).

Fourteen cases of ruptured renal artery aneurysm associated with pregnancy had been reported prior to 1982 (Barrett et al 1982): nearly all the ruptures occurred antepartum and 10 of the patients died. In more recently reported instances, however, there has been a favourable maternal outcome (Dayton et al 1990; Richardson et al 1990; Rijbroek et al 1994). Four cases of pregnancy-related rupture of an ovarian artery aneurysm have also been recorded, all rupturing in the immediate postpartum period (Barrett et al 1982). Rupture of a cerebral artery aneurysm during pregnancy is discussed in Chapter 45.

Hypertensive disease of pregnancy

Death due to eclampsia is now very rare in Western countries and demise due to cardiac failure in this condition is extremely rare. There has, in the past, been some debate as to the existence or otherwise of a specific 'toxaemic cardiomyopathy' but it is now agreed that cardiac failure in pre-eclampsia or eclampsia is solely, and directly, attributable to hypertension. In fatal cases, the typical changes of hypertensive heart disease are found with concentric hypertrophy of the left ventricular wall (Fig. 46.6), often to a striking degree: there is not usually any marked dilatation. Histologically, the myocardial fibres are hypertrophied but in normal alignment: focal fibrous replacement may be noted (Fig. 46.7). Ultrastructurally, there is an increase in the number of myocardial mitochondria (Fig. 46.8), above the normal of one per two sarcomeres, together with folding of the nuclear membrane, enlargement of the Golgi apparatus and hypertrophy of the T tubular system. The amount of glycogen is increased and intramitochondrial glycogen deposits may be encountered (Maron & Ferrans 1975; Olsen 1980a).

Peripartal cardiomyopathy

Peripartal cardiomyopathy has, for many years, been defined as heart failure occurring for the first time either

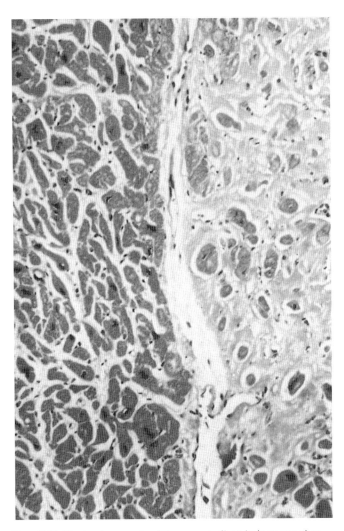

Fig. 46.7 Photomicrograph of the myocardium in hypertension showing fibre hypertrophy. There is an increase in diameter of the cardiocytes as well as nuclear changes of hypertrophy. A focus of replacement fibrosis is clearly seen.

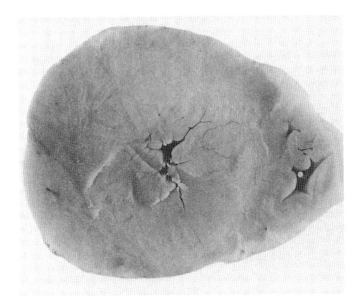

Fig. 46.6 Cross-section of the ventricles in hypertensive heart disease, showing concentric hypertrophy of the left ventricle.

in the last trimester of pregnancy or during the first six months after delivery in the absence of any pre-existing heart disease and in the absence of any determinable cause for the cardiac failure, such as eclampsia, hypertension or rheumatic heart disease (Demakis et al 1971; Demakis & Rahimtoola 1971; Goodwin 1975). Recently, however, a further criterion has been added, namely that there should be echographic evidence of impairment of left ventricular systolic function (Heider et al 1999; Hibbard et al 1999). The incidence of the disease is difficult to ascertain but estimates range from 1:15 000 in the United States (Cunningham et al 1986) to 1:6000 in Japan (Hsieh et al 1992) and 1:1000 in South Africa (Desai et al 1995). Data recording the incidence of this disease should, however, be treated with some sceptism for the clinical diagnosis often turns out to be incorrect (Cunningham et al 1986). Despite this caveat it does appear clear that the condition occurs most commonly in older, multiparous black women (Vielle 1984).

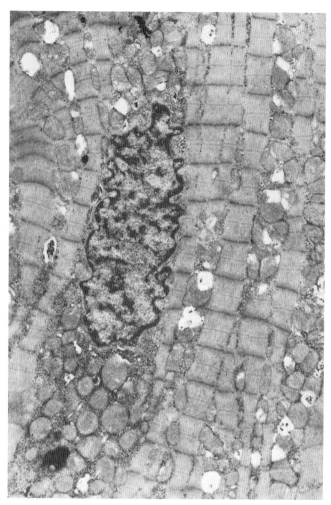

Fig. 46.8 Electronmicrograph of hypertrophy due to hypertension. The wall of the nucleus is slightly folded. An increase of mitochondria of up to 3 per 2 sarcomeres (normal 1 mitochondrion per 2 sarcomeres) between the myofibrils in parallel alignment can be observed. An increase in glycogen, best seen between the mitochondria in the perinuclear areas, is also present. Lead citrate and uranyl acetate.

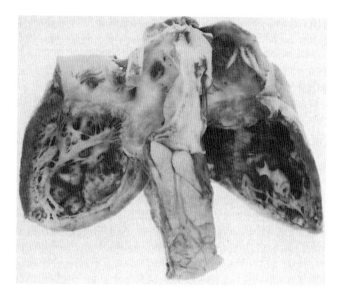

Fig. 46.9 Peripartal cardiomyopathy. The ventricular cavities have been displayed. Despite hypertrophy the myocardial walls are normal in thickness. This is due to severe dilatation masking the degree of hypertrophy that is present. Note the intracavitary thrombus. From a 27-year-old Nigerian woman who, following the onset of symptoms three weeks after a second uneventful pregnancy, died three months later. (By courtesy of Dr J F Geddes from the Department of Histopathology, Royal Free Hospital, London.)

Typically, patients present with left heart failure late in pregnancy or during the puerperium: dyspnoea, tachycardia, oedema, embolism or pulmonary oedema make up the clinical picture whilst angina-like pain is not uncommon (Gilchrist 1963; Lee & Cotton 1989). Physical signs include a soft mitral systolic murmur, a third heart sound and cardiomegaly whilst an electrocardiogram shows evidence of left ventricular hypertrophy and non-specific S–T changes.

In fatal cases there is a uniform pathological appearance. The heart weight is considerably increased, up to twice its normal size, and there is dilatation of all the chambers. Because of this latter change the myocardial wall measurements may be normal despite the hypertrophy (Fig. 46.9). The myocardium appears pale and flabby whilst the endocardium is thickened: mural thrombi are commonly present, particularly in the apical region of the ventricles. The coronary arteries are usually normal.

Histologically, the myocardial fibres are in normal alignment and the nuclear abnormalities typical of hypertrophy, such as pyknosis or vesicular change, are seen: because of attenuation the diameter of the myocardial fibres is usually normal (Fig. 46.10). Varying degrees of fibrosis are usually present and there is an increase in interstitial connective tissue. The small intramural vessels are normal whilst the thickened endocardium shows a prominent smooth muscle component.

With the advent of the bioptome, histochemical and electronmicroscopic studies have been made possible in peripartal cardiomyopathy. Histochemical studies have shown a patchy decrease in myocardial glycogen and succinic dehydrogenase whilst ultrastructural studies have shown only the typical features of hypertrophy together with a number of non-specific degenerative changes.

The overall pathological picture is therefore totally non-specific and identical to that which has been described in dilated (congestive) cardiomyopathy (Olsen 1972, 1980a). This resemblance further extends to the frequent finding, common to both conditions, of a significant increase in the number of chronic inflammatory cells in the interstitium of the myocardium together with fraying of adjacent myocardial fibres (Balchum et al 1956; Meadows 1960).

The aetiology, or aetiologies, of peripartal heart disease are unknown and it is still not clear whether this is a condition which is aetiologically linked to pregnancy or whether the gravid state simply unmasks pre-existent subclinical heart muscle disease which is made overt by the physiological stress imposed by pregnancy (Witlin et al

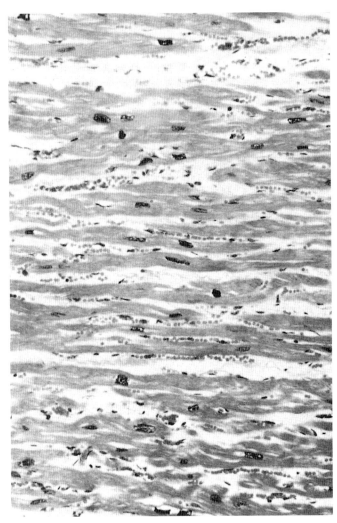

Fig. 46.10 From a patient with peripartal cardiomyopathy. The tissue had been obtained by means of the King's bioptome. The myocardial fibres are in parallel alignment, nuclear changes of hypertrophy (vesicular or pyknotic changes or blunting of the nuclear poles) are present but the diameter of cardiocytes is normal. This dissociation is due to stretching of the fibres.

1997). This latter view is, however, unlikely for the prognosis in dilated cardiomyopathy is usually poor whilst most women with peripartal heart disease recover.

Suggested aetiological factors for peripartal cardiomyopathy have included malnutrition, viral myocarditis, an immune mediated myocarditis, small vessel disease and excess alcohol intake but none of these theories has withstood either the passage of time or the test of critical scrutiny (Lang et al 1998) though the belief that the disease is a form of myocarditis currently finds favour (Brown & Bertolet 1998).

The outcome of peripartal cardiomyopathy is variable. Most patients recover fully with a return of their heart size to normal, usually within six months from the time of initial diagnosis (Lang et al 1998). Some patients, however, die suddenly and unexpectedly whilst heart failure persists in others; the poor prognosis for these latter patients has been much improved by cardiac transplantation (Joseph et al 1987; Hess & Hess 1992; Keogh et al 1994; Aziz et al 1999; Heider et al 1999). Many patients who have made a full recovery from peripartal cardiomyopathy have uncomplicated further pregnancies (Sutton et al 1991) but the disease can recur in subsequent pregnancies (Ceci et al 1998).

Idiopathic pericarditis

A few cases of apparently idiopathic acute pericarditis during pregnancy have been reported (Adams 1959; Probst & Mier 1963; Kraus et al 1978; Simpson et al 1989; Hagley & Shaub 1993; Mecacci et al 2000): in all cases the pregnancies proceeded to term and the pericarditis resolved.

Idiopathic myocarditis

There have been a few reports of this condition complicating pregnancy (Mendelson 1951; Faruque 1965; Hibbard 1975). The disease tends to occur during the third trimester and is associated with a very high maternal mortality.

Pregnancy after cardiac transplantation

There have now been a significant number of reports of successful pregnancies in women who have had a previous cardiac transplantation (Key et al 1989; Camann et al 1991; Darbois et al 1991; Kirk 1991; Carvalho et al 1992; Wagoner et al 1993; Branch et al 1998; Haugen et al 1998; Morini et al 1998).

The cardiovascular changes associated with pregnancy appear to be well tolerated by the transplanted heart.

REFERENCES

Abildgaard U, Gjestvang F T, Lossius P, Hodne E 1999 Low molecular heparin in a pregnant woman with heart valve prosthesis. Tidsskrift for den Norske-laegeforening 119: 4319–4320

Adams C W 1959 Postviral myopericarditis associated with the influenza virus: report of 8 cases. American Journal of Cardiology 4: 56–67

Ahronheim J H 1977 Isolated coronary periarteritis: report of a case of unexpected death in a young pregnant woman. American Journal of Cardiology 40: 287–290

Alpert M A 1993 Mitral valve prolapse: mostly benign. British Medical Journal 306: 943–944

Alpert M A, Mukerju V, Sabeti M, Russell J, Beitman B D 1991 Mitral valve prolapse, panic disorder and chest pain. Medical Clinics of North America 75: 1119–1133

Angelakis E J, Bair W E, Barone J E, Lincer M 1993 Splenic artery aneurysm rupture during pregnancy. Obstetrical and Gynecological Survey 48: 145–148

Antoine J M, Bonnardot J P, Vitoux B, Salat-Baroux J 1991 Eisenmenger syndrome and pregnancy. European Journal of Obstetrics, Gynecology and Reproductive Biology 20: 79–82

Aoyama T, Francke U, Gasner C, Furthmayr H 1995 Fibrillin abnormalities and prognosis in Marfan syndrome and related disorders. American Journal of Medical Genetics 58: 169–176

Arias F, Pineda J 1978 Aortic stenosis and pregnancy. Journal of Reproductive Medicine 20: 229–232

Artal R, Greenspoon J S, Rutherford S 1988 Transient ischaemic attack: a complication of mitral valve prolapse in pregnancy. Obstetrics and Gynecology 71: 1028–1030.

Avila W S, Grinberg M, Snitcowsky R et al 1995 Maternal and fetal outcome in pregnant women with Eisenmenger's syndrome. European Heart Journal 16: 460–464

Ayhan A, Yapar E G, Yuce K, Kisnisci H A, Nazil N, Ozmen F 1991 Pregnancy and its complications after cardiac valve replacement. International Journal of Gynaecology and Obstetrics 35: 117–122

Aziz T M, Burgess M I, Acladious N N et al 1999 Heart transplantation for peripartum cardiomyopathy: a report of three cases and a literature review. Cardiovascular Surgery 7: 565–567

Badalian S S, Silverman R K, Aubry R H, Longo J 2000 Twin pregnancy in a woman on long-term epoprostenol for primary pulmonary hypertension: a case report. Journal of Reproductive Medicine 45: 149–152

Badduke B R, Jamieson W R, Miyagishima R T et al 1991 Pregnancy and childbearing in a population with biologic valvular prostheses. Journal of Thoracic and Cardiovascular Surgery 102: 179–186

Badui E, Enciso R 1996 Acute myocardial infarction during pregnancy and puerperium: a review. Angiology 347: 739–756

Bagga R, Sawhney H, Saxena S V, Aggarwal N, Vasishta K 2001 Intracranial bleed in a pregnant woman on oral anticoagulants for prosthetric heart valve. Acta Obstetricia et Gynecologica Scandinavica 80: 766–767

Balchum O J, McCord M C, Blount S G Jr 1956 The clinical and hemodynamic pattern in non-specific myocarditis; a comparison with other entities also impairing myocardial efficiency. American Heart Journal 52: 430–443

Banning A P, Pearson J F, Hall R J C 1993 Role of balloon dilatation of the aortic valve in pregnant patients with severe aortic stenosis. British Heart Journal 70: 544–545

Barlow J B, Bosman C K, Pocock W A, Marchand P 1968 Late systolic murmur and non-ejection ('mid-late') systolic clicks: an analysis of 90 patients. British Heart Journal 30: 203–218

Barrett J M, Hooydonk J E van, Boehm F H 1982 Pregnancy-related rupture of arterial aneurysms. Obstetrical and Gynecological Survey 37: 557–566

Bascou V, Ferrandis J, Bauer V, Bouret J M, de Meeus J B Magnin G 1993 Obstructive myocardiopathy and pregnancy. European Journal of Gynecology, Obstetrics and Reproductive Biology 22: 309–311

Bassa A, Desai D K, Moodley J 1995 Takayasu's disease and pregnancy: three case studies and a review of the literature. South African Medical Journal 85: 107–112

Becker A E, DeWit A P M 1979 Mitral valve apparatus: a spectrum of normality relevant to mitral valve prolapse. British Heart Journal 42: 680–689

Ben-Ami M, Battino S, Rosenfeld T, Marin G, Shalev E 1990 Aortic valve replacement during pregnancy: a case report and review of the literature. Acta Obstetricia et Gynecologica Scandinavica 69: 651–653

Benham G H H 1949 Pregnancy and coarctation of the aorta. Journal of Obstetrics and Gynaecology of the British Empire 56: 606–618

Bergh P A, Hollander D, Gregori C, Breen J 1988 Mitral valve prolapse and thromboembolic disease in pregnancy: a case report. International Journal of Gynaecology and Obstetrics 27: 133–137

Bloechle M, Bollmann R, Chaoui R, Birnbaum M, Bartho S 1995 Schwangerschaft bei Takayasu-Arteritis. Zeitschrift fur Geburtshilfe und Neonatologie 199: 116–119

Boccio R V, Chung J H, Harrison D M 1986 Anaesthetic management of cesarean section in a patient with idiopathic hypertrophic subaortic stenosis. Anaesthesiology 65: 663–665

Born D, Martinez E E, Almeida P A et al 1992 Pregnancy in patients with prosthetic heart valves: the effect of anticoagulants on mother, fetus and neonate. American Heart Journal 124: 413–417

Boudoulas H, Wooley C F 1988 Mitral valve prolapse: prevalence. In: Boudoulas H, Wooley C F (eds) Mitral valve prolapse and the mitral valve prolapse syndrome. Fortuna, Mount Kisco, NY, pp 161–170

Branch K R, Wagoner L E, McGrory C H et al 1998 Risks of subsequent pregnancies on mother and newborn in female heart transplant recipients. Journal of Heart and Lung Transplantation 17: 698–702

Brown C S, Bertolet B D 1998 Peripartum cardiomyopathy: a comprehensive review. American Journal of Obstetrics and Gynecology 178: 409–414

Camann W F, Jarcho J A, Mintz K J, Greene M F 1991 Uncomplicated vaginal delivery 14 months after cardiac transplantation. American Heart Journal 121: 939–941

Caraballo V 1997 Fetal myocardial infarction resulting from coronary artery septic embolism after abortion: unusual cause and complication of endocarditis Annals of Emergency Medicine 29: 175–177

Caruso A, deCarolis S, Ferrazzani S, Paradisi F, Pomini F, Pompei A 1994 Pregnancy outcome in women with cardiac valve prosthesis. European Journal of Obstetrics, Gynecology and Reproductive Biology 54: 7–11

Carvalho A C, Almeida D, Cohen M 1992 Successful pregnancy, delivery and puerperium in a heart transplant patient with previous peripartum cardiomyopathy. European Heart Journal 13: 1589–1591

Ceci O, Beradesca C, Caradonna F, Corsano P, Guglielmi R, Nappi L 1998 Recurrent peripartum cardiomyopathy. European Journal of Obstetrics, Gynecology and Reproductive Biology 76: 29–30

Chen H 1998 Genetic causes of cardiac diseases. In: Elkayam U, Gleicher N (eds) Cardiac problems in pregnancy, 3rd edn. Wiley-Liss, New York, pp 671–708

Chia Y, Yeoh S, Lim M, Viegas O, Ratnam S 1994 Pregnancy outcome and mitral valve prolapse. Asia-Oceania Journal of Obstetrics and Gynaecology 20: 383–388

Clarke S L 1991 Cardiac disease in pregnancy. Obstetrics and Gynecology Clinics of North America 18: 237–256

Clarkson P M, Wilson N J, Neutze J M, North R A, Calder A L, Barratt-Boyes B G 1994 Outcome of pregnancy after the Mustard operation for transposition of the great arteries. Journal of the American College of Cardiology 24: 190–193

Cleland W P, Counihan T B, Goodwin J F, Steiner R E 1956 Coarctation of the aorta. British Medical Journal 2: 379–390

Colman J M, Sermer M, Seaward P G, Siu S C 2000 Congenital heart disease in pregnancy. Cardiology Reviews 8: 166–173

Connolly H M, Warnes C A 1994 Ebstein's anomaly: outcome of pregnancy. Journal of the American College of Cardiology 23: 1194–1198

Connolly H M, Grogan M, Warnes C A 1999 Pregnancy among women with congenitally corrected transposition of the great arteries. Journal of the American College of Cardiology 33: 1692–1695

Corone S, Davido A, Lang T, Corone P 1992 Outcome of patients with Eisenmenger syndrome: a report of 62 cases followed up for an average of 16 years. Archives des Maladies du Coeur et des Vaisseaux 85: 521–526

Coulson C C, Kuller J A, Bowes S A 1995 Myocardial infarction and coronary artery dissection in pregnancy. American Journal of Perinatology 12: 328–330

Coven G, Zizzi S, Cimino F et al 1994 Electric cardioversion in pregnant patients with obstructive hypertrophic cardiomyopathy: a clinical case. Minerva Anestesiologica 60: 725–728

Cox S M, Leveno K J 1989 Pregnancy complicated by bacterial endocarditis. Clinical Obstetrics and Gynecology 32: 48–53

Cunningham F G, Pritchard J A, Hankins G D V et al 1986 Peripartum heart failure: idiopathic cardiomyopathy or compounding cardiovascular events. Obstetrics and Gynecology 67: 157–167

Daliento L, Somerville J, Presbitero P et al 1998 Eisenmenger syndrome: factors relating to deterioration and death. European Heart Journal 19: 1845–1855

Dalvi D B, Chaudhuri A, Kulkarni H L, Kale P A 1992 Therapeutic guidelines for congenital complete heart block presenting in pregnancy. Obstetrics and Gynecology 79: 802–804

Darbois Y, Seebacher J, Vauthier-Brouzes O et al 1991 Transplantations cardiaques: repercussions sur la fecondite feminine. Bulletin de l'Academie National de la Medecine 175: 531–540

Dave S P, Reis E D, Hossain A et al 2000 Splenic artery aneurysm in the 1990's. Annals of Vascular Surgery 14: 223–229

Davies M J, Parker D J, Bonella D 1981 Collagen synthesis in floppy mitral valve. Abstract, Proceedings of the British Cardiac Society. British Heart Journal 45: 345

Dayton H, Helgerson R B, Sollinger H W, Archer C W 1990 Ruptured renal artery aneurysm in a pregnant uninephric patient: successful ex vivo repair and auto transplantation. Surgery 107: 708–711

De Andrade J, Maldonado M, Pontes S 2001 Papel de la valvuloplastia por cateter-balon durante el embarazo en mujeres portadoras de estenosis mitral reumatica. Revista Espanola de Cardiologia 54: 573–579

De Backer T L, De Buyzere M L, De Potter C R, Gheeraert P J, Clement D L 1999 Primary pulmonary hypertension with fatal outcome in a young woman and review of the literature. Acta Cardiologica 54: 31–39

Deal K, Wooley C F 1973 Coarctation of aorta and pregnancy. Annals of Internal Medicine 78: 706–710

Deiml R, Hess W, Bahlmann E 2000 Primare Sectio caesara Vorgehen bei einer Patientin mit Hypertropher Obstruktiver Kardiomyopathie unter Verwendung von Pheyleohrin. Anaesthesist 49: 527–531

Demakis J G, Rahimtoola S H 1971 Peripartum cardiomyopathy. Circulation 44: 964–968

Demakis J G, Rahimtoola S H, Sutton G C et al 1971 Natural course of peripartum cardiomyopathy. Circulation 44: 1053–1061

Desai D, Moodley J, Naidoo D 1995 Peripartum cardiomyopathy: experience at King Edward VIII Hospital, Durban, South Africa and review of the literature. Tropical Doctor 25: 118–123

Desai D K, Adanlawo M, Naidoo D P, Moodley J, Kleinschmidt I 2000 Mitral stenosis in pregnancy: a four year experience at King Edward VIII Hospital, Durban, South Africa. British Journal of Obstetrics and Gynaecology 107: 953–958

Dietz H C, Cutting G R, Pyeritz R E et al 1991 Marfan syndrome caused by a recurrent de novo missense mutation in the fibrillin gene. Nature 352: 337–339

Donnelly J E, Brown J M, Radford D J 1991 Pregnancy outcome and Ebstein's anomaly. British Heart Journal 66: 368–371

Easterling T R, Chadwick H S, Otto C M, Benedetti C J 1988 Aortic stenosis in pregnancy. Obstetrics and Gynecology 72: 113–118

Easterling T R, Ralph D D, Schmucker B C 1999 Pulmonary hypertension in pregnancy: treatment with pulmonary vasodilators. Obstetrics and Gynecology 93: 494–498

Ebrahami R, Leung C Y, Elkayam U, Reid C L 1998 Infective endocarditis. In: Elkayam U, Gleicher N (eds) Cardiac problems in pregnancy, 3rd edn. Wiley-Liss, New York, pp 191–198

Eddy W A, Frankenfeld R H 1977 Congenital complete heart block in pregnancy. American Journal of Obstetrics and Gynecology 128: 223–225

Edwards J E 1960 In: Gould S E (ed) Pathology of the heart, 2nd edn. Thomas, Springfield, Ill, p 449

Ehrenfeld E N, Brezizinsky I A, Braon K, Sadowsky E, Sadowski A 1964 Heart disease in pregnancy. Obstetrics and Gynecology 23: 363–371

Elkayam U, Dave R 1998 Hypertrophic cardiomyopathy and pregnancy. In: Elkayam U, Gleicher N (eds) Cardiac problems in pregnancy, 3rd edn. Wiley-Liss, New York, pp 101–109

Elkayam U, Gleicher N 1998 Hemodynamics and cardiac function during normal pregnancy and the puerperium. In: Elkayam U, Gleicher N (eds) Cardiac problems in pregnancy, 3rd edn. Wiley-Liss, New York, pp 3–19

Elkayam U, Hameed A 1998a Vascular dissections and aneurysms during pregnancy. In: Elkayam U, Gleicher N (eds) Cardiac problems in pregnancy, 3rd edn. Wiley-Liss, New York, pp 201–209

Elkayam U, Hameed A 1998b Takayasu's arteritis and pregnancy. In: Elkayam U, Gleicher N (eds) Cardiac problems in pregnancy, 3rd edn. Wiley-Liss, New York, pp 237–245

Elkayam U, Kahn, S S 1998 Pregnancy in the patient with artificial heart valve. In: Elkayam U, Gleicher N (eds) Cardiac problems in pregnancy, 3rd edn. Wiley-Liss, New York, pp 61–78

Elkayam U, Dave R, Bokhari W H 1998a Primary pulmonary hypertension and pregnancy. In: Elkayam U, Gleicher N (eds) Cardiac problems in pregnancy, 3rd edn. Wiley-Liss New York, pp 183–190

Elkayam U, Ostrzega E, Shotan A, Mehra A 1998b Marfan syndrome and pregnancy. In: Elkayam U, Gleicher N (eds) Cardiac problems in pregnancy, 3rd edn. Wiley-Liss, New York, pp 211–221

Esteves C A, Ramos A I, Braga S L et al 1991 Effectiveness of percutaneous balloon mitral valvotomy during pregnancy. American Journal of Cardiology 68: 930–934

Faruque A A 1965 Acute fulminating puerperal myocarditis. British Heart Journal 27: 139–143

Fawzy M E, Kinsara A J, Stefadouros M et al 2001 Long term outcome of mitral balloon valvotomy in pregnant women. Journal of Heart Valve Disease 10: 153–157

Felice P V, Salom I L, Levine R 1995 Bivalvular endocarditis complicating pregnancy: a case report and literature review. Angiology 46: 441–444

Fletcher E, Knox E W, Morton P 1967 Acute myocardial infarction in pregnancy. British Medical Journal 3: 586–588

Fletcher A P, Alkjaersig N K, Burstein R 1979 The influence of pregnancy upon blood coagulation and plasma fibrinolytic enzyme function. American Journal of Obstetrics and Gynecology 134: 743–751

Frenkel Y, Barkai G, Reisin L, Rath S, Mashiach S, Battler A 1991 Pregnancy after myocardial infarction: are we playing safe? Obstetrics and Gynecology 77: 822–825

Fulton R M, Hutchinson E C, Jones A M 1952 Ventricular weight in cardiac hypertrophy. British Heart Journal 14: 413–420

Garcia Leon J F, von der Meden-Alarcon W, Buganza del Castillo A, Ibarrola-Buenabad E, Kably-Ambe A 1993 Hypertrophic cardiomyopathy and pregnancy: presentation of a case and review of the literature. Ginecologia y Obstetricia de Mexico 61: 160–162

Garini O, Astorri E, Cimolato B, Bonifazi C, Bianchi C, Ferrari O 1995 Bacterial endocarditis in pregnancy: report of a clinical case diagnosed postpartum. Minerva Cardioangiologie 43: 443–447

Genoni M, Jenni R, Hoerstrup S P, Vogt P, Turina M 1999 Pregnancy after atrial repair for transposition of the great arteries. Heart 81: 276–277

Gilchrist A R 1963 Cardiological problems in younger women: including that of pregnancy and the puerperium. British Medical Journal 1: 209–216

Glantz J C, Pomerantz R M, Cunningham M J, Woods J R 1993 Percutaneous balloon valvulotomy of severe mitral stenosis during pregnancy: a review of the therapeutic options. Obstetrical and Gynecological Survey 48: 503–508

Gleicher N, Midwall I, Hoenberger D, Jaffin H 1979 Eisenmenger's syndrome and pregnancy. Obstetrical and Gynecological Survey 34: 721–741

Goodwin J F 1958 Pregnancy and coarctation of the aorta. Lancet 1: 16–20

Goodwin J F 1975 Peripartal heart disease. Clinical Obstetrics and Gynecology 18: 125–131

Gordon C F, Johnson M D 1993 Anaesthetic management of the pregnant woman with Marfan syndrome. Journal of Clinical Anaesthesia 5: 248–251

Gupta A, Lokhandwala Y Y, Satoskar P R, Salvi V S 1998 Balloon mitral valvotomy in pregnancy: maternal and fetal outcomes. American Journal of Cardiology 82: 786–788

Hagley M T, Shaub T F 1993 Acute pericarditis with a symptomatic pericardial effusion complicating pregnancy. Journal of Reproductive Medicine 38: 813–814

Hanania G, Thomas D, Michel P L et al 1994 Grossesses chex les porteuses de prostheses valvularies: etude cooperative retrospective francais (155 cas). Archives des Maladies du Coeur et des Vaisseaux 87: 429–437

Hankins G D V, Wendel D G, Leveno K J, Stoneham J 1985 Myocardial infarction in pregnancy: a review. Obstetrics and Gynecology 65: 139–146

Haugen G, Aass H, Ihlen H et al 1998 Pregnancy in heart and heart–lung transplant recipients. Acta Obstetricia et Gynecologica Scandinavica 77: 574–576

Hauth J C, Cunningham G J, Young B K 1977 Takayasu's syndrome in pregnancy. Obstetrics and Gynecology 59: 373–374

Heider A L, Kuller J A, Strauss R A, Wells S R 1999 Peripartum cardiomyopathy: a review of the literature. Obstetrical and Gynecological Survey 54: 526–531

Hennessy T G, MacDonald D, Hennessy M S et al 1996 Serial changes in cardiac output during normal pregnancy: a Doppler ultrasound study. European Journal of Obstetrics, Gynecology and Reproductive Biology 70: 117–122

Hess D B, Hess L W 1992 Management of cardiovascular disease in pregnancy. Obstetrics and Gynecology Clinics of North America 19: 679–695

Hibbard L T 1975 Maternal mortality due to cardiac disease. Clinical Obstetrics and Gynecology 18: 27–36

Hibbard J U, Lindheimer M, Lang R M, 1999 A modified definition for peripartum cardiomyopathy and prognosis based on endocardiography. Obstetrics and Gynecology 94: 311–316

Holdsworth R J, Gunn A 1992 Ruptured splenic artery aneurysm in pregnancy: a review. British Journal of Obstetrics and Gynaecology 99: 595–597

Hsieh C C, Chiang C W, Hsieh T T, Soong Y K 1992 Peripartum cardiomyopathy. Japanese Heart Journal 33: 343–349

Irons D W, Pollard K P 1993 Post partum haemorrhage secondary to Marfan's disease of the uterine vasculature. British Journal of Obstetrics and Gynaecology 100: 279–281

Ishikawa K, Matsuura S 1982 Occlusive thromboaortopathy (Takayasu's disease) and pregnancy: clinical course and management of 33 pregnancies and deliveries. American Journal of Cardiology 50: 1293–1300

Jana N, Vasishta K, Khunnu B, Dhall G I, Grover A 1993 Pregnancy in association with mitral valve prolapse. Asia-Oceania Journal of Obstetrics and Gynaecology 19: 61–65

Jones A M, Howitt G 1965 Eisenmenger syndrome in pregnancy. British Medical Journal 1: 1627–1631

Jonge M J M de, Knipscheer R J J L, Weigel H M 1983 Takayasu's or pulseless disease in pregnancy. European Journal of Obstetrics, Gynecology and Reproductive Biology 14: 241–249

Joseph S G 1987 Peripartum cardiomyopathy: successful treatment with cardiac transplantation. Western Journal of Medicine 146: 230–232

Kainulainen K, Sakai L Y, Child A et al 1992 Two mutations in Marfan syndrome resulting in truncated fibrillin polypeptides. Proceeding of the National Academy of Sciences USA 89: 5917–5921

Kangavari S, Collins J, Cereek B, Atar S, Siegel R 2000 Tricuspid valve group B streptococcal endocarditis after an elective termination of pregnancy. Clinical Cardiology 23: 301–303

Kazimuddin M, Vashist A, Basher A W, Brown E J, Alhaddad I A 1998 Pregnancy-related severe left ventricular systolic dysfunction in a patient with hypertrophic cardiomyopathy. Clinical Cardiology 21: 848–850

Keene R J, Steiner R E, Olsen E G J, Oakley C 1971 Aortic root aneurysm — radiographic and pathologic features. Clinical Radiology 22: 330–340

Keogh A, McDonald P, Spratt P, Marshman D, Larbalestier R, Kaan A 1994 Outcome in peripartum cardiomyopathy after heart transplantation. Journal of Heart and Lung Transplantation 13: 202–207

Key T C, Resnik R, Dittrich H C, Reisner L S 1989 Successful pregnancy after cardiac transplantation. American Journal of Obstetrics and Gynecology 160: 367–371

Kirk E P 1991 Organ transplantation and pregnancy: a case report and review. American Journal of Obstetrics and Gynecology 164: 1629–1634

Kolibash A J Jr 1988 Natural history of mitral valve prolapse. In: Boudoulas H, Wolley C F (eds) Mitral valve prolapse and the mitral valve prolapse syndrome. Futura, Mount Kisco, New York, pp 257–275

Konishi Y, Tatsuta N, Kumada K et al 1980 Dissecting aneurysm during pregnancy and the puerperium. Japanese Circulation Journal 44: 726–733

Knapp R C, Arditi L I 1968 Closed mitral valvulotomy in pregnancy. Clinical Obstetrics and Gynecology 11: 928–931

Koul A K, Hollander G, Moskovits N, Frankel R, Herrera L, Shani J 2001 Coronary artery dissection during pregnancy and the postpartum period: two case reports and review of the literature. Catheterization and Cardiovascular Interventions 50: 280–284

Kraus Z Y, Naparstek E, Eliakim M 1978 Idiopathic pericarditis and pregnancy. Australian and New Zealand Journal of Obstetrics and Gynaecology 18: 86–89

Kulka P J, Scheu C, Tryba M, Grunewald R, Wiebalck A, Oberheiden R 2001 Myokardinfarke in der Schwangerschaft. Anaesthesist 50: 280–284

Leading Article 1976 Peripartum cardiac failure. British Medical Journal 1: 302–303

Lang R M, Lampert M B, Poppas A, Hameed A, Elkayam U 1998 Peripartal cardiomyopathy In: Elkayam U, Gleicher N (eds) Cardiac problems in pregnancy, 3rd edn. Wiley-Liss, New York, pp 87–100

Lao T T, Sermer M, McGee L et al 1993a Congenital aortic stenosis. American Journal of Obstetrics and Gynecology 169: 540–545

Lao T T, Adelman A G, Sermer M, Colman J M 1993b Balloon valvuloplasty for congenital aortic stenosis in pregnancy. British Journal of Obstetrics and Gynaecology 100: 1141–1142

Lao T T, Sermer M, Colman J M 1994 Pregnancy following surgical correction for transposition of the great arteries. Obstetrics and Gynecology 83: 665–668

Lecuru F, Taurelle R, Desnos M 1993 Anticoagulant treatment and pregnancy: a propos of 47 cases. Annales de Cardiologie et de l'Angiologie 42: 465–470

Lee C N, Wu C C, Lin P Y, Hsieh F J, Chen H Y 1994 Pregnancy following cardiac prosthetic valve replacement. Obstetrics and Gynecology 83: 353–356

Lee W, Cotton D B 1989 Peripartum cardiomyopathy: current concepts and clinical management. Clinical Obstetrics and Gynecology 32: 54–67

Low J, Grange C 1999 Anaesthesia for caesarean section in severe pulmonary hypertension. British Journal of Anaesthesia 82: 809

Lung B, Cormier B, Elias J et al 1994 Usefulness of percutaneous balloon commissurotomy for mitral stenosis during pregnancy. American Journal of Cardiology 73: 398–400

Lynch-Salamon D I, Maze S S, Combs C A 1993 Pregnancy after Mustard repair for transposition of the great arteries. Obstetrics and Gynecology 82: 676–679

Maarek-Charbit M, Corone P 1986 Consultation de medicine: Hospital de ia Pitie. Arch Maladies Coeur 79: 733–740

McAnulty J H, Metcalfe J, Ueland K 1981 General guidelines in the management of cardiac disease. Clinical Obstetrics and Gynecology 24: 773–788

McAnulty J H, Metcalfe J, Ueland K 1982 Cardiovascular disease. In: Burrow G N, Ferris T F (eds) Medical complications during pregnancy. Saunders, Philadelphia, pp 145–168

McColgin S W, Martin J N, Morrison J C 1989 Pregnant women with prosthetic heart valves. Clinical Obstetrics and Gynecology 32: 76–88

McIvor R A 1991 Percutaneous balloon aortic valvuloplasty during pregnancy. International Journal of Cardiology 32: 1–4

MacMahon S W, Roberts J K, Kramer-Fix R, Zucker D M, Roberts R B, Devereux R B 1987 Mitral valve prolapse and infective endocarditis. American Heart Journal 113: 1281–1290

Mandel W, Evans E W, Walford R L 1954 Dissecting aortic aneurysm during pregnancy. New England Journal of Medicine 251: 1059–1061

Markiewizc W, Stoner J, London E, Hunt S A, Popp R L 1976 Mitral valve prolapse in one hundred presumably healthy young females. Circulation 53: 464–473

Marks A R, Choong C U, Sanfilippo S J 1989 Identification of high risk and low risk subgroups of patients with mitral valve prolapse. New England Journal of Medicine 320: 1032

Maron B J, Ferrans V J 1975 Intramitochondrial glycogen deposits in hypertrophied human myocardium. Journal of Molecular and Cellular Cardiology 7: 697–702

Mayet J, Steer P, Somervile J 1998 Marfan syndrome, aortic dilatation, and pregnancy. Obstetrics and Gynecology 92: 713

Meadows W R 1960 Postpartum heart disease. American Journal of Cardiology 6: 788–802

Mecacci F, La Torre P, Parretti E et al 2000 Pericardite acuta in gravidanza: descrizione di un caso. Minerva Ginecologica 52: 259–262

Megerian G, Bell J G, Huhta J C, BoHallico J N, Weimer S 1994 Pregnancy outcome following Mustard procedure for transposition of the great arteries: a report of five cases and review of the literature. Obstetrics and Gynecology 83: 512–516

Mendelson C L 1951 Acute isolated myocarditis in pregnancy. American Journal of Obstetrics and Gynecology 61: 1341–1347

Meyer E C, Tulsky A S, Sigmann P, Silber E N 1964 Pregnancy in the presence of tetralogy of Fallot: observations on the patients. American Journal of Cardiology 14: 874–879

Milewcz D M, Pyeritz R E, Crawford E S, Byers P H 1991 Marfan syndrome: defective synthesis, secretion and extracellular formation of fibrillin by cultured dermal fibroblasts. Journal of Clinical Investigation 88: 79–86

Minnich M E, Quirk J G, Clark R B 1987 Epidural anaesthesia for vaginal delivery in a patient with idiopathic hypertrophic subaortic stenosis. Anesthesiology 67: 590–592

Mokaddem A, Bachraoui K, Selmi K, Kachboura S, Boujnah M R 2000 Cardiomyopathie hypertrophique et grossesse. Tunisie Medical 78: 682–684

Morini A, Spina V, Aleandri V, Cantonetti G, Lambiasi A, Papalia U 1998 Pregnancy after heart transplant: update and case report. Human Reproduction 13: 749–757

Mortensen J D, Ellsworth H S 1965 Coarctation of the aorta and pregnancy. Journal of the American Medical Association 191: 596–598

Naeye R, Hagstrom J W C, Talmadge B A 1967 Postpartum death with maternal congenital heart disease. Circulation 36: 304–312

Nolan T E, Hankins G D V 1989 Myocardial infarction in pregnancy. Clinical Obstetrics and Gynecology 32: 68–75

Oakley G D G, McGarry K, Limb D G, Oakley C M 1979 Management of pregnancy in patients with hypertrophic cardiomyopathy. British Medical Journal 1: 1749–1750

O'Driscoll M K, Coyle C F V, Drury M I 1962 Rheumatic heart disease complicating pregnancy: the remote prospect. British Medical Journal 2: 767–768

O'Grady J P, Day E J, Toole A L, Paust J C 1977 Splenic artery aneurysm rupture in pregnancy. Obstetrics and Gynecology 50: 627–630

O'Hare R, McLoughlin C, Milligan K, McNamee D, Sidhin H 1998 Anaesthesia for caesarean section in the presence of severe primary pulmonary hypertension. British Journal of Anaesthesia 81: 790–792

Oliver M F, Boyd C S 1955 Plasma lipid and serum lipoprotein patterns during pregnancy and the puerperium. Clinical Science 14: 15–23

Olofsson C, Bremme K, Forsesell G, Ohqvist G 2001 Caesarean section under epidural ropivacaine 0.75% in a parturient with severe pulmonary hypertension. Acta Anaesthesiologica Scandinavica 45: 258–260

Olsen E G J 1972 Cardiomyopathies. In: Edwards J E, Brest A N (eds) Cardiovascular clinics. Clinical-pathologic correlations 1. Davis, Philadelphia, pp 239–261

Olsen E G J 1975a Cardiovascular system. In: Harrison C V, Weinbren K (eds) Recent advances in pathology, vol 9. Churchill Livingstone, London, pp 1–15

Olsen E G J 1975b Marfan's disease. Pathologica et Microbiologica 43: 120–123

Olsen E G J 1980a The pathology of the heart, 2nd edn. Macmillan Press, Basingstoke

Olsen E G J 1980b The pathology of idiopathic hypertrophic subaortic stenosis (hypertrophic cardiomyopathy): a critical review. American Heart Journal 100: 553–562

Olsen E G J, Al-Rufaie H K 1980 The floppy mitral valve: study on pathogenesis. British Heart Journal 44: 674–683

Onderoglu L, Tuncer Z S, Oto A, Durukan T 1995 Balloon valvuloplasty during pregnancy. International Journal of Gynaecology and Obstetrics 49: 181–183

Oskoui R, Lindsay J Jr 1994 Aortic dissection in women < 40 years of age and the unimportance of pregnancy. American Journal of Cardiology 73: 821–823

Pavankumar P, Venugopal P, Kaul U et al 1988 Pregnancy in patients with prosthetic cardiac valve: a 10-year experience. Scandinavian Journal of Thoracic and Cardiovascular Surgery. 8: 221–224.

Payne D C, Fishburne J I, Rufty A J, Johnston F R 1982 Bacterial endocarditis in pregnancy. Obstetrics and Gynecology 60: 247–250

Pelliccia F, Cianfrocca L, Gaudio C, Reale A 1992 Sudden death during pregnancy in hypertrophic cardiomyopathy. European Heart Journal 13: 421–423

Penning S, Thomas N, Arwal D, Nageotte M, McConnell D 2001 Cardiopulmonary bypass support for emergency cesarean delivery in a patient with severe pulmonary hypertension. American Journal of Obstetrics and Gynecology 184: 225–226

Perloff J K 1994 Congenital heart disease and pregnancy. Clinical Cardiology 17: 579–587

Piacenza J M, Kirkorian G, Audra P H, Mellier G 1998 Hypertrophic cardiomyopathy and pregnancy. Euopean Journal of Obstetrics, Gynecology and Reproductive Biology 80: 17–23

Pitkin R M, Perloff J K, Koos B J, Beall M H 1990 Pregnancy and congenital heart disease. Annals of Internal Medicine 112: 445–454

Presbitero P, Somerville J, Stone S, Aruta E, Spiegelhalter D, Rabajoli F 1994 Pregnancy in cyanotic congenital heart disease: outcome of mother and fetus. Circulation 89: 2673–2676

Presbitero P, Rabajoli F, Somerville J 1995 Pregnancy in patients with congenital heart disease. Schweizerische Medizineische Wochenschrift 125: 311–315

Pritchard J A 1953 Coarctation of the aorta and pregnancy. Obstetrical and Gynecological Survey 8: 775–791

Probst R, Mier T 1963 Acute pericarditis complicating pregnancy. Obstetrics and Gynecology 22: 393–395

Procacci P M, Savran S V, Schreiter S L, Bryson A L 1976 Prevalence of clinical mitral-valve prolapse in 1169 young women. New England Journal of Medicine 294: 1086–1088

Pyeritz R E 1981 Maternal and fetal complications of pregnancy in the Marfan syndrome. American Journal of Medicine 71: 784–790

Ramin S M, Maberry M C, Gilstrap L C 1989 Congenital heart disease. Clinical Obstetrics and Gynecology 32: 41–47

Rao K 1992 Pregnancy and Takayasu's aorto-arteritis. Journal of the Indian Medical Association 90: 107

Rayburn W F 1998 Mitral valve prolapse and pregnancy. In: Elkayam U, Gleicher N (eds) Cardiac problems in pregnancy, 3rd edn. Wiley-Liss New York, pp 175–182

Rayburn W F, Fontana M E 1981 Mitral valve prolapse and pregnancy. American Journal of Obstetrics and Gynecology 141: 9–11

Rayburn W F, LeMire M S, Bird J L, Buda A 1987 Mitral valve prolapse: echocardiographic changes during pregnancy. Journal of Reproductive Medicine 32: 185–187

Richardson A J, Liddington M, Jaskowski A, Murie J A, Gillmer M, Morris P J 1990 Pregnancy in a renal transplant recipient complicated by rupture of a transplant renal artery aneurysm. British Journal of Surgery 77: 228–229

Rijbroek A, Van Dijk H A, Roex A J 1994 Rupture of renal artery aneurysm during pregnancy. European Journal of Vascular Surgery 8: 375–376

Robinson J N, Banerjee R, Landzberg M J, Thiet M P 1999 Inhaled nitric oxide therapy in pregnancy complicated by pulmonary hypertension. American Journal of Obstetrics and Gynecology 180: 1045–1046

Rosenthal L 1955 Coarctation of the aorta and pregnancy: report of 5 cases. British Medical Journal 1: 16–18

Rossiter J P, Repke J T, Morales A J, Murphy E A, Pyeritz R R E 1995 A prospective longitudinal evaluation of pregnancy in the Marfan syndrome. American Journal of Obstetrics and Gynecology 173: 1599–1606

Roth A, Elkayam U 1996 Acute myocardial infarction associated with pregnancy. Annals of Internal Medicine 125: 751–762

Roth A, Elkayam U 1998 Acute myocardial infarction and pregnancy. In: Elkayam U, Gleicher N (eds) Cardiac problems in pregnancy, 3rd edn. Wiley-Liss, New York, pp 131–155

Rousseil M P, Irion O, Begium F et al 1995 Successful term pregnancy after Mustard operation for transposition of the great arteries. European Journal of Obstetrics, Gynecology and Reproductive Biology 59: 111–113

Rubin L J 1997 Primary pulmonary hypertension. New England Journal of Medicine 336: 111–117

Sadler L, McCowan L, White H, Stewart A, Bracken M, North R 2000 Pregnancy outcomes and cardiac complications in women with mechanical, bioprosthetic and homograft valves. British Journal of Obstetrics and Gynaecology 107: 245–253

Saidi A S, Bezold L I, Altman C A, Ayres N A, Bricker J T 1998 Outcome of pregnancy following intervention for coarctation of the aorta. American Journal of Cardiology 82: 786–788

Salazar E, Izaguirre R, Verdejo J, Mutchinick O 1996 Failure of adjusted doses of subcutaneous heparin to prevent thromboembolic phenomena in pregnant patients with mechanical cardiac valve prostheses. Journal of the American College of Cardiology 27: 1698–1703

Samuels L E, Kaufman M S, Morris R J, Brockman S K 1998 Postpartum coronary artery dissection: emergency coronary artery bypass with ventricular assist device support. Coronary Artery Disease 9: 457–460

Sareli P, England M J, Berk M R 1989 Maternal and fetal sequelae of anticoagulation during pregnancy in patients with mechanical heart valve prostheses. American Journal of Cardiology 63: 1462–1465

Sawhney H, Suri V, Vasishta K Gupta N, Devi K, Grover A 1998 Pregnancy and congenital heart disease — maternal and fetal outcome. Australian and New Zealand Journal of Obstetrics and Gynaecology 3: 266–271

Sbarouni E, Oakley C M 1993 Outcome of pregnancy in women with valve prostheses. British Heart Journal 71: 196–201

Schmaltz A A, Neudorf U, Winkler U H 1999 Outcome of pregnancy in women with congenital heart disease. Cardiology of the Young 9: 88–96

Shaper A G 1966 Fibrinolytic activity in pregnancy, during parturition and the puerperium. Lancet ii: 874–876

Shaper A G 1968 Platelet function. Lancet i: 642–643

Shaper A G, Macintosh D M, Kyobe J 1965 Fibrinolysis and plasminogen levels in pregnancy and the puerperium. Lancet 2: 706–708

Shapiro E, Trimble E, Robinson J, Estruch M, Gottlieb S 1985 Safety of labor and delivery in women with mitral valve prolapse. American Journal of Cardiology 56: 806–807

Sharma B K, Jain S, Vasishta K 2000 Outcome of pregnancy in Takayasu's arteritis. International Journal of Cardiology 75: Supplement 1, S159–S162

Shaver P J, Carrig T F, Baker W P 1978 Postpartum coronary artery disease. British Heart Journal 40: 83–86

Shime J, Mocarski E J M, Hastings O et al 1987 Congenital heart disease in pregnancy: short and long term implications. American Journal of Obstetrics and Gynecology 156: 313–322

Simpson W G, DePriest P D, Conover W B 1989 Acute pericarditis complicated by cardiac tamponade during pregnancy. American Journal of Obstetrics and Gynecology 160: 415–416

Singh H, Bolton P J, Oakley C M 1982 Pregnancy after surgical correction of tetralogy of Fallot. British Medical Journal 285: 168–170

Smith V C, Eckenbrecht P D, Hankins D V, Leach C I 1989 Marfan's syndrome, pregnancy and the cardiac surgeon. Military Medicine 154: 404–406

Stewart R, Tuazon D, Olson G, Duarte A G 2001 Pregnancy and primary pulmonary hypertension: successful outcome with epoprostenol therapy. Chest 119: 973–975

Sutton M S, Cole P, Piappert M, Saltzman D, Goldhaber S 1991 Effects of subsequent pregnancy on left ventricular cardiomyopathy. American Heart Journal 121: 1776–1778

Szekely P, Turner R, Snaith L 1973 Pregnancy and the changing pattern of rheumatic heart disease. British Heart Journal 35: 1293–1303

Takeuchi K, Yokota H, Moryama T, Ideta K, Maruo T 1998 Two cases of primary pulmonary hypertension diagnosed during pregnancy. Journal of Perinatal Medicine 26: 248–251

Tang L, Chang S, Wong V, Ma H 1985 Pregnancy in patients with mitral valve prolapse. International Journal of Gynaecology and Obstetrics 23: 217–221

Therrien J, Barnes I, Somerville J 1999 Outcome of pregnancy in patients with congenitally corrected transposition of the great arteries. American Journal of Cardiology 84: 820–824

Tessler M J, Hudson R, Naugler M A, Biel D R 1990 Pulmonary oedema in two parturients with hypertrophic obstructive cardiomyopathy (HOCM). Canadian Journal of Anaesthesia 37: 469–473

Thomas D, Boubrit K, Darbois Y, Seebacher J, Seirafi D, Hannania G 1994 Pregnancy in patients with heart valve prosthesis: retrospective study a propos of 40 pregnancies. Annales de Cardiologie et Angiologie 43: 313–321

Trastek V F, Pairolero P C, Bernatz P E 1985 Splenic artery aneurysms. World Journal of Surgery 9: 378–383

Ueland K 1978 Cardiovascular diseases complicating pregnancy. Clinical Obstetrics and Gynecology 21: 429–442

Ueland K 1984 Cardiac diseases. In: Creasy R K, Resnik R (eds) Maternal fetal medicine. W B Saunders, Philadelphia, p 691

Ueland K, Metcalfe J 1975 Circulatory changes in pregnancy. Clinical Obstetrics and Gynecology 18: 41–50

Uetsuka Y, Higashidate N, Aosaki M et al 1990 Fifteen year experience with 24 pregnancies associated with prosthetic valve replacement. Journal of Cardiology 20: 929–935

Van Kasteren Y M, Kleinhout J, Smit M A, van Vugt J M G, van Geijn H P 1991 Hypertrophic cardiomyopathy and pregnancy: report of three cases. European Journal of Obstetrics, Gynecology and Reproductive Biology 38: 63–67

Vassalotti S B, Schaller J A 1967 Spontaneous rupture of splenic artery aneurysm during pregnancy: report of first known antepartum rupture with maternal and fetal survival. Obstetrics and Gynecology 30: 264–268

Vielle J C 1984 Peripartum cardiomyopathies: a review. American Journal of Obstetrics and Gynecology 148: 805–818

Vongpatanasin W, Brickner M E, Hillis L D, Lange R A 1998 The Eisenmenger syndrome in adults. Annals of Internal Medicine 128: 745–755

Vosloo S, Reichart B 1987 The feasibility of closed mitral valvotomy in pregnancy. Journal of Thoracic and Cardiovascular Surgery 93: 675–679

Wagoner L, Taylor D, Olson S et al 1993 Immunosuppressive therapy, management and outcomes of heart transplant recipients during pregnancy. Journal of Heart and Lung Transplantation 12: 993–1000

Warnes C A, Elkayam U 1998 Congenital heart disease and pregnancy. In: Elkayam U, Gleicher N (eds) Cardiac problems in pregnancy, 3rd edn. Wiley-Liss, New York, pp 39–53

Watson H, Emslie-Smith D, Herring J, Hill I G W 1960 Myocardial infarction during pregnancy and puerperium. Lancet 2: 523–526

Weiss B M, Zemp L, Seifert B, Hess O M 1998 Outcome of pulmonary vascular disease in pregnancy: a systematic overview from 1978 through 1996. Journal of the American College of Cardiology 31: 1650–1657

Westaby S, Parry A J, Forfar J C 1992 Reoperation for prosthetic valve endocaritis in the third trimester of pregnancy. Annals of Thoracic Surgery 53: 363–365

Wilansky S, Belcic T, Osborn R, Carpenter R 1998 Hypertrophic cardiomyopathy in pregnancy: the use of two-dimensional and Doppler echocardiography during labor and delivery. Journal of Heart Valve Disease 7: 355–357

Winn H N, Setaro J F, Mazor M, Reece E A, Black H R, Hobbins J C 1988 Severe Tayakasu's arteritis in pregnancy: the role of central hemodynamic monitoring. American Journal of Obstetrics and Gynecology 159: 1135–1136

Witlin A G, Mabie W C, Sibai B M 1997 Peripartum cardiomyopathy: an ominous diagnosis. American Journal of Obstetrics and Gynecology 176: 182–188

Wooley C F, Sparks E H 1992 Congenital heart disease, heritable cardiovascular disease, and pregnancy. Progress in Cardiovascular Diseases 35: 41–60

Wooley R F, Hugh V R, Ryan J M 1961 Pregnancy and congenital heart disease (abstract). Circulation 24: 1075

Wong V, Cheng C H, Chan K C 1993 Fetal and neonatal outcome of exposure to anticoagulants during pregnancy. American Journal of Medical Genetics 45: 17–21

Yaryura R A, Carpenter R J, Duncan J M, Wilansky S 1996 Management of mitral valve stenosis in pregnancy: case presentation and review of the literature. Journal of Heart Valve Disease 5: 251–253

Zamprogno R, Neri G, Alitto F, Moro E, Sandri R 1990 Bacterial endocarditis in pregnancy: description of 2 cases and review of the literature. Minerva Cardioangiologie 38: 85–88

Zeek P M 1942 Heart weight I. The weight of the normal heart. Archives of Pathology 34: 820–832

Zeira M, Zohar S 1993 Pregnancy and delivery in women with coarctation of the aorta. Harefuah 124: 765–758

Zuber M, Gautschi N, Oechslin E, Widmer V, Kowski W, Jenni R 1999 The outcome of pregnancy in women with congenital shunt disease. Heart 81: 271–275

47

Pathology of maternal death

H. Fox

Introduction   1559

Classification of maternal deaths   1560

Direct obstetric deaths   1560
Specific causes of direct maternal death   1561

INTRODUCTION

The World Health Organization defines a maternal death as 'the death of a woman while pregnant or within 42 days of termination of pregnancy, irrespective of the duration or site of the pregnancy, from any cause related to or aggravated by the pregnancy or its management but not from accidental or incidental causes'. The Report on Confidential Enquiries into Maternal Deaths in the United Kingdom 1994–1996 (1998) adds to this definition a category of 'late maternal death' which applies to deaths occurring between 43 days and one year after delivery or miscarriage, this being necessary because of the current frequent prolongation of existence by life-support systems.

There can be no doubt that, in Western countries, maternal deaths have now declined to a very low rate, though it is difficult to obtain exact figures. This is due to a number of factors which include the use of different denominators (such as the number of women of reproductive age, the number of live births, the number of pregnancies), poor denominator data, a failure to identify maternal deaths because of coding errors, failure to include late maternal deaths, the inclusion of fortuitous deaths and the exclusion of deaths occurring in early pregnancy. Bouvier-Colle et al (1991) found that in France there was an under-reporting of 56% in the official statistics and that in other countries in Western Europe and the USA the underestimation of maternal deaths ranged from 17–63%. Clearly, therefore, official data and international comparisons have to be regarded with some scepticism but within these restraints the current maternal death rate in the United Kingdom is 12.2 per 100 000 maternities (Report on Confidential Enquiries into Maternal Deaths in the United Kingdom 1994–1996, 1998), a maternity being defined as 'a pregnancy that results in a live birth at any gestation or a stillbirth occurring at or after 24 completed weeks of gestation'. The quoted, but not strictly comparable, rates for other countries are 8.8 in the Netherlands, 9.1 in the

United States, 30 in all developed countries, 270 in Latin America, 420 in Asia and 640 in Africa (Hogberg 1985; Editorial 1987; Schuitemaker et al 1991; Grimes 1994).

In England and Wales the number of maternal deaths per million of the female population aged 15–44 years has fallen from 9.0 in 1973–75 to 4.3 in 1994–96 whilst the maternal mortality rate per 100 000 maternities appears to have risen from 9.9 in 1991–93 to 12.2 in 1994–96: the figures in 1994–1996 are, however, not strictly comparable to those in previous reports for the use of improved computer-based ascertainment systems has led to detection of extra cases which would not otherwise have been considered.

Because maternal deaths are now so uncommon in most Western countries few pathologists will have more than an extremely limited experience of conducting autopsies on such cases. Pathologists required to undertake such a post-mortem examination will, however, find a very useful guide in the reviews of this topic by Rushton & Dawson (1982), Shanklin et al (1991) and Toner (1992); in these, the authors point out that there is no special mystique to autopsies on maternal deaths, stress the importance of taking adequate material for histological examination and review the more important causes of death associated with pregnancy.

CLASSIFICATION OF MATERNAL DEATHS

Maternal deaths can be classified into three broad groups:

1. *Direct maternal deaths.* These are defined as 'those resulting from obstetric complications of the pregnant state (pregnancy, labour and puerperium), from interventions, omissions, incorrect treatment or from a chain of events resulting from any of the above'.
2. *Indirect maternal deaths.* Deaths in this category are defined as 'those resulting from previous existing disease, or from disease which developed during pregnancy and which was not due to direct obstetric causes, but was aggravated by the physiologic effects of pregnancy'.
3. *Fortuitous maternal deaths.* This group is formed of 'deaths which occur during pregnancy or the puerperium from causes not related to the pregnancy or its complications or its management'.

It should be noted that this classification is dependent upon accurate establishment of the cause of death, usually by autopsy study. In some countries, however, accurate data of this type can not be obtained and the category of *pregnancy-related death* applies to 'the death of a woman while pregnant or within 42 days of termination of pregnancy, irrespective of the cause of death', this categorisation being intended for those cases in which the cause of death can not be identified with precision.

The latest Report on Confidential Inquiries into Maternal Deaths in the United Kingdom (1998) covers the years 1994–96 and during this period there were complete details of 376 maternal deaths of which 134 (36%) were classed as direct, 134 (36%) as indirect, 36 (9%) as fortuitous and 72 (19%) as late. In this chapter only direct maternal deaths are considered. A majority of indirect maternal deaths are due to cardiovascular, hepatic, renal or neurological disorders and the pathology of these conditions is discussed in Chapters 43–46. Occasional indirect deaths are related to endocrine disorders, autoimmune diseases, blood dyscrasia and gastrointestinal disease: the interrelationships between medical conditions of this type and pregnancy are detailed in several comprehensive volumes (Burrow & Ferris 1982; de Swiet 1989; Reece et al 1992).

Little point would be served by considering fortuitous maternal deaths. The pregnant woman can fall prey to any of the ills that beset humanity and many of these diseases neither influence the pregnancy nor are themselves influenced by the gravid state. Suffice it to say that trauma is the commonest cause of fortuitous maternal death, both in the United Kingdom (Confidential Report 1998) and in the USA (Fildes et al 1992), and that malignant disease is the second commonest (Dinh & Warshal 2001).

DIRECT OBSTETRIC DEATHS

The main causes of direct maternal death in the United Kingdom during the years 1994–96 are detailed in Table 47.1: in many instances, of course, multiple factors were present which may have contributed to the demise of a particular woman but the table indicates the single factor which was thought to play the predominant rôle.

A comparison of the figures for 1994–96 with those in previous Confidential Reports shows that there has been a marked increase in deaths due to thromboembolism, an increase in deaths due to amniotic fluid embolism and sepsis, and a slight increase in deaths from uterine rupture and pregnancy-related hypertension since the early 1980s but a decrease in deaths related to anaesthesia and haemorrhage.

The figures for maternal deaths in the United Kingdom represent the most detailed analysis of maternal

Table 47.1 Main causes of direct maternal death in the United Kingdom 1994–96

Thrombosis and thromboembolism	48
Hypertensive diseases of pregnancy	20
Amniotic fluid embolism	17
Sepsis	14
Haemorrhage	12
Ectopic pregnancy	12
Anaesthetic-associated	1
Abortion	3
Ruptured uterus	2

mortality in any Western country; there are, almost certainly, minor differences in the pattern of disorders contributing to maternal mortality in other Western countries but nevertheless the figures for the United Kingdom are probably roughly representative for contemporary industrialised (or post-industrialised) Western countries. They are, however, far from being representative of the pattern encountered in lesser developed countries where there is a particularly high mortality rate from haemorrhage and sepsis (Duley 1992; Drife 2001).

SPECIFIC CAUSES OF DIRECT MATERNAL DEATH

Pulmonary thromboembolism

Approximately one-third of fatal cases of obstetric pulmonary thromboembolism occur during pregnancy and about two-thirds during the puerperium. About half of the puerperal deaths from this cause take place during the first two weeks after delivery (particularly during the first seven days) but nearly half occur between two and six weeks after delivery: occasional cases of fatal embolism are encountered more than six weeks after delivery.

Factors predisposing to thromboembolism during pregnancy and the puerperium include advancing age, increasing parity, obesity, a history of previous thromboembolism and delivery by Caesarean section (Tindall 1971; Ruckley 1992); some patients with a history of previous thromboembolic disease may have deficiencies of antithrombin III, protein C or protein S. Two groups of women thought to be at particular risk are those undergoing a surgical procedure, such as tubal ligation, during the puerperium and those in whom lactation has been suppressed by the administration of oestrogens (Daniel et al 1967; Jeffcoate et al 1968).

The pathological findings in obstetric cases of fatal pulmonary thromboembolism do not differ from those of this catastrophe in the non-pregnant patient. It is, however, mandatory that not only the legs be carefully examined for evidence of thrombosis but that attention also be directed towards the pelvic and ovarian veins.

Haemorrhage

Maternal death from haemorrhage is usually due to abruptio placentae, placenta praevia, postpartum bleeding or ruptured ectopic pregnancy; less common causes include a tear of the uterine wall, a tear of the cervix or a laceration of the vagina (Chamberlain 1992). In most autopsies on fatal cases of obstetric haemorrhage the pathological findings are quite straightforward, but in performing such an autopsy several points should be kept in mind:

1. In cases of known or suspected placenta praevia in which the placenta is still in situ the uterus and vagina should be removed as a single block and the uterus subsequently opened from the fundus, this allowing for a clear demonstration of a placenta covering the lower uterine segment or internal cervical os. If the fetus and placenta have been delivered the lower uterine segment should be carefully examined histologically for evidence of a placental site reaction.

2. In women thought to have died from abruptio placentae it is necessary to confirm the presence of retroplacental bleeding. If the placenta has been delivered it should be examined for either adherent thrombus or a depressed empty crater on the maternal surface. If the placenta is still within the uterus the blood may have tracked from the retroplacental area to extend widely into the myometrium, this producing one variety of the so-called 'Couvelaire uterus'.

3. In cases of postpartum bleeding with retained placenta the placental implantation site should be examined histologically for evidence of placenta accreta.

4. Postpartum bleeding after the placenta has been delivered is usually due to uterine atony (Watson 1980; Varner 1991; Chamberlain 1992) and the presence of small retained fragments of placental tissue should not be afforded undue significance.

5. Postpartum bleeding may be due to a coagulopathy. In most cases this is a consequence of a particular complication of pregnancy but occasionally postpartum bleeding is a manifestation of von Willebrand's disease or thrombocytopenic purpura (Watson 1980).

6. Relatively minor degree of postpartum blood loss per vaginam may be associated with large pelvic haematomas (Pieri 1958; Flegner 1971); these not uncommonly prove fatal because the internal nature of the haemorrhage results in late diagnosis.

7. Unrecognised amniotic fluid embolism may be responsible for severe postpartum bleeding. Careful histological study of the pulmonary vessels for evidence of amniotic fluid embolism is therefore essential in all cases of fatal postpartum haemorrhage.

8. Disseminated intravascular coagulation may complicate abruptio placentae and thus accentuate the severity of the haemorrhage. Histological evidence of intravascular fibrin deposition should therefore be sought for in all cases of fatal abruption.

Sepsis

Sepsis may complicate abortion, vaginal delivery or Caesarean section. Until relatively recently postabortal sepsis accounted for most obstetric deaths attributable to infection; the incidence of septic abortion has, however, fallen dramatically in England and Wales during the last few decades and there is now an approximately equal distribution of septic obstetric deaths between abortions, vaginal deliveries and Caesarean sections. In the United

States, however, maternal deaths from sepsis occur twice as commonly after Caesarean section as they do after vaginal delivery (Eschenbach & Wager 1980).

In many cases of maternal death from sepsis the autopsy findings are quite straightforward and include septic endometritis, myometrial abscesses, purulent salpingitis, pelvic peritonitis and septicaemia.

Several particular forms of obstetric sepsis do, however, merit further comment:

1. Puerperal sepsis. This, in its classical form, is now a rare complication of pregnancy in the Western world though the number of deaths from streptococcal puerperal sepsis in the United Kingdom appears to be slowly increasing (Drife 2001). More commonly, when infection complicates a vaginal delivery, sepsis is due to organisms which ascend from the birth canal: in many such cases there has been a prolonged rupture of the membranes and chorioamnionitis (Stevenson 1969) and it is therefore necessary in all cases of fatal puerperal sepsis to examine the placenta and membranes for evidence of an inflammatory process. When diagnosing a puerperal endometritis it is prudent to bear in mind that an apparently physiological leucocytic infiltration of the decidua occurs after most uncomplicated deliveries.

Although many cases of fatal puerperal sepsis are a result of infection with Gram-negative bacteria a minority are due to Clostridia: these organisms can produce a gas gangrene of the uterus and their entry into the bloodstream results in an acute haemolytic anaemia with jaundice, haemoglobinuria and renal failure.

2. Purulent pelvic phlebitis. This condition has a high mortality and is found in a significant proportion of women who die from puerperal infection. It is not related to phlebitis or phlebothrombosis of the leg veins or to bland thrombosis of the pelvic veins but is due to direct bacterial invasion of the pelvic venous plexuses. The bacteria damage the venous intima and this results in thrombosis (Collins et al 1951): the thrombi subsequently become colonised by bacteria and undergo partial liquefaction. The infection spreads directly along the venous wall and also along the perivenous lymphatics and can cause a rapidly spreading purulent phlebitis and a pelvic cellulitis. The infected pelvic veins are filled with a mixture of partially liquefied thrombus, tissue debris and inflammatory cells and there is a tendency for showers of small septic emboli to be thrown off to produce multiple metastatic abscesses (Collins et al 1951). Many emboli lodge in the pulmonary vasculature and, because they are small and multiple, produce a purulent pneumonitis rather than a typical pulmonary infarct.

Clinically, purulent pelvic phlebitis often develops between seven and 21 days after delivery, either in a woman who until then has appeared to be having a normal puerperium or in one who has persistent post-delivery infection. There is a sudden onset of chills, tachycardia and a swinging pyrexia, these symptoms soon being followed by respiratory complaints due to the multiple pulmonary emboli. Some patients present, however, with an acute onset of lower abdominal pain between two and five days after delivery (Eschenbach & Wager 1980).

3. Superficial fascial necrosis. This is an extremely dangerous complication of an episiotomy wound infection; the infecting organisms are usually either haemolytic streptococci or anaerobic bacteria whilst some cases are infected by both these groups of organisms. The superficial fascia in the region in which an episiotomy incision is made is continuous with that of the abdominal wall, buttocks and legs: hence infection and necrosis of the superficial fascia may extend to any, or all, of these sites, a situation associated with severe toxic symptoms and terminating, not uncommonly, in death (Golde & Ledger 1977; Ewing et al 1979; Shy & Eschenbach 1979). The involved areas are markedly oedematous and the overlying skin is discoloured and sometimes gangrenous. The necrotic fascia appears dull and grey.

4. Septic shock. This may complicate puerperal sepsis, gestational pyelonephritis or septic abortion. It is due to the entry of Gram-negative organisms into the bloodstream with subsequent release of endotoxins: these endotoxic substances are thought to be polysaccharide–lipid–protein complexes which are derived from the bacterial cell wall. The pregnant uterus offers extremely favourable conditions for the development of septic shock in so far as the dilated uterine veins and sinuses afford a readily accessible portal of entry for organisms into the maternal circulation.

The pathophysiology of septic shock is not yet fully understood but two important mechanisms appear to be implicated. Firstly, there is generalised vasoconstriction and impaired regional tissue perfusion, this being possibly due to the release of biogenic amines and kinins. Secondly, disseminated intravascular coagulation develops.

Clinically, septic shock is characterised by high fever and shock: in the early stages the patient is alert and flushed but later develops cold, clammy skin, mental confusion and progressive cardiac insufficiency.

At autopsy in such cases the principal findings are pelvic sepsis, fibrin thrombi in the renal glomerular capillaries, bilateral adrenal haemorrhage (a frequent but far from constant feature) and centrilobular hepatic necrosis (McCally & Vasicka 1962). In cases which have followed a vaginal delivery there is usually a chorioamnionitis, and Studdiford & Douglas (1956) have described a characteristic placental bacteraemia in which clumps of organisms are seen in the intervillous space.

Some patients appear to recover from the acute episode of shock but then develop progressive respiratory distress, this being due to the development of the adult respiratory distress syndrome (Hasleton 1983; Weiner-Kronish et al 1990). In fatal cases (Fig. 47.1) the lungs are heavy and show focal areas of airlessness and cerise discoloration (Corrin & Spencer 1981). Histologically

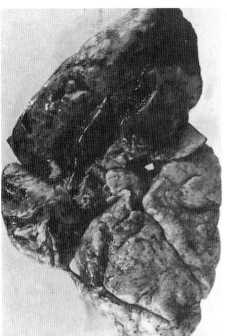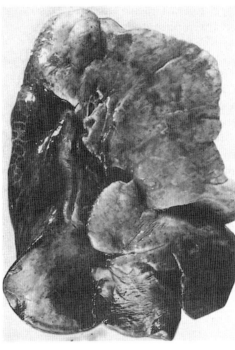

Fig. 47.1 Post-mortem appearances of the lungs in a case of septic shock. There are irregular areas of congestion and collapse. (From Corrin & Spencer 1981, courtesy of Professor B Corrin.)

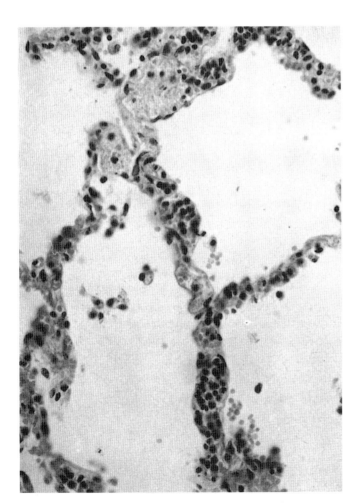

Fig. 47.2 Lungs in a case of septic shock. There is marked sequestration of polymorphs within the pulmonary capillaries. (From Corrin & Spencer 1981, courtesy of Professor B Corrin.)

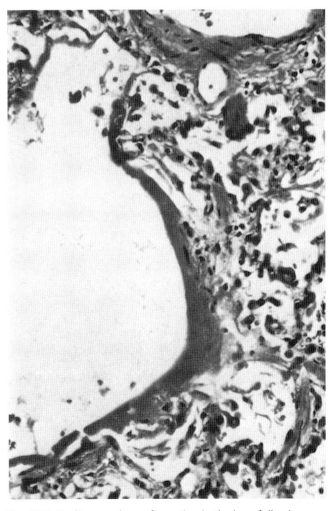

Fig. 47.3 Hyaline membrane formation in the lung following shock.(Courtesy of Dr P Hasleton and the Editor of Histopathology.)

there is, in the acute stage, intense congestion of the pulmonary capillaries, focal alveolar collapse and patchy oedema. The pulmonary capillaries contain sequestrated polymorphonuclear leucocytes (Fig. 47.2) and platelets, often in association with microthrombi. In the later stages of the adult respiratory distress syndrome there is diffuse alveolar damage with hyaline membrane formation (Fig. 47.3) and pulmonary oedema. If the patient survives this phase there is a subsequent proliferation of alveolar and bronchiolar epithelium together with interstitial fibrosis. The pathogenesis of these pulmonary changes is far from being fully understood but it is postulated that the sequestration of red blood cells within the pulmonary capillaries leads to the release of free radicals (with subsequent lipid peroxidation) and to lysosomal degranulation (Corrin & Spencer 1981).

Hypertensive disease of pregnancy

Many of the pathological changes found in pre-eclampsia and eclampsia have been described in Chapters 40, 41, and 43–46 but it is appropriate to summarise here, in very brief form, the salient findings in fatal cases (Sheehan & Lynch 1973; Govan 1976; Fox 1987):

1. Petechial haemorrhages may be found in the cerebral cortex, cerebellum and pons. Massive intracerebral haemorrhage is not uncommon and is a major cause of death in this disease.
2. Subcapsular haemorrhages and areas of infarction are often seen in the liver, these usually being most prominent in the right lobe (Fig. 47.4): occasionally there may be subcapsular rupture of the liver with a haemoperitoneum. Histologically the liver shows periportal necrosis and haemorrhage.

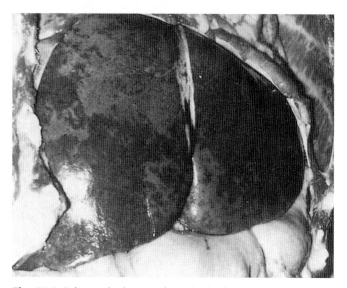

Fig. 47.4 Subcapsular haemorrhage in the liver of a patient dying from eclampsia.

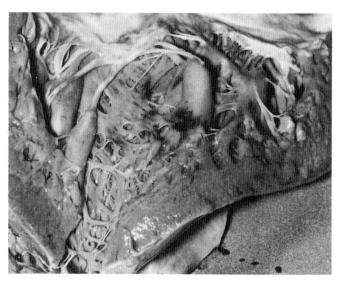

Fig. 47.5 Subendocardial haemorrhages in a fatal case of eclampsia.

3. Subendocardial haemorrhages are found in the heart, particularly on the left side of the interventricular septum (Fig. 47.5).
4. In the lungs there is characteristically a bilateral haemorrhagic pneumonia.
5. The kidneys show glomerular abnormalities and the lower nephron is often obstructed by protein casts. Bilateral renal cortical necrosis may be found.
6. Acute ulceration of the stomach, oesophagus and duodenum is not uncommon.
7. Haemorrhages are frequently seen within the splenic pulp. The lymphoid tissue around branches of the arterial vessels within the spleen is often necrotic.
8. Streak haemorrhages are frequently seen in the adrenal cortex. Very occasionally there is massive bilateral intra-adrenal haemorrhage.

In the HELLP syndrome pre-eclampsia is associated with a haemolytic anaemia, elevated liver enzymes and low platelet counts (Weinstein 1982). This condition usually resolves but a rebound thrombocytosis may develop and can predispose to thrombosis, a fatal case of carotid artery occlusion having been recorded under these circumstances (Katz & Cefalo 1989).

Amniotic fluid embolism

It has traditionally been thought that during a normal pregnancy, labour and delivery there is no escape of liquor into the maternal circulation but that in a few patients an infusion of amniotic fluid occurs which results in a syndrome combining acute cardiopulmonary failure with a haemorrhagic tendency due to a coagulation defect. In recent years, however, this belief has been challenged by the suggestion that amniotic fluid may routinely enter the venous circulation and that the clinical picture of amniotic fluid embolism could be due to infusion of abnormal amniotic fluid into the maternal circulation rather than to amniotic fluid per se (Clark 1990, 1991). This view is based on the fact that studies of pregnant women undergoing pulmonary artery catheterisation have shown that squames can commonly be detected in the maternal pulmonary arterial circulation (Plauche 1983; Clark et al 1986; Lee et al 1986): this finding does not, however, in itself prove that amniotic fluid routinely enters the circulation for squames are introduced during venepuncture: hence this contention still awaits proof.

The portal of entry of amniotic fluid into the maternal circulation is not always clear though in a proportion of cases a definite uterine laceration, which presumably affords a site of ingress, is found. Attwood (1972) has emphasised that small lower segment tears, either incomplete or complete with an intact but ballooned broad ligament, are more likely to be associated with a fatal amniotic fluid embolism than are large uterine lacerations. Amniotic fluid infusion occurs through a small lower segment tear if the membranes have ruptured and the head, in crowning, forms a plug behind which each uterine contraction pumps fluid into the maternal bloodstream. When, by contrast, there is a large uterine laceration, amniotic fluid tends to leak principally into the peritoneal cavity whilst uterine contractions cease. It has been suggested that in those cases in which no uterine tear is apparent the route of entry may be through the small lacerations which normally occur in the endocervical veins during cervical dilatation (Anderson 1967).

The cardiopulmonary failure in the amniotic fluid embolism syndrome has for many years been attributed to severe pulmonary hypertension with acute cor pulmonale, the pulmonary hypertension being variously attributed to mechanical obstruction of the pulmonary vasculature, reflex vasoconstriction of the pulmonary vessels, an anaphylactoid reaction or the presence of a vasoactive substance in the emboli. Morgan (1979) did not think that anaphylaxis played a rôle in the production of this syndrome but Clark et al (1995) were sufficiently impressed by the anaphylaxis-like nature of amniotic fluid embolism that they suggested renaming it as 'anaphylactoid syndrome of pregnancy'; this view has won some support by the demonstration of a marked increase in pulmonary mast cells in women dying of amniotic fluid embolism (Fineschi et al 1998). Experimental studies, using a variety of techniques on a variety of animals under a variety of circumstances and yielding a variety of results (Steiner & Lushbaugh 1941; Cron et al 1952; Hunter et al 1956; Halmagyi et al 1962; Attwood & Downing 1965; Stolte et al 1967; Macmillan 1968; Reis et al 1969; Rodgers et al 1969, 1971; Adamsons et al 1971; Kitzmiller & Lucas 1972; Reeves et al 1974; Hankins et al 1993; Petroianu et al 1999), have on balance tended to suggest that a vasoactive substance plays a key rôle in the haemodynamic changes. Trypsin

has been proposed as a candidate for this rôle (Attwood 1972) but a more plausible suggestion is that the prostaglandin $PGF_{2\alpha}$, a substance present in amniotic fluid in significant amounts only during labour, precipitates the haemodynamic changes. Thus, Kitzmiller & Lucas (1972) showed that the vascular changes observed in amniotic fluid embolism could be reproduced in cats only by the injection of fluid from women who were actually in labour and noted that these changes could be replicated by injection of $PGF_{2\alpha}$. Reeves et al (1974) found that the haemodynamic effects of amniotic fluid injection could be prevented by aspirin, a potent inhibitor of prostaglandin synthesis. Clark (1990) has proposed that leucotrienes, also metabolites of arachidonic acid, may be involved as vasoactive agents.

The classical concept of an acute cor pulmonale being fully responsible for the clinical features of the amniotic fluid embolism syndrome has, however, not been confirmed by haemodynamic studies in humans. These have, without exception, shown little or no increase in pulmonary arterial pressure (Dolyniuk et al 1983; Clark et al 1985, 1988; Girard et al 1986; Noble & St Amand 1993; Koegler et al 1994) but have yielded conflicting results about left ventricular output, some finding depression of left ventricular function (Clark et al 1985, 1988) and others demonstrating a normal (Koegler et al 1994) or increased (Noble & St Amand 1993) left ventricular output. It has been suggested that the failure to detect an elevated pulmonary arterial pressure may be because the pulmonary arterial vasoconstriction is short lived (less than 30 minutes) and has been dissipated before catheter studies can be undertaken and further claimed that, despite its transient nature, the pulmonary vasoconstriction produces severe hypoxia which damages the myocardium of the left ventricle (Clark et al 1985; Clark 1990, 1991). This view is given some credence by the finding that, in a woman who developed the clinical features of an amniotic fluid embolism whilst having her arterial oxygen saturation continuously measured, there was a drop in oxygen saturation from 98–100% to 70% within 30 seconds (Fava & Galizia 1993).

There is disagreement as to the nature of the coagulation defect which is a prominent feature of the clinical syndrome of amniotic fluid embolism. Attwood (1972) has pointed out that fibrin thrombi are very rarely seen in autopsies on women dying from amniotic fluid embolism but nevertheless most believe that the bleeding diathesis is due to disseminated intravascular coagulation, resulting from the presence within the emboli of a thromboplastic substance (Beller 1974). Amniotic fluid can activate factor X and has a thromboplastin-like effect when added to normal plasma, properties suggesting that the fluid may contain tissue factor, a primary biological initiator of coagulation. Lockwood et al (1991) have indeed confirmed that tissue factor is present in amniotic fluid, that the presence of this substance accounts for virtually all the procoagulant activity of the fluid and that the quantity of this substance in the fluid increases progressively with increasing gestational age.

It is widely believed that advancing age, high parity, a large fetus, tumultuous labour, intrauterine fetal death and the use of uterine stimulants all predispose to the amniotic fluid embolism syndrome (Peterson & Taylor 1970; Courtney 1970; Gregory & Clayton 1973). Morgan (1979), in his review of 272 reported cases of amniotic fluid embolism, was unable to confirm that there was any true association with the use of uterine stimulants, large babies or intrauterine fetal death. A tumultuous or hypertonic labour, though associated with an unduly high incidence of the amniotic fluid embolism syndrome, is by no means an essential prerequisite for this complication which may also occur during the course of an entirely normal labour, in women being delivered by Caesarean section and in women who have not yet gone into labour (Clark et al 1995). Amniotic fluid embolism may also occur immediately after labour, i.e. within 5 minutes of delivery, but reports of the syndrome occurring as late as 36 hours postpartum (Devriendt et al 1995) are probably based upon an incorrect diagnosis. Amniotic fluid embolism syndrome can also complicate intrauterine injection of hypertonic saline for termination of pregnancy (Goldstein 1968), intra-amniotic glucose infusion (Lee & Frampton 1964), amniocentesis (Krause 1969) and therapeutic saline amnioinfusion (Dragich et al 1991; Dibble & Elliott 1992; Maher et al 1994). Surgical termination of pregnancy can be complicated by amniotic fluid embolism and, indeed, it has been claimed that approximately 12% of all deaths following legal termination of pregnancy are attributable to this cause (Guidotti et al 1981).

Clinically, the onset of symptoms in the amniotic fluid embolism syndrome is usually abrupt. There is a sudden onset of dyspnoea, cyanosis and shock: convulsions are not uncommon and are sometimes the presenting feature. Frequently the patient dies within a few minutes but if she survives this acute episode a haemorrhagic tendency soon supervenes and this often leads to severe, sometimes catastrophic, uterine bleeding: occasionally a coagulopathy is the sole clinical feature of the syndrome (Choi & Duffy 1995; Bastien et al 1998; Locksmith 1999). The mortality rate has been traditionally thought to be very high, in the region of 90% (Morgan 1979): until recently the true death rate has, however, been difficult to determine, largely because of the paradoxical situation that the mere fact of survival was commonly regarded as proof that an individual did not have amniotic fluid embolism (Benson 1993) and because of the belief that the diagnosis could only be proven at autopsy. It is certainly true that absolute proof of the diagnosis does rest upon the autopsy findings but the clinical features have now been defined and analysed to a point where they have a sufficient degree of specificity to allow for a diagnosis on clinical grounds alone (Clark 1990, 1991; Clark et al 1995; Locksmith 1999; Fletcher & Parr 2000): using the clinical criteria proposed by the amniotic fluid national registry in the United States a maternal mortality rate of 61% was noted (Clark et al 1995). It was at one time hoped that the detection of squamous cells in pulmonary artery blood would allow for the confirmation of the diagnosis during life (Dolyniuk et al 1983) but, as already remarked, squames can be found in the pulmonary blood of perfectly healthy pregnant women (Clark et al 1986).

At autopsy the macroscopic findings in a case of amniotic fluid embolism syndrome are commonly nonspecific: the lungs are usually oedematous and show patchy atelectasis with marked dilatation of the right side of the heart and acute congestion of the liver. Occasionally a macroscopic diagnosis can be achieved by allowing blood from the pulmonary arteries to collect within the pericardial sac after removal of the heart: vernix, lanugo hairs and greenish staining due to meconium may be seen (Attwood 1972). Essentially, however, the diagnosis of amniotic fluid embolism rests upon the histological demonstration of amniotic fluid debris in the pulmonary vasculature. Four points require to be stressed:

1. Multiple blocks of lung tissue should be taken for histological examination.
2. If amniotic fluid debris is not detected in the pulmonary vasculature the diagnosis of amniotic fluid embolism cannot be substantiated.
3. Although fetal squames have been detected in the blood of healthy women it would be unwise to assume that amniotic fluid debris in the pulmonary vasculature is a physiological event.
4. Trophoblastic emboli are not uncommonly found in the lung: these are evidence of a physiological process and are not indicative of amniotic fluid embolism.

The particulate matter that may be found in the pulmonary vessels includes epithelial squames (Fig. 47.6) from the fetal skin, lanugo hairs, fat from the vernix caseosa, bile and mucin (Figs 47.7, 47.8), the latter two constituents being derived from fetal meconium passed into the liquor. Attwood (1972) has stressed the inadequacy of the haematoxylin and eosin stain for detecting amniotic debris; a better staining method for the demonstration of the various components of the emboli is the Alcian Blue phloxine technique which stains mucin green and squames red (Attwood 1958). A superior technique for detecting squames in amniotic fluid emboli (Fig. 47.9) is, however, to use an anti-keratin antibody (Garland & Thompson 1983) and it is worth noting that the amniotic squames also stain intensely for endothelin-1 (Khong 1998). More recently it has been shown that immunostaining with the monoclonal antibody TKH-2, which reacts with meconium- and amniotic fluid-derived mucin-type glycoprotein, produces a strongly positive reaction to

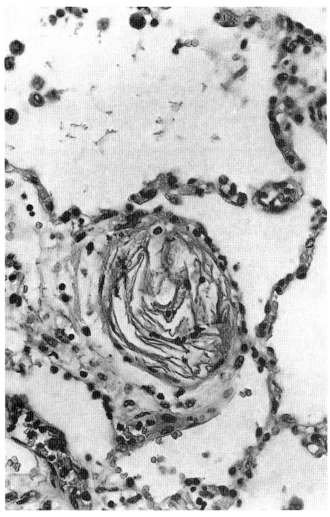

Fig. 47.6 An amniotic fluid embolus in a pulmonary vessel. This consists almost entirely of squames. (Courtesy of Dr D I Rushton, Birmingham.)

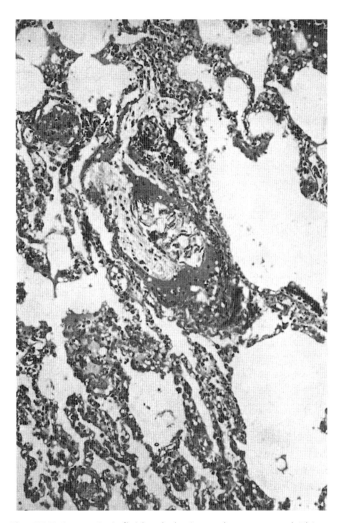

Fig. 47.7 An amniotic fluid embolus in a pulmonary vessel. This consists of a mixture of squames, mucus and meconium. Alcian Blue phloxine.

mucinous material in amniotic fluid emboli within the pulmonary vasculature (Kobayashi et al 1997; Ooi et al 1998) and this is now probably the stain of choice.

Using the Attwood stain, Peterson & Taylor (1970) studied 40 patients who had died of amniotic fluid embolism and found that although squames could be demonstrated in the pulmonary vessels in 80% of cases they were the major constituent of the emboli in only 20%: in the other 80% mucin was the most prominent particulate matter. Mucin was found principally in the small pulmonary arteries whilst squames tended to be more commonly seen in the arterioles and capillaries. Amniotic emboli may be found in capillaries in many organs outside the lungs but are usually few and small and of apparently little clinical importance.

The histological diagnosis of amniotic fluid embolism is usually straightforward but confusion may occasionally arise between epithelial squames and endothelial cells which have been shed from the walls of the pulmonary vessels; these latter cells are, however, usually nucleated (as compared to the generally anuclear squames) and do not take up the Alcian Blue phloxine stain (Attwood 1972).

Air embolism

The pregnant uterus is particularly vulnerable to air embolism because of the large venous sinuses that are exposed at placental separation. Air embolism may complicate a termination of pregnancy, particularly an illegal termination (Bryans 1963; Fox 1967), internal version, manual exploration of the uterus, replacement of an inverted uterus or manual removal of the placenta: it has been suggested that air embolism following intrauterine manipulations is due to air within the uterus becoming trapped by the operator's arm which occludes the vagina, any sudden increase in intrauterine pressure then tending to force the air into the venous sinuses (Nelson 1960). Air entry into the maternal circulation may, very exceptionally, occur during an otherwise

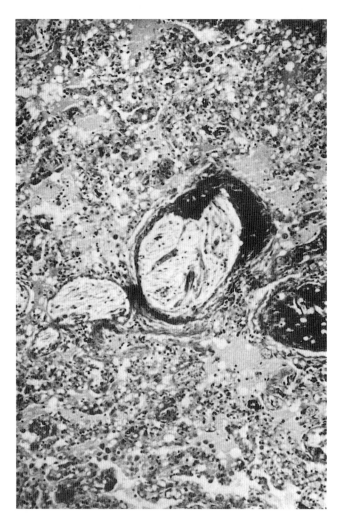

Fig. 47.8 An amniotic fluid embolus in a pulmonary vessel. This consists almost entirely of mucus and meconium. Alcian Blue phloxine.

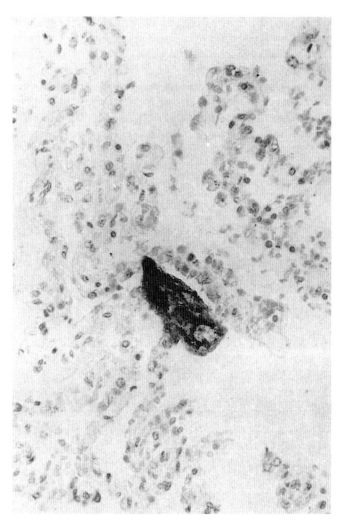

Fig. 47.9 Squames in an amniotic fluid embolus in a pulmonary vessel: these have been stained with an immunoperoxidase-linked antikeratin antibody. (Courtesy of Dr I W C Garland, Aberdeen.)

normal labour, vaginal delivery or Caesarean section. Air embolism can also occur during pregnancy, well before the onset of labour (Ragan 1981); this event may appear to develop spontaneously but is usually due to orogenital sexual activity (Bray et al 1983). The practice of blowing into the vagina is one which is devoid of danger in the non-pregnant woman; however, the capacity of the vagina is considerably increased during pregnancy and under these circumstances this somewhat unusual sexual manoeuvre carries a serious risk of air embolism.

Air embolism during the puerperium is thought to be particularly associated with the performance by the patient of knee–chest exercises; the vagina has, during the puerperium, a capacity of about 1000 ml and this quantity of air may be trapped intravaginally by approximation of the thighs whilst in the knee–chest position and subsequently forced into the uterine veins when the patient returns her legs to the horizontal position.

The clinical picture of an air embolism is dependent upon the amount of air entering the maternal circulation but it is generally accepted that entry of 500–600 ml of air is usually fatal. In such cases there is a sudden onset of cyanosis, shock and acute cor pulmonale with a rapid progression to convulsions, coma and death. At autopsy, the cardinal finding is of dark, frothy, bubble-studded blood in the right side of the heart and also, often, in the inferior vena cava and in the uterine veins.

Acute uterine inversion

This is an uncommon complication of the puerperium occurring in about 1 in 6400 deliveries (Shah-Hosseini & Evrard 1989); it may follow attempted manual removal of the placenta, particularly in cases of placenta accreta, but can also occur spontaneously and without warning (Kitchin et al 1975; Watson et al 1980): very occasionally inversion can occur in association with a uterine rupture

(Grischke et al 1999). A patient with this complication tends to suffer severe haemorrhage and shock and a mortality rate of between 13% and 18% has traditionally been quoted (Bell et al 1953; Bunke & Hofmeister 1965; Moldavsky 1967). The more recent trend towards prompt replacement of the uterus has dramatically reduced this death rate (Watson et al 1980; Shah-Hosseini & Evrard 1989; Phillippe et al 1991; Rasmussen 1992; Ogueh & Ayida 1997; Hostetler & Bosworth 2000).

Acute uterine torsion

This is an extremely rare, but potentially fatal, catastrophe in pregnancy (Piot et al 1973; Smith 1975; Visser et al 1983). Dextrorotation of the gravid uterus is common but axial rotation amounts to torsion if it exceeds 45°. Torsion usually occurs during labour, may lead to uterine rupture and is of unknown pathogenesis.

Rupture of the uterus

The incidence of uterine rupture during pregnancy is not known with any degree of certainty but it has been estimated that in Western countries this catastrophe complicates about 1 in 2000 to 2500 pregnancies (Garnet 1964; Schrinsky & Benson 1978). In other parts of the world uterine rupture is, however, much more common occurring, for example, in 1 in 546 deliveries in a black South African population (Mokgokong & Marivate 1976), in 1 in 425 deliveries in Kenya (Lema et al 1991), in 1 in 119 deliveries in Conakry/Guinea (Balde et al 1990) and in 1 in 97 pregnancies in a rural Turkish population (Kafkas & Taper 1991).

Uterine rupture may be classified as traumatic, spontaneous or scar-associated and in most series between 30 and 60% have been due to rupture of a uterine scar. In the vast majority of these patients the scar has been due to a previous Caesarean section but scars resulting from a previous myomectomy, including laparoscopic myomectomy (Harris 1992; Dubuisson et al 1995; Friedmann et al 1996; Pelosi & Pelosi 1997; Hockstein 2000; Nkemayim et al 2000), or cornual resection may also undergo rupture. Rupture has also occurred at the site of a previous invasive mole (Kaczmarek et al 1994), following reimplantation into the uterus of the Fallopian tubes (Brandt & Larsen 1989) and after surgical treatment of Asherman's syndrome (Deaton et al 1989).

The scar of a previous classical Caesarean section is much more susceptible to rupture than is that following a lower segment section, Garnet (1964) estimating that a classical scar is ten times more likely to rupture than is a lower segment scar. This does not imply, however, that most cases of scar rupture seen today follow a classical section for this operation is now performed so infrequently that the vast majority of scar ruptures occur in women who have had a lower segment section. It is important when dealing with a scar rupture to differentiate between a true rupture, which is usually associated with severe haemorrhage and can lead to maternal death, and simple dehiscence of the scar. In the latter condition the peritoneum overlying the scar is intact and separates the membranes, which bulge through the gaping edges of the dehiscent scar, from the peritoneal cavity: dehiscence is rarely associated with bleeding and is not a cause of maternal death (Yussman & Haynes 1970). The absolute risk of uterine rupture following a lower segment section is extremely low, being in the range of 0.2–1.4% (Meehan et al 1989; Farmer et al 1991; Jones et al 1991; Lurie et al 1992; Ravasia et al 2000) though this increases to 3.7% in women who have had two previous sections (Caughey et al 1999).

The commonest causes of traumatic uterine rupture in Western countries are probably internal version and forceful delivery through an incompletely dilated cervix (O'Driscoll 1966): other precipitating factors include instrumentation whilst performing an illegal abortion, failed forceps delivery, shoulder dystocia, cephalopelvic disproportion and transverse lie (Schrinsky & Benson 1978). Obstructed labour is by far the commonest cause in developing countries.

Spontaneous rupture should, by definition, occur in a normal uterus during a normal pregnancy or labour but, by convention, this diagnostic term is extended to include rupture of a congenitally abnormal uterus, rupture of a cornual pregnancy and rupture complicating placenta accreta. In the absence of these latter factors the cause of spontaneous uterine rupture is largely unknown. The rôle of oxytocic stimulation has been much debated for, whilst a proportion of cases of uterine rupture do follow administration of oxytocin (Golan et al 1980), it has been doubted if use of this substance in a normal labour carries any risk of this complication, rupture only becoming a real possibility if oxytocin is administered in an already complicated labour. There has, however, been an increasing number of reports of uterine rupture following vaginal administration of prostaglandin E_2 for induction of labour (Sawyer et al 1981; Larue et al 1991; Maymon et al 1992; Prasad & Ratnam 1992; Azem et al 1993; Lydon-Rochelle et al 2001), though the absolute risk of this complication is low. There are anecdotal reports of an association between cocaine usage and spontaneous uterine rupture (Gonsoulin et al 1990; Trive et al 1994) whilst rupture has occurred, probably coincidentally, in a woman exposed prenatally to DES (Adams et al 1989).

Rupture of a lower segment section scar usually occurs during labour whilst rupture of a classical scar may occur at any time during pregnancy. Rupture of a myomectomy scar has been noted as early as the 16th week of pregnancy (Report on Confidential Enquiries into Maternal Deaths in England and Wales 1976–1978, 1982). Clearly, traumatic rupture usually occurs during labour and whilst most cases of spontaneous rupture also occur during labour (Milon et al 1983), rupture of this type can occur at any stage of gestation (Taylor & Canning 1979), the earliest recorded case being at the 19th week of pregnancy (de Wane & McCubbin 1981).

The death rate associated with uterine rupture has been variously estimated as between 6.5 and 10% (Golan et al 1980) though in most Western centres the currently expected mortality rate would be much lower than this; in developing countries the mortality rate is in the range of 7.5–21% (Balde et al 1990; Konje et al 1990). There is general agreement that the mortality rate is highest in cases of spontaneous uterine rupture and lowest in scar ruptures (Schrinsky & Benson 1978): this view may, however, be misleading in so far as many cases classed as scar ruptures are, in fact, examples of scar dehiscence, a condition not associated with maternal death.

Anaesthetic deaths

Anaesthesia-related deaths in pregnant women do not, in general, differ in any specific manner from those occurring during, or after, general surgical procedures. Obstetrical patients are, however, unduly prone to pulmonary aspiration of gastric contents, partly because of the increased intragastric pressure resulting from compression of the abdominal contents by the gravid uterus and partly because of the progesterone-induced relaxation of the gastro-oesophageal sphincter (Baggish & Hooper 1974; Cohen 1982). The clinical and pathological features of pulmonary aspiration depend very considerably on whether liquid or solid material is aspirated, the former being the more common.

Acid fluid aspiration

The clinical features resulting from aspiration of acid gastric juice into the lungs were first described by Mendelson (1946) and his name is usually applied to this syndrome. Aspiration may occur silently and, whilst quite severe symptoms may result from inhalation of relatively trivial quantities of fluid, it is generally estimated that a serious hazard to the patient is only presented when the volume of the aspirate exceeds 25 ml (Cohen 1982). The pulmonary reaction to the highly acid gastric juice may develop immediately after aspiration or may be delayed for two to five hours, becoming apparent at a time when the patient is making an apparently satisfactory recovery from anaesthesia. There is a rapid onset of tachypnoea, cyanosis, tachycardia, hypotension and bronchospasm; this latter symptom may be an inconspicuous feature but can be sufficiently marked as to mimic an acute asthmatic attack. Most patients recover but a few progress to convulsions, coma and death.

Aspirated fluid damages the pulmonary vascular epithelium with consequent intra-alveolar haemorrhage and pulmonary oedema: the surfactant-producing cells are destroyed and there is an intra-alveolar exudate of oedema fluid, erythrocytes, polymorphonuclear leucocytes and fibrin, often with the formation of hyaline membranes. These changes result in alveolar collapse and consolidation which initiates a significant degree of shunting and hypoxia (Cohen 1982). In fatal cases the lungs are heavy, congested and oedematous: there may be subpleural haemorrhages and serosanguinous fluid in the pleural cavities. The heart is dilated and may show subpericardial haemorrhages whilst the abdominal viscera are deeply congested (McCormick 1967). Histologically, the alveolar changes described above will be present and there may also be extensive necrosis and desquamation of the bronchial epithelium.

These pulmonary changes are widely thought to be directly due to the acid nature of the inhaled liquid (Bartlett & Gorbach 1975; Stewardson & Nyhus 1977) and indeed the effects of aspiration of gastric juice have been likened to an acute chemical burn (Stewardson & Nyhus 1977; Cohen 1982). This view has been largely based upon experimental studies in which it has been shown that the severity of the lung lesions is related to the pH of the fluid and that pulmonary oedema is inevitable only if the pH of the aspirate is below 2.5 (Teabeaut 1952; Awe et al 1966; Wynne & Modell 1977). Alexander (1968) has, however, maintained that the development of pulmonary oedema is independent of the pH of the inhaled liquid, suggesting that fluid alone can damage the alveolar capillary membrane and that acidity only potentiates the exudative reaction. Support has been given to this contention by Schwartz et al (1980) who showed that instillation of gastric juice at a pH value of 5.9 into the lungs of dogs produced changes which were just as severe as those resulting from the use of fluid at a pH value of 1.8.

Faecal fluid aspiration

In patients with prolonged labour there is depression of intestinal peristalsis, increased intra-abdominal pressure and delayed emptying of the stomach: the gastric contents thus come to resemble those found in intestinal obstruction and not only have a high pH but may also contain numerous organisms (McCormick 1967). Aspiration of this material may produce acute respiratory distress which can be accompanied by profound hypotension, the latter probably being due to toxic shock resulting from entry of bacteria into the circulation from the lungs.

Aspiration of solid material

This, depending on the size and consistency of the inhaled particles, may cause variable degrees of airway obstruction: if the particulate matter is sufficiently large the patient may asphyxiate whilst collapse of a lobe or a segment may occur. Smaller particles appear to accentuate the effects of inhaled fluid and elicit an acute peri-bronchial inflammatory reaction which later becomes granulomatous in nature.

Pneumomediastinum

During labour the intense Valsalva manoeuvre associated with 'bearing down' causes a marked, transient elevation of pulmonary intra-alveolar pressure which may result in rupture of marginally situated alveoli with subsequent tracking of air, along perivascular tissue planes, towards the hilum and into the mediastinum (Bard & Hassini 1975; Brandfass & Martinez 1976). In most such cases the air is resorbed over a few days whilst in others escape of air from the mediastinum into the subcutaneous tissues relieves the build-up of pressure. Occasionally, however, a tension-pneumomediastinum develops and this may prove fatal.

Hyperemesis gravidarum

Death during pregnancy from hyperemesis gravidarum is now exceedingly rare. Sheehan (1939), at a time when this condition was more commonly fatal, studied the pathological changes in 19 autopsied cases and was unable to find any that could not be directly attributed to prolonged vomiting and starvation. The most consistent abnormalities were cardiac atrophy, centrilobular fatty change in the liver and fatty change in the renal tubules. A less common finding was a Wernicke's encephalopathy whilst rarely there may be bilateral retinal haemorrhages and degenerative changes in the peripheral nerves (Fairweather 1968).

Salt poisoning

A number of deaths have, largely if not entirely in the past, followed injection of hypertonic saline into the gravid uterus for termination of pregnancy. The autopsy findings in such cases are characteristic and consist of symmetrical haemor-rhagic infarction of the brain, involving particularly the region of the amygdaloid nuclei and a Y-shaped area in the pons (Cameron et al 1969). It is thought that these lesions are due to a sudden change in plasma osmolarity, either because of accidental intraperitoneal or intravenous injec-tion of saline or by leakage of salt solution through tears in the amnion into the maternal tissues.

Water intoxication

Administration of oxytocin is occasionally followed by severe fluid retention and water intoxication. In a woman dying from this complication Lilien (1968) found only pulmonary and cerebral oedema at autopsy. Fatal water intoxication can also complicate the use of beta-agonists as a tocolytic therapy, i.e. to inhibit uterine contractions (RCOG Guideline 1997).

Ectopic pregnancy

This important cause of maternal death is considered in Chapter 31.

REFERENCES

Adams D M, Druzin M L, Cederqvist L L 1989 Intrapartum uterine rupture. Obstetrics and Gynecology 73: 471–473

Adamsons K, Mueller-Heubach E, Myers R E 1971 The innocuousness of amniotic fluid infusion in the pregnant rhesus monkey. American Journal of Obstetrics and Gynecology 109: 977–984

Alexander I G S 1968 The ultrastructure of the pulmonary alveolar vessels in Mendelson's (acid pulmonary aspiration) syndrome. British Journal of Anaesthesia 40: 408–414

Anderson D G 1967 Amniotic fluid embolisms: a re-evaluation. American Journal of Obstetrics and Gynecology 98: 336–346

Attwood H D 1958 The histological diagnosis of amniotic fluid embolism. Journal of Pathology and Bacteriology 76: 211–215

Attwood H D 1972 Amniotic fluid embolism. In: Sommers S C (ed) Pathology annual. Appleton-Century-Crofts, New York, pp 145–172

Attwood H D, Downing S E 1965 Experimental amniotic fluid and meconium embolism. Surgery, Gynecology and Obstetrics 120: 255–262

Awe W B, Fletcher W S, Jacob S W 1966 The pathophysiology of aspiration pneumonitis. Surgery 60: 232–239

Azem F, Jaffa A, Lessing J B, Peyser M R 1993 Uterine rupture with the use of a low-dose vaginal PGE2 tablet. Acta Obstetricia et Gynecologica Scandinavica 72: 316–317

Baggish M S, Hooper S 1977 Aspiration as a cause of maternal death. Obstetrics and Gynecology 43: 327–336

Balde M D, Breitbach G P, Bastert G 1990 Uterine rupture — an analysis of 81 cases in Conakry/Guinea. International Journal of Gynaecology and Obstetrics 32: 223–227

Bard R, Hassini N 1975 Pneumomediastinum complicating pregnancy. Respiration 32: 185–188

Bartlett J G, Gorbach S L 1975 The triple threat of aspiration pneumonia. Chest 65: 580–586

Bastien J L, Graves J R, Bailey S 1998 Atypical presentation of amniotic fluid embolism. Anesthesia and Analgesia 87: 124–126

Bell E J, Wilson G F, Wilson L A 1953 Puerperal inversion of the uterus. American Journal of Obstetrics and Gynecology 66: 767–777

Beller F K 1974 Disseminated intravascular coagulation and consumption coagulopathy in obstetrics. Obstetrics and Gynecology Annual 3: 267–281

Benson M D 1993 Non-fatal amniotic fluid embolism: three possible cases and a new clinical definition. Archives of Family Medicine 2: 989–994

Bouvier-Colle M-H, Varnoux N, Costes P, Hatton F 1991 Reasons for the underreporting of maternal mortality in France as indicated by a survey of all deaths among women of childbearing age. International Journal of Epidemiology 20: 717–721

Brandfass R T, Martinez D M 1976 Mediastinal and subcutaneous emphysema in labor. Southern Medical Journal 69: 1554–1555

Brandt C A, Larsen B 1989 Uterine rupture after re-implantation of fallopian tubes. Acta Obstetricia et Gynecologica Scandinavica 68: 281–282

Bray P, Myers R A M, Cowley R A 1983 Orogenital sex as a cause of non-fatal air embolism in pregnancy. Obstetrics and Gynecology 61: 553–557

Bryans F E 1963 Vascular accidents in maternal mortality. Clinical Obstetrics and Gynecology 6: 861–873

Bunke J W, Hofmeister F J 1965 Uterine inversion — obstetrical entity or oddity? American Journal of Obstetrics and Gynecology 91: 934–939

Burrow G N, Ferris T F (eds) 1982 Medical complications during pregnancy, 2nd edn. Saunders, Philadelphia

Cameron J M, Morgan A G, Robinson A E, Urich H 1969 Brain damage following therapeutic abortion by amniotic fluid replacement: an experimental approach. Journal of Obstetrics and Gynaecology of the British Commonwealth 76: 168–175

Caughey A B, Shipp T D, Repke J T, Zelop C M, Cohen A, Lieberman E 1999 Uterine rupture during induced or augmented labor in gravid women with one prior cesarean delivery. American Journal of Obstetrics and Gynecology 181: 882–886

Chamberlain G V P 1992 The clinical aspects of massive haemorrhage. In: Patel N (ed) Maternal mortality — the way forward. Royal College of Obstetricians and Gynaecologists, London, pp 54–62

Choi D M A, Duffy B L 1995 Amniotic fluid embolism. Anaesthetics and Intensive Care 23: 741–743

Clark S L 1990 New concepts of amniotic fluid embolism: a review. Obstetrical and Gynecological Survey 45: 360–368

Clark S L 1991 Amniotic fluid embolism. Critical Care Clinics 7: 877–882

Clark S L, Montz P J, Phelan J P 1985 Hemodynamic alterations associated with amniotic fluid embolism: a reappraisal. American Journal of Obstetrics and Gynecology 151: 617–621

Clark S L, Pavlova Z, Greenspoon J et al 1986 Squamous cells in the maternal pulmonary circulation. American Journal of Obstetrics and Gynecology 154: 104–106

Clark S L, Cotton D B, Gonik B et al 1988 Central hemodynamic alterations in amniotic fluid embolism. American Journal of Obstetrics and Gynecology 158: 1124–1126

Clark S L, Hankins D V, Dudley D A, Dildy G A, Porter T F 1995 Amniotic fluid embolism: analysis of the national registry. American Journal of Obstetrics and Gynecology 172: 1158–1169

Cohen S E 1982 The aspiration syndrome. Clinics in Obstetrics and Gynaecology 9: 235–254

Collins C G, MacCallum E A, Nelson E W, Weinstein B B, Collins J H 1951 Suppurative pelvic thrombophlebitis. I. Incidence, pathology and etiology. Surgery 30: 298–310

Corrin B, Spencer H 1981 Some aspects of pulmonary pathology. In: Anthony P P, MacSween R N M (eds) Recent advances in histopathology 11. Churchill Livingstone, Edinburgh, pp 83–98

Courtney L D 1970 Amniotic fluid embolism. British Medical Journal 1: 545

Cron R S, Kilkenney G S, Wirthwein C, Evrard J R 1952 Amniotic fluid embolism. American Journal of Obstetrics and Gynecology 64: 1360–1363

Daniel D G, Campbell H, Turnbull A C 1967 Puerperal thromboembolism and suppression of lactation. Lancet 2: 287–289

Deaton J L, Maier D, Andreoli J 1989 Spontaneous uterine rupture during pregnancy after treatment of Asherman's syndrome. American Journal of Obstetrics and Gynecology 160: 1053–1054

De Swiet M 1989 Medical disorders in obstetric practice, 2nd edn. Blackwell Scientific, Oxford

De Wane J C, McCubbin J H 1981 Spontaneous rupture of an unscarred uterus at 19 weeks gestation. American Journal of Obstetrics and Gynecology 141: 222–224

Devriendt J, Machayekhi S, Staroukine M 1995 Amniotic fluid embolism: another case with non-cardiogenic pulmonary oedema. Intensive Care Medicine 21: 698–699

Dibble L A, Elliott J P 1992 Possible amniotic fluid embolism associated with amnioinfusion. Journal of Maternal and Fetal Medicine 1: 263–266

Dinh T A, Warshal D P 2001 The epidemiology of cancer in pregnancy. In: Barnea E R, Jauniaux E, Schwartz P E (eds) Cancer and pregnancy. Springer, London, pp 1–5

Dolyniuk M, Oriel E, Vania H, Karlman R, Tomich P 1983 Rapid diagnosis of amniotic fluid embolism. Obstetrics and Gynecology 61: 28s–30s

Dragich D A, Ross A F, Chestnut D H, Wenstrom K D 1991 Respiratory failure associated with amnioinfusion during labor. Anesthesia and Analgesia 72: 549–551

Drife J 2001 Infection and maternal mortality. In: MacLean A, Regan L, Carrington D (eds) Infection and pregnancy. RCOG Press, London, pp 355–364

Dubuisson J B, Chavet X, Chapron C et al 1995 Uterine rupture during pregnancy after laparoscopic myomectomy. Human Reproduction 10: 1475–1477

Duley I 1992 Maternal mortality associated with hypertensive disorders of pregnancy in Africa, Asia, Latin America and the Caribbean. British Journal of Obstetrics and Gynaecology 99: 547–553

Editorial 1987 Maternal health in Subsaharan Africa. Lancet i: 255–257

Eschenbach D A, Wager G P 1980 Puerperal infections. Clinical Obstetrics and Gynecology 23: 1003–1037

Ewing T C, Smale L E, Elliott F A 1979 Maternal deaths associated with postpartum vulvar edema. American Journal of Obstetrics and Gynecology 134: 173–177

Fairweather D V I 1968 Nausea and vomiting in pregnancy. American Journal of Obstetrics and Gynecology 102: 135–175

Farmer R M, Kirschbaum T, Potter D et al 1991 Uterine rupture during trial of labor after previous cesarean section. American Journal of Obstetrics and Gynecology 163: 996–1001

Fava S, Galizia A C 1993 Amniotic fluid embolism. British Journal of Obstetrics and Gynaecology 100: 1049–1050

Fildes J, Reed L, Jones N et al 1992 Trauma: the leading cause of maternal death. Journal of Trauma 32: 643–645

Fineschi V, Gambassi R, Gherardi M, Turillazzi E 1998 The diagnosis of amniotic fluid embolism: an immunohistochemical study for the quantification of pulmonary mast cell tryptase. International Journal of Legal Medicine 111: 238–243

Flegner J R H 1971 Postpartum broad ligament haematomas. Journal of Obstetrics and Gynaecology of the British Commonwealth 78: 184–189

Fletcher S J, Parr M J A 2000 Amniotic fluid embolism: a case report and review. Resuscitation 43: 141–146

Fox H 1987 Histopathology of pre-eclampsia and eclampsia. In: Sharp F, Symonds M E (eds) Hypertension in pregnancy. Perinatology Press, Ithaca, New York, pp 119–130

Fox L P 1967 Abortion deaths in California. American Journal of Obstetrics and Gynecology 98: 645–651

Friedmann W, Maier R F, Luttkus A et al 1996 Uterine rupture after laparoscopic myomectomy. Acta Obstetricia et Gynecologica Scandinavica 75: 683–684

Garland I W C, Thompson W D 1983 Diagnosis of amniotic fluid embolism using an antiserum to human keratin. Journal of Clinical Pathology 36: 625–627

Garnet J D 1964 Uterine rupture during pregnancy: an analysis of 133 patients. Obstetrics and Gynecology 23: 898–905

Girard P, Mal H, Laine J F, Petitpretz P, Rain B, Duroux P 1986 Left heart failure in amniotic fluid embolism. Anesthesiology 64: 262–265

Golan A, Sandbank O, Rubin A 1980 Rupture of the pregnant uterus. Obstetrics and Gynecology 56: 549–554

Golde S, Ledger W J 1977 Necrotizing fasciitis in postpartum patients: a report of four cases. Obstetrics and Gynecology 50: 670–673

Goldstein P J 1968 Amniotic fluid embolism complicating intrauterine saline abortion. American Journal of Obstetrics and Gynecology 101: 858–859

Gonsoulin W, Borge D, Moise K J 1990 Rupture of unscarred uterus in association with cocaine abuse. American Journal of Obstetrics and Gynecology 163: 526–527

Govan A D T 1976 The histology of eclamptic lesions. Journal of Clinical Pathology 29: Supplement (Royal College of Pathologists) 10: 63–69

Gregory M G, Clayton E M 1973 Amniotic fluid embolism. Obstetrics and Gynecology 42: 236–244

Grimes D A 1994 The morbidity and mortality of pregnancy: still risky business. American Journal of Obstetrics and Gynecology 170: 1489–1494

Grischke E M, Wallwiener D, Bastert G 1999 Inversio uteri puerperalis bei gedeckter Uterusruptur. Zeitschrift fur Geburtshilfe und Neonatalogie 203: 123–125

Guidotti R J, Grimes D A, Cates W 1981 Fatal amniotic fluid embolism during surgically induced abortion, United States, 1972 to 1978. American Journal of Obstetrics and Gynecology 141: 257–261

Halmagyi D F J, Starzecki B, Shearman R P 1962 Experimental amniotic fluid embolism. American Journal of Obstetrics and Gynecology 84: 251–256

Hankins J D V, Snyder R R, Clark S L et al 1993 Acute hemodynamic and respiratory effects of amniotic fluid embolism in the pregnant goat model. American Journal of Obstetrics and Gynecology 168: 1113–1118

Harris W J 1992 Uterine dehiscence following laparoscopic myomectomy. Obstetrics and Gynecology 80: 545–546

Hasleton P S 1983 Adult respiratory distress syndrome — a review. Histopathology 7: 307–332

Hockstein S 2000 Spontaneous uterine rupture in the early third trimester after laparoscopically assisted myomectomy. Journal of Reproductive Medicine 45: 139–141

Hogberg U 1985 Maternal mortality — a worldwide problem. International Journal of Gynaecology and Obstetrics 23: 463–470

Hostetler D R, Bosworth M F 2000 Uterine inversion: a life-threatening obstetric emergency. Journal of the American Board of Family Practice 13: 120–123

Hunter R M, Scott J C, Schneider J P, Krieger J A 1956 Experimental amniotic fluid infusion: a preliminary report. American Journal of Obstetrics and Gynecology 72: 75–78

Jeffcoate T N A, Miller J, Roos R F, Tindall V R 1968 Puerperal thromboembolism in relation to the inhibition of lactation by oestrogen therapy. British Medical Journal 4: 19–25

Jones R O, Nagashima A W, Hartnett-Goodman M M, Goodlin R C 1991 Rupture of low transverse cesarean scars during trial of labor. Obstetrics and Gynecology 77: 815–817

Kaczmarek J C, Kates R, Rau F et al 1994 Intrapartum uterine rupture in a primiparous patient previously treated for invasive mole. Obstetrics and Gynecology 83: 842–844

Kafkas S, Taper C E 1991 Ruptured uterus. International Journal of Gynaecology and Obstetrics 34: 41–44

Katz V L, Cefalo R C 1989 Maternal death from carotid artery thrombosis associated with the syndrome of hemolysis, elevated liver function and low platelets. American Journal of Perinatology 6: 360–362

Khong T Y 1998 Expression of endothelin-1 in amniotic fluid embolism and possible pathophysiological mechanism. British Journal of Obstetrics and Gynaecology 105: 802–804

Kitchin J D, Thiacarajah S, May H V, Thornton W N 1975 Puerperal inversion of the uterus. American Journal of Obstetrics and Gynecology 123: 51–56

Kitzmiller J L, Lucas W E 1972 Studies on a model of amniotic fluid embolism. Obstetrics and Gynecology 39: 626–627

Kobayashi H, Ooi H, Hayakawa H et al 1997 Histological diagnosis of amniotic fluid embolism by monoclonal antibody TKH-2 that recognizes NeuAc alpha 2-6GalNAc epitope. Human Pathology 28: 428–433

Koegler A, Sauder P, Marolf A, Jaeger A 1994 Amniotic fluid embolism: a case report with non-cardiogenic pulmonary edema. Intensive Care Medicine 20: 45–46

Konje J C, Odukoya O A, Ladipo A O 1990 Ruptured uterus in Ibadan — a twelve year review. International Journal of Gynaecology and Obstetrics 32: 207–213

Krause W 1969 Erfahrungen mit der transabdominalen Amniozentese. Zentralblatt fur Gynakologie 91: 1561–1566

Larue L, Marpeau L, Percque M et al 1991 Rupture d'un uterus sain lors d'une interruption de grossesse par prostaglandines au deuxieme trimestre. Journal de Gynecologie et Obstetrique et de la Biologie de Reproduction 20: 269–272

Lee H A, Frampton J 1964 Case of intra-amniotic glucose induction followed by non-fatal amniotic fluid embolism and acute renal failure. American Journal of Gynecology 90: 554–555

Lee W, Ginsburg K A, Cotton D B et al 1986 Squamous and trophoblastic cells in the maternal pulmonary circulation identified by invasive hemodynamic monitoring during the peripartum period. American Journal of Obstetrics and Gynecology 155: 999–1002

Lema V M, Ojwang S B, Wanjala S H 1991 Rupture of the gravid uterus: a review. East African Medical Journal 68: 430–441

Lilien A A 1968 Oxytocin-induced water intoxication: a report of a maternal death. Obstetrics and Gynecology 32: 171–173

Locksmith G J 1999 Amniotic fluid embolism. Obstetrics and Gynecology Clinics of North America 26: 435–444

Lockwood C J, Bach R, Guha A et al 1991 Amniotic fluid contains tissue factor, a potent initiator of coagulation. American Journal of Obstetrics and Gynecology 165: 1335–1341

Lurie S, Hagay Z, Goldschmitt R, Insler V 1992 Routine previous cesarean scar exploration following successful vaginal delivery: is it necessary? European Journal of Obstetrics, Gynecology and Reproductive Biology 45: 185–196

Lydon-Rochelle M, Holt V L, Easterling T R, Martin D P 2001 Risk of uterine rupture during labor among women with a prior cesarean delivery. New England Journal of Medicine 345: 3–8

McCally M, Vasicka A 1962 Generalized Schwartzman reaction and hypofibrinogenemia in septic abortion: report of a case. Obstetrics and Gynecology 19: 359–364

McCormick P W 1967 Pulmonary aspiration in obstetrics. Hospital Medicine 2: 163–171

Macmillan D 1968 Experimental amniotic fluid embolism. Journal of Obstetrics and Gynaecology of the British Commonwealth 75: 849–852

Maher J E, Wenstrom K D, Hauth J C, Meis P J 1994 Amniotic fluid embolism after saline amnioinfusion: two cases and review of the literature. Obstetrics and Gynecology 83: 851–854

Maymon R, Haimovich L, Shulman A et al 1992 Third trimester uterine rupture after prostaglandin E2 use for labor induction. Journal of Reproductive Medicine 37: 449–452

Meehan F P, Burke G, Kehoe J T 1989 Update on delivery following prior cesarian section: a 15 year review 1972–1987. International Journal of Gynaecology and Obstetrics 30: 205–212

Mendelson C L 1946 The aspiration of stomach contents into the lungs during obstetric anesthesia. American Journal of Obstetrics and Gynecology 52: 191–204

Milon D, Chevrant-Breton O, Tekam S, Peton J, Saint-Marc C, Giraud J R 1983 Rupture of the uterus during labor without apparent cause. European Journal of Obstetrics, Gynecology and Reproductive Biology 15: 1–4

Mokgokong E T, Marivate M 1976 Treatment of the ruptured uterus. South African Medical Journal 50: 1621–1624

Moldavsky L F 1967 Management of inversion of the uterus: report of four cases. Obstetrics and Gynecology 29: 488–494

Morgan M 1979 Amniotic fluid embolism. Anaesthesia 34: 20–32

Nelson P K 1960 Pulmonary gas embolism in pregnancy and the puerperium. Obstetrical and Gynecological Survey 15: 449–481

Nkemayim D C, Hammadeh M E, Hippach M, Mink D, Schmidt W 2000 Uterine rupture in pregnancy subsequent to previous laparoscopic eletromyolysis: case report and review of the literature. Archives of Gynecology and Obstetrics 264: 154–156

Noble W H, St Amand J 1993 Amniotic fluid embolism. Canadian Journal of Anaesthesia 40: 871–880

O'Driscoll R 1966 Rupture of the uterus. Proceedings of the Royal Society of Medicine 59: 65–66

Ogueh O, Ayida G 1997 Acute uterine inversion: a new technique of hydrostatic replacement. British Journal of Obstetrics and Gynaecology 104: 951–952

Ooi H, Kobayashi H, Hirashima Y, Yamazaki T, Kobayashi T, Terao T 1998 Serological and immunohistochemical diagnosis of amniotic fluid embolism. Seminars in Thrombosis and Hemostasis 24: 479–484

Pelosi M, Pelosi M A 1997 Spontaneous uterine rupture at thirty-three weeks subsequent to previous superficial laparoscopic myomectomy. American Journal of Obstetrics and Gynecology 177: 1547–1549

Peterson E W, Taylor H B 1970 Amniotic fluid embolism: an analysis of forty cases. Obstetrics and Gynecology 35: 787–793

Petroianu G A, Altmannsberger S H, Maleck W H et al 1999 Meconium and amniotic fluid embolism: effects on coagulation in pregnant MINI-pigs. Critical Care Medicine 27: 348–355

Philippe H J, Goffinet F, Jacquemard F et al 1991 Les traitements des inversions uterines obstetricales: a propos de trois observations. Journal de Gynecologie et Obstetrique et Biologie de la Reproduction 20: 843–849

Pieri R I 1958 Pelvic hematomas associated with pregnancy. Obstetrics and Gynecology 12: 244–258

Piot D, Gluck M, Oxorn H 1973 Torsion of the gravid uterus. Canadian Medical Association Journal 109: 1010–1011

Plauche W C 1983 Amniotic fluid embolism. American Journal of Obstetrics and Gynecology 147: 982–985

Prasad R N, Ratnam S S 1992 Uterine rupture after induction of labour for intrauterine death using the prostaglandin E2 analogue sulprostone. Australian and New Zealand Journal of Obstetrics and Gynaecology 32: 282–283

Ragan W D 1981 Antepartum air embolism. Journal of the Indiana State Medical Association 74: 30–32

Rasmussen O B 1992 Puerperal inversion of the uterus. Acta Obstetricia et Gynecologica Scandinavica 71: 558–559

Ravasia D J, Wooo S L, Pollarro J K 2000 Uterine rupture during induced trial of labor among women with previous cesarean delivery. American Journal of Obstetrics and Gynecology 183: 1176–1179

RCOG Guideline 1997 Beta-agonists for the care of women in preterm labour. Royal College of Obstetricians and Gynaecologists, London

Reece E A, Hobbins J C, Mahoney M J, Petrie R H 1992 Medicine of the fetus and mother. Lippincott, Philadelphia

Reeves T, Daoud F S, Estriole M, Stone W H, McGary D 1974 Pulmonary pressor effects of small amounts of bovine amniotic fluid. Respiration Physiology 20: 231

Reis R L, Pierce W S, Behrendt D M 1969 Hemodynamic effects of amniotic fluid embolism. Surgery, Gynecology and Obstetrics 129: 45–48

Report on Confidential Enquiries into Maternal Deaths in England and Wales 1976–1978 1982 Her Majesty's Stationery Office, London

Report on Confidential Enquiries into Maternal Deaths in the United Kingdom 1994–1996 1998 Her Majesty's Stationery Office, London

Rodgers B M, Staroscik R N, Reis R L 1969 Amniotic fluid embolism: effects of myocardial contractility and systemic and pulmonary vascular resistance. Surgical Forum 20: 203–205

Rodgers B M, Staroscik R N, Reis R L 1971 Effects of amniotic fluid on cardiac contractility and vascular resistance. American Journal of Physiology 220: 1979–1982

Ruckley C A 1992 Diagnosis and management of thromboembolic disease during pregnancy and the puerperium. In: Patel N (ed) Maternal mortality — the way forward. Royal College of Obstetricians and Gynaecologists, London, pp 41–50

Rushton D I, Dawson I M P 1982 The maternal autopsy. Journal of Clinical Pathology 35: 909–921

Sawyer M M, Lipshitz J, Anderson G D, Dilts P V 1981 Third trimester uterine rupture associated with vaginal prostaglandin E$_2$. American Journal of Obstetrics and Gynecology 140: 710–711

Schrinsky D C, Benson R C 1978 Rupture of the pregnant uterus: a review. Obstetrical and Gynecological Survey 33: 217–232

Schuitemaker N W, Gravenhorst J B, Van Geijn H P et al 1991 Maternal mortality and its prevention. European Journal of Obstetrics, Gynecology and Reproductive Biology 42 (suppl): s31–s35

Schwartz O J, Wynne J W, Gibbs C P, Hood C I, Kuck E J 1980 The pulmonary consequences of aspiration of gastric contents of pH values greater than 2.5. American Review of Respiratory Disease 121: 119–126

Shah-Hosseini M, Evrard J R 1989 Puerperal uterine inversion. Obstetrics and Gynecology 73: 367–370

Shanklin D R, Sommers S C, Brown D A et al 1991 The pathology of maternal death. American Journal of Obstetrics and Gynecology 165: 1126–1155

Sheehan H L 1939 Pathology of hyperemesis and vomiting in late pregnancy. Journal of Obstetrics and Gynaecology of the British Empire 46: 685–699

Sheehan H L, Lynch J B 1973 Pathology of toxaemia of pregnancy. Churchill Livingstone, Edinburgh

Shy K K, Eschenbach D A 1979 Fatal perineal cellulitis from an episiotomy site. Obstetrics and Gynecology 54: 292–298

Smith C A 1975 Pathologic uterine torsion: a catastrophic event in late pregnancy. American Journal of Obstetrics and Gynecology 123: 32–33

Steiner P E, Lushbaugh C C 1941 Maternal pulmonary embolism by amniotic fluid as a cause of obstetric shock and unexpected death in obstetrics. Journal of the American Medical Association 117: 1245–1254

Stevenson C A 1969 Maternal death from puerperal sepsis following vaginal surgery: a 17 year study in Michigan (1950–1966). American Journal of Obstetrics and Gynecology 104: 699–710

Stewardson R H, Nyhus L M 1977 Pulmonary aspiration — an update. Archives of Surgery 112: 1192–1197

Stolte L, van Kessel H, Seelen J, Eskes T, Wagatsuma T 1967 Failure to produce the syndrome of amniotic fluid embolism by infusion of amniotic fluid and meconium into monkeys. American Journal of Obstetrics and Gynecology 98: 694–697

Studdiford W E, Douglas G W 1956 Placental bacteremia: a significant finding in septic abortion accompanied by vascular collapse. American Journal of Obstetrics and Gynecology 71: 842–858

Taylor P J, Canning D C 1979 Spontaneous rupture of primigravid uterus. Journal of Reproductive Medicine 22: 168–170

Teabeaut J R 1952 Aspiration of gastric contents — an experimental study. American Journal of Pathology 28: 50–67

Tindall V R 1971 The aetiology and pathology of pulmonary embolism. In: Macdonald R R (ed) Scientific basis of obstetrics and gynaecology, 1st edn. Churchill Livingstone, London, pp 385–414

Toner P G 1992 The role of the histopathologist in maternal death. In: Patel N (ed) Maternal mortality — the way forward. Royal College of Obstetricians and Gynaecologists, London

Trive B K, Bristwo R E, Hsu C D et al 1994 Uterine rupture associated with recent antepartum cocaine abuse. Obstetrics and Gynecology 83: 840–841

Varner M 1991 Postpartum hemorrhage. Critical Care Clinics 7: 883–897

Visser A A, Giesteira M V K, Heyns A, Marais C 1983 Torsion of the gravid uterus: case reports. British Journal of Obstetrics and Gynaecology 90: 89–97

Watson P 1980 Postpartum hemorrhage and shock. Clinical Obstetrics and Gynaecology 23: 985–1001

Watson P, Besch N, Bowes W A 1980 Management of acute and subacute puerperal inversion of the uterus. Obstetrics and Gynecology 55: 12–16

Weiner-Kronish J P, Gropper M A, Matthay M A 1990 The adult respiratory distress syndrome: definition and prognosis, pathogenesis and treatment. British Journal of Anaesthesia 65: 107–129

Weinstein L 1982 Syndrome of hemolysis, elevated liver enzymes, and low platelet count: a severe consequence of hypertension in pregnancy. American Journal of Obstetrics and Gynecology 142: 159–167

Wynne J W, Modell J H 1977 Respiratory aspiration of stomach contents. Annals of Internal Medicine 87: 466–474

Yussman M A, Haynes D M 1970 Rupture of the gravid uterus: a 12 year study. Obstetrics and Gynecology 36: 115–120

48

The pathology of multiple pregnancy

H. Fox

Twin pregnancy   1575
Incidence of twinning   1575
Zygosity of twinning   1576
Aetiology of twin pregnancy   1576
Twin placentation   1576
Specific clinical features of the various forms of twin
    placentation   1580
Twin transfusion syndrome   1581
Discordant growth in twin pregnancies   1585
Fetus papyraceous   1585
The vanishing twin syndrome   1585
Twin pregnancy with hydatidiform mole   1586
Conjoined twins   1586
Pathological examination of the twin placenta   1587

Triplet placentation   1588

Higher multiple births   1589

TWIN PREGNANCY

INCIDENCE OF TWINNING

The incidence of twin conception is very much higher than the incidence of twin births for ultrasound studies have suggested that about 12% of all conceptions are twins, as many as 70% of these being converted to singleton pregnancies by early asymptomatic loss of one of the conceptuses, the so-called 'vanishing twin syndrome' (see later).

Amongst white Caucasians the incidence of twinning is usually said to be in the region of one in 80 births (Strong & Corney 1967; Benirschke & Kim 1973a); in both Europe and the USA this rate appeared to be decreasing during the first half of the 20th century (Elwood 1973) but, for reasons that are far from fully clear, has since quite markedly increased (Bryan 1994; Derom et al 1995; Jewell & Yip 1995; Taffel 1995; Keith et al 2000). The rate of twinning is higher amongst individuals of African origin, being approximately one in 70 amongst black Americans and reaching an apogee in Nigeria where reported rates have ranged from one in 20 births (Nylander 1969, 1973) to one in 35 (Aisien et al 2000). By contrast, the twinning rate is low in Orientals (Baldwin 1994), though the incidence in India and Pakistan is similar to that in Europe (Bulmer 1970; Nylander 1975b).

ZYGOSITY OF TWINS

Twins may be either monozygotic or dizygotic. The former are produced from a single fertilised ovum which replicates during the very early stages of development, whilst the latter are due to the independent release, and subsequent fertilisation, of two separate ova. Monozygotic twins are of the same sex and are, with very rare exceptions, genetically identical. The commonest, albeit still extremely rare, form of genetic discordance in monozygotic twins is in the sex chromosomes, usually absence of one X chromosome in one twin, most obvious with male twins where one becomes monosomy X with Ullrich– Turner syndrome (Perlman et al 1990; Machin 1996). Other patterns of numerical sex chromosome and autosome discordance (Dallpiccola et al 1985; Nieuwint et al 1999) and discordance of chromosomal structure (Juberg et al 1981) are even less common. Cytogenetically discordant monozygotic twin pairs may arise from either post-zygotic non-disjunction or anaphase lag, followed or accompanied by twinning, and are sometimes known as heterokaryonts. Clear confirmation of monozygosity in phenotypically and cytogenetically discordant twins is essential to diagnose heterokaryonts, and tissue as well as blood must be sampled for chromosome analysis to differentiate them from blood chimeras due to vascular mixing.

Dizygotic twins are no more genetically similar than any other pair of siblings and may or may not be of the same sex; it is even possible, if coitus occurs with two men in a short period of time, for apparently dizygotic twins to have separate fathers (Gedda 1961; Hafez 1974; Terasaki et al 1978; Majsky & Kout 1982; Wenk et al 1992; Ambach et al 2000), though superfecundation, as this phenomenon is known, is very rare. It has been suggested that superfetation, in which a second fertilised ovum is implanted in a uterus containing a month-old pregnancy, can occur (Scrimgeour & Baker 1974; Walter et al 1975), but there is no conclusive proof that this actually happens (Corney & Robson 1975; Baldwin 1994).

The possibility of a third type of twinning in which a single ovum is fertilised by two separate spermatozoa (monovular dispermic twinning) has long been entertained (Bulmer 1970): the resulting twins would be neither dizygotic nor monozygotic but a combination of the two. There is now evidence, derived from DNA analysis, that twinning of this type does occur as a result of fertilisation of a polar body as well as an oocyte from the same ovum (Baldwin 1994, 1999). Fertilisation of the diploid first polar body leads to a triploid twin (Bieber et al 1981) whilst fertilisation of the haploid second polar body leads to a diploid twin (Boklage 1987). The incidence of polar body twinning is not known because it requires detailed molecular analysis to determine the parent of origin of the components of the genetic material of the twins, and may be suspected only when a normal boy and normal girl have a proven monochorionic placenta (Baldwin 1994).

Amongst white Caucasians about a third of twins are monozygotic (Potter 1963; Cameron 1968; Fujikura & Froehlich 1971; Corney et al 1972; Cameron et al 1983), but where the twinning rate is very high, as amongst the Yoruba of Nigeria, monozygotic twins constitute only about 8% of the total (Nylander 1971a, 1973); conversely, where the twinning rate is low, as in the Far East, monozygotic twins tend to predominate (Chun 1970; Dawood et al 1975). These findings are in accord with the view that the incidence of monozygotic twinning is roughly uniform in all parts of the world, the very marked national and ethnic variations in twinning rate

being due entirely to differences in the incidence of dizygotic twins (Bulmer 1970; Bortolus et al 1999).

AETIOLOGY OF TWIN PREGNANCY

The cause of twinning is uncertain, but there is a strong hereditary element, predominantly but not entirely confined to the maternal side, in dizygotic twinning, and there is a good deal of circumstantial evidence to suggest that this form of twinning may be related to a high follicle stimulating hormone (FSH) level with resulting polyovulation (Benirschke & Kim 1973a; Nylander 1975a; Bomsel Helmreich & Al Mufti 1995; Lambalk et al 1998a,b). There is now evidence that maternal, but not paternal, hereditary factors also play a role in some cases of monozygotic twinning (Lichtenstein et al 1996, 1998); it has nevertheless been suggested that such twinning is a form of abnormal development similar in aetiology and pathogenesis to a congenital malformation (Benirschke & Kim 1973a,b; Nylander 1975a).

TWIN PLACENTATION

Dizygotic twin placentation

If the two ova of dizygotic twins are implanted at some distance from each other there will be two separate and discrete placentas, each having its own amniotic sac; the placentation is therefore clearly of the dichorionic–diamniotic type. If the two ova implant in close proximity to each other there will be two amniotic sacs but the two placentas may show varying degrees of fusion to form what appears to be a single chorionic mass (Fig. 48.1); more

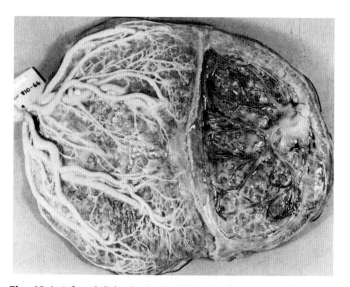

Fig. 48.1 A fused dichorionic placenta. The amnions have been stripped off from the fetal surface but a ridge of chorionic tissue remains at the site of the base of the septum between the two amniotic cavities. The vessels of one cord have been injected with barium mixture and there is no evidence of any communication between the two vascular systems.

detailed examination reveals, however, that this is formed by two placentas and hence the form of placentation is still dichorionic and diamniotic. The theoretical possibility exists that the two placentas of dizygotic twins may show true complete fusion to form a monochorionic placenta, but nearly all the claimed examples of twins of opposite sex having a monochorionic form of placentation have been based more upon anecdotal maternal reminiscences than on any scientific evidence (Strong & Corney 1967). Occasional reported exceptions to this rule can with hindsight be seen to have been examples of dispermic monovular twinning rather than true dizygotic twins. Therefore for all practical purposes the finding of a monochorionic placenta excludes any possibility of the twins being dizygotic, a view occasionally disputed (Mortimer 1987), but confirmed by genetic studies (Husby et al 1991).

Monozygotic twin placentation

The form of placentation of monozygotic twins depends upon the stage at which duplication occurs (Fig. 48.2). It is believed (Corner 1955) that if the single fertilised ovum separates into two during the first three days after fertilisation, that is, before the differentiation of the trophoblast, two separate embryos will develop, each having its own placenta and amniotic sac, and the subsequent placentation of these will be exactly similar to that seen in dizygotic twins. Thus if the two embryos implant at some distance from each other there will be two separate placentas and amniotic sacs and placentation will obviously be of the dichorionic–

diamniotic variety. If the two developing embryos implant in close proximity to each other there may be fusion of the two placentas but there will be two amniotic sacs; as with dizygotic twins, the fusion is not absolute and placentation is still of the dichorionic–diamniotic type.

If splitting occurs during the blastocyst stage, i.e. between the third and eighth day after fertilisation, when the trophoblast, but not the amniotic cavity, has differentiated, the twins will develop a single placenta (Fig. 48.3) with two amniotic sacs; the placentation is then categorised as monochorionic–diamniotic.

The amniotic cavity differentiates between the 8th and 13th day after fertilisation and it is thought that if splitting occurs during this period there will be only one placenta and one amniotic sac, the placentation being of the monochorionic–monoamniotic form. Not all workers, however, are persuaded that monoamniotic placentation is produced in this fashion; some claim that in all, or most, of such cases there were originally two amniotic cavities which were converted into one by the breaking down and disappearance of the dividing membranes between the two cavities. There is good evidence that, on occasion, there may be a spontaneous or traumatic disruption of the dividing septum, the remnants of which appear as a plica on the surface of the monochorionic placenta (Foglmann 1974; Megory et al 1991). Benirschke & Kaufmann (2000) suggest however that a plica of this type is due, not to the almost total disintegration of a previously present septum, but to the splitting of the blastomere at the very moment when the amnion was forming but was as yet incomplete. This is a rather

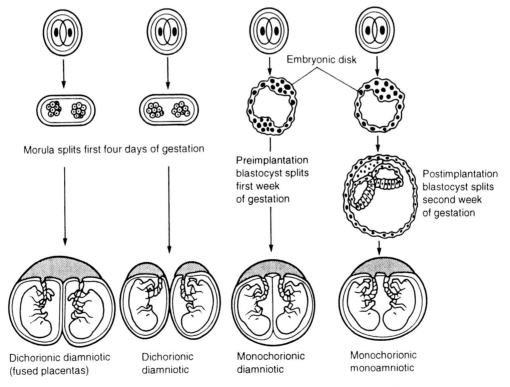

Fig. 48.2 Diagrammatic representation of the development and placentation of monozygotic twins.

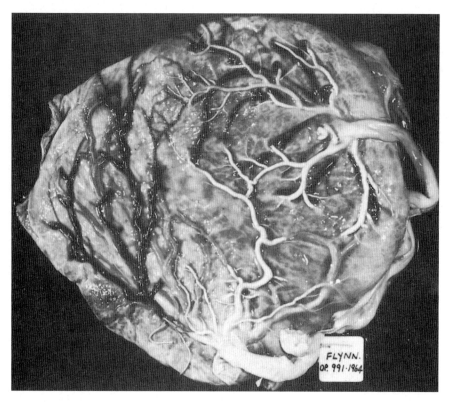

Fig. 48.3 A monochorionic twin placenta. The amnion has been stripped off from the fetal aspect to leave a smooth continuous surface. The arteries of cord 1 (no label) have been injected with barium solution and this shows a direct communication with an artery from cord 2. A major artery of cord 2 has been injected with Indian ink and this substance is seen to have passed to the veins of placenta 1, this indicating the presence of a deep vascular communication.

recondite dispute to which no firm answer is as yet available, and which is of theoretical rather than practical importance.

If splitting occurs at or after the 13th day of development this will result in conjoined twins, the earliest and simplest stage of which is monoamniotic twins whose umbilical cords fuse before inserting into the placenta (Larson et al 1969).

Incidence of various forms of placentation and relationship to zygosity

The various studies on this topic from Britain and the USA (Potter 1963; Strong & Corney 1967; Cameron 1968; Fujikura & Froehlich 1971; Corney et al 1972) and from Nigeria (Nylander & Corney 1969; Nylander 1970a,b, 1971a) have been collated by Corney (1975).

For all practical purposes all twins having a monochorionic placenta are monozygotic; twins with dichorionic placentation may, however, be either monozygotic or dizygotic. Hence the proportion of twins with dichorionic placentation will be higher than the proportion of dizygotic twins. In white Caucasian populations about 80% of twins have a dichorionic form of placentation; in Nigeria, where the proportion of monozygotic twins is low, 95% of twin placentas are dichorionic. The proportions of dichorionic placentas that are separate or fused are very roughly equal; between 10 and 15% of dichorionic placentas will be from monozygotic twins, there being in most, but not all, studies a greater tendency for monozygotic dichorionic placentas to be fused rather than separate.

Looking at the situation in the reverse fashion, the proportion of monozygotic twins having a dichorionic form of placentation is between 20 and 40%.

Vascular anastomoses in twin placentas

Monochorionic placentas

It was well established in the 19th century that vascular communications between the two territories of monozygotic twins are often found in monochorionic placentas (Hyrtle 1870; Schatz 1900); indeed so complete were these early descriptions that relatively little new information on this topic has since emerged. It is agreed that such anastomoses are present in nearly all monochorionic placentas, their reported incidence varying from 76 to 100% (Benirschke 1961a; Bleisch 1965; Strong & Corney 1967; Cameron 1968; Arts & Lohman 1971; Galea et al 1982; Robertson & Neer 1983; Ramos-Arroyo et al 1988), and that these communications may be either superficial or deep. The superficial anastomoses are between relatively large vessels on the fetal surface of the placenta (Fig. 48.3) and the vast majority are direct arterio-arterial communications between a chorionic artery of one fetus and a chorionic artery of the other; a minority are of the veno-venous type, and in a few placentas both varieties of superficial communication may be present. Of perhaps greater pathological significance are arterio-venous anastomoses between the two circulatory systems; these are deep, i.e. within the placental substance, and form what Schatz (1900) referred to as the 'third circulation' (the other two being those of the two fetuses). These

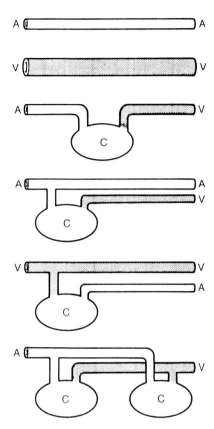

Fig. 48.4 Diagrammatic representation of the various forms of vascular communication that can occur in monochorionic twin placentae. A=artery; V=vein; C=shared lobule with capillary anastomoses.

arterio-venous anastomoses occur in shared lobules (Fig. 48.4), which are supplied by an artery from one twin and drain into a vein from the other twin; the anastomosis is via the capillary system of the villi and there are no direct pre-capillary arterio-venous communications. Such shared lobules are often multiple and are situated along the equator separating the individual territories of the two twins. In some placentas in which there are multiple shared lobules the arterio-venous communications may be all in the same direction, but in others some of the shared lobules may be supplied by an artery from the first twin and drain into a vein of the second twin, whilst others may be supplied by an artery from the second twin and drain into a vein from the first twin.

In many, probably most or even all, monochorionic twin placentas both deep and superficial anastomoses are present; indeed, the arterial supply to a shared lobule is not uncommonly from a branch which arises from a superficial arterio-arterial communication (Arts & Lohman 1971); occasionally venous drainage from a shared lobule is into a superficial veno-venous anastomosis.

Dichorionic placentas

Vascular communications between dichorionic placentas which are totally separate from each other have never

been described: one placenta which macroscopically appeared to be dichorionic with superficial vascular anastomoses between the two placental masses was considered to be actually a bilobate monochorionic placenta (Kim & Lage 1991) and a similar bilobate monochorionic placenta has been described by Altshuler & Hyde (1993). There is, however, some dispute as to whether anastomoses between the two circulatory systems ever occur in fused dichorionic placentas. Occasional claims in the earlier literature to have demonstrated such communications (Scipiades & Burg 1930; Szendi 1938; Perez et al 1947; Gedda 1961) were regarded with some scepticism by Strong & Corney (1967), who did not find any anastomoses in dichorionic placentas, an experience they shared with Benirschke (1961a), Bleisch (1964), and Arts & Lohman (1971). However, Cameron (1968) was able to prove the presence of vascular communications in two of the 500 dichorionic placentas which he studied; in each case the twins appeared to be monozygotic, and both arterio-arterial and veno-venous anastomoses were present on the placental surface. Bhargava & Chakravarty (1975) have reported finding vascular communications in seven out of 143 dichorionic placentas; even more surprisingly they claimed that in six of these the anastomoses were of the deep arterio-venous type. It is difficult to evaluate this report, for a corrosion technique, which is probably less reliable than an injection method, was used, and all the illustrations of vascular communications were of such structures in monochorial placentas. Robertson & Neer (1983) described anastomoses in one of 68 fused dichorionic placentas whilst Lage et al (1989) also reported an example of both deep and superficial anastomoses across fused dichorionic placentas: a rather similar case of anatomoses in a fused dichorionic placenta was described by Molnar-Nadasdy & Altschuler (1996). A fully convincing report of proven anastomoses with substantial functional interfetal transfusion between dichorionic placentas with fusion only of the membranes has been reported by King et al (1995) whilst an equally convincing case of vascular anastomoses within a fused dichorionic placenta of opposite sex dizygotic twins has been documented (Phelan et al 1998). There is, therefore, evidence that anastomoses between the two circulatory systems may sometimes occur in fused dichorionic placentas, a conclusion bolstered by the occasional finding of blood group chimerism in dizygotic twins of opposite sex (Baldwin 1994; van Djik et al 1996), a finding which suggests, albeit indirectly, some degree of vascular mixing during fetal life.

Associated pathological features of twin placentas

Strong & Corney (1967) noted a very high incidence of single umbilical artery in twins; however, this has not been everyone's experience and a number of workers have specifically denied that any association exists between the two conditions (Fox 1997). Velamentous insertion of the cord appears to be unduly common in twin placentas (Robinson et al 1983; Bardawil et al 1988; Ramos-Arroyo et al 1988; Fries et al 1993; Baldwin 1994; Machin 1997; Di Salvo et al 1998; Benirschke & Kaufmann 2000); this high incidence has been attributed, very unconvincingly, to intrauterine crowding and a secondary distortion of placental growth.

SPECIFIC CLINICAL FEATURES OF THE VARIOUS FORMS OF TWIN PLACENTATION

Monochorionic–diamniotic twin placentation

Twins with this form of placentation have a much higher perinatal mortality than do those with dichorionic placentas (Gaziano et al 2000); the perinatal mortality rate has, however, varied considerably in different series, ranging from just over 7% (Gruenwald 1970) to 22 to 25% (Benirschke & Driscoll 1967; Myrianthopoulos 1970). Perhaps the most important factor contributing to this high death rate is premature onset of labour, an event often attributed to polyhydramnios (Bajoria & Kingdom 1997); there must, however, be some doubt as to whether polyhydramnios is particularly prone to complicate monochorionic placentation in the absence of the twin-transfusion syndrome, for Nylander & MacGillivray (1975), although not noting the form of placentation, found that excessive accumulation of liquor occurred with equal frequency in monozygotic and dizygotic twin pregnancies. Nevertheless, polyhydramnios does develop unduly often as an accompaniment, or complication, of the 'twin–twin transfusion syndrome', which is an important cause of perinatal mortality in monochorionic twins, particularly those that are diamniotic (see below).

Monochorionic–monoamniotic twin placentas

This is the least common form of twin pregnancy but despite, or perhaps because of, its relative rarity it has been the subject of a considerable number of studies, outstanding amongst which have been those of Quigley (1935), Raphael (1961), Timmons & de Alvarez (1963), Wharton et al (1968), and Pauls (1969): more recent, but less comprehensive, reviews include those of Hollingsworth (1973), Israelstam (1973), Tagawa (1974), Lumme & Saarikoski (1986), Rodis et al (1987), Sutter et al (1986), Tessen & Zlatnik (1991), Dorum & Nesheim (1991), Olsen (1992) and Drack et al (1993).

The incidence of monoamniotic twins is a matter of some dispute, their reported frequency in multiple pregnancies having ranged from one in 65 (Librach & Terrin 1957) to one in 666 (Acosta-Sison et al 1946). Wenner (1956) claimed, however, that four of the hundred twins in his series had a monoamniotic placentation, and,

although this figure has often been considered as grossly atypical, it has not markedly conflicted with those noted in careful prospective studies, which have shown an incidence of between 1 and 3% (Strong & Corney 1967); particularly striking in this respect was the finding of 18 monoamniotic twins in a series of 581 twin pregnancies investigated in Birmingham, UK, by Wharton et al (1968).

Monoamniotic placentation is associated with a high fetal mortality. Quigley (1935) found that nearly 70% of fetuses died, but more recent figures are somewhat less dismal and suggest that between 50 and 70% of monoamniotic twins now survive (Raphael 1961; Wensinger & Daly 1962; Wharton et al 1968; Baldwin 1994; Benirschke & Kaufmann 2000). The reasons for what is still an alarmingly high fetal death rate are not fully clear, but there is no doubt that an important contributory factor is the tendency for the two umbilical cords to become twisted and entangled with each other (Fig. 48.5), with the formation of true knots, these latter being found in about 40 to 70% of cases (Salerno 1959; Zuckerman & Brzezinski 1960; Krussel et al 1994): although cord entanglement is a potent cause of fetal death in monoamniotic pregnancies a few twins do spontaneously survive this complication (Annan & Hutson 1990). Cord entanglement can now be recognised antenatally by colour flow Doppler ultrasound (Belfort et al 1993; Abuhamad et al 1995; Rodis et al 1997; Shahabi et al 1997; Arabin et al 1999) and amnioreduction to prevent fetal movements and worsening cord entanglement has proved successful in some cases (Overton et al 1999). A rare event, but one that can cause considerable obstetrical embarrassment, is for the neck of the first delivered twin to be tightly encircled by the cord of the other twin; division of the cord may then lead to exsanguination of the undelivered twin (Hagood & Stokes 1953; Goplerud 1964; Tagawa 1974; Ong et al 1976; McLeod & McCoy 1981). There is also an increased risk of obstructed labour because of interlocking of the twins.

Perhaps rather unexpectedly the transfusion syndrome is not a significant cause of fetal mortality or morbidity in monochorionic–monoamniotic twins and, indeed, there is some doubt as to the frequency with which placental vascular anastomoses between the two twins occur in this form of placentation. At first sight it would appear logical to expect that such anastomoses occur with at least the same frequency as in monochorionic–diamniotic placentas, but Wenner (1956) maintained that conjoined twins (which are always monoamniotic) may not have placental vascular communications, whilst Benirschke (1965) has suggested that such anastomoses occur less commonly in monoamniotic than in diamniotic placentas; this view appears to be supported by the fact that both Benirschke & Driscoll (1967) and Strong & Corney (1967) have each studied monoamniotic placentas in which no vascular anastomoses were present. On the other hand, Wharton et al (1968) found such anastomoses in 16 of their 18 monoamniotic

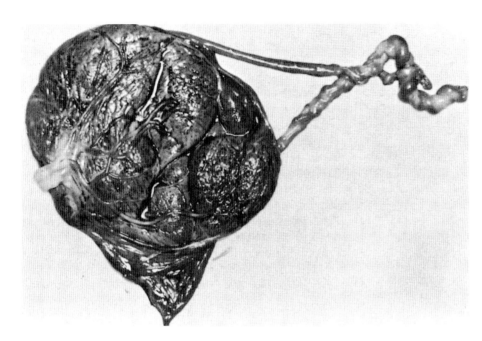

Fig. 48.5 A twin placenta (presumed to have been monoamniotic) with entanglement and knotting of the two umbilical cords.

placentas, whilst Bhargava et al (1971) demonstrated communications in all six monoamniotic placentas in their study. Bajoria (1998a) found a higher incidence of vascular anastomoses in monoamniotic–monochorionic placentas than in diamniotic–monochorionic placentas and it is possible that this relatively rich anastomotic network reduces the risk of unidirectional shunts. Certainly a chronic transfusion syndrome is exceptionally rare in monoamniotic twins, the only acceptable reports of such a complication being those of Hollander (1969), Meyer et al (1970) and Lumme & Saarikoski (1986).

Dichorionic–diamniotic twin placentation

The perinatal mortality rate of dichorionic twins is in the region of 7 to 10% (Potter 1963; Benirschke & Driscoll 1967; Myrianthopoulos 1970), but, in contrast to the situation in monochorionic twins, placental or cord factors are rarely, if ever, of importance in fetal or neonatal death. The pathology of separate dichorionic placentas can be considered as identical to that of placentas from singleton pregnancies, but in fused dichorionic placentas a transfusion syndrome may occur in exceptional cases, for, as discussed previously, such placentas can very occasionally have vascular anastomoses.

TWIN TRANSFUSION SYNDROME

The term 'twin to twin transfusion syndrome' is now known to encompass a variety of clinical syndromes which includes not only the classical chronic transfusion syndrome but also the acute transfusion syndrome, the effects on the surviving fetus of death of one twin and the development of an acardiac fetus. With very few exceptions all these complications are restricted to monochorionic twins.

Chronic twin-to-twin transfusion

The chronic twin–twin transfusion (or 'feto-fetal transfusion') syndrome was defined and largely elucidated by Schatz (1900) and has been reviewed by, amongst others, Conway (1964), Corney & Aherne (1965), Rausen et al (1965), Anger & Ring (1972), Hollander & Backmann (1974), Sekiya & Hafez (1977), Tan et al (1979), Galea et al (1982), Brown et al (1989), Giles et al (1990), Urig et al (1988), Blickstein (1990), Bruner & Rosemond (1993), Machin & Still (1995) and Machin & Keith (1998). The frequency with which this complicates monochorionic–diamniotic placentation has been estimated at about 15% (Rausen et al 1965; Arts & Lohman 1971), though Strong & Corney (1967) consider that its true incidence is probably over 30%. A chronic twin-to-twin transfusion occurs as a result of a long-standing haemodynamic imbalance and a slow net transfusion from one fetus to the other. The classically described clinical features of the chronic transfusion syndrome are an excessive amount of fluid in the amniotic sac of the recipient twin and a paucity of fluid in that of the donor (the 'oligohydramnios–polyhydramnios sequence') with one twin (the donor) being pale and anaemic whilst the other (the recipient) is plethoric and polycythaemic (Fig. 48.6); there is a substantial difference in haemoglobin levels between the two twins, and increased numbers of normoblasts are seen in the peripheral blood of the anaemic infant. The anaemic twin is smaller and lighter than the plethoric one and there may be a marked difference in organ weights between the two; cardiomegaly is often present in the polycythaemic infant (Naeye 1965). The placenta also shows marked changes (Fig. 48.7), the maternal surface of the placental territory of the anaemic, or donor, twin being pale and bulky and thus contrasting markedly with the placental substance of

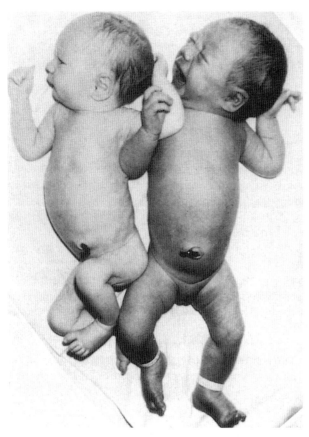

Fig. 48.6 Chronic twin–twin transfusion syndrome. The larger recipient twin, on the right, is still more plethoric than the considerably smaller donor twin, on the left, despite exchange transfusion. At birth: twin I 3.6 kg, twin II 2.2 kg.

the plethoric, or recipient, twin. Histological examination shows that the villi in the placenta of the recipient twin have large, engorged fetal vessels but are otherwise normal, whilst those of the donor twin's placenta are oedematous and bulky with small inconspicuous vessels (Aherne et al 1968). More recent fetal studies have, however, pointed out that haemoglobin and birth weight discrepancies are by no means universal in the twin–twin transfusion syndrome and that polyhydramnios, oedema and cardiac hypertophy in the recipient twin and oligohydramnios in the donor twin are the defining, and cardinal, clinical features of the syndrome (Bajoria et al 1995); furthermore there may be little difference, either grossly or histologically, between donor and recipient placentas in prenatally diagnosed cases (Wigglesworth 1995).

Schatz (1900) proposed that the twin–twin transfusion syndrome was due to 'a dynamic asymmetry of the third circulation', i.e. that there was a shunt of arterial blood from the donor twin through arterio-venous anastomoses in shared lobules into the venous circulation of the recipient twin. This state of affairs can be compensated for if superficial large vessel anastomoses are present to correct a unidirectional haemodynamic imbalance in the deep anastomoses or if there are arterio-venous anastomoses that run in the reverse direction. This concept has been widely

accepted, and indeed recently confirmed (Bajoria et al 1995; Machin 1996; Bajoria 1998a; Denbow et al 2000), but it is doubtful if it explains all of the features of the syndrome, and it must further be allowed that the detailed pathophysiology of the haemodynamic shunt remains obscure. Sebire et al (2001) have suggested, in a somewhat complex paper, that an asymmetric anastomotic pattern is of importance, attributing this to a discordant loss of the anastomoses that develop in a random fashion at the stage of connection of embryonic and extra-embryonic circulations. Kloosterman (1963) has maintained that the communications between the two circulatory systems are too small to allow for the transfer of any appreciable amount of blood and has suggested that many of the features of the syndrome are due to hyperproteinaemia in the heavier twin; it is true that IgG levels are usually higher in the recipient than in the donor twin (Bryan & Slavin 1974; Bryan et al 1976), but it is not clear how this difference arises or how it could be responsible for the observed clinical and pathological features. It is, nevertheless, the case that the oligohydramnios–polyhydramnios sequence can occur in the absence of intertwin transfusion (Bruner & Rosemond 1993; Bruner et al 1998) and that, conversely, substantial intertwin transfusion can occur without any evidence of the twin-to-twin transfusion syndrome (King et al 1995). The polyhydramnios in the recipient twin in cases of twin–twin transfusion has traditionally been attributed to polyuria as a consequence of circulatory overload (Bajoria et al 1995; Bajoria 1998a,b) and indeed fetal polyuria has been confirmed by the demonstration of an increased hourly urine production (Rosen et al 1990) and a chronically enlarged bladder (Kilby et al 1997) in the recipient twin. Wieacker et al (1992) suggested that the polyuria in the recipient twin was due to a high level of atrial natriuretic polypeptide and this has recently been confirmed by Bajoria et al (2001) who showed high plasma levels of this substance and immunohistochemical evidence of up-regulation of atrial natriuretic polypeptide in the kidneys and heart of the recipient twin. The cause of the increased synthesis and secretion of atrial natriuretic polypeptide is far from clear though it may be related to chronic cardiac overload and atrial stretching (Fig. 48.8), cardiac chamber enlargement being frequently detectable in the recipient twin by fetal echocardiography (Simpson et al 1998).

Because a chronic twin-to-twin transfusion can lead to the death of one or both twins several therapeutic techniques have been utilised, including removal of one twin (Urig et al 1988), repeated amniocentesis (Pinette et al 1993; Trespidi et al 1997; Garry et al 1998, division of the amniotic septum (Pistorius & Howarth 1999; Suzuki et al 1999) and fetoscopic laser ablation of placental vessels (De Lia et al 1995, 1999; Ville et al 1998; Quintero et al 2001): such techniques have met with varying degrees of success with laser surgery probably achieving the best results (Hecher et al 1999; van Gemert et al 2001).

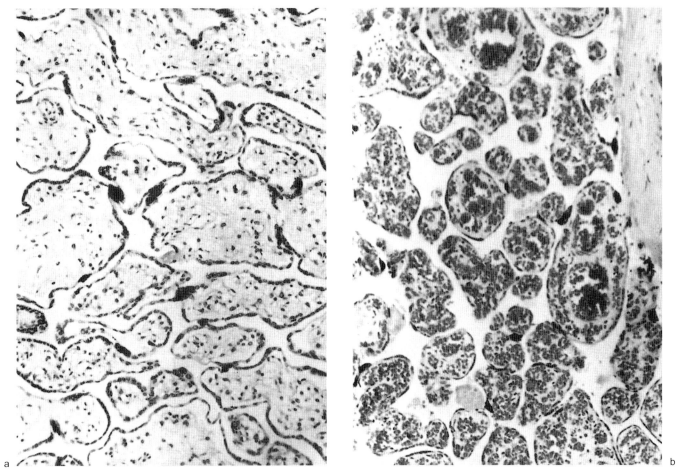

Fig. 48.7 Chronic twin–twin transfusion syndrome. The villi of the donor's placenta (**a**) are large and have small inconspicuous vessels whilst those of the recipient's placenta (**b**) have large engorged vessels.

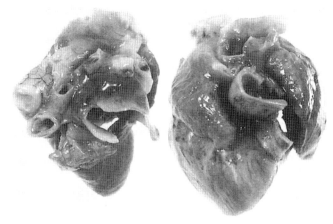

Fig. 48.8 Chronic twin–twin transfusion syndrome. The recipient heart, on the right weighs 13 g whilst the donor heart, on the left, weighs 7 g.

Acute twin transfusion

In an acute twin-to-twin transfusion, which is uncommon and usually occurs during birth, the fetuses are of roughly equal size but the donor twin is pale and the recipient twin plethoric. The haemoglobin levels and red cell counts of the twins are normal at birth but within a few hours anaemia becomes apparent in the donor and polycythaemia in the recipient. It is believed that in the acute syndrome the transfusion is usually through the superficial vessels, flow through which had been previously balanced (Baldwin 1994). The factor causing the sudden haemodynamic imbalance may be one twin going into shock because, for instance, of hypoxia due to cord compression.

Although most cases of acute transfusion occur at, or near to, birth (Uotila & Tammela 1999) some may complicate a chronic transfusion when operative interventions are undertaken (Baldwin & Wittmann 1990) and an acute transfusion may complicate the death of one twin (Fusi et al 1990, 1991; Baldwin 1999).

Acardiac fetus

A twin-transfusion syndrome, albeit of an unusual type, appears to be responsible for the development of acardiac fetuses; certainly, this malformation only occurs in monozygotic multiple pregnancies with monochorionic placentation (Moore et al 1990; Kunz & Arnaboldi 1991; Pinet et al 1994). Acardiac fetuses occur in about 1% of monozygotic twin gestations (Gillim & Hendricks 1953;

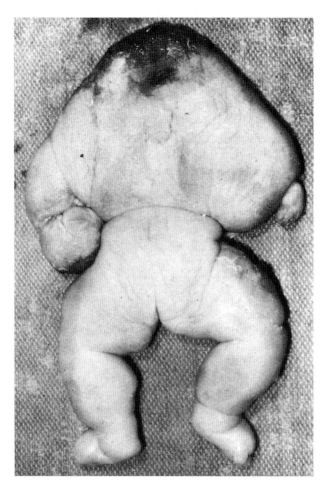

Fig. 48.9 An acardiac twin. There is no head and the upper limbs are poorly formed.

Napolitani & Schreiber 1960; Amatuzio & Gorlin 1981; Sogaard et al 1999), i.e. once in 35 000 pregnancies and vary considerably in gross appearance and in their degree of organogenesis, ranging from a large but grossly deformed fetus to an amorphous mass (Fig. 48.9): there is commonly a vertebral axis with some attempt at limb formation and internally the heart is either absent or rudimentary. Acardiac fetuses have been the basis of many complicated classifications (Lachman et al 1980; Sato et al 1984) which Baldwin (1994) has described as more confusing than helpful and are, as Benirschke & Kim (1973a) have commented, all virtually meaningless in view of their common pathogenesis. An acardiac twin usually has the same karotype as the normal twin (Benirschke & Kaufmann 2000) but there have been two examples of trisomy 2 restricted to the acardiac fetus (Chalia et al 1999; Blaicher et al 2000).

In the past the aetiology of acardia was uncertain with two contrasting theories holding sway, one maintaining that the defect was a primary one, the fetus never having had a heart, and the other proposing that the fetus did have a heart, which became atrophied as a result of an imbalance in the placental vascular communications (Keith et al 1967; Wilson 1972; Alderman 1973; Severn

& Holyoke 1973). Currently, it is believed that a placental vascular malfunction lies at the root of this anomaly, the abnormal twin having no placental parenchymal circulation of its own but having an arterial system which anastomoses with branches of the umbilical artery of the normal twin and a venous drainage into the umbilical veins of the normal twin. The fetal circulation is thus the reverse of normal, the abnormal twin receiving unoxygenated blood that has already perfused the normal twin, a situation known as 'twin reversed arterial perfusion' (van Allen 1981; van Allen et al 1983; Stephens 1984; Benson et al 1989; Shalev et al 1992; Schwarzler et al 1999) and which leads to altered cardiovascular development with secondary abnormalities in the other tissues. Acardiac fetuses can therefore be regarded as a form of conjoined twin in which the conjunction is of the chorionic circulation (Baldwin 1994), hence the resurrection of the term 'chorangiopagus parasiticus twin' to describe this anomaly. It should be noted that the normal, or 'pump' twin, has also to circulate its blood through the abnormal twin and that this may lead to cardiomegaly, high output cardiac failure and polyhydramnios (Baldwin 1994): it is because of this that attempts, usually successful, have been made to ligate or coagulate the cord vessels of the acardiac twin (Quintero et al 1994; Foley et al 1995; Arias et al 1998; Rodeck et al 1998; Sergi et al 2000).

Death of one twin

A further consequence of the vascular anastomoses in monochorionic placentas is that the death of one fetus may be associated with, and probably cause, abnormalities in the surviving co-twin, a situation which does not occur with dichorionic placentas. Death of one twin in the third trimester of pregnancy may be associated with visceral, and especially cerebral, lesions in the survivor (Benirschke 1961b; Yoshioka et al 1979; Enbom 1985; Szymonwicz et al 1986; Yoshida & Soma 1986; Bulla et al 1987; Anderson et al 1990; Fusi et al 1991; Gaucherand et al 1994; Murphy 1995; Nicolini & Poblete 1999; Vial & Hohlfeld 1999; Saito et al 1999; Pharoah & Adi 2000). These have been attributed to the release of thromboplastic material from the dead fetus which passes into the circulation of the living twin and there triggers off disseminated intravascular coagulation (Moore et al 1969; Enbom 1985; Yoshida & Soma 1986). An alternative, and currently more widely held, view is, however, that the damage to the surviving twin is due to hypovolaemic shock as a consequence of the dead fetus acting as a 'vascular sink', the live fetus effectively haemorrhaging into its co-twin's resistance-free blood vessels by an acute transfusion through superficial anastomatic arterioarterial or venovenous vessels (Fusi et al 1991; Liu et al 1992; Benirschke 1993; Baldwin 1994; Vial & Hohfeld 1999). Bajoria et al (1999) showed that this was indeed the case in pregnancies which had not been complicated by a chronic transfusion syndrome whereas in pregnancies complicated by a chronic transfusion death of the recipient twin will put the still living donor twin at considerable risk of death because of the unidirectional nature of the arteriovenous connections. Despite these risks to the surviving fetus there have been some series in which the only complications found in the surviving twin have been those due to prematurity (Petersen & Nyholm 1999).

DISCORDANT GROWTH IN TWIN PREGNANCIES

In twin pregnancies complicated by a chronic twin–twin transfusion syndrome there is, as already discussed, a marked difference in fetal weights. However, dichorionic twins often show marked differences in size as may also monochorionic twins in whom there has been no obvious transfusion syndrome. Indeed, the discordance in monochorionic twins may be such that the twin–twin transfusion syndrome is mimicked despite the absence of functional interfetal vascular anastomoses (Blickstein & Lancet 1988; Bruner et al 1998). Such a disparity in growth in monochorionic twins has been attributed to asymmetric 'placental insufficiency' (Bruner et al 1998),

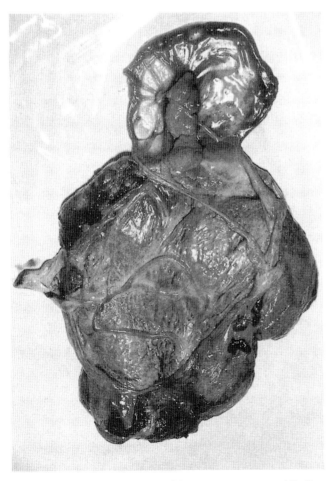

Fig. 48.10 A fetus papyraceous. This was an unsuspected finding in the placenta of an apparent singleton pregnancy.

asymmetric placental development (Victoria et al 2001), unequal vascular sharing (van Gemert & Umur 2000) or to a subclinical transfusion syndrome without changes in amniotic fluid (Bajoria 1998b). More recently, however, Sooranna et al (2001) have shown that, for reasons which are not fully clear, in cases of twin–twin transfusion the plasma leptin levels are much higher in the recipient twin than in the donor: as leptin appears to be a growth factor for both fetus and placenta this finding may be of importance in our understanding of the pathogenesis of the discordant growth pattern.

FETUS PAPYRACEOUS

This forms when one twin dies at a relatively early stage of pregnancy, i.e. during the second trimester, and becomes compressed and mummified as the gestation proceeds: a fetus papyraceous may be easily apparent at delivery but can appear only as a localised area of thickening within the membranes. Occasionally a fetus papyraceous is sufficiently large to cause obstruction during labour (Leppert et al 1979; Lau & Rogers 1999). A fetus papyraceous (Fig. 48.10) can be associated with anatomical defects, such as intestinal atresia, in the surviving co-twin (Baldwin 1994): under these circumstances transfer of thromboplastic material or emboli through vascular anatomoses appears the most plausible mechanism (Jauniaux et al 1998a; Wagner et al 1990).

THE VANISHING TWIN SYNDROME

This term is applied to the situation when there is a singleton birth following a pregnancy in which there was, during its early stages, ultrasound evidence of a twin gestation (Robinson & Caines 1977; Varma 1979; Brown 1982; Landy et al 1982, 1986; Boklage 1990; Landy & Nies 1995; Landy & Keith 1998). It should be noted that this term is only applied to very early death of a twin and does not refer to the presence of an obvious second fetus which takes the form of a fetus papyraceous, death in such cases having occurred during the early second trimester.

A twin may indeed vanish completely leaving no morphological residue though genetic evidence of an absorbed twin is occasionally detectable in the form of a restricted placental chimerism, i.e the presence of both 46,XX and 46,XY cell lines in a singleton placenta (Callen et al 1991; Reddy et al 1991; Falik-Borenstein et al 1994); this differs from a restricted placental mosaicism for which there is no conceptual necessity to invoke the prior presence of a second fetus.

Morphological remnants of a second gestation may, however, be found, albeit often with some difficulty, in placentas from pregnancies complicated by a vanishing twin. Sulak & Dodson (1986) noted a collapsed gestational sac within the membranes of a placenta from such a case, this appearing macroscopically as a plaque-like thickening within the membranes. Jauniaux et al (1988b) examined 10 placentas from pregnancies complicated by the vanishing twin phenomenon and found in one case remnants of an embryonic vertebral column immediately adjacent to a peripheral plaque of perivillous fibrin; they noted peripherally situated and well-delineated plaques of perivillous fibrin deposition in four other cases and implied, but did not clearly state, that they considered these plaques to be the remains of the placental tissue of the vanished fetus. Others have detected fetal tissue remnants, degenerate placental villi or empty gestational sacs either at the placental margin, within the membranes or on the fetal surface of the surviving twin's placenta in a high proportion of placentas from pregnancies in which a twin had apparently vanished (Yoshida & Soma 1986; Huter et al 1990; Rudnicki et al 1991; Nerlich et al 1992; Baldwin 1994), these usually being visible, on careful examination, as small nodules or foci of thickening (Yoshida 1995; Mathelier & Karachorlu 1999).

TWIN PREGNANCY WITH HYDATIDIFORM MOLE

A number of twin pregnancies have been reported in which one of the twins was a normal fetus and the other a complete hydatidiform mole. Fox (1997) reviewed 22 examples of this form of twin pregnancy that had been documented up to 1995 and a number of further cases have subsequently been reported (Bhutta 1996; Eblen & Richards 1996; Soyal et al 1996; Harada et al 1997; Hurteau et al 1997; Fishman et al 1998; Ishi et al 1998; Hirose et al 1999; Kauffman et al 1999; Matsui et al 1999; Montes de Oca Valero et al 1999; Vandeginste et al 1999; Benirschke et al 2000; Bruchim et al 2000; Japaraj & Sivalingam 2000; Matsui et al 2000; Albers et al 2001; Kashimura et al 2001; Malhotra et al 2001), the report of Matsui et al (2000) being particularly striking insofar as it was a Japanese national collaborative study of no less than 72 cases. In some of the reported pregnancies one of a pair of fused dichorionic twin placentas was converted into a complete hydatidiform mole whilst in others one of two separated dichorionic placentas was molar. Complete molar change in one of a fused pair of dichorionic twin placentas should not be, but has been, confused with and described as a partial hydatidiform mole: a true example of a twin gestation in which one fetus and placenta were normal whilst the other was a triploid fetus with a partial hydatidiform mole has been reported (Steller et al 1994b). A remarkable twin pregnancy in which one conceptus was a complete mole and the other a partial mole (with a fetus) has also been described (Ozumba & Ofodile 1994). Interestingly, there is an unusually high incidence of persistent trophoblastic disease and of maternal complications, such as pre-eclampsia, in twin gestations with a complete mole, much higher than is the case with a singleton molar pregnancy (Vejerslev 1991; Steller et al 1994a,b; Fishman et al 1998; Matsui et al 2000).

CONJOINED TWINS

The pathogenesis of conjoined twins is far from clear: it was at one time postulated that they arose as a result of fusion of homologous developed parts but it is now thought that the fault occurs at 13 to 15 days postfertilisation either because of incomplete fission of the developing embryo or because of the development of codominant axes with apposition of parts of the axes (Baldwin 1994).

The twins may be united in either the sagittal plane with the duplicated parts facing in the same direction or in the coronal plane with the twins facing either towards or away from each other. The former range from an apparent singleton with severe hypertelorism to a double headed twin with duplication of the upper half of the trunk. Fusion in the coronal plane varies similarly in degree. The commonest forms are the face to face twins (Fig. 48.11) joined in the sternal region (thoracopagus) or umbilical area (xiphopagus) and the back to back twins joined in the lumbosacral region (pygopagus). Conjoined twins usually show extensive sharing of common viscera.

The placenta of a conjoined twin is always monochorionic and monoamniotic; there may be a single cord from the placental surface which may divide before inserting

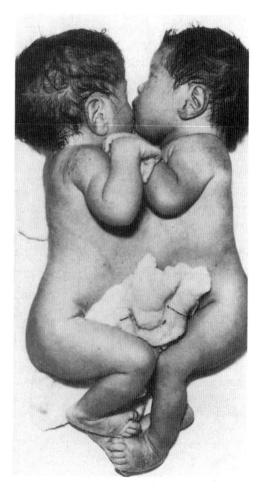

Fig. 48.11 Conjoined twins.

into the twins or two cords that originate separately and fuse closer to the infant(s): a single umbilical artery is common but far from universal.

PATHOLOGICAL EXAMINATION OF THE TWIN PLACENTA

When examining a placenta from a twin pregnancy particular attention should be paid to the position of insertion of the cords and to the number of arteries in each cord; in this respect the pathologist should insist that the cords are correctly and separately labelled in the delivery room, it being made quite clear which cord is from the first and which from the second delivered twin.

From the discussion in the earlier part of this chapter it will be apparent that the pathologist is required to examine a twin placenta for one, or both, of the following two specific reasons:

1. To establish the form of placentation and hence, in some cases, the zygosity of the twins.
2. To determine whether placental vascular anastomoses are present between the two fetal circulatory systems.

Identification of type of placentation and zygosity

If the two placentas are quite separate from each other they are clearly dichorionic, and if the infants are of opposite sex they are dizygotic; if the infants are of the same sex they may be either di- or monozygotic, and placental examination will be of no help in determining which. If the placenta is monoamniotic then it is also monochorionic and the twins are monozygotic. The principal task of the pathologist is, therefore, to distinguish between a monochorionic–diamniotic placenta and a fused dichorionic–diamniotic placenta. It is often suggested that the first step in this investigation is to try and separate the two placental masses from each other by gentle traction: no separation will occur in monochorionic placentas, but a proportion of fused dichorionic placentas can be cleaved from each other. It should be stressed that this is the crudest possible technique of examining twin placentas; it gives no information if separation is not obtained, may make eventual identification of the nature of the septum between the two amniotic sacs more difficult, and can obviate subsequent attempts to inject the placental vasculature.

The real crux of the differentiation between monochorionic and fused dichorionic placentas is the presence in the latter, but not in the former, of chorionic tissue in the septum between the two amniotic cavities, and attention should first be directed to the septum itself. If the placenta is monochorionic the septum will be translucent, but in dichorionic placentas the presence of chorionic tissue makes the septum appear relatively opaque. A piece of septum should be taken for histological examination, and Benirschke & Driscoll's (1967) technique of taking a

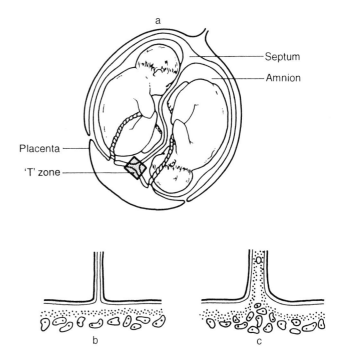

Fig. 48.12 (**a**) Diagrammatic representation of the site of the 'T-zone' in diamniotic twin placentas. (**b**) Diagrammatic representation of the histology of the 'T-zone' in a monochorionic–diamniotic twin placenta; the septum consists solely of two layers of amnion. (**c**) Diagrammatic representation of the histology of the 'T-zone' in a dichorionic–diamniotic twin placenta. Chorionic tissue is present in the septum between the two layers of amnion.

longitudinal strip of the septum which is then rolled and sectioned has much to commend it. Next, the base of the septum should be examined; in dichorionic placentas an elevated ridge, which is at the base of the chorionic tissue in the septum, will invariably be present (Fig. 48.1), whilst in monochorionic placentas this ridge will be absent. A block for histological examination should also be taken from the 'T-zone' (Fig. 48.12), i.e. from the point at which the septum joins the surface of the placenta (Allen & Turner 1971). The amnion should then be stripped off from the fetal surface of the placenta; in monochorionic placentas the amnion peels off easily, leaving a smooth continuous surface, but in dichorionic placentas there will be tearing of the placental substance at the base of the septum, at the site of the ridge.

Subsequent histological examination of the membrane roll from the septum should give a good indication of the type of placentation, for in monochorionic placentas it will consist solely of two layers of amnion (Fig. 48.13), whilst in dichorionic placentas the two layers of amnion will be separated by two layers of chorionic tissue (Fig. 48.14). In practice, unfortunately, a clear-cut answer will not always be obtained, because by the time the placenta is received in the laboratory the septal membranes may be distorted and their relationships disturbed (Bleisch 1964). Under such circumstances the histology of the 'T-zone' may be more rewarding, for this will show more clearly the extension of the chorion into the septum.

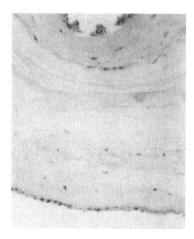

Fig. 48.13 Histological appearances of the septum separating the two amniotic cavities of a monochorionic–diamniotic twin placenta: this consists solely of two layers of amnion. H & E X150.

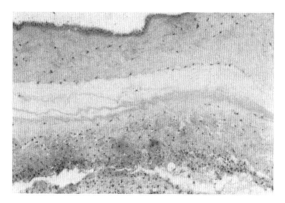

Fig. 48.14 Histological appearances of the septum separating the two amniotic cavities of a dichorionic–diamniotic twin placenta. The two layers of amnion are separated from each other by chorionic tissue. H & E X120.

Demonstration of vascular anastomoses

Theoretically, an attempt should be made to demonstrate the possible presence of vascular communications in all monochorionic or fused dichorionic placentas. In practice, most pathologists will simply content themselves with noting whether or not there are any superficial anastomoses between large vessels which are easily visible to the naked eye, and only those with a special interest in the topic will routinely proceed to injection studies. Nevertheless, any pathologist who is prepared to examine twin placentas must also be prepared to study their vascular systems under certain specific circumstances. These are:

1. If, after gross and microscopic examination, the type of placentation still remains in doubt.
2. If there is any suspicion of the twin-transfusion syndrome.
3. If there is any abnormality in the surviving twin following death of one infant in utero.
4. In any case in which intrauterine or neonatal death of a twin has occurred for no obvious reason.

Large superficial anastomoses may be relatively easy to detect, for they are often visible on the fetal surface of the placenta; the nature of such communications is not, however, always obvious, for, in the placenta, it may be quite difficult to distinguish between veins and arteries. Some workers inject air bubbles into the superficial vessels and show that they can be pushed from the vessels of one twin to those of the other; unfortunately the inherent vagaries of this technique, which are largely due to the surface tension properties of air bubbles, restrict considerably its value. A number of other substances have been suggested for the demonstration of large superficial anastomoses, these including milk and Indian ink. The former has been used by some workers (Coen & Sutherland 1970) and can give a quite clear demonstration of the vascular communications (50 ml being injected into a superficial vessel). Perhaps the simplest and best substance to use routinely is coloured saline (Benirschke 1961a).

The identification of the deep arterio-venous anastomoses is, of course, of more importance in investigating a case of possible twin–twin transfusion syndrome, in which superficial anastomoses are frequently absent. For this purpose two methods are available; the first is to inject a radio-opaque dye and then trace the vascular communications by radiological study, and the other is to inject a coloured plastic substance and then prepare a corrosion specimen. It cannot be claimed that accurate results are achieved by either technique without a considerable amount of experience, and if one is content simply to show that communications exist, is not concerned with their actual physical demonstration, and is satisfied by showing that fluid injected into one twin's vascular territory will appear in that of the other twin, it is probable that injection of coloured saline will suffice.

TRIPLET PLACENTATION

In white Caucasians and in a Japanese population triplets occur in about one in 10 000 deliveries, but in Ibadan, Nigeria, their frequency is one in 563 deliveries (Nylander 1971b, 1975b; Shanklin & Perrin 1984; Imaizumi 1990). Triplets may be trizygotic, dizygotic or monozygotic. Trizygotic triplets are due to the fertilisation of three ova, whilst dizygotic triplets are produced by the fertilisation of two ova, one of which subsequently replicates; monozygotic triplets result from the fertilisation of a single ovum which then undergoes replication, a further replication then occurs in one of the already replicated zygotes.

The placentation of triplets (Fig. 48.15) has been discussed by Boyd & Hamilton (1970), Nylander & Corney (1971), Corney (1975) and Baldwin (1994), and follows the same principles as those already described for dizygotic and monozygotic twin placentation. Thus trizygotic triplets have a trichorionic–triamniotic placentation, but

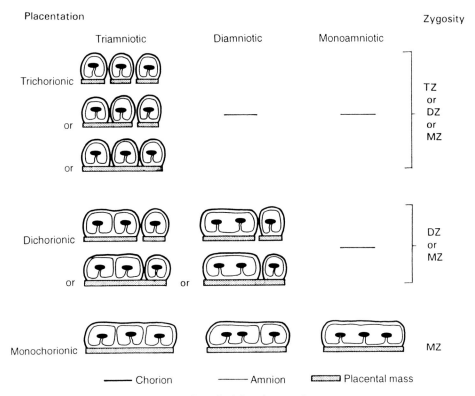

Fig. 48.15 Diagrammatic representation of triplet placentation.

there may be three separate placentas, two fused placentas and one separate placenta, or fusion of the three placentas to form a single mass. Dizygotic triplets may have a placentation identical to that of trizygotic triplets, or may be dichorionic; if dichorionic, the two placentas may be separate or fused and there may be two or three amniotic sacs. Monozygotic triplets may show any of the forms of placentation seen in dizygotic or trizygotic triplet placentation, or may be monochorionic, in which case they may be monoamniotic, diamniotic or triamniotic.

In practice, in white Caucasian populations, about 16% of triplets are monochorionic, 42% dichorionic and 42% trichorionic; in Nigeria, however, 72.5% of triplets are trichorionic and only 2.5% are monochorionic (Nylander & Corney 1971).

HIGHER MULTIPLE BIRTHS

It would be merely repetitious to detail here the possible permutations of forms of placentation found in higher multiple births. Suffice it to say that the principles of monozygotic and dizygotic placentation apply to these with equal cogency, that quadruplet placentation is discussed in some detail by Boyd & Hamilton (1970) and Hafez (1974), and that case reports of placentation in still higher multiple pregnancies include those of Hamblen et al (1937), Gibbs et al (1960), Neubecker et al (1962), Berbos et al (1964), Turksoy et al (1967), Cameron et al (1969), Lachelin et al (1972), Bender & Brandt (1974), Metler et al (1974), Garrett et al (1976), Giovannucci-Uzielli et al (1981), Serreyn et al (1984) and Egwuato et al (1992).

REFERENCES

Abuhamad A Z, Mari G, Copel J A, Cantwell C J, Evans A T 1995 Umbilical artery flow velocity waveforms in monoamniotic twins with cord entanglement. Obstetrics and Gynecology 86: 674–677

Acosta-Sison H, Aragon G T, de la Paz A 1946 Monoamniotic twins: danger to the life of at least one twin (First case report in Philippines). Journal of the Philippine Medical Association 22: 43–46

Aherne W, Strong S J, Corney G 1968 The structure of the placenta in the twin transfusion syndrome. Biologia Neonatorum 12: 121–135

Aisien A O, Olarewaju R S, Imade G E 2000 Twins in Jos Nigeria: a seven-year retrospective study. Medical Sciences Monitor 6: 945–950

Albers E, Daneshmand S, Hull A 2001 Placental pathology casebook: complete hydatidiform mole with coexistent twin pregnancy. Journal of Perinatology 73: 151–154

Alderman B A 1973 Foetus acardius amorphus. Postgraduate Medical Journal 49: 102–105

Allen M S, Turner U G 1971 Twin birth — identical or fraternal twins? Obstetrics and Gynecology 37: 538–542

Altshuler G, Hyde S 1993 Placental pathology casebook: a bidiscoid monochorionic placenta. Journal of Perinatology 13: 492–493

Amatuzio J C, Gorlin R J 1981 Conjoined acardiac monsters. Archives of Pathology and Laboratory Medicine 105: 253–255

Ambach E, Parson W, Brezinka C 2000 Superfecundation and dual paternity in a twin pregnancy ending with placental abruption. Journal of Forensic Sciences 45: 181–183

Anderson R L, Golbus M S, Curry C J R, Callen P W, Hastrup W H 1990 Central nervous system damage and other anomalies in surviving fetus following second trimester antenatal death of co-twin: report of four cases and literature review. Prenatal Diagnosis 10: 513–518

Anger H, Ring A 1972 Die fetofetale Transfusion bei Zwillingen. Zeitschrift für Geburtshilfe und Perinatologie 176: 164–167

Annan B, Hutson R C 1990 Double survival despite cord entwinement in monoamniotic twins: case report. British Journal of Obstetrics and Gynaecology 97: 950–951

Arabin B, Laurini R N, van Eyck J 1999 Early prenatal diagnosis of cord entanglement in monoamniotic multiple pregnancies. Ultrasound in Obstetrics and Gynecology 13: 181–186

Arias F, Sunderji S, Gimpelson R, Colton E 1998 Treatment of acardiac twinning. Obstetrics and Gynecology 91: 818–821

Arts N F Th, Lohman A H M 1971 The vascular anatomy of monochorionic diamniotic twin placentas and the transfusion syndrome. European Journal of Obstetrics and Gynecology 3: 85–93

Bajoria R 1998a Abundant vascular anastomoses in monoamniotic versus diamniotic monochorionic placentas. American Journal of Obstetrics and Gynecology 179: 788–793

Bajoria R 1998b Vascular anatomy of monochorionic placenta in relation to discordant growth and amniotic fluid volume. Human Reproduction 13: 2933–2940

Bajoria R, Kingdom J 1997 The case for routine determination of chorionicity and zygosity in multiple pregnancy. Prenatal Diagnosis 17: 1207–1225

Bajoria R, Wigglesworth J, Fisk N M 1995 Angioarchitecture of monochorionic placentas in relation to the twin–twin transfusion syndrome. American Journal of Obstetrics and Gynecology 172: 856–863

Bajoria R, Wee L Y, Anwar S, Ward S 1999 Outcome of twin pregnancies complicated by single intrauterine death in relation to vascular anatomy of the monochorionic placenta. Human Reproduction 14: 2124–2130

Bajoria R, Ward S, Sooranna S R 2001 Atrial natruiretic peptide mediated polyuria: pathogenesis of polyhydramnios in the recipient twin of twin–twin transfusion syndrome. Placenta 22: 716–724

Baldwin V J 1994 Pathology of multiple pregnancy. Springer Verlag, New York

Baldwin V J 1999 Placental pathology and multiple gestation. In: Lewis H L, Perrin E (eds) Pathology of the placenta, 2nd edn. Churchill Livingstone, New York, pp 213–257

Baldwin V J, Wittmann B K 1990 Pathology of intragestational intervention in twin-to-twin transfusion syndrome. Pediatric Pathology 10: 79–93

Bardawil W A, Reddy R L, Bardawil L W 1988 Placental considerations in multiple pregnancy. Clinics in Perinatology 15: 13–40

Belfort M A, Moise K J, Kirshon B, Saade G 1993 The use of color flow Doppler ultrasonography to diagnose umbilical cord entanglement in monoamniotic twin gestation. American Journal of Obstetrics and Gynecology 168: 601–604

Bender H G, Brandt G 1974 Morphologie und Morphometrie der Fünflings-Placenta. Archiv fur Gynakologie 216: 61–72

Benirschke K 1961a Accurate recording of twin placentation — a plea to the obstetrician. Obstetrics and Gynecology 18: 334–347

Benirschke K 1961b Twin placenta in perinatal mortality. New York State Journal of Medicine 61: 1499–1508

Benirschke K 1965 Major pathologic features of the placenta, cord and membranes. Birth Defects Original Articles Series 1: 52–56

Benirschke K 1972a Multiple births. In: Barnett H L, Einhorn A H (eds) Pediatrics, 15th edn. Appleton-Century-Crofts, New York, pp 117–125

Benirschke K 1972b Origin and clinical significance of twinning. Clinical Obstetrics and Gynecology 15: 220–235

Benirschke K 1993 Intrauterine death of a twin: mechanisms, implications for surviving twin, and placental pathology. Seminars in Diagnostic Pathology 10: 222–231

Benirschke K, Driscoll S G 1967 The pathology of the human placenta. Springer-Verlag, New York

Benirschke K, Kaufmann P 2000 Pathology of the human placenta, 4th edn. Springer-Verlag, New York

Benirschke K, Kim C K 1973a Medical progress: multiple pregnancy. New England Journal of Medicine 288: 1276–1284

Benirschke K, Kim C K 1973b Medical progress: multiple pregnancy. New England Journal of Medicine 288: 1329–1336

Benirschke K, Spinosa J C, McGinnis M J, Marchevsky A, Sanchez J 2000 Partial molar transformation of the placenta of presumably monozygotic twins. Pediatric and Developmental Pathology 3: 95–100

Benson C B, Bieber F R, Genest D R, Doubilet P M 1989 Doppler demonstration of reversed umbilical blood flow in an acardiac twin. Journal of Clinical Ultrasound 17: 291–295

Berbos J D, King B F, Janusz A 1964 Quintuple pregnancy. Journal of the American Medical Association 188: 813–816

Bhargava I, Chakravarty A 1975 Vascular anastomoses in twin placentae and their recognition. Acta Anatomica 93: 471–480

Bhargava J, Chakravarty A, Raja P T K 1971 An anatomical study of the foetal blood vessels on the chorial surface of the human placenta. III. Multiple pregnancies. Acta Anatomica 80: 465–479

Bhutta S Z 1996 Twin pregnancy with complete hydatidiform mole and coexistent fetus. Journal of the Pakistan Medical Association 46: 180–181

Bieber F R, Nance W E, Morton C C et al 1981 Genetic studies of an acardiac monster: evidence of polar body twinning in man. Science 213: 775–777

Blaicher W, Repa C, Schaller A 2000 Acardiac twin pregnancy associated with trisomy 2: case report. Human Reproduction 15: 474–475

Bleisch V R 1964 Diagnosis of monochorionic twin placentation. American Journal of Clinical Pathology 42: 277–284

Bleisch V R 1965 Placental circulation of human twins: constant arterial anastomoses in monochorionic placentas. American Journal of Obstetrics and Gynecology 91: 862–869

Blickstein I 1990 The twin–twin transfusion syndrome. Obstetrics and Gynecology 76: 714–722

Blickstein I, Lancet M 1988 The growth discordant twin. Obstetrical and Gynecological Survey 43: 509–515

Boklage C E 1987 Twinning, nonrighthandedness, and fusion malformations: evidence for heritable causal elements held in common. American Journal of Medical Genetics 28: 67–84

Boklage C E 1990 Survival probability of human conceptus from fertilization to term. International Journal of Fertility 35: 75–94

Bomsel-Helmreich O, Al Mufti W 1995 The mechanism of monozygosity and double-ovulation. In: Kieth L G, Papiernik E, Kieth D M, Luke B (eds) Multiple pregnancy: epidemiology, gestation and perinatal outcome. Parthenon, New York, pp 25–40

Bortolus R, Parazzini F, Chatenoud L, Benzi G, Bianchi M M, Marini A 1999 The epidemiology of multiple births. Human Reproduction Update 5: 179–187

Boyd J D, Hamilton W J 1970 The human placenta. Heffer, Cambridge

Brown B St J 1982 Disappearances of one gestational sac in the first trimester of multiple pregnancies — ultrasonographic findings. Journal of the Canadian Association of Radiologists 33: 273–275

Brown D L, Benson C B, Driscoll S G, Doubilet P M 1989 Twin transfusion syndrome: sonographic findings. Radiology 170: 61–63

Bruchim I, Kidron D, Amiel A, Altaras M, Fejgin M D 2000 Complete hydatidiform mole and a coexistent viable fetus: report of two cases and review of the literature. Gynecologic Oncology 77: 197–202

Bruner J P, Rosemond R L 1993 Twin-to-twin transfusion syndrome: a subset of the twin oligohydramnios–polyhydramnios sequence. American Journal of Obstetrics and Gynecology 169: 925–930

Bruner J P, Anderson T L, Rosemond R L 1998 Placental pathophysiology of the twin oligohydramnios–polyhydramnios sequence and the twin–twin transfusion syndrome. Placenta 19: 81–86

Bryan E 1994 Trends in twinning rates. Lancet 343: 1151–1152

Bryan E M, Slavin B 1974 Serum IgG levels in feto-fetal transfusion syndrome. Archives of Disease in Childhood 49: 908–910

Bryan E M, Slavin B, Nicholson E 1976 Serum immunoglobulins in multiple pregnancy. Archives of Disease in Childhood 51: 354–359

Bulla M, von Lilien T, Goecke H, Roth B, Ortmann M, Heising J 1987 Renal and cerebral necrosis in survivors after in utero death of co-twin. Archives of Gynecology 240: 119–124

Bulmer M G 1970 The biology of twinning in man. Clarendon Press, Oxford

Callen D F, Fernandez H, Hull Y J et al 1991 A normal 46, XX infant with a 46, XX/69, XXY placenta: a major contribution to the placenta is from a resorbed twin. Prenatal Diagnosis 11: 437–442

Cameron A H 1968 The Birmingham twin survey. Proceedings of the Royal Society of Medicine 61: 229–234

Cameron A H, Robson E B, Wade-Evans J, Wingham J 1969 Septuplet conception: placental zygosity studies. Journal of Obstetrics and Gynaecology of the British Commonwealth 76: 692–698

Cameron A H, Edwards J H, Derom R, Thiery M, Bolaert R 1983 The value of twin surveys in the study of malformations. European Journal of Obstetrics, Gynecology and Reproductive Biology 14: 347–356

Chalia C, Schwarzler P, Booker M et al 1999 Trisomy 2 in an acardiac twin in a triplet in-vitro fertilization pregnancy. Human Reproduction 14: 1378–1380

Charlton A, Winston H G, Chomke M 1953 Monoamniotic twin pregnancy. Obstetrics and Gynecology 2: 148–151

Chun F Y 1970 Some data on twinning in Singapore. Journal of the Singapore Paediatric Society 12: 44–58

Coen R W, Sutherland J M 1970 Placental vascular communications between twin fetuses: a simplified technique for demonstration. American Journal of Diseases of Children 120: 332

Conway C F 1964 Transfusion syndrome in multiple pregnancy. Obstetrics and Gynecology 23: 745–751

Corner G W 1955 The observed embryology of human single-ovum twins and other multiple births. American Journal of Obstetrics and Gynecology 70: 933–951

Corney G 1975 Placentation. In: MacGillivray I, Nylander P P S, Corney G (eds) Human multiple reproduction. W B Saunders, London, pp 40–76

Corney G, Aherne W 1965 The placental transfusion syndrome in monozygous twins. Archives of Disease in Childhood 40: 264

Corney G, Robson E B 1975 Types of twinning and determination of zygosity. In: MacGillivray I, Nylander P P S, Corney G (eds) Human multiple reproduction. W B Saunders, London, pp 16–39

Corney G, Robson E B, Strong S J 1972 The effect of zygosity on the birth weight of twins. Annals of Human Genetics 36: 45–59

Dallpiccola B, Stomeo C, Ferranti G, Di Lecce A, Purpura M 1985 Discordant sex in one of three monozygotic triplets. Journal of Medical Genetics 22: 6–11

Dawood M Y, Ratnam S S, Lim Y C 1975 Twin pregnancy in Singapore. Australian and New Zealand Journal of Obstetrics and Gynaecology 15: 93–98

De Lia J E, Kuhlmann R S, Harstad T W, Cruikshank D P 1995 Fetoscopic laser ablation of placental vessels in severe previable twin–twin transfusion syndrome. American Journal of Obstetrics and Gynecology 172: 1202–1211

De Lia J E, Kuhlmann R S, Lopez K P 1999 Treating the previable twin–twin transfusion syndrome with fetoscopic laser surgery: outcomes following the learning curve. Journal of Perinatal Medicine 27: 61–67

Denbow M L, Cox P, Taylor M, Hammal D M, Fisk N M 2000 Placental angioarchitecture in monochorionic twin pregnancies: relationship to fetal growth, fetofetal transfusion syndrome and pregnancy outcome. American Journal of Obstetrics and Gynecology 182: 417–426

Derom R, Orlebeke J, Eriksson A, Thiery M 1995 The epidemiology of multiple births in Europe. In: Keith L G, Papiernik E, Keith D M, Luke B (eds) Multiple pregnancy: epidemiology, gestation and perinatal outcome. Parthenon, New York, pp 145–162

Di Salvo D N, Benson C B, Laing F C, Brown D L, Frates M C, Doubilet P M 1998 Sonographic evaluation of the placental cord insertion site. American Journal of Roentgenology 170: 1295–1298

Dorum A, Nesheim B I 1991 Monochorionic monoamniotic twins — the most precarious of twin pregnancies. Acta Obstetricia et Gynecologica Scandinavica 70: 381–383

Drack G, Kind C, Lorenz U 1993 Management monoamnioter Zwillingsschwangerschaften. Geburtshilfe und Frauenheilkunde 53: 100–104

Eblen A C, Richards D S 1996 Favourable outcome in a twin pregnancy with complete hydatidiform mole and coexisting fetus. Journal of Maternal and Fetal Medicine 5: 345–347

Egwuato V E, Iloabachie G C, Okezie O, Ibe B C 1992 Quintuplet pregnancy: case report. West African Journal of Medicine 11: 154–157

Elwood J M 1973 Decline in dizygotic twinning. New England Journal of Medicine 289: 486

Enbom J A 1985 Twin pregnancy with intrauterine death of one twin. American Journal of Obstetrics and Gynecology 152: 424–429

Falik-Borenstein T C, Korenberg J R, Schreck R R 1994 Confined placental chimerism: prenatal and postntal cytogenetic and molecular analysis, and pregnancy outcome. American Journal of Medical Genetics 50: 51–56

Fishman D A, Padila L A, Keh P, Cohen L, Frederiksen M, Lurain J R 1998 Management of twin pregnancies consisting of a complete hydatidiform mole and normal fetus. Obstetrics and Gynecology 91: 546–550

Foglmann R 1974 Monoamniotic twins. Acta Geneticae Medicae et Gemellologiae 23: Supplement 17

Foley M R, Clewell W H, Finberg H J, Mills M D 1995 Use of Foley cordostat grasping device for selective ligation of the umbilical cord of an acardiac twin: a case report. American Journal of Obstetrics and Gynecology 172: 212–214

Fox H 1997 Pathology of the placenta, 2nd edn. W B Saunders, London

Fries M H, Goldstein R B, Kilpatrick S J, Golbus M S, Callen P W, Filly R A 1993 The role of velamentous cord insertion in the etiology of twin–twin transfusion. Obstetrics and Gynecology 81: 569–574

Fujikura T, Froehlich L A 1971 Twin placentation and zygosity. Obstetrics and Gynecology 37: 34–43

Fusi L, McParland P, Fisk N, Nicolini U, Wigglesworth J 1991 Acute twin–twin transfusion: a possible mechanism for brain damaged survivors after intrauterine death of a monochorionic twin. Obstetrics and Gynecology 78: 517–520

Galea P, Scott J M, Goel K M 1982 Feto-fetal transfusion syndrome. Archives of Disease in Childhood 57: 781–794

Garrett W J, Carey H M, Stevens L H, Climie C R, Osborn R A 1976 A case of nonuplet pregnancy. Australian and New Zealand Journal of Obstetrics and Gynaecology 16: 193–202

Garry D, Lysikiewicz A, Mays J, Canterino J, Tejani N 1998 Intra-amniotic pressure reduction in twin–twin transfusion syndrome. Journal of Perinatology 18: 284–286

Gaucherand P, Rudigoz R C, Piacenza J M 1994 Monofetal death in multiple pregnancies: risks for the co-twin, risk factors and obstetrical management. European Journal of Obstetrics, Gynecology and Reproductive Biology 55: 111–115

Gaziano E P, De Lia J E, Kuhlmann R S 2000 Diamnionic monochorionic twin gestations: an overview. Journal of Maternal Fetal Medicine 9: 89–96

Gedda L 1961 Twins in history and science. Charles C Thomas, Springfield, Illinois

Gibbs C E, Boldt J W, Daly J W, Morgan H C 1960 A quintuplet gestation. Obstetrics and Gynecology 16: 464–468

Giles W B, Trudinger B J, Cook C M, Connelly A J 1990 Doppler umbilical studies in the twin–twin transfusion syndrome. Obstetrics and Gynecology 76: 1097–1099

Gillim D M, Hendricks C H 1953 Holocardius: a review of the literature and case report. Obstetrics and Gynecology 2: 647–653

Giovannucci-Uzielli M L, Vecchi G, Donzelli G P, D'Ancona V L, Lapi E 1981 The history of the Florence sextuplets: obstetric and genetic considerations. Progress in Clinical Biology Research 69: 217–220

Goplerud C P 1964 Monoamniotic twins with double survival: report of a case. Obstetrics and Gynecology 23: 289–290

Gruenwald P 1970 Environmental influence on twins apparent at birth: a preliminary study. Biology of the Neonate 15: 79–93

Hafez E S E 1974 Physiology of multiple pregnancy. Journal of Reproductive Medicine 12: 88–98

Hagood M, Stokes R H 1953 Double survival of monoamniotic twins. American Journal of Obstetrics and Gynecology 65: 1152–1154

Hamblen D C, Baker R D, Derieux G D 1937 Roentgenographic diagnosis and anatomic studies of quintuple pregnancy. Journal of the American Medical Association 109: 10–12

Harada I, Tsutsumori O, Takai Y et al 1997 DNA polymorphism analysis of complete hydatidiform mole coexisting with a fetus. Human Reproduction 12: 2563–2566

Hecher K, Plath H, Bregenzer T, Hansmann M, Hackeloer B J 1999 Endoscopic laser surgery versus serial amniocenteses in the treatment of severe twin–twin transfusion syndrome. American Journal of Obstetrics and Gynecology 180: 717–724

Hirose M, Kimura T, Mitsuno N et al 1999 DNA flow cytometric quantification and DNA ploymorphism analysis in the case of a complete mole with a coexisting fetus. Journal of Assisted Reproduction and Genetics 16: 263–267

Hollander H-J 1969 Monoamniotische Zwillinge. Zeitschrift für Gebürtshilfe und Gynakologie 171: 292–300

Hollander H-J, Backmann R 1974 Das Transfusionssyndrom bei Zwillingen. Gebürtshilfe und Frauenheilkunde 34: 931–936

Hollingsworth W C 1973 Monoamniotic twin pregnancy: a case report. North Carolina Medical Journal 34: 443–444

Hurteau A, Roth L M, Schildler M, Summers J 1997 Complete hydatidiform mole coexisting with a twin live fetus: clinical course. Gynecologic Oncology 66: 156–159

Husby H, Holm N V, Gernow A, Thomsen S G, Kock K, Gurtler H 1991 Zygosity, placental membranes and Weinberg's rule in a Danish consecutive twin series. Acta Geneticae Medicae et Gemellologiae 40: 147–152

Huter O, Brezinka C, Busch G, Pfaller C 1990 Zur Frage der 'Vanishing Twin'. Geburtshilfe und Frauenheilkunde 50: 989–992

Hyrtle J 1870 Die Blutgefasse der menschlichen Nachgeburt. Braumüler, Vienna

Imaizumi Y, 1990 Triplets and higher order births in Japan. Acta Geneticae Medicae et Gemellologiae 37: 295–306

Ishii J, Iituka Y, Takano H, Matsui H, Osada H, Sekiya S 1998 Genetic differentiation of complete hydatidiform moles coexisting with normal fetuses by short tandem repeat derived deoxyribonucleic acid polymorphism analysis. American Journal of Obstetrics and Gynecology 179: 628–634

Israelstam D M 1973 Mono-amniotic twin pregnancy: a case report. South African Medical Journal 47: 2026–2027

Japaraj R P, Sivalingam N 2000 Complete hydatidiform mole and surviving coexistent twin — a case report. Singapore Medical Journal 41: 126–128

Jauniaux E, Elkhazen N, Vanrysselberge M, Leroy F 1988a Aspects anatomo-cliniques du syndrome du foetus papyrace. Journal de la Gynecologie, Obstetrique et Biologie de la Reproduction 17: 653–659

Jauniaux E, Elkhazen N, Leroy F, Wilkin P, Rodesch F, Hustin, J 1988b Clinical and morphologic aspects of the vanishing twin phenomenon. Obstetrics and Gynecology 72: 577–581

Jewell S E, Yip R 1995 Increasing trends in plural births in the United States. Obstetrics and Gynecology 85: 229–232

Juberg R C, Stallard R, Straughen W J, Avotri K J, Washington J W 1981 Clinicopathological conference: a newborn monozygotic twin with abnormal facial appearance and respiratory insufficiency. American Journal of Medical Genetics 10: 193–200

Kashimura Y, Tanaka M, Harada N et al 2001 Twin pregnancy consisting of 46, XY heterozygous complete mole coexisting with a live fetus. Placenta 22: 323–327

Kauffman D E, Sutkin G, Heine R P, Watt-Morse M, Price F V 1999 Metastatic complete hydatidiform mole with a surviving coexistent twin: a case report. Journal of Reproductive Medicine 44: 131–134

Keith L, Cestaro A, Elias I 1967 Fetus holoacardius: a complication of monochorial twinning. Chicago Medical School Quarterly 27: 30–35

Keith L G, Oleszczuk J J, Keith D M 2000 Multiple gestation: reflections on epidemiology, causes and consequences. 45: 206–214

Kilby M D, Howe D T, McHugo J M, Whittle M J 1997 Bladder visualisation as a prognostic sign in oligohydramnios–polyhydramnios sequence in twin pregnancies treated using therapeutic amniocentesis. British Journal of Obstetrics and Gynecology 104: 939–942

Kim K, Lage J M 1991 Bipartite diamnionic monochorionic twin placenta with superficial anastomoses: report of a case. Human Pathology 22: 501–503

King A D, Soothill P W, Montemagno R, Young M P, Sams V, Rodeck C H 1995 Twin-to-twin blood transfusion in a dichorionic pregnancy without the oligohydramnios–polyhydramnios sequence. British Journal of Obstetrics and Gynecology 102: 334–335

Klebe J G, Ingomar C J 1972 The fetoplacental circulation during parturition illustrated by the interfetal transfusion syndrome. Pediatrics 49: 112–116

Kloosterman G J 1963 The 'third circulation' in identical twins. Nederlands Tijdschrift voor Verloskunde en Gynaecologie 63: 395–412

Krussel J S, von Eckardstein S, Schwenzer T 1994 Doppelter Nabelschnurknoten bei monoamniotischer Geminigravidität als Ursache des intrauterinen Fruchttods beider Zwillinge. Zentralblatt fur Gynakologie 116: 497–499

Kunz J, Arnaboldi M 1991 Acardiacus bei Zwillingsschwangerschaft. Zeitschrift fur Geburtshilfe und Perinatologie 195: 275–279

Lachelin G C L, Brant H A, Swyer G I M, Little V, Reynolds E O R 1972 Sextuplet pregnancy. British Medical Journal i: 787–790

Lachman R, McNabb M, Furmanski M, Karp L 1980 The acardiac monster. European Journal of Pediatrics 134: 195–200

Lage J M, Vanmarter L J, Mikhael E 1989 Vascular anastomoses in fused, dichorionic twin placenta resulting in twin transfusion syndrome. Placenta 10: 55–59

Lambalk C B, Boomsma D, De Boer L et al 1998a Increased levels of and pulsatility of FSH in mothers of hereditary DZ twins. Journal of Clinical Endocrinology and Metabolism 83: 481–486

Lambalk C B, De Koning C H, Braat D D 1998b The endocrinology of dizygotic twinning in the human. Molecular and Cellular Endocrinology 145: 97–102

Landy H J, Keith L G 1998 The vanishing twin: a review. Human Reproduction Update 4: 177–183

Landy H J, Nies B M 1995 The vanishing twin. In: Keith L G, Papiernik E, Keith D M, Luke B (eds) Multiple pregnancy: epidemiology, gestation and perinatal outcome. Parthenon, New York, pp 59–72

Landy H J, Keith L G, Keith D 1982 The vanishing twin. Acta Geneticae Medicae et Gemellologiae 31: 179–194

Landy H J, Weiner S, Corson S L, Batzer F R, Bolognese R J 1986 The 'vanishing twin'; ultrasonographic assessment of fetal disappearance in the first trimester. American Journal of Obstetrics and Gynecology 155: 14–19

Larson S L, Kempers R D, Titus J L 1969 Monoamniotic twins with a common umbilical cord. American Journal of Obstetrics and Gynecology 105: 635–636

Lau W C, Rogers M S 1999 Fetus papyraceous: an unusual cause of obstructed labour. European Journal of Obstetrics, Gynecology and Reproductive Biology 86: 109–111

Leading article 1976 Worldwide decline in dizygotic twinning. British Medical Journal i: 1553

Leppert P C, Wartel L, Lowman R 1979 Fetus papyraceus causing dystocia: inability to detect blighted twin antenatally. Obstetrics and Gynecology 54: 381–384

Librach S, Terrin A J 1957 Monoamniotic twin pregnancy. American Journal of Obstetrics and Gynecology: 74: 440–443

Lichtenstein P, Olausson P O, Kallen A T 1996 Twin births to mothers who are twins: a registry based study. British Medical Journal 312: 879–881

Lichenstein P, Hallen B, Kuster M 1998 No paternal effect in MZ twins in the Swedish Twin Registry. Twin Research 1: 212–215

Liu S, Benirschke K, Scioscia A L, Mannino F L 1992 Intrauterine death in multiple gestation. Acta Geneticae Medicae et Gemellologiae 41: 5–26

Lumme R H, Saarikoski S V 1986 Monoamniotic twin pregnancy. Acta Geneticae Medicae et Gemellologiae 35: 99–105

Machin G A 1996 Some causes of genotypic and phenotypic discordance in monozygotic twin pairs. American Journal of Medical Genetics 61: 216–228

Machin G A 1997 Velamentous cord insertion in monochorionic twin gestation: an added risk factor. Journal of Reproductive Medicine 42: 785–789

Machin G A, Keith L G 1998 Can twin-to-twin transfusion syndrome be explained, and how is it treated? Clinical Obstetrics and Gynecology 41: 104–113

Machin G A, Still K 1995 The twin–twin transfusion syndrome: vascular anatomy of monochorionic placentas and their clinical outcome. In: Keith L G, Papiernik E, Keith D M, Luke B (eds) Multiple pregnancy: epidemiology, gestation and perinatal outcome. Parthenon, New York, pp 367–394

Majsky A, Kout M 1982 Another case of occurrence of two different fathers of twins by HLA typing. Tissue Antigens 20: 305

Malhotra N, Deka D, Takkar D, Kochar S, Goel S, Sharma M C 2001 Hydatidiform mole with coexisting live fetus in dichorionic twin gestation. European Journal of Obstetrics, Gynecology and Reproductive Biology 94: 301–303

Mari G, Roberts A, Detti L et al 2001 Perinatal morbidity and mortality rates in severe twin–twin transfusion syndrome: results of the International Amnioreduction Registry. American Journal of Obstetrics and Gynecology 185: 708–715

Mathelier A C, Karachorlu K 1999 Vanished twin and fetal alcohol syndrome in the surviving twin: a case report. Journal of Reproductive Medicine 44: 394–398

Matsui H, Iitsuka Y, Ishii J, Osada H, Seki K, Sekiya S 1999 Androgenetic complete mole coexistent with a twin live fetus. Gynecologic Oncology 74: 217–221

Matsui H, Sekiya S, Hando T, Wake N, Tomoda Y 2000 Hydatidiform mole coexistent with a twin live fetus: a national collaborative study in Japan. Human Reproduction 15: 608–611

McLeod F, McCoy D R 1981 Monoamniotic twins with an unusual cord complication: case report. British Journal of Obstetrics and Gynaecology 88: 774–775

Megory E, Weiner E, Shalev E, Ohel G 1991 Pseudoamniotic twins with cord entanglement following genetic funipuncture. Obstetrics and Gynecology 78: 915–918

Metler S, Meyer J, Rudzinski L 1974 Morphology of the afterbirth of the Danzig quintuplets. Acta Geneticae Medicae et Gemellologiae 22: 164–167

Meyer W C, Keith L, Webster A 1970 Monoamniotic twin pregnancy with the transfusion syndrome: a case report. Chicago Medical School Quarterly 29: 42–51

Molnar-Nadasdy G, Altshuler G 1996 Perinatal pathology case book: a case of twin transfusion syndrome with dichorionic placentas. Journal of Perinatology 16: 507–509

Montes de Oca Valero F, Macara L, Shaker A 1999 Twin pregnancy with a complete hydatidiform mole and co-existing fetus following in-vitro fertilization. Human Reproduction 14: 2905–2907

Moore C M, McAdams A J, Sutherland J M 1969 Intrauterine disseminated intravascular coagulation: a syndrome of multiple pregnancy with a dead twin fetus. Journal of Pediatrics 74: 523–528

Moore T R, Gate S A, Bewirschke K 1990 Perinatal outcome of forty-nine pregnancies complicated by acardiac twinning. American Journal of Obstetrics and Gynecology 163: 907–912

Mortimer G 1987 Zygosity and placental structure in monochorionic twins. Acta Geneticae Medicae et Gemellologiae 36: 417–420

Murphy K W 1995 Intrauterine death in a twin: implications for the survivor. In: Ward R H, Whittle M (eds) Multiple pregnancy. RCOG Press, London, pp 218–231

Myrianthopoulos N C 1970 An epidemiologic survey of twins in a large prospectively studied population. American Journal of Human Genetics 22: 611–629

Naeye R L 1965 Organ abnormalities in a human parabiotic syndrome. American Journal of Pathology 46: 829–842

Napolitani F D, Schreiber L 1960 The acardiac monster: a review of the world literature and presentation of two cases. American Journal of Obstetrics and Gynecology 80: 582–589

Nerlich A, Wiser J, Krone S 1992 Flazentabefunde bei 'Vanishing Twins'. Geburtshilfe und Frauenheilkunde 52: 230–234

Neubecker R D, Blumberg J M, Townsend F M 1962 A human monozygotic quintuplet placenta: report of a specimen. Journal of Obstetrics and Gynaecology of the British Commonwealth 69: 137–139

Nicolini U, Poblete A 1999 Single intrauterine death in monochorionic twin pregnancies. Ultrasound in Obstetrics and Gynecology 14: 297–301

Nieuwint A, van Zalen-Sprock R, Hummel P, Pals G, Van Vugt J, van der Harten H 1999 'Identical' twins with discordant karotypes. Prenatal diagnosis 19: 72–76

Nylander P P S 1969 The value of the placenta in the determination of zygosity — a study of 1052 Nigerian twin maternities. Journal of Obstetrics and Gynaecology of the British Commonwealth 76: 699–704

Nylander P P S 1970a Placental forms and zygosity determination of twins in Ibadan, Western Nigeria. Acta Geneticae Medicae et Gemellologiae 19: 45–54

Nylander P P S 1970b Twinning in Nigeria. Acta Geneticae Medicae et Gemellologiae 19: 457–464

Nylander P P S 1971a Biosocial aspects of multiple births. Journal of Biosocial Science, Supplement 3: 29–38

Nylander P P S 1971b The incidence of triplets and higher multiple births in some rural and urban populations in Western Nigeria. Annals of Human Genetics 34: 409–415

Nylander P P S 1973 The placenta and zygosity of twins. Acta Geneticae Medicae et Gemellologiae 22: 234–237

Nylander P P S 1975a The causation of twinning. In: MacGillivray I, Nylander P P S, Corney G (eds) Human multiple reproduction. W B Saunders, London, pp 77–86

Nylander P P S 1975b Frequency of multiple births. In: MacGillivray I, Nylander P P S, Corney G (eds) Human multiple reproduction. W B Saunders, London, pp 87–97

Nylander P P S, Corney G 1969 Placentation and zygosity of twins in Ibadan, Nigeria. Annals of Human Genetics 33: 31–38

Nylander P P S, Corney G 1971 Placentation and zygosity of triplets and higher multiple births in Ibadan, Nigeria. Annals of Human Genetics 34: 417–426

Nylander P P S, MacGillivray I 1975 Complications of twin pregnancy. In: MacGillivray I, Nylander P P S, Corney G (eds) Human multiple reproduction. W B Saunders, London, pp 137–146

Nylander P P S, Osunkoya B O 1970 Unusual monochorionic placentation with heterosexual twins. Obstetrics and Gynecology, 36, 621–625

Olsen M E 1992 Monoamniotic twin gestations. Journal of the Tennessee Medical Association 85: 511–512

Ong H C, Puvan I S, Chan W F 1976 An unusual complication of a twin pregnancy — umbilical cord of twin 2 around the neck of twin 1. Australian and New Zealand Journal of Obstetrics and Gynaecology 16: 57–58

Overton T G, Denbow M L, Duncan K R, Fisk N M 1999 First-trimester cord entanglement in monoamniotic twins. Ultrasound in Obstetrics and Gynecology 13: 140–142

Ozumba B C, Ofodile A 1994 Twin pregnancy involving complete hydatidiform mole and partial mole after five years of amenorrhoea. European Journal of Obstetrics, Gynecology and reproductive Biology 53: 230–234

Patignat P, Senn A, Hohlfeld P, Blant S A, Laurini R, Germond M 2001 Molar pregnancy with a coexistent fetus after intracytoplasmic sperm injection: a case report. Journal of Reproductive Medicine 46: 270–274

Pauls F 1969 Monoamniotic twin pregnancy: a review of the world literature and a report of two new cases. Canadian Medical Association Journal 100: 254–256

Perez M L, Firpo J R, Baldi E M 1947 Sobre las anastomosis circulatorias de las placentas dizigoticas. Obstetricia y Ginecologia Latino-Americans 5: 5–22

Perlman E J, Stetten G, Tuck-Muller C M et al 1990 Sexual discordance in monozygotic twins. American Journal of Medical Genetics 37: 551–557

Petersen I R, Nyholm H C 1999 Multiple pregnancies with single intrauterine demise: description of 38 pregnancies. Acta Obstetricia et Gynecologica Scandinavica 78: 202–206

Pharoah P O D, Adi Y 2000 Consequences of in-utero death in a twin pregnancy. Lancet 355: 1597–1602

Phelan M C, Geer J S, Blackburn W R 1998 Vascular anastomoses leading to amelia and cutis aplasia in a dizygotic twin pregnancy. Clinical Genetics 53: 126–130

Pinet C, Colau J C, Delezoide A L, Menez F 1944 Les jumeaux acardiaques. Journal de Gynecologie, Obstetrique et Biologie de la Reproduction 23: 85–92

Pinette M G, Pan Y M M, Pinette S G, Stubblefield P G 1993 Treatment of twin–twin transfusion syndrome. Obstetrics and Gynecology 82: 841–846

Pistorius L R, Howarth G R 1999 Failure of amniotic septostomy in the management of 3 subsequent cases of severe previable twin-twin transfusion syndrome. Fetal Diagnosis and Therapy 14: 337–340

Potter E L 1963 Twin zygosity and placental form in relation to the outcome of pregnancy. American Journal of Obstetrics and Gynecology 87: 566–577

Quigley J K 1935 Monoamniotic twin pregnancy: a case record with review of the literature. American Journal of Obstetrics and Gynecology 29: 354–362

Quintero R A, Reich H, Puder K S et al 1994 Brief report: umbilical cord ligation of an acardiac twin by fetoscopy at 19 weeks of gestation. New England Journal of Medicine 330: 469–471

Quintero R A, Bornick P W, Allen M H, Johnson P K 2001 Selective laser photocoagulation of communicating vessels in severe twin–twin transfusion syndrome in women with an anterior placenta. Obstetrics and Gynecology 97: 477–481

Ramos-Arroyo M A, Ulbright T M, Christian J C 1988 Twin study: relationship between birth weight, zygosity, placentation, and pathologic placental changes. Acta Geneticae Medicae et Gemellologiae 37: 229–238

Raphael S I 1961 Monoamniotic twin pregnancy: a review of the literature and a report of 5 new cases. American Journal of Obstetrics and Gynecology 81: 323–330

Rausen A R, Seki M, Strauss L 1965 Twin transfusion syndrome: a review of 19 cases studied at one institution. Journal of Pediatrics 66: 613–628

Reddy K S, Petersen M B, Antonarakis S E, Blakemore K J 1991 The vanishing twin: an explanation for discordance between chorionic villi karotype and fetal karotype. Prenatal Diagnosis 11: 679–684

Robertson E G, Neer K J 1983 Placental injection studies in twin gestation. American Journal of Obstetrics and Gynecology 147: 170–174

Robinson H P, Caines J S 1977 Sonar evidence of early pregnancy failure in patients with twin conceptions. British Journal of Obstetrics and Gynaecology 84: 22–25

Robinson L K, Jones K L, Benirschke K 1983 The nature of structural defects associated with velamentous and marginal insertion of the umbilical cord. American Journal of Obstetrics and Gynecology 146: 199–204

Rodeck C, Deans A, Jauniaux E 1998 Thermocoagulation for the early treatment of pregnancy with an acardiac twin. New England Journal of Medicine 339: 1293–1295

Rodis J F, Vintzileos A M, Campbell W A, Deaton J L, Fumia F, Nochimson J 1987 Antenatal diagnosis and management of monoamniotic twins. American Journal of Obstetrics and Gynecology 157: 1255–1257

Rosen D J, Rabinowitz R, Beyth Y, Fejgin M D, Nicolaides K M 1990 Fetal urine production in normal twins and in twins with acute polyhydramnios. Fetal Diagnosis and Therapy 5: 57–60

Rudnicki M, Vejerslev L O, Junge J 1991 The vanishing twin: morphologic and cytogenetic evaluation of an ultrasonographic phenomenon. Gynecological and Obstetrical Investigation 31: 141–145

Saito K, Ohtsu Y, Amano K, Nishijima M 1999 Perinatal outcome and management of single fetal death in twin pregnancy: a case series and review. Journal of Perinatal Medicine 27: 473–477

Salerno L J 1959 Monoamniotic twinning: a survey of the American literature since 1935 with a report of four new cases. Obstetrics and Gynecology 14: 205–213

Sato T, Kaneko K, Konuma S, Sato I, Tamada T 1984 Acardiac anomalies: review of 88 cases in Japan. Asia and Oceania Journal of Obstetrics and Gynaecology 10: 45–52

Schatz F 1900 Klinische Beitrage zur Physiologie des Fetus. Hirschwald, Berlin

Schwarzler P, Ville Y, Moscoso G, Tennstedt C, Bollmann R, Chaoui R 1999 Diagnosis of twin reversed arterial perfusion sequence in the first trimester by transvaginal color Doppler ultrasound. Ultrasound in Obstetrics and Gynecology 13: 143–146

Scipiades E, Burg E 1930 Uber die Morphologie der menschlichen Placenta mit besonderer Rücksicht auf unsere eigenen Studienen. Archiv für Gynakologie 141: 577–619

Scrimgeour J B, Baker T G 1974 A possible case of superfetation in man. Journal of Reproduction and Fertility 36: 69–73

Sebire N J, Talbert D, Fisk N M 2001 Twin-to-twin transfusion syndrome results from dynamic asymmetrical reduction in placental anastomoses: a hypothesis. Placenta 22: 383–391

Sekiya S, Hafez E S E 1977 Physiomorphology of twin transfusion syndrome: a study of 86 twin gestations. Obstetrics and Gynecology 50: 288–292

Sergi C, Grischke E M, Schnabel P A et al 2000 Akardius oder 'Twin-Reversed-Arterial-Perfusion' Sequenz: Bericht uber 4 Geminigravidaten und Ubersicht uber den aktuellen Stand der therapeutischen Moglichkeiten. Pathologe 21: 308–314

Serreyn R, Thiery M, Vandekerckhove D 1984 Outcome of an octuplet pregnancy. Archives of Gynaecology 234: 283–293

Severn C B, Holyoke E A 1973 Human acardiac anomalies. American Journal of Obstetrics and Gynecology 116: 358–365

Shahabi S, Donner C, Wallond J, Schlikker I, Avni E F, Rodesch F 1997 Monoamniotic twin cord entanglement: a case report with color flow Doppler ultrasonography for antenatal diagnosis. Journal of Reproductive Medicine 42: 740–742

Shalev E, Zalel Y, Ben-Ami M, Weiner E 1992 First trimester ultrasonic diagnosis of twin reversed arterial perfusion sequence. Prenatal Diagnosis 12: 219–222

Shanklin D R, Perrin E V D K 1984 Multiple gestation. In: Perrin E V D K (ed) Pathology of the placenta. Churchill Livingstone, New York, pp 165–182

Simpson L L, Marx G R, Elkadry E A, D'Alton M E 1998 Cardiac dysfunction in twin-twin transfusion syndrome: a prospective, longitudinal study. Obstetrics and Gynecology 92: 557–562

Sogaard K, Skibsted L, Brocks V 1999 Acardiac twins: pathophysiology, diagnosis, outcome and treatment: six cases and review of the literature. Fetal Diagnosis and Therapy 14: 53–59

Sooranna S R, Ward S, Bajoria R 2001 Discordant fetal leptin levels in monochorionic twins with chronic midtrimester twin–twin transfusion syndrome. Placenta 22: 392–398

Soyal M, Kara S, Ekici E 1996 Twin pregnancy with a fetus and a complete hydatidiform mole. Archives of Gynecology and Obstetrics 259: 41–44

Steller M A, Genest D R, Bernstein M R, Lage J M, Goldstein D P, Berkowitz R S 1994a Natural history of twin pregnancy with complete hydatidiform mole and coexisting fetus. Obstetrics and Gynecology 83: 35–42

Steller M A, Genest D R, Bernstein M R, Lage J M, Goldstein D P, Berkowitz R S 1994b Clinical features of multiple conception with partial or complete molar pregnancy and coexisting fetuses. Journal of Reproductive Medicine 39: 147–154

Stephens T D 1984 Muscle abnormalities associated with the twin-reversed-arterial-perfusion (TRAP) sequence (acardia). Teratology 30: 311–318

Strong S J, Corney G 1967 The placenta in twin pregnancy. Pergamon Press, Oxford

Sulak L E, Dodson M G 1986 The vanishing twin: pathologic confirmation of an ultrasound phenomenon. Obstetrics and Gynecology 68: 811–815

Sutter J, Arab H, Manning F A 1986 Monoamniotic twins: antenatal diagnosis and management. American Journal of Obstetrics and Gynecology 155: 836–837

Suziki S, Ishikawa G, Sawa R, Yoneyama Y, Otsubo Y, Araki T 1999 Iatrogenic monoamniotic twin gestation with progressive twin–twin transfusion syndrome. Fetal Diagnosis and Therapy 14: 98–101

Szendi B 1938 Uber die Bedeutung der Struktur der Eihute und des Gefassnetzes der Placenta auf Grund von 112 Zwillingsgeburten. Archiv für Gynakologie 167: 108–129

Szymonowicz W, Preston H, Yu Y Y H 1986 The surviving monozygotic twin. Archives of Disease in Childhood 61: 454–458

Tafell S M 1995 Demographic trends in twin births: USA. In: Keith L G, Papiernik E, Keith D M, Luke B (eds) Multiple pregnancy: epidemiology, gestation and perinatal outcome. Parthenon, New York, pp 133–144

Tagawa T 1974 Monoamniotic twins with double survival: report of a case with a peculiar cord complication. Wisconsin Medical Journal 73: 131–132

Tan K L, Tan R, Tan S H, Tan A M 1979 The twin transfusion syndrome, clinical observations in 35 affected pairs. Clinical Pediatrics 18: 111–114

Terasaki P I, Gjertson D, Bernoco D, Perdue S, Mickey M R, Bond J 1978 Twins with two different fathers identified by HLA. New England Journal of Medicine 299: 590–592

Tessen J A, Zlatnik F J 1991 Monoamniotic twins: a retrospective controlled study. Obstetrics and Gynecology 77: 832–834

Timmons J D, de Alvarez R R 1963 Monoamniotic twin pregnancy. American Journal of Obstetrics and Gynecology 86: 875–881

Trespidi L, Boschetto C, Caravelli E, Villa L, Kustermann A, Nicolini U 1997 Serial amniocenteses in the management of twin-twin transfusion syndrome: when is it valuable? Fetal Diagnosis and Therapy 12: 15–20

Turksoy R N, Toy B L, Rogers J, Papageorge W 1967 Birth of septuplets following human gonadotrophin administration in Chiari–Frommel syndrome. Obstetrics and Gynecology 30: 692–698

Uotila J, Tammela O 1999 Acute intrapartum fetoplacental transfusion in monochorionic twin pregnancy. Obstetrics and Gynecology 94: 819–821

Urig M A, Simpson G F, Elliott J P, Clewell W H 1988 Twin-twin transfusion syndrome: the surgical removal of one twin as a treatment option. Fetal Therapy 3: 185–188

Urig M A, Clewell W M, Elliott J P 1990 Twin-twin transfusion syndrome. American Journal of Obstetrics and Gynecology 163: 1522–1526

van Allen M I 1981 Fetal vascular disruptions: mechanisms and some resulting birth defects. Pediatric Annual 10: 219–233

van Allen M I, Smith D W, Shepard T H 1983 Twin reversed arterial perfusion (TRAP) sequence: a study of 14 twin pregnancies with acardius. Seminars in Perinatology 7: 285–293

Vandeginste S, Vergote I B, Hanssenns M et al 1999 Malignant trophoblastic disease following a twin pregnancy consisting of a complete hydatidiform mole and a normal fetus and placenta: a case report. European Journal of Gynaecological Oncology 20: 105–107

van Dijk B A, Boomsma D I, de Mann A J M 1996 Blood group chimerism in human multiple births is not rare. American Journal of Medical Genetics 61: 264–268

van Gemert M J, Umur A 2000 Trends of discordant fetal growth in monochorionic twin pregnancies. Physics in Medicine and Biology 45: 85–93

van Gemert M J, Umur A, Tijssen J G, Ross M G 2001 Twin-twin transfusion syndrome: etiology, severity and rational management. Current Opinion in Obstetrics and Gynecology 13: 193–206

Varma T R 1979 Ultrasound evidence of early pregnancy failure in patients with multiple conceptions. British Journal of Obstetrics and Gynaecology 86: 290–292

Vejerslev L O 1991 Clinical management and diagnostic possibilities in hydatidiform mole with coexistent fetus. Obstetrical and Gynecological Survey 46: 577–588

Vial Y, Hohlfeld P 1999 Mort in utero d'un jumeau. Schweizerische Rundschau fur Medizin Praxis 88: 1435–1438

Victoria A, Mora G, Arias F 2001 Perinatal outcome, placental pathology, and severity of discordance in monochorionic and dichorionic twins. Obstetrics and Gynecology 97: 310–315

Ville Y, Hecher K, Gagnon A, Sebire N, Hyett J, Nicolaides K 1998 Endoscopic laser coagulation in the management of severe twin-to-twin transfusion syndrome. British Journal of Obstetrics and Gynaecology 105: 446–453

Wagner D S, Klein R L, Robinson H B, Novak R W 1990 Placental emboli from a fetus papyraceous. Journal of Pediatric Surgery 25: 538–542

Walter A, Hasenohr G, Kerin J F P 1975 Superfetation in man. Australian and New Zealand Journal of Obstetrics and Gynaecology 15: 240–246

Wenk R E, Houtz T, Brooks M, Chiafari F A 1992 How frequent is heteroparental superfecundation? Acta Geneticae Medicae et Gemellologiae 41: 43–47

Wenner R 1956 Les examens vasculaires des placentas gemellaires et le diagnostic des jumeaux homozygotes. Bulletin de la Société Belge de Gynécologie et Obstétrique 26: 773–781

Wensinger J A, Daly R F 1962 Monoamniotic twins. American Journal of Obstetrics and Gynecology 83: 1254–1256

Wharton B, Edwards J H, Cameron A H 1968 Monoamniotic twins. Journal of Obstetrics and Gynaecology of the British Commonwealth 75: 158–163

Wieacker P, Wilhelm C, Prompeler H, Petersen P G, Schillinger H, Breckwoldt M 1992 Pathophysiology of polyhydramnios in twin transfusion syndrome. Fetal Diagnosis and Therapy 7: 87–92

Wigglesworth J S 1995 The placenta in twins. In: Ward R H, Whittle M (eds) Multiple pregnancy. RCOG Press, London, pp 48–55

Wilson E A 1972 Holoacardius. Obstetrics and Gynecology 40: 740–748

Yoshida K 1995 Documenting the vanishing twin by pathological examination. In: Kieth L G, Papiernik E, Kieth D M, Luke B (eds) Multiple pregnancy: epidemiology, gestation and perinatal outcome. Parthenon, New York, pp 51–58

Yoshida K, Soma H 1986 Outcomes of the surviving co-twin of a fetus papyraceous or of a dead fetus. Acta Geneticae Medicae et Gemellologiae 35: 91–98

Yoshioka H, Kadomoto Y, Mino M, Morikawa Y, Kasubuchi Y, Kusunok T 1979 Multicystic encephalomacia in liveborn twin with a stillborn macerated co-twin. Journal of Pediatrics 95: 798–800

Zuckerman H, Brzezinski A 1960 Monoamniotic twin pregnancy: report of two cases with review of the literature. Gynaecologia 150: 290–298

49

The application of new techniques to gynaecological pathology

A. N. Y. Cheung   H. Fox   M. Wells

Introduction   1595

Molecular and genetic studies   1595
Studies of oncogene expression   1595
Studies of tumour suppressor genes   1597
Study of *FHIT* gene   1600
Studies of apoptosis-related genes   1601
Study of DNA mismatch genes and microsatellite instability   1601
Study of telomerase activity   1601
Studies of clonality   1602
In situ hybridisation   1603
Study of chromosomal imbalances by comparative genomic hybridisation   1604
Arrays   1605
Study of imprinted genes   1605
Detection and typing of HPV   1606

Studies of cell proliferation and of apoptotic markers   1606
Studies of cell proliferation   1606
Studies of apoptosis   1607

Determination of tumour ploidy   1608
Introduction   1608
Ovarian carcinoma   1609
Ovarian epithelial tumours of borderline malignancy   1610
Non-epithelial tumours of the ovary   1610
Carcinoma of Fallopian tube   1610
Endometrial adenocarcinoma   1610
Uterine sarcomas   1611
Carcinoma of the cervix   1611
Carcinoma of the vagina   1611
Carcinoma of the vulva   1611
Gestational trophoblastic disease   1611
Conclusions   1611

Morphometry   1612
Introduction   1612
Vulva   1612
Cervix   1612
Endometrium   1613
Ovary   1613

INTRODUCTION

Some of the newer techniques introduced into pathology during the past few decades have not only left the confines of the research laboratory but have passed fully into standard diagnostic practice. Thus, for instance, immunohistochemistry has become a routine technique in virtually all laboratories and information about the use and validity of this diagnostic tool has been integrated into the various chapters in this volume. In this chapter we discuss a number of techniques, some quite well established and others only recently introduced, which can no longer be considered simply as research tools but which have not yet been extensively employed in diagnostic laboratories outside of major academic centres and critically consider their value in gynaecological pathology.

MOLECULAR AND GENETIC STUDIES

STUDIES OF ONCOGENE EXPRESSION

Oncogenes are altered proto-oncogenes that are related to the development of neoplasia. Proto-oncogenes play a major rôle in the control of cell proliferation and abnormalities in the expression of their products may result from gene amplification, point mutation or rearrangement. As a result the gene product may be produced in excess or in abnormally stabilised form and such abnormalities may be detected by immunocytochemistry. A direct demonstration of gene amplification can be achieved by the use of the fluorescent differential polymerase chain reaction.

Oncogenes related to the type-1 growth factor family

This family encompasses oncogene encoded transmembrane phosphoglycoproteins with tyrosinate activity and their ligands. It includes epidermal growth factor receptor (*EGFR*), *c-erbB-2* (or *HER2/neu* gene) and *c-erb-3* which share considerable structural homology with each other.

Ovarian carcinoma

Both *EGFR* and *c-erbB-2* expression are detectable in many ovarian tumours of borderline malignancy (van Haaften Day et al 1996). In ovarian carcinomas overexpression of *c-erbB-2*, with or without gene amplification, is found in about 20% of cases of early-stage disease but is more common in advanced-stage disease (Felip et al 1995; Leeson et al 1995; Anreder et al 1999; Ross et al 1999). Whilst some studies have not found *c-erbB-2* overexpression or amplification to be a significant prognostic marker in ovarian carcinoma (Wilkinson et al 1991; Rubin et al 1993; Makar et al 1994; Rubin et al 1994; Singleton et al 1994; Leeson et al 1995; Ross et al 1999; Skirnisdottir et al 2001a) others have found it to be associated with large postoperative tumour bulk, resistance to chemotherapy or poor survival (Berchuck et al 1990; Meden et al 1994; Felip et al 1995).

EGFR expression is detectable in about 12% of ovarian carcinomas and overexpression of *EGFR*, to a degree greater than that seen in the original tumour, is found in persistent or recurrent disease after chemotherapy and is an independent adverse prognostic factor (van Dam et al 1994; Skirnisdottir et al 2001a).

c-erbB-3 expression in ovarian carcinoma is not significantly associated with tumour stage, differentiation, ploidy, S-phase fraction or post-operative tumour bulk (Simpson et al 1995).

Endometrial carcinoma

The incidence of *c-erbB-2* amplification or overexpression in endometrial carcinoma has varied between 9 and 52% in different studies (Bigsby et al 1992; Wang et al 1993; Khalifa et al 1994; Monk et al 1994; Czerwenka et al 1995; Saffari et al 1995; Rolitsky et al 1999). Endometrial papillary serous adenocarcinoma is more likely to exhibit immunoreactivity for *c-erbB-2* than is conventional endometrioid carcinoma of the endometrium (Prat et al 1994). Overexpression of *c-erbB-2* has been found to correlate with high histological grade, vascular-lymphatic space invasion and cell turnover indices (Khalifa et al 1994; Czwerwenka et al 1995; Ioffe et al 1998) emerging as an indicator of poor survival in some studies (Hetzel et al 1992; Saffari et al 1995; Riben et al 1997; Rolitsky et al 1999) but not in others (Reinartz et al 1994; Czerwenka et al 1995; Pisani et al 1995).

EGFR expression has been detected in 70–90% of endometrial carcinomas (Esteller et al 1995; Salomon et al 1995). The prognostic significance of *EGFR* expression in endometrial carcinoma is controversial. Khalifa et al (1994) showed that such expression correlated with tumour metastasis and decreased survival in endometrioid, serous papillary and clear cell carcinomas, whilst others could find no correlation between *EGFR* immunoreactivity and survival or indeed any other prognostic variable (Reinartz et al 1994; Santini et al 1994).

Cervical carcinoma

Frequent amplification of *c-erbB-2* has been documented in cervical carcinoma (Sharma et al 1999). *c-erbB-2* immunostaining was found by Nevin et al (1999) to be significantly associated with poor survival and was considered to be a marker of high-risk disease: *c-erbB-2* immunostaining was also found to be an important prognostic factor for predicting tumour recurrence in cervical carcinomas treated by radiotherapy (Nakano et al 1997; Nishioka et al 1999).

Demonstrable *EGFR* in cervical carcinomas appeared to be associated with a poor prognosis in two studies (Hale et al 1993; Kristensen et al 1996) but was of no prognostic value in another (Oka et al 1997).

Overexpression of *c-erbB-3* oncoprotein in squamous, adenosquamous and adenocarcinomas of the cervix shows no association with clinical outcome (Hunt et al 1995).

Both *c-erbB-2* and *EGFR* are activated in CIN (Ngan et al 1999a) and this raises the possibility that antibodies or antigenes targeted against these oncogenes may alter the progress of CIN to invasive disease.

K-ras oncogene

Ovarian carcinoma

Mutations or amplifications of the *ras* oncogene occur in 20–40% of ovarian carcinomas (van Dam et al 1994; Park et al 1995): they occur far more frequently in mucinous than in non-mucinous tumours (Cuatrecasas et al 1997). In one series *K-ras* point mutations were more frequently found in advanced-stage disease and in tumours associated with nodal metastases and hence activation of *K-ras* oncogene was thought to be a major factor in tumour progression (Teneriello et al 1993). Other studies have, however, shown that *K-ras* mutations occur in borderline tumours with the same frequency as in invasive adenocarcinomas, the rate of such mutation being considerably higher in borderline mucinous tumours than in their serous counterparts (Mok et al 1993; Cuatracasas et al 1997; Caduff et al 1999). In a recent study Garrett et al (2001) confirmed the high incidence of *K-ras* mutations in ovarian borderline mucinous tumours and showed that the same mutations were also frequently present in adjacent histologically benign epithelium: in one case the same *K-ras* mutation was present in contiguous benign, borderline and carcinomatous epithelia. These findings suggest that *K-ras* mutation is an early event in ovarian carcinogenesis but may not alone be sufficient for malignant transformation.

Endometrial hyperplasia and carcinoma

Point mutations in codon 12 or 13 of the *K-ras* oncogene have been found in between 6 and 16% of cases of atypical hyperplasia of the endometrium and in between 10 and 37% of cases of endometrioid carcinoma of the endometrium: mutations are not found in simple or complex hyperplasia and are rarely detectable in either serous or clear cell carcinomas (Enomoto et al 1993, 1995; Sasaki et al 1993; Caduff et al 1995). The frequency of mutation of this oncogene seems to demonstrate geographical variation with a two-to three-fold higher prevalence in endometrial carcinomas from Japan compared with those from the USA (Sasaki et al 1993; Enomoto et al 1995). Such differences in K-ras mutation may be related to the differences in incidence and histopathological features of endometrial carcinoma between the two countries. The similar incidence of K-ras mutations in atypical hyperplasia and adenocarcinoma suggests that K-ras activation is an early event in endometrial carcinogenesis and this has been confirmed in a more recent study which demonstrated K-ras mutation in both premalignant microsatellite stable and unstable endometrial neoplasia, sometimes before the development of histological features diagnostic of atypical endometrial hyperplasia (Mutter et al 1999).

The prognostic significance of K-ras mutations in endometrial carcinoma is debatable. Sasaki et al (1993) found no correlation between such mutations and depth of myometrial invasion, histological grade or stage though considered that ras mutations were asociated with a good prognosis whilst Caduff et al (1995) found no relationship of any sort between K-ras mutations and clinical outcome. By contrast, Ito et al (1996) found a correlation between K-ras mutations and an adverse outcome but only in postmenopausal patients.

Cervical carcinoma

Mutations in the K-ras oncogene have not been identified in cervical carcinomas (Falcinelli et al 1993) but it has been claimed that positive staining for the ras oncogene product, p21, is correlated with nodal metastases and a poor prognosis (Hayashi et al 1991); this has, however, not been everyone's experience (Symonds et al 1992).

c-myc oncogene

In ovarian neoplasms p62c-myc, which is the product of the c-myc oncogene, has been detected in serous and mucinous adenocarcinomas (Polacarz et al 1989; Sasano et al 1992). It has been suggested that in ovarian carcinomas c-myc overexpression is indicative of aggressive tumour behaviour (Bauknecht et al 1990) and that amplification of the c-myc gene correlates with poor survival.

Amplification of c-myc occurs in about 10% of endometrial carcinomas and is particularly found in high-grade and high-stage neoplasms (Monk et al 1994). The c-myc oncogene product is expressed in a high proportion of endometrial adenocarcinomas (Sato et al 1991; Bai et al 1994) and intense staining is related to high grade and deep myometrial invasion.

c-myc amplification has been demonstrated in CIN and invasive cevical carcinoma (Dellas et al 1997; Aoyama et al 1998; Ngan et al 1999a), suggesting that it is important in early cervical carcinogenesis. Moreover, c-myc over-expression correlates with high-risk HPV positive neoplasia and with cellular proliferation (Dellas et al 1997). It has been claimed that an increased level of c-myc transcripts is strongly indicative of a poor prognosis in early-stage cervical carcinoma (Iwasaka et al 1992) but not in late stage disease (Symonds et al 1992).

Colony stimulating factor (CSF) and receptor (c-fms) oncogenes

The c-fms oncogene encodes a protein that transduces signals via tyrosine kinases and stimulates cell proliferation. High levels of transcripts of CSF and its receptor have been found in 10–20% of ovarian carcinomas and a positive correlation has been found between CSF and c-fms mRNA expression levels (Bauknecht et al 1994; Kommoss et al 1994). Thus, the co-expression of CSF and its receptor may regulate the growth of ovarian carcinomas via an autocrine loop. Further, high levels of c-fms transcripts correlate with predictors of poor outcome such as high-grade carcinoma and late-stage disease.

STUDIES OF TUMOUR SUPPRESSOR GENES

p53

The p53 tumour suppressor gene (tp53), located on chromosome 17p, plays a regulatory role in cell growth by inducing a G1 arrest for DNA repair and controlling the initiation of apoptosis. Normal, or wild type, tp53 gene product is normally rapidly degraded and not detectable by immunohistochemistry. Mutations in the tp53 gene are common in gynaecological cancers (Manek & Wells 1996) and mutant p53 protein, which is resistant to degradation, can accumulate in the nucleus and can be demonstrated by immunohistochemical techniques. However, mutation of the tp53 gene is not always associated with overexpression of the mutant protein (Wynford-Thomas 1992) and overexpression of wild type p53 protein can also occur and be detectable by immunocytochemistry and hence DNA sequencing is necessary to confirm mutation.

Ovarian carcinoma

tp53 mutations have been found in about 50% of ovarian carcinomas: benign epithelial tumours and tumours of borderline malignancy usually, though not invariably, stain negatively for p53 or show only weak immunoreactivity (Kohler et al 1993; Teneriello et al 1993; Klemi et al 1994; Kappes et al 1995; Kupryjanczyk et al 1995; van Haaften et al 1996; Anreda et al 1999; Chan et al 2000).

Mutations of *tp53* in ovarian carcinomas are found particularly in advanced-stage tumours (Kupryjanczyk et al 1995). Overexpression of p53 protein has, however, also been noted in atypical surface epithelium adjacent to a carcinoma or within inclusion cysts (Hutson et al 1995) and mutations of *tp53* in the epithelium of borderline tumours immediately adjacent to a carcinoma (Kupryjanczyk et al 1995), suggesting that *tp53* mutation may be an early event in ovarian carcinogenesis. Nevertheless, no increase in the expression of *p53* has been found in the surface epithelium of ovaries removed prophylactically from women with a family history of ovarian cancer (Werness et al 1999a). Although Schildkraut et al (1997) found that mutant *p53* overexpression correlated with the total number of ovulations this was not confirmed in a later study (Webb et al 1998).

In a number of studies *p53* expression has emerged as an adverse prognostic factor in cases of ovarian carcinoma (Hartmann et al 1994; Henriksen et al 1994; Levesque et al 1995; Allan et al 1996; Geisler et al 2000; Skirnisdottir et al 2001b) though this has not been an invariable finding (Niwa et al 1994). The chemosensitivity of ovarian carcinomas may be related to *p53* dependent apoptosis (Sato et al 1999) and to the expression of *p21*$^{WAF1/cip1}$ which is the major downstream effector of *p53* (Costa et al 1999; Werness et al 1999b).

p53 overexpression in borderline ovarian tumours was not predictive of tumour recurrence in two series (Kupryjanczyk et al 1995; Eltabbakhet al 1997) but was a predictive factor in one (Gershenson et al 1999).

Carcinoma of Fallopian tube

Immunoreactivity for *p53* is found in about 50% of tubal carcinomas. An early study reported that *p53* immunoreactivity was associated with a poor survival rate (Zheng et al 1997) but more recent studies have found that *p53* immunoreactivity and/or *tp53* mutation did not correlate with tumour progression, response to treatment or patient survival (Rosen et al 1998; Hellstrom et al 2000).

Endometrial carcinoma

The reported incidence of overexpression of p53 protein has varied widely but anything up to 50% of endometrioid adenocarcinomas and virtually 100% of serous papillary carcinomas stain positively for *p53* protein (Tashiro et al 1997a; Burton & Wells 1998); only about 25% of clear cell carcinomas stain positively for *p53* (Lax et al 1998b). Histological variants of endometrioid adenocarcinomas, such as mucinous, secretory or ciliated cell carcinomas, have a low incidence of positive staining for *p53* (Lax et al 1998a). It is important to note that positive immunostaining for p53 protein may be found in endometrial adenocarcinomas in the absence of *tp53* mutation, possibly because of abnormal stabilisation of

the wild p53 protein by mdm 2 (Stewart et al 1998; Burton et al 1999). Overexpression of *p53* is more common in endometrioid adenocarcinoma than in atypical hyperplasia suggesting that *tp53* mutation may be a late event in the histogenesis of this neoplasm (Yu et al 1993). By contrast serous papillary carcinomas show *p53* overexpression, associated with mutation, at all stages and the precursor lesion of this form of endometrial neoplasm also shows *p53* overexpression (Tashiro et al 1997a; Zheng et al 1998): hence *tp53* mutation is an early event in the histogenesis of serous papillary carcinoma.

In endometrioid adenocarcinomas *p53* overexpression tends to be associated with high grade, proliferative activity, lack of PR expression, advanced stage and deep myometrial invasion (Yamauchi et al 1996; Taskin et al 1997; Ioffe et al 1998; Lax et al 1998a). However, though some have found *p53* overexpression to be an independent and strong indicator of a poor prognosis (Pisani et al 1995; Hamel et al 1996; Sorbe et al 1997; Lax et al 1998a), even in early-stage disease (Kohlberger et al 1996; Athanassiodou et al 1999), others have not found it to emerge only from multivariate analysis as an independent adverse prognostic factor (Hachisuga et al 1993; Lukes et al 1994; Reinartz et al 1994; Strang et al 1996). In a recent and probably definitive study, in which all confounding factors were taken into account, patients with endometrial carcinomas who had *p53* overexpression were found to have a seven-fold higher risk of dying from the disease compared to those without *p53* overexpression (Sung et al 2000).

Cervical carcinoma

Inactivation of *tp53* appears to play a key rôle in the development of cervical squamous cell carcinoma (Manek & Wells 1996; Helland et al 1998; Thomas et al 1999), either because it is inactivated by binding with the E6 protein of oncogenic HPV types or because it undergoes mutation: patterns of *p53* immunoreactivity suggest also that *tp53* inactivation plays a key rôle in the progression from intraepithelial to invasive neoplasia (Troncone et al 1998; Lie et al 1999; Ngan et al 1999a). There has, however, been some dispute about the significance of a common polymorphism that occurs in the *p53* amino acid sequence which results in the presence of either a proline or an arginine at position 72. Storey et al (1998) found that individuals homozygous for arginine 72 were about seven times more susceptible to HPV-associated tumorigenesis than were heterozygotes. However, subsequent studies have shown no relationship between the *tp53* genotype and the risk of cervical cancer (Rosenthal et al 1998; Giannoudis et al 1999; Ngan et al 1999b; Yamashita et al 1999; Malcolm et al 2000).

In cervical adenocarcinoma the rôle of *p53* and HPV is more controversial but *p53* reactivity has been demonstrated in endocervical carcinoma in situ (Cina et al

1997; McCluggage et al 1997). *tp53* gene alterations are rare in minimal deviation adenocarcinoma (Toki et al 1999) and are not found in villoglandular adenocarcinomas (Jones et al 2000).

The prognostic value of *p53* immunoreactivity in cervical carcinoma is controversial. Some have found no association between *p53* overexpression or the presence of mutant p53 protein and clinical outcome (Hunt et al 1996; Pillai et al 1999) whilst others have reported that *p53* expression identifies a subset of cervical carcinomas with a poor prognosis (Uchiyama et al 1997).

Vulvar carcinoma

tp53 gene mutations are present in about a half of HPV-negative vulvar carcinomas (Kim et al 1996; Ngan et al 1999c) and is commonly present in differentiated VIN (Yang & Hart 2000). Immunostaining of p53 protein or detection of *tp53* point mutations in vulvar squamous cell carcinomas have been variously reported as indicative of a poor prognosis (Kohlberger et al 1995; Sliutz et al 1997) and devoid of any useful prognostic value (Kagie et al 1997).

Uterine sarcomas

Abnormal expression of *p53* is common in uterine leiomyosarcomas (Liu et al 1994; Zhai et al 1999): tumours with *tp53* mutation or p53 protein overexpression tend to have a high histological grade and and be at a high stage on initial presentation and are at higher risk of recurrence (Hall et al 1997; Blom et al 1998b).

Gestational trophoblastic disease

No mutational changes in hot spots of *tp53* can be found in hydatidiform moles (Chen et al 1994; Cheung et al 1994a, 1999a; Shi et al 1996) and only wild type p53 protein can be demonstrated in trophoblastic tissue. Nevertheless, higher expression of wild type *p53* mRNA and protein are found in choriocarcinoma and hydatidform moles when compared with normal placenta (Chen et al 1994; Cheung et al 1994a, 1999a; Lee 1995; Shi et al 1996; Fulop et al 1998): p53 protein expression correlates with proliferative activity in all forms of trophoblastic disease but does not, in hydatidiform moles, correlate with the development of persistent trophoblastic disease requiring chemotherapy (Cheung et al 1998, 1999a).

Loss of heterozygosity (LOH)

LOH is defined as deletion of a portion of a chromosome that contains a putative tumour suppressor gene and implies loss of the normal polymorphism present at a given locus. LOH is therefore taken as a marker of a mutation in or loss of a tumour suppressor gene.

Ovarian tumours

LOH occurs only occasionally in benign or borderline ovarian tumours but has frequently been demonstrated in multiple chromosomal loci, including those on chromosomes 6q, 13q, 17p, 17q and 22q, in nearly all histological types of ovarian carcinoma and is especially common in advanced-stage disease (Cliby et al 1993; Liu et al 1994; Bryan et al 1996; Saretzki et al 1997; Dion et al 2000). Because most carcinomas show LOH at more than one locus it is reasonable to infer that multiple genetic alterations are involved in ovarian tumorigenesis. Candidate tumour suppressor genes have been localised to chromosome 17p (Phillips et al 1996; Schutz et al 1996; Bruening et al 1999), 17q (Garcia et al 2000) 22q (Bryan et al 1996) and 13q (Liu et al 1994). Liu et al (1994) found only infrequent mutations of the retinoblastoma (*RB*) gene in a group of patients having high frequency of LOH at 13q, implying the involvement of other tumour suppressor genes than *Rb* on 13q in ovarian carcinogenesis. In a more recent study, however, Gras et al (2001) detected LOH at the Rb-1 locus in nearly 25% of ovarian carcinomas, this being particularly common in those of serous type. The LOH on 17q that is found quite commonly in sporadic ovarian carcinomas is thought to be related to a tumour suppressor gene other than *BRCA-1* and tends to be associated with high-grade serous carcinomas (Jacobs et al 1993; Pieretti et al 1995; Garcia et al 2000). Interestingly, LOH on chromosome 17 increases with age except in elderly women (Pieretti et al 1995; Garcia et al 2000) and it has been suggested that the repetitive repair and remodelling of the ovarian serosa during ovulation might predispose to LOH (Pieretti & Turker 1997).

Endometrial carcinoma

Allelotypic analysis of endometrial carcinomas has demonstrated frequent LOH or allelic imbalance in multiple chromosomal loci (Fujino et al 1994; Jones et al 1994; Nagase et al 1996; Tritz et al 1997). LOH is encountered most frequently on chromosome 10q25–10q26 and there is a strong correlation between LOH on chromosome 14 and death from disease (Fujino et al 1994). LOH is more frequently found in non-endometrioid endometrial carcinomas than in endometrioid carcinomas, suggesting diverse tumorigenic pathways (Tritz et al 1997).

Cervical neoplasia

LOH has been recurrently detected in multiple chromosomal regions in CIN (3p, 5p, 5q, 6p, 6q, 11q, 13q, 17q), invasive carcinoma (3p, 6p, 6q, 11q, 17p, 18q) and lymph node metastases from cervical carcinomas (3p, 6p, 11q, 17p, 18q, X) (Hampton et al 1994; Bethwaite et al 1995;

Larson et al 1997; Kersemaekers et al 1998, 1999; Luft et al 1999; Lu et al 2000; Chuaqui et al 2001). These changes accumulate in a fashion that parallels the progresson of cervical carcinoma and indicate the stepwise fashion of cervical carcinogenesis. The finding of a strong association between the number of chromosomes associated with LOH in CIN and its grade lends further support to the concept of progressive genetic changes (Larson et al 1997). Chromosomal instability is probably an early event in cervical carcinogenesis for Chatterjee et al (2001) have demonstrated at least two tumour suppressor genes on 6p related to invasive cervical carcinoma in 50% of low-grade CIN and in 90% of high-grade CIN. The detection of LOH in chromosome 3p and 6p loci in CIN suggests that identification of a specific marker panel encompassing this region might be of value in the assessment of possible regression, persistence or progression of the lesion (Luft et al 1999; Chatterjee et al 2001).

The prognostic significance of LOH in cervical carcinoma is still controversial. Kersemaekers et al (1998) noted no relationship between clinical or histological parameters and losses on chromosomes 3p, 11q, and 17p. Harima et al (1999) found, however, that LOH on 17p13 was associated with bulky tumours that responded poorly to radiotherapy.

PTEN gene

The gene *PTEN* (phosphate and tensin homologue deleted on chromosome 10) is located on the 10q23–24 region, negatively regulates the function of integrins and plays a rôle in the control of cell growth, apoptosis and cytoskeletal organisation; it is a candidate tumour suppressor gene which is frequently deleted or mutated in human cancers (Tamura et al 1999).

Ovarian carcinoma

In most studies alterations in *PTEN* have been very uncommon in ovarian carcinomas (Tashiro et al 1997b; Maxwell et al 1998a; Yokomizo et al 1998). Obata et al (1998) demonstrated, however, frequent *PTEN* mutations in endometrioid adenocarcinomas of the ovary especially those of low grade and stage, this suggesting that in this form of ovarian carcinoma *PTEN* inactivation is an early event in tumorigenesis.

Endometrial carcinoma

PTEN mutations are found in about 50% of endometrioid carcinomas of the endometrium but are rarely present in serous papillary or clear cell adenocarcinomas (Risinger et al 1997; Tashiro et al 1997b; Lin et al 1998; Bussaglia et al 2000). *PTEN* mutations are present in endometrioid adenocarcinomas with or without microsatellite instability although the spectrum of *PTEN* mutation differs between those with microsatellite instability and those without (Bussaglia et al 2000). The prevalence of *PTEN* mutation is similar amongst high-grade and low-grade tumours and amongst early-stage and late-stage disease and *PTEN* mutations are found in 23% of cases of endometrial atypical hyperplasia (Levine et al 1998; Maxwell et al 1998b): these findings suggest that *PTEN* mutation plays an early significant rôle in the pathogenesis of the endometrioid type of endometrial carcinoma. *PTEN* mutation can even be detected in histologically normal endometria and immunostaining for PTEN protein may be a marker for premalignant endometrial disease (Mutter et al 2000a, 2001).

BRCA1 gene

The *BRCA1* gene, situtated on chromosome 17q, is thought to be a tumour suppressor gene and germline mutations in this gene are associated with familial ovarian cancer (a topic discussed in Chapter 18). Somatic mutations of *BRCA1* in sporadic ovarian carcinoma are generally considered as uncommon (Hosking et al 1995; Matsushima et al 1995; Merajver et al 1995) but recently Khoo et al (1999) have reported a number of instances of somatic mutation in exon 11 of the *BRCA1* gene amongst sporadic cases of ovarian carcinoma with no age selection. *BRCA1* gene mutations have also been reported in a surprisingly high proportion of cases of CIN, involving 76% of such cases in one study (Park et al 1999). The mutations did not correlate with the type of CIN or with the presence or absence of HPV.

STUDY OF THE *FHIT* GENE

Recent studies have found that abnormalities of the *FHIT* (fragile histidine triad) gene, including loss of heterozygosity, homozygous deletions and aberrant transcripts, are common in cervical carcinomas, implicating this gene in cervical carcinogenesis (Hendricks et al 1997; Muller et al 1998; Su et al 1998; Yoshino et al 1998): *FHIT* abnormalities have been observed in various histological types of cervical carcinomas (Segawa et al 1999).

Nakagawa et al (1999) found *FHIT* gene abnormalities in both CIN and invasive carcinoma but the incidence did not increase with progression to invasion or with advancing clinical stage: they suggested that aberrant expression of the gene may play a critical rôle in early cervical carcinogenesis but not in the progression of cervical cancer, a view supported by Wu et al (2000) from their studies of cervical carcinoma cell lines. By contrast, Yoshino et al (2000) found aberrations of *FHIT* to be more common in invasive carcinomas than in CIN suggesting that *FHIT*-gene inactivation occurred as a late event in cervical carcinogenesis, after the tumour had acquired an invasive character.

The relationship between HPV infection and *FHIT* gene aberrations has not been established. At first, HPV 16 was found to be associated with loss of heterozygosity in the *FHIT* region (Muller et al 1998). More recent studies have, however, found no relationship between *FHIT* abnormalities and HPV infection (Su et al 1998; Yoshino et al 2000). Segawa et al (1999) have suggested that whilst the E6–E7 genes of oncogenic HPV are important for the development of cervical neoplasia, they may not be required for the development of cervical carcinoma in cells that have abnormal *FHIT* genes.

STUDIES OF APOPTOSIS-RELATED GENES

Some of these genes, such as *Bcl-2*, merit consideration in their own right as possible prognostic markers but as they are inextricably interlinked with studies of apoptosis they are considered under the later section on studies of cell proliferation and loss.

STUDY OF DNA MISMATCH GENES AND MICROSATELLITE INSTABILITY

A number of genes are known to encode proteins involved in DNA mismatch repair, these including *hMSH2*, *hMLH1* and *hPMS2*: mutations in these genes lead to genetic instability and an increased susceptibility to cancer (Fishel & Kolodner 1995; Kolodner 1995). The genetic instability phenotype associated with defective mismatch repair genes is most readily observed through somatic length alterations in simple repeat sequences which are located throughout the genome and are known as microsatellites: replication errors in these repeat sequences are probably common and their inefficient repair results in microsatellite instability.

Germline mutations in DNA mismatch genes are linked with the hereditary non-polyposis colon cancer syndrome (Marra & Boland 1995) of which endometrial carcinoma is a feature (Millar et al 1999). Cases associated with the hereditary non-polyposis colon cancer syndrome make up only a tiny minority of endometrial neoplasms but nevertheless microsatellite instability is found in about 20–30% of endometrial carcinomas (Risinger et al 1993; Burks et al 1994; Duggan et al 1994; Wong et al 1999b). In fact, mutations in DNA mismatch genes are rarely found in sporadic endometrial carcinomas (Katabuchi et al 1995), but there are epigenetic changes in these genes with hypermethylation and inactivation of the *hMLH1* promoter gene in 71% of cases in which there was microsatellite instability, as compared to only 10% in cases without microsatellite instability (Simpkins et al 1999). Microsatellite instability is found before and during clonal expansion in endometrial carcinoma suggesting that the expression of genomic instability contributes to, and is not a consequence of, malignant transformation (Duggan et al 1994). This view is reinforced by the finding that hypermethylation of the *hMLH1* promoter

gene is found in microsatellite instability negative endometrial hyperplasia coexisting with microsatellite instability positive endometrial carcinoma indicating that the epigenetic change is the earliest event in endometrial carcinogenesis (Esteller et al 1999). There are no significant clinical differences between those endometrial carcinomas that show microsatellite instability and those which lack this feature (Wong et al 1999b).

STUDY OF TELOMERASE ACTIVITY

Telomerase is a ribonucleoprotein complex that adds telomeric DNA repeats onto the ends of chromosomes during cell proliferation thus replacing the loss of sequences from each DNA strand that occurs with each replication. Since most normal cells lack this activity, successive cell divisions normally result in progressive shortening of telomeres which may result in cellular senescence and leads to cell death. It is suggested that activation of telomerase is necessary for the sustained proliferation of tumour cells and for their 'immortalisation' (Kim et al 1994; Feng et al 1995). It should be noted that telomerase activity is not confined to malignant cells for it is also found in normal highly regenerative tissues such as intestinal crypt cells and haematopoietic precursors (Kyo et al 1999). Several components of telomerase have been identified including the telomerase RNA component (hTR), telomerase catalytic subunit gene (hTERT) and telomerase associated protein (TP1/TLP1). Telomerase activity is usually assessed by the telomeric repeat amplification protocol (TRAP) assay whilst hTR, hTERT and TP can be studied using the reverse-transcriptase polymerase chain reaction (RT–PCR), in situ hybridisation (ISH) and the RNase-protection assay.

Ovary

By TRAP assay there is a high prevalence of telomerase activity in borderline tumours and invasive carcinomas of the ovary but high activity is only seen in invasive tumour (Datar et al 1999). Assaying for telomerase has proved to be a more sensitive tool for detecting cancer cells in the peritoneal fluid of patients with ovarian carcinoma than has cytology (Duggan et al 1998).

Endometrium

Telomerase activity has been detected in normal endometrium during the proliferative phase of the cycle with activity mainly being localised to the glands (Brien et al 1997; Saito et al 1997; Shroyer et al 1997; Tanaka et al 1998; Kyo et al 1999). Activity has also been detected in all endometrial hyperplasias and in most endometrial carcinomas. Telomerase activity is low in the endometrium of pregnant and normal post-menopausal women and in the endometrium exposed to anti-oestrogen drugs. Detection of telomerase activity in postmenopausal endometrium reflects abnormal proliferative activity and can provide a novel marker for early endometrial cancer (Brien et al 1997; Saito et al 1997; Shroyer et al 1997; Tanaka et al 1998; Oshita et al 2000). In endometrial carcinomas the detection of telomerase activity is not associated with architectural grade, depth of myometrial invasion, stage or ploidy (Brien et al 1997; Shroyer et al 1997).

Cervix

A number of studies have demonstrated a relationship between telomerase activity in cervical neoplasia with increasing telomerase activation paralleling increasingly advanced histological changes (Anderson et al 1997; Pao et al 1997; Iwasaka et al 1998; Kyo et al 1998; Nakano et al 1998; Shroyer et al 1998; Snijders et al 1998; Takakura et al 1998; Wisman et al 1998; Riethdorf et al 2001): there have, however, been conflicting reports about an association between telomerase activation and high-risk HPV infection (Snijders et al 1998; Yashima et al 1998). Advanced cervical cancers have a wider range of variation of telomeric restriction fragment length than do early lesions (Zhang et al 1999) but there is no relationship between telomerase activity and any other clinical or pathological parameters.

Telomerase activity has also been reported in normal cervical tissue and in cases of reactive atypia (Pao et al 1997) and it is still unsettled whether assessment of telomerase activity in cervical smears is useful in primary screening for cervical neoplasia. Some have found it to be of value (Kyo et al 1997; Takakura et al 1998; Zheng et al 2000; Reddy et al 2001) but others have found such assessment to have a low sensitivity for high-grade CIN and/or invasive carcinoma (Wisman et al 1998).

It is important to note that telomerase activity in cervical tissue is inhibited by 5% acetic acid. Thus applying acetic acid prior to colposcopically directed biopsy of tissue to be submitted for telomerase activity should be avoided (ChangChien et al 1998).

Trophoblastic disease

The presence of telomerase activity in hydatidiform moles has been found to be associated with the development of persistent trophoblastic disease, particularly those cases which progress to choriocarcinoma (Bae & Kim 1999; Cheung et al 1999b).

STUDIES OF CLONALITY

The clonality of carcinomas may be assessed by analysing chromosome X inactivation patterns, restriction length polymorphism (RFLP) and genetic deletions or mutations (Enomoto et al 1994; Sawada et al 1994): the X

chromosome linked phosphoglycerokinase gene and androgen receptor (AR) gene are frequently studied for this purpose. Small DNA samples prepared from either frozen or paraffin sections of tumours may be used for PCR-based techniques.

Ovary and peritoneum

The interrelationships and origin of disseminated serous carcinoma involving the ovary and peritoneum may not be clear from histological examination. The monoclonal nature of such cases has, however, been demonstrated by studying the patterns of LOH, *tp53* mutations and X chromosome inactivation (Jacobs et al 1992; Li et al 1993b; Kupryjanczyk et al 1996), this strongly suggesting that the peritoneal lesions are metastases from the ovarian tumour. By contrast, a multifocal origin of at least some cases of papillary serous carcinoma of the peritoneum has been observed in a study analysing the AR gene locus for patterns of LOH and X chromosome inactivation (Schorge et al 1998). Similarly, bilateral ovarian serous borderline tumours or extraovarian lesions in association with serous borderline tumours are found to be multifocal in origin (Lu et al 1998). In high-stage ovarian papillary serous borderline tumours a study by Gu et al (2001) demonstrated different non-random inactivation patterns of the X chromosome in most peritoneal and ovarian tumours from the same patient, again suggesting independent origins of these tumours.

Endometriotic cysts of the ovary have been demonstrated to be monoclonal in a number of studies (Nilbert et al 1995; Jimbo et al 1997; Tamura et al 1998; Yano et al 1999). This may mean that such cysts are in reality endometrioid cystadenomas but monoclonality does not necessarily equate with neoplasia: thus in the case of endometriosis a focus of the disease may derive from implantation of a single endometrial gland which would be physiologically monoclonal because all of its cells were derived from a single stem cell. Ovarian carcinomas can arise in ovarian endometriosis and by studying the LOH patterns on 12 chromosome arms, X inactivation and *tp53* mutation, common genetic abnormalities have been detected in most cases of ovarian carcinoma and associated endometriosis, this indicating their common lineage (Jiang et al 1998).

Endometrium

Using a PCR assay for non-random X chromosome inactivation, endometrial carcinomas, endometrial polyps and atypical hyperplasia of the endometrium were found to be monoclonal whilst normal and non-ovulatory endometrium were polyclonal (Mutter et al 1995; Jovanovic et al 1996; Mutter et al 2000a): it is also known that the vast majority of simple and complex hyperplasias of the endometrium are polyclonal (Inoue 2001). Clonality can be determined in small endometrial biopsies and may thus be of value in the diagnosis of atypical hyperplasia or adenocarcinoma in such samples (Esteller et al 1997).

A difficult situation arises when uterine papillary serous carcinoma of the endometrium is showing no myometrial invasion but is nevertheless associated with extensive extrauterine disease: clonal studies of four such cases were based on *tp53* gene analysis and showed, in each case, identical mutational patterns in the non-myoinvasive endometrial tumour and the extrauterine lesions, this indicating that the latter were metastases (Baergen et al 2001).

Cervix and vulva

The monoclonality of invasive cervical carcinomas has been demonstrated in microdissected tissues by PCR-based analysis of X chromosome inactivation of the AR gene (Guo et al 1998). The finding that early invasive carcinoma is monoclonal supports the view that monoclonality is not a late event due to clonal competition or selection. Nearly all cases of high-grade CIN have been found to be monoclonal whilst a relatively small proportion of cases of low-grade CIN are monoclonal (Park et al 1996; Enomoto et al 1997; Chuaqui et al 2001): X chromosomal inactivation patterns suggests that CIN develops into a monoclonal lesion during progression from CIN1 to CIN3. In view of these findings it is not suprising that there is a clear association between infection with high-risk types of HPV and monoclonality (Park et al 1996). In cases of mutifocal CIN the pattern of X chromosome inactivation is the same in most of the lesions suggesting that they were derived from a single cell with intraepithelial extension within the cervical mucosa (Enomoto et al 1997). A local field effect of genomic instability that progressively affects the clonal evolution of CIN to invasive cancer has been proposed (Chu et al 1999).

Most cases of VIN are monoclonal and in one study some cases of vulvar hyperplasia and lichen sclerosus were also found to be monoclonal, suggesting that clonal expansion may evolve in presumed pre-neoplastic precursors before the development of morphological atypia in the vulvar epithelium (Tate et al 1997). However, in another study whilst all invasive carcinomas were monoclonal, hyperplastic and histologically normal squamous epithelium were polyclonal, implying that squamous hyperplasia might not serve as a direct precursor of invasive carcinoma (Kim et al 1996).

Synchronous or metachronous tumours and mixed neoplasms

Simultaneous involvement of the endometrium and ovary by a carcinoma, usually an endometrioid adenocarcinoma, may be considered either as a single primary lesion with a metastasis or as two independent synchronous primary neoplasms. Genetic studies may prove helpful in resolving such cases (Matias-Guiu et al 2002). Fujita et al (1996) studied five such cases and found identical patterns of X chromosome inactivation, mutations in the *k-ras* oncogene, mutations and allelic loss of the *tp53* gene in three cases, indicating that they were primary tumours with a metastasis, whilst in the other two cases the patterns of X chromosome inactivation clearly demonstrated the presence of independent primary neoplasms. Shenson et al (1995) and Emmert-Buck et al (1997) also used genetic techniques to demonstrate a lack of shared genetic alterations in synchronously occurring endometrial and ovarian endometrioid tumours, indicating independent pathways for these tumours in their cases.

Coexisting mucinous tumours of the appendix and ovary pose a similar problem. Cuatrecasas et al (1996) analysed the pattern of *K-ras* mutations in such tumours and found them to arise from the same clone, thus indicating that one originated from the other. Chuaqui et al (1996) compared patterns of LOH on chromosomes 17q and 3p in synchronous appendicular and ovarian mucinous neoplasms and found identical patterns in each of the two tumours in three cases and quite different patterns in two further cases, this clearly allowing for a distinction between two independent primary neoplasms and a primary tumour with a metastasis.

Kushima et al (2001) recently studied three cases of cervical CIN and two of invasive squamous cell carcinoma of the cervix, all of which were associated with either intraepithelial or invasive squamous neoplasia in the endometrium, Fallopian tube or ovary. LOH analyses with a panel of microsatellite markers revealed a monoclonal process in four of these cases.

In a study of gynaecological carcinosarcomas Fujii et al (2000), after microdissection and isolation of the carcinomatous and sarcomatous components, found shared allelic losses between the two malignant tissues in 41 microsatellite markers, this being strongly supportive of a monoclonal origin for these neoplasms. Similarly, clonal loss of wild type *BRCA2* allele and identical *tp53* mutations were evident in both carcinomatous and sarcomatous components of an ovarian carcinosarcoma suggesting that both histological elements of this tumour arose from the same progenitor cell (Sonoda et al 2000).

IN SITU HYBRIDISATION

Probes to repetitive sequences of a particular chromosome allow numerical and structural chromosome aberrations to be detected in non-mitotic cells. The technique has been particularly applied to the detection of monosomies and trisomies in material from miscarriages (van Lijnschoten et al 1994; Mark et al 1997) and has been used for distinguishing between partial hydatidiform moles, complete hydatidiform moles and hydropic miscarriages (van de Kaa et al 1991). However, chromosomal studies have not been found to have any value in predicting the prognosis of hydatidiform moles (Cheung et al 1994b; van de Kaa et al 1997).

STUDY OF CHROMOSOMAL IMBALANCES BY COMPARATIVE GENOMIC HYBRIDISATION

Comparative genomic hybridisation (CGH) allows for the detection of chromosomal imbalances in a comprehensive fashion in so far as entire genomes are examined and regions of DNA gain or loss identified. It can effectively identify chromosomal alterations as targets for the characterisation of pathogenetically relevant genes, can analyse chromosomal imbalances during tumour progression and can detect prognostic markers.

Ovarian tumours

Ovarian carcinomas and borderline tumours frequently display numerous consistent chromosomal imbalances, including gains in 8q, 20q and 3q and loss in 5q, 9q and 17q (Sonoda et al 1997a; Blegen et al 2000; Suehiro et al 2000a) (Fig. 49.1). Some changes, such as underrepresentation of 17p and over-representation of 3q are observed only in advanced stage carcinomas indicating that these are late events in tumour progression. Some of these chromosomal alterations appear to be of prognostic value. Thus, in ovarian clear cell adenocarcinomas two

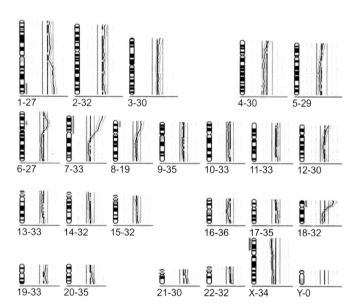

Fig. 49.1 CGH aberrations detected in a case of ovarian mucinous borderline tumour. The central black graph bar represents a ratio of 1.0, i.e. equal binding of the tumour and reference DNA. On the left and right sides of this are the loss (0.75) and gain (1.25) threshold bars, respectively. Overlying the graph are the mean ratios and the 95% confidence intervals from analysis of more than 20 metaphase spreads. Areas of increased copy number are represented on the right of the chromosome ideogram, and areas of decreased copy number are represented on the left. The CGH profile of this specimen suggests copy gains of 1q32.1-qter, 6p21.1–p22.1, 7p, 8p21.1-pter, 18p and loss of Xp.

subtypes can be found, one associated with an increase in copy numbers of 8q and the other with increases in copy numbers of 17q and 20q: there appears to be overrepresentation of the 8q subset in those cases that did well whilst the 17q and 20q subset occurred more frequently in cases with a poor prognosis (Suehiro et al 2000a). Development of acquired resistance to chemotherapy has been found to be associated with substantial genomic instability (Waseniu et al 1998).

Comparative genomic hybridisation of ovarian borderline tumours has shown that chromosomal imbalances are present in less than 50% (Sonoda et al 1997a; Blegen et al 2000; Wolf et al 2000): the chromosomal abnormalities found are of the same nature and order as those in early invasive carcinomas.

Endometrial carcinomas and hyperplasia

Chromosome changes, most commonly gains of 1p, 1q and 8q, are detectable in many endometrial carcinomas, there being a correlation between tumour stage and grade and the degree of genomic imbalance (Sonoda et al 1997b; Suzuki et al 1997). It is of interest from a pathogenetic point of view that genomic imbalances detected by CGH were not observed in tumours showing microsatellite instability (Sonoda et al 1997b). The average number of genetic aberrations was significantly greater in the tumours of non-surviving patients than in those from disease-free patients (Suehiro et al 2000b).

The incidence of aberrant CGH profiles in endometrial hyperplasia tends to parallel the degree of cytological atypia (Kiechle et al 2000). The most frequent imbalances are 1p, 16p, and 20q under-representations and 4q over-representation, these being quite different to those seen in endometrial adenocarcinoma. This suggests that transition to an invasive carcinoma proceeds through the accumulation of a series of genetic alterations.

Cervical neoplasia

Recurrent chromosome aberrations have been demonstrated in both invasive cervical squamous carcinoma and high-grade CIN, there being a consistent chromosome gain at 3q and deletions at 3p (Kirchoff et al 1999; Hidalgo et al 2000). Interestingly, purely HPV 18 positive carcinomas are associated with a high incidence of imbalances at specific loci coinciding with known HPV integration sites suggesting that the development and progression of these alterations is triggered by integration of the viral DNA into the host genome (Hidalgo et al 2000).

Miscellaneous tumours

The chromosomal anomalies found in uterine leiomyomas and leiomyosarcomas were found to be quite different, arguing against there being a benign–malignant continuum (Levy et al 2000).

Consistent chromosomal imbalances have been found in choriocarcinomas, these being amplification of 7q21–q31 and loss of 8p12–p21 (Ahmed et al 2000): by contrast, all hydatidiform moles have normal CGH profiles.

ARRAYS

Comparative hybridization of cDNA arrays is a powerful tool for the measurement of expression of large numbers of genes among different tissues (Fig. 49.2). Differential gene expression has been demonstrated in carcinomas of the cervix (Shim et al 1998), ovary (Schummer et al 1999; Welsh et al 2001) and endometrium (Smid-Koopman et al 2000) and also in gestational trophoblastic disease (Vegh et al 1999) as compared to normal tissues. Array study of ovarian tumours has also demonstrated significant differences in gene expression between benign and malignant serous ovarian tumours as well as in malignant tumours at different stages and of differing histological grade (Tapper et al 2001).

The applications of array technology, for the pathologist, are only just beginning to emerge. The immediately obvious advantages of the technique are that it will allow for the genetic profiling of tumour subtypes and the iden-

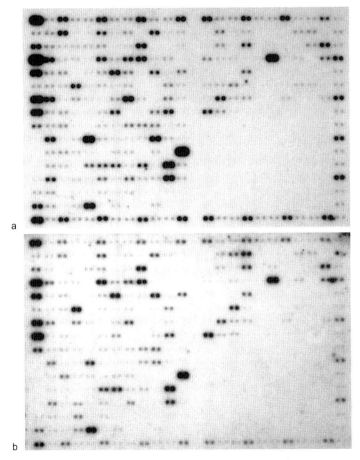

a

b

Fig. 49.2 Gene expression profiling of human cervical cancer **(a)** and normal cervical tissue **(b)** using cDNA expression array. (Courtesy of Professor H Y S Ngan.)

tification of genes associated with tumour progression or resistance to chemotherapy.

STUDY OF IMPRINTED GENES

Genomic imprinting is defined as a gamete-specific modification causing differential expression of two alleles of a gene in somatic cells and is becoming increasingly recognised as playing an important rôle in many diseases. Both genetic and epigenetic targets are associated with imprinted gene expression (Li et al 1993a).

Imprinted genes can be involved in carcinogenesis in several ways. LOH at an imprinted region may result in the deletion of the only functional copy of the gene. On the other hand, loss of imprinting of an imprinted gene that promotes cell growth may allow gene expression to be inappropriately increased. Mutational inactivation of an imprinting centre might result in aberrant expression of several imprinted oncogenes and tumour suppressor genes present in an imprinted chromosomal region. Inactivation of an imprinted gene by allelic hypermethylation is also an important mechanism.

The imprinted genes most commonly studied include the insulin-like growth factor-2 gene (*IGF2*) and the *H19* gene. *IGF2* is expressed by the paternal allele and *H19* by the maternal allele and both genes are located close to each other on chromosome 11p15.5 in a region subject to LOH. Studies of imprinted genes in ovarian cancer have yielded variable results. One early study demonstrated monoallelic expression of the *IGF2* gene in both normal ovaries and in ovarian carcinoma suggesting that any increased *IGF2* expression in ovarian cancer may be achieved by a mechanism other than loss of imprinting (Yun et al 1996). Subsequently, LOH of *H19* and *IGF2* was found to be different in different types of ovarian epithelial tumours suggesting that alteration of *H19* and *IGF2* imprinting plays differing rôles in carcinogenesis and in tumour progression (Kim et al 1998). Chen et al (2000) reported that LOH of both *IGF2* and *H19* genes was associated with advanced ovarian cancer whilst loss of imprinting of these genes appeared to play a rôle in the early development of ovarian malignant disease.

Ovarian teratomas also demonstrate variable patterns of loss of imprinting involving *H19*, *IGF2* and *SNRPN* (Miura et al 1999; Ross et al 1999). This may indicate differences in the timing of tumorigenesis in germ cells and that imprinting is a progressively organised process involving mechanistically linked genes.

A high incidence of LOH and abnormal imprinting of *H19* and *IGF2* genes has been demonstrated in cervical carcinomas (Douc-Rasy et al 1996). The data suggest that *H19* and *IGF2* genes, via deletions and/or abnormal imprinting, could play a crucial rôle in cervical carcinogenesis.

There is loss of imprinting of *H19* in the androgenetic tissue of complete hydatidiform moles and it has been suggested that this may be related to their malignant potential (Ariel et al 1994; Walsh et al 1995). On the other hand, a low expression of *IGF2* and a high expression of *H19* is frequently found in choriocarcinomas (Arima et al 1997).

DETECTION AND TYPING OF HPV

Several techniques are now available for the detection and typing of HPV. HPV DNA techniques based on signal amplification are standardised, commercially available and can detect several high-risk HPVs at low viral burden (Cope et al 1997). HPV DNA typing by in situ hybridisation in cervical smears (Autillo-Touati et al 1998) or paraffin embedded tissues are also available. The hybrid capture (HC) assays, especially the new generation, are now being widely used (Cope et al 1997; Poljak et al 1999). The current HC-II has an expanded number of high-risk HPV types and a lower threshold for HPV, giving it a level of sensitivity similar to that of PCR (Peyton 1998).

The techniques for the detection and typing of HPV are therefore well established. The clinical value of the use of these techniques in primary screening, triage and follow-up are, however, highly controversial and outside the scope of this chapter.

STUDIES OF CELL PROLIFERATION AND OF APOPTOTIC MARKERS

Cell accumulation in tumours is determined by the balance of cell proliferation and cell loss due to necrosis and apoptosis. Besides estimation of mitotic and apoptotic figures in haematoxylin and eosin stained histological sections other measures have been used to assess the state of cellular proliferation (Quinn & Wright 1992; Cheung 1997) and cell loss related to apoptosis (Heatley 1995; Mundle et al 1995) in tissues. In studying cell proliferation the use is made of antigens which are specifically expressed by proliferating cells and which can be demonstrated immunocytochemically with monoclonal antibodies. Proliferating cell nuclear antigen (PCNA), which is expressed during the G1 and early S phases of the cycle and Ki-67, which is recognised by the antibody MIB-1, and is expressed during the G2 and mitotic phases of the cycle are the most widely studied proliferation antigens, though it is thought that Ki-67 gives a more reliable indication of the growth fraction of a tumour. Topoisomerase II alpha (TopoIIa), which can be demonstrated by immunocytochemistry, is a nuclear protein which plays a rôle in the separation of chromosomes and DNA replication and can therefore also be used as a marker for cell proliferation.

Apoptotic cells are identified by the in situ identification of DNA strand breaks or broken ends by nick translation or end labelling (TUNEL): it should be noted that although this technique is widely employed it has been subject to criticism on the grounds of possible nonspecific reactivity with necrotic and inflammatory cells (Burton & Wells 1999). In addition the apoptosis regulatory genes, the bcl-2 family, can be studied: this family contains pro-apoptotic members, such as Bax, and anti-apoptotic genes, such as bcl-2.

STUDIES OF CELL PROLIFERATION

Ovarian neoplasms

Studies of PCNA expression in ovarian carcinoma have yielded conflicting results, one study finding PCNA staining to be an independent indicator of an adverse prognosis (Schonborn et al 1996) and two finding it to be of no prognostic value at all (Guo et al 1993). The Ki-67 index is, unsurprisingly, higher in ovarian cystadenocarcinomas than in cystadenomas or tumours of borderline malignancy, is highest in undifferentiated carcinomas, correlates with histological grade (Garzetti et al 1995a; Kuwashima et al 1995) and increases in recurrent carcinoma when compared to the primary tumour (Geisler et al 1995). There is a good correlation between TopoIIa and Ki-67 indices and TopIIa also correlates with histological grade, though not with histological type (Tanoguchi et al 1998; Costa et al 2000). There has been a significant inverse relationship between the proliferative index, as assessed by MIB-1 immunostaining of Ki-67, and survival in most studies (Kerns et al 1994; Garzetti et al 1995a; Layfield et al 1997; Viale et al 1997; Anttila et al 1998; Geisler et al 1998a) though de Nictolas et al (1996) were unable to confirm that the Ki-67 index was an independent prognostic variable in serous carcinomas. TopoIIa expression is also inversely related to patient survival (Costa et al 2000).

In primary granulosa cell tumours a wide spectrum of proliferative activity has been demonstrated and the Ki-67 correlates only weakly with a disease-free course: however, in recurrent tumours the Ki-67 index was higher and correlated with *p53* immunoreactivity (Costa et al 1996).

Tumours of the uterine body

Whether assessment of cell proliferation is helpful in distinguishing endometrial carcinoma from hyperplasia is controversial though proliferation indices tend to be higher in carcinoma than in hyperplasia (Mora et al 1999): possibly the apoptotic index/proliferation index ratio may serve as a better indicator of potential progression (Ioffe et al 1998).

Endometrial carcinomas show, perhaps as would be expected, Ki-67 indices that generally correlate with other morphological prognostic factors: thus a low Ki-67 index is found in well-differentiated endometrioid carcinomas and those with low-grade squamous differentiation whilst a high Ki-67 index is found in poorly differentiated endometrioid carcinomas, those showing high-grade squamous differentiation and those with a serous papillary or clear cell histology (Lax et al 1998a,b). Ki-67 expression has been identified as a prognostic factor for recurrence and survival in some studies (Geisler et al 1996, 1999; Salvesen et al 1998) as has immunostaining for PCNA (Garzetti et al 1996a,b): however, two studies have found staining for neither PCNA nor Ki-67 to be of any prognostic value in endometrial neoplasms (Hamel et al 1996; Nordstrom et al 1996b).

Ki-67 antigen expression was found at higher levels in the highly malignant carcinosarcomas of the uterus than in the less aggressive adenosarcomas and a high Ki-67 index correlated with decreased survival in patients with carcinosarcomas (Swisher et al 1996).

Neoplasia of the cervix and vulva

A positive correlation between histopathological grading in cervical neoplasia and the proliferation index has been noted in several studies (Mittal et al 1993; Shurbaji et al 1993; McCluggage et al 1994, 1998; Raju 1994; Amortegui et al 1995; Isaacson et al 1996; Resnick et al 1996; Dellas et al 1997; ter Harmsel et al 1997). In normal cervical squamous epithelium PCNA and Ki-67 are expressed only in the basal and parabasal layers but in CIN expression extends to the upper levels of the epithelium or even throughout its full thickness: the degree of proliferation parallels the grade of the CIN. There is little or no proliferative activity in atrophic cervical epithelium and staining with MIB-1 is therefore useful in distinguishing intraepithelial neoplasia from atrophy in both cervical biopsies and smears (Mittal et al 1999; Bulten 2000): similarly MIB-1 differentiates between cervical adenocarcinoma and benign glandular lesions of the cervix (Cina et al 1997).

There has been some disagreement about the value of proliferation indices as prognostic markers in invasive squamous carcinoma of the cervix. One study of the PCNA index found it to be of considerable import (Oka et al 1992) whilst another was unable to show that this index was of any prognostic value (Al Nafussi et al 1993). In one study of stage I tumours there was a correlation between the Ki-67 index and tumour size, presence of lymphatic spread and disease-free interval (Garzetti et al 1995a): this same group suggested that the more aggressive behaviour of cervical carcinomas in women below the age of 40 was related to the high Ki-67 indices found in cervical carcinomas in this age group (Garzetti et al 1997). Others have, however, found that the Ki-67 index did not, in itself, have any prognostic value (Cole et al 1992; Levine et al 1995; Oka et al 1996). Oka & Arai (1996) could not find any relationship between the Ki-67 index and the response of cervical carcinomas to radiotherapy but Suzuki et al (2000) reported that tumours with a high Ki-67 index were more radiosensitive than those with lower indices and were associated with a better survival rate.

In the normal vulvar epithelium staining for PCNA and Ki-67 is confined to the basal and parabasal layers and, as with CIN, there is an extension of staining into the upper layers of the epithelium in VIN (van Hoeven & Kovatich 1996). In a study of invasive squamous cell carcinomas of the vulva the percentage of cells staining positively for Ki-67 was not of prognostic value but the survival time for patients with tumours showing a diffuse pattern of Ki-67 labelling was shorter than for those whose neoplasms had a focal pattern of staining (Hendricks et al 1994).

Gestational trophoblastic disease

PCNA and Ki-67 expression in hydatidiform moles is seen predominantly in villous cytotrophoblast (Cheung et al 1993, 1994c; Suresh et al 1993; Cheville & Robinson 1996; Schammel & Bocklage 1996). Most studies have agreed that analyses of PCNA and Ki-67 indices does not allow for a distinction to be made between hydatidiform moles and hydropic miscarriages (Cheung et al 1993; Cheville & Robinson 1996) (Fig. 49.3) but Schammel et al (1996) reported that the Ki-67 index, though not the PCNA index, was significantly higher in moles than in hydropic miscarriages. Neither the PCNA nor the Ki-67 index has been found to be of any value in predicting possible progression of hydatidiform moles to persistent trophoblastic disease (Cheung et al 1994c; Cheville & Robinson 1996; Jeffers et al 1996).

STUDIES OF APOPTOSIS

Ovarian neoplasms

Apoptotic activity, as assessed by the TUNEL technique, is low in normal ovarian surface epithelium and in benign ovarian tumours but is increased in borderline and malignant neoplasms, with the highest apoptotic index being

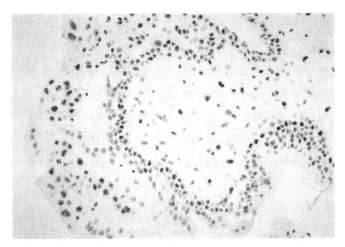

Fig. 49.3 Immunoreactivity for Ki-67 is confined to the nuclei of the cytotrophoblast of a hydatidiform mole.

found in grade III carcinomas (Diebold et al 1996b; Chan et al 2000). Bcl-2 positivity is present in 54–80% of ovarian carcinomas but expression of this gene is stronger in benign and borderline tumours than in malignant neoplasms (Henriksen et al 1995; Diebold et al 1996b; Herod et al 1996; Chan et al 2000). Expression of Bax is increased in ovarian carcinoma above the levels found in normal ovaries and in benign ovarian neoplasms (Marone et al 1998; Wehrli et al 1998; Witty et al 1998). There have been conflicting findings as to the prognostic significance of bcl-2 expression in ovarian carcinomas, some finding bcl-2 expression to be a strong independent factor indicating a relatively good prognosis (Henriksen et al 1995; Herod et al 1996) whilst others were unable to demonstrate any correlation between survival and bcl-2 expression (Diebold et al 1996b).

Cytotoxic chemotherapeutic drugs act, in part at least, by inducing apoptosis but the rôle of the apoptotic index as an assay of chemotherapeutic effectiveness is uncertain (Burton & Wells 1999). It has been suggested that expression of bcl-2 in ovarian carcinomas is a predictor of a poor response to chemotherapy (Mano et al 1999) but Beale et al (2000) found that bcl-2 expression correlated with a sensitivity to platinum drugs.

Endometrial carcinoma

Ioffe et al (1998) showed that the apoptotic index in endometrial adenocarcinoma was three-fold greater than that in normal proliferative endometrium whilst Heatley (1997) found that the less well differentiated the endometrial carcinoma the higher was the apoptotic index. Expression of bcl-2 is increased in simple endometrial hyperplasia, but is weaker in atypical hyperplasia and further reduced in endometrial carcinoma (Chieng et al 1996; Henderson et al 1996; Nakamura et al 1997; Sakuragi et al 1998; Mora et al 1999). Bcl-2 expression is more common in endometrioid than in non-endometrioid adenocarcinomas of the endometrium and is inversely correlated with depth of invasion, histological grade and FIGO stage (Yamauchi et al 1996; Taskin et al 1997; Geisler et al 1998b; Athanassiadou et al 1999; Morsi et al 2000).

Cervical neoplasia

The apoptotic index in a spectrum of CIN and invasive squamous cell carcinoma was, as assessed with the TUNEL technique, found to increase with histological grade (Resnick et al 1996; Shoji et al 1996) though Arends (2000) stated that there was a general pattern of decreasing frequency of apoptosis in the CIN–carcinoma sequence. There is, however, general agreement that Bcl-2 expression increases with progression of CIN through to invasive carcinoma (ter Harmsel et al 1996; Dellas et al 1997; Arends 2000) whilst the expression of Bax decreases (Arends 2000).

Studies of the prognostic significance of apoptosis in cervical carcinoma have yielded somewhat conflicting results; thus, Sheridan et al (1999) found that a high apoptotic index, especially when associated with a low proliferative index, was indicative of a good prognosis in cervical adenocarcinoma whilst Liu et al (2001) found, in a heterogenous group of cervical carcinomas, that low apoptotic activity was an index of improved survival. Immunohistochemical expression of Bcl-2 was found to correlate with tumour stage and with the presence of vascular/lymphatic permeation by Tjalma et al (1998). Harima et al (1998) found that, whilst neither Bax nor Bcl-2 protein expression prior to radiotherapy correlated with response or survival, post-radiotherapy expression of these proteins was of prognostic significance. Thus, after radiotherapy Bax-positive tumours were associated with a better prognosis than Bax-negative tumours and Bcl-2-positive tumours had a worse prognosis than Bcl-2-negative tumours.

Gestational trophoblastic disease

Using the TUNEL technique Wong et al (1999a) showed that the apoptotic index in hydatidiform moles was inversely correlated with Bcl-2 expression but did not correlate in any way with Bax expression: the apoptotic index of moles that did not progress to persistent trophoblastic disease was statistically higher than in those which did progress to the stage of requiring chemotherapy. Another recent study using another apoptotic marker, the M30 CytoDeath antibody, also came to the conclusion that apoptotic activity was a significant prognostic marker for the clinical progress of hydatidiform moles (Chiu et al 2001).

DETERMINATION OF TUMOUR PLOIDY

INTRODUCTION

Ploidy is usually assessed by flow cytometry, a technique that can also be used to measure the number of cells in the S phase of the mitotic cycle. This latter measurement is, however, best considered under the heading of 'proliferation indices' and only the use of flow cytometry for ploidy determination will be considered here. Ploidy can also be evaluated by the currently less commonly used technique of static image cytometry in which the DNA content of Feulgen-stained nuclei in histological sections or touch preparations is measured via an image analysis system. Although there is a good correlation between ploidy results obtained from flow and static image cytometry (Bauer et al 1990; Kaern et al 1992a), the static image technique allows for the identification of small subpopulations of aneuploid tumour cells that may be missed on flow cytometry; static cytometry also has the advantage that tissue morphology is retained. It is possible that static digital image cytometry will be more widely utilised in the future but most reported studies of ploidy in gynaecological tumours have been based upon flow cytometric data.

Flow cytometry is a relatively simple and rapid technique for the measurement of cellular DNA content which can be used on both fresh and archival tissue and allows for tumours to be classed, in general terms, as either diploid or aneuploid. In essence, either cells are disassociated from tumours by mechanical or enzymatic techniques or recovered from paraffin blocks, stained with a fluorochrome dye that binds specifically and stoichiometrically with nucleic acids and then passed through a flow cytometer in a liquid suspension medium as a laminar flow jet. The flow cytometer measures and records fluorescence and light scatter in the cells and the fluorescence of the stained cells is converted into a digital electronic signal: the results are shown as a histogram in which the number of stained cells is plotted as a function of the intensity of the fluorescence. If the main peak of the DNA histogram centres around the 2C region and the overall DNA distribution is comparable to that of normal somatic cells the tumour is classified as diploid. Populations of cells with a DNA content dissimilar to that of normal cells are classed as aneuploid and these may be hypodiploid, hyperdiploid or tetraploid (van Dam et al 1992). The DNA index (DI) is calculated by dividing the modal DNA content of the tumour cells in G0/G1 by the modal DNA content of normal cells in the G0/G1 phases of the mitotic cycle: diploid cells will therefore have a DI of 1 whilst aneuploid cells will have a DI of less than 1, more than 1 or, if tetraploid, 2.

The technique is not, however, without its pitfalls and difficulties and can detect DNA aneuploidy only if a significant proportion of the tumour cells have lost or duplicated several chromosomes (van Dam et al 1992; van Dam 1995). Other variables that have to be taken into consideration are the method of extraction and staining of the nuclei, delays in tissue fixation, intra- and interlaboratory variability, the minimum number and proportion of tumour cells analyzed, the choice of the reference cell population, the programme for debris correction and, very importantly, tumour heterogeneity (Koss et al 1989; McCarthy & Fetterhoff 1989; Heiden et al 1990; Arbor et al 1992; Robinson 1992; Coon et al 1994; van Dam 1995; Rosenberg et al 1997; Tirindelli-Danesi et al 1997). Furthermore, the interpretation of DNA histograms is not always straightforward for there is a grey area between DNA diploidy and DNA aneuploidy and it can be difficult to define what constitutes a true diploid histogram and when aneuploidy begins (Koss et al 1989; Werst et al 1991). In studies utilising the DNA index there has been little agreement in defining cut-off values. If care is paid to detail in references, these difficulties can be largely overcome (Elavathil et al 1996; Tirindelli-Danesi et al 1997) but their neglect must be an important factor in the conflicting results that occur with

some frequency in the literature on the value of ploidy determination in gynaecological cancer.

OVARIAN CARCINOMA

About 45% of stage I ovarian carcinomas are aneuploid as are about 75% of stage III–IV tumours (van Dam 1995). Tumour aneuploidy has been clearly demonstrated in many studies to be an independent adverse prognostic factor in both early and late stage ovarian epithelial cancer (Friedlander et al 1984, 1988; Baak et al 1987; Rodenberg et al 1987; Iversen 1988; Kallioniemi et al 1988; Klemi et al 1989; Volm et al 1989; Barnabei et al 1990; Khoo et al 1990, 1993; Jakobsen et al 1991; Vergote et al 1993; Gajewski et al 1994; Kaern et al 1994; Schueler et al 1996; Zanetta et al 1996; Kimball et al 1997; Bakshi et al 1998; Pietrzak & Olszewski 1998; Silvestrini et al 1998; But & Gorisek 2000; Valverde et al 2001) but there has been a significant number of dissenters from this view (Erba et al 1985; Kigawa et al 1993; Scambia et al 1993; Pfisterer et al 1994; Rice et al 1995; Resnik et al 1997; Curling et al 1998; Reles et al 1998; Meyer et al 2001). In general terms tumour aneuploidy correlates with serous or clear cell histology, advanced stage, large tumour bulk, presence of residual tumour and retroperitoneal lymph node metastases (van Dam 1995): DNA ploidy has also correlated with histological grade in some but not all studies (Friedlander et al 1988; Kaern et al 1994; Reles et al 1998) whilst aneuploidy correlates well with *tp53* mutation (Diebold et al 1996a; McManus et al 1996). Ploidy appears to be of particular significance in patients with stage III disease who have been optimally debulked: in these cases the survival rate for those with diploid tumours was four times that of women with aneuploid neoplasms (Khoo et al 1990). It is of interest that, in cases of advanced disease, whilst the peritoneal metastases from an aneuploid primary tumour are usually also aneuploid, the nodal metastases are frequently diploid (Kimball et al 1997). No clear relationship has been demonstrated between ploidy and response to chemotherapy in ovarian carcinoma.

It is difficult to envisage a significant clinical rôle for the use of flow cytometry in cases of advanced ovarian cancer for all patients who have been debulked, optimally or otherwise, will receive chemotherapy irrespective of the ploidy of their tumour.

There is a possible, but as yet far from fully proven, rôle for flow cytometry to play in stage I ovarian carcinoma, particularly as an aid for the selection of those patients who can be safely treated by conservative surgery without adjuvant therapy. In the only study of the significance of ploidy in stage I well-differentiated ovarian carcinomas treated without adjuvant therapy, tumour aneuploidy did not predict recurrent disease but a DI of above 1.4 was associated with a significantly worse 5-year survival rate (Schueler et al 1993).

OVARIAN EPITHELIAL TUMOURS OF BORDERLINE MALIGNANCY

Most (over 90%) ovarian tumours of borderline malignancy are diploid but there has been quite marked disagreement about the prognostic value of flow cytometry and ploidy determination in these neoplasms. Tumour aneuploidy has been found to be a highly significant prognostic indicator of a poor clinical outcome in some studies (Padberg et al 1992a; Kaern et al 1993), of no value in others (Harlow et al 1993; Demirel et al 1996; Kuoppala et al 1996; Sykes et al 1997) and of only equivocal importance in yet others (Lai et al 1996). It is difficult to reconcile these disparate findings especially as in one very large series of cases with long follow-up aneuploidy proved to be *the* most important independent indicator of a poor prognosis (Kaern et al 1993). It has to be borne in mind, however, that these studies did not take into account the now widely accepted view that many apparent high-stage mucinous tumours of borderline malignancy are in reality metastases from an appendicular carcinoma: inclusion of such cases in the 'borderline' category will clearly lead to bias. Further, it is also now widely thought that patients who die from tumours of borderline malignancy do so because of progressive peritoneal disease and that stage I tumours rarely, if ever, cause death. This being so, there seems little point in determining the ploidy of borderline tumours limited to the ovary. In stage III tumours it would be of value to assess the ploidy of the ovarian tumour if its ploidy was always the same as was that of the peritoneal lesions: this is, however, not necessarily the case and diploid ovarian tumours may be associated with aneuploid peritoneal lesions (Padberg et al 1992b). If flow cytometry has any role in assessing prognosis in tumours of borderline malignancy it is therefore logical to suggest that this may lie in assessing the ploidy of the peritoneal lesions in women with stage III disease.

NON-EPITHELIAL TUMOURS OF THE OVARY

The results of flow cytometric studies in sex cord–stromal tumours of the ovary have provided conflicting results; some finding DNA cellular content to be predictive of the clinical behaviour of these neoplasms (Klemi et al 1990; Holland et al 1991) but others being unable to confirm any clear relationship between ploidy and prognosis (Hitchcock et al 1989; Swanson et al 1990; Wabersich et al 1998; Miller et al 2001).

Amongst germ cell tumours, DNA ploidy does not appear to be a prognostic factor in ovarian dysgerminomas (Oud et al 1988) whilst immature teratomas in a paediatric population are, irrespective of grade, diploid (Baker et al 1998); yolk sac tumours, by contrast, are aneuploid and combined immature teratomas/yolk sac tumours show a diploid teratomatous component and an aneuploid yolk sac component (Baker et al 1998).

It is of considerable interest, when considering the significance of aneuploidy in ovarian tumours, that one of the most aggressive of all ovarian neoplasms, the small cell carcinoma with hypercalcaemia, is almost invariably diploid (Eichhorn et al 1992), there having been only two reported exceptions to this general rule (Fukunaga et al 1997a; Meganck et al 1998). By contrast, neuroendocrine ovarian tumours, whether of small or non-small type, appear to be usually aneuploid (Eichhorn et al 1996; Fukunaga et al 1997b).

CARCINOMA OF FALLOPIAN TUBE

In a study of 53 cases of primary carcinoma of the Fallopian tube all the tumours were found to be aneuploid (Hellstrom et al 1994): clearly, therefore, determination of DNA ploidy plays no role in the assessment of tubal carcinomas.

ENDOMETRIAL ADENOCARCINOMA

About 15% of stage I endometrial carcinomas are aneuploid, the incidence of aneuploidy rising with increasing stage. In endometrial carcinoma it has been repeatedly shown that patients with diploid tumours have a better prognosis than do those with aneuploid tumours and that on multivariate analysis aneuploidy and the mitotic index are independent prognostic indicators (Lindahl et al 1987a,b; Iversen et al 1988; Rosenberg et al 1989; van der Putten et al 1989; Britton et al 1990; Newbury et al 1990; Lindahl & Gulberg 1991; Ambros & Kurman 1992; Dyas et al 1992; Ikeda et al 1993; Melchiorri et al 1993; Sorbe et al 1994; von Minckwitz et al 1994; Braly 1995; Pfisterer et al 1995; Susini et al 1995; Nordstrom et al 1996a; Zaino et al 1998; Larson et al 1999; Susini et al 1999) with aneuploidy being significantly related to an increased risk of nodal metastases, recurrence and disease-related death. There have been only a few dissenting voices from this consensus (Konski et al 1996; Mariani et al 2000; Pasini et al 2000) but these have been sufficiently emphatic to indicate that the last word on this topic may not yet have been spoken. In most studies ploidy has been a stronger prognostic factor than any other tumour-associated variable with the possible exception of positive immunostaining for *p53* (Sorbe & Risberg 1997). In general, though not absolute, terms aneuploid endometrial neoplasms are usually either G3 endometrioid adenocarcinomas, clear cell carcinomas or uterine papillary serous adenocarcinomas, strongly *p53* positive and oestrogen receptor negative (Heinonen et al 1994; Sorbe & Risberg 1997; Zaino et al 1998): it has to be stressed, however, that ploidy appears to be a prognostic factor that is independent of histological type (Zaino et al 1998).

The principal clinical rôle for flow cytometry in endometrial adenocarcinoma is probably in the subset of patients in whom the need for adjuvant therapy after hysterectomy is unclear, i.e. those with grade 1 or 2 node-negative endometrioid carcinomas with inner- or middle-third myometrial invasion (Zaino et al 1998). There appears little justification for the use of flow cytometry in those cases in which there are other clear indications for adjuvant therapy such as deep myometrial involvement or a papillary serous histology.

UTERINE SARCOMAS

Aneuploidy was a highly significant indicator of poor survival for patients with endometrial stromal sarcomas in one series (Nola et al 1996) but was devoid of prognostic significance in another (Nordal et al 1996). In a recent study endometrial stromal sarcomas classed as 'low grade' were all diploid whilst most of those categorised as 'high grade' were aneuploid (Blom et al 1999): perhaps not surprisingly aneuploidy correlated with poor survival but it was also apparent that ploidy estimation played no rôle in identifying those low-grade endometrial stromal sarcomas which were likely to recur or metastasize.

In a study of 11 uterine adenosarcomas, three were found to be aneuploid (Kerner et al 1997): there was no obvious relationship between ploidy and survival. A majority of uterine carcinosarcomas are aneuploid but ploidy does not appear to be an independent prognostic factor for survival (Blom et al 1998a).

Taken overall, aneuploidy is an independent indicator of poor survival in uterine leiomyosarcomas (Blom et al 1998b): however, when considering only those tumours which are stage I and stage II, ploidy does not achieve prognostic significance in a multivariate analysis.

CARCINOMA OF THE CERVIX

A high proportion of invasive cervical neoplasms show DNA aneuploidy (van Dam et al 1992) but attempts to demonstrate that aneuploid carcinomas have a worse prognosis than diploid ones have either proved wholly unsuccessful or have yielded equivocal, and usually not statistically significant, results (Davis et al 1989; Kenter et al 1990; Leminen et al 1990; Ji et al 1991; Strang et al 1991; Jarrell et al 1992; Zanettta et al 1992; Connor et al 1993; Pfisterer et al 1996; Kaspar et al 1997; Magtibay et al 1999; Tsang et al 1999), this applying equally to squamous and glandular carcinomas. Studies of ploidy as a prognostic factor for responsiveness of cervical carcinomas to radiotherapy have yielded contradictory results (Anton et al 1997; Gasinska et al 1999) but it has been claimed that the DNA index, though not ploidy, is a good predictor of response to adjuvant chemotherapy (Lai et al 1997).

CARCINOMA OF THE VAGINA

Squamous cell carcinomas of the vagina are usually aneuploid and flow cytometry does not provide information of any prognostic value.

CARCINOMA OF THE VULVA

In vulvar squamous cell carcinomas tumour ploidy was shown to be one of the most important prognostic factors in one study, even to the extent that patients with aneuploid tumours but without lymph node metastases had a lower five-year survival rate than did those with diploid tumours and lymph node metastases (Kaern et al 1992b). Others have, however, failed to show that ploidy is of any prognostic value in vulvar carcinoma (Ballouk et al 1993; Dolan et al 1993; Drew et al 1996). It is difficult to reconcile these disparate findings but in all these studies vulvar squamous cell carcinoma has been considered as a single entity and it would be of interest to know if the prognostic value of flow cytometry in the classical keratinising type of vulvar squamous cell carcinoma differs from that in carcinomas of basaloid or warty (Bowenoid) type: in a recent study it was found that whilst 83% of HPV-positive vulvar carcinomas (which are usually basaloid or warty) were aneuploid only 59% of HPV-negative carcinomas (which are usually keratinising) were aneuploid (Scurry et al 1999).

GESTATIONAL TROPHOBLASTIC DISEASE

Cytometric determination of ploidy is of considerable value in the recognition of partial hydatidiform moles and in distinguishing between complete and partial moles (Hemming et al 1987; Lage et al 1992; Lage & Popek 1993; Lage & Bagg 1996; Fukunaga et al 1993; Berezowsky et al 1995; Topalovsky et al 1995; Paradinas et al 1996; Gschwendtner et al 1998; Fukunaga 2000) (Fig. 49.4). Some have found that ploidy determination was not of any predictive value in identifying those cases of molar disease likely to progress to, or persist as, persistent trophoblastic disease (Hemming et al 1988; van de Kaa et al 1996): however, in a recent study Fukunaga (2001) found, perhaps rather surprisingly, that aneuploid complete moles were at lesser risk of progression to persistent disease than were diploid moles.

Nearly all placental site trophoblastic tumours are diploid and flow cytometry is of no value in assessing the degree of malignancy in these neoplasms (How et al 1995).

CONCLUSIONS

Despite the many studies of the value of determination of ploidy in gynaecological neoplasms remarkably little of realistic clinical value has emerged. There are currently no grounds for suggesting that ploidy determination has any value in the clinical assessment of carcinoma of the cervix, vulva or Fallopian tube. The independent prognostic value of ploidy determination in ovarian carcinoma has not yet been fully proven and any prognostic niche this technique may eventually come to occupy in these neoplasms is probably confined to the assessment of well-differentiated stage I tumours. Conflicting views have

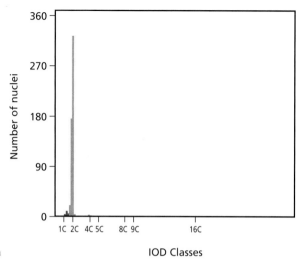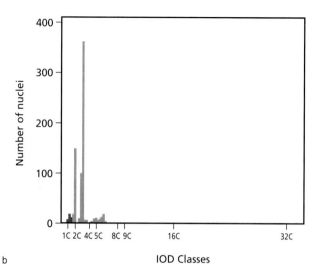

Fig. 49.4 Ploidy determination by digital image analysis in diploid complete (**a**) and triploid partial (**b**) hydatidiform mole. Note the 2C diploid peak only in the complete mole. (Courtesy of Fairfield Imaging.)

been expressed about the significance of ploidy in ovarian tumours of borderline malignancy and in ovarian granulosa cell tumours and in neither group of neoplasms has ploidy determination achieved an agreed rôle in prognostic assessment. Only in endometrial carcinoma has ploidy clearly emerged as an independent indicator of an adverse clinical outcome but even in these neoplasms the practical clinical value of ploidy determination is probably limited to stage I cases where there is some doubt about the necessity for adjuvant therapy.

MORPHOMETRY

INTRODUCTION

In the fourth edition of this book a detailed historical account was given of the application of quantitative techniques to human cells and tissues in general and to gynaecological neoplasia in particular (Baak et al 1995). The application of cytometry in the determination of the ploidy status of tumours has been discussed above and the final section of this chapter concerns itself with the geometric analysis of tissue components (morphometry and stereology). It is not the intention to reiterate here the detail and complexity of the 1995 chapter. Despite persuasive arguments for the introduction of these techniques into routine histopathological practice, seven years on from publication of the last edition, it is fair to say that this has not been realised except in a few laboratories, from which many of the original publications in the field emanate. Nevertheless, there is now a convincing evidence base, particularly in endometrial and ovarian epithelial neoplasia, that such parameters can provide useful prognostic information. Whether the failure of the profession to embrace these techniques more widely is due to misconceptions relating to their technical com-

plexity and the additional requirement of staff and time in a discipline that is under-resourced, or to the realisation that the added value accruing to the individual patient is limited is a matter for conjecture. Advocates of quantitative image analysis would argue that these are quick, inexpensive, reliable and reproducible techniques, which can improve the prognostic accuracy and prowess of the light microscopist.

The emphasis here will be on those areas where there is a strong case for routine application of morphometry which, by virtue of the status of the current literature and experience, means predominantly endometrial hyperplasia and neoplasia, ovarian epithelial neoplasia and, to a lesser extent, cervical neoplasia. Only brief mention will be made of the application of morphometry to vulval pathology. It is not considered that morphometry has made an important contribution to other facets of diagnostic gynaecological pathology. No attempt is made here to assess the relative merits of morphometry over ploidy analysis for individual tumour types; there are many factors that may influence which particular technique or techniques are incorporated into diagnostic practice in an individual laboratory.

VULVA

It has been suggested that the use of morphometry to determine nuclear area and other parameters is effective in identifying the two distinct groups of vulval squamous cell carcinoma (Okon et al 1998).

CERVIX

Image analysis has mostly been applied in the field of cervical cytology, which is beyond the scope of this chapter. Very few studies have addressed cervical intraepithelial or invasive neoplasia and little has emerged of diagnostic or prognostic utility (Syrjanen et al 2001). Studies have focused predominantly on relative tumour volume (Yorukoglu et al 2001) or nuclear volume as an objective means of tumour grading in cervical squamous carcinoma (Sorensen et al 1992). The measurement of density of cancer cell nuclei has proved to be an independent prognostic indicator with increased nuclear density being associated with an unfavourable prognosis (Tosi et al 1992). A recent study has confirmed that quantitative analysis using a semi-automated image analysis system based on nuclear morphology and chromatin texture can be a reliable predictor of survival, recurrence and response (Weyn et al 2000).

Nuclear morphometry, including nuclear area, has also been applied in an attempt to predict response to radiotherapy and/or chemotherapy (Yacoub et al 1994; Poulin et al 1999).

Studies of cervical intraepithelial neoplasia have been few in number (Orille et al 1993). Syntactic structure analysis, which is based on graph theory and provides quantitative data on the spatial distribution of points in two-dimensional space, has been used to evaluate nuclear crowding as a criterion in the diagnosis of cervical intraepithelial neoplasia by an automated machine vision system (Keenan et al 2000). Discriminant analysis of geometric data revealed significant discriminatory variables from which a classification score was derived. The scoring system distinguished between normal and CIN 3 in 98.7% of cases and, interestingly, between koilocytosis and CIN 1 in 76.5% of cases, but only 62.3% of the CIN cases were classified into the correct group, with CIN 2 showing the highest rate of misclassification.

Image analysis has also been combined with immunohistochemistry for Ki-67 and was found to be a useful diagnostic tool to distinguish between different grades of CIN and may indicate an apparently low-grade lesion that has a greater likelihood of progression (Kruse et al 2001). This potentially interesting finding clearly needs further study. Similarly, quantitative image analysis of MIB-1 reactivity has been applied to endocervical lesions to distinguish between neoplastic and non-neoplastic lesions (van Hoeven et al 1997).

ENDOMETRIUM

The value of morphometry (in contrast to ploidy determination) has been the identification by quantitative analysis, of a subset of objectively measured morphometric parameters, which predict the subsequent development of endometrial adenocarcinoma from a pre-existing 'hyperplasia'. Image analysis on haematoxylin and eosin stained sections has allowed the analysis of various architectural and cytological features. These have been weighted in a predictive formula to yield a calculated 'D-score' which when applied to endometrial biopsy or curettage material

predicts the likelihood of there being coexisting carcinoma of progression to carcinoma (Baak et al 1988a; Baak 1995; Dunton et al 1996). A further recent and exciting development has been the demonstration that a number of apparently 'non-atypical hyperplasias' are monoclonal and that computerised morphometry was effective in resolving cases of endometrial hyperplasia into monoclonal and polyclonal subgroups (Mutter et al 2000). An important component of the D-score, the volume percentage stroma, appears to be the most sensitive morphometric discriminant of monoclonal growth. Thus, this architectural feature of putative precancers may prove to be a highly useful discriminant in cases where cytological atypia is equivocal. It implies that endometrial precancer can be identified by architectural criteria alone whereas nuclear atypia is, by conventional histology, an essential criterion of atypical hyperplasia or intraendometrial neoplasia. Whether it is appropriate to equate monoclonality with precancer, which seems to be the fundamental premise on which this work is based, is a moot point.

OVARY

Borderline tumours

Evidence has accrued for a role for morphometry in identifying the small proportion of borderline tumours that have a poor prognosis, by allowing the detection of details which may elude the conventional light microscopist (Burton & Wells 1999). Baak et al (1985) investigated 32 quantitative features in 20 borderline tumours, including mitotic activity index (number of mitoses per 25 high-power fields at × 400 magnification), volume percentage of epithelium, nuclear perimeter, nuclear area, shortest nuclear axis, longest nuclear axis, and nuclear axes ratio. The measurements were performed on areas with the highest cellularity and mitotic count, the greatest atypicality and avoiding areas of necrosis, inflammation, or calcification. Using multivariate analysis, neoplasms with a mitotic activity index greater than 30 and a volume percentage of epithelium greater that 70 were associated with a poor prognosis. Extraovarian extension was not seen in tumours with a volume percentage of epithelium less than 50. The predictive power of morphometric analysis was greater than that of unaided light microscopy.

Ovarian cancer

Early ovarian cancer

In patients with early ovarian carcinoma (FIGO stages I and II) Haapasalo et al (1989, 1990) observed that morphometric parameters are highly reproducible, objective and may have greater prognostic value than the FIGO stage. They found that the volume-corrected mitotic index (the number of mitotic figures in one square millimetre of neoplastic epithelium) was found to have significant prognostic value being, in their hands, the best predictor of prognosis for FIGO stage I tumours. Baak et al (1986) found that the volume percentage of epithelium, standard deviation of the shortest nuclear axis and the mitotic activity index showed strong correlation with tumour grade and prognosis. They suggested that patients with FIGO stage I ovarian cancer fall into three morphometrically determined prognostic groups: 1) mitotic activity index <30 and percentage volume of epithelium <65, 2) mitotic activity index <30 and percentage volume of epithelium >65 and 3) mitotic activity >30. The mitotic activity index was the strongest prognostic factor: the five-year survival rates were 89% (group 1), 71% (group 2) and 52% (group 3).

In a study of 102 patients with FIGO IA, IB and IC ovarian cancer who had not undergone postoperative treatment, Brugghe et al (1998) performed morphometric analysis on the most poorly differentiated areas of the tumours. The strongest prognostic factors for survival were the mean nuclear area and volume-weighted mean nuclear volume. Survival was 100% in patients with a mean nuclear volume smaller than 55.6 mm², whereas 20% of patients with a mean nuclear volume greater than 55.6 mm² died of their disease.

In contrast to studies on borderline tumours Brugghe et al (1998) were unable to demonstrate any prognostic value in the measurement of the mitotic activity index or volume percentage of epithelium. However, multivariate analysis demostrated that mean nuclear area and FIGO stage have additional prognostic value. These factors were combined (precise details are not given here) to produce an 'early carcinoma of the ovary prognostic score' (ECOPS). Ninety-eight per cent of patients with an ECOPS less than 5.4 (the 66th centile) survived, whilst 25% of patients with an ECOPS greater than 5.4 died. Patients with an ECOPS >5.4 had a 29.2 times greater risk of death than patients with an ECOPS <5.4. Furthermore, compared to the FIGO stage or mean nuclear area alone, ECOPS had a greater accuracy, specificity and positive predictive value. The authors assert that the mean nuclear area can be reproducibly assessed in ten minutes per case.

Advanced ovarian cancer

In studying morphometric prognostic factors in advanced tumours, it must be remembered that cisplatin chemotherapy may itself alter nuclear morphometry through an unknown mechanism (Baak et al 1988b). Morphometric prognostic groups demonstrated for early ovarian cancer remain valid for advanced disease. In a study of 73 patients with stage III and IV disease who had undergone treatment with cisplatin, the mean and standard deviation of nuclear area showed a significant correlation with prognosis, a value of <56.3 mm² being associated with a better prognosis. Cox regression analysis revealed that mean nuclear area is the strongest prognostic factor, followed by FIGO stage and the presence or absence of bulky disease (Baak et al 1988b). These factors can be combined to produce an 'advanced carcinoma of the ovary prognostic score' (the precise details are not given here) or ACOPS. Patients with an ACOPS > -2.520 have a favourable prognosis, those with an ACOPS < -3.255 have a poor prognosis. The results of Wils et al (1988) support the role of the ACOPS in determining the prognosis of patients after platinum-based combination chemotherapy.

The difficult issue remains, however, as to how far knowledge of such parameters would determine management in the individual patient. It is highly questionable whether any medical oncologist would withhold or modify therapy in a patient with advanced ovarian cancer merely on the basis of morphometric indices. The clinical situations in which there is a strong case for morphometric analysis of an ovarian tumour are probably analogous to those already described in the context of ploidy analysis.

REFERENCES

Ahmed M N, Kim K, Haddad B, Berchuck A, Qumsiyeh M B 2000 Comparative genomic hybridization studies in hydatidiform moles and choriocarcinoma: amplification of 7q21–q31 and loss of 8p12–p21 in choriocarcinoma. Cancer Genetics Cytogenetics 116: 10–15

Allan L A, Campbell M K, Eccles R C F et al 1996 The significance of p53 mutation and over-expression in ovarian cancer prognosis. International Journal of Gynecological Cancer 6: 483–490

Al-Nafussi A I, Klys H S, Rebello G, Kelly C, Kerr G, Cowie V 1993 The assessment of proliferating cell nuclear antigen (PCNA) immunostaining in the uterine cervix and cervical squamous neoplasia. International Journal of Gynecological Cancer 3: 154–158

Ambros R A, Kurman R J 1992 Identification of patients with stage I uterine endometrioid adenocarcinoma at high risk of recurrence by DNA ploidy, myometrial invasion, and vascular invasion. Gynecologic Oncology 45: 235–239

Amortegui A J, Meyer M P, Elborne V L, Amin R M 1995 P53, retinoblastoma gene product, and cyclin protein expression in human papillomavirus DNA positive cervical intraepithelial neoplasia and invasive cancer. Modern Pathology 8: 907–912

Anderson S, Shera K, Ihle J et al 1997 Telomerase activity in cervical cancer. American Journal of Pathology 151: 25–31

Andreda M B, Freeman S M, Halabi S, Marrogi A J 1999 p53, c-erbB2, and PCNA status in benign, proliferative and malignant ovarian surface epithelial neoplasms: a study of 75 cases. Archives of Pathology and Laboratory Medicine 123: 310–316

Anton M, Nenutil R, Rejhar A, Kopecny J, Ptackova B, Zaloudik J 1997 DNA flow cytometry: a predictor of a high-risk group in cervical cancer. Cancer Detection and Prevention 21: 242–246

Anttila M, Kosma VM, Ji H et al 1998 Clinical significance of a-catenin, collagen-IV, and Ki-67 expression in epithelial ovarian cancer. Journal of Clinical Oncology 16: 2591–2600

Aoyama C, Peters J, Senadheera S, Liu P, Shimada H 1998 Uterine cervical dysplasia and cancer: identification of c-myc status by quantitative polymerase chain reaction. Diagnostic Molecular Pathology 7: 324–330

Arbor D, Cook P, Moser L, Speights V 1992 Variations in reference cells for DNA analysis of paraffin-embedded tissue. American Journal of Clinical Pathology 97: 387–392

Arends M J 2000 Assessment of apoptosis in gynaecological tumours. CME Journal of Gynecologic Oncology 5: 164–170

Ariel I, Lustig O, Oyer C E et al 1994 Relaxation of imprinting in trophoblastic disease. Gynecologic Oncology 53: 212–219

Arima T, Matsuda T, Takagi N, Wake N 1997 Association of IGF2 and H19 imprinting with choriocarcinoma development. Cancer Genetics and Cytogenetics 93: 39–47

Athanassiadou P, Petrakakou E, Liossi A et al 1999 Prognostic significance of p53, Bcl-2 and EGFR in carcinoma of the endometrium. Acta Cytologica 43: 1039–1044

Autillo-Touati A, Joannes M, d'Ercole C et al 1998 HPV typing by in situ hybridization on cervical cytologic smears with ASCUS. Acta Cytologica 42: 631–638

Baak J P A 1995 The role of computerized and cytometric feature analysis in endometrial hyperplasia and cancer prognosis. Journal of Cell Biochemistry 59 (Suppl 23): 137–146

Baak J P A, Fox H, Langley F A, Buckley C H 1985 The prognostic value of morphometry in ovarian epithelial tumors of borderline malignancy. International Journal of Gynecological Pathology 4: 186–191

Baak J P A, Wisse-Brekelmans E C M, Langley F A, Talerman A, Delemarre J F M 1986 Morphometric data to FIGO stage and histological type and grade for prognosis of ovarian tumours. Journal of Clinical Pathology 39: 1340–1346

Baak J P A, Wisse-Brekelmans E C, Uyterlinde A M, Schipper N 1987 Evaluation of the prognostic value of morphometric features and cellular DNA content in FIGO I ovarian cancer patients. Annals of Quantitative Cytology and Histology 9: 287–290

Baak J P A, Meijer G J Brinkhuis M, Belien J A M, Brugghe J, Broeckaerts M 1995 Quantitative pathology of gynaecological tumours. In: Fox H, Wells M (eds) Haines and Taylor Obstetrical and Gynaecological Pathology, Fourth Edition, Churchill Livingstone, 1333–1358

Baak J P A, Nauta J, Wisse-Brekelmans E, Bezemer P 1988a Architectural and nuclear morphometrical features together are more important prognosticators in endometrial hyperplasias than nuclear morphometrical features alone. Journal of Pathology 154: 335–341

Baak J P A, Schipper N W, Wisse-Brekelmans E C M et al 1988b The prognostic value of morphometrical features and cellular DNA-content in cis-platin treated late ovarian cancer patients. British Journal of Cancer 57: 503–508

Bae S N, Kim S J 1999 Telomerase activity in complete hydatidiform mole. American Journal of Obstetrics and Gynecology 180: 328–333

Baergen R N, Warren C D, Isacson C, Ellenson L H 2001 Early uterine serous carcinoma: clonal origin of extrauterine disease. International Journal of Gynecological Pathology 20: 214–219

Bai M K, Costopoulos J S, Christofiridou B P, Papadimitrou C S 1994 Immunochemical detection of the c-myc oncogene product in normal, hyperplastic and carcinomatous endometrium. Oncology 51: 314–319

Baker B A, Frickey L, Yu I T et al 1998 DNA content of ovarian immature teratomas and malignant germ cell tumors. Gynecologic Oncology 71: 14–18

Bakshi N, Rajwanshi A, Patel F, Ganguly N K 1998 Prognostic significance of DNA ploidy and S-phase fraction in malignant serous cystadenocarcinoma of the ovary. Analytical and Quantitative Cytology and Histology 20: 215–220

Ballouk F, Ambros R A, Malfetano J H, Ross J S 1993 Evaluation of prognostic indicators in squamous carcinoma of the vulva including nuclear DNA content. Modern Pathology 6, 371–375

Barnabei V M, Scott-Miller D, Bauer K D et al 1990 Flow cytometric evaluation of epithelial ovarian cancer. American Journal of Obstetrics and Gynecology 162: 1584–1592

Bauer T W, Tubbs R R, Edinger M G, Suit P F, Gephardt G N, Levin H S 1990 Prospective comparison of DNA quantitation by image and flow cytometry. American Journal of Clinical Pathology 93: 322–326

Bauknecht T, Bermelin G, Kommoss F 1990 Clinical significance of oncogenes and growth factors in ovarian carcinoma. Journal of Steroid Biochemistry and Medical Biology 37: 855–862

Bauknecht T, Kiechle, Schwarz M, du Bois A, Wolfle J, Kacinski B, 1994 Expression of transcripts for CSF-1 and for the 'macrophage' and 'epithelial' isoforms of the CSF-1R transcripts in human ovarian carcinomas. Cancer Detection Preview 18: 231–239

Beale P J, Rogers P, Boxall F, Sharp S Y, Kelland L R 2000 BCL-2 family gene expression and platinum drug resistance in ovarian carcinoma. British Journal of Cancer 82: 436–440

Berchuck A, Kamel A, Whitaker R et al 1990 Overexpression of HER-2/neu is associated with poor survival in advanced epithelial ovarian cancer. Cancer Research 50: 4087–4091

Berezowsky J, Zbieranowski I, Demers J, Murray D 1995 DNA ploidy of hydatidiform moles and nonmolar conceptuses: a study using flow and tissue section image cytometry. Modern Pathology 8: 775–781

Bethwaite P B, Koreth J, Herrington C S, McGee J O'D 1995 Loss of heterozygosity occurs at the D11S29 locus on chromosome 11q23 in invasive cervical carcinoma. British Journal of Cancer 71: 814–818

Bigsby R M, Aixin L I, Bomalaski J, Stehman F B, Look K Y, Sutton G P 1992 Immunohistochemical study of HER-2/neu, epidermal growth factor receptor, and steroid receptor expression in normal and malignant endometrium. Obstetrics and Gynecology 79: 95–100

Blegen H, Einhorn N, Sjovall K et al 2000 Prognostic significance of cell cycle proteins and genomic instability in borderline, early and advanced stage ovarian carcinoma. International Journal of Gynecological Cancer 10: 477–487

Blom R, Guerrieri C, Stal O, Malmstrom H, Sullivan S, Simonsen E 1998a Malignant mixed Müllerian tumors of the uterus: a clinicopathologic, DNA flow cytometric, p53, and mdm-2 analysis of 44 cases. Gynecologic Oncology 68: 18–24

Blom R, Guerrieri C, Stal O, Malmstrom H, Simonsen E 1998b Leiomyosarcoma of the uterus: a clinicopathologic, DNA flow cytometric, p53, and mdm-2 analysis of 49 cases. Gynecologic Oncology 68: 54–61

Blom R, Malmstrom H, Guerrieri C 1999 Endometrial stromal sarcoma of the uterus: a clinicopathologic, DNA flow cytometric, p53, and mdm-2 analysis of 17 cases. International Journal of Gynecological Cancer 9: 98–104

Braly P 1995 Flow cytometry as a prognostic factor in endometrial cancer — what does it add? Gynecologic Oncology 58: 145–147

Brien T P, Kallakury B V, Lowry C V et al 1997 Telomerase activity in benign endometrium and endometrial carcinoma. Cancer Research 57: 2760–2764

Britton I C, Wilson T O, Gaffey T A, Cha S S, Wieand H S, Podratz K C 1990 DNA ploidy in endometrial carcinoma: major objective prognostic factor. Mayo Clinic Proceedings 65: 643–650

Bruening W, Prowse A H, Schultz D C, Holgado-Madruga M, Wong A, Godwin A K 1999 Expression of OVCA1, a candidate tumor suppressor, is reduced in tumors and inhibits growth of ovarian cancer cells. Cancer Research 59: 4973–4983

Brugghe J, Baak J P A, Wiltshaw E, Brinkhuis M, Meijer G A, Fisher C 1998 Quantitative prognostic features in FIGO I ovarian cancer patients without postoperative treatment. Gynecologic Oncology 68: 47–53

Bryan E J, Watson R H, Davis M, Hitchcock A, Foulkes W D, Campbell I G 1996 Localization of an ovarian cancer tumor suppressor gene to a 0.5-cM region between D22S284 and CYP2D, on chromosome 22q. Cancer Research 56: 719–721

Bulten J, de Wilde P C, Boonstra H, Gemmink J H, Hanselaar A G 2000 Proliferation in "atypical" atrophic pap smears. Gynecologic Oncology 79: 225–229

Burks R T, Kessis T D, Cho K R, Hedrick L 1994 Microsatellite instability in endometrial carcinoma. Oncogene 9 (Suppl. 4): 1163–1166

Burton J L, Wells M 1998 Recent advances in the histopathology and molecular pathology of carcinoma of the endometrium. Histopathology 33: 297–303

Burton J L, Wells M 1999 The role of apoptosis in the prognosis of epithelial ovarian carcinoma. CME Journal of Gynecologic Oncology 4: 238–242

Burton J L, Stewart R L, Heatley M K, Royds J A, Wells M 1999 p53 expression, p21 expression and the apoptotic index in endometrioid endometrial adenocarcinoma. Histopathology 35: 221–229

Bussaglia E, del-Rio E, Matias-Guiu X, Prat J 2000 PTEN mutations in endometrial carcinomas: a molecular and clinicopathologic analysis of 38 cases. Human Pathology 31: 312–317

But I, Gorisek B 2000 DNA-ploidy as an independent prognostic factor in patients with serous ovarian carcinoma. International Journal of Gynaecology and Obstetrics 71: 259–262

Caduff R F, Johnston C M, Frank T S 1995 Mutations of the Ki-ras oncogene in carcinoma of the endometrium. American Journal of Pathology 146: 182–188

Caduff R F, Svoboda-Newman S M, Ferguson A W, Johnston C M, Frank T S 1999 Comparison of mutations of Ki-ras and p53 immunoreactivity in borderline and malignant epithelial ovarian tumors. American Journal of Surgical Pathology 23: 323–328

Chan W Y, Cheung K K, Schorge J O et al 2000 Bcl-2 and p53 protein expression, apoptosis, and p53 mutation in human epithelial ovarian cancers. American Journal of Pathology 156: 409–417

ChangChien C C, Lin H, Leung S W et al 1998 Effect of acetic acid on telomerase activity in cervical intraepithelial neoplasia. Gynecologic Oncology 71: 99–103

Chatterjee A, Pulido H A, Koul S et al 2001 Mapping the sites of putative tumor suppressor genes at 6p25 and 6p21.3 in cervical carcinoma: occurrence of allelic deletions in precancerous lesions. Cancer Research 61: 2119–2123

Chen C A, Chen Y H, Chen T M et al 1994 Infrequent mutation in tumour suppressor gene p53 in gestational trophoblastic disease. Carcinogenesis 15: 2221–2223

Chen C L, Ip S M, Cheng D, Wong L C, Ngan H Y 2000 Loss of imprinting of the IGF-II and H19 genes in epithelial ovarian cancer. Clinical Cancer Research 6: 474–479

Cheung A N Y 1997 The use of markers of cell proliferation and cell loss in gynaecological cancers. Current Opinion in Obstetrics and Gynaecology 9: 32–36

Cheung A N Y, Ngan H Y S, Chen W Z, Loke S L, Collins R J 1993 The significance of proliferating cell nuclear antigen in human trophoblastic disease — an immunohistochemical study. Histopathology 22: 565–568

Cheung A N Y, Srivastava G, Chung I P et al 1994a Expression of the p53 gene in trophoblastic cells in hydatidiform moles and normal human placentas. Journal of Reproductive Medicine 39: 223–227

Cheung A N Y, Sit A S Y, Chung L P et al 1994b Detection of heterozygous X Y complete hydatidiform mole by chromosome in situ hybridization. Gynecologic Oncology 55: 386–392

Cheung A N Y, Ngan H Y S, Collins R J, Wong Y L 1994c Assessment of cell proliferation in hydatidiform mole using monoclonal antibody MIB1 to Ki-67 antigen. Journal of Clinical Pathology 47: 386–392

Cheung A N Y, Shen D H, Khoo U S, Wong L C, Ngan H Y S 1998 p21$^{WAF1/CIP1}$ expression in gestational trophoblastic disease: correlation with clinicopathological parameters and Ki-67 and p53 gene expression. Journal of Clinical Pathology 51: 159–162

Cheung A N Y, Shen D H, Khoo U S et al 1999a Immunohistochemical and mutational analysis of p53 tumor suppressor gene in gestational trophoblastic disease — correlation with mdm2, proliferation index and clinicopathological parameters. International Journal of Gynecological Cancer 9: 123–130

Cheung A N Y, Zgang D K, Ngan H Y S, Shen D H, Tsao S W 1999b Telomerase activity in gestational trophoblastic disease. Journal of Clinical Pathology 52: 588–592

Cheville J C, Robinson R 1996 Evaluation of Ki-67 (MIB-1) in placentas with hydropic change and partial and complete hydatidiform mole. Pediatric Pathology and Laboratory Medicine 16: 41–50

Chieng D C, Ross D S, Ambros R A 1996 BCL-2 expression and the development of endometrial carcinoma. Modern Pathology 402–406

Chiu P M, Ngan H Y S, Khoo U S, Cheung A N Y 2001 Apoptotic activity in gestational trophoblastic disease correlates with clinical outcome — assessment by M30 CytoDeath antibody which recognises caspase cleavage site within cytokeratin 18. Histopathology 38: 243–249

Chu T Y, Shen C Y, Lee H S, Liu H S 1999 Monoclonality and surface-lesion specific microsatellite alterations in premalignant and malignant neoplasia of uterine cervix: a local field effect of genomic instability and clonal evolution. Genes Chromosomes and Cancer 24: 127–134

Chuaqui M F, Zhuang Z, Emmert-Buck N R et al 1996 Genetic analysis of synchronous mucinous tumors of the ovary and appendix. Human Pathology 27: 165–171

Chuaqui R, Silva M, Emmert-Buck M 2001 Allelic deletion mapping on chromosome 6q and X chromosome inactivation clonality patterns in cervical intraepithelial neoplasia and invasive carcinoma. Gynecologic Oncology 80: 364–371

Cina S J, Richardson M S, Austin R M, Kurman R J 1997 Immunohistochemical staining for Ki-67 antigen, carcinoembryonic antigen, and p53 in the differential diagnosis of glandular lesions of the cervix. Modern Pathology 10: 176–180

Cliby W, Ritland S, Hartmann L et al 1993 Human epithelial ovarian cancer allelotype. Cancer Research 53: 2393–2398

Cole D J, Brown D C, Crossley F, Alcock C J, Gatter K C 1992 Carcinoma of the cervix uteri: an assessment of the relationship of tumour proliferation to prognosis. British Journal of Cancer 65: 783–785

Connor J P, Miller D S, Bauer K D, Murad T M, Rademaker A W, Lurain J R 1993 Flow cytometric evaluation of early invasive cervical cancer. Obstetrics and Gynecology 81: 367–371

Coon J, Paxton H, Lucy L, Homberger H 1994 Interlaboratory variation in DNA flow cytometry. Archives of Pathology and Laboratory Medicine 118: 681–685

Cope J U, Hildesheim A, Schiffman M H et al 1997 Comparison of the hybrid capture tube test and PCR for detection of human papillomavirus DNA in cervical specimens. Journal of Clinical Microbiology 35: 2262–2265

Costa M J, Walls J E, Ames P, Roth I M 1996 Transformation in recurrent ovarian granulosa cell tumors: Ki-67 (MIB-1) and p53 immunohistochemistry demonstrates a possible molecular basis for the poor histopathologic prediction of clinical behaviour. Human Pathology 27: 274–291

Costa M J, Hansen C L, Walls J E Scudder S A 1999 Immunohistochemical markers of cell cycle control applied to ovarian and primary peritoneal surface epithelial neoplasms: p21 (WAF1/C1P1) predicts survival and good response to platinin-based chemotherapy. Human Pathology 30: 640–647

Costa M J, Hansen C L, Holden J A, Guinee D 2000 Topoisomerase II alpha: prognostic predictor and cell cycle marker in surface epithelial neoplasms of the ovary and peritoneum. International Journal of Gynecological Pathology 19: 248–257

Cuatrecasas M, Matias-Guiu X, Prat J 1996 Synchronous mucinous tumors of the appendix and the ovary associated with pseudomyxoma peritonei: a clinicopathologic study of six cases with comparative analysis of c-Ki-ras mutations. American Journal of Surgical Pathology 20: 739–746

Cuatrecasas M, Villanueva A, Matias-Guiu X, Prat J 1997 K-ras mutations in mucinous ovarian tumors: a clinicopathologic and molecular study of 95 cases. Cancer 79: 1581–1586

Curling M, Stenning S, Hudson C N, Watson J V 1998 Multivariate analyses of DNA index, p-63myc and clinicopathological status of patients with ovarian cancer. Journal of Clinical Pathology 51: 455–461

Czerwenka K, Lu Y, Heuss F 1995 Amplification and expression of the c-erbB-2 oncogene in normal, hyperplastic and malignant endometria. International Journal of Gynecological Pathology 14: 98–106

Datar R H, Naritoku W Y, Li PL et al 1999 Analysis of telomerase activity in ovarian cystadenomas, low malignant potential tumors, and invasive carcinomas. Gynecologic Oncology 74: 338–345

Davis J R, Aristizabal S, Way D L, Weines S A, Hicks M J, Hagaman R M 1989 DNA ploidy, grade, and stage in prognosis of uterine cervical cancer. Gynecologic Oncology 32: 4–7

Dellas A, Schultheiss E, Holzgreve W, Oberholzer M, Torhorst J, Gudat F 1997 Investigation of the Bcl-2 and C-myc expression in relation to the Ki-67 labelling index in cervical intraepithelial neoplasia. International Journal of Gynecological Pathology 16: 212–218

Demirel D, Laucirica R, Fishman A et al 1996 Ovarian tumors of low malignant potential: correlation of DNA index and S-phase fraction with histopathologic grade and clinical outcome. Cancer 77: 1494–1500

de Nictolas M, Garbisa S, Lucarini G et al 1996 72 kilo-dalton type IV collagenase, type IV collagen and Ki-67 in serous tumors of the ovary: a clinicopathologic, immunohistochemical, and serological study. International Journal of Gynecological Pathology 15: 102–109

Diebold J, Suchy B, Baretton G B et al 1996a DNA ploidy and MYC DNA amplification in ovarian carcinomas: correlation with p53 and bcl-2 expression, proliferative activity and prognosis. Virchows Archiv 429: 221–227

Diebold J, Baretton G B, Felchner M et al 1996b Bcl-2 expression, p53 accumulation, and apoptosis in ovarian carcinomas. American Journal of Clinical Pathology 105: 341–349

Dion F, Mes-Masson A M, Seymour R J, Provencher D, Tonin P N 2000 Allelotyping defines minimal imbalance at chromosomal region 17q25 in non-serous epithelial ovarian cancers. Oncogene 19: 1466–1472

Dolan J R, McCall A R, Gooneratne S, Walter S, Lansky D M 1993 DNA ploidy, proliferation index, grade, and stage as prognostic factors for vulvar squamous cell carcinomas. Gynecologic Oncology 48: 232–235

Douc-Rasy S, Barrois M, Fogel S et al 1996 High incidence of loss of heterozygosity and abnormal imprinting of H19 and IGF2 genes in invasive cervical carcinomas: uncoupling of H19 and IGF2 expression and biallelic hypomethylation of H19. Oncogene 12: 423–430

Drew P A, Al-abbadi M A, Orlando C A, Hendricks J B, Kubilis P S, Wilkinson E J 1996 Prognostic factors in carcinoma of the vulva: a clinicopathologic and DNA flow cytometric study. International Journal of Gynecological Pathology 15: 235–241

Duggan B D, Felix J C, Muderspach L I, Tourgeman D, Zheng J, Shibata D 1994 Microsatellite instability in sporadic endometrial carcinoma. Journal of the National Cancer Institute 86: 1216–1221

Duggan B D, Wan M, Yu M C et al 1998 Detection of ovarian cancer cells: comparison of a telomerase assay and cytologic examination. Journal of the National Cancer Institute 90: 238–242

Dunton C, Baak J, Palazzo J et al 1996 Use of computerized morphometric analyses of endometrial hyperplasias in the prediction of coexistent cancer. American Journal of Obstetrics and Gynecology 174: 1518–1521

Dyas C H, Simmons T K, Ellis C M et al 1992 Effect of desoxyribonucleic acid ploidy status on survival of patients with carcinoma of the endometrium. Surgery Gynecology and Obstetrics 174: 133–136

Eichhorn J H, Young R H, Scully R E 1992 DNA content and proliferative activity in ovarian small cell carcinomas of the hypercalcemic type: implications for diagnosis, prognosis and histogenesis. American Journal of Clinical Pathology 98: 579–586

Eichhorn J H, Lawrence W D, Young R H, Scully R E 1996 Ovarian neuroendocrine carcinomas of non-small-cell type associated with surface epithelial adenocarcinomas: a study of five cases and review of the literature. International Journal of Gynecological Pathology 15: 303–314

Elavathil L J, Celebre G, McFarlane D 1996 Reproducibility of DNA ploidy and S-phase values from paraffin-embedded tissues. Analytical and Quantitative Cytology and Histology 18: 316–322

Eltabbakh G H, Belinson J L, Kennedy A W, Biscotti C V, Casey G, Tubbs R R 1997 p53 and HER-2/neu overexpression in ovarian borderline tumors. Gynecologic Oncology 65: 218–224

Emmert-Buck M R, Chuaqui R, Zhuang Z, Nogales F, Liotta L A, Merino M J 1997 Molecular analysis of synchronous uterine and ovarian endometrioid tumors. International Journal of Gynecological Pathology 16: 143–148

Enomoto T, Fujita M, Inoue M et al 1993 Alterations of the p53 tumor suppressor gene and its association with activation of the c-K-ras-2 protooncogene in premalignant and malignant lesions of the human uterine endometrium. Cancer Research 53: 1883–1888

Enomoto T, Fujita M, Inouee M, Tanizawa O, Nomura T, Shroyer K R 1994 Analysis of clonality by amplification of short tandem repeats: carcinomas of the female reproductive tract. Diagnostic Molecular Pathology 3: 292–297

Enomoto T, Fujita M, Inoue M, Nomura T, Shroyer K R 1995 Alteration of the p53 tumor suppressor gene and activation of c-k-ras-2 protooncogene in endometrial adenocarcinoma from Colorado. American Journal of Clinical Pathology 103: 224–230

Enomoto T, Haba T, Fujita M et al 1997 Clonal analysis of high-grade squamous intra-epithelial lesions of the uterine cervix. International Journal of Cancer 73: 339–344

Erba E, Ubezio P, Pepe S et al 1989 Flow cytometric analysis of DNA content in human ovarian cancer. British Journal of Cancer 60: 45–50

Esteller M, Garcia A, Palones J M M, Cabero A, Reventos J 1995 Detection of c-erbB-2/neu and fibroblast growth factor-3INT/-2 but not epidermal growth factor receptor gene amplification in endometrial cancer by differential polymerase chain reaction. Cancer 75: 2139–2146

Esteller M, Garcia A, Martinez-Palones J M, Xercavins J, Reventos J 1997 Detection of clonality and genetic alterations in endometrial pipelle biopsy and its surgical specimen counterpart. Laboratory Investigation 76: 109–116

Esteller M, Catasus L, Matias-Guiu X et al 1999 hMLH1 promoter methylation and gene silencing is an early event in human endometrial carcinogenesis, American Journal of Pathology 155: 1767–1772

Falcinelli C, Luzi P, Alberti P et al 1993 Human papillomavirus infection and Ki-ras oncogene in paraffin-embedded squamous carcinomas of the cervix. Gynecological and Obstetrical Investigation 40: 147–151

Felip E, Del Campo J M, Rubio D, Vidal M T, Colomer R, Bermejo B 1995 Overexpression of c-erbB-2 in epithelial ovarian cancer. Cancer 75: 2147–2152

Feng J, Funk W D, Wang S S et al 1995 The RNA component of human telomerase. Science 269: 1236–1241

Fishel R, Kolodner R D 1995 Identification of mismatch repair genes and their role in the development of cancer. Current Opinion in Genetic Development 5: 382–395

Friedlander M L, Hedley D W, Taylor I W, Russell P, Coates A S, Tattersall M H 1984 Influence of cellular DNA content on survival in advanced ovarian cancer. Cancer Research; 44: 397–400

Friedlander M L, Hedley D H, Swanson C, Russell P 1988 Prediction of long term survivals by flow cytometric analysis of cellular DNA content in patients with advanced ovarian cancer. Journal of Clinical Oncology 6: 282–290

Fujii H, Yoshida M, Gong Z X 2000 Frequent genetic heterogeneity in the clonal evolution of gynecological carcinosarcoma and its influence on phenotypic diversity. Cancer Research 60: 114–120

Fujino T, Risinger J I, Collins N K et al 1994 Allelotype of endometrial carcinoma. Cancer Research 54: 4294–4298

Fujita M, Enomoto T, Wada H, Inoue M, Okudaira Y, Shroyer K R 1996 Application of clonal analysis: differential diagnosis for synchronous primary ovarian and endometrial cancers and metastatic cancer. American Journal of Clinical Pathology 105: 350–359

Fukunaga M 2000 Early partial hydatidiform mole: prevalance, histopathology, DNA ploidy, and persistence rate. Virchows Archiv 437: 180–184

Fukunaga M 2001 Flow cytometric and clinicopathologic study of complete hydatidiform mole with special reference to the significance of cytometric aneuploidy. Gynecologic Oncology 81: 67–70

Fukunaga M, Ushigome S, Fukunaga M, Sugishita M 1993 Application of flow cytometry in diagnosis of hydatidiform moles. Modern Pathology 6: 353–359

Fukunaga M, Endo Y, Nomura K, Ushigome S 1997a Small cell carcinoma of the ovary: a case report of large cell variant. Pathology International 47: 250–255

Fukunaga M, Endo Y, Miyazawa Y, Ushigome S 1997b Small cell neuroendocrine carcinoma of the ovary. Virchows Archiv 430: 343–348

Fulop V, Mok S C, Genest D R, Gati I, Doszpod J, Berkowitz R S 1998 p53, p21, RB and mdm2 oncoproteins: expression in normal placenta, partial and complete mole, and choriocarcinoma. Journal of Reproductive Medicine. 43: 118–127

Gadducci A, Ciancia E M, Campani D et al 1994 Immunohistochemical detection of p-185 product, p21 product, and proliferating nuclear cell antigen (PCNA) in formalin-fixed, paraffin-embedded tissues from ovarian carcinomas: preliminary data. European Journal of Gynaecological Oncology 15: 359–368

Gajewski W H, Fuller A F, Pastel-Ley C et al 1994 Prognostic significance of DNA content in epithelial ovarian cancer. Gynecologic Oncology 53: 5–12

Garcia A, Bussaglia E, Machin P, Matias-Guiu X, Prat J 2000 Loss of heterozygosity on chromosome 17q in epithelial ovarian tumors: association with carcinomas of serous differentiation. International Journal of Gynecological Pathology 19: 152–157

Garrett A P, Lee K R, Colitti C R, Muto M G, Berkowitz R S, Mok S C 2001 k-ras mutation may be an early event in mucinous ovarian tumorigenesis. International Journal of Gynecological Pathology 20: 244–251

Garzetti G G, Ciavattini S, Goteri G et al 1995a Ki-67 antigen immuno-staining (MIB-1 monoclonal antibody) in serous ovarian tumors: index of proliferative activity with prognostic significance. Gynecologic Oncology 56: 169–174

Garzetti G G, Ciavattini A, Lucarini G et al 1995b MIB1 imunostaining in stage 1 squamous cervical carcinoma: relationship with natural killer cell activity. Gynecologic Oncology 58: 28–33

Garzetti G G, Ciavattini A, Goteri G et al 1996a Proliferating cell nuclear antigen (PCNA) immunoreactivity in stage I endometrial cancer: a new prognostic factor. International Journal of Gynecological Cancer 6: 186–192

Garzetti C G, Ciavattini A, Goteri G, de Nictolis M, Romanini G 1996b Proliferating cell nuclear antigen in endometrial adenocarcinoma: pretreatment identification of high risk patients. Gynecologic Oncology 61: 16–21

Garzetti G G, Ciavattini A, Lucarini G, Goteri G, de Nictolis M, Biagini G 1997 MIB 1 immunostaining in cervical carcinoma of young women. Gynecologic Oncology 67: 184–187

Gasinska A, Urbanski K, Jakubowicz J, Klimek M, Biesaga B, Wilson G D 1999 Tumour cell kinetics as a prognostic factor in squamous cell carcinoma of the cervix treated with radiotherapy. Radiotherapy and Oncology 50: 77–84

Geisler J P, Wiemann M C, Miller G A, Zhou Z, Geisler H E 1995 Change in MIB-1 staining between primary and recurrent epithelial ovarian cancer. European Journal of Gynaecological Oncology 16: 343–345

Geisler J P, Wiemann M C, Zhou Z, Miller G A, Geisler H E 1996 Proliferation index determined by MIB-1 and recurrence of endometrial carcinoma. Gynecologic Oncology 61: 373–377

Geisler J P, Zhou Z, Miller G A et al 1998a MIB-1: a predictor of survival in patients with ovarian carcinoma. International Journal of Gynecological Cancer 8: 392–396

Geisler J P, Geisler H E, Wiemann M C, Zhou Z, Miller G A, Crabtree W 1998b Lack of Bcl-2 persistence: an independent prognostic indicator of poor prognosis in endometrial carcinoma. Gynecologic Oncology 71: 305–307

Geisler J P, Geisler H E, Miller G A, Wiemann M C, Zhou Z, Crabtree W 1999 MIB-1 in endometrial carcinoma: prognostic significance with 5-year follow-up. Gynecologic Oncology 75: 432–436

Geisler J P, Geisler H E, Miller G A, Wiemann M C, Zhou Z, Crabtree W 2000 p53 and Bcl-2 in epithelial ovarian carcinoma: their value as prognostic indicators at a median follow-up of 60 months. Gynecologic Oncology 77: 278–282

Gershenson D M, Deavers M, Diaz S et al 1999 Prognostic significance of p53 expression in advanced-stage ovarian serous borderline tumors. Clinical Cancer Research 5: 4053–4058

Giannoudis A, Graham D A, Southern S A, Herrington C S 1999 p53 codon 72arg/pro polymorphism is not related to HPV type or lesion grade in low- and high-grade squamous intra-epithelial lesions and invasive squamous carcinoma of the cervix. International Journal of Cancer 83: 66–69

Gras E, Pons C, Machin P, Matias-Guiu X, Prat J 2001 Loss of heterozygosity at the RB-1 locus and pRB immunostaining in epithelial ovarian tumors: a molecular, immunohistochemical, and clinicopathologic study. International Journal of Gynecological Pathology 20: 335–340

Gschwendtner A, Neher A, Kreczy A, Muller-Holzner E, Volgger B, Mairinger T 1998 DNA ploidy of early molar pregnancies by image analysis: comparison to histologic classification. Archives of Pathology and Laboratory Medicine 122: 1000–1004

Gu J, Roth L M, Younger C et al 2001 Molecular evidence for the independent origin of extra-ovarian papillary serous tumors of low malignant potential. Journal of the National Cancer Institute 93: 1122–1123

Guo L-N, Wilkinson N, Buckley C H, Fox H, Hale R J, Chawner L 1993 Proliferating cell nuclear antigen (PCNA) immunoreactivity in ovarian serous and mucinous neoplasms: diagnostic and prognostic value. International Journal of Gynecological Cancer 3: 391–394

Guo Z, Thunberg U, Sallstrom J, Willander E, Ponten J 1998 Clonality analysis of cervical cancer on microdissected archival materials by PCR-based X-chromosome inactivation approach. International Journal of Oncology 12: 1327–1332

Haapasalo H, Collan Y, Atkin N B, Pesonen E, Seppa A 1989 Prognosis of ovarian carcinomas: prediction by histoquantitative methods. Histopathology 15: 167–178

Haapasalo H, Collan Y, Seppa A, Gidlund A L, Atkin N B, Pesonen E 1990 Prognostic value of ovarian carcinoma grading methods — a method comparison study. Histopathology 16: 1–7

Hachisuga T, Fukuda K, Uchiyama M, Matsuo N, Iwasaka T, Sugimori H 1993 Immunohistochemical study of p53 expression in endometrial carcinomas; correlation with markers of proliferating cells and clinicopathologic features. International Journal of Gynecological Cancer 3: 363–368

Hale R J, Buckley C H, Gullick W J et al 1993 Prognostic value of epidermal growth factor receptor expression in cervical carcinoma. Journal of Clinical Pathology 46: 149–153

Hall K L, Teneriello M G, Taylor R R et al 1997 Analysis of Ki-ras, p53, and MDM2 genes in uterine leiomyomas and leiomyosarcomas. Gynecologic Oncology 65: 333–335

Hamel N W, Sebo T U, Wilson T O et al 1996 Prognostic value of p53 and proliferating cell nuclear antigen expression in endometrial carcinoma. Gynecologic Oncology 62: 192–198

Hampton G M, Penny L A, Baergen R N et al 1994 Loss of heterozygosity in cervical carcinoma: subchromosomal localization of a putative tumor-suppressor gene to chromosome 11q22–q24. Proceedings of the National Academy of Sciences USA 91: 6953–6957

Harima Y, Harima K, Shikata N, Oka A, Ohnishi T, Tanaka Y 1998 Bax and Bcl-2 expressions predict response to radiotherapy in human cervical cancer. Journal of Cancer Research and Clinical Oncology 124: 503–510

Harima Y, Shirahama S, Harima K, Aoki S, Ohnishi T, Tanaka Y 1999 Genetic alterations on chromosome 17q associated with response to radiotherapy in bulky cervical cancer. British Journal of Cancer 81: 108–113

Harlow B L, Fuhr J E, McDonald T W, Schwartz S M, Beuerlein F J, Weiss N S 1993 Flow cytometry as a prognostic indicator in women with borderline epithelial ovarian tumors. Gynecologic Oncology 50: 305–309

Hartmann R C, Podratz K C, Keeney G L et al 1994 Prognostic significance of p53 immunostaining in epithelial ovarian cancer. Journal of Clinical Oncology 12: 64–69

Hayashi Y, Hachisuga T, Iwasaka T et al 1991 Expression of ras oncogene product and EGF receptor in cervical squamous cell carcinomas and its relationship to lymph node involvement. Gynecologic Oncology 40: 147–151

Heatley M K 1995 Association between the apoptotic index and established prognostic parameters in endometrial adenocarcinoma. Histopathology 27: 469–472

Heatley M K 1997 A high apoptotic index occurs in subtypes of endometrial adenocarcinoma associated with a poor prognosis. Journal of Pathology 29: 272–275

Heiden T, Strang P, Stendhal U, Tribukait B 1990 The reproducibility of flow cytometric analysis in human tumours. Anticancer Research 10: 49–54

Heinonen P K, Isola J, Kuoppala T 1994 Immunohistochemical determination of estrogen and progesterone receptors and DNA flow cytometry in endometrial cancer. International Journal of Gynecological Cancer 4: 169–173

Helland A, Karlsen F, Due E U, Holm R, Kristensen G, Borresen Dale A I 1998 Mutations in the TP53 gene and protein expression of p53, MDM2 and p21/WAF-1 in primary cervical carcinomas with no or low human papillomavirus load. British Journal of Cancer 78: 69–72

Hellstrom A C, Hue J, Silfversward C, Auer G 1994 DNA-ploidy and mutant p53 overexpression in primary fallopian tube cancer. International Journal of Gynecological Cancer 4: 408–413

Hellstrom A C, Blegen H, Malec M et al 2000 Recurrent fallopian tube carcinoma: TP53 mutation and clinical course. International Journal of Gynecological Pathology 19: 145–151

Hemming J D, Quirke P, Womaack C, Wells M, Elston C E 1987 Diagnosis of molar pregnancy and persistent trophoblastic disease by flow cytometry. Journal of Clinical Pathology 40: 615–620

Hemming J D, Quirke P, Womack C, Wells M, Elston C E, Pennington G W 1988 Flow cytometry in persistent trophoblastic disease. Placenta 9: 615–621

Henderson G S, Brown K A, Perkins S L, Abbott T M, Clayton F 1996 BCL-2 is down-regulated in atypical endometrial hyperplasia and adenocarcinoma. Modern Pathology 9: 430–438

Hendricks D T, Taylor R, Reed M, Birrer M J 1997 FHIT gene expression in human ovarian, endometrial, and cervical cancer cell lines. Cancer Research 57: 2112–2115

Hendricks J B, Wilkinson E J, Kubilis P, Drew P, Blaydes S M, Munakata S 1994 Ki-67 expression in vulvar carcinoma. International Journal of Gynecological Pathology 13: 205–210

Henriksen R, Strang P, Wilander E, Backstrom T, Tribukait B, Oberg K 1994 p53 expression in epithelial ovarian neoplasms; relationship to clinical and pathological parameters, Ki-67 expression and flow cytometry. Gynecologic Oncology 53: 301–306

Henriksen R, Wilander E, Oberg K 1995 Expression and prognostic significance of Bcl-2 in ovarian tumours. British Journal of Cancer 72: 1324–1329

Herod J J O, Eliopoulos A G, Warwick J et al 1996 The prognostic significance of Bcl-2 and p53 expression in ovarian carcinoma. Cancer Research 56: 2178–2184

Hetzel D J, Wilson T O, Keeney G L et al 1992 HER-2/neu expression: a major prognostic factor in endometrial cancer. Gynecologic Oncology 47: 179–185

Hidalgo A, Schewe C, Petersen S et al 2000 Human papillomavirus status and chromosomal imbalances in primary cervical carcinomas and tumour cell lines. European Journal of Cancer 6: 542–548

Hitchcock C L, Norris H J, Khalifa M A, Wargotz E S 1989 Flow cytometric analysis of granulosa cell tumors. Cancer 64: 2127–2132

Holland D R, Le Riche J, Swenerton K D, Elit L 1991 Flow cytometric assessment of DNA ploidy is a useful prognostic factor for patients with granulosa cell ovarian tumors. International Journal of Gynecological Cancer 1: 227–232

Hosking L, Trowsdale J, Nicolai H et al 1995 A somatic BRCA1 mutation in an ovarian tumour. Nature Genetics 9: 343–344

How J, Scurry J, Grant P et al 1995 Placental site trophoblastic tumor: report of three cases and review of the literature. International Journal of Gynecological Cancer 5: 241–249

Hunt C R, Hale R J, Armstrong C, Rajkumar T, Gullick W J, Buckley C H 1995 c-erbB-3 proto-oncogene expression in uterine cervical carcinoma. International Journal of Gynecological Cancer 5: 282–285

Hunt C R, Hale R J, Buckley C H, Hunt J 1996 p53 expression in carcinoma of the cervix. Journal of Clinical Pathology 49: 971–974

Hutson R, Ramsdale J, Wells M 1995 p53 protein expression in putative precursor lesions of epithelial ovarian cancer. Histopathology 27: 367–371

Ikeda M, Watanabe Y, Nanjoh T, Noda K 1993 Evaluation of DNA ploidy in endometrial cancer. Gynecologic Oncology 50: 25–29

Inoue M 2001 Current molecular aspects of the carcinogenesis of the uterine endometrium. International Journal of Gynecological Cancer 11: 339–348

Ioffe O B, Papadimitriou J C, Drachenberg C B 1998 Correlation of proliferation indices, apoptosis, and related oncogene expression (Bcl-2 and c-erbB-2) and p53 in proliferative, hyperplastic, and malignant endometrium. Human Pathology 29: 1150–1159

Isaacson C, Kessis T D, Hedrick L, Cho K R 1996 Both cell proliferation and apoptosis increases with lesion grade in cervical neoplasia but do not correlate with human papillomavirus type. Cancer Research 56: 669–674

Ito K, Watanabe K, Karim S et al 1996 k-ras point mutation in endometrial carcinoma: effect on outcome is dependent on age of patients. Gynecologic Oncology 63: 238–246

Iversen O E 1988 Prognostic value of the flow cytometric DNA index in human ovarian carcinoma. Cancer 6: 971–975

Iversen O E, Utaaker E, Skaarland E 1988 DNA ploidy and steroid receptors as predictors of disease course in patients with endometrial carcinoma. Acta Obstetricia et Gynecologica Scandinavica 67: 531–537

Iwasaka T, Yokoyama M, Oh-Uchida M et al 1992 Detection of human papillomavirus genome and analysis of c-myc and Ha-ras oncogenes in invasive cervical carcinomas. Gynecologic Oncology 46: 298–303

Iwasaka T, Zheng P S, Yokoyama M et al 1998 Telomerase activation in cervical neoplasia. Obstetrics and Gynecology 91: 260–262

Jacobs I J, Kohler M F, Wiseman R W et al 1992 Clonal origin of epithelial ovarian carcinoma: analysis by loss of heterozygosity, p53 mutation, and X-chromosome inactivation. Journal of the National Cancer Institute 84: 1793–1798

Jacobs I J, Smith S A, Wiseman R W et al 1993 A deletion unit on chromosome 17q in epithelial ovarian tumors distal to the familial breast/ovarian cancer locus. Cancer Research 53: 1218–1221

Jakobsen A, Bichel P, Stornes 1991 Prognostic significance of DNA index in advanced ovarian cancer. International Journal of Gynecological Cancer 1: 195–197

Jarrell M A, Heintz N, Howard P et al 1993 Squamous cell carcinoma of the cervix: HPV 16 and DNA ploidy as predictors of survival. Gynecologic Oncology 46: 361–366

Ji H K, Syrjanen S, Klemi P, Chang F, Tosi P, Syrjanen K 1991 Prognostic significance of human papillomavirus (HPV) type and nuclear DNA content in invasive cervical cancer. International Journal of Gynecological Cancer 1: 59–67

Jiang X, Morland S J, Hitchcock A, Thomas E J, Campbell I G 1998 Allelotyping of endometriosis with adjacent ovarian carcinoma reveals evidence of a common lineage. Cancer Research 58: 1707–1712

Jimbo H, Hitomi Y, Yoshikawa H et al 1997 Evidence for monoclonal expansion of epithelial cells in ovarian endometrial cysts. American Journal of Pathology 150: 1173–1178

Jones M H, Koi S, Fujimoto I, Hasumi K, Kato K, Nakamura Y 1994 Allelotype of uterine cancer by analysis of RFLP and microsatellite polymorphisms: frequent loss of heterozygosity on chromosome arms 3p, 9q, 10q, and 17p. Genes Chromosomes and Cancer 9: 119–123

Jones M W, Kounelis S, Papadaki H et al 2000 Well-differentiated villoglandular adenocarcinoma of the uterine cervix: oncogene/tumor suppressor gene alterations and human papillomavirus genotyping. International Journal of Gynecological Pathology 19: 110–117

Jovanovic A S, Boynton K A, Mutter G L 1996 Uteri of women with endometrial carcinoma contain a histopathological spectrum of monoclonal putative precancers, some with microsatellite instability. Cancer Research 56: 1917–1921

Kaern J, Wetteland J, Trope C et al 1992a Comparison between flow cytometry and image cytometry in ploidy distribution assessments in gynecologic cancer. Cytometry 13: 314–321

Kaern J, Iversen T, Trope C, Pettersen E O, Nesland J M 1992b Flow cytometric DNA measurements in squamous cell carcinoma of the vulva: an important prognostic method. International Journal of Gynecological Cancer 169–174

Kaern J, Trope C G, Kristensen G B, Abeler V M, Pettersen E O 1993 DNA ploidy: the most important prognostic factor in patients with borderline tumors of the ovary. International Journal of Gynecological Cancer 3: 349–358

Kaern J, Trope C G, Kristensen C B et al 1994 Evaluation of DNA ploidy and S-phase fraction as prognostic parameters in advanced epithelial ovarian carcinoma. American Journal of Obstetrics and Gynecology 170: 479–487

Kagie M J, Kenter G G, Tollenaar R A E M, Hermans J, Trimbos J B, Fleuren G J 1997 p53 protein overexpression, a frequent observation in squamous cell carcinoma of the vulva and in various synchronous vulvar epithelia, has no value as a prognostic parameter. International Journal of Gynecological Pathology 16: 124–130

Kallioniemi O P, Punnonen R, Mattila J et al 1988 Prognostic significance of DNA index, multiploidy and S-phase fraction in ovarian cancer. Cancer 61: 334–339

Kappes S, Milde-Langosch K, Kressin P et al 1995 p53 mutations in ovarian tumors, detected by temperature-gradient gel electrophoresis, direct sequencing and immunohistochemistry. International Journal of Cancer 64: 633–634

Kaspar H G, Dinh T V, Hanningan E V 1997 Flow cytometry in cervical adenocarcinoma: correlating DNA content with clinical picture. Journal of Reproductive Medicine 42: 170–172

Katabuchi H, van Rees B, Lambers A R et al 1995 Mutations in DNA mismatch repair genes are not responsible for microsatellite instability in most sporadic endometrial carcinomas. Cancer Research 55: 5556–5560

Keenan S J, Diamond J, McCluggage G W, Bharucha H, Thompson D, Bartels P H, Hamilton P W 2000 An automated machine vision system for the histological grading of cervical intraepithelial neoplasia (CIN). Journal of Pathology 192: 351–362

Kenter G G, Cornelisse C J, Aartsen J L et al 1990 DNA ploidy level as prognostic factor in low stage carcinoma of the uterine cervix. Gynecologic Oncology 39: 181–185

Kerner H, Levy R, Friedman M, Beck D 1997 Uterine and extrauterine Müllerian adenosarcoma: a histopathologic and flow cytometric study. International Journal of Gynecological Cancer 7: 318–324

Kerns B J M, Jordan P A, Faerman L L et al 1994 Determination of proliferation index with MIB-1 in advanced ovarian cancer using quantitative image analysis. American Journal of Clinical Pathology 101: 192–197

Kersemaekers A M F, Hermans J, Fleuren G J, van de Vijver M J 1998 Loss of heterozygosity for defined regions on chromosomes 3, 11 and 17 in carcinomas of the uterine cervix. British Journal of Cancer 77: 192–200

Kersemaekers A M F, van de Vijver M J, Kenter G G, Fleuren G J 1999 Genetic alterations during the progression of squamous cell carcinomas of the uterine cervix. Genes Chromosomes and Cancer 26: 346–354

Khalifa M A, Manuel R S, Haraway S D, Walker J, Min K W 1994 Expression of EGFR, HER-2/neu, p53, and PCNA in endometrioid, serous papillary, and clear cell endometrial adenocarcinomas. Gynecologic Oncology 53: 346–354

Khoo S K, Hurst T, Kearsley G D et al 1990 Prognostic significance of tumor ploidy in patients with advanced ovarian cancer. Gynecologic Oncology 39: 284–288

Khoo S K, Battistutta D, Hurst T, Sanderson B, Ward B G, Free K 1993 The prognostic value of clinical, pathologic, and biologic parameters in ovarian cancer. Cancer 72: 479–481

Khoo U S, Ozcelik H, Cheung A N Y et al 1999 Somatic mutations in the BRCA1 gene in Chinese sporadic breast and ovarian cancer. Oncogene 18: 4643–4646

Kiechle M, Hinrichs M, Jacobsen A et al 2000 Genetic imbalances in precursor lesions of endometrial cancer detected by comparative genomic hybridization. American Journal of Pathology 156: 1827–1833

Kigawa J, Minagawa Y, Ishihara H, Kanamori Y, Terakawa N 1993 Tumor DNA ploidy and prognosis of patients with serous cystadenocarcinoma of the ovary. Cancer 72: 804–808

Kim H T, Choi B H, Nikawa N, Lee T S, Chang S I 1998 Frequent loss of imprinting of the *H19* and IGF-II genes in ovarian tumors. American Journal of Medical Genetics 80: 391–395

Kim N W, Piatyszek M A, Prowse K R et al 1994 Specific association of human telomerase activity with immortal cells and cancer. Science 266: 2011–2015

Kim Y T, Thomas N F, Kessis T D, Wilkinson E J, Hedrick L, Cho K R 1996 p53 mutations and clonality in vulvar carcinomas and squamous hyperplasias: evidence suggesting that squamous hyperplasias do not serve as direct precursors of human papillomavirus-negative vulvar carcinomas. Human Pathology 27: 389–395

Kimball R E, Schlaerth J B, Kute T et al 1997 Flow cytometric analysis of lymph node metastases in advanced ovarian cancer: clinical and biologic significance. American Journal of Obstetrics and Gynecology 176: 1326–1327

Kirchoff M, Rose H, Petersen B L et al 1999 Comparative genomic hybridization reveals a recurrent pattern of chromosomal aberrations in severe dysplasia/carcinoma in situ of the cervix and in advanced-stage cervical carcinoma. Genes Chromosomes and Cancer 24: 144–150

Klemi P J, Joensuu H, Naenpaa J, Kiiholma P 1989 Influence of cellular DNA content on survival in ovarian carcinoma. Obstetrics and Gynecology 74: 200–204

Klemi P J, Joensuu H, Tuala S 1990 Prognostic value of flow cytometric DNA content analysis in granulosa cell tumors of the ovary. Cancer 65: 1189–1193

Klemi P J, Takahashi S, Joensuu H, Kiilholma P, Narimatsu E, Mori M 1994 Immunohistochemical detection of p53 protein in borderline and malignant serous ovarian tumors. International Journal of Gynecological Pathology 13: 228–233

Kohlberger P, Kainz C, Breiteneker G et al 1995 Prognostic value of immunohistochemically detected p53 expression in vulvar carcinoma. Cancer 76: 1786–1789

Kohlberger P, Gitsch G, Loesch A, Reinthaler A, Kainz C, Breiteneker G 1996 p53 protein overexpression in early stage endometrial carcinoma. Gynecologic Oncology 62: 213–217

Kohler M F, Marks J R, Wiseman R W et al 1993 Spectrum of mutation and frequency of allelic deletion of the p53 gene in ovarian cancer. Journal of the National Cancer Institute 85: 979–983

Kolodner R D 1995 Mismatch repair: mechanisms and relationship to cancer susceptibility. Trends in Biochemical Sciences 20: 397–401

Kommoss F, Wofle H, Bauknecht T et al 1994 Co-expression of M-CSF transcripts and protein, FMS (M-CSF receptor) transcripts and protein, and steroid receptor content in adenocarcinoma of the ovary. Journal of Pathology 174: 111–119

Konski A, Domenico D, Tyrkus M et al 1996 Prognostic characteristics of surgical stage 1 endometrial adenocarcinoma. International Journal of Radiation Oncology Biology and Physics 35: 935–940

Koss L G, Czerniak B, Herz F, Westro R P 1989 Flow cytometric measurements of DNA and other cell components in human tumors: a critical appraisal. Human Pathology 20: 528–548

Kristensen G B, Holm R, Abeler V M, Trope C G 1996 Evaluation of the prognostic significance of cathpepsin-D, epidermal growth factor receptor and c-erbB-2 in early cervical squamous cell carcinoma. Cancer 78: 433–440

Kruse A J, Baak J P, de Bruin P C et al 2001 Ki-67 immunoquantitation in cervical intraepithelial neoplasia (CIN): a sensitive marker for grading. Journal of Pathology 193: 48–54

Kuoppala T, Heinola M, Aine R, Isola J, Heinonen P K 1996 Serous and mucinous borderline tumors of the ovary: a clinicopathologic and DNA-ploidy study of 102 cases. International Journal of Gynecological Cancer 6: 302–308

Kupryjanczyk J, Bell D A, Dimeo D, Beauchamp R, Thor A D, Yandell D W 1995 p53 gene analysis of ovarian borderline tumors and stage I carcinomas. Human Pathology 26: 387–392

Kupryjanczyk J, Thor A D, Beauchamp R, Poremba C, Scully R E, Yandell D W 1996 Ovarian, peritoneal, and endometrial serous carcinoma: clonal origin of multifocal disease. Modern Pathology 9: 166–173

Kushima M, Fujii H, Murakami et al 2001 Simultaneous squamous cell carcinomas of the uterine cervix and upper genital tract: loss of heterozygosity analysis demonstrates clonal neoplasms of cervical origin. International Journal of Gynecological Pathology 20: 353–358

Kuwashima Y, Uehara T, Kurosumi M, Shiromizu K, Matsuzawa M, Kishi K 1995 Cell dynamics of undifferentiated carcinoma of the ovary: immunohistochemical estimation of their growth fraction and apoptotic status. European Journal of Gynaecological Oncology 16: 268–273

Kyo S, Takakura M, Ishikawa H et al 1997 Application of telomerase assay for the screening of cervical lesions. Cancer Research 57: 1863–1867

Kyo S, Takakura M, Tanaka M et al 1998 Telomerase activity in cervical cancer is quantitatively distinct from that in its precursor lesions. International Journal of Cancer 79: 66–70

Kyo S, Kanaya T, Takakura M et al 1999 Human telomerase reverse transcriptase as a critical determinant of telomerase activity in normal and malignant endometrial tissues. International Journal of Cancer 80: 60–63

Lage J M, Bagg A 1996 Hydatidiform moles: DNA flow cytometry, image analysis and selected topics in molecular biology. Histopathology 28: 379–382

Lage J M, Mark S D, Roberts D J, Goldstein D P, Bernstein M R, Berkowitz R S 1992 A flow cytometric study of 137 fresh hydropic placentas: correlation between types of hydatidiform moles and nuclear DNA ploidy. Obstetrics and Gynecology 79: 403–410

Lage J M, Popek E J 1993 The role of DNA flow cytometry in evaluation of partial and complete hydatidiform moles and hydropic abortions. Seminars in Diagnostic Pathology 10: 267–274

Lai C H, Hsueh S, Chang T C et al 1996 The role of DNA flow cytometry in borderline malignant ovarian tumors. Cancer 78: 794–802

Lai C H, Hsueh S, Chang T C et al 1997 Prognostic factors in patients with bulky stage IB or IIA cervical carcinoma undergoing neoadjuvant chemotherapy and radical hysterectomy. Gynecologic Oncology 64: 456–462

Larson A A, Liao S Y, Stanbridge E J, Cavenee W K, Hampton G M 1997 Genetic alterations accumulate during cervical tumorigenesis and indicate a common origin for multifocal lesions. Cancer Research 57: 4171–4176

Larson D M, Berg R, Shaw G, Krawisz B R 1999 Prognostic significance of DNA ploidy in endometrial cancer. Gynecologic Oncology 74: 356–360

Lax S F, Pizer E S, Ronnett B M, Kurman R J 1998a Comparison of estrogen and progesterone receptor, Ki-67, and p53 immunoreactivity in uterine endometrioid carcinoma with squamous, mucinous, secretory, and ciliated cell differentiation. Human Pathology 29: 924–931

Lax S F, Pizer E S, Ronnett B M, Kurman R J 1998b Clear cell carcinoma of the endometrium is characterized by a distinctive profile of p53, Ki-67, estrogen and progesterone receptor expression. Human Pathology 29: 551–558

Layfield L J, Saria E A, Berchuck A et al 1997 Prognostic value of MIB-1 in advanced ovarian cancer as determined using automated immunohistochemistry and quantitative image analysis. Journal of Surgical Oncology 66: 230–237

Layfield L J, Liu K, Dodge R, Barsky S H 2000 Uterine smooth muscle tumors: utility of classification by proliferation, ploidy, and prognostic markers versus traditional histopathology. Archives of Pathology and Laboratory Medicine 124: 221–227

Lee Y S 1995 p53 expression in gestational trophoblastic disease. International Journal of Gynecological Pathology 14: 119–124

Leeson S C, Morphopoulos G, Buckley C H, Hale R J 1995 c-erbB-2 oncogene expression in stage I epithelial ovarian cancer. British Journal of Obstetrics and Gynaecology 102: 65–67

Leminen A, Paavonen J, Vesterinen E et al 1990 Deoxyribonucleic acid cytometric analysis of cervical adenocarcinoma: prognostic significance of deoxyribonucleic acid ploidy and S-phase fraction. American Journal of Obstetrics and Gynecology 162: 848–853

Levesque M A, Katsaros D, Yu H et al 1995 Mutant p53 protein overexpression is associated with poor outcome in patients with well or moderately differentiated ovarian carcinoma. Cancer 75: 1327–1338

Levine E L, Renehan A, Gossiel R et al 1995 Apoptosis, intrinsic radiosensitivity and prediction of radiotherapy response in cervical carcinoma. Radiotherapy Oncology 37: 1–9

Levine R L, Cargile C B, Blazes M S, van Rees B, Kurman R J, Ellenson L H 1998 PTEN mutations and microsatellite instability in complex atypical hyperplasia, a precursor lesion to uterine endometrioid carcinoma. Cancer Research 58: 3254–3258

Levy B, Mukherjee T, Hirschhorn K 2000 Molecular cytogenetic analysis of uterine leiomyoma and leiomyosarcoma by comparative genomic hybridization. Cancer Genetics and Cytogenetics 121: 1–8

Li E, Beard C, Jaenisch R 1993 Role for DNA methylation in genomic imprinting. Nature 366: 362–365

Li S, Han H, Resnik E, Carcangiu M L, Schwartz P E, Yang-Feng T L 1993 Advanced ovarian carcinoma: molecular evidence of unifocal origin. Gynecologic Oncology 51: 21–25

Lie A K, Skarsvag S, Skomedal H, Haugen O A, Holm R 1999 Expression of p53, MDM2, and p21 proteins in high-grade cervical intraepithelial neoplasia and relationship to human papillomavirus infection. International Journal of Gynecological Pathology 18: 5–11

Lin W M, Forgacs E, Warshal D P et al 1998 Loss of heterozygosity and mutational analysis of the PTEN/MMAC1 gene in synchronous endometrial and ovarian carcinomas. Clinical Cancer Research 4: 2577–2583

Lindahl B, Gullberg B 1991 Flow cytometrical DNA-ploidy and clinical parameters in the prediction of prognosis in Stage I–II endometrial cancer. Anticancer Research 11: 397–401

Lindahl B, Alm P, Killander D, Langstrom E, Trope C 1987a Flow cytometric DNA analysis of normal and cancerous human endometrium and cytological–histopathological correlations. Anticancer Research 7: 781–789

Lindahl B, Alm P, Ferno M, Killander D, Langstrom E, Norgren A, Trope C 1987b Prognostic value of flow cytometrical DNA measurements in stage I–II endometrial carcinoma: correlations with steroid receptor concentration, tumor myometrial invasion, and degree of differentiation. Anticancer Research 7: 791–798

Liu F S, Kohler M F, Marks J R, Bast R C, Boyd J, Berchuck A 1994 Mutation and overexpression of the p53 tumor suppression gene frequently occurs in uterine and ovarian sarcomas. Obstetrics and Gynecology 83: 118–124

Liu S S, Tsang B K, Cheung A N Y et al 2001 Anti-apoptotic proteins, apoptotic and proliferative parameters and their prognostic significance in cervical carcinoma. European Journal of Cancer 37: 1104–1110

Liu Y, Heyman M, Wang Y et al 1994 Molecular analysis of the retinoblastoma gene in primary ovarian cancer cells. International Journal of Cancer 58: 663–667

Lu K H, Bell D A, Welch W R, Berkowitz R S, Mok S C 1998 Evidence for the multifocal origin of bilateral and advanced human serous borderline ovarian tumors. Cancer Research 58: 2328–2330

Lu X, Nikaido T, Toki T et al 2000 Loss of heterozygosity among tumor suppressor genes in invasive and situ carcinoma of the uterine cervix. International Journal of Gynecological Cancer 10: 452–458

Luft F, Gebert J, Schneider A, Melsheimer P, Doeberitz M V 1999 Frequent allelic imbalance of tumor suppressor gene loci in cervical dysplasia. International Journal of Gynecological Pathology 18: 374–380

Lukes A S, Kohler M F, Pieper C F et al 1994 Multivariate analysis of DNA ploidy, p53 and HER-2/neu as prognostic factors in endometrial carcinoma. Cancer 73: 2380–2385

Magtibay P M, Perrone J F, Stanhope R, Katzmann J A, Keeney G L, Li H 1999 Flow cytometric analysis of early stage adenocarcinoma of the cervix. Gynecologic Oncology 75: 242–247

Makar A P, Holm R, Kristensen G B, Nesland J M, Trope O G 1994 The expression of c-erbB-2 (HER-2/neu) oncogene in invasive ovarian malignancies. International Journal of Gynecological Cancer 4: 194–199

Malcolm E K, Baber G B, Boyd J C, Stoler M H 2000 Polymorphism at codon 72 of p53 is not associated with cervical cancer risk. Modern Pathology 13: 373–378

Manek S, Wells M 1996 The significance of alterations in p53 expression in gynaecological neoplasms. Current Opinion in Obstetrics and Gynecology 8: 52–55

Mano Y, Kikuchi Y, Yamamoto K et al 1999 Bcl-2 as a predictor of chemosensitivity and prognosis in primary epithelial ovarian cancer. European Journal of Cancer 35: 1214–1219

Mariani L, Conti L, Antenucci A, Vercillo M, Atlante M, Gandolfo G M 2000 Predictive value of cell kinetics in endometrial adenocarcinoma. Anticancer Research 20: 3569–3574

Mark H F, Jenkins R, Miller W A 1997 Current applications of molecular cytogenetic technologies. Annals of Clinical Laboratory Science 27: 47–56

Marone M, Scambia G, Mozzetti S et al 1998 BCL-2, BAX, BCL-XL, and BCL-XS expression in normal and neoplastic ovarian tissues. Clinical Cancer Research 4: 517–524

Marra G, Boland C R 1995 Hereditary nonpolyposis colorectal cancer: the syndrome, the genes, and historical perspectives. Journal of the National Cancer Institute 87: 1114–1125

Matias-Guiu X, Lagarda H, Catasus L et al 2002 Clonality analysis in synchronous or metachronous tumors of the female genital tract. International Journal of Gynecological Pathology 21: 205–211

Matsushima M, Kobayashi K, Emi M et al 1995 Mutation analysis of the BRCA1 gene in 76 Japanese ovarian cancer patients: four germline mutations, but no evidence of somatic mutation. Human Molecular Genetics 4: 1953–1956

Maxwell G L, Risinger J I, Tong B et al 1998a Mutation of the PTEN tumor suppressor gene is not a feature of ovarian cancers. Gynecologic Oncology 70: 13–16

Maxwell G L, Risinger J I, Gumbs C et al 1998b Mutation of the PTEN tumor suppressor gene in endometrial hyperplasia. Cancer Research 58: 2500–2503

McCarthy R, Fetterhoff T 1989 Issues for quality assurance in clinical flow cytometry. Archives of Pathology and Laboratory Medicine 21: 551–558

McCluggage W G, Buhidma M, Tang L, Maxwell P Bharucha H 1996 Monoclonal antibody MIB-1 in the assessment of cervical squamous intraepithelial lesions. International Journal of Gynecological Pathology 15: 131–136

McCluggage W G, McBride H, Maxwell P, Bharucha H 1997 Immunohistochemical detection of p53 and Bcl-2 proteins in neoplastic and non-neoplastic endocervical glandular lesions. International Journal of Gynecological Pathology 17: 29–35

McCluggage W G, Maxwell P, Bharucha H 1998 Immunohistochemical detection of metallothionein and MIB1 in uterine cervical squamous lesions. International Journal of Gynecological Pathology 17: 29–35

McManus D T, Murphy M, Arthur K, Hamilton P W, Russell S E, Toner P G 1996 p53 mutation, allele loss on chromosome 17p, and DNA content in ovarian carcinoma. Journal of Pathology 179: 177–182

Meden H, Marx D, Rath W et al 1994 Overexpression of the oncogene c-erbB-2 in primary ovarian cancer: evaluation of the prognostic value in a Cox proportional hazards multiple regression. International Journal of Gynecological Pathology 13: 45–53

Meganck G, Moerman Ph, Schrijver D de, Berteloot P, Vergote I 1998 A non-diploid, small cell carcinoma of the ovary of the hypercalcemic type. International Journal of Gynecological Cancer 8: 430–433

Melchiorri C, Chieco P, Lisignoli G, Marabini A, Orlandi C 1993 Ploidy disturbance as an early indicator of intrinsic malignancy in endometrial carcinoma. Cancer 72: 165–172

Merajver S D, Pham T M, Caduff R F et al 1995 Somatic mutations in the BRCA1 gene in sporadic ovarian tumours. Nature Genetics 9: 439–443

Meyer J S, Gersell D J, Yim S 2001 Cell proliferation in ovarian carcinoma: superior accuracy of S-phase fraction (SPF) by DNA labelling index versus flow cytometric SPF, lack of independent prognostic power for SPF and DNA ploidy, and limited effect of SPF on tumor growth rate. Gynecologic Oncology 81: 466–476

Millar A L, Pal T, Madlensky L et al 1999 Mismatch repair gene defects contribute to the genetic basis of double primary cancers of the colorectum and endometrium. Human Molecular Genetics 8: 823–829

Miller B E, Barron B A, Dockter M E, Delmore J E, Silva E G, Gershenson D M 2001 Parameters of differentiation and proliferation in adult granulosa cell tumors of the ovary. Cancer Detection and Prevention 25: 48–54

Minckwitz G von, Kuhns W, Kaufmann M, Feichter G E, Heep J, Schmid, H, Bastert G 1994 Prognostic importance of DNA-ploidy and S-phase fraction in endometrial cancer. International Journal of Gynecological Cancer 4: 250–256

Mittal A L, Mesia A, Demopoulos R I 1999 MIB-1 expression is useful in distinguishing dysplasia from atrophy in elderly women. International Journal of Gynecological Pathology 18: 122–124

Mittal K R, Demopoulos R J, Goswami S 1993 Proliferating cell nuclear antigen (cyclin) expression in normal and abnormal squamous epithelia. American Journal of Surgical Pathology 17: 117–122

Miura K, Obama M, Yun K et al 1999 Methylation imprinting of H19 and SNRPN genes in human benign ovarian teratomas. American Journal of Human Genetics 65: 1359–1367

Mok S C, Bell D A, Knapp R C et al 1993 Mutation of K-ras protooncogene in human ovarian epithelial tumors of borderline malignancy. Cancer Research 53: 1489–1492

Monk B J, Chapman J A, Johnson G A et al 1994 Correlation of C-myc and HER-2/neu amplification and expression with histopathologic variables in uterine corpus cancer. American Journal of Obstetrics and Gynecology 171: 1193–1198

Mora L B, Diaz J L, Cantor A B, Nicosia S V 1999 Differential diagnosis of endometrial hyperplasia and carcinoma by computerized image cytometry of cell proliferation, apoptosis and BCL-2 expression. Annals of Clinical Laboratory Science 29: 308–315

Morsi H M, Leers M P G, Radespiel-Troger M et al 2000 Apoptosis, Bcl-2 expression and proliferation in benign and malignant endometrial epithelium: an approach using multiparameter flow cytometry. Gynecologic Oncology 77: 11–17

Muller C Y, O'Boyle J D, Fong K M et al 1998 Abnormalities of fragile histidine triad genomic and complementary DNAs in cervical cancer: association with human papillomavirus type. Journal of the National Cancer Institute 90: 433–439

Mundle S D, Gao X Z, Khan S, Gregory S A, Preisler H D, Raza A 1995 Two in situ labelling techniques reveal different patterns of DNA fragmentation during spontaneous apoptosis in vivo and induced apoptosis in vitro. Anticancer Research 15: 1895–1904

Mutter G L, Chaponot M L, Fletcher J A 1995 A polymerase chain reaction assay for non-random X chromosome inactivation identifies monoclonal endometrial cancers and precancers. American Journal of Pathology 146: 501–508

Mutter G L, Wada H Faquin W C, Enomoto T 1999 K-ras mutations appear in the premalignant phase of both microsatellite stable and unstable endometrial carcinogenesis. Molecular Pathology 52: 257–262

Mutter G L, Lin M C, Fitzgerald J T et al 2000a Altered PTEN expression as a diagnostic marker for the earliest endometrial precancers. Journal of the National Cancer Institute 92: 924–930

Mutter G L, Baak J P A, Crum C P, Richart R M, Ferenczy A, Faquin W C 2000b Endometrial precancer diagnosis by histopathology, clonal analysis and computerized morphometry. Journal of Pathology 190: 462–469

Mutter G L, Ince T A, Baak J P A, Kust G A, Zhou X P, Eng C 2001 Molecular identification of latent precancers in histologically normal endometrium. Cancer Research 61: 4311–4314

Nagase S, Sato S, Tezuka F, Wada Y, Yajima A, Horii A 1996 Deletion mapping on chromosome 10q25–q26 in human endometrial cancer. British Journal of Cancer 74: 1979–1983

Nakagawa S, Yoshikawa H, Kimura M et al 1999 A possible involvement of aberrant expression of the FHIT gene in the carcinogenesis of squamous cell carcinoma of the uterine cervix. British Journal of Cancer 79: 589–594

Nakamura T, Nomura S, Sakai T, Nariya S 1997 Expression of BCL-2 oncoprotein in gastrointestinal and uterine carcinomas and their premalignant lesions. Human Pathology 28: 309–315

Nakano K, Watney E, McDougall J K 1998 Telomerase activity and expression of telomerase RNA component and telomerase catalytic subunit gene in cervical cancer. American Journal of Pathology 153: 857–864

Nakano T, Oka K, Ishikawa A, Morita S 1997 Correlation of cervical carcinoma c-erbB-2 oncogene with cell proliferation parameters in patients treated with radiation therapy for cervical carcinoma. Cancer 79: 513–520

Nevin J, Laing D, Kaye P et al 1999 The significance of Erb-b2 immunostaining in cervical cancer. Gynecologic Oncology 73: 354–358

Newbury R, Schuerch C, Godspeed N, Fanning J, Glidewell O, Evans M 1990 DNA content as a prognostic factor in endometrial carcinoma. Obstetrics and Gynecology 76: 251–257

Ngan H Y S, Liu S S, Yu H, Liu K L, Cheung A N Y 1999a Proto-oncogenes and p53 protein expression in normal cervical stratified squamous epithelium and cervical intra-epithelial neoplasia. European Journal of Cancer 35: 1546–1550

Ngan H Y S, Liu V W, Liu S S 1999b Risk of cervical cancer is not increased in Chinese carrying homozygous arginine at codon 72 of p53. British Journal of Cancer 80: 1828–1829

Ngan H Y S, Cheung A N Y, Liu S S, Yip P S, Tsao S W 1999c Abnormal expression or mutation of TP53 and HPV in vulvar cancer. European Journal of Cancer 35: 481–484

Nilbert M, Pejovic T, Mandahl N et al 1995 Monoclonal origin of endometriotic cysts. International Journal of Gynecological Cancer 5: 61–63

Nishioka T, West C M, Gupta N et al 1999 Prognostic significance of c-erbB-2 protein expression in carcinoma of the cervix treated with radiotherapy. Journal of Cancer Research and Clinical Oncology 125: 96–100

Niwa K, Itoh M, Murase T 1994 Alterations of p53 gene in ovarian carcinoma: clinicopathologic correlation and prognostic significance. British Journal of Cancer 70: 1191–1197

Nola M, Babic D, Ilic S et al 1996 Prognostic parameters for survival in patients with mesenchymal tumors of the uterus. Cancer 78: 2543–2550

Nordal R R, Kristensen G B, Kaern J, Stenwic A E, Pettersen E O, Trope C G 1996 The prognostic significance of surgery, tumor size, malignancy grade, menopausal status, and DNA ploidy in endometrial stromal sarcoma. Gynecologic Oncology 62: 254–259

Nordstrom B, Strang P, Lindgren A, Bergstrom R, Tribuukait B 1996a Carcinoma of the endometrium: do the nuclear grade and DNA ploidy provide more prognostic information than do the FIGO and WHO classifications? International Journal of Gynecological Pathology 15: 191–201

Nordstrom B, Strang P, Bergstrom R, Nilsson S, Tribukait B 1996b A comparison of proliferation markers and their prognostic value for women with endometrial carcinoma: Ki-67, proliferating cell nuclear antigen and flow cytometric S-phase factor. Cancer 78: 1942–1951

Obata K, Morland S J, Watson R H et al 1998 Frequent PTEN/MMAC mutations in endometrioid but not serous or mucinous epithelial ovarian tumours. Cancer Research 58: 2095–2097

Oka K, Arai T 1996 MIB1 growth fraction is not related to prognosis in cervical squamous cell carcinoma treated with radiotherapy. International Journal of Gynecological Pathology 15: 23–27

Oka K, Hoshi T, Arai T 1992 Prognostic significance of the PC10 index as a prospective assay for cervical cancer treated with radiation therapy alone. Cancer 70: 1545–1550

Oka N, Nakano T, Arai T 1997 Expression of cathpepsin-D and epidermal growth factor receptor in stage III cervical carcinomas. International Journal of Gynecological Cancer 7: 122–126

Okon D, Basta A, Stachura J 1998 Morphometry separates squamous cell carcinoma of the vulva into two distinct groups. Polish Journal of Pathology 49: 293–295

Orille V, Sampedro A, Ferrer-Barriendos J, Corral N, Martinez A 1993 Quantitative pathology of the cervical intraepithelial neoplasia. European Journal of Gynaecological Oncology 14: 491–500

Oshita T, Nagai N, Ohama K 2000 Expression of telomerase reverse transcriptase mRNA and its quantitative analysis in human endometrial cancer. International Journal of Oncology 17: 1225–1230

Oud P S, Soeters R P, Pahlplatz M M M et al 1988 DNA cytometry of pure dysgerminomas of the ovary. International Journal of Gynecological Pathology 7: 258–267

Padberg P-C, Arps H, Franke U et al 1992a DNA cytophotometry and prognosis in ovarian tumors of borderline malignancy: a clinicopathological study of 80 cases. Cancer 69: 2510–2514

Padberg P-C, Stegner H E, von Sengbusch S, Arps H, Schroder S 1992b DNA cytophotometry and immunocytochemistry in ovarian tumours of borderline, malignancy and related peritoneal lesions. Virchows Archiv A Pathological Anatomy 421: 497–503

Pao C C, Tseng C J, Lin C Y et al 1997 Differential expression of telomerase activity in human cervical cancer and cervical intraepithelial neoplasia lesions. Journal of Clinical Oncology 15: 1932–1937

Paradinas F J, Browne P, Fisher R A, Foskett M, Bagshawe K D, Newlands E 1996 A clinical, histological and flow cytometric study of 149 complete moles, 146 partial moles and 107 non-molar hydropic abortions. Histopathology 28: 101–109

Park J S, Kim H K, Han S K, Lee J M, Namkoong S E, Kim S J 1995 Detection of c-K-ras point mutation in ovarian cancer. International Journal of Gynecological Cancer 5: 107–111

Park S J, Chan P J, Seraj I M, King A 1999 Denaturing gradient gel electrophoresis screening of the BRCA1 gene in cells from precancerous cervical lesions. Journal of Reproductive Medicine 44: 575–580

Park T W, Richart S M, Sun X W, Wright T C Jr 1996 Association between human papillomavirus type and clonal status of cervical squamous intraepithelial lesions. Journal of the National Cancer Institute 88: 355–358

Pasini A, Corbella P, Colombo E, Redaelli L, Belloni C 2000 Carcinoma endometriale: significato prognostico della ploidia cellulare. Minerva Ginecologica 52: 179–184

Peyton C L 1998 Comparison of PCR- and hybrid capture-based human papillomavirus detection systems using multiple cervical specimen collection strategies. Journal of Clinical Microbiology 36: 3248–3254

Pfisterer J, Kommoss F, Sauerbrei A et al 1994 Cellular DNA content and survival in advanced ovarian cancer. Cancer 74: 2509–2515

Pfisterer J, Kommos, Sauerbrei W et al 1995 Prognostic value of DNA ploidy and S phase fraction in stage I endometrial carcinoma. Gynecologic Oncology 58: 149–156

Pfisterer J, Kommoss F, Sauerbrei W et al 1996 DNA flow cytometry in stage IB and II cervical carcinoma. International Journal of Gynecological Cancer 6: 54–60

Phillips N J, Ziegler M R, Radford D M et al 1996 Allelic deletion on chromosome 17p13.3 in early ovarian cancer. Cancer Research 56: 606–611

Pieretti M, Turker M S 1997 Mutation, ageing, and ovarian cancer. Lancet 349: 700–701

Pieretti M, Powell D, Gallion H H, Caze E, Conway P S, Turker M S 1995 Genetic alterations on chromosome 17 distinguish types of epithelial ovarian tumors. Human Pathology 26: 393–397

Pietrzak K, Olszewski W 1998 DNA ploidy as a prognostic factor in patients with ovarian carcinoma. Polish Journal of Pathology 49: 141–144

Pillai M R, Jayaprakash P G, Nair M K 1999 Bcl-2 immunoreactivity but not p53 accumulation associated with tumour response to radiotherapy in cervical carcinoma. Journal of Cancer Research and Clinical Oncology 125: 55–60

Pisani A L, Barbuto D A, Chen D, Ramos L, Lagasse L D, Karlan B Y 1995 HER-2/neu, p53 and DNA analyses as prognosticators for survival in endometrial carcinoma. Obstetrics and Gynecology 85: 729–734

Polacarz S V, Hey N A, Stephenson T J, Hill A S 1989 c-myc oncogene product P62c-myc in ovarian mucinous neoplasms: immunohistochemical study correlated with malignancy. Journal of Clinical Pathology 42: 896–899

Poljak M, Brencic A, Seme K et al 1999 Comparative evaluation of first- and second-generation digene hybrid capture assays for detection of human papillomaviruses associated with high or intermediate risk for cervical cancer. Journal of Clinical Microbiology 37: 796–797

Poulin N, Boiko I, MacAulay C 1999 Nuclear morphometry as an intermediate endpoint biomarker in chemoprevention of cervical carcinoma using alpha-diflouromethylornithine. Cytometry 38: 214–223

Prat J, Oliva E, Lerma E, Vaquero M, Matias-Guiu X 1994 Uterine papillary serous adenocarcinoma: a 10-case study of p53 and c-erbB-2 expression and DNA content. Cancer 74: 1778–1783

Quinn C M, Wright N A 1992 The usefulness of clinical measurements of cell proliferation in gynecological cancer. International Journal of Gynecological Pathology 11: 361–369

Raju G C 1994 Expression of the proliferating cell nuclear antigen in cervical neoplasia. International Journal of Gynecological Pathology 13: 337–341

Reddy V G, Khanna N, Jain S K, Dash B C, Singh N 2001 Telomerase — a molecular marker for cervical cancer screening. International Journal of Gynecological Cancer 11: 100–106

Rienartz J J, Goerge E, Lindgren B R. Niehans G A 1994 Expression of p53, transforming growth factor alpha, epidermal growth factor receptor, and c-erbB-2 in endometrial carcinoma and correlation with survival and known predictors of survival. Human Pathology 25: 1075–1083

Reles A E, Gee C, Schellschmidt I et al 1998 Prognostic significance of DNA content and S-phase fraction in epithelial ovarian carcinomas analyzed by image cytometry. Gynecologic Oncology 71: 3–13

Resnik E, Trujillo Y P, Taxy J B 1997 Long term survival and DNA ploidy in advanced epithelial ovarian cancer. Journal of Surgical Oncology 64: 299–303

Resnik M, Lester S, Tate J E, Sheets E E, Sparks C, Crum C P 1996 Viral and histopathologic correlates of MN and MIB-1 expression in cervical intraepithelial neoplasia. Human Pathology 27: 234–239

Riben M W, Malfetano J H, Nazeer T, Muraca P J, Ambros R A, Ross J S 1997 Identification of HER-2/neu oncogene amplification by fluorescence in situ hybridization in stage I endometrial carcinoma. Modern Pathology 10: 823–831

Rice L W, Mark S D, Berkowitz R S, Goff B A, Lage J M 1995 Clinicopathologic variables, operative characteristics, and DNA ploidy in predicting outcome in ovarian epithelial carcinoma. Obstetrics and Gynecology 86: 379–385

Riethdorf S, Riethdorf L, Schulz G et al 2001 Relationship between telomerase activation and HPV 16/18 oncogene expression in squamous intraepithelial lesions and squamous cell carcinomas of the uterine cevix. International Journal of Gynecological Pathology 20: 177–185

Risinger J I, Berchuck A, Kohler M F, Watson P, Lynch H T, Boyd J 1993 Genetic instability of microsatellites in endometrial carcinoma. Cancer Research 53 (Suppl 21): 5100–5103

Risinger J I, Hayes A K, Berchuck A, Barrett J C 1997 PTEN/MMAC1 mutations in endometrial cancers. Cancer Research 57: 4736–4738

Robinson R 1992 Defining the limits of DNA cytometry. American Journal of Clinical Pathology 26: 275–277

Rodenberg C J, Cornelisse C J, Heintz P A, Hermans J, Fleuren G J 1987 Tumor ploidy as a major prognostic factor in advanced ovarian cancer. Cancer 59: 317–323

Rolitsky C D, Theil K S, McGaughy V R, Copeland L J, Niemann T H 1999 HER-2/neu amplification and overexpression in endometrial carcinoma. International Journal of Gynecological Pathology 18: 138–143

Rosen A C, Ausch C, Hafner E et al 1998 A 15-year overview of management and prognosis in primary fallopian tube carcinoma. Australian Cooperative Study Group for Fallopian Tube Carcinoma. European Journal of Cancer 34: 1725–1729

Rosenberg P, Wingren S, Simonsen E, Stal O, Risberg O, Nordenskjold B 1989 Flow cytometric measurements in DNA index, and S-phase on paraffin embedded early stage endometrial carcinoma: an important prognostic indicator. Gynecologic Oncology 35: 50–54

Rosenberg P, Wingren S, Guerrieri C 1997 Flow-cytometric DNA heterogenicity in paraffin-embedded endometrial cancer. Acta Oncologica 36: 23–26

Rosenthal A N, Ryan A, Al Jehani R M, Storey A, Harwood C A, Jacobs I J 1998 p53 codon 72 polymorphism and risk of cervical cancer in UK. Lancet 352: 871–872

Ross J A, Schmidt P T, Perentesis J P, Davies S M 1999 Genomic imprinting of *H19* and insulin-like growth factor 2 in pediatric germ cell tumors. Cancer 85: 1389–1394

Ross J S, Yang F, Kallakury B V, Sheehan C E, Ambros R A, Muraca P J 1999 HER-2-neu oncogene amplification by fluorescence in situ hybridization in epithelial tumors of the ovary. American Journal of Clinical Pathology 111: 311–316

Rubin S C, Finstad C L, Wong G Y et al 1993 Prognostic significance of HER-2/neu expression in advanced epithelial ovarian cancer: a multivariate analysis. American Journal of Obstetrics and Gynecology 168: 162–169

Rubin S C, Finstad C L, Federici M G et al 1994 Prevalance and significance of HER-2/neu expression in early epithelial ovarian cancer. Cancer 73: 1456–1459

Saffari B, Jones L A, el-Naggar A, Felix J C, George G, Press M F 1995 Amplification and overexpression of HER-2/neu (c-erbB-2) in endometrial cancers: correlation with overall survival. Cancer Research 55: 5693–5698

Saito T, Schneider A, Martel N et al 1997 Proliferation-associated regulation of telomerase activity in human endometrium and its potential implication in early cancer diagnosis. Biochemical Biophysics Research Communication 231: 610–614

Sakuragi N, Ohkouchi T, Hareyama H et al 1998 Bcl-2 expression and prognosis of patients with endometrial carcinoma. International Journal of Cancer 79: 153–158

Salomon D S, Brandt R, Ciardiello F, Normanno J 1995 Epidermal growth factor-related peptides and their receptors in human malignancies. Critical Reviews in Oncology/Hematology 19: 183–232

Salvesen H B, Iversen O E, Akslen L A 1998 Identification of high risk patients by assessment of nuclear Ki-67 expression in a prospective study of endometrial carcinomas. Clinical Cancer Research 4: 2779–2785

Santini D, Ceccarelli C, Martinelli G N et al 1994 Immunocytochemical study of epidermal growth factor receptor, transforming growth factor alpha, and 'squamous differentiation' in human endometrial carcinoma. Human Pathology 25: 1319–1323

Saretzki G, Hoffmann U, Rohlke P et al 1997 Identification of allelic losses in benign, borderline, and invasive epithelial ovarian tumors and correlation with clinical outcome. Cancer 80: 1241–1249

Sasaki H, Nishi H, Takahashi H et al 1993 Mutation of the Ki-ras protooncogene in human endometrial hyperplasia and carcinoma. Cancer Research 53: 1906–1910

Sasano H, Nagura H, Silverberg S G 1992 Immunolocalization of c-myc oncoprotein in mucinous and serous adenocarcinomas of the ovary. Human Pathology 23: 491–495

Sato S, Ito K, Ozawa N et al 1991 Expression of c-myc, epidermal growth factor receptor and c-erbB-2 in human endometrial carcinoma and cervical adenocarcinoma. Tohoku Journal of Experimental Medicine 165: 137–145

Sato S, Kigawa J, Minagawa Y et al 1999 Chemosensitivity and p53-dependent apoptosis in epithelial ovarian carcinoma. Cancer 86: 1307–1313

Sawada M, Azuma C, Hashimoto K et al 1994 Clonal analysis of human gynecologic cancers by means of the polymerase chain reaction. International Journal of Cancer 58: 492–496

Scambia G, Panici P B, Ferrandina G et al 1993 Expression of HER-2/neu oncoprotein, DNA-ploidy and S-phase fraction in advanced ovarian cancer. International Journal of Gynecological Cancer 3: 271–278

Schammel D P, Bocklage T 1996 P53, PCNA and Ki-67 in hydropic molar and nonmolar placentas: an immunohistochemical study. International Journal of Gynecological Pathology 15: 156–166

Schildkraut J M, Bastos E, Berchuck A 1997 A relationship between lifetime ovulatory cycles and overexpression of mutant p53 in epithelial ovarian cancer. Journal of the National Cancer Institute 89: 932–938

Schonborn I, Minguillon C, Reles A et al 1996 Significance of PCNA proliferating fraction for prognosis of ovarian carcinoma. Geburtshilfe und Frauenheilkunde 56: 357–364

Schorge J O, Muto M G, Welch W R et al 1998 Molecular evidence for multifocal papillary serous carcinoma of the peritoneum in patients with germline BRCA1 mutations. Journal of the National Cancer Institute 90: 841–845

Schueler J A, Cornelisse C J, Hermans J, Trimbos J B, van der Burg M E L, Fleuren G J 1993 Prognostic factors in well-differentiated early stage epithelial ovarian cancer. Cancer 71: 787–795

Schueler J A, Trimbos J B, Burg M, Cornelisse C J, Hermans J, Fleuren G J 1996 DNA index reflects the biological behaviour of ovarian carcinoma stage I–IIa. Gynecologic Oncology 62: 59–66

Schultz D C, Vanderveer L, Berman D B, Hamilton T C, Wong A J, Godwin A K 1996 Identification of two candidate tumor suppressor genes on chromosome 17p13.3. Cancer Research 56: 1997–2002

Schummer M, Ng W V, Bumgarner R E et al 1999 Comparative hybridization of an array of 21,500 ovarian cDNAs for the discovery of genes overexpressed in ovarian carcinomas. Gene 238: 375–385

Scurry J, Hung J, Flowers L, Kneafsays P, Gazdar A 1999 Ploidy in human papillomavirus positive and negative squamous cell carcinomas and adjacent skin lesions. International Journal of Gynecological Cancer 9: 187–193

Segawa T, Sasagawa T, Yamazaki H, Sakaike J, Ishikawa H, Inoue M 1999 Fragile histidine triad transcription abnormalities and human papillomavirus E6-E7 mRNA expression in the development of cervical carcinoma. Cancer 85: 2001–2010

Sharma A Pratap M, Sawhney V M et al 1999 Frequent amplification of C-erbB2 (HER-2/neu) oncogene in cervical carcinoma as detected by non-fluorescence in situ hybridization technique on paraffin sections. Oncology 56: 83–87

Shenson D L, Gallion H H, Powell D E, Pieretti M 1995 Loss of heterozygosity and genomic instability in synchronous endometrioid tumors of the ovary and endometrium. Cancer 76: 1052–1060

Sheridan M T, Cooper R A, West C M 1999 A high ratio of apoptosis to proliferation correlates with improved survival after radiotherapy for cervical adenocarcinoma. International Journal of Radiation Oncology, Biology and Physics 44: 507–512

Shi Y F, Xie X, Zhao C L et al 1996 Lack of mutation in tumour-suppressor gene p53 in gestational trophoblastic tumours. British Journal of Cancer 73: 1216–1219

Shim C, Zhang W, Rhee C H, Lee J H 1998 Profiling of differentially expressed genes in human primary cervical cancer by complementary DNA expression array. Clinical Cancer Research 4: 3045–3050

Shoji Y, Saegusa M, Takano Y, Ohbu M, Okayasu I 1996 Correlation of apoptosis with tumour cell differentiation, progression, and HPV infection in cervical carcinoma. Journal of Clinical Pathology 49: 134–138

Shroyer K R, Stephens J K, Silverberg S G et al 1997 Telomerase expression in normal endometrium, endometrial hyperplasia, and endometrial adenocarcinoma. International Journal of Gynecological Pathology 16: 225–232

Shroyer K R, Thompson L C, Enomoto T et al 1998 Telomerase expression in normal epithelium, reactive atypia, squamous dysplasia, and squamous cell carcinoma of the uterine cervix. American Journal of Clinical Pathology 109: 153–162

Shurbaji M S, Brooks S K, Thurmond T S 1993 Proliferating cell nuclear antigen: immunoreactivity in cervical intraepithelial neoplasia and benign cervical epithelium. American Journal of Clinical Pathology 100: 22–26

Silvestrini R, Daidone M G, Veneroni S et al 1998 The clinical predictivity of biomarkers of stage III–IV epithelial ovarian cancer in a prospective randomized treatment protocol. Cancer 82: 159–167

Simpkins S B, Bocker T, Swisher E M et al 1999 MLH1 promoter methylation and gene silencing is the primary cause of microsatellite instability in sporadic endometrial cancers. Human Molecular Genetics 8: 661–666

Simpson B J B, Weatherill J, Miller E P, Lessells A M, Langson S P, Miller W R 1995 c-erbB-3 protein expression in ovarian tumours. British Journal of Cancer 71: 758–762

Singleton T P, Perrone T, Oakley G et al 1994 Activation of c-erbB-2 and prognosis in ovarian carcinoma. Cancer 73: 1460–1466

Skirnisdottir I, Sorbe B, Seidal T 2001a The growth factor receptors HER-2/neu and EGFR, their relationship, and their effects on the prognosis in early stage (FIGO I–II) epithelial ovarian carcinoma. International Journal of Gynecological Cancer 11: 119–129

Skirnisdottir I, Sorbe B, Seidal T 2001b P53, bcl2, and bax: their relationship and effect on prognosis in early stage epithelial ovarian carcinoma. International Journal of Gynecological Cancer 11: 147–158

Sliutz G, Schmidt W, Tempfer C et al 1997 Detection of p53 point mutation in primary human vulvar cancer by PCR with temperature gradient gel electrophoresis. Gynecologic Oncology 64: 93–98

Smid-Koopman E, Blok L J, Chadha-Ajwani S, Helmerhorst T J M, Brinkmann A O, Huikeshoven F J 2000 Gene expression profiles of human endometrial cancer samples using a cDNA-expression array technique: assessment of an analysis method. British Journal of Cancer 83: 246–251

Snijders P J, van Duin M, Walboomers J M et al 1998 Telomerase activity exclusively in cervical carcinomas and a subset of cervical intraepithelial neoplasia grade III lesions: strong association with elevated messenger RNA levels of its catalytic subunit and high risk human papillomavirus DNA. Cancer Research 58: 3812–3818

Sonoda G, Palazzo J, du Manoir S et al 1997a Comparative genomic hybridization detects frequent overrepresentation of chromosomal material from 3q26, 8q24, and 20q13 in human ovarian carcinomas. Genes Chromosomes and Cancer 20: 320–328

Sonoda G, du Manoir S, Godwin A K et al 1997b Detection of DNA gains and losses in primary endometrial carcinomas by comparative genomic hybridization. Genes Chromosomes and Cancer 18: 115–125

Sonoda Y, Saigo P E, Federici M G, Boyd J 2000 Carcinosarcoma of the ovary in a patient with a germline BRCA2 mutation: evidence for monoclonal origin. Gynecologic Oncology 76: 226–229

Sorbe B, Risberg B 1997 Prognostic importance of the nuclear proteins p53 and Rb in conjunction with DNA, nuclear morphometry and grading in endometrial carcinoma. International Journal of Gynecological Cancer 7: 34–41

Sorbe B, Risberg B, Thornwaite J 1994 Nuclear morphometry and DNA flow cytometry as prognostic methods for endometrial carcinoma. International Journal of Gynecological Cancer 4: 94–100

Sorensen F B, Bichel P, Jakobsen A 1992 DNA levels and stereologic estimates of nuclear volume in squamous cell carcinomas of the uterine cervix. A comparative study with analysis of prognostic impact. Cancer 69: 187–199

Stewart R L, Royds J A, Burton J L, Heatley M K, Wells M 1998 Direct sequencing of the p53 gene shows absence of mutations in endometrioid endometrial adenocarcinomas expressing p53 protein. Histopathology 33: 440–445

Storey A, Thomas M, Kalita A, Harwood C, Gardiol D, Mantovani F 1998 Role of a p53 polymorphism in the development of human papillomavirus-associated cancer. Nature 393: 229–234

Strang P, Stendhal U, Bergstrom R, Frankendal B, Tribuait R 1991 Prognostic flow cytometric information in cervical squamous cell carcinoma: a multivariate analysis of 307 patients. Gynecologic Oncology 43: 3–8

Strang P, Nordstrom B, Nilsson S, Bergstrom R, Tribukait B 1996 Mutant p53 protein as a predictor of survival in endometrial carcinoma. European Journal of Cancer 32: 598–602

Su T H, Wang J C, Tseng H H et al 1998 Analysis of FHIT transcripts in cervical and endometrial cancers. International Journal of Cancer 76: 216–222

Suehiro Y, Sakamoto M, Umayahara K et al 2000a Genetic aberrations detected by comparative genomic hybridization in ovarian clear cell adenocarcinoma. Oncology 59: 50–56

Suehiro Y, Umayahara K, Ogata H et al 2000b Genetic aberrations detected by comparative genomic hybridization predict outcome in patients with endometrioid carcinoma. Genes Chromosomes and Cancer 29: 75–82

Sung C J, Zheng Y, Quddus M R et al 2000 p53 as a significant prognostic marker in endometrial carcinoma. International Journal of Gynecological Cancer 10: 119–127

Susini T, Rapi S, Savino L, Boddi V, Berti P, Massi G 1995 Prognostic value of flow cytometric deoxyribonucleic acid index in endometrial cancer: comparison with other clinical-pathologic parameters. American Journal of Obstetrics and Gynecology 170: 527–534

Susini T, Rapi S, Massi D et al 1999 Preoperative evaluation of tumor ploidy in endometrial carcinoma: an accurate tool to identify patients at risk for extrauterine disease and recurrence. Cancer 86: 1005–1012

Suzuki A, Fukushige S, Nagase S, Ohuchi N, Satomi S, Horii A 1997 Frequent gains on chromosome arms 1q and/or 8q in human endometrial cancer. Human Genetics 100: 629–636

Suzuki M, Tsukagoshi S, Saga Y, Ohwada M, Sato I 2000 Assessment of proliferation index with MIB-1 as a prognostic factor in radiation therapy for cervical cancer. Gynecologic Oncology 79: 300–304

Swanson S A, Norris H J, Kelsten M L, Wheeler J E 1990 DNA content of juvenile granulosa cell tumors determined by flow cytometry. International Journal of Gynecological Pathology 9: 101–109

Swisher E M, Gown A M, Skelly M et al 1996 The expression of epidermal growth factor, HER-2/Neu, p53, and Ki-67 antigen in uterine malignant mixed mesodermal tumors and adenosarcoma. Gynecologic Oncology 60: 81–88

Sykes P, Quinn M, Rome R 1997 Ovarian tumors of borderline malignancy: a retrospective study of 234 patients. International Journal of Gynecological Cancer 7: 218–226

Symonds R P, Habeshaw T, Paul J et al 1992 No correlation between ras, c-myc and c-jun proto-oncogene expression and prognosis in advanced carcinoma of the cervix. European Journal of Cancer 28: 1616–1617

Syrjanen K J, Erzen M, Costa S 2001 Histological and quantitative pathological prognostic factors in cervical cancer. CME Journal of Gynecologic Oncology 6: 279–301

Takakura M, Kyo S, Kanaya T et al 1998 Expression of human telomerase subunits and correlation with telomerase activity in cervical cancer. Cancer Research 58: 1558–1561

Tamura M, Fukaya T, Murakami T, Uehara S, Yajima A 1998 Analysis of clonality in human endometriotic cysts based on evaluation of X chromosome inactivation in archival formalin-fixed, paraffin embedded tissue. Laboratory Investigation 78: 213–218

Tamura M, Gu J, Tran H, Yamada M 1999 PTEN gene and integrin signalling in cancer. Journal of the National Cancer Institute 91: 1820–1828

Tanaka M, Kyo S, Takakura M et al 1998 Expression of telomerase activity in human endometrium is localized to epithelial glandular cells and regulated in a menstrual phase-dependent manner correlated with cell proliferation. American Journal of Pathology 153: 1985–1991

Tanoguchhi K, Sasano H, Yabuki N et al 1998 Immunohistochemical and two-parameter flow cytometric studies of DNA topoisomerase II alpha in human epithelial ovarian carcinoma and germ cell tumor. Modern Pathology 11: 186–193

Tapper J, Kettunen E, El Rifai W, Seppala M, Andersson L C, Knuutila S 2001 Changes in gene expression during progression of ovarian carcinoma. Genes Chromosomes and Cancer 128: 1–6

Tashiro H, Isacson C, Levine R, Kurman R J, Cho K R, Hedrick L 1997a p53 gene mutations are common in uterine serous carcinoma and occur early in their pathogenesis. American Journal of Pathology 150: 177–185

Tashiro H, Blazes M S, Wu R et al 1997b Mutations in PTEN are frequent in endometrial carcinoma but are rare in other common gynecological malignancies. Cancer Research 57: 3935–3940

Taskin M, Lallas T A, Barber H R, Shevchuk M M 1997 Bcl-2 and p53 in endometrial adenocarcinoma. Modern Pathology 10: 728–734

Tate J E, Mutter G L, Boynton K A, Crum C P 1997 Monoclonal origin of vulvar intraepithelial neoplasia and some vulvar hyperplasias. American Journal of Pathology 150: 315–322

Teneriello M G, Ebina M, Linnoila R I et al 1993 p53 and Ki-ras gene mutations in epithelial ovarian neoplasms. Cancer Research 53: 3103–3108

Ter Harmsel B, Smedts F, Kuijpers J, Jeunink M, Trimbos B, Ramaekers F 1996 BCL-2 immunoreactivity increases with severity of CIN: a study of normal cervical epithelia, CIN, and cervical carcinoma. Journal of Pathology 179: 26–30

Ter Harmsel B, Kuijpers J, Jeunink M, Trimbos B, Ramaekers F 1997 Progressing imbalance between proliferation and apoptosis with increasing severity of cervical intraepithelial neoplasia. International Journal of Gynecological Pathology 16: 206–211

Thomas M, Pim D, Banks L 1999 The role of the E6-p53 interaction in the molecular pathogenesis of HPV. Oncogene 18: 7690–7700

Tirindelli-Danesi D, Spano M, Altavista P et al 1997 Quality control study of the Italian Group of Cytometry on flow cytometry DNA content measurements. II. Factors affecting inter- and intralaboratory variability. Cytometry 30: 85–97

Tjalma W, Weyler J, Goovaerts G, De Pooter C, van Marck E, van Dam P 1998 Prognostic value of Bcl-2 expression in patients with operable carcinoma of the uterine cervix. Journal of Clinical Pathology 50: 33–36

Toki T, Zhai Y L, Park J S, Fujii 1999 Infrequent occurrence of high-risk human papillomavirus and of p53 mutation in minimal deviation adenocarcinoma of the cervix. International Journal of Gynecological Pathology 18: 215–219

Topalovsky M, Hankin R C, Michael C, Hunter S V, Edwards A M, Chen J C 1995 Ploidy analysis of products of conception by image and flow cytometry with cytogenetic correlation. American Journal of Clinical Pathology 103: 409–414

Tosi P, Cintorino M, Santopietro R et al 1992 Prognostic factors in invasive cervical carcinomas associated with human papillomavirus. Quantitative data and cytokeratin expression. Pathology Research and Practice 188: 866–873

Tritz D, Pieretti M, Turner S, Powell D 1997 Loss of heterozygosity in usual and special variant carcinomas of the endometrium. Human Pathology 28: 607–612

Troncone G, Martinez J C, Palombini L et al 1998 Immunohistochemical expression of mdm2 and p21WAF1 in invasive cervical cancer: correlation with p53 protein and high risk HPV infection. Journal of Clinical Pathology 51: 754–760

Tsang R W, Wong C S, Fyles A W et al 1999 Tumour proliferation and apoptosis in human uterine cervix carcinoma II: correlations with clinical outcome. Radiotherapy and Oncology 50: 93–101

Uchiyama M, Iwasaka T, Matsuo N, Hachisuga T, Mori M, Sugimori H 1997 Correlation between human papillomavirus positivity and p53 gene overexpression in adenocarcinoma of the uterine cervix. Gynecologic Oncology 65: 23–29

Valverde J J, Martin M, Garcia-Asenjo J A, Casado A, Vidart J A, Diaz-Rubio E 2001 Prognostic value of DNA quantification in early epithelial ovarian carcinoma. Obstetrics and Gynecology 97: 409–416

van Dam P A 1995 Ploidy in ovarian cancer and prognosis. In: Leake R, Gore M, Ward R H (eds) The biology of gynaecological cancer. RCOG Press, London, pp 258–273

van Dam P A, Watson J V, Lowe D G, Shepherd J H 1992 Flow cytometric DNA analysis in gynecological oncology. International Journal of Gynecological Cancer 2: 57–65

van Dam P A, Vergote I B, Lowe D G et al 1994 Expression of c-erbB-2, c-myc, and c-ras oncoproteins, insulin-like growth factor receptor I, and epidermal growth factor receptor in ovarian carcinoma. Journal of Clinical Pathology 47: 914–919

van de Kaa C A, Nelson K A, Ramaekers F C et al 1991 Interphase cytogenetics in paraffin sections of routinely processed hydatidiform moles and hydropic abortions. Journal of Pathology 165: 281–287

van de Kaa C A, Schjf C P, de Wilde P C et al 1996 Persistent gestational trophoblastic disease: DNA image cytometry and interphase cytogenetics have limited predictive value. Modern Pathology 9: 1007–1014

van de Kaa C A, Schijf C P, de Wilde P C et al 1997 The role of deoxyribonucleic acid image cytometric and interphase cytogenetic analyses in the differential diagnosis, prognosis, and clinical follow-up of hydatidiform moles: a report from the Central Molar Registration in the Netherlands. American Journal of Obstetrics and Gynecology 177: 1219–1229

van der Putten H W, Baak J P A, Koenders T J, Kurver P H, Stolk H G, Stolte L A 1989 Prognostic value of quantitative pathological features and DNA content in individual patients with stage I endometrial carcinoma. Cancer 63: 1378–1387

van Haaften Day C, Russell P, Boyer C M et al 1996 Expression of cell regulatory proteins in ovarian borderline tumors. Cancer 77: 2092–2098

van Hoeven K H, Kovatich A J 1996 Immunohistochemical staining for proliferating cell nuclear antigen, Bcl-2 and Ki-67 in vulval tissues. International Journal of Gynecological Pathology 15: 10–16

Van Hoeven K H, Ramondetta L, Kovatich A J, Bibbo M, Dunton C J 1997 Quantitative image analysis of MIB-1 reactivity in inflammatory, hyperplastic, and neoplastic endocervical lesions. International Journal of Gynecological Pathology 16: 15–21

van Lijnschoten G, Albrechts J, Vallinga M et al 1994 Fluorescence in situ hybridization on paraffin-embedded abortion material as a means of retrospective chromosome analysis. Human Genetics 94: 518–522

Vegh G L, Fulop V, Liu Y et al 1999 Differential gene expression pattern between normal human trophoblast and choriocarcinoma cell lines: downregulation of heat shock protein-27 in choriocarcinoma in vitro and in vivo. Gynecologic Oncology 75: 391–396

Vergote I B, Kaern J, Abeler V M et al 1993 Analysis of prognostic factors in stage I epithelial ovarian carcinoma: importance of degreee of differentiation and DNA ploidy in predicting relapse. American Journal of Obstetrics and Gynecology 169: 40–52

Viale G, Maisonneuve P, Bonoldi E et al 1997 The combined evaluation of p53 accumulation and Ki-67 (MIB1) labelling index provides independent information on overall survival of ovarian carcinoma patients. Annals of Oncology 8: 469–476

Volm M, Kleine W, Pfleiderer A 1989 Flow cytometric prognostic factors for the survival of patients with ovarian carcinoma: a 5 year follow-up study. Gynecologic Oncology 35: 84–89

Wabersich J, Fracas M, Mazzer S, Marchetti M, Altavilla G 1998 The value of the prognostic factors in ovarian granulosa cell tumors. European Journal of Gynaecological Oncology 19: 69–72

Walsh C, Miller S J, Flam F, Fisher R A, Ohlsson R 1995 Paternally derived *H19* is differentially expressed in malignant and nonmalignant trophoblast. Cancer Research 55: 1111–1116

Wang D P, Konishi I, Koshiyama M et al 1993 Expression of c-erb-B-2 protein and epidermal growth factor receptor in endometrial carcinomas. Cancer 72: 28–37

Wasenius V M, Jekunen A, Monni O et al 1997 Comparative genomic hybridization analysis of chromosomal changes occurring during development of acquired resistance to cisplatin in human ovarian carcinoma lines. Genes Chromosomes Cancer 18: 286–291

Webb P M, Green A, Cummings M C, Purdie D M, Walsh M D, Chevenix-Trench G 1998 Relationship between number of ovulatory cycles and accumulation of mutant p53 in epithelial ovarian cancer. Journal of the National Cancer Institute 90: 1729–1734

Wehrli B M, Krajewski S, Gascoyne R D et al 1998 Immunohistochemical analysis of BCL-2, BAX, mcl-1, and BCL-X expression in ovarian surface epithelial tumors. International Journal of Gynecological Pathology 17: 255–260

Welsh J B, Zarrinkar P P, Sapinoso I M et al 2001 Analysis of gene expression profiles in normal and neoplastic ovarian tissue samples identifies candidate molecular markers of epithelial ovarian cancer. Proceedings of the National Academy of Sciences USA 98: 1176–1181

Werness B A, Afify A M, Eltabbakh G H, Huelsman K, Piver M S, Paterson J M 1999a P53, c-erbB, and Ki-67 expression in ovaries removed prophylactically from women with a family history of ovarian cancer. International Journal of Gynecological Pathology 18: 338–343

Werness B A, Freedman A N, Piver M S, Romero-Gutierrez M, Petrow E 1999b Prognostic significance of p53 and p21 (waf1/cip1) immunoreactivity in epithelial cancers of the ovary. Gynecologic Oncology 75: 413–418

Werst R, Liblit R, Koss L 1991 Flow cytometric DNA analysis of human solid tumors: a review of the interpretation of DNA histograms. Human Pathology 22: 1085–1098

Weyn B, Tjalma W, Van de Wouwer G et al 2000 Validation of nuclear texture, density, morphometry and tissue syntactic structure analysis as prognosticators of cervical carcinoma. Analytic and Quantitative Cytology and Histology 22: 373–382

Wilkinson N, Todd N, Buckley C H, Gusterson B A, Fox H 1991 An immunohistochemical study of the incidence and significance of c-erbB-2 oncoprotein overexpression in ovarian neoplasia. International Journal of Gynecological Cancer 1: 285–289

Wils J, van Geuns H, Baak J P A 1988 Proposal for therapeutic approach based on prognostic factors including morphometric and flow-cytometric features in stage III-IV ovarian cancer. Cancer 61: 1920–1925

Wisman G B, Hollema H, de Jong S et al 1998 Telomerase activity as a biomarker for (pre)neoplastic cervical disease in scrapings and frozen sections from patients with abnormal cervical smear. Journal of Clinical Oncology 16: 2238–2245

Witty J P, Jensen R A, Johnson A L 1998 Expression and localization of BCL-2 related proteins in human ovarian cancer. Anticancer Research 18: 1223–1230

Wolf N G, Abdul-Karim F W, Farver C, Schrock E, du Manoir S, Schwartz S 2000 Analysis of ovarian borderline tumors using comparative genomic hybridization and fluorescence in situ hybridization. Genes Chromosomes Cancer 25: 307–315

Wong S Y, Ngan H Y S, Chan C C W, Cheung A N Y 1999 Apoptosis in gestational trophoblastic disease — correlated with clinical outcome and Bcl-2 expression but not bax expression. Modern Pathology 12: 1025–1033

Wong Y F, Ip T Y, Chung T K H et al 1999 Clinical and pathologic significance of microsatellite instability in endometrial cancer. International Journal of Gynecological Cancer 9: 406–410

Wu R, Connolly D C, Dunn R L, Cho K R 2000 Restored expression of fragile histidine triad protein and tumorigenicity of cervical carcinoma cells. Journal of the National Cancer Institute 92: 338–344

Wynford-Thomas D 1992 p53 in tumour pathology: can we trust immunocytochemistry? Journal of Pathology 166: 329–330

Yacoub S F, Shaeffer J, El-Mahdi A M, Faris L, Zhu A 1994 Nuclear morphometry as a predictor of response to neoadjuvant chemotherapy plus radiotherapy in locally advanced cervical cancer. Gynecologic Oncology 54: 327–332

Yamashita T, Yaginuma Y, Saitoh Y et al 1999 Codon 72 polymorphism of p53 as a risk factor for patients with human papillomavirus-associated squamous intraepithelial lesions and invasive cancer of the uterine cervix. Carcinogenesis 20: 1733–1736

Yamauchi N, Sakamoto A, Uozaki H, Iihara K, Machinami R 1996 Immunohistochemical analysis of endometrial adenocarcinoma for Bcl-2 and p53 in relation to expression of sex steroid receptor and proliferative activity. International Journal of Gynecological Pathology 15: 202–208

Yang B, Hart W R 2000 Vulvar intraepithelial neoplasia of the simplex (differentiated) type: a clinicopathologic study including analysis of HPV and p53 expression. American Journal of Surgical Pathology 24: 429–441

Yano T, Jimbo H, Yoshikawa H, Tsutsumi O, Taketani Y 1999 Molecular analysis of clonality in ovarian endometrial cysts. Gynecological and Obstetric Investigation 47: 41–45

Yashima K, Ashfaq R, Nowak J et al 1998 Telomerase activity and expression of its RNA component in cervical lesions. Cancer 82: 1319–1327

Yokomizo A, Tindall D J, Hartmann L, Jenkins R B, Smith D I, Liu W 1998 Mutation analysis of the putative tumour suppressor gene PTEN/MMAC1 in human ovarian cancer. International Journal of Oncology 13: 101–105

Yorukoglu K, Sayhan S, Dicle N 2001 Tumour volume estimation by the percentage carcinoma method in uterine carcinoma. Analytical and Quantitative Cytology and Histology 23: 89–92

Yoshino K, Enomoto T, Nakamura T et al 1998 Aberrant FHIT transcripts in squamous cell carcinoma of the uterine cervix. International Journal of Cancer 76: 176–181

Yoshino K, Enomoto T, Nakamura T 2000 FHIT alterations in cancerous and non-cancerous cervical epithelium. International Journal of Cancer 85: 6–13

Yu C C, Wilkinson N, Brito M J, Buckley C H, Fox H, Levison D A 1993 Patterns of immunohistochemical staining for proliferating cell nuclear antigen and p53 in benign and neoplastic human endometrium. Histopathology 23: 367–371

Yun K, Fukumoto M, Jinno Y 1996 Monoallelic expression of the insulin-like growth factor-2 gene in ovarian cancer. American Journal of Pathology 148: 1081–1087

Zaino R J, Davis A T L, Ohlsson-Wilhelm B M, Brunetto V L 1998 DNA content is an independent prognostic indicator in endometrial adenocarcinoma: a Gynecology Oncology Group study. International Journal of Gynecological Pathology 17: 312–319

Zanetta G M, Katzmann J A, Keeney G L, Kinney W K, Cha S S, Podratz K C 1992 Flow-cytometric DNA analysis of stages IB and IIA cervical carcinoma. Gynecologic Oncology 46: 13–19

Zanetta G, Keeney G L, Cha S S, Wieand H S, Katzmann J A, Podratz K C 1996 DNA index by flow cytometric analysis: an additional prognostic factor in advanced ovarian carcinoma without residual disease after primary operation. Gynecologic Oncology 62: 208–212

Zhai Y L, Kobayashi Y, Mori A et al 1999 Expression of steroid receptors, Ki-67, and p53 in uterine leiomyosarcomas. International Journal of Gynecological Pathology 18: 20–28

Zhang D K, Ngan H Y, Cheng R Y et al 1999 Clinical significance of telomerase activation and telomeric restriction fragment (TRF) in cervical cancer. European Journal of Cancer 35: 154–160

Zheng P S, Iwasaka T, Zhang Z M, Pater a, Sugimori H 2000 Telomerase activity in Papanicolaou smear-negative exfoliated cervical cells and its association with lesions and oncogenic human papillomaviruses. Gynecologic Oncology 77: 394–398

Zheng W, Sung C J, Cao P et al 1997 Early occurrence and prognostic significance of p53 alteration in primary carcinoma of the fallopian tube. Gynecologic Oncology 64: 38–48

Zheng W, Khurana R, Farahmand S, Wang Y, Zhang Z F, Felix J C 1998 p53 immunostaining as a significant diagnostic marker for uterine surface carcinoma — precursor lesion of uterine papillary serous carcinoma. American Journal of Surgical Pathology 22: 1463–1473

Index

Note: Page numbers in **bold** indicate major discussion; those in *italics* refer to figures and tables. *vs* denotes differential diagnosis, or comparison.
To save space in subentries the following abbreviations have been used:
   HRT—Hormone replacement therapy
   IUCD—Intrauterine contraceptive device

A
Abdominal lymph node, endometriosis *971*
Abdominal pain
  endometritis 419
  genital tract malformations 46
  intra-abdominal desmoplastic small round cell
    tumour 919
  ovarian fibroma 859
  ovarian follicle cysts 663
  ovarian lymphomas 940
  small cell ovarian tumours 904
  tubal adenocarcinoma 609
Abdominal pregnancy **1062–1063**
  blood supply 1063
  intraligamentous gestation 1063
  placental removal 1063
  primary, criteria for diagnosis 1062
  secondary to tubal rupture 1059
Abdominal surgery, ectopic pregnancy 1050
Abortion
  septic 1503
  spontaneous *see* Miscarriage
  see also Termination of pregnancy
Abruptio placentae **1503**
  acute renal failure **1503**
  antepartum haemorrhage 1350
  maternal death 1561
  placental haemangioma 1453
  pre-eclampsia 1342
Abscess
  amoebic, pregnancy 1479
  Bartholin's gland 58
  listeriosis 1315, *1315*, 1532
  Monro's 73
  ovary 683, *683*
  tubo-ovarian
    acute salpingitis *621*
    enterobiasis 1142
Acantholytic disorders, vulval genetic disorders
  60–62
Acanthosis nigricans *68*
  ovarian cancer **1193**
  stromal luteoma and 846
  vulvar hyperpigmentation 68
Acanthotic rete pegs *269*
Acardiac fetus *1584*
  twin transfusion syndrome 1583–1584
  see also Fetus acardius
Accessory lobe, placental *1275*, 1275–1276
  see also Placenta, accessory lobe
Acetowhite cervical epithelium *322*
  cervical intraepithelial neoplasia 322
Achlorhydria, vulvar dermatosis **1181**
Acid fluid aspiration, maternal death 1570
Acidophilic cells 1022
Acne, in polycystic ovary disease 667
Acquired immunodeficiency syndrome
    see HIV/AIDS

Acrodermatitis enteropathica, vulvar conditions
    associated 63–64
Acromegaly, menstrual irregularity **1182**
Acrosome reaction 1007
  impairment 994
ACTH *see* Adrenocorticotropic hormone (ACTH)
Actin
  placental villi smooth muscle cells 1244
  sclerosing stromal tumours (ovarian) 766
Actinomyces, infections associated with IUCD use
    1113, 1115
Actinomyces israelii 1113
  endometritis 431
  IUCD use and 1113
Actinomyces-like organisms, in cervix/vagina, IUCD
    use effect 1112–1113
Actinomycosis 1186
  cervical 282, 1113
  endometritis 431, *431*
  IUCD association 170, 1113
  ovarian involvement 683, *683*
  tuberculous salpingitis vs 618
  vaginitis 170
  vulvar 57–58
Activated protein C (APC) resistance 1103
  miscarriage 1434
Acute abdomen, cavernous haemangioma in
    Fallopian tube 605
Acute atherosis, pre-eclampsia 1339
Acute fatty liver of pregnancy (AFLP) 1469–1474,
    1470–1473
  acute renal failure **1503**
  auxiliary liver transplantation 1472
  clinical features 1469
  histological features 1470–1471
  incidence and risk factors 1469
  laboratory investigations 1469–1470
  liver rupture 1476
  maternal and fetal complications 1471–1472
  pathogenetic mechanisms 1472–1474
'Acute Meigs' syndrome' 676–677
Acute post-infectious glomerulonephritis, in
    pregnancy *1515*, **1516**
Acute renal failure, in pregnancy *see* Renal failure,
    acute
Acute tubular necrosis **1500**, *1501*
Addison's disease, autoimmune oophoritis 680, 681
Adenoacanthosis, endometrial 449, *452*
Adenocarcinoid (amphicrine) tumour 111
Adenocarcinoma
  Bartholin's gland 130
  cervical *see* Cervical adenocarcinoma
  clear cell *see* Clear cell adenocarcinoma
  colon, vulvar metastases *126*
  endocervical *see* Endocervical (mucinous)
    adenocarcinoma
  endocervix, microglandular hyperplasia 289
  endometrial *see* Endometrial carcinoma

  enteric *343*
  gastric, uterine cervix metastases *386*
  hyperplasia sequence 606
  metastatic, vs endosalpingiosis 922
  ovarian *see* Ovarian tumours, adenocarcinoma
  tubal *see* Fallopian tube, adenocarcinoma
  vaginal *see* Vagina, adenocarcinoma
  vulvar 111
  see also specific tumours
Adenocarcinoma in situ
  cervical glandular intraepithelial neoplasia
    (CGIN) 351–353
  cervical large cell neuroendocrine carcinoma and
    373
  cone biopsy, residual presence *355*
  endocervical curettage 323–324
  see also Carcinoma in situ
Adenocystadenofibroma, clear cell 727, *727*
Adenofibroma
  clear cell 727, *727*
  endometrioid 715, *716*
    with epithelial atypia 725–727, *726*
  Fallopian tube 602, *602*
  mucinous 714–715
  ovarian 714–715
  tubal fimbriae 602, *602*
  uterine *551*, **551–552**
    adenosarcoma vs 557
    atypical polypoid adenomyoma vs 575
    invasion of myometrium and pelvic veins 552
Adenofibromatous polyp
  endometrial 417
  Fallopian tube 1009, *1009*
Adenoid basal carcinoma, cervix 345–346, *346*
Adenoid cystic carcinoma
  Bartholin's gland 131
  cervix 345, *345*
  ovarian **909**
  vulvar 131
Adenoma
  Bartholin's gland 129–130
  cervical villoglandular papillary 383
  corticotroph 1024
  gonadotroph cell 1024
  hepatic, steroid contraceptives and 1101, 1103,
    1103
  hepatocellular 1455
  pituitary gland *see* Pituitary gland
  rete ovarii *902*, 902–903
  Sertoli cell 1219
  thyroid, Sertoli–Leydig cell tumours 1190
  tubular, ovarian tumours and *755*, 755–756
  urethral 132
  villous *see* Villous adenoma
Adenoma malignum, of cervix
  endocervical variant 342–343
  endometrioid variant 344
Adenomatoid mesothelioma, uterine *539*, **539**

Adenomatoid tumour
  Fallopian tubes 603, *603*
  ovarian **873**, *907*, **907–908**
    tumours of probable Wolffian origin vs 902
  uterus *539*, **539**
Adenomyolipoma **577**
  uterine **577**, *577*
Adenomyoma 498
  atypical polypoid 498, **573–575**
    adenofibroma vs 552
    adenosarcoma vs 557
    clinical features 573
    clinical outcome 575
    differential diagnosis 462, 466, 574–575
    endometrium 418, *418*
    gross and histological features *573*, 573–574, *574*
    oestrogen therapy link 1074
    peritoneal keratin granulomas association 574
    uterine cervix 384
  definition 576
  differential diagnosis 531
  ovarian round ligament *626*
  uterine 576
  uterine cervix 384
Adenomyomatosis, endometrium 576
Adenomyomatous polyp, endometrial 417–418
Adenomyosis, uterine **497–499**, *498*
  clinicopathological correlation 499
  definition 497
  diffuse 498
  endometrial carcinoma involving 459, 498
  endometrial stromal sarcoma vs 510
  focal/localised 498, *499*
  histology 498, *498*
  'internal endometriosis' and 963
  intravascular, endometrial stromal sarcoma vs 509–510
  menstrual endometrium vs 499
  polypoid 499
  symptoms 499
  tamoxifen and 498, 1080
  in tropics **1151**
Adenosarcoma
  cervix, embryonal rhabdomyosarcoma 378
  Müllerian 530
  Müllerian with sex-cord-like elements **559**
  ovarian 731
  uterine **552–559**
    adenofibroma vs 557
    atypical polypoid adenomyoma vs 575
    cambium layer 566, *566*, 570
    clinical outcome and recurrence 558
    differential diagnosis 557–558
    endometrial stromal tumours vs 514
    epidemiology and aetiology 552–553
    gross pathology *553*, 553–554
    microscopic pathology *554*, 554–557, *556*
    myometrial invasion *553*, 557, 558
    with sarcomatous overgrowth 558–559
    spread and outcome 570–571
    therapy 558
    types *555*
  vaginal 559
Adenosis, vaginal *see* Vagina, adenosis
Adenosquamous carcinoma 111
  Bartholin's gland 130
  cervix *348*, 348–349
    clear cell 349
    human papillomavirus infection 341
    microinvasive 356
  vagina 208
  vulval 107, 111
Adenovirus infection, cervix 287
Adhesion molecules
  endometriosis 965
  malaria 1319
  trophoblast penetration 1347
Adhesions
  Fallopian tube 1010, *1011*, 1011–1012
    postoperative 1011–1012, 1028
  intrauterine (Asherman's syndrome) 396, 432–433, *433*, 1002, 1027
  ovarioligamentous 1018, *1019*
  pelvic fibrous, endosalpingiosis with *921*, 921–922
  periovarian 1018, *1019*
  perisalpingeal *1011*
  peritoneal serous borderline tumours and 923

tubo-ovarian *1018*
  fimbrial occlusion and infertility 1010, *1010*
  uterine 1002
ADH secretion, inappropriate 370, **1195**
'Adipocytic infiltration,' ovarian 868
Adipose metaplasia 415
'Adipose prosoplasia' 868
Adnexal tumours
  carcinoma, Paget's disease of vulva 98
  in mature teratoma 803
Adolescence **1157–1180**
  cervical adenocarcinoma *1174*, **1174–1175**
  cervical cancer and HPV **1175**
  cervical metaplasia 261
  genital tract pathology **1157–1180**
  germ cell tumours **1163–1177**
  Klinefelter's syndrome 1220
  ovarian sex cord–stromal tumours 1164, **1169–1172**
  pregnancy 1163
  squamous neoplasia **1175**
  sterility 991
  vaginal adenocarcinoma **1174–1175**
  vaginitis 159
Adrenal cortex
  hypo-/hyper-function and infertility 1026
  streak haemorrhages, hypertensive disease of pregnancy 1564
Adrenal cortical rests, in ovary 685
Adrenal hyperandrogenism 1026
Adrenal hyperplasia 1026
  acquired 1026
  congenital 1026
    adrenogenital syndrome 855, 1212
    cytochrome P450c21 1213
    lipoid 1216
    pseudohermaphroditism, male 1216–1217
    sexual ambiguity **1158–1159**
  polycystic ovary disease and 668
  see also Adrenogenital syndrome
Adrenal steroids, hypersecretion 1017, 1026
Adrenal-type tissue, ovarian 685
Adrenarche, 'exaggerated' 1026
Adrenocortical rests 845, 855
  broad ligament 845, 855
Adrenocorticotropic hormone (ACTH)
  cervical small cell carcinoma 370
  ectopic production 1194
  neoplastic hypersecretion 1022, 1024
Adrenogenital syndrome
  11-beta-hydroxylase 1212–1213
  congenital 855, 1212
    degree of virilisation 1213
  female pseudohermaphroditism 1212–1214
  males 1214
  tumour development 1213
  see also Adrenal hyperplasia
Adrenoreceptors, isthmic muscle 1007
Adult polycystic renal disease *1519*, **1519**
Adult respiratory distress syndrome, septic shock 1562–1564
AFP *see* Alphafetoprotein (AFP)
Age
  cervical adenocarcinoma prognosis 351
  cervical glandular intraepithelial neoplasia 354
  cervical physiology 276–277
  cervical small cell carcinoma 370
  ectopic pregnancy 1046
  at first coitus *see* Sexual activity, age at onset
  hydatidiform moles risk factors **1365**
  infertility and 991
  menarchal 653
  at menopause 657, 990
  miscarriage rate 991
  oocyte competency loss with 991
  yolk sac tumours 777
  see also other specific tumours
Aging, reproductive 990, 991
AgNORs
  endometrial adenocarcinoma 483
  hydatidiform moles 1383, **1386**
AIDS *see* HIV/AIDS
Air embolism
  maternal death 1567–1568
  orogenital sexual activity 1568
Airway obstruction, aspiration of solid material 1570
Alanine transferase (ALT), pregnancy 1466
Albright's syndrome **1189**

Alcohol abuse, maternal, placental examination 1309
Aldosterone, production, steroid cell tumours 850
Alkaline phosphatase (AP) 1466
  dysgerminoma 776
  gonadoblastoma in mixed gonadal dysgenesis 1227
  intrahepatic cholestasis of pregnancy 1467
  placental, trophoblastic disease 1381, 1393, 1415
  placental, yolk sac tumours 784
  toxaemia of pregnancy 1474
  yolk sac tumours 784
Allantoic remnants, umbilical cord 1293
Allantoic vessels
  fetal-placental circulation 1255
  placental vascularisation 1255
Allantois
  umbilical cord cysts 1300
  umbilical cord development 1255
Allen–Masters syndrome 996
Allergens, causing vaginal hypersensitivity 155
Allergic dermatitis, vulvar 74, *74*
Allergy
  seminal fluid 155, 993
  vaginal candidiasis association 172
  vulvar 74, *74*
Alloimmune-mediated graft rejection process, miscarriage 1433
Alopecia, vulvar 82
Alopecia areata 82
Alpha1–antitrypsin
  embryonal carcinoma 788
  immature teratoma 791
  ovarian granulocytic sarcoma 947
  yolk sac tumours 784
Alphafetoprotein (AFP)
  embryonal carcinoma 788
  germ cell tumours, vaginal 216
  haemangiomas of umbilical cord 1301
  hydatidiform moles 1368–1369
  immature teratoma 791, 792–793
  intervillous thrombosis 1285
  maternal floor infarction 1279
  maternal levels and uterine malformations 48
  mucinous cystadenoma (ovarian) *783*
  non-gestational carcinomas with trophoblastic metaplasia 1412
  peritoneal gliomatosis 793
  placental haemangioma 1453
  in pregnancy, causes 793
  Sertoli–Leydig cell tumours 753
  tumoral vs hepatic 785
  uterine carcinosarcoma 563, 566
  uterine malformations 48
  yolk sac tumours 784, 785
5–Alpha reductase
  fetal testis 1212
  synthesis failure and male differentiation 20–21
5–Alpha reductase 2 deficiency, pseudohermaphroditism, male 1219–1220
ALT (alanine transferase) in pregnancy 1466
Alveolar rhabdomyosarcoma
  embryonal rhabdomyosarcoma of uterine cervix 378
  metastases in ovary 890
Alveolar soft part sarcoma
  cervix 379, *379*
  vulva 124
Ambiguous genitalia
  gonadoblastoma association 823
  testicular regression syndrome 1215
  see also Sexual ambiguity
Amenorrhoea
  endometrial tuberculosis 427
  HIV/AIDS 1152
  IUCD use and 1117
  in polycystic ovary disease 667
  primary
    androgen resistance syndromes 1160
    gonadoblastoma 823
    hypogonadism 678
    imperforate transverse vaginal septum 46
    testicular feminisation, complete 1217
    Turner's syndrome 1159
  resistant ovary syndrome (Savage syndrome) 679
  secondary, hypogonadism 678
  stress-induced 1020
AMH gene over–expression, paramesonephric ducts in male differentiation 14
Aminotransferases, pregnancy 1466

Ammonia, serum levels, acute fatty liver of
    pregnancy 1469
Amniocentesis, diagnostic, amniotic band syndrome
    1307
Amnion
    epithelial cells 1302
    meconium staining 1303
    squamous metaplasia *1301*, 1301–1302
    umbilical cord development 1253,
        1254
    see also Membranes, fetal
Amnion nodosum 1302–1303
    congenital abnormalities 1303
    nodule appearance 1302, *1302*
Amniotic band formation *1308*
    extra-amniotic pregnancy 1306
Amniotic bands and strings 1307–1308
    amniotic rupture early pregnancy 1308
    extra-amniotic pregnancy 1307
Amniotic cavity
    floor 6
    fluid accumulation 1255
    formation 5
    inner cell mass 5
Amniotic fluid
    accumulation 1255
    debris 1566
    infection
        inflammation of membranes 1303
        vaginal examinations during labour 1305
Amniotic fluid embolism 1564–1567
    acute renal failure **1503**
    macroscopic findings at autopsy 1566
    maternal death 1564–1567
    onset of symptoms 1566
    postpartum haemorrhage 1561
    pulmonary vessels *1567*
    renal diseases in pregnancy **1503**
Amniotic inclusions, umbilical cord cysts 1301
Amniotic sac infection 1305
Amniotic strings *see* Amniotic bands and strings
Amniotic vesicle 1254
Amoebae, IUCD use and 1113
Amoebiasis 1140–1141
    liver abscess, pregnancy 1479
    vaginal 175–176
    vulvar 55
Amoebic abscess, pregnancy 1479
Amphetamines, infertility and 996
Amphicrine tumour, vulvar 111
Ampulla of fallopian tube *see* Fallopian tube
Amputations, intrauterine
    amniotic bands and strings 1307
    constriction rings 1308
Amylase, endocervical neoplasias 360
Amyloid, deposition in uterine smooth muscle
    tumours *520*
Amyloidosis
    cervix **1182**
    ovarian 685, 1193
    pituitary 1021
    renal involvement 1193
    tubal 622
    vulva 65, **1182**
Amyloid stroma, in strumal carcinoid tumour 810
Anaemia
    aplastic in pregnancy, *Clostridium perfringens* 431
    fetal infective haemolytic, syphilis 1314
    haemolytic *see* Haemolytic anaemia
    maternal, placental villi 1251
    megaloblastic, cervical changes 1188
    neonatal, placental haemangioma 1453
Anaerobic infections
    salpingitis 620
    vaginitis 167, 169
Anaesthesia-related maternal deaths 1570
Anal canal *36*
    anatomy 35
Anal membrane, external genitalia development 19
Anal sphincters 35–36
    external 35–36
    internal 35
Anaphylactoid syndrome of pregnancy 1565
Anaplastic variant, dysgerminoma *775*, 776
Anastomoses, placental *see* Placental anastomoses
Anatomical defects, fetus papyraceous 1585
Anatomy **1–40**
    anal canal 35
    broad ligament *654*
    cervical epithelium **251–268**

cervix **247–272**, *248*
    developmental **249–251**
    coccyx 21
    embryonic pelvis 21–38
    Fallopian tubes *see* Fallopian tube
    female genital tract **1–40**
    fimbriae (tubal) *586*, 587
    follicles (ovarian) *655*, 655–656
    frenulum of labia 38
    innominate bone 21
    ischiorectal fossa 36–37
    labia majora/minora 37–38
    ovary **650–657**, *654*
        see also Ovary, anatomy
    perineum 35
    placenta **1233–1272**
    sacrum 21
    uterotubal junction 587
    uterus 32–34, *654*
    vagina 35, 147, **147–152**
    vulva 37–38
Androblastoma
    diffuse nonlobular 758
    Fallopian tube 605
    mixed germ cell sex cord–stromal tumours vs 840
Androgen(s)
    deficiency, pseudohermaphroditism, male 1216
    overproduction
        infertility and 1026
        pregnancy luteoma association 675
        see also Hyperandrogenism
    receptor 1161
    receptor disorders 1217–1219
        classification 1217
    see also Testosterone
Androgen insensitivity syndromes 1217–1219
    testes *1218*
Androgen resistance syndromes **1160–1161**
    genotype 1160
Aneuploidy 1608, 1609
    cervical carcinoma 358, **1611**
    endometrial carcinoma **1610–1611**
    endometrial stromal sarcomas 1611
    fallopian tube carcinoma **1610**
    flow cytometry 1608, 1609
    infertility and 992
    ovarian carcinoma **1609**
        prognosis 736
    ovarian endometriosis, atypical 975
    ovarian epithelial/non-epithelial tumours **1610**
    Paget's disease of vulva recurrence 100
    persistent trophoblastic disease **1386**
    trophoblastic neoplasms 1395
    uterine sarcomas **1611**
    vulvar squamous cell carcinoma **1611**
    see also Ploidy analysis
Aneurysms
    arterial **1550–1553**
    berry, of circle of Willis *1528*, **1528–1529**
    combined steroid contraceptives and 1105
    hemiplegic migraine 1531
    ovarian artery 1551
    pregnancy-related 1550–1551
    renal artery 1550–1551
    splenic artery 1550
Angiitis of umbilical vessels, chorioamnionitis 1304
Angiofibroma, cellular, vulvar 120
Angiofollicular lymph node hyperplasia 71–72
Angiogenesis
    cervical cancer 332
    endometrial adenocarcinoma 483
    placental and Hofbauer cells 1244
Angiogenic factors, endometriosis 966
Angiography, cervical 274
Angiokeratoma, vulvar 118–119, *119*
Angiolymphoid hyperplasia with eosinophilia, vulvar
    involvement 81
Angiomas *1529*, 1530, *1530*
Angiomyofibroblastoma
    Fallopian tube 605
    urethral 132
    vulvar 120
Angiomyxoma
    aggressive 120–121, 1172, *1173*
        vulval 120–121
    superficial 121
Angiosarcoma
    ovarian *869*, **869–870**
    uterine 538
    vulvar 121–122

Ann Arbor system, Hodgkin's disease staging *938*,
    938–939
Annular tubules, sex cord–stromal tumours with
    757, **758–760**, *759*
Anorexia nervosa 1021
Anovulation 1014–1015, 1018
    stress-induced 1020
Anovulatory menstrual cycle, endometrial
    hyperplasia 444
Antecedent infertility, ectopic pregnancy 1046
Ante-mortem torsion, umbilical cord
    see Umbilical cord
Antepartum haemorrhage 1349–1352, *1350*
    abruptio placentae 1350
    marginal haematoma 1284
    pre-eclampsia 1342
    recurrent, placenta membranacea 1275
    velamentous insertion of umbilical cord 1296
Antibodies
    anticardiolipin *see* Anticardiolipin antibodies
    anti-endometrial and endometriosis 980
    antiphospholipid *see* Antiphospholipid antibodies
    endometrial adenocarcinoma detection 482
    in immunohistochemistry
        see Immunohistochemistry
    MIB-1 proliferation marker
        cervical lesions 290
        endocervical neoplasia 358
    monoclonal *see* Monoclonal antibody
    T-cells 944
    villous component markers 1244
Anticardiolipin antibodies 995
    fetal artery thrombosis 1282
    miscarriage 1434
    systemic lupus erythematosus in pregnancy 1345
Anticoagulants, prosthetic heart valves 1549
Anticonvulsants, dosage in pregnancy
    1533
Anti-cytokeratin, trophoblast 1244
Anti-desmin, fibroblasts of placental villi 1244
Antidiuretic hormone (ADH), inappropriate
    secretion 370, **1195**
Anti-gamma-smooth muscle actin, placental villi
    1244
Antigen-presenting cells
    cervical epithelium 266
    ectocervix 274
Anti-βhCG, syncytiotrophoblast 1244
Anti-hPL, syncytiotrophoblast 1244
Anti-Müllerian hormone (AMH)
        see Müllerian inhibiting substance (MIS)
Anti-oestrogens **1075–1081**
        see also Clomiphene; Tamoxifen
Antiovarian antibodies 680, 1016
Antioxidants, in semen, infertility and 995
Antiphospholipid antibodies
    HELLP syndrome 1476
    miscarriage 1434
    thrombosis and miscarriage 1434
Antiphospholipid syndrome
    chorea gravidarum **1524**
    co-existence with SLE in pregnancy 1345
    venous thrombosis 1526
Anti-progestins **1086–1087**
Antithrombin III deficiency, thromboembolism
    1561
Anti-vimentin, stromal cells of placental villi 1244
Anus *see Entries beginning anal*
Aorta
    coarctation **1543–1544**
    dissection
        Marfan's syndrome 1546
        pregnancy-associated 1550
Aortic plexus 657
Aortic stenosis **1544–1545**
    rheumatic origin 1548
Aphthous ulcers, vulvar 67
Aplasia, female genital tract 42–43
    cervix 42, 996
    Fallopian tube 42
    unilateral, of Müllerian duct 42
    vagina 42, 996
Aplastic anaemia in pregnancy, *Clostridium
    perfringens* 431
Apocrine miliaria, vulvar involvement 84
Apoplectic leiomyoma 525–526
Apoptosis
    cascade interruption, secondary necrosis of
        syncytiotrophoblast 1241
    cervical stroma 249

Apoptosis (cont'd)
  endometrial stromal cells 397
  inhibition by Bcl-2 483
  inhibitors, syncytial fusion 1240
  Müllerian tract modelling 391
  oocytes 649, 656
Apoptotic markers 483, 1606, **1607–1608**
  bax 1608
  bcl-2 1608
  cervical carcinoma **1608**
  endometrial carcinoma **1608**
  hydatidiform moles 1608
  M30 CytoDeath antibody 1608
  ovarian carcinoma **1607–1608**
Apoptotic nuclei, syncytial knots 1241
Appendiceal tumours
  metastatic
    to Fallopian tubes 613
    in ovary 884–885
  mucinous carcinoid, differential diagnosis 809
APUDoma, malignant *see* Small cell carcinomas
Arcuate arteries 998
  postpartum involution 1354
  pregnancy 1332
Arcuate nucleus, damage 1020
Arcuate uterus 44, *44*
Argentaffin granules, insular carcinoid tumour 808
Argyrophilia, large cell neuroendocrine tumours of
    uterine cervix 374
Argyrophilic carcinoma *see* Small cell carcinomas
Argyrophilic granules, small cell carcinomas of
    uterine cervix 372
Arias–Stella reaction
  cervical epithelium 275–276
  clear cell adenocarcinoma vs 471
  endocervix *276*
  endometrium
    clear cell metaplasia 413
    cytomegalovirus infection 426
    pregnancy 1329, *1329*
  tubal pregnancy, uterine response 1056, *1058*
Aromatase
  congenital increase of activity 1016
  cytochrome P450 966, 1005
  gene, placental aromatase defect 1214
  uterine endometrium in endometriosis 966
Arrays **1605**
Arterial aneurysms **1550–1553**
Arteriopathy, pre-eclampsia 1339
Arteriosclerosis, acute atherosis in
    pre-eclampsia 1343
Arterio-venous anastomoses
  in vulvar glomus tumours 119–120
  see also Placental anastomoses
Arterio-venous communications, antepartum
    haemorrhage and 1351
Arterio-venous malformations *1529*, 1529–1530
  angiomas *1529*, 1530, *1530*
  antepartum haemorrhage and 1351
  hemiplegic migraine 1531
  proton beam therapy 1530
  uterine *538*, *539*
Arterio-venous shunts, antepartum haemorrhage
    and 1352
Arteritis
  granulomatous 619
  necrotising **1191**
  obliterative, fetal stem arteries 1310
  uterine 291
Artery–artery communication, twin pregnancy
    1578, *1579*
Arthritis
  acute, gonorrhoea 1193
  rheumatoid *see* Rheumatoid arthritis
Articulated pelvis 21–22
Asbestos, diffuse malignant mesothelioma of
    peritoneum 916–917
Ascaris 1143, 1148
  vaginitis 176
Ascending infection, fetal membranes 1303
Ascites
  diffuse malignant mesothelioma of peritoneum
    917
  Krukenberg tumours 892
  ovarian fibroma association 860
  steroid cell tumours association 850
  theca cell tumour with 762
Asherman's syndrome (intrauterine adhesions)
    432–433, *433*, 1002, 1027
  basal endometrium 396

Aspartate transaminase (AST), pregnancy 1466
Aspiration
  acid fluid 1570
  faecal fluid 1570
  solid material 1570–1571
Aspirin, amniotic fluid embolism syndrome
    prevention 1565
'Assisted hatching' 5
Assisted reproductive technology (ART) **1029**
  complications 1029
  ectopic pregnancy 1050
  hormonal therapy effects 1090, *1090*
  see also In vitro fertilisation
AST (aspartate transaminase) 1466
Asthenospermia 994
Astrocytoma 1535
  epileptic fits 1533–1534, *1534*
Ataxia-telangiectasia
  dysgerminoma association 773
  gonadoblastoma association 823
  tumours **1182**
  yolk sac tumours association 777
Atherosis, acute, pre-eclampsia 1339, *1340*
Atrial naturetic peptide, polyuria in twin transfusion
    syndrome 1582
Atrial septal defects 1544
Atypical gonadoblastoma *see* Mixed germ
    cell sex cord–stromal tumours (ovarian)
Atypical polypoid adenomyoma
    see Adenomyoma, atypical polypoid
Auditory defects, uterine malformations 48
Autoantibodies
  infertility and 1025
  sperm-coating 997
Autoantigen, steroid cell, 3β-hydroxysteroid
    dehydrogenase as 681
Autofluorescence, pseudoxanthoma cells 969
Autoimmune diseases
  hepatitis, pregnancy 1483
  infertility and 1025
  lichen planus 78
  lichen sclerosis 75
  neuropathy 1536
  oophoritis 680–681, *681*, 1016
  thyroiditis 805
Autoimmune mechanism, endometriosis-associated
    infertility 980
Autoimmunity
  premature ovarian failure due to 1016
  sperm 992
Autonomic innervation of fallopian tube 32
Autonomic plexuses, pelvic innervation 25
Autosomal trisomy, miscarriage, spontaneous 1435
Auxiliary liver transplantation, acute fatty liver of
    pregnancy 1472
Azygos arteries 35

B
Bacteraemia, IUCDs and 1106
Bacterial flora
  vagina *see* Vagina, microflora
  vulva **54**
Bacterial infections
  cervix 281–283
  chorioamnionitis 1305
  endometritis 427–431
  placental villi 1291
  in tropics **1134–1139**
  tubal 617–618
  vaginal 165–170
    see also Vaginitis, bacterial
  vulvar 56–59
  see also individual infections
Bacterial vaginosis *see* Vaginosis, bacterial
Bacteriuria
  asymptomatic, in pregnancy 1495
  prevalence, in pregnancy 1497
  urine collection 1497
Bacteroides
  salpingitis 620
  vulvar flora 54
Barium sulphate, vaginal lesions due to 154
Barr body 642
Barrier contraception
  cervical adenocarcinoma 340
  ectopic pregnancy 1050
Bartholin's gland
  abscess, mycoplasma infection 58
  adenoma 129–130
  adenosquamous carcinoma 130

carcinoma 130–131
  duct cysts 84, *84*
  malacoplakia 66
  mucinous cystadenoma 130
  papilloma 130
  tuberculosis 57
  tumours **129–131**
    benign 129–130
    malignant 130–131
Basal cell(s)
  endometrium 393
  Fallopian tubes 587
  squamous epithelium of cervix 252
    transmission electronmicrograph image 254
Basal cell carcinoma
  adenoid, of cervix 345–346, *346*
  Gorlin's syndrome *1171*, **1171**
  lichen sclerosis 78
  in mature teratoma 803
  vagina 210
  vulva 109–111, *110*
Basal cell hyperplasia
  cervical epithelium 267, 288, *289*
  cervical trichomoniasis 284
Basal cell-like carcinoma, vagina 210
Basal cell naevus syndrome (Gorlin's syndrome)
    1171, **1171, 1184**
  multiple ovarian fibromas *858*, *859*
  ovarian fibrosarcoma and 861
Basal cell papilloma, vulvar 96, *96*
Basal layer
  cervical stratified squamous epithelium 273
  endometrium 395–396
    isthmic endometrium 396
Basaloid carcinomas 106–107
  squamous cell 110–111
Basal plate of placenta 1257–1259, *1258*
  fibrin deposition and maternal floor infarction
    1278–1279
Basement membrane
  cervical adenocarcinoma prognosis 351
  cervical epithelium 253
  glomerular, pre-eclampsia 1508, *1509*
  trophoblastic, thickening 1287
  vaginal epithelium 149, *149*
Basidiobolus haptosporus 1140
  vulvar infection 56
Basilar cells, ciliated, vaginal 150
bax
  cervical carcinoma 1608
  ovarian carcinoma 1608
B-cell lymphomas *see* Non-Hodgkin's lymphoma
B-cells
  cervical epithelium 267
  ectocervix 274
  endometrium 395
  lymphoid infiltration in uterine leiomyoma 532
  mucosal, migration to female genital tract 938
BCGosis (disseminated granulomatous disease)
    1193
Bcl-2, syncytial fusion 1240
bcl-2 gene
  cervical carcinoma 1608
  chemotherapy sensitivity 1608
  endometrial carcinoma 483, 1608
  expression, uterine leiomyosarcoma 523
  hydatidiform moles 1608
  ovarian carcinoma 1608
  uterine carcinosarcoma 572
Beckwith–Wiedemann syndrome 1363, 1364
Behçet's syndrome
  cervix 291
  genital ulceration 291
  vaginal changes 154
  vulva 66–67, *67*
Bell's palsy 1536
Benign intracranial hypertension **1527**
Benign lymphangiomatous papules **1193**
Benign melanotic pigmentation *see* Melanosis
'Benign strumosis' 806
Benign tumours
  Bartholin's gland 129–130
  cervix
    epithelial 382–383
    mesenchymal 383–384
    mixed mesenchymal–epithelial 384
  Fallopian tube **602–605**
    epithelial 602–603
    mesodermal 603–605
  ovarian

epithelial–stromal *see* Epithelial–stromal
  tumours, ovarian
germ cell tumours 772, 773
  serous 713–714
urethral 132
uterus *550*, 551–552
  endometrial stromal 502–503
  smooth muscle *515*, 515–519
vagina **192–198**
  see also Vagina, benign neoplasms
vulvar
  granular cell 122–123
  mixed 131
  skin adnexal tumours 126–128
  see also specific tumour types
Berry aneurysm of circle of Willis *1528*, **1528–1529**
  pathology 1529
Beta-agonists, water intoxification 1571
11–Beta-hydroxylase, adrenogenital syndrome
  1212–1213
Bethesda classification system, cervical and vaginal
  diseases 306–308
Bicarbonate, seminal fluid 994
Bicornuate uterus
  non-communicating rudimentary horn *44*
  twin pregnancy and antepartum haemorrhage
    1352
Bile
  cholesterol saturation index in pregnancy 1485
  composition in pregnancy **1484–1485**
Bile acids
  composition and pregnancy 1485
  enterohepatic circulation and pregnancy 1485
  intrahepatic cholestasis of pregnancy 1467
  sulphation, in pregnancy 1468
Bilharzial salpingitis, ectopic pregnancy 1048
Bilharziasis *see* Schistosomiasis
Bilharzioma 1144
Biliary tract, rupture (spontaneous) in pregnancy
  1481
Biliary transport proteins, gene mutation and
  intrahepatic cholestasis in pregnancy 1468
Bilirubin
  elevated, by steroid contraceptives 1100
  intrahepatic cholestasis of pregnancy 1467
  serum levels in pregnancy 1466
Bilobate placenta 1276, *1276*
  monochorionic, vascular anastomoses 1579
  velamentous insertion umbilical cord 1276
Biopsy
  cervical carcinoma and radiotherapy 332
  colposcopic punch 323
  cone *324*, 324–325
    see also Cone biopsy
  endometrial *see* Endometrium, biopsy
  liver *see* Liver biopsy
  placental bed
    intrauterine fetal growth retardation *1344*
    pre-eclampsia *1341*
  punch, cervix *261*, *262*, 267
  specimen examination *323*
  trophoblastic lesion 1412
  vaginal *219*, 220
  wedge 333
Birth *see* Delivery; Labour; Preterm delivery
Bladder 29–31
  arterial supply 30
  carcinoma, metastatic, to ovary 888
  nerve supply 30
  stability 30
  venous drainage 30
  voiding initiation 30–31
Blastocyst(s)
  implantation *see* Implantation
  retention 999
    failure due to leiomyoma 999
  X chromosome inactivation 642
Blastocyst cavity 5
Blastomyces dermatitidis, endometritis 432
Blastomycosis, tuberculous salpingitis vs 618
Bleeding, gastrointestinal, variceal 1483
Bleeding, vaginal/uterine
  abnormal, arteriovenous malformation of uterus
    539
  cervical carcinoma 326
  cervical polyps 290
  dysfunctional uterine **408–409**
  endometrial adenocarcinoma 456
  endometrial biopsy 392
  endometritis, chronic non-specific 419

fetal, velamentous insertion of umbilical cord
  1296
first-trimester, bilobate placenta 1276
hormone withdrawal 398
Klippel–Trenaunay–Weber syndrome 1187
leiomyosarcoma 520
lymphoma presentation 953
metastatic tumours 218
perimenopausal 409
postcoital, vaginal tumours 189
postmenopausal 409, *409*
  granulosa cell tumours 945
  Krukenberg tumours 892
  uterine lymphoma 949
  vaginal tumours 189
postpartum 1276
reproductive years 409
retroplacental 1350
uterine adenosarcoma 553
uterine carcinosarcoma 561
withdrawal 398
  after withdrawal of oestrogen therapy 1072
  after withdrawal of prostagens 1082
  combined oral contraceptives 1092
  hormone replacement therapy 1088
  see also Haemorrhage; Menstruation
Blepharophimosis syndrome **1182**
Blepharophimosis type I 1015
Blighted ovum
  hydatidiform moles and 1361
  villous appearances in tubal pregnancy 1053
Blood–brain barrier
  hypertensive encephalopathy 1525
  permeability in pregnancy 1523
Blood coagulation *see* Coagulation
Blood groups
  antigens, endocervical neoplasia 359
  chimerism, dizygotic twins 1579
Blood pressure
  measurement
    pre-eclampsia 1505
    in pregnancy 1505
  pregnancy 1336
  see also Hypertension
Blood supply
  abdominal pregnancy 1063
  Fallopian tube 32
  ovary 657
  pelvic 26–27
  pregnant uterus 1332
  uterus 998, *1332*
Blood vessels
  cervical epithelium 274
  endometrial basalis 395
  haemangioma, placental 1450
  myometrial 1333, *1334*
  pelvic 26–28
  transposition of great vessels **1545**
  uterine in pregnancy 1331–1332
  uteroplacental 1257–1259
  villous, endothelium 1242
  see also Entries beginning vascular
Blue naevus
  cervix 279, *279*, 282, 382
  vagina 193
B lymphocytes *see* B-cells
Body stalk, primitive 5
Bone
  density, steroid contraceptives and 1105
  heterotopic formation, ovary 684
  tumours, ovarian **866**
Bowenoid papulosis *see* Vulvar intraepithelial
  neoplasia (VIN)
Bowen's disease *see* Vulvar intraepithelial neoplasia
  (VIN)
Brain
  damage in pregnancy 1532
  petechial haemorrhages 1532
  tumours, WHO classification 1535
  tumours in pregnancy **1535**
BRCA1 gene 702
  germline mutations
    hereditary ovarian cancer 702
    serous ovarian carcinoma 702
  mutations
    Fallopian tube adenocarcinoma 605
    frequency 702
    primary peritoneal carcinoma 627
    primary peritoneal serous carcinoma 925
  tumour suppressor gene studies involving **1600**

BRCA2 gene 702
  germline mutations, hereditary ovarian cancer
    702
  mutations, frequency 702
Breast
  benign disease, decreased risk with steroid
    contraceptives 1100
  development, puberty 652–653
  ectopic tissue *see* Ectopic breast tissue
  steroid contraceptives effect 1100
Breast carcinoma
  gonadotrophin treatment association 1029
  hormone replacement therapy and 1089
  increased risk with steroid contraceptives 1100
  lobular
    cervical metastases 385, *386*
    metastatic vs small cell undifferentiated ovarian
      carcinoma 905
    uterine metastases 510
  metastatic
    to cervix 385, *386*
    ovarian lymphomas vs 945
    to ovary 880, 881, *881*, 881–882
    placental 1455
    to uterus 510
    to vagina 219
  ovarian tumours association 1081
  prevention, tamoxifen 1076
  tamoxifen treatment
    endometrial carcinoma and 1078–1080
    ovarian cysts association 1081
  unopposed oestrogen therapy and 1074
Breast feeding
  'contraceptive failure' of 997
  ovarian carcinoma risk decreased 700
  postpartum infertility 989
Brenner cells, uroepithelial nature 699
Brenner tumours (transitional cell)
  broad ligament 625
  ovarian *694*, 697, 699, *716*, 716–717
    borderline malignancy *727*, 727–728
    cystic changes 717, *717*
    epidemiology 716
    histiogenesis 699
    histology 716, *716*, 717
    of low malignant potential 727–728
    malignant *732*, 732–733
    metaplastic 717
    mucinous tumours associated 697
    'proliferating' 727
    recurrence and metastases 728
    size 716
  peritoneal 927
Breslow thickness, vulvar melanoma 114
Breus's mole (subchorial haematoma) *1284*,
  1285
Broad ligament *32*, **623–627**, 653
  anatomy *654*
  cysts 623–624, *624*
    secondary neoplasia 624–625
  embryology 623, 897
  ependymoma 625
  epithelial lesions 623–625
    tumours 625
  hyperplasia 627
  leiomyosarcoma 626
  lipoma 626, *626*
  mesodermal lesions 626
  mesothelial lesions 627
  metaplastic lesions 627
  papillary cystadenoma 625
  pseudomyxoma peritonei 625
  tumours *624*, 624–625, 627
    miscellaneous 627
    steroid cell 855
  vascular lesions 626–627
Broders' system, grading of ovarian carcinoma
  735–736
Bromocriptine
  adverse effects 1029
  prolactinomas 1022, 1024
Bromsulphthalein (BSP) excretion tests, pregnancy
  1466
Bronchial carcinoid tumours, metastatic to ovary
  886, 886–887
Bronchial carcinoma
  metastatic, to ovary 885–886
  placental metastatic disease 1455
  uterine cervix metastases 386
Brown bowel syndrome 500

BRST2 (GCDFP-15) immunostaining, uterine
  leiomyoma with tubules 530
Brugia malayi 1142
Buccal smear, Turner's syndrome 1222
Buccopharyngeal membrane 6
Budd–Chiari syndrome 1100–1101
  pregnancy 1481
Bullous (blistering) diseases, vulvar 69–72
Bullous erythema multiforme, vaginal changes 154
Bullous pemphigoid, vulvar 70
Burkitt's lymphoma
  granulosa cell tumour vs 945
  histology *943*, 943–944
  ovarian *942*, 942–944
  staging 938
  in tropics **1150**
Burkitt-type lymphoma, vaginal involvement 954
Buschke–Lowenstein tumour *see* Cervical
  carcinoma, verrucous

C
C1q deposition, SLE in pregnancy 1345
C3 deposition
  decidual arteries in pre-eclampsia 1340
  diabetes mellitus in pregnancy 1344
  mesangiocapillary glomerulonephritis in
    pregnancy 1514, *1514*
  SLE in pregnancy 1345
CA19–9, endocervical neoplasia 359
CA125
  endocervical neoplasia 359
  Meigs' syndrome 1196–1197
  ovarian carcinoma 733
  ovarian fibroma 860
  pregnancy luteoma association 675
  sarcoidosis 1189
  SLE 1190
  uterine carcinosarcoma 562
  yolk sac tumours 785
Caecovaginal fistula 185
Caesarean section
  maternal death after 1561, 1569
  placenta creta 1347
  uterine rupture 1569
Calcification
  corpus luteum, misinterpretation as malignant
    change 685
  gonadoblastoma 826, 829, *829*, 830
  intervillous thrombosis 1285
  ovarian
    bilateral 684
    immature teratoma 789
    mature teratoma 796–797
    theca cell tumour 763
  placental 1285
Calcinosis, vulva 81–82
Calcium oxalate, in struma ovarii 806
h-Caldesmon *see* h-Caldesmon
Call–Exner bodies
  adult-type granulosa cell tumour *747*, 748, *749*,
    751
  cystic granulosa cell tumour *747*
  hyaline type, gynandroblastoma 760, *760*
  'starry sky' macrophage vs 945
  types 748, *749*
Call–Exner-like bodies
  endometrial stromal tumours 513
  gonadoblastoma 827, *827*, 828–829
  mixed germ cell sex cord–stromal tumours 835,
    837
Calymmatobacterium granulomatis, vulvar infection
  57
Cambium layer 212
  adenosarcoma (uterine) 556, *556*, 570
  sarcoma botryoides 212, *213*
Campylobacter, miscarriage 1432
Canalisation failure, female genital tract
  malformation 45
Canal of Nuck cysts, vulvar involvement 85
Cancer
  hereditary syndromes 702
  see also Tumour(s): *specific tumours/anatomical
    regions*
Candida
  detection 171
  species and infection sites 172
  in tropics 1140
  vaginal flora 170
    IUCD use effect 1112
  vulvar flora 54

Candida albicans 172
  vaginal flora 170
  vaginitis 170–172
Candidiasis (*Candida* infections)
  cervical 283
  chorioamnionitis 1303
  ectocervix *283*
  endometritis 432
  in tropics 1140
  vaginal 170–172
    diabetes mellitus 1183
    diagnosis 171
    HIV/AIDS 1152
    recurrent 172
    risk factor and epidemiology 171
    transmission 171–172
  vulvar 55
Capacitation 1007
Capillary haemangiomas, uterine 538
Capsular chorion frondosum 1256
Capsular decidua 1257
Carbonic anhydrase, stimulation by sperm 994
Carcinoembryonic antigen (CEA)
  endocervical neoplasia 359
  endometrioid adenocarcinoma 463, *463*
  immature teratoma 791
  Paget's disease of vulva 99
  primary ovarian carcinoma vs colonic metastases
    884
  uterine cervix
    small cell carcinoma 370
    villoglandular papillary adenomas 383
    villous adenomas 383
  yolk sac tumours 784
Carcinofibroma, uterine 559, *560*
Carcinogenesis
  field theory 189
  human papillomavirus (HPV) 299–300
Carcinogens, ovarian tumours 702
Carcinoid heart disease 807
Carcinoid syndrome 807, **1194**
  atypical carcinoid tumours of cervix 375
  small cell carcinoma of cervix 370
Carcinoid tumours
  cervix 375
    atypical 375
  gastrointestinal/bronchial/pancreatic, metastatic to
    ovary 886, 886–887
  goblet cell/mucinous, metastatic to ovary *810*,
    886, 886–887
  ovarian **806–811**
    classification 806–807
    clinical features 807
    histogenesis 807
    incidence and age 807
    insular 807, *808*, 808–809, *809*
    macroscopic appearance 807–808, *808*
    microscopic appearance *808*, 808–811, *809*,
      810
    mucinous 807, 809–810, *810*
    mucinous cystadenoma association 807
    strumal 807, *810*, 810–811
    trabecular 807, 809, *810*
    treatment and prognosis 811
  see also Small cell carcinomas
Carcinoma *see specific types and sites*
Carcinoma, clear cell *see* Clear cell adenocarcinoma
Carcinoma in situ
  Fallopian tube 607, *607*
  in mature teratoma 802–803, *803*
  vagina 201–203, *202*
  see also Adenocarcinoma in situ
Carcinomesenchymoma, uterine **559**
Carcinosarcoma
  alternative terminology 550
  cervical 561
  Fallopian tube 611, *611*
  HPV aetiological role 561
  ovarian 731
  prevalence 550
  spontaneous heterologous, female genital tract
    550
  uterine **559–573**
    adenosarcoma vs 557
    aetiology and clinical features 559, 561
    alternative terminology 550
    cytological evaluation 561–563
    differential diagnosis 570
    endometrial stromal tumours vs 514
    extrauterine spread 561

gross pathology 562, 564
    heterologous 565, 566, *567*, 567–569, *568*,
      569, 571
    homologous *563*, *564*, 565, *566*
    microscopic pathology 562, *563*, *564*, 564–570,
      565
    myometrial invasion 564, 571
    predictors of outcome 571–572
    prognostic factors 572
    risk factors 561
    role of carcinomatous component 572
    treatment 572–573
    vascular invasion 569
  see also Mixed Müllerian tumours
Cardiac arrest 1027
Cardiac failure
  amniotic fluid embolism syndrome 1565
  eclampsia *1551*, **1551**
  haemorrhagic endometrial infarction 408
  in pregnancy 1550
Cardiac transplants, in pregnancy **1553**
Cardinal ligaments of Mackenrodt 24, 248, *248*
Cardiomegaly, transient neonatal 1453
Cardiomyopathy
  dilated (congestive) 1552
  hypertrophic **1549**
  peripartal **1551–1553**
Cardiovascular system
  diseases in pregnancy **1541–1558**
    acquired disease 1547–1550
    blood coagulation changes 1543
    cardiac transplantation 1553
    disease arising during 1550–1553
    haemodynamic changes 1543
    hypertensive disease 1551
    myocardial infarction 1550
    pre-existing conditions 1543–1550
    see also individual diseases
  normal heart in pregnancy 1542–1543
  steroid contraceptives effect 1103
Carneous mole (massive subchorial haematoma)
  1284, 1285
Carney complex (CNC) **1182**
Carpal tunnel syndrome 1536
Cartilage
  cervical heterotopic 279
  tumours, ovarian **866**
  in uterine carcinosarcoma 566, *568*
Cartilaginous metaplasia, endometrium
  414
Castleman's disease 71–72
Cave of Retzius 28
Cavernous haemangioma *see* Haemangioma
Cavernous lymphangiomas, vulvar lymphangiomas
  122
CD1a, Langerhans' cell histiocytosis 957
CD4 T cells *see* T-cells
CD10
  endometrial stromal sarcoma differentiation 509
  uterine cellular leiomyoma 525
  uterine leiomyoma differential diagnosis 518
  uterine mesenchymal tumours 501
CD15 (Leu-M1), ovarian granulocytic sarcoma 948
CD20, ovarian lymphomas 944
CD30, embryonal carcinoma 788
CD34 staining, endometrial stromal sarcoma
  differentiation 509
CD44 expression
  cervical adenocarcinoma 358
  cervical cancer 332
  high-grade CGIN 358
CD56, endometrial granulocytes 1329
CD68
  endometrial hyperplasia 448
  ovarian granulocytic sarcoma 947, *947*
CD99 immunoreactivity
  adult-type granulosa cell tumour 751
  endometrial stromal tumours 512
Cell adhesion molecules, endometriosis 965
Cell columns, placenta 1259–1260
Cell islands, placenta *1259*, 1259–1260
Cell proliferation studies **1606–1607**
  cervical carcinoma 1607
  endometrial carcinoma **1606–1607**
  gestational trophoblastic disease 1607
  ovarian carcinoma **1606**
  vulvar carcinoma **1607**
Cellular differentiation, cervical intraepithelial
  neoplasia 312
Cellular fibromas *860*, 860–861

Central nervous system
  embryology 7–8
  in pregnancy *see* Nervous system diseases, in
    pregnancy
  trauma in pregnancy **1532**
Central pontine myelinosis **1531**
Centromeres 638
c-*erbB-2* oncogene
  cervical cancer 332
  endocervical neoplasia 360
  overexpression
    Fallopian tube adenocarcinoma 611
    ovarian adenocarcinoma 697
    ovarian carcinoma prognosis 736
    persistent trophoblastic disease 1386
    type-1 growth factor family oncogenes **1595–1596**
    uterine carcinosarcoma 572
Cerebellar degeneration, subacute **1198**
Cerebral angiopathy, postpartum 1524
Cerebral venous thrombosis **1525–1527**
Cerebrovascular accident *see* Stroke
Cerebrovascular disease, steroid contraceptives and
  1105
Cervical adenocarcinoma **339–351**
  aneuploidy 358
  barrier contraception 340
  in childhood/adolescence *1174*, **1174–1175**
  classification 341–349, *342*
  clear cell 344, 1174
    diethylstilboestrol 344, 1075
  cytomegalovirus 341
  endocervical 342, *342*, 473
    minimal deviation 342–343
    ovarian neoplasia and 350
  endometrioid 344
  Epstein–Barr virus 341
  herpes simplex virus 341
  hormones 340–341
  human papillomavirus 339
  incidence 339
  in situ 323–324, 373
  intestinal (enteric) type 343–344
  invasive, villous adenoma of cervix 348
  lymph node metastases 332, 350
  mesonephric 278, 348
  metastatic 349–350
    to ovary 889
  microinvasive 356–357
  minimal deviation 342, *342*, 759
  mucinous 473
    see also Cervical adenocarcinoma, endocervical
  non-neuroendocrine type 373
  prognostic indicators 350–351
  secondary 384
  stage 350
  tumours mimicking 290
  viruses and 339, 341
  see also Cervical carcinoma
Cervical canal 33
Cervical carcinoma
  adenocarcinoma *see* Cervical adenocarcinoma
  adenoid basal 345–346, *346*
  adenoid cystic 345, *345*
  adenosquamous *see* Adenosquamous carcinoma
  aetiology **298–303**
  amyloidosis and 1193
  aneuploidy **1611**
  apoptotic marker studies **1608**
  bax 1608
  bcl-2 1608
  cell proliferation studies **1607**
  chromosomal imbalances **1604**
  clear cell *see* Cervical adenocarcinoma, clear cell
  clonality studies **1603**
  c-*myc* **1597**
  comparative genomic hybridisation **1604**
  diethylstilboestrol (DES) exposure **1174–1175**
  DNA arrays 1605, *1605*
  DNA index 1611
  EGFR oncogenes **1596**
  epidemiology **298–303**
  FHIT 1600
  FIGO staging 319–320
  genetic factors 302–303
  glassy cell 349
  histological prognostic indicators **331–333**
  HIV/AIDS 1187
  human papillomavirus (HPV) *see* Human
    papillomavirus (HPV)
  immunological factors 302–303

invasive 297, **326–331**
  steroid contraceptives and 1098–1099
K-ras **1597**
large cell neuroendocrine 373–375
loss of heterozygosity (LOH) **1599–1600**
metastases **384–386**
  lung 1197
  ovary 881, 889
  placental 1455
  vagina 217, *217*
microinvasive 316–321, *317–320*
  definition 319–321
  distribution 357
  growth pattern 319
  histology of early invasive growth 317–318
  lymphatic channel involvement 318
  lymph node metastases 318, 332
  tumour dimensions 318–319
morphometry **1612–1613**
National Health Service Cervical Screening
  Programme 298
natural history **310–312**
p53 **1598–1599**
placental metastatic disease 1455
pregnancy 333
prognostic factors 331–332
radiotherapy 332
risk factors for different histological types *340*
schistosomiasis 1146–1147
screening *see* Cervical smears
sexual activity 298
small cell 369–373, *371*, *374–375*
  argyrophilic granules 372
  carcinoid syndrome 370
  clinical features 370
  differential diagnosis 372–373
  gross examination 370
  microscopic examination 370–372
  prognostic indicators 373
  special techniques 372
  ultrastructural features 372
squamous cell *291*, 297, 326–329, *327*, *328*
  age at first coitus 298
  FIGO international classification
    326
  histogenesis *309*
  keratinising type 327
  metastatic to ovary 889
  microscopic findings 326
  nodulo-infiltrative type 326
  number of sexual partners 298
  parity 298
  post radiotherapy *332*
  sexual intercourse 298
  spread 328–329
  ulceroinfiltrative type 326
telomerase activity **1601**
therapy, infertility after 996
trichomonal vaginitis association 175
  in tropics **1149**
vaginal intraepithelial neoplasia (VAIN)
  association 201
verrucous 329, 329–330
  biopsy 330
  human papillomavirus infection 329
Cervical epithelial–stromal interface 297
Cervical epithelium **247–272**
  abnormalities 267, 310–312, *311*
    basal abnormalities of uncertain significance
      (BAUS) 315
  atypical 267–268
    colposcopic appearance 267
    histological appearance 267–268
  basal cells 252, *253*, 254
    hyperplasia 267, 288, *289*
  changes, types/nomenclature 305
  columnar *257*
  congenital transformation zone 265, 267–268
  distribution *252*
  dynamic anatomy **251–268**
  functional cells 266–267
  intermediate layer *254*
  Langerhans' cells, epithelial 266
  metaplastic, atypical 267
  metaplastic cell origin 265–266
  metaplastic squamous 251, *259–265*, 274–275,
    287
    atypical immature 267
    colposcopic appearance 259–261
    histological appearance 262–265

original columnar 256–259, *260*
  gross morphological appearance 256–257
  histological appearance 257–258
  ultrastructural appearance 258–259
original squamous *252*, 252–256, *253*, *254*, *255*
  Basker-weave pattern *306*
  histological appearance 252–253
  parabasal layer *254*
  ultrastructural appearance 253–255
physiological changes **247–272**
physiological transformation zone *256*, *261*
stratified squamous 273
superficial squamous cell *255*
transformation zone 250, 251–252, 259, 275
types *251*
vacuolation by glycogen and koilocytic change
  285–286
see also Cervico–vaginal epithelium
Cervical ganglion *see* Uterovaginal plexus
Cervical glandular intraepithelial neoplasia (CGIN)
  351–356
  adenocarcinoma 353–354
  cervical surgery 354
  differential diagnosis 354–355
  high grade (H-CGIN) 351–353, *353*
  histology 352–353
  intestinal differentiation *344*
  low grade (L-CGIN) 351–353, *352*, *353*
  mimics 290
  taxonomy scheme *351*
  treatment and prognosis 355–356
Cervical intraepithelial neoplasia (CIN) 267,
  310–312
  ablative therapy, infertility after 996
  apoptotic marker studies **1608**
  BRCA1 1600
  cell proliferation studies **1607**
  chromosomal imbalances **1604**
  CIN 1 *313*
    histological features 313
  CIN 2 *314*
    histological features 314
  CIN 3 *314*
    high-grade CGIN 352
    histological features 314
  clonality studies 1603, **1603**
  criteria for diagnosis in pregnancy 276
  genetic abnormalities 310
  glandular *see* Cervical glandular intraepithelial
    neoplasia (CGIN)
  histogenesis 309–310
  histology **312–316**
  human papillomavirus infection 285, 1175
    and HIV 1153, 1187
    subclinical *306*, *307*
  Ki-67/MIB-1 reactivity 1613
  loss of heterozygosity (LOH) **1599–1600**
  morphometry **1612–1613**
  natural history **310–312**
  progression 311
  squamous, steroid contraceptives and 1098
  syntactic structure analysis 1613
  telomerase activity 1601
  terminology 305–306
  vaginal intraepithelial neoplasia relationship 201,
    202
Cervical lip, anterior, metaplastic transformation
  process *260*
Cervical mucus 277, **277**, 996–997
  abnormalities 997
  arborisation 277
  composition 277, 997
    changes 997
    changes in infections 997
    cyclical changes 997
    fatty acid and IUCD use 1113
  fertility promotion 997
  functions 277
  G-type 997
  hydrogel (E-type mucus) 997
  inadequate secretion 997
  lecithin 1113
  non-inflammatory hyperacidity 997
  periovulatory change 997
  postpartum 997
  sperm incompatibility 997
Cervical pregnancy 280, **1062**
  criteria for diagnosis 1062
  miscarriage 1062
  ovum transport 1062

Cervical smears
  cervical lymphoma detection 949
  Darier's disease 1183
  oestrogen therapy effect on 1074
  parasites **1148**
  radio/chemotherapy effects 1193
  schistosome eggs 1148, *1148*
  tamoxifen-associated changes 1081
  uterine lymphomas and leukaemia detection 949
Cervicitis
  acute 280, *280*
  bacterial, infertility and 994
  cervical mucus 277
  chronic 280–281
    morphology 281
    non-specific and chlamydial infection 283
    papillary 290
    plasma cell 281
  follicular 281, *284*
  granulomatous 281
  non-specific non-infectious, IUCD use and 1112
Cervicitis emphysematosa, trichomoniasis of cervix 284
Cervico–vaginal epithelium
  early fetal life 249–250
  early postnatal life 251
  late fetal life 250–251
  see also Cervical epithelium
Cervico-vaginal fistula 185
Cervix
  actinomycosis, IUCD use and 1113
  adenocarcinoma *see* Cervical adenocarcinoma
  adenoma, villoglandular papillary 383
  adenoma malignum *see* Adenoma malignum
  adenosarcoma 378
    embryonal rhabdomyosarcoma 378
  amyloidosis **1182**
  anatomy 247–272
  angiography 274
  aplasia 42, 996
  atresia, congenital 277
  benign epithelial tumours **382–383**
  benign mesenchymal tumours **383–384**
  benign mixed mesenchymal–epithelial tumours **384**
  blue naevus 279, *279*, 282, 382
  carcinoma *see* Cervical carcinoma
  choriocarcinoma 382
  combined steroid contraceptives effect 1097–1099, *1098*
  condylomata, human papillomavirus infection 303–304
    cervical intraepithelial neoplasia 304
    colposcopic appearance 303–304
  cone biopsy *324*, 324–325
    see also Cone biopsy
  congenital abnormalities **277–278**, 998
  congenital aplasia 996
  Cowden's disease (multiple hamartoma syndrome) **1182**
  cysts **287**
    epithelial inclusion 287
  deformities, diethylstilboestrol association 1075
  developmental abnormalities **277–278**
  development from paramesonephric duct 17
  diagnosis of premalignant disease, technical aspects 321–323
  dilatation and curettage *see* Dilatation and curettage
  discharge, lobular endocervical glandular hyperplasia 289
  diseases, Bethesda classification system 306–308
  dyskaryosis, IUCD use and 1114
  ectopic pregnancy *see* Cervical pregnancy
  ectopy 1097
  effect of steroid contraceptives 1097–1099, *1098*
  embryonal rhabdomyosarcoma
    see Embryonal rhabdomyosarcoma
  endocrine tumours **369–375**
    classification *374*
  endometrial carcinoma metastases 349
  endometriosis 278, *980*
  epithelium *see* Cervical epithelium
  eversion
    cervical squamous neoplasia 309
    transformation zone 323
  germ cell tumours 380
  glandular lesions **339–368**
    see also Cervical glandular intraepithelial neoplasia (CGIN)

  glandular neoplasia *see* Cervical adenocarcinoma
  glucose supply for sperm 994
  granulocytic sarcoma (myelosarcoma) 951–952, *952*
  heterotopia **278–280**
  Hodgkin's disease 951
  hyperplasia **288–290**
    see also Endocervical hyperplasia
  implantation of metastasis 384
  incompetence 997–998
    aetiological classification 997–998
    diagnosis 998
    miscarriage, second-trimester 1433
    prematurity 48
  infections **281–287**
  infertility due to abnormalities 996–998
  inflammation **280–281**
    neoplasia 292
    radiotherapy 292
  inflammatory lesions, lymphoma vs 952
  internal os 247
  intrauterine contraceptive device (IUCD) effect 1112–1114
  laceration, intrauterine contraceptive device 1106
  leiomyomas 383–384
  leiomyosarcoma 378–379
  ligaments 248, *248*
  ligneous (pseudomembranous) inflammation 996
  lipoma 384
  local immune response 274
  lymphomas 949
  malignant melanoma **380–382**
    differential diagnosis 381–382
  malposition, infertility 996
  MALT lymphomas 950, *950*
  mechanical lesions, infertility due to 996
  megaloblastic anaemia 1188
  melanosis 279, 382
  menstrual cycle changes 275
  mesenchymal tumours 383–384
  metaplasia *253, 264*, **287–288**
  metastases **384–386**
    from endometrial stromal sarcoma 510–511
    from extragenital sites 385–386
    from genital tract sites 384
    from lobular carcinoma of breast 385, *386*
    signet-ring carcinoma *385*
    small cell carcinoma 373
  microglandular hyperplasia 1098
    endometrial adenocarcinoma vs 463
    progestagens causing 1084
    steroid contraceptives causing 1097–1098, *1098*
  mucosal immunity 274
  mucous barrier, endometritis 419
  Müllerian papilloma *1176*, **1176**
  neurofibroma 384
  non-Hodgkin's lymphoma **948–953**
    see also Non-Hodgkin's lymphoma
  non-neoplastic conditions **273–296**
  normal histology **273–274**
    endocervical epithelium 274
  obstruction, pyometra 420
  occlusion 277
  oestrogen and 340
  oestrogens therapy effect 1074
  physiological changes **274–277**
    epithelium **247–272**
  physiology **274–277**
    and aging 276–277
  polyarteritis nodosa 291
  polyps 290
    endometrial polyp risk 415
    see also Endocervical polyps
  pregnancy *262*
  premalignant and malignant squamous lesions **297–338**
  premalignant disease *see* Cervical intraepithelial neoplasia (CIN)
  primary tumours **369–384**
  progestagen effect 1084, 1192
  pseudosarcomatous lesions 380
  pubertal 261
  radiotherapy effect 292, *292*
  reserve cell hyperplasia 1097
  Rosai–Dorfman disease 953
  sarcoidosis 281
  sarcomas **375–380**
  schistosomiasis 1144–1145, 1146, *1147*
  secondary disease **290–291**

  sperm transport 1007
  squamous cell carcinoma *see* Cervical carcinoma, squamous
  squamous lesions **297–338**
  squamous metaplasia 274, *274*
  squamous neoplasia, histogenesis **309–310**
  stenosis, endometrial squamous cell carcinoma 473
  stroma **248–249**
    decidualisation *276*
    fetal 275
    histology 274
  stromal sarcoma *see* Endocervical stromal sarcoma
  structural abnormalities and in utero exposure to diethylstilboestrol 278
  supravaginal 33, 248
  systemic diseases **290–292**
  teratoma
    imprinted genes 1605
    mature 380
  transformation zone *see* Transformation zone
  trichomoniasis, basal cell hyperplasia 284
  trophoblastic tumours 382
  tuberculosis 281, 282
  ulceration, pemphigus vulgaris 291
  undifferentiated neoplasms 952
  vaginal 33
  villoglandular papillary adenoma 383
  warts, multiple, cytomegalovirus infection 286
  wedge biopsy 333
  Wilm's tumour 382
  see also Entries beginning endocervical
Cervix uteri 33
Cestode infections **1143–1144**
c-fms (CSF receptor), oncogene expression studies **1597**
Chancre
  cervical 282
  vaginal 168, *168, 169*
  vulvar 58
Chancroid, vulvar infection 57
Charcot–Böttcher crystals 704
Charcot–Böttcher filaments, sex cord–stromal tumours with annular tubules 759
Chédiak-Higashi syndrome, ovarian tumours **1182**
Chemical lesions, vagina 154
Chemotherapy
  adult-type granulosa cell tumours 751–752
  choriocarcinoma 1405
  dysgerminoma 776–777
  follicular damage 1015
  gonadoblastoma 832
  immature teratoma 793–794
  ovarian changes due to 679
  ovarian tumours
    borderline serous tumours 723
    mixed germ cell sex cord–stromal tumours 839, 841
    resistance 1604
  in pregnancy 958
  primary peritoneal serous carcinoma 925
  resistance, chromosomal imbalances 1604
  sensitivity, *Bcl-2* 1608
  uterine carcinosarcoma 573
  uterine leiomyosarcoma 523
  vaginal cancer 192
  yolk sac tumours 785
Childbirth *see* Delivery; Labour; Preterm delivery
Children
  chlamydial infections, vaginal 165
  follicle cysts 664
  genital tract pathology **1157–1180**
  gonococcal-like vaginitis 168
  herpetic vulvo-vaginitis 163
  linear IgA disease 71
  neoplasms of ovarian/genital tract **1163–1177**
    epithelial **1174–1175**
    germ cell tumours **1164–1169**
    mesenchymal **1172–1174**
    mixed germ cell sex cord–stromal tumours **1172**
    pattern 1163–1164, *1164*
    sex cord–stromal tumours **1169–1172**
  non-neoplastic ovarian lesions **1162–1163**
    miscellaneous **1175–1177**
  syphilis, sexual abuse and 168
  tubular torsion 594
  vaginal epithelium 159
  vaginal foreign bodies 153

vulvo-vaginitis 159
see also Adolescence
Chimerism
    blood group in dizygotic twins 1579
    placental in vanishing twin syndrome 1585
Chlamydia
    detection 158
    inclusion bodies 426
Chlamydial infections (*Chlamydia trachomatis*)
    cervical 283–284
    chorioamnionitis 1305
    detection, cervico-vaginal smears 164, *164*
    ectopic pregnancy 1049
    endometritis 426–427, 993–994, 1003
        chronic 1134
    follicular cervicitis *284*
    inclusions *164*
    infertility and 993–994, 1010
    lymphogranuloma venereum
            see Lymphogranuloma venereum
    miscarriage 1432
    salpingitis 616, 620, 622
    transmission 165
    vagina *164,* 164–165
        steroid contraceptives and 1099
    vaginitis 158, 165
    vulvar 58
Chloroma *see* Granulocytic sarcoma
Chlorpromazine
    drug-induced hepatic injury in pregnancy 1480
    postpartum depression 1523
Chocolate cysts *see* Endometriotic cysts
Cholangiocarcinoma, steroid contraceptives and
            1101
Cholecystectomy, pregnancy 1485
Cholecystokinin, levels reduced by combined oral
            contraceptives 1092
Cholelithiasis, pregnancy **1484–1485**
Cholestasis, intrahepatic *see* Intrahepatic cholestasis
Cholesterol
    steroid contraceptives effect 1103
    Tibolone and combined HRT effects
            1090
Cholesterol gallstones, pregnancy 1484
Cholesterol saturation index of bile, pregnancy
            1485
Chondroitin sulphate A, malarial parasites 1319
Chondroma, ovarian *865,* **866**
Chondrosarcoma
    ovarian *866,* **866**
    in uterine carcinosarcoma *568, 569*
    vulvar extraskeletal mesenchymal 125
Chorangiomas, placental *see* Placental haemangioma
Chorangiomatosis 1449
    chorangiosis vs 1451
Chorangiopagus parasiticus twin *see* Acardiac fetus
Chorangiosis 1289, *1290*
Chorea gravidarum **1524**
    antiphospholipid syndrome **1524**
    contraceptive pill 1524
    oestrogen 1524
Chorioamnionitis 1303, *1303*
    congenital pneumonia 1306
    HIV/AIDS 1152
    human immunodeficiency virus infection 1318
    listeriosis 1314
    membrane rupture, premature 1306
    necrotising funisitis 1300
    organisms involved 1305
Chorioangiomas, placental *see* Placental
            haemangioma
Choriocarcinoma 1384, *1385,* **1398–1405**
    aetiology and pathogenesis 1394–1395
        environmental factors 1396
    antecedent gestation types *1397*
    cervix 382
    clinical features 1398
    differential diagnosis 1414
    epithelioid trophoblastic tumours **1409–1411**
    Fallopian tube 1398
    genetic polymorphisms **1405**
    genetics 1395
    gestational, non-gestational vs 786
    gonadoblastoma association 830
    hydatidiform moles 1384, 1385
    hyperreactio luteinalis association 676
    immunocytochemistry **1404**
    incidence 1396–1397
    Ki-67 index 1404
    macroscopic appearances **1398,** *1399*

metastases 1401, **1402–1403**
    prevalence and sites *1397*
        vaginal deposits 218, *218,* 221–222, *222*
    microscopic appearances **1398–1402,** *1400–1404*
    myometrial invasion 1401
    non-gestational **785–787,** *786*
    pathology **1398–1405**
    placental defects 1347
    post-ectopic pregnancy 1060
    in pregnancy 1535
    prognosis 1405
    pure non-gestational 1167, *1167*
    in tropics **1150**
    ultrastructure **1403–1404**
Chorion 5
    formation 5
Chorionic gonadotrophin *see* Human chorionic
            gonadotrophin (hCG)
Chorionic plate
    definitive 1256
    development 1253–1257, *1255*
    placenta extrachorialis 1274
    primary
        layers day 14 post-conception 1256
        placental development 1235
Chorionic vein tears, subamniotic haematoma 1284
Chorionic villi *see* Placental villi
Chorionic villus sampling, amniotic band syndrome
            1307
Chorion laeve
    formation 1257
    paraplacental exchange organ 1257
Chromidrosis, vulvar involvement 84
Chromoblastomycosis (chromomycosis), vulvar
            infection 56
Chromogranin, small cell ovarian tumours 904, *904*
Chromophobe cells 1022
Chromosomal abnormalities
    age at conception and 991
    behavioural 992
    cervical carcinoma **1604**
    comparative genomic hybridisation **1604–1605**
    endometrial carcinoma 1604
    fetal
        placental villous histology 1440
        sporadic miscarriage 1431–1432
    gonadoblastoma 824
    granulosa cell tumours and thecomas 705
    infertility and 992
    in situ hybridisation 1603
    miscarriage, spontaneous sporadic 1435
    mutations 992
    ovarian carcinoma *1604,* **1604**
    ovarian failure 1015
    ovarian tumours 702
    types/groups 992
Chromosomal instability, female infertility 995
Chromosomal translocation 992
    Burkitt's lymphoma 943
    intra-abdominal desmoplastic small round cell
            tumour 920
Chromosome 3p14, cervical intraepithelial neoplasia
            (CIN) 310
Chromosome 11, aggressive angiomyxoma 121
Chromosome 12, aggressive angiomyxoma 121
Chromosomes
    centromere 638
    marker, vaginal squamous cell carcinoma
            200–201
    sex *see* Sex chromosomes
    sex determining 3
    terminology 638
Chromosome Y specific genes, hermaphrodite, true
            1228
Chronic bullous disease of childhood
            see Linear IgA disease
Chronic plasma cell balanoposthitis 79–80
Chronic twin–twin transfusion *see* Twin–twin
            transfusion
Cicatricial pemphigoid *70,* 70–71
Cigarette smoking *see* Smoking
Cilia
    activity depression, Fallopian tube 1008
    endometrial cells 1005
    endometrial glandular cells 462
Ciliated cells
    basilar, vaginal 150
    endometrial epithelium 394, 411, *412*
    Fallopian tubes 587
    immature teratoma *791*
CIN *see* Cervical intraepithelial neoplasia (CIN)

Circinate ulcerative vulvitis 73
Circumcision, female 1151
Circummarginate placenta 1274, *1274*
Circumvallate placenta 1274, *1274*
    congenital malformations 1275
    extramembranous pregnancy 1306
    low birth weight 1275
Cirrhosis
    pregnancy in 1483
    primary biliary, fetal microchimerism 1481–1482
c-kit gene
    dysgerminoma 773, 776
    gonadoblastoma in mixed gonadal dysgenesis
            1227
Clear cell(s), endometrial stromal tumours 503
Clear cell adenocarcinoma
    cervix 345, *345*
    diethylstilboestrol (DES) exposure 204, *207,*
            1075, **1174–1175**
    endometrial *see* Endometrial carcinoma, clear cell
    endometriosis 976
    extragonadal endometriosis 978
    Fallopian tube 611
    Krukenberg tumours vs 732
    Müllerian, ovarian tumours of probable Wolffian
            origin vs 902
    ovarian *731,* 731–732
        endometriosis and 977
    ovarian and endometriosis 977
    signet ring cells 732
    vagina 204, 344
        diethylstilboestrol association 204, *207,* 1075
        see also Vagina, adenocarcinoma
    vulvar endometriosis 132
Clear cell adenosquamous carcinoma of cervix 349
Clear cell hidradenoma, vulvar 127
Clear cell hyperplasia, Fallopian tube 607
Clear cell lesions, peritoneal 927
Clear cell metaplasia of endometrium 413
Clear cell pattern, epithelioid smooth muscle
            tumour (uterine) 530
Clear cell tumours, ovarian *694, 696, 699*
    adenocarcinoma *731,* 731–732
    benign 716
    borderline 727, *727*
Cleavage division 2
Cleft palate, anti-epileptics 1533
Clitoris
    development 19–20
    haemangioma, neonatal *119*
    neurofibroma 1172
Clitoromegaly, gonadoblastoma 826
Cloacal dysgenesis sequence 1158
Cloacal membrane 6
Cloacogenic carcinoma, vagina 208
Clomiphene (clomiphene citrate) **1075–1076**
    adverse effects 1028, 1075–1076
    endometrial appearance after 405
    increased ovarian carcinoma risk 700
    indications 1075
    mechanism of action 1075
Clonality, cervical squamous neoplasia 309
Clonality studies **1602–1603**
    cervical carcinoma **1603**
    endometrial carcinoma **1602–1603**
    mixed neoplasms **1603**
    ovarian carcinoma **1602**
    ovarian endometriosis 1602
    synchronous/metachronous tumours
            1603
    vulvar carcinoma **1603**
Clostridium infection
    gangrene 58
    puerperal sepsis 1562
    salpingitis 620
Clostridium perfringens
    aplastic anaemia in pregnancy 431
    endometritis 431
Clostridium vaginale see Gardnerella vaginalis
            (*Clostridium vaginale*)
Clue cells 157, 166
    bacterial vaginosis 157
    detection methods 157
    Gardnerella vaginalis infection *166*
CMV *see* Cytomegalovirus (CMV)
c-myc oncogene
    endocervical neoplasia 359–360
    expression studies **1597**
    overexpression, ovarian carcinoma prognosis 736
    uterine carcinosarcoma 572

Coagulation
  changes in pregnancy **1543**
  defect, amniotic fluid embolism 1565
  disseminated intravascular
      see Disseminated intravascular coagulation
  intravascular, pre-eclampsia 1506
Coagulative tumour cell necrosis
  mitotically active leiomyoma (uterine) 524, *524*
  uterine leiomyosarcoma 521, 522, *522*
Coagulopathy
  maternal, fetal artery thrombosis 1282
  postpartum haemorrhage 1561
Coarctation of aorta **1543–1544**
Cocaine, infertility and 996
Coccidioides immitis, endometritis 432
Coccidioidomycosis, tuberculous salpingitis vs 618
Coccygeus muscle, pelvic floor 23
Coccyx, anatomy 21
Coelomic epithelial cells 637, *637*, 647
  proliferation 645
Coelomic metaplastic theory, endometriosis 964
'Coffee bean' nuclei, of Langerhans' cells 957
Coitus see Sexual intercourse
Cold knife cones
  margins, cervical glandular intraepithelial
      neoplasia 355
  microinvasive glandular lesions of cervix 357
Collagen
  cervical stroma 249
  intercellular hyalinised, endometrial stromal
      tumours 502
  synthesis, myometrium in pregnancy 1330
  vaginal 151
Collagen III deficiency, premature membrane
      rupture 1306
Colon, vaginal fistula 185
Colon cancer
  hereditary non-polyposis see Hereditary non-
      polyposis colon carcinoma (HNPCC)
  metastatic
      to ovary 881, *882*, 882–884, *883*, *884*
      to vagina 219, *219*
  reduced risk after HRT 1089
Colony-stimulating factor (CSF), oncogene
      expression studies **1597**
Colposcopic punch biopsy 323
Colposcopy *321*
  abnormal cervical findings 321–323
  biopsy specimen examination 323
  cervical carcinoma in pregnancy 333
  cervical epithelial abnormalities 321
  cervical examination 321–323
  chlamydial infection of cervix 283
  normal cervical findings 321
  postmenopausal women 323
Columnar epithelium of cervix *257*
Combined steroid contraceptives (oral) 1091
  accelerated metabolism 1192–1193
  adverse effects 1092
  candidiasis of cervix 283
  cerebrovascular disease and 1105
  cervical carcinoma and 302, 340
      invasive 1098–1099
  cervical mucus 277
  cervical physiology 275
  chorea gravidarum 1524
  Crohn's disease 1186
  ectopic pregnancy 1050
  effect on breast and breast cancer 1100
  effect on cardiovascular system 1103
  effect on cervix 1097–1099, *1098*
  effect on endometrium 1092–1095, *1093*, *1094*
  effect on myometrium 1097
  effect on other tissues 1105–1106
  effect on ovary 1099–1100
  effect on vagina 1099
  effects on liver 1100–1103
  endometrial carcinoma and 455, 1091, 1094
  failure rate 1092
  haemolytic uraemic syndrome 1505
  haemorrhagic cellular leiomyoma (apoplectic)
      525, 526
  hypertension and 1105
  idiopathic postpartum acute renal failure 1505
  increased mid-cycle oestrogen 1093
  infertility and 989
  ischaemic heart disease and 1104–1105
  leiomyosarcoma and 1095
  mechanism of action and ovulation failure 1017,
      1091

  monophasic, biphasic and triphasic 1091
  ovarian carcinoma risk reduced 700–701
  pelvic inflammatory disease risk 620
  persistent trophoblastic disease 1384
  sex cord–stromal tumours risk 705
  smoking 1186
  squamous cervical intraepithelial neoplasia (CIN)
      and 1098
  systemic consequences 1196
  third generation 1091, 1092
      contraindications 1104
      thromboembolic disease and 1104
  thromboembolic disease and 1103–1104
  trichomonal vaginitis and 175
  uterine sarcomas and 1095
  vaginal candidiasis association 172
  villoglandular papillary adenocarcinoma of cervix
      347
  see also Contraception, steroid
Comparative genomic hybridisation
  cervical carcinoma **1604**
  chromosomal imbalances **1604–1605**
  endometrial carcinoma 1604
  ovarian carcinoma *1604*, **1604**
Complement deposition
  decidual arteries in pre-eclampsia 1340
  diabetes mellitus in pregnancy 1344
  mesangiocapillary glomerulonephritis in
      pregnancy 1514, *1514*
  SLE in pregnancy 1345
Compression necrosis 1151
Conceptus
  abnormal, ectopic pregnancy 1051
  immune tolerance 1006
  maturation, endometrial secretory activity 1328
  maturation delay, cervical pregnancy
      1062
Condensation zone, squamous epithelium of cervix
      253
Condyloma *304*
  giant (proliferative) 162
  see also Verrucous carcinoma, vulvar
Condyloma acuminata **1175**
  cervical 303, *303*
  'flat' vaginal *163*
  human papillomavirus infection 299, 303
  vagina *161*, **161–162**, *162*, *163*
  vulvar (warts) 59, 97, *97*
      epithelium 98
Condylomata lata, vulva 58
Cone biopsy *324*, 324–325
  cervical *324*, 324–325
  cervical carcinoma
      microinvasive 318–319
      in pregnancy 333
  endometrial curettage 325
Confidential Enquiries into Maternal Deaths in the
      United Kingdom, Report 1559, 1560
Confluent growth, microinvasive carcinoma of
      cervix 319
Congenital abnormalities/malformations
  amnion nodosum 1303
  cervical atresia 277
  cervix 277–278, 998
  circumvallate placentas 1275
  Fallopian tube
      congenital inguinal ectopia 594
      infertility due to 1009
  female genital tract **41–52**
      aetiology and pathogenesis 45
      classification and types 42–45
      clinical features and significance 46–48
      complications 48
      incidence 45–46
  intestinal atresia, umbilical cord ulceration 1299
  ovary
      absent/reduced follicle pool due to 1014–1015
      congenital inguinal ectopia 594
  tubal pregnancy 1046–1047
  Turner's syndrome 1222
  uterine
      endometriosis 964
      see also Uterus, malformations
  vagina 148
      infertility due to 995–996
  vulva 995–996
  see also Fetus, malformations; Genital tract,
      malformations
Congenital adrenal hyperplasia see Adrenal
      hyperplasia, congenital

Congenital adrenogenital syndrome 855
Congenital heart disease
  anti-epileptics 1533
  heart block **1547**
Congenital pneumonia, chorioamnionitis 1306
Congenital syphilis see Syphilis
Congenital transformation zone, cervical epithelium
      265, 267–268
Congenital tuberculosis 427
Conisation, cervical incompetence due to 998
Conjoined twins *1586*, 1586–1587
  coronal plane 1586
Conjunctivitis, ligneous (pseudomembranous) **1187**
Connecting stalk, umbilical cord development 1255
Constriction rings
  amniotic bands and strings 1307
  intrauterine amputations 1308
Contarini's syndrome 1197
Contraception 989, **1090–1118**
  barrier see Barrier contraception
  ectopic pregnancy 1049–1050
  failure, genital tract malformations 48
  intrauterine devices see Intrauterine contraceptive
      device (IUCD)
  oral see Combined steroid contraceptives (oral)
  pathology **1090–1118**
  pelvic inflammatory disease risk factor
      993
  steroid **1091–1106**
      Budd–Chiari syndrome 1481
      cerebrovascular disease and 1105
      combined see Combined steroid contraceptives
          (oral)
      contraindications 1100
      effect on cardiovascular system 1103
      effect on cervix 1097–1099, *1098*
      effect on endometrium 1092–1097
      effect on myometrium 1097
      effect on other tissues 1105–1106
      effect on vagina 1099
      effects on breast 1100
      effects on liver 1100–1103
      effects on ovary 1099–1100
      high-dose oestrogen 1091, *1096*
      hypertension and 1105
      ischaemic heart disease and 1104–1105
      pelvic inflammatory disease and 1099
      progestagen-only see Progestagen-only
          contraceptives ('mini-pill')
      thromboembolic disease and 1103–1104
      see also Combined steroid contraceptives (oral)
  tubal sterilisation and see Sterilisation, tubal
Copper
  intrauterine contraceptive device 1106, 1107,
      1109
      ectopic pregnancy and 1117
      menstrual blood loss 1117
      pregnancy (intrauterine) and 1117
  serum levels after IUCD use 1117
Cornstarch powder, granulomatous reaction 1011
Cornual obstruction, by leiomyoma 999
Coronary artery disease, steroid contraceptives and
      1104–1105
Corpora lutea, pregnancy 677
Cor pulmonale, acute, amniotic fluid embolism
      syndrome 1565
Corpus albicans 657
Corpus luteum
  calcific deposits, misinterpretation as malignant
      change 685
  cysts *665*, **665**, 1017
  deficiency see Luteal phase defect
  dysfunction 1000
  formation 656–657, **1014**
      premature 1017–1018
  function defects 405
      see also Luteal phase deficiency
  luteal-placental shift 1014
  plasma progesterone 1328
  premature failure 407–408
  steroid production 1014
Cortical stromal hyperplasia 670, 671
Corticotroph adenoma 1024
Corticotropin-releasing hormone (CRF) 1020
Cortisol, ectopic production 850, 1194
Corynebacterium diphtheriae, vaginitis 169
Corynebacterium minutissimum, vulvar infections 56
Corynebacterium vaginale 157
Cotinine, cervical cancer 302
Coumarin derivatives 1549

Covarian tumours, serous, histiogenesis 696–697
Cowden's disease (multiple hamartoma syndrome)
    1182
    vulvar genetic disorders 62
Cowpox, vulvar infection 60
Coxsackie virus, miscarriage 1432
Cribriform glands, microinvasive glandular lesions
    of cervix 356
Crohn's disease *64*, **1184–1186**
    anogenital lesions 64
    Fallopian tubes 1185, *1185*
    fistulae 1185, 1186
    granuloma 684, 1185, 1186, *1186*
    hidradenitis suppurativa 82
    ovarian granuloma 684, 1185, *1186*
    ovarian involvement 684
    in pregnancy 1185
    steroid contraceptives and 1106, 1186
    vulvitis granulomatosa 1188
    vulvo-vaginal, vaginal intraepithelial neoplasia
        with 203
Cryptococcus glabratus, endometritis 432
Curettage
    endocervical 323–324, 325
    endometrial 325
        see also Uterus, curettage
    hydatidiform moles 1384
    trophoblastic lesion biopsy 1412
    see also Dilatation and curettage
Cushing's syndrome **1194**
    carcinoid tumours with 807
    cervical small cell carcinoma 370
    mature teratoma association 797
    steroid cell tumours causing 850
Cycle length variation 393
Cyclophosphamide, ovarian changes due to 679
Cylindroma, vagina 210
Cyst(s)
    Bartholin's gland duct 84, *84*
    canal of Nuck 85
    cervical **287**
    cervical epithelial inclusion 287
    chocolate *see* Endometriotic cysts
    corpus luteum 665, *665*, 1017
    dermoid *see* Dermoid cyst
    emphysematous, vaginal *178*, 178–179, *179*
    endometriotic 287, 968, *974*
        of ovary 715
    epidermal 83
    epidermoid, ovarian 717
    epithelial inclusion 287
    fluid filled inside placental cell islands 1260
    follicle *see* Follicle cysts
    Gartner's 180
    hydatid 287
    hydatid of Morgagni 624
    inclusion, peritoneal 914–915, *915*, 922
    luteal 665, **665**, 1017
    lutein, nonspecific 677
    mesonephric *see* Mesonephric cysts
    mucinous 84–85, *85*
    Müllerian duct 278
    multiloculated peritoneal inclusion 914–915, *915*
    myometrial 500–501
    Nabothian *see* Nabothian cysts (follicle)
    ovarian *see* Ovary, cysts
    paraintroital 182, *182*
    paramesonephric 623–624, *624*
    paraovarian/paratubal *624*
    postoperative peritoneal 914, 915
    rete ovarii 903
    septal, intervillous thrombosis 1285
    umbilical cord *see* Umbilical cord, cysts
    vaginal *see* Vagina, cysts
    vaginal cuff 180
    vulvar 85, *85*
    Walthard rest 592, *593*
Cystadenofibroma
    endometrial, ovarian endometriosis 976
    endometrioid 715
    papillary (uterine) *551*, **551–552**
    serous papillary 624, *625*
        in paratubal cyst 624, *624*
Cystadenoma
    broad ligament, papillary 625
    endometrioid 699
    mucinous *see* Mucinous cystadenoma
    serous
        ovarian 713–714
        papillary 714, *714*

Cysticercosis, tuberculous salpingitis vs 618
Cystic granulosa cell tumour 746–747, *747*
    unilocular 677
Cystic hyperplasia, endometrial
        see Endometrial hyperplasia
Cystic teratoma 1149, 1198
    benign, vaginal 216
    exophytic papillary growth *802*
    extraovarian teratoma association 795
    Fallopian tube 605
    macroscopic appearance *797*, 798, *798*, *802*
    malignant change *802*, 802–803, *803*
    microscopic appearance *798*, *799*, *800*, *802*
    mucinous tumours association 697
    ovarian 939
    reactive phenomena 800, *801*
    tissue types found *798*
    vaginal (benign) 216
Cytochrome P450 enzymes
    aromatase 1005
        uterine endometrium in endometriosis 966
    cervical expression and smoking 302
    P450c21, 21–hydroxylase deficiency 1213
Cytogenetics
    abnormalities, miscarriage 1435
    Fallopian tube adenocarcinoma 611
    Turner's syndrome 1221
    uterine leiomyoma 516–517
Cytokeratin(s)
    aberrant expression, uterine leiomyosarcoma 522
    cervical epithelium 265
    cervical tumours 348
    CK7
        ovarian metastases from appendiceal carcinoma
            884
        primary ovarian carcinoma 884
    CK20
        ovarian metastases from appendiceal carcinoma
            884
        primary ovarian carcinoma (negative) 884
    endometrial stromal tumours 502
    Fallopian tube 587
    ovarian tumours of Wolffian origin 899
    Paget's disease of vulva 99
    primary ovarian carcinoma vs colonic metastases
        884
    small cell ovarian tumours 904, *904*
    uterine adenomatoid mesothelioma 539, *539*
    uterine carcinosarcoma 566–567
Cytokines
    changes in endometrium 1006
    chorioamnionitis and premature onset of labour
        1305
    endometriosis 965
    peritoneal fluid in endometriosis 1019
Cytomegalovirus (CMV)
    cervical adenocarcinoma 341
    cervical infection 286–287
    endometritis 426
    focal cortical necrosis of ovary 683
    inclusion bodies, placental infection 1317
    liver allograft recipients and pregnancy 1484
    miscarriage 1432
    placental examination 1317, *1317*
    vulvar infection 59
Cytoplasmic inclusions, uterine leiomyoma with
        bizarre nuclei 526, 526–527
Cytosol protein receptors, high affinity 20
Cytotoxic T cells, human papillomavirus infection
    302
Cytotrophoblast
    apoptosis 1241
    extravillous *see* Extravillous cytotrophoblast
    placental development 1233
    proliferation
        decidual spiral arteries 1335
        trophoblastic ischaemia in pre-eclampsia 1310
    syncytial fusion 1239
    villous, proliferation 1239
Cytotrophoblast cells
    hyperplasia, trophoblastic membrane thickening
        1287
    placental barrier 1236
    villous trophoblast 1236
Cytotrophoblastic cells, villous, maternal
        uteroplacental blood flow reduction 1287

D
D9B1 monoclonal antibody 1110
Danazol (Danocrine)

adverse effects 1028
    effect on endometrium 1083, *1085*
    pseudopregnancy therapy in endometriosis 982
Darier's disease *62*, 1183
    vulvar genetic disorders 61–62
Dating, endometrial 1000
DAX1 gene 641
    mutation 1016
    ovarian development 1210
    sex determination 1210
Deafness, sensorineural deafness (Perrault
        syndrome) **1190**
Decay accelerating factor 1006
Decidua
    capsular 1257
    changes
        endometriosis 971
        tubal pregnancy 1055–1056, *1056*
    ectopic 682, **682**, 927–928, *928*
        ovary 682, *682*
        peritoneum **927–928**, *928*
    metaplasia, ectopic pregnancy *591*
    necrosis, pre-eclampsia 1342
    placenta creta 1347
    vaginal squamous cell carcinoma vs 220, *221*
Decidual arteries
    C3 deposition in pre-eclampsia 1340
    cytotrophoblast proliferation 1335
    IgM deposition in pre-eclampsia 1340
Decidual cast, ectopic pregnancy *1058*
Decidualisation
    cervical epithelium 276
    endocervical stroma *276*
Decidual-myometrial junction, multinucleated giant
        cells 1334–1335
Decidual response, defective 1025
Decidual veins, pregnancy 1336
Deciduoid mesothelioma *918*, 918–919
Deciduosis 590–591, *591*
Deep perineal pouch 37
Deep vein thrombosis, oral contraceptives and
    1104
Defibrination syndrome 1503
Delivery (birth)
    caesarean *see* Caesarean section
    vaginal *see* Vaginal delivery
Dense-core granules, small cell carcinoma of uterine
        cervix 372
Depigmentation, vulvar 69
Depression, postpartum 1523
Dermatitis, vulvar 74, *74*
Dermatitis herpetiformis, vulvar 71
Dermatofibromas, vulvar 116
Dermatofibrosarcoma, vulvar *117*
Dermatofibrosarcoma protuberans, vulvar
        116–117
Dermatomyositis **1193–1194**
Dermatophyte fungi, vulvar infection 55
Dermatoses, vagina 154–155
Dermoid cyst
    Fallopian tube 605
    ovarian 1164
DES *see* Diethylstilboestrol
Desmin
    expression, endometrial stromal tumours 512
    immunoreactivity
        carcinosarcoma (uterine) 567–568
        cellular leiomyoma (uterine) 525
Desmoid tumour, vulvar 85
17,20–Desmolase deficiency 1216
20,22–Desmolase deficiency 1216
Desmoplastic small round cell tumour
    extrauterine stromal sarcoma vs 514
    intra-abdominal *919*, 919–920
    ovarian 906, 906–907, *907*
Desonorgestrel, thromboembolic disease and
        1104
Desquamative inflammatory vaginitis 179–180
Desquamative vaginitis 79
Detrusor muscle 30
Development, sexual *see* Sexual development
Developmental anatomy, cervix **249–251**
Developmental disorders
    cervix 277–278
    female infertility 995
    gonads/genital tract **1157–1162**
    see also Congenital abnormalities/malformations
Development of external genitalia 18–21
    mechanism of differentiation 20–21
DHT *see* Dihydrotestosterone (DHT)

Diabetes mellitus **1183**
  endometrial adenocarcinoma risk factor 455,
    456, 1183
  gestational 1025, 1092
  infertility and 1025
  insulin-dependent, infective vaginitis 160
  miscarriage 1433
  placental examination 1308
  polycystic ovarian disease 1183
  pregnancy 1344
  vulvovaginitis 1183
Diabetic glomerulopathy in pregnancy **1517–1519,**
    1518
  diffuse/nodular glomerulosclerosis 1518
  Kimmelstiel–Wilson nodules 1518, *1518*
  pre-eclampsia 1517
Dialysis, pregnancy 1511
Diathermy, pin and ball, cervical glandular
    intraepithelial neoplasia 356
Diathermy heat artifact, large loop excision
    specimen 325
Dichorionic–diamniotic twin placentation 1576,
    1581
  chorionic tissue in septum 1587
  monochorionic–diamniotic placentation vs 1587
  monozygotic twins 1577
Dichorionic placenta *1576*
  fused 1579
  twin placentas, complete molar change 1586
  vascular communications 1579
Diet, ovarian tumours association 703
Diethylstilboestrol (DES) **1074–1075**
  cervical carcinoma association 1174
    clear cell adenocarcinoma 344, **1174–1175**
  cervical deformities 1075
  cervical incompetence due to 998
  prenatal exposure effects 1074–1075
    ectopic pregnancy 1047
    vaginal development 16
  tubal defects due to 1009
  uterine problems 1075
  vaginal adenosis and 1075
  vaginal carcinoma association 188, 204, 207, *207*,
    1075, 1174
    clear cell adenocarcinoma **1174–1175**
  vaginal deformities 1075
  vulvo-vaginal adenosis 82
Diffuse laminar endocervical hyperplasia 289
Diffuse peritoneal leiomyomatosis **537–538**, *928*,
    928–929
Diffuse uterine leiomyomatosis *533*, **533**
Dihydrotestosterone (DHT)
  fetal testis 1212
  male differentiation of urogenital sinus and
    external genitalia 20
  sexual development of embryo 1212
  sexual differentiation 20
Dilatation and curettage
  cervical incompetence due to 998
  complications 1027
  endometrial sampling 392
  see also Curettage
Dilated (congestive) cardiomyopathy 1552
  peripartal cardiomyopathy 1552
Diphtheria
  cervical infection 282
  vulvar infection 57
Diploid tumours, endometrial adenocarcinoma 482
'Dirty necrosis,' ovarian metastasis 883, *883*
Disseminated granulomatous disease (BCGosis)
    1193
Disseminated intravascular coagulation
  acute fatty liver of pregnancy 1469
  hepatitis E infection in pregnancy 1478
  postpartum haemorrhage 1561
Diverticular disease **1184**
Dizygotic triplets 1588
Dizygotic twin placentation 1576–1577
Dizygotic twins 1575–1576
  blood group chimerism 1579
DNA arrays **1605**
DNA content *see* Aneuploidy; Ploidy analysis
DNA index
  cervical carcinoma 1611
  flow cytometry 1609
DNA mismatch repair **1601**
DNA ploidy *see* Aneuploidy; Ploidy analysis
Döderlein bacillus *see Lactobacillus acidophilus*
Donahue syndrome 1162
Donavan bodies 1137

Donavanosis (granuloma inguinale) **1136–1138**
  histology 1137, *1138*
  vulvar infection 57
Dosage compensation 642
Dosage-sensitive sex reversal (DSS) 1158
Down's syndrome, ovarian dysgerminoma 1183
Drash syndrome, gonadoblastoma association 823
Drosophila melangaster, sex chromosomes 3
Drug abuse, maternal, placental examination 1309
Drugs
  adverse effects 1192–1193
    see also Diethylstilboestrol (DES)
  cervical mucus hyperacidity due to 997
  infertility and 996
  inflammatory disease of vagina due to 155
DSS (dosage-sensitive sex reversal) 1158
DTM1 gene, deletions 641
Dubin–Johnson syndrome 1100
  pregnancy 1484
Ductus arteriosus, patent 1544
Duval sinus pattern, yolk sac tumours *779*,
    779–780, *780*
Dwarfism, Laron-type 1020
Dysfunctional uterine bleeding **408–409**
  progestagen therapy, endometrial changes 1083
Dysgenetic gonadoma *see* Gonadoblastoma
Dysgerminoma 705, **773–777**, *1165*, **1165**
  anaplastic variant *775*, 776
  clinical features 773–774
  differential diagnosis 776
    clear cell adenocarcinoma vs 732
    ovarian lymphomas vs 945
  Down's syndrome and 1183
  gonadoblastoma association 822, 826, *826*, 829,
    829, 832
  incidence and age 773
  macroscopic appearances 774, *774*
  microscopic appearances *774*, 774–776, *775*
  mixed germ cell sex cord–stromal tumours
    association *840*, 841
  syncytiotrophoblastic giant cells with *775*, 776
  treatment and prognosis 776–777
  tumour markers 776
Dyskeratosis, papillomavirus infection, subclinical
    305
Dyskeratosis congenita, vulvar genetic disorders 63
Dyskeratotic leukoplakia, acquired, vulvar genetic
    disorders 63
Dysovulation 1017–1018
Dyspareunia, organic 996
Dystrophy with atypica *see* Vulvar intraepithelial
    neoplasia (VIN)

E
E2 protein expression, human papillomavirus
    (HPV) 299
Early embryogenesis 4–9
Ebstein's anomaly **1545**
E-cadherin, endometriosis 965–966
Eccrine milliaria, vulvar involvement 83–84
Eccrine poroma, malignant, vulvar *129*
Echinococcosis (*Echinococcus granulosus*) 1143
  endometritis 432
  hydatid cysts 287
  vaginitis 176
  vulvar 54
Eclampsia
  CNS changes 1524–1525, *1525*
  encephalopathy **1524–1525**
  heart failure *1551*, **1551**
  HELLP syndrome 1524
  hypertensive encephalopathy 1525
  reversible posterior leukoencephalopathy
    syndrome 1524
  see also Pre-eclampsia
Ectocervical hyperplasia 288, *288*
Ectocervical polyps 290
Ectoderm and neural plate formation *7*
Ectoparasites, vulvar infection 54
Ectopia
  congenital inguinal 594
  Fallopian tube 594
  ovary 594
  vagina **186**
  vulva 81–82
Ectopic breast tissue
  tumours in vulvar region 131–132
  vulva 81
Ectopic decidua *see* Decidua, ectopic
Ectopic pregnancy **1045–1070**

  abdominal *see* Abdominal pregnancy
  aetiology and pathogenesis 1046–1051
  cervical *see* Cervical pregnancy
  chronic 1058
  contraception 1049–1050
  decidual metaplasia *591*
  demography 1046
  ectopic moles 1369–1370
  extratubal factors 1049–1051
  incidence 1045–1046
    IUCD use and 1117
  IUCD use and 1116–1117
  liver 1477
  maternal death 1571
  ovarian *see* Ovarian pregnancy
  paratubal haemorrhage 592
  pelvic inflammatory disease and 1048, 1117
  placenta creta 1348
  pregnancy 1306, *1307*
  in tropics 1150, **1151**
  tubal *see* Tubal pregnancy
  tubal adenomatoid tumour association 603
  tubal factors 1046–1049
  tubo-ovarian 1051
Ectopic production, hormones 850, 1194
Ectopic prostatic tissue, cervical 280
Ectopic salivary tissue, vulva 81
Ectopic tissue origin tumours, vulvar **131–132**
Eczema, vulvar 74, *74*
EGF receptors *see* Epidermal growth factor
    receptors (EGFR)
Ehlers–Danlos syndrome 998
  vulvar genetic disorders 62–63
Eisenmenger's syndrome **1544**
Elastic tissue, cervix 248
Elderly
  uterine leiomyosarcoma 520
  see also Postmenopausal women
Electronmicroscopy
  Fallopian tube 588, *588*, 589
  vaginal tumours diagnosis 189
Electrosurgical cone margins, cervical glandular
    intraepithelial neoplasia 355
Elephantiasis, vulvar filariasis infection 54
Ellis–van Creveld syndrome, genital tract
    malformation 45
Embolism
  air *see* Air embolism
  amniotic fluid *see* Amniotic fluid embolism
  pulmonary 1561
  tumour, Krukenberg tumours 891
Embryo 636, 644
  coelomic epithelial cells 637, *637*
  death, determination 1442
  early 4–9
  excretory system 18
  flexion 7–9, 644
  implantation *see* Implantation
  indifferent **9–13**
  length, developmental stage 1
  preimplantation 4
    tubal role in immune protection 1008
  sexual development 1212
  transfer, ovarian pregnancy 1062
Embryogenesis
  Carnegie stage 1 2
  early **4–9**
Embryoid body 788, *788*
Embryology **1–40**
  broad ligament 623, 897
  central nervous system 7–8
  endometrium **391**
  epithelial–stromal tumours 695
  Fallopian tube 586–587
  female genital tract **1–40**
  follicles, ovarian 638
  granulosa cells 637
  hymen 148
  mesonephric duct 897
  mesonephros 644, 897
  ovarian *see* Ovary, embryology
  rete system 637
  sexual development, abnormal **1209–1212**
  testis 636, 646, 898
  vagina 148
Embryonal carcinoma 1167
  cells 706, *787*, 788
  gonadoblastoma association 830
  ovarian *787*, **787–788**, *788*, 1167
  vagina 216

Embryonal rhabdomyosarcoma
cervix *376*, 376–378, *377*
  differential diagnosis 378
  microscopic appearance 377
  microscopic examination 377
  prognosis 378
  strap cells 377
ovarian *864*, 864–865, *865*
vagina 1172, *1173*
vulvar 115–116
see also Sarcoma botryoides
Embryonic death, determination 1442
Embryonic disk, double layered 1254
Embryonic length, developmental stage 1
Embryonic pelvis *10*
Embryonic plasticity, paramesonephric (Müllerian)
  ducts 587
Embryonic pole 4
Embryonic stem cells, harvesting 650
Embryo transfer, ovarian pregnancy 1062
Emphysematous vaginitis *178*, **178–179**, *179*
Empty sella syndrome 1021, 1535
Encephalopathy of pre-eclampsia/eclampsia
  1524–1525
Enchondromatosis **1183**
see also Maffucci's syndrome; Ollier's disease
Endarteritis, necrotising, rubella infection
  1315–1316
Endarteritis obliterans 1313
  fetal stem arteries *1292*, 1292–1293
  intrauterine fetal growth retardation 1311
Endarteritis villous stem vessels, maternal syphilis
  infection 1314
Endocarditis, infective **1548**
Endocervical (mucinous) adenocarcinoma
  cervix *see* Cervical adenocarcinoma
  ovarian neoplasia 350
Endocervical canal 247–248, *256*
Endocervical crypts, squamous metaplasia *276*
Endocervical curettage 323–324
  cone biopsy 325
Endocervical epithelium *259*, 274
  columnar *257*
  see also Cervical epithelium
Endocervical hyperplasia 288–290
  diffuse laminar 289
  glandular, lobular 289
  microglandular, differential diagnosis 450
Endocervical neoplasia
  carcinomas, appearance 326
  cell proliferation markers 358
  tumour markers **357–360**
  see also Cervical carcinoma
Endocervical polyps 279
  benign, cervical embryonal rhabdomyosarcoma
    378
  tamoxifen treatment 290
  see also Cervix, polyps
Endocervical squamous metaplasia 274, *274*
Endocervical stroma, decidualisation *276*
Endocervical stromal sarcoma *375*, 375–376
  differential diagnosis 376
  embryonal rhabdomyosarcoma of uterine cervix
    378
  gross examination 376
  histological examination 376
  mitotic activity 376
Endocervicosis 278–279, **925–926**, *926*
Endocrine carcinoma *see* Small cell carcinomas
Endocrine disorders **1194–1195**
  carcinoid syndrome *see* Carcinoid syndrome
  Cushing's syndrome *see* Cushing's syndrome
  hyperaldosteronism **1194**
  hypercalcaemia **1194**
  hyperchorionic gonadotrophinism **1194–1195**
  hyperprolactinaemia **1195**
  infertility and 1025
Endocrine failure, infertility 991
Endocrine tumours, uterine cervix *see* Cervix,
  endocrine tumours
Endoderm
  flexion phase of embryogenesis 8
  primary 5
Endodermal derivatives, immature teratoma 791,
  793, *794*
Endodermal sinus tumour
  endometrial, clear cell adenocarcinoma vs 471
  terminology 777
  vagina 216
  see also Yolk sac tumours

Endometrial adenocarcinoma *see* Endometrial
  carcinoma (adenocarcinoma)
Endometrial basilis 393
  blood vessels 395
  stromal cells 395
Endometrial biopsy *see* Endometrium, biopsy
Endometrial carcinoma (adenocarcinoma)
  455–488
  adenocanthoma, new terminology 465
  adenomyosis vs 498
  adenomyosis with 459
  adenosquamous, new terminology 465
  angiogenesis and VEGF 483
  antidiuretic hormone (ADH) 1195
  apoptosis markers 483, 1608
  apoptotic marker studies **1608**
  bcl-2 483, 1608
  benign lymphangiomatous papules **1193**
  capillary invasion 481
  cell proliferation studies **1606–1607**
  cell types 478–479
  chromosomal imbalances **1604**
  ciliated cell 462
  clear cell **469–471**, 479
    differential diagnosis 471
    epidemiology 470
    histology 470–471, *471*
      hobnail appearance 470, *471*
      patterns/types 470
      survival time *484*
  clinical presentation 409, 456
  clonality studies **1602–1603**
  c-myc **1597**
  combined oral contraceptives and 1091, 1094
  comparative genomic hybridisation **1604**
  curettings/biopsy correlation with hysterectomy
    specimens 456–457
  cytological criteria *458*, 458–459
  diagnostic criteria 458
  differential diagnosis 462–463
  diffusely infiltrative *461*, 462
  diploid tumours 482
  D-score *1613*
  EGFR **1596**
  endocervical gland involvement 475
  endometrial hyperplasia coexistent 447, 459
  endometrial hyperplasia vs 457–459
  endometrioid *461*, **461–463**, *462*
    ciliated cells 462
    differential diagnosis 457–459, 462–463
    grade 1 *476*, *476*
    grade 2 *476*, *477*
    grade 3 *476*, *477*, *478*
    histological classification 478, 479
    histology *461*, 461–462, *462*, *1085*
    immunohistochemistry 463, *463*
    oestrogen therapy and 1073, *1074*
    papillary 466, 467
    papillary serous carcinoma with 467
    progestagen therapy 1083, *1085*
    psammoma bodies 469
    survival time *484*
    variants 461–462
    villoglandular adenocarcinoma with 464, *464*
  endometritis 421
  epidemiology 455–456
  FIGO staging 476, 477, 483–484
  flow cytometry 1610–1611
  genetic predisposition 995
  gross pathology *459*, 459–460, *460*
  high-grade adenocarcinoma with sarcomatous
    metaplasia 568
  histological classification *460*, 460–474
  histological grades 476–478
  hormonal therapy of 486, *487*, 1083–1084
    histological effects 486–488
  infectious pneumoperitoneum 1198
  intraepithelial (EIC) 455, 467, *468*, 469
  invasion
    depth 479–480
    myometrial *see Below*
    specimens for assessment 457
    vascular and lymphatic 480–481, *481*
  IUCD use and 1112
  K-ras **1596–1597**
  loss of heterozygosity (LOH) **1599**
  lymphatic invasion 481
  lymph node sampling 457
  Lynch type II syndrome **1184**
  metastatic

  to cervix 349
  endometrial stromal tumours vs 514
  to Fallopian tubes 614, *615*
  to ovary 881, 888–889
  to vagina *217*, 217–218
microsatellite instability 1601
mixed carcinomas 460
molecular alterations in pathogenesis 485–486
morphometry **1613**
mucinous **471–473**, 479
  differential diagnosis 473
  histology *472*, 472–473
myometrial invasion 459, 475, *479*, **479–480**
  of adenomyosis 480
  survival time *484*
nuclear grading 478
oestrogens and 455–456, 1073–1074
  prevention by progestagen therapy 1074, 1084
  unopposed 1073–1074
oncocytic 462
ovarian cancer coexistence 488
p53 **1598**
papillary serous 466–467, *468*
pathogenesis, molecular alterations 485–486
pathology
  gross *459*, 459–460, *460*
  microscopic 460–474
patterns of spread 486, *486*
peritoneal cytology 481–482
Pipelle sampling 392
ploidy 482, **1610–1611**
polycystic ovarian disease and 1026
postmenopausal bleeding 409
primary vs metastatic 488
prognosis, pathological models 483–485, *484*
prognostic features 475–476
  Bcl-2 loss 483
prognostic indicators 1610, 1612
progression, molecular alterations 485–486
proliferating cell nuclear antigen (PCNA) 1607
proliferation markers 482–483
PTEN **1600**
radiation therapy 486
  histological effects 486–488
rare cell types 474
risk factors 455, 561
secretory *462*, 462
  clear cell adenocarcinoma vs 471
  elements in carcinosarcoma *563*
serous **466–469**, *467*, 479
  differential diagnosis 468–469
  histology 467–468, *468*, *469*
  papillary 466–467, *468*
  papillary, elements in carcinosarcoma *563*
  prognosis and spread 466–467
  survival time *484*
Sertoliform 474
small cell (neuroendocrine) 474, 510
squamous cell *411*, *473*, 473–474
with squamous differentiation **464–466**, *465*,
  478–479
  differential diagnosis 466
  histology *465*, 465–466, *466*
  terminology change 465
stage II *475*
staging *474*, 474–475
steroid receptors 482
subtypes (pathogenetic) 455
superior vena cava syndrome 1197
surgical stage *474*, 474–475
surgicopathological staging *474*, 474–475, *476*
survival time by stage *484*
synchronous/metachronous tumours 1603
systemic hypertension 1190
tamoxifen-associated polyps and 1078
tamoxifen association *see* Tamoxifen
telomerase activity **1601**
therapy 486
Torre–Muir syndrome **1184**
trophoblastic differentiation 474
in tropics **1149**
vaginal vault recurrence 486
vascular invasion **480–481**, *481*
villoglandular **463–464**, *464*, 469, 479
  survival time *484*
well-differentiated, diagnostic criteria *458*, *458*
Endometrial cycle
  control 396
  functional changes 396–397
  menstrual phase 398–399

Endometrial cycle (*cont'd*)
  morphological changes 397–401
  postmenopausal and proliferative (follicular)
    phase 399–400
  proliferative phase 397–398
  secretory phase *see* Secretory phase of endometrial
    cycle
  see also Menstrual cycle
Endometrial functionalis 393
Endometrial gliomatosis 415, *415*
Endometrial granulocytes 395, 1329, *1330*
Endometrial hyperplasia 443, **444–455**
  adenocarcinoma coexistent 447, 459
  adenocarcinoma vs 457–459
  adenomatous 445
  atypical 445, 446, *1074*
    cytological criteria *458*, 458–459
    cytology *449, 450, 1074*
    with mucinous metaplasia 473
    treatment 459
  classification 445–446, *446*
  clinical detection and sampling 446–447
  coexisting lesions 451
  comparative genomic hybridisation 1604
  complex 445, 446, 448, *448*, *1073*
  complex atypical (CAH) 445–446
    cytology *449, 450*
  cystic *449*, *451*
    progression to carcinoma 451–452
  diagnosis, reproducibility 445–446
  diagnostic problems 443
  differential diagnosis 450–451
    artifactual simulation *453*
    endometrial adenocarcinoma 457–459
  endometrial intraepithelial neoplasia and 455
  endometrial polyps 415
  endometritis 420
  epidemiology 444–445
  focal *452*
  gland to stromal ratio 447–448
  glandular proliferation 443, 447–448, *457*
  gross pathology 447, *447*
  K-ras **1596–1597**
  microscopic pathology *447*, 447–449, *448, 449*
    gland structures 448
  morphometry 454
  natural history 451–453
  oestrogen levels 404
  oestrogen therapy causing 1073, *1073*
  pathogenesis, molecular alterations 454–455
  progression 451, 452, *457*
    prediction 454
  regression 451, 452
  reversal by progestagens 1073
  simple 445, 446, *447*, 448, *1073*
  simple atypical (SAH) 445, *449*
  spectrum 444, *444*, 445, 448, 457
  squamous metaplasia with *452*
  stromal nodular 505
  tamoxifen association 1076–1077
  terminology changes 445
  therapy 453–454
    progestational agents effect on pathology
      447
Endometrial intraepithelial neoplasia (EIN) 455,
  467, 468, *469*
Endometrial polyps
  differential diagnosis
    adenofibroma vs 552
    adenosarcoma vs 557
    hyperplasia vs 450
  hormonal replacement therapy and 1089
  hyperplasia within 449
  hysteroscopic diagnosis 415
  infertility and 1002
  non-neoplastic **415–418**, *416*
  simple 416–417
    functional component 416
    glands 416
    postmenopausal 416
    stroma 416
    structure 416
  tamoxifen association *1077*, 1077–1078, *1078*
    carcinoma development 1078
    differential diagnosis 1078
    epithelial components *1078, 1079*
  tubal and papillary oxyphil metaplasia *1078*
'Endometrial stromal sarcoma,' vagina 216
Endometrial stromal tumours **502–515**
  classification, controversies 503–504

with epithelial elements **575–576**
  focal (non-dominant) 576
with glandular differentiation 512, *512*
high-grade sarcoma 502, 503–504, **511–512**
  clinicopathological correlation 512
  cytogenetic findings 509
  differential diagnosis 511–512
  histological features 502–503
low-grade sarcoma 502, 503, *504*, **506–511**
  clinical features 506
  clinicopathological correlation 510–511
  cytogenetic findings 509
  differential diagnosis 506, 509–510, 514
  glandular differentiation 514
  gross pathology 506
  metastases 510–511
  microscopic pathology 506–509, *507, 508*
  rhabdoid differentiation 508
  spindle cell lesions vs 509–510
  'star-burst pattern' 508, *508*
  therapy 511
metastases 510–511
mixed smooth muscle tumours 576–577
pseudodecidualisation by progestagen therapy
  510
pulmonary metastases, differential diagnosis 509
sarcomas
  adenosarcoma vs 557
  aneuploidy 1611
  extrauterine **514–515**
  pure heterologous 538
  sex cord-like features 512, 512–513, *513*
    differential diagnosis 513–514
  smooth muscle cell tumours vs *501*
  stromal fragments vs 506
  stromal nodules 503, *504*, **504–506**
    differential diagnosis 506
    gross pathology 504–505
    microscopic appearance 505, *505*
  'stromomyoma' 508
  tamoxifen association 1080
  tubular elements 513, *513*
  undifferentiated sarcoma 504
  uterine leiomyoma vs 518
Endometrioid adenocarcinoma
  carcinoembryonic antigen (CEA) 463, *463*
  cervical 344
  endometrium *see* Endometrial carcinoma
  minimal deviation 344
  ovarian *see* Ovarian tumours, endometrioid
    adenocarcinoma
  see also Endometrioid carcinoma
Endometrioid adenofibroma 715, *716*
  with epithelial atypia 725–727, *726*
  ovarian endometriosis 976
Endometrioid carcinoma
  endometriosis 976
  extraovarian endometriosis 978
  Fallopian tube 611
  pelvic extraovarian endometriosis 977
  yolk sac tumours vs 731, 777
  see also Endometrioid adenocarcinoma
Endometrioid cystadenofibroma 715
Endometrioid cystadenoma 699
Endometrioid neoplasia 446
Endometrioid pattern, metastatic ovarian tumours
  883, *883*
Endometrioid stromal sarcoma, ovarian *870*,
  870–872, *871*
  endometriosis 978
Endometrioid tumours, ovarian *see* Ovarian tumours
Endometriosis **963–988**, 1195
  adhesion molecules and 965
  aetiology and pathogenesis **963–966**
  aggressive 513
  atypical 513
    ovarian intraepithelial neoplasia 975
    precancerous significance 974
  black lesions 967
  cervical 278, *980*
  cervical superficial, endometrial stromal sarcoma
    vs 510
  classification 967
  clear cell adenocarcinoma and 976
  clinical aspects 979–982
  decidual changes 971
  definition 497
  early lesions 966
  E-cadherin 965–966
  ectocervix *278*

ectopic endometrial-type glands vs 974
epidemiology 966–967
epithelial component 971–972
extraovarian, malignant tumours 978
Fallopian tube *see* Fallopian tube
familial 965
genetic predisposition 995
gross and microscopic appearances 967–974
histological diagnosis 969
infertility and 979, 995
interleukins 965
intestinal obstruction 979
intussusception 979
laparotomy scars 965
maternal inheritance 965
mixed mesodermal (Müllerian) tumours and
  978
neoplasia relationship 974–979
neoplastic transformation 972
oestrogen and 963, 966
oestrogen therapy sensitivity 1074
ovarian *see* Ovarian endometriosis
pelvic lymph nodes 969–970
peritoneal fluid excess 1019
polypoid 968–969
  adenosarcoma vs 557–558
post-pill 989
post-salpingectomy 598–599, *599*
pregnancy-induced changes 973, *973*
progestagens effect 1086
progestagen therapy *591*
pseudopregnancy therapy 981–982
red lesions 967
salpingitis isthmica nodosa (SIN) vs 601
serosal 499
sites of occurrence 963
steroid contraceptives and 1105
'stromal' 510–511, 971
  differential diagnosis 515
tamoxifen effects 1081
in tropics **1151**
tubal, infertility 1013
tuberculosis 423
urinary tract 979
uterine malformations 48, 964
uterus 966
vagina 220, *220*, 979
  biopsy 220, *220*
vaginal cysts 182
vulva 81
vulvar tumours arising in 132
white lesions 967
Endometriotic cysts 968, *974*
  cervical 287
  endometrioid adenocarcinoma *978*
Endometriotic disease 966
  see also Endometriosis
Endometritis 418, **418–425**
  Actinomyces israelii 431
  bacterial 431, 1134
  chlamydial 993–994, 1003, 1134
  chronic
    after combined oral contraceptives
      1093–1094
    Chlamydia 1134
    gonorrhoea 1134
    granulomatous 423
    infertility due to 1002–1005
    Neisseria gonorrhoea 431
    non-specific non-tuberculous 421–423, *422,
      423*, 1003, 1093–1094
    non-tuberculous 1003–1005
    in tropics **1134–1136**
    tuberculous 1003, *1004*, **1134–1136**
  focal necrotising 425
  gonococcal 1003
  granulomatous 423
  histiocytic 423, *424*
  infertility and 1003–1005
  mycoplasmal 994, 1003–1005, *1004*
  Neisseria meningitidis 431
  non-specific 418–423, *424*
    aetiology 419–421
    chronic non-tuberculous 421–423, *422, 423*
    clinical correlates 419
    diagnosis 421–423
    incidence 419
  post-caesarean 160
  subacute focal 1005
  transient acute superficial, gonorrhoea 430–431

Endometritis–salpingitis–peritonitis, *Neisseria meningitidis* 431
Endometrium
  abnormalities
    causing infertility 1000–1006
    due to HRT 1089
  abnormally sited in pelvis 964
  adenoacanthosis 449, *452*
  adenocarcinoma *see* Endometrial carcinoma (adenocarcinoma)
  adenofibroma 551
  adenomyomatosis 576
  adenosarcoma *see* Adenosarcoma, uterine
  adhesions 1002
  anatomical aspects 392–396
  atrophy
    cystic, tamoxifen causing 1077
    depot progestagens causing 1097
    high-dose steroid contraceptives causing *1096*
    hypo-oestrogenic states 403–404
    prolonged progestagens causing 1083, *1084*
    submucous leiomyoma and 999, *999*
    terminology and 1077
  atypical polypoid adenomyoma *see* Adenomyoma, atypical polypoid
  basal *394*, 395
  basal cell layer 393
  biochemical defects causing infertility 1005
  biopsy 392, 1027
    abnormal bleeding 392
    adenocarcinoma diagnosis 456–457
    after depot progestagens 1097
    Asherman's syndrome 433
    infertile patients 409
    instruments for 1000
    isthmic 396
    luteal phase deficiency diagnosis 1000–1001
    postmenopausal 402
    postmenopausal bleeding *409*
    premature failure of corpus luteum 407
    timing 392
    timing for dating 1000
    tuberculosis 428
  bleeding, abnormal 409
    see also Bleeding, vaginal/uterine
  breakdown, factors affecting 397
  carcinoma *see* Endometrial carcinoma
  cilia on glandular cells 462
  ciliary structure abnormalities 1005
  clear cell metaplasia 413
  constituents, normal 393–395
  contraceptives effect
    combined oral contraceptives 1092–1095, *1093*, *1094*
    compression artefact due to IUCDs 1108, *1108*
    IUCDs *1107*, 1107–1112, *1108*, *1109*, *1110*, *1111*
    progestagen-only 1095–1097, *1096*
  curettage, cone biopsy 325
  cyclical changes 393, 1000–1001
    morphological 397–402
    see also Endometrium, proliferative phase; Endometrium, secretory phase
  cyclical vascular proliferation 399
  cystadenofibromatous tumours, ovarian endometriosis 976
  cystic atrophy, tamoxifen causing 1077
  cytokines 1006
    endometrial re-shaping 397
  dating, histological vs chronological 1000
  development
    homeobox genes role 1005
    from paramesonephric duct tissue 15
  disordered proliferative 444, *444*
    differential diagnosis 450
    oestrogen therapy causing 1072, *1072*
  disorders
    delayed/prolonged or irregular shedding 408
    functional 403–408
  dysfunction in luteal phase defect *see* Luteal phase defect
  embryology 391
  epithelial cells *394*
    interanastomosing bridges in endometrioid adenocarcinoma 461
    'lobster-claw pattern' 551
    postmenopausal 402
  epithelial ulceration, IUCD use and 1110

  epithelium *394*
  fibrosis
    endometritis 422
    postinflammatory *see* Endometrium, postinflammatory fibrosis
  foreign body granulomata 1108, *1109*
  functional disorders 403–408
  gestational *1001*, 1001–1002
  gestational hyperplasia 1001
  glands 393, 394, *394*
    adenomyosis 498
    combined oral contraceptives effect 1092, *1093*
    cystic dilatation 449, *451*
    HRT effect 1088, *1088*
    hypersecretory *1082*
    IUCD use and *1109*, 1110
    microscopic appearance 448
    in myometrium *see* Adenomyosis, uterine
    oestrogens effect 1072, *1072*, *1073*, *1074*
    progestagens effect 1082, *1082*
    proliferation 443, 447–448, *457*
  glandular secretory changes, progesterone 396
  growth
    modelling and breakdown 397
    oestrogen 397
  hobnail metaplasia 413
  Hodgkin's disease 951
  hormonal therapy of infertility and 1090
  hormone replacement therapy (HRT) effects *1088*, 1088–1089, *1089*
    Tibolone 1090
  hostility, cervical pregnancy 1062
  hyperplasia *see* Endometrial hyperplasia
  hypertrophic 1002
  immune cells/response 1006
  implantation in *see* Implantation
  infarction, haemorrhagic 408
  infection, IUCD use and 1111, *1111*, 1114
  infertility and 409, 1000–1006
  inflammation 418–432
    chronic, osseous metaplasia 414, *414*
    IUCD use and 1111
    postmenopausal bleeding 409
  intraepithelial carcinoma (EIC) 455, 467, 468, *469*
  intravascular leiomyomatosis 509
  intravascular thrombi *405*
  late proliferative *399*
  leiomyoma 506
    differential diagnosis 509
    see also Leiomyoma, uterine
  lesions causing infertility 1002–1005
  lining, structural abnormalities 391
  luteal phase
    defect/insufficiency 406, 406–407, *407*, 1000, 1018
    pregnancy diagnostic criteria *1001*, 1001–1002, *1002*
    see also Luteal phase deficiency
  lymphoma 950–951
  menstrual
    adenomyosis vs 499
    endometrioid adenocarcinoma vs 462–463
    menstrual cycle changes 399, 1000–1001
  metaplasia 409–415, 450
    hyperplasia vs 450
    mucinous 412–413, 473
    mucinous, atypical endometrial hyperplasia with 473
    serous, oestrogen therapy causing 1073
    squamous *see* Endometrium, squamous metaplasia
    tamoxifen-associated polyps *1078*, *1079*
  metaplastic squamous epithelium, oestrogen therapy causing 1073
  micropapillae, IUCD use and *1110*
  microvascular density, progestagen-only pill 1097
  molecular defects, infertility due to 1005
  myometrium junction 497
  non-proliferative conditions 391–442
  normal 391–442, 392–403
    constituents 393–395
    newborn 393
    reproductive years 393
  oedema
    IUCD use and 1110
    see also Endometrium, stromal oedema
  oestrogen therapy effect *1072*, 1072–1074, *1073*
  osseous metaplasia 1005

  ossification 414
    endometritis 420
  in ovarian dysfunction 1002–1005
  papillary syncytial metaplasia 469
  partial shedding 405
  perimenopausal, 'snouted' apocrine-like cells *394*
  in polycystic ovarian disease 667
  polyps *see* Endometrial polyps
  postinflammatory fibrosis 432–433
    Asherman's syndrome 432–433
    IUCD use and *1109*
  postmenopausal 402, 402–403
  predecidualised stroma 1328
  pregnancy 1328–1329, *1329*
  progestagens effect *1082*, 1082–1084, *1083*, *1084*, *1085*
  progestagen therapy 1192
  progesterone receptors 1082
  proliferation
    disordered *see* Endometrium, disordered proliferative
    oestrogen therapy causing 1072, *1072*
    spectrum 444, *444*, 445, 448, *457*
    see also Endometrial carcinoma; Endometrial hyperplasia
  proliferative phase 393, 393–394, *394*
    oestrogens effect 1072
    progestagens effect 1082
  regrowth 399
  response to irradiation 487
  sampling 392, 446–447
    hyperoestrogenic states 405
    infertility investigation 1027
  sarcoidosis 425, 1189, *1190*
  saw-tooth appearance 1328, *1328*
  schistosomiasis 1147
  secretion, conceptus maturation 1328
  secretory phase *400*, 400–401, *401*, 1001, 1002, *1003*
    oestrogens effect 1072
    progestagens effect 1082–1083
    see also Secretory phase of endometrial cycle
  serous metaplasia, oestrogen therapy causing 1073
  shedding 393, *408*
    delayed/prolonged or irregular 408
    partial 405
    spontaneous miscarriage 408
  small cell (neuroendocrine) carcinoma 474, 510
  sperm interaction 994
  squamous cell carcinoma *411*, *473*, 473–474
  squamous metaplasia 1005
    endometrial hyperplasia with *452*
    IUCD use and 1108, *1109*
    oestrogen therapy causing 1073
  stomal cells of basilis 395
  stroma
    in carcinosarcoma 565, *565*
    cells, 'bare-nucleus' appearance 1092
    fragments vs stromal nodules 506
    nodules *see* Endometrial stromal tumours, stromal nodules
    oestrogen effect 1072
    placentation 1235
    pleomorphism in adenofibroma 551–552
    smooth muscle metaplasia 1005
    tumours *see* Endometrial stromal tumours
  stromal nodular hyperplasia 505
  stromal oedema
    in hyperplasia 448
    IUCD use and 1110, *1111*
  stromal sarcoma, endometrial adenocarcinoma vs 463
  transformation, coordinated delayed 406
  tubal pregnancy 1057, *1057*
  tuberculosis 427–430, 1003, *1004*
    biopsies 428
    caseation 427
    granulomas 428
    intrauterine adhesions 433
  unresponsiveness to oestrogen 1002
  vascular disturbances, leiomyoma and infertility association 999
  vascular regeneration 397
Endosalpingeal hyperplasia, focal, tubal pregnancy 1056
Endosalpingiosis 593, 598, *921*, 921–922
  atypical 721, 922
  cervix 279
  cystic 921

Endosalpingiosis (*cont'd*)
  differential diagnosis 720–721, 922
  endometrial 412
  endometriosis vs 972
  histiogenesis 922
  histology *921*, 921–922
Endosalpingitis
  IUCD use and 1115, *1115*
  non-granulomatous 623, *623*
  suppurative *622*
  see also Salpingitis
Endosalpinx
  granulomatous inflammation 618, *618*
  tuberculous infection 618
Endothelial necrosis
  spiral arteries and veins 1258
  villous fetal vessels in rubella infection 1316
Endothelial vacuolation, uteroplacental arteries in
    hypertensive state 1343
Endotoxic shock, chorioamnionitis 1306
Endovascular trophoblast 1261
  luminal, uteroplacental arteries in pre-eclampsia
    1339
  migration waves, uteroplacental vasculature 1336
Entamoeba dispar 1140
Entamoeba gingivalis, in uterus, IUCD use and
    1113
Entamoeba histolytica 1140
  amoebiasis 55
  amoebic abscess in pregnancy 1479
  cervical smears 1148
  endometritis 432
Enteric adenocarcinoma, cervical 343, *343*
Enterobacter agglomerans, vaginitis 169
Enterobiasis **1142–1143**
Enterobius vermicularis 1142, *1143*, 1163
  cervical smears 1148
  endometritis 432
  ovarian infection 684
  vaginal infection 176
  vulvar infection 54
Enteropathy, protein-losing, endometriosis 979
Entero-vaginal fistulas 184–185
Entrapped villi, perivillous fibrin deposition 1277
Environmental sex determination 3
Eosinophilic inclusion bodies, rubella infection
    1316
Eosinophilic metaplasia, endometrial 413
Eosinophilic myometritis 500
Eosinophilic salpingitis 616
Eosinophils, cervix 281
Ependymoma, broad ligament 625
Epicanthus inversus syndrome (blepharophimosis)
    1182
Epidermal cysts, vulvar involvement 83
Epidermal growth factor (EGF), endometriosis 966
Epidermal growth factor receptors (EGFR)
  cervical carcinoma 332, **1596**
  endometrial carcinoma **1596**
  ovarian carcinoma **1596**
  type-1 growth factor family oncogenes **1595–1596**
Epidermisation, cervical epithelium 264, *264*
Epidermoid carcinoma, vagina 200
Epidermoid cysts
  ovarian 717
  vulva *83*
Epidermolysis bullosa, vulvar infection 60
Epidermolysis bullosa acquisita, vulvar 70
Epidermophyton floccosum, vulvar infection 55
Epilepsy in pregnancy **1533–1534**
  anticonvulsant levels 1533
  drug teratogenicity 1533
  fluid retention 1533
  folate demand 1533
Epithelial cells
  budding, villoglandular papillary adenocarcinoma
    of cervix 347
  coelomic *see* Coelomic epithelial cells
  endometrium *see* Endometrium, epithelial cells
  metaplasia, endometrial 410–414
  see also Epithelium
Epithelial hyperplasia, lichen sclerosis 76
Epithelial inclusion cysts
  cervical 287
  ovarian 697
Epithelial inclusion glands, hydropic change in ovary
    685, *685*
Epithelial membrane antigen (EMA)
  aberrant expression, uterine leiomyosarcoma 522
  endocervical neoplasia 359

negativity, adult-type granulosa cell tumours 751
  ovarian tumours of Wolffian origin 899
Epithelial–mesenchymal neoplasms (mixed)
  benign, cervix **384**
  uterine 549, 577–578
    see also Mixed Müllerian tumours
  vaginal
    benign 197–198, *198*
    malignant **216**
  vulva 131
Epithelial–stromal tumours, ovarian **695–703,**
    713–743
  aetiology and pathogenesis **699–703**
  benign **713–717**
    clear cell 716
    endometrioid 715, *716*
    mucinous *714*, 714–715, *715*
    serous 713–714
    squamous 717
    transitional cell *see* Brenner tumours, ovarian
  borderline **717–728**
    Brenner tumours *727*, 727–728
    clear cell 727, *727*
    definition 717, *718*
    endometrioid 725–727, *726*
    extraovarian spread 718
    mucinous *see* Ovarian tumours, mucinous
      Müllerian (endocervical) type 725, *726*
    serous *see* Serous tumours
    steroid contraceptives and 1100
    stromal invasion 718
  endometriosis and 976
  histiogenesis 695–699
  malignant **728–736**
    see also Ovarian tumours, carcinoma
    prevalence 713
    steroid contraceptives and 1099
    tumours included *694*, 713
  see also specific tumours (listed page 594)
Epithelial tubules, uterine leiomyoma with
    576–577, *577*
Epithelial tumours
  benign
    cervix 382–383
    Fallopian tube 602–603
    ovarian *see* Epithelial–stromal tumours, ovarian
    vaginal 193, 197–198
  in childhood/adolescence **1174–1175**
    diethylstilboestrol (DES) exposure **1174–1175**
    squamous neoplasia **1175**
    vaginal/cervical adenocarcinoma **1174–1175**
  ovarian *see* Epithelial–stromal tumours, ovarian
  sarcoma combined, ovarian **873**
  trophoblast
    epithelioid **1409–1411**, 1415
    placental site nodules 1415, 1416, *1416*
  vulva **95–111**
Epithelioid sarcoma, vulvar 124
  histology 124
Epithelioid tumours
  haemangioendothelioma, vulvar 121
  trophoblastic, uterine cervix 382
  uterine smooth muscle *529*, **529–530**, 530, *530*
Epithelioma pflugerien *see* Mixed germ cell sex
    cord–stromal tumours (ovarian)
Epithelium
  cervical *see* Cervical epithelium
  endometrium 394
  Fallopian tube 590
  types, cervix 251
  vaginal *see* Vagina, epithelium
  see also Epithelial cells
Epoophoron 897
Epstein–Barr virus (EBV)
  Burkitt's lymphoma and 943
  cervical adenocarcinoma 341
  cervical infection 287
  interaction with human papillomavirus (HPV)
    301
  lymphoepithelioma-like carcinoma of cervix 331
  nasopharyngeal carcinoma 331
  vulval lymphoma and 956
  vulvar infection 59
Erosive vulvitis 58
Erythema multiforme, bullous, vaginal changes
    154
Erythrasma, vulvar infection 56
Erythroblastosis fetalis with hydrops 676
Erythrocytes, nucleated, maternal syphilis infection
    1314

Erythrocytosis **1195**
  steroid cell tumours association 850
Erythroplasia of Queyrat *see* Vulvar intraepithelial
    neoplasia (VIN)
Erythropoietin **1195**
Escherichia coli
  acute pyelonephritis 1497
  malacoplakia 424
  vaginitis 160
Essential hypertension, pre-eclampsia 1337, *1342*,
    1343–1344
Estes procedure 1008
Ethinyloestradiol, combined oral contraceptives,
    effect on endometrium 1092–1095, *1093*,
    1094
Ethnic factors
  hydatidiform mole **1365–1367**
  ovarian adenocarcinoma risk and 701
Evacuation, hydatidiform moles 1384
Eversion, cervical *see* Cervix, eversion
Ewing's sarcoma, vulvar 124
Exercise
  fertility and 990
  reproductive dysfunction due to 1020
Exocoelom cavity
  formation 1255
  occlusion 1256
Exocoelomic membrane 5
Exocytosis, misplaced 1022
External anal sphincter 35–36
External genitalia
  development *18*, **18–21**, *19*
    failure 1212
  feminisation 19–20
  gonadal dysgenesis, mixed 1225
  gonadoblastoma 826
  male pseudohermaphroditism 1215
  masculinisation 19
  see also specific anatomical structures
External trauma to uterus, miscarriage 1433
Extra-amniotic pregnancy 1306–1307, *1307*
Extrachorial placentation, clinical significance 1275
Extra-embryonic coelom formation 5, *6*
Extra-embryonic mesoblast 1253–1254
Extragenital tumours
  carcinomas, cervix metastases 385–386
  cervical metastases 349
  see also specific tumours/sites
Extragonadal yolk sac tumours, uterine cervix 380
Extrahepatic bile duct carcinoma, metastatic, to
    ovary 885
Extramedullary haemopoiesis, acute fatty liver of
    pregnancy 1470
Extramembranous pregnancy 1306, *1307*
  amnion nodosum 1302
Extravillous cytotrophoblast
  endovascular trophoblast 1261
  interstitial trophoblast 1261
  tubal placentation 1053
Extravillous trophoblast 1260–1261
  extravillous cytotrophoblast 1261
  extravillous syncytiotrophoblast 1261
  formation 1258
  function in pre-eclampsia 1337
  interstitial 1261
    placentation in tubal pregnancy 1052
    uteroplacental arteries 1335
  nomenclature 1260–1261

F
Factitial lesions, vagina 153
Factor V gene, point mutation and miscarriage
    1434
Factor V Leiden 1103
  Budd–Chiari syndrome and pregnancy 1481
Factor X activation, amniotic fluid 1565
Faecal fluid aspiration, maternal death 1570
Fallopian tube **585–622**
  absent 1009
  adenocarcinoma **605–611**
    aetiology/pathogenesis 606
    epidemiology 605
    gross pathology *610*
    histological grades 609
    histology 607–609, *608*, *609*
    metastatic to ovary 889
    patterns 607–608
    spread 610
    staging system 609–610
    see also Fallopian tube, carcinoma

adenofibroma 602, *602*
adenofibromatous polyp 1009, *1009*
adenomatoid tumour 603, *603*
adhesions 1010, *1011*
  postoperative 1011–1012, 1028
ampulla 32, *587*
  anatomy 587, *587*
  carcinoma 607
  fibropapilloma 602, *602*
  localised diverticulum of 601
  ovum movement 1006
  sperm 1007
  zygote entrapment 1008
ampullosthmic junction, ovum at 1007
amyloidosis 622
anatomy 31–32, *585*, 585–586, *586*, 587–588, 654
  segmental 32, *586*, 587
aplasia, bilateral 42
arterial supply 32
atresia 1009
autonomic innervation 32
average length 31
biochemistry and physiology 589
  segmental *586*
biology **586–589**
carcinoma
  p53 **1598**
  ploidy **1610**
  primary, criteria 605, *605*
  see also Fallopian tube, adenocarcinoma
carcinoma in situ 607, *607*
choriocarcinoma 1398
chronic spasm 1008
ciliary activity depression 1008
clear cell hyperplasia 607
congenital defects, infertility due to 1009
congenital inguinal ectopia 594
Crohn's disease 1185, *1185*
cystic teratoma (dermoid cyst) 605
cytology, normal 587, *587*, 588
deciliation, ectopic pregnancy 1048
ectopic pregnancy
  endometrium 420
  IUCD use and 1117
  tubal factors 1046–1049
electronmicroscopy 588, *588*, 589
embryology 586–587
embryotrophic role 1007–1008
endometriosis *971*, *981*
  ectopic pregnancy 1047
  infertility 1013
epithelial tumours, benign 602–603
epithelium 590
  oestrogen therapy effect 1074
fimbriae *see* Fimbriae, tubal
fluid 589
formation 14
functions 585–586, 589, 1006
  perifertilisation events 1007–1008, 1018
  protection of preimplantation embryo 1008
gamete transport 1006
glassy cell carcinoma 611
haematosalpinx **596–597**
herniations 594
hydrosalpinx **596–597**, 598, 617
hyperplasia 607
hyperplasia–adenocarcinoma sequence 606
immunohistochemistry 587–588
implantation 1051–1053
  tubal sterilisation 1047
infections, infertility due to 1009–1011
infertility due to 1006–1013
inflammation, IUCD-induced and ectopic pregnancy 1049
inflammatory disease **615–622**
  ectopic pregnancy 1048
  see also Salpingitis
inflammatory disease of ovary and 682
intramural segment 587
intussusception **596**
isthmus 32, *586*, 587
  adenomatoid tumour 603, *603*
  adrenoreceptor activity 1007
  metastatic carcinoma *612*
  occlusion and infertility 1010, *1011*
  ovum transport 1007
  polyspermy prevention 1007

IUCD use and 1114–1115
leiomyoma 603–604
  hypercellular 1074
length 1006
lesions after sterilisation reversal 1012
lesions causing infertility 1008–1013
  anatomical 1009–1013
  functional 1008–1009
ligation, ovarian carcinoma risk reduced 701
ligneous (pseudomembranous) inflammation 996
lymphoma *948*, **948**
macrophage hyperactivity 1008
malignant tumours **605–615**
  adenocarcinoma *see Above*
  borderline 605–611
  lymphomas *612*, 613
  metaplastic primary epithelial 611
  metastatic *612*, *613*, 613–615, *614*, *615*
  metastatic leukaemia 613
  mixed Müllerian tumours 611, *611*
  non-epithelial 611–613
mechanical disorders **594–596**
mesodermal tumours, benign 603–605
mesothelium 592–594
metaplasia 288, 587, 589–594
  endocervix *279*
  endometrium 411–412
  mesothelial 592–594
  mucinous 590, *590*
  primary malignancies 611
  serosal 590
  stromal 590–591
  transitional cell 590, *590*
metaplastic papillary tumour 602–603
morbid anatomy **589–601**
mucinous adenocarcinoma 611
mucosal epithelial proliferation (MEP) *606*, 606–607
mucosal polyps, infertility due to 1009
muscle invasion, placentation tubal pregnancy 1052
neonatal auto-amputation 594, 596
neoplasms **601–615**
  benign **602–605**
    ectopic pregnancy 1047
    malignant *see* Fallopian tube, malignant tumours
occlusion, midtubal and infertility 1010
oocyte–cumulus pick-up 1006
  inhibition 1008
ovary functional co-operation 1006
  interference and infertility 1008
paramesonephric duct 14
parasympathetic innervation 32
patency 1006
perfusion pressure increase 1008
perifertilisation events, role 1007–1008
physiology *586*
placental site nodule 605
placentation 1053
polyps 602–603
  infertility due to 1009
postmenopausal changes 587
prolapsed **594**
  differential diagnosis 220–221, *221*
  vaginal cysts 181–182
proximal occlusion 1010, *1011*
response to pregnancy 1055–1056
rupture 1059
  abdominal pregnancy secondary to 1059
sarcoma 611
schistosomiasis 1011, 1147, *1148*
secretion, endometriosis associated infertility 980
segmental anatomy/physiology *586*, 587
sliding hernia **594**
spasm, chronic 1008
sperm transport 994
sterilisation *see* Sterilisation, tubal
stroma (lamina propria) 590
  metaplasia 590–592
  ovarian stromal metaplasia 591, *592*
subserosal fibromuscular connective tissue 591–592
surgery
  in infertility, complications 1028
  reconstructive, ectopic pregnancy 1048
torsion
  aetiology/pathogenesis 595–596
  isolated **594–596**

neonatal 594, *595*
  pathology 596
transitional cell carcinoma 611
transportation capacity 1006–1007
  impairment 1008
tuberculosis 1135–1136
venous infarction *595*, 596
wall, ectopic tissues in 591
Fallot's tetralogy **1544**
Falls, trauma in pregnancy 1532
Familial cancer syndromes 702
Familial endometriosis 965
Familial renal agenesis 1158
Familial XX gonadal dysgenesis 641
Fascia of Waldeyer 24
Fat
  accumulation, acute fatty liver of pregnancy 1470
  ovarian tumours *868*, **868**
  vulvar tumours 118
Fatty acid oxidation capacity, acute fatty liver of pregnancy 1472
Fatty change metaplasia 415
Fatty liver of pregnancy *see* Acute fatty liver of pregnancy (AFLP)
Febrile neutrophilic dermatosis, vulvar involvement 64
Fecundability 990
Fecundity rate, monthly 990
Female circumcision 1151
  vaginal fistulas association 184
Female differentiation 14–18
Female infertility *see* Infertility
Female intersex *see* Pseudohermaphroditism, female
Female isoimmunisation 992
Feminisation of external genitalia 19–20
Fenestrate placenta 1276, *1276*
Ferritin
  embryonal carcinoma 788
  yolk sac tumours 784
Fertilisation **2–4**
  Fallopian tube role 1007–1008, 1018
  sex chromosomes 2–3
Fertility
  behavioural factors influencing 989–990
  biological factors affecting 990
  control by contraceptives 989
  definition 989
  diseases depressing 995
  IUCD use effect 1117–1118
  see also Infertility
Fetal arteries and veins, villous trees 1249
Fetal artery thrombosis 1282, *1282*
Fetal death 990
  determination 1442
  fetal artery thrombosis 1282
  maternal floor infarction 1278–1279
  necrotising funisitis 1300
  parvovirus B 19 infection 1317
  perivillous fibrin deposition 1278
  placental changes 1313
    tubal pregnancy 1054
  placental examination 1313–1314
  placental haemangioma 1453
  placental infarction 1279
  placental villi changes 1288, *1288*
  retroplacental haematoma 1284
  sudden, bile acid levels, maternal serum 1469
  umbilical cord examination 1313
  umbilical cord torsion 1298
  umbilical vessel thrombosis 1299
  uteroplacental blood flow 1314
  see also Fetus, mortality
Fetal distress
  intrahepatic cholestasis of pregnancy 1468
  meconium staining 1303
  placental haemangioma 1453
  umbilical cord knots 1297
  velamentous vessel compression 1296
Fetal stem arteries
  abnormalities 1292–1293
  maternal uteroplacental blood flow reduction 1293
  pre-eclampsia and obliterative arteritis 1310
  thrombosis, villous abnormalities 1288
Fetiform teratoma 799
Feto–fatal transfusion syndrome
  see Twin–twin transfusion, chronic
Feto–maternal circulatory unit 1252
Feto-placental circulation 1236

Fetus
  abnormalities, amniotic bands and strings
      1307–1308
  blood flow
      cessation, fibromuscular sclerosis 1292
      reduction, placental villi abnormalities 1288
  brain damage, chorioamnionitis 1306
  capillaries, placental development 1236
  cervix, cervical stroma 275
  chromosomal abnormalities
      placental villous histology 1440
      sporadic miscarriage 1431–1432
      see also Chromosomal abnormalities
  death see Fetal death
  distress see Fetal distress
  DNA synthesis, viruses, inhibitory effect of 1292
  factor V Leiden mutation, miscarriage 1434
  growth
      defect, circumvallate placentation 1275
      malarial infection 1319
      retardation see Intrauterine fetal growth
          retardation
  gut maturation, meconium passage 1303
  haemorrhage
      insertion funiculi furcata 1296
      intervillous thrombosis 1285
      omphalomesenteric duct remnants in umbilical
          cord 1294
      placental accessory lobe 1276
      velamentous insertion of umbilical cord 1296
  hydrops, parvovirus B 19 infection 1317
  hypoxia
      chronic, chorangiosis 1289
      meconium staining 1303
      placental infarction 1279
      retroplacental haematoma 1284
      villous oedema 1289
  leucocytes, chorioamnionitis 1304
  leukaemia, placental involvement 1460, 1460
  lymphoma, placental involvement 1460
  macrophages, Hofbauer cells 1242
  malformations
      placental haemangiomas 1453
      umbilical artery, single 1294
      see also Congenital
          abnormalities/malformations; Genital tract,
          malformations
  membranes see Membranes, fetal
  microchimerism, primary biliary cirrhosis
      1481–1482
  mobility, umbilical cord length 1293
  mortality 990
      monochorionic–monoamniotic twin
          placentation 1580–1581
      see also Fetal death
  motilin secretion, meconium staining 1303
  ovary development see Ovary, embryology
  perfusion patterns, placental, intrauterine fetal
      growth retardation 1311
  polyuria, polyhydramnios in twin transfusion
      syndrome 1582
  red cells, nucleation status and fetal death 1442
  squames, amniotic fluid embolism syndrome
      1566
  testicular hormones, genital duct differentiation
      13
  vagina and cervix, epithelial boundaries at birth
      250
  villous vessels, necrotising endarteritis in rubella
      infection 1315–1316
Fetus acardius, teratoma of umbilical cord vs 1301
Fetus acardius amorphus, placental teratomas 1454
Fetus papyraceous 1585, 1585
FHIT gene studies 1600–1601
  cervical carcinomas 1600
  HPV infection 1600–1601
Fibrillin-1 gene 1546
Fibrin deposition
  intrasinusoidal, acute fatty liver of pregnancy
      1470
  maternal floor infarction 1278–1279
  periportal intrasinusoidal, toxaemia of pregnancy
      1474, 1475
  perivillous 1276–1278
Fibrinoid
  fibrin-type 1261
  matrix-type 1261
  Nitabuch's 1261
  placental 1261
Fibrinoid change

Leydig cell tumours 849, 849
  uterine leiomyoma with bizarre nuclei 527
Fibrinoid deposition
  cell columns of placenta 1259–1260
  placental development 1261
Fibrinoid necrosis
  arteriopathy in pre-eclampsia 1339
  idiopathic postpartum acute renal failure 1504,
      1504
  myometrial necrobiotic granulomas 500
  placental villi 1288–1289, 1289
Fibrin-type fibrinoid 1261
Fibroadenomas of vulva 132, 132
Fibroepithelial polyps of cervix 380
Fibroepitheliomatous stromal polyp, vulvar 95,
      95–96
  histological appearance 96
Fibrohistiocytic origin tumours, vulvar 116–117
Fibroma(s)
  cellular 860, 860–861
  ovarian 765, 858–860
      cellular 860, 860–861
      histogenesis 858
      macroscopic appearance 858, 858
      multiple 858, 859
      origin 704
      thecomas and 704
  vulvar 116
      extirpated 116
Fibromatosis, ovary 672–673, 673
Fibromuscular sclerosis, fetal stem arteries 1292,
      1292
Fibropapilloma, Fallopian tube 602, 602
Fibrosarcoma
  ovarian 861, 861, 873
  vulvar 116
Fibrosarcoma ovarii mucocellulares
      (carcinomatoides) see Krukenberg tumours
Fibrosis
  endometrial 422
  retroperitoneal 1189
  stromal, cervical polyps 290
  villous, fetal death 1313
Fibrothecoma 858, 1017, 1171
Fibrous histiocytoma, malignant, vulvar
      117
Fibrous tissue tumours
  ovarian 858–861
  vulva 116
FIGO international classification/staging
  cancer definition, vaginal 187, 187, 190
  cervical carcinoma 326
  endometrial adenocarcinoma 476, 477, 483–484
  lymphoma staging 938–939
  microinvasive glandular lesions of cervix 356
  vaginal cancer staging 190, 191
Filariasis 1141–1142
  vulvar 54
Filshie clip 597
Fimbriae, tubal 31
  adenofibroma 602, 602
  anatomy 586, 587
  carcinoma 607
  implantation, tubal pregnancy 1051
  metastatic carcinoma 612, 613
  occlusion 1010, 1010
  ostial phimosis 1010
  ovarian stromal metaplasia 591, 592
  ovum transport/interaction 1006, 1018
  serosal metaplasia 590
  transitional cell metaplasia 590, 590
Fimbriectomy 598
Fine needle aspiration biopsy (FNAB)
  carcinosarcoma (uterine) 562
  vaginal tumours 189
First mitotic division 2
First-trimester bleeding, bilobate placenta 1276
'Fish flesh' pattern, sarcoma 520
Fistula
  caecovaginal 185
  Crohn's disease 1185, 1186
  gastrointestinal-vaginal 184–185
  HIV infection 1152, 1153
  ileo-vaginal 1185
  large and small bowel with vagina 185
  pathology, vaginal 185–186
  postpartum 1151
  rectovaginal 184–185
  sigmoidovaginal 185
  tubointestinal 1012

  vaginal 183–186
      see also Vagina, fistulas
  vaginal-urinary 184
  vesicovaginal 184, 185
Fitz–Hugh–Curtis syndrome 622
Fixed drug eruption, vulvar 69–70
Flagellate infections, Trichomonas
      see Trichomonas vaginalis
Flexion phase of embryogenesis 7–9, 644
Florid condylomata of vulva 97
Flow cytometry
  endometrial adenocarcinoma detection 483
  low-grade endometrial stromal sarcoma 511
  ovarian carcinoma prognosis 736
  primary peritoneal serous carcinoma 925
  tumour ploidy determination 1608, 1609
Fluid retention, epilepsy in pregnancy 1533
Fluke infection, vulvar 54–55
5–Fluorouracil, topical, vaginal lesions due to 153
Foam cells
  endometrial hyperplasia 448, 450
  endometrial stromal tumours 503
Focal aplasia within Müllerian duct system 42
Focal necrotising villitis, rubella infection 1315
Folate
  deficiency
      cervical epithelium 290
      hyperhomocysteinaemia, acquired 1434
  epilepsy in pregnancy 1533
Follicle cysts
  autonomous 664
  children 664, 1162–1163
  cytology 664
  Donahue syndrome 1162
  McCune–Albright syndrome 1162
  multiple 668, 668, 669
  polycystic ovaries 666
  solitary 663, 663–664
  solitary luteinized, of pregnancy/puerperium 677,
      677
Follicles, ovarian
  absent/reduced pool 1014–1015
  accelerated depletion 1016
  aromatase activity increase 1016
  atresia 650, 656
      steroid contraceptives effect 1099
  cysts see Follicle cysts
  depletion rate 657
  development, hypo-oestrogenic state 403
  developmental abnormalities, luteal phase defects
      405
  dominant, selection 1013
  dysfunction due to enzyme defects 1016
  embryology/development 638
  Graafian 655, 656
  growth, endometrial cycle control 396
  maturation stages 655, 655–656
  number 649, 650
  ovulatory 1014
  perinatal period 648
  preovulatory, development 1013
  prepubertal 650
  primary, anatomy 655, 655–656
  primordial 647, 650, 651, 655
      maturation 655
      structure 655–656
  recruitment 1013
  recurrent empty follicle syndrome 1015
  rupture with failure of ovum release
      1017
  secondary, anatomy 655, 656
  tertiary
      anatomy 655, 656
      steroid contraceptives effect 1099
  see also Ovulation
Follicle stimulating hormone (FSH)
  defective 1016
  normal menstrual cycle 1013
  prostaglandin E$_2$ relationship 1013
  receptor, antibodies to 680
  receptor binding, inhibition in resistant ovary
      syndrome 680
  release 1013
  surge 1013, 1014
  twin pregnancy 1576
Follicular cervicitis 281
Follicular hyperthecosis 667
Follicular phase, luteal phase insufficiency 405
Follicular salpingitis 623, 1010
Folliculitis, vulvar infection 56

Folliculopathy 1015–1016
Folliculostatin 1013
Food, reproductive dysfunction and 1020
Foreign bodies
   granulomata in uterus due to IUCDs 1108, *1109*
   ovarian inflammation 684
   vagina 153
Foscarnet, vaginal lesions due to 154
Fourchette 38
Fox–Fordyce disease 84, *84*
Fractures, steroid contraceptives and 1105
Fragile X gene 642
Frankenhauser's ganglion/ plexus
     see Uterovaginal plexus
Fraser's (cryptophthalmos) syndrome 1158, 1168,
   1183
Frenulum of labia, anatomy 38
Friedrich's ataxia 500
Fulminant hepatitis, pregnancy 1478
Functional endometrium 396–397
Functional villi, lesions reducing mass 1276–1284
Fungal infections
   cervix 283
   chorioamnionitis 1305
   endometritis 432
   in tropics **1140**
   vaginal 170–173
   see also Candidiasis (*Candida* infections)
Funiculitis, chorioamnionitis of umbilical cord
   1305
Funisitis
   acute 1300
   necrotising 1300
Furcate insertion, umbilical cord 1296
Fusion defects
   amniotic bands and strings 1308
   female genital tract malformation 43–44
   non-obstructed 46
Fusospirochaetosis, vaginal 168–169

G
Galactosaemia **1183**
Gallbladder
   carcinoma, metastatic, to ovary 885
   function in pregnancy **1484–1485**
   pathology in pregnancy **1465–1494**
   volume in pregnancy 1485
Gallstones
   cholesterol, pregnancy 1484
   intrahepatic cholestasis of pregnancy 1469
   steroid contraceptives and 1103
Gamete intrafallopian transfer (GIFT) 1090
   ovarian disease 1062
Gametes, transport, tubal 1006
Gamma glutamyl transpeptidase (GGT), pregnancy
   1466
Ganglioneuroma, ovarian **867**
Gardnerella vaginalis (*Clostridium vaginale*)
   cervical infection 282
   chorioamnionitis 1305
   epidemiology 167, *167*
   genitourinary infections 996
   transmission (sexual) 167, *167*
   vaginitis 158, 165–167
      pregnancy 166
   vulva, microbial flora 54
'Garland' pattern, ovarian metastasis 883, *883*
Gartner's cysts, vaginal 180
Gartner's duct 18, 897
   cysts *see* Mesonephric cysts
Gastric carcinoma
   ovarian metastases 881
      Krukenberg tumours 891
   uterine cervix metastases 385, *386*
Gastric contents, aspiration 1570
Gastric MALT lymphoma 938
Gastrointestinal carcinoid tumours, metastatic to
   ovary *886,* 886–887
Gastrointestinal-vaginal fistula **184–185**
Gaucher's disease 1183–1184
GCDFP-15 (BRST2), uterine leiomyoma with
   tubules 530
Gender identification disorders
   abnormal sex chromosome constitution
      1220–1228
   normal chromosome constitution **1212–1220**
Genes, imprinted *see* Imprinted genes
Genetic abnormalities
   cervical intraepithelial neoplasia (CIN)
      310

cervical neoplasia 310
   hydatidiform moles *see* Hydatidiform mole
   miscarriage 1435
   trophoblastic neoplasms **1395–1396**
   see also Genetic factors
Genetic disorders
   vulva 60–63
   see also Entries beginning familial, hereditary
Genetic factors
   cervical carcinoma 302–303
   choriocarcinoma 1395
   endometrial carcinoma 995
   genital tract malformations 45
   gonadoblastoma 824
   infertility 992, 995
   miscarriage 1435
   ovarian tumours 702
   polycystic ovarian disease 995
   see also Genetic abnormalities
Genetic imprinting *see* Imprinted genes
Genetic screening programmes, Klinefelter's
   syndrome 1220
Genetic studies *see* Molecular pathology
Genital canal development *16*
   paramesonephric duct 15
Genital duct differentiation **13–18**
   female differentiation 14–18
Genital herpesvirus infection, vulvar 59
Genitalia
   ambiguous *see* Ambiguous genitalia
   development 18–21
   external *see* External genitalia
   feminisation 19–20
   masculinisation 19
Genital membrane
   external genitalia development 19
   rupture 19
Genital pox virus infections, vulvar 59–60
Genital ridge, transplantation, animal model of
   teratoma 706
Genital tract (female)
   carcinoma, metastases to uterine cervix 384
   classification of malformations **42–45**
   congenital malformations *see* Congenital
      abnormalities/malformations
   embryology 41–42
   local immune response in 993
   malformations
      aetiology and pathogenesis **45**
      classification **42–45**
      clinical features **46–48**
      complications **48**
      failure of surgical termination of pregnancy 48
      genetic factors 45
      incidence **45–46**
Genital ulceration, Behçet's syndrome 291
Genital warts *see* Condyloma acuminata
Genomic imprinting **1605–1606**
   see also Imprinted genes
Genomic instability, female infertility 995
Germ cell(s)
   aberrant migration, placental teratomas 1454
   mixed germ cell sex cord–stromal tumours 834,
      835, 836
   mutations 679
   neoplasias of vulva 125
   primordial 635–636
      embryogenesis 1211
      migration 636
      number 638
      proliferation in indifferent gonad 636
      teratoma origin 706
      vulnerability 679
   uterine cervix tumours 380
   see also Oocytes
Germ cell tumours **1164–1169**
   androgen resistance syndromes 1161
   bimodal age distribution 1164
   childhood/adolescence **1163–1177**
   endodermal sinus tumour of vagina **1168–1169**
   epidemiology **1164**
   Fallopian tube 611
   familial cancer syndromes **1168**
   gonadoblastoma 1167–1168, *1168,* 1172
   metastatic, to vagina 218
   mixed **794,** 1172
      see also Mixed germ cell sex cord–stromal
      tumours (ovarian)
   non-gestational carcinomas with trophoblastic
      metaplasia **1411–1412**

ovarian *see* Ovarian germ cell tumours
   sex cord–stromal tumours with *see* Mixed germ
      cell sex cord–stromal tumours (ovarian)
   teratomas *see* Teratoma
   vagina **216**
   see also Choriocarcinoma; Dysgerminoma; Yolk sac
      tumours
Germinoma, hermaphroditism, true 1229
Gestational diabetes 1025, 1092
Gestational hypertension 1505, 1506
Gestational trophoblastic diseases **1359–1430**
   miscarriage material 1442
Gestodene, thromboembolic disease and 1104
GGT (gamma glutamyl transpeptidase)
   1466
Giant cells
   epithelial, carcinosarcoma (uterine) *563*
   intraglandular, IUCD use and *1109*
   multinucleated
      emphysematous colpitis 179, *179*
      uterine leiomyosarcoma 521, *521*
   osteoclast-like, uterine leiomyosarcoma 521
Giant cell tumour, ovarian **866**
Giant condyloma acuminatum *see* Cervical
   carcinoma, verrucous
Giant skin naevi, benign, placental metastases 1459
Giemsa banding
   X chromosome 642, *642*
   Y chromosome 639, *639*
Giemsa stain, *C. trachomatis* inclusion bodies 426
GIFT *see* Gamete intrafallopian transfer (GIFT)
Gilbert's syndrome, pregnancy 1484
'Gishiri cutting' *see* Female circumcision
Glandular lesions of cervix 339–368
Glandular secretory activity exhaustion, endometrial
   401
Glassy cell carcinoma
   cervix 349
   Fallopian tube 611
Glial fibrillary acidic protein (GFAP)
   immature teratoma 791
   uterine carcinosarcoma 566
Glial implants, immature teratoma 792, *795*
Glial polyp 290
Glioblastoma 1535
Gliomatosis peritonei 792, 793, *795, 796*
Glomerular capillary endotheliosis, pre-eclampsia
   1506, *1507,* 1511
Glomerular diseases, coexisting with pregnancy
   1512–1519
Glomerulonephritis, in pregnancy
   acute post-infectious, *1515,* **1516**
   membranous *1512,* **1512–1513**
   mesangiocapillary **1513–1515,** *1514*
   see also Mesangiocapillary glomerulonephritis
Glomerulonephropathy, minimal change *1513,*
   1513
Glomus tumour of vulva 119–120
Gloves, granulomatous reaction to cornstarch
   powder 1011
Glucagonoma syndrome 63
Glucocorticoid biosynthesis *1213*
Glucose
   cervical supply 994
   tolerance impairment, by combined oral
      contraceptives 1092
Glucose-6-phosphate dehydrogenase (G6PD) 642
α-Glutathione S-transferase, sclerosing stromal
   tumours (ovarian) 766
Glycogen
   metabolic defects, endometrial, infertility and
      1005
   storage, urogenital sinus epithelium 148
   in vaginal epithelial cells 150
Gnathostoma 1143
Goblet cells, mucinous carcinoid tumour of ovary
   810, 886–887, *887*
Goldberg–Maxwell–Morris syndrome (testicular
   feminisation) **1184**
   see also Testicular feminisation
Gonad(s)
   development/differentiation **1157–1158**
   differentiation mechanisms 638–643, 645
      supporting cells role 640–641
   DSS (dosage-sensitive sex reversal) 1158
   indifferent 636–637, *644*
      development 638, 897–898
      transformation to embryonic ovary 638, 646
      transformation to embryonic testis 638, 646
   induction 644–645

Gonad(s) (cont'd)
  intersex disorders **1160**
  mixed gonadal dysgenesis **1160**
  Müllerian anomalies **1158**, 1160
  sex differentiation 638–643
  SRY 1157
  streak 1015, *1015*, 1160
    gonadal dysgenesis, mixed 1226, *1226*
    gonadoblastoma in 826
    Turner's syndrome and 1015, *1015*, 1160
  see also Ovary; Testes
Gonadal defects, primary, pseudohermaphroditism, male 1215–1217
Gonadal dysgenesis
  familial XX 641
  gonadoblastoma association 823–824
  mixed *1224*, 1225–1228, *1226*
    genetic and karyotypic abnormalities 1225
    hermaphroditism, true vs 1229
    Müllerian duct derived organs 1225
    Wolffian duct derived organs 1225
  pure
    46, XY type 1223
    46,XX type 1223
    genetic identification disorders 1223–1224
Gonadal ridge *636*, 645
  genital duct differentiation 13
Gonadal tissue, hermaphroditism, true 1229
Gonadal tumours
  hermaphroditism, true 1229
  malignant, androgen insensitivity disorders 1219
  Turner's syndrome 1222
Gonadectomy
  gonadoblastoma 831–832
  testicular feminisation, incomplete 1219
Gonadoblastoma **821–832, 1167–1168**, *1168*, **1172**
  atypical *see* Mixed germ cell sex cord–stromal tumours (ovarian)
  behaviour and prognosis 832
  'burnt out' 823, 829, *830*
  calcification 826, 829, *829*, *830*
  clinical findings 823
  differential diagnosis 831, 840
  dysgerminoma association 822, 826, *826*, 829, *829*, 832
  familial aspects 823–824
  genetic findings 824
  gonadal dysgenesis, mixed 1226, *1227*
  hormonal findings 824–825
  incidence 822–823
  in male pseudohermaphrodites 821
  metastatic lesions 830
  neoplasms associated 830
  neoplastic germ cell elements 829, 830, 832
  neoplastic nature 822
  pathology 825–831
    histology 826–831, *826–831*
    macroscopic *825*, 825–826
    ultrastructure 828, *828*
  sex-cord derivatives 827, 829
  terminology and early descriptions 821–822
  therapy 831–832
    chemotherapy 832
Gonadoblastoma Y gene locus (GBY) 1227
Gonadoma, dysgenetic *see* Gonadoblastoma
Gonadotroph cell adenoma 1024
Gonadotrophin(s)
  elevated, gonadoblastoma 825
  follicle cyst pathogenesis 663, 664
  maternal chorionic, fetal testosterone secretion 14
  ovarian adenocarcinoma risk and 701
  ovarian hypersensitivity 1017
  secretion inhibition by stress 1020
  therapeutic, complications 1029
  see also Follicle stimulating hormone (FSH); Human chorionic gonadotrophin (hCG); Luteinizing hormone (LH)
Gonadotrophin releasing hormone (GnRH)
  ovulation control 1013, 1014
  pulsatile release 1013, 1020
  receptors 1013
Gonadotrophin releasing hormone (GnRH) agonists **1087**
  haemorrhagic cellular leiomyoma (apoplectic) association 526
  indications 1087
  lymphoid infiltration in uterine leiomyoma 533
  uterine leiomyoma regression 516

Gonadotrophin releasing hormone (GnRH) neurons
  damage 1020
  nutritional effects on 1021
Gonium *see* Germ cell(s), primordial
Gonochorism 3
Gonococcal endometritis 1003
Gonocytoma
  classification 821
  type 2 *see* Mixed germ cell sex cord–stromal tumours (ovarian)
  see also Gonadoblastoma
Gonorrhoea
  acute arthritis 1193
  cervix 281–282
  distribution of lesions 165
  endometritis *430*, 430–431
    chronic 1134
  vaginitis 167–168
  vulvar infection 56
  vulvovaginitis 1163
  see also Neisseria gonorrhoeae
Gorlin's syndrome *see* Basal cell naevus syndrome
Goserelin 1087
Graafian follicle *655*, 656
Gram-negative bacilli, vulvar infections 57–58
Gram-negative cocci, vulvar infections 56
Gram-positive bacilli, vulvar infections 56–57
Gram-positive cocci, vulvar infections 56
Gram staining, vaginal fluids 157
Granular cells, endometrial stromal tumours 503
Granular cell tumours (myoblastoma)
  cervix 384
  vagina 197
  vulvar *122*, 122–123, *123*, *123*
    benign 122–123
    malignant 123
Granulation tissue, vaginal biopsy *219*, 220
Granules, prolactinoma 1022, *1023*
Granulocyte colony stimulating factor, chorioamnioitis 1305
Granulocyte-macrophage colony-stimulating factor, IUCD use and 1111
Granulocytes, endometrial 395, 1329, *1330*
Granulocytic sarcoma
  cervix 951–952, *952*
  ovarian **946–948**, *947*
  uterus 951–952, *952*
  vaginal 954
Granuloma
  cortical, ovarian 684
  Crohn's disease 684, 1185, 1186, *1186*
  endometrium 428
  enterobiasis 1143
  foreign body, ovarian 684
  infantile gluteal 80
  leishmaniasis 1141
  ovarian
    infections 683–684
    non-infectious 684
  peritoneal keratin 574
    granulomatous salpingitis vs 619
  postoperative necrobiotic, myometrium 500
  postoperative necrobiotic palisading, granulomatous salpingitis vs 619, *619*
  pyogenic, vulvar involvement 80
  renal tuberculosis *1499*, 1499–1500
  sarcoid-like, endometrial tuberculosis 429
Granuloma inguinale (donavanosis) **1136–1138**
  histology 1137, *1138*
Granulomatous arteritis, localised, granulomatous salpingitis vs 619
Granulomatous disease
  cervicitis 281
  disseminated (BCGosis) 1193
  endometritis, endometrial oblation 421
Granulomatous nodules, endometriosis 969
Granulomatous reaction, to cornstarch powder 1011
Granulomatous salpingitis 617–619, 1010–1011, *1012*
  ectopic pregnancy 1048
  see also Salpingitis, tuberculous
Granulomatous vasculitis **1190–1191**, *1191*, *1192*
Granulosa cells 685
  anti-Müllerian hormone (AMH) secretion 14
  artifacts misinterpreted as malignant 685–686
  corpus luteum formation and 1014
  embryology 637
  gonadoblastoma 827, *827*
  gynandroblastoma 760, *760*

oocytes as organisers 703
origin 703
proliferations 677–678, *678*
Sertoli cells homology 745
unilocular cystic tumour 677
Granulosa cell tumours
  adult-type **746–752**
    biological behaviour and therapy 751–752
    Call–Exner bodies *747*, 748, *749*, 751
    cystic variant 746–747, *747*
    differential diagnosis 748, 945
    gross pathology 746–747, *747*
    heterologous elements 749, 751
    immunohistochemistry 751
    incidence and clinical features 746
    intermediate differentiation 748
    metastatic *747*, 748
    microscopic pathology *747*, 747–751, *748*, *749*, *750*
    ovarian lymphomas vs 945
    pathology 746–751
    poorly differentiated 749
    sarcomatoid pattern 749, *750*
    sarcomatous change 751
    Sertoli cell tumour vs 748, *748*
    small cell undifferentiated ovarian carcinoma vs 905
    theca element *747*, 747–748, 751
    trabecular pattern 748, *749*
    ultrastructure 751
    watered-silk pattern 749, *750*
    well-differentiated 748, *749*
  aetiology and pathogenesis 705
  blepharophimosis **1182**
  experimental induction 704–705
  histogenesis 703
  juvenile-type **752–753**, *761*, **1169**, *1169*, 1171
    clinical features and differential diagnosis 945
    leprechaunism 1183, 1187
    pathology *752*, 752–753, *753*
    small cell undifferentiated ovarian carcinoma vs 905
  origin 704
  ovarian lymphomas vs 945
  ovarian tumours of probable Wolffian origin vs 902
  pancytopenia 1196
  unilocular cystic 677
Granulosa–theca cell tumours 704, 746
Greater sciatic foramen, piriformis muscle 23
Grimelius reaction, insular carcinoid tumour 809
Group B haemolytic streptococci, chorioamnionitis 1305
Growth
  discordant, twin pregnancy 1585
  fetal *see* Fetus, growth
Growth hormone (GH), deficiency 1020
Grzybowski's generalised eruptive keratoacanthoma **1184**
Guillain–Barré syndrome 1536
Gummas
  cervical 282
  vulva 58
Gupta bodies 170, *170*
Gynandroblastoma *760*, **760**

H
H19, imprinted genes 1605, 1606
Haemangioblastic progenitor cells, fetal capillaries 1236
Haemangioendothelioma, epithelioid, vulvar 121
Haemangioendotheliomatosis, diffuse, ovarian 869
Haemangioma
  capillary, uterine 538
  cavernous
    ampulla (Fallopian tube) *604*, 605
    ovarian 869
  cervix 384
  clitoris, neonatal *119*
  Fallopian tube *604*, 604–605
  histocytoid, vagina 197
  ovarian **868–869**
  placental *see* Placental haemangioma
  thrombocytopenia **1196**
  umbilical cord 1301
  uterine, Klippel–Trenaunay–Weber syndrome 1187
  vaginal 197
  vulvar 118

Haemangiopericytoma
  ovarian **869**
  uterine 510, 538
  vulvar 120
Haematogenous spread
  endometriotic tissue 965
  extragonadal tumours to ovary 879–880
Haematoma
  formation, antepartum haemorrhage 1350
  marginal 1284–1285
  pelvic, postpartum haemorrhage 1561
  placental *see* Placenta, haematoma
  retroplacental *see* Retroplacental haematoma
  subamniotic 1284
  subchorial, massive *1284*, 1285
  umbilical cord *see* Umbilical cord, haematomas
Haematometrocolpos, genital tract malformations
  46
Haematosalpinx **596–597**
Haematoxylin bodies, small cell carcinomas of
  cervix 372
Haematuria, hermaphroditism, true 1228
Haemochorial placentation, migratory trophoblast
  1332
Haemochromatosis 1021, **1186**
Haemodilution in pregnancy, serum protein levels
  1465
Haemodynamic imbalance, chronic twin–twin
  transfusion syndrome 1581
Haemoglobin levels, chronic twin–twin transfusion
  1581–1582
Haemolytic anaemia 797, **1196**
  microangiopathic 1503
Haemolytic uraemic syndrome
  idiopathic postpartum acute renal failure 1505
  pregnancy 1480
Haemoperitoneum
  immature teratoma 792
  solitary follicle cysts 663
Haemophilus ducreyi, vulvar infection 57
Haemophilus influenzae, endometritis in pregnancy
  427
Haemophilus vaginalis (Corynebacterium vaginale)
  157
Haemorrhage
  adrenal cortex 1564
  antepartum *see* Antepartum haemorrhage
  fetal *see* Fetus, haemorrhage
  intracerebral *see* Intracerebral haemorrhage
  intraluminal, endometriosis 966
  Kline's *see* Intervillous thrombosis
  maternal death 1561
  paratubal 592
  petechial
    of brain 1532
    hypertensive diseases of pregnancy 1564
  pituitary gland 1024
  postpartum *see* Postpartum haemorrhage
  stellate, haemorrhagic cellular leiomyoma 526
  vagina 173, 174
Haemorrhagic endometrial infarction 408
Haemorrhagic nodules, vagina 221–222, *222*
Haemorrhoidal plexus 25
Haemosiderin
  carcinogenicity 699
  endometriosis 974
  extramembranous pregnancy 1306
  vulvar pigmentation disorders 67
Haemosiderosis 1021
Hailey–Hailey disease *see* Pemphigus, chronic
  benign familial
Hair
  axillary, development 653
  loss, vulvar 82
  pubic, development 653
HAM 56 antibody, primary ovarian carcinoma vs
  colonic metastases 883
Hamartoma, multiple hamartoma syndrome
  (Cowden's disease) **1182**
Hand–foot–uterus syndrome 45
Hashimoto's thyroiditis 1182
h-Caldesmon
  cellular leiomyoma (uterine) 525
  uterine leiomyoma differential diagnosis 518
  uterine mesenchymal tumours 501
Head and tail fold formation *9*
Head injuries, in pregnancy **1532**
Heart
  block, congenital **1547**
  blood coagulation changes in pregnancy **1543**

haemodynamic changes in pregnancy **1543**
  in pregnancy **1542–1543**
  size/weight *1542*, **1542–1543**
  wall measurements 1542, *1542*
Heart disease
  carcinoid 807
  congenital *see* Congenital heart disease
  coronary, steroid contraceptives and 1104–1105
  ischaemic, combined steroid contraceptives
    1104–1105
  rheumatic *see* Rheumatic heart disease
Heart failure *see* Cardiac failure
Heart valves, prosthetic **1548–1549**
  anticoagulants 1549
  thromboembolism risk 1548–1549
Hedgehog signalling pathway, Gorlin's syndrome
  1171, **1171**
Helicobacter pylori 938
HELLP syndrome **1503**, 1524
  acute fatty liver of pregnancy 1473
  acute renal failure **1503**
  criteria 1475
  hypertensive disease of pregnancy 1564
  liver involvement 1475–1476
  liver rupture 1476
  maternal complications 1475
  maternal mortality rates 1475
  neonatal complications 1476
Helminth infections, in tropics **1141–1148**
Hemiplegic migraine 1531
  aneurysms 1531
Hepatic adenoma, steroid contraceptives and 1101,
  1103, *1103*
Hepatic blood flow, pregnancy 1465
Hepatic dysfunction, toxaemia 1474
Hepatic function *see* Liver function
Hepatic injury in pregnancy, drug-induced
  1479–1480
Hepatic sinusoidal dilatation 1100, *1101*
Hepatic tumours, steroid contraceptives and
  1101–1102
Hepatitis
  acute viral in pregnancy 1478–1479
  autoimmune in pregnancy 1483
  chronic viral in pregnancy 1482–1483
  herpes simplex in pregnancy 1479
Hepatitis A, pregnancy 1478
Hepatitis B
  pregnancy 1478, 1482
    vertical transmission 1482
  vaccination of newborn infants 1482
Hepatitis C, pregnancy 1482–1483
Hepatitis D, pregnancy 1483
Hepatitis E, pregnancy 1478–1479
  vertical transmission of infection 1479
Hepatitis G, pregnancy 1483
Hepatitis of pregnancy *see* Intrahepatic cholestasis,
  of pregnancy
Hepatoblastoma
  fetal, placental metastases 1459
  steroid contraceptives and 1101
Hepatocellular adenoma, placental 1455
Hepatocellular carcinoma
  metastatic, to ovary 887, *887*
  pregnancy 1480
  steroid contraceptives and 1101
Hepatocellular disease, steroid contraceptives
  contraindicated 1100
Hepatocyte(s)
  ballooning, acute fatty liver of pregnancy 1470
  elements in adult-type granulosa cell tumours
    749, 751
  elements in Sertoli–Leydig cell tumours 755
Hepatocyte growth factor, endometriosis
  966
Hepatoid carcinoma, ovarian *908*, **908–909**, *909*
HER-2/neu proto-oncogene, overexpression,
  endometrial adenocarcinoma 485
Hereditary breast/ovarian cancer syndrome 702
Hereditary non-polyposis colon carcinoma
  (HNPCC) 702, **1184**
  DNA mismatch repair 1601
  endometrial adenocarcinoma risk factor 456
Hereditary site-specific ovarian cancer syndrome
  702
Hermaphroditism, true 640, **1228–1229**
  clinical presentation 1228
  gonadal dysgenesis, mixed vs 1229
  gonadoblastoma association 823
  phenotype 1228

Hernia, sliding, Fallopian tube **594**
Hernia uteri inguinalis *see* Persistent Müllerian duct
  syndrome
Herpes simplex virus (HSV)
  cervical adenocarcinoma 341
  cervical infection 286
  cervical lesions 286
  chorioamnionitis 1305
  endometrial infection, necrotising funisitis 1300
  hepatitis, pregnancy 1479
  interaction with human papillomavirus 301
  miscarriage 1432
  neoplasia and 163–164
  transmission 162
  type 2, vaginitis 162–164
Herpesvirus hominis, endometrial infection
  425–426
Herpes zoster, HIV/AIDS 1152, *1152*
Herpetic lesions of cervix 286
Herpetic ulcers 163
HerW-env protein 1240
Heterokaryonts 1576
Heteroploidy, IUCD use and 1116
Heterotopia in cervix 278–280
Heterotropic cartilage, cervical 279
Heterotropic pregnancy 1051
Heterozygosity, loss, borderline mucinous ovarian
  tumours 698
Hiatus of Schwalbe 24
Hidradenitis suppurativa, vulvar 82
Hidradenoma
  clear cell, vulvar 127
  papillary, vulvar 127–128
High altitude, placental villi 1251
High-density lipoprotein (HDL) cholesterol
  combined steroid contraceptives and 1103,
    1104
  HRT and 1090
High-grade endometrial stromal sarcoma,
  cytogenetic findings 509
Hilus cells 848
  in endosalpinx/perisalpinx 591
  hyperplasia, ovarian *673*, **673–674**, 847
Hilus cell tumours **757**, 848, *848*
Hind gut
  embryogenesis 10
  primitive *10*
Hirsutism, in polycystic ovary disease 667
Histiocytic endometritis 423
Histiocytic malignant lymphoma 937
Histiocytoma, malignant fibrous, vulvar 117
Histiocytosis
  Langerhans' cell (histiocytosis X) **957**, **1187**
    vulvar *65*, 65–66
  mucicarminophilic, ovarian 685
Histiocytoid haemangioma, vagina 197
HIV/AIDS **1186–1187**
  cervical infection 287
  cervical intraepithelial neoplasia (CIN) 1153
  cervical neoplasia 301, 303
  chorioamnionitis 1152
  endometritis 420, 426
  epidemiology **1151–1152**
  fistulae 1152, **1153**
  genital tract **1551–1153**
  genital ulcers 1152, **1153**, 1551
  herpes zoster 1152, *1152*
  human papillomavirus (HPV) and 301, **1153**
  lymphoma 1533
  menstrual irregularity 1152
  nervous system **1532–1533**
  non-Hodgkin's lymphoma 1153
  opportunistic infections 1533
  pathology **1152–1153**
  pelvic inflammatory disease (PID) 1152
  placental examination 1318
  pre-AIDS 1532
  pregnancy 1152
  transmission, bacterial vaginosis association 164
  tuberculosis 1152
  vaginal changes 164
  vertical transmission 1318
  vulvo-vaginal candidiasis 1152
HLA (human leukocyte) antigens
  persistent trophoblastic disease **1384–1385**
  sperm antibodies and 993
  trophoblastic neoplasms 1395
HLA-BW35, sperm antibodies and 993
HLA-DQw3 antigen, squamous cell carcinoma of
  cervix 303

HMB-45
  melanoma 888
  steroid cell tumours 853, 854
HMF62, Fallopian tube 588
HMGIC gene, angiomyxoma 121
hMLH1 gene, germline mutation, hereditary ovarian cancer 702
hMSH2 gene, germline mutation, hereditary ovarian cancer 702
Hobnail appearance, clear cell endometrial carcinoma 470, *471*
Hobnail metaplasia, endometrium 413
Hodgkin's disease
  cervix 951
  classification *936, 937*
  ovarian involvement 945–946
  primary, of female genital tract 935
  staging *938, 938–939*
  vulval 954
Hoeppli–Splendore reaction 1143
Hofbauer cells
  immunological aspects 1243
  maternal syphilis infection 1314
  placenta 1242
  placental angiogenesis 1244
Homeobox genes, *HOXA 10* and *HOXA 11*, functions 1005
Hormodendron compatum, vulvar infection 56
Hormonal factors, intrahepatic cholestasis in pregnancy 1468
Hormonal polypeptides, small cell carcinomas of cervix 370
Hormonal responses, endometriosis 973
Hormonal therapy **1071–1087**
  anti-oestrogens **1075–1081**
    see also Clomiphene; Tamoxifen
  anti-progestins **1086–1087**
  cytological changes 1192
  diethylstilboestrol *see* Diethylstilboestrol (DES)
  endometrial adenocarcinoma 486, *487*
  endometrial hyperplasia 453–454
  endometritis, focal necrotising 425
  fracture risk 1196
  GnRH agonists **1087**
  histological effects, on endometrial adenocarcinoma 486–488
  hormone replacement therapy *see* Hormone replacement therapy (HRT)
  infertility treatment **1090**
  low-grade endometrial stromal sarcoma 511
  oestrogens **1071–1074**
    see also Oestrogen(s)
  progestagens **1082–1086**
    see also Progestagens
Hormone(s)
  cervical adenocarcinoma 340–341
  effect on uterine leiomyomata 536
  withdrawal bleeding *see* Bleeding, withdrawal
  see also specific hormones
Hormone receptor status
  prognosis cervical adenocarcinoma 351
  see also Oestrogen receptors; Progesterone receptors
Hormone replacement therapy (HRT) **1087–1090,** 1196
  combined hormones 1087–1089
    combined daily 1088
    effect on breast and ovary 1089
    effects on endometrium *1088,* 1088–1089, *1089*
    sequential 1088
    systemic effects 1089
  ovarian carcinoma risk and 701
  Tibolone 1090
Host defenses
  vaginal candidiasis 171
  see also Immune response
HOX gene, endometriosis 966
HPV *see* Human papillomavirus (HPV)
HSV *see* Herpes simplex virus (HSV)
Human AMH gene over-expression, paramesonephric ducts in male differentiation 14
Human chorionic gonadotrophin (hCG)
  epithelioid trophoblastic tumour, misdiagnosis 1411
  hydatidiform moles 1359, 1368, **1386–1387,** 1413
  hyperchorionic gonadotrophinism **1194–1195**

immature teratoma 793
non-gestational choriocarcinoma 787
non-molar miscarriage 1379
ovulation induction 1090
persistent trophoblastic disease 1385
pregnancy luteoma association 675
secretion, corpus luteum rescue 1014
solitary luteinized follicle cyst of pregnancy/puerperium association 677
systemic lupus erythematosus (SLE) 1190
trophoblastic neoplasms 1412
uterine carcinosarcoma 566
Human development, Carnegie stages 1
Human Fertilisation and Embryology Act (1990) 649
Human immunodeficiency virus (HIV) *see* HIV/AIDS
Human papillomavirus (HPV) 299
  antigen, cervical infection 285
  Bartholin's gland carcinoma 130
  basaloid carcinomas 107
  carcinogenesis 299–300
  carcinosarcoma aetiology 561
  cellular immune response 302
  cervical adenocarcinoma 339, 340, 341
    prognosis 351
    villoglandular papillary 347
  cervical carcinoma 297, 300
    adenoid basal 346
    adenoid cystic 345
    in adolescents **1175**
    clear cell adenosquamous 349
    HPV types 299
    small cell 372
    in tropics 1149
  cervical epithelium *305–308*
  cervical infection 285–286
    histological features **303–305**
    subclinical 304–305
  condyloma acuminata 97, **1175**
    vagina 161
  detection/typing **1606**
  endometrial squamous metaplasia 411
  epidemiology 300–301
  FHIT 1600–1601
  genetic damage 310
  HIV/AIDS 1153, **1186–1187**
  hybrid capture assays 1606
  immunosuppressive treatment 1188
  infection 299
  intrapartum infection of newborn 161
  mechanisms of oncogenesis 299–300
  non-oncogenic 299
  oncogenic 299
  p53 overexpression 358
  permissive infection 299
  persistence 300–301
  schistosomiasis 1146
  squamous-type vaginal carcinoma 188
  structure 298
  type 6 161
  type 11 161
  type 18 161
  vaginal cancer pathogenesis 188
    squamous cell carcinoma 188, 201
  vegetative viral replication 299
  viral interaction 301
  vulvar infection 59
  vulvar intraepithelial neoplasia (VIN) 100
  vulvar squamous cell carcinoma 105
  warty carcinomas 107
Human placental lactogen, embryonal carcinoma 788
Humoral immunity, human papillomavirus infection 302
Hürthle cells, in struma ovarii 806
Hyaline, gonadoblastoma in mixed gonadal dysgenesis 1227
Hyaline bodies, gonadoblastoma 826, *826,* 827, *827*
Hyaline droplets, carcinosarcoma (uterine) 569
Hyaline globules
  plasma proteins within 784
  yolk sac tumours 778, *778,* 781, *781,* 784
Hyaline necrosis, uterine leiomyosarcoma vs 522
Hyalinisation
  adenosarcoma (uterine) 556
  gonadoblastoma 828
  intravenous leiomyomatosis (uterine) 535
  theca cell tumour 762, *762*
  uterine leiomyosarcoma 522

Hyalinosis, in pregnancy **1513**
Hyaluronic acid, mesenchymal villi 1247
H-Y antigen, in gonadoblastoma 824
Hydatid cysts, cervical 287
Hydatid cysts of Morgagni 624
Hydatid disease **1143–1144,** 1187
Hydatidiform mole **1361–1388**
  aetiology/pathogenesis **1361–1367**
  AgNORs 1383, **1386**
  alphafetoprotein (AFP) **1368–1369**
  apoptotic marker studies 1608
  bcl-2 1608
  cell proliferation studies 1607
  choriocarcinoma (invasive mole) and 1384, 1385
    see also Choriocarcinoma
  classification 1360–1361
  clinical presentation **1368–1370**
  complete
    clinical presentation 1368, 1369
    genetic abnormalities 1361–1363
    hydropic change 1373, *1373*
    microscopic appearances **1371–1376**
    persistent trophoblastic disease **1384–1387,** 1396
    placental development 1346
    pleiomorphic trophoblast 1372–1373, *1374*
    prognosis **1384–1387**
    twin pregnancy 1586
    see also Trophoblastic disease, persistent
  differential diagnosis, trophoblastic lesions 1413, **1413–1416**
  DNA polymorphisms **1383**
  ectopic moles 1369–1370
  genetic abnormalities
    complete moles 1361–1363
    non-molar hydropic miscarriages 1364
    partial moles 1363–1364
  histochemistry **1381**
  histological grading systems **1385–1386**
  historical aspects 1359–1361
  human chorionic gonadotrophin (hCG) 1359, 1368, **1386–1387,** 1413
  hyperreactio luteinalis association 676
  immunocytochemistry **1381**
  imprinted genes 1605–1606
  incidence *1366,* **1367–1368**
  interphase cytogenetics **1383**
  invasive moles **1388–1392**
    accreta type *1389,* 1390, *1390*
    choriocarcinoma and 1384, 1385
    clinical presentation **1388–1389**
    incidence **1388–1389**
    increta type 1390, *1391*
    macroscopic appearances 1389, *1389*
    metastases **1390–1391,** *1391*
    microscopic appearances *1389,* 1389–1390
    molar villi 1389, *1389*
    pathogenesis **1388**
    pathology **1389–1391**
    percreta type 1390
    prognosis **1391–1392**
  IUCD use and 1116–1117
  Ki-67 indices 1607, *1607*
  linear IgA disease 1193
  M30 CytoDeath antibody 1608
  macroscopic appearances *1370,* **1370–1371,** *1371*
  microscopic appearances
    complete mole **1371–1376,** 1413
    non-molar miscarriages **1379–1380**
    partial mole **1376–1379**
  molar placenta 1370
  p53 expression **1599**
  partial
    clinical presentation 1368, **1369**
    genetic abnormalities 1363–1364
    hydropic change 1377, *1377*
    microscopic appearances **1376–1379**
    missed miscarriage 1369
    persistent trophoblastic disease **1387–1388**
    polyploidy 1363–1364
    twin pregnancy 1586
  pathology **1370–1380**
  PCNA 1607
  pemphigoid gestationis 1193
  prognosis **1383–1388**
    clinical indicators **1385**
    complete moles **1384–1387**
  risk factors **1364–1367**
    environmental factors **1367**
    family history 1365

geographical distribution **1365–1367**, *1366*
  maternal/paternal age **1365**
  nutrition 1367
  socioeconomic factors 1367
in situ hybridisation 1603
in tropics **1150**
twin pregnancy 1586
Hydrometrocolpos, transverse vaginal septum, imperforate 46
Hydronephrosis
  bilateral and genital tract malformations 46
  Turner's syndrome 1222
Hydropic change
  ovary 685, *685*
  placenta and miscarriage 1438, *1439*
  tubal pregnancy 1054, *1056*
Hydropic degeneration, uterine leiomyoma 529, *536*, 536–537, *537*
Hydrops, fetal 676, 1317
Hydrops tubae profluens 606
Hydrosalpinx 586, **596–597**, 598
  fimbrial occlusion and infertility 1010, *1010*
  pregnancy rate depression 1008
  tuberculous salpingitis 617
Hydrothorax, Krukenberg tumours 892
5–Hydroxyindoleacetic acid (5HIAA), carcinoid syndrome 807
11β-Hydroxylase, adrenogenital syndrome 1212–1213
21–Hydroxylase
  adrenogenital syndrome 1212–1213
  cytochrome P450c21 1213
3β-Hydroxylase dehydrogenase, deficiency, adrenal hyperplasia, congenital 1216
3β-Hydroxysteroid dehydrogenase 648
  steroid cell autoantigen 681
17–Hydroxysteroid dehydrogenase 1216
17β-Hydroxysteroid dehydrogenase deficiency 1216
H-Y gene 639–640
Hymen
  embryology 148
  imperforate **1158**
  tampon-induced changes 153
Hymeneal clefts, 'horizontal,' tampon-related 153
Hyperaldosteronism **1194**
Hyperamylasaemia **1196**
Hyperandrogenism
  infertility and 1026
  stromal luteoma and 846
  see also Androgen(s), overproduction
Hyperbilirubinaemia syndromes, pregnancy 1484
Hypercalcaemia **1194**
  dysgerminoma association 773
  malignant change in mature teratomas 802
  small cell undifferentiated carcinoma of ovary 903–905, *904*
  steroid cell tumours association 850
Hyperchorionic gonadotrophinism **1194–1195**
Hyperchromasia, condyloma acuminatum of vagina *162*
Hypercoagulability **1196**
Hypercoagulable state in fetus, fetal artery thrombosis 1282
Hyperemesis gravidarum 1531
  central pontine myelinosis **1531**
  liver involvement 1477
  maternal death 1571
Hypergonadotrophic hypogonadism *678*, **679–682**
  congenital lipoid adrenal hyperplasia 1216
Hyperhomocysteinaemia 995
  miscarriage 1434
Hyperinsulinaemia
  chronic reactive, infertility and 1025
  polycystic ovarian disease 666
Hypermethylation, mismatch repair gene, endometrial hyperplasia 455
Hyperoestrinism, Sertoli cell tumours 757
Hyperoestrogenic state
  endometrial disorders 404–405
  simple endometrial polyps 415
Hyperparathyroidism, in pregnancy 1026
Hyperpigmentation, vulvar 67–68
Hyperplasia
  basal cell 288
  cervical 288–290
  ectocervical 288
  endocervical *see* Endocervical hyperplasia
  endometrial *see* Endometrial hyperplasia
  epithelial, lichen sclerosis 76
  mesothelial *see* Mesothelial hyperplasia

microglandular 289–290
  ovarian *see under* Ovary
  polypoid microglandular 290
  reserve cell *see* Reserve cell hyperplasia
  tubal 607
Hyperprolactinaemia 1024–1025, **1195**
  polycystic ovary disease 668
  surgical treatment 1028
Hyperproteinaemia, chronic twin–twin transfusion 1582
Hyperreactio luteinalis 675–677, *676*
  virilisation 1214
Hypertension
  essential, pre-eclampsia 1337, *1342, 1343*–1344
  in pregnancy
    benign intracranial **1527**
    cardiac failure **1551**
    gestational hypertension 1505
    idiopathic postpartum acute renal failure 1503
    pre-eclampsia **1505–1511**
    pyelonephritis 1499
    renal tubular acidosis **1519**
    sub-intimal proliferation 1343.
    see also Pre-eclampsia
  primary pulmonary, in pregnancy **1549–1550**
  steroid contraception and 1105
  systemic **1190, 1197**
Hypertensive disease of pregnancy 1336–1344, 1564
Hypertensive encephalopathy 1525
Hyperthecosis
  follicular 667
  stromal 666, **668–670**, *669*, 673
Hyperthyroidism 1026
  struma ovarii and 805
Hypertonic labour, amniotic fluid embolism 1566
Hypertrophic cardiomyopathy **1549**
Hypertrophic pulmonary osteoarthropathy **1196**
Hypogastric artery 26–27
Hypogastric plexus, pelvic innervation 26
Hypoglycaemia **1195**
  acute fatty liver of pregnancy 1469
  dysgerminoma and 773
  ovarian fibroma association 860
  small cell carcinoma of uterine cervix 370
Hypogonadism **678–682**
  classification *678*
  hypergonadotrophic *678*, **679–682**, 1216
  hypogonadotrophic 678, 679
  pituitary adenomas causing 1022
Hypogonadotrophic hypogonadism 678, 679
Hypomenorrhoea, endometrial appearance 403
Hypo-oestrogenic states
  endometrial appearance 403
  endometrial atrophy 403–404
  endometrial disorders 403–404
Hypopigmentation, vulvar 69
Hypopituitarism 1025
Hypoprolactinaemia 1025
Hypospadias, pseudovaginal perineoscrotal 1219–1220
Hypothalamo-hypophysial system
  disconnection 1025
  disturbances causing infertility 1020–1025
  functional disorders 1024–1025
Hypothalamo-hypophysio-ovarian relationship, abnormal 1017
Hypothalamus 1020
  disorders 1020–1021
  medial basal, selective dysgenesis 1020
  nutritional suppression/effects 1020–1021
  tumours 1020
Hypothalamus–pituitary–ovary (HPO) axis
  abnormal feedback 1017
  dysfunction in luteal phase defect 1018
  feedback mechanisms 1013–1014
Hypothyroidism **1195**
  polycystic ovarian disease 1184
  primary 668
    infertility and 1026
Hypovolaemic shock, twin transfusion syndrome 1584
Hypoxia
  fetal *see* Fetus, hypoxia
  severe, amniotic fluid embolism 1565
Hysterectomy
  adenofibroma treatment 552
  apical vaginal granulation tissue 154
  biopsy/curettage specimens correlation in endometrial adenocarcinoma 456–457

complications, tubal prolapse 594
  for endometrial hyperplasia 453
  gonadoblastoma 832
  granulation tissue at vaginal vault *219, 220*
  hydatidiform mole in situ 1346
  ovarian carcinoma risk reduced 701, 702
  placental site trophoblastic tumour 1409
  specimen 326
    luteal phase insufficiency 407
  total abdominal, uterine carcinosarcoma 572
  vaginal, prolapsed Fallopian tube after 181, 220–221, *221*
Hysterosalpingography, complications 1027
Hysteroscope, endometrial sampling and resection 392
Hysteroscopic lysis, intrauterine lesions 433
Hysteroscopy, complications 1027

I
ICAM-1, mononuclear cells in malarial infection 1319
Ichthyosis linearis circumflexa 63
Icterus gravidarum *see* Intrahepatic cholestasis, of pregnancy
Idiopathic hypertrophic subaortic stenosis **1549**
Idiopathic postpartum acute renal failure **1503–1505**, *1504*
  accelerated hypertension 1503
  fibrinoid necrosis 1504, *1504*
  haemolytic uraemic syndrome 1505
  microangiopathic haemolytic anaemia 1503
Idiopathic vulvar melanosis 111
IgA
  linear IgA disease 1193
  mesangial IgA disease, in pregnancy *1516*, **1516**
  pemphigus 73–74
  pustulosis, vulvar involvement 73–74
  secretion in Fallopian tube 589
IgM deposition
  in decidual arteries, pre-eclampsia 1340
  diabetes mellitus in pregnancy 1344
  systemic lupus erythematosus in pregnancy 1345
Iliac arteries *27*
  pelvic supply 26
Iliococcygeus muscle, pelvic floor 23
Image analysis
  cytometry 1608
  morphometry **1612–1614**
Imaging techniques, acute fatty liver of pregnancy 1469
Immature intermediate villi 1247
Immune complex formation, pre-eclampsia 1341
Immune response
  cellular, human papillomavirus infection 302
  to conceptus 1006
  deficient, vaginal candidiasis association 172
  to ejaculate constituents 993
  in genital tracts 993
  humoral, human papillomavirus infection 302
  preimplantation embryo protection from 1008
Immune system, secretory, Fallopian tube 589
Immune tolerance, pre-eclampsia 1506
Immunobullous disorders
  differential diagnosis 72
  vulvar 70
Immunoglobulin A *see* IgA
Immunoglobulins, IUCD use and 1113
Immunohistochemistry
  B-cell lymphoma 950
  desmoplastic small round cell tumour
    intra-abdominal 920
    ovarian 906
  diffuse malignant of peritoneum mesothelioma 918
  endometrial metaplasia 410
  endometrioid adenocarcinoma, endometrial 463, *463*
  lipoleiomyoma (uterine) 531, *531*
  lymphoepithelioma-like carcinoma of cervix 330
  ovarian granulocytic sarcoma 946
  ovarian tumours 944–945
  ovarian tumours of Wolffian origin *900*
  small cell carcinomas of ovary 904, *904*
  steroid cell tumours not otherwise specified 853
  stromal hyperthecosis 670
  villous components of human placenta 1244–1245
  vulval lymphoma 955–956
Immunological factors, infertility 992–993

Immunoreactivity, small cell carcinomas of uterine cervix 372
Immunostimulators, sperm immunogenicity 993
Immunosuppression, cervical neoplasia risk 303
Immunosuppressive factors, decreased in recurrent miscarriage 1006
Immunosuppressive treatment 1188
  liver transplantation and pregnancy 1484
Imperforate hymen **1158**
Imperforate transverse vaginal septum 46
Implantation
  erosion of maternal tissue 1235
  failure in infertility 995, *1003*
    endometrial biochemical defects causing 1005
    prevalence 1002
  fimbrial, tubal pregnancy 1051
  intrauterine ovarian 1008
  mural, tubal pregnancy 1051, *1052, 1053*
  placental accessory lobe 1276
  placental development 1233
  placenta membranacea 1275
  plial, tubal pregnancy 1051, *1052*
  site 1233
  tolerance of semi-allogeneic conceptus 1006
  trophoblastic tissue, laparoscopic treatment tubal gestation 1060
Implantation phase embryogenesis 4–5
Implantation pole
  lacuna formation 1234
  trophoblastic wall 1234
Imprinted genes **1605–1606**
  Beckwith–Wiedemann syndrome 1363, 1364
  cervical teratomas 1605
  H19 1605, 1606
  hydatidiform moles 1362, 1605–1606
  insulin-like growth factor-2 (IGF2) 1605
  loss of heterozygosity 1605
  ovarian teratomas 1605
Imprinting, genomic **1605–1606**
'Incessant ovulation' hypothesis 701
Inclusion bodies, chlamydial infection 426
Incontinence, urinary 31
Indian-file arrangement of tumour cells, uterine cervix metastases 385
Indian ink, placental vascular anastomoses 1588
Indifferent embryo **9–13**
Indifferent gonads *see* Gonad(s), indifferent
Induction theory endometriosis 964–965
Infantile gluteal granuloma 80
Infants
  liveborn, placental haemangioma 1453
  low birth weight *see* Low birth weight
  vulvar inflammatory conditions 80
  see also Neonates
Infarction
  endometrial haemorrhagic 408
  Fallopian tube *595, 596*
  maternal floor *see* Maternal floor infarction
  myocardial *see* Myocardial infarction in pregnancy
  placental *see* Placenta, infarction
  villous, fibromuscular sclerosis 1292
Infection(s)
  cervical *see* Cervix, infections
  cervical inflammation 280
  childhood, ovarian cancer risk and 703
  human papillomavirus (HPV) *see* Human papillomavirus (HPV)
  infertility due to 994
  IUCD use and *see* Intrauterine contraceptive device (IUCD)
  listeriosis **1532**
  maternal, placental examination 1314–1319
  miscarriage 1432–1435
  nervous system **1532**
  non-granulomatous, ovarian 682–683
  placental villitis 1291
  salpingitis *see* Salpingitis
  in tropics **1134–1148**
  vaginal *see* Vagina, infective disease
  vulvar *see* Vulva, infections
  see also specific infections and sites
Infectious mononucleosis, vulvar involvement 954–955, *957*
Infective haemolytic anaemia, fetal, syphilis 1314
Inferior haemorrhoidal nerve, ischiorectal fossa 37
Infertile male syndrome, androgen insensitivity syndrome 1219
Infertile phenotypic male, XX male syndrome 1222
Infertility **989–1043**
  after IUD removal 989

anovulatory, polycystic ovarian disease 666
cervical factors 996–998
cervical incompetence causing 997–998
complications of diagnosis and treatment **1026–1029**
  of investigations 1027
  of surgery 1028
  of treatment 1027–1029, 1075–1076
definition **990**
ectopic pregnancy and 1046
endometrial abnormalities 1000–1006
endometrial tuberculosis 427
endometriosis 979, 995
Fallopian tube and 1006–1013
  lesions causing 1008–1013
female **995–1026**
  genetic causes 995
genital tract malformations 47
hypothalamo-hypophysial system causing 1020–1025
  see also Hypothalamus; Pituitary gland
immunological 992–993
interactive **991–995**
  age and 991
  biochemical factors 994–995
  biophysical factors 994
  genetic factors 992
  immunological factors 992–993
  microbiological factors 993–994
  physical factors 991
  psychological factors 991–992
involuntary, definition 990
IUCD use and 1117–1118
lactational, 'failure' 997
male **990–991**
  causes 991
  microdeletions in Y chromosome 641
Mycoplasma hominis 427
myometrial abnormalities 998–1000
ovarian causes 1013–1018
ovarian tumours association 700
pelvic tuberculosis 1134
peritoneal disorders 1018–1019
physical factors 991
in polycystic ovary disease 667
postpartum 989
post-pill 989
prevalence **990**
sperm antibodies and 993
stress of 992
subfertility 1016
systemic diseases associated 1025–1026
treatment
  complications of 1027–1029, 1075–1076
  hormonal **1090**
tubal 993
vulval/vaginal factors 995–996
see also Fertility
Infibulation 1151
Inflammation
cervical 280–281
chronic
  cervical mucus 277
  lymphoepithelioma-like carcinoma 330
endometrium 418–432
neoplasia associated in cervix 292
Inflammatory bowel disease
  fistulas involving vagina 185
  steroid contraceptives and 1106
  see also Crohn's disease; Ulcerative colitis
Inflammatory cell infiltrate
  endometritis 418
  villitis 1290
Inflammatory dermatoses, vulva 72–80
Inflammatory disease
  cervix 952
  Fallopian tube **615–622**, 1048
  ovary **682–684**
    see also Ovary, inflammatory disease
  pelvic *see* Pelvic inflammatory disease (PID)
  vaginal *see* Vagina, inflammatory disease
  vulva **72–80**
Inflammatory lesions, placental villi 1290–1292
Inflammatory pseudotumour
  lymphoid infiltration in uterine leiomyoma vs 532
  of uterus 952
Infundibulo-pelvic ligament 653
Infundibulum of fallopian tube 32
Inguinal hernia, ectopic adnexa 594

Inguinal node metastases, microinvasive squamous cell carcinoma of vulva 104
Inhibin
  antibodies, immunostaining in fibrosarcoma 861
  functions 1013
  gonadoblastoma in mixed gonadal dysgenesis 1227
  juvenile-type granulosa cell tumour 753
  levels in adult-type granulosa cell tumour 746, 751
  theca cell tumour 763
Inhibin-α
  ovarian tumours of Wolffian origin 899
  sex cord-like features of endometrial stromal tumours 512
Inhibin-B 1017
Inner cell mass 4
  embryogenesis 5–7
Innominate bone, anatomy 21
Insertion funiculi furcata 1296
In situ hybridisation 1603–1604
  chromosome aberrations 1603
  interphase cytogenetics **1383**
Insular carcinoid tumour 807, *808,* 808–809, *809*
Insulin 666
  metabolism defect, polycystic ovarian disease 666
  resistance 670
    polycystic ovarian disease 666, 670
    stromal luteoma 846
  secreting tumours 1195
Insulin-like growth factor-2 (IGF2)
  Beckwith–Wiedemann syndrome 1364
  imprinted genes 1364, 1605
Integrins, endometriosis 965–966
Intercellular adhesion molecule 1, mononuclear cells in malarial infection 1319
Intercellular IgA dermatoses (pustulosis), vulvar involvement 73–74
Intercourse-related vaginitis 180
Interleukin 1
  chorioamnionitis 1305
  endometriosis 965
  Hofbauer cells 1243
Interleukin 2, chorioamnionitis 1305
Interleukin 6
  chorioamnionitis 1305
  endometriosis 965
  endometrium in endometritis 966
Interleukin 8
  chorioamnionitis 1305
  endometriosis 966
Intermediate filament proteins, cervical epithelium 265
  see also Cytokeratin(s)
Intermediate mesoderm 8–9
Intermediate trophoblast *see* Extravillous trophoblast, interstitial
Internal iliac artery, pelvic supply 26–27
Internal os 247
Internal version
  air embolism 1567
  uterine rupture 1569
International Federation of Gynecology and Obstetrics *see* FIGO
International Society for Study of Vulvovaginal Disease (ISSVD), classification of non-neoplastic disease of vulva 53–54
Interposito velamentosa 1296
Intersex disorders **1209–1232**
  with abnormal gonads **1160**
  abnormal sex chromosome constitution **1220–1224**
  classification *1210*
  normal chromosome constitution **1212–1220**
  see also Pseudohermaphroditism
Interstitial nephritis, in pregnancy **1499**
Interstitial trophoblast 1261
  see also Extravillous trophoblast
Intertrigo, vulvar involvement 72
Intertwin transfusion, twin transfusion syndrome 1582
Intervillositis, chronic, miscarriage 1439
Intervillous space 1251–1253
  blood supply in pre-eclampsia 1337
  lacunar system 1235
  malarial infection 1319
  maternal arterial inflow 1252
Intervillous thrombosis 1285, *1285*
  macroscopic abnormalities 1285
Intervillous tumour cells 1456

Intestinal metaplasia
  cervical 288
  endometrial 412–413
Intestinal (enteric) type cervical adenocarcinoma
  343–344
Intestine
  atresia, congenital, umbilical cord ulceration
    1299
  carcinoid tumours, metastatic to ovary *886,*
    886–887
  carcinoma
    metastatic, to ovary 880, *882,* 882–884, *883,*
      884
    see also Colon cancer
  inflammatory disease **1184–1186**
  large, endometriosis 979
  obstruction, endometriosis 979
  small
    endometriosis 979, *980*
    fistulas connecting to vagina 185
Intra-abdominal desmoplastic small round cell
  tumour *919,* 919–920
Intracerebral haemorrhage **1528–1529**
  berry aneurysm of circle of Willis *1528,*
    1528–1529
  petechial haemorrhage 1532
Intracytoplasmic sperm injection (ICSI) 1029
Intraduct papilloma of vulvar 132
Intra-embryonic coelom formation 6, *7*
Intraepidermal neutrophilic IgA dermatosis 73–74
Intraepithelial neoplasia
  cervical *see* Cervical intraepithelial neoplasia
    (CIN)
  endometrial 455, 467, 468, *469*
  ovarian 696, 718, 975
  vaginal *see* Vagina, intraepithelial neoplasia
    (VAIN)
  vulvar *see* Vulvar intraepithelial neoplasia (VIN)
Intraepithelial zone, squamous epithelium of cervix
  253
Intrahepatic cholestasis
  benign recurrent 1468
  of pregnancy 1467–1469
    biochemical changes 1467
    clinical features 1467
    fetal effects 1468–1469
    histological features 1467–1468
    incidence and risk factors 1467
    maternal outcome 1469
    pathogenetic mechanisms 1468
  steroid contraceptives and 1100, *1101*
Intrahepatic lesions, benign, pregnancy 1480
Intraligamentous gestation, abdominal pregnancy
  1063
Intralumenal haemorrhage, miscarriage tubal
  pregnancy 1058
Intraluminal haemorrhage, endometriosis 966
Intramural haemorrhage, miscarriage tubal
  pregnancy 1058
Intramural segment of fallopian tube 32
Intranuclear inclusions, uterine leiomyoma with
  bizarre nuclei *526,* 526–527
Intrapartum fetal death, umbilical cord knots 1297
Intraplacental oxygenation, capillary development
  1251, *1251*
Intrasplenic grafting technique, granulosa cell
  tumours induction 705
Intrauterine adhesions 433
Intrauterine amputations
  amniotic bands and strings 1307
  constriction rings 1308
Intra-uterine arteries and pre-eclampsia *1343*
Intrauterine contraceptive device (IUCD)
  1106–1118
  actinomycosis association 282
    vaginal 170
  complications 1106
  composition and structure 1106
  ectopic 1106
  ectopic pregnancy and 1049–1050, 1061,
    1116–1117
  effect on cervix 1112–1114
  effect on Fallopian tube 1114–1115
  effect on ovary 1114–1115
  effect on vagina 1112–1114
  effects on endometrium *1107,* 1107–1112, *1108,*
    1109, 1110, 1111
  endosalpingitis and 1115, *1115*
  expulsion rates 1106–1107
  fertility after 1117–1118

infections associated
  endometrial 1111
  pelvic inflammatory disease and 1114–1115
  in pregnancy 1116
  tubal 1114–1115, *1115*
  vaginal/cervical 1112–1113, *1113*
infertility after 989
levonorgestrel-releasing device 1111, 1117
medicated 1114
multiple insertion 1106
myometrial hypertrophy association 500
ovarian pregnancy 1061
pelvic inflammatory disease and 1114–1115
pelvic sepsis 1196
pregnancy and 1116–1117
  ectopic 1049–1050, 1061, 1116–1117
pregnancy rate 1116
removal, early in pregnancy 1116
systemic effects 1117
tail-string and infections 1114
timing of insertion and type 1116
uterine perforation 1106
uterine tumours and 1112
Intrauterine decapitation, amniotic bands 1308
Intrauterine fetal death *see* Fetal death
Intrauterine fetal distress *see* Fetal distress
Intrauterine fetal growth retardation
  absence of pre-eclampsia 1344
  fetal perfusion patterns, placental 1311
  hypertension in pregnancy 1344
  maternal floor infarction 1279
  necrotising funisitis 1300
  perivillous fibrin deposition 1277–1278
  placental bed biopsy *1344*
  placental examination 1310–1312
  placental infarction 1279
  pregnancy hypertension with proteinuria 1344
  uterine malformations 48
  villitis 1291
  villous immaturity 1286
Intrauterine fetal hypoxia *see* Fetus, hypoxia
Intrauterine infection, IUCD use and 1111, *1111*
Intrauterine mortality *see* Fetal death
Intrauterine ovarian implantation 1008
Intrauterine synechiae, basal endometrium 396
Intravascular leiomyomatosis
  see Leiomyomatosis
Intravascular papillary endothelial hyperplasia,
  vulvar 81
Intravascular trophoblastic plugs, spontaneous
  miscarriage 1345
Intravenous leiomyomatosis
  see Leiomyomatosis
Intussusception
  in endometriosis 979
  Fallopian tube **596**
In vitro fertilisation
  diffuse peritoneal leiomyomatosis association 537
  endometrial polyps 415
  first cleavage division 2
  hormonal therapy 1090, *1090*
  hydrosalpinx effect on 1008
  ovarian pregnancy 1062
  vasculitis **1198**
Involution of pregnant uterus, postpartum
  haemorrhage 1353
Irradiation, therapeutic *see* Radiotherapy
Ischaemic heart disease, combined steroid
  contraceptives 1104–1105
Ischaemic placenta, maternal effects 1310
Ischiococcygeus muscle 23
Ischiorectal fossa *36*
  anatomy 36–37
Isoimmunisation, genetic predisposition 992–993
Isosexual precocious pseudopuberty
  see Pseudopuberty, isosexual precocious
Isthmic communications 44
Isthmic endometrium 396
Isthmus *see* Fallopian tube, isthmus
IUGR *see* Intrauterine fetal growth retardation
IVF *see* In vitro fertilisation

J
Jaundice
  cholestatic in pregnancy *see* Intrahepatic
    cholestasis, of pregnancy
  hepatitis, acute viral in pregnancy 1478
  idiopathic of pregnancy 1100
  of late pregnancy *see* Intrahepatic cholestasis, of
    pregnancy

toxaemia of pregnancy 1474
Juvenile dermatitis herpetiformis *see* Linear IgA
  disease
Juvenile-type granulosa cell tumour
  see Granulosa cell tumours

K
Kallmann's syndrome 679, 1016, 1020
Kaposi's sarcoma, vulvar 121
Kartagener's syndrome 1005
  endometrium 394
Karyorrhexis, villous intravascular 1313
Karyotype
  acardiac fetus 1584
  endometrial polyps 415–416
  hermaphrodite, true 1228
  Klinefelter's syndrome 1220
  Turner's syndrome 1221
K cell (Kornchenzellen) *see* Endometrial
  granulocytes
Keratin 253
  expression, cervical epithelium 266
  low molecular weight, in dysgerminoma 774
  see also Cytokeratin(s)
Keratinisation
  cervical epithelium *306*
  squamous epithelium of cervix 253
  see also Dyskeratosis
Keratinising carcinomas, cervix 327
Keratinocytes, immortalised 'basal-like' 300
Keratin pearls, endometrial squamous cell
  carcinoma 474
Keratoacanthoma, vulvar *96,* 96–97
Keratosis follicularis *see* Darier's disease
17-Ketosteroid, excretion, gonadoblastoma 825
17-Ketosteroid reductase 1216
Ki-67 1606
  cervical adenocarcinoma 358
  cervical carcinoma 1607, 1613
  choriocarcinoma 1404
  endometrial adenocarcinoma detection 482
  endometrial carcinoma 1606–1607
  hydatidiform moles 1386, 1387–1388, 1607,
    1607
  ovarian carcinoma 1606
    prognosis 736
  placental cell proliferation 1287
  placental site trophoblastic tumour 1415
  squamous cell carcinoma 108
Kidney disease *see Entries beginning renal;* Renal
  diseases
Kiel classification 953
  lymphomas 936
Kimmelstiel–Wilson nodules 1518, *1518*
Ki-S5, endometrial adenocarcinoma detection 482
Klinefelter's syndrome 638
  gender identification disorders 1220–1221
  genetic screening programmes 1220
  neoplasms 1221
Kline's haemorrhages *see* Intervillous thrombosis
Klippel–Trenaunay–Weber syndrome **1187**
Knee–chest exercises, air embolism 1568
Koebner phenomenon 76
Kogan endocervical speculum, cervical examination
  323
Koilocytes
  condyloma acuminata of vagina *162*
  papillomavirus infection 285
    subclinical 304
Koilocytic change *305*
Koilocytosis *268*
  flat, papillomavirus infection of cervix 285, *285*
  papillomavirus 285
Korsakoff's psychosis 1531
KP1, ovarian granulocytic sarcoma 947
K-ras
  cervical carcinoma **1597**
  endocervical neoplasia 357–358
  endometrial adenocarcinoma 485
  endometrial hyperplasia/carcinoma **1596–1597**
  Fallopian tube adenocarcinoma 611
  mucinous tumours (ovarian) 698
  oncogene expression studies **1596–1597**
  ovarian carcinoma **1596**
  primary peritoneal serous carcinoma 925
Krukenberg tumours **890–892**
  age and symptoms 892
  benign signet ring stromal tumours vs 767
  bladder carcinoma metastatic to ovary as 888
  cervix 386

Krukenberg tumours (cont'd)
  clear cell adenocarcinoma vs 732
  diagnosis 890, 892
  histology 890, 890–892, 891
  metastatic nature 890, 891, 892
  mucinous carcinoid of ovary vs 809
  natural history and prognosis 892
  as primary tumour 892
  'pseudosarcomatous' pattern 891
  terminology 890
  tumour emboli 891
Kupffer cell hyperplasia, acute fatty liver of
    pregnancy 1470

L
L26 (CD20), ovarian lymphomas 944
Labia majora
  anatomy 37
  development 19–20
Labia minora
  anatomy 37–38
  development 19–20
Labour
  amniotic infection and 1305
  hypertonic, amniotic fluid embolism 1566
  obstructed see Obstructed labour
  premature onset see Preterm labour
  tumultuous, amniotic fluid embolism 1566
  vaginal examinations during 1305
Lactic dehydrogenase, elevated, dysgerminoma 776
Lactobacillus, vaginal 158
Lactobacillus acidophilus
  vagina 151
  vulvar microbial flora 54
Lactoferrin overexpression, endocervical neoplasias
    358
Lacunae, placental development 1234
Lacuna formation, trophoblast subdivision 1235
Lacunar stage placental development 1234–1235
Lacunar system 1235
LAMB syndrome, vulvar hyperpigmentation 68
Lamina propria, vagina 150
Langerhans' cell(s)
  counts, cigarette smoking 266
  nuclei 957
Langerhans' cell histiocytosis
            see Histiocytosis, Langerhans' cell
            (histiocytosis X)
Langhans cells
  choriocarcinoma metastases 221, 222
  tuberculous salpingitis 1012
  see also Cytotrophoblast cells
Langier–Hunziker disease, vulvar
            hyperpigmentation 68
Laparoscopy
  complications 1027
  infertility investigation 1027
Laparotomy
  scars, endometriosis 965
  tubal pregnancy, ruptured 1060
Large bowel see Colon cancer; Intestine
Large cell neuroendocrine carcinoma, uterine cervix
    373–375
Large loop excision of transformation zone
            see LLETZ
Large loop excision specimen 325
Laser vaporisation, colposcopy 323
Lateral fold formation 9
Lateral ligaments
  cervical 248, 248
  uterus 24
Lateral mesoderm 8
Lecithin, cervical mucus 1113
Lectin histochemistry, endocervical neoplasias 359
LEEP, cervical intraepithelial neoplasia 323
Left to right shunts 1544
Leiomyoblastoma, uterine 530
Leiomyoma, uterine 530
  apoplectic 525–526
  broad ligament 626, 626
  cervical 383–384
  cotyledenoid ('dissecting') 509, 533–534, 534
  Fallopian tubes 603–604
    hypercellular 1074
  haemorrhagic cellular (apoplectic) 525–526
  mitotically active cellular 525
    ovarian 863
  ovarian 862
  placental 1455
  urethral 195

uterus see Leiomyoma, uterine
  vaginal 195–196
  vulvar 114–115
Leiomyoma, uterine 501, 506, 516–519, 952,
    952–953
  ataxia-telangiectasia 1182
  clinical features 517
  combined oral contraceptives effect 1097
  cytogenetics 516–517
  degeneration types 518
    cystic 519
    hyaline 536, 537
    hydropic 529, 536, 536–537, 537
    'red degeneration' 519, 519, 536
  differential diagnosis 509, 518–519
  epidemiology and aetiology 516
  with epithelial tubules 576–577, 577
  epithelioid smooth muscle tumours 529,
    529–530, 530
  erythrocytosis 1195
  fascicular pattern 520
  GnRH agonists effect 1087
  'grape-like' 534
  gross pathology 517, 517, 519
  hormone effects 536
  infections 517
  infertility due to 999
  leiomyosarcoma vs 522, 1000
  low-grade stromal sarcoma vs 509
  Meigs' syndrome 1196–1197
  microscopic features 517–518, 519
  myometrial 999
  neurilemmomatous pattern 519
  'parasitic' 517
  perinodular hydropic (perinodular hyaline) 537
  progestagens effect 1084
  'sago pudding' ('in aspic') pattern 537, 537
  small vs large 517
  stromal nodules vs 506
  submucous 999
  treatment and results 999–1000
  variants 515, 524–538
    atypical 522, 524, 526, 526–527
    benign metastasising 527
    with bizarre nuclei 522, 526, 526–527
    cellular 525, 525
    diffuse 533, 533
    dissecting 509, 533–534, 534
    haemorrhagic cellular (apoplectic) 525–526
    lipoleiomyoma 531, 531
    with lymphoid infiltration 531–533, 532
    mitotically active 524, 524–525
    'symplastic'/'bizarre' 522, 526, 526–527
    with tubules 530–531
  with vascular invasion 534, 534
Leiomyomatosis
  diffuse peritoneal 537–538, 928, 928–929
  diffuse uterine 533, 533
  intravascular (intravenous), uterine 509, 529,
    534, 534–536, 535
    differential diagnosis 535
    management 535–536
Leiomyomatosis peritonealis disseminata 592
Leiomyosarcoma
  broad ligament 626
  cervix 378–379
  combined oral contraceptives and 1095
  diffuse peritoneal leiomyomatosis development
    928–929
  metastatic, diffuse peritoneal leiomyomatosis vs
    929
  ovarian 862–864, 863
    epithelioid 863
    myxoid 863
    prognosis 864
    spread 864
  uterine 501, 519–523
    ataxia-telangiectasia 1182
    in carcinosarcoma 566
    clinical/epidemiological features 519–520
    clinicopathological correlation 523
    epithelioid 530
    gross pathology 520, 520–521
    histological features 519, 521–522, 522, 523
    leiomyoma vs 522, 1000
    myxoid 527–529, 528
    therapy 523
    xanthomatous variant 521
  vaginal 213, 215, 215–216
  vulvar 115

Leishmaniasis 1141
  vulvar 55
Leishmania tropica 55
Lentigines, vulvar 68
Lentigo of vulva 111
Lentigo simplex, vulvar 111–112
Leprechaunism, juvenile granulosa cell tumour
    1183, 1187
Leprosy, vulvar infection 57
Leptin, plasma levels, twin transfusion syndrome
    and discordant growth 1585
Leptothrix vaginalis, vaginal infection 169
Leucoplakia
  cervical intraepithelial neoplasia 322
  cervix 316
Leucorrhoea, vaginal 157
Leukaemia
  acute lymphoblastic, ovarian involvement 946,
    946
  endometrial stromal sarcoma vs 510
  fetal, placental involvement 1460, 1460
  metastatic, Fallopian tube 613
  ovarian involvement 946, 946
  pregnancy 1457
  small cell undifferentiated ovarian carcinoma vs
    905
  staging 938
  vaginal deposits 954
  vulvar ulceration 125
  yolk sac tumours association 785
Leukaemia inhibitory factor (LIF) 1005, 1019
  secretion changes by xeno-oestrogens 1008
Leu M1 marker, yolk sac tumour negativity 785
Levator ani, pelvic floor 23
Levonorgestrel-releasing IUCD 1111, 1117
Leydig cells 848
  agenesis
    luteinizing hormone levels 1216
    phenotype 1216
    pseudohermaphroditism, male 1215–1216
  development 638
  fetal testis 1212
  fetal type, testicular feminisation, complete 1218
  in gonadoblastoma 825
  in hilus cell tumour 848, 848
  Klinefelter's testis 1221, 1221
Leydig cell tumours, of ovary 704, 746, 757
  differential diagnosis 853–855
  hilus cell type 757, 848, 848
  non-hilar type 757, 848, 849
  not further classified types 757
  Reinke's crystals 757, 758, 848, 849, 850
Leydig-like cells, gonadoblastoma 827
Lichenification, vulvar involvement 74
Lichen planus 78, 79
  vulvar involvement 78–79
Lichen sclerosus, vulvar 75, 76, 77, 79
  aetiology and pathogenesis 75–77
  differential diagnosis 77
  histology 76–77
  malignancy 78
  squamous cell carcinoma 105
  vestibular involvement 76
Lichen simplex, vulvar involvement 74, 75
Liesegang rings
  chronic salpingitis 619
  endometriosis 973, 977
Lifestyle, fertility and 990
Li-Fraumeni syndrome 1168, 1187
Ligaments
  cervix 248, 248
  uterine 24
  uterosacral 24, 34, 248
  see also Broad ligament
Ligneous (pseudomembranous) conjunctivitis 1187
Ligneous disease, vulvar 66
Ligneous (pseudomembranous) inflammation,
    genital tract 425, 996
Linear-dense deposit disease 1514
Linear IgA disease 1193
  vulvar involvement 71
Lipid cell tumours see Steroid (lipid) cell tumours
Lipids
  serum levels, pregnancy 1466
  see also Cholesterol
Lipoadenofibroma, uterine 577
Lipochrome granules, gonadoblastoma 827
Lipochrome pigment
  Leydig cell tumours 849
  steroid cell tumours not otherwise specified 851

Lipodystrophy, polycystic ovarian disease **1188**
Lipofuschin deposits, uterus 500
Lipoid adrenal hyperplasia, congenital 1216
Lipoid cell tumours *see* Steroid (lipid) cell tumours
Lipoleiomyoma, uterine *531*, **531**, 577
Lipoma
  broad ligament 626, *626*
  cervix 384
  ovarian 868
  uterine 531, *532*
  vulvar 118, *118*
Lipophages, arteriopathy in pre-eclampsia 1339
Liposarcoma
  ovarian 868, *868*
  in uterine carcinosarcoma *569*
  vulvar 118
Listerial meningitis 1532
Listeria monocytogenes 1532
  miscarriage 1432
Listeriosis **1532**
  placental examination 1314–1315
Lithiasis, vaginal **186**
Liver
  adenoma, steroid contraceptives and 1101, 1103, *1103*
  allograft function in pregnancy 1484
  blood flow, pregnancy 1465
  drug metabolism in pregnancy 1465
  dysfunction, toxaemia 1474
  failure, acute fatty liver of pregnancy **1503**
  focal nodular hyperplasia, steroid contraceptives and 1102, *1102*
  injury in pregnancy, drug-induced 1479–1480
  pathology, pregnancy **1465–1494**
  rupture, acute fatty liver of pregnancy (AFLP) 1476
  spontaneous rupture in pregnancy 1476–1477, *1477*
  steroid contraceptives effect 1100–1103
  toxaemia of pregnancy 1474–1475
  transplantation
    acute fatty liver of pregnancy 1472
    pregnancy 1484
Liver biopsy
  HELLP syndrome 1476
  herpes simplex hepatitis 1479
Liver cell death, acute fatty liver of pregnancy 1470–1471
Liver disease
  chronic and pregnancy 1482
  coexistent development with pregnancy **1478–1482**
    hepatic injury, drug-induced 1479–1480
    hepatitis, acute viral 1478–1479
    hepatitis, herpes simplex 1479
    neoplasms and tumour-like lesions 1480
  pre-existing and pregnancy **1482–1484**
    cirrhosis 1483
    hepatitis, autoimmune 1483
    hepatitis, chronic viral 1482–1483
    metabolic 1483–1484
  specific to pregnancy **1467–1477**
    acute fatty liver 1469–1474
    HELLP syndrome 1475–1476
    intrahepatic cholestasis of pregnancy 1469–1474
    spontaneous rupture of liver 1476–1477
    toxaemia in pregnancy 1474–1475
Liver function, in pregnancy
  biochemical changes 1466
  clinical manifestations 1466
  morphological changes 1466–1467
  normal **1465–1467**
  steroid hormone levels 1465
Liver function tests
  intrahepatic cholestasis of pregnancy 1467
  normal pregnancy 1466, *1466*
  toxaemia of pregnancy 1474
Liver pregnancy 1477
LLETZ
  cervical intraepithelial neoplasia 323
  diathermy artifact and cervical glandular intraepithelial neoplasia 355
  infertility after 996
  specimen 325
Lobular endocervical glandular hyperplasia 289
Long-chain 3-hydroxyacyl-coenzyme A dehydrogenase (LCHAD) 1472
Long coiled terminal capillary loops, mature intermediate villi 1250

Loop biopsies, microinvasive adenocarcinoma of cervix 357
Loop electrosurgical excisional procedure 323
Loss of heterozygosity (LOH) **1599–1600**
  cervical carcinoma **1599–1600**
  cervical intraepithelial neoplasia (CIN) **1599–1600**
  endocervical neoplasia 358
  endometrial carcinoma **1599**
  imprinted genes 1605
  ovarian carcinoma **1599**
  ovarian endometriosis, atypical 975
Low birth weight
  antenatal intrauterine infection, subclinical 420
  circumvallate placenta 1275
  malarial infection 1319
  subamniotic haematoma 1284
  umbilical artery, single 1294
Low-density lipoprotein (LDL) cholesterol
  combined steroid contraceptives and 1103
  HRT and 1090
Lower genital tract neoplastic syndrome (LGTNS) **189–190**
Low-grade endometrial stromal sarcoma, cytogenetic findings 509
Lumbarisation, sacrum 21
Lumbosacral plexus *25*
  obturator internus muscle 22
  pelvic nerve supply 24–25
Lung carcinoma *see* Bronchial carcinoma
Lupus anticoagulant
  miscarriage 1434
  pregnancy 1345
Lupus erythematosus
  systemic *see* Systemic lupus erythematosus (SLE)
  vulvar 66
Lupus nephritis, pregnancy 1345, *1515*, **1515–1516**
Luteal cysts *665*, **665**, 1017
Luteal phase, menstrual cycle 1013
Luteal phase defect 1018
  clomiphene therapy 1076
  endometrium 1000
  IUCD use and 1110–1111
  miscarriage 1433
Luteal phase deficiency 1000
  coordinated delayed endometrial transformation 406
  diagnosis 1000–1001
  endometrial disorders 405–407
  endometrium *406*, 406–407, *407*, 1000
  generally inadequate secretory phase 406–407
  infertility due to 1000
  oestrogen deficiency 406
Luteal-placental shift 1014
Lutein cells
  solitary luteinized follicle cyst of pregnancy/puerperium 677
  stromal hyperthecosis *669*, 670
Lutein cysts, nonspecific 677
Luteinization
  Brenner tumours 717
  premature, infertility due to 1017–1018
Luteinized cells, benign mucinous tumours 715
Luteinized unruptured follicle (LUF) syndrome 1017
  infertility and mild endometriosis 981
Luteinizing hormone (LH)
  defective 1016
  erratic release, polycystic ovary disease 667
  levels, Leydig cell agenesis 1216
  LH:FSH ratio, polycystic ovarian disease 667
  midcycle surge 1013, 1014
    premature luteinization and 1017–1018
  normal menstrual cycle 1013
  receptors 1014
  release 1013
Luteinizing hormone releasing hormone (LHRH)
  agonists 1087
  infertility treatment 1090
  pseudopregnancy therapy in endometriosis 982
Lutein-like cells, gonadoblastoma 827
Luteoma
  differential diagnosis 853–855
  ovarian stromal *846*, **846–847**, *847*
  pregnancy *see* Pregnancy, luteoma
Lymphadenectomy, verrucous carcinoma 109
Lymphangioleiomyomatosis 533, 1190
  endometrial stromal sarcoma vs 509
Lymphangioma
  cavernous, vulvar 122

multiloculated peritoneal inclusion cyst vs 915
  ovarian **870**
  vulvar 122
Lymphangioma circumscripta, vulvar lymphangiomas 122
Lymphangioma simplex, vulvar lymphangiomas 122
Lymphangiosarcoma, ovarian **870**
Lymphatic abnormalities, vulva **80–81**
Lymphatic anastomoses, vaginal 149
Lymphatic channels, microinvasive carcinoma of cervix 318
Lymphatic drainage
  ovary 657
    interference leading to massive oedema 672
  rectum 29
  vagina *148*, 149, 190
Lymphatic spread
  cervical cancer 332
  endometriotic tissue dissemination 965
  extragonadal tumours to ovary 879
Lymphatic tumours
  ovarian **870**
  vulvar 122
Lymph nodes
  abdominal, endometriosis *971*
  metastases
    cervical adenocarcinoma/carcinoma 318, 350
    cervical carcinoma, prognosis 332
    para-aortic, sampling, endometrial adenocarcinoma 457
    pelvic *see* Pelvic lymph nodes
    spread, squamous cell carcinoma of vulva 108
Lymphocytes
  endometrium 395
  see also B-cells; T-cells
Lymphoedema, vulvar 81
Lymphoepithelioma,like carcinoma, cervix *330*, 330–331, *331*
Lymphoepithelioma-like carcinoma
  cervix
    cell-mediated immune response 330
    Epstein–Barr virus 331
    microscopic features 330
  vaginal 954
Lymphogranuloma venereum *1139*, **1139**
  inguinal lymphadenitis 58
  vaginal involvement 164
Lymphoid follicles, endometrium 395
Lymphoid infiltration
  dysgerminoma 776
  mycoplasmal endometritis 1004
  struma ovarii 806
  uterine leiomyoma **531–533**, *532*
Lymphoma 935
  brain, HIV/AIDS 1533
  Burkitt's *see* Burkitt's lymphoma
  cervix *see* Non-Hodgkin's lymphoma
  classification 936, *936*, *937*
  endometrial stromal sarcoma vs 510
  Fallopian tube *612*, 613
  fetal and placental involvement 1460
  Hodgkin's *see* Hodgkin's disease
  malignant and placental involvement 1457
  MALT *see* MALT lymphomas
  non-Hodgkin's *see* Non-Hodgkin's lymphoma
  ovary *see* Non-Hodgkin's lymphoma, ovary
  pregnancy and **957–958**
  primary, of female genital tract 935
  small cell undifferentiated ovarian carcinoma vs 905
  staging *938*, 938–939
  uterine *see* Non-Hodgkin's lymphoma, uterus
  vulvar 125
Lymphoplasmacytic infiltrate
  cervicitis, chronic 280
  endometrial, cytomegalovirus endometritis 426
Lymphoplasmacytic villitis, placental cytomegalovirus infection 1317
Lymphoproliferative disease **935–961**
  classification 936, *936*
  definition 935
  see also Lymphoma
Lynch type II syndrome *see* Hereditary non-polyposis colon carcinoma (HNPCC)

M
M30 CytoDeath antibody 1608
McCune–Albright syndrome 664, 1162, 1189, 1196

Macrophages
  arteriopathy of pre-eclampsia 1340
  cervical epithelium 266
  hyperactive tubal 1008
  meconium-laden 1303
  peritoneal, sperm phagocytosis in endometriosis
      981
  peritoneal and endometriotic lesions 965
  peritoneal fluid in endometriosis 1019
  premature ovarian failure and 1017
  'starry sky' 943, 943–944, 945
  uteroplacental arteries in pre-eclampsia
      1342–1343
Maffucci's syndrome 1171, 1183
  juvenile-type granulosa cell tumour 752
  ovarian fibrosarcoma association 861
Major histocompatibility antigens
  cervical neoplasia 303
  class II antigens, inappropriate expression,
      premature ovarian failure and 1017
  distribution in tubal gestation 1055
  see also HLA (human leukocyte) antigens
Malacoplakia 1196
  Bartholin's gland 66
  endometrial 423–424, 425
  granulomatous salpingitis vs 619
  Michaelis–Gutmann bodies 424
  vulvar lesions 66
Malaria 1188
  placental examination 1319
Malassezia furfur, vulvar infection 55–56
Male autoimmunisation 992
Male differentiation, genital ducts 13–14
Male infertility 990–991
  causes 991
Male intersex see Pseudohermaphroditism, male
Male sex organs, gonadoblastoma 826
Malformations see Congenital
      abnormalities/malformations; Genital tract
      (female)
Malformation syndromes, genital tract anomalies
      1158
'Malignant endometrioid tumour of ovary' 731
Malouf syndrome 1188
MALT lymphomas 937, 938
  of cervix 950, 950
  therapy and survival 951
Mammary-type adenocarcinomas of vulva 132
Manchester Children's Tumour Registry
      1163–1164, 1164
Marfan forme fruste 1546
Marfan's syndrome 1545–1547
  aortic regurgitation 1546
  complications 1546
  fibrillin-1 gene 1546
  'Marfan forme fruste' 1546
  postpartum haemorrhage risk 1547
  vaginal delivery 1546
Marginal haematoma 1284–1285
Marginal insertion, umbilical cord 1295
Marital customs, fertility and 990
Masculinisation
  androgen ingestion in pregnancy 1214
  external genitalia 19
  ovarian tumours 1195
Masson's tumour 81
Mast cell infiltration
  lymphoid infiltration in uterine leiomyoma vs
      533
  myometrium 500
Mast cells, cervix 281
Maternal blood flow, perivillous fibrin deposition
      1278
Maternal coagulopathy, fetal artery thrombosis
      1282
Maternal death 1559–1574
  abruptio placentae 1561
  classification 1560
  definition 1559
  direct 1560, 1560–1571
  fortuitous 1560
  indirect 1560
Maternal floor infarction 1278–1279, 1279
  intrauterine fetal growth retardation 1310–1311
  miscarriage 1438
Maternal pyrexia, chorioamnionitis 1306
Maternal tachycardia, chorioamnionitis 1306
Maternal vasculopathy, preterm delivery 1312
Materno-fetal 'battle-field' 1258
  basal plate 1258

Materno-fetal blood flow, malarial infection 1319
Matrix-type fibrinoid 1261
Mature intermediate villi 1246
'Maturitas praecox placentae,' preterm delivery
      1312, 1312
Mayer–Rokitansky–Kuster–Hauser syndrome 43
  clinical features 46
Mcl-1 syncytial fusion. 1240
mdm 2, p53 stabilisation 1598
Meconium aspiration syndrome 1303
Meconium-induced necrosis, umbilical cord
      1299–1300
Meconium staining, fetal membranes 1303
  fetal gut maturation 1303
Median sacral artery, pelvic supply 27
Medroxyprogesterone acetate
  bone density reduced 1105
  depot, endometrial carcinoma and 1094
Megakaryocytes, identification 948
Megaloblastic anaemia, cervical changes 1188
Megaloblastic disease, cervix 290–291
Megaloblasts, cervical epithelium 290
Meigs' syndrome 1196–1197
  acute 676–677
  dysgerminoma and 774
  ovarian fibroma association 860
  theca cell tumour with 762
Meiosis 643
  oogonia, control/initiation 647
  stages 643
Melanin
  Paget's disease of vulva 99
  vulvar pigmentation disorders 67
Melanocytes, in vagina 208
Melanocytic lesions/neoplasms, vulva 111–114
Melanocytic naevi, vulvar 111–112
Melanoma, malignant
  amelanotic, vaginal 209, 209
  cervical 380–382, 381
  fetal, placental metastases 1459
  in situ uterine cervix 381
  lichen sclerosus 78
  in mature teratoma 803, 803
  metastatic
      glial implants in immature teratoma vs 792
      to ovary 881, 888
      small cell undifferentiated ovarian carcinoma vs
          905
  placental metastatic disease 1455, 1456
      fetal 1459
      macroscopic and histological appearance
          1455
  steroid cell tumours vs 854
  steroid contraceptives and 1105
  superficial spreading, Paget's disease 99
  urethral 133
  vagina see Vagina, malignant melanoma
  vulvar 112, 112–114, 113, 113
      histological microstaging 114
      incidence 113
      staging 113
      surgery 114
      survival rates 113
Melanosis
  cervical 279, 382
  vaginal 208, 209
  vulvar 68, 111
Melkersson–Rosenthal syndrome 1188
  vulvar involvement 65
Membranes, fetal
  development 1253–1257, 1256
  inflammation 1303–1306
  meconium staining 1303
  pathology 1301–1308
  premature rupture 1305, 1306
      chorioamnionitis 1306
      necrotising funisitis 1300
  rupture and chorioamnionitis 1305
  squamous metaplasia 1301–1302
  structure at term 1257
Membranous glomerulonephritis, in pregnancy
      1512, 1512–1513
Menarche, age of 653
  ovarian carcinoma risk 700
Mendelson syndrome 1570
Meningiomas 1535
Meningitis
  chorioamnionitis 1306
  listerial 1532
Meningococcal infection, cervical 282

Menopause
  age 657, 990
      ovarian carcinoma risk 700
  late, endometrial adenocarcinoma risk factor
      455, 456
  premature 681–682, 682, 1016, 1197
      blepharophimosis 1182
      galactosaemia 1183
      hypogonadism 678
      see also Ovary, premature failure
  sterility after 990
  symptom relief, Tibolone therapy 1090
  see also Postmenopausal women
Menstrual cycle
  anovulatory, endometrial hyperplasia 444
  cervical mucus changes 277
  cervical physiology 275
  endometrial changes and dating 1000
      see also Endometrial cycle; specific phases under
          endometrium
  Fallopian tube changes 587, 589
  follicular phase 1013
  hormones and feedback mechanisms 1013, 1014
  luteal phase 1013
      defect see Luteal phase defect
  non-granulomatous salpingitis risk factor 620
  ovulation see Ovulation
  proliferative phase
      cervical changes 248
      cervical mucus 277
      endometrium see Endometrium, proliferative
          phase
  secretory phase 400–401
      cervical mucus 277
      endometrium see Endometrium, secretory
          phase
  vaginal changes 150
      lamina propria 150
      microflora 151
  see also Endometrial cycle
Menstrual disturbances
  atypical polypoid adenomyoma 573
  corpus luteum cysts 665
  follicle cysts 663–664
  irregularity
      acromegaly 1182
      HIV/AIDS 1152
  IUCD use and 1107, 1108, 1117
  Krukenberg tumours 892
  ovarian fibroma 859
  polycystic ovary disease 666, 667
  systemic disorders 1021
Menstrual endometrium 398
Menstrual toxic shock syndrome (TSS)
      see Toxic shock syndrome (TSS)
Menstruation 398
  blood loss increased by IUCD use 1117
  evolutionary significance 990
  onset 398
  retrograde, haematosalpinx 597
  see also Menstrual cycle
Mental and motor impairment, childhood, umbilical
      cord length 1293
Meralgia paraesthetica 1536
Merkel cell tumour, vulvar 111
Mesangial cells
  pre-eclampsia 1508, 1508, 1509
  proliferation in mesangial IgA disease 1516, 1516
Mesangial IgA disease, in pregnancy 1516, 1516
Mesangiocapillary glomerulonephritis, in pregnancy
      1513–1515, 1514
  linear-dense deposit disease 1514
  serum C3 1514, 1514
Mesenchymal–epithelial tumours
      see Epithelial–mesenchymal neoplasms
      (mixed)
Mesenchymal metaplasia of endometrium 414–415
Mesenchymal tissue, immature teratoma 791
Mesenchymal tumours
  cervix, benign 383–384
  in childhood 1172–1173
      aggressive angiomyxoma 1172, 1173
      mixed Müllerian tumours 1172
      neurofibroma of clitoral region 1172
      rhabdomyosarcoma 1172
      sarcoma botryoides 1172
  epithelial–mesenchymal mixed
      see Epithelial–mesenchymal neoplasms
  ovarian 857–877
      see also Ovarian tumours

uterine **501–502**
  mixture of elements **577–578**
  myometrium involvement 501
vaginal
  benign 193–197
  malignant 211–216
vulvar **114–125**
  uncertain origin 124–125
Mesenchymal villi 1247
Mesenchyme
  components in yolk sac tumours *783*, 783–784
  subcoelomic 578, *578*
Mesenteric thrombosis 1104
Mesoderm
  extraembryonic 5, *6*
  gonadal differentiation 1211
  intermediate 8–9, 644
  intraembryonic 6, *7*
  lateral 8
  paraxial 8
Mesodermal lesions, broad ligament 626
Mesodermal stromal polyps 290
Mesodermal tumours, Fallopian tube, benign 603–605
Mesonephric adenocarcinoma, cervix 278, 348
Mesonephric blastema 898
Mesonephric cysts
  congenital vaginal *182*, 182–183, 183, *183*
  vulvar 85, *85*
Mesonephric (Wolffian) duct(s) 41
  congenital vaginal cysts *182*, 182–183, 183, *183*
  convoluted 625
  embryogenesis *11*, 11–12, 897
  excretory system for developing embryo 18
  female adnexal tumour originating 208
  female differentiation 18
  male differentiation 14
  paramesonephric duct growth and development 12
  remnants *see* Mesonephric (Wolffian) remnants
Mesonephric hyperplasia
  cervix 278
  mesonephric adenocarcinoma of cervix 348
Mesonephric (Wolffian) remnants 625, 897
  cervix 278
  cystic 183
  ectocervix *278*
  ovarian tumours of Wolffian origin from 901–902
Mesonephric structures 695
Mesonephric tumours
  cervix 278, 348
  vagina 208
Mesonephric vesicles, embryogenesis 11
Mesonephros
  embryology 644, 897
  urinary system development 11
Mesothelial hyperplasia **913–914**
  differential diagnosis 914
    adenocarcinoma vs 914
  ovarian 685
  peritoneal **913–914**, *914*
Mesothelial inclusions in ovaries, endometriosis 970, *972*
Mesothelial lesions
  broad ligament 627
  'mural mesothelial proliferation' 915
  peritoneum **913–920**
    multiloculated peritoneal inclusion cysts 914–915, *915*
  see also Mesothelial hyperplasia; Mesothelioma
Mesothelioma
  adenomatoid, uterine 539, *539*
  broad ligament 627
  cystic, uterine 501
  deciduoid malignant *918*, 918–919
  diffuse malignant of peritoneum 916–918
    adenocarcinoma vs 918
    biphasic (mixed) 917
    differential diagnosis 918
    epithelial 917–918
    immunohistochemistry 918
    mesothelial hyperplasia vs 914
    peritoneal serous carcinoma vs 925
    pure sarcomatous 917
    spread and histology 917, *917*
  genital and peritoneal, benign, morphology 916
  multicystic (peritoneal) 914–915, *915*
  papillary
    broad ligament 627

well-differentiated peritoneal 915–916, *916*
  tumour markers 627
'Mesothelioma,' vagina 211
Mesovarium 653
Metanephros, urinary system development 11
Metaplasia
  adipose 415
  broad ligament 627
  cervical *253*, *264*, 287–288
  decidual, ectopic pregnancy *591*
  endometrial *see* Endometrium, metaplasia
  eosinophilic, endometrial 413
  Fallopian tube 288, 589–594
    see also Fallopian tube
  fimbrial *see* Fimbriae, tubal
  intestinal 288
  mucinous *see* Mucinous metaplasia
  osseous, endometrium 414
  ovary 695
  sebaceous, ectocervix 279
  squamous epithelium of cervix *263*
  stromal *see* Stromal metaplasia
  transitional cell 288
  tuboendometrioid 287–288
  vagina *186*, **186**
Metaplastic cell origin, cervix 265–266
Metaplastic papillary tumour, Fallopian tube 602–603
Metaplastic squamous epithelium of cervix *see* Cervical epithelium, metaplastic squamous
Metastases **1188**
  of Brenner tumours (transitional cell) 728
  of cervical carcinoma *see* Cervical carcinoma
  in cervix *see* Cervix, metastases
  from choriocarcinoma *see* Choriocarcinoma
  from endometrial carcinoma
    see Endometrial carcinoma (adenocarcinoma)
  in Fallopian tube *612*, *613*, 613–615, *614*, *615*
  in fimbriae (tubal) *612*, *613*
  from germ cell tumours 218
  from gonadoblastoma 830
  from immature teratoma 792
  from invasive hydatidiform mole **1390–1391**, *1391*
  Krukenberg tumours and 890, 891, 892
  to lymph nodes *see* Lymph nodes
  from melanoma *see* Melanoma, malignant
  from mixed germ cell sex cord–stromal tumours (ovarian) 838–839
  in ovary *see* Ovarian tumours, metastatic
  placental *see* Placenta, metastases
  in uterus 510
  in vagina *see* Vagina, metastatic tumours
  vulva **125–126**
  see also individual tumours and sites
Metazoan diseases, vaginal 176
Methotrexate, tubal pregnancy 1060
MHC *see* HLA (human leukocyte) antigens; Major histocompatibility antigens
MIB-1 staining (proliferation marker antibody)
  cervical intraepithelial neoplasia (CIN) 1613
  cervical lesions 290
  endocervical neoplasia 358
  endometrial adenocarcinoma detection 482
Mice
  F1 hybrid^{W/Wv} 705
  SWR/J 705
  teratoma induction 706
Michaelis–Gutmann bodies, malacoplakia 424
Microangiopathic haemolytic anaemia 1503
Microcystic endocervical adenocarcinoma 346
Microflora
  vaginal *see* Vagina, microflora
  vulva **54**
Microglandular hyperplasia
  cervical 289–290
  endocervix *290*
Microinvasive adenocarcinoma of cervix 356–357
Microinvasive carcinoma of cervix
  see Cervical carcinoma, microinvasive
Microinvasive squamous cell carcinoma of vulva 104–105
  measurement of depth of invasion 104
Microsatellite instability **1601**
  endometrial adenocarcinoma 485
  endometrial carcinoma 1601, 1604
  endometrial hyperplasia 454, 455
  ovarian borderline tumours 697
  PTEN, endometrial carcinoma **1600**

Microvesicular steatosis, acute fatty liver of pregnancy 1470
Microvessel density, cervical adenocarcinoma prognosis 350
Midzone cells, cervical stratified squamous epithelium 273
Mifepristone 1086
Migraine **1530–1531**
  hemiplegic 1531
Migratory cytotrophoblast *1333*
  myometrial blood vessels 1333, *1334*
  placental bed giant cells 1333
Migratory trophoblast 1332–1335
  non-villous interstitial, function 1333
  pre-eclampsia 1337
  uterine tissue invasion 1332
Mineralocorticoid biosynthesis *1213*
Minimal change glomerulonephropathy *1513*, **1513**
Minimum deviation adenocarcinoma of cervix 342, *342*, 759
Miscarriage
  activated protein C resistance 1434
  aetiological factors **1432–1435**
    congenital abnormalities of fetus 1435
    endocrinological abnormalities 1433
    genetic abnormalities 1435
    immunological factors 1433–1434
    infections 1432
    physical 1432–1433
    psychological factors 1433
    thrombophilias 1434–1435
  age-related increase in rate 991
  cervical pregnancy 1062
  confirmation of pregnancy 1442
  Coxsackie virus 1432
  definition 1431–1432
  early 1431
    endometrial bleeding 409
  endometritis, acute non-specific 419
  first-trimester, amnion nodosum 1302
  habitual
    Mycoplasma hominis 427
    Toxoplasma gondii 432
  hydatidiform moles *see* Hydatidiform mole
  hydropic 1383
  incidence 1432
  incomplete first trimester, syphilitic endometritis 431–432
  induction, sharp curettage and subsequent cervical pregnancy 1062
  late 1431
  massive subchorial thrombosis 1285
  material
    anatomico-pathological classification 1436–1437
    morphological classification 1441
  missed 1369
  nephrolithiasis and 1026
  non-molar
    genetic abnormalities **1364**, 1379
    microscopic appearances **1379–1380**
  osseous metaplasia 414
  ovarian pregnancy 1062
  pathogenesis **1435–1436**
  pathology **1431–1448**
  placenta membranacea 1275
  prolonged intrauterine death **1503**
  recurrent spontaneous 992, 995, 1431
    definition 1431
    hyperprolactinaemia and 1024
    polycystic ovary syndrome 1433
    procoagulant disorders 1434
    reduced immunosuppressive factors 1006
    second-trimester 998
  septic, IUCD use and 1107
  spontaneous 1367, 1370, 1413, 1431
    anatomical malformations of fetus 1435
    autosomal trisomy 1435
    cervical pregnancy 1062
    defective placentation 1345, *1346*
    definition 1431
    early, endometrial bleeding 409
    endometrial shedding 408
    endometrium 420
    histological examination of tissue 1442
    iatrogenic 1442
    IUCD use and 1116
    systemic lupus erythematosus 1190
    sporadic, fetal chromosomal abnormalities 1431–1432

Miscarriage (cont'd)
　stillbirth vs 1313
　triploidy 1367–1368
　tubal pregnancy without tubal rupture
　　1058–1059
　uterine malformations 47
Misoprostol (Cytotec) 1193
Mites, vaginitis 176
Mitochondria
　beta-oxidation pathway of fatty acid metabolism,
　　defects 1472
　DNA, deletion, infertility due to endocrine failure
　　991
Mitosis 643
Mitotic activity (index)
　adenosarcoma with sarcomatous overgrowth
　　558–559
　cervical intraepithelial neoplasia 313, 313,
　　313–316
　endocervical stromal sarcomas 376
　endometrial polyps, simple 416–417
　gonadoblastoma 827
　intravenous leiomyomatosis (uterine) 535
　mesenchymal uterine tumours 501, 502
　mitotically active leiomyoma (uterine) 524, 524
　placental haemangiomas 1451
　uterine adenosarcoma 556
　uterine leiomyoma with bizarre nuclei 527
　uterine leiomyosarcoma 521
　uterine smooth muscle tumours 515, 516
Mitotically active leiomyoma, uterine 524,
　524–525
Mitral valve prolapse 1545
Mitral valve stenosis 1547, 1547–1548
Mixed carcinoma–sarcoma elements
　see Carcinosarcoma
Mixed epithelial–mesenchymal tumours
　see Epithelial–mesenchymal neoplasms
　　(mixed)
Mixed germ cell sex cord–stromal tumours
　(ovarian) 794, 821, 832–841, 1172
　behaviour and prognosis 840–841
　clinical findings 833
　differential diagnosis 840
　dysgerminoma association 840, 841
　epidemiology 832–833
　genetic findings 833
　gonadoblastoma vs 831, 840
　hormonal findings 833–834
　hyaline bodies 835, 837
　incidence 832–833
　metastatic 838–839
　pathology 834–840
　　connective tissue 836, 837, 838
　　cystic spaces 838
　　germ cell component 834, 835, 836
　　histological patterns 835
　　histology 834–840, 835–840
　　macroscopic 834, 834
　　sex-cord derivative component 834, 835, 835,
　　　836
　　ultrastructure 839
　terminology and synonyms 832
　therapy 841
　　chemotherapy 839, 841
　trabecular pattern 835, 835, 836, 837, 839
　tubular pattern 835, 837
　see also Gonadoblastoma
Mixed germ cell tumours (ovarian) 794
Mixed gonadal dysgenesis 1160
Mixed mesodermal tumour
　see Carcinosarcoma; Mixed Müllerian
　　tumours
Mixed Müllerian tumours
　cervix 379, 379
　endometriosis and 978
　extrauterine 578
　Fallopian tube 611, 611
　uterine 549–573
　　benign 550
　　　see also Adenofibroma; Adenosarcoma
　　carcinofibroma 559, 560
　　carcinomesenchymoma 559
　　classification 550, 550–551
　　heterologous types 550
　　histogenesis 549–550
　　history 549
　　homologous types 550
　　malignant see Carcinosarcoma
Mixed tumours, vulvar 131

MMMT see Mixed Müllerian tumours
Mobiluncus, bacterial vaginosis 158
Molar pregnancies see Hydatidiform mole
Molecular pathology 1595–1606
　apoptosis-related genes 1601
　arrays 1605
　chromosomal imbalance 1604–1605
　clonality 1602–1603
　comparative genomic hybridisation 1604–1605
　DNA mismatch repair/microsatellite instability
　　1601
　FHIT 1600–1601
　HPV detection/typing 1606
　imprinted genes 1605–1606
　in situ hybridisation 1603–1604
　loss of heterozygosity (LOH) 1599–1600
　oncogene expression 1595–1597
　telomerase activity 1601–1602
　tumour suppressor gene 1597–1600
Molluscum contagiosum, vulvar infection 59, 59–60
Monochorionic–diamniotic twin placentation 1580
　1577
　chronic twin–twin transfusion 1581
　fused dichorionic–diamniotic placenta vs 1587
Monochorionic–monoamniotic twin placentation
　1577, 1580–1581
Monochorionic placentation
　vascular anastomoses 1578–1579, 1579
　vascular anastomoses and death of one twin
　　1584
Monochorionic twins, twin transfusion syndrome
　1581
Monoclonal antibody
　1C5, endocervical neoplasia 359
　D9B1 1110
　see also specific antibodies
Monocyte-chemotactic protein-1, uterine
　　endometrium in endometriosis 966
Mononuclear cells, cervical epithelium 266
Monovular dispermic twinning 1576
Monozygotic triplets 1588
Monozygotic twins 1575–1576
　development and placentation 1577
　genetic discordance 1575
　placentation 1577–1578
Monro's abscess, psoriasis 73
Morgagni, hydatid cysts 624
Morphometry 1612–1614
　cervical cancer 1612–1613
　endometrial carcinoma 1613
　ovarian cancer 1613–1614
　squamous cell carcinoma of vulva 108
　vulvar carcinoma 1612
Morula, preimplantation phase embryogenesis 4
Morules, metaplastic squamous epithelium of
　endometrium 410–411
Mosaicism, placental see Placenta, mosaicism
MUC2 apomucin, primary ovarian carcinoma vs
　colonic metastases 884
MUC5AC apomucin, primary ovarian carcinoma vs
　colonic metastases 884
Mucicarminophilic histiocytosis, ovarian 685
Mucin(s)
　amniotic fluid embolism syndrome 1567
　cervical mucus 277
　endocervical neoplasia 358
　neutral, adenosarcoma (uterine) 554
　primary ovarian carcinoma vs colonic metastases
　　884
　secretion by vaginal cysts 182, 182, 183
　staining 472
Mucinous adenocarcinoma
　cervical 473
　endometrial see Endometrial carcinoma,
　　mucinous
　Fallopian tube 611
　ovarian see Ovarian tumours, mucinous
　　adenocarcinoma
Mucinous adenofibroma, ovarian 714–715
Mucinous borderline tumours of Müllerian type,
　endometriosis 978
Mucinous cystadenoma
　Bartholin's gland 130
　carcinoid tumour association 807
　ovarian 714, 714–715, 715, 783
　　fibrosarcoma association 873
　Sertoli–Leydig cell tumours vs 715
Mucinous cysts, vulva 84, 84–85
Mucinous lesions, secondary Müllerian system
　925–926

Mucinous metaplasia
　endometrium 412–413, 473
　Fallopian tube 590, 590
Mucinous tumours
　adenofibroma, ovarian 714–715
　benign, luteinized cells 715
　Brenner tumours (transitional cell) associated
　　697
　carcinoid 810, 886, 886–887
　　appendiceal tumours vs 809
　　of ovary 807, 809–810, 810
　cystic, of retroperitoneum 926
　cystic teratoma association 697
　ovarian see Ovarian tumours
　peritoneal 926
　see also Mucinous adenocarcinoma
Mucoid adenocarcinoma, cervical 342
Mucometra, mucinous metaplasia of endometrium
　412
Mucosa-associated lymphoid tissue (MALT)
　lymphoma see MALT lymphomas
Mucosal epithelial proliferation (MEP), Fallopian
　tube adenocarcinoma 606, 606–607
Mucosal immunity
　cervix 274
　HIV infection of cervix 287
Mucous membrane pemphigoid, vulvar 70–71
Mucus
　cervical see Cervical mucus
　isthmus 1007
Mucus-related antigens, endocervical neoplasia
　358–359
Müllerian adenofibroma 551, 551–552
Müllerian adenosarcoma 530
　with sex cord-like features 559
Müllerian anomalies 1158, 1160, 1163, 1193
Müllerian clear cell carcinoma, ovarian tumours of
　probable Wolffian origin vs 902
Müllerian ducts see Paramesonephric (Müllerian)
　ducts
Müllerian epithelia, adenosarcoma (uterine) 554,
　555
Müllerian inhibiting substance (MIS)
　　(anti-Müllerian hormone)
　defects, pseudohermaphroditism, male 1217
　gene
　　male sex determination 1210
　　mutations, persistent Müllerian duct syndrome
　　　1217
　granulosa cells 14
　male sexual development 1211
　oocyte meiosis 1211
　paramesonephric duct regression 13
　synthesis 638
　testicular descent 1211
Müllerian metaplasia, peritoneum 922
Müllerian mixed tumours see Mixed Müllerian
　tumours
Müllerianosis 964
Müllerian papilloma 290, 1176, 1176
　uterine cervix 382–383, 383
　　clinical examination 383
　　differential diagnosis 383
　　microscopic examination 383
　vaginal 193
Müllerian stromal sarcoma, vaginal 216
Müllerian system, secondary 578, 920–929
　clear cell lesions 927
　diffuse, differentiation pathways 695
　diffuse peritoneal leiomyomatosis 928, 928–929
　ectopic decidua 927–928, 928
　mucinous lesions 925–926
　serous lesions 921–926
　squamous lesions 927
　transitional-like lesions 926–927
　see also Peritoneum
Multiloculated peritoneal inclusion cysts 914–915,
　915
Multinucleation, human papillomavirus infection
　305
Multiparity
　HELLP syndrome 1475
　liver rupture in pregnancy 1476–1477
　pregnancy luteoma association 674–675,
　　1214
　splenic artery rupture 1481
Multiple angiokeratomas of vulva 119
Multiple births see Multiple pregnancy
Multiple endocrine neoplasia syndrome type I
　1022, 1188

Multiple hamartoma syndrome (Cowden's disease) 62, **1182**
Multiple pregnancy **1575–1594**
　acute fatty liver of pregnancy 1472
　hyperreactio luteinalis 676
　monozygotic, monochorionic placentation and acardiac fetus 1583–1584
　placentation **1589**
　pre-eclampsia risk 1505
　velamentous insertion of umbilical cord 1295
Multiple sclerosis 1021, **1534–1535**
　aetiology 1535
　pathology 1534–1535
　protective factors 1534
　relapse rate 1534
Multipolar mitotic figure, cervical intraepithelial neoplasia 313
Mumps
　follicular damage 1015
　oophoritis 679
Mural implantation, tubal pregnancy 1051, *1052, 1053*
'Mural mesothelial proliferation' 915
Muramidase, ovarian granulocytic sarcoma 947, *947*
Muscle tumours *see* Smooth muscle, tumours
Mutations, infertility and 992
Myasthenia gravis **1536**
　carcinosarcoma association 561
Mycobacterium leprae, vulvar infection 57
Mycobacterium tuberculosis
　chronic endometritis 1134
　endometrial tuberculosis 427
　granulomatous salpingitis 1010–1011
　vulvar infection 57
　see also Tuberculosis
Mycobacterium tuberculosis var *hominis,* cervical tuberculosis 282
Mycoplasma
　endometritis 427, 994, 1003–1005, *1004*
　vaginal infection 165
　vulvar infection 58
　vulvar microbial flora 54
Mycoplasma hominis
　bacterial vaginosis 160
　ectopic pregnancy 1049
　endometritis 427
　genitourinary infections 996
　miscarriage 1432
　　habitual 427
　salpingitis 620
Mycoses *see* Fungal infections
Mycosis fungoides 937
Mycotic chorioamnionitis 1305
Myelinosis, central pontine myelinosis **1531**
Myelocytes, granulated 946
Myelosarcoma, uterus and cervix 951–952
Myoblastoma, granular cell *see* Granular cell tumours (myoblastoma)
Myocardial infarction in pregnancy **1550**
　coronary artery morphology 1550
Myocarditis, idiopathic **1553**
Myofibroblastoma, polypoid, vaginal 194
Myointimal cells, pre-eclampsia arteriopathy 1340
Myometrial blood vessels, interstitial migratory cytotrophoblast 1333
Myometrial radiate arteries
　physiological changes in pregnancy 1339, *1339*
　pre-eclampsia 1343, *1343*
Myometrial veins, pregnancy 1336
Myometritis, eosinophilic 500
Myometrium
　abnormalities, infertility due to 998–1000
　adenofibroma invasion 552
　adenomyosis *see* Adenomyosis
　adenosarcoma invasion *553, 557,* 558
　carcinosarcoma invasion 564, 571
　chronic subinvolution 499–500
　combined oral contraceptives effect 1097
　cysts 500–501
　discoloration 500
　endometrial carcinoma invasion *see* Endometrial carcinoma
　endometrial glands within *see* Adenomyosis, uterine
　endometrial junction 497
　hypertrophy 497
　idiopathic (diffuse) hypertrophy 499–500
　leiomyoma 999
　mast cell infiltration 500

　mesenchymal tumours involvement 501
　non-neoplastic conditions **497–501**
　postoperative necrobiotic granulomas 500
　pregnancy 1330, *1331*
　progestagens effect 1084
　vascular malformations 500
　vasculitis 500
Myosalpinx, tuberculous infection 618
Myospherulosis 800
Myxoid leiomyosarcomas of vulva 115
Myxoid stromal zone, vagina 150
Myxoma
　ovarian *867,* **867–868**
　vagina 195

N
Nabothian cysts (follicle), cervix 287, *288*
　columnar epithelium 257
Naevoid basal cell carcinoma syndrome (Gorlin's syndrome) *see* Basal cell naevus syndrome
Naevus
　blue *see* Blue naevus
　vulvar 111–112
　white sponge, vulvar 63
Napkin rashes, vulvar involvement 80
Nasopharyngeal carcinoma, Epstein–Barr virus 331
National Health Service Cervical Screening Programme 298
Natural killer (NK) cells
　cervical epithelium 267
　endometriosis 965
　increased in endometrium 1006
　premature ovarian failure and 1017
Necrolytic migratory erythema 63
Necrosis
　coagulative *see* Coagulative tumour cell necrosis
　compression 1151
　decidual 1342
　'dirty necrosis,' ovarian metastasis 883, *883*
　endothelial *see* Endothelial necrosis
　fibrinoid-type *see* Fibrinoid necrosis
　hyaline, uterine leiomyosarcoma vs 522
　meconium-induced, umbilical cord 1299–1300
　superficial, gonorrhoea induced endometritis 431
　superficial fascial, sepsis 1562
　umbilical cord 1299–1300
　villitis 1290
Necrotic pseudoxanthomatous nodules, endometriosis 969, *970*
Necrotising arteritis **1191**
Necrotising endarteritis, rubella infection 1315–1316
Necrotising fasciitis, vulvar 58–59
Necrotising funisitis *1299,* 1300, *1300*
Necrotising subcutaneous infection, vulvar 58–59
Neisseria gonorrhoeae
　cervical infection 281–282
　endometritis 430–431
　infertility and 993
　salpingitis 620
　vaginitis due to 167–168
　see also Gonorrhoea
Neisseria lactamica, vaginitis 169
Neisseria meningitidis
　endometritis 431
　endometritis–salpingitis–peritonitis 431
　vaginitis 169
Nelson's syndrome 855
Nematode infections
　in tropics **1141–1143**
　vulvar 54–55
Neonates
　anaemia, placental haemangioma 1453
　asphyxia, umbilical cord knots 1297
　chlamydial infections 165
　gonococcal vaginitis 168
　herpes hepatitis 1479
　intrapartum infection, human papillomavirus (HPV) 161
　oedema, placental haemangioma 1453
　sexual ambiguity **1158–1162**
　thrombocytopenia, placental haemangioma 1454
　trichomonal vaginitis 175
　tubular torsion 594, *595*
　Turner's syndrome 1221–1222
　vaginal epithelium 150
Neoplasms (neoplasia) *see* Tumour(s)
Neovascularisation *see* Angiogenesis
Nephritis
　interstitial, in pregnancy **1499**

　lupus, pregnancy 1345, *1515,* **1515–1516**
　see also Glomerulonephritis
Nephrogenic adenoma, urethral neoplasms, benign 132, *132*
Nephrolithiasis, spontaneous miscarriage and 1026
Nephrotic syndrome **1197**
　mesangiocapillary glomerulonephritis in pregnancy **1513–1515**
　ovarian cancer 1197
　placental site trophoblastic tumour 1197
Nerves, pelvic 24–26
Nerve supply
　bladder 30
　lumbrosacral plexus 24–25
　obturator internus muscle 22
　ovary 657
　rectum 29
Nervi erigentes 25
Nervous system, embryology 7–8
Nervous system diseases, in pregnancy **1523–1539**
　arterial obstruction 1527–1528
　benign intracranial hypertension 1527
　blood–brain barrier permeability 1523
　central pontine myelinosis 1531
　cerebral venous thrombosis 1525–1527
　chorea gravidarum 1524
　cranial/peripheral nerve lesions 1536
　epilepsy 1533–1534
　HIV/AIDS 1532–1533
　infections 1532
　intracerebral haemorrhage 1528–1529
　migraine 1530–1531
　multiple sclerosis 1534–1535
　myasthenia gravis 1536
　neoplasms 1535
　pituitary gland ischaemia 1535
　postpartum depression 1523
　pre-eclampsia/eclampsia encephalopathy 1524–1525
　puerperal psychosis 1523
　trauma 1532
　tumours 1535
　vascular disorders 1524–1530
　vascular malformations 1529–1530
　Wernicke's encephalopathy 1531, *1531*
Netherton's syndrome, vulvar genetic disorders 63
Neural fold formation 7
Neural groove formation 7
Neural origin tumours, vulvar 122–124
Neural plate ectoderm, longitudinal groove *8*
Neural tube
　closure and growth 7–8
　formation *8*
Neural tumours
　cervix 384
　ovarian **867**
　vagina 197
　vulvar 122–124
Neuroblastoma
　placental involvement 1458, *1458*
　vagina 211
Neuroblastoma cells
　fetal vessel plugging 1458
　placental immunological defense mechanism 1459
Neuroectodermal tumours
　immature teratoma *792*
　malignant 1167
　ovarian (primary), small cell undifferentiated ovarian carcinoma vs 905
Neuroendocrine carcinoma *see* Small cell carcinomas
Neuroendocrine tumours of vulva 111
Neuroepithelial tubules, in immature teratoma *790, 791*
Neuroepithelioma, vagina 210, 211
Neurofibroma
　of clitoral region 1172
　ovarian **867**
　uterine cervix 384
　vulva 123–124
Neurofibromatosis type 1 (Von Recklinghausen's syndrome) **1191–1192,** 1536
Neurohormonal peptides, immature teratoma 791
Neuroma
　traumatic, vaginal 154
　uterine cervix 384
Neuromyopathy **1197**
Neurone-specific enolase (NSE), small cell ovarian tumours 904, *904*

Neuropathies **1197**
  acute inflammatory demyelinating polyneuropathy 1536
  autoimmune 1536
  chronic inflammatory demyelinating polyradiculoneuropathy 1536
  entrapment 1536
  Guillain–Barré syndrome 1536
  trigeminal 1536
Neurovascular pedicle, lateral cervical ligament 34
Neurovascular sheaths and ligaments, pelvis 24
Neutrophils *see* Polymorphonuclear leucocyte infiltrate
Newborn *see* Neonates
Nicotine, cervical cancer 302
Nitabuch's fibrinoid 1261
Nodular fasciitis, vulva 85
Nodular hyperthecosis 670
Non-gestational choriocarcinoma **785–787,** *786*
Non-granulomatous endosalpingitis 623, *623*
Non-granulomatous infectious disease, ovary 682–683
Non-granulomatous salpingitis *see* Salpingitis, non-granulomatous
Non-Hodgkin's lymphoma
  B-cell *936*
    cervix *949*
    classification 937, *937*
    endometrial 950–951
    follicle centre *944*
    high-grade 937, 940, 941, *941, 949*
    immunohistochemistry 944–945, 950
    low-grade 937, 940
    ovarian 940, 941, *941*
    vaginal 953–954
    vulval *955*
  Burkitt's *see* Burkitt's lymphoma
  cervix *see* Non-Hodgkin's lymphoma, uterus and cervix
  classification 936, *936, 937*
  Fallopian tube *948,* **948**
  follicular
    Fallopian tube 948, *948*
    ovary 941, *942*
  histiocytic 937, 939
    well-differentiated, ovarian 941
  HIV/AIDS 1153
  lymphoblastic 936
  lymphoplasmacytic, vaginal *953,* 954
  MALT *see* MALT lymphomas
  ovary **939–945**
    age range 940
    clinical features 940
    diagnostic criteria 939
    differential diagnosis 945
    gross pathology 940
    histology 940–942, *941*
    immunohistochemistry 944–945
    incidence and pathogenesis 939–940
    prognosis and survival 945
    sclerosis 942
    subtypes 940–942, *942*–944
  plasmacytoma, ovarian 942
  pregnancy and **957–958**
  primary, of female genital tract 935
  putative NK-cell *936*
  staging *938,* 938–939
  subtypes 937–938
  T-cell *936,* 937
    classification 937, *937*
    immunohistochemistry 944–945
    ovarian 942
    vulval *956*
  uterus and cervix **948–953**
    clinical features 949
    detection by cervical smears 949
    differential diagnosis 952–953
    gross pathology 949, *949*
    histology *949,* 949–951, *950*
    incidence 948–949
    sclerosis 951
    stage, therapy and survival 951
  vaginal *953,* **953–954**
    sclerosis 951
  vulval **954–956,** *955, 956*
    inflammatory lesions mimicking 954–956
Non-neoplastic conditions
  cervix **273–296**
  myometrium **497–501**

ovary **663–692**
vulva and related structures **53–94**
Norethindrone, haemorrhagic cellular leiomyoma (uterine) association 526
Norethisterone
  combined oral contraceptives, effect on endometrium 1092–1095, *1093, 1094*
  effect on endometrium 1082, *1082*
Norplant 1097
19–Nortestosterone, endometrial atrophy 1083
Notochordal process 6
Nuclear inclusions, parvovirus B 19 infection 1317
Nuclear palisading, ovarian fibroma 859
Nucleated erythrocytes, maternal syphilis infection 1314
Nuclei
  abnormalities, cervical intraepithelial neoplasia 312–313
  atypia, mucinous adenocarcinoma of endometrium 472
  bizarre, adult-type granulosa cell tumours 748, *749, 750*
  cigar-shaped, uterine leiomyoma *519*
  'coffee bean,' of Langerhans' cells 957
  grooves, in Brenner tumours 716, *716*
  pleomorphism, adenosarcoma (uterine) 556–557
Nucleolar organiser regions
  endocervical neoplasia 360
  proteins (AgNORs) *see* AgNORs
Nulliparity, endometrial adenocarcinoma risk factor 455, 456
Nulliparous state, adult, uterus 32
Nuptiality, fertility and 990
Nutrition, fertility and 990

O

Oat cell carcinoma *see* Small cell carcinomas
Obesity
  endometrial adenocarcinoma risk factor 455, 456
  oestrogen levels and anovulatory infertility 1017
  in polycystic ovary disease 667
Obliteration, placental blood supply 1258
Obliterative arteritis, fetal stem arteries 1310
Obliterative endarteritis, fetal stem arteries *1292,* 1292–1293
Obstetrical trauma
  vagina 152
  vesicovaginal fistulas 184
Obstructed labour
  monochorionic–monoamniotic twin placentation 1580
  uterine rupture 1569
Obturator foramen 22
Obturator internus muscle
  nerve supply 22
  pelvic wall 22–23
Obturator nerve 25
Oedema
  diabetic glomerulopathy in pregnancy 1517
  endometrial, IUCD use and 1110
  massive, of ovary *671,* **671–672,** *672,* 1163
  neonatal, placental haemangioma 1453
  pre-eclampsia 1505
  stromal (endometrial) *see* Endometrium, stromal oedema
  villous 1289, *1289*
Oestrogen(s)
  anti-oestrogens **1075–1081**
  cervical adenocarcinoma 340
  chorea gravidarum 1524
  in combined oral contraceptives 1091
    effect on endometrium 1092–1095, *1093, 1094*
    thromboembolic disease and 1103–1104
    see also Combined steroid contraceptives (oral)
  deficiency, luteal phase insufficiency 406
  effect on endometrium
    normal 1072
    oral contraceptives 1092–1095, *1093, 1094*
    therapeutic administration *1072,* 1072–1074, *1073*
    see also Endometrium
  effect on spiral arteries 1072
  endometrial adenocarcinoma aetiology 455
    see also Endometrial carcinoma
  endometrial disorders (levels) 403, 404
  endometrial growth 397
  endometrial unresponsiveness 1002
  endometriosis 963, 966
  high-dose, contraceptives 1091, *1096*
  in HRT 1087

see also Hormone replacement therapy (HRT); Oestrogen(s), unopposed excess
  hypothalamus and pituitary inhibition 1013
  levels in pregnancy, hepatic function 1465
  loss, vaginal atrophy 155–156, *156*
  paramesonephric ducts and normal development 17
  periovulatory rise 1007
  prenatal exposure, teratoma of testis 707
  production, gonadoblastoma 825
  stimulation, uninterrupted, endometrial disorders 404–405
  therapeutic **1071–1074**
    atypical polypoid adenomyoma link 1074
    cervical smear changes 1074
    effect on cervix 1074
    effect on endometrium *1072,* 1072–1074, *1073*
    effect on Fallopian tube 1074
    endometrial hyperplasia after 445
    indications 1071
    sex cord–stromal tumours risk 705
    testicular feminisation, incomplete 1219
    types 1071
    uterine adenosarcoma after 552
    withdrawal, effects *1072*
  unopposed excess
    breast cancer and 1074
    endometrial carcinoma link 455–456, 1073–1074
    endometrial hyperplasia link 445
    uterine leiomyoma aetiology 516
    vaginal epithelium proliferation 149–150
  see also Hyperoestrogenic state; Hypo-oestrogenic states
Oestrogen receptors
  benign metastasising uterine leiomyoma 527
  ectocervical epithelial cells 273
  endometrial adenocarcinoma 482
  low-grade endometrial stromal sarcoma 511
  ovarian carcinoma prognosis 736
  peritoneal expression 1028
  reduced by copper IUCD 1110
  vaginal epithelium 149
Oligodendroglioma, immature teratoma *793*
Oligohydramnios
  amnion nodosum 1302
  placental haemangiomas 1453
Oligohydramnios–polyhydramnios sequence, chronic twin–twin transfusion 1581
Oligomenorrhoea, hypo-oestrogenic states 403
Oligo-ovulation 1014–1015
Ollier's disease **1171, 1183**
  juvenile-type granulosa cell tumour 752
Omphalomesenteric duct remnants
  differentiation into gastrointestinal type structures 1294, *1294*
  umbilical cord 1293, *1293*
    cysts 1300
Onapristone 1086, 1087
Oncocytic carcinoma, endometrial 462
Oncocytic metaplasia
  endometrial 413
  ovarian 909
Oncocytic tumours (oncocytoma), ovarian 909
Oncogenes
  c-erbB-2 / c-erb-3 **1595–1596**
  cervical carcinoma 1596
  c-fms (CSF receptor) **1597**
  c-myc **1597**
  colony-stimulating factor (CSF) **1597**
  endocervical neoplasia 359–360
  endometrial carcinoma 1596
  epidermal growth factor receptors (EGFR) **1595–1596**
  expression studies **1595–1597**
  hydatidiform moles **1386**
  K-ras **1596–1597**
  ovarian carcinoma **1596**
  trophoblastic neoplasms 1395
  type-1 growth factor family **1595–1596**
  see also C-erbB-2 oncogene; C-myc oncogene; K-ras
Oocytes
  absence, Turner's syndrome 1222
  apoptosis 649, 656
  competency loss with age 991
  defective 1015
  degeneration 1016
  development, perinatal period 648
  donation programmes, Turner's syndrome 1222

fetal ovary 648–649
  maturation 1014
  meiosis, Müllerian inhibiting substance (MIS) 1211
  numbers 648–649
  organisers of granulosa cells 703
  ovulation 1014
  parthenogenetic reduplication, teratoma origin 706
  sperm interaction
    abnormal 993, 995
    normal 1007
  sperm penetration, preparation 1007
  see also Germ cell(s)
Oogonia
  arrangement in fetal ovary 646–647
  number 648
  proliferation
    early fetal period 646–647
    embryonic period 646
    late fetal period 647
Oophorectomy
  borderline serous tumours 722
  paradoxical 1008
  prophylactic, in colon cancer 882
Oophoritis
  autoimmune 680–681, *681*, 1016
  mumps 679
Oral contraceptives *see* Combined steroid contraceptives (oral); Contraception, steroid
Orf, vulvar infection 60
Organogenesis, acardiac fetus 1584
Organ transplantation *see* Transplantation
Organ weights, chronic twin–twin placentation 1581–1582
Orgasm, vaginal physiology 151
Orogenital sexual activity, pregnancy and air embolism 1568
Osseous metaplasia, endometrium 414
Ossification, endometrial 414, 420
Osteoclastoma, ovarian **866**
Osteogenesis imperfecta **1188**
Osteogenic sarcoma, ovarian **866**
Osteoma, ovarian **866**
Osteoporosis
  hormonal therapy effect 1089, 1090
  steroid contraceptives and 1105
Osteosarcoma, in uterine carcinosarcoma 568
Ovarian artery 657
  aneurysms 1551
  pregnancy 1331
Ovarian cancer *see* Ovarian tumours
Ovarian descent 15
Ovarian endometriosis 698, 870, *972, 976*
  clonality studies 1602
  epithelial atypica 972
  tumours and 974
Ovarian follicles *see* Follicles, ovarian
Ovarian germ cell tumours 705–707, 771–820, 821, **1164–1167**
  aetiology and pathogenesis 707
  age/ethnic distribution 773
  benign 772, 773
  classification *694–695*
  common features in all types 773
  comparison with testicular germ cell tumours 772–773
  cytogenetics **1167**
  distribution 772
  Down's syndrome and 1183
  dysgerminoma *see* Dysgerminoma
  embryonal carcinoma *787*, **787–788**, *788*, 1167
  familial cancer syndromes **1168**
  groups 705
  histiogenesis 705–707, 771–772
    animal studies 706
    classical concept 771, *772*
    human studies 706
    human vs mouse teratomas 706–707
    normal embryogenesis relationship 772
    objections to histiogenetic hypothesis 771–772
    tridimensional tetrahedron model 772
  immature teratoma *see* Ovarian teratoma, immature
  malignant 773
  malignant neuroectodermal tumours 1167
  malignant potential assessment 772
  mature teratomas *see* Ovarian teratoma, mature
  non-gestational choriocarcinoma **785–787**

ploidy 1610
  pure non-gestational choriocarcinoma 1167, *1167*
  serum tumour markers 1167
  yolk sac *see* Yolk sac tumours
  see also Dysgerminoma; Teratoma
Ovarian hyperstimulation syndrome 675–677
  causes 1029, 1075
Ovarian intraepithelial neoplasia 696, 718
  endometriosis, atypical 975
Ovarian ligament 653–654
Ovarian nerves, in ovulation process 1014
Ovarian pedicle, torsion 671–672
Ovarian pregnancy 678, *1061*, **1061–1062**
  extrafollicular 1061
  intrafollicular 1061–1062
  IUCD use and 1117
  primary 1061
  secondary 1061
Ovarian remnant syndrome **665**
Ovarian sex cord–stromal tumours *694*, **1169–1172**
  with annular tubules *1170*, **1170–1171**, 1188
  childhood/adolescence 1164, **1169–1172**
  fibrothecomas 1171, 1172
  juvenile granulosa cell tumour *1169*, **1169**
  ovarian myxoma 1172
  Peutz–Jeghers syndrome 1188
  ploidy 1610
  sclerosing stromal tumour 1172
  Sertoli–Leydig cell tumours *1169*, **1169–1170**, *1170*
  steroid cell neoplasms 1171–1172
Ovarian sex-cord tumours *see* Ovarian tumours, sex-cord tumours
Ovarian teratoma 705
  aetiology and pathogenesis 707, 795
  animal models 706
  childhood 1164
  cystic *see* Cystic teratoma
  extraovarian disease 795, 1166
  fetiform 799
  growing teratoma syndrome 793–794
  haemolytic anaemia 1196
  histiogenesis 706, 795
    human vs mouse 706–707
  hyperprolactinaemia 1195
  immature **788–794**, *1165*, **1165–1166**, 1610
    AFP levels 791, 792–793
    calcification 789
    clinical features 789
    endodermal 791, *793, 794*
    gonadoblastoma association 830
    histological grading 790, *790*
    incidence and age 789
    macroscopic appearances 789, *789*
    metastases 792
    microscopic appearances 789–792, *790, 791, 792, 795*
    spontaneous capsular rupture 789
    treatment and prognosis 793–794
    tumour markers 792–793
  imprinted genes 1362, 1605
  mature **794–801, 1164–1165**
    clinical features 796–797
    complications 797
    cystic *see* Cystic teratoma
    dermoid protuberance *798*, 798–799
    incidence and age 796
    macroscopic appearance *797*, 797–799, *798*
    malignant tumours arising in **801–804**, *802, 803*, 857
    microscopic features *799*, 799–800, *800*
    parthenogenetic origin 795
    solid 795, 798
    torsion 797
    treatment and prognosis 800–801
  mature cystic teratoma (dermoid cyst) 1164
  mature solid teratoma 1164, 1165
  monodermal (monophyletic) **804–806**
  risk factors 707
  thyroid tissue within *805*, 805–806
Ovarian tumours **693–712**
  acanthosis nigricans **1193**
  ACOPS 1614
  adenocarcinoma
    bilateral involvement 733
    borderline endometrioid adenofibroma evolution 726
    cervical metastases 349
    clear cell *731*, 731–732
    endometrioid 729–731, *730, 733*

focal invasive in borderline mucinous tumours 724
    genetic predisposition 995
    gonadotrophin treatment association 1029
    low-grade vs borderline 721–722
    mucinous 695–696, 729, *729*
    protective effect of pregnancies 700
    serosal origin 696
    serous *see* Serous tumours, ovarian
    steroid contraceptives and 1099
    vulvar metastases 126
    see also Ovarian tumours, carcinoma
  adenoid cystic carcinoma **909**
  adenomatoid 873, *907*, **907–908**
    tumours of probable Wolffian origin vs 902
  adenosarcoma 731
  advanced **1614**
  aetiology and pathogenesis **699–703**
    genetic factors 702
    hypergonadotrophic hypothesis 701
    'incessant ovulation' hypothesis 701
    miscellaneous factors 702–703
    reproductive factors 700–702
  amyloidosis 1193
  angiosarcoma *869*, **869–870**
  apoptotic marker studies **1607–1608**
  ataxia-telangiectasia **1182**
  Bax 1608
  Bcl-2 1608
  benign signet ring stromal **766–767**, *767*
  of bone **866**
  borderline 697, **1613**
  BRCA1 1600
    breast cancer association 1081
  Brenner tumours *see* Brenner tumours
  carcinoid *see* Carcinoid tumours
  carcinoid syndrome **1194**
  carcinoma 728
    clinical features and staging *734*, 734–735
    forms 728
    haematogenous spread 734
    histological grading 735–736
    lymphatic spread 734
    mixed epithelial tumours 733
    nulliparity as risk factor 700
    pathology 728–733
    prognostic pathological factors 735–736
    risk factors 700–701
    risk reduced by breast feeding 700
    spread and staging 733–734
    squamous cell 728, 733
    transperitoneal spread 733–734
    undifferentiated 733
    see also Epithelial–stromal tumours, ovarian; Ovarian tumours, adenocarcinoma
  carcinoma cells 696
  carcinosarcoma 731
  Carney complex (CNC) **1182**
  of cartilage **866**
  cell proliferation studies **1606**
  cellular fibromas *860*, **860–861**
  Chédiak-Higashi syndrome **1182**
  chemotherapy resistance 1604
  childhood **1163–1177**
  chondroma *865*, **866**
  chondrosarcoma *866*, **866**
  chromosomal imbalances *1604*, **1604**
  classification **693–695**
    histological *694*
  clear cell *694*, 696, 699
    adenocarcinoma *731*, 731–732
    benign 716
    borderline malignancy *727*, *727*
    clonality studies 1602
  c-myc **1597**
  combined sarcoma and epithelial 873
  common epithelial *see* Epithelial–stromal tumours
  Cowden's disease (multiple hamartoma syndrome) **1182**
  CSF/*c-fms* (CSF receptor) **1597**
  Cushing's syndrome **1194**
  cystic teratoma 939
  dermatomyositis **1193–1194**
  disseminated granulomatous disease (BCGosis) 1193
  DNA arrays 1605
  dysgerminoma *see* Dysgerminoma
  early (FIGO stages I and II) **1613–1614**
  ECOPS 1614
  EGFR oncogenes **1596**

Ovarian tumours *(cont'd)*
embryonal rhabdomyosarcoma *864,* 864–865, *865*
endocervical adenocarcinoma 350
endometrial adenocarcinoma coexistence 488
endometrioid *694,* 698–699
  benign 715, *716*
  borderline malignancy 725–727, *726*
  proliferative 726
endometrioid adenocarcinoma 698, 729–731,
   730, 733, 978
  differential diagnosis 729, 730–731
  endometriosis 975–976
  metastatic intestinal tumour vs 883, *883,* 884
  squamous metaplasia 730, *731*
  yolk sac tumour pattern 777
endometrioid stromal sarcoma *870,* 870–872, *871*
endometriosis 974
epithelial/non-epithelial tumour ploidy **1610**
epithelial–stromal (surface)
   see Epithelial–stromal tumours, ovarian
familial, *BRCA1* **1600**
of fat *868,* **868**
fibroma *see* Fibroma(s)
fibrosarcoma *861,* **861,** 873
fibrous tissue **858–861**
ganglioneuroma **867**
germ cell *see* Ovarian germ cell tumours
giant cell tumour **866**
gonadoblastoma *see* Gonadoblastoma
granulocytic sarcoma **946–948,** *947*
granulosa cell *see* Granulosa cell tumours
haemangioma **868–869**
haemangiopericytoma **869**
hepatoid carcinoma *908,* 908–909, *909*
hereditary types 702
Hodgkin's disease 945–946
hyperamylasaemia **1196**
hypercoagulability **1196**
hypertrophic pulmonary osteoarthropathy **1196**
hypothyroidism 1195
K-ras **1596**
Krukenberg *see* Krukenberg tumours
leiomyoma **862**
leiomyosarcoma *see* Leiomyosarcoma
leukaemia **1176**
Leydig cell tumours *see* Leydig cell tumours
Li-Fraumeni syndrome 1187
lipoma 868
liposarcoma 868, *868*
loss of heterozygosity (LOH) **1599**
lymphangioma **870**
lymphangiosarcoma **870**
of lymphatic vessels **870**
lymphoma **1176**
lymphosarcoma 1150
Lynch type II syndrome 1184
malignant schwannoma **867**
Manchester Children's Tumour Registry
   1163–1164, *1164*
masculinisation **1195**
Meigs' syndrome 1196–1197
mesenchymal **857–877**
  histiogenesis problems 857–858
metastases, in vagina *217,* 218
metastatic **879–896,** 1188
  from appendiceal carcinoma 884–885
  from bladder/ureteric/urethral carcinoma 888
  from breast cancer 880, *881,* 881–882
  from bronchial carcinoma 885–886
  from carcinoid tumours *886,* 886–887
  from cervical carcinoma 881, 889
  clinical aspects 881–891
  from colon cancer 880, *882,* 882–884, *883, 884*
  'dirty necrosis' 883, *883*
  from endometrial adenocarcinoma 888–889
  endometrioid pattern 883, *883*
  from extrahepatic bile duct carcinoma 885
  to Fallopian tube *614,* 614–615
  from gallbladder carcinoma 885
  'garland' pattern 883, *883*
  from hepatocellular carcinoma *887,* 887
  incidence 881
  mechanisms of spread (to ovary) 879–880
  from melanomas 888
  mistaken for primary tumours 881–882
  from pancreatic adenocarcinoma 885
  pathological features *880,* 881–891
  primary ovarian tumours vs *883,* 883–884
  primary tumours with 881

from renal adenocarcinoma *887,* 887–888
from sarcomas 889–890
specific forms 881–890
from tubal carcinoma 889
from tumours in unusual sites 890
see also Krukenberg tumours
mixed epithelial 733
mixed germ cell sex cord–stromal *see* Mixed germ
   cell sex cord–stromal tumours (ovarian)
morphometry **1613–1614**
mucinous **694**
  adenofibroma 714–715
  benign *714,* 714–715, *715*
  carcinoid tumours 807, 809–810, *810*
  cystadenoma *see* Mucinous cystadenoma
  cystic teratoma with 697
  cystic tumour with rhabdomyosarcoma 873
  gastrointestinal type 698
  histiogenesis 697–698
  metastatic vs appendiceal tumours 885
  pseudomyxoma ovarii 724
mucinous, borderline 698, **723–725**
  extraovarian spread 724–725
  intestinal type *723,* 723–725, *724*
  with intraepithelial carcinoma 724
  Müllerian (endocervical) type 725, *726*
mucinous adenocarcinoma 695–696, 729, *729*
  colon cancer metastases vs 882
  pelvic endometriosis 977
Müllerian 697
myxoma *867,* **867–868**
nephrotic syndrome 1197
of neural origin 867
neurofibroma **867**
non-Hodgkin's lymphoma **939–945**
  see also Non-Hodgkin's lymphoma
oncocytic 909
oral contraceptives and 700–701
osteoclastoma **866**
osteogenesis imperfecta **1188**
osteogenic sarcoma **866**
osteoma **866**
p53 **1597–1598**
palmar fasciitis **1197**
Peutz–Jeghers syndrome 1182
phaeochromocytoma 853, 854, **867**
ploidy **1609,** 1610
polyarthritis **1197**
polycystic ovarian disease associated 667
polymyositis 1193–1194
of possible mesonephric origin **897–903**
primary, metastases masquerading as 881–882
of probable Wolffian origin **898–902,** *898–902,*
   898–902
  clinical features and behaviour 901
  differential diagnosis 902
  histiogenesis 901–902
  morphology *899,* 899–901, *900, 901*
prognostic indicators 1613–1614
PTEN **1600**
of rete ovarii *902,* 902–903
rhabdomyosarcoma **864–865,** *865,* 873
sarcoma
  combined epithelial tumour 873
  stromal, with thecomatous features 763
  undifferentiated 'stromal' 872–873, *873*
schwannoma **867**
sclerosing stromal **765–766,** *766*
serous *see* Serous tumours, ovarian
serous carcinoma, metastatic to Fallopian tube
   614, 614–615
serous cystadenocarcinoma, metastases in vagina
   217, 218
serous cystadenoma 713–714
Sertoli cell *see* Sertoli cell tumours, of ovary
Sertoli–Leydig cell tumours 704
  see also Sertoli–Leydig cell tumours
sex cord–stromal tumours *see* Ovarian sex
   cord–stromal tumours
sex-cord tumours
  with annular tubules, gonadoblastoma vs
   831
  uterine tumours resembling *575,* **575–576**
situs inversus totalis **1190**
small cell (carcinoma) **903–907**
  desmoplastic small round *906,* 906–907, *907*
  differential diagnosis 905
  hypercalcaemic type *1175,* **1175–1176**
  immunohistochemistry 904, *904*
  pulmonary type 905–906

undifferentiated carcinoma (hypercalcaemic
   type) 903–905, *904*
of smooth muscle **862–864**
squamous, benign 717
squamous cell carcinoma 728, 733
steroid (lipid) cell *see* Steroid (lipid) cell tumours
steroid contraceptives and 1099–1100
of striated muscle **864–865,** *865*
stromal sarcoma with thecomatous features 763
stromal tumours with minor sex-cord elements **765**
subacute cerebellar degeneration **1198**
surface epithelial–stromal **694**
synchronous/metachronous tumours 1603
telomerase activity **1601**
teratomas *see* Ovarian teratoma
of testicular cell type 746
theca cell *see* Theca cell tumour
thecoma–fibroma group tumours 703–704
transitional cell *see* Brenner tumours, ovarian
transitional cell carcinoma, pure 732–733
in tropics **1149–1150**
of uncertain origin **897–911**
undifferentiated 'stromal' sarcoma 872–873, *873*
of vascular origin **868–870,** *869*
Wilms' tumour 903, *903*
Ovarian veins 657
Ovary **635–661**
abscess 683, *683*
accessory, steroid cell tumours arising from 855
actinomycosis 683, *683*
adrenal-type tissue 685
amyloidosis 685, 1193
anatomy **650–657,** *654*
  mature 653–657
  postmenopausal 657
  prepubertal 650, 652
  puberty and 652–653
antibodies to 680, 1016
artifacts misinterpreted as malignant 685–686
blood supply 657
calcification, bilateral 684
carcinoma *see* Ovarian tumours
chemotherapy-induced changes 679
congenital anomalies, absent/reduced follicle pool
   due to 1014–1015
congenital inguinal ectopia 594
cortex 654
  embryology 637
cortical stromal hyperplasia 670, *671*
in Crohn's disease 684
cystic, chronic adnexal torsion 595
cysts 968
  causes 663
  cortical inclusion, serous tumours arising from
   697
  follicle *see* Follicle cysts
  haemorrhagic, endometriosis 968, *968*
  hydropic changes 685, *685*
  hyperreactio luteinalis 675–677, *676*
  multilocular in borderline mucinous tumours
   723
  multiple 668, *668*
  polycystic disease *see* Polycystic ovarian disease
  reduced after HRT 1089
  reduced after steroid contraceptives 1099
  serous cystadenoma 713–714
  solitary **663–665**
  solitary luteinized follicle, of pregnancy 677,
   677
  tamoxifen association 1080–1081
  tumours of Wolffian origin 899
  yolk sac tumours 778, *778*
descent 15
development **643–650**
  see also Ovary, embryology
developmental disorders **1159–1160**
  mixed gonadal dysgenesis **1160**
  Turner's syndrome *see* Turner's syndrome
  see also Ovary, embryology
differentiation **641–643**
dimensions 650
  mature ovary 653
  postmenopausal 657
  during puberty 653
diminished reserve and subfertility 1016
dysfunction
  endometrial bleeding, abnormal 409
  endometrial disturbances 1002–1005
  in luteal phase defect 1018
  oligomenorrhoea 403

dysplasia 696
ectopic 1018
ectopic decidua 682, *682*
ectopic pregnancy within 678
   IUCD use and 1117
   see also Ovarian pregnancy
embryology **635–650**, 897
   early fetal period 646–647, *649*
   embryonic period 646, *647*, *648*
   indifferent gonad transformation 638, 646, 898
   induction 644–645
   late fetal period 647–648, *650*, *651*
   perinatal period 648–650, *652*
endometriosis *see* Ovarian endometriosis
enlargement, primary hypothyroidism 1026
Enterobius vermicularis infection 684
failure
   autoimmune oophoritis 680–681, *681*
   chemo-/radiotherapy causing 1015
   chromosomal abnormalities causing 1015
   hypo-oestrogenic states 403
   premature *see* Ovary, premature failure
Fallopian tube functional co-operation 1006
   interference and infertility 1008
fibromatosis **672–673**, *673*, 1163
fibrothecoma 1017
focal cortical necrosis after CMV infection 683
follicles *see* Follicles, ovarian
functional components 654, 654–655
gonadotrophin-induced hyperstimulation 1029
hermaphrodite, true 1228
heterotopic bone formation 684
hilus cell hyperplasia *673*, **673–674**
   stromal luteoma 847
hilus cells, in endosalpinx/perisalpinx 591
Hodgkin's disease 945–946
hormone function disturbance, endometriosis 963
hydropic change 685, *685*
'hyper-responsive' 1017
hyperstimulation *see* Ovarian hyperstimulation syndrome
hypoplasia 1015
infarction 684
infertility due to 1013–1018
inflammatory disease **682–684**
   infectious granulomatous *683*, 683–684
   non-granulomatous infectious disease 682–683
   non-infectious granulomatous 684
IUCD use and 1114–1115
leukaemia involving 946, *946*
lymphatic drainage 657
   interference leading to massive oedema 672
lymphoblastic leukaemia involving 946, *946*
malignant changes, artifacts misinterpreted as 685–686
malposition 1018
mass, uterus-like 684
massive oedema *671*, **671–672**, *672*, 1163
mesothelial hyperplasia 685
mesothelium 696
metaplasia 695
mixed germ cell sex cord–stromal tumours *see* Mixed germ cell sex cord–stromal tumours
mucicarminophilic histiocytosis 685
myxoma 1172
nerve supply 657
nodular hyperthecosis 846
non-Hodgkin's lymphoma **939–945**
   see also Non-Hodgkin's lymphoma
non-neoplastic disorders **663–692**
   childhood **1162–1163**
pathology, obturator nerve 25
in pelvic inflammatory disease 682–683
pituitary disease **1188–1189**
position 653
   abnormal 1018
pregnancy in *see* Ovarian pregnancy; Ovary, ectopic pregnancy
pregnancy-related lesions **674–678**
premature failure 679, **1016–1017**
   autoimmune oophoritis and 681
   causes 1016–1017
   definition 1016
   idiopathic **681–682**, *682*
   see also Menopause, premature
preovulatory events 1013
progestagens effect 1086, *1086*
pseudoxanthomatous inflammation, granulomatous salpingitis vs 619

radiation-induced changes 679
resistant ovary syndrome (Savage syndrome) 679–680, *680*
sarcoidosis 684, 1189
schistosomiasis 684, 1147
serosa 696
size *see* Ovary, dimensions
splenic–gonadal fusion 684
steroid contraceptives effect 1099–1100
stroma
   decrease in chronic illness 671
   diffuse luteinization 666
   luteoma *846*, **846–847**, *847*
   tumours *see* Epithelial–stromal tumours, ovarian
stromal cells
   enzymes 671
   luteinized 673, 846
   steroid cell tumours 845
stromal hyperplasia 666, **670–671**, *671*, 673
   theca cell tumour 762, 764
stromal hyperthecosis 666, *668*, **668–670**, *669*, 673
   stromal luteoma and 846
stromal luteoma 684
   tubal fimbriae 591, *592*
stromatosis 870
supernumerary, mature teratomas from 795
superovulation, vasculitis **1198**
surface epithelium 696
surgery for infertility, complications 1028
tamoxifen effects 1080–1081
theca-lutein cysts, bilateral, haemangioma 1452
torsion 684
   in absence of tumour 1163
   in massive ovarian oedema 1163
tuberculosis 683–684
vascularisation 650–651
Ovotestis, hermaphrodite, true 1228
Ovulation 656, *656*, 1013
   disorders 1014–1018
      ectopic pregnancy 1049
   dysovulation 1017–1018
   endometrial cycle control 396
   failure 1018
      see also Anovulation
   growth hormone and 1020
   'incessant ovulation' hypothesis 701
   induction 1017, 1090
      complications 1028
   infertility and 991
   inhibition
      by antiprogestins 1087
      by stress 1020
   mechanics 1013–1014
   oestrogen effect after 1072
   prevention by combined steroid contraceptives 1017, 1091, 1099
   timing 1013–1014
Ovulatory agents, ectopic pregnancy 1050
Ovum
   blighted 1053, 1361
   Brownian movement 1006
   pick-up 1006
      failure 1018
      inhibition 1008
      normal 1018
   preparation for sperm penetration 1007
   release failure 1017
   transport 1006
      cervical pregnancy 1062
      isthmic 1007
Oxidative stress, sperm sensitivity 994–995
Oxygen
   concentration, placental villi 1251
   levels, high, placental villi 1251
   supply, normal, pregnancy 1251
Oxyphilic metaplasia 1078, *1078*
   endometrial 413
Oxytocin, water intoxication 1571
Oxyuriasis, vulva 54

P
p53 gene **1597–1599**
   cervical adenocarcinoma 357
   cervical carcinoma 303, **1598–1599**
   endometrial carcinoma 485, **1598**
   endometrial hyperplasia 457
   endometrial intraepithelial carcinoma (EIC) 468

endometrial stromal sarcoma 509
Fallopian tube carcinoma 611, **1598**
Fallopian tube carcinoma in situ 607
high-grade endometrial stromal sarcoma 511
human papillomavirus infection 358
hydatidiform moles **1599**
mdm 2 stabilisation 1598
mesothelioma 627
ovarian carcinoma 702, **1597–1598**
   prognosis 736
primary peritoneal serous carcinoma 925
squamous cell carcinoma of vulva 105
tumour suppressor gene studies **1597–1599**
uterine carcinosarcoma 572
uterine sarcomas **1599**
vulvar carcinoma 105, **1599**
P53 protein, overexpression
   ovarian adenocarcinoma 697
   ovarian carcinoma relationship 701, 702
   squamous cell carcinoma of vulva 108
P185cerbB-2, endocervical neoplasias 360
P185erb-2, endometrial adenocarcinoma 485
Paget's disease
   melanoma, superficial spreading 99
   sweat gland carcinomas of vulva 129
   vulvar 97–100, *98*, *99*
      histological appearance 99
      macroscopic appearance 99
      prognosis 99
      recurrence 100
      regional malignant disease 98
      treatment 100
Palmar fasciitis **1197**
Pampiniform plexus 657
Pancreatic adenocarcinoma, metastatic, to ovary 885
Pancreatic carcinoid tumours, metastatic to ovary *886*, 886–887
Pancreatitis, acute fatty liver of pregnancy 1472
Pancytopenia 1196
Panhypopituitarism 1025
Papanicolaou-stained smears
   clue cells detection 157
   Fallopian tube adenocarcinoma 606
   vaginal tumours 189
   see also Cervical smears
Papillary adenocarcinoma
   cervical 347
      serous 346–347
      villoglandular *347*, 347–348
   endometrial *see* Endometrial carcinoma (adenocarcinoma)
   ovarian 719, 721
Papillary adenofibroma *551*, **551–552**
   uterine cervix 384
Papillary cervicitis, chronic 290
Papillary cystadenofibroma, uterine *551*, **551–552**
Papillary cystadenoma
   broad ligament 625
   serous, ovarian 713–714, *714*
Papillary hidradenoma, vulvar *127*, 127–128
Papillary mesothelioma *see* Mesothelioma, papillary
Papillary serous carcinoma, uterus 349, *349*
'Papillary serous cystadenocarcinoma,' vagina 211
Papillary synctial change, endometrium *413*
Papillary syncytial metaplasia of endometrium 413–414
Papillary tumours
   Fallopian tube 602–603
   serous, ovarian 714, *714*
   see also Papillary adenocarcinoma
Papilloma
   basal cell, vulvar 96, *96*
   Müllerian *see* Müllerian papilloma
   squamous *see* Squamous papilloma
   vagina 193
Papillomatosis, vestibular *87*, 87–88
PAP smears *see* Cervical smears; Papanicolaou-stained smears
Papulo-erosive dermatitis of Jacquet, napkin rash 80
Para-aortic lymph nodes, sampling, endometrial adenocarcinoma 457
Parabasal cell layer, cervical stratified squamous epithelium 252–253, 273
Paraganglioma, of vulva 123
Paragonimus 1148
Paraintroital cysts 182, *182*

Paramesonephric (Müllerian) ducts 41, 695
  aplasia 42
  cysts 623–624, *624*
    cervix 278
  embryonic plasticity 587
  endometrial development 391
  Fallopian tube embryology and 587
  female differentiation 14–17
  fusion defects 43–44
  hyperplasia, endometrium 391
  indifferent embryo 12–13
  male differentiation 13–14
  mesonephric duct involvement in development
      12
  oestrogens and normal development 17
  origin 587
  persistence 13–14
  regression 13
  vaginal cysts 183
  vaginal origin 148
Paraneoplastic pemphigus, vulvar involvement
      71–72
Paraovarian cysts *624*
Paraovarian tumours, of Wolffian origin 901
Parasites, cervical smears **1148**
Parasitic infections
  cervix 284
  endometritis 432
  vulvar 54–55
  see also Protozoal infections
Parasympathetic system, pelvic innervation 26
Parathyroid hormone related protein, small cell
      ovarian tumours 904
Paratubal cysts *624*
Paratubal haemorrhage 592
Paratubal tumours 625
Paraurethral ducts, urethra 31
Paravascular net, villous trees 1249
Paraxial mesoderm 8
Parietal fascia, pelvic floor/walls 24
Parity
  squamous cell carcinoma of cervix 298
  see also Multiparity
Parvovirus B19 infection, placental examination
      1317
Patent ductus arteriosus 1544
PCNA *see* Proliferating cell nuclear antigen (PCNA)
PCR *see* Polymerase chain reaction (PCR)
Peg cells
  benign papillary serous tumours of ovary 714
  Fallopian tubes 587, *587*
Peliosis, steroid contraceptives and 1100
Pelvic bones
  embryonic development 21
  sex differences 21
Pelvic ectopic kidney **1519**
Pelvic floor *22, 23,* 23–24
  parietal fascia 24
Pelvic haematomas, postpartum haemorrhage 1561
Pelvic inflammatory disease (PID)
  causative agents 996
  diagnostic curettage causing 1027
  ectopic pregnancy and 1048, 1117
  endometritis 420
  HIV/AIDS 1152
  infertility 993–994
  inflammatory disease of ovary and 682
  IUCD use and 1114–1115
    causative organisms 1114–1115
    risk factors 1114
  Mycoplasma hominis 427
  ovulation failure 1018
  risk factors 620, 993
  steroid contraceptives and 1099
  terminology 617
  in tropics **1134**
  see also Salpingitis
Pelvic irradiation, vaginal cancer pathogenesis 188
Pelvic lymph nodes 28
  adenosarcoma (uterine) spread 570–571
  endometriosis 969–970
  sampling, endometrial adenocarcinoma 457
Pelvic mesothelium, metaplastic potential 964
Pelvic nerves 24–26
Pelvic plexuses 26
'Pelvic relaxation' syndrome 150, 152
Pelvic sepsis, intrauterine contraceptive device
      (IUD) 1196
Pelvic splanchnic nerves 25
Pelvic ureter 29

Pelvic veins 27–28
  adenofibroma invasion 552
Pelvic venous plexuses, bacterial invasion 1562
Pelvic vessels 26–28
Pelvic viscera 28–38
  bladder 29–31
  pelvic ureter 29
  rectum 28–29
  urethra 31
Pelvic walls *22,* 22–23
  parietal fascia 24
Pelvis
  anatomy **28–38**
  fascia 24
  fractures, vaginal damage association 152
  midline section *20*
  nerves 24–26
  peritoneum 28
    midline section *28*
  tuberculosis, infertility 1134
Pemphigoid
  bullous, vulvar 70
  cicatricial *70,* 70–71
Pemphigoid gestationis **1193**
Pemphigus, chronic benign familial *61*
  vulvar genetic disorders 60–61
Pemphigus, IgA 73–74
Pemphigus vegetans *71–72*
Pemphigus vulgaris 71
  cervical ulceration 291
  vaginal changes 154, 1183
Pentastomiasis 1148
Peptostreptoccus, salpingitis 620
Perianal dermatitis of newborn 80
Pericarditis, idiopathic **1553**
Perifolliculitis, eosinophilic 1016
Perimenopausal bleeding 409
Perinatal mortality
  circumvallate placentation 1275
  dichorionic–diamniotic twin placentation 1581
  group B haemolytic streptococci 1305
  intrahepatic cholestasis of pregnancy 1468–1469
  monochorionic–diamniotic twin placentation
      1580
  umbilical artery, single 1294
  umbilical cord haematomas 1299
Perineal membrane 37, *37*
Perineal pouch
  deep 37
  superficial 37
Perineum *37*
  abnormalities **1158**
  anatomy 35
  development of external genitalia 19
Perinuclear clearing, condyloma acuminatum of
      vagina *162*
Perinuclear haloes, trichomoniasis of cervix 284
Periovarian adhesions 1018, *1019*
Peripartal cardiomyopathy **1551–1553,** *1552*
  dilated (congestive) cardiomyopathy 1552
  histology 1552, *1553*
  outcome 1553
Perisalpingitis 1010
  chronic lymphofollicular 616
Peritoneal cytology
  carcinosarcoma (uterine) 562
  endometrial adenocarcinoma 481–482
Peritoneal field defect 925
Peritoneal fluid 1018, *1019*
Peritoneotubal exchange, Fallopian tube
      development 586–587
Peritoneum
  carcinoma
    primary 627, *924,* 924–925
    serous (low-grade) *923, 924,* 924–925
  clear cell lesions 927
  diffuse leiomyomatosis **537–538,** *928,* **928–929**
  ectopic decidua **927–928,** *928*
  endocervicosis and 925–926, *926*
  endometriotic lesions 965
  gliomatosis 792, 793, *795, 796*
  inclusion cysts
    endosalpingiosis vs 922
    multiloculated 914–915, *915*
  infertility due to disorders 1018–1019
  keratin granulomas
    atypical polypoid adenomyoma association 574
    granulomatous salpingitis vs 619
  Müllerian metaplasia 922
  'Müllerianosis' 921

nodules, immature teratoma 792
oestrogen/progesterone receptors 1028
pathology **913–920**
  see also Mesothelial lesions
postoperative cysts 914, *915*
pseudoxanthomatous inflammation,
    granulomatous salpingitis vs 619
secondary Müllerian system 920
  see also Müllerian system, secondary
serous tumours
  borderline 922–923, *923*
  broad ligament 627
  carcinoma *924,* 924–925
  squamous lesions 927
  transitional cell tumours 927
  Walthard nests **926–927,** *927*
Peritonitis
  chemical 797
  Neisseria meningitidis 431
  pelvic lipogranulomatous, granulomatous
      salpingitis vs 619
  recurrent, diffuse malignant mesothelioma of
      peritoneum after 917
  sclerosing 764
Perivaginal plexus, vaginal lymphatics 149
Perivascular stromal cells, predecidual change 395
Perivasculitis villous stem vessels, maternal syphilis
      infection 1314
Perivillous fibrin deposition *1276, 1278*
  miscarriage 1437
  placental villi function 1276–1278
Perivillous fibrin plaques, functional villous tissue
      1277
Permissive infection, human papillomavirus 299
Perrault syndrome **1190**
Persistent Müllerian duct syndrome
  MIS gene mutations 1217
  pseudohermaphroditism, male 1217
Persistent trophoblastic disease
  see Trophoblastic disease, persistent
Pessaries, chronic placement, vaginal lesions 153
Pessary ulcer, vaginal *219,* 220
Petechial haemorrhages 1532
  hypertensive diseases of pregnancy 1564
Peutz–Jeghers syndrome **1188**
  Carney complex (CNC) **1182**
  lipid-rich Sertoli cell tumours, of ovary 757
  metastatic adenocarcinoma 350
  ovarian neoplasms in 759
  ovarian sex cord–stromal tumours with annular
      tubules 758, 759, 1170–1171, 1188
Pflüger's tubes 832
PG-MN1, ovarian granulocytic sarcoma 948
pH
  vaginal *see* Vagina, pH
  vaginal fluids 151
Phaeochromocytoma, ovarian 853, 854, **867**
Phenotype, hermaphrodite, true 1228
Phenotypic female, gonadal dysgenesis 1223
Phenotypic male
  gonadal dysgenesis *1226*
  hermaphroditism, true, haematuria 1228
Phosphatase and tensin homologue deleted on
      chromosome ten gene *see* PTEN gene
Phthirius pubis (crab louse), vulvar infection 54
Phyllodes tumours of vulva 132
Phyto-oestrogens, effect on Fallopian tubes 1008
Piedra (trichosporosis nodosa), vulvar infection 56
Pigmentation, vulvar
  disorders 67–69
  miscellaneous causes 69
Pigmentosis tubae 622
Pilar tumour, vulva 128
'Pill-induced' cholestasis, intrahepatic cholestasis of
      pregnancy 1468
Pilomatrixoma, in mature teratoma 803
Pilosebaceous unit disorders, vulvar involvement 82
Pineal gland, dysfunction 1021
Pinwheel effect, endometritis 423
Pin-worm *see* Enterobius vermicularis
Pipelle cannula, endometrial sampling 446, 456
Pipelle sampler, endometrial sampling 392
Piriformis muscle, pelvic wall 23
Pituitary gland 1020
  adenomas 1021, 1022, *1022,* 1024
    complications 1024
    surgery 1028
    vasculature 1024
  amyloidosis 1021
  anatomical lesions 1021–1022

disease **1188–1189**
ischaemia, in pregnancy **1535**
disorders 1021–1024
failure 1025
haemorrhage 1024
infarction 1021, 1024
inflammation 1021
surgery for infertility, complications 1028
tumours 1021–1022
see also Hypothalamus–pituitary–ovary (HPO)
axis
Pityriasis versicolor, vulvar infection 55–56
Placenta
abdominal pregnancy 1063
abnormalities, miscarriage 1437–1438
abruption *see* Abruptio placentae
accessory lobe *1275*, 1275–1276
blastocyst implantation 1276
fetal haemorrhage 1276
postpartum bleeding 1276
vascular supply 1275
anastomoses *see* Placental anastomoses
anatomy **1233–1272**
barrier, layers 1236
bilobate *see* Bilobate placenta
calcification 1285
cell columns and islands 1259–1260
chimerism, vanishing twin syndrome 1585
chronic twin–twin transfusion 1581–1582
circummarginate 1274
circumvallate *see* Circumvallate placenta
conjoined twin 1586–1587
development **1233–1272**
abnormalities 1274–1276
early **1233–1236**, *1234*
early villous stages 1235–1236
stages *1237*, **1261–1268**
see also Placentation
dichorionic *see* Dichorionic placenta
dysfunction 1025
examination, indications 1309
extramembranous pregnancy 1306
fetal death 1313
fetal vasculature, increased resistance and
intrauterine growth retardation 1311
fibrinoid 1261
functional reserve capacity 1283
growth, primary defect 1282–1284
haemangioma *see* Placental haemangioma
haematoma 1284–1285
marginal, miscarriage 1437
sites of occurrence *1283*
hepatocellular adenoma 1455
histological abnormalities 1285–1293
miscarriage 1438–1442
hyperoxia, fetal hypoxia 1311
hypoxic hypercapillarised, villi 1253
immunological defence mechanism,
neuroblastoma cells 1459
infarction 1279–1282, *1280, 1281*
antepartum haemorrhage 1351
histology early infarct 1279
histology old infarct 1279
inadequate transformation of spiral arteries
1282
pre-eclampsia 1309, 1342
thrombosis 1280
insufficiency, intrauterine fetal growth retardation
1344
ischaemic damage 1310
lacunae 1234
leiomyoma 1455
leukaemia *1458*
listeriosis, microabcesses 1315, *1315*
macroscopic abnormalities 1273–1285
manual removal
air embolism 1567
placenta creta 1349
mass, fetal growth 1283
maternal blood flow 1235
mesenchymal dysplasia, haemangioma 1452
metastases
from fetal neoplasms **1457–1460**
from maternal neoplasms **1455–1457**
of non-melanotic neoplasms 1455
monochorionic, vascular anastomoses *1578,*
1578–1579
death of one twin 1584
mosaicism
aneuploid fetus 1436

miscarriage, spontaneous 1435
vanishing twin syndrome 1585
non-villous parts **1253–1261**, *1257*
pathology **1273–1293**
peripheral extension 1336
potential for further growth 1283
premature aging, accelerated villous development
1286
prematurely delivered 1312
preterm maturation 1252
schistosomiasis 1148
septa 1259
structure **1236–1246**
mature *1238, 1239*
teratomas *1454*, 1454–1455
fetus acardius amorphus 1454
thrombi 1285
tissue, intratubal, tubal rupture 1059
toxoplasmosis *1318*
hydropic form 1318
materno-fetal rhesus incompatibility vs 1318
trabeculae 1234
tubal pregnancy 1054
tumours, non-trophoblastic **1449–1464**
primary 1449–1454
tumours, trophoblastic *see* Placental site,
trophoblastic tumour; Trophoblastic
neoplasms
twin
pathological examination 1587–1588
pathological features 1579–1580
placentation type and zygosity 1587
septum *1588*
vascular anastomoses 1578–1579, 1588
vascular malfunction, acardiac fetus 1584
vaso-regulation 1242
villous structure **1236–1246**
water content, villous oedema 1289
Placenta accreta 1347, *1347*
maternal death 1561
Placenta creta 1347–1349
ectopic pregnancy 1348
primiparae 1349
Placenta extrachorialis *1274,* 1274–1275
Placenta increta 1347
Placental abruption *see* Abruptio placentae
Placental anastomoses
arterio-venous 1578
chronic twin–twin transfusion 1582
identification 1588
superficial 1578
identification 1588
Placental aromatase defect
female pseudohermaphroditism 1214
virilisation, maternal 1214
Placental bed 1258, *1334*
biopsy *see* Biopsy
giant cells, early placentation 1333
pathology **1336–1345**
spiral arteries, pre-eclampsia 1337
vascular malformations, retroplacental
haematoma 1284
Placental disc, placental membranacea 1275
Placental:fetal weight ratio
intrauterine fetal growth retardation 1310
pre-eclampsia 1309
primary defect in placental growth 1283
Placental haemangioma 1449–1454, *1450, 1451,*
1452
abruptio placentae 1453
atypical 1451
changes associated 1452
classification 1451
clinical effects 1452–1454
complications
affecting fetus and neonate 1453–1454
during labour 1453
during pregnancy 1452–1453
degenerative changes 1450–1451
histology *1450*, 1450–1451
nature and origin 1452
recurrence 1454
Placental lactogen, embryonal carcinoma 788
Placental membrane roll examination 1587
Placental site
giant cells, early placentation 1333
nodules 1415, 1416, *1416*
reaction, detection in miscarriage material
1442
trophoblastic tumour

differential diagnosis 1414, 1415, 1416
genetic polymorphisms **1407–1408**
immunocytochemistry **1407**
Ki-67 1415
macroscopic appearances *1405,* **1405–1406**
metastases 1406–1407
microscopic appearances **1406–1407,**
1406–1408
nephrotic syndrome 1197
ovarian involvement 1409
pathology **1405–1409**
prognosis **1408–1409**
treatment 1409
ultrastructure **1407**
uterine cervix 382
Placental substance tears 1587
Placental villi *1244, 1245, 1250*
abnormalities 1285–1292
fetal blood flow reduction 1288
maternal uteroplacental blood supply, reduced
1287
pathogenesis unknown 1288–1290
villous maturation 1285–1286
avascular, fetal artery thrombosis 1282, *1282*
components, immunohistochemical markers
1244–1245
cross-sectional features 1253
development, pregnancy *1247*
differentiation 1249
fetal vessels, endothelial necrosis 1316
fibrinoid necrosis 1288–1289, *1289*
fibrosis, fetal death 1313
formation in early placentation 1332
histological appearance 1438, *1438*
placenta and fetal chromosomal abnormalities
1440
hypoxic hypercapillarised 1253
immaturity
fetal growth retardation 1286
syphilis infection 1314
infarction, fibromuscular sclerosis 1292
infiltrate 1291
maturation
abnormalities 1285–1287
accelerated, pre-eclampsia 1286
normal 1253
morphology, post-mortem changes 1313
normal mature 1253
oedema 1289, *1289*
villous immaturity vs 1289
parenchyma, listeriosis 1314
placenta membranacea 1275
pre-eclampsia 1309, *1309*
'pulse,' fetal death 1314
stroma 1242–1244
inflammatory damage due to placental CMV
infection 1317
structure **1236–1246**
tangential sectioning 1253
terminal *see* Terminal villi
tertiary villi formation 1236
tissue of placenta
from miscarriages, morphological classification
1441
morphometric analysis 1440
trophoblastic neoplasms **1413**, *1413–1414*
tubal pregnancy 1053–1054
Placental villitis *see* Villitis, placental
Placental villous trees **1246–1253**
angioarchitecture 1249–1251
development 1247–1249
early expansion 1236
maternal venous outlets 1252
maturation, placenta function 1286
mature placental *1243*
placenta **1246–1253**
primary villi branching 1235
types *1248, 1249*
structure 1246–1247
Placenta membranacea 1275
placenta praevia 1275
Placenta percreta 1347
Placenta praevia
maternal death 1561
placenta creta 1347
placenta membranacea 1275
Placentation
defects **1345–1354**
spontaneous miscarriage 1345, *1346*
trophoblastic disease 1346–1347

Placentation (cont'd)
dichorionic–diamniotic twin
   see Dichorionic–diamniotic twin
   placentation
dizygotic twin 1576–1577
early **1332–1336**
   migratory trophoblast 1332–1335
extrachorial, clinical significance 1275
Fallopian tube 1052, 1053
haemochorial, migratory trophoblast 1332
inadequate, miscarriage 1436
migratory trophoblast 1332–1335
monochorionic–diamniotic type
   see Monochorionic–diamniotic twin
   placentation
monochorionic–monoamniotic type 1577,
   1580–1581
monochorionic type 1577
monozygotic twins see Monozygotic twins
multiple pregnancy **1589**
trichorionic–triamniotic, trizygotic triplets
   1588–1589
triplet **1588–1589**, *1589*
tubal pregnancy 1052–1053, *1057*
twin, clinical features 1580–1581
Virchow's triad and 1351
zygosity 1578
see also Placenta, development
Placentomegaly, haemangioma 1452
Placentone 1252
architecture 1251–1253
centres 1249, 1252
perilobular zone 1252
Plasma cell cervicitis, chronic 281
Plasma cell orificial mucositis 80
Plasma cells, ectocervix 274
Plasmacytoma
ovarian 942
vaginal 954
Plasmacytosis circumorificialis 80
Plaster of Paris pelvis 1134
Platelets
adhesion, perivillous fibrin plaque formation
   1278
adhesiveness, post-delivery 1543
Pleomorphic rhabdomyosarcomas, cervix 378
Plexiform tumourlets, epithelioid smooth muscle
   tumours 529
Plexiform tumours, epithelioid smooth muscle
   tumours 529
Plial implantation, tubal pregnancy 1051, *1052*
Ploidy analysis **1382–1383, 1608–1612, 1611, *1612***
AgNORs 1383, **1386**
cervical carcinoma **1611**
endometrial carcinoma 482, **1610–1611**
endometrial stromal sarcomas 1611
fallopian tube carcinoma **1610**
flow cytometry 1608, 1609
hydatidiform moles **1382–1383, 1386, 1611, *1612***
   partial 1363–1364
miscarriage 1367–1368
ovarian carcinoma **1609**
ovarian epithelial tumours **1610**
ovarian non-epithelial tumours **1610**
persistent trophoblastic disease **1386**
squamous cell carcinoma of vulva 108
uterine sarcomas **1611**
vulvar squamous cell carcinoma **1611**
see also Aneuploidy
Pneumomediastinum, maternal death
   1571
Pneumonia
bilateral haemorrhagic, hypertensive disease of
   pregnancy 1564
congenital, chorioamnionitis 1306
Polar body twinning 1576
Polyarteritis nodosa
cervical lesions 291
necrotising arteritis **1191**
Polyarthritis **1197**
Polycystic liver disease, pregnancy 1484
Polycystic ovarian disease **666–668**
clomiphene effect 1076
continuum of disorders 666
diabetes mellitus 1183
endometrial carcinoma and 1026
endometrial hyperplasia link 445
genetic predisposition 995
gross pathology 666, *667*
histology 667, *667*

hyperprolactinaemia and 1024
hypothyroidism 1184
insulin resistance 666, 670
lipodystrophy **1188**
masculinisation 1195
miscarriage, recurrent 1433
ovarian tumours associated 667
pathophysiology 667
surgery, complications 1028
terminology 665, 666
see also Stein-Leventhal syndrome
Polycystic renal disease **1189**
adult *1519*, **1519**
Polycythaemia, uterine leiomyoma 517
Polyembroma 788
Polyhydramnios
monochorionic–diamniotic twin placentation
   1580
placental haemangiomas 1452–1453
Polymerase chain reaction (PCR)
reverse transcriptase, Ewing's sarcoma of vulva
   124
spirochaetal DNA 1314
Polymorphonuclear leucocyte infiltrate
endometritis 421
extraplacental membranes 1303, *1304*
Polymyositis **1536–1537**
ovarian cancer 1193–1194
Polyneuropathy, acute inflammatory demyelinating
   1536
Polyostotic fibrous dysplasia 664, **1189**
Polyp(s)
adenofibromatous, endometrial 417
adenomyomatous, endometrial 417–418
cervical see Cervix, polyps
ectocervical 290
endocervical see Endocervical polyps
endometrial see Endometrial polyps
Fallopian tube 602–603
   infertility due to 1009
fibroepithelial stromal, vaginal 193–195, *194*
glial 290
malignant cervical 290
mesodermal stromal 290
postmenopausal bleeding 409
tamoxifen-associated 417
vaginal 193–195, *194, 195*
Polypoid adenomyoma, atypical see Adenomyoma,
   atypical polypoid
Polypoid stroma, simple endometrial polyps 416
Polypoid endometriosis 968–969
Polypoid microglandular hyperplasia 290
Polysomies, high-grade endometrial stromal
   sarcoma 509
Polyspermy, prevention by isthmus 1007
Polyvinylpyrrolideone, mucicarminophilic
   histiocytosis of ovary 685
Pomeroy technique, tubal sterilisation 596,
   597–598
Porphyria, hereditary hepatic, pregnancy
   1483–1484
Porphyria cutanea tarda, steroid contraceptives and
   1106
Portal hypertension, pregnancy in 1483
splenic artery rupture 1481
Posterior femoral cutaneous nerve, pelvic nerve
   supply 25
Post-hysterectomy pregnancy **1063**
Postinflammatory hypopigmentation, vulvar 69
Postinflammatory pigmentation, vulvar 67–68
Postmenopausal bleeding see Bleeding,
   vaginal/uterine
Postmenopausal women
adenofibromas 551
adenomyosis 498
atrophic vaginitis 155–156, *156*
carcinosarcoma, uterine 559
clear cell adenocarcinoma of endometrium 470
colposcopy 323
endometrial hyperplasia 444–445
endometrial tuberculosis 430
endometrium *402*, 402–403
Fallopian tube changes 587
hormonal therapy see Hormone replacement
   therapy (HRT)
hydrosalpinx 596–597
infectious vaginitis 160
malignant change in mature teratomas 801
oestrogens effect on endometrium 1072, *1072*
osseous metaplasia 414

ovary anatomy 657
stromal luteoma 846
tamoxifen effect 1076
Tibolone therapy 1090
uterine adenosarcoma 552
vaginal trichomoniasis 173
Postoperative spindle cell nodule
pseudosarcomatous lesions of cervix 380
vulvar 85
Postpartum atrophic vaginitis 180
Postpartum cerebral angiopathy 1524
Postpartum depression 1523
Postpartum endometritis
acute non-specific 419
Mycoplasma hominis 427
Postpartum fistulae **1151**
Postpartum haemorrhage *1352*, 1353–1354
cirrhosis 1483
intrahepatic cholestasis of pregnancy 1469
Marfan's syndrome 1547
pituitary infarction 1021
placental accessory lobe 1276
secondary 1353, *1353*
Postpartum pelvic sepsis, chorioamnionitis 1306
Postpartum pyrexia, *Mycoplasma hominis* 427
Postpartum sterilisation, ectopic pregnancy 1047
Potter's syndrome, juvenile-type granulosa cell
   tumour 752
Pouch of Douglas, recto-uterine 28
Pox virus infections, vulvar 59–60
Prader–Willi syndrome **1189**
Prechordal plate 6
Precocious pseudopuberty, isosexual
   see Pseudopuberty, isosexual precocious
Precocious puberty see Puberty, precocious
Predecidual change in endometrium 401
Prednisone, adverse effects 1029
Pre-eclampsia 1337, **1503**, 1505, **1505–1511**, *1506*
abruptio placentae 1342
acute atherosis 1339–1341, *1340*
blood pressure measurement 1505
diabetic glomerulopathy in pregnancy 1517
encephalopathy **1524–1525**
epithelial cells 1508
gestational hypertension 1505, 1506
glomerular basement membrane 1508, *1509*
glomerular capillary endotheliosis 1506, *1507*,
   1511
glomerular tuft/capsule adhesions 1510–1511
heart failure *1551*, **1551**
HELLP syndrome 1475–1476
hydatidiform moles 1505
immune tolerance 1506
intrauterine fetal growth retardation 1344
intravascular coagulation 1506
mesangial cells 1508, *1508, 1509*
multiple pregnancy 1505
oedema 1505
pathogenesis **1506**
perivillous fibrin deposition 1277
placenta 1309–1310
placental examination 1308–1309
placental infarction 1280
predisposing factors 1505
proteinuria 1505, 1512
recurrent and latent renal disease 1344
renal changes **1506–1511**
spiral arteries, physiological changes 1337–1339,
   1338, 1339
subendothelial space 1508, *1510*
thromboplastin 1506
tubules 1511
uterine malformations 48
vascular changes 1511
see also Eclampsia
Pregnancy
abdominal see Abdominal pregnancy
acute fatty liver **1469–1474**
   see also Acute fatty liver of pregnancy (AFLP)
adenomyosis and 498
adolescence 1163
aneurysms 1550–1551
aplastic anaemia and *Clostridium perfringens* 431
Asherman's syndrome 433
basal endometrium 396
cardiovascular system see Cardiovascular system,
   diseases in pregnancy
cervical see Cervical pregnancy
cervical carcinoma 333
cervical cytology 247, *262*

cervical physiology 275–276
chemotherapy 958
in childhood and adolescence 1163
cirrhosis 1483
complete molar *see* Hydatidiform mole
complications and placental haemangiomas
    1452–1453
confirmation following miscarriage 1442
corpora lutea 677
diabetes mellitus 1344
diffuse peritoneal leiomyomatosis 928, 929
ectopic *see* Ectopic pregnancy
endometrial bleeding, abnormal 409
endometrial glandular secretion 401
endometritis 419
extra-amniotic 1306–1307
extramembranous 1306
gallbladder pathology **1465–1494**
Gardnerella vaginalis infection of vagina 166
granulosa cell proliferations 677–678, *678*
haemorrhagic nodule 221–222, *222*
hepatitis, acute viral 1478–1479
herpetic infections 163
heterotropic 1051
high altitude and chorangiomas 1452
hilus cell hyperplasia *673*, 673–674
HIV/AIDS 1152
hyperparathyroidism 1026
hyperreactio luteinalis 675–677, *676*
hypertensive disorders 1336–1344
idiopathic jaundice 1100
increased AFP, causes 793
intravenous leiomyomatosis (uterine) 534
IUCD use and 1116–1117
kidney *see* Renal diseases, in pregnancy
Krukenberg tumours and 892
late luteal phase endometrial biopsy *1001*,
    1001–1002, *1002*
liver function **1465–1467**
liver function tests 1466
liver pathology **1465–1494**
liver transplantation 1484
loss *see* Miscarriage; Termination of pregnancy
luteoma *674*, 674–675, *675*
    steroid cell tumours vs 854–855
    virilisation 1214
lymphoma and **957–958**
mature teratoma association 797
metaplastic papillary tumour (tubal) 602–603
molar *see* Hydatidiform mole
multiple *see* Multiple pregnancy
nervous system *see* Nervous system diseases, in
    pregnancy
non-gonorrhoeal vaginosis, bacterial 159–160
ovarian 678
ovarian lesions **674–678**
ovarian lymphomas and 940, 945
ovarian tumour risk and 700
protective effect on ovarian adenocarcinoma 700
rate after IUCD use 1118
rate after tubal sterilisation reversal 990
rate during IUCD use 1116
recurrent loss 995
    see also Miscarriage
risk after tubal sterilisation 597
Sertoli cell proliferations 677–678
sex cord–stromal tumours (ovarian) **760–761**,
    761
solitary luteinized follicle cyst 677, *677*
termination *see* Termination of pregnancy
tubal ectopic, endometrium 420
twin *see* Twin pregnancy
uterine adaptions **1328–1332**
uterine leiomyoma 536
vaginal candidiasis 172
vaginitis 159
yolk sac tumours association 777
Pregnancy-associated plasma protein A (PAPP-A),
    tubal pregnancy 1055
Preimplantation phase embryogenesis 4
Prelacunar stage placental development 1233–1234
Premature delivery *see* Preterm delivery
Premature onset of labour *see* Preterm labour
Premature ovarian failure *see* Ovary, premature
    failure
Preterm delivery
    before 28 weeks gestation 1312
    chorioamnionitis 1305
    intrahepatic cholestasis of pregnancy 1468
    placental examination 1312–1313

premature rupture of membranes 1306
villous maturation, accelerated 1286
Preterm labour
    chorioamnionitis 1305
    infective species associated 160
    IUCD use and 1116
    marginal haematoma 1284–1285
    monochorionic–diamniotic twin placentation 1580
    necrotising funisitis 1300
    perivillous fibrin deposition 1277–1278
    placental haemangioma 1453
    placenta membranacea 1275
Preterm maturation of placenta, mature placentone
    centres 1252
Prickle cell layer (parabasal) 252–253, 273
Primary biliary cirrhosis, fetal microchimerism
    1481–1482
Primary endoderm 5
Primary villi, placental development 1235
Primiparae, placenta creta 1349
Primitive body stalk 5
Primitive streak 5–6
Primordial germ cells *see* Germ cell(s)
Procidentia, vaginal carcinoma aetiology 188
Products of conception *see* Conceptus
Progestagen-only contraceptives ('mini-pill')
    1091–1092, **1095–1106**
    effect on endometrium 1095–1097, *1096*
Progestagens **1082–1086**
    antagonists 1086–1087
    contraceptives
        combined oral 1091
        depot injection 1092, 1097
        effect on endometrium 1092–1095, *1093*, *1094*
        implants 1092
        IUCD devices 1108–1109, *1109*, *1110*
        progestagen-only *see* Progestagen-only
            contraceptives ('mini-pill')
        see also Combined steroid contraceptives (oral)
    effect on endometriosis 1086
    effect on endometrium *1082*, 1082–1084, *1083*,
        1084, *1085*
    prolonged usage 1083
    effect on myometrium 1084
    effect on ovary 1086, *1086*
    effects on cervix 1084
    effects on extragenital sites 1086
    for endometrial hyperplasia therapy 453, *453*,
        453–454
    in HRT 1087
    hypospadias in male offspring 1214
    pseudohermaphroditism, female 1214
    therapeutic
        cervix changes 1192
        endometrial adenocarcinoma 486, 487, *487*
        endometriosis *591*
        endometrium 1192
        intrauterine, endometrial adenocarcinoma 488
        low-grade endometrial stromal sarcoma 511
        miscarriage prevention 1433
        reversal of endometrial hyperplasia 1073
Progesterone
    endometrial cycle control 396
    endometrial secretory phase 400
    hypothalamus inhibition 1013
    levels in pregnancy, hepatic function 1465
    measurement, mid-luteal phase 405
    plasma, endometrium in pregnancy 1328
    role in uterine leiomyoma aetiology 516
    secretion
        luteal phase insufficiency 405
        by luteinized thecal cells 1014
    squamous epithelium of cervix 253
Progesterone receptors
    benign metastasising uterine leiomyoma 527
    defect, endometrial disorders 408
    endometrial adenocarcinoma 482
    low-grade endometrial stromal sarcoma 511
    ovarian carcinoma prognosis 736
    peritoneal expression 1028
    reduced by copper IUCD 1110
Progestins *see* Progestagens
Progressive familial intrahepatic cholestasis 1468
Prolactin, excess secretion 1024
Prolactinaemia, mature teratoma and 797
Prolactinoma 1022, *1022*
    bromocriptine treatment 1022, 1024
Prolapse
    ectocervical hyperplasia 288
    mitral valve **1544**

tubal *see* Fallopian tube
urethral mucosa *86*, *87*
uterus, non-stromal lesions 510
Proliferating cell nuclear antigen (PCNA) 1381,
    1606
    cervical carcinoma 1607
    endometrial carcinoma 482–483, 1607
    hydatidiform moles 1381, 1386, 1607
    ovarian carcinoma 1606
        prognosis 736
    vulvar carcinoma 1607
Proliferating trichilemmal tumour, vulvar 128
Proliferative cells, endometrial epithelium 394
Proliferative phase *see* Endometrial cycle;
    Endometrium, proliferative phase
Pronephros, urinary system development 11
Prostacyclin (PGI$_2$), endometriosis 981
Prostaglandin E$_2$
    follicle stimulating hormone interaction 1013
    vaginal administration and uterine rupture 1569
Prostaglandin F
    amniotic fluid embolism syndrome 1565
    tubal motility and endometriosis 981
Prostaglandins
    chorioamnionitis and premature onset of labour
        1305
    endometriosis associated infertility 981
    ovulation process 1014
Prostatic plexus, autonomic innervation of pelvis 25
Prostatic tissue, ectopic in cervix 280
Prosthetic heart valves *see* Heart valves
Protease inhibitor enzyme secretion, cervical mucus
    277
Protein, serum concentration, pregnancy 1466
Protein C deficiency 1103
    fetal artery thrombosis 1282
    thromboembolism 1561
Protein S deficiency, thromboembolism 1561
Proteinuria, pre-eclampsia 1511, 1512
Proteus mirabilis, malacoplakia 424
Prothrombin gene mutation, miscarriage 1435
Proton beam therapy, arteriovenous malformations
    1530
Protozoal infections
    in tropics **1140–1141**
    vaginal 173–176
        see also Trichomonas vaginalis
    vulvar 55
    see also Parasitic infections
Pruritus
    intrahepatic cholestasis of pregnancy 1467
    vulval, candidiasis 171
Pruritus gravidarum *see* Intrahepatic cholestasis, of
    pregnancy
Prussian blue stain, amniotic macrophages 1303
Psammocarcinoma 729
    serous, of peritoneum 923–924, *924*
Psammoma bodies
    cervical smears 281
    endometrioid adenocarcinoma 730
    endometrioid carcinoma 469
    endosalpingiosis 593, 922
    primary peritoneal serous carcinoma 925
    serous adenocarcinoma (ovarian) 728–729, *729*
    serous borderline ovarian tumours 718, *719*
    well-differentiated papillary mesothelioma
        (peritoneal) 916
Pseudoacanthosis nigrans, vulvar hyperpigmentation
    68
'Pseudoactinomycotic radiate granules' 683
Pseudocarcinomatous hyperplasia, vulvar *123*
Pseudodecidualisation, of stromal tumours 510
Pseudofolliculitis, vulvar 82
Pseudohermaphroditism
    female 1212–1214
        danazol association 1028
        fetal defects 1212–1214
        maternal influence 1214
    male 1160, 1161, *1162*, 1214–1220
        end-organ defects 1217–1219
        gonadal defects, primary 1215–1217
        gonadoblastoma 821, 823, 824
Pseudohypoparathyroidism 1016
Pseudomembranous inflammation, genital tract
    425, 996
Pseudomyxoma ovarii 724, 729
Pseudomyxoma peritonei 725, *725*
    broad ligament involvement 625
    Fallopian tube metastases 613
    ovarian metastases vs 885

Pseudopregnancy
  dysgerminoma and 773
  therapy, endometriosis 981–982
Pseudopuberty
  heterosexual, steroid cell tumours association 850
  isosexual precocious
    dysgerminoma and 773
    juvenile-type granulosa cell tumour 752
    mixed germ cell sex cord–stromal tumours and 833
    non-gestational choriocarcinoma 786
Pseudosarcoma botryoides
  cervical 380
  vaginal 193–195, 194, 197
Pseudosarcomatous lesions of uterine cervix 380
'Pseudosarcomatous' pattern, Krukenberg tumours 891
Pseudo-sulphur granules 1113, 1113
Pseudovaginal perineoscrotal hypospadias 1219–1220
Pseudoxanthoma cells, endometriosis 969, 969
Pseudoxanthoma elasticum, vulvar genetic disorders 62
Pseudoxanthomatous inflammation, ovary/peritoneum, granulomatous salpingitis vs 619
Psoriasis 72, 73
Psychogenic hypothesis, infertility 991–992
Psychological factors, infertility 991–992
Psychomotor abnormalities, short umbilical cord 1293
Psychosis
  Korsakoff's 1531
  puerperal 1523
PTEN gene 465, 1600
  mutations
    endometrial adenocarcinoma 485
    endometrial hyperplasia 454, 457
    endometrioid tumours of ovary 698
    ovarian endometriosis, atypical 975
  as tumour suppressor 455
Ptosis (blepharophimosis) 1182
Pubertal cervix, metaplasia 261
Puberty 652–653
  5 alpha-reductase 2 deficiency 1219
  breast development 652–653
  precocious 1189
    hyperaldosteronism 1194
  precocious, theca cell tumour 762
  spontaneous, Turner's syndrome 1222
  see also Pseudopuberty
Pubic hair, development 653
Pubococcygeus muscle, pelvic floor 23
Puborectalis muscle, pelvic floor 23–24
Pudendal nerve
  anal canal innervation 36
  ischiorectal fossa 36
  pelvis 25
Puerperal psychosis 1523
Puerperal venous thrombosis 1526
Puerperium
  solitary luteinized follicle cyst 677, 677
  see also Entries beginning postpartum
Pulmonary aspiration of gastric contents, maternal death 1570
Pulmonary carcinoma see Bronchial carcinoma
Pulmonary hypertension, primary 1549–1550
  maternal mortality rate 1550
Pulmonary metastases
  endometrial stromal sarcoma 509, 511
  non-gestational choriocarcinoma 786
Pulmonary stenosis 1545
Pulmonary thromboembolism, maternal death 1561
Punctation, cervical epithelium 322
Pyelography, renal tuberculosis in pregnancy 1499
Pyelonephritis
  acute 1495–1497
    E. coli 1497
    histology 1496, 1496
    kidney scarring 1497, 1498, 1498
  chronic 1497–1499
    causes 1498–1499
    histology 1498, 1498
    hypertension 1499
    kidney scarring 1497, 1498, 1498
    prognosis 1499
    renal tubule destruction 1498, 1498
Pyoderma gangrenosum, vulvar involvement 64–65
Pyogenic granuloma, vulvar involvement 80

Pyometra, endometrial squamous cell carcinoma 473
Pyrexia of unknown origin 1197
Pyrrhocoris apterus, sex chromosomes 2–3

R
Racial factors see Ethnic factors
'Racquet cells,' carcinosarcoma (uterine) 565, 567
Radial arteries of uterus, pregnancy 1332
Radiation
  injury in endocervix 292
  ovary, changes 679
  pelvic, vaginal cancer pathogenesis 188
  salpingitis 622
Radiation salpingitis 622
Radio-opaque dye, placental anastomoses 1588
Radiotherapy
  adenosarcoma (uterine) after 552
  cervical carcinoma 332
  cervical inflammation 292, 292
  diffuse malignant mesothelioma of peritoneum after 917
  endometrial adenocarcinoma 486
  endometritis 421
  endometrium response 487
  histological effects, on endometrial adenocarcinoma 486–488
  immature teratoma 793
  ovarian changes due to 679
  pelvic, carcinosarcoma risk after 561
  uterine carcinosarcoma 572–573
  vaginal lesions due to 154
  vesicovaginal fistulas due to 185
  yolk sac tumours 785
ras proto-oncogene
  activation, endometrial adenocarcinoma 485
  see also K-ras
Reactive oxygen species (ROS)
  peritoneal fluid 1019
  in semen, infertility and 995
Rectal plexus 25
Recto-uterine pouch of Douglas 28
Rectovaginal endometriotic nodules 965
Rectovaginal fistula 184–185
Rectum, anatomy 28–29
Recurrent empty follicle syndrome 1015
Recurrent jaundice of pregnancy
    see Intrahepatic cholestasis, of pregnancy
Recurrent miscarriage see Miscarriage, recurrent spontaneous
Red degeneration, uterine leiomyoma 519, 519, 536
Red lesions, endometriosis 967
5α-Reductase 1013
Reifenstein phenotype, androgen receptor disorders 1217
Reifenstein's syndrome, androgen insensitivity syndromes 1219
Reinke's crystals 704
  electronmicroscopy 849
  Leydig cell tumours 757, 758, 848, 849, 850
    hilus cell tumour 757, 848
    non-hilus cell tumour 757, 849
    stromal–Leydig cell tumour 765, 765
Reiter's disease, vulvar involvement 73
Renal adenocarcinoma, metastatic, to ovary 887, 887–888
Renal agenesis
  familial 1158
  fetal, amnion nodosum 1302
Renal anomalies, clinically silent, umbilical artery, single 1294
Renal artery aneurysms 1550–1551
Renal blood flow, acute renal failure 1500
Renal cell carcinoma, metastatic
  to ovary 881, 887, 887–888
  to vagina 218, 218
Renal cortical necrosis, bilateral 1501–1503, 1502
  causes 1502–1503
  prognosis 1503
Renal diseases, in pregnancy 1495–1558
  acute post-infectious glomerulonephritis 1515, 1516
  acute renal failure see Renal failure, acute, in pregnancy
  adult polycystic renal disease 1519, 1519
  amniotic fluid embolism 1503
  asymptomatic bacteriuria 1495
  defibrination syndrome 1503
  diabetic glomerulopathy 1517–1519, 1518

  dialysis patients 1511
  focal/segmental sclerosis and hyalinosis 1513
  hypertension 1505–1511
  infection 1495–1500
  interstitial nephritis 1499
  lupus nephritis 1515, 1515–1516
  membranous glomerulonephritis 1512, 1512–1513
  mesangial IgA disease 1516, 1516
  mesangiocapillary glomerulonephritis 1513–1515, 1514
  minimal change glomerulonephropathy 1513, 1513
  pelvic ectopic kidney 1519
  pre-eclampsia 1337, 1343, 1505–1511
  pre-existing diseases 1511–1519
  pyelonephritis
    acute 1495–1497
    chronic 1497–1499
  renal function test variation 1495
  renal transplant patients 1511
  renal tuberculosis 1499–1500
  renal tubular acidosis 1519
  scleroderma 1516, 1517
  urolithiasis 1519
Renal failure, acute
  idiopathic postpartum 1503–1505, 1504
    see also Idiopathic postpartum acute renal failure
  in pregnancy 1500–1505
    abruptio placentae 1503
    acute fatty liver of pregnancy 1503
    adult polycystic renal disease 1519, 1519
    amniotic fluid embolism 1503
    bilateral renal cortical necrosis 1501–1503, 1502
    causative factors 1500
    HELLP syndrome 1503
    idiopathic postpartum 1503–1505, 1504
    pre-eclampsia 1503
    prerenal failure 1500
    prolonged intrauterine death 1503
    renal blood flow 1500
    renal function tests 1500
    septicaemia 1503
  prerenal failure 1500
Renal failure, chronic, infertility and 1021
Renal transplant
  cervical neoplasia 303
  in pregnancy 1511
Renal tuberculosis
  granulomas 1499, 1499–1500
  in pregnancy 1499–1500
Renal tubular acidosis 1519
Renin substrate 1105
Repetitive moles 1362, 1365
Report on Confidential Enquiries into Maternal Deaths in the United Kingdom 1559, 1560
Reproduction, assisted see Assisted reproductive technology (ART)
Reproductive aging 990, 991
Reproductive capacity, genital tract malformations 46–48
Reserve cell(s)
  cervical epithelium 265, 275
  Fallopian tubes 587
  hyperplasia after steroid contraceptives 1097
Reserve cell hyperplasia 288
  atypical, cervical glandular intraepithelial neoplasia 354
  cervical 288
  cervical squamous neoplasia 309
  endocervix 275
Resistant ovary syndrome (Savage syndrome) 679–680, 680
Respiratory distress, acute, faecal fluid aspiration 1570
Rete ovarii 897
  adenocarcinoma 903
  adenomatous hyperplasia 902, 902–903
  cysts 903
  tumours 902, 902–903
Rete pegs, acanthotic 269
Rete system, embryology 637
Reticulin
  adenosarcoma (uterine) 556, 556
  carcinosarcoma (uterine) 570
  endometrial stromal tumours 502
  stromal nodules 505

Retiform differentiation
  Sertoli–Leydig cell tumours
    see Sertoli–Leydig cell tumours
    stromal nodules 505
Retinal vein thrombosis 1104
Retrograde lymphatic permeation, metastatic spread
    of adenocarcinoma 349
Retrograde menstruation, endometrial fragments
    964
Retroperitoneal fibrosis **1189**
Retroperitoneum, cystic mucinous tumours 926
Retroplacental bleeding, antepartum haemorrhage
    1350
Retroplacental haematoma 1284–1285
  antepartum haemorrhage 1350, *1350*
  miscarriage 1437
  pre-eclampsia 1309
Retropubic space 28
Reverse transcriptase PCR, Ewing's sarcoma of
    vulva 124
Reversible posterior leukoencephalopathy syndrome
    1524
Rhabdoid differentiation, endometrial stromal
    tumours 503
  low-grade sarcoma 508
Rhabdoid tumour, malignant
  epithelioid sarcoma of vulva 124
  vulvar 124–125
Rhabdomyoblasts *865*
  carcinosarcoma (uterine) *567*
Rhabdomyoma
  ovarian **864**
  vagina *196*, 196–197
  vulvovaginal 115
Rhabdomyosarcoma
  alveolar 378
    metastatic to ovary 890
    vulvar 115–116
  in childhood **1172**
  clinical group staging system *215*
  element in uterine carcinosarcoma 565
  embryonal *see* Embryonal rhabdomyosarcoma
  histiogenesis 858
  ovarian **864–865**, *865*
    embryonal *864*, 864–865, *865*
    mucinous cystic tumour with 873
    pleomorphic 865
    small cell undifferentiated ovarian carcinoma vs
      905
  pleomorphic
    embryonal rhabdomyosarcomas of uterine
      cervix 378
    vulvar 115–116
  steroid contraceptives and 1101
Rhesus incompatibility, materno-fetal
  immature intermediate villi 1247
  placental toxoplasmosis vs 1318
Rheumatic fever, chorea gravidarum **1524**
Rheumatic heart disease **1547–1548**
  arterial obstruction 1528
  mitral valve stenosis *1547*, 1547–1548
Rheumatoid arthritis 1089, **1189**
  steroid contraceptives and 1105
Right to left shunts **1544**
Robertsonian translocation 992
Rokitansky–Küstner–Hauser syndrome 996
Rosai–Dorfman disease of cervix 953
Rosenthal fibres 792, 800
Rotor syndrome 1100
  pregnancy 1484
Round ligaments of uterus, pelvis 24, 34
Roundworms, vaginitis 176
Rubella infection
  cervix 287
  miscarriage 1432
  placental examination 1315–1317, *1316*
Rudimentary horn pregnancy 47

S
S-100 protein
  adult-type granulosa cell tumours 751
  Langerhans' cell histiocytosis 957
  melanoma 888
  steroid cell tumours not otherwise specified 853
Saccharomyces cerevisiae, vaginitis 173
Sacralisation, sacrum 21
Sacral sympathetic trunks, pelvic innervation 26
Sacroilliac joint 21–22
Sacrum, anatomy 21
Sagittal plane conjoined twins 1586

Saline
  coloured, placental anastomoses 1588
  hypertonic, pregnancy termination 1566
  poisoning, maternal death 1571
Salivary MALT lymphoma 938
Salpingectomy
  distal 598, *599*
  partial, for sterilisation 598–599
  specimen, tubal pregnancy 1059
  tubal pregnancy, ruptured 1060
Salpingitis **615–622**
  asymptomatic endosalpingeal 616
  bilharzial, ectopic pregnancy 1048
  chlamydial 616, 622
  chronic
    endometriosis-associated infertility 980, *981*
    Liesegang rings 619
  chronic lipoid 1011, *1012*
  definition 617
  endometritis 420
  eosinophilic 616
  Fallopian tube adenocarcinoma risk 606
  follicular *623*, 1010
  granulomatous 617–620
    differential diagnosis 619–620
    infertility due to 1010–1011, *1012*
    see also Salpingitis, tuberculous
  infectious **617–622**
    causative agents 620
    complications 621–622
    spread 620
  infertility due to 980, *981*, 1009–1011
    mechanisms 1010–1011
  myometrial leiomyoma association 999
  non-granulomatous 617, 620–622, *623*
    causative agents and spread 620–621, 1010
    ectopic pregnancy 1048–1049
    infertility due to 1009–1010
    risk factors 620
  physiological menstrual 615–616
  physiological puerperal 616
  radiation **622**
  transmural lymphocytic 616, *616*
  tubal allograft rejection 616
  tuberculous 427, 617, *617*, 617–618
    diagnosis and differential diagnosis 618
    infertility due to 1010–1011, *1012*
    pathology/histology *617*, 617–618, *618*
  xanthogranulomatous 618–619
  see also Pelvic inflammatory disease (PID)
Salpingitis isthmica nodosa (SIN) **599–601**, *600*,
    601
  differential diagnosis 601
  ectopic pregnancy 1047
  tubal spasm causing 1008
Salpingo-oophorectomy
  borderline serous tumours 722
  carcinoid tumours of ovary *811*
Salt poisoning, maternal death 1571
Sarcoidosis **1189**, *1190*
  cervical 281
  endometrium 425, 1189, *1190*
  Fallopian tube 1189
  ovarian involvement 684, 1189
  uterus 1189
  vulvar 65
Sarcoma
  alveolar soft part, uterine cervix 379
  cervix 375–380
  endometrial stromal *see* Endometrial stromal
    tumours
  endometrioid stromal, of ovary *870*, **870–872**,
    871
  epithelioid *see* Epithelioid sarcoma
  Ewing's, vulvar 124
  Fallopian tube 611
  'fish flesh' pattern *520*
  granulocytic *see* Granulocytic sarcoma
  Kaposi's 121
  metastatic, to ovary 889–890
  osteogenic, ovarian **866**
  ovarian *see* Ovarian tumours, sarcoma
  pure heterologous, uterine **538**
  synovial, vulva 125
  uterine *see* Uterus, sarcoma
  vaginal *see* Vagina, sarcoma
Sarcoma botryoides **1172**
  cells of origin 150
  embryonal rhabdomyosarcoma of uterine cervix
    376

  vaginal 211–213, *212*, *213*, *214*
    presentation 189
  see also Embryonal rhabdomyosarcoma
Sarcomatous change, adult-type granulosa cell
    tumours 751
Sarcoptes scabiei, vulvar infection 54
Savage syndrome (resistant ovary syndrome)
    679–680, *680*
Scanning electronmicroscopy (SEM) 588, *588*
  cervical stroma 248
  columnar epithelium of cervix 258–259
  squamous epithelium of cervix 255
Schistosoma haematobium 1144, 1147
  endometritis 432
  vaginitis 176
Schistosoma mansoni, vaginitis 176
Schistosomiasis **1144–1148**
  bilharzioma 1144
  cervical 1144–1145, 1146, *1147*
  cytology 1148
  endometrial 1147
  endometritis 432
  Fallopian tubes 1147, *1148*
  lesion distribution *1144*
  ovarian 684, 1147
  placental 1148
  tubal infertility 1011
  vaginal 1145, 1146
  vaginal carcinoma aetiology 188
  vulvar 54–55, *1145*, 1145–1146, *1146*
Schwannoma
  cervix 384
  intracranial 1535
  malignant
    ovarian **867**
    vulvar 122
  ovarian **867**
  uterine leiomyoma with similar features *520*
  vulvar 122
Sciatica 1536
Scleroderma, renal, in pregnancy **1516**, *1517*
Sclerosing stromal tumour 1172
  ovarian **765–766**, *766*
Sclerosis, focal/segmental, in pregnancy 1513
Sebaceous carcinoma of vulva 129
Sebaceous gland disorders, vulvar area involvement
    82–83
Sebaceous gland hyperplasia, vulvar 82
Sebaceous metaplasia, ectocervix 279
Seborrhoeic dermatitis, vulvar 72–73
Secondary Müllerian system *see* Müllerian system,
    secondary
Secretory cells, endometrial epithelium 394
Secretory phase of endometrial cycle 400–401
  early phase 400
  late phase 401
  mid-secretory phase 400–401
  see also Endometrium, secretory phase
Segmentation cavity, preimplantation phase
    embryogenesis 4
Semen, abnormalities 995
Seminal fluid
  abnormalities 994, 995
  allergy 155, 993
  bicarbonate 994
  buffering capacity 994
Seminiferous tubules, immature, testicular
    feminisation, complete 1218
Seminoma, dysgerminoma relationship 773
Senile cystic atrophy, endometrium,
    postmenopausal 403
Sensorineural deafness (Perrault syndrome) **1190**
Sepsis
  maternal death 1561–1564
  puerperal 1562
  purulent pelvic phlebitis 1562
  superficial fascial necrosis 1562
Septal cysts, intervillous thrombosis 1285
Septate uterus 45
Septic abortion 1503
Septicaemia
  acute renal failure in pregnancy **1503**
  septic abortion 1503
Septic shock, maternal death 1562–1564, *1563*
Septum dissolution failure, female genital tract
    malformation 44–45
Serous adenocarcinoma
  endometrial *see* Endometrial carcinoma, serous
  ovarian *see* Serous tumours, ovarian
  papillary, of cervix *346*, 346–347

Serous carcinoma, peritoneal 923, *924,* 924–925
Serous cystadenoma
  ovarian 713–714
  papillary 713–714, *714*
Serous lesions, secondary Müllerian system
    921–926
Serous psammocarcinoma, of peritoneum 923–924,
    924
Serous tumours, ovarian *694,* 840
  adenocarcinoma 728–729, *729*
    histiogenesis 697
    micropapillary 719, 721
  benign 713–714
    papillary 714, *714*
  borderline malignancy 717–723
    adenocarcinoma appearance of 720
    bilateral 723
    clinical features and management 722–723
    endosalpingiosis with 921
    extraovarian, management 723
    extraovarian spread 719–720, *720,* 721, 722
    mesothelial hyperplasia vs 914
    metastases 721
    pathology 718–722, *719, 720*
    prognostic features 722
    stromal microinvasion 719, *719*
    survival rates 721
Serous tumours, peritoneal
  borderline 922–923, *923*
  carcinoma 923, *924,* 924–925
Sertoli cells
  adenomas, androgen insensitivity disorders 1219
  development 638, 641
  genes involved in differentiation and function
      1210
  granulosa cell homology 745
  proliferations 677–678
  sex-cord differentiation to 703
Sertoli cell tumours, of ovary 704, **756–757**
  adult-type granulosa cell tumours vs 748, *748*
  lipid-rich 757
Sertoliform endometrial carcinoma 474
Sertoli–Leydig cell tumours 704, 746, **753–756,**
    1169–1170
  biological behaviour 756
  categories 755
  differential diagnosis 756
    nodule in mucinous cystadenoma 715
    ovarian tumours of probable Wolffian origin
        902
    unclassified sex cord–stromal tumours 758
  hyperaldosteronism 1194
  immunohistochemistry 756
  incidence and clinical features 753
  intermediate differentiation *755,* 756, *756*
  masculinisation 1195
  molecular pathology 756
  mucinous tumours and 697
  pathology 753–756, *754, 755, 1169, 1170*
  poorly differentiated 756, *756*
  prognosis 1170
  retiform *755,* 756–757
    mixed germ cell sex cord–stromal tumours vs
        840
  retiform differentiation 755
  thyroid adenoma 1190
  ultrastructure 756
  well-differentiated (tubular adenoma) *755,*
      755–756
Sex
  ambiguous *see* Ambiguous genitalia; Sexual
      ambiguity
  determination 3–4, 635–636, **638–643**
    chromosomes 3
    DAX 1 gene 1210
    environmental 3
    SRY gene role 640–641
    testis-determining factor (TDF) 1209
  differences, anatomy of pelvic bones 21
  differentiation 3–4
    female 641–643
    male 638–641
Sex chromatin 642
Sex chromosomes 2–3, 3, 635
  abnormalities 638
  cytogenetic disorders **1182**
  see also X chromosome; Y chromosome
Sex-cord cells
  differentiation into granulosa cells 703
  differentiation into Sertoli cells 703

Sex-cord derivatives
  gonadoblastoma 827
  mixed germ cell sex cord–stromal tumours 834,
      835, *835,* 836
  ovarian fibroma *859*
Sex cord-like features
  endometrial stromal tumours *512,* 512–513
  Müllerian adenosarcoma **559**
  uterine tumours with *575,* **575–576**
Sex-cords
  cellular origin 645
  epithelial origin 703
  folliculogenous 647
  formation 637, 645
  minor, in stromal tumours **765**
  ovary 745
Sex cord–stromal tumours
  broad ligament 626
  gonadoblastoma **1167–1168,** *1168*
    see also Gonadoblastoma
  Gorlin's syndrome *see* Basal cell naevus syndrome
  hyperaldosteronism 1194
  juvenile granulosa cell tumour *1169,* **1169,** 1171
  Maffucci's syndrome *see* Maffucci's syndrome
  mixed germ cell *see* Mixed germ cell sex
      cord–stromal tumours (ovarian)
  Ollier's disease **1171,** 1183
  ovarian *see* Ovarian sex cord–stromal tumours
  testicular, androgen resistance syndromes 1161
Sex cord–stromal tumours, ovarian *694,* **703–705,**
    745–770
  aetiology and pathogenesis 704–705
  classification 745–746, *746, 746*
  germ cells with *see* Mixed germ cell sex
      cord–stromal tumours (ovarian)
  histiogenesis 703–705
  risk factors 705
  with sex-cord component **746–761**
    with annular tubules (SCTAT) 757, **758–760,**
        759
    gynandroblastoma *760,* 760
    indeterminate (mixed cell) types 757–760, *758*
    Leydig cell tumours 757
    in pregnancy **760–761,** *761*
    unclassified types **758**
    see also Granulosa cell tumours; Sertoli cell
        tumours; Sertoli–Leydig cell tumours
  of specialised gonadal stroma **761–767**
    benign signet ring stromal tumour **766–767,**
        767
    classification *762*
    fibroma **765**
    sclerosing stromal tumour **765–766,** *766*
    stromal–Leydig cell tumour *764,* **764–765,** *765*
    stromal tumours with minor sex-cord elements
        765
    theca cell tumour *see* Theca cell tumour
Sex determination *see* Sex, determination
Sex-determining region Y (SRY) gene
    see SRY (sex determining region Y) gene
Sex steroid biosynthesis *1213*
    see also Oestrogen(s); Testosterone
Sexual abuse
  condyloma acuminata **1175**
  syphilis in children 168
  vaginitis due to 159
Sexual activity
  age at onset
    cervical cancer 1149
    cervical squamous cell carcinoma 298
    pelvic inflammatory disease risk 1134
    squamous cell carcinoma of cervix 298
  cervical cancer 298, 1175
  pelvic inflammatory disease risk 620, 1134
    see also Sexual intercourse
Sexual ambiguity
  frequent, genetic identification disorders
      1224–1228
  infrequent 1220–1224
    Klinefelter's syndrome 1220–1221
    pure gonadal dysgenesis 1223–1224
    Turner's syndrome 1221–1222
    XX male syndrome 1222–1223
  in neonates **1158–1162**
    androgen resistance syndromes **1160–1161**
    congenital adrenal hyperplasia **1158–1159**
    ovarian developmental disorders **1159–1160**
    Turner's syndrome **1159–1160**
    see also Ambiguous genitalia
Sexual behaviour, fertility and 989

Sexual development
  abnormal **1209–1232**
  female internal organs 1212
  male 1211, *1211*
Sexual differentiation 3–4
  see also Sex, differentiation
Sexual dimorphism 3
Sexual intercourse
  age at first *see* Sexual activity, age at onset
  frequency, infertility and 991
  inflammatory disease of vagina after 155
  multiple partners and squamous cell carcinoma of
      cervix 298
  squamous cell carcinoma of cervix 298
  vaginal hypersensitivity 155
  vaginal physiology 151
  vaginal trauma 152–153
  see also Sexual activity
Sexually transmitted diseases (STDs)
  incidence of ectopic pregnancy 1051
  infertility and 993
  vaginal involvement 167–169
  vulvar intraepithelial neoplasia 100
  see also Chlamydial infections (*Chlamydia
      trachomatis*); Condyloma acuminata;
      Gonorrhoea; Syphilis
Sexual precocity, follicle cysts and 664,
    1162
Sexual transmission
  vaginal candidiasis 171–172
  vaginitis aetiology 159
Sezary's syndrome 937
SF-1 receptor, sertoli cell differentiation and
    function 1210
Sheehan's syndrome 1535
Shigella sonnei, cervical infection 282–283
Shigella species, vaginal infection 169
Shock, septic, maternal death 1562–1564, *1563*
Shunts **1544**
Siamese twins *see* Conjoined twins
Sigmoidovaginal fistula 185
Signet ring carcinoma, bladder, metastatic to ovary
    888
Signet ring cells
  clear cell adenocarcinoma 732
  Krukenberg tumours 890–891, *891*
  uterine cervix metastases 385
Signet ring stromal tumour, of ovary **766–767,** *767*
Simple polyps, endometrial *see* Endometrial polyps
Sinovaginal bulbs 16
Sinusoidal dilatation, hepatic 1100, *1101*
sis oncogene, uterine carcinosarcoma 572
Situs inversus totalis **1190**
Sjögren's syndrome
  vaginal changes 154
  vulvar involvement 66
Skene's ducts 31
Skene's gland, cystic lesions 182
Skin adnexal tumours, vulvar **126–129**
  benign 126–128
  malignant 129
Skin appendage disorders, vulva 82–84
Small bowel *see* Intestine, small
Small cell carcinomas
  behaviour and prognostic factors 373
  cervix *see* Cervical carcinoma, small cell
  endometrium 474, 510
  lung
    metastatic, small cell undifferentiated ovarian
        carcinoma vs 905
    ovarian small cell carcinoma resembling
        905–906
  ovary *see* Ovarian tumours, small cell
  squamous, of vulva *104*
  vagina 210
Small cell tumours
  desmoplastic round cell tumour
      see Desmoplastic small round cell tumour
  ovary *see* Ovarian tumours, small cell
Small cell undifferentiated carcinoma
    see Small cell carcinomas
Small round cell tumours
  of childhood 920
  desmoplastic *see* Desmoplastic small round cell
      tumour
Smith–Lemli–Opitz syndrome **1190**
  pseudohermaphroditism, male 1220
Smoking
  cervical carcinogenesis and HPV infection 300
  cervical neoplasia 301–302

Crohn's disease and contraceptive pill 1186
ectopic pregnancy 1050
HPV-transformed cell proliferation 302
ischaemic heart disease and contraceptives 1104
Langerhan's cell counts 266
oocyte–cumulus pick-up (tubal) inhibition 1008
supernumerary umbilical vessels 1295
Smooth chorion see Chorion laeve
Smooth muscle
actin, sclerosing stromal tumours (ovarian) 766
cervical stroma 249
hyperplasia
myometrium in pregnancy 1330
uterus in pregnancy, vessel involvement 1331
hypertrophy
myometrium in pregnancy 1330
uterus in pregnancy, vessel involvement 1331
metaplasia, endometrial 414–415
tumours
ovarian **862–864**
uterine see Uterine smooth muscle tumours
vulvar 114–115
Sneddon–Wilkinson disease 74
Solitary luteinized follicle cyst of pregnancy 677,
677
Sox9 gene, sertoli cell differentiation and function
1210
SP1, embryonal carcinoma 788
Special investigations **1381–1383**
Sperm (spermatozoa)
abnormalities (biophysical) 994
antibodies 993, 997
antigens
cell-mediated response 993
immune response 993
autoimmunity 992
carbonic anhydrase stimulation 994
cervical mucus incompatibility 997
chemotaxis 995
chromatin stability impairment 994
chromosomes 635
endometrium interaction 994
glucose supply 994
motility impairment 993, 994
number reaching tubes 994
oocyte interaction abnormality 993, 995
phagocytosis, endometriosis associated infertility
981
preparation for oocyte penetration 1007
preparation of ovum for penetration 1007
transport 1007
infertility due to 994
leiomyoma causing infertility by 999
normal 1007
passage through isthmus 1007
regulation by cervical mucus 277
Spindle cell epithelioma, vagina 198
Spiral arteries
changes due to IUCD use 1110
conversion to sinusoid vessels 1335
cytotrophoblast proliferation 1335, 1335
endometrium 395
inadequate transformation and placental
infarction 1282
maturation, cycle dating 407
oestrogen effect 1072
premature development 1090
regressive changes 1258
term placenta 1258
Spirochaetal infections
endometritis 431–432
vulvar 58
Spirometra 1144
Splenic artery
aneurysms 1550
spontaneous rupture in pregnancy
1481
Splenic-gonadal fusion 684
Spontaneous miscarriage see Miscarriage,
spontaneous
Sports, vaginal injury due to 152
Squamous cell(s), vaginal epithelium 149
Squamous cell carcinomas
Bartholin's gland 130
basaloid 110–111
cervix see Cervical carcinoma, squamous cell
common 265
endometrial 411, 473, 473–474
Fallopian tube 611
in situ see Vulvar intraepithelial neoplasia (VIN)

lichen sclerosis 78
in mature teratoma 801, 803
microinvasive, vulvar 104–105
non-keratinising type 328
ovarian 728, 733
ovarian endometriosis 978
typical keratinising 106–107
vagina see Vagina, squamous cell carcinoma
vulvar see Vulva, squamous cell carcinoma
vulvar intraepithelial neoplasia, differentiated 103
Squamous epithelium
cervix see Cervical epithelium, original squamous
ectocervical and herpesvirus infection
286
metaplastic 259–265
stratified, cervical 273
Squamous lesions, peritoneum 927
Squamous metaplasia
cervical epithelium 251, 274–275, 287
atypical immature 267
cervical squamous neoplasia 309
early phase 275
endocervical crypts 276
endometrium 410, 452
hypoplastic endometrium 410–411
newly metaplastic epithelium 275
peritoneum 927
Squamous morule, endometrium 410
Squamous papilloma
cervix 382
vaginal 193
vulvar 96
Squamous tumours, benign, ovarian 717
SRY (sex determining region Y) gene 639, **640–641**,
1157
Sertoli–Leydig cell tumours 756
sexual development 1209–1210
Staphylococcal infections
cardiac 1541, 1542, 1542
cervix 282
scalded skin syndrome, vulva 69
tampon use association 177, 178
vulvar 56
Staphylococcus aureus
penicillinase-producing, toxic shock syndrome
177
toxic shock syndrome 176–178
vulvar infection 56
Staphylococcus epidermidis
vulva, microbial flora 54
vulvar infection 56
Staphylococcus saprophyticus, vulvar infection 56
StAR gene mutations 1216
Static image cytometry 1608
Steatocystoma, vulvar involvement 83, 83
Steatorrhoea, intrahepatic cholestasis of pregnancy
1469
Stein–Leventhal syndrome 665
see also Polycystic ovarian disease
Stem villi 1246
Sterilisation, tubal **597–599**
anatomical effects 597–598
ectopic pregnancy 1047–1048
partial salpingectomy 598–599
Pomeroy technique 596, 597–598
pregnancy after 597
pregnancy rate after reversal 990
recanalisation after 597, 597
reversal, tubal lesions causing infertility after
1012
sequelae 596, 597–598
tubal implantation 1047
Sterility
adolescent 991
postmenopausal 990
Steroid cell neoplasms 1171–1172
Steroid (lipid) cell tumours (ovarian) 745, **845–856**
classification 746, 746, 845–846
clinical/pathological features 846
differential diagnosis 853–855
extraovarian 855
Leydig cell tumours see Leydig cell tumours
not otherwise specified 850–853, 851, 852, 853
immunohistochemistry 853
stromal luteoma 846, **846–847**, 847
terminology 845
Steroid contraception see Combined steroid
contraceptives (oral); Contraception
Steroid hormones
human papillomavirus oncogene expression 302

localisation in Sertoli–Leydig cell tumours 756
therapy see Hormonal therapy
see also specific hormones
Steroidogenic acute regulatory gene mutations
1216
Stevens–Johnson syndrome 69
Stillbirth
fibromuscular sclerosis 1292
intrahepatic cholestasis of pregnancy 1468
miscarriage vs 1313
placental examination 1313
supernumerary umbilical vessels 1295
umbilical cord stricture 1298
Stomach ulceration, hypertensive disease of
pregnancy 1564
Stones, vagina **186**
Straight sinus 1527
Strap cells, embryonal rhabdomyosarcoma of
uterine cervix 377
Stratified Mucin–producing Intraepithelial Lesion
(SMILE) 354
Stratified squamous epithelium, endometrial
metaplasia 411
Stratum corneum, squamous epithelium of cervix
253
Stratum cylindricum see Basal cell(s)
Stratum granulosum, secondary follicle 656
Stratum spinosum profundum (parabasal cell layer)
252–253, 273
Stratum spinosum superficiae cells, squamous
epithelium of cervix 253
Streak gonad see Gonad(s), streak
Streptococcal infections
cervix 282
puerperal sepsis 1562
vaginitis 169
vulvar 56
Streptococcus, group A haemolytic, endometritis,
acute non-specific 419
Stress
adrenal stimulation 1026
amenorrhoea/anovulation 1020
Stress incontinence, urinary 31
Striated muscle tumours
ovarian **864–865**, 865
vulvar 115–116
Stroke
combined steroid contraceptives and 1105
postpartum cerebral angiopathy 1524
risk in pregnancy 1524
Stroma, endometrium, postmenopausal 402
Stromal cells
cervical epithelium 266, 274
endometrial see Endometrium, stroma
ovarian see Ovary, stromal cells
perivascular and predecidual change 395
pinwheel effect in endometritis 423
uterine, differentiation 550
Stromal fibrosis, cervical polyps 290
Stromal hyperplasia see Ovary, stromal hyperplasia
Stromal hyperthecosis see Ovary, stromal
hyperthecosis
Stromal infiltrate, endometrium, late secretory
phase 401
Stromal invasion
microinvasive glandular lesions of cervix 356
vulvar intraepithelial neoplasia 104
Stromal–Leydig cell tumour 764, **764–765**, 765
Stromal luteoma 846, **846–847**, 847
differential diagnosis 853–855
Stromal melanocytic foci (blue naevus) 279, 279,
282, 382
Stromal metaplasia
endometrium 410, 414–415
fimbriae, tubal 591, 592
ovarian 684
Stromal nodules, endometrial see Endometrial
stromal tumours, stromal nodules
Stromal oedema, endometrial cycle secretory phase
401
see also Endometrium, stromal oedema
Stromal reaction
adenoid cystic carcinoma of cervix 345
microinvasive carcinoma of cervix 317
squamous cell carcinoma of cervix 328
Stromal sarcoma
differential diagnosis 509, 510
endocervical see Endocervical stromal sarcoma
'endometrial,' in vagina 216
endometrioid, of ovary 870, **870–872**, 871

Stromal sarcoma (cont'd)
  low-grade, endometriosis vs 971
  Müllerian, vaginal 216
  with thecomatous features, ovarian 763
  undifferentiated, of ovary 872–873, *873*
Stromomyoma, endometrial 508, 525, 576–577
  differential diagnosis 513–514
Strongyloides 1148
Strumal carcinoid tumour 807, *810*, 810–811
Struma ovarii *805*, **805–806**
  prognostic indicators 806
  tumours associated 806
Struma salpingii 605
Subamniotic haematoma 1284
Subarachnoid haemorrhage, combined oral
      contraceptives and 1105
Subchorial haematoma, massive *1284*, 1285
Subchorial intervillositis 1303
Subchorial thrombosis, placental, miscarriage 1437,
    1437, 1438
Subchorionic fibrin plaques, intervillous thrombosis
    1285
Sub-columnar basal cells, cervical epithelium 265
Subcorneal pustular dermatosis, vulvar involvement
    74
Subendocardial haemorrhages, in pregnancy 1564,
    1564
Subinvoluted vessels, endovascular trophoblast
    1353
Subnuclear vacuoles, endometrial early secretory
    phase 400
Subscapular haemorrhage in liver, in pregnancy
    1564, *1564*
Sulphation of bile acids 1468
Sulphur granules
  actinomycosis of ovary 683, *683*
  pseudo- 1113, *1113*
Superfecundation, dizygotic twins 1576
Superfetation, dizygotic twins 1576
Superficial invasion patterns, microinvasive
    glandular lesions of cervix 357
Superficial perineal pouch 27
Superficial spreading melanoma, Paget's disease 99
Superficial zone cells, cervical stratified squamous
    epithelium 273
Superior rectal artery, pelvic supply 27
Superior rectal (haemorrhoidal) plexus, pelvic
    innervation 26
Superior sagittal sinus thrombosis **1526–1527**
Superior vena cava syndrome 1197
Supporting cells, gonadal differentiation role
    640–641
Supravaginal cervix 33, 248
Surgery, endometrial adenocarcinoma 486
Surgical termination of pregnancy, failure and
    genital tract malformation 48
Suspensory ligament of ovary 653
Sustenaculum of Bonney 24
Sutton's ulcers, vulvar involvement 67
Sweat gland
  adenocarcinoma of vulva *129*
  carcinomas of vulva 129
  disorders, vulvar involvement 83–84
Sweet's syndrome 64
Swyer syndrome 1160
Sydenham's chorea, chorea gravidarum **1524**
Sympathetic system, pelvis 25–26
Symphysis pubis 22
Synctial giant cell formation *1333*
Syncytial fusion
  apoptotic extrusion 1241
  controls 1240
  transfer of RNA 1239
Syncytial giant cells of junctional zone, formation
    1258
Syncytial growth, cytotrophoblastic cells 1237
Syncytial knots 1239
  apoptotic nuclei 1241
  true, syncytial sprouts vs 1288
Syncytial papillary change 413–414
Syncytial protrusions 1253
Syncytin 1240
Syncytiotrophoblast
  apoptosis 1241
  focal degeneration 1236
  growth and regeneration 1242, *1242*
  prelacunar stage placental development 1233
  secondary necrosis due to apoptosis cascade
    interruption 1241
  ultrastructural and enzyme patterns 1239

Syncytiotrophoblastic cells
  embryonal carcinoma 788
  giant, dysgerminoma with *775*, 776
Syndactyly, amniotic bands and strings 1308
Syndrome of inappropriate ADH secretion 370,
    1195
Synovial sarcoma of vulva 125
Syntactic structure analysis, cervical intraepithelial
    neoplasia (CIN) 1613
Syphilis
  cervical infection 282
  congenital *1314*
    necrotising funisitis 1300
  distribution of lesions 165
  placental examination 1314
  secondary 282
  in tropics **1136**
  vaginal involvement 168
  verrucous carcinoma of vulva 108
  vulvar infection 58
Syringoma of vulva *126*, 126–127
Systemic diseases
  infertility associated 1025–1026
  placental bed pathology 1344–1345
  secondary conditions of cervix 290–292
  vulva-associated conditions 63–67
Systemic lupus erythematosus (SLE) **1190**
  antibody to FSH receptor 680
  antiphospholipid syndrome 1190, 1526
  dysgerminoma and 774
  lupus nephritis in pregnancy *1515*, **1515–1516**
  pregnancy 1345
Systemic sclerosis (scleroderma), renal, in
    pregnancy **1516**, *1517*

T
Tachycardia, chorioamnionitis 1306
Takayasu's disease **1549**
Talc, ovarian tumours association 702–703
Tamoxifen **1076–1081**
  adenomyosis and 498, 1080
  carcinosarcoma risk after 561
  cervical smear changes 1081
  effect on endometrium 1076–1080
  effect on vaginal epithelium 150, 156
  effects on endometriosis 1081
  effects on ovary 1080–1081
  endocervical polyps 290
  endometrial adenocarcinoma link 456, 486,
    1078–1080
    dosage relationship 1079
    prognosis 1080
    serous type 1080
  endometrial epithelial metaplasia 410
    mucinous metaplasia and polyps 413
  endometrial hyperplasia 1076–1077, 1192
  endometrial polyps 417, *1077*, 1077–1078, *1078*,
    1079
    see also Endometrial polyps
  endometrium, postmenopausal 403
  indications 1076
  polyps
    adenosarcoma vs 558
    endometrial *see Above*
  uterine stromal tumours 1080
Tampons
  staphylococcal infections 178
  superabsorbent, toxic shock syndrome and
    177–178
  toxic shock syndrome (TSS) association 176, 177
  vaginal trauma 153
Tangential sectioning of cervical canal 356
Tapeworm (*Echinococcus granulosus*) 1143
  vulvar infection 54–55
T-cells
  abnormalities at implantation 1006
  antibodies 944
  cervical epithelium 266
  cervical stroma 274
  cytotoxic 302
  human papillomavirus infection 302
  IUCD use andpregnancy 1116
  premature ovarian failure and 1017
Teenage pregnancy 1163
Teeth, in mature teratoma *798*, 799
Telomerase 1599, **1601–1602**
  activation, endocervical neoplasia 358
  cervical carcinoma **1601**
  endometrial carcinoma **1601**
  hydatidiform moles **1599**

  ovarian carcinoma **1601**
  persistent trophoblastic disease 1386
  trophoblastic disease **1599**
Tenascin, mesenchymal villi 1247
Tenebrio molitor, sex chromosomes 3
Tenesmus, endometriosis 979
Tenny-Parker changes, placental villi 1253
Tension-pneumomediastinum, maternal death 1571
Teratogenic drugs
  anti-epileptics 1533
  coumarin derivatives 1549
Teratoma 705
  cervical 380, 1605
    mature 380
  extraovarian 795, 1166
  ovarian (mature/immature) *see* Ovarian teratoma
  placental *1454*, 1454–1455
  risk factors 707
  testis, aetiology 707
  umbilical cord 1301
    fetus acardius vs 1301
Terminal villi 1246–1247
  capillary sinusoids 1250
  deficiency and fetal growth retardation 1286,
    1286
  protrusion 1250
  ultrastructural features *1240*
Termination of pregnancy
  actinomycotic endometritis 431
  air embolism 1567
  amniotic fluid embolism after 1566
  chlamydial endometritis 426
  effect on fertility 989
  endometritis after 420
  failure, uterine malformations and 48
  hydatidiform mole 1384
  hypertonic saline, intrauterine injection 1566
  infective salpingitis after 620
  IUCD use and 1116
  pelvic inflammatory disease 1134
  previous, ectopic pregnancy 1050
  prior, ectopic pregnancy after 1050
  salt poisoning 1571
  surgical
    amniotic fluid embolism 1566
    failure and genital tract malformation 48
  see also Miscarriage
Tertiary villi, differentiation/formation 1236
Testes
  central zone (medulla), gonadal dysgenesis, mixed
    1225
  descent, initiation and Müllerian inhibiting
    substance (MIS) 1211
  development 13
  differentiation 639–640
  embryology 898
    indifferent gonad transformation 638, 646, 898
  enlargement, mixed germ cell sex cord–stromal
    tumours and 833
  fetal, meiosis absence 647
  gonadal dysgenesis, mixed 1225
  hermaphrodite, true 1228
  hilar region, gonadal dysgenesis, mixed
    1225–1226
  intersex disorders 1160
  Klinefelter's syndrome 1220, *1221*
  microscopic appearances 1161, *1161*
  in mixed germ cell sex cord–stromal tumours
    833, 834, 838, 841
  superficial cortex, gonadal dysgenesis, mixed
    1225
  testicular feminisation, complete 1218
  XX male syndrome 1223
Testicular cords, development 638
Testicular feminisation **1184**
  androgen receptor disorders 1217
  complete, male pseudohermaphroditism
    1217–1219
  incomplete, androgen insensitivity syndrome
    1219
Testicular germ cell tumours, ovarian germ cell
    tumours comparison 772–773
Testicular regression syndrome *1211*
  genital appearance 1215
  male pseudohermaphroditism 1215
  phenotype affected individual 1215
Testis-determining factor 638
  sex determination 1209
Testosterone
  fetal testis 1212

levels in female, adrenogenital syndrome 1213
in Leydig (hilus) cell tumours 848
male differentiation of mesonephric ducts 20
metabolism, disordered, male
    pseudohermaphroditism 1219–1220
production
    gonadoblastoma 825
    mesonephric duct stabilisation 14
sexual differentiation in embryogenesis 20
synthesis defects, male pseudohermaphroditism
    1216
Tetracycline
drug-induced hepatic injury in pregnancy 1479
vaginal lesions due to 154
Tetraploidy, miscarriage, spontaneous 1435
Theca cells, function 1014
Theca cell tumour **761–764**
calcified 763
clinical features 761–762
partly luteinized 763, 763–764, *764*
pathology 762, 762–763
Theca element, adult-type granulosa cell tumours
    747, 747–748, 751
Thecoma
aetiology and pathogenesis 705
'burnt out' 858
luteinized *763*, 763–764, *764*
origin 704
Thecoma–fibroma group tumours, histiogenesis
    703–704
Thread worm *see Enterobius vermicularis*
Three-group metaphase, cervical intraepithelial
    neoplasia 313
Thrombocytopenia **1196**
neonatal, placental haemangioma 1454
Thrombocytopenic purpura
postpartum haemorrhage 1561
steroid contraceptives and 1105
thrombotic, pregnancy 1480
Thromboembolic disease, steroid contraceptives and
    1103–1104
Thromboembolism, progestagens and 1086
Thrombophilia 1103
miscarriage 1434–1435
Thromboplastins, pre-eclampsia 1506
Thrombosis
deep vein, oral contraceptives and 1104
occlusive, pre-eclampsia 1342
straight sinus 1527
superior sagittal sinus thrombosis **1526–1527**
umbilical vessels 1299
vein of Galen 1527
venous *see* Venous thrombosis
Thrombotic microangiopathy (TMA), pregnancy
    1480–1482
Thrombotic thrombocytopenic purpura, pregnancy
    1480
Thymectomy model, granulosa cell tumours
    induction 705
Thyroid gland
abnormalities, Sertoli–Leydig cell tumours 753
adenoma, Sertoli–Leydig cell tumours 1190
autoantibodies, miscarriage, recurrent 1433
MALT lymphoma 938
Thyroiditis, autoimmune (Hashimoto's) 805
Thyroid replacement therapy, miscarriage 1433
Thyroid stimulating hormone (TSH),
    macroadenoma secreting 1024
Thyroid tissue
in ovarian teratomas *805*, 805–806
in strumal carcinoid tumour 810, *811*
Thyrotoxic crisis 805
Tibolone 1090
Tinctorial stains, endometrial stromal cells vs
    muscle cells 502
Tissue necrosis *see* Necrosis
T lymphocytes *see* T-cells
TNM system, vaginal neoplasms 190, *191*
Topoisomerase II alpha (Topo IIa) 1606
Torre–Muir syndrome **1184**
Torulopsis glabrata 173
cervical infection 283
vaginal infection 172–173
vulvar infection 55
Toxaemia of pregnancy
acute fatty liver of pregnancy 1472
liver involvement *1474*, 1474–1475
Toxic epidermal necrolysis, vulva 69
Toxic shock syndrome (TSS) 176–178
epidemiology 176, 177

menstrual (mTSS) 176
epidemiology 177
pathogenesis 177–178
pathology 177
Toxic shock syndrome toxin 1 (TSST-1) 176–177
vaginal carrier rate of organisms producing 177
Toxoplasma cysts, vaginal 176
Toxoplasma gondii
endometritis 432
miscarriage 1432
placental infection 1318
Toxoplasmosis, placental examination 1318
tp53 mutation
mucinous tumours (ovarian) 698
serous tumours (ovarian) 697
Trabeculae
mixed germ cell sex cord–stromal tumours 835,
    835
placental development 1234
Trabecular carcinoid tumour 807, 809, *810*
Transaminases, elevated, by steroid contraceptives
    1100
Transformation zone
cervical epithelium *251*, 251–252, 259, 275
    congenital 265, 267–268
cervical squamous neoplasia 309
Transfusion syndrome,
    monochorionic–monoamniotic twin
    placentation 1580
Transitional cell carcinoma
Bartholin's gland carcinoma 131
Fallopian tube 611
ovarian 732–733
    see also Brenner tumours (transitional cell)
peritoneum 927
urinary tract, metastatic to ovary 888
vagina 210, 211
Transitional cell metaplasia
ectocervical 288
peritoneum 927
tubal fimbriae 590, *590*
vaginal epithelium 186
Transitional cell papilloma, urethral neoplasms,
    benign 132
Transitional cell tumours
ovarian *see* Brenner tumours, ovarian
peritoneum 927
Transketolase, Wernicke's encephalopathy 1531
Transmission electronmicroscopy (TEM) 588,
    589
columnar epithelium of cervix 258
squamous epithelium of cervix 253–255.
Transplacental infection, herpesvirus 425–426
Transplacental spread, neoplasm (maternal to fetus)
    1456
Transplantation **1188**
cardiac, in pregnancy **1553**
liver *see* Liver, transplantation
renal *see* Renal transplant
Transposition of great vessels **1545**
Transvaginal falloposcopy 587
Transvaginal ultrasound, endometrial hyperplasia
    detection 446–447
Transverse cervical ligaments 248, *248*
Transverse ligaments of uterus 24
Transverse vaginal septum 43
imperforate 46
TRAP assays 1601
Trauma
head injuries in pregnancy **1532**
liver rupture in pregnancy 1476
uterine and miscarriage 1433
Trematode infections **1144–1148**
Treponema pallidum
cervical infection 282
endometritis 431–432
miscarriage 1432
vulvar infection 58
Treponema pertenue, vulva infection 58
Triangular ligament (urogenital diaphragm) 37, *37*
Trichoepithelioma of vulva 128
Trichomonas, cervical smears 1148
Trichomonas vaginalis 174
cervical infection 284
characteristics 174, *174*
strains 175
transmission 174–175
vaginitis 173–175
    cervical cancer association 175
    diagnosis and clinical features 173–174

epidemiology 173, 175
vulvar 55
Trichomoniasis
cervical 284
vulvar 55
Trichomycosis, vulvar infection 56–57
Trichophyton rubrum, vulvar infection 55
Trichorionic–triamniotic placentation, trizygotic
    triplets 1588–1589
Trichosporon beigelii, vaginitis 173
Tricuspid atresia **1545**
Trigeminal neuropathy 1536
Triplet placentation **1588–1589**, *1589*
Triple X syndrome 1015
Triploidy
cervical adenocarcinoma 358
miscarriage, spontaneous 1435
Trisomy 8, ovarian fibrosarcoma and 861
Trisomy 12
cellular fibroma and 860
granulosa–stromal cell tumours 746
Trisomy 13, uterine fusion defects 45
Trisomy 18
umbilical cord cysts 1301
uterine fusion defects 45
Trisomy 21 (Down's syndrome), ovarian
    dysgerminoma 1183
'Triton' tumour 197
Trizygotic triplets 1588
Trophoblast
basement membrane thickening, maternal
    uteroplacental blood flow reduction 1287
emboli, amniotic fluid embolism syndrome 1566
endovascular *see* Endovascular trophoblast
implantation, laparoscopic treatment tubal
    gestation 1060
membrane antigens, tubal pregnancy 1055
migratory *1332*
    placentation 1332–1335
    uterine tissue invasion 1332
normal development 1392–1393, *1393*, *1394*
postpartum 1353
primary, migratory trophoblast 1332
proliferation, chorionic plate growth 1256
suspicious 1414, *1414*
tubal pregnancy 1055
villous *see* Villous trophoblast
Trophoblastic apoptotic index, miscarriage 1440
Trophoblastic disease
persistent
    AgNORs **1386**
    clinical prognostic indicators **1385**
    combined oral contraceptives and 1092
    complete moles **1384–1387**
    differential diagnosis 1414
    evacuation/curettage 1384
    factors influencing **1384–1387**
    growth factors **1386**
    heterozygosity **1385**
    histological grading systems **1385–1386**
    HLA antigens **1384–1385**
    human chorionic gonadotrophin (hCG) 1385,
        1386–1387
    hyperdiploidy/aneuploidy **1386**
    immunological aspects **1384–1385**
    invasive moles *see under* Hydatidiform mole
    maternal environment **1384–1385**
    oncogenes **1386**
    partial moles **1387–1388**
    placentation defects 1346
    proliferative activity **1386**, 1387
    risk 1384
    telomerase activity 1386
    twin pregnancy with hydatidiform mole 1586
placentation defects 1346–1347
Trophoblastic neoplasms **1392–1412**
aetiology/pathogenesis **1394–1396**
    environment factors 1396
    genetic abnormalities 1395–1396
    HLA antigens 1395
    maternal environment 1394–1395
biopsy **1412–1416**
cervix 382
choriocarcinoma *see* Choriocarcinoma
differential diagnosis **1412–1416**
    lesions containing chorionic villi **1413**
    lesions not containing chorionic villi
        1413–1416
differentiation 1393
epithelioid **1409–1411**, 1415

Trophoblastic neoplasms (cont'd)
 gestational trophoblastic diseases **1359–1430**
 hCG see Human chorionic gonadotrophin (hCG)
 hydatidiform moles see Hydatidiform mole
 incidence/clinical presentation **1396–1398**, *1397*
 metastases *1397*, **1397–1398**
 non-gestational carcinomas with trophoblastic
  metaplasia **1411–1412**
 normal trophoblast 1392–1393, *1393, 1394*
 persistent trophoblastic disease
  see Trophoblastic disease, persistent
 placental site see Placental site, trophoblastic
  tumour
 in tropics **1150**
Trophoblastic shell
 formation 1257–1258
 placental development 1235
Trophoblastic tissue absorption, ectopic gestation
 1058
Trophotropism, velamentous insertion umbilical
 cord 1295
Tropical pathology **1133–1156**
 infections **1134–1148**
 neoplastic disease **1148–1150**
Tubal carcinoma see Fallopian tube,
 adenocarcinoma
Tubal pregnancy 587, **1051–1061**, *1054, 1055, 1059*
 implantation and placentation in tube
  1051–1053, *1057*
 natural history 1058–1059, *1060, 1061*
 pathological findings 1059–1060
 placental villi morphology 1053–1054
 sterilisation as predisposing factor 597
 treatment, complications and effects 1060
 trophoblast 1055
 uterine response 1056–1058
Tubal sterilisation see Sterilisation, tubal
Tube, Fallopian see Fallopian tube
Tuberculosis
 Bartholin's gland 57
 BCGosis (disseminated granulomatous disease)
  1193
 cervical 281, 282
 cervix 281, 282
 congenital 427
 endometrial 427–430, 1003, *1004*
  see also Endometrium
 endometriosis 423
 endometritis, chronic granulomatous 423
 endometritis 427–430, *428–430*, 1003, *1004*,
  1134–1136
 endosalpinx 618
 Fallopian tube 1135–1136
 Fallopian tubes 1135–1136, 1186
 genital 617–620
  complications and presentation 619–620
 granulomas see Granuloma
 granulomatous infection of ovary 683–684
 histological diagnosis **1135**
 HIV/AIDS 1152
 intestinal spread 1186
 ovary 683–684
 pelvis 1134
 renal, in pregnancy *1499*, **1499–1500**
 salpingitis see Salpingitis
 tubal see Salpingitis, tuberculous
 vaginal 170
 vulvar infection 57
 see also Mycobacterium tuberculosis
Tuberous sclerosis **1190**
Tuboendometrioid metaplasia 287–288
 cervical glandular intraepithelial neoplasia 354
Tubointestinal fistula 1012
Tubo-ovarian abscess, acute salpingitis *621*
Tubo-ovarian absence 1009
Tubo-ovarian adhesions *1018*
 fimbrial occlusion and infertility 1010, *1010*
Tubo-ovarian carcinoma 889
Tubo-ovarian interference, infertility due to 1008
Tubo-ovarian pregnancy, fimbrial implantation
 1051
Tubo-ovarian relationships *1018*
 disturbed 1017, *1018*
Tuboperitoneal complex 586
Tubular adenoma
 of Pick see Sertoli cell tumours
 Sertoli–Leydig cell tumours *755*, 755–756
Tubular differentiation, uterine leiomyoma
 530–531
Tubular elements

endometrial stromal tumours 513, *513*
 uterine leiomyoma with 576–577, *577*
Tubular necrosis, acute, in pregnancy **1500**, *1501*
Tumour(s)
 arising in endometriosis, vulvar 132
 ataxia-telangiectasia **1182**
 of dysgenetic gonad see Gonadoblastoma
 of ectopic breast tissue, vulvar 131–132
 fibrous tissue, vulvar 116
 lymphatic origin, vulvar 122
 mechanisms of spread to ovary 879–880
 metastases see Metastases
 neural origin, vulvar 122–124
 placenta, non-trophoblastic **1449–1464**
  primary 1449–1454
 size, cervical cancer 331, 350
 smooth muscle, vulvar 114–115
 striated muscle, vulvar 115–116
 volume
  cervical adenocarcinoma 350
  cervical cancer 331
  microinvasive carcinoma of cervix 318–319
 see also specific tumours, sites
Tumour emboli, Krukenberg tumours 891
Tumour markers
 dysgerminoma 776
 endocervical neoplasia 357–360
 endometrial adenocarcinoma 482–483
 human chorionic gonadotrophin (hCG) 1167,
  1359
 immature teratoma 792–793
 mesothelioma 627
 ovarian germ cell tumours 1167
 vaginal squamous cell carcinoma 200–201
 yolk sac tumours 784, 785
Tumour necrosis factor alpha (TNF-α)
 chorioamnionitis 1305
 cytotrophoblast 1239
 endometriosis 966
 fetal villous macrophages 1239
Tumour necrosis factor-receptor 1 (TNF-R1),
 cytotrophoblast 1239
Tumour suppressor genes **1597–1600**
 BRCA1 **1600**
 loss of heterozygosity (LOH) **1599–1600**
 p53 see P53 gene
 PTEN see PTEN gene
Tumultuous labour, amniotic fluid embolism 1566
TUNEL technique see Apoptotic markers
Tunnel clusters
 cystic (type B) 289
 endocervical hyperplasia 288–289
 non-cystic (type A) 289, 343
Turner's syndrome 638, 641, **1159–1160**, 1182
 atypical polypoid adenomyoma association 573
 cardiac malformations 1160
 gender identification disorders 1221–1222
 gonadoblastoma association 823, 824
 karyotype 1159, *1159*
 ovarian atresia 1159
 phenotype 1160
 renal tract anomalies 1160
 streak gonads 1015, *1015*, 1160
Twin conception, incidence 1575
Twin molar pregnancies 1369, 1416
Twin placentas, pathological features 1579–1580
Twin placentation 1576–1580
 clinical features 1580–1581
 dizygotic twin 1576–1577
 monozygotic twin 1577–1578
 see also Placentation
Twin pregnancy **1575–1588**
 aetiology 1576
 discordant growth 1585
 hydatidiform mole 1586
 incidence 1575
 placentas, pathological features 1579–1580
Twin reversed arterial perfusion, acardiac fetus
 1584
Twin to twin transfusion syndrome see Twin
 transfusion syndrome
Twin transfusion, acute 1583
Twin transfusion syndrome 1581–1585
 acardiac fetus 1583–1584
 acute 1583
 chronic twin–twin transfusion 1581–1582
 death of one twin 1584–1585
 discordant growth 1585
 fetus papyraceous 1585
 vanishing twin syndrome 1585–1586

Twin–twin transfusion 1580
 acute 1583
 chronic 1581–1582, *1582*
  therapeutic techniques 1582
Typical keratinising squamous cell carcinoma
 106–107
T-zone diamniotic twin placentas *1587*

U
Ulceration/ulcers
 cervix, pemphigus vulgaris 291
 endometrium epithelial, IUCD use and 1110
 genital
  Behçet's syndrome 291
  HIV/AIDS 1152, **1153**, 1551
 herpetic 163
 linear, umbilical cord 1299
 pessary, vagina *219*, 220
 stomach, hypertensive disease of pregnancy 1564
 umbilical cord 1299–1300
 vulvar see Vulva, ulceration
Ulcerative colitis **1186**
 anogenital skin manifestations 64
 steroid contraceptives and 1106
Ultrasound
 mature teratoma 797
 placental haemangioma diagnosis 1453
 transvaginal, endometrial hyperplasia detection
  446–447
Umbilical angiitis 1304, *1304*
Umbilical artery, single 1294–1295
 conjoined twins 1587
 miscarriage 1437
 primary aplasia 1294
 renal anomalies 1294
 secondary atrophy 1294
 twin placentas 1579–1580
Umbilical cord **1293–1301**
 abnormalities, miscarriage 1437
 amniotic bands and strings 1308
 cysts 1300–1301
  amniotic inclusions 1301
  vestigial remnants 1300–1301
  Wharton's jelly degeneration 1301
 development 1253–1257, *1254*
  connecting stalk 1255
 developmental abnormalities 1293–1297
  interposito velamentosa 1296
 eccentric insertion 1295
 entanglement, monochorionic–monoamniotic
  twin placentation 1580
 examination, intrauterine fetal death 1313
 furcate insertion 1296
 haemangioma 1301
 haematomas 1298–1299
  simple 1298–1299
  spontaneous 1298
 inflammation 1300
 insertion *1295*
  squamous metaplasia 1301
 interposito velamentosa 1296
 knots 1297
  formation *1296*
  functional significance 1297
  intrapartum fetal death 1297
  monochorionic–monoamniotic twin
   placentation 1580, *1581*
  true/false 1297
 length 1293
  haematomas and 1299
  long 1293, 1299
  short 1293
 marginal insertion 1295
 mechanical lesions 1297–1298
 meconium-induced necrosis 1299–1300
 pathology **1293–1301**
 rupture 1297–1298
  complete 1297
  incomplete 1297
 stricture 1298, *1298*
 teratoma 1301
 torsion *1297*, 1298
  ante-mortem 1298
  ante-mortem vs post-mortem 1298
 traction, excessive, subamniotic haematoma 1284
 tumours 1301
 ulceration and necrosis 1299–1300
 vascular lesions 1298–1299
 vascular profiles 1295
 velamentous insertion 1295–1296, *1296*

bilobate placenta 1276
  twin placentation 1580
  vestigial remnants 1293–1294
Umbilical vessels
  angiitis, chorioamnionitis 1304
  supernumerary 1295
  thrombosis 1299
Undervirilised male syndrome, androgen
    insensitivity syndrome 1219
Unilateral aplasia of Müllerian duct 42
Uninuclear cytotrophoblast 1334
Unruptured term pregnancy, tubal gestation 1059
Ureaplasma urealyticum
  endometritis due to 994, 1003–1005,
    1004
  miscarriage 1432
  pelvic inflammatory disease 993
  salpingitis 620
Ureter, pelvic, anatomy 29
Ureteric bud, mesonephric ducts 11
Ureteric carcinoma, metastatic, to ovary 888
Urethra 31
  anatomy 31
  angiomyofibroblastoma 132
  carcinoma 133
    metastatic to ovary 888
  caruncle 85–86, *86*
  cavernous 19
  leiomyoma 195
  mycoplasmal diseases 165
  neoplasms
    benign 132
    malignant 133
    vulvar involvement **132–133**
  prolapse 86
Urethral crest, posterior *31*
Urinary incontinence 31
Urinary tract
  development 11
  endometriosis 979
  fistulas **184**
  infections
    Mycoplasma hominis 996
    vaginitis association 160
  stones, in pregnancy **1519**
  transitional cell carcinoma, metastatic to ovary
    888
Urogenital diaphragm 37, *37*
Urogenital sinus
  epithelium, vaginal origin 148
  epithelium, glycogen storage 148
  external genitalia development 18
Urolithiasis, in pregnancy **1519**
Urorectal septum, indifferent embryo 10–11
Uterine arteries *29*, 34, 998
  pregnancy 1331
Uterine blood vessels, pregnancy 1331–1332
Uterine cervix *see* Cervix
Uterine smooth muscle tumours **515–538**
  amyloid formation *520*
  benign *515*
  coagulative tumour cell necrosis 515
  diagnostic algorithm *524*
  differential diagnosis, endometrial stromal
    tumours vs *501*
  epithelioid *529*, **529–530**, *530*
    malignant 530
  fixation and sampling 516
  leiomyoma *see* Leiomyoma
  leiomyoma variants *see* Leiomyoma, uterine
  leiomyosarcoma *see* Leiomyosarcoma
  malignant *515*
  mitotic activity 515, 516
  mixed endometrial stromal tumours 576–577
  myxoid **527–529**, *528*
    hydropic degeneration of uterine leiomyoma vs
      537
  of uncertain malignant potential ('stump') *515*,
    523–524
  variants *515*
Uterine tube
  formation 14
  see also Fallopian tube
Uteroplacental arteries
  atherosclerotic lesions and intrauterine growth
    retardation 1344
  endothelial vacuolation 1343
  extravillous interstitial trophoblast cells 1335
  physiological changes in pregnancy *1339*
  pre-eclampsia 1339–1340, *1340*, *1343*

luminal endovascular trophoblast 1339
  reduced blood flow (ischaemia), syncytial knotting
    1288
  spiral artery conversion 1335
  see also Uteroplacental vasculature
Uteroplacental blood flow
  maternal in fetal death 1314
  pre-eclampsia 1310
Uteroplacental ischaemia, syncytial knotting 1288
Uteroplacental vasculature 1257–1259, *1339*
  development 1335–1336
  diabetes mellitus 1344
  placenta creta 1349
  pre-eclampsia 1337
  pregnancy changes 1259
  see also Uteroplacental arteries
Uterosacral ligament 24, 34, 248
Uterotubal junction, anatomy 587
Utero-vaginal anlage 249
Uterovaginal canal, development from
    paramesonephric duct 16
Uterovaginal plexus 34
  autonomic innervation of pelvis 25
Uterovesical pouch 28
Uterus *32*
  acute inversion 1568–1569
  acute torsion 1569
  adaptions to pregnancy **1328–1332**
  adenocarcinoma *see* Endometrial carcinoma
  adenofibroma *551*, **551–552**
  adenomatoid mesothelioma *539*, **539**
  adhesions 1002, 1027
  adult nulliparous state 32
  anatomy 32–34
    posterior surface *654*
  angiosarcoma 538
  arcuate 44
  arteritis 291
  atony, postpartum haemorrhage 1561
  bicornis bicollis 43, *43*, 277
  bicornuate (bicornis unicollis) 43, *44*
    non-communicating rudimentary horn *44*
    twin pregnancy and antepartum haemorrhage
      1352
  bleeding
    dysfunctional *see* Dysfunctional uterine
      bleeding
    see Bleeding, vaginal/uterine
  blood supply 998, *1332*
  body 33
  cavity 33
  congenital hypovascularity 998
  contraction postpartum, postpartum haemorrhage
    1353
  curettage 325
    endometritis 420
    placenta creta 1347
    tubal pregnancy 1057
  decidual cast, ectopic pregnancy *1058*
  didelphys 43, *43*, 277
    septate vagina *43*
  discoloration 500
  endometrial stromal tumours
    see Endometrial stromal tumours
  endometriosis pathogenesis 966
  endo-myomerial junction 497
  enlargement, carcinosarcoma 561
  external trauma, miscarriage 1433
  formation, paramesonephric duct 15
  function 998
  functional problems due to diethylstilboestrol
    1075
  fusion defects 45
  granulocytic sarcoma (myelosarcoma) 951–952
  growth, postpubertal 998
  hypoplastic, gonadoblastoma 826
  infections, IUCD and 1111, 1114
  infertility due to 998–1006
  inflammatory lesions, lymphoma vs 952
  inflammatory pseudotumour 952
  inversion, acute 1568–1569
  involution, postpartum haemorrhage
    1353
  isthmus, epithelium *396*
  laceration
    amniotic fluid infusion 1565
    see also Uterus, perforation
  leiomyoma *952*, 952–953, *999*
    infertility due to 999
    see also Leiomyoma

leiomyomas
  endometritis 421
  miscarriage 1432
leiomyosarcoma *see* Leiomyosarcoma
lipoma 531, *532*
lymphoid infiltration, leiomyoma **531–533**, *532*
lymphoma **948–953**
  see also Non-Hodgkin's lymphoma, uterus and
    cervix
malformations
  auditory defects 48
  endometriosis 48, 964
  fetal intrauterine growth retardation 48
  infertility 47
  miscarriage 47, 1432
  neoplasia 48
  pre-eclampsia 48
  prematurity 47–48
  serum alpha-fetoprotein levels 48
manual exploration and air embolism 1567
mesenchymal tumours **501–502**
metastases, from lobular breast carcinoma 510
mixed Müllerian tumours *see* Mixed Müllerian
    tumours
mixed tumours **549–584**
  atypical polypoid adenomyoma
      see Adenomyoma
  carcinofibroma **559**, *560*
  carcinomesenchymoma **559**
  mesenchymal elements (mixture) 549, **577–578**
  miscellaneous **576–577**
  ovarian sex-cord tumour resemblance **575–576**
  stromal with epithelial elements **575–576**
non-Hodgkin's lymphoma **948–953**
  see also Non-Hodgkin's lymphoma
papillary serous carcinoma, metastases 349, *349*
perforation 1027
  intrauterine contraceptive device 1106, *1107*
  partial 1106
positional disturbances 998
pregnant **1327–1358**
  blood supply 1332
pure heterologous sarcomas 538
rare tumours 474
response, tubal pregnancy 1056–1058
rupture, maternal death 1569–1570
sarcoidosis 1189
sarcoma
  aneuploidy **1611**
  ataxia-telangiectasia **1182**
  chromosomal imbalances **1604**
  clinical staging 502
  combined oral contraceptives and 1095
  p53 **1599**
  pure heterologous **538**
  tamoxifen association 1080
  see also Endometrial stromal tumours
smooth muscle cell tumours *see* Uterine smooth
    muscle tumours
spindle cell lesions **509–510**
stromomyoma *see* Stromomyoma, endometrial
structural abnormalities, infertility due to 998
surgery for infertility, complications 1028
torsion, acute, pregnancy 1569
tumours associated with IUCD use 1112
tumours resembling ovarian sex-cord tumours
    512, 512–513, *513*, *575*, **575–576**
undifferentiated neoplasms 952
unicornis unicollis 42, *42*
vascular abnormalities, infertility due to 998
vascular insufficiency 998
vascular tumours/malformations **538–539**
weight, parity-induced increase 499
see also Endometrium; *Entries beginning
    endometrial;* Myometrium
Uterus-like masses, endometriosis 973

V
Vaccinial vaginitis 164
Vagina **147–245**
  adenocarcinoma **204–208**
    aetiology 206
    biopsy 221
    in childhood/adolescence **1174–1175**
    DES-associated 187, 188, 204, 207, *207*, 1075,
      1174–1175
    epidemiology 206–207
    histology 206
    mesonephric origin 207, *207*
    non-DES association 204–205, 207

Vagina (*cont'd*)
    paramesonephric origin 207, *207*
    primary spontaneous 206–207
    variants *207*
  adenosarcoma 559
  adenosis
    aetiology 206
    clear cell carcinoma association 1075
    diethylstilboestrol association 1075
    endocervical-type *205*
    histology *205*
    spontaneous (non-DES-associated) *205,*
      205–206
    squamous cell carcinoma association 201
  adenosquamous carcinoma 208
  agenesis 996
  anatomy 35, 147, **147–152**
  aplasia 42, 996
  atresia 996, **1158**
  atrophic, absorptive capability 151
  atrophy
    postmenopausal 155–156, *156*
    steroid contraceptives and 1099
  basal cell-like carcinoma 210
  benign cystic teratoma 216
  benign mixed tumour 197–198, *198*
  benign neoplasms **192–198**
    epithelial 193
    mesenchymal 193–197
    mixed epithelial–mesenchymal 197–198, *198*
    range/types *192*
    symptoms *192*
  biopsy
    differential diagnosis *219,* **219–222**
    granulation tissue *219,* 220
  bleeding *see* Bleeding, vaginal/uterine
  blue naevus 193
  Burkitt-type lymphoma 954
  candidiasis 170–172
    see also Candidiasis
  carcinoma *in situ* 201–203, *202*
  chemical lesions 154
  clear cell carcinoma
    diethylstilboestrol association 204, *207,* 1075
    see also Vagina, adenocarcinoma
  cloacogenic carcinoma 208
  compartments 148, *148*
  condyloma acuminatum *161,* **161–162,** *162, 163*
  congenital anomalies 148
    diethylstilboestrol association 278, 1075
    infertility due to 995–996
  cuff cysts 180
  cylindroma 210
  cysts **180–183**
    acquired *180,* 180–182, *181*
    classification *180*
    congenital *182,* 182–183
    emphysematous *178,* 178–179, *179*
    endometriotic 182
    Gartner's 180
    intraepithelial *179*
    paraintroital 182, *182*
    paramesonephric ducts 183
    prolapsed Fallopian tube 181–182
    squamous *180,* 180–181
    toxoplasma 176
  degenerative lesions 155–156
  dermatoses 154–155
  development 1158
  discharge
    abnormal, vaginitis 156
    candidiasis of cervix 283
    endometrial adenocarcinoma 456
    fishy malodour 166
    Trichomonas vaginalis infection 173
  diseases, Bethesda classification system 306–308
  ectopia **186**
  embryological development from
    paramesonephric duct 16–17
  embryology 148
  embryonal cell carcinoma 216
  embryonal rhabdomyosarcoma 1172, *1173*
  endodermal sinus tumour 216, **1168–1169**
  'endometrial stromal sarcoma' 216
  endometriosis 220, *220,* 979
  epidermoid carcinoma 200
  epithelial tumours
    benign 193
    children 1174–1175
    malignant 199–211

  epithelium
    children 159
    epitopes 148
    glycogen accumulation 150
    hormone-dependent changes 150
    layers 149, *149*
    in neonates 150
    normal organisation *149,* 149–150
    oestrogen-induced proliferation 149–150, 156
    oestrogen loss effect 155–156, *156*
    thickness 150
    Tibolone effect 1090
    transitional cell metaplasia 186
    ultrastructure 150–151
  examinations during labour, amniotic infection
    1305
  factitial lesions 153
  fetal, oestrogen levels, maternal 17
  fibroepithelial polyp, origin 150
  fistulas **183–186**
    non-congenital 184
    pathology 185–186
  fluid *see* Vaginal fluids
  foreign bodies 153
  fornices *29,* 247
  function **147–152**
  germ cell tumours **216**
  granular cell myoblastoma 197
  granulocytic sarcoma 954
  haemangioma 197
  haemorrhages, punctate in *Trichomonas vaginalis*
    infection 173, *174*
  haemorrhagic nodules 221–222, *222*
  histiocytoid haemangioma 197
  histology *149,* 149–150
  hypersensitivity 155
  iatrogenic lesions 153–154
  'inclusion dermoid' 181
  infective disease 156–176
    bacterial 165–170
    chlamydial *164,* 164–165
    fungal 170–173
    metazoan (helminths) 176
    mycoplasmal 165
    protozoal 173–176
    symptoms 156–157
    toxic shock syndrome 176–178
    viral 160–164
    see also Vaginitis, infective
  inflammatory disease **154–176**
    infective *see* Vagina, infective disease
    local 154
    primary non-infective **154–155**
    secondary non-infective **155–156**
    systemic disease association 155
  insufflation 152–153
  intraepithelial neoplasia (VAIN) **201–204**
    behaviour 202
    cervical cancer association 201
    cervical intraepithelial neoplasia (CIN)
      relationship 201, 202
    cytology 202–203, *203*
    summary of features 203–204
    IUCD effect 1112–1114
  lacerations 152
  lamina propria 150
  leiomyoma 195–196
  leiomyosarcoma 213, *215,* 215–216
  leucorrhoea 157
  leukaemic deposits 954
  ligneous (pseudomembranous) inflammation
    996
  local immune response 993
  lymphatic drainage *148, 149,* 190
  lymphoepithelioma-like carcinoma 954
  lymphoma, non-Hodgkin's 951, *953,* **953–954**
  malignant melanoma 208–210, *209,* 221
    behaviour and spread 210
    non-pigmented *209,* 209
    prognostic factors 210
  melanocytes 208
  melanosis 208, *209*
  mesenchymal tumours
    benign 193–197
    malignant 211–216
    mixed epithelial *see Below*
  mesonephric tumours 208
  'mesothelioma' 211
  metaplasia *186,* **186**
  metastatic tumours 187, 188, 189, **216–219,** *219*

    from cervical carcinoma 217, *217*
    from endometrial carcinoma *217,* 217–218
    from ovarian carcinoma *217,* 218
    primary tumours (mechanism of spread) *217*
    from renal cell carcinoma 218, *218*
  microbiology 151
  microflora 151, *151,* 158, 170
    alterations due to tampon use 178
    IUCD use effect 1112
  mixed epithelial and mesenchymal tumours
    benign 197–198, *198*
    malignant **216**
  mucous membrane 149
  Müllerian papilloma 193
  myxoid stromal zone 150
  myxoma 195
  neoplasms **187–219**
    aetiology 187–189
    benign *see* Vagina, benign neoplasms
    classification *189,* 189
    definition 187
    DES role 187, 188
    diagnosis 189
    epidemiology 187–189
    FIGO definition 187, *187,* 190
    grading and staging 190, *191, 192*
    HPV role 188
    incidence 187
    metastatic *see* Vagina, metastatic tumours
    method of spread 190
    pathogenesis 190
    presentation 189
    primary malignant 187, 189, *198,* **198–216**
    prognosis *192*
    treatment 190, 192
    vulval lesions with 190
    see also individual tumours under 'vagina'
  neovagina 1186, 1197
  neural tumours 197
  neuroblastoma 211
  neuroepithelioma 210, 211
  obstetrical trauma 152
  oestrogen loss effect 155–156, *156*
  oral contraceptives effect 1099
  'papillary serous cystadenocarcinoma' 211
  papillary 'squamo-transitional' cell carcinoma
    211
  pemphigus vulgaris 1183
  pessary ulcer *219,* 220
  pH
    normal 151
    squamous metaplasia of cervical epithelium
      274
  physiology 151–152
  plasmacytoma 954
  polypoid myofibroblastoma 194
  polyps (fibroepithelial stromal) 193–195, *194,*
    195
  'popping sounds' 178
  post-hysterectomy lesions 154
  proteins secreted 151
  rhabdomyoma *196,* 196–197
  rhabdomyosarcoma 1172, *1173*
  sarcoma 211
    pleomorphic 212
    rare, of paramesonephric origin 216, *216*
  sarcoma botryoides **211–213,** *212, 213, 214*
    presentation 189
    recurrence, grading and staging 213
  schistosomiasis 1145, *1146*
  septum, complete transverse 995
  small cell neuroendocrine carcinoma 210
  soft tissue lesions 154
  solitary fibrous tumour (pseudosarcoma
    botryoides) 193, 197
  spindle cell epithelioma 198
  squamous cell carcinoma 199, **199–201**
    adenosis association 201
    aetiology and pathogenesis 187–188, 201
    aneuploidy 1611
    behaviour and VAIN phase 202
    biopsy 221
    clinical features 189, 199–200
    decidua vs 220, *221*
    differential diagnosis 220, 221, *221*
    epidemiology 199
    invasive *199,* **199–201**
    marker chromosomes 200–201
    spread 200
    survival rates 201

squamous papilloma 193
squamous-type carcinoma
    epidemiology 187–188
    HPV association 188
steroid contraceptives effect 1099
stones **186**
structural abnormalities, and in utero DES
    exposure 278, 1075
transitional cell carcinoma 210, 211
traumatic lesions **152–154**
    chemical 154
    obstetrical 152
    sexually-related 152–153
    sports-related 152
traumatic neuromas 154
tuboendometrioid adenosis, atypical 344
tumours *see* Vagina, neoplasms
ulceration 155
    herpetic 163
    non-syphilitic 168–169
    pessary *219, 220*
    syphilitic (chancre) 168, *168, 169*
    tampon-related 153
ultrastructure 150–151
vault, granulations *219, 220*
verrucous carcinoma 204
Vaginal cervix 33
    see also Cervix
Vaginal delivery
    Marfan's syndrome 1546
    vaginal trauma 152
Vaginal fluids 151
    Gram staining 157
    pH 151
    pyogenic bacterial growth inhibition 158
Vaginal plate
    canalisation failure 45
    cavitation 17
    development 16
    female genital tract development 42
Vaginal-urinary fistula **184**
Vaginal vault 247
Vaginismus 996
Vaginitis
    adolescent 159
    anaerobic 167, 169
    atrophic
        postmenopausal 155–156, *156*
        postpartum 180
    bacterial 165–170
        actinomycosis 170
        anaerobic 167, 169
        complications 170
        Gardnerella vaginalis 165–167
        gonorrhoea 167–168
        miscellaneous genera 169–170
        tuberculous 170
    'candidiasis' 157, 170–172
    chlamydial 165
    desquamative inflammatory 179–180
    emphysematous *178,* **178–179,** *179*
    fungal 170–173
        candidiasis 170–172
        Torulopsis glabrata 172–173
        uncommon organisms causing *173*
        see also Candidiasis
    'haemophilus' 157, 165, 166
        diagnosis 166–167
        epidemiology 167, *167*
        transmission 167, *167*
        see also Gardnerella vaginalis (Clostridium
            vaginale)
    infective **156–176**
        aetiological agents 157–158, 159, *159*
        factors promoting growth patterns *159*
        pathogenesis 158
        postmenopausal 160
        see also Vagina, infective disease
    intercourse-related 180
    mites causing 176
    mycoplasmal 165
    non-specific 157, 165
        Gardnerella vaginalis causing 165, 166, 167
        see also Vaginitis, 'haemophilus'
    postmenopausal atrophic 155–156, *156*
    postpartum atrophic 180
    pregnancy 159
    protozoal 173–176
        see also Trichomonas vaginalis
    risk factors 156

'scarlet fever' 173, 174
'strawberry' 173, 174
toxic shock syndrome and 176–178
'trichomoniasis' 157, 173–175
types 157
viral **160–164**
    condyloma acuminatum (HPV infection) *161,*
        161–162, *162, 163*
    herpes simplex virus (HSV) type 2 162–164
    HIV 164
    vaccinial 164
Vagino-ovarian fistula 185
Vagino-peritoneal fistula 185
Vaginosis, bacterial 157, 165
    causative organisms 167, 996
    complications 170
    definition 157, 167
    diagnostic criteria 157
    diagnostic methods 157
    epidemiology 158
    Gardnerella vaginalis causing 165–167
    HIV-1 transmission 164
    infertility due to 996
    IUCD use effect 1112
    miscarriage 1432
    non-gonorrhoeal, pregnancy 159–160, 166
    see also Vaginitis
VAIN *see* Vagina, intraepithelial neoplasia (VAIN)
Vanishing twin syndrome 1575, 1585–1586
    morphological remnants 1585
Variceal bleeding, cirrhosis in pregnancy 1483
Varicella-zoster virus, vulvar infection 59
Vasa praevia, velamentous insertion of umbilical
        cord 1296
VASA protein, expression, germ cells 636
Vascular anastomoses
    placentas, twin 1578–1579, 1588
    see also Vascular communications
Vascular communications
    dichorionic placentas 1579
    monochorionic placentas 1578
    twin placentas 1588
Vascular disorders, in pregnancy
    cardiovascular *see* Cardiovascular system
    nervous system **1524–1530**
Vascular endothelial growth factor (VEGF)
    endometrial adenocarcinoma 483
    endometriosis 966
    endometrium 399
    pre-eclampsia 1337
    sclerosing stromal tumours (ovarian) 766
Vascular insufficiency, uterus 998
Vascular invasion
    endometrial adenocarcinoma 480–481, *481*
    microinvasive glandular lesions of cervix 356
    uterine adenosarcoma 557
    uterine leiomyoma **534,** *534*
Vascular lesions/malformations **1529–1530**
    antepartum haemorrhages 1351
    arteriovenous *1529,* 1529–1530
    broad ligament 626–627
    endometrium 999
    myometrium 500
    umbilical cord 1298–1299
    uterine **538–539,** 998
    vulva 80–81
Vascular permeation, cervical cancer 332
Vascular regeneration, endometrium 397
Vascular tumours
    Fallopian tubes *604,* 604–605
    ovarian **868–870,** *869*
    uterine **538–539**
Vasculitis **1190–1191**
    fetal vessels *1304*
        chorioamnioitis 1304
    granulomatous **1190–1191,** *1191, 1192*
    myometrium 500
    necrotising arteritis **1191**
    ovarian superovulation **1198**
Vasculogenesis, placental and Hofbauer cells 1244
Vasculopathies, acute, diabetes mellitus in
        pregnancy 1344
Vasoactive intestinal polypeptide 1007
Vasoconstriction, obliterative endarteritis in fetal
        stem arteries 1293
Vaso-regulation, placenta 1242
Vein of Galen 1527
Velamentous insertion of cord *see* Umbilical cord,
        velamentous insertion
Velamentous vessel compression 1296

Veno-occlusive disease *see* Budd–Chiari syndrome
Venous infarction
    Fallopian tube *595, 596*
    tubal adenocarcinoma *606*
Venous thrombosis
    antiphospholipid syndrome 1526
    cerebral **1525–1527**
    deep, oral contraceptives and 1104
    oral contraceptives and 1104
    outcomes 1527
    puerperal 1526
    reduced risk with Tibolone 1090
    superior sagittal sinus 1526–1527
Ventricular septal defects 1544
Vernix caseosa, amnion nodosum 1303
Verruciform xanthoma, vulvar 85
Verrucous carcinoma
    cervical *see* Cervical carcinoma, verrucous
    vagina 204
    vulvar 108, *108,* 108–109, *109*
        clinical presentation 108
        histology 108–109
        natural history 109
Vesical plexus 25
Vesicourethral canal, urogenital sinus 18
Vesicovaginal fistula **184,** 185
Vestibular gland disorders, vulva 84–85
Vestibular papillae, vulvar 86
Vestibular papillomatosis, vulvar 86–87, *87*
Vestibulitis 72
Vestibulodynia 72
Vestigial remnants, umbilical cord cysts 1300
Villi
    avascular, fetal artery thrombosis 1282, *1282*
    placental *see* Placental villi
    trophoblastic mantle 1237
Villitis, placental 1290–1292
    basal 1291, *1291*
    chronic 1291
        placental toxoplasmosis 1318
        pre-eclampsia 1341
    cytomegalovirus infection 1317
    focal 1291, *1290*
        necrotising, rubella infection 1315
        proliferative, maternal syphilis infection 1314
    immune response 1291
    incidence 1291
    lymphoplasmacytic, placental cytomegalovirus
        infection 1317
    non-basal 1291
    placental, intrauterine fetal growth retardation
        1311
    recurrence in subsequent pregnancies 1292
Villoglandular adenocarcinoma, endometrial
        463–464, *464,* 469, 479
Villoglandular adenoma, uterine cervix 383, *383*
Villoglandular papillary adenocarcinoma of cervix
        347, 347–348
Villoglandular papillary adenoma, uterine cervix 383
Villous *see Entries under* placental villi
Villous adenoma
    cervix 348
    urethral neoplasms, benign 132
    uterine cervix 383
Villous cytotrophoblast
    cells, maternal uteroplacental blood flow
        reduction 1287
    proliferation 1239
Villous intravascular karyorrhexis 1313
Villous oedema *see* Placental villi, oedema
Villous 'pulse,' fetal death 1314
Villous stem arteries, changes following fetal death
        1313
Villous trees *see* Placental villous trees
Villous trophoblast 1236–1239
    role of apoptosis in turnover *1244*
    syncytial fusion and apoptosis cascade 1240
    turnover and apoptosis 1239–1241
Villous vessels
    endothelium 1242
    fetal 1315–1316
    vaso-regulation 1242
Vimentin staining
    adult-type granulosa cell tumours 751
    dysgerminoma 774
    endometrioid adenocarcinoma 463, *463,* 488
    juvenile-type granulosa cell tumour 753
    ovarian tumours of Wolffian origin 899
    small cell ovarian tumours 904, *904*
    theca cell tumour 763

Vincent's infection, vaginal 168–169
Viral infections
  acute hepatitis, pregnancy 1478–1479
    see also specific hepatitis viruses
  cervical 285–287
  cervical adenocarcinoma 341
  endometrium 425–426
  infertility and 994
  vaginitis **160–164**
  vulvar 59–60
    see also Viruses; *specific virus infections*
Virchow's triad, thrombogenesis and placentation
    1351
Virilisation
  adrenogenital syndrome 1213
  gonadoblastoma 824–825
  maternal during pregnancy 1214
  Sertoli–Leydig cell tumours 753
Virilising tumours, pseudohermaphroditism, female
    1214
Viruses
  capsid proteins, human papillomavirus 298
  inhibition fetal DNA synthesis 1292
  interaction, human papillomavirus 301
  typing, human papillomavirus 298
    see also Viral infections
Vitamin B₁₂ deficiency, cervical epithelium 290
Vitamin B deficiency, hyperemesis gravidarum
    1531
Vitamin E supplements, Norplant and 1097
Vitiligo, vulvar hypopigmentation 69, *69*
Vitronectin receptor, endometrial 1005
Voiding bladder, initiation 30–31
Volvulus, endometriosis 979
Von Hippel-Lindau disease **1191**
  papillary cystadenoma of broad ligament 625
Von Recklinghausen's disease **1191–1192**, 1536
  malignant schwannoma of ovary 867
Von Willebrand's disease, postpartum haemorrhage
    1561
Vulva 53–94
  adenocarcinoma 111
  adenosquamous carcinoma 107, 111
  alopecia 82
  amoebiasis *1140, 1141*
  amyloidosis **1182**
  anatomy 37–38
  angiokeratomas 118–119
  angiomyofibroblastoma 120
  angiomyxoma
    aggressive 120–121
    superficial 121
  angiosarcoma 121–122
  atrophy with introital stenosis 996
  Bartholin's gland benign tumours 129–130
  basal cell carcinoma 109–111, *110*
  benign epithelial tumours 95–97
  bullous (blistering) diseases **69–72**
  carcinoma
    cell proliferation studies **1607**
    clinical and pathological staging 106, *106*
    clonality studies **1603**
  cellular angiofibroma 120
  chancroid 57
  childhood neoplasms 1177
  classification of non-neoplastic disease 53, *54*
  conditions associated with systemic disease
    63–64
  congenital malformations, infertility due to
    995–996
  dermatosis, achlorhydria **1181**
  dystrophy with atypia *see* Vulvar intraepithelial
    neoplasia (VIN)
  ectopias **81–82**
  elephantiasis 54
  embryonal rhabdomyosarcoma 115–116
  epithelial tumours
    benign 95–97
    malignant 104–111
  extraskeletal mesenchymal chondrosarcoma 125
  fibroadenomas 132, *132*
  fibrohistiocytic origin tumours 116–117
  fibromas 116
  fibrosarcoma 116
  fibrous tissue tumours 116
  folliculitis 56
  genetic disorders **60–63**
    acantholytic conditions 60–62
  germ cell neoplasias 125
  glomus tumour 119–120

granular cell tumours *see* Granular cell tumours
    (myoblastoma)
haemangiopericytoma 120
Hodgkin's disease 954
hyperpigmentation, acanthosis nigricans 68
infancy, inflammatory conditions **80**
infections **54–60**
  bacterial 56–59
  differential diagnosis 60
  fungal 55–56
  parasites 54–55
  protozoan 55
  viral 59–60
infectious mononucleosis involving 954–955, *957*
inflammatory conditions
  infancy **80**
  lymphoma mimicked by 954–956
inflammatory dermatoses **72–80**
intraepithelial neoplasia *see* Vulvar intraepithelial
    neoplasia (VIN)
Langerhans' cell (histiocytosis X) 65, *65–66*
leiomyomas 114–115
  histology 114
leiomyosarcoma 115
ligneous (pseudomembranous) inflammation 996
lipoma 118, *118*
liposarcoma 118
lymphangioma 122
lymphoedema 81
lymphogranuloma venereum *1139*,
    1139
lymphoma **954–956**, *955, 956*
  malignant rhabdoid tumour 124–125
  melanoma *see* Melanoma, malignant
melanosis 68, 111
mesenchymal tumours **114–125**
    uncertain origin 124–125
metastases **125–126**
microflora 54
microinvasive squamous cell carcinoma 104–105
mixed tumours 131
naevi 63, 111–112
neoplastic disease *see* Vulva, tumours
neuroendocrine tumours 111
neurofibroma 123–124
non-Hodgkin's lymphoma **954–956**, *955, 956*
non-mesenchymal non-epithelial neoplasms 125
normal flora 54
papilloma, basal cell 96
paraganglioma 123
pigmentation disorders 67–69, **67–69**
pruritus, candidiasis 171
pseudocarcinomatous hyperplasia *123*
rhabdoid tumour, malignant 124–125
rheumatoid arthritis 1189
sarcoidosis 65
sebaceous carcinoma 129
skin adnexal tumours *see* Skin adnexal tumours,
    vulvar
skin appendage disorders 82–84
smooth muscle tumours 114–115
squamous cell carcinoma 104–108, *106, 107*
  aetiology 105
  aneuploidy **1611**
  basaloid or warty (Bowenoid) types 1611
  clinical features and gross pathology 105–106
  epidemiology 105
  histopathology 106–107
  microinvasive 104–105
  morphometry **1612**
  p53 1611
  pathogenesis 105
  ploidy **1611**
  prognosis and prognostic factors 107–108
  spread 106
  staging 106
striated muscle tumours 115–116
superficial spreading melanomas 113
sweat gland carcinomas 129
synovial sarcoma 125
syphilis 1136, *1137*
syringoma *126*, 126–127
systemic disease affecting **63–67**
tinea cruris 55
tuberculosis 57
tumour-like lesions 85–87, **85–87**
tumours **95–146**
  arising in endometriosis 132
  childhood 1177
  of ectopic breast tissue 131–132

of fat 118
of lymphatic origin 122
of neural origin 122–124
sebaceous differentiation 128
of vascular tissue 118–122
ulceration
  Behçet's syndrome *67*
  junctional epidermolysis bullosa *60*
  leukaemia 125
  non-infective 67
vascular and lymphatic abnormalities **80–81**
verrucous carcinoma *see* Verrucous carcinoma
vestibular gland disorders **84–85**
yolk sac tumours 125
Vulvar intraepithelial neoplasia (VIN) 100–103
  aetiology 100–101
  basaloid type 101, *101*
  Bowenoid 101, *101*
  cell proliferation studies 1607
  clinical aspects 101
  clonality studies 1603
  epidemiology 100
  grading 102
  histological appearance 101–102
  management and prognosis 103
  natural history 103
  undifferentiated 101–102
Vulvitis 156
  erosive 58
  Zoon's plasma cell 79–80
Vulvitis circumscripta plasmacellularis 79–80
Vulvitis granulomatosa 1188
Vulvodynia, dysaesthetic 72
Vulvo-vaginal adenosis 82
Vulvo-vaginal candidiasis
  diabetes mellitus 1183
  HIV/AIDS 1152
Vulvo-vaginal-gingival syndrome 79
Vulvovaginal rhabdomyoma 115
Vulvovaginitis 156
  children, viral 163, 164
  chronic, infertility due to 996
  diabetes mellitus 1183
  gonorrhoeal 1163
  herpetic 163
  paediatric 159

W
Waldeyer fascia 24
Walthard nests **926–927**, *927*
Walthard rest 592, *592*
  cysts 592, *593*
Warthin-Starry stain, spirochaetal placental
    infection 1314
Warts, genital *see* Condyloma acuminata
Warty carcinoma 106–107
Warty squamous cell carcinoma, vulvar 1611
Water intoxication, maternal death 1571
Wedge biopsy, cervical carcinoma in pregnancy 333
Well-differentiated peritoneal mesothelioma
    915–916, *916*
Wernicke's encephalopathy *1531*, **1531**
Wharton's jelly
  deficiency
    umbilical cord haematomas 1299
    umbilical cord stricture 1298
  degeneration, umbilical cord cysts 1301
  false knots 1297
  funisitis, acute 1300
  insertion funiculi furcata 1296
White lesions, endometriosis 967
White sponge naevus, vulvar genetic disorders 63
Wickham's striae, lichen planus 79
Wilms' tumour
  cervix 382
  extrarenal **1176–1177**
  ovary 903, *903*
Wilms' tumour suppressor gene *(WT-1)*, expression,
    granulosa cell tumours 705
Wilson's disease **1192**
  pregnancy 1483
Wolffian bodies, mesonephros 11
Wolffian ducts *see* Mesonephric (Wolffian) duct(s)
Wolffian origin, ovarian tumours *898–902*, **898–902**
  see also Ovarian tumours, of probable Wolffian
    origin
Wolffian structures 695
World Health Organization
  lymphoid neoplasm classification 936, *937*
  ovarian tumour classification 693, *695*

Wuchereria bancrofti 1141–1142, *1142*, *1143*
  vulvar infection, 54

X

Xanthine oxidase, pre-eclampsia 1337
Xanthoma, verruciform 85
X cells *see* Extravillous trophoblast
X chromosome 635, **641–643**
  abnormalities, accelerated follicular depletion
    1016
  functions 641
  Giemsa banding 642, *642*
  inactivation **642–643**
    familial skewed, recurrent pregnancy loss due to
      995
    ovary meiosis onset and 647
    pseudoautosomal region 642
Xeno-oestrogens, environmental, effect on tubes
  1008
XIST gene 643
X-linked lethal syndromes 992
45 XO monosomy, miscarriage, spontaneous 1435
XX male syndrome
  genetic identification disorders 1222–1223
  mechanisms of occurrence 1223

Y

Yaws, vulvar infection 58
Y chromosome **638–639**

Giemsa banding *630*, 639
  in gonadoblastoma 824
  length 639
  microdeletions and infertility 641
  sex-determining region 639, **640–641**
Yeasts, vulvar infections 55
Yolk sac
  extragonadal tumours, uterine cervix 380
  formation *5*
  primary, umbilical cord development 1254–1255
Yolk sac tumours **777–785**, *1166*, **1166–1167**, *1167*
  clinical features 777
  endometrioid carcinoma vs 731, 777
  glandular *782*, 782–783
  gonadoblastoma association 830
  hepatic hepatoid 783, *783*
  immunohistochemistry 784–785
  incidence and age 777
  intestinal *781*, 782
  leukaemia association 785
  macroscopic appearance 777–778, *778*
  mesenchyme-like components *783*, 783–784
  microscopic features 778–784
    classical patterns 778–782
    endodermal (Duval sinus) pattern *779*,
      779–780, *780*
    parietal patterns 782
    polyvesicular vitelline pattern *780*,
      781

reticular (microcystic) pattern *780*, 780–781
solid patterns *781*, 781–782
special differentiated 782–784
somatic differentiated varieties 783–784
terminology and tumour types 777
treatment and prognosis 785
tumour markers 784, 785
vaginal 216
vulvar 125
Y(+) XX male syndrome 1223
Y(-) XX male syndrome 1223

Z

ZFY (zinc finger Y) gene 639, **640**
Ziehl-Neelsen-stained sections, endometrial
    tuberculosis 429
Zinc deficiency, acrodermatitis enteropathica 63
Zoladex 1087
Zollinger–Ellison syndrome 715, **1195**
Zona pellicida
  dissolution 4, *4*
  oocyte 2
Zoon's plasma cell vulvitis 79–80
Zygomycosis
  subcutaneous 1140, *1140*
  vulvar infection 56
Zygosity of twins 1575–1576
Zygote 2, *2*, 3
  tubal entrapment 1008